Unit 10
Integumentary Disorders.....................1261
Anatomy and Physiology Review:
The Integumentary System 1262
48 Assessment of the Integumentary System 1267
49 Management of Clients with Integumentary
    Disorders 1279
50 Management of Clients with Burn Injury....... 1331

Unit 11
Circulatory Disorders........................1361
Anatomy and Physiology Review:
The Circulatory System 1362
51 Assessment of the Vascular System 1368
52 Clients with Hypertensive Disorders: Promoting
    Positive Outcomes........................... 1379
53 Management of Clients with Vascular
    Disorders 1399

Unit 12
Cardiac Disorders............................1433
Anatomy and Physiology Review: The Heart 1434
54 Assessment of the Cardiac System 1447
55 Management of Clients with Structural Cardiac
    Disorders 1481
56 Management of Clients with Functional Cardiac
    Disorders 1515
57 Management of Clients with Dysrhythmias..... 1550
58 Management of Clients with Myocardial
    Infarction 1579

Unit 13
Oxygenation Disorders 1611
Anatomy and Physiology Review:
The Respiratory System 1612
59 Assessment of the Respiratory System 1623
60 Management of Clients with Upper Airway
    Disorders 1651
61 Management of Clients with Lower Airway and
    Pulmonary Vessel Disorders 1685
62 Management of Clients with Parenchymal and
    Pleural Disorders 1710
63 Management of Clients with Acute Pulmonary
    Disorders 1746

Unit 14
Sensory Disorders 1777
Anatomy and Physiology Review:
The Eyes and Ears.............................. 1778
64 Assessment of the Eyes and Ears.............. 1787
65 Management of Clients with Visual
    Disorders 1809

66 Management of Clients with Hearing and
    Balance Disorders 1831

Unit 15
Cognitive and Perceptual Disorders............1855
Anatomy and Physiology Review:
The Neurologic System 1856
67 Assessment of the Neurologic System 1874
68 Management of Comatose or Confused
    Clients..................................... 1905
69 Management of Clients with Cerebral
    Disorders 1923
70 Management of Clients with Stroke 1953
71 Management of Clients with Peripheral
    Nervous System Disorders................... 1983
72 Management of Clients with Degenerative
    Neurologic Disorders 2002
73 Management of Clients with Neurologic
    Trauma..................................... 2026

Unit 16
Protective Disorders 2071
Anatomy and Physiology Review:
The Hematopoietic System....................... 2072
74 Assessment of the Hematopoietic System 2089
75 Management of Clients with Hematologic
    Disorders 2103
76 Management of Clients with Immune
    Disorders 2129
77 Management of Clients with Autoimmune
    Disease..................................... 2140
78 Management of the Client with Leukemia and
    Lymphoma.................................. 2165

Unit 17
Multisystem Disorders........................2183
79 Management of Clients with Acquired
    Immunodeficiency Syndrome 2185
80 Management of Clients Requiring
    Transplantation 2213
81 Management of Clients with Shock and
    Multisystem Disorders 2231
82 Management of Clients in the Emergency
    Department 2261
Appendix A Religious Beliefs and Practices
            Affecting Health Care 2291
Appendix B A Health History Format That
            Integrates the Assessment of
            Functional Health Patterns.......... 2298
Appendix C Laboratory Values of Clinical
            Importance in Medical-Surgical
            Nursing 2301
Index...2311

GET CONNECTED

To Content Updates, Study Tools, and More!

Meet SIMON   Your free online website companion

sign on at:

http://www.wbsaunders.com/SIMON/Black/medsurg

what you'll receive:

Whether you're a student or an instructor, you'll find information just for you. Things like:
- Content Updates
- Links to Related Publications
- Author Information . . . and more

plus:

WebLinks

Access hundreds of active websites keyed specifically to the content of this book. The WebLinks are continually updated, with new ones added as they develop.

Free Study and Tutorial CD-ROM

with every copy of Black's *Medical-Surgical Nursing*
Clinical Management for Positive Outcomes, 6th Edition

With a Strong Emphasis on Clinical and Functional Relevance, this Valuable CD-ROM Features:

- Detailed discussions for the "Thinking Critically" questions found in the book provide examples of appropriate answers.
- 10 case studies from the text—plus 2 bonus case studies—are presented with discussions for each of the questions as well as 7 to 10 multiple choice questions for further review. Answers include rationales for incorrect answers. Finally, a nursing care plan based on the case study pulls it all together.
- Over **700** NCLEX review questions provide you with an opportunity for review before exams and for additional review before your licensure exam.

W.B. SAUNDERS COMPANY

Medical-Surgical Nursing

CLINICAL MANAGEMENT for POSITIVE OUTCOMES

VOLUME 1

6th EDITION

Joyce M. Black, PhD, RN, CPSN, CCCN, CWCN
Assistant Professor
College of Nursing
University of Nebraska Medical Center
Omaha, Nebraska

Jane Hokanson Hawks, DNSc, MSN, RN, C
Associate Professor of Nursing
Midland Lutheran College
Fremont, Nebraska

Annabelle M. Keene, MSN, RN, C
Bellevue Public Schools
Bellevue, Nebraska
Formerly, Associate Professor
College of Saint Mary
Omaha, Nebraska

W.B. SAUNDERS COMPANY
An Imprint of Elsevier Science
Philadelphia   London   New York   St. Louis   Sydney   Toronto

W.B. SAUNDERS COMPANY
An Imprint of Elsevier Science

The Curtis Center
Independence Square West
Philadelphia, Pennsylvania 19106

NOTICE

Nursing is an ever-changing field. Standard safety precautions must be followed, but as new research and clinical experience broaden our knowledge, changes in treatment and drug therapy may become necessary or appropriate. Readers are advised to check the most current product information provided by the manufacturer of each drug to be administered to verify the recommended dose, the method and duration of administration, and contraindications. It is the responsibility of the treating physician, relying on experience and knowledge of the patient, to determine dosages and the best treatment for each individual patient. Neither the Publisher nor the editor assumes any liability for any injury and/or damage to persons or property arising from this publication.

The Publisher

Library of Congress Cataloging-in-Publication Data

Medical-surgical nursing: clinical management for positive outcomes / edited by Joyce M. Black, Jane Hokanson Hawks, Annabelle Keene.—6th ed.

    p.;   cm.

Includes bibliographical references and index.

ISBN 0–7216–8198–0 (single volume)

ISBN 0–7216–8197–2 (2 vol set)

  1. Nursing. 2. Surgical nursing. 3. Psychophysiology.   I. Black, Joyce M.   II. Hawks, Jane Hokanson.   III. Keene, Annabelle.
    [DNLM: 1. Nursing Care. 2. Perioperative Nursing.   WY 150 M489365 2001]

RT41.L87 2001
610.73—dc21   99–089356

Vice-President and Nursing Editorial Director: Sally Schrefer

Executive Editor: Thomas Eoyang

Production Managers: Linda Garber, Natalie Ware

Developmental Editor: Victoria Legnini

Manuscript Editor: Carol J. Robins

Illustration Coordinator: Rita Martello

Design Coordinator: Karen O'Keefe Owens

MEDICAL-SURGICAL NURSING: Clinical Management   Single volume 0–7216–8198–0
for Positive Outcomes   Two-volume set: 0–7216–8197–2

Printed in the United States of America.

Last digit is the print number: 9   8   7   6   5   4   3

There are several people at the University of Nebraska who seemingly never tire of my questions on how to explain or teach something more clearly. Thank you, Drs. Janet Cuddigan, Louise LaFramboise, and Barbara Manz. I also appreciate the countless students and patients who taught me the value of caring and teaching. I appreciate the expertise of the contributors to this text. And I thank my family for their ongoing understanding of the considerable strain on my time and energy.

J. M. B.

I want to thank my family, parents, and nursing friends from my doctoral and master's programs; my colleagues at Midland Lutheran College, Fremont, Nebraska; and my peers from the Iowa Nurses' Association and Society of Urologic Nurses and Associates (SUNA) who helped me with words of encouragement and support.

J. H. H.

To Chuck, Alice, and Clair. Words cannot express my thanks for your support of my projects, including this book. May you have similar support to pursue your dreams.

A. M. K.

At the time of publication of the fifth edition, **Joyce M. Black, PhD, RN, CPSN, CCCN, CWCN,** was a Nursing Specialist with the Adult Health and Illness Department of the University of Nebraska Medical Center (UNMC). In December 1999 she received her Doctorate from the University of Nebraska College of Nursing. Her dissertation research focused on patient, wound, treatment, and health care system risk factors affecting the rate of pressure ulcer healing. Since graduation, she has returned to her position as Assistant Professor at UNMC, where she teaches medical-surgical nursing. She received her Master's degree from UNMC and her undergraduate degrees from Winona State University in Winona, Minnesota, and Rochester Community College in Rochester, Minnesota.

Dr. Black has also had several years of experience as a medical-surgical nurse at Saint Mary's Hospital, which is affiliated with the Mayo Clinic in Rochester, Minnesota. Her practice has included critical care, burns, respiratory disorders, orthopedics, and plastic surgery. She is certified by the American Society of Plastic and Reconstructive Surgical Nurses and Wound, Ostomy, and Continence Nurses, and she serves as editor of *Plastic Surgical Nursing*. Her area of research concerns pressure ulcers.

Jane Hokanson Hawks, DNSc, RN, C, is an Associate Professor of Nursing at Midland Lutheran College, Fremont, Nebraska. She teaches sophomore students in medical-surgical nursing and senior students in advanced medical-surgical nursing and nursing management. Dr. Hawks received her Doctorate of Nursing Science in collegiate nursing education from Widener University in Chester, Pennsylvania; her Master of Science degree in Nursing in medical-surgical nursing and nursing administration from UNMC in Omaha, Nebraska; and her Bachelor of Science degree in Nursing from St. Olaf College in Northfield, Minnesota.

Dr. Hawks has worked in and taught medical-surgical nursing for more than 22 years. She has practiced in a variety of areas, including critical care, renal transplantation, orthopedics, general surgery, and urology. She serves as the editor of *Urologic Nursing*. Her areas of research include empowerment and alcoholism. She and her colleagues developed the NANDA nursing diagnosis Altered Family Process: Alcoholism.

Annabelle M. Keene, MSN, RN, C, is a School Nurse with Bellevue Public Schools in Bellevue, Nebraska. She directs the health offices of several school buildings (approximately 2000 students and staff) and is certified by the State of Nebraska as a school nurse for grades K through 12. She also is a data analysis consultant for nursing graduate students who are studying nurses' perceptions of ethical problems across various specialty areas. Ms. Keene received her Master's degree from UNMC and her B.S.N. from Cornell University–New York Hospital School of Nursing, New York, New York.

Anne Keene has worked in and taught medical-surgical nursing for more than 25 years. She has been a staff nurse, a head nurse, a staff development instructor, and a nursing instructor in a multitude of clinical areas. She has been Assistant Professor at the University of Nebraska College of Nursing, teaching health assessment and medical-surgical nursing to undergraduate students. Anne also has been Associate Professor at the College of Saint Mary, Omaha, Nebraska, teaching in the undergraduate program. Ms. Keene is certified in medical-surgical nursing by the American Nurses Credentialing Center.

Contributors

Mary A. Allen, MS, RN
Clinical Trials Specialist, National Institute of Allergy and Infectious Diseases, National Institutes of Health, Bethesda, Maryland

Chris Stewart Amidei, MSN, RN, CNRN, CCRN
Clinical Nurse Specialist, University of Chicago, Chicago, Illinois

Helen Andrews, RN, BSN
Care Manager, Alegent Health Bergan Mercy Medical Center, Omaha, Nebraska

Jane Allen Austgen, RN, BSN, CRNH
Hospice Nurse Care Manager, Alegent Health Home Care & Hospice, Omaha, Nebraska

Susan Baker, DNS, RN
Instructor, Indiana University School of Nursing, Indianapolis, Indiana

Patricia McCallig Bates, BSN, CURN
Clinical Urology Nurse, Urology Department, Kaiser-Permanente, Portland, Oregon

Deborah L. Bayliss, MS, RN
Community Nurse Care Manager, Poudre Valley Health System, Fort Collins, Colorado

Francie Bernier, BSN, RN, C
Clinical Consultant for Continence Care, Independent Urologic/Urogynecologic Clinical Consultant, Specialist in Continence Care, Leesburg, Virginia

Deborah S. Bjerstedt, MSN, RN, CS, FNP
Family Nurse Practitioner, Allina Medical Group, Shoreview, St. Paul, Minnesota

Hilary S. Blackwood, MSN, RN
Clinician III, Surgical Nutrition Support Services, University of Virginia Health System, Charlottesville, Virginia

Meg Blair, BA, BSN, MSN
Assistant Professor, Nebraska Methodist College of Nursing and Allied Health; Staff Nurse, Emergency Department, St. Joseph's Hospital, Omaha, Nebraska

R. B. Boley, PhD
Professor (Ret.), Biology Department, University of Texas at Arlington, Arlington, Texas

Cynthia A. Bolin, RN
Program Coordinator, Congestive Heart Failure Management Center, St. Luke's Hospital, St. Louis, Missouri

Shawnda Braun, RN
Case Manager, Allied Health Alternatives, Inc., Faribault, Minnesota

Sarah Jo Brown, PhD, RN
Principal and Consultant, Practice-Research Integrations, Norwich, Vermont

Terri Sellin Brown, BSN, RN
School Nurse, Omaha Public Schools, Omaha, Nebraska

Mary Vorder Bruegge
Clinician IV, Nerancy Neuro ICU, University of Virginia Health System, Charlottesville, Virginia

Candace Cantwell, RD
Clinical Dietitian, Clinical Nutrition Support Services, University of Pennsylvania Health System, Philadelphia, Pennsylvania

Robert G. Carroll, PhD
Professor of Physiology, Brody School of Medicine, East Carolina University, Greenville, North Carolina

Bernice B. Christopher, BSN, RN
Keystone Mercy Health Plan, Philadelphia, Pennsylvania

Linda K. Clarke, MS, RN, CORLN
Head and Neck Nurse Specialist, Greater Baltimore Medical Center, Towson, Maryland

Marsha E. Cloud, BSN, RN
Clinician II, Surgical Services, University of Virginia Health System, Charlottesville, Virginia

Linda Carman Copel, PhD, RN, CS, DAPA, ACFE, CGP, CFLE
Associate Professor, Villanova University, Villanova, Pennsylvania; Psychotherapist, Private Practice, Ardmore, Pennsylvania

Pamela Cornwell, MA, RN
Manager, Intensive and Intermediate Care Units, Shriners Hospitals for Children, Northern California, Sacramento, California

Sherill Nones Cronin, PhD, RN, C
Professor of Nursing, Bellarmine College; Nurse Researcher, Jewish Hospital, Louisville, Kentucky

Janice Z. Cuzzell, MA, RN
Vice President, Island Home Care, Inc., Savannah, Georgia

Jean Elizabeth DeMartinis, PhD, APRN, FNP-C
Assistant Professor and Director of the Masters in Cardiac Health and Rehabilitation CNS/ANP Program, Creighton University School of Nursing, Omaha, Nebraska

Kaye M. Dietrich, MS, RN, C
Consultant, Kiel, Wisconsin

Peggy Doheny, PhD, MSN, RN
Associate Professor, Kent State University College of Nursing, Kent, Ohio

Rebecca M. Dudley, RN
Staff Nurse, Fairview Lakes HomeCaring & Hospice, Chisago City, Minnesota

Kimberly Elgin, BSN, RN
Clinician III, Clinical Manager, Surgical Services, University of Virginia Health System, Charlottesville, Virginia

Charlotte Eliopoulos, PhD, MPH, RN, C
President, Health Education Network, Glen Arm, Maryland

James A. Fain, PhD, RN, FAAN
Associate Professor and Director, PhD Nursing Program,
University of Massachusetts Graduate School of Nursing,
Worcester, Massachusetts

Kathryn Fiandt, DNS, ARNP
Associate Professor, University of Nebraska College of Nursing;
Coordinator, Family Nurse Practitioner Program, University of
Nebraska Medical Center; Clinical Director, Family Health Care
Center, Omaha, Nebraska

Mary L. Fisher, PhD, RN, CNAA
Associate Professor, Nursing Administration, Indiana University
School of Nursing, Indianapolis, Indiana

Susan Flannigan, MPH, RN, ANP
Adult Nurse Practitioner, Fairview Lakes Medical Center,
Chisago City, Minnesota

Ann K. Frantz, BSN, RN
Independent Health Care Consultant, Pontiac, Michigan

Anne Marie Johnson Fredrichs, MSN, RN, CPNP
Research Coordinator, Nebraska Foundation for Spinal
Research, Omaha, Nebraska

Peggy Gerard, DNSc, RN
Professor, School of Nursing, Purdue University, Calumet,
Hammond, Indiana

Nancy Girard, PhD, MSN, RN
Associate Professor and Chair, Acute Nursing Care Department,
University of Texas Medical School at San Antonio, School of
Nursing, San Antonio, Texas

Elizabeth W. Good, MSN, RN, C
Clinician III, Urology Care Coordinator, Surgical Services,
University of Virginia Health System, Charlottesville, Virginia

Michelle Goodman, MS, RN, OCN
Assistant Professor of Nursing, Rush University College of
Nursing; Oncology Clinical Nurse Specialist, Section of Medical
Oncology, Rush Cancer Institute, Rush Presbyterian–St. Luke's
Medical Center, Chicago, Illinois

Lisa A. Gorski, MS, RN
Clinical Nurse Specialist, Covenant Home Health and Hospice,
Milwaukee, Wisconsin

Maribeth Guzzo, MSN, RN, CRNP
Nurse Practitioner, Division of Cardiology, the Hospital of the
University of Pennsylvania, Philadelphia, Pennsylvania

Sheila A. Haas, PhD, RN
Dean and Professor, Loyola University of Chicago Marcella
Niehoff School of Nursing, Chicago, Illinois

Diana P. Hackbarth, PhD, RN
Professor, Department of Community, Mental Health, and
Administrative Nursing, Loyola University of Chicago Marcella
Niehoff School of Nursing, Chicago, Illinois

Linda R. Haddick, MSN, RN
Clinical Nurse Specialist, Alegent Health Home Care &
Hospice, Omaha, Nebraska

Margie Hansen, PhD, RN
Clinical Associate Professor, Family Nurse Practitioner Program,
University of North Dakota College of Nursing, Grand Forks,
North Dakota

Karen A. Hanson, MS, RN, CNP
Urology Nurse Practitioner, Mayo Clinic, Rochester, Minnesota

Tammi G. Hardiman, BSN, RN
Nurse Consultant, Community Services Quality Assurance,
Department of Social and Health Services, State of Washington,
Arlington, Washington

Jeannine Mueller Harmon, MSN, RN, FNP, CS
Family Nurse Practitioner, Metropolitan State University, St.
Paul, Minnesota

Debra E. Heidrich, MSN, RN, AOCN, CHPN
Nursing Consultant, West Chester, Ohio

Esther A. Hellman, PhD, RN
Assistant Professor, Creighton University School of Nursing,
Omaha, Nebraska

Beverley E. Holland, PhD, MSN, ARNP
Associate Professor, Lansing School of Nursing, Bellarmine
College, Louisville, Kentucky

Rhonda Holloway, BSN, RN, MBA, NP
Women's Wellness Center, Lone Tree, Colorado

Roberta Jorgensen, BSN
Gastrointestinal Nurse Coordinator, Mayo Clinic, Rochester,
Minnesota

Juanita Fogel Keck, DNS, BSN
Associate Professor, Indiana University School of Nursing,
Indianapolis, Indiana

Catherine A. Kernich, MSN, RN
Clinical Faculty, Frances Payne Bolton School of Nursing, Case
Western Reserve University; Director, Ambulatory Practice,
Department of Medicine; University Faculty Services,
University Hospitals Health Systems, Cleveland, Ohio

Helene J. Krouse, PhD, ARNP, CORLN
Associate Professor of Nursing, University of Florida College of
Nursing, Gainesville, Florida

Kim K. Kuebler, MN, RN, ANP-CS
Adjunct Faculty, College of Nursing and Health Sciences,
Saginaw Valley State University, University Center, Michigan;
Adult Nurse Practitioner, Oncology/Palliative Care, Private
Practice, Adjuvant Therapies, Inc., Lake, Michigan

Joanie J. Kush, MS, RN
Director of Hospice, Visiting Nurse Association of Omaha,
Omaha, Nebraska

Louise Nelson LaFramboise, PhD, RN
Assistant Professor, University of Nebraska College of Nursing,
Omaha, Nebraska

Joan Lappe, PhD, RN
Associate Professor, Creighton University Schools of Nursing
and Medicine, Omaha, Nebraska

Anne Larson, PhD, MS, BA, RN, C
Associate Professor of Nursing, Midland Lutheran College,
Fremont, Nebraska

Joyce Larson-Presswalla, PhD, RN
President, "Culture Counts," Marketing Coordinator, James A. Haley Veterans Hospital, Tampa, Florida

Cindi Leo-Gofta, BSN, RN
Operations Director, Resource and Referral/Business Development, Alegent Health Home Care & Hospice, Omaha, Nebraska

James Higgy Lerner, RN, LAc
Private practice of acupuncture, traditional Oriental medicine, and biofeedback, Chico, California

Cindy Ludwig, MS, RN
Nurse Manager, Providence Saint Joseph Medical Center, Burbank, California

Cyndy Hunt Luzinski, MS, RN
Community Nurse Case Manager, Poudre Valley Health System, Fort Collins, Colorado

Donna W. Markey, MSN, RN, ACNP-CS
Clinician IV, Surgical Services, University of Virginia Health System, Charlottesville, Virginia

Karen S. Martin, MSN, RN, FAAN
Health Care Consultant, Martin Associates, Omaha, Nebraska

Cynthia McCurren, PhD, MSN
Associate Professor, University of Louisville School of Nursing; Nurse Researcher, University of Louisville Hospital, Louisville, Kentucky

James McLean, BSN, RN, WOCN
Enterostomal Therapist, Fort Worth, Texas

Norma D. McNair, MSN, RN, CCRN, CNRN, CS
Assistant Clinical Professor, University of California, Los Angeles, School of Nursing; Clinical Nurse III, Liver Transplant and Surgical Subspecialties, Intensive Care Unit, UCLA Medical Center, Los Angeles, California

Mary E. McQuinn, RPT
Physical Therapist, Visiting Nurse Association of Omaha, Omaha, Nebraska

Colette H. McVaney, BSN, RN
Lead Nurse, Geriatric Clinic, Nebraska Health System, Omaha, Nebraska

Patricia Meier, MA, BSN, RN, AOCN
Nurse Manager, Shady Grove Adventist Hospital, Rockville, Maryland

Stephanie Mellon-Reppen, MSN, RN, ACNP, OCN
Acute Care Nurse Practitioner and Oncology Certified Nurse, Section of Bone Marrow Transplant and Cell Therapy, Rush Presbyterian–St. Luke's Medical Center, Chicago, Illinois

Melanie Minton, BSN, RN, MBA, CNRN
Lead Adjunct Faculty, Le Tourneau University; Nurse Specialist, Nursing Support and Patient Education, The Methodist Hospital, Houston, Texas

Kim Miracle, MSN, RN, C
Clinical Nurse Specialist, Outcomes Manager, Jewish Hospital, Louisville, Kentucky

Anita E. Molzahn, PhD, MN
Professor, School of Nursing, and Dean, Faculty of Human and Social Development, University of Victoria, Victoria, British Columbia, Canada

Bernadette K. Mruz, RN
Clinical Manager, Visiting Nurse Association of Omaha, Omaha, Nebraska

Elizabeth A. Murphy-Blake, MSEd, MS, RN, ARNP
Assistant Professor of Nursing, Midland Lutheran College, Fremont, Nebraska

Pamela J. Nelson, MS, RN
Assistant Professor of Nursing, Bethel College, St. Paul, Minnesota

Noreen Heer Nicol, MS, RN, FNP
Clinical Senior Instructor, University of Colorado School of Nursing; Director of Nursing, Dermatology Clinical Specialist and Nurse Practitioner, National Jewish Medical and Research Center, Denver, Colorado

Cheryl Noetscher, MS, RN
Director of Case Management, Crouse Hospital and Community–General Hospital, Syracuse, New York

Janice D. Nunnelee, PhD, RN, CS/ANP, CRN
Clinical Associate Professor of Nursing, University of Missouri–St. Louis. Adult Nurse Practitioner, Vascular Nurse Practitioner, Unity Medical Group, St. Louis, Missouri

Barbara B. Ott, PhD, RN, CCRN
Associate Professor, Villanova University College of Nursing, Villanova, Pennsylvania

Arlene L. Polaski, MEd, MSN, RN
Program Director (Ret.), York Technical College/University of South Carolina Lancaster Cooperative Program in Associate Degree Nursing, Rock Hill, South Carolina

Kathleen Popelka, DNSc, CFNP
Family Nurse Practitioner, Women's Veterans Coordinator, Veterans Administration Medical Center, Omaha, Nebraska

David Porta, PhD
Associate Professor, Bellarmine University; Adjunct Faculty, University of Louisville School of Medicine, Louisville, Kentucky

Kathleen Rea, BSN, RN
Clinician III, Clinical Manager, Surgical Services, University of Virginia Health System, Charlottesville, Virginia

Marlene Reimer, PhD, RN, CNN(C)
Associate Dean, Research and Graduate Programs, University of Calgary Faculty of Nursing, Calgary, Canada

Roxanne Rivard, BSN, RN, CWOCN
Enterostomal Therapy Nurse, Fairview Lakes, HomeCaring & Hospice, Chisago City, Minnesota

Dottie Roberts, MSN, MACI, RN, C, ONC, CNS
Medical-Surgical Clinical Nurse Specialist, Penrose–St. Francis Health Services, Colorado Springs, Colorado

Helen Murdock Rogers, BS, MS, DNSc
Associate Professor, Adult Health, Research, and Physical
Assessment, Department of Nursing, Worcester State College;
Community Nurse, University of Massachusetts, Memorial
Home Health, Worcester, Massachusetts

Amy Perrin Ross, MSN, RN, CNRN
Neuroscience Program Coordinator, Loyola University Medical
Center, Maywood, Illinois

Vicki M. Ross, MSN, RN
Nurse Clinician, Nutritional Support Services, Truman Medical
Center, Kansas City, Missouri

Pamela K. Schaid, MA, RN
Administrator, Seasons Hospice, Rochester, Minnesota

Nancy J. Scheet, MSN, RN
Compliance Officer, Visiting Nurse Association of Omaha,
Omaha, Nebraska

Linda Ludy Scott, MS, CFNP
Nurse Practitioner, National Institute of Allergy and Infectious
Diseases, Laboratory of Allergic Diseases, National Institutes of
Health, Bethesda, Maryland

Carol Sedlak, PhD, MSN, RN
Assistant Professor, Kent State University College of Nursing,
Kent, Ohio

Judy Selfridge-Thomas, MSN, RN, CEN, FNP
Nurse Practitioner, Department of Emergency Medicine, St.
Mary Medical Center, Long Beach, California; General Partner,
Selfridge, Sparger, Shea and Associates, Ventura and Orange
Counties, California

Carol Sharkey, MSN, PhD
Associate Professor, Department of Nursing, Regis University,
Denver, Colorado

Sandra Sharma, PhD, ARNP, CS
James A. Haley Veterans Hospital, Tampa, Florida

Suzanne Shaw, BSN, RN
Director, Walls Regional Hospital Home Health, Cleburne, Texas

Nancy Shoemaker, MS, RN, CS-P
Nursing Program Consultant, State of Maryland, Department of
Public Safety and Correctional Services, Jessup, Maryland

Mary Sieggreen, MSN, RN, CS, NP, CUN
Assistant Professor, Wayne State University; Clinical Nurse
Specialist/Nurse Practitioner, Vascular Surgery, Harper Hospital,
Detroit Medical Center, Detroit, Michigan

Pamela Singh, CS, MSN, RN, FNP
Family Nurse Practitioner, San Diego, California

Dianne Smolen, PhD, MSN, RN, C
Associate Professor and Director of Continuing Nursing
Education, Medical College of Ohio School of Nursing, Toledo,
Ohio

Debra A. Solomon, MSN, RN, FNP-C
Clinical Coordinator, Fairview Lakes HomeCaring & Hospice,
Chisago City, Minnesota

Kimberly Stallo, BSN, RN, CETN
Wound, Ostomy, and Continence Nurse, Fort Worth, Texas

Mary M. Stasiak, MA, BSN, RN, PHN
Case Manager, Allied Health Alternatives, Inc., Rochester,
Minnesota

Eleanor M. Stockbridge, MS, CRRN, FNP
Community Nurse Case Manager, Poudre Valley Health System,
Fort Collins, Colorado

Nancy Evans Stoner, MSN, RN, CNSN
Education Manager, Clinical Nutrition Support Services,
University of Pennsylvania Health System, Philadelphia,
Pennsylvania

Linda J. Svatora, OTR/L, MBA
Occupational Therapist, Visiting Nurse Association of Omaha,
Omaha, Nebraska

Janice Tazbir, MS
Assistant Professor, Purdue University Calumet, Hammond,
Indiana

Jill E. Timm, BAN, RN, PHN
Public Health Nurse II, Washington County Department of
Public Health and Environment, Stillwater, Minnesota

Peter J. Ungvarski, MS, RN, FAAN, ACRN
Clinical Associate Professor, City University of New York,
Hunter College–Bellevue School of Nursing; Clinical Nurse
Specialist, HIV/AIDS, and Clinical Director, AIDS Services, The
Visiting Nurse Service of New York, New York, New York

Linda A. Vader, BS, RN, CRNO
Head Nurse, W. K. Kellogg Eye Center, University of
Michigan, Ann Arbor, Michigan

Amy Verst, MSN, RN, CPNP, ATC
Assistant Professor, Bellarmine College; Pediatric Nurse
Practitioner, Jefferson County Health Department, Louisville,
Kentucky

Bernadette White, MSN, RN
Assistant Professor, Creighton University School of Nursing,
Omaha, Nebraska

Connie White-Williams, MSN, RN, FNP
Affiliate Faculty and Cardiothoracic Transplant Coordinator,
University of Alabama, Birmingham, Alabama

Gail F. Wilkerson, MSN, RN, CS
Disease Management Specialist, Heart Failure, Group Health
Plan, St. Louis, Missouri

Linda Yoder, MSN, MBA, PhD
Colonel, United States Army Nurse Corps, McDonald Army
Community Hospital, Fort Eustis, Virginia

Nancy York, MSN, RN
Assistant Professor of Nursing, Bellarmine College, Lansing
School of Nursing, Louisville, Kentucky

Bridget A. Young, BSN, RN, MBA
Vice President of Clinical Services, Visiting Nurse Association
of Omaha, Omaha, Nebraska

Reviewers

Jan Anderson, MSN, RN, CNS
Assistant Director, ADN Program, Santa Barbara City College, Santa Barbara, California

Linda J. Becker, MSN, RN, C
Department Chair, St. Clair County Community College, Port Huron, Michigan

Barbara J. Benz, MS
Roswell Park Cancer Institute, Buffalo, New York

Veronica K. Casey, MA, RN, C
Assistant Professor, Norwalk Community-Technical College, Norwalk, Connecticut

Joy Churchill, MSN, RN
Northern Kentucky University, Highland Heights, Kentucky

Betty R. Ferrell, PhD, RN, FAAN
City of Hope National Medical Center, Duarte, California

Kay Fitterer, MA, RN
Central Lakes College, Brainerd, Minnesota

Gloria J. Green, PhD, MSN, RN
Southeast Missouri State University, Cape Girardeau, Missouri

Angie B. Greer, MSN, RN, CS
Henderson State University, Arkadelphia, Arkansas

Joyce Harris, MA, RN
Director, Butler County Program of Practical Nursing Education, Hamilton, Ohio

JoAnn Romanzi Herne, MS, RNC, FNP-CS
Student Health Supervisor, Crouse Hospital School of Nursing, Syracuse, New York

Robin Higley, MSN
Fairview Hospital, Cleveland, Ohio

Sheilagh Helen Hunt, BA, RN
Certificate in Palliative Care and Thanatology; Professor, Fanshawe College, London, Ontario, Canada

Mary Jane Jones, MN, RN
Associate Professor, Henderson Community College, Henderson, Kentucky

Elizabeth A. Kassel, MSN, RN
Assistant Professor, Syracuse University, Crouse Hospital School of Nursing, University Hospital, Syracuse, New York

Anne Larson, PhD, RN, C
Associate Professor, Midland Lutheran College, Fremont, Nebraska

Suzanne K. Marnocha, MSN, RN, CCRN
Assistant Professor, University of Wisconsin, Oshkosh, Oshkosh, Wisconsin

Jeanette A. McNeill, DrPH, RN, AOCN
Associate Professor/Department Chair, School of Nursing, University of Texas, Houston, Houston, Texas

Captain John J. Melvin, BSN, RN, CCRN
Brooke Army Medical Center, Fort Sam Houston, Texas

Christine C. Mihal, MS, RN, CS
Lecturer, Fairleigh Dickinson University, Teaneck, New Jersey

Carla Mueller, MS, RN
Associate Professor, Department of Nursing, University of Saint Francis, Fort Wayne, Indiana

Elizabeth A. O'Connor, MSN, RNCS, FWP, CCRN
Montana State University at Bozeman, College of Nursing, Great Falls, Montana

Netha O'Meara, MS, RN, CNS
Former Director of Associate Degree Nursing, Wharton County Junior College, Wharton, Texas

Kay B. O'Neal, MSN, RN
El Centro Community College, Dallas, Texas

Molly R. Parker, MHR, BSed, RN
Practical Nursing Program Director, Green Country Area Vocational-Technical School, Okmulgee, Oklahoma

Diana Reding, MS, RN
El Centro College, Parkland Hospital, Dallas, Texas

Lisa Anderson Shaw, DrPH, MSN, MA, RN, CS
Clinical Instructor, Medical/Surgical Nursing, University of Illinois at Chicago College of Nursing; Clinical Ethics Consultant, University of Illinois at Chicago Medical Center, Chicago, Illinois

Beth Ann Stevenson, MSN, RN, CS
School Nurse, Columbus Public Schools; Nurse Clinician, Ohio Department of Health, Columbus, Ohio

Martha Summers, MSN, C-FNP
West Virginia University, Morgantown, West Virginia

Janice M. Thompson, PhD, MSN, RN, C
Associate Professor, Quinnipiac College, Hamden, Connecticut

Lieutenant Michael Welker, BSN, RN, AN
Brooke Army Medical Center, Fort Sam Houston, Texas

Charlene A. Winters, DNSc, RNCS
Montana State University, Missoula, Montana

Preface

It is our conviction that a book is not a static document. Certainly, a book—bound and printed—portrays health care at a given moment in time. The sixth edition of *Medical-Surgical Nursing* is our best attempt to provide instructors and students with a guide to delivering safe and appropriate nursing care. To that end, we see this book as a "work in progress." Future editions will continue to improve, and we appreciate your comments, questions, and corrections to guide our ongoing work. We can improve only with your input. We also realize that educators and students must share in the task of bringing the book to life.

PHILOSOPHY AND APPROACH

This text grows out of the belief that nurses and physicians do not compete with each other but instead collaborate to reach certain outcomes in cooperation with the client and family. Nonetheless, nursing and medicine are separate disciplines. Consequently, in this text nursing and medical content are not intermingled. However, because nursing and medicine are collaborative efforts, it is often difficult for nursing students to understand one without having an understanding of the other. We therefore present thorough coverage of both nursing management and medical management.

With the increased emphasis on outcomes in health care, we have organized client care under the heading of Outcome Management. Several headings appear under this heading, including: Medical Management, Nursing Management of the Medical Client, Surgical Management, and Nursing Management of the Surgical Client, as appropriate.

In this text, we use the nursing process to describe nursing management but we do not apply the nursing process to every disorder. Instead, we have designated the nursing process for major or prototypical disorders. Within the presentation of the nursing process for those disorders, we have developed nursing diagnoses and collaborative problems, as appropriate, with their own outcomes and interventions. Collaborative problems define those client problems that are not resolvable through independent nursing actions; they are potential complications that may develop because of a disorder, a surgical procedure, or a nonsurgical treatment. Collaborative problems complete the picture of nursing care and eliminate the need to force-fit every client problem into the framework of nursing diagnosis. We have written Outcomes and Intervention sections for *each* identified nursing diagnosis and collaborative problem because we have found, from our teaching experience, that students cannot easily pull apart lists of diagnoses, followed by lists of outcomes and interventions, and rebuild them into care plans.

ORGANIZATION

This edition is organized from simple to complex and from common to uncommon disorders. The early portion of the text focuses on care of clients usually assigned to beginning students. The book then progresses to address care of clients with more complex disorders, which are more commonly taught in upper division classes.

Another change in organization is the use of separate chapters for complex disorders, such as renal failure, the need for transplantation, AIDS/HIV, respiratory failure, myocardial infarction, and central nervous system trauma. These disorders are complex and more commonly addressed in upper division course work. We also separate some other material on fluids and electrolytes, stroke, immune disorders, and nutrition to provide adequate coverage and to differentiate major concepts for these disorders.

The sixth edition is divided into 17 units. The first three units are devoted to content that is applicable to all medical-surgical clients. The material in this first portion of the book will guide the student in learning to provide comprehensive care regardless of the specific diagnosis or problem. Concepts that span medical-surgical practice, such as health promotion, care delivery settings, pain, perioperative care, and oncology, are found in this portion of the book. The remainder of the text is divided into common responses to health disorders. Most of these units begin with a review of anatomy and physiology, followed by a chapter on health and diagnostic assessment; thereafter, one or more "Nursing Care" chapters present the nursing care of clients with specific disorders.

Unit 2 presents an overview of nursing and health care today. Chapter 4 describes the "stakeholders" in health care delivery, because medical-surgical nurses (not just managers) in all areas of practice must be increasingly aware of how health care is financed. Because the practice of medical-surgical nursing is not confined to certain areas, more material has been added to this edition on nursing care and philosophy in various care settings. Chapters 5 through 8 address nursing care in ambulatory, acute, home health, and long-term care settings.

Unit 3 covers health assessment, physical examination, and diagnostic testing. The format for health assessment and physical examination that is introduced in Chapters 9 and 10 is carried through in the Assessment chapters for each body system. This structure helps the student to become familiar with one form of thorough assessment and then to apply it in a focused way for clients with specific disorders.

Unit 4 looks at concepts that are common to many medical-surgical clients. Fluid and electrolyte disorders have been separated into two chapters. Other chapters address acid-base disorders, the surgical experience, wound healing, infectious disorders, cancer, psychosocial and mental health concerns, and sleep and sensory disorders, including new material on fatigue and pain. New to this edition is a chapter on end-of-life concerns (Chapter 22). Material on substance abuse has been moved forward into the introductory material because of the increasing numbers of people with substance abuse problems. Chapter 24 discusses the effects of substance abuse on major body systems. It also identifies populations at risk for substance abuse and presents strategies for care.

Units 5 through 16 focus on management of clients with specific disorders. Each unit begins with a structure and function overview of the pertinent body systems as well as a nursing assessment chapter. The structure and function overview has been shortened and redesigned, with more artwork added for each body system.

Discussion of specific disorders generally includes headings for Etiology, Pathophysiology, Clinical Manifestations, and Outcome Management. Because more and more nursing care is being directed toward health promotion, in this edition we have added content focusing on health promotion, health maintenance, and health restoration to the Risk Factors and Etiology topics in chapters on disorders. To emphasize the importance of understanding pathophysiology and its relationship to treatment of a disorder, we have incorporated headings in the management sections that will help the student see the relationship between the pathophysiologic changes and specific strategies to promote positive outcomes in nursing management. The term "clinical manifestations" has been selected to encompass signs and symptoms along with diagnostic findings. The term "manifestations" replaces "signs and symptoms" in all chapters except one; in Chapter 22, "end-of-life symptom management" is the preferred term.

The major content areas for Units 5 through 16 are mobility disorders (Unit 5); nutritional disorders, including ingestive and digestive disorders as well as a new chapter on malnutrition (Unit 6); elimination disorders, including urinary and intestinal problems (Unit 7); sexuality and reproductive disorders (Unit 8); metabolic disorders (Unit 9); integumentary disorders (Unit 10); circulatory disorders (Unit 11); cardiac disorders (Unit 12); oxygenation disorders (Unit 13); sensory disorders (Unit 14); cognitive and perceptual disorders (Unit 15); and protective disorders (Unit 16).

Unit 17 presents care of clients with multisystem disorders. A new chapter, Chapter 79, covers care of the client with HIV infection and AIDS. Chapter 80, also new, looks at organ donation issues, the transplantation process, quality of life issues, and specific interventions for clients requiring organ transplantation. Shock and multisystem disorders are discussed in Chapter 81. Chapter 82 examines the basic concepts of triage, ethical issues, and maintaining the chain of custody of medicolegal evidence. The chapter organizes emergency conditions by various nursing diagnoses identified and treated.

SPECIAL FEATURES

Bridging the gap between classroom instruction and clinical nursing care is difficult. We find that students often think, "I learned that for a test last year," and question how the material is relevant to the clinical situations that they face today. To address those questions, Joyce Black has devised a method of clinical teaching in which the pathophysiology of a disorder is presented graphically and is then overlaid with corresponding clinical manifestations and treatments. The overlays allow students to visualize how changes in pathophysiology lead to certain

manifestations and how a particular treatment is designed to block the progression of the pathophysiologic changes into the development of clinical manifestations. Underlying this teaching method is the assumption that it is easier to "transfer" material if you can visualize the links among pathophysiology, clinical manifestations, and interventions. The fifth edition incorporated this teaching method in special features called **Pathophysiology/Treatment Algorithms (PTAs).** These features are presented on such topics as "Understanding Asthma and Its Treatment." A new PTA on Cushing's disease has been added because of the positive response to the PTAs from the fifth edition.

As another way to help students, particularly at the upper level, to integrate material that they have learned in many courses over the span of a number of years, we have retained all six **Case Studies** from the fifth edition and have added four new ones. The Case Studies, some of which are illustrated, present complex client scenarios that are typical of the situations that students will encounter in clinical practice. Following each scenario is a series of questions for students to consider. The discussions for these questions are included on the CD-ROM packaged with the text.

More and more, students are recognizing the importance of providing quality nursing care to clients with backgrounds different from their own. To help them, this edition includes **Diversity in Health Care** boxes about such topics as "Cultural Perspectives on Pain," "Cultural Aspects of Death and Dying," and "Cultural Influences on Nutrition."

The increased use of alternative and complementary therapies by clients affects their health care management. A new feature, **Alternative Therapies,** has been added to help the student understand what complementary therapies may be used by their clients and the impact that these treatments might have on prescribed therapy ordered by the health care provider. Although many of the alternative therapies are not scientifically supported, they are widely endorsed and should be considered as part of the nursing assessment.

Client Education Guides are presented throughout the text. This important feature helps nurses teach clients how to collaborate in their own care and are worded in client-centered language.

Unlicensed assistive personnel continue to provide direct client care in hospitals. We also recognize that few nursing students have had the opportunity to learn how to delegate care safely. In this edition, we have added 10 additional **Management and Delegation** features, for a total of 19. These discuss assessments and interventions that can, under certain circumstances, be delegated to assistive personnel. They also provide guidance about how to decide whether a particular aspect of care is safe to delegate, and they emphasize that in all cases the responsibility for client care, analysis of client data, and the safety of the client rests squarely on the nurse.

Case management is another area of ongoing change in hospital nursing, and one of the hallmarks of case management is the use of clinical pathways. Two features in this revision highlight the importance of this content area. The first is Case Management. This feature, written by a practicing case manager, presents key coordination and anticipatory issues under consistent headings of "Assess," "Advocate," and "Prevent Readmission," thus linking nursing care with patient-focused case management. Many textbooks now incorporate clinical pathways. In this book we have gone a step further by including a group of **Clinical Pathway Guides** (or CareMap) that have been carefully selected by two experts in case management as among the best in use today. We have included portions of the clinical pathway and a guide to orient the student to the value and important components of each pathway.

The growing use of standardized language in nursing has been addressed by including a list of appropriate **Nursing Outcomes Classification (NOC)** labels at the start of each nursing management chapter. The outcomes chosen include those that may apply to clients with any of the conditions presented within the chapter.

Critical Monitoring features highlight for the student those clinical manifestations that must be reported to the physician without delay. **Care Plans** summarize the nursing diagnoses, outcomes, interventions and rationales, and evaluation criteria for selected disorders.

We have found that students often struggle with how to record normal assessment findings. This edition again includes **Physical Assessment Findings in the Healthy Adult** features, which serve both to remind students of the relevant normal findings for each body system and to demonstrate how to chart those findings with clinical precision.

Bridging the distance from the theoretical to the practical, and from the hospital to the home, is essential in nursing today. To that end, we have asked practicing home care nurses to write new **Bridge to Home Health Care** features for this edition. These features provide practical suggestions on the ever more critical skill of adapting medical-surgical care to the home.

Nursing research is providing evidence to guide practice decisions for all nurses. No longer can just one study be summarized and included in a chapter. We have examined nursing research findings and have incorporated them into the discussion of nursing care. A new feature has been designed to help the student gain a sense of the "state of the science" in selected areas of practice. The **Bridge to Evidence-Based Practice** features examine an integrative review of research evidence for a specific topic by identifying the research questions, studies examined, findings of the studies, limitations, and application to practice. These features appear at the end of units in which the content is related.

Another feature, the **Bridge to Critical Care,** highlights common treatment modalities and assessments performed in critical care. Rather than attempt to discuss all of critical care nursing in these features, we have tried to impart through them a basic understanding of hospital-based critical care treatments as they are used in inpatient care. Some examples are the use of pulmonary pressure monitors, ventilators, and arterial lines.

The prevalence of many diseases in older adults and the special needs of older adults prompted retention of sections called **Modifications for Elderly Clients** for many disorders. Because it is often difficult to differentiate normal manifestations of aging from pathologic conditions in the elderly, we have also included content on normal aging for each body system.

Because of the growing importance of being able to "think critically" as a nurse, we have concluded each nursing care chapter in the book with a series of **Thinking Critically** exercises. Each of these exercises presents a typical client scenario and poses several questions about what actions to take. To give the student clues about how to think through these clinical problems, each exercise includes one or more *Factors to Consider.* On the enclosed CD-ROM, we provide a brief discussion of each of these exercises. Because there is no one right answer to a *Thinking Critically* question, these are *discussions* rather than hard-and-fast *answers.*

SUPPLEMENT PACKAGE

Student Study CD-ROM

Packaged with each copy of the text, this new feature provides students with a wealth of study materials. All of the Case Studies from the text, plus two *bonus* Case Studies, are presented with the corresponding questions and a discussion for each question. Each Case Study also provides 7 to 10 multiple choice questions for further review and presents a nursing care plan in summary. The Thinking Critically questions, with discussions written by the authors, are also included. Students will also benefit from the more than 700 NCLEX-style test questions included for study and review. Icons throughout the text provide reminders for students to refer to the CD-ROM.

Study Guide

The *Study Guide* is designed to improve understanding of each chapter of the textbook. Learning objectives are provided to help the student focus on critical content in each chapter. In addition, *Study Guide* chapters include the following sections, as appropriate:

- Learning the Language
- Critical Thinking: Understanding Rationales
- Thinking Clinically: Knowing What to Do and Why
- Client Education: Knowing What to Teach and Why
- Putting It All Together
- Diagnostic Tests: Knowing Why You Do What You Do
- At-a-Glance Worksheets

Instructor's Electronic Resource

The *Instructor's Electronic Resource* (IER) is designed to help faculty develop lectures, assignments, and clinical assignments based on the content of the textbook and is free to textbook adopters. The IER is a CD-ROM composed of four components:

- A 2000 multiple-choice question test bank in the ExaMaster format
- Image Collection of approximately 200 illustrations from the text
- NEW! LectureView composed of more than 1000 Powerpoint slides
- Instructor's Manual

ExaMaster, a computer test bank, provides approximately 2000 NCLEX-style questions from which instructors can automatically or manually generate examinations. Provided for each question is the correct answer, the rationale for the correct answer, the cognitive level according to Bloom's taxonomy, and the corresponding learning objective in the *Study Guide* and *Instructor's Manual.* These questions are also available to textbook adopters in printed form.

Approximately 300 color illustrations from the text are available through the **Image Collection** and provide exciting visual aids to help the instructor with classroom presentations.

LectureView presents more than 1000 Powerpoint slides organized by each unit of the text. These slides provide instructors with ready-made lectures and are an effective teaching tool.

The **Instructor's Manual** repeats the Learning Objectives from the Student Study Guide and includes Facilitating Student Learning ideas and Critical Points to Emphasize summaries.

SIMON WEB SITE

The SIMON Web site provides instructors and students who are using this textbook with several tools to enhance teaching and learning. It acts as an "Internet"-based ancillary that includes Web links that connect the content of each chapter to numerous Web sites. These linkages are updated during the life of the book so that the content is always current. The Web site also provides content updates, ethics challenges, and other relevant and helpful material.
(http://www.wbsaunders.com/SIMON/Black/medsurg/)

ACKNOWLEDGMENTS

We have been asked several times, "Isn't a revision a lot less work than a new book?" You would think so, but it's amazing—a revision is no less work than a new book.

A project of this size certainly could not be accomplished without the collaboration of many people. First and foremost, we recognize the importance of the clinical expertise of our many contributing authors, which enables

us to present a new edition that continues to be the "gold standard" for textbooks of medical-surgical nursing. We would also like to thank the special feature contributors and to acknowledge Anne Larson for her contribution of the Case Studies.

There are also many people at W. B. Saunders Company who have made this monumental task a "do-able" task. Thank you, Thomas Eoyang, former Editorial Manager, Nursing Books, for your ongoing encouragement, help, and support. Thank you, Terri Ward, former Developmental Editor, and Victoria Legnini, Developmental Editor; without your help and day-to-day management, we would still be behind on the deadlines. Your organization made this project move well. Thank you, Ceil Roberts and Rita Martello, for your meticulous coordination of a massive art program. Thank you, Observatory Group, for your stunning new full-color illustrations. Thank you, Karen O'Keefe Owens, Designer, for your fresh, appealing, full-color design. Thank you, Carol J. Robins, Manuscript Editor, for finding just the right words when we could not, for coordinating the work of other copy editors, and for fielding countless changes, additions, and deletions with unfailing grace. Thank you, Linda Garber and Natalie Ware, Production Managers, for keeping the book on schedule against overwhelming odds. Thank you, Fran Murphy, for coordinating the peer reviews of the book, and Adrienne Simon for handling the countless administrative tasks associated with the publication of the book. Thank you, Barbara Nelson Cullen, Executive Editor, for developing and producing the book's supplement package.

Finally, we want to thank *you*—educators and students—for allowing us to join you in the teaching and learning of medical-surgical nursing. We trust that you will find the sixth edition of *Medical-Surgical Nursing: Clinical Management for Positive Outcomes* a valuable asset.

JOYCE M. BLACK
JANE HOKANSON HAWKS
ANNABELLE M. KEENE

Contents

UNIT 1

Promotion of Self-Care 1

1 Theories of Health Promotion and Illness Management 3

Esther A. Hellman

History of Health Care, 3
  Theories of Disease Causation, 3
  Concept of Health, 3
  Concept of Wellness, 7
  Relationship Between Disease, Illness, Health, and Wellness, 8

Concept of Health Promotion, 9
  Evolution of the Concept of Health Promotion, 9
  Epidemiologic Concepts, 10
  Models of Health Promotion, 11
  Teaching and Motivating Clients, 12

Chronic Conditions or Illnesses, 13
  Multifactorial Aspects of Chronic Disease, 13
  Management of Chronic Conditions and Illness, 16

Outcome Management in Chronic Conditions, 21
  Identifying Client Strengths, 21
  Nursing Diagnosis, 21
  Expected Outcomes, 22
  Evaluation, 22
  Interventions, 22

Health Promotion and Illness Prevention Interventions, 24
  Modifying Behavioral Health Risk Factors, 24
  Modifying Environmental Health Risk Factors, 28

2 Health Promotion in Young and Middle-Aged Adults 30

Kathryn Fiandt

Health Risks, 30
Health Promotion, 30
  Healthy Eating, 30
  Healthy Activity, 33
  Stress Management, 35

Prevention of Injury and Illness, 36
  Accidents, 37
  Alcohol Abuse, 37
  Drug Abuse, 37
  Smoking Cessation, 37
  Domestic Abuse, 39
  Infectious Diseases, 40

Screening for Disease, 40
  Recommendations for Screening, 40
  Breast Self-Examination, 41
  Testicular Self-Examination, 41
  Prostate Cancer, 41
  Colorectal Cancer, 42

3 Health Promotion in Older Adults 45

Beverley E. Holland
Cynthia McCurren

Nursing and the Study of Aging, 45
The Older Population, 46
  Trends Among the Elderly, 46
  Cultural Aspects of Aging, 47
  Health Promotion, Maintenance, and Restoration in Older Clients, 48

Normal Aging and Commonly Occurring Pathologic Processes, 52
Presentation of Illness, 52
Functional Status, 52
  Physiologic Factors That Influence Functional Status, 53
  Psychosocial Factors That Influence Functional Status, 55

Mental Health Disorders in the Elderly, 57
  Dementia, Delirium, and Depression, 57
  Substance Use Disorders, 58

Medication Use in the Elderly, 60
  Pharmacokinetics, 60
  Pharmacodynamics, 61
  Polypharmacy, 61

Health Care for the Elderly Client, 61
  Resources, Services, and Options for Older People, 61
  Managed Care, 63
  Acute Care, 64
  Long-Term Care, 64

Legislation Affecting the Elderly Population, 65
Ethical Issues That Affect the Elderly, 65
  Autonomy, 65
  Competence, 66
  Self-Determination, 67

UNIT 2

Health Care Delivery Systems 71

4 Overview of Health Care Delivery 73

Mary L. Fisher

Major Stakeholders in the Health Care System, 73
  Government, 73
  Physicians, 75
  Hospital Administrators and Governing Boards, 76
  Business and Industry, 76
  The Public, 76
  Nurses, 76

Financing of Health Care Services, 77
Funding Mechanisms, 77
Period of Expansion, 77
Period of Regulation and Cost Containment, 79
Period of Reform, 81

5   Ambulatory Health Care 83
Sheila A. Haas
Diana P. Hackbarth
Definition and Characteristics of Ambulatory Care
Nursing, 83
Conceptual Models That Influence Ambulatory Care
Nursing Practice, 84
The Clinical Model, 84
Levels of Prevention Model, 84
Primary Health Care, Primary Care, and Managed
Care Models, 85
Ambulatory Care Nursing Conceptual
Framework, 85
Ambulatory Care Practice Settings, 86
Characteristics of Ambulatory Care Client
Population, 88
Research in Ambulatory Care Nursing, 89
Dimensions Unique to Nursing Practice in
Ambulatory Care, 89
Ambulatory Care Interdisciplinary Team, 91
Professional and Legal Considerations, 91
Trends and Directions for the Future, 92

6   Acute Health Care 95
Cindy Ludwig
History of Hospital Nursing, 95
Acute Care Hospitals, 95
Roles of Nurses in Hospitals, 98
Nursing Care Delivery Systems, 99
Management and Delegation, 100
Ensuring Quality Health Care Delivery, 100
Monitoring Health Care Outcomes, 102
Regulatory Requirements and Issues, 102
Performance Improvement and Goals, 104
Risk Management, 105
The Future of Acute Care Hospital Nursing, 106

7   Home Health Care 107
Karen S. Martin
Trends, 107
Perspectives, 109
Community-Focused Philosophy, 110
Risks, 111
Resources, 111
Providing Care, 111
The Omaha System, 111
Automation and the Nightingale Tracker, 116

8   Long-Term Care 118
Charlotte Eliopoulos
Growth of Long-Term Care Facilities, 118
Residents of Long-Term Care Facilities, 119
Staff of Long-Term Care Facilities, 121
Nursing Responsibilities, 121
Assessment, 121
Care Planning, 121
Caregiving, 121
Communication, 123
Management, 123
Other Forms of Long-Term Care, 125

UNIT
3

Health Assessment 127

9   Health History 129
Annabelle M. Keene
The Health History, 129
Accuracy, 129
Depth, 130
Guidelines for the Health History Interview, 130
Preparation of the Environment, 130
Preparation of the Client, 130
Preparation of the Interviewer, 135
Components of the Health History, 135
Biographical and Demographic Information, 135
Current Health, 136
Past Health History, 137
Family Health History, 137
Psychosocial History, 137
Review of Systems, 145
Health Promotion and Health Risk Appraisal, 145
Health Promotion Across the Life Span, 155
Screening Tests and Procedures, 155
Organizing the Health History Interview, 160
Recording the Health History Interview, 160
Applying the Nursing Process to Health
Assessment, 160

10   Physical Examination 163
Annabelle M. Keene
Purpose of the Examination, 163
Levels of Physical Examination, 163
Accuracy of Physical Examination, 163
Physical Examination and the Nursing
Process, 163
Techniques of Physical Examination, 174
Inspection, 174
Palpation, 174
Percussion, 177
Auscultation, 178
Olfaction, 179
Guidelines for Physical Examination, 179
Preparation of the Environment, 179
Preparation of Equipment, 179
Preparation of the Client, 180
Preparation of the Examiner, 180
Adult General Screening Physical Examination, 180
General Survey, 180
Processing the Data, 185
Comparison of Findings, 185
Comparison with Known Standards, 185
Suspected Problem Areas, 185
Health Teaching, 185
Terminating the Health Assessment, 185
Recording the Findings, 185
Health Assessment, Nursing Diagnosis, and Nursing
Process, 185

11 Diagnostic Assessment........................ 187
  Annabelle M. Keene
    General Nursing Management, **187**
      Assessment, **187**
      Nursing Interventions, **187**
    Specificity and Sensitivity of Diagnostic Tests, **187**
    *Measurements Used to Report Laboratory Test
      Results,* **188**
      Reference Values, **188**
      International System of Units, **188**
    Laboratory Diagnostic Testing, **188**
      Microbiology Studies, **189**
      Blood Studies, **190**
      Urine Studies, **191**
    Diagnostic Imaging, **192**
      X-ray Studies, **192**
      Magnetic Resonance Imaging, **196**
      Positron Emission Tomography, **197**
      Angiography, **198**
      Ultrasonography, **198**
      Radionuclide Imaging, **199**
    Endoscopy, **200**
      Arthroscopy, **200**
      Bronchoscopy, **200**
      Endoscopy of the Gastrointestinal Tract, **200**
    Cytologic Studies, **200**
      Closed Biopsy, **200**
      Open Biopsy, **200**
      Sections, **201**

UNIT 4

Foundations of Medical-Surgical Nursing... 205

Anatomy and Physiology Review: The Cell... 206
  R. B. Boley
  Arlene L. Polaski
  David Porta

12 **Clients with Fluid Imbalances: Promoting
  Positive Outcomes.......................... 215**
  Bernadette White
    Overview, **215**
      Fluid Movement from Pressure Changes, **215**
      Fluid Movement by Diffusion and Osmolality, **216**
      Hormonal Regulation of Fluid Balance, **217**
    Extracellular Fluid Volume Deficit, **217**
    Intracellular Fluid Volume Deficit, **225**
    Extracellular Fluid Volume Excess, **225**
    Intracellular Fluid Volume Excess: Water
      Intoxication, **228**
    Extracellular Fluid Volume Shift: Third-Spacing, **229**

13 **Clients with Electrolyte Imbalances:
  Promoting Positive Outcomes................ 233**
  Bernadette White

    Electrolyte Balance, **233**
      Dietary Intake, **233**
      Regulated Output, **233**
    Electrolyte Imbalances, **233**
      Sodium Imbalances, **235**
        Hyponatremia, **236**
        Hypernatremia, **239**
      Potassium Imbalances, **242**
        Hypokalemia, **243**
        Hyperkalemia, **246**
      Calcium Imbalances, **248**
        Hypocalcemia, **249**
        Hypercalcemia, **252**
      Phosphate Imbalances, **254**
        Hypophosphatemia, **254**
        Hyperphosphatemia, **254**
      Magnesium Imbalances, **255**
        Hypomagnesemia, **255**
        Hypermagnesemia, **256**

14 **Acid-Base Balance........................... 259**
  Margie Hansen
    Regulation of Acid-Base Balance, **259**
      *Modulation of Serum pH by Blood Buffer
        Systems,* **259**
      Regulation of Volatile Acid by the Lungs, **260**
      *Regulation of Fixed Acids and Bicarbonate by the
        Kidneys,* **260**
    Interaction of Acid-Base Regulatory Systems, **263**
      Acid-Base Compensation, **263**
      Acid-Base Correction, **263**
      Analysis of Arterial Blood Gases, **264**
    Disorders of Acid-Base Balance, **264**
      Respiratory Alkalosis, **264**
      Respiratory Acidosis, **265**
      Metabolic Alkalosis, **266**
      Metabolic Acidosis, **267**
      Complex Acid-Base Disorders, **268**

15 **Clients Having Surgery: Promoting Positive
  Outcomes................................... 273**
  Nancy Girard
    Perioperative Nursing, **273**
    Basic Concepts of Perioperative Nursing, **273**
    Preoperative Period, **274**
      Preoperative Assessment, **274**
      Physical Examination, **276**
      Educational Assessment **282**
    Immediate Preoperative Care, **282**
      Physical Care, **282**
      Nutritional Care, **284**
      Preoperative Teaching, **284**
      Components of Preoperative Teaching, **285**
      Preoperative Teaching for Older Adults, **287**
      Informed Consent, **287**
      Preparing the Client on the Day of Surgery, **288**
      *Preoperative Preparation Immediately Before
        Surgery,* **289**
      Preoperative Medications, **289**
      Transporting the Client to Surgery, **289**
      *Preparing the Client's Room for Postoperative
        Care,* **289**
      Caring for Significant Others, **289**

Intraoperative Period, 290
  Members of the Surgical Team, 290
  Anesthesia, 292
  Intraoperative Nursing Care, 298
Postoperative Period, 302
  Post-Anesthesia Care Unit Nursing, 303
  Postoperative Nursing Care, 308

16 Clients with Wounds: Promoting Positive Outcomes 315
Joyce M. Black
  Normal Wound Healing, 315
    Phases of Wound Healing, 316
    Wound Healing Intention, 320
    Nutrition and Wound Healing, 321
  Clients with Acute Inflammation, 321
  Clients with Chronic Inflammation, 324
  Clients with Incisions, 324
  Clients with Open Wounds, 324
  Disorders of Wound Healing, 330
    Delayed Wound Healing, 330
      Intrinsic Factors, 331
      Extrinsic Factors, 332
    Wound Infection, 332
    Wound Disruption, 333
    Altered Collagen Synthesis, 333

17 Perspectives on Infectious Disorders 335
Carol Sharkey
  The Process of Infection, 335
    Agent, 335
    Environment, 336
    Host, 336
  Risks of Hospitalization, 338
    Urinary Tract Infections, 338
    Pneumonia, 338
    Surgical Wound Infections, 339
    Device-Related Infections and Bacteremias, 339
    Antibiotic-Resistant Microorganisms, 339
    Other Nosocomial Infections, 340
  Preventing and Controlling Infection, 340
    Immunization Programs, 341
    Infection Control in Hospitals, 343
    Infection Control in Long-Term Care Facilities, 346
    Infection Control in Community-Based Settings, 346

18 Perspectives in Oncology 349
Patricia Meier
  Terminology, 349
  Epidemiology, 349
    Incidence and Prevalence, 350
    Mortality, 350
    Trends, 350
  Pathophysiology, 353
    Carcinogens, 354
    Carcinogenesis: Transformation of Normal Cells into Cancer Cells, 355
    Inability of Immune System to Recognize Cancer Cells, 360
    Apoptosis, 361
  Genetics and Cancer, 362
  Classification of Neoplasms, 362
    Benign Versus Malignant, 362
    Tissue of Origin, 362

19 Clients with Cancer: Promoting Positive Outcomes 367
Patricia Meier
  Health Promotion and Maintenance, 367
    Cancer Prevention and Control, 367
  Health Restoration, 370
    Maintaining Wellness During Treatment, 370
    Rehabilitation, 370
  Outcome Management, 371
    Diagnosis of Cancer, 371
    Grading and Staging Cancer, 371
    Identifying Treatment Goals, 373
    Determining Treatment Modalities, 373
    Radiation Therapy, 377
    Clinical Trials, 389
    Evaluation of Treatment Response, 390
    Myelosuppression, 392
    Gastrointestinal Effects, 393
    Integumentary Effects, 394
    Effects on the Reproductive System, 395
    Oncologic Emergencies, 395
  Psychosocial Aspects of Cancer Care, 397
    Providing Support for Clients, 397
    Providing Support for Family, 398
    Promoting Positive Self-Concept, 398
    Promoting Coping Throughout the Cancer Continuum, 399

20 Clients with Psychosocial and Mental Health Concerns: Promoting Positive Outcomes 405
Nancy Shoemaker
  Universal Issues, 407
    Anxiety, 407
    Stress, 407
    Coping Mechanisms, 408
    Self-Esteem, 409
  Additional Needs of Clients with Concurrent Mental Illness, 409
    Comprehensive Nursing Assessment, 409
    Awareness of Communication, 410
    Client and Family Teaching, 411
    Specialized Referrals, 411
    Summary, 411
  Anxiety, 412
    Possible Causes, 414
    Outcome Management, 415
    Intervention, 415
  Schizophrenia, 416
    Possible Causes, 417
    Outcome Management, 417
    Intervention, 419
  Mood Disorders, 420
    Possible Causes, 421
    Outcome Management, 422
    Intervention: Major Depression, 422
    Intervention: Depression, 424
    Intervention: Bipolar Disorder, 426

21 Clients with Sleep and Rest Disorders and Fatigue: Promoting Positive Outcomes 431
Marlene Reimer
  Sleep and Sleep Pattern Disturbances, 431
    Chronobiology, 432
    Physiology of Sleep and Arousal, 432

Sleep Disorders, **434**

Dyssomnias, **434**

Intrinsic Sleep Disorders, **434**

Extrinsic Sleep Disorders, **436**

Circadian Rhythm Sleep Disorders, **437**

Arousal Disorders, **437**

Sleep-Wake Transition Disorders, **437**

Parasomnias Associated with Rapid Eye Movement
Sleep, **437**

Other Parasomnias, **437**

*Sleep Disorders Associated with Medical and
Psychological Disorders,* **437**

Neurotransmitter Imbalances, **437**

Head Injury, **438**

Hormonal Imbalances, **438**

Respiratory Disorders, **438**

Cardiovascular Disorders, **439**

Gastrointestinal Disorders, **439**

Other Disorders, **439**

Hospital-Acquired Sleep Disturbances, **439**

Sleep Onset Difficulty, **439**

Sleep Maintenance Disturbance, **439**

Early-Morning Awakening, **440**

Sleep Deprivation, **440**

Diagnostic Assessment, **440**

Fatigue, **442**

Sensory Disturbances, **442**

Classification, **443**

Sensory Overload, **443**

Sensory Deprivation, **443**

Diagnosis and Prevention, **443**

Diagnosis, **443**

Prevention, **443**

22   Perspectives on End-of-Life Care 447

Kim K. Kuebler
Debra E. Heidrich

End-of-Life Care, **447**

Hospice, **447**

Continued Unmet Needs of the Dying, **448**

Palliative Care, **448**

Symptoms at the End of Life, **449**

Pain, **449**

Dyspnea, **451**

Delirium, **453**

Depression, **453**

Fatigue and Weakness, **454**

Sleep Disturbances, **454**

Cachexia-Anorexia Syndrome **455**

Indicators of Imminent Death, **456**

Communication, **456**

Care for the Caregivers, **456**

Support of the Grieving Family, **457**

**23   Clients with Pain: Promoting Positive
Outcomes 461**

Juanita Fogel Keck
Susan Baker

The Problem of Pain, **461**

Definition of Pain, **462**

Perception of Pain, **463**

Misconceptions and Myths, **463**

Misinformation About Pain, **463**

Types of Pain, **464**

Acute Pain, **464**

Chronic Pain, **465**

Physiology, **466**

Physiologic Basis of Pain Perception, **466**

Gate Control Theory of Pain, **470**

Sources of Pain, **471**

Classification, **471**

Referred Pain, **472**

Inflammation, **472**

Neuropathy, **473**

Phantom Limb Sensation, **473**

Headache, **473**

Malignancy, **473**

Human Immunodeficiency Virus Infection, **473**

Factors Affecting Pain, **474**

Situational Factors, **474**

Sociocultural Factors, **474**

Age, **476**

Gender, **476**

Meaning of Pain, **476**

Anxiety, **476**

Past Experience with Pain, **476**

Expectation and the Placebo Effect, **477**

Medications to Control Pain, **483**

Anesthetic Agents, **483**

Analgesics, **484**

Negative Effects of Pain, **496**

Nonpharmaceutical Interventions, **496**

Cutaneous Stimulation, **496**

Transcutaneous Electrical Nerve Stimulation
(TENS), **497**

Massage, **497**

Heat and Cold Applications, **498**

Acupuncture, **498**

Acupressure, **498**

Music, **498**

Progressive Relaxation Training, **498**

Deep Breathing for Relaxation, **499**

Guided Imagery, **499**

Rhythmic Breathing, **499**

Meditation, **499**

Hypnosis, **499**

Humor, **499**

Biofeedback, **499**

Therapeutic Touch, **500**

Distraction, **500**

Magnets, **500**

Evaluation and Documentation, **500**

Evaluation, **500**

Documentation, **503**

**24   Clients with Substance Abuse Disorders:
Promoting Positive Outcomes 507**

Linda Carman Copel

Frameworks for Explaining Addictive Behaviors, **508**

Biologic Framework, **508**

Psychological Framework, **508**

Sociocultural Framework, **509**

Definitions and Terminology, **509**

General Assessment, **511**

*Assessment and Management of Substance-Abusing
Clients,* **513**

Alcohol, **513**

Amphetamines, **516**

Caffeine, **517**

Cannabis, **517**

Cocaine, **517**

Hallucinogens, **517**

Inhalants, **518**
Nicotine, **518**
Opioids, **518**
Phencyclidine, **518**
Sedatives, Hypnotics, and Anxiolytics, **519**
Drug and Alcohol Intervention, **519**
Confrontation About Drug Abuse, **519**
Treatment Options, **519**
Prevention of Relapse, **522**
Surgery and Substance Abuse, **523**
The Impaired Health Care Professional, **524**

UNIT
5

Mobility Disorders 529

Anatomy and Physiology Review: The Musculoskeletal System..................... **530**
David Porta
Joyce M. Black

25 Assessment of the Musculoskeletal System.... 537
Peggy Doheny
Carol Sedlak

History, **537**
Biographical and Demographic Data, **537**
Current Health, **537**
Past Health History, **538**
Family Health History, **539**
Psychosocial History, **539**
Review of Systems, **540**
Physical Examination, **540**
General Musculoskeletal Examination, **540**
Neurovascular Assessment, **542**
Diagnostic Tests, **545**
Noninvasive Tests of Structure, **545**
Invasive Tests of Structure, **546**
Laboratory Studies, **548**

26 Management of Clients with Musculoskeletal Disorders **551**
Dottie Roberts
Joan Lappe

Osteoarthritis, **551**
Metabolic Bone Disorders, **565**
Osteoporosis, **566**
Paget's Disease, **572**
Osteomalacia, **575**
Gout and Gouty Arthritis, **575**
Spinal Column Deformities, **576**
Scoliosis, **577**
Kyphosis, **578**
Lordosis, **578**
Bone Infections, **578**
Osteomyelitis, **578**
Septic Arthritis, **579**

Bone Tumors, **580**
Malignant Bone Tumors, **581**
Disorders of the Foot, **582**
Hallux Valgus (Bunions), **582**
Morton's Neuroma (Plantar Neuroma), **582**
Hammer Toe, **583**
Muscular Disorders, **583**
Muscular Dystrophy, **583**

27 Management of Clients with Musculoskeletal Trauma or Overuse **587**
Dottie Roberts

Fractures, **587**
Specific Fractures, **607**
Hip Fractures, **607**
Condylar Fractures, **616**
Pelvic Fractures, **616**
Patellar Fractures, **617**
Tibial and Fibular Fractures, **617**
Foot Fractures, **617**
Upper Extremity Fractures, **617**
Dislocations and Subluxations, **619**
Sports Injuries, **619**
Overuse Syndromes, **619**
Lower Extremities, **620**
Upper Extremities, **620**
Strains, **621**
Sprains, **621**
Rotator Cuff Tears, **622**
Anterior Cruciate Ligament Injuries, **623**
Meniscal Injuries, **623**
Remobilization After Traumatic Injury, **623**

UNIT
6

Nutritional Disorders...................... 629

Anatomy and Physiology Review: The Nutritional (Gastrointestinal) System......... **630**
Robert G. Carroll

28 Assessment of Nutrition and the Digestive System..................................... **638**
Vicki M. Ross

Screening and Assessment of Nutritional Status, **638**
Nutritional Health, **638**
Malnutrition, **639**
Nutrition Screen or Assessment? **640**
History, **640**
Biographical and Demographic Data, **640**
Current Health, **645**
Past Health History, **646**
Family Health History, **648**
Psychosocial History, **648**
Review of Systems, **649**

Physical Examination, **649**
  Anthropometric Measures, **649**
  Mouth, **650**
  Abdomen, **652**
Diagnostic Tests, **655**
  Laboratory Tests, **655**
  Radiography, **656**
  Computed Tomography, **657**
  Ultrasonography, **657**
  Endoscopy, **657**
  Exfoliative Cytologic Analysis, **658**
  Gastric Analysis, **658**
  Acid Perfusion Test, **659**
  Esophageal Manometry, **659**
  Ambulatory Esophageal pH Monitoring, **659**

29 Management of Clients with Malnutrition 661
Nancy Evans Stoner
Candace Cantwell
Protein-Energy Malnutrition, **661**
Eating Disorders, **677**
  Obesity, **677**
  Anorexia Nervosa and Bulimia Nervosa, **679**

30 Management of Clients with Ingestive
Disorders 683
Elizabeth A. Murphy-Blake
Dental Disorders, **683**
Oral Disorders, **684**
  Stomatitis, **684**
    Aphthous Stomatitis, **684**
    Herpes Simplex, **684**
    Vincent's Angina, **684**
  Candidiasis, **685**
  Tumors of the Oral Cavity, **686**
    Benign Tumors of the Oral Cavity, **686**
    Premalignant Tumors of the Oral Cavity, **686**
    Malignant Tumors of the Oral Cavity, **686**
Disorders of the Salivary Glands, **690**
  Inflammation, **690**
  Calculi, **690**
  Tumors, **690**
Disorders of the Esophagus, **690**
  Dysphagia, **690**
    Dysphagia Caused by Mechanical Obstructions, **690**
    Dysphagia Caused by Cardiovascular
      Abnormalities, **690**
    Dysphagia Caused by Neurologic Diseases, **690**
    Dysphagia from Other Causes, **691**
  Regurgitation, **691**
  Pain, **691**
  Heartburn, **691**
  Achalasia, **691**
  Gastroesophageal Reflux Disease, **695**
  Hiatal Hernia, **697**
  Diverticula, **698**
  Esophageal Cancer, **699**
Vascular Disorders, **702**
Trauma, **702**

31 Management of Clients with Digestive
Disorders 705
Elizabeth A. Murphy-Blake
  General Clinical Manifestations of Gastrointestinal
  Disorders, **705**
    Pain, **705**

Anorexia, **705**
Nausea and Vomiting, **705**
Bleeding, **706**
Diarrhea, **706**
Belching and Flatulence, **706**
Indigestion, **706**
Gastrointestinal Intubation, **706**
  Types of Tubes, **706**
  Inserting Gastrointestinal Tubes, **707**
  Suctioning Gastrointestinal Tubes, **707**
  Nursing Management of Clients with Gastrointestinal
  Tubes, **708**
Gastritis, **708**
  Acute Gastritis, **708**
  Chronic Gastritis, **709**
Peptic Ulcer Disease, **712**
  Duodenal Ulcers, **712**
  Gastric Ulcers, **712**
  Stress-Induced and Drug-Induced Ulcers, **712**
Gastric Cancer, **724**

UNIT

7

Elimination Disorders 731

Anatomy and Physiology Review: The
Elimination Systems 732
Robert G. Carroll

32 Assessment of Elimination 739
Roberta Jorgensen
Karen A. Hanson
Bowel Elimination, **739**
  History, **739**
    Biographical and Demographic Data, **739**
    Current Health, **739**
    Past Health History, **740**
    Family Health History, **741**
    Psychosocial History, **741**
    Review of Systems, **742**
  Physical Examination, **742**
    Abdomen, **742**
    Anus and Rectum, **743**
  Diagnostic Tests, **743**
    Laboratory Tests, **745**
    Fecal Analysis, **745**
    Radiography, **746**
    Endoscopy, **746**
Urinary Elimination, **747**
  History, **747**
    Biographical and Demographic Data, **747**
    Current Health, **747**
    Past Health History, **751**
    Family Health History, **752**
    Psychosocial History, **753**
    Review of Systems, **754**
  Physical Examination, **754**
    Abdomen, **754**

Genitalia, 755
Rectum, 756
Lymph Nodes, 756
Related Body Systems, 756

Diagnostic Tests, 756

Laboratory Tests, 756
Radiography, 758
Ultrasonography, 759
Radionuclide Studies, 759
Endoscopy, 760
Biopsy, 760
Urodynamic Studies, 762

**33 Management of Clients with Intestinal
Disorders** 765

Helen Murdock Rogers

General Clinical Manifestations, 765

Disorders of the Large and Small Bowel, 766

Inflammatory Disorders, 766

Infections and Infestations, 766
Viral and Bacterial Infections: Gastroenteritis, 766
Parasitic Infections, 767

Appendicitis, 768
Peritonitis, 769
Inflammatory Bowel Disease, 770

Neoplastic Disorders, 780

Benign Tumors of the Bowel, 780
Cancer of the Bowel, 780
Cancer of the Small Bowel, 780
Colorectal Cancer, 780

Other Disorders of the Large and Small Bowel, 787

Herniations, 787
Diverticular Disease, 789
Meckel's Diverticulum, 790
Obstruction, 790
Irritable Bowel Syndrome, 793

Disorders of the Anorectal Area, 795

Hemorrhoids, 795
Pilonidal Cyst, 797
Anal Fissure, 797
Anal Fistula, 797
Anorectal Abscess, 797
Cancer 797
Bowel Incontinence, 797

Blunt or Penetrating Trauma, 798

**34 Management of Clients with Urinary
Disorders** 801

Francie Bernier

Infectious and Inflammatory Disorders, 802

Cystitis, 802
Interstitial Cystitis, 807
Urosepsis, 808
Urethritis, 809
Ureteritis, 809

Obstructive Disorders, 809

Bladder Cancer, 809
Ureteral Tumors, 821
Urinary Calculi, 821
Urinary Reflux, 829

Voiding Disorders, 829

Urinary Retention, 829
Urinary Incontinence, 833
Neurogenic Bladder, 841

Traumatic Disorders, 846
Bladder Trauma, 846
Urethral Trauma, 846
Ureteral Trauma, 846
Congenital Anomalies, 847

**35 Management of Clients with Renal
Disorders** 851

Anita E. Molzahn

Extrarenal Conditions, 851

Diabetes Mellitus, 851
Hypertension, 852
Hypotension, 852
Rhabdomyolysis, 852
Cardiovascular Disease, 852
Peripheral Vascular Disease, 853
Sepsis, 853
Pregnancy, 853
Other Causes, 853

Nephrotoxins, 853

Acquired Disorders, 854

Nephrolithiasis, 854
Pyelonephritis, 854
Renal Candidiasis, 856
Renal Tuberculosis, 857
Renal Abscess, 857
Perinephric Abscess, 858
Hydronephrosis, 858
Renal Cancer, 858
Tubulointerstitial Disease, 862
Glomerulonephritis, 862
Nephrotic Syndrome, 862
Nephritic Syndrome, 863

Types of Glomerulonephritis, 863

Renal Vascular Abnormalities, 869

Renal Artery Disease, 869
Renal Vein Disease, 870

Congenital Disorders, 870

Anomalies Involving Kidney Number and
Position, 870
Anomalies Involving Kidney Form and Size, 871
Anomalies Involving Cystic Disease, 871
Polycystic Kidneys, 871
Adult-Onset Medullary Cystic Disease, 872
Medullary Sponge Kidney, 872

Other Hereditary Renal Disorders, 872

36 Management of Clients with Renal Failure ... 875

Anita E. Molzahn

Uremic Syndrome, 875
Acute Renal Failure, 876
Chronic Renal Failure, 882

UNIT

8

Sexuality and Reproductive Disorders **903**

**Anatomy and Physiology Review: The
Reproductive Systems** **904**

Robert G. Carroll

37   Assessment of the Reproductive System 915

Rhonda Holloway

The Female Reproductive System, **915**

> *History,* **915**
>
> > *Biographical and Demographic Data,* **916**
> > *Current Health: The Chief Complaint,* **916**
> > *Past Health History,* **916**
> > *Gynecologic History,* **916**
> > *Family Health History,* **917**
> > *Psychosocial History,* **917**
> > *Review of Systems,* **919**
>
> *Physical Examination,* **919**
>
> > *Breasts and Axillae,* **919**
> > *Pelvis,* **922**
> > *Vaginal Speculum Examination,* **924**
>
> *Diagnostic Tests,* **926**
>
> > *Gynecologic Studies,* **926**
> > *Breast Studies,* **931**

The Male Reproductive System, **934**

> *History,* **934**
>
> > *Biographical and Demographic Data,* **934**
> > *Current Health: The Chief Complaint,* **934**
> > *Past Health History,* **934**
> > *Sexual and Reproductive History,* **935**
> > *Family Health History,* **935**
> > *Psychosocial History,* **935**
> > *Review of Systems,* **936**
>
> *Physical Examination,* **936**
>
> > *Breasts and Axillae,* **936**
> > *External Genitalia,* **936**
> > *Prostate,* **939**
>
> *Diagnostic Tests,* **939**
>
> > *Laboratory Studies,* **940**
> > *Radiography,* **941**
> > *Ultrasonography,* **941**
> > *Radionuclide Imaging,* **942**
> > *Cystoscopy,* **942**
> > *Urodynamic Assessment,* **942**
> > *Prostatic Biopsy,* **942**
>
> *Prevention of Male Reproductive Problems,* **942**

38   Management of Men with Reproductive Disorders 945

Patricia McCallig Bates

Prostate Disorders, **945**

> *Benign Prostatic Hyperplasia,* **945**
> *Prostate Cancer,* **958**
> *Prostatitis,* **962**

Testicular and Scrotal Disorders, **964**

> *Testicular Cancer,* **964**
> *Testicular Torsion,* **966**
> *Orchitis,* **966**
> *Epididymitis,* **966**
> *Hydrocele, Hematocele, and Spermatocele,* **966**
> *Varicocele,* **966**
> *Vasectomy (Elective Sterilization),* **967**
> *Undescended or Mispositioned Testicles,* **967**
> *Infertility,* **968**

Penile Disorders, **970**

> *Phimosis,* **970**
> *Paraphimosis,* **970**
> *Posthitis and Balanitis,* **970**
> *Urethritis,* **971**
> *Urethral Stricture,* **971**
> *Epispadias,* **971**
> *Hypospadias,* **971**
> *Peyronie's Disease,* **971**
> *Priapism,* **972**
> *Penile Cancer,* **972**
> *Penile and Scrotal Injuries,* **972**

Erectile Dysfunction, **972**

39   Management of Women with Reproductive Disorders 979

Francie Bernier

Menstrual Disorders, **979**

> Cultural Influences, **979**
> Reactions to Manifestations, **980**
>
> > *Dysmenorrhea,* **980**
> > *Premenstrual Syndrome,* **981**
> > *Abnormal Uterine Bleeding,* **982**
> >
> > > *Amenorrhea,* **982**
> > > *Menorrhagia,* **983**
> > > *Metrorrhagia,* **984**
> >
> > *Menopause,* **984**
> >
> > > *Surgical Menopause,* **984**
> > > *Perimenopausal Changes,* **984**
> > > *Postmenopausal Bleeding,* **986**

Pelvic Inflammatory Disease, **986**

> *Chronic Pelvic Inflammatory Disease,* **989**

Uterine Disorders, **989**

> *Endometriosis,* **989**
> *Benign Uterine Tumors (Leiomyomas),* **991**
> *Endometrial (Uterine) Cancer,* **994**
> *Cervical Cancer,* **995**
> *Urogenital Displacement and Prolapse,* **998**
>
> > *Cystocele and Urethrocele,* **998**
> > *Rectocele and Enterocele,* **999**
> > *Vaginal or Uterine Prolapse,* **999**
>
> *Polyps,* **1000**

Ovarian Disorders, **1000**

> *Benign Ovarian Tumors,* **1000**
> *Ovarian Cancer,* **1001**

Vaginal Disorders, **1002**

> *Vaginal Discharge and Pruritus,* **1002**
> *Vaginitis,* **1002**
> *Toxic Shock Syndrome,* **1003**
> *Atrophic Vaginitis,* **1003**
> *Vaginal Fistulae,* **1003**
> *Vaginal Cancer,* **1004**

Vulvar Disorders, **1005**

> *Vulvitis,* **1005**
> *Vulvar Cancer,* **1005**
> *Bartholinitis,* **1008**
> *Female Genital Mutilation,* **1008**

40   Management of Clients with Breast Disorders 1011

Michelle Goodman
Stephanie Mellon-Reppen

Breast Cancer in Women, **1011**

> *Primary Breast Cancer,* **1019**
> *Breast Reconstruction,* **1029**
> *Local Recurrence,* **1034**
> *Metastatic Breast Cancer,* **1035**

Breast Cancer in Men, **1036**
Benign Breast Disease, **1036**

> *Fibrocystic Breasts,* **1037**
> *Hyperplasia and Atypical Hyperplasia,* **1037**
> *Fibroadenoma,* **1037**

Papilloma, **1037**
Duct Ectasia, **1037**
Mastodynia and Mastalgia, **1037**
Gynecomastia, **1037**
Mammaplasty, **1037**
Breast Augmentation, **1037**
Reduction Mammaplasty, **1038**
Mastopexy, **1039**

41 Management of Clients with Sexually Transmitted Diseases **1041**
Meg Blair
Sexually Transmitted Diseases: An Overview, **1041**
Diseases Characterized by Urethritis or Cervicitis, **1047**
Chlamydial Infections, **1047**
Gonorrhea, **1048**
Diseases Characterized by Ulcerations, **1050**
Syphilis, **1050**
Genital Herpes, **1051**
Chancroid, **1053**
Lymphogranuloma Venereum, **1053**
Granuloma Inguinale, **1053**
Infection with Human Papillomavirus, **1053**
Genital Warts (Condylomata Acuminata), **1053**
Diseases Characterized by Vaginal Discharge, **1054**
Trichomoniasis, **1054**
Bacterial Vaginosis, **1055**
Acquired Immunodeficiency Syndrome, **1055**
Vaccine-Preventable Diseases, **1056**
Hepatitis A and B, **1056**
Diseases Caused by Infestations, **1056**
Pediculosis Pubis and Scabies, **1056**
Sexually Transmitted Enteric Infections, **1056**
Management of Clients Reporting Sexual Assault, **1056**

UNIT 9

Metabolic Disorders **1059**

Anatomy and Physiology Review: The Metabolic Systems **1060**
Robert G. Carroll

42 Assessment of the Endocrine and Metabolic Systems **1070**
Dianne Smolen
History, **1070**
Biographical and Demographic Data, **1070**
Current Health, **1070**
Past Health History, **1071**
Family Health History, **1072**
Psychosocial History, **1072**
Review of Systems, **1073**
Physical Examination, **1073**
General Appearance and Nutritional Status, **1074**
Vital Signs, **1074**

Integument, **1074**
Head, **1074**
Eyes, **1074**
Nose, **1074**
Mouth, **1074**
Neck, **1074**
Extremities, **1074**
Thorax, **1075**
Abdomen, **1075**
Genitalia and Rectum, **1078**
Modifications for Older Adults, **1078**
Diagnostic Tests, **1078**
Endocrine Function Studies, **1078**
Metabolic Function Studies, **1080**

43 Management of Clients with Thyroid and Parathyroid Disorders **1089**
Anne Larson
Thyroid Disorders, **1089**
Goiter, **1089**
Hypothyroidism, **1090**
Hyperthyroidism, **1099**
Thyroiditis, **1106**
Thyroid Cancer, **1107**
Parathyroid Disorders, **1109**
Hyperparathyroidism, **1109**
Hypoparathyroidism, **1114**

44 Management of Clients with Adrenal and Pituitary Disorders **1119**
Anne Larson
Adrenocortical Disorders, **1119**
Adrenal Insufficiency, **1119**
Primary Adrenal Insufficiency, **1120**
Secondary Adrenal Insufficiency, **1126**
Adrenocortical Hyperfunction, **1126**
Hypercortisolism, **1126**
Hyperaldosteronism, **1133**
Adrenomedullary Disorders, **1135**
Pheochromocytoma, **1135**
Anterior Pituitary Disorders, **1137**
Hyperpituitarism and Hyperprolactinemia, **1139**
Sexual Disturbances, **1142**
Hypopituitarism, **1142**
Posterior Lobe (Neurohypophyseal) Disorders, **1143**
Gonadal Disorders, **1143**

45 Management of Clients with Diabetes Mellitus **1149**
James A. Fain
Acute Complications of Diabetes Mellitus, **1172**
Hyperglycemia and Diabetic Ketoacidosis, **1172**
Hyperglycemic, Hyperosmolar, Nonketotic Syndrome, **1177**
Hypoglycemia, **1177**
Other Hypoglycemic Disorders, **1180**
Hypoglycemic Unawareness, **1180**
Hypoglycemia with Rebound Hyperglycemia, **1180**
Dawn Phenomenon, **1180**
Chronic Complications of Diabetes Mellitus, **1180**
Macrovascular Complications, **1182**
Coronary Artery Disease, **1184**
Cerebrovascular Disease, **1184**

Hypertension, **1184**
Peripheral Vascular Disease, **1184**
Infections, **1184**

Microvascular Complications, **1186**
Diabetic Retinopathy, **1186**
Nephropathy, **1187**
Neuropathy, **1188**

46 Management of Clients with Exocrine Pancreatic and Biliary Disorders............1193
Dianne Smolen

Disorders of the Exocrine Pancreas, **1193**

Acute Pancreatitis, **1194**
Chronic Pancreatitis, **1200**
Pancreatic Pseudocysts, **1201**
Pancreatic Cancer, **1202**
Pancreatic Trauma, **1202**
Cystic Fibrosis, **1202**

Biliary Tract Disorders, **1203**

Cholelithiasis (Gallstones), **1203**
Acute Cholecystitis, **1212**
Acute Acalculous Cholecystitis, **1213**
Chronic Cholecystitis, **1213**
Choledocholithiasis and Cholangitis, **1214**
Sclerosing Cholangitis, **1215**
Carcinoma of the Gallbladder, **1215**

47 Management of Clients with Hepatic Disorders 1219
Dianne Smolen

Jaundice, **1220**
Hepatitis, **1223**
Viral Hepatitis, **1223**
Complications of Hepatitis, **1229**
Fulminant Hepatitis, **1229**
Chronic Hepatitis, **1229**
Chronic Persistent Hepatitis, **1229**
Chronic Active Hepatitis, **1229**
Chronic Carrier State, **1230**
Aplastic Anemia, **1230**
Toxic Hepatitis, **1232**
Alcoholic Hepatitis, **1232**
Cirrhosis, **1232**
Complications of Cirrhosis, **1240**
Portal Hypertension, **1240**
Ascites, **1245**
Hepatic Encephalopathy, **1250**
Fatty Liver (Hepatic Stenosis), **1253**
Liver Neoplasms, **1254**
Benign Hepatic Tumors, **1254**
Malignant Hepatic Tumors, **1254**
Primary Hepatocellular Cancer, **1254**
Metastatic Hepatic Cancers, **1255**
Liver Transplantation, **1256**
Liver Abscess, **1257**
Hemochromatosis, **1258**
Amyloidosis, **1258**
Congenital Conditions, **1258**
Wilson's Disease, **1259**
Caroli's Syndrome, **1259**
Congenital Hepatic Fibrosis, **1259**
Liver Trauma, **1259**

UNIT 10

Integumentary Disorders 1261

Anatomy and Physiology Review: The Integumentary System......................1262
Robert G. Carroll

48 Assessment of the Integumentary System....1267
Noreen Heer Nicol

History, **1267**
Current Health, **1267**
Past Health History, **1267**
Family Health History, **1268**
Psychosocial History, **1268**
Review of Systems, **1269**

Physical Examination, **1269**
Terminology, **1269**
Types of Lesions, **1269**
Examination Environment, **1269**
Depth of Examination, **1269**
Inspection and Palpation, **1271**
Skin Self-Examination, **1276**

Diagnostic Tests, **1276**
Skin Culture and Sensitivity, **1276**
Potassium Hydroxide Examination and Fungal Culture, **1276**
Tzanck's Smear, **1276**
Scabies Scraping, **1276**
Wood's Light Examination, **1276**
Patch Testing, **1276**
Biopsy, **1277**

49 Management of Clients with Integumentary Disorders 1279
Noreen Heer Nicol
Joyce M. Black

Topical Medications, **1279**
Topical Therapy, **1279**
Topical Vehicles, **1280**
Topical Corticosteroids, **1281**

Wound Dressings, **1282**
Unna Boot, **1282**

Soaks and Wet Wraps, **1282**
Skin Lubricants, **1283**
Ultraviolet Light Therapy, **1283**
Ultraviolet B Therapy, **1284**
Photochemotherapy, **1284**
Combination Therapies, **1284**

Psychosocial Aspects of Skin Disorders, **1284**
Common Skin Disorders, **1286**
Pruritus, **1286**
Eczematous Disorders, **1286**
Atopic Dermatitis, **1287**
Xerotic Eczema, **1290**
Stasis Dermatitis, **1290**
Contact Dermatitis, **1291**
Intertrigo, **1291**

Psoriasis Vulgaris, **1292**
Acne Vulgaris, **1293**
Acne Rosacea, **1294**

Skin Tears, **1294**
Pressure Ulcers, **1295**
Precancerous Changes in the Skin, **1302**
   Sunburn, **1302**
   Actinic Keratosis, **1303**

Skin Cancer, **1305**
   Basal Cell Carcinoma, **1306**
   Squamous Cell Carcinoma, **1306**
   Malignant Melanoma, **1307**
   *Cutaneous T-Cell Lymphoma (Mycosis
    Fungoides),* **1309**
   Kaposi's Sarcoma, **1309**

Bullous Disorders: Pemphigus, **1310**

Infectious Disorders, **1310**
   Erysipelas and Cellulitis, **1310**
   Herpes Zoster (Shingles), **1310**

Plastic Surgery and Other Cosmetic/Restorative
Procedures, **1313**

Basic Principles of Plastic Surgery, **1314**

Achieving Minimal Scarring, **1314**
   Skin Lines, **1314**
   Elliptical Incisions, **1314**
   Suturing Techniques, **1314**
   Other Variables, **1314**

Selecting Clients, **1314**
   Understanding Motivations for Surgery, **1314**
   Determining Realistic Expectations, **1315**
   Documentation Through Photography, **1316**

Facial Rejuvenating Surgery, **1316**

Rhytidectomy (Face Lift), **1316**
Blepharoplasty, **1318**
Facial Resurfacing, **1318**
   Alpha-Hydroxy Peels, **1318**
   Trichloroacetic Acid Peels, **1318**
   Laser Resurfacing, **1318**
   Dermabrasion, **1319**
   Collagen Injection, **1319**
Rhinoplasty, **1319**

Body-Contouring Surgery (Lipectomy), **1319**

Suction-Assisted Lipectomy, **1319**
Abdominoplasty, **1320**
Panniculectomy, **1320**

Reconstructive Plastic Surgery, **1321**

Reconstructive Modalities, **1321**
   Skin Grafts, **1321**
   Flaps, **1322**
   Implants, **1325**
   Skin Expansion, **1325**
   Lasers, **1326**

Repair of Traumatic Injuries, **1326**

Facial Injuries, **1326**
   Lacerations, **1326**
   Facial Fractures, **1326**

Traumatic Amputations, **1328**

Nail Disorders, **1328**

50 **Management of Clients with Burn Injury ... 1331**
Pamela Cornwell
   Emergent Phase, **1338**
   Acute Phase, **1346**
   Rehabilitation Phase, **1354**

UNIT
11

Circulatory Disorders **1361**

**Anatomy and Physiology Review: The
Circulatory System** **1362**
Robert G. Carroll

51 **Assessment of the Vascular System** **1368**
Mary Sieggreen
   History, **1368**
    Biographical and Demographic Data, **1368**
    Current Health, **1368**
    Past Health History, **1369**
    Family Health History, **1370**
    Psychosocial History, **1370**
    Review of Systems, **1370**
   Physical Examination, **1370**
    Inspection, **1370**
    Palpation, **1373**
    Auscultation, **1375**
   Diagnostic Tests, **1375**
    Noninvasive Vascular Laboratory Techniques, **1375**
    Invasive Techniques, **1376**

52 **Clients with Hypertensive Disorders: Promoting
Positive Outcomes** **1379**
Jean Elizabeth DeMartinis
   Hypertension, **1379**
    *Hypertensive Crises: Urgency Versus
    Emergency,* **1395**
   Syncope, **1397**

53 **Management of Clients with Vascular
Disorders** **1399**
Janice D. Nunnelee
   Peripheral Artery Disorders, **1399**
    Acute Arterial Occlusion, **1415**
    Arterial Ulcers, **1416**
    Aneurysms, **1416**
     Classification, **1416**
     Abdominal Aortic Aneurysms, **1416**
    Aortic Dissection, **1419**
     Thoracic Aortic Aneurysms, **1420**
    Raynaud's Syndrome, **1421**
    *Thromboangiitis Obliterans (Buerger's
    Disease),* **1421**
     Peripheral Aneurysms, **1422**
    Subclavian Steal Syndrome, **1422**
    Thoracic Outlet Syndromes, **1422**
   Venous Disorders, **1422**
    Acute Venous Disorders, **1422**
    Chronic Venous Disorders, **1426**
     Varicose Veins, **1426**
     Chronic Venous Insufficiency, **1427**
     Venous Stasis Ulceration, **1429**
   Lymphatic Disorders, **1429**
    Lymphedema, **1429**

Congenital Disorders, **1501**
Cardiac Surgery, **1501**

Types of Heart Surgery, **1501**

Valvular Surgery, **1501**
Heart Transplantation, **1502**
Assisted Circulation and Mechanical Hearts, **1504**
Open Heart Surgery, **1504**

UNIT
12

Cardiac Disorders........................ **1433**

Anatomy and Physiology Review:
The Heart **1434**

Robert G. Carroll

54   Assessment of the Cardiac System **1447**

Kathleen Popelka

History, **1447**

Risk Factor Analysis, **1447**
Biographical and Demographic Data, **1448**
Current Health, **1448**
Past Health History, **1453**
Family Health History, **1454**
Psychosocial History, **1454**
Review of Systems, **1455**

Physical Examination, **1455**

General Appearance, **1455**
Level of Consciousness, **1456**
Head, Neck, Nails, and Skin, **1456**
Edema, **1456**
Blood Pressure, **1456**
Pulse, **1457**
Respirations, **1457**
Head and Neck, **1457**
Chest, **1458**
Abdomen, **1462**

Diagnostic Tests, **1464**

Laboratory Tests, **1464**
Electrocardiogram, **1466**
Electrophysiologic Studies, **1472**
Cardiac Diagnostic Imaging, **1472**
Hemodynamic Studies, **1476**

55   Management of Clients with Structural Cardiac
Disorders **1481**

Barbara B. Ott

Infectious Disorders, **1481**

Rheumatic Fever, **1481**
Infective Endocarditis, **1484**
Myocarditis, **1487**
Pericarditis, **1488**

Acute Pericarditis, **1488**
Acute Pericarditis with Effusion, **1489**
Chronic Constrictive Pericarditis, **1489**
Cardiac Tamponade, **1489**

Cardiomyopathy, **1490**

Dilated Cardiomyopathy, **1490**
Hypertrophic Cardiomyopathy, **1492**
Restrictive Cardiomyopathy, **1493**

Valvular Heart Disease, **1495**

Mitral Valve Disease, **1495**
Aortic Valve Disease, **1498**
Tricuspid Valve Disease, **1500**
Pulmonic Valve Disease, **1500**

56   Management of Clients with Functional Cardiac
Disorders **1515**

Peggy Gerard
Janice Tazbir

Coronary Heart Disease, **1515**
Heart Failure, **1529**

57   Management of Clients with
Dysrhythmias **1550**

Maribeth Guzzo

Dysrhythmias, **1550**
Atrial Dysrhythmias, **1552**
Disturbances in Automaticity, **1552**

Sinus Tachycardia, **1552**
Sinus Bradycardia, **1553**
Sinus Dysrhythmia, **1554**
Premature Atrial Contractions, **1554**

Disturbances in Conduction, **1554**

Sinoatrial Node Conduction Defects, **1554**

Reentry of Impulses, **1555**

Paroxysmal Atrial Tachycardia, **1555**
Atrial Flutter, **1556**
Atrial Fibrillation, **1556**

Atrioventricular Junctional Dysrhythmias, **1556**
Disturbances in Automaticity, **1557**

Premature Junctional Contractions, **1557**
Paroxysmal Junctional Tachycardia, **1557**

Disturbances in Conduction, **1557**

First-Degree Atrioventricular Block, **1557**
Second-Degree Atrioventricular Block, **1558**

Mobitz Type I Block (Wenckebach
Phenomenon), **1558**
Mobitz Type II Block, **1558**

Third-Degree Atrioventricular Block, **1559**

Disturbances in Conduction, **1559**

Bundle Branch Block, **1559**

Ventricular Dysrhythmias, **1559**
Disturbances in Automaticity, **1560**

Premature Ventricular Contractions, **1560**
Ventricular Fibrillation, **1564**
Ventricular Asystole, **1565**
Pulseless Electrical Activity, **1565**

Reentry of Impulses, **1565**

Ventricular Tachycardia, **1565**
Torsades de Pointes, **1565**
Pre-excitation Syndromes, **1565**
Other Forms of Defibrillation, **1568**

58   Management of Clients with Myocardial
Infarction **1579**

Janice Tazbir
Peggy Gerard

Angina Pectoris, **1579**
Acute Myocardial Infarction, **1585**

UNIT
13

Oxygenation Disorders 1611

Anatomy and Physiology Review: The
Respiratory System........................ 1612
Robert G. Carroll

59   Assessment of the Respiratory System....... 1623
Amy Verst
General Respiratory Assessment, 1623
History, 1623
Biographical and Demographic Data, 1623
Current Health, 1623
Past Health History, 1625
Family Health History, 1626
Psychosocial History, 1626
Review of Systems, 1627
Physical Examination, 1627
Inspection, 1627
Palpation, 1629
Percussion, 1631
Auscultation, 1632
Assessment of the Nose, Pharynx, and Sinuses, 1635
History, 1635
Current Health, 1635
Past Health History, 1635
Physical Examination, 1635
Nose, 1635
Nasopharynx, 1636
Paranasal Sinuses, 1636
Smell, 1636
Diagnostic Tests, 1637
Tests to Evaluate Respiratory Function, 1637
Tests to Evaluate Anatomic Structures, 1643
Specimen Recovery and Analysis, 1647

60   Management of Clients with Upper Airway
Disorders 1651
Linda K. Clarke
Methods of Controlling the Airway, 1651
Tracheostomy, 1651
Tracheostomy Tubes, 1652
Potential Problems Associated with Tracheostomy
Tubes and Cuffs, 1654
Weaning, Removal, and Rescue Breathing, 1655
Weaning From a Tracheostomy Tube, 1655
Removing a Tracheostomy Tube, 1656
Performing Rescue Breathing, 1656
Neoplastic Disorders, 1660
Benign Tumors of the Larynx, 1660
Cancer of the Larynx, 1661
Hemorrhagic, Infectious, and Inflammatory
Disorders, 1672
Epistaxis, 1672
Sinusitis, 1676
Pharyngitis, 1678
Acute Tonsillitis, 1678
Chronic Tonsillitis, 1679
Peritonsillar Abscess (Quinsy), 1679

Rhinitis, 1679
Laryngitis, 1680
Diphtheria, 1680
Obstructions of the Upper Airway, 1681
Acute Laryngeal Edema, 1681
Chronic Laryngeal Edema, 1681
Laryngospasm, 1681
Laryngeal Paralysis, 1681
Laryngeal Injury, 1682
Chronic Airway Obstruction, 1682
Nasal Polyps, 1682
Deviated Nasal Septum and Nasal Fracture, 1682

61   Management of Clients with Lower Airway
and Pulmonary Vessel Disorders............ 1685
Sherill Nones Cronin
Kim Miracle
Disorders of the Lower Airways, 1685
Asthma, 1685
Chronic Obstructive Pulmonary Disease, 1691
Chronic Obstructive Bronchitis, 1695
Emphysema, 1695
Tracheobronchitis, 1705
Bronchiectasis, 1705
Disorders of the Pulmonary Vasculature, 1706
Pulmonary Embolism, 1706
Pulmonary Hypertension, 1708

62   Management of Clients with Parenchymal
and Pleural Disorders 1710
Nancy York
Atelectasis, 1710
Infectious Disorders, 1711
Influenza, 1711
Pneumonia, 1711
Lung Abscess, 1716
Pulmonary Tuberculosis, 1716
Extrapulmonary Tuberculosis, 1722
Nontuberculous Mycobacterial Infection, 1723
Fungal Pulmonary Infections 1723
Cystic Fibrosis, 1724
Interstitial Lung Disease, 1725
Sarcoidosis, 1726
Neoplastic Lung Disorders, 1726
Malignant Lung Tumors, 1726
Benign Lung Tumors, 1739
Occupational Lung Diseases, 1739
Restrictive Lung Disorders, 1740
Lung Transplantation, 1741
Disorders of the Pleura and Pleural Space, 1742
Pleural Pain, 1742
Pleural Effusion, 1742
Primary Pleural Effusion, 1742
Recurrent Pleural Effusion, 1743
Bronchopleural Fistula, 1743
Metastatic Pleural Tumors, 1743
Disorders of the Diaphragm, 1743
Subdiaphragmatic Abscess, 1743
Diaphragmatic Paralysis, 1744

63   Management of Clients with Acute Pulmonary
Disorders 1746
Joyce M. Black
Respiratory Failure, 1746
Hypoxemic Respiratory Failure, 1747
Pulmonary Edema, 1747

Acute Ventilatory Failure, **1749**
Adult Respiratory Distress Syndrome, **1761**
Chest Trauma, **1764**

Pneumothorax, **1765**

Open Pneumothorax and Mediastinal Flutter, **1767**
Tension Pneumothorax and Mediastinal Shift, **1767**

Hemothorax, **1768**
Chest Fractures, **1768**

Flail Chest, **1768**

Fractured Ribs, **1769**
Fractured Sternum, **1770**
Near-Drowning, **1770**
Carbon Monoxide Poisoning, **1770**

UNIT 14

Sensory Disorders.........................1777

Anatomy and Physiology Review: The Eyes and Ears....................................1778
Robert G. Carroll

64 Assessment of the Eyes and Ears 1787
Linda A. Vader
Helene J. Krouse
Assessment of the Eye, **1787**

History, **1787**

Biographical and Demographic Data, **1787**
Current Health, **1787**
Past Health History, **1788**
Family Health History, **1789**
Psychosocial History, **1789**
Review of Systems, **1789**

Physical Examination, **1789**

External Eye, **1789**
Internal Eye, **1794**

Diagnostic Tests, **1796**

Fundus Photography, **1796**
Exophthalmometry, **1796**
Ophthalmic Radiography, **1796**
Ophthalmodynamometry, **1797**
Electroretinography, **1797**
Visual Evoked Response, **1797**
Fluorescein Angiography, **1797**

Assessment of the Ear, **1798**

History, **1798**

Biographical and Demographic Data, **1799**
Current Health, **1799**
Past Health History, **1799**
Family Health History, **1800**
Psychosocial History, **1800**
Review of Systems, **1800**

Physical Examination, **1800**

Inspection and Palpation, **1800**
Tests for Auditory Acuity, **1802**
Tests for Vestibular Acuity, **1804**

Diagnostic Tests, **1804**

Tests for Aural Structure, **1804**
Tests for Auditory Function, **1804**
Laboratory Tests, **1806**

65 Management of Clients with Visual Disorders 1809
Linda A. Vader
Glaucoma, **1809**
Cataracts, **1814**
Retinal Disorders, **1817**

Retinal Detachment, **1817**
Diabetic Retinopathy, **1820**
Retinitis Pigmentosa, **1821**
Age-Related Macular Degeneration, **1821**
Retinal Artery Occlusion, **1821**

Corneal Disorders, **1821**

Corneal Dystrophies, **1821**
Corneal Infection: Keratitis, **1823**

Uveal Tract Disorders: Uveitis, **1824**
Malignant Ocular Tumors, **1825**

Ocular Melanoma, **1825**
Retinoblastoma, **1826**

Eyelid Tumors, **1826**
Eyelid, Lacrimal, and Conjunctival Disorders, **1826**

Dry Eye Syndrome, **1826**

Refractive Disorders, **1826**

Myopia, **1827**
Hyperopia, **1827**
Astigmatism, **1828**

Ocular Manifestations of Systemic Disorders, **1828**

Endocrine Disorders: Graves' Disease, **1828**
Rheumatoid and Connective Tissue Disorders, **1829**
Neurologic Disorders, **1829**
Circulatory Disorders, **1829**
Immunologic Disorders, **1829**
Lyme Disease, **1829**

66 Management of Clients with Hearing and Balance Disorders.........................1831
Helene J. Krouse

Hearing Impairment, **1831**
Otalgia, **1840**
Balance Disorders, **1847**

UNIT 15

Cognitive and Perceptual Disorders 1855

Anatomy and Physiology Review: The Neurologic System.........................1856
Joyce M. Black

67 Assessment of the Neurologic System........1874
Mary Vorder Bruegge
History, **1874**

Biographical and Demographic Data, **1874**
Current Health, **1874**

Past Health History, **1874**
Family Health History, **1879**
Psychosocial History, **1879**
Review of Systems, **1879**

Physical Examination, **1879**

Vital Signs, **1880**
Mental Status, **1880**
Head, Neck, and Back, **1883**
Cranial Nerves, **1883**
Motor System, **1886**
Sensory Function, **1888**
Reflex Activity, **1889**
Autonomic Nervous System, **1892**
Functional Assessment, **1893**
Clinical Applications, **1893**

Diagnostic Tests, **1894**

Noninvasive Tests of Structure, **1894**
Invasive Tests of Structure, **1896**
Noninvasive Tests of Function, **1901**
Invasive Tests of Function, **1903**

68 Management of Comatose or Confused Clients **1905**

Chris Stewart Amidei

Disorders of Consciousness, **1905**
Confusional States, **1918**

69 Management of Clients with Cerebral Disorders **1923**

Melanie Minton

Seizure Disorders, **1923**

Epilepsy, **1923**
Seizures, **1931**
Status Epilepticus, **1931**

Brain Tumors, **1931**
Hemorrhagic Cerebrovascular Disorders, **1939**

Subarachnoid Hemorrhage, **1940**

Arteriovenous Malformations, **1944**

Infections, **1944**

Bacterial Meningitis, **1944**
Bacterial Toxins, **1945**
Brain Abscess, **1946**
Viral Infections, **1946**
Viral Meningitis, **1946**
Viral Encephalitis, **1947**

Arbovirus Encephalitis, **1947**
Herpes Simplex Virus Encephalitis, **1947**

Fungal Infections, **1947**
Parasitic Infestations, **1948**
Toxoplasmosis, **1948**

Headache, **1948**

70 Management of Clients with Stroke **1953**

Catherine A. Kernich

Stroke—Scope of the Problem, **1953**
Transient Ischemic Attacks, **1978**

71 Management of Clients with Peripheral Nervous System Disorders **1983**

Anne Marie Johnson Fredrichs

Lower Back Pain, **1983**
Cervical Disc Disorders, **1991**
Post-Polio Syndrome, **1993**
Syringomyelia, **1993**
Spinal Tumors, **1994**

Vascular Spinal Cord Lesions, **1994**

Myelomalacia, **1994**
Hematomyelia, **1994**

Neurosyphilis, **1995**
Disorders of the Cranial Nerves, **1995**

Trigeminal Neuralgia, **1995**
Bell's Palsy, **1996**

Upper Motor Neuron Lesions, **1997**
Lower Motor Neuron Lesions, **1997**
Disorders of the Peripheral Nerves, **1997**

Peripheral Neuropathies, **1998**

Cumulative Trauma Disorders, **1998**
Carpal Tunnel Syndrome, **1998**
Ulnar Nerve Syndrome, **1998**
Tarsal Tunnel Syndrome, **1998**

Dupuytren's Contracture, **2000**
Ganglion, **2000**
Peripheral Nerve Injuries, **2000**
Peripheral Nerve Tumors, **2001**

72 Management of Clients with Degenerative Neurologic Disorders **2002**

Amy Perrin Ross

Alzheimer's Disease, **2002**
Creutzfeldt-Jakob Disease, **2009**
Huntington's Disease, **2009**
Multiple Sclerosis, **2012**
Guillain-Barré Syndrome, **2016**
Parkinson's Disease, **2017**
Myasthenia Gravis, **2020**
Eaton-Lambert (Myasthenic) Syndrome, **2023**
Amyotrophic Lateral Sclerosis, **2023**

73 Management of Clients with Neurologic Trauma **2026**

Norma D. McNair

Increased Intracranial Pressure, **2026**
Traumatic Brain Injury, **2039**
Spinal Cord Injury, **2046**

UNIT
16

Protective Disorders **2071**

Anatomy and Physiology Review: The Hematopoietic System **2072**

Joyce M. Black

74 Assessment of the Hematopoietic System **2089**

Mary A. Allen

History, **2089**

Biographical and Demographic Data, **2089**
Current Health, **2089**
Past Health History, **2090**
Family Health History, **2091**
Psychosocial History, **2092**
Review of Systems, **2092**

Physical Examination, 2093
Diagnostic Tests, 2094

Hematologic Tests, **2094**
Immunologic Status Tests, **2100**

75 **Management of Clients with Hematologic Disorders** 2103
Linda Yoder

Disorders Affecting Red Blood Cells, 2103

The Anemias, **2103**
Iron Deficiency Anemia, **2112**
Megaloblastic Anemia, **2113**
Pernicious Anemia, **2113**
Anemia Caused by Folic Acid Deficiency, **2114**
Aplastic Anemias, **2115**
Hemolytic Anemia, **2115**
Sickle Cell Anemia and Sickle Cell Trait, **2116**
Polycythemia Vera, **2118**

Disorders Affecting White Blood Cells, 2119

Agranulocytosis, **2119**
Multiple Myeloma, **2120**
Infectious Mononucleosis, **2121**
Splenic Rupture and Hypersplenism, **2121**

Disorders of Platelets and Clotting Factors, 2122

Hemorrhagic Disorders, **2122**
Idiopathic Thrombocytopenic Purpura, **2122**
Coagulation Disorders, **2123**

Hypoprothrombinemia, **2123**
Disseminated Intravascular Coagulation, **2123**
The Hemophilias, **2126**

76 **Management of Clients with Immune Disorders** 2129
Linda Ludy Scott

Hypersensitivity Disorders, 2129
Allergic Disorders, 2135

Food Allergy, **2135**
Atopic Dermatitis, **2135**
Urticaria, **2136**
Anaphylaxis, Insect Sting Allergy, and Latex Allergy, **2137**
Allergic Rhinitis, **2138**
Asthma, **2138**

77 **Management of Clients with Autoimmune Disease** 2140
Joyce M. Black

Autoimmunity, **2141**

Theories on Autoimmunity, **2141**

Rheumatoid Arthritis, **2142**
Systemic Lupus Erythematosus, **2156**
Progressive Systemic Sclerosis (Scleroderma), **2159**
Ankylosing Spondylitis, **2160**
Sjögren's Syndrome, **2161**
Fibromyalgia Syndrome, **2161**
Polymyositis and Dermatomyositis, **2162**
Vasculitis, **2162**
Reiter's Syndrome, **2163**
Polymyalgia Rheumatica and Cranial Arteritis, **2163**
Mixed Connective Tissue Disease, **2163**
Lyme Disease, **2163**
Secondary Arthritis, **2163**

Whipple's Disease, **2163**
Other Disorders Causing Arthritis, **2163**

78 **Management of the Client with Leukemia and Lymphoma** 2165
Linda Yoder

Leukemia, **2166**
Lymphomas, **2173**

Hodgkin's Disease, **2173**
Non-Hodgkin's Lymphoma, **2176**

Bone Marrow Transplantation, **2179**
Graft-Versus-Host Disease, **2180**

Acute Graft-Versus-Host Disease, **2180**
Chronic Graft-Versus-Host Disease, **2181**

UNIT
17

Multisystem Disorders **2183**

79 **Management of Clients with Acquired Immunodeficiency Syndrome** 2185
Peter J. Ungvarski

80 **Management of Clients Requiring Transplantation** 2213
Connie White-Williams

Historical Perspective, **2213**
Related Issues, **2214**

Cost, **2214**
Shortage of Organ Donors, **2215**
Ethical Considerations, **2215**

Outcome Management **2215**

Clients with End-Stage Organ Disease, **2215**
Postoperative Transplantation Clients, **2222**
Clients Receiving a Specific Organ Transplant, **2225**

Self-Care, **2227**
Quality of Life After Transplantation, **2228**

81 **Management of Clients with Shock and Multisystem Disorders** 2231
Louise Nelson LaFramboise

Shock, **2231**
Multiple Organ Dysfunction Syndrome, **2255**

82 **Management of Clients in the Emergency Department** 2261
Judy Selfridge-Thomas

Emergency Medical Services, **2262**
Emergency Nursing, **2262**
Legal Issues, **2262**

Federal Legislation, **2262**
Consent to Treat, **2262**
Restraints, **2263**
Mandatory Reporting, **2263**
Evidence Collection and Preservation, **2263**
Violence, **2263**

Ethical Issues, **2264**

  Unexpected Death, **2264**
  Advance Directives, **2264**
  Organ and Tissue Donation, **2265**

Components of Emergency Care, **2265**

  Triage, **2265**
  Nursing Assessment, **2265**
  Diagnosis, **2266**
  Outcome Management, **2267**
  Evaluation, **2267**
  Client Disposition, **2267**
  Nursing Documentation, **2267**

Emergency Conditions, **2267**

  Ineffective Airway Clearance, **2267**
  Ineffective Breathing Patterns, **2269**

    Hyperventilation, **2269**
    Hypoventilation, **2270**

  Impaired Gas Exchange, **2270**

    Traumatic Pneumothorax, **2271**
    Flail Chest, **2272**

  Fluid Volume Deficit, **2273**
  Fluid Volume Excess, **2274**
  Decreased Cardiac Output, **2275**
  Pain, **2275**

Acute Confusion, **2276**
Sensory Perceptual Alterations, **2277**
Infection, **2278**
Impaired Physical Mobility, **2278**
Impaired Skin Integrity, **2279**
Poisoning, **2281**

  Accidental and Intentional Poisonings, **2281**
  Snake Bite, **2282**

Hyperthermia, **2282**
Hypothermia, **2282**

  Frostbite, **2283**

Ineffective Individual Coping, **2283**

Appendix A **Religious Beliefs and Practices Affecting Health Care** **2291**

Appendix B **A Health History Format That Integrates the Assessment of Functional Health Patterns** **2298**

Appendix C **Laboratory Values of Clinical Importance in Medical-Surgical Nursing.** **2301**

Index **2311**

Special Features

Alternative Therapies

Alternative and Complementary Modalities
Used by Clients 136
Spirituality and Health 413
Alternative Treatments for Irritable Bowel
Syndrome 794
Urinary Disorders 833
Benign Prostatic Hyperplasia 946
Female Reproductive System: Premenstrual
Syndrome and Menopause 1009
Integumentary Disorders 1281
Vascular Disorders 1405
Cardiac Disorders 1525

Bridges to Critical Care

Swan-Ganz Monitoring 1477
Intra-aortic Balloon Pumping–Counterpulsation
Device 1510
Example of a Ventilator Control Panel and
Troubleshooting Alarms 1753
Intracranial Pressure Monitoring 2032

Bridges to Evidence-Based Practice

The Trait and Process of Resilience 69
Patient-Centered Communication 202
Decision-Making: Withholding or Withdrawing Life
Support 527
Falls Among the Elderly 626
Feeding Tube Placement Errors 728
The Implantable Cardioverter-Defibrillator and
Quality of Life 1607
Arterial Oxygen Saturation Monitoring by Pulse
Oximetry 1772
Respiratory Care of Older Adults after Cardiac
Surgery 1774
Fever-Related Interventions 2285
Quality of Life After Organ Transplantation 2288

Bridges to Home Health Care

Detecting Elder Abuse 57
Managing Multiple Medications 60
Finding Financial Help 108
Medicare and Medicaid Coverage of Home Health
Services 109
Managing Intravenous Therapy 242
Recovering from Surgery 312
Infection Control 345
Dealing with Grief Related to a New Cancer
Diagnosis 398
Providing Hospice Care 449
Controlling Pain 484

Addressing Substance Abuse 512
Managing the Immobile Client 618
Managing Swallowing Difficulties 667
Managing Tube Feedings 675
Adjusting to Life with a Colostomy 787
Managing an Ileal Conduit 818
Inserting Urinary Catheters 845
Living with Peritoneal Dialysis 890
Intermittent Self-Catheterization for Men 948
Teaching About Sexually Transmitted
Infections 1048
Diabetic Foot Care 1187
Managing Pressure Ulcers 1303
Managing After Burns 1355
Managing Peripheral Vascular Disease 1428
Recovery After Heart Surgery 1512
Managing Heart Failure 1546
Heart-Healthy Living After a Myocardial
Infarction 1598
Living with a Tracheostomy 1660
Conserving Oxygen with Chronic Obstructive
Pulmonary Disease 1705
Living with a Ventilator 1762
Coping with Failing Vision 1819
Living with a Severe Hearing Loss 1838
Safety Solutions for People with Alzheimer's
Disease 2007
Respite Care for Caregivers of People with
Alzheimer's Disease 2008
Managing Immunosuppression and Nutrition 2136
Increasing Independent Living with Rheumatoid
Arthritis 2151
Living with HIV/AIDS 2208

Care Plans

The Older Client at Risk for Relocation Stress
Syndrome 56
Side Effect Management for the Client Receiving
Chemotherapy 383
The Client with Degenerative Joint Disease and
Concurrent Panic Disorder: Mrs. James 416
The Client with Hiatal Hernia and Concurrent
Schizophrenia: Mr. Barnes 420
The Client with Diabetic Ketoacidosis and
Concurrent Depression: Mrs. Conners 423
The Client with Stroke and Concurrent Depression:
Mr. Moore 425
The Client with Dehydration and Concurrent
Bipolar Disorder: Miss Howard 427
The Client with Osteoporosis 574
The Client in Traction 610
Foot Infections in the Client with Diabetes
Mellitus 1186
Management of the Client with Hepatic Failure ... 1248
The Client with Atopic Dermatitis 1289

Postoperative Care of the Client Who Has Had
 Arterial Bypass Surgery of the Lower
 Extremity 1408
The Client with Cardiomyopathy 1494
The Client with Heart Failure 1542
The Client with a Myocardial Infarction 1599
The Client with Chronic Obstructive Pulmonary
 Disease 1702
The Client Undergoing Thoracic Surgery 1733
The Mechanically Ventilated Client 1757
The Client with Vertigo 1852
The Client Who Has Undergone Craniotomy 1938
The Client with Stage I Graft-Versus-Host
 Disease 2181

Case Management

The Elective Surgery Client 283
The Client with Cancer 376
Hip Fracture 616
Diabetes 1170
The Client with Impaired Skin Integrity 1302
Heart Failure 1547
Acute Myocardial Infarction 1593
Chronic Obstructive Pulmonary Disease 1686
Pneumonia 1715
Stroke 1970
The Older Adult 2020

Case Studies

Perforated Ulcer Managed Surgically 723
Acute Renal Failure and Abdominal Aortic
 Aneurysm Resection 880
Breast Cancer with Mastectomy 1026
Hyperthyroidism and Postmenopausal
 Osteoporosis 1102
Diabetes and Pneumonia 1153
Cirrhosis 1238
Cardiogenic Shock, Tachycardia, and Heart
 Failure 1594
Meningioma, Fractured Hip, and Possible
 Cerebrovascular Accident 1966
Spinal Cord Injury 2056
Human Immunodeficiency Virus (HIV) 2207

Client Education Guides

Skin Care Within the Treatment Field 380
Living with Obstructive Sleep Apnea Syndrome.... 436
Diet for Dumping Syndrome 721
Colostomy Irrigation 786
Ostomy Supplies 786
Learning to Care for a Urinary Diversion 820
Preventing Recurrence of Urinary Stones 826
Preventing Vaginitis 1003
Recovering from Radical Vulvectomy 1007
Postmastectomy Exercises 1027
Arm Care After Axillary Lymph Node
 Dissection 1028
Sexually Transmitted Diseases 1045
How to Use a Condom 1046

Thyroid Supplements 1098
Self-Injection of Insulin 1168
Visual Complications of Diabetes 1188
Sick Day Management for Diabetes Mellitus 1190
Skin Self-Examination 1285
Simple Guidelines to Help Protect You from the
 Damaging Rays of the Sun 1304
Postoperative Care After Rhinoplasty 1319
Low-Sodium Diet 1393
Low-Fat, Low-Cholesterol Diet 1393
Calorie-Restriction Diet 1394
Foot Care 1403
Stump and Prosthesis Care 1414
Stress Testing 1471
Infective Endocarditis 1487
The Client with a Permanent Pacemaker 1596
Swallowing Technique After a Partial
 Laryngectomy 1668
Care of a Tracheoesophageal Puncture Wound 1671
Exercises After Radical Neck Surgery 1673
Asthma 1693
Tuberculosis 1722
Care After Cataract Removal 1817
Infection of the Tympanic Membrane, Middle Ear,
 or Mastoid Cavity 1846
Precautions After Ear Surgery 1847
When a Loved One Is in an Altered State of
 Consciousness 1917
Epilepsy 1928
Migraine Headache 1949
Transfer from Bed to Wheelchair by a Hemiplegic
 Client 1972
Low Back Care 1991
Home Care After Cervical Laminectomy or
 Fusion 1993
Home Care After Carpal Tunnel Release 2000
Caring for Family Members with Alzheimer's
 Disease 2006
Parkinson's Disease 2021
Monitoring Family Members After Head Injury 2046
Use of a Halo Vest 2062
Using Topical Pain Relievers 2152
Shock 2255

Clinical Pathway Guides

Total Hip Replacement 562
GI Hemorrhage 715
Mastectomy 1021
Coronary Bypass Grafting 1529
Chronic Obstructive Pulmonary Disease 1700
Pneumonia 1716
Stroke 1968

Critical Monitoring

Fluid and Electrolyte Imbalance Secondary
 to Any Disorder/Condition 236
Acid-Base Imbalances 270
The Client in a Cast 605
Postoperative Monitoring After Urinary Diversion
 Procedures 817
Hypothyroidism 1097

Hyperthyroidism 1099
Hyperparathyroidism and Hypoparathyroidism 1109
Does Your Client Have an Antidiuretic Hormone
  (ADH) Imbalance? 1142
The Rehydration Process 1175
Manifestations of Adult Respiratory Distress
  Syndrome Secondary to Acute Pancreatitis...... 1198
Esophageal Bleeding Secondary to Portal
  Hypertension 1241
Musculocutaneous Reconstruction 1323
Cardiac Tamponade 1490
Asthma 1689
Manifestations of Changes in Neurologic Status.... 1912
Respiratory Distress with Guillain-Barré
  Syndrome 2016
Features of Autonomic Dysreflexia 2064
Postoperative Brachial Plexus Compromise 2155
Worsening Shock 2242

Diversity in Health Care

Health and Illness Beliefs and Practices 19
Health Care Practitioners 74
Introduction to Cultural Aspects of Health Care ... 146
Communicating with Culturally Diverse Clients ... 147
The Significance of Cultural Assessment 412
Cultural Aspects of Death and Dying 457
Cultural Perspectives on Pain 475
Cultural Influences on Nutrition 643
Ethnopharmacology and Hypertension 1391
HIV and AIDS in Minority Populations 2187

Management and Delegation

Measuring and Recording Vital Signs and Other
  Client Data 183
Performing Specimen Collection and Testing 188
Care of Clients with Fluid Volume Deficit 222
Postoperative Care: Dressings and Drains 310
Infection Control 344
Assisting with Mobility and Use of Splints 573
Application of Heat and Cold 614
Care of Nasogastric Tubes, Small-Bore Feeding
  Tubes, and Gastrostomy and Jejunostomy
  Tubes...................................... 677
Stoma Care and Application of Ostomy
  Appliances 778

Application and Care of Rectal Pouches and
  Rectal Tubes 799
Helping Clients with Urinary Incontinence 840
Measuring and Recording Blood Glucose Levels ... 1167
Skin Inspection 1295
Care of Clients with Pressure Ulcers 1301
Care of Clients Recovering from Plastic Surgery ... 1320
Assisting with Respiratory Care 1657
Hearing Aids 1839
Preparing Enteral Nutrition 1915
Physical Restraints 1921

Physical Assessment Findings in the Healthy Adult

Musculoskeletal System 540
Gastrointestinal System 655
Urinary System 754
Female Reproductive System 921
Male Reproductive System 941
Thyroid Gland 1075
Integumentary System 1269
Peripheral Vascular System 1370
Cardiovascular System 1456
Respiratory System 1629
The Eye 1790
The Ear 1801
Neurologic System 1882
Hematopoietic System 2094

Pathophysiology/Treatment Algorithms

Understanding Inflammation and Its Treatment 317
Understanding Chronic Renal Failure and Its
  Treatment 884
Understanding Hypercortisolism (Cushing's Disease)
  and Its Treatment 1128
Understanding Diabetes Mellitus and Its
  Treatment 1152
Understanding Cirrhosis and Its Treatment 1236
Understanding Myocardial Infarction and Its
  Treatment 1586
Understanding Asthma and Its Treatment 1687
Understanding ARDS and Its Treatment 1763
Understanding DIC and Its Treatment 2125
Understanding Rheumatoid Arthritis and Its
  Treatment 2143

UNIT 1

Promotion of Self-Care

1 Theories of Health Promotion and Illness Management

2 Health Promotion in Young and Middle-Aged Adults

3 Health Promotion in Older Adults

CHAPTER

1

Theories of Health Promotion and Illness Management

Esther A. Hellman

As a result of the growing prevalence of chronic conditions and related cost burden, health promotion and illness prevention will be increasingly important. This chapter describes epidemiologic concepts and health promotion theories and shows how these concepts and theories are used in managing chronic conditions, which can occur across the life span. Health promotion concepts in two groups of the adult population are described in Chapters 2 and 3.

HISTORY OF HEALTH CARE

Disease and illness have plagued humans since the beginning of time. Familiarity with dominant ideas about the health care and diseases of each era is useful in understanding the antecedents of the current health care system. Through the ages, people have wondered why some individuals become sick while others remain healthy. When the populace of early civilizations had little knowledge of disease processes, magic and superstition were the mainstays in treating illness. As medical knowledge increased, treatment became more science-based. Table 1–1 presents an overview of health care history from prehistoric times to the 19th century.

During prehistoric times, diseases were thought to be caused by the stars, angry spirits, or demons. Sorcerers and priests treated disease by exorcism or by placating the evil spirits. As medical knowledge progressed, Asians in India and China and Greeks believed that a body fluid imbalance caused illness. Early forms of immunizations, medications, and surgeries were developed during this period. During the Dark Ages, physicians could not stop smallpox, cholera, or bubonic plague from killing millions of people. People believed that they had no control over disease and illness. During the Dark Ages, minimal progress was made toward understanding health or illness; medical care consisted of magic and superstitious practices. During the Renaissance, interest in science revived and medical knowledge advanced through direct observation during autopsies and analyses of urine and blood. It

was not until the late 19th century that scientists began to discover causes of infectious diseases.

■ THEORIES OF DISEASE CAUSATION

Scientific concepts about the causes of disease and illness are relatively new ideas. Table 1–2 describes some theories of disease causation. One of the earliest theories, Pasteur's *germ theory,* described microorganisms, such as viruses and bacteria, as the causative factor in infectious disease. Although the germ theory helped to increase medical knowledge and to reduce deaths from infection, it did not explain the causes of all diseases.

The *biomedical model* described disease as malfunctioning cells or organs with consistent signs and symptoms. This model focused on cause-and-effect relationships while ignoring psychosocial components of disease.

Multicausal theories, such as Bernard and Cannon's Theory of Homeostasis and Selye's Theory of the General Adaptation Syndrome, explained the influence of lifestyle, genetic background, diet, and stress response on disease and illness.

Psychosocial theories integrate physiologic, psychological, and sociologic factors to better explain disease development. Examples of psychosocial theories are Mason's Theory of Specificity of the Stress Response; Lazarus' Theories of Stress Response; Wolff's Theory of Stress, Organ Maladaptation, and Disease; and Holmes and Rahe's Theory of Life Change and the Onset of Illness.

Multicausal and psychosocial theories of disease causation more closely approximate reality and increase the likelihood of discovering factors susceptible to intervention.

■ CONCEPT OF HEALTH

The word "health," as it is used today, did not appear in writing until about 1000 A.D. Until the 19th century, being healthy was the norm and sick people were ostracized. The dawn of the 19th century scientific era led to new discoveries and better understanding of human physi-

TABLE 1-1	THE HISTORY OF HEALTH CARE	
Time Period	**Theories of Disease Development**	**Health Care Practices**
Prehistoric	Illnesses are sent from the angry spirits of dead animals or people	Sorcerers claimed to be able to placate evil spirits with herbs or potions. They practiced trephining (perforation of the skull). The skull holes supposedly enabled evil spirits to leave the body

Early civilizations
  Sumerians (Mesopotamia)
  Egyptians
	Medicine is based on astronomy
	  A person's destiny is told in the stars
	  Demons, infesting the earth, produced diseases
		Priests treated disease by exorcism. A wide range of drugs, obtained from plants, fruits, animals, and minerals, were also used

Asian civilizations
  India
 	
  China
	Illness is described as an imbalance
	  Belief that imbalance occurs between three physical humors: spirit, bile, and phlegm
	  Imbalance occurs between *Yin* (negative, passive, feminine) and *Yang* (positive, active, masculine)
		Physicians specialized in plastic surgery, especially rhinoplasty (reshaping of the nose)
		Chinese physicians were the first to vaccinate against smallpox and to prescribe iron for anemia; developed acupuncture

Israelite civilization	Illness represents a visible sign of God's wrath on sinful people who have broken rules of faith related to food preparation and hygiene. Dietary and other religious practices promote health	Faith brought health. Priests treated disease (e.g., leprosy treated with isolation and cleansing); then the recovered person was reintroduced into the community

Greek civilization
  Hippocrates, the "Father of Medicine," author of the Hippocratic Oath
  Aristotle described body's organs in elaborate detail
	Nature has power to heal. Health and illness are due to balance or imbalance between blood, phlegm, yellow bile, and black bile. Human suffering and disease can be reduced through good hygiene, not magic. Proven cures for diseases are used, not relying on religious and demonic explanations	The body had the means to cure itself. Fevers, inflammation, boils, and diarrhea were seen as the body's way of purging itself

Roman civilization Galen wrote 22 massive volumes on health, illness, and health care	Superstition and magic are central to health care	Various gods were called on to help people through specific troubles (Opigena called on to help women in childbirth) Animal liver was used to cure various ailments Public health improvements were introduced (sewers, aqueducts)
Dark Ages	Superstitions prevail	Plagues killed millions of people. Physicians powerlessness to help. Society moved away from reason and back to superstition. The common practice of bloodletting allowed the body to get rid of bad "humors"

The Renaissance
  Leonardo da Vinci described muscles and arteries
  Vesalius described human anatomy
  Paré developed principles of surgery
  Harvey discovered how blood circulates
	Culture is revived, and science begins again. Direct observation of the natural world leads to knowledge	Diagnosis of illness made by analyses of urine and bloodletting; physicians, educated in universities

18th and 19th centuries
  Florence Nightingale established the profession of nursing
 	
  Semmelweis thought puerperal fever was contagious
  Lister and Pasteur
	Germ theory is developed
	  Believed that controlling the environment promotes health and healing and prevents disease
	  Ordered hand-washing and disinfection practices
	  Introduced disinfection techniques into hospitals and operating rooms
		Basic means to inhibit spread of disease by hand-washing and disinfection began

TABLE 1–2	THEORIES OF DISEASE CAUSATION	
Theory	**Description**	**Components**
Germ theory	Pasteur proposed that a specific microorganism was capable of causing infectious disease	Antibiotics, vaccinations, and other treatments were developed as a result of this theory. *Weakness of theory:* Does not explain causes of all diseases (i.e., most diseases today are not infectious).
Biomedical model	Disease is a result of malfunctioning organs or cells	Diseases are observable and quantifiable, in that most findings are objective (called "signs") and symptoms are subjective reports of disease. *Weakness of model:* Does not account for many other factors specific to each individual (lifestyle, diet, genetic background, stress response) that may also contribute to disease.
Multicausal theories (factors specific to each client must be examined; an individual's lifestyle and genetic background play an underlying role in development of disease)	1. Bernard and Cannon's *Theory of Homeostasis* a. Bernard hypothesized that if an organism is to live, it must have the capacity to maintain its internal environment b. Canon developed the concept of *feedback mechanisms* to explain Bernard's theory of regulation of the internal environment	a. Illness occurs as the result of an imbalance in the body's internal environment, and disease is an adaptive effort by the body to restore its balance. b. Homeostasis is a dynamic equilibrium, flexible and ongoing, that maintains certain factors within a given range, e.g., body temperature, blood pressure, fluid and electrolyte balances. The fight-or-flight response prepares the body to react in an emergency and to move quickly away from danger.
	2. Selye's *Theory of the General Adaptation Syndrome:* A framework to describe how people respond to stress; involves generalized changes that affect several body systems *Local Adaptation Syndrome* takes place in a single organ or specific section of the body (e.g., inflammation)	2. Both syndromes develop in three distinct stages: (a) alarm reaction, or fight-or-flight response, (b) resistance, and (c) exhaustion. The most important regulators are the central and autonomic nervous systems and pituitary and adrenal glands. Disease occurs when the adaptive capacity of the body is exceeded.
Psychosocial theories (integrate physiologic, psychological, and sociologic factors that explain disease development)	1. Mason's *Theory of Specificity of the Stress Response:* The stress response is dependent on psychological factors (e.g., a person's perception of the stressor rather than the stressor itself)	1. Cortisol hormonal responses to stress increase when (a) we first experience a new stimulus, (b) we learn to avoid noxious stimuli, and (c) we receive punishment. We can modify the cortisol response by coping effectively with a stressor.
	2. Lazarus' *Theories of the Stress Response:* The degree of resistance to infection depends on how well a person copes with stress and general life experiences	2. The brain, through one's perception of the stressor, appears to be the mediating influence on how the body responds to stress. Daily hassles are irritating, frustrating, minor life events that everyone experiences, such as losing things and being delayed in traffic. Daily uplifts are buffers to daily hassles. People who cope poorly with stress have significantly impaired immune responses, as shown by diminished leukocyte activity levels.

Table continued on following page

TABLE 1–2	THEORIES OF DISEASE CAUSATION *Continued*	
Theory	**Description**	**Components**
	3. Wolff's *Theory of Stress, Organ Maladaptation, and Disease:* It is hypothesized that disease often results from adaptive attempts to restore homeostasis that were appropriate in kind but incorrect in magnitude. Inappropriate adaptation attempts occur because: a. Humans can symbolize, recall the past, and project themselves into the future; therefore, threats of possible danger and symbols of danger are just as important a cause of disease as noxious chemicals, microbes, and mechanical forces b. People depend on others for much of their satisfaction in life	3. Stressors are created by the need to be successful at work and with other people. Some individuals consistently respond to frustrating situations through a response by a particular body system or organ, perhaps the stomach, back muscles, colon, or nasal mucous membranes. Pathologic changes that occur regularly and that are combined with other chemical, biologic, or physical stressors can eventually lead to tissue damage.
	4. Roy's *Adaptation Model:* Health is a state of being and a process of becoming an integrated whole	4. Human behavior is a result of adaptation to internal and external stimuli. The model provides a framework to help understand human adaptive responses and interventions that can be used to foster adaptation and minimize stress. The four modes of adaptation are (a) physiologic responses, (b) self-concept responses, (c) role function, and (d) interdependent relations.
	5. Holmes and Rahe's *Theory of Life Change and the Onset of Illness:* Life changes (both positive and negative) are a form of stress to which people must learn to adapt, both psychologically and physically	5. If we must adapt to too many significant changes over a short period of time, we expend too much energy trying to adapt, which may result in illness. Minor ailments, serious disease, depression, and suicide attempts typically follow a cluster of both positive and negative life changes.
Biopsychosociospiritual theories	A person's body, mind, and environment all function together to determine whether illness develops 1. Wolf's *Concept of Disease as a Way of Life:* The brain has a role in regulating bodily processes and in causing disease when it defines situations that can evoke chemical and nervous system reactions	1. The body needs high levels of epinephrine, blood glucose, and other hormones during times of physical threat when a person must literally fight or flee. When these responses occur inappropriately or chronically, the excess hormones can cause harm, including disease. Disease can arise from evoked reaction patterns that are meant to be protective when a person is physically threatened but that are destructive when used inappropriately to fight symbolic battles.
	2. Schwartz's *Model of the Brain as an Adaptive Regulator:* The brain is an adaptive system for regulation of the body through a feedback system with the peripheral organs	2. The brain is central to any change in health because it is the mediator between the external and internal environments. Through the brain's interpretation, a person can (a) change an environment, (b) leave it, (c) engage in it, or (d) rest, exercise, or diet. People have the ability to regulate themselves and move toward health on the health care continuum.

TABLE 1–2	THEORIES OF DISEASE CAUSATION *Continued*	
Theory	**Description**	**Components**
Mediators of the stress response: 1. Internal variables (personality, personal resources, temperament, history, genes)	1. Behavior Patterns a. Friedman and Rosenman described two behavior types: (1) *Type A* personality is characterized by constant mobilization of inner resources to combat real or imagined stresses (2) *Type B* personality characteristically takes life with all its stresses in stride	(1) People with a type A personality are described as aggressive, often hostile, hard-driving, and deadline-ridden, with a chronic sense of urgency. Between ages 35 and 60 years, they are almost three times more likely to have coronary artery disease than type B people. (2) Although often intelligent and ambitious, type B people do not allow activity to become self-destructive. They can relax without feeling guilty and can work without a sense of time urgency.
	b. Kobasa's *Model of Hardiness:* A personality component that moderates or buffers the response to stress. Hardy clients can remain healthy under stressful situations and can view the stressor as an opportunity to practice mastery and undergo personal growth	Concepts of hardiness have been associated with health maintenance in the following areas: (1) *Control:* The sense of mastery or self-confidence needed to appraise and interpret health stressors appropriately (2) *Commitment:* Presence of active involvement in efforts to maintain or improve health (3) *Challenge:* Presence of flexibility and persistence in coping with health stressors
2. Environment (social supports, physical setting, organizational factors)	2. Social support: More socially isolated or less socially integrated people are less healthy psychologically and physically and are more likely to die than more socially oriented people	2. Physiologic studies show a link between the amygdala and the hypothalamus in the brain and positive social relationships. Social contact decreases hormones such as cortisol, epinephrine, and norepinephrine.

ology and disease origins. At the same time, society began to treat illness with less disgust and defined health simply as the absence of disease.

In 1947, the World Health Organization (WHO) definition of health emphasized several holistic qualities: "Health is a state of complete physical, mental, and social well-being and not merely the absence of disease or infirmity."[44] Since 1947, alternate definitions of health have been proposed. Some definitions portray health and illness on an interactive continuum, with multiple configurations ranging from depletion of health (death) to high-level wellness.[29] High-level wellness is further conceptualized as self-actualization and maximization of an individual's potential. Other definitions describe health as a unidirectional developmental process consisting of a unitary patterning of person and environment. When each person is viewed as being part of a complex, interconnected social, biologic, and environmental system, health can be better understood. Table 1–3 lists various definitions of health.

In general, today's definitions of health reflect a multidimensional, holistic, and subjective view. Individual definitions and perceptions of health are taken into account. The meaning of health can be viewed in many contexts, such as historical, social, personal, scientific, philosophical, and spiritual. These meanings will always exist in the various contexts of individual human experience, are sometimes contradictory, and often overlap. Cultural ideologies and tradition also influence one's image of health.

Support client participation in the process of actualizing a defined image of health, and do not negate the ability of clients to form their own image of health. Include clients' perceptions when assessing their health to fully understand the priority of their values and perceptions of these very complex interactions.

■ CONCEPT OF WELLNESS

Dunn was the first to define and describe wellness, a term and an ideal that was the precursor to the health promotion movement.[10] His now-classic definition of what he termed *high-level wellness* is "an integrated method of functioning which is oriented toward maximizing the potential of which the individual is capable within the environment where he is functioning." Dunn stressed that wellness is an ongoing process directed toward higher potential, not a static goal; and that high-level wellness is a feeling of being "alive to the tips of the fingers, with energy to burn, tingling with vitality."[10] He postulated

TABLE 1–3	DEFINITIONS OF HEALTH
Nursing Model	**Definition**
King's goal attainment theory	Health is a dynamic life experience. "Dynamic" implies a continuous adjustment to stressors in internal and external environments and the use of one's resources to achieve maximum potential.
Leininger's transcultural model	Health refers to "beliefs, values, and action patterns that are culturally known and used to preserve and maintain personal or group well-being, and to perform daily role activities."[23a]
Levine's conservation principles	Health is defined in terms of an Anglo-Saxon word meaning "whole." Patterns of wholeness change with growth and development. Health and disease patterns reflect adaptive change.
Neuman's systems model	Health is a condition in which the parts and subparts of the whole person are in harmony.
Orem's self-care model	Health is a state of wholeness, including a person's parts and modes of functioning.
Pender's health promotion model	"Health is a manifestation of evolving patterns of person-environment interaction throughout the life span."[31]
Rogers' unitary person model	Health and illness are seen as expressions of the interaction of a person and the environment in the process of unfolding consciousness.
Roy's adaptation model	Health is a process or state of being and a process of becoming an integrated whole.
Watson's model of human caring	Health is more than the absence of disease. It is a harmony within the mind, body, and soul.
World Health Organization	Health is a "state of complete physical, mental, and social well-being and not merely the absence of disease or infirmity."[44]

that health professionals tend to focus on disease rather than on wellness because their training is disease-focused rather than wellness-oriented or prevention-oriented. It is easier to fight against disease than to fight for a condition of greater wellness.

Travis popularized the theoretical concept of wellness through development and teaching of the wellness model (Fig. 1–1). The effect of this model resulted in the recognition that wellness requires attention; it does not happen automatically. The left side of the figure represents the biomedical model. The client exhibits manifestations of a disease, is treated, and is brought back to a neutral point where disease manifestations have been alleviated. In the case of chronic illness, disease manifestations are con-

trolled and minimized. The right side represents the wellness model and the potential for high-level health and wellness. The nurse can use the wellness model at any point by directing clients beyond the neutral point and encouraging them to move as far toward high-level wellness as possible. The biomedical and wellness models can work in harmony. For example, if clients are ill, treatment is important, but clients should not stop there. After recovery, clients should practice healthy behaviors (such as regular exercise and eating a low-fat, balanced diet) to minimize future illnesses.

Wellness is the quality or condition of being well, even among people with chronic illness, especially of being robust, healthy, and fit. Wellness is not simply the absence of clinical manifestations; it incorporates positive mental, physical, and spiritual well-being. High-level wellness is a method of functioning oriented toward maximizing individual potential within the environment. High-level wellness involves (1) progression toward a higher level of functioning, (2) integration of the whole being, and (3) an open-ended future with the challenge of fuller potential.

■ RELATIONSHIP BETWEEN DISEASE, ILLNESS, HEALTH, AND WELLNESS

In the biomedical model, disease is a biomedical term, identified by clinical manifestations. A person who has a disease has a medically defined condition similar to that suffered by others (e.g., diabetes mellitus or hepatitis).[8] From a multicausal perspective, disease may be defined as "the failure of a person's adaptive mechanisms to adequately counteract stimuli and stresses, resulting in functional or structural disturbances."[12] As mentioned earlier, multicausal and psychosocial theories of disease causation more closely approximate reality and increase the chances of discovering factors that are amenable to intervention.

In contrast to the concept of disease, illness has a broader meaning and includes the perception and the response of clients and those around them. Illness is a state of being with social and psychological as well as biomedical components. Illness is a disenabling response, a mismatch between a person's needs and the resources available to meet those needs; it signals that the present balance is not working.[12] A person can have a disease without feeling ill. A seemingly healthy person may have an early form of disease without clinical manifestations. For example, young people in their 20s may already have heart disease, such as atherosclerosis (or "hardening of the arteries"), without evidence of disease. Although such people appear healthy, if they continue unhealthy habits such as smoking, eating a high-fat diet, and not exercising, the heart disease will progress until clinical manifestations appear. Similarly, injury changes the balance on the wellness continuum (see Fig. 1–1). Injuries usually require treatment; after recovery or rehabilitation, people can achieve higher levels of wellness by practicing healthy behaviors.

In summary, disease, illness, health, and wellness are related concepts. Disease and health must be considered together because without disease, there is no need to discuss health.[12] Disease is a state of disequilibrium, whereas health is a state of equilibrium, or balance.[14]

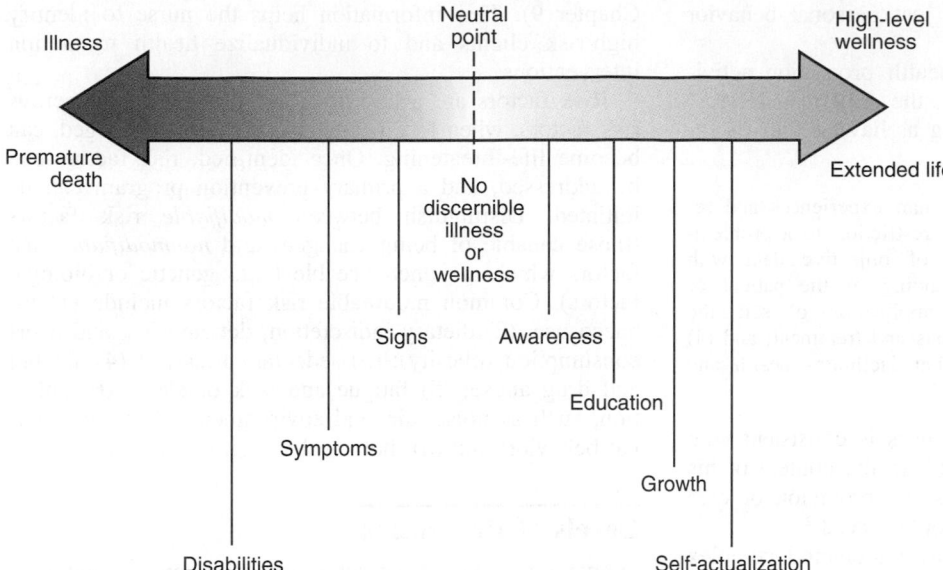

FIGURE 1–1 Travis' wellness model.

Health and illness are dynamic patterns that change with time and social circumstances; they are not mutually exclusive. There are degrees of health and illness; clients with cancer and others with chronic diseases can achieve personal levels of wellness. Health is a resource for everyday living. High-level wellness maximizes one's potential capacity and is a component of the highest level of health.

CONCEPT OF HEALTH PROMOTION

Health promotion is the process of fostering awareness, influencing attitudes, and identifying alternatives so that people can make informed choices and change behavior to achieve an optimal level of physical and mental health and improve their physical and social environments. According to WHO, health promotion includes activities that encourage healthy lifestyles, create supportive environments for health, strengthen community action, reorient health service, and build healthy public policy. Health promotion has to do with acquiring mental, physical, and spiritual assets to protect and buffer people from disease as well as to move them along a continuum toward high-level wellness.

Health promotion programs are designed to improve the health and well-being of individuals and communities through empowerment. Clients are empowered through the provision of information, skills, services, and support needed to undertake and maintain positive lifestyle changes. Health promotion activities are geared toward individuals, families, and communities. WHO defines *community* as a social group determined by geographical boundaries or common values and interests. Community members know and interact with one another. The community within a particular social structure creates norms, values, and social institutions.

Health is affected by the extent of control or mastery people have over their lives or by the amount of power or powerlessness felt. Health promotion involves empowering the client. *Empowerment* gives the client power by

transferring from the nurse knowledge, skills, resources, access, and language. The nurse can empower the client by teaching about self-care.

■ EVOLUTION OF THE CONCEPT OF HEALTH PROMOTION

During the 1970s and 1980s, the field of health promotion grew alongside the emerging ideology and practice of wellness. Initially, it found expression in Canada with the Lalonde Report[21] and in the United States in the Surgeon General's Report, *Healthy People.*[38] Both documents discussed the significance of environmental factors in influencing health and were not limited to mention of individual lifestyle or personal behavior issues, which are hallmarks of the wellness movement. The Lalonde Report made recommendations in four equally weighted areas: (1) human biology, (2) environment, (3) lifestyle, and (4) health care organization. The Surgeon General's Report noted that lifestyle influenced health more than the other categories did. The Surgeon General's Report argued that Americans are killing themselves, not only by careless habits but also by polluting the environment and permitting harmful social conditions to exist. For the first time, attention was directed toward environmental issues such as control of toxic agents and occupational health and safety.

In 1991, *Healthy People 2000* was published.[39] This report introduced a set of clearly articulated, measurable goals for improving the health of the nation by the year 2000. Three broad goals were identified: (1) increasing the span of healthy life for Americans, (2) reducing health disparities among Americans, and (3) achieving access to preventive services for all Americans. Specific goals, objectives, and strategies were delineated for achieving 22 priorities in health promotion, health protection, and preventive services. More recently, *Healthy People 2000: Review 1997*[41] was published and work on objectives for the next decade is under way. These reports prompted agencies to focus on prevention and promotion through institutional change strategies, legislation, and public policy, and not just personal behavior change.

Nurses have long conducted health promotion activities. In its social policy statement, the American Nurses' Association (ANA) defined nursing as having four essential features[2]:

(1) attention to the full range of human experiences and responses to health and illness without restriction to a problem-focused orientation; (2) integration of objective data with knowledge gained from an understanding of the patient or group's subjective experience; (3) application of scientific knowledge to the processes of diagnosis and treatment; and (4) provision of a caring relationship that facilitates health and healing.

Therefore, a focus on health behaviors is consistent with nursing's focus on a person's health in the context of his or her total life. Nursing involves the provision of care that promotes well-being in the people served.[2]

To promote health, nurses must understand complex social, political, and economic forces that shape clients' lives. A nurse who is active socially and politically models the ANA social policy statement that delineates involvement in social reform as being a part of nursing practice. The policy states, among other concerns, the "provision for the public health through use of preventive and environmental measures and increased assumption of responsibility by individuals, families, and other groups."[2] Labonte, a health educator, believed that the ultimate challenge is to create social and health conditions that allow all of the world's citizens to achieve a state of good health.

■ EPIDEMIOLOGIC CONCEPTS

Epidemiology is the study of patterns of health, disease, disability, death, and other problems in a population. Epidemiology focuses on how diseases originate and spread.[24] A major epidemiologic goal is identifying aggregates, or subpopulations, at high risk for acquiring a disease and then modifying or reducing those risks. For example, smokers have a three-fold higher risk for development of cardiac disease compared with nonsmokers. Nurses can modify or reduce a smoker's risk of cardiac disease by counseling about how to accomplish smoking cessation. Risk factors and levels of prevention are epidemiologic concepts.

Risk Factors

Risk factors are factors whose presence is associated with increased probability of the occurrence of an illness or disease. Health risk factors can be categorized:

- *Genetic* or *biologic* (age, race, family history)
- *Behavioral* (health habits, such as eating a high-fat diet, not exercising, smoking)
- *Environmental* (living in an area with frequent smog warnings)

The risk level for disease or illness is assessed through health risk appraisal. Health risk appraisal identifies potential health threats prior to illness or disease development and provides clients with a way to evaluate their vulnerability to identified potential health threats (see Chapter 9). This information helps the nurse to identify high-risk clients and to individualize health promotion interventions.

Risk factors are a key to health promotion. Numerous risk factors, when left unattended or unacknowledged, can become life-threatening. Once identified, risk factors can be addressed, and a primary prevention program can be initiated. Distinguish between *modifiable* risk factors (those capable of being changed) and *nonmodifiable* risk factors which are unchangeable (e.g., genetic or biologic factors). Common modifiable risk factors include (1) tobacco use; (2) dietary indiscretion, deficiencies, and overconsumption (obesity); (3) sedentary lifestyle; (4) alcohol and drug abuse; (5) fatigue and lack of sleep; (6) pollution, such as noise, air, and environment; (7) unsafe sexual behavior; and (8) motor vehicle and firearm misuse.

Levels of Prevention

"Prevention" means averting the development and progression of disease.[23] Preventive health care is more dynamic than health maintenance. Prevention deals with health enhancement and promotion, whereas health maintenance is concerned with maintaining the status quo. Thinking about the levels of prevention implies a commitment to wellness and a conscious desire to prevent illness and disease. The levels of prevention are primary, secondary, and tertiary. Table 1–4 identifies selected behaviors associated with these levels.

PRIMARY PREVENTION
Primary prevention involves health promotion activities that provide protection against the occurrence of a specific illness or disease.[23] Primary prevention does not include therapeutic treatment or identification of symptoms. It does include health promotion (e.g., teaching clients about healthy lifestyle behaviors) and specific protection interventions (e.g., immunizations) to decrease vulnerability to illness or dysfunction. A health promotion program or enhancement activities can be developed to increase immunity and strengthen the body and mind. Everyday behavior can be examined in order to guide primary prevention. The objective is to achieve maximum functioning in each health potential.

For example, impaired mobility is usually preventable. If a client is at risk for impaired mobility, nursing intervention can prevent impairment. For the client who has arthritis and currently does not have mobility problems but is at risk for impaired mobility, for example, encouraging the client to eat a well-balanced diet and to engage in specific exercises may help delay the development of mobility problems.

SECONDARY PREVENTION
Secondary prevention refers to health behavior that promotes the early detection (case-finding or screenings) and treatment of disease, and limitation of disability[23] (also known as "health maintenance"). Screening primarily identifies cases in an early stage of disease, when treatment is more effective.

When working with a client:

1. Identify risk factors that cannot be modified but that leave the client vulnerable to disease.

TABLE 1–4	BEHAVIORS ASSOCIATED WITH EACH LEVEL OF PREVENTION
Level of Prevention	**Type of Behavior***
PRIMARY	Stop smoking, or do not start smoking
	Avoid overexposure to the sun
	Support antipollution legislation
	Practice safe sex, monogamy, or abstinence
	Obtain genetic counseling for family-linked disorders
	Design and follow a regular exercise plan
	Maintain ideal body weight
	Maintain a low-cholesterol, low-fat, high-fiber nutritious diet
	Wear a seat belt and helmet
	Identify and eliminate stressors
	Limit alcohol intake, and never drink and drive
	Have regular dental care
SECONDARY	Obtain genetic counseling for family-linked disorders
	Undergo screening for tuberculosis
	Obtain tonometry yearly after age 40 for glaucoma screening
	Have yearly Papanicolaou smears and mammograms per recommended guidelines
	Have eye examinations every 2 years
	Practice monthly self-breast, self-testicular, self-skin, and self-oral examinations
	Undergo a physical examination yearly after age 40
	Self-monitor blood pressure for hypertension
TERTIARY	Have a complete blood count before chemotherapy
	Have speech therapy after a stroke
	Participate in cardiac rehabilitation
	Have breast reconstruction
	Participate in stroke or coma rehabilitation

*Preventive behaviors identified are representative and not intended to be inclusive.

2. Using secondary prevention, analyze assessment data in order to derive nursing diagnoses and to identify problems common to target populations that exhibit nonmodifiable risk factors.
3. Rank intervention priorities, identify nursing management approaches within the secondary prevention mode, and evaluate outcomes.
4. Obtain assessment data by interview, observation, and physical examination.
5. Proceed to work with the client to develop a means of early detection, such as screening for the disease.

Using the immobility example to examine secondary prevention, consider subconcepts that emerge if immobility is thought of as the prescribed or unavoidable restriction of movement in any area. Immobility can be (1) physical, (2) emotional or psychological, (3) intellectual, or (4) social.

Causes of physical immobility may be (1) decreased energy from ischemia, hypoxia, malnutrition, and electrolyte imbalance; (2) lack of innervation, as in central nervous system or peripheral nerve impairment; (3) decreased musculoskeletal strength, as in endocrine diseases, disuse syndrome, and scar tissue formation; and (4) pain, which inhibits movement and the desire to move.

When looking at problems of immobility, consider individual norms. Although complications may not always be preventable, manifestations can be detected early and thus some complications can be avoided. Nursing interventions, such as applying heat, balancing exercise and rest, and administering prescribed anti-inflammatory drugs, can help prevent a serious mobility problem.

TERTIARY PREVENTION

Tertiary prevention is directed toward rehabilitation after a disease or condition already exists to minimize disability and help the client learn to live productively with limitations. Tertiary prevention is used when disability is permanent and irreversible. It minimizes effects of disease and disability by surveillance and maintenance aimed at preventing complications and deterioration. Incorporate creative problem-solving approaches in the design, implementation, and evaluation of nursing intervention to support the client's achievement of successful adaptation to known risks, optimal reconstitution, or establishment of high-level wellness.

Continuing the immobility example, muscle and joint degeneration and metabolic and circulatory disturbances occur when a client is immobile for any length of time. Identifying immobility as an actual diagnosis permits development of a rehabilitation plan and restoration to high-level wellness. The plan would implement (1) active exercise, (2) passive mobilization, and (3) frequent position changes. Tertiary preventive outcome goals are optimal rehabilitation within parameters that the client can achieve.

■ MODELS OF HEALTH PROMOTION

Social scientists have worked on models of health-related behavior change or health promotion behavior. The models look at factors that affect individual readiness to take health action. Nurses use health promotion models to motivate clients to make health behavior changes.

Social Cognitive Theory

Bandura developed the Social Cognitive Theory to explain human behavior. The model is based on the premise that human behavior is influenced by "reciprocal determinism" between cognition, behavior, and environment.[4] According to this theory, both efficacy and outcome expectations are crucial for behavioral change. The central concept is self-efficacy. Perceived self-efficacy or efficacy expectation is a judgment of one's ability to execute a specific behavior.

People with high self-efficacy are more confident of their abilities to maintain behavioral change (e.g., exercise adherence, smoking cessation, or achievement of ideal weight). They will attempt to execute the behavior more readily, with greater intensity, and with greater perseverance in response to initial failure than people with comparatively weaker self-efficacy. Interventions to increase self-efficacy include (1) *performance attainment*—having clients successfully execute the behavior; (2) *vicarious experiences*—watching others successfully enact the behavior; (3) *verbal persuasion*—convincing clients of their capability to execute the behavior; and (4) *physiologic states*—helping clients to expect and interpret various physiologic states (e.g., stress, anxiety, fatigue, pain) that may occur when the behavior is executed.

Interventions to increase perceived self-efficacy may be beneficial when the nurse is encouraging health-protecting and health-promoting behaviors. Social Cognitive Theory affects behavior change through phases:

1. Promoting and motivating clients to change a target behavior
2. Providing skills training so that clients can acquire the specific behavioral change skills
3. Developing support networks to help maintain the new behavior
4. Maintaining the behavior through reinforcement
5. Generalizing to other levels of interaction, from the family to the community

Health Belief Model

The Health Belief Model attempts to explain why some people who are illness-free take actions to avoid illness, whereas others do not. This model is based on the idea that people want to avoid negatively valued outcomes or personal threats, such as illness, disability, nonproductivity, discomfort, and death. The Health Belief Model includes five factors, identified and illustrated in Box 1–1. Cognitive and emotional beliefs identify an individual's readiness to change behavior.[36] Before people take action to change a behavior, they must decide that the selected behavior (whether it is smoking, not being immunized, or engaging in unprotected sexual activity) creates a serious

---

BOX 1–1   The Health Belief Model: Client Characteristics and Starting an Exercise Program

1. *Perceived susceptibility to a problem.* Negative effects of not exercising (identified as threatening) include difficulty managing weight, lack of energy, and increased risk of coronary artery disease.
2. *Perceived seriousness of a problem.* The client feels that the identified negative effects of not exercising are serious problems.
3. *Perceived benefits and barriers to taking action.* If an exercise program is started, the benefits (weight loss and maintenance, more energy, better health) will be greater than any barriers (lack of time, cost of equipment, lack of an exercise partner).
4. *Cues to action.* The client has been exposed to action cues. An exercise room is available to employees at work, and the company's nurse practitioner has advised the client to begin an exercise program.
5. *Self-efficacy* (the behavior is doable). The client is confident that he or she will be able to begin and continue a regular exercise program.

---

health harm and that moderating or stopping the behavior will be beneficial.[14]

Health Promotion Model

Pender's Health Promotion Model emphasizes developing individual resources to enhance well-being.[31] This model demonstrates complex biopsychosocial processes that motivate people to engage in behaviors directed toward health enhancement.[14] The model links individual characteristics and experiences, and behavior-specific cognitions and affects (including benefits of and barriers to action and interpersonal and situational influences), to a commitment to a health-promoting behavior. The final behavioral outcome is also influenced by the immediate competing demands and preferences, which can derail an intended health-promoting action (e.g., selecting a meal with a high-fat rather than a low-fat content because of taste preferences).

Transtheoretical Model

The Transtheoretical Model, developed by Prochaska and DiClemente,[33] identifies stages of change: The individual moves from (1) not thinking about change in the near future *(precontemplation)*, (2) to seriously thinking about making a change *(contemplation)*, (3) to actively planning and starting a behavior change *(preparation)*, (4) to overtly making changes *(action)*, and (5) to taking steps to maintain changes and avoid relapse *(maintenance)*. This model stages the client's readiness to change and incorporates (1) pros and cons of a behavior change, (2) self-efficacy, and (3) change processes. For example, a client who states no intention of beginning an exercise program would be in the precontemplation stage for exercise. The model is a guide for assessing a client's readiness to change and for developing stage-specific health interventions.

■ TEACHING AND MOTIVATING CLIENTS

Nurses encounter clients during times of major health changes and are in key positions to help them make decisions and adopt behaviors that greatly alter health. To effectively assist others in making healthy decisions and changes, nurses must teach about healthy behaviors, function as role models, and understand the concepts of motivation. The previously described health promotion models can be used as client teaching guides to identify potential areas for assessment and crucial teaching content to facilitate desired behavioral changes. An example of health behavior client teaching, using the Transtheoretical Model, follows.[33] This example can be applied to any health behavior change, such as quitting smoking, starting a regular exercise program, or eating a low-fat, balanced diet.

According to the Transtheoretical Model, assessment of the client's readiness to change must be done before any health behavior change instruction is initiated. First determine the stage of change and by assessing the client's willingness to modify or reduce health risk by making the desired healthy behavior change and by assessing the client's progress toward making the change. Then use an intervention that is appropriate for the client's stage of change. Both practice and research have demonstrated that giving information to clients does not in itself bring about healthy behaviors. Nurses frequently give up trying to teach because of a lack of client motivation. When this occurs, the client may be labeled as "noncompliant" or "difficult." Instead, it may be that the client cannot relate to the intervention because it is not directed at the client's specific stage of behavioral change, situation, or cultural perspective. Ask clients about their perceived benefits of changing the behavior as well as about barriers to changing the behavior.

Motivating others to change health behaviors involves the following:

- Clients must believe that the problem is solvable.
- Clients must view the solution as something they want to do.
- Clients must feel competent to successfully carry out the behavior.
- Clients must feel able to overcome barriers to change.
- Clients must experience positive feedback and consequences.

The nurse's role is to use multiple skills to empower clients to engage in healthy behaviors. Approaches include helping clients to identify their values and to explore feelings about themselves, with emphasis on identifying strengths. Helping clients set goals (developing intrinsic motivation) greatly enhances the likelihood of achieving the desired behavioral changes. Nurses assist clients in differentiating perceived from actual barriers and in promoting behaviors to overcome the actual barriers. Whenever possible, nurses should act as models of health with a joyful zest for living, thus providing a living example.

CHRONIC CONDITIONS OR ILLNESSES

Since the 1920s, chronic conditions have become an increasingly larger challenge to health care providers and health care delivery systems.[16] In the ensuing 80 years, chronic conditions replaced infectious diseases as the dominant health care challenge. The number of people who have chronic conditions is increasing with the ever-growing number of older people and the increasing number of people who survive major illness. In 1995, it was estimated that 99 million people in the United States had chronic conditions.[16] Of these, 41 million were limited in their daily activities, and 12 million were unable to go to school or work or to live independently. By the year 2030, it is estimated that nearly 150 million Americans will have a chronic condition; 42 million of these will be limited in their ability to go to school or work or to live independently. In addition, the lives of family members and others are affected by the related caregiving responsibilities.

A *chronic illness* or *condition* has been defined as a long-term health problem caused by an irreversible disorder (e.g., a severe spinal cord injury), an accumulation of disorders (e.g., neuropathy and retinopathy as complications of diabetes), or a latent disease (e.g., development of lung cancer after years of exposure to asbestos). A *chronic condition* is a general term that includes both

chronic illnesses and impairments, such as developmental disabilities or impairments caused by injuries. From this broad definition, it is apparent that chronic conditions are prevalent. Whether in an acute care, an ambulatory, or a long-term care setting or in the community, nursing care is provided to clients who have chronic conditions. A "chronic condition" is consistent with the concept of health as multidimensional, so that some dimensions of health exist until death. Health promotion, illness prevention, and health maintenance interventions are extremely important for people who have a chronic condition.

In 1995, chronic conditions cost the economy $470 billion (in 1990 dollars)[18] in direct medical costs and more than $230 billion in lost productivity.[16] These estimated costs would be even higher if they were expressed in the current year's dollars as a result of inflation. The cost of chronic conditions increases daily and affects the health care system. The health care system is undergoing a paradigm shift involving changes in philosophies about health, chronic illness, disability, and the roles of health care professionals, clients, and families in the management of chronic conditions. Increased emphasis is being given to prevention of chronic conditions and finding ways to help people live with and shape the course of such conditions.

◼ MULTIFACTORIAL ASPECTS OF CHRONIC DISEASE

As mentioned earlier, a century ago our ancestors fought infectious and communicable diseases. Although serious infectious diseases are still a public health threat, most life-threatening diseases today are those that become chronic as a result of metabolic abnormalities induced by health risk factors such as genetic or biologic (aging), behavioral (nutrition), and environmental influences. Figure 1–2 shows the association between multiple risk factors and chronic diseases. Health risk factors reflect a multicausal disease causation theory. The relationships among health risk factors and disease are examined in the following text.

Genetic or Biologic Health Risk Factors

HEREDITY AND DISEASE

Genetic aspects of disease have been recognized for many years. Recent technology has allowed researchers to identify the actual gene that is faulty in some disorders. Most recently, therapy has been developed to treat altered gene structures and to clone a new being.

More than one fifth of the human genes differ in form from one person to another. This remarkable degree of genetic variation among normal people is what accounts for natural variations in attributes such as height, hair color, intelligence, personality, and blood pressure. These genetic differences also affect each person's ability to handle environmental challenges, including those that produce disease. In every disease, there is some degree of genetic interaction with the environment. For example, lung cancer may develop in many smokers, but not in all. In 1990, medical researchers identified a single gene linked to lung cancer risk. Perhaps a person's genetic makeup allows the body to kill early cancer cells.

More than 5000 diseases are known to have a genetic

FIGURE 1–2 Multiple risk factors have been linked to most of the chronic diseases. NIDDM, non–insulin-dependent diabetes mellitus. (From Whitney, E. N., & Rolfes, S. R. [1993]. *Understanding nutrition* [6th ed., p. 93]. Belmont, CA: West Publishing Company. Reprinted by permission of Wadsworth Publishing Co.)

	Genetics	Age	High-fat diet or overweight	Sedentary lifestyle	Stress	Smoking	Excessive alcohol intake	Low complex carbohydrate/fiber intake	Low fluoride intake	High sugar intake	Low calcium intake	Low vitamin and/or mineral intake	High salt intake or salt-preserved foods	Environmental contaminants
Cancers	✓		✓	✓	✓	✓	✓	✓				✓	✓	✓
Hypertension	✓	✓	✓	✓	✓	✓	✓					✓	✓	✓
Diabetes (NIDDM)	✓	✓	✓	✓						✓				
Osteoporosis	✓	✓		✓		✓	✓			✓		✓		
Atherosclerosis	✓	✓	✓	✓	✓	✓	✓							
Obesity	✓		✓	✓						✓				
Stroke	✓	✓	✓		✓	✓	✓							
Diverticulosis			✓	✓	✓			✓	✓				✓	
Dental disease	✓								✓	✓	✓		✓	

component. In certain diseases, however, the genetic component is so overwhelming that the disease occurs in a predictable manner. Such diseases are termed *genetic disorders;* an example is Huntington's chorea, which is a progressive neurologic disease.

New approaches to the treatment of genetic disease include gene therapy. *Gene therapy* involves the injection of deoxyribonucleic acid (DNA) fragments into cells. The fragments find their way to the nucleus and repair enzymes to restore normal function to the cell. Today research is being conducted on the use of gene therapy in the treatment of Alzheimer's disease, muscular dystrophy, cystic fibrosis, and some forms of primary and secondary epilepsy. Gene therapy is a rapidly evolving form of treatment, and other new approaches include the promotion of new blood vessel growth *(angiogenesis)* for clients who have impaired circulation.

AGING AND DISEASE

There is an increased risk for all diseases with aging, especially cancer. Older clients tend to attribute aches and pains to aging itself and often are less likely to have routine preventive screenings. Older clients are more prone to injury, acute infections (especially respiratory), and other acute illnesses than younger clients. Contributing to this are the increased occurrence of chronic illness, decreased reserves of energy, and decreased ability to respond physiologically to stress. It is common to see an older client who is mentally competent become confused during the stress of acute illness often resulting from renal and hepatic changes. Recovery from acute illness takes longer than in a younger client, and it is possible that the previous level of functioning will not be regained.

Common problems in the care of the older client include promotion of physical safety, prevention of alterations in skin integrity, promotion of social interactions, and promotion of adequate nutrition. Do not presume that all elderly clients are weak and debilitated. The older client and the nurse's role are described in Chapter 3.

Behavioral Health Risk Factors

NUTRITION AND DISEASE

Heart disease, cancer, stroke, and liver disease are associated with nutritional factors. These disorders are four of the 10 leading causes of death in the United States (Box 1–2). The role of nutrition in these diseases is discussed, and more information is presented later.

LIPIDS. There are three types of lipids, or fats: (1) triglycerides and their component fatty acids, (2) phospholipids, and (3) sterols. Triglycerides are an energy source, and stored fat is used as body insulation. Triglycerides contain one molecule of glycerol and three fatty acid molecules. The fatty acids can be saturated, monounsaturated, or polyunsaturated. The polyunsaturated and monounsaturated fats lead to a lower blood cholesterol level. Fatty acids are used as starting points for the manufacture of hormonal regulators. Phospholipids and sterols build cell membranes and manufacture hormones, vitamin D, and bile.

LIPOPROTEINS. As fats are digested, they must be "packaged" for transport in the blood because they are not soluble in water. Fats cluster together with special proteins, forming lipoproteins. There are four types: chy-

---

BOX 1–2   Ten Leading Causes of Death

1. Heart disease
2. Cancer
3. Stroke
4. Unintentional injuries
5. Chronic obstructive lung disease
6. Pneumonia and influenza
7. Diabetes mellitus
8. Suicide
9. Chronic liver disease and cirrhosis
10. Homicide

lomicrons, very-low-density lipoproteins (VLDLs), low-density lipoproteins (LDLs), and high-density lipoproteins (HDLs). High HDL levels and low LDL levels are associated with reduced risk of heart disease. Laboratory values for VLDLs and LDLs are found in Appendix C. Lipoproteins are explained in Chapter 56.

CHOLESTEROL. Cholesterol is carried in several lipoproteins, primarily in LDLs. A high level of cholesterol carried in LDL is directly correlated with atherosclerosis. A *direct correlation* means that as one factor rises, so does the other; in this case, the higher the cholesterol and LDL, the higher the incidence of heart disease from atherosclerosis. High blood cholesterol in HDL correlates *inversely* with risk of heart disease. Appendix C describes the range of normal laboratory values for cholesterol. The pathophysiology of atherosclerosis and heart disease is discussed in Chapter 56.

ALCOHOL. Alcohol intake plays several roles in health. Research indicates that moderate alcohol intake (one glass of red wine per day) raises HDL levels and reduces the risk of heart disease.[43] A high intake of alcohol, however, is associated with hypertension, stroke, liver disease, and several types of cancer, including some found in the head, neck, and reproductive system.

OBESITY. Obesity has been associated with increased risk of heart disease, stroke, hypertension, and diabetes (see Chapters 28 and 29). The pathophysiology of these disorders is discussed in Chapters 45 (diabetes), 52 (hypertension, 56 (heart disease), and 70 (stroke).

NUTRITION AND CANCER

Cancer is a disease of multiple origins, such as heredity, smoking, and environmental exposure. Some cancers have dietary links. Many people fear that food additives are *carcinogens* (cancer-causing substances). In fact, food additives have little to do with cancer. Contaminants of food, entities that get into foods by accident, may be powerful carcinogens, such as pesticides and bacteria. Fat has been implicated in cancer. Fat does not cause cancer; however, animals that have been exposed to a carcinogen and given a high-fat diet appear to have greater numbers of tumors than animals given a low-fat diet. Thus, fat appears to be a cancer promoter, perhaps by (1) causing the body to secrete more hormones, such as estrogen; (2) promoting the secretion of bile into the intestine, where organisms can convert the bile into compounds that cause cancer; or (3) incorporating into cell membranes and changing them so they offer less resistance to carcinogenic invaders. It is thought that fiber and vegetables might help reduce the risk of some forms of cancer by speeding excretion of bile from the body, decreasing transit time of food through the colon, and reducing exposure.

Beta-carotene (vitamin A) regulates cellular differentiation, a process that goes awry in cancer. Some people think that if they take vitamin A supplements, their risk of cancer will be reduced. This area is still being studied, but it appears that the fiber in foods containing vitamin A is more important than the vitamin itself. Other antipromoters of cancer include vitamin B_6, folate, pantothenic acid, vitamin B_{12}, iron, zinc, selenium, and antioxidants, such as vitamins C and E. Some non-nutrient compounds are found in foods from the cabbage family. These foods produce chemicals that activate enzymes that destroy carcinogens. The research base for the synthetic form of antioxidants and other cancer-preventing vitamin supplements is less conclusive. Dietitians recommend eating vegetables and consuming various foods to dilute the effects of harmful cancer promoters but may or may not recommend taking vitamin supplements.

OXYGEN FREE RADICALS AND DISEASE

Oxygen free radicals, or superoxide radicals, are by-products of energy production. Superoxide radicals are atoms or molecules with one or more pairs of unpaired, free electrons that are reactive. The radicals commonly bind to oxygen for stabilization. The oxygen then binds to hydrogen for stabilization. The product of this reaction is hydrogen peroxide, which is toxic to cells. The most unbalanced form of free radicals is free hydroxy radicals. The free hydroxy radicals bind to polyunsaturated fatty acids, which are commonly found in cell membranes and membranes of organelles within the cell. If the free radical binds to the lysosome, the cell is destroyed.

The body is equipped to handle some of these radicals with antioxidants for the conversion of the radical back to usable oxygen. The antioxidants include vitamins C and E and beta-carotene (vitamin A). Vitamin E and selenium in cell membranes are oxidized by the free radicals, much as fatty acid is. Vitamin E neutralizes the free radical and prevents it from attaching to a fatty acid. In the process, vitamin E is damaged. The damaged vitamin E is restored by vitamin C. The role of beta-carotene is not clear in free radical antioxidation. Vitamins A and E are carried by the LDLs.

Environmental Health Risk Factors

Studies in cancer causation have revealed that chemicals in the workplace are responsible for specific cancers. Such discoveries have left the impression that most human cancers are associated with environmental chemical contamination. This opinion has led to public pressure on government to control chemical contamination as a key means of cancer prevention. In most of today's industrialized world, however, work-related cancer is rare and should remain infrequent if regulations are followed. A careful analysis of the causative elements in each type of cancer has shown that prevailing lifestyles in a given population (especially tobacco use, nutritional variations, and physical activity) account for the incidence of cancer.

Sun exposure increases the risk of skin cancers. The populations most sensitive to the sun's effects are those with fair skin, such as people of Celtic descent. The chief cause of skin cancer is damage to DNA from ultraviolet light. An allegedly "healthy" look (tanned skin) can have unhealthy consequences. The belief that sun exposure is needed for vitamin D absorption is obsolete in most countries, because milk is supplemented with vitamin D. Children who have no sun exposure and do not drink milk can be at risk for rickets from low vitamin D levels. Adults who do not consume adequate vitamin D develop osteomalacia. Arabic women constitute a high-risk group because they shield their skin from the sun and do not drink milk.

Air and water pollution can lead to disease. Water pollution has caused endemic infections with various microorganisms throughout the world. Air pollution increases the risk of asthma and lung cancer.

Interrelationship of Health Risk Factors

A person's body, mind, and environment all function together to determine whether illness develops. The brain helps maintain an internal milieu and assists the body in adapting to the external environment. The response can affect the body's functioning. The way the brain defines a situation can evoke chemical and nervous system reactions. When people habitually respond to every frustration, disappointment, or loss as if it is a matter of life and death, the endocrine, musculoskeletal, and autonomic nervous systems respond. If people view life as requiring constant domination of things and people, they can have excessive production of cholesterol, triglycerides, norepinephrine, adrenocorticotropic hormone (ACTH), and insulin. This attitude may contribute to deficient levels of pituitary growth hormone.

The function and balance of neurotransmitters (chemical messengers, such as enkephalins and endorphins) can be influenced by drugs, viruses, bacteria, poor nutrition, defective genes, aging, or the perception of stress. Tissue damage can result from normal bodily processes that go awry or are disrupted; these processes include (1) neurotransmitter activity in the brain, (2) the stress hormones of the adrenal glands and nervous system, and (3) the helper and suppressor cells of the immune system. For example, excessive stress hormones (corticosteroids, catecholamines) can lead to artery damage or may suppress the action of antibodies and natural killer cells, which protect the body from foreign invaders and tumor development. Deficient suppressor cells may permit overaction of the immune system to the point at which the body starts attacking itself, such as in rheumatoid arthritis. Autoimmune disorders are discussed in Chapter 77.

The brain is central to any change in health because it is the mediator between the external and internal environments. Through the brain's interpretation, we can change an environment, leave it, or engage in it, or we can decide to rest, exercise, or diet. Ultimately, illness involves a combination of mind-body factors. These factors interact to produce symptoms. It is not uncommon to experience depression with physical illness or to have physical manifestations of mental or emotional illness.

Increasingly, scientific study is directed toward the mind-body interactions. The increase in chronic conditions and the disillusion with medical care have led to increased use of alternative, or complementary, practices which are often based on mind-body connection theory, are wellness-oriented, are less intrusive, and have fewer side effects. The Office of Alternative Medicine within the National Institutes of Health (NIH) funds research to evaluate the effectiveness of alternative medical treatment. This research provides support for the interactive nature of systems (the mind-body connection) and presents evidence other than the biomedical model.

■ MANAGEMENT OF CHRONIC CONDITIONS AND ILLNESS

Nursing management can strengthen the client's and family's ability to live with, and can shape the course of, chronic conditions. For effective management of chronic conditions it is essential to know (1) the time pattern of chronic conditions; (2) commonalities in physical, psychological, and social adaptation to different chronic conditions; (3) health promotion and illness prevention nursing interventions in the care of people with chronic conditions; and (4) patterns of health care delivery for people with chronic conditions. This chapter addresses these aspects.

Stages of a Chronic Condition

In general, chronic conditions evolve in a typical pattern. Various terms are used to describe this process; it can be called the *course of illness,* the *trajectory,*[4] or *time phases.*[44] Awareness of the effect of time on chronic disease creates an appreciation for the challenges experienced by clients and their families living with chronic conditions. Awareness of the pattern also promotes an appreciation that management of chronic conditions is accomplished largely by clients and families in the home. Knowledge of the time pattern of chronic conditions helps broaden the focus of health care to include all levels of prevention and to increase the percentage of health care dollars allocated to prevention.

The three stages of the pattern in all chronic conditions are (1) *prediagnostic,* (2) *diagnostic,* and (3) *chronic.* Some chronic conditions also have a *terminal stage.*

PREDIAGNOSTIC STAGE

In the prediagnostic stage, manifestations of chronic conditions are vague or absent. Risk factors common to one or more chronic conditions may be present. This chapter presents an overview, and several other chapters are devoted to specific chronic conditions.

Some risk factors are modifiable, and others are not. Modifying behavioral and environmental risk factors can prevent the development or may extend the prediagnostic phase of some chronic conditions. For example, not smoking or stopping smoking is a controllable behavior that decreases the risk for development of a chronic condition in the respiratory, cardiovascular, or other systems. These chronic conditions include asthma, emphysema, bronchiectasis, coronary artery disease, angina, myocardial infarction, hypertension, and cancer. A low-fat diet appears to decrease the risk of obesity, coronary disease, diabetes, hypertension, stroke, and cancer. Seat belts protect against injury in vehicular accidents. Reducing high stress levels may help lower the risk of cardiovascular disease, peptic ulcers, asthma, ulcerative colitis, multiple sclerosis, cancer, and accidental trauma. Specific immunizations can prevent the development of certain diseases.

DIAGNOSTIC STAGE

In the diagnostic stage, the client recognizes that something is wrong and seeks medical attention, and a disorder is diagnosed. In some cases, chronic conditions are sequelae to acute illness, trauma, or treatment. In these instances, the health care provider may simply inform the client that he or she has a given disorder. This stage occurs in all cases because chronic disorders affect all ages.

Clinical manifestations range from vague to severe or even life-threatening. Manifestations differ because the client may have ignored early warning signs or may have been able to cope with early clinical manifestations, or the condition's course may be variable. Hypertension, for example, is called a "silent killer" because most people have no clinical manifestations. Thus, hypertension may be diagnosed incidentally when a client has a routine physical examination, receives treatment for another problem, or has suffered a stroke from untreated hypertension.

CHRONIC STAGE

The chronic stage has been referred to as the "long haul" because the client must live with the condition for a prolonged time. In fact, this stage may last for the rest of the client's life.

Clinical manifestations may be controlled or out of control. Changes in function may be stable or may be marked by remissions and exacerbations, or function may progressively decline. If the onset has been acute (i.e., stroke, spinal cord injury, myocardial infarction), the greatest return of function frequently occurs within the first 6 months. Remissions and exacerbations may be frequent or infrequent. Progressive decline may be rapid or slow. Changes in function and the rate of change are more predictable for some chronic conditions than for others. Acute episodes of illness during this stage frequently relate to exacerbations, sudden decline in body system function, or side effects or complications of treatment. With medical and surgical advances (i.e., liver and heart transplants, chemotherapy), life spans have been extended but new health problems may develop. Some acute episodes can be managed at home; others must be managed in the hospital. When death occurs at this stage, it is sudden and unexpected.

TERMINAL STAGE

Transition to the terminal stage occurs (1) when changes in body systems become irreversible and the loss of these functions is incompatible with life and (2) when death is expected within 6 months.

For many chronic conditions (e.g., arthritis), there is no terminal stage. Death for these clients is due to other causes. Technological advances have eliminated the terminal stage for other chronic conditions. For example, organ transplants in clients with organ failure may reverse this stage to the chronic stage. Recent cure for some types of childhood cancers has changed the time pattern from terminal to an "at-risk" stage.

Process of Adaptation

Adaptation to chronic conditions is complex and continuous and involves physiologic, psychological, social, technological, and time factors. Knowledge related to adaptation factors has been generated by many disciplines. Adaptation is pivotal for the client with a chronic condition. In this chapter, *adaptation* refers to the body's or mind's response to a chronic condition. However, some adaptations are not positive and can worsen the condition. The nurse's role is to monitor and prevent adaptations that are not beneficial and to assist the client and family to adapt their lifestyles to the condition.

PHYSIOLOGIC ADAPTATION

Chronic conditions can interfere with physiologic functions. The body's intake, digestion, and expenditure of physical energy for cellular metabolism and protein synthesis can be altered. When physical energy demands exceed the intake and processing of physical energy, general resistance to physiologic stressors is impaired. Neuroendocrine responses to psychological distress have been implicated in adaptation to (1) anorexia, pain, fatigue, shortness of breath, and decreased immune response; (2) progressive decline or exacerbations of chronic conditions; and (3) delayed recovery from acute episodes of illness during the chronic stage. It is thought that adaptive energy from neuroendocrine sources becomes exhausted over time.

Another physiologic adaptation is the loss of coordinated function of various body systems. Clients whose levels of mobility become limited because of self-imposed inactivity, progression of chronic health problems, surgery, trauma, or acute episodes of medical treatment are at high risk for experiencing changes in body system functions. Collectively, these adaptive responses are commonly referred to as "hazards of immobility" or the "disuse syndrome." Clearly, these adaptive responses increase levels of disability.

PSYCHOLOGICAL ADAPTATION

Psychological adaptation to a chronic condition is difficult and demanding. This adaptation process is ongoing and overlaps other biologic and psychosocial processes associated with gains, losses, and challenges throughout the remaining life span. Box 1–3 identifies common concerns, fears, and events of personal change associated with a chronic condition.

As with other ongoing processes, psychological adaptation to a chronic condition is characterized by periods of changing demands and transitions. Some of these are predictable; others are not. Predictable periods of changing demands and transitions include onset and diagnosis, hospitalizations for treatment, exacerbation of illness, treatment failures, and loss of self-care abilities. These times can be expected to be especially stressful. Some periods are marked by depression when clients realize they may not get better and may get worse. The client and family must redefine their roles, expectations, and life goals. Clients in the terminal stage must adapt to a shortened life span and to the process of dying.

Although chronic diseases, such as acquired immunodeficiency syndrome (AIDS), cancer, diabetes mellitus, and multiple sclerosis, may differ in their impact on each client, psychological adaptation to various chronic conditions, over varying lengths of time, has many similar characteristics. Therefore, some general statements can be made. The incidence of clinical depression in persons living with chronic conditions ranges from "no difference from" to "higher than" that of community-dwelling adults without chronic health problems. Risk factors for depression have been identified as (1) biologic changes, (2) medications (e.g., digoxin, droperidol, ethanol), and (3) psychological vulnerability. Some cases of depression may be resolved with medical treatment or by a change in medication. If these interventions are not effective, the client should receive psychiatric evaluation and treatment.[1]

Different clients adapt to the same diagnosis and stage of illness in different ways. During the diagnostic stage, one client may appear overwhelmed and may assume a

---

BOX 1-3 Common Concerns, Fears, and Events of Personal Change Associated with Chronic Conditions

Concerns and Fears

Loss of sense of self
Loss of control and predictability
Heightened sense of mortality
Loss of productivity
Loss of valued roles
Loss of relationships
Loss of opportunity or ability for sexual expression or reproduction
Uncertainty about the future
Loss of purpose and meaning in life
Fear of procedures
Fear of death

Events of Personal Change

Life plans and goals
Established roles and patterns of interacting within family and outside the home
Relationships with others
Work (job) or school roles, relationships, and patterns of interaction
Daily routines
Loss of gratifying behaviors
Changes in health maintenance and management behaviors
Activity and sleep patterns
Financial resources
Appearance

---

lower level of physical, psychological, or social functioning than the physical condition warrants. Another client may evidence minimal distress and may regain or maintain a high level of physical, psychological, and social functioning.

GENERAL PATTERN OF ADAPTATION. A general pattern of psychological adaptation to personal change perceived as a loss or threat of loss has been described by sociologists, psychologists, physicians, and nurses. Phases of this pattern have been labeled in various ways by different authors. The pattern has been referred to as the *grief process* and the *mourning process.*

Disbelief. The first phase is commonly referred to as disbelief or *resistance.* Denial (unconscious refusal to acknowledge painful realities) of the changes or the need for personal change is characteristic. This phase is similar to the "fight-or-flight" response and is believed to protect the client from being psychologically overwhelmed.

Developing Awareness. The second phase, commonly referred to as the *anger* phase, is developing awareness. It is characterized by withdrawal, preoccupation with self, crying, depression, expression of anger toward others, and feelings of guilt for having brought the disease on oneself, being different, and being alone. In this phase, the client experiences acute awareness of what has been lost and grieves for it.

Integration. The third phase is characterized by rational acceptance that a physical or psychological change

has occurred and by attempts to keep emotional distress within manageable limits. Other cognitive behaviors associated with this phase are reestablishing a sense of self, meaning, and purpose; revising life goals; learning to live with uncertainty; and acquiring new strategies for coping with one's environment.

Some people describe experiencing intermittent chronic sorrow.[11] Triggers of sadness include the anniversary date of the condition's onset, special events, birthdays, and losses in physical function. Knowledge that feelings of sorrow are commonly felt may help mitigate the distress associated with the experience.

COPING BEHAVIORS. Clients with the same medical diagnosis and in the same phase of chronic illness use a variety of physical, cognitive, and verbal behaviors to manage distress. The type of behaviors used and their effectiveness are highly individual. Some coping behaviors are passive; others are active. *Emotion-focused (affective)* behaviors have been defined as thoughts or actions that make a person feel better but do not alter the distressing situation. *Problem-focused* behaviors are efforts taken to change or resolve distressing situations. A number of behaviors fall into both categories. The prevailing assumption is that problem-focused behaviors are more efficacious, but some research suggests that a combination of both behaviors may be most efficacious, especially when the problem cannot be resolved and must be managed.

Interestingly, some clients report that talking about their illness helps them cope.[22] Others report that *not* talking about their illness helps them cope. Strategies reported as being effective in managing distressful situations include avoiding, ignoring, accepting, thinking out, and changing the situation. Shopping, driving, going out to eat, and exercising are types of activities that some people find helpful in relieving stress. Other reported helpful strategies include taking naps; seeking information and advice; changing values, attitudes, and goals; hope; prayer; putting the problem in God's hands; humor; positive thinking; positive self-talk; trying to maintain some control over the situation; trying to look at the problem objectively; and drawing on past experiences.[27] Although many strategies are constructive, others can be destructive, such as imagining the worst, taking anger out on others, blaming others, taking illegal drugs, overeating, smoking, and abusing alcohol.

SOCIAL ADAPTATION

The roles of clients with chronic conditions overlap social roles related to age, sex, family, work, and recreation. The impact of health and illness roles on social roles ranges from minimal to severe, with health and illness roles being dominant. The degree to which clients adapt socially is influenced by (1) changes in physical appearance, (2) ability to communicate, (3) ability to navigate the physical environment, (4) social resources (e.g., people, money, and community services), and (5) societal values and attitudes. Society responds more favorably to clients who have less apparent chronic conditions than to those with more visible signs of illness. Beliefs and values influence social acceptance related to attractiveness,

DIVERSITY IN HEALTH CARE

Health and Illness Beliefs and Practices

Whether we consider ourselves well or ill is primarily a matter of cultural definition. Kleinman and colleagues[3] describe illness as culturally shaped, in that it is individually perceived. What is important is how one explains one's illness, such as:

- How it was caused
- How long it will last
- What type of treatment should be received
- What type of practitioner should deliver the treatment

Illness includes the subjective experiences of the person who is ill and how the illness is perceived and experienced by the social group also.

In many cultures, illnesses are defined as "natural" or "unnatural."[2] In the folk health tradition, *natural* illnesses are those that occur because of some known external factors in the environment, such as bad air, night air, bad food, bad water, or infestations. An example of a folk illness or culture-bound syndrome that is considered to be the result of natural factors is *Empacho,* an illness recognized by Hispanics in which pain and cramping in the abdomen are believed to be due to food forming into a ball and clinging to the stomach or intestines.[1] Another example of a natural illness is "high blood," believed among some African Americans and Haitians to be the result of eating too many rich foods or red meat.[1] Treatment may involve consuming an astringent substance to promote "sweating out" the excess blood nutrients.

Unnatural illnesses are believed to be caused by supernatural forces, such as punishment from God or a hex or curse by a witch, a root doctor, or other practitioner. An unnatural illness that shows up in many cultures around the world is the Evil Eye, known as *Mal Ojo* in Spanish or as other names in other languages. The Evil Eye is usually considered to be a disorder in which a child falls ill as a result of a stranger's attention or admiration. In *Mal Ojo,* the practice of touching a child by one who is admiring him or her is believed to prevent the disorder.[2] *Susto,* or magical fright, is another unnatural illness and is believed to result from the loss of the spirit from the body. Treatment at times includes the use of ceremonies along with herbs.[4]

The concept of "balance" is also important in many cultures in understanding and maintaining health and treating illnesses. For health, a balance must exist among a person's psychological, physical, social and spiritual realms. If imbalance is present, illness results. The "hot-cold" theory related to the balance needed for health exists in many cultures and is a classification in which illnesses, treatments, and foods are identified as to their hot and cold qualities; these qualities are not related to temperature.[6] If an illness is considered "cold," a "hot"

treatment, such as particular herbal tea, food (e.g.,meat), or a medication is given to help restore balance. The opposite is done with a "hot" illness. Whether or not a particular illness or substance is considered hot or cold varies across cultures.

In Asian cultures following Taoist philosophy, the concepts of the opposing forces in nature of *Yin* and *Yang* are the bases for determining balance.[1] *Yin* is considered to be all that is female, dark, cold, quiet, empty, and negative; *Yang* is all that is male, light, warm, and positive. What is especially important to nurses and other caregivers about these belief systems is that clients may not want to follow a treatment regimen if they consider that the wrong treatment is being given for the illness and thus that balance will not be achieved. If a client identifies the illness as hot, such as in an infection, and the medication is also considered hot, such as an antibiotic, the client may throw away the medication in favor of a cold treatment. If a nurse elicits the client's belief system, the nurse can then help to make the treatment more acceptable, such as by adding a substance (e.g., herbal tea) that is considered cold to a regimen that includes a hot treatment.

In relation to her theory of culture care, Leininger emphasizes the need for the nurse to understand the client's view of illness in order to provide culturally congruent care. One of the theory-based modes of nursing action identified by Leininger is that of cultural care *repatterning,* which refers to the supportive and facilitative professional actions and decisions that help clients reorder or modifiy their health care patterns in a more health-promoting direction while respecting their cultural values and beliefs.[5] By understanding the client's view of illness and providing care that respects and incorporates the beliefs of the client, the nurse can improve the probability that the client will achieve the most positive health outcomes possible.

References

1. Andrews, M. M., & Boyle, J. S. (1999). *Transcultural concepts in nursing care* (3rd ed.). Philadelphia: Lippincott–Williams & Wilkins.
2. Giger, J. N., & Davidhizar, R. E. (1999). *Transcultural nursing: Assessment and intervention* (3rd ed.). St. Louis: Mosby.
3. Kleinman, A., Eisenberg, L., & Good, B. (1978). Clinical lessons from anthropologic and cross-cultural research. *Annals of Internal Medicine, 88,* 251–258.
4. Purnell, L. D., & Paulanka, B. J. (1998). *Transcultural health care: A culturally competent approach.* Philadelphia: F. A. Davis.
5. Reynolds, C. L., & Leininger, M. (1993). *Madeleine Leininger: Cultural care diversity and universality theory.* Newbury Park, CA: Sage.
6. Spector, R. E. (1996). *Cultural diversity in health and illness* (4th ed.). Stamford, CT: Appleton & Lange.

Sandra Sharma, PhD, ARNP, CS, *James A. Haley Veterans Hospital, Tampa, Florida*

productivity, independence, self-reliance, normality, individual rights, and health and illness. These beliefs and values also influence the availability of social resources and health services as well as job, recreational, and housing opportunities.

SOCIAL BELIEFS. Social beliefs and expectations about behavior appropriate for people experiencing physi-

cal illness have changed since the 1950s when Parsons described the "sick role" in our society.[30] Parsons stated that people are not responsible for their illness. This pattern of thinking has shifted to an idea that a client may have a role in the development of some illnesses. Parsons also stated that society believed that all clients should be released from the usual role responsibilities. The belief today is shifting to one in which clients try to maintain responsibility for personal, family, and social activities that they are capable of doing or learning. The expectation that clients should view illness as undesirable and try to get well is shifting to one in which cure is not possible for all illnesses and that clients should maintain an active role in managing incurable health problems. The expectation persists that clients should seek medically competent help; however, clients are more actively involved in decision-making related to care options and management of health problems than they were 50 years ago. Differences in beliefs and expectations about clients who have chronic conditions and how they respond to their sick role are a frequent source of conflict among caregivers, clients, and families. See Diversity in Health Care.

SOCIAL CHANGE EVENTS. Events of social change commonly associated with a chronic condition relate to roles and interaction patterns, mobility patterns, employment, living arrangements, recreation, finances, time and place for vacations, and health insurance.

FAMILY ADAPTATION

Because of the long-term nature of chronic conditions and the role of the family in maintaining the health of its members, a chronic condition is also a family condition. Families must cope with unusual ongoing adaptive challenges related to the presence of a chronic condition. Some families are more effective than others in meeting adaptive challenges. Types of physical impairments, family resources, family perception, the developmental stage of family members and the family unit, behaviors of the client, the health care environment, and society's expectation are interrelated factors that affect family adaptation. Some family units become stronger, whereas others disintegrate.

Challenges to family adjustment vary with different stages of the condition. Adaptive challenges during the *diagnostic* stage are the same as those related to acute illness, such as (1) pulling together, (2) learning to cope with the acute care environment and treatment, and (3) establishing relationships with caregivers. Other challenges include (1) identifying the meanings of health and illness, (2) assessing potential changes in the family, (3) moving toward integration of temporary and permanent changes while maintaining a sense of continuity between past and present, and (4) developing an attitude of flexibility toward future personal and family goals.

Adaptive challenges during the *chronic* stage include (1) maintaining a sense of normality, (2) adjusting to changing expectations of each family member, (3) striving to balance family resources, and (4) maintaining autonomy of all family members despite the pull toward mutual dependency, caretaking, or focus on the family member who has the chronic condition. Some demands during the chronic stage result from treatment, for example, changing work schedules to accommodate treatment, or loss of strength related to treatment side effects. Similarly, the client's roles may have to be assumed by other family members or friends. If the client is the primary wage earner, the tasks of earning a living may have to be undertaken by another. Initially, the condition may generate a lot of support from extended family members and friends; after several months, support may decline.

When a family has a member with a long-term disabling condition and limited financial resources, complex issues must be managed. Some couples divorce so that they can qualify for funding to care for a family member. If the family member has impaired judgment or reduced ability to conduct personal business, another family member may need to obtain power of attorney. If the chronic condition is terminal, families must also manage issues related to the family member's death and to resuming a normal family life after the death.

Health Care and Chronic Conditions

Health care management after the diagnostic stage occurs in various settings, such as (1) rehabilitation centers, units, and programs; (2) home health care agencies; (3) long-term health care facilities; (4) nurse-managed clinics; (5) case management; (6) hospice care; and (7) community service agencies. During the other phases of chronic conditions, care may be provided in acute care hospitals, rehabilitation units, nursing homes, or the client's home.

Chronic care is different from *acute* care.[18] The goal of acute care is to restore a person to the previous level of functioning. The goal of chronic care is to maintain independent living, facilitate successful personal and social adjustment, and minimize further deterioration of physical and mental health. The aim of chronic care is not to "fix" or "cure." Chronic care requires interdisciplinary collaboration and multidisciplinary approaches. Medical management varies with the type and stage of the chronic condition and the technology available. Management and management outcomes are better defined for some conditions than others. Medical management includes prevention, diagnosis, treatment of acute episodes, and helping clients manage and shape the course of their chronic condition. Multidisciplinary approaches are employed in promoting maximal use of the client's functional abilities and adaptation to deficits. Increasingly, goals for management are established in conjunction with other health team members, the client, and family.

In the United States, chronic conditions are the leading cause of illness, disability, and death.[18] Today's health care system is not very effective in treating chronic conditions, because available care is often fragmented, inappropriate, and difficult to obtain. New health problems may result when clients who have chronic conditions face barriers in accessing services such as preventive care, durable medical equipment, medications, or home nursing care. These secondary health problems might have been prevented through better coordination of health care services and more preventive care. Managed care or the case management approach has the potential to provide the range of integrated services required by people with chronic conditions.

FUNDING ISSUES

Chronic conditions cost $470 billion (in 1990 dollars) in direct medical costs.[18] This cost has the potential to be reduced. Table 1–5 demonstrates how more health promotion and illness prevention interventions might be cost-effective in chronic care.

TABLE 1–5	THE OPPORTUNITY COSTS OF CHRONIC CARE

America's lack of investment in an adequate system of chronic care carries an *opportunity cost;* that is, when money is spent on "X"—usually acute care services—it is not available to spend on "Y"—early, up-front prevention and treatment of chronic conditions, or coordinated systems of supportive services.

Examples:

More money spent on	*May mean less money spent on*
1. Screening, nutrition, and education to prevent heart attacks	1. Emergency department treatment and subsequent care for a heart attack victim
2. Relatively inexpensive preventive care for a client with diabetes	2. Complications leading to amputation and lifelong disability
3. Breast cancer screening for early detection, when treatment is less expensive and more effective than later detection	3. Chemotherapy, radiation, or surgery for breast cancer
4. Modest cost of installing a handrail to prevent falls	4. Hip replacement surgery
5. Adult day care	5. Nursing home care

From The Institute for Health and Aging, University of California, San Francisco.

One example of the current chronic care system's fragmentation is the lack of distribution of assistive technology (e.g., wheelchair, walker, hearing aid, brace, or artificial limb) among those in need. The 1990 National Health Interview survey showed that more than 2.5 million people reported a need for assistive technology but did not receive it.[18] Of these, nearly half were adults of working age (25 to 64 years old), and more than half reported that they could not afford a device. Clients with physical disabilities benefit from assistive devices and techniques that compensate or substitute for lost function. Acquiring skills in using these devices improves functional levels. Unfortunately, many clients and families who would benefit are not referred because some health care professionals lack knowledge about rehabilitation services, or third-party payers may not reimburse clients for these services.

OUTCOME MANAGEMENT IN CHRONIC CONDITIONS

The focus of the health history varies with the stage of the chronic condition. In the *prediagnostic* phase, emphasis is on obtaining the history, determining the client's current health status, and identifying risk factors. In the *diagnostic* phase, the emphasis is on manifestations and the client's related experiences, for example:

- When did they start?
- What makes them better or worse?
- To what degree are they interfering with sleep and the activities and demands of daily living?

In the *chronic* phase, assessment focuses on several aspects of the major manifestations: (1) change or stability, (2) frequency and severity, (3) triggers, and (4) means of relief. Manifestations common to a number of chronic conditions are anorexia, fatigue, pain, shortness of breath, and sleep and sexual disturbances.

Ask about (1) facilitators and barriers encountered in carrying out prescribed health care regimens in the home, (2) recreational and work environments, (3) general energy level, (4) sleep pattern, (5) activity level and amount of assistance needed in conducting activities, and (6) demands of daily living. Levels of mobility and self-care are on a continuum ranging from complete or modified independence to modified or complete dependence.

Assess the client for treatment-related, environmental, and psychological factors as well as illness-related factors that may be contributing to physical symptoms and immobility. Self-reported symptoms are better predictors of functioning than objective measurements of physical function. Assessing the client's strengths is beneficial and provides a positive starting point for health promotion interventions. Assessment is described in Chapters 9 and 10.

■ IDENTIFYING CLIENT STRENGTHS

Everyone has both strengths and weaknesses. Help the client to recognize this fact, and encourage the client to take the necessary time to identify them. Consider questions such as the following:

- What do I like best about myself?
- What are my personal strengths?
- What goals do I set for myself?
- Am I able to complete goals I set for myself?
- How do I perceive my personal strengths as a way of understanding these patterns?

Evaluating one's strengths can help build an individual's belief system. Gaining knowledge of strengths and weaknesses fosters a sense of personal worth, which may be severely tested or destroyed during periods of stress or crisis. Our thoughts affect our life patterns. Working on acknowledging one's strengths allows them to be called into consciousness during stressful periods. Positive cognitive thoughts connect with all the human potentials so that the body responds positively. When activating and acting from one's strengths, a person is more likely to develop positive attitudes. Developing positive attitudes enhances one's ability to cope effectively with stress during the inevitable everyday life struggles that confront us all. Active interventions, such as recognizing strengths, enable individuals to call up inner resources to combat stress on the journey toward becoming healthy.

■ NURSING DIAGNOSIS

A number of interrelated physiologic, psychological, and sociologic nursing diagnoses are associated with chronic conditions (Box 1–4). Etiologic factors for the diagnoses

---

BOX 1–4 Physiologic, Psychological, and Social Nursing Diagnoses Commonly Associated with Chronic Conditions

Physiologic Diagnoses

Activity intolerance
Constipation
Disuse syndrome, risk for
Fatigue
Fluid volume deficit
Fluid volume excess
Health maintenance, altered
Impaired physical mobility
Incontinence, bowel
Infection, risk for
Injury, risk for
Nutrition: less than body requirements, altered
Nutrition: more than body requirements, altered
Pain
Pain, chronic
Self care deficit (bathing/hygiene, dressing/grooming, feeding, toileting)
Urinary elimination, altered

Psychological Diagnoses

Anxiety

Body image disturbance
Decisional conflict (specify)
Fear
Grieving, anticipatory
Grieving, dysfunctional
Growth and development, altered
Hopelessness
Knowledge deficit (specify)
Powerlessness
Self-esteem disturbance
Spiritual distress

Social Diagnoses

Communication, impaired verbal
Diversional activity deficit
Family processes, altered
Parenting, altered
Role performance, altered
Sexuality patterns, altered
Social interaction, impaired
Social isolation

---

differ according to individual characteristics, stage of chronic condition, changes in physiologic structure or function, treatment, and environment.

■ EXPECTED OUTCOMES

The expected outcomes for the client with a chronic condition are directly related to the specific diagnosis, physiologic changes, treatment, and adaptive energy. In general, a cure is not expected and some outcomes are more predictable than others. *Long-term* outcomes are usually written with months allowed for achievement. *Short-term* outcomes that are achievable and measurable provide positive feedback to clients, families, and caregivers. This feedback is believed to decrease the potential for caregiver burnout. The client, family, and other health team members should be involved in determining long-term and short-term outcomes.

When clients and families identify seemingly unrealistic goals, tell them that they may not achieve them and that most people with similar problems have not done so. Then identify incremental goals that can be achieved. For example, for the client with a spinal cord injury who has a goal of walking, the work would be on maintaining range of motion, which is necessary for walking. As clients and families work toward more modest goals, they will, with time, readjust their goals. In some cases, clients and families have achieved goals that were perceived as unrealistic by others.

■ EVALUATION

Expected outcomes for clients living with chronic conditions are achieved over time. Evaluation examines outcome achievement and movement to another level of care. For example, a client in acute care may become physiologically stable and may be discharged to the home for home care, to a skilled or long-term care facility, or to an acute rehabilitation center.

When gains in physical function stabilize with or without assistive devices, the client can be moved to less skilled care areas or discharged to the home. Of course, the original goals may not have been met. In these instances, determine the cause, keeping in mind that the condition may have worsened and that the expected outcome and interventions may require revision.

■ INTERVENTIONS

Nursing interventions should strengthen the client's and family's ability to live with and shape the course of the chronic condition. General strategies used in the care of clients with chronic conditions include providing direct care, teaching, counseling, working things out, making arrangements, and advocating. Interventions must be specific to the client and the setting. Use the health promotion theories presented earlier as a guide to motivate health behavior change.

Providing Client Education

Most chronic illnesses exist in a balance between control and crisis. Client education includes teaching how to determine when an illness is becoming uncontrolled, how to treat it, and when to contact the health care provider; for example:

1. Teach diabetic clients to recognize the clinical manifestations of hyperglycemia and hypoglycemia,

how to begin treatment, and when to notify the health care provider.

2. Instruct diabetic clients to carry a blood glucose testing device, a fast-acting carbohydrate, and insulin at all times.
3. Advise asthmatic clients to carry a rescue bronchodilator and angina clients to carry nitroglycerin.

Preventive actions (e.g., annual influenza vaccinations) and healthy behaviors (e.g., regular exercise) will help the client with chronic illness achieve the highest possible level of wellness.

Most chronic illnesses require some degree of daily treatment. These treatments can range from taking medication to receiving multiple injections to running a home dialysis unit. Assess the client's and the family's ability to follow the treatment guidelines, and ask whether they have experienced problems in carrying out the treatment regimen. When formulating your questions, consider these characteristics:

- *Degree of difficulty in learning the regimen.* Are there several steps involved? What complications might result from using equipment or giving medications incorrectly? Does the client or family member have the dexterity required to complete the regimen successfully? Does the client or a family member have limitations that can interfere with performing tasks?
- *Amount of time required to implement the regimen.* How much time does the treatment regimen require? How many times each day must the regimen be performed?
- *The monetary cost.* Can the client afford this regimen? Are there alternatives?
- *Amount of discomfort and exertion associated with the regimen.* How painful or inconvenient is the treatment? Do you believe the client will comply or that a family member will be persuasive enough to ensure compliance?
- *Visibility of the regimen to other people, and its social acceptance.* Will the client need to take equipment everywhere, as with oxygen? Does the client have a disfiguring condition, such as a tracheostomy or a fistula?
- *Effectiveness and speed of the regimen in controlling the condition or its manifestations.* Will the client or family members have to wait a long time for results of the regimen? What complications might occur because of the regimen (e.g., drug side effects)?

On the basis of these and other questions, develop a comprehensive teaching plan to help the client implement the treatment regimen successfully.

Controlling Clinical Manifestations

In addition to implementing a treatment regimen properly, the client and family may need to learn ways to control the chronic condition's influence on their lives. Some clients must plan ahead so that needed items will be available. For example, they may need to buy adequate supplies before leaving on a trip. The client may need to hand-carry supplies when traveling or may need adaptive

equipment. Clients with arthritis, for example, may benefit from using fastening tape (Velcro) closures rather than zippers or buttons.

Restructuring Time

Assess the client's time requirements. A client who is unemployed because of a chronic condition may have too much free time; a client who spends hours each day undergoing a medical regimen may have little time to enjoy life.

Focus the teaching plan on helping the client maintain enough free time to enjoy a high-quality life. Examine areas of the client's life that include wasted time. Encourage a hobby or a support group, which may help to build a support system and to cultivate interests. Consult a recreational therapist at a local physical rehabilitation center about recreational activities in the home or community.

Adjusting to Changes

The teaching plan can provide invaluable assistance in helping clients cope with the course of a chronic disorder. With some disorders, the course is stable; for others, it is unpredictable. For example, the course of chronic ulcerative colitis usually is stable, whereas that of multiple sclerosis can be erratic.

Inform the client and the family about predictable flare-ups. For example, depression is common 4 to 6 months after a cerebrovascular accident or a myocardial infarction. Educate the client and family ahead of time, so that they can watch for signs of depression and can consult a health care provider if necessary. Support groups exist for many chronic conditions and should be included in the teaching plan along with instruction on how to access a local group.

Promoting Physiologic Adaptation

Physical adaptation to a chronic condition can be improved by a change in medication, dosages, or schedules or diet and activity patterns. Identifying environmental or behavioral factors that trigger manifestations, improve sleep, increase energy levels, or substitute for lost function can increase feelings of wellness. Early detection of complications, knowledge about the condition and its management, and how to substitute and compensate for changes in physical function facilitate physiologic adaptation.

Promoting Psychological Adaptation

Interventions to enhance psychological adaptation during the diagnostic stage include (1) encouraging the client's active involvement in the diagnostic process and treatment decisions, (2) facilitating the client's expressions of feelings, and (3) helping a client to seek appropriate information.

Some clients may perceive hospitalization during the *chronic* stage as a crisis episode; other clients may view hospitalization during this stage as a reprieve from day-to-day hassles and concerns or as a period of hope because new treatments may be available. In the *terminal* stage, one client may fear death whereas another may view death as a preferable alternative to suffering and disability. Personal factors that may contribute to the individual nature of psychological adaptation include hope, commitment, confidence, appraisal of changes, perception of the effectiveness of management, coping strategies, and personal, spiritual, and social resources. Appraisals of change are based on an individual's beliefs, knowledge, skills, previous losses, and threat of loss. Each client's ability to manage loss, the threat of loss, and challenges also differs. Spiritual adaptation can positively affect the mental and physical health of clients during this time of adjustment to the chronic illness. Relaxation, meditation, distraction, social support, spiritual guidance, and cognitive therapies are interventions that may promote psychological adaptation.

Promoting Sociologic Adaptation

Interventions that promote sociologic adaptation include teaching and counseling related to management of the chronic condition in home, work, and recreational environments and assisting the client and family in locating professional and community resources to lower barriers to social integration. Vocational rehabilitation and job skills training may help a client gain employment. Interventions that foster and support role changes include (1) *role-playing* in anticipated situations; (2) imaginative *role-taking,* in which the client imagines how another person would respond to behaviors; and (3) *role-modeling,* in which the individual is introduced to another person who has the same chronic condition and has adapted positively to enforced changes. Role-modeling may help the client gain practical tips about hunting for a job, finding accessible housing, and meeting new friends.

Role clarification is a strategy in which the client is given information about behaviors necessary to play a particular role. Reference group interaction brings together people with similar problems and concerns. These groups are helpful for exchanging ideas for solving problems and relieving feelings of isolation and helplessness.

Encourage clients to normalize their lives and to resume social activities. Some visible deformities can be disguised with clothing, such as scarves, or make-up to reduce self-consciousness. Similarly, clients with dyspnea, by looking in a store window, can disguise the fact that they are stopping to catch their breath. If a condition cannot be disguised, prepare the client to sometimes be the object of rude stares and comments. Encourage the client to educate others. Eventually, the client will learn to ignore the stares and comments.

HEALTH PROMOTION AND ILLNESS PREVENTION INTERVENTIONS

Health promotion and illness prevention interventions are essential for everyone, including people who have chronic conditions. Chronic conditions account for approximately 80% of all medical expenses.[13] Chronic conditions usually cannot be cured, but health promotion and illness prevention interventions can improve the quality of life for those with chronic conditions and have the potential to reduce medical expenses. A health risk appraisal should be done, with risk reduction interventions tailored to each individual's need. A general discussion of health promotion follows. Health promotion for young and middle-aged adults is described in Chapter 2; for older clients, see Chapter 3.

■ MODIFYING BEHAVIORAL HEALTH RISK FACTORS

Nutrition and exercise are addressed together because they work synergistically to promote high-level wellness. Sedentary living and the lack of sound nutrition contribute to major risk factors, such as hypercholesterolemia, obesity, and muscular atrophy. When people begin to modify one of these two areas, the other area often receives attention at the same time.

Nutrition

Nutrition has moved into the forefront as a prominent component of health promotion and disease prevention. A correlation exists between what we eat and how we feel; the potential for development of disease is also correlated with nutritional status and habits. Cardiovascular disease, cancer, and osteoporosis are three common afflictions that are directly related to nutrition to some degree. Scores of other conditions related to poor nutrition may be less crippling, but they clearly affect how we feel (e.g., dental caries, constipation, and acne). The U.S. Department of Agriculture (USDA) has revised its dietary recommendations and has created the "food pyramid" (see Chapter 2), which includes food groupings and provides suggested servings from each group.

NUTRITIONAL DEFICITS
Deficits in nutritional intake can result in stunted growth, reduced metabolic function, delayed or premature cessation of reproductive function, and increased risk for less serious illnesses. Mechanisms of homeostasis protect the body from temporary deficits, but chronic nutritional deprivation creates a susceptible host for the diseases of malnutrition. Three classic deficiency diseases are scurvy (vitamin C deficiency), beriberi (thiamin deficiency), and pellagra (niacin deficiency). Malnutrition also increases susceptibility to infection (see Chapter 17) and decreases wound-healing ability (see Chapter 16).

NUTRITIONAL EXCESSES
Overeating or eating too many of the wrong foods can also cause illness and disease. Many people, especially those in the lowest socioeconomic group, eat foods that are high in fat, sugar, protein, simple carbohydrates, caffeine, and alcohol. Over time, diseases of overconsumption or malconsumption appear. Obesity, atherosclerosis, alcoholism, constipation, hypertension, cardiorespiratory disorders, and some cancers are, to some extent, thought to be related to nutritional imbalance (see Chapter 2).

BALANCED NUTRITION
Healthy nutrition is defined as a balance of nutrients, fiber, fluids, vitamins, and minerals. Whenever possible, foods should be free of chemicals, additives, preserva-

tives, and toxins. Clients should eat fresh foods, fruits, vegetables, legumes, and lean meats and should avoid high-fat, overprocessed, and fried foods. The U.S. government recommends a diet with less fat and more complex carbohydrates (see Chapter 2). Clients can use a food diary (see Chapter 28) to assess their food intake.

Exercise

Until recently, physical fitness was directed primarily toward building muscle groups for the purpose of preparing for competition. A new way of thinking about fitness is depicted in Chapter 2. Exercise, like nutrition, should be balanced and performed on a regular basis; it cannot be effective if it is performed sporadically. Exercise tones and strengthens internal organs and the circulatory, respiratory, and musculoskeletal systems. It is more than calisthenics. The components of fitness are multiple, and all aspects should be part of a routine.

Exercise does not reverse pathophysiologic changes but is believed to condition muscles to work more efficiently and to use less oxygen. Exercise also stimulates the production of endorphins (which promote the feelings of well-being), increases production of high-density lipoproteins (HDLs), assists in weight control, decreases risk of some cancers, and increases activity tolerance.

A physical exercise program coupled with a balanced nutritional diet is the most effective way to actualize promotion of physical health. Eating and exercising wisely develop strength and endurance, a more youthful appearance, increased vitality, straight posture, and general physical stamina (see Chapters 2 and 3).

Empowerment

Empowerment involves helping clients assume control and mastery over all aspects of their lives. This involves health care as well as social and political environments. Accept clients as the experts in their own experience and definition of health. At the basic level, empowerment means a transfer of skills, resources, access, and language, so that the client with a chronic condition can be as independent as possible. Empowerment can occur only in a supportive environment. Learn how to establish and maintain an empowering environment in which the client sees the potential and value in seizing power and being independent.

In the United States, changing social beliefs about individual rights and normality have influenced state and federal laws. This legislation has contributed to a decrease in attitudinal and architectural barriers to social integration as well as to increased availability of health care, housing, employment, recreation, and transportation for ill people. Nurses can encourage clients to be politically active and can also be active themselves in advocating for the health care rights of those with chronic conditions.

Developing Human Potential

Current definitions of health refer to the achievement of maximum potential, or *self-actualization* (see Table 1–3).

In the domain of health promotion, people develop and maintain life potentials, becoming the best and healthiest that they can. The more time and energy devoted to developing strengths, the less likely problems are to develop. The physical potentials of nutrition and exercise have been discussed earlier.

Figure 1–3 represents the circle of human potentials, each of which needs to be developed to maximize health. Each physical body is unique. Through the senses of sight, hearing, touch, taste, and smell, we gather experience of the world. When the body is nurtured, it increases in strength, vitality, energy, sexuality, and the capacity to communicate and connect with other potentials.

Our picture of the world is created uniquely from mental stimuli. It is through logical processes that we learn to fully understand, enjoy, and appreciate many of life's greatest pleasures. Growth is possible when we are receptive to information, suggestions, and help.

Emotions are feelings, the inner and outer responses to the events encountered in life. One of the greatest challenges is to acknowledge, own, express, and understand one's emotions. Increasing attention to the development and balancing of this potential allows spontaneity and positive zest for living to emerge.

Spirit comes from one's roots and inner core of being. It is related to the universal need to understand the human experience of life on Earth. Where did we come from? Where are we going? What is our purpose? Why do good and evil exist? What occurs after death? Who or what put this life form together? Development of the spiritual potential allows for the transcendence of the experience of oneness, peace, harmony, and connection with the universe.

We cannot live purposeful lives without meaningful relationships. We may not share a house with anyone, but many of us live in neighborhoods and all of us are part

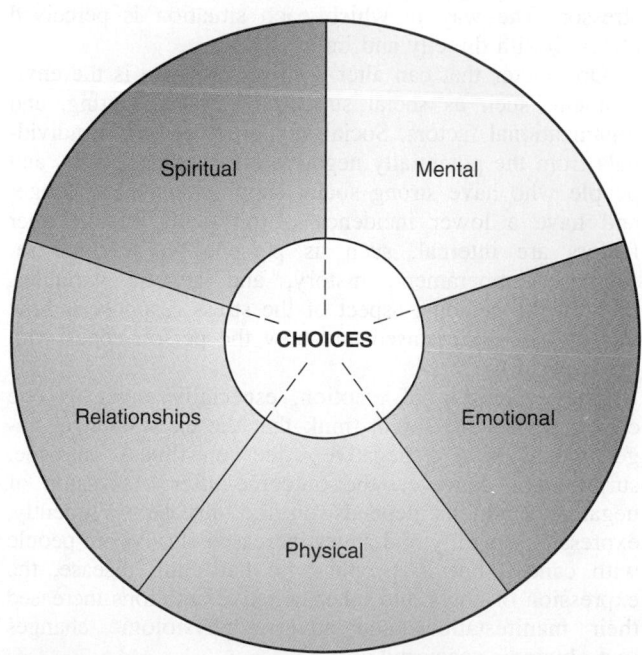

FIGURE 1–3 The circle of human potentials.

of communities, cities, and states. Our relationships extend to our nation and to the whole of planet Earth. The challenge in relationships is to extend ourselves and to learn how to exchange feelings of honesty, trust, intimacy, compassion, openness, and harmony. When we share our feelings and experiences, true interchange occurs. It is through our attitude and orientation that we affect the outcome of all of our encounters.

People have enormous capacity for making choices either consciously or unconsciously. Health and balance occur when we use the skill of effective choice-making. Each of us is responsible for assessing our values and desires. No one else can make decisions for us.

Milio[26] contends that the focus on choice is paramount in shaping the overall health for the person as well as for the society as a whole. Our range of choices is affected by personal resources, which include awareness, knowledge, our own beliefs, and our family's beliefs. Time, money, support of family and friends, and the urgency of other priorities influence what choices are made. Milio notes that "most human beings, professional or nonprofessional, provider or consumer, make the easiest choices available to them most of the time."[26] Try to recognize this tendency when working with clients. Lifestyle behavioral patterns are not isolated choices unrelated to social, personal, or economic circumstances.

Stress Management

All of us have experienced stress, but each of us has different perceptions and thoughts about it. What are your perceptions? Think of a recent stressful event at home or at work that involved you and someone else. How did you react? How did the other person react? Was there a different reaction to the same event? Stress is an individual matter. No two people respond in completely the same manner. In a given situation, one person may perceive a challenge whereas the other perceives a serious stressor. The way in which each situation is perceived affects health directly and indirectly.

One factor that can alter a stress response is the environment, such as social supports, physical setting, and organizational factors. Social supports can buffer individuals from the potentially negative effects of stressors, and people who have strong social supports may live longer and have a lower incidence of physical illness. Other factors are internal, such as personality, personal resources, temperament, history, and genetic variables. (Within the personal aspect of the stress response is how the stressor is appraised and how the person copes with the stressor.)

The expression of emotion, especially anger, is one coping style. One might think that the expression of anger would have a negative effect on illness outcome; surprisingly, however, the outcome after expression of negative emotions depends on the disease. Frequently, expressing hostility and anger increased survival in people with cancer, but in people who had lung disease, the expression of anger and other negative emotions increased their manifestations and adverse physiologic changes (e.g., hypoxia) occurred.

SOCIAL SUPPORT

Scientists have long noted a link between social relationships and health. Socially isolated people are less healthy, psychologically and physically, and are more likely to die than people who are more socially integrated; however, the actual cause and effect are not clear. Are unhealthy people less likely to have and maintain social relationships, or does the lack of social relationships cause people to become ill and die? Do people in a social network provide a basis of health?

As we learn more about chronic illnesses, the role of social support seems even stronger. Physiologic studies have shown a link between the amygdala and the hypothalamus in the brain and positive social relationships. Social contact decreases levels of hormones such as cortisol, epinephrine, and norepinephrine. From a psychological standpoint, social relationships provide a sense of meaning or coherence that promotes a healthy lifestyle. Social support may help a client adhere to medical treatment and seek of medical care. Marriage, a widely studied area of social support, may be simultaneously a source of stress and support, but regardless of the quality of the interaction, marriage is a form of support. Frequently, a quick deterioration in the health of a survivor is seen after the death of a spouse. Health care providers must make use of a client's social support network, including the network in the treatment regimen and assessing the impact of illness on the partner.

SELF-HELP GROUPS

Self-help groups are growing in industrialized nations. It is estimated that there are at least 500,000 to 750,000 self-help groups in the United States, with at least 10 to 15 million members. Some groups are approved by various organizations. Reach for Recovery, an organization for women who have had a mastectomy, is approved by the American Cancer Society. Informal groups also exist, such as people caring for older, infirm parents in their homes, who meet to discuss common problems. Self-help groups are recognized and accepted as a form of assistance to meet people's needs. The largest groups help people with mental illnesses, and the second largest groups help people with AIDS.

There are two types of self-help groups. One is the Twelve-Step program, of which Alcoholics Anonymous is the prototype. The other is a group whose members share common experiences. Characteristics of both types of groups include (1) helping with cognitive restructuring of an event or experience, (2) instructing in adaptive skills, and (3) fostering emotional support, personal disclosure, socialization, taking actions together, empowerment, self-reliance, and self-esteem.

DEVELOPING COPING SKILLS

Many practical methods exist to cope with stress. Planning is one effective way to reduce adverse effects. For example, we prepare for predictable life changes, such as marriage, job change, or retirement. We plan by establishing goals. Through planning, we develop a belief system that allows us to dictate our life and our experience. Setting goals facilitates this belief system because it serves as a reminder that we have the power to create new experiences in our lives. Goals should include areas such as meaning and purpose, fun and play, exercise, nutrition, work, and relaxation.

The most widely practiced and possibly the most effective exercise for immediate stress reduction is to evoke the relaxation response:

1. When first learning to do this, remove yourself from the source of stress, assume a relaxed posture, and begin taking deep breaths through your nose.
2. Consciously and progressively relax all of your muscles.
3. Begin thinking of your strengths and imagining a successful outcome.
4. Realize that, in the great scheme of things, this event, whatever its nature, is only a minor event. Evoking the relaxation response induces a decrease in sympathetic nervous system activity and produces an altered, quieted state of consciousness.
5. As you begin to appreciate the effects of the simple progressive relaxation technique, you may want to explore and develop more long-term stress management techniques, such as biofeedback training, yoga, *Tai Chi,* meditation, and guided imagery.

Mind-Body Views and Alternative Therapies

Various mind-body therapies have been introduced to Western medicine. Biofeedback, autogenic training, therapeutic touch, guided imagery, and focused thought are examples. Mind-body therapies can influence the immune system, help manage pain, and reduce stress and anxiety. An example of the positive influences of a mind-body therapy is teaching a client to slow down, simplify, and fully relax, so that the client might experience enhanced life satisfaction and beneficial immune system changes.

Alternative medicine (complementary medicine) refers to a wide range of treatments that include mind-body therapies, homeopathy, and herbal medicine. In 1992, Congress established the Office of Alternative Medicine within the National Institutes of Health to evaluate alternative medicine therapies. Table 1–6 lists seven fields of alternative and complementary medicine.

About 40% of Americans surveyed in 1997 reported using some form of alternative health care. There is a growing demand for these therapies, but more needs to be

---

TABLE 1–6   CATEGORIES OF COMPLEMENTARY AND ALTERNATIVE MEDICINE

1. *Alternative systems of medical practice.* Seventy per cent to 90% of world health care ranges from self-care based on folk principles to organized health care that is based on an alternative tradition or practice
   a. *Popular* (informal practices in the home, such as using herbal teas for a cold)
   b. *Community-based* (care that reflects the natural environment, health needs, and health beliefs of those who use it, such as nonprofessional practices occurring in many urban and rural communities)
   c. *Professionalized* (a health care delivery system based on theories of health and disease, including traditional oriental medicine, acupuncture, Ayurvedic medicine, homeopathy, anthroposophically extended medicine, naturopathy, and environmental medicine)
2. *Mind-body interventions.* Therapies that make use of the interconnectedness of the mind and body and of the power of each to affect the other
   a. Psychotherapy
   b. Meditation
   c. Hypnotherapy
   d. Yoga
   e. Prayer and mental efforts
   f. Support groups
   g. Guided imagery and relaxation
   h. Dance, music, and art therapy
   i. Biofeedback
   j. Humor
3. *Manual healing methods.* Therapy that includes touch and manipulation of soft tissues or realignment of body parts to correct a dysfunction that affects the function of other body parts
   a. Osteopathic medicine
   b. Massage and other physical healing methods
   c. Chiropractic
   d. Biofield therapeutics (laying on of hands)
   e. Acupuncture
   f. Reflexology
   g. Rolfing
4. *Bioelectromagnetic applications.* Based on the ways living organisms interact with electromagnetic fields
   a. *Nonthermal non-ionizing radiation* (includes bone repair, nerve stimulation, wound healing, osteoarthritis treatment, electroacupuncture, tissue regeneration, and immune system stimulation)
   b. *Thermal non-ionizing radiation* (includes radiofrequency [RF], hyperthermia, laser and RF surgery, RF diathermy)
5. *Herbal medicine.* The use of plants and plant products as remedies, often self-administered and purchased through herbalists, health food stores, and certain practitioners. In the United States, these products are marketed as food supplements without specific health claims because of the lack of Food and Drug Administration (FDA) approval related to insufficient standards for safety and efficacy of herbal remedies
6. *Pharmacologic and biologic treatments.* The use of drugs, vaccines, and other agents (including antioxidants, oxidizing agents, chelation treatments, cell treatment, and metabolic therapy) not yet accepted by conventional medicine; clinical safety and effectiveness trials to meet FDA approval have not been fully investigated because of lack of sponsors and funding
7. *Diet, nutrition, and lifestyle changes.* Therapy that uses foods to affect biochemical and physiologic processes in the body. This field includes orthomolecular medicine (high-dose vitamins, a Macrobiotic diet, nutritional supplements, and dietary and other lifestyle changes in the treatment of chronic diseases such as AIDS; bronchial asthma; cancer; cardiovascular diseases, heart attacks, and stroke; lymphedema; and mental and neurologic disorders)

Modified from U.S. Office of Alternative Medicine. (1994). *Alternative medicine: Expanding medical horizons* (pp. 3–206). Washington, DC: National Institutes of Health.
AIDS, acquired immunodeficiency syndrome.

known about their effectiveness. Recently, there has been a call for higher standards in the evaluation of alternative medicine, especially in regard to herbal medicine.[3] Herbs are considered to be dietary supplements that are exempt from U.S. Food and Drug Administration (FDA) guidelines for prescribed medications. Some authorities claim that alternative therapies should be subjected to the same scientific testing as conventional treatments.[3]

The Office of Alternative Medicine recently reviewed the use of acupuncture for treatment of chronic conditions. Acupuncture was found to be effective for addictions and psychiatric disorders; allergy and immunology; general pain; headaches; and nausea, vomiting, and postoperative problems.[28] Another effective therapy was the integration of behavioral and relaxation approaches into the treatment of chronic pain and insomnia (see also Chapters 21 and 23).[28]

■ MODIFYING ENVIRONMENTAL HEALTH RISK FACTORS

Environment is one of the four primary determinants of health. It is not enough to think solely in terms of self or of our immediate surroundings when we think of health promotion. We are not just members of families, communities, states, or regions; we are intertwined with one another and linked as a global family. What affects one of us now has a ripple effect and affects us all. Because of the population explosion and congested urban living conditions, it is easy to affect another person's living environment. For example, it is possible to pollute the air by driving a car with a defective exhaust pipe, to impinge on auditory air space by playing loud music, or to create an eyesore by littering. Collectively, we can pollute the environment to such a great degree that life itself is threatened.

Health promotion, because it addresses the whole self and the whole human family, must also address protection of the environment. It is not within the scope of this chapter to delineate ways to do this; its purpose is to stimulate an awareness that each of us can play a role in cleaning, maintaining, and striving to improve environmental conditions to the best of our ability.

CONCLUSIONS

Health promotion is a key watch phrase for the 21st century. Nurses are encouraged to develop a consciousness that includes attention to the social, political, and economic aspects of the environment. Once we recognize that establishing health-promoting behaviors can alter the presence or absence of good health, specific interventions must be delineated and disseminated to the subsets of the population that can benefit. Clients with chronic conditions are a subset of the population that has potential to achieve improvements in quality of life and health care savings with interventions of health promotion and illness prevention. Appraisal of health risk can reveal which risk reduction interventions would be helpful. Models of health promotion serve as a guide for motivating clients to make health behavioral changes. A broad understanding of chronic conditions will widen the nurse's role and will assist the nurse in providing holistic nursing care to facilitate client and family adaptation and ameliorate the course of a chronic condition.

BIBLIOGRAPHY

1. Agency for Health Care Policy and Research. (1993). *Clinical practice guideline No. 5: Depression in primary care.* Rockville, MD: U.S. Department of Health and Human Services.
2. American Nurses' Association. (1995). *Nursing's social policy statement.* Washington, DC: Author.
3. Angell, M., & Kassirer, J. (1998). Alternative medicine: The risks of untested and unregulated remedies. *New England Journal of Medicine, 339*(12), 839–841.
4. Bandura, A. (1986). *Social foundations of thought and action: A social cognitive theory* (p. 22). Englewood Cliffs, NJ: Prentice-Hall.
5. Cassileth, B. R. (1998). *The alternative medicine handbook: The complete reference guide to alternative and complementary therapies.* New York: W. W. Norton.
6. Clark, C. (1996). *Wellness practitioner: Concepts, research, and strategies* (2nd ed.). New York: Springer.
7. Dossey, B. (1998). Holistic modalities and healing moments. *American Journal of Nursing, 98*(6), 44–47.
8. Downie, R., Tannahill, C., & Tannahill, A. (1996). *Health promotion models and values* (2nd ed.). New York: Oxford University Press.
9. Duke, J. A. (1997). *The green pharmacy.* Emmaus, PA: Rodale Press.
10. Dunn, H. (1961). *High-level wellness.* Arlington, VA: R. W. Beatty.
11. Eakes, G., Burke, M., & Hainsworth, M. (1998). Middle-range of chronic sorrow. *Image: Journal of Nursing Scholarship, 30,* 179–184.
12. Edelman, C., & Mandle, C. (Eds.). (1997). *Health promotion throughout the life span* (4th ed.). St. Louis: Mosby–Year Book.
13. Fox, P., & Fama, T. (1996). *Managed care and chronic illness: Challenges and opportunities.* Gaithersburg, MD: Aspen.
14. Gochman, D. (Ed.). (1997). *Handbook of health behavior research: I: Personal and social determinants.* New York: Plenum Press.
15. Gorin, S., & Arnold, J. (1998). *Health promotion handbook.* St. Louis: Mosby–Year Book.
16. Hoffman, C., Rice, D., & Sung, H. (1996). Persons with chronic conditions: Their prevalence and costs. *Journal of the American Medical Association, 276,* 1473–1479.
17. Hover-Kramer, D. (1996). *Healing touch: A resource for health care professionals.* Albany, NY: Delmar.
18. Institute for Health and Aging, University of California–San Francisco. (1996). *Chronic care in America: A 21st century challenge.* Princeton, NJ: The Robert Wood Johnson Foundation.
19. Kobasa, S., Maddi, S., & Zola, M. (1983). Type A and hardiness. *Journal of Behavioral Medicine, 6,* 41–51.
20. Labonte, R. (1994). Health promotion and empowerment: Reflections on professional practice. *Health Education Quarterly, 21*(2), 253–268.
21. Lalonde, M. (1974). *A new perspective on the health of Canadians.* Ottawa: Government of Canada.
22. Lazarus, R., & Folkman, S. (1984). *Stress, appraisal, and coping.* New York: Springer.
23. Leavell, H., & Clark, E. (1965). *Preventative medicine for the doctor in his community: An epidemiologic approach.* New York: McGraw-Hill.
23a. Leininger, M. (1978). *Transcultural nursing: Concepts, theories and practices.* New York: John Wiley and Sons.
24. Lilienfeld, A. (1976). *Foundations of epidemiology.* New York: Oxford University Press.
25. Micozzi, M. S. (Ed.). (1996). *Fundamentals of complementary and alternative medicine.* New York: Churchill Livingstone.
26. Milio, N. (1976). A framework for prevention: Changing health damaging to health-generating life patterns. *American Journal of Public Health, 66,* 435–439.
27. Morse, J., & Doberneck, B. (1995). The concept of hope. *Image, 27,* 227–286.
28. National Institutes of Health, Office of Alternative Medicine. Grant award and research data. Bethesda, MD: Office of Alternative Medicine. Available: *http://altmed.od.nih.gov.*
29. Newman, M. (1987). Health conceptualizations: Nursing emergency paradigm: The diagnosis of pattern. In McLean (Ed.), *Class of*

nursing diagnosis. St. Louis: Proceedings of the Seventh Conference.

30. Parsons, T. (1951). *The social system*. New York: Free Press.
31. Pender, N. (1996). *Health promotion in nursing practice* (3rd ed.). Stamford, CT: Appleton & Lange.
32. Portnoy, B., et al. (1989). Application of diffusion theory to health promotion research. *Family Community Health, 12,* 63–71.
33. Prochaska, J., Redding, C, & Evers, K. (1996). The Transtheoretical Model and stages of change. In K. Glanz, F. Lewis, & B. Rimer (Eds.), *Health behavior and health education: Theory, research, and practice* (2nd ed., pp. 60–84). San Francisco: Jossey-Bass.
34. Randall, J., & Lazar, J. (1997). Complementary and alternative therapies in primary care. *Primary Care: Clinics in Office Practice, 24*(4).
35. Roy, C., & Andrews, H. (1998). *The Roy adaptation model* (2nd ed.). Englewood Cliffs, NJ: Prentice-Hall.
36. Strecher, V., & Rosenstock, I. (1996). The Health Belief Model. In K. Glanz, F. Lewis, & B. Rimer (Eds.), *Health behavior and health education: Theory, research, and practice* (2nd ed., pp. 41–59). San Francisco: Jossey-Bass.
37. Turner, J. (1986). World Health Organization: Charter for health promotion. *Lancet, 2,* 1407.
38. U.S. Department of Health and Human Services. (1979). *Healthy people: The Surgeon General's report on health promotion and disease prevention.* Washington, DC: U.S. Government Printing Office.
39. U.S. Department of Health and Human Services. (1991). *Healthy people 2000: National health promotion and disease prevention objectives.* (PHS No. 91-50213.) Washington, DC: U.S. Government Printing Office.
40. U.S. Department of Health and Human Services. (1996). *Physical activity and health: A report of the Surgeon General.* Atlanta: National Center for Chronic Disease Prevention and Health Promotion.
41. U.S. Department of Health and Human Services. (1997). *Healthy people 2000: Review 1997.* (DHHS No. 98-1256.) Hyattsville, MD: U.S. Government Printing Office.
42. U.S. Office of Alternative Medicine. (1994). *Alternative medicine: Expanding medical horizons.* Washington, DC: National Institutes of Health.
43. Wannamethee, S., & Shaper, A. (1999). Type of alcoholic drink and risk of major coronary heart disease events and all-cause mortality. *American Journal of Public Health, 89,* 685–690.
44. World Health Organization. (1947). Constitution of the World Health Organization. *Chronicle of the World Health Organization, 1*(1–2), 29–43.

CHAPTER

2

Health Promotion in Young and Middle-Aged Adults

Kathryn Fiandt

It is essential that nurses be knowledgeable regarding health promotion and disease prevention. When providing holistic care, think beyond current health problems to the client's general well-being and future risk for illness or injury. This can be particularly important when you are working with young and middle-aged adults who rarely visit health care providers except for family planning, child-bearing needs, acute illness, or injury episodes. It is not uncommon for young and middle-aged adults to go 10 years between health care visits. Because of the rarity of contacts with this population, take every opportunity to address health risks and risk management in these age groups.

HEALTH RISKS

The leading causes of death in young adults are motor vehicle and other unintentional injuries, homicide, suicide, malignant neoplasms, and heart disease. In middle-aged adults, the risk of premature death from cancer or heart disease increases.[47] In both age groups, death from human immunodeficiency virus (HIV) infection has increased; of the more than 1 million people with acquired immunodeficiency syndrome (AIDS) in the United States, the majority are 20 to 40 years old.[12]

Healthy People 2000, the federal population-based health objectives (1995 revisions), identified health-related goals that apply to young and middle-aged adults (Table 2–1). Nurses can assist in achieving these goals by assessing the client's lifestyle and risk status and by intervening to modify poor habits and to reduce risk. This chapter describes the components of a healthy lifestyle, including health promotion (primary prevention), risk assessment, and risk management, specifically disease prevention (*primary* prevention) and early detection (*secondary* prevention) in the young and middle-aged populations.

HEALTH PROMOTION

Health promotion involves activities that promote general well-being. These activities are categorized as patterns of healthy eating, healthy activity, and effective coping with stress. The concept of health promotion is described in Chapter 1. The following topics describe specific health promotion activities.

■ HEALTHY EATING

Healthy eating is a cornerstone of a healthy lifestyle. The U.S. Department of Agriculture (USDA) and the U.S. Department of Health and Human Services (USDHHS) developed the *Dietary Guidelines for Americans* (Table 2–2). Be familiar with these guidelines as the foundation for healthy eating. A useful tool for explaining these guidelines to clients is the *Food Guide Pyramid,* a pictorial representation of the principles described in the dietary guidelines (Fig. 2–1).

To use the guidelines effectively for achieving healthy eating patterns, clients must be able to identify a serving size and to read nutrition labels. The food labeling system mandated by the U.S. Food and Drug Administration (FDA) is designed to assist consumers in making informed decisions regarding the foods they purchase. The Nutrition Facts label (Fig. 2–2) is a tool to identify both serving size and the nutritional components of the food item.

Nurses who are knowledgeable regarding the Dietary Guidelines for Americans, the Food Guide Pyramid, and the Nutrition Facts label can assist clients to adopt healthy eating patterns. Young and middle-aged adults are often in excellent health but may have poor eating patterns that lay the foundation for future health problems. In addition, these clients may already have health problems as a result of poor eating patterns. Health patterns of concern include obesity, cancer risk, osteoporosis, and cardiovascular disease. Obesity and cancer risk are discussed here. Chapter 26 covers osteoporosis; Chapters 55 and 58 cover heart disease; and Chapter 52 covers hypertension.

Obesity

Although the *Healthy People 2000* goals include reducing the number of overweight Americans to 20%, the per-

TABLE 2–1	*HEALTHY PEOPLE 2000* GOALS FOR YOUNG AND MIDDLE-AGED ADULTS

1. Decrease motor vehicle deaths to no more than 14.2/100,000
2. Reduce motor vehicle deaths caused by alcohol to no more than 5.5/100,000
3. Reduce prevalence of overweight to no more than 20%
4. Reduce coronary heart disease deaths to no more than 100/100,000
5. Reduce cancer deaths to no more than 130/100,000
6. Reduce diabetes to a prevalence of 25/1,000
7. Confine the prevalence of HIV infection to no more than 400/100,000
8. Reduce the incidence of vaccine-preventable disease
9. Reduce suicide deaths to no more than 10.5/100,000
10. Increase to 30% the proportion of people who exercise regularly
11. Reduce cigarette smoking to no more than 15% of people 18+ years old
12. Reduce alcohol consumption to an annual average of no more than 2 gallons/person
13. Reduce unplanned pregnancies to no more than 30% of all pregnancies
14. Increase to at least 20% the proportion of people who seek help in coping with personal and emotional problems
15. Increase the number of people who meet U.S. Preventive Services Task Force guidelines for screening, vaccinations, and counseling services
16. Reduce deaths caused by unintentional injuries to 29.3/100,000

HIV, human immunodeficiency virus.
Modified from U.S. Department of Health and Human Services. (1996). *Healthy People 2000: Midcourse review and 1995 revisions.* Sudbury, MA: Jones & Bartlett.

TABLE 2–2	DIETARY GUIDELINES FOR AMERICANS

1. Eat a variety of foods
2. Maintain a healthy weight
3. Choose a diet low in fat, saturated fat, and cholesterol:
   a. 30% or less of calories from fat
   b. Less than 10% of calories from saturated fat
4. Choose a diet with plenty of vegetables, fruit, and grain products:
   a. 3 or more daily servings of various vegetables
   b. 2 or more daily servings of fruit
   c. 6 or more servings of grain products per day
5. Use sugar only in moderation
6. Use salt and sodium only in moderation
7. If you drink alcohol, do so in moderation:
   a. 1 drink per day for women
   b. 2 drinks per day for men

Modified from U.S. Department of Health and Human Services. (1994). *Clinician's handbook of preventive services.* Washington, DC: U.S. Government Printing Office.

centage of overweight people has actually increased from 26% (1976–1980 data) to 34% (1988–1991 data).[45] Obesity poses serious health risks. Obese people have an increased risk for heart disease, hypertension, type 2 diabetes, degenerative joint disease, sleep apnea, and gallbladder disease. When obesity is associated with a high-fat diet, the risk of breast, colon, rectum, and prostate cancer increases. Take every opportunity to measure height and weight, and calculate body mass index (BMI) (see Chapter 28). Obesity is defined as a BMI of 30 or greater. Advise clients when they fall outside the range of healthy weight.

FIGURE 2–1 The USDA Food Guide Pyramid. (From U.S. Department of Agriculture and U.S. Department of Health and Human Services, Washington, DC.)

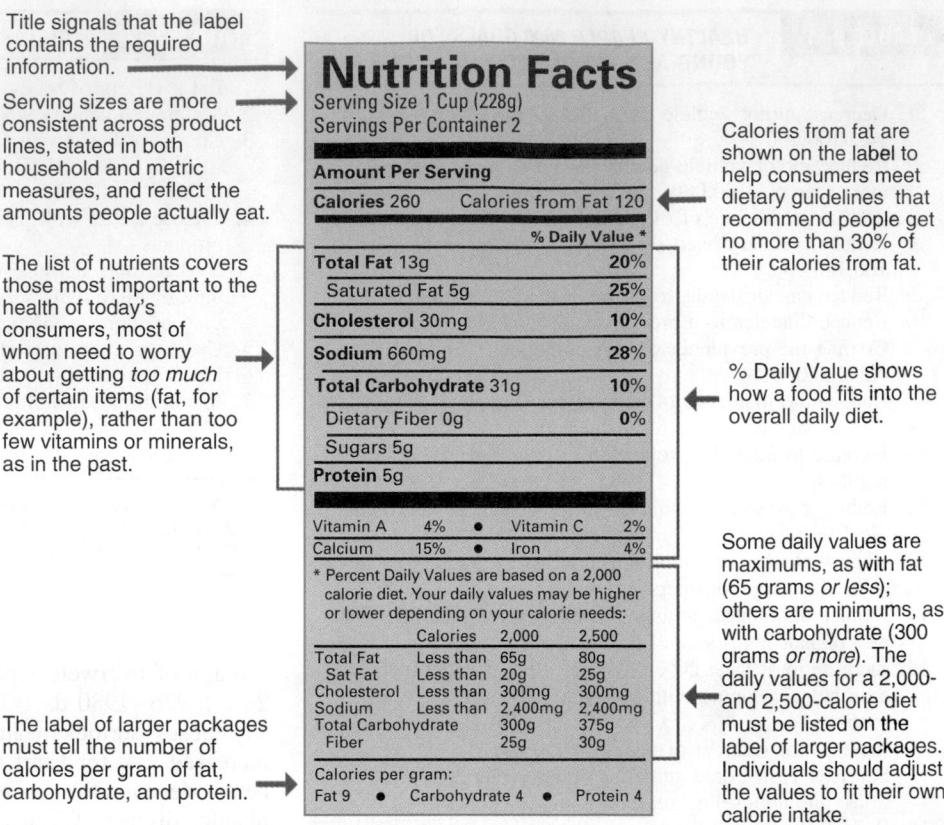

Title signals that the label contains the required information.

Serving sizes are more consistent across product lines, stated in both household and metric measures, and reflect the amounts people actually eat.

The list of nutrients covers those most important to the health of today's consumers, most of whom need to worry about getting *too much* of certain items (fat, for example), rather than too few vitamins or minerals, as in the past.

Calories from fat are shown on the label to help consumers meet dietary guidelines that recommend people get no more than 30% of their calories from fat.

% Daily Value shows how a food fits into the overall daily diet.

Some daily values are maximums, as with fat (65 grams *or less*); others are minimums, as with carbohydrate (300 grams *or more*). The daily values for a 2,000- and 2,500-calorie diet must be listed on the label of larger packages. Individuals should adjust the values to fit their own calorie intake.

FIGURE 2–2 Guide to using a food label. (Modified from U.S. Food and Drug Administration. [December 10, 1992]. The new food label. *FDA Backgrounder,* 1–9.)

The label of larger packages must tell the number of calories per gram of fat, carbohydrate, and protein.

This label is only a sample.

MANAGEMENT OF THE OBESE CLIENT

The basic therapeutic approach to obesity is to modify eating patterns through improving the *quality* (versus *quantity*) of foods eaten. The focus is on making positive changes in eating patterns. Specific modifications include (1) decreasing portion size, (2) modifying the composition of the diet through substitution and modification of foods consumed, and (3) changing eating behaviors. The second therapeutic component of obesity management is improving activity patterns (see later).

ASSESSMENT. Before recommending diet modifications, assess the client's current eating patterns. Simple dietary assessment tools include a 24-hour diet recall and use of a 3-day dietary log in which the client records all food and drink for 3 days, one of which should be a weekend day. The 24-hour diet recall is ideal for obtaining information at the time of the nurse-client encounter. The 3-day dietary log includes not only what food was eaten but when, why, and how the client ate. This tool assists both the nurse and the client in recognizing eating patterns and problematic eating behavior. Chapter 28 discusses nutritional assessment.

INTERVENTION. Once eating patterns have been assessed, collaboratively develop a list of problems and a mutually agreed-on, realistic plan for addressing these problems with the client. Focus interventions on changing foods eaten through substitution (e.g., carrots for candy), increasing certain foods (e.g., fruits and vegetables), or decreasing other foods (e.g., fats). Interventions can also include modifying the eating circumstances, for example, adding a breakfast meal, not eating after the evening

meal, setting the eating utensil down between bites, and eating only at the table.

Eating behavior has a strong emotional component. Poor eating patterns are used to cope with emotional discomfort such as depression or anger. Understanding circumstances under which the client eats helps to identify interventions specifically designed to address these problems. For example, if the client recognizes that anger or fatigue leads to eating, a more appropriate coping behavior, such as taking a walk around the block, may be identified.

Although weight loss can greatly affect a client's health and well-being, it can also seem to be a hopeless task, especially for the seriously overweight and for adults with a lifetime of poor eating patterns. Assist the client in setting small achievable goals (see Chapter 1). Reassure the client that a 10% weight loss can have a substantial positive effect on health.[15]

Diet and Management of Risk for Disease

Diets high in fat, even in the absence of obesity, are associated with increased risk of coronary heart disease and cancer of the breast, colon, rectum, and prostate. Cancer risk can be managed by following the Dietary Guidelines for Americans. These recommendations include choosing a diet with less than 30% of calories from fat and with plenty of fruits, vegetables, and grain products. For clients who are at increased risk for coronary heart disease, as determined by borderline or elevated serum cholesterol levels, a cholesterol-lowering diet is recommended by the National Cholesterol Education Panel (NCEP).[30] The NCEP Step I diet includes decreasing dietary cholesterol to less than 300 mg/day and decreasing total dietary calories from saturated fat to between 8% and 10%. Step II includes a reduction of dietary cholesterol to below 200 mg/day and an intake of less than 7% of total daily calories from saturated fat. Referral to a dietitian is recommended for clients needing a Step II cholesterol-lowering diet.

■ HEALTHY ACTIVITY

Another cornerstone of a healthy lifestyle is healthy activity. People who are active throughout life live longer and are healthier than their less active counterparts.[33] However, more than 60% of adults do not achieve the recommended level of regular physical activity and 25% of adults get no activity. Physical inactivity increases with age, and women are more inactive than men.[46] Physical inactivity is a serious, nationwide problem resulting in a significant burden of unnecessary illness and premature death. It is associated with increased risk for coronary heart disease, type 2 diabetes, hypertension, and obesity.

Benefits of physical activity include (1) weight maintenance, (2) lower blood pressure, (3) improved mood, (4) relief from depression, (5) improved sense of well-being, (6) decreased risk of type 2 diabetes, (7) reduced mortality from coronary heart disease, and (8) increased levels of peak bone mass. In people with chronic, disabling conditions, activity improves stamina, muscle strength, and quality of life[17] (see Chapter 1). Given these benefits, take every opportunity to assess clients' activity patterns and work with them to improve activity levels.

MANAGEMENT OF THE INACTIVE CLIENT

Current activity recommendations are that every adult in the United States should accumulate "30 minutes or more of moderate-intensity physical activity on most, preferably, all days of the week."[34] Activity can be accumulated, but it should occur in blocks of at least 8 minutes and should be perceived as moderate or difficult in intensity.[4, 21] Simple walking is an excellent initial activity that requires no special equipment and can be done anywhere. Although this is a minimum standard, important benefits can be obtained through modest amounts of daily physical activity.[34]

Most research indicates that counseling individuals to increase their physical activity is rarely effective in initiating behavioral change. However, a trial of the effect of brief counseling suggests that highly structured and specific programs might, with minimal expense or time, be effective in promoting healthy patterns of physical activity in clients (see Chapter 1).[5]

ASSESSMENT. Intervention to improve activity patterns begins with assessment of the client's current activity pattern. Two effective tools are the 24-hour recall and a 3-day activity log. In the 24-hour recall, help the client identify all forms of activity during that day. Focus on activity that was sustained for at least 8 minutes and perceived as moderate to heavy exertion. Encourage the client to be thorough by giving examples, such as time spent doing housework. Then sum the total number of minutes spent in moderate or heavy activity per day.[4] During assessment, begin developing ideas for new activity opportunities. This information will be useful later for developing an intervention plan.

Benefits outweigh the risks with the current recommendation for moderate physical activity. Before beginning an activity program, however, all clients should be screened for risks that contraindicate unsupervised activity. People with known health problems, especially those involving cardiac risk including hypertension, elevated serum cholesterol, cigarette smoking, diabetes, and a family history of early heart disease, should be evaluated by their health care provider before increasing physical activity levels.[44]

INTERVENTION. Once the activity pattern has been assessed and there are no evident risks requiring further evaluation, work with the client to identify problem areas and develop a plan to increase physical activity. The *Activity Pyramid* is an excellent tool for beginning instruction (Fig. 2–3). Like the Food Guide Pyramid, the Activity Pyramid is a pictorial representation of the principles of healthy activity and can be used during nurse-client encounters to provide basic information.

Another tool for counseling clients regarding physical activity is the Project PACE (Physician-Based Assessment and Counseling for Exercise).[25, 35] Project PACE, a system of materials initially developed for physicians, is designed to assess a client's readiness to modify physical activity, to screen for activity contraindications, and to develop and implement an individualized activity program. Whichever tools are used, the intervention program should include a personalized exercise prescription and a plan for identifying and overcoming probable barriers to implementation and maintenance of the plan (see Chapter 1).

The Exercise Prescription. A written exercise prescription specifies recommended activity. The exercise prescription has four major components:

- *Mode,* or the type of activity engaged in
- *Intensity* with which the activity is performed
- *Duration* of time
- *Frequency*

As noted earlier, the minimum goal for an exercise program is a moderate-intensity (intensity) physical activity performed for a total of at least 30 minutes (duration) most days of the week (frequency). Many activities (Table 2–3) that are a part of most people's daily routine can serve as the mode of a physical activity program, including walking, housework, child care, and gardening.

Intensity is an essential component of an activity. Instruct clients how to assess exertion level. One simple means of measuring perceived exertion is the *talk test;* clients should be able to talk but only a few words at a time when engaged in the activity. If they can carry on a normal conversation they are not working hard enough; if they cannot talk at all, they are working too hard. Another measure of intensity is the *Borg rating* of perceived exertion (Fig. 2–4).

Overcoming Barriers. Research indicates that people who successfully incorporate physical activity into their daily lives are confident in their ability to perform the activity, find it pleasurable, and have social support.[2, 4] Activities should also be convenient and realistic.

Simple strategies can increase the likelihood of success in implementing an activity program. On the basis of the

THE ACTIVITY PYRAMID

EACH WEEK, TRY TO INCREASE YOUR PHYSICAL ACTIVITY USING THIS GUIDE. HERE'S HOW TO START...

IF YOU ARE INACTIVE
(Rarely do activity)
Increase daily activities at the *base* of the Activity Pyramid by
– taking the stairs instead of the elevator
– hiding the TV remote control
– making extra trips around the house or yard
– stretching while standing in line
– walking whenever you can

CUT DOWN ON
WATCHING TV
COMPUTER GAMES
SITTING FOR MORE THAN 30 MINUTES AT A TIME

IF YOU ARE SPORADIC
(Active some of the time, but not regularly)
Become consistent with activity by increasing activity in the *middle* of the pyramid by
– finding activities you enjoy
– planning activities in your day
– setting realistic goals

2-3 TIMES A WEEK

LEISURE ACTIVITIES
GOLF
BOWLING
SOFTBALL
YARDWORK

FLEXIBILITY AND STRENGTH
STRETCHING/YOGA
PUSH-UPS/CURL-UPS
WEIGHT LIFTING

IF YOU ARE CONSISTENT
(Active most of the time, or at least four days each week)
Choose activities from the *whole* pyramid by
– changing your routine if you start to get bored
– exploring new activities

**ABOVE ALL...
HAVE FUN AND GOOD LUCK!**

3-5 TIMES A WEEK

AEROBIC EXERCISE
(20+ MINUTES)
BRISK WALKING
CROSS-COUNTRY SKIING
BICYCLING
SWIMMING

RECREATIONAL
(30+ MINUTES)
SOCCER   HIKING
BASKETBALL   TENNIS
MARTIAL ARTS DANCING

EVERYDAY
(AS MUCH AS POSSIBLE)

WALK THE DOG
TAKE LONGER ROUTES
TAKE THE STAIRS INSTEAD OF THE ELEVATOR

BE CREATIVE IN FINDING A VARIETY OF WAYS TO STAY ACTIVE

WALK TO THE STORE OR THE MAILBOX
WORK IN YOUR GARDEN
PARK YOUR CAR FARTHER AWAY
MAKE EXTRA STEPS IN YOUR DAY

Copyright © 1999 Park Nicollet Medical Foundation

FIGURE 2–3 The activity pyramid. (Copyright © 1999, Park Nicollet *HealthSource* ® Institute for Research and Education.)

assessment of the client's activity level, (1) advise the client to increase time spent in current moderate-intensity activities, (2) help the client identify pleasurable activities to incorporate into the current routine, and (3) encourage the client to identify friends or family members who can serve as a support system and, ideally, who can join in the planned activity.

Activity plans should include a monitoring method, such as a log, and a reward system. Help clients identify potential barriers and assist them in developing a plan to overcome them (Table 2–4). Although the primary goal

of a regular activity plan is to improve physical health, many benefits relate to feelings of well-being. When working with a client to improve activity patterns, use interventions that increase self-efficacy by choosing realistic activities and goals.

TABLE 2–3	EXAMPLES OF MODERATE LEVELS OF ACTIVITY

AROUND THE HOUSE

Washing windows or floors
Washing and waxing the car
Walking and running with children
Climbing stairs
Pushing a stroller
Raking leaves
Shoveling snow
Digging and weeding in the garden

SPORTS AND LEISURE ACTIVITIES

Volleyball or basketball
Bicycling
Social dancing (fast)
Walking (briskly)
Skiing
Swimming

PERCEIVED EXERTION

Category Scale

6	
7	**VERY, VERY LIGHT**
8	
9	**VERY LIGHT**
10	
11	**FAIRLY LIGHT**
12	
13	**SOMEWHAT HARD**
14	
15	**HARD**
16	
17	**VERY HARD**
18	
19	**VERY, VERY HARD**
20	

FIGURE 2–4 The Borg perceived exertion scale. (From Strauss, R.H. [Ed.]. [1991]. *Sports medicine* [2nd ed.]. Philadelphia: W. B. Saunders.)

TABLE 2-4	OVERCOMING BARRIERS TO EXERCISE
Barrier	**Suggested Response**
Exercise is hard work.	Pick an activity that you enjoy and that is easy for you.
I do not have the time.	We are talking about only three 20-minute sessions per week. Could you do without three television shows each week?
I am usually too tired for exercise.	Tell yourself, "This activity will give me more energy." See if it happens.
I hate to fail, so I will not start.	Physical activity is not a test. You will not fail if you choose an activity you like and start off slowly.
I do not have anyone to work out with.	Maybe you have not asked. A neighbor or coworker may be a willing partner, or you can choose an activity that you enjoy doing by yourself.
There is not a convenient place.	Pick an activity you can do at a convenient place. Walk around your neighborhood or do exercises with a television show or a videotape at home.
I am afraid of being injured.	Walking is a safe and excellent exercise. Choose a safe and well-lit area.
The weather is too bad.	There are many activities that you can do in your home, in any weather.
Exercise is boring.	Listening to music during your activity keeps your mind occupied. Walking, biking, or running can take you past lots of interesting things.
I am too overweight.	You can benefit regardless of your weight. Pick an activity that you are comfortable with, such as walking.
I am too old.	It is never too late to start. People of any age, including older people, can benefit from physical exercise.

Modified from Project PACE. (1991). *Physician-based assessment and counseling for exercise.* San Diego, CA: San Diego State University. Project PACE material is available from San Diego State University, Student Health Services, 550 Campanile Dr., San Diego, CA, 92182 (619-594-5949).

One successful strategy for increasing physical activity is to increase social support within the community as well as within the client's social circle. Use every opportunity to support community projects that promote physical activity, such as developing hiking, walking, and biking trails or opening schools for community recreation. If security is a concern, support efforts to organize a community watch unit or to develop a walking club to take advantage of safety in numbers. Occupational health nurses can encourage employers to develop on-site programs to support employee health. Nurses who regularly work with clients to develop activity programs can maintain a comprehensive listing of community resources available to support activity plans. Community nursing organizations can develop a volunteer pool to work with walking clubs in area malls, perform blood pressure screenings, and provide health education classes.

■ STRESS MANAGEMENT

Stress, the body's response to demands, seems to be increasing in today's world. Physical demands for adaptation are compounded by the adaptive responses required by the volume of information and decisions required for existence in today's society. Stress is usually the result of an imbalance between the demands placed on a person and one's ability to adapt. Stress management, the final cornerstone of a healthy lifestyle, is the ability to cope with these adaptive demands effectively.

Dysfunction in one's ability to adapt and manage stress has a negative effect on health[6]:

1. *Behavioral* responses to stress include decreased ability to think clearly and function, increased tobacco and alcohol use, overeating, and disrupted sleep patterns.
2. *Emotional* responses include depression, anger, decreased self-esteem, apathy, and impatience.
3. *Physical* responses to stress can include tight, sore neck and shoulder muscles, increased blood pressure and heart rate, palpitations, chest discomfort, headaches, gastrointestinal upset, and fatigue.

MANAGEMENT OF STRESS

ASSESSMENT. Today it seems that people are always "stressed," often blaming stress for their physical and mental problems. As a result, clients may request help in coping with stress. Assessment of the problem is the first step in intervention. Include a thorough history of the cognitive, emotional, and physical manifestations that lead clients to conclude that they are stressed. Assess the problems or situations that seem to precipitate stress and the behavioral and emotional response (i.e., how clients feel and act when the problem is present). Also evaluate how clients currently cope with the problem (see discussion of coping in Chapters 1 and 20). Help the person recognize ineffective coping and develop a plan to cope effectively with the stress.

INTERVENTION. Stress management has three components: stress resistance, cognitive reappraisal, and effective coping skills.

Stress Resistance. Stress resistance involves decreasing the body's response to stress, healthy eating and activity, and relaxation techniques. Physical activity can be a *positive* stressor; that is, activity requires an adaptive response, and when performed properly, it results in physical changes that counter the normally negative effects of stress. Physical activity improves mental function, decreases depression, and increases physical endurance.

Healthy eating can increase resistance to stress, and unhealthy eating adds to stress. Healthy eating, based on the Dietary Guidelines for Americans, aids stress resistance; however, some foods are associated with effective or ineffective coping. Complex carbohydrates (e.g., breads, beans, grains) provide a sustained source of energy and have a relaxing effect, whereas fruits, vegetables, and protein provide energy and increased physiologic ability to cope. Intake of simple carbohydrates (e.g., sugar) can temporarily increase energy, but this rise is then quickly followed by weakness and lethargy as the blood glucose level drops. Overeating, an ineffective means of coping, can result in decreased energy and lowered self-esteem. The stimulant caffeine induces the fight-or-flight biologic response and can exacerbate the physical damage that results from stress when it is consumed in excess.

Sleep and rest are natural forms of relaxation that are essential for healing and repairing the physiologic consequences to stress. Inadequate rest worsens stress, especially through impaired mental functioning. Chapter 21 discusses promoting positive outcomes in clients with sleep and rest disorders. In addition to sleep and rest, people can practice techniques to facilitate physical and mental relaxation. *Progressive relaxation* is a technique of slowly focusing on each muscle group, tensing the muscles for 5 to 7 seconds, and then relaxing them. This process promotes learning how to relax the entire body and particularly benefits people with muscle tension or spasm, insomnia, and neck or back pain. Many forms of relaxation involve *breathing techniques,* such as breath awareness, deep breathing, and the purifying breath.[9]

Meditation, once considered an alternative practice, is an established form of relaxation therapy. Research has shown that physiologic changes, such as lowering blood pressure and decreasing heart disease risk, occur as a result of meditation. There are several active or passive forms of meditation, including focusing on breath awareness or a *mantra,* meditative movement such as *yoga* or *Tai Chi,* mindfulness, and prayer.

Cognitive Reappraisal. The goal of cognitive reappraisals or restructuring is to change the perception or interpretation of events as stressors. Cognitive reappraisal is based on the assumption that a major factor in stress is the individual's perception of the event or experience as a stressor.[26] Three common techniques are presented.

Thought stopping is an ideal intervention for "worriers" (i.e., people who obsessively maintain ongoing inner dialogues of "what if". . . or "I can't"). Clients identify the obsessive thought and allow the self to imagine a situation involving the thought. As the obsessive dialogue begins, the person interrupts the dialogue with a loud "STOP!" and substitutes a positive thought. The goal of this process is to learn to automatically disrupt obsessive and nonproductive thoughts with a positive message.

Refuting irrational ideas, like thought stopping, involves interventions designed to disrupt obsessive, nonproductive thoughts. The intervention derives from Rational Emotive Therapy. It is based on the belief that much stress is related to common irrational beliefs such as "I must be perfect in everything I do" and "It's absolutely necessary that I have love and approval from my peers and family at all times." To overcome these stressful beliefs, the client first identifies the irrational idea and then identifies the facts, such as "no one is perfect all the time." Clients also need to explore their emotional response to stressful thoughts. The client then substitutes rational self-talk for the previous irrational self-talk. This particular intervention is very effective for self-directed, empowered people.

Guided imagery, a form of relaxation, is an excellent method of cognitive reappraisal. Guided imagery is usu-

ally practiced under the direction of a trained therapist. The therapist assists the client to visualize a stressful event, become worried, and then to switch to a relaxing event or to rework the situation so that it is less stressful. Alternatively, the therapist may help the client into a guided dialogue with his or her inner self or may act as a guide to help with problem-solving.

Effective Coping. Effective coping involves recognition of the problem causing stress and, through problem-solving skills, development and implementation of an effective strategy to cope with or solve the problem. Effective coping skills include time management, assertiveness, solution-oriented therapy, and development of a support system.[9, 26] Often clients use ineffective coping strategies, usually designed to avoid the problem, resulting in repression of associated unpleasant emotions. Addictive behaviors, such as alcohol abuse and overeating, often begin as ineffective coping strategies.

Effective coping starts with identifying the problem. Help the client to differentiate the problem from the emotional response to the problem. Once the problem is identified, several issues must be addressed before one can work on problem-solving skills.

First, does the problem really exist, or is it imagined? People often worry about imagined problems. Help the client assess validity of the problem before working on a solution.

Second, is the problem really important or just a nuisance? If the problem is not important, use cognitive reappraisal techniques to put the problem in perspective.

Third, does the problem have feasible solutions? Some problems (an untimely death or catastrophic illness) are beyond control. In these cases, the goal is not problem resolution but acceptance. The individual will need support to learn from the problem and to develop an ongoing support system for assistance through the crisis.

Important, controllable problems are amenable to intervention or action responses using standard problem-solving, assertiveness, and time management skills. Nurses often assist people in distress. Mastering effective coping skills can be an asset in clinical practice. However, nurses often work with people experiencing crises in which basic coping strategies are not enough. Develop a network of counseling and support resources to which clients can be referred.

PREVENTION OF INJURY AND ILLNESS

The greatest causes of injury and premature death in young and middle-aged adults include accidents, particularly motor vehicle accidents, and violence, particularly suicide and homicide.[47] Risk identification and risk management counseling can prevent illness and injury in these populations. Place particular emphasis on preventable causes of accidents, specifically the use of drugs and alcohol, and preventable causes of cancer, specifically smoking. In addition, always be aware of the risk for domestic or spouse abuse.

■ ACCIDENTS

Because motor vehicle accidents are the leading cause of death in young adults, focus prevention counseling on regular use of lap and shoulder belts and refraining from drug or alcohol use while driving. Because of the significant impact drugs, alcohol, and tobacco have on health, most prevention measures are devoted to screening and intervening in alcohol, drug, and tobacco abuse. The following discussion focuses on screening and primary prevention measures. Chapter 24 describes secondary intervention for clients who have abuse problems.

■ ALCOHOL ABUSE

Alcohol abuse results in specific health problems, including withdrawal syndrome; hepatitis, cirrhosis, and pancreatitis; and cancers of the liver, oropharynx (especially in smokers), and esophagus as well as an increased risk of breast cancer. In addition to diseases clearly associated with alcohol abuse, "problem drinkers" have increased mortality from all causes, beginning with four drinks per day for men and two drinks per day for women. Alcohol is associated with more than 50% of all injuries (44% of all traffic accidents), fires, drownings, homicides, and suicides.[47]

Problem drinkers are more likely to be seen in primary care clinics and hospitals. They often do not present with manifestations of dependence that would immediately result in identification of the problem. All clients, not just those with obvious problems, should be screened for problem drinking. Nurses are in a position to identify problem drinking because their role includes obtaining a comprehensive psychosocial history (see Chapter 9).

A variety of tools are available to screen for problem drinking. The mnemonic CAGE is a useful popular 4-item tool[47]:

- *C* = Have you ever felt you ought to *Cut* down on drinking?
- *A* = Have people *Annoyed* you by criticizing your drinking?
- *G* = Have you ever felt bad or *Guilty* about your drinking?
- *E* = Have you ever had a drink first thing in the morning to steady your nerves or get rid of a hangover (*Eye-opener*)?

If problem drinking is suspected or if the client answers "yes" to any item, the Alcohol Use Disorders Identification Test (AUDIT) may be administered. The AUDIT is a 10-item tool developed by a six-nation team in conjunction with the World Health Organization (WHO). The AUDIT is highly sensitive and specific[22, 40] and can easily be included in a social history format. Score the AUDIT tool (Table 2–5) by summing the total points for all answers. Drinking is considered problematic if the score is 8 points or more.

Do not hesitate to screen for problem drinking. If you suspect that a client has a drinking problem (based on screening), briefly state so to the client. Be sure to have an established support and referral network of clinical specialists to assist the client and family with acceptance and management of problem drinking.[47] Chapter 24 details interventions for clients who have substance abuse problems.

■ DRUG ABUSE

Unfortunately since 1992, after years of decline in drug use, abuse of illicit and legal drugs has been on the increase. More than 5.5 million Americans are affected by drug abuse, and 50% of these people are in the criminal justice system. Drug abuse is more common among men, the unemployed, and people without a high school education. Although drug abuse is more prevalent in urban communities, rural communities are not immune. Drug abusers are at increased risk for HIV infection and other communicable diseases. Drug abuse is a significant factor in homicides, suicides, and motor vehicle accidents.[47]

Be aware of the hazards of drug abuse and of the possibility of drug abuse in clients. Several standardized tools can be used to screen for drug abuse, but none has well-established validity or reliability.[47] Take every opportunity to assess for drug abuse. Ask the client about drug use as a routine part of lifestyle assessment, following questions regarding tobacco and alcohol use (see Chapter 9). State questions directly ("Do you currently use any other drugs such as marijuana ['pot,' 'weed'] or cocaine ['crack']?"). If the answer is "no," follow with "Have you ever used any other drugs?" If the client indicates current or past use of illicit drugs, further explore the patterns of use.

Advise abusing and high-risk clients (adolescents, males, people exposed to users of drugs) of the hazards of substance abuse. Advise users to stop or cut down, and offer help through referral. See Chapter 24 for interventions for substance abuse problems.

■ SMOKING CESSATION

More than 25% of Americans smoke, and thousands of children begin smoking every day.[32] Smoking is directly linked to many forms of cancer, heart disease, and hypertension. It is a risk factor in health problems as diverse as osteoporosis, ulcer disease, and low birth weight in babies. Smoking accounts for one of every five deaths in the United States.[47] All nurses should have the skills necessary to help people who are ready to stop smoking and to help motivate people who are not at a point where they can stop. The Agency for Health Care Policy and Research (AHCPR) has published guidelines for smoking cessation intervention (Table 2–6).[1]

INTERVENTION. Smoking cessation intervention can be seen as a stepped process. First, ask all clients if they smoke or are exposed to secondary smoke. When a person who smokes or is regularly exposed to smoke is identified, advise him or her to stop or to avoid exposure. Personalize the need to stop smoking. For example, remind parents of young children of the increased risk for ear infections and asthma the child may have or of the type of role model the parent is presenting. Remind women that smoking increases the risk of osteoporosis and premature aging of the skin. Remind asymptomatic men of the increased risk for emphysema, heart disease, and lung cancer.

Once the client is identified as a smoker and is advised

| TABLE 2-5 | THE ALCOHOL USE DISORDERS IDENTIFICATION TEST (AUDIT) STRUCTURED INTERVIEW |

	Score*				
Question	0	1	2	3	4
How often do you have a drink containing alcohol?	Never	Monthly or less	2–4 times/mo	2–3 times/wk	4 or more times/wk
How many drinks do you have on a typical day when you are drinking?	None	1 or 2	3 or 4	5 or 6	7–9†
How often do you have 6 or more drinks on one occasion?	Never	Less than monthly	Monthly	Weekly	Daily or almost daily
How often during the last year have you found that you were unable to stop drinking once you had started?	Never	Less than monthly	Monthly	Weekly	Daily or almost daily
How often last year have you failed to do what was normally expected from you because of drinking?	Never	Less than monthly	Monthly	Weekly	Daily or almost daily
How often during the last year have you needed a first drink in the morning to get yourself going after a heavy drinking session?	Never	Less than monthly	Monthly	Weekly	Daily or almost daily
How often during the last year have you had a feeling of guilt or remorse after drinking?	Never	Less than monthly	Monthly	Weekly	Daily or almost daily
How often during the last year have you been unable to remember what happened the night before because you had been drinking?	Never	Less than monthly	Monthly	Weekly	Daily or almost daily
Have you or has someone else been injured as a result of your drinking?	Never	Yes, but not in last year (2 points)		Yes, during the last year (4 points)	
Has a relative, doctor, or other health worker been concerned about your drinking or suggested you cut down?	Never	Yes, but not in last year (2 points)		Yes, during the last year (4 points)	

*Score of greater than 8 (out of 41) suggests problem drinking and indicates need for more in-depth assessment. Cut-off of 10 points recommended by some to provide greater specificity.
†Five points if response is 10 or more drinks on a typical day.
From U.S. Preventive Services Task Force. (1996). *Guide to clinical preventive services* (2nd ed.). Baltimore: Williams & Wilkins.

| TABLE 2-6 | RECOMMENDATIONS FOR SUCCESSFUL SMOKING CESSATION TREATMENT |

1. Every person who smokes should be offered smoking cessation treatment at every office visit.
2. Clinicians should ask and record tobacco-use status of every client.
3. Cessation treatments even as brief as 3 minutes per visit are effective.
4. More intense treatment is more effective in producing long-term abstinence from tobacco.
5. Nicotine replacement therapy (patches or gum or nasal spray), clinician-delivered social support, and skills training are the three most effective components of treatment.
6. Health care systems should make institutional changes that result in the systematic identification of, and intervention with, all tobacco users at every visit.

From Agency for Health Care Policy and Research. (1996). *Smoking cessation: Information for specialists.* Washington, DC: U.S. Government Printing Office, AHCPR Pub. No. 96-0694.

of the need to stop smoking, assess motivation to change (see Chapter 1). If a client expresses any interest in changing the smoking behavior, from cutting down to stopping, ask what can be done to help. Success is more likely if people spend thoughtful time planning the behavior change in preparation to quit. Help the client evaluate his or her smoking patterns to personalize the plan. Suggestions include (1) cleaning the house to rid tobacco odor just prior to stopping; (2) getting rid of all cigarettes; and (3) setting up a support network. Advise the client to inform friends who smoke that he or she is trying to quit and that they should respect this by not smoking around the client or not offering cigarettes. If the client's history indicates a high degree of nicotine addiction, offer advice about or referral for nicotine replacement.

Finally, address how the client will manage "triggers" to smoking (e.g., alcohol or anxiety-producing situations) and alternatives to smoking. When the urge to smoke strikes, advise the client to walk and learn deep breathing

TABLE 2–7	THINGS TO DO INSTEAD OF SMOKING

Take a slow deep breath of fresh air.
Take a walk.
Chew on a piece of gum or a carrot or hard candy.
Drink a glass of water.
Think about your children.
Brush your teeth.
Play with worry beads.
Pray or meditate.
Think about the money you are saving.
Smile.

to work through the urge. Table 2–7 lists suggested activities to substitute instead of smoking.

In addition to explaining smoking cessation, be aware of community resources to which clients can be referred for assistance. Provide a variety of motivational literature to clients, such as the excellent materials by the American Cancer Society and the American Lung Association. Support community-based smoking cessation interventions. These include a smoke-free work environment and participation in such community programs as the National Smoke-Off day. Whatever the practice environment, seek out ways to support smoking cessation.

Passive Smoking

Passive smoking, or exposure to second-hand smoke, also places people at increased risk for heart disease and cancer. The Atherosclerosis Risk in the Community (ARIC) study in 1994 indicated that non-smokers who are regularly exposed to environmental tobacco smoke have a 20% increase in progression of atherosclerosis compared with non-smokers who are not exposed to tobacco smoke.[22] Identify people who are exposed to environmental tobacco smoke, and help them devise ways to modify their risk. Ideally, risk modification involves smoking cessation on the part of a family member. However, people are often exposed to tobacco smoke in their work environment (e.g., bars, casinos), and the client may have to make difficult decisions regarding risk management versus livelihood and family.

■ DOMESTIC ABUSE

The Surgeon General's report in the mid-1980s identified domestic violence as a public health issue. Estimates range from 1 million[47] to 4 million[18] women as victims of assault, robbery, or rape by a spouse, ex-spouse, or intimate partner each year. Too often, this violence escalates to murder; 50% of murders are committed by an intimate partner.[18] It is estimated that 35% of women are seen in emergency departments for abuse and that 30% of women seen in primary care are abuse victims.[39] One study of inpatient female psychiatric clients found that 64% reported abuse as adults.[39] Although men are not immune from domestic abuse, most victims are women; therefore, this discussion focuses on abuse of women.

Nurses in all clinical settings see women who are abused; they must, therefore, be aware of the risk of violence and must be comfortable addressing abuse risk issues in client encounters. The American Nurses' Association position paper, *Physical Violence Against Women,*[7] supports the need to (1) increase nurses' awareness of and sensitivity to the problem of physical violence against women; (2) work to reduce injuries, psychological trauma, and cost that are a result of such violence; and (3) increase nurses' awareness of their role in assessing, intervening for, and preventing physical violence against women.[39]

ASSESSMENT. Although nurses often work with women who are victims of abuse, this text emphasizes (1) identification of risk for abuse and (2) interventions to prevent abuse before it starts. Identification begins with recognizing characteristics common to abused women. Characteristics of women at increased risk for violence include living in households with high degrees of stress, being abused as a child, and marrying young.[39, 47] Abused women often display low self-esteem and experience helplessness.[18, 39] In addition, certain characteristics in the woman's partner can increase her risk, such as having been abused or observed abuse as a child, abusing drugs or alcohol, having controlling behaviors, and pathologic jealousy. In addition, men who repetitively abuse women verbally often escalate to physical violence over time, during periods of high stress, or when a woman is pregnant.[39] Remember, any woman can be a victim of abuse, and any man can be an abuser. Routine screening for a history of abuse or current abuse in all women is an appropriate component of a psychosocial history (see Chapter 9).

The Partner Violence Screen (PVS)[13] is brief, easy to use, and accurate in identifying abuse. The tool consists of three questions:

1. Have you been hit, kicked, punched, or otherwise hurt by someone within the past year? If so, by whom?
2. Do you feel safe in your current relationship?
3. Does a partner from a previous relationship make you feel unsafe now?

INTERVENTION. Once a woman is identified as being at risk for violence either through having established risk factors or having been abused in the past, work with her to develop an individualized plan designed to prevent future violence. The plan may include assertiveness training, participation in a woman's empowerment or support group, self-esteem work, and social services assistance to improve her educational and economic status.[19, 27] Additional prevention strategies include community health nurse visits to high-risk families and community-wide media campaigns to enhance public awareness of the problem.[39] Explain stress management strategies, especially effective coping (see earlier), to help the client to avoid violence.

If a woman is identified as being in a currently violent relationship, focus intervention on safety. This woman is at high risk for sustaining significant injury or death. Therefore, nurses who screen for domestic violence must have a clearly established protocol for ensuring that every effort has been made to protect the woman. This protocol should be developed in collaboration with local law enforcement agencies and women's safety groups (e.g., YWCAs or other agencies).[10]

■ INFECTIOUS DISEASES

With the exception of HIV disease, infectious diseases are not a major cause of illness or premature death in young and middle-aged adults. However, these groups are not immune to problems related to infectious diseases. Two activities are essential for protection from infectious diseases in these populations: maintaining up-to-date immunizations and practicing safe sex.

Immunization

The U.S. Preventive Services Task Force (USPSTF)[47] recommends that all young and middle-aged adults have a tetanus-diphtheria booster vaccination every 10 years and that women of child-bearing age who do not have proven immunity to rubella have a rubella vaccination. In addition, people at risk for hepatitis B (Table 2–8) should receive the hepatitis B vaccination series.

Safe Sex

There are dozens of infectious sexually transmitted diseases (STDs). Of these, HIV infection and hepatitis B and C can result in significant morbidity and premature death; others result in permanent infection (e.g., herpes simplex) or infertility (e.g., gonorrhea). Risk factors for contracting a STD include:

1. Having a high number of sex partners.
2. Having sex with a person who engages in high-risk behavior (e.g., multiple partners).
3. Having sex for money.
4. Having sex with an intravenous (IV) drug user.

People who abuse drugs and alcohol are at increased risk, even if they do not abuse IV drugs, because they are more likely to engage in high-risk sexual behaviors while in an impaired state.

Do not hesitate to screen for high-risk sexual behavior, and advise clients about the risks and behaviors to protect from infection. Safe sex behavior includes:

1. Abstaining from sex
2. Maintaining a mutually monogamous relationship with a non-infected partner

TABLE 2–8	PEOPLE AT HIGH RISK FOR HEPATITIS B

1. Recipients of blood products (including hemodialysis clients)
2. People with frequent occupational exposure to blood or blood products
3. Men who have sex with men
4. Injection drug users and their sex partners
5. People with multiple sexual partners
6. People with a history of sexually transmitted diseases
7. Travelers to countries where hepatitis B is endemic

From U.S. Preventive Services Task Force. (1996). *Guide to clinical preventive services* (2nd ed.). Baltimore: Williams & Wilkins.

3. Avoiding sexual contact with casual or high-risk partners
4. Using male or female condoms consistently and appropriately.

Present information regarding referral sources in the community to assist clients with free or low-cost screening and treatment for STDs and information regarding sources of low-cost condoms. If you work in an ambulatory clinic or a community-based practice, consider finding a source of low-cost condoms and making them available at little or no cost to people at high risk.[47] Chapters 41 and 79 cover working with clients who have STDs, including AIDS.

SCREENING FOR DISEASE

Secondary prevention includes early detection of illness. Early identification is key to preventing premature death from many catastrophic illnesses, including coronary heart disease, cancer, and type 2 diabetes mellitus. Be aware of the risks for diseases and the current recommendations regarding screening, and take every opportunity to advise clients of the need for regular screening (see Chapter 9). Facilitating early detection of disease saves lives.

■ RECOMMENDATIONS FOR SCREENING

The Preventive Services Task Force issued its landmark report regarding the effectiveness of preventive services in 1989 and updated its recommendations in 1996. These recommendations are the "gold standard" regarding screening services, and you should be familiar with them. In addition to screening, the Task Force recommends the counseling, immunization, and chemoprophylaxis measures discussed earlier in this chapter. The recommendations are specific to age groups (except for pregnant women) and differentiate screenings recommended for all people in the group from screenings recommended for those with high-risk characteristics.

Screening recommendations are based on several factors that apply to populations rather than to individuals. The screening test must be reasonably priced, sensitive, and specific to the problem. In addition, there is generally no value to screening for diseases for which there is no treatment or when treatment does not improve either the quality of life or longevity. As a result, many tests do not meet requirements for an effective screening program.

Screenings recommended for the general population between the ages of 11 and 24 years are listed in Table 2–9. Screenings recommended for the general population between the ages of 25 and 64 years are listed in Table 2–10.

Many other organizations, particularly the American Cancer Society and the American Academy of Family Physicians, publish additional screening guidelines that have been addressed by the Task Force but that do not meet its criteria for recommendation. The American Cancer Society recommends that all women over age 20 perform breast self-examination (BSE) on a monthly basis.[42, 47] Although the American Cancer Society does not formally recommend that men practice regular testicular self-examination (TSE), its literature does support the practice.[43] Nurses can teach individuals how to do these self-examinations.

TABLE 2–9	RECOMMENDED SCREENINGS FOR THE GENERAL POPULATION AGES 11 TO 24 YEARS

Screening	Frequency	For
Height and weight	Periodic*	Obesity
Blood pressure	Periodic*	Hypertension
Papanicolaou (Pap) test (females)	At least every 3 years	Cervical cancer
Chlamydia screen (females)	With Pap test	*Chlamydia trachomatis*
Rubella serology (females)†	Once	Non-immune status
Assess for problem drinking	Periodic	Problem drinking

*Clinician discretion.
†In women with childbearing potential with incomplete vaccination history.
Modified from U.S. Preventive Services Task Force. (1996). *Guide to clinical preventive services* (2nd ed.). Baltimore: Williams & Wilkins.

BREAST SELF-EXAMINATION

BSE is a technique that women can use to assess their breasts. When women perform BSE properly and regularly, they can note early changes in their breasts and seek further evaluation. A major barrier to BSE is lack of confidence. Take time when working with the woman to ensure that she is confident of her skill and has had all her questions addressed. The BSE technique is described in Figure 2–5.

When teaching, emphasize that the examination should be done every month and at the end of menses in all menstruating women. Advise nonmenstruating women to pick one day a month (e.g., the first day of the month) to do BSE. Inform women that most breast lumps are benign but it is essential that they seek professional evaluation if they find anything that concerns them. Chapter 37 discusses physical assessment of the breast, including the clinical breast examination.

TESTICULAR SELF-EXAMINATION

TSE is a simple technique that men can use to assess for changes in their testicles that may signal testicular cancer. The risk is highest in adolescents and in men under age 35 years. As with BSE, the man should become familiar with the normal appearance and feel of his genitals to feel confident of his ability to perform TSE. Advise the man to schedule a regular time each month to assess his genitals. The best time is after bathing, because the warm water causes the scrotum to relax and makes the testicles easier to examine.

Teach the client to perform TSE as follows (Fig. 2–6):

1. Hold the scrotum in the palms of your hands, and examine each testicle with the thumbs and fingers of both hands. The index and middle fingers should be on the underside of each testicle with the thumbs on the top.
2. The testicle is rolled between your thumb and fingers. A normal testicle is shaped like an egg and is about 4 cm (1⅗ inches) long. It feels firm but not hard (like an ear lobe) and should be smooth without lumps.
3. After examining the testicles, examine the epididymides (behind the testicles); they should be soft and may feel sponge-like.
4. Examine the spermatic cords, which ascend from the epididymides up into the body. They are normally firm, smooth tubular structures.

PROSTATE CANCER

Nearly 40,000 men die annually of prostate cancer. Men at increased risk include those who have a first-degree relative (e.g., father, brother, son) with prostate cancer and African Americans. Despite the prevalence of the disease, both the Task Force and the American Academy of Family Physicians do not recommend screening for prostate cancer because early screening and treatment have not proved beneficial. However, the American Cancer Society and American Urological Association recommend screening for prostate cancer using a prostate-specific antigen (PSA) test and a digital rectal examination for all men over age 50 (over age 40 for African American men) (see Chapter 37).

When advising men about screening, keep in mind the man's prostate cancer risk factors, his general health, and his desires. Generally, prostate cancer screening should not be done in men over 70 years or who have significant underlying illness that would result in a life expectancy of less than 10 years.[29]

TABLE 2–10	RECOMMENDED SCREENINGS FOR THE GENERAL POPULATION AGES 25 TO 64 YEARS

Screening	Frequency	For
Blood pressure	Periodic*	Hypertension
Height and weight	Periodic*	Obesity
Total blood cholesterol†	Every 5 years	Coronary heart disease risk
Papanicolaou (Pap) test (females)	At least every 3 years	Cervical cancer
Fecal occult blood test‡	Annually	Colorectal cancer
Mammogram and clinical breast exam§	Annually	Breast cancer
Rubella serologic testing (females)‖	Once	Non-immune status
Assessment for problem drinking	Periodic*	Problem drinking

*Clinician discretion.
†Males age 35–64; females age 45–64.
‡Over age 50, or sigmoidoscopy less often.
§Females ≥ 50 years.
‖In women of childbearing age with an inaccurate vaccination history.
From U.S. Preventive Services Task Force. (1996). *Guide to clinical preventive services* (2nd ed.). Baltimore: Williams & Wilkins.

A

B

C

D

E

F

G

H

I

J

FIGURE 2-5 Self-examination of female breasts and axillae. Accomplished by observation and palpation. The client assumes various positions for observation while standing in front of a mirror. *A*, Arms relaxed at sides. Next, lean forward. *B*, Raise arms high overhead. Press arms behind head. *C*, Rest palms on hips, and firmly press inward to flex chest muscles. *D*, In shower, examine breast contours. *E*, Method of palpating breast. With fingers flat, gently press with small circular motions around an imaginary clock face; begin at 12 o'clock. Move an inch at a time toward the nipple. *F*, As a final step, squeeze the nipple gently between the thumb and index finger. Palpation of the breast is accomplished while lying down. *G*, Position to examine inner breast. *H*, Position to examine axilla. *I*, Position to examine outer breast. *J*, Repeat entire process for opposite breast and axilla. (See text and Chapter 37 for discussion of technique and observations.)

■ COLORECTAL CANCER

Colorectal cancer is the second most common form of cancer in the United States and accounts for more than 55,000 deaths per year. If the disease is found while still localized, survival rates are at 91%. If the disease is found when it has spread, the survival rate is much lower.[47] Therefore, early detection of the disease is essential. Risk factors include uncommon hereditary familial polyposis syndromes and ulcerative colitis of greater than 10 years' duration. More common risk factors include a

Lump

FIGURE 2–6 Testicular self-examination.

family history of colorectal cancer, especially in young and middle-aged adults, and possibly high-fat and low-fiber diets.[47]

Current recommendations are for annual screening using fecal occult blood testing (FOBT) for adults over 50 years of age.[47] People who are at increased risk would benefit from beginning screening at age 40. Fecal occult blood testing is easily done at home, but the client should be instructed on dietary restrictions, specifically, no raw meat; no aspirin or nonsteroidal anti-inflammatory agents (NSAIDs), and no vitamin C in doses over 250 mg for 48 hours prior to and during specimen collection. Specimens should be kept away from heat and should be tested within 2 weeks of collection. Advise clients at increased risk to discuss the benefits of regular sigmoidoscopy screening with a health care provider. Current Task Force recommendations include consideration of a sigmoidoscopy at age 50.

CONCLUSIONS

Health promotion and disease prevention activities are at the core of health care for young and middle-aged adults. Be familiar with current recommendations regarding healthy eating and activity patterns and with strategies for coping with daily stressors. Take every opportunity to work with clients to assist them to implement healthy lifestyles. Include risk assessment, risk management, and appropriate screening for diseases when working with these populations. Based on assessment results, provide education and appropriate referral.

BIBLIOGRAPHY

1. Agency for Health Care Policy and Research. (1996). *Smoking cessation: Information for specialists.* Washington, DC: U.S. Government Printing Office, AHCPR Pub. No. 96-0694.
2. Bonheur, B., & Young, S. (1991). Exercise as a health-promoting life-style choice. *Applied Nursing Research, 4*(1), 2–6.
3. Burns, C. M. (1993). Assessment and screening for substance abuse: Guidelines for the primary care nurse practitioner. *Nurse Practitioner Forum, 4*(4), 199–206.
4. Burns, K. (1996). A new recommendation for physical activity as a means of health promotion. *Nurse Practitioner, 21*(9), 18, 21–22, 26, 27.
5. Calfas, K., et al. (1996). A controlled trial of physician counseling to promote the adoption of physical activity. *Preventive Medicine, 25,* 225–233.
6. Chrousos, G., & Gold, P. (1992). The concepts of stress and stress system disorders. *Journal of the American Medical Association, 267*(9), 1244–1252.
7. Council of Community Health Nurses. (1991). *Physical violence against women: ANA position statement.* Kansas City, MO: American Nurses' Association.
8. Daughton, D., et al. (1994, September). Confronting cigarette addiction: A guide to efficient clinical intervention. *Internal Medicine,* 68–70, 73–77.
9. Davis, M., Eshelman, E., & McKay, M. (1995). *The relaxation and stress reduction workbook* (4th ed.). Oakland, CA: New Harbinger Publications.
10. Domestic violence: Ending the cycle of abuse. (1998). *Clinician Reviews, 8*(1), 55–57, 61–62, 67–68, 71.
11. Edmunds, M. (1991). Strategies for promoting physical fitness. *Nursing Clinics of North America, 26*(4), 855–866.
12. Ferri, R. (1998, June 25). Treating HIV infection. *The Clinical Advisor,* 30–36.
13. Feldhaus, K., et al. (1997). Accuracy of three brief questions for detecting partner violence in the emergency department. *Journal of the American Medical Association, 277,* 1357–1361.
14. Franklin, B., Buchal, M., & Hollingsworth, V. (1991). Exercise prescription. In R. Strauss (Ed), *Sports medicine* (2nd ed.). Philadelphia: W. B. Saunders.
15. Goldstein, D. J. (1992). Beneficial effects of modest weight loss. *International Journal of Obesity, 16,* 397–415.
16. Gorin, S. S. (1998). Smoking cessation. In S. S. Gorin & J. Arnold (Eds.), *Health promotion handbook.* St. Louis: Mosby–Year Book.
17. Grubbs, L. (1993). The critical role of exercise in weight control. *Nurse Practitioner, 18*(4), 20, 22, 25–26, 29.
18. Hoff, L. A. (1992). Battered women: Understanding, identification, and assessment. *Journal of the American Academy of Nurse Practitioners, 4*(4), 148–155.
19. Hoff, L. A. (1993). Battered women: Intervention and prevention. *Journal of the American Academy of Nurse Practitioners, 5*(1), 34–39.
20. Howard, G., et al. (1998). Cigarette smoking and progression of atherosclerosis: The Atherosclerosis Risk in Communities (ARIC) study. *Journal of the American Medical Association, 279*(2), 119–124.
21. Jones, K. D., & Jones, J. M. (1997). Physical activity and exercise. *Clinician Reviews, 7*(3), 81–83, 86–88, 93–94, 97–98, 101–102, 104.
22. Isaacson, J., Butler, R., & Zackarek, M. (1994). Screening with the Alcohol Use Disorders Identification Test (AUDIT) in an inner-city population. *Journal of General Internal Medicine, 9,* 550–553.
23. Krawiec, J. V., & Pohl, J. M. (1998). Smoking cessation and nicotine replacement therapy: A guide for primary care providers. *American Journal of Nurse Practitioners, 2*(1), 15–16, 19–22, 27–33.

24. Kushner, R., & Hopson, S. (1998). Obesity therapy: What works—what doesn't? *Consultant, 38*(3), 511–518.

25. Long, B. J., et al. (1996). A multisite field test of the acceptability of physical counseling in primary care: Project PACE. *American Journal of Preventive Medicine, 12*(2), 73–81.

26. McCloskey, J. C., & Bulechek, G. M. (1996). *Nursing intervention classification* (2nd ed.). St. Louis: Mosby–Year Book.

27. McWhirter, E. H. (1994). *Counseling for empowerment.* Alexandria, VA: American Counseling Association.

28. Melkus, G. D. (1994). Obesity: Assessment and intervention in primary care practice. *Nurse Practitioner Forum, 5*(1), 28–33.

29. Naitoh, J., Zeiner, R. L., & Dekernion, J. B. (1998). Diagnosis and treatment of prostate cancer. *American Family Physician, 57*(7), 1531–1539.

30. National Cholesterol Program. (1993). *Second report of the National Cholesterol Education Expert Panel on detection, evaluation, and treatment of high blood cholesterol in adults (Adult Treatment Panel II),* NIH Pub. No. 93-3085. Bethesda: National Institutes of Health, National Heart, Lung, and Blood Institute.

31. National Institutes of Health Consensus Panel on Optimal Calcium Intake. (1992). Optimal calcium intake. *Journal of the American Medical Association, 272*(24), 1942–1948.

32. Novak, J. C. (1998). Effective smoking cessation strategies. *Clinical Letter for Nurse Practitioners, 2*(1), 1–6.

33. Paffenbarger, R. S., et al. (1986). Physical activity, all-cause mortality, and longevity in college alumni. *New England Journal of Medicine, 314*(10), 605–613.

34. Pate, R. R., et al. (1995). Physical activity and public health. *Journal of the American Medical Association, 273*(5), 402–407.

35. Patrick, K., et al. (1994). A new tool for encouraging activity. *The Physician and Sportsmedicine, 22*(11), 45–55.

36. Peddicord, K. (1991). Strategies for promoting stress reduction and relaxation. *Nursing Clinics of North America, 26*(4), 867–874.

37. Pender, N. J. (1996). *Health promotion in nursing practice* (3rd ed.). Stamford, CT: Appleton & Lange.

38. Pi-Sunyer, F. X. (1993). Medical hazards of obesity. *Annals of Internal Medicine, 119*(7), 655–660.

39. Quillian, J. P. (1995). Domestic violence. *Journal of American Academy of Nurse Practitioners, 7*(7), 351–358.

40. Saunders, J., et al. (1993). Development of the Alcohol Use Disorders Identification Test (AUDIT): WHO collaboration project on early detection of persons with harmful alcohol consumption. II. *Addiction, 88,* 791.

41. Schussheim, D. H., & Siris, E. S. (1998). Osteoporosis: Update on prevention and treatment. *Women's Health in Primary Care, 1*(2), 133–140.

42. Strauss, R. H. (1991). *Sports medicine* (2nd ed.). Philadelphia: W. B. Saunders.

43. Sugg, N. K., & Inui, T. (1992). Primary care physicians' response to domestic violence. *Journal of the American Medical Association, 267*(23), 3157–3160.

44. U.S. Department of Health and Human Services. (1998). *Clinician's handbook of preventive services* (3rd ed.). Washington, DC: U.S. Government Printing Office.

45. U.S. Department of Health and Human Services. (1996). *Healthy People 2000: Midcourse review and 1995 revisions.* Sudbury, MA: Jones & Bartlett.

46. U.S. Department of Health and Human Services. (1996). *Physical activity and health,* S/N 017-023-00196-5. Washington, DC: U.S. Government Printing Office.

47. U.S. Preventive Services Task Force. (1996). *Guide to clinical preventive services* (2nd ed.). Baltimore: Williams & Wilkins.

CHAPTER 3

Health Promotion in Older Adults

Beverley E. Holland
Cynthia McCurren

NURSING OUTCOMES CLASSIFICATION (NOC)
for Nursing Diagnoses—Clients at Risk for Relocation Stress Syndrome

Relocation Stress Syndrome	Loneliness
Anxiety Control	Mood Equilibrium
Caregiver Adaptation to Patient Institutionalization	Psychosocial Adjustment: Life Change
Coping	Quality of Life
Depression Control	Sleep
Depression Level	Social Support
Grief Resolution	

As a result of the phenomenon of the aging of the United States population and related issues, health promotion in older adults merits special attention. According to the American Association of Retired Persons,[28] almost 34 million Americans were age 65 years or older in 1996. This figure represents 12.8% of the population, about one in every eight Americans. The older population will continue to grow (Fig. 3–1). The most rapid increase is expected between the years 2010 and 2030, when the "baby boom" generation (those born between 1946 and 1964) reach age 65. By 2030, there will be about 70 million elderly, more than twice the number in 1996; they will represent 20% of the population. The elderly population is currently the fastest-growing segment in the nation. Concern for rapidly increasing aging populations is an international dilemma.

The aging of America has profound implications for nursing practice across all settings, including acute care, the community, and long-term care. Among all hospital admissions in the United States, nearly 60% involve clients over age 65.[10] Nurse experts on aging agree that nurses need information to provide appropriate care to older people. Nurses who care for older clients must be aware of the unique physical, psychosocial, legal, ethical, and economic issues surrounding the aging process.

Knowing what resources, services, and options are available at the federal, state, and local levels is essential.

Nurses must understand the normal aging process and must be prepared to care for clients who have chronic disorders and complex acute conditions. Normal aging changes the structure and function of various organ systems. Pathologic processes often present and progress differently in the elderly, necessitating adaptation of interventions. Selected effects of aging as they relate to assessment, disease presentation, and nursing intervention appear throughout this book in discussions of the different body systems and their disorders.

This chapter examines late adulthood and the implications for nursing practice from a holistic perspective. The focus is on issues associated with health promotion and disease prevention in older adults.

NURSING AND THE STUDY OF AGING

Two terms are used in the study of aging[8]:

1. *Geriatrics,* from Greek *geras* (old age) and *iatrike* (medicine), is the branch of medicine concerned with medical problems and care of older people. Geriatrics pertains to all health care disciplines, and

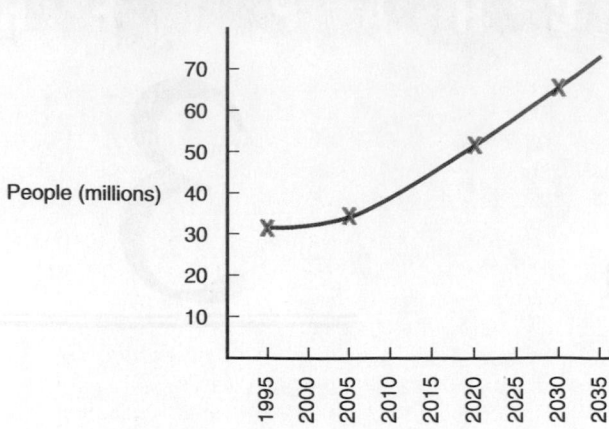

FIGURE 3–1 Projected rise in America's 65-and-older population.

professionals who care for these clients should be familiar with the illnesses that affect them.

2. *Gerontology* takes a broader perspective. It is the scientific study of the process and problems of aging and focuses on the biologic, sociologic, and psychological aspects of normal aging.

Ebersole and Hess studied aging within the discipline of nursing.[10] They assert that *geriatric nursing* occurs primarily with the ill elderly in a medical setting. These authors use the term *gerontic nursing,* defined as the specialized nursing care of older adults that occurs in any setting in which nurses use knowledge, expertise, and caring abilities to promote optimal functioning. Gerontic nursing includes a comprehensive understanding of aging within a holistic perspective. It is more than the medical or scientific approach and encompasses nursing's concept of the spiritual biopsychosocial person.

The American Nurses' Association (ANA) identifies standards of *gerontological nursing* practice.[1] "Gerontological nursing" is the ANA's term for nursing specializing in the care of older adults. These standards include practice guidelines for health promotion, health maintenance, disease prevention, and self-care, with a goal of restoring and maintaining optimal physical, psychological, and social functioning. Organizational standards for nursing service, research, ethics, and professional development are also included. *Standards of Gerontological Nursing Practice* defines what gerontological nurses can do and outlines their unique contributions by describing and prescribing professional nursing practice related to care of older adults.

The ANA provides three levels of gerontological nursing certification:

- Gerontological nurse
- Gerontological clinical nurse specialist (GCNS)
- Gerontological nurse practitioner (GNP)

Advanced-practice nurses (GNPs and GCNSs) have diverse opportunities for practice. They can manage many health problems that occur among residents in skilled nursing facilities, retirement communities, day care settings, ambulatory care settings, hospitals, and private practice. Gerontological nurse specialists can also assume roles in education, counseling, case management, and long-term care administration.

THE OLDER POPULATION

■ TRENDS AMONG THE ELDERLY

Aging trends have profound implications for nursing practice and the delivery of health care. The Pew Health Professions Commission report, *Healthy America: Practitioners for 2005,*[31] summarized the aging population growth trends. The 65-and-older group was expected to increase between 1995 and 2005. After 2010, there will be rapid growth to the year 2030 as baby boomers age. Figure 3–1 depicts this rapid rise. Not only is the total U.S. population aging; the elderly population is aging too. In 1987, 9.6% of the elderly population was older than 85 years; by 2010, this percentage will increase to 15.5%. There are now 36,000 centenarians in the United States. If present trends continue, there may be 266,000 centenarians by the year 2020.

Ethnicity

In 1997, 15.3% of persons 65 years and older in the United States were minorities. By 2030, this percentage is expected to increase to 25%.[28] It is projected that Hispanics will represent 13%; blacks, 17%; Asians and Pacific Islanders, 12%; and Native Americans, Eskimos, and Aleuts, 11% of the older population. Whites will make up 47% of the total elder population.[28] Caregivers who work with diverse older Americans must consider ethnic origin in relation to health and illness issues, family and social support, and interaction within the health care system.

Aging, Sex, and Marital Status

Of the 33.9 million Americans over age 65 years, nearly 20 million are women and 13.9 million are men.[28] Life expectancy for men is 80 years, and 84 years for women. Among people 65 years and older, 76% of men live with their spouses, compared with only 43% of women.[10] The implications for nursing practice are evident. Most older women living alone are an at-risk population, frequently encountering problems accessing and obtaining quality health care. Traditionally, women assumed dependent roles, letting others make their decisions, including treatment choices. In general, these women are vulnerable; nurses need to ensure that they receive their share of medical resources and quality health care.

Economic Forces

The largest single income source for an older adult is the Social Security benefit, about 40%. Other contributing sources include earnings, property income, pensions, and public assistance. In 1997, the median yearly income for older men was $17,768; for older women, it was $10,062.[28] The poverty and near-poverty rate was 16.9% among all elderly in 1997.[28] Among minority ethnic groups, poverty levels are even higher. Approximately 26% of elderly black Americans currently fall below the federal poverty line, compared with 9% of elderly white Americans and nearly 51% of elderly Native Americans.

Although most older adults receive Medicare benefits, Medicare does not provide comprehensive coverage of health care expenses. Medicare does not cover most preventive care, including vision, hearing, or dental examinations. For a person living at or near poverty level, supplemental health insurance is not an option. Medicare reimburses only for limited home health care services and does not cover a large part of nursing home costs.

Educational Issues

In 1987, fewer than half of the elderly population were high school graduates.[11] Current trends indicate that by the year 2000, 66% of all elders will have completed high school and more older adults will have advanced degrees.[8] There is great disparity in educational levels among various ethnic groups. Many blacks older than 65 years of age have not had a formal education. Hispanic elderly people have the least amount of formal education, whereas Asians are the most educated minority.

■ CULTURAL ASPECTS OF AGING

Diverse Definitions of "Elderly"

The United States has many ethnocultural groups interacting within one society. Culture defines who is old, establishes rituals for identifying the elderly, sets socially acceptable roles and expectations for behavior of older adults, and influences attitudes toward aged members.

The definitions of functional and chronological aging indicate that there are no arbitrary or widely accepted markers for old age. The prevailing definition of old age in the United States is considered to be age 65; there are diverse perceptions of old age in various cultures. People may be recognized as elders as early as age 40 among Southeast Asian and Native American groups. Social changes, such as becoming grandparents and retirement, or changes in functional status rather than chronological age, mark entrance into old age in different cultures. Clients may be chronologically old but, in functional terms, are active and productive.

When working with older people, use a holistic approach. Holistic care encompasses understanding the interaction of culture, socioeconomic background, and spirituality as well as the physiological and psychological processes of the person. Chapter 9 discusses psychosocial and cultural assessment. A holistic approach takes into account the complexities of the interactions and delivers individualized care to meet each client's needs.[24]

Family Support

Nurses who care for older clients and families from different cultural backgrounds notice that family relationships vary within a cultural context. The availability of physical and personal support from family members can facilitate the older person's ability to maintain independence, cope effectively with acute and chronic illnesses, remain functional and productive despite disability, and experience a peaceful death.

Since decision-making in the Hispanic culture usually includes the family, the following guidelines apply:

1. Involve the relatives in the plan of care and consult with them.

2. In the inpatient setting, do not be surprised to see a room full of guests visiting the client. Be sensitive to this, and know that Hispanic elders value close family contact.

3. Encourage this if it is not contraindicated by the current therapy, and view it as a necessary integral part of the client's recovery.[24]

Some older adults from culturally diverse backgrounds who have given material and social support to children and grandchildren may expect reciprocity during their aging years. In many Hispanic, Native American, Asian American, Amish, Arab American, and first-generation immigrant ethnic groups, the cultural norm is to care for aging parents, grandparents, and extended family members.

The importance of family support is compounded for older refugees. In instances of forced migration, the traditional family structure may have been altered or destroyed in the country of origin, sometimes in extremely violent ways. When older refugees arrive in the new host country, they may be isolated. Older refugees may have limited or no English language skills and have lost their social status, their country, and their home. The psychological stress related to cultural change is more intense. The older refugee is more likely to rely on younger family members for economic and social support, housing, and access to health services.[24]

Older adults from cultures that highly value independence and self-reliance may refuse offers of assistance from their children, grandchildren, and extended family members. Depending on personal finances, these individuals may have planned carefully for their aging in ways that rely on personal resources. They may seek assistance on a fee-for-service basis from organizations that provide services and homes for the elderly but may refuse help from relatives.

A national sample of older Hispanics revealed that 30% reported providing child care to younger family members, 50% reported assisting in family decisions, and 12% provided financial assistance to family members. This compares with a national average of 19% of older Americans providing child care regularly, and 15% occasionally caring for their grandchildren. More grandparents in Japan and France (51%) provide regular care than grandparents in Great Britain (19%).[24] In black American households, the grandmother often takes a direct role in childrearing. More than twice as many young blacks live in households headed by elderly family members compared with whites.

Cultural Influences on Caregiving

Historically, a higher proportion of older adults among minority ethnic groups have been cared for in home environments than older white Americans have. Research indicates that family care of the elderly in other cultures is supportive for several reasons: as a substitute for formal services, as a more affordable alternative, as a caring option that is consistent with cultural values and preferences, and as an effective strategy for overcoming language barriers. In large extended families, more relatives are likely to be available to provide partial services and care for an older family member.[24]

In Hispanic families, the elder has a position of respect and is usually cared for at home by the family. Should institutionalization occur, a Hispanic elder may suffer feelings of isolation, anguish, and perhaps betrayal by loved ones. The Hispanic male in a traditional authority role may be greatly affected by the transition to a dependent, passive role.[24]

Economic Issues

The work histories of cultural groups, including long careers in agricultural and domestic labor, often preclude coverage within the Social Security or Medicare system. For this reason, many elderly members from diverse cultural backgrounds face out-of-pocket health care expenses on limited incomes and have difficulty paying health care costs. Nurses who work with aged clients in their homes often find them also unable to afford these costs. In many cases, family members of culturally diverse older adults bear the burden of such expenses.[24]

Older adults who have made major lifestyle adjustments from their homelands to the United States and from rural to urban settings may be unaware of health care alternatives (e.g., preventive programs, benefits, and screening programs) for which they are eligible. The nurse can help clients in evaluating their social networks, seeking assistance for health care needs, activating social contacts for support, and developing culturally competent care plans.

■ HEALTH PROMOTION, MAINTENANCE, AND RESTORATION IN OLDER CLIENTS

Older adults are more likely to suffer from multiple chronic and disabling illnesses than younger adults (see Chapter 2). Approximately 80% of elderly people in the United States have one or more chronic diseases.[28] Chronic conditions result in limitations in *activities of daily living* (ADL) for 50%, major limitations in activities for 18%, and home confinement for 5%. Heart disease, cancer, and strokes account for 80% of deaths in people older than age 65. Clients with hypertension, arthritis, pulmonary disorders, diabetes, visual and hearing problems, dementia, and depression require ongoing care and rehabilitation.[10]

A traditional definition of *health* as the absence of disease or disability is clearly not applicable to most older people. A more appropriate focus is on health as a state of mind and on the ability to live and function effectively in society. Health encompasses an interaction of physical, functional, and psychosocial factors. Health promotion goals, therefore, must include individual and group efforts related to spiritual, emotional, psychosocial, and physical concerns (see Chapter 1). Desired outcomes of health promotion programs should include:

1. Maximizing functional independence, thereby reducing dependency.
2. Decreasing mortality.
3. Decreasing morbidity, including impairment.
4. Maintaining or improving quality of life.
5. Promoting behavioral change when necessary.
6. Increasing productivity.

Elders can make efforts to control aspects of their health and move toward wellness (Table 3–1). Nursing

TABLE 3-1	HEALTH PROMOTION, MAINTENANCE, AND RESTORATION ACTIVITIES FOR OLDER ADULTS	
Promotion*	**Maintenance†**	**Restoration‡**
Primary Prevention (prevents occurrence of specific disease and provides specific protection)	*Secondary Prevention* (early detection and treatment and limitation of disability)	*Tertiary Prevention* (rehabilitation after disease)

Smoking cessation programs
Diet low in fat, high in fiber
Regular weight-bearing exercise
Weight control
Limiting alcohol ingestion
 	
Testicular self-examination
Breast self-examination
Education in osteoporosis:
   calcium and vitamin D intake
Use of seat belt
 	
Vaccinations
   Tetanus-diphtheria toxoid
   Pneumococcus
   Influenza
	Complete physical examination
	   Blood pressure
	   Electrocardiogram
	   Total cholesterol with high-density lipoprotein
	   Clinical breast examination
	   Mammography
	   Digital rectal examination
	   Fecal occult blood testing
	   Thyroid-stimulating hormone test
	   Pelvic examination with Papanicolaou smear
	   Prostate examination
	   Sigmoidoscopy
	
	Counseling
	   Sexuality
	   Urinary incontinence
	   Depression/life satisfaction
	
	Counseling and referral
	   Hearing examination
	   Visual examination with glaucoma test
	   Dental examination and cleaning
		Post-stroke rehabilitation
		Cardiac rehabilitation
		Pulmonary rehabilitation
		Orthopedic rehabilitation

*Health promotion activities for older adults are similar to recommendations for all adults.

†Recommendations on frequency of examinations vary, depending on the recommending organization (American College of Physicians, American Cancer Society, U.S. Preventive Services Task Force, and American Geriatrics Society) and the risk factors and presenting manifestations of the individual.

‡Rehabilitation programs are interdisciplinary and developed to meet the specific needs and deficits of the person.

has a prominent role in helping elders practice health promotion, including self-care, physical activity, nutritional awareness, and stress management.

Self-Care and Self-Responsibility

As older adults become better informed and increasingly aware of the self-help movement, health care expectations also rise. There is an increasing desire to be in control of one's body, mind, and spirit and to assume responsibility for one's own wellness. This does not mean that traditional health care providers are ignored. Instead, strategies are taught that enable people to respond to their body signals and to take action accordingly. You can help the aging person understand this shared role (between the individual and health care professionals) for maintaining wellness, counsel elders about factors that can alter wellness, and provide information about available alternatives (see Chapter 1). Given adequate information, elders can practice effective self-care through a process of examining choices and making informed, meaningful decisions.

Most older people want to have as much control as possible over their body, mind, and spirit. Assessment should include an evaluation of self-care, with an emphasis on abilities rather than disabilities. Suggested preventive practices are discussed in Chapters 1, 2, and 9. Physical activity, nutrition, and stress management are also factors in geriatric wellness.

Physical Activity

Exercise and activity are essential for health promotion and maintenance and for achieving an optimal level of functioning (see Chapters 1 and 2). Approximately half of the physical deterioration in the elderly population is caused by disuse rather than by the aging process or disease. Positive effects of exercise on health include (1) increased energy, (2) improved eating and sleeping, (3) decreased discomfort and stress, and (4) decreased smoking and alcohol use.[10]

Physiologically, benefits to the cardiopulmonary, vascular, and musculoskeletal systems result in (1) improved oxygen transport, (2) decreased blood pressure and pulse rate, (3) increased vital lung capacity, (4) decreased body fat and increased lean body mass, (5) reduced osteoporosis, and (6) increased muscle strength and joint flexibility. Positive psychological changes occur as well, including improved cognitive functioning and a heightened sense of well-being.

Before beginning an exercise program, older clients should have a physical examination, which may include an exercise stress test. One of the best exercises for an older adult is walking, with progression to 30-minute sessions three to five times each week (Fig. 3–2). Swimming and dancing are also beneficial. Age alone does not preclude older people from pursuing a range of physical activities; the issue is simply one of physical tolerance. Elders confined to a chair or with limited mobility can perform adapted exercises. At many senior centers, wellness programs, and fitness clubs, consultants, instructors, or physical therapists can help the client establish an individualized exercise program (Fig. 3–3).

FIGURE 3–2 Walking provides a multitude of physiologic benefits for the older person.

Nutrition

Nutritional status is important to an older person's ability to remain healthy, to maintain structural integrity, think clearly, and to possess the necessary energy to engage in social and fitness activities. Several physiologic changes related to aging can affect nutritional status (Table 3–2).

FIGURE 3–3 Today's older adult is interested in maintaining strength and endurance.

TABLE 3-2	STRUCTURAL AND FUNCTIONAL CHANGES AND COMMON HEALTH PROBLEMS IN OLDER ADULTS	
System	**Normal Changes Associated with Aging**	**Common Health Problems**
Cardiovascular	Decreased contractility, impaired coronary artery blood flow, altered preload and afterload, increased atherosclerotic plaques	Hypertension, ischemic heart disease, heart failure, cardiac dysrhythmia, valvular heart disease, peripheral vascular disease, varicose veins, dehydration, stroke/transient ischemic attack
Neurologic/behavioral	Decreased speed of neural conduction, decreased number of brain cells, decreased neurotransmitters, decreased rapid eye movement sleep, decreased cerebral circulation	Parkinsonism, essential tremor, Alzheimer's disease or dementia, depression, anxiety, psychosis or paranoid state, sleep disturbance, subdural hematoma, trigeminal neuralgia
Respiratory	Increased rigidity of thoracic cage, decreased elasticity, decreased vital capacity, increased residual volume, decreased cough efficiency, decreased ciliary action	Pneumonia, chronic obstructive pulmonary disease, dyspnea
Gastrointestinal	Decreased secretion of gastric acid, delayed gastric emptying, decreased gastrointestinal motility, altered nutrient digestion, altered bowel function, weakening of lower esophageal sphincter	Diverticula or diverticulitis, constipation, diarrhea, gastroesophageal reflux or hiatus hernia, fecal incontinence, colorectal cancer, rectal prolapse, dysphagia, anorexia, gallbladder disease
Genitourinary	Decreased bladder capacity, decreased concentrating and diluting abilities, decreased creatinine clearance, increased prostate size	Renal insufficiency, urinary incontinence, urinary tract infection, enlarged prostate or prostate cancer, sexual dysfunction
Endocrine/metabolic	Decreased basal metabolism, altered pancreatic function, decreased testosterone, estrogen, progesterone	Diabetes mellitus, hyperthyroidism or hypothyroidism, thyroid cancer, hypercalcemia or hypocalcemia, hyperlipidemia, hypokalemia, hyponatremia, gout
Musculoskeletal	Decreased bone density, decreased muscle size and strength, degenerated joint cartilage	Paget's disease, osteoporosis, osteomalacia, rheumatoid arthritis, osteoarthritis, polymyalgia rheumatica, spondylosis, fractures, foot pathology, gait disturbance, falls
Autonomic nervous system	Decreased reaction time and coordination, decreased temperature regulation, decreased sensitivity of baroreceptors	Falls, accidental injuries, orthostatic hypotension, impaired body temperature regulation
Hematologic and immune	Decreased erythropoietin production, decreased intrinsic factor, decreased functioning T and B cells and monocytes	Iron deficiency anemia, pernicious anemia, anemia of chronic disease, cancer, autoimmune disorders
Oral	Decreased salivary secretion, decreased oral motor apparatus, loss of teeth	Periodontal disease; problems with speech, chewing, and swallowing
Sensory	Decreased accommodation, decreased visual acuity, decreased hearing of high-pitched frequencies	Visual impairment, hearing impairment, diminished smell or taste
Dermatologic	Decreased elasticity, decreased secretion of natural oil and perspiration, thinning of skin, decreased heat regulation, decreased epidermal renewal, decreased inflammatory response	Pressure sores, basal cell and squamous carcinoma, herpes zoster, seborrheic and actinic keratosis, stasis dermatitis, pruritus, hypothermia or hyperthermia
Reproductive	Female: vaginal mucosa thinning, atrophy, decreased breast tissue, sexual dysfunction Male: decreased sexual desire	Female: cervical cancer, breast cancer Male: prostate cancer, impotence

Socioeconomic factors can contribute to malnutrition. With reduced income, some elders may restrict food intake to near-starvation levels because they may choose to pay rent and buy medicine over spending for food. Diets may be unbalanced because of the expense of fresh fruits, vegetables, and meats. Lack of transportation and the inability to carry heavy quantities of groceries can prohibit some people from obtaining food. Living alone can also be associated with poor nutrition, since many older adults may lose the motivation to prepare a balanced diet for just themselves.

Psychologically, depression and stress can affect nutritional status. Both conditions can lead to overeating or undereating. Medications can influence nutrition, producing side effects of increased or decreased appetite, constipation, nausea, or decreased absorption. Additionally, drugs such as diuretics can affect fluid and electrolyte balance, leading to problems with dehydration and constipation.

Physiologically, energy requirements lessen with age because of a decline in basal metabolic rate and often a reduction in physical activity. There is an increased need for vitamin D, vitamin B_6, and calcium to protect against osteoporosis. Increased fiber intake is recommended to reduce the apparent risk of some forms of cancer and to promote bowel function. Unexplained weight loss of more than 5% in 1 month or more than 10% in 6 months is cause for concern. Clients at risk for nutritional problems should be identified (Box 3–1; see also Chapter 28). When no physical cause can be identified, elders with altered nutrition should be referred to community resources for assessment and assistance related to food, finances, and dental care.

Stress Management

Any real or perceived threat to one's physical, emotional, and social well-being can create stress (see Chapters 1 and 2). Life's later years can include changes such as acute or chronic illness, retirement, death of significant others, financial hardship, or relocation resulting in stress that can be overwhelming. Although the sources of stress may vary, the physiologic outcomes are similar. Stimulation of the sympathetic nervous system results in the release of epinephrine, norepinephrine, and adrenal glucocorticoids. Prolonged stress can result in serious consequences, including heart disease, hypertension, cerebrovascular accident, cancer, gastric ulcers, skin problems, complications of underlying disorders, and numerous social and emotional problems.

The way in which an older person adapts to change and stress is influenced by personality traits, past coping strategies, and spirituality. Spirituality extends beyond religion to include contemplation, experiential learning, recognition through growth, discovery and acceptance, new connections, and letting go. Growth, self-discovery, and connecting with others support older people in times of stress, reinforce a sense of self-worth, and provide confidence to overcome obstacles.

Encourage the client to respond to stress in a healthy manner. Balancing nutrition, rest, and exercise, remaining connected with others, and having a sense of inner peace help with stress management. Explain methods of relaxation, including biofeedback, meditation, progressive relaxation, breathing control exercises, physical activity, and involvement in pastimes that provide respite from stressful demands should also be emphasized (see Chapters 1 and 2).

Teaching

Encouraging health promotion and disease prevention among elders requires effective teaching. Teaching elders is similar to teaching members of any age group, in that individual characteristics and learning needs must be considered. General guidelines for teaching older adults are listed in Box 3–2.

BOX 3–1   Risk Factors for Malnutrition in the Elderly Population

*D*isease
*E*ating poorly
*T*ooth decay or oral pain
*E*conomic hardship
*R*educed social contact
*M*ultiple medications
*I*nvoluntary weight loss or gain
*N*eeds assistance with self-care
*E*lder older than 80 years

From the Nutrition Screening Initiative in conjunction with the American Academy of Family Physicians, the American Dietetic Association, and the National Council on the Aging.

BOX 3–2   Guidelines for Effectively Teaching Older Adults

Vision
1. Provide large, easy-to-read typeface
2. Emphasize contrasting colors: black and white
3. Avoid blues and greens
4. Use nonglare paper
5. Write short, simple paragraphs
6. Make sure eyeglasses are in place and clean

Hearing
1. Speak slowly
2. Enunciate clearly
3. Lower the pitch of your voice
4. Eliminate background noise
5. Face the learner
6. Use nonverbal cues
7. Make sure client's hearing aid is in place and working properly

Energy Level/Attention
1. Use short teaching sessions
2. Offer liquid refreshment and bathroom breaks
3. Promote comfort

Information Processing and Memory
1. Present most important information first
2. Clarify information with use of examples that the client can relate to
3. Motor skills: Teach one step at a time, demonstrate, allow for return demonstration
4. Encourage association between items
5. Be concrete and specific
6. Eliminate distractions
7. Encourage verbal interactions
8. Correct wrong answers and reinforce correct answers
9. Offer praise and encouragement

NORMAL AGING AND COMMONLY OCCURRING PATHOLOGIC PROCESSES

Aging has been defined as a universal, internally predictable biologic process following maturity. It is characterized by changes accumulated over time that increase susceptibility to disease and ultimately lead to death. Physiologically, aging in the absence of disease involves a steady decline in the functional reserve of organ systems and homeostatic controls, especially when a person is under stress. In addition to disease, nutritional status and other extrinsic factors (i.e., environment, activity, medication, depression) are superimposed on the basic process of aging and create individual differences in how one experiences aging.

PRESENTATION OF ILLNESS

With advanced age, the body does not respond as vigorously to illness or disease because of diminished physiologic reserve. People often attribute discomforts to "old age" and accept the changes as inevitable, thus failing or refusing to seek help for potentially treatable conditions. A frequent complicating factor in identifying and treating disease in older people is the presence of multiple ailments. The number of pathologic conditions that a person has at one time is strongly correlated with age.[14] The presenting picture may be further complicated by atypical or altered presentation of disease (i.e., weakness, weight loss, confusion, or failure to thrive). Each of these factors presents a challenge; conduct careful and thorough assessments and analyses of manifestations to promote appropriate treatment.

Atypical or altered presentation of disease can be displayed in various ways. For example, an older adult with pneumonia may exhibit confusion, have an increased respiratory rate, and generalized weakness instead of the classic symptoms of productive cough, fever, and chest pain. Frequently, manifestations in one organ system may cause abnormality in another system. This results in manifestations unrelated to the actual problem, such as confusion accompanying a urinary tract infection. Chronic conditions can mask the presence of acute illness. This can be seen in new-onset heart failure, when orthopnea might be hidden if a person regularly uses multiple pillows because of gastroesophageal reflux, arthritis, or obesity.

Finally, expected manifestations may not be present at all, as in the case of a myocardial infarction unaccompanied by chest pain. Table 3–2 summarizes common structural and functional changes associated with normal aging and presents common diseases, disorders, and injuries frequently seen in older adults. Risk factors for many chronic diseases in old age are manifested in early-to-middle adulthood (see Chapters 45, 52, 61, and 70). Increasing age and chronic disease, functional disabilities, and hospitalization intensify the demand and need for health care services. This has implications in any health care setting.

FUNCTIONAL STATUS

Assessment of functional status of the older adult is important when one is considering the client's level of inde-

pendence within the environment. Assess basic and instrumental activities of daily living, balance and mobility, cognitive abilities, vision and hearing, bowel and bladder function, nutritional status, and environmental factors. Research has found that functional impairments (both physical and psychosocial) are reliable early indicators of active illness in older people.[5, 10]

Basic activities of daily living (BADL) are the essential activities and tasks performed to get through the day. BADL can be remembered by the mnemonic DEATH: *d*ressing, *e*ating, *a*mbulating, *t*oileting, and *h*ygiene. BADL assessment helps to determine the need for daily personal care and to plan long-term care. There is a corresponding rise in functional dependency related to BADL with increasing age (Fig. 3–4).[28]

Instrumental activities of daily living (IADL) are more complex and are essential to community living situations. IADL include all the daily activities of BADL and SHAFT (*s*hopping, *h*ousework, *a*ccounting (managing money), *f*ood preparation, and *t*ransportation. Evaluation of IADL is used to decide what type of assistance is needed by people in independent or semi-independent settings. The ability to perform IADL is less important in institutional settings than in community settings, although the assessment can prove important for discharge planning when the client is returning to the home environment.

Upon completion of a functional assessment, the individual's problems can be categorized as "functional," "medical," or "support" issues, and a management plan

FIGURE 3–4 Use of a grabber to retrieve a dropped object from the floor.

can be developed. This plan may include coordination of environmental changes, facilitation for the use of assistive devices (Figs. 3–5 and 3–6), and arrangements for community referrals (Table 3–3) for services that would allow the person to remain in the chosen environment.

Functional assessment instruments generally include scales for measuring BADL and IADL. The Barthel,[21] Katz,[17] and Older Americans Resources and Services (OARS) indexes[16] are commonly used. Observation, interview, mental status screening,[12] and a screen for depression can assess psychosocial functioning. These provide information about cognitive functioning, perceptual-motor skills, insight, reasoning, and contact with reality. Chapters 9 and 67 describe mental status assessment.

■ PHYSIOLOGIC FACTORS THAT INFLUENCE FUNCTIONAL STATUS

Sleep

Older adults fall asleep with more difficulty, awaken more readily and more frequently, spend more time in the drowsiness stage, and spend less time in deep sleep than do younger adults.[34] Functionally, these changes have little impact on the daily life of the older adult. However,

FIGURE 3–6 A sock slide allows a person to put on socks independently.

adverse reactions can occur when these changes coincide with illness, stress, daily demands, or certain medications, such as hypnotic, antidepressant, diuretic, and some antihypertensive medications. Sleep disorders and their treatment are discussed in Chapter 21.

Sensory Impairments

Normal aging results in some sensory impairment (see Table 3–2). Vision and hearing are senses that individuals rely on to communicate and to function in the environment. Sensory impairments can affect safety, communication with others, performance of daily activities, and quality of life. Assessment suggests that limitations in ADL are more likely to occur in older people with sensory impairments than in those without sensory loss. Vision changes can affect the performance of a variety of daily activities: driving a vehicle; shopping for groceries; negotiating stairs; maneuvering safely in dark or unfamiliar environments; seeing markings on clocks, radios, thermostats, appliances, and televisions; and reading newspapers, signs, directories, and labels on food items and medication containers. Besides influencing daily activities, impaired vision increases the risk of falling. Impairments and treatment for vision and hearing disorders are discussed in Chapters 65 and 66.

FIGURE 3–5 An electric recliner lifts a person from a sitting to standing position or assists in lowering a person from a standing to sitting position.

Mobility and Balance

Mobility is essential for maintaining independence. Serious consequences occur when mobility declines. Older

TABLE 3-3	CONTINUUM OF CARE: COMMUNITY RESOURCES, SERVICES, AND HOUSING OPTIONS*			

Functional Level of Care	Nursing Functions	Services Needed		Living and Housing Options
		In the Home	*In the Community*	
Older adults of all functional levels	Support individual in achieving highest level of autonomy possible in situation. Provide health surveillance. Identify health, social, spiritual, and economic need. Make clients and families aware of options and resources		Support groups (e.g., for illness or bereavement). Advocacy services. Outpatient nurse-run clinics. Mental health clinics. Private physicians	
Older adults who are functionally independent	Assist client and family to modify patterns detrimental to health. Evaluate deviations from normal and advise clients of appropriate action. Identify existing or impending illness. Educate clients regarding self-responsibility for health	Gatekeepers	All of the above, *plus:* Senior centers Meal sites	Own home Retirement community House-sharing
Older adults who need some help with IADL	Teach clients and families. Consult and collaborate with agencies and multiprofessional representatives. Provide appropriate information to clients and families about treatment plan, medications, and diagnosis in collaboration with physician	Chore services Housekeeping Escort Transportation Emergency response system Home modifications Home-delivered meals Friendly visitors Telephone reassurance Gatekeepers	All of the above, *plus:* Adult day care Case management Respite care Outpatient rehabilitation	Retirement community Assisted-living facilities Congregate or shared housing Sheltered living Family care homes
Older adults who need help with IADL and BADL	Promote health through clinic and home contact. Provide appropriate resources. Counsel clients and family members	All of the above, *plus:* Personal care services Home health aides Public health nurse Respite care at home	All of the above	Assisted-living facilities Sheltered living
Older adults who need help with most IADL and BADL	Give treatments, medications, and rehabilitative exercises. Observe and evaluate response to treatment and medication	All of the above	All of the above, *plus:* Adult day care Case management	Nursing homes
Older adults who are acutely ill, need rehabilitation, or are dying	Keep physician aware of changes in client's conditions. Ensure adequate medical, dental, and podiatric care. Maintain hydration, nutrition, aeration, and pain management. Provide emotional support	All of the above, *plus:* Visiting nurse Visiting rehabilitation therapist Hospice care at home	Case management	Hospitals Rehabilitation facilities Nursing homes

*Availability of resources and services varies from community to community.
IADL, instrumental activities of daily living; BADL, basic activities of daily living.

people use mobility and balance to assess whether they are in relatively good or poor health. At least half of older adults have some limitation in function that prevents them from being fully independent.

Mobility depends on the ability to maintain balance and strength. Decreased functioning of various body systems can affect balance and strength and may place the person at risk. Decreases in functional status can be caused by impaired sensory ability (vision and hearing), cardiopulmonary disorders (dysrhythmia, postural hypotension, chronic obstructive pulmonary disease), neurologic disorders (parkinsonism and problems that affect gait, balance, sway, and reaction time), and depression. Side effects from medications also increase risk. The side effects of hypovolemia, postural hypotension, excessive sedation, decreased cognitive functioning, and loss of postural control can negatively affect mobility and balance.[35] Chronic disorders that increase with age and affect functional ability include osteoporosis, osteoarthritis, and rheumatoid arthritis (see Chapters 26 and 77).

Unstable balance is of concern because the risk of falling increases with age. Falls occur in 32% of 65- to 74-year-olds, 35% of 75- to 84-year-olds and 51% of those aged 85 years and older.[35] In hospitals, falls make up the largest category of reported incidents.

The effect of falls in the elderly is far-reaching. Falls contribute to significant morbidity and mortality.[35] Consequences of falls consume a large portion of health care dollars in the United States, and fear of subsequent falls contributes to restricted activity and mobility and to reduced independence. This self-restriction contributes to functional decreases and social isolation, thus setting up a spiral of downward decline. Up to 40% of all nursing home admissions are related to falls and instability.[35]

■ PSYCHOSOCIAL FACTORS THAT INFLUENCE FUNCTIONAL STATUS

Although physiologic changes and chronic illnesses associated with aging may affect functional abilities, psychosocial changes are often the most challenging and demanding. Some challenges arise from physical changes, but many are caused by changes in roles, relationships, and living environments. These changes tax coping abilities and energies.

Ageism

"Ageism" refers to the prejudices and stereotypes applied to older people purely because of their age. Ageism, like racism and sexism, is a way of labeling a group of people and not allowing them to be individuals with unique ways of living. Prejudice toward the elderly is often an attempt by younger generations to shield themselves from their own eventual aging and death. Such stereotyping allows younger individuals to see older people as different from themselves, and they ultimately cease to identify with older people as human beings. An awakening comes when these younger people age and find themselves the victims of the same stereotypes and attitudes.

The significance of ageism is considerable. Ageism can affect a person's self-confidence, disempower by limiting potential, and cause early or excessive dependency. It can also affect well-being by influencing the attitudes of health care providers and political powers. Typically, diagnosis and treatment of disease in the elderly are less aggressive; programs are generally underfunded; and the ability of older people to remain a contributing force, as perceived by society, is reduced simply because of chronological age.[10]

Negativism can have a devastating effect and cause the elder to adopt modes of dependency, helplessness, and a negative self-image. This can lead to increased vulnerability to biopsychosocial stressors.[32] Images of older persons as being dependent, deteriorating beyond rehabilitative efforts, and being physically and mentally unappealing can lead to reluctance among professionals to care for them. This can result in carelessness about the quality of care delivered. However, each elderly person has potential for rehabilitation, treatment, self-actualization, or improvement in quality of life and well-being, regardless of how small that potential may be.

Multiple Losses

Many losses inevitably occur in later life. Assessing the impact of the losses and supporting the elder are major goals. Aging persons experience personal, social, and economic losses. Among the most devastating are "people" losses—parents, friends, spouse, or children (Fig. 3–7). Other typical losses may include loss of one's home, possessions, pets, employment, social position, or financial security. An "overload" state can result when losses become multiple; the emotional upheaval becomes a catalyst, and the result is mental confusion, withdrawal, helplessness, and depression.

King and coworkers[18] examined the loss of one's traditional dwelling and the effect of relocation. Central to the reaction and adjustment to relocation was whether the move was voluntary or involuntary. Individuals at high risk for poor relocation adjustment have low self-esteem, no friends or support, many worries, high levels of alienation, poor self-perception of health, and depression. Interventions to help with relocation include assessing for risk factors, empathizing with the difficulties of the move,

FIGURE 3–7 Loss of loved ones may result in an emotional burden accompanied by mental and physical effects.

■ THE OLDER CLIENT AT RISK FOR RELOCATION STRESS SYNDROME

Nursing Diagnosis. Risk for Relocation Stress Syndrome related to changes associated with health care facility transfer or admission to long-term care facility as evidenced by anxiety, insecurity, and changes in health status.

Outcomes. (1) Resident will verbalize feelings, expectations, and disappointments with staff and/or family. (2) Resident will react in a positive manner to staff efforts to assist in adjustment to new facility. (3) Resident will socialize with staff and/or other residents. (4) Resident will maintain stable preadmission weight, appetite, and sleep patterns.

Interventions	Rationales
1. Assess for low self-esteem, anxiety, feeling of insecurity, and disorientation related to move.	1. These are risk factors associated with poor adjustment to relocation.
2. Assess resident's current health status, medications, and needs for additional health services after move.	2. Provides a current baseline of health status and opportunity to review medication, chronic health conditions, and need for additional services.
3. Encourage resident to express emotions associated with the relocation.	3. Allowing resident to express emotions provides an opportunity to correct misconceptions, answer questions, and reduce anxiety.
4. Assist resident and family to prepare for the move by providing information, arranging a visit to the new facility, and introducing them to the new staff if possible.	4. Allows the resident and family to become familiar with the new environment and reduce the stress of relocation.
5. Educate family members about relocation stress syndrome and its potential effects.	5. Family needs to know that family member may exhibit anxiety and other stress-related symptoms and that visiting and providing emotional support during transition period are helpful.
6. Communicate all aspects of the resident's care plan to appropriate staff members at the new location.	6. Communication with staff allows for continuity of care and reduces stress for the resident.

Evaluation. Accomplishment of expected outcomes may require considerable time. Reassessment and revision of plan are important.

and suggesting positive resources to effectively cope. The accompanying Care Plan offers additional information. Adjustment to loss is a challenge at any age. For older adults, resolution of grief loss may not always be achieved but can be integrated into their lives without causing dysfunction.

Neglect and Abuse

Neglect and abuse are complex, serious issues affecting older adults. Research suggests that *elder abuse* is widespread. It occurs among all subgroups of the population and affects up to two million older people a year. Elder abuse encompasses physical, psychological, and financial abuse or neglect by oneself or by a caregiver. It is not uncommon for adults to experience several types of abuse simultaneously. Without intervention, abuse tends to escalate. See Bridge to Home Health Care: Detecting Elder Abuse.

The typical abuse victim is a woman of advanced age with few social contacts, who has a history of mental illness, cognitive impairment, and poor health. These factors often limit her ability to perform BADL. In addition, she frequently lives alone or with the abuser and depends on the abuser for care.[2, 38]

Elder abuse has emerged as a significant aspect of family violence for several reasons. One is the increased number of older adults. As more people live to an advanced age, more adult children are assuming the caregiver role. If the adult child is unprepared for this responsibility, abuse and neglect may occur. Because an older person's dependency needs increase with time, the stress and burden of caregiving also increase, thus raising the risk of abuse. It is the responsibility of the health care provider, both ethically and legally, to be aware of the obvious and subtle signs of abuse and neglect. As a client

advocate, encourage and coordinate assistance for victims and abusers. The passage of elder abuse and adult protective services laws has led to increased reporting of mistreatment and self-neglect. This has resulted in greater recognition of the problem.

MENTAL HEALTH DISORDERS IN THE ELDERLY

■ DEMENTIA, DELIRIUM, AND DEPRESSION

Dementia (specifically Alzheimer's disease) and delirium (also known as "confusion") are discussed in Chapter 72 along with their pathophysiology, clinical manifestations, assessment, and management. The focus here is on three important conditions in the elderly: dementia, delirium, and depression. Clinically, the presenting manifestations of these conditions in older clients can be very similar. A differential diagnosis is essential.

Disorders associated with cognitive decline are among the most common and frightening problems faced by the elderly. A common myth is that older adults inevitably experience cognitive decline as a consequence of aging. Serious difficulties with thinking clearly and remembering are abnormal consequences at any age and are manifestations of medical illness or altered psychosocial well-being.[29]

The stereotypical view that cognitive decline is a normal part of aging prevails. For this reason, an acute deterioration in cognition is frequently overlooked; undetected cases of cognitive disorders have ranged from 16% to 72%.[13] Because many older adults believe that cognitive decline is part of aging, they do not seek medical attention when they notice changes in processing stimuli

---

BRIDGE TO HOME HEALTH CARE

Detecting Elder Abuse

In the home care setting, factors beyond the physical condition of the client—such as the environment of care, relationships, and support systems—are crucial to the achievement of positive outcomes. This is especially true when abuse of a client is suspected. When you suspect abuse, you must incorporate the client, family, and caregiver into your total assessment and care plan.

When providing home care, listen carefully to the client and observe overt and covert behaviors. In addition to completing a history and physical assessment related to the client's current condition, confirm the caregiver's report of the client's condition. For example, if the caregiver attributes bruises to a fall, determine whether gait instability is consistent with the client's condition.

It may be difficult for a client to admit that a caregiver is abusive. Many times, abusive caregivers provide assistance with activities of daily living (ADL), financial assistance, or emotional support, which allows the client to continue to live in the community.

Situations can appear to indicate abuse when, in real-

ity, a caregiver is simply uninformed about providing care. Inform the client and family about nutrition, transfers, ambulation, and positioning so that caregivers can adequately meet the needs of clients. In addition, the frustration of providing care can contribute to abuse. Encourage caregivers to arrange for regular absences from care.

When you suspect abuse, a multidisciplinary plan of care is essential. Inform the physician of the situation and of any clinical manifestations. A social worker can coordinate family counseling, make referrals to community resources, and facilitate day care. Homemakers and home health aides can help to relieve the burden of care. Volunteers can provide respite for the caregiver. In most states, reporting abuse is mandatory for health care professionals; contact the local Adult Protection Service department for investigation of suspected abusive situations.

Do not be reluctant to confront suspicious situations for fear of jeopardizing rapport with the client and family. Although maintaining a relationship is important, client safety and advocacy are your first priorities.

Bridget A. Young, RN, BSN, MBA, Vice President of Clinical Services, Visiting Nurse Association of Omaha, Omaha, Nebraska or in responding to stressful life events. Family members may react to acute cognitive changes as the "beginning of the end" and may prematurely plan for alternative living arrangements and entertain other actions and thoughts that may be unnecessary.[3]

Dementia

Dementia is a clinical syndrome characterized by severe intellectual deterioration that interferes with one's ability to cope with daily life. It is gradually progressive and *irreversible*. Deficits occur in memory, language, perception, praxis, learning, problem-solving, abstract thinking, and judgment. Approximately 3% of people 65 to 74 years of age have dementia; the prevalence increases to 47.2% for those older than 85 years.[32] Dementia can be *primary*, as with Alzheimer's disease, multi-infarct dementia, alcoholism, and Pick's disease, or *secondary* to other causes, as with Parkinson's disease and trauma. Causes of dementia can vary, but the clinical presentation is similar regardless of cause. Therefore, the descriptive term *dementia of Alzheimer's type* (DAT) is generally used.

Before a diagnosis of dementia is made, all potential physical and psychosocial causes of cognitive decline should be ruled out. The onset and progressive nature of the cognitive decline should be documented, and serial neuropsychological testing should be performed. The diagnosis can be complicated when delirium, depression, or both are superimposed on dementia.

Delirium

Delirium is a syndrome characterized by global cognitive impairment of abrupt onset that is *reversible*. This condition becomes irreversible only if underlying causes are undetected or treated unsuccessfully. Delirium is also known as acute confusion, reversible dementia, pseudosenility, acute brain failure, and clouded state. Attention deficits are the most salient feature of delirium. Other diagnostic criteria include disorganized thinking, reduced level of consciousness, perceptual disturbances, disturbances of the sleep-wake cycle, increased or decreased psychomotor activity, disorientation, and memory impairment.

Delirium is one of the most prevalent cognitive disorders among hospitalized older clients. It is associated with higher mortality, prolonged hospital stays, a greater nursing time than necessary for the admitting diagnosis, and a higher rate of nursing home placement.[6, 23] Delirium is often the presenting manifestation of physical illness in an older person, exceeding the indicators of fever, pain, and tachycardia. It has been associated with a variety of conditions, especially adverse drug reactions, metabolic disorders (e.g., electrolyte disorders, renal failure, respiratory failure, and endocrinopathies), cardiac failure, cerebrovascular disorders, infection (especially pulmonary, renal, or neurologic), anemia, and surgery. Psychosocial factors can also cause or contribute to a delirious state; these include bereavement, relocation, and sensory deprivation or overstimulation.

The key to differentiating delirium from dementia is the assessment of the onset of the cognitive manifestations. Onset of delirium is rapid, occurring within hours to days; dementia onset is slower and more gradual. It is imperative that reversible delirium not be classified as dementia. A comprehensive investigation of all possible physical and psychosocial factors that might cause altered cognition must be conducted.

Depression

Research suggests that significant manifestations of depression occur in approximately 10% to 15% of all community-dwelling elders over 65 years; among institutionalized elders, the prevalence rate increases to 50% to 75%.[32] Depression is a complex syndrome that manifests itself in a variety of ways in older people. The most common manifestations are *vegetative*, which include insomnia, fatigue, weight loss, constipation, preoccupation with physical health, and thoughts of death. Elders suffering from depression may also exhibit sadness, crying, anxiety, irritability, or paranoia.

Depression can also lead to cognitive impairment. It is estimated that depression-associated cognitive disorders occur in 10% to 29% of depressed elderly clients.[29] Therefore, differentiation between depression-related cognitive alteration and dementia may be difficult. Depressed clients often look and act demented, and they perform poorly on mental status tests; however, the vegetative signs of depression are not usually seen in demented people. Features supporting a diagnosis of depression versus dementia include recent onset of depressive symptoms and inconsistencies with actual functional performance and cognitive testing. Table 3–4 contrasts the primary clinical features of delirium, dementia, and depression.

Treatment Strategies

Several strategies are used to help older clients who have dementia, delirium, or depression. Four strategies are commonly used by gerontological nurses: (1) reality orientation, (2) validation therapy, (3) remotivation therapy, and (4) reminiscence therapy. Treatment modalities and their specific application are described in gerontological nursing and psychiatric literature.[10]

■ SUBSTANCE USE DISORDERS

Substance use disorders refer to ingestion of any compound in quantities that may be harmful to health or well-being. This includes overindulgence in legal drugs, alcohol, nicotine, caffeine, nonprescription over-the-counter (OTC) drugs and preparations, prescription drugs, controlled drugs (e.g., meperidine or codeine), and illegal drugs (see Chapter 24). Dependence on alcohol, nicotine, and prescription and OTC drugs is far more common among the elderly population than is generally thought. The addictive experience includes alterations in mood and sensation, immediate gratification, and enhanced sense of control and power. These are elements that may be missing in the lives of some elders.

As many as 15% of community-dwelling elders and 18% to 44% of hospitalized elders have serious problems

TABLE 3–4	COMMON MENTAL HEALTH DISORDERS IN THE ELDERLY: CLINICAL FEATURES		
	Delirium	**Dementia**	**Depression**
DESCRIPTION	A reversible, acute confusional state	A gradually progressive, irreversible cognitive decline	A reversible affective feeling associated with sadness, which may vary from mild downheartedness or a feeling of indifference to a feeling of great despair beyond hope
ONSET	Rapid, acute, often at night	Slow, gradual	Gradual or sudden
DURATION	Days to weeks, but usually less than 1 month	Continuous, ongoing, months to years	Varies from weeks to years
DISORIENTATION	Present, especially for time; tendency to mistake unfamiliar for familiar persons, place	May be absent in mild states of dementia	May seem disoriented to place or time
THINKING	Slow or accelerated; may be dream-like, impoverished	Impoverished; poor abstracting ability	Slowed thinking, indecisiveness
MEMORY	Short-term memory impaired; long-term memory intact	Short-term memory impaired; long-term memory may be affected	May seem impaired for recent and remote events
ATTENTION	Consistently impaired; easily distracted; fluctuates	Typically intact	Complaints or evidence of diminished ability to concentrate
ALERTNESS	Reduced or increased, but awareness always affected	Typically normal; may be reduced	Psychomotor agitation or retardation
PERCEPTION	Invariably affected, especially at night; often have hallucinations	May be intact; usually no hallucinations	May have auditory hallucinations
SLEEP	Sleep-wake cycle altered	Usually normal for age	Insomnia or hypersomnia
COURSE	Typically fluctuates with lucid intervals and exacerbations	Relatively stable over course of a day	Usually rapid progression
AFFECT	Intermittent fear, perplexity, bewilderment	Flat or indifferent	Sad, worried, anxious, hopeless; may show agitation or apathy
CAUSE	Multiple potential causes (e.g., surgery, infection, drugs)	Unknown, possible environmental, hereditary, chemical	Secondary to other mental illness; related to loss, physical illness, medications, loneliness

Data from American Psychiatric Association. (1994). *Diagnostic and statistical manual of mental disorders* (4th ed.). Washington, DC: Author.

related to alcohol use.[40] Alcohol abusers can be divided into two types: (1) long-term and (2) recent-onset. Long-term drinkers who live to old age can be called survivors. They may be at risk for serious medical problems and generally have alienated their families and social support systems.

Drinkers who have a relatively recent onset of problems with alcohol may be reacting to some event, such as loss of a loved one, or they may have general negative feelings, such as helplessness or depression stemming from role losses in later life.[40] The recent-onset alcohol abuser is more successful in substance abuse treatment than the long-term abuser. Learning new coping skills and increasing socialization often help the recent-onset drinker to overcome problems.

Older individuals who drink are at risk for developing medical, relationship, and social problems. Medical problems include:

- Liver and pancreatic disease
- Gastrointestinal problems (gastritis, ulcers and hemorrhage, malnutrition, nausea and vomiting, electrolyte disturbance, dehydration, hypoglycemia)
- Central nervous system damage
- Cognitive changes of impairment and confusion
- Cardiac problems (cardiomyopathy, dysrhythmia, systolic hypertension, peripheral edema)
- Injuries and accidents because of decreased tolerance to alcohol and the normal changes in dexterity, balance, and proprioception associated with aging

Psychosocially, these people may have alienated family and friends, exhausted their funds, and estranged themselves from health care and social service providers.[40]

It is difficult to determine the extent of prescription drug abuse by older people. Researchers contend that thousands of older Americans are "hooked" on their prescription drugs in an "inadvertent addiction."[27] The cycle of addiction usually begins benignly with a medication or a drink for pain or anxiety. Physicians often are unaware of the problem, and they may also be unaware of the number of medications that a client may be taking because the prescriptions may be issued by several different physicians.

MEDICATION USE IN THE ELDERLY

In the United States, adults age 65 years and over consume 30% of all prescription medications and 40% to 50% of all OTC medications.[10, 33] Elders who live in long-term care facilities typically take four to seven different medications,[32] or approximately 4.5 medications at any one time. Among Medicare beneficiaries who rate their health as poor, an average of 31 prescriptions per year is reported. Of community-dwelling elders, 90% took an average of three OTC and five prescription drugs daily (Fig. 3–8). See Bridge to Home Health Care: Managing Multiple Medications.

The most commonly prescribed and used drugs are cardiovascular, anti-infective, antipsychotic, antidepressant, and diuretic agents.[9, 33] Analgesics, laxatives, and antacids are the most frequently used OTC drugs. The trend of multiple drug use will continue as more sophisticated drug therapies are developed. When used properly,

drugs can be beneficial; when used inappropriately, they threaten one's functional abilities and health.

■ PHARMACOKINETICS

Age-related changes affect a medication's pharmacokinetics, or how the body handles the drug. The term includes (1) absorption of the medication into the systemic circulation, (2) distribution of the drug to the tissues, (3) metabolism (breakdown) of the medication, and (4) elimination (removal) of the drug from the body.

Absorption refers to the movement of a drug from the site of administration into the circulation. Absorption is not greatly affected by age, but the rate of absorption is. Age-related changes in stomach emptying, changes in gastric pH, gastrointestinal motility, and nutritional status may influence absorption rate.

Distribution is the movement of the drug throughout the body. This activity depends on the adequacy of the circulatory system and the ability of the drug to exit the circulation and enter the cell. Altered cardiac output and sluggish circulation can delay the arrival of medication at the target receptors. Age-related changes in body composition influence drug distribution. Total body water decreases with age and adipose tissue or fat content increases; the result can be higher than usual blood levels of water-soluble drugs and storage of lipid-soluble drugs in the fatty tissue. This can result in higher concentration of drug levels (toxicity), with less drug reaching the site

BRIDGE TO HOME HEALTH CARE

Managing Multiple Medications

Clients who take several medications often need help to understand the best procedures and follow instructions as closely as possible. Failure to take the right drug at the right time and in the proper way often results in relapses, rehospitalizations, or nursing home placement.

Nurses play a crucial role when they foster client independence and assess and facilitate the client's ability to follow a prescribed medication regimen. Review all prescription and nonprescription medications, and carefully explain the administration schedule to the client and family members. Tailoring the schedule to the client's lifestyle increases the likelihood that the instructions will be followed. For example, if the client goes to bed at 7:00 P.M., be sure that the last dose is scheduled at that hour.

Some people need minimal help with organizing their drugs and dosages. They may benefit from any number of compliance aids that can be purchased at pharmacies, such as containers with separate compartments for each day of the week. The challenge is greater when the client has a complex medication program; reduced strength and dexterity; or a visual, hearing, cognitive, or other impairment in functional status. These clients may need to purchase an automated medication dispenser that emits visual cues, such as flashing strobe lights, or audible cues, such as beeps. Dispensers that beep are ideal for people with visual impairments, whereas dispensers that flash a strobe light are good for people with hearing impairments.

Although units vary, an automated dispenser must be simple to use. One such dispenser can be programmed easily to provide a reminder at the right time for up to four times a day for a week. This dispenser helps the client manage complex schedules, is tamper-proof, and dispenses only the pills needed from a supply cassette in a removable drawer. Other automated dispensers have light-emitting diode (LED) screens on which preprogrammed messages, such as "Take with food" or "Take 30 minutes before food," serve as additional reminders.

Determine how and when the client will obtain refills. If the client has no transportation, a pharmacy may have a delivery service or a family member can obtain them. A social service referral is needed if the client cannot pay for prescriptions.

Monitor the client for side effects. Many people stop taking essential medications because of unpleasant side effects. Sometimes the client can manage this problem effectively by changing the times of doses or by taking the medication with food.

Instruct the client on drug storage. Some drugs are sensitive to light; others must be secured to decrease the risk of overdoses. All medications must be safely kept away from any children who visit or live in the household.

Simplicity is the key to successful medication management. Regularly evaluate the client's regimen and household routines, and discuss any changes that would make things easier with the client, family members, and physician.

Kaye M. Dietrich, RN,C, MS, *Consultant, Kiel, Wisconsin*

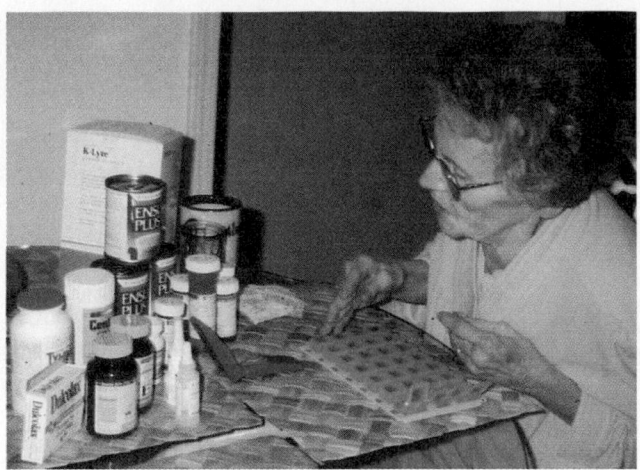

FIGURE 3–8 Use of a medication planner assists older people in managing multiple medications.

of action because of storage in the adipose tissue, thereby reducing the drug's effect.

Metabolism occurs primarily in the liver. There is an age-related decrease in liver size and blood flow, contributing to decreased hepatic clearance. As a result of this slowed metabolism, the drug remains in the body longer, with prolonged responses.

Elimination of the drug from the body occurs primarily through the renal system but also through bile, feces, sweat, and saliva. Age-related changes in renal function include reductions in renal blood flow, glomerular filtration rate, and tubular secretion. These changes affect both the duration and intensity of the drug responses in the body.

■ PHARMACODYNAMICS

Pharmacodynamics, or drug activity, refers to the actual effects of the drug in the body. An altered pharmacodynamic response is considered an adverse effect. An interaction occurs when drugs with similar actions or similar adverse effects are administered together. Drug interactions increase with age and the number of drugs taken. The interactive effect may be (1) additive, (2) synergistic, (3) antagonistic, or (4) potentiated. These effects can be beneficial or harmful. Nearly one third of elderly clients report adverse reactions to medications, accounting for as many as 10% of their hospitalizations.[10]

An *additive* effect occurs when two drugs with same or similar adverse effects are combined, resulting in a summative effect from the doses taken. The additive effects for an older person taking a diuretic (e.g., furosemide) for a cardiovascular disorder and an aminoglycoside antibiotic (e.g., tobramycin) for an infection can be adverse, resulting in increased damage to the organs of hearing and balance *(ototoxicity)* and to the kidneys *(nephrotoxicity)*.

A *synergistic* effect occurs when two drugs with or without the same effects are combined for an outcome that is greater than the sum of the individual drugs. The effect is greater than that seen in additive effects. Positive synergistic interaction is experienced when hypertension is treated with a diuretic (e.g., hydrochlorothiazide) and a beta-adrenergic blocker (e.g., atenolol). This combination lowers blood pressure better than either drug alone.

An *antagonistic* reaction occurs when the combined effect of two drugs is less than that of either active drug alone (the opposite of a synergistic effect). Often the addition of a second drug diminishes or eliminates the effect of the first. Protamine sulfate (an anticoagulant antagonist) is given as an antidote when a person is bleeding as a result of the anticoagulant action of heparin. The protamine binds with the heparin to form a stable compound with no anticoagulant effect. A thiazide diuretic can counter the hypoglycemic action of an antidiabetic medication.

Potentiation describes a synergistic effect in which the effect of only one of the two drugs is made greater by the presence of the second drug. When acetaminophen is given with codeine, the result is increased analgesia.

■ POLYPHARMACY

Polypharmacy, the use of large quantities of different drugs to relieve symptoms of illness or symptoms resulting from drug therapy, has become one of the major causes of *iatrogenic* (treatment-acquired) illness and complications in the elderly. The use of generic drugs or the substitution of OTC drugs compounds it. Polypharmacy occurs because of the multiple medications prescribed by different specialists for treating concurrent conditions, the beliefs and practices of older clients, and the use of multiple pharmacies for prescription filling.[34] Table 3–5 presents suggestions for helping elders to manage medication regimens.

HEALTH CARE FOR THE ELDERLY CLIENT

In the United States, older people historically did not use as many health care services as they do today. Before Medicare and Medicaid, only a small proportion of the federal budget went toward health care for older people, and government agencies paid little attention to their health and medical needs. Today, older people constitute the largest group of health care consumers, and it is projected that by the year 2040, they will account for 45% of health care expenditures.[39]

In this current period of health care reform, the political climate is one of change. Legislatures are looking for ways to reduce government spending. Government health insurance (Medicare) and government health assistance (Medicaid) programs will change, and these changes will have ramifications for all Americans.

■ RESOURCES, SERVICES, AND OPTIONS FOR OLDER PEOPLE

An outgrowth of gerontology has been development of programs and services designed to address the unique needs of older adults. These programs and services recognize that these adults have varied individual needs and health conditions that call for different service options at different stages of aging as the clients move along the health-illness continuum.

The continuum of care refers to services designed to provide diagnostic, preventive, therapeutic, rehabilitative, supportive, and maintenance care. These services can be

TABLE 3–5	HELPING OLDER CLIENTS TO MANAGE MEDICATION REGIMENS
Potential Problem	**Strategy**
Motivation	▪ Assess the client's understanding of need for medication and desire to take medication. Provide information as needed to promote informed decision-making
Knowledge deficit related to drug regimen	▪ Assess vision, hearing, comprehension, and best learning style ▪ Teach the client about medication's purpose, correct dosage, and administration instructions ▪ Identify common side effects for each drug. If side effects occur, advise what to do, what changes in administration to make, and when to notify the physician ▪ Reinforce information with written instructions when appropriate ▪ Include family members and other support persons in teaching sessions

Safety	▪ Assess for any over-the-counter drugs being used to avoid possible interaction effects; advise the client to avoid any over-the-counter drugs unless approved by the physician
	▪ Basic rules to teach the client:
	  ▪ Take only the amount of drug prescribed by the physician
	  ▪ Never take medication prescribed for someone else
	  ▪ Do not share medication with others
	  ▪ Dispose of outdated medications in a sink or toilet, never in the trash within reach of children
	  ▪ Keep drugs in the original, labeled container

Physiologic limitations ▪ Swallowing	▪ Assess need for liquids versus pills or thickened liquids for administration of drugs ▪ Discuss which drugs cannot be chewed or crushed
▪ Vision	▪ Larger label for medication bottles ▪ Color coding (e.g., red heart for heart medication) ▪ Braille labels where appropriate
▪ Memory impairment	▪ Memory aids include calendars; day, week, month pill containers; timers or voice mail reminders
▪ Fine motor coordination deficit	▪ Teach about availability and use of non-childproof caps and organization containers or any automated medication dispenser
Economic limitations	▪ Assess for transportation or monetary problems ▪ Use social services to identify community resources for financial assistance with pharmaceutical needs and transportation and delivery of medications
Information overload	▪ Keep the number of medications to a minimum, and keep instructions clear, concise, and simple

provided in a variety of institutional, non-institutional, and community health care settings. The continuum also includes an expanded variety of living arrangements. The goal behind the concept of continuum of care services is to ensure that clients have control over their environment by offering services that are supportive, preserve health, and counteract dependency. Table 3–3 presents a variety of available services to help people maintain independence and live in their chosen environment as long as possible.

The changing economy promotes structural changes in health care institutions that affect the continuum of care. Many institutions, facilities, and services are merging into integrated systems. An *integrated* system provides a seamless delivery of services and encompasses the entire range of health, community-based, and in-home services. Advantages of an integrated system include a single point of access and entry, assessment and coordination of appropriate care services, and assured quality of care in a cost-effective, time-efficient system.

In the United States, approximately 32 million people over age 65 years have a current or potential need for more assistance and support in their living environment.[10] These individuals frequently choose alternative living arrangements. The continuum of housing, or alternative living arrangements, offers choices to meet a variety of needs. Options include:

1. Retirement communities for the older person who is fully independent but wants socialization, security, emergency medical services, and some supplemental services without homeowner responsibilities.
2. Sheltered living environments (rest homes, family care homes, shared congregate housing), which provide minimal assistance with BADL in a family setting environment.
3. Nursing facilities (nursing homes, intermediate care, skilled care) for the person who needs long-term sheltered care and cannot function independently.

Intermediate care facilities (ICFs) do not provide round-the-clock professional nursing care but do provide medication and BADL assistance and safety supervision. *Skilled care facilities* (SNFs) provide care for a person requiring 24-hour observation and highly technical care of unstable medical conditions; this may include rehabilitative services. Nursing home facilities rarely have only intermediate or skilled care; there is usually a mixture of both types of services (see Table 3–3). Not all programs, services, and housing options are available in every community. Area agencies on aging or the American Associa-

tion of Homes and Services for the Aging can provide information about what is available in individual communities (Box 3–3).

■ MANAGED CARE

The way in which health care is delivered is changing. Among the major shifts taking place is the rapid growth

---

BOX 3–3　Aging Resources

Administration on Aging
330 Independence Ave., SW
Cohen Building, Room 4760
Washington, DC 20201
(202) 619-0556
http://www.aoa.dhhs.gov

Aging Network
http://www.mfaaa.org/agingnet.html

Alzheimer's Association
919 N. Michigan Ave.
Suite 1000
Chicago, IL 60657-1676
(312) 335-8870 or 1/800-272-3900
http://www.alz.org

American Association of Homes and Services for the Aging
901 E St. NW
Suite 500
Washington, DC 20004
(202) 783-2242
http://www.aahsa.org

American Association of Retired Persons
601 E Street NW
Washington, DC 20049
(202) 434-2277
http://www.aarp.org

American Geriatrics Society
770 Lexington Ave.
Suite 400
New York, NY 10021
(212) 308-1414
http://www.americangeriatrics.org

American Society on Aging
833 Market St.
Suite 511
San Francisco, CA 94103-1824
(415) 882-2910

Area Agencies on Aging
http://www.mfaaa.org/aging_aaa.html

Family Caregiver Alliance
425 Bush St.
Suite 500
San Francisco, CA 94108
(415) 434-3508
http://www.caregiver.org

Gerontological Society of America
1275 K St. NW
Suite 350
Washington, DC 20005-4006
(202) 842-1275
http://www.gsa.iog.wayne.edu

Gray Panthers
1424 16th St. NW
Suite 602
Washington, DC 20036
(202) 387-1111

Internet and e-mail Resources on Aging
http://www.aoa.dhhs.gov/aoa/pages/jpost1st.html

National Association of State Units on Aging
2033 K St. NW
Suite 304
Washington, DC 20006
(202) 785-0707
http://www.mfaaa.org/aging_state.html

National Citizen's Coalition for Nursing Home Reform
1424 16th St. NW
Suite 202
Washington, DC 20036
(202) 332-2275
http://www.aoa.dhhs.gov/aoa/dir/144.html

National Council on Aging
409 3rd St. SW
Suite 200
Washington, DC 20027
(202) 479-1200

National Council of Senior Citizens
1311 F St. NW
Suite 200
Washington, DC 20004-1174
(202) 347-8800
http://www.ncscinc.org

National Institute on Aging/National Institutes of Health
Federal Bldg. 31-C, Room 5C27
9000 Rockville Pike
Bethesda, MD 20892
http://www.senior.com/npolnia.html

National Senior Citizens Law Center
1815 H St. NW
Suite 700
Washington, DC 20006
(202) 887-5280

Older Women's League (OWL)
666 11th St. NW
Suite 700
Washington, DC 20001
(202) 783-6686
http://www.scn.org

of managed care. This transition represents a fundamental change. Managed care is a system that provides generalized structure and focus for overseeing the use, cost, quality, and effectiveness of health care services. The basic concept revolves around accountability and standardization of care for a given disorder or for a specific population. The increasing number of frail older persons with chronic disorders has resulted in pressure to move Medicare into a managed care system. The thrust of services will be to coordinate and integrate health services and resources in order to improve quality, to provide service flexibility, to contain cost, and to help the older person maintain function and independence as long as possible.

■ ACUTE CARE

Most nurses who care for older adults provide care in an inpatient hospital setting. This setting can be for an emergency or acute illness, such as a stroke or hip fracture (see Chapter 6). These facilities are driven by diagnosis-related group (DRG) assessment. DRGs determine the length of stay (LOS) according to the diagnosis. Medicare generally pays for most necessary and appropriate treatments, tests, and equipment after a deductible is met. Medicare provides for 150 days of hospitalization.

Hospitals are developing new ways of delivering care to older adults in order to improve both quality and efficiency. Some hospitals are establishing geriatric units with specially trained staff who work together as an interdisciplinary team. The team typically includes nurses, a geriatrician, a pharmacist, a social worker, various rehabilitation therapists (e.g., speech, physical, and occupational), and mental health professionals (e.g., psychologists or psychiatrists). These programs focus on helping older adults with complex problems to remain at their highest possible level of functioning. Geropsychiatric and geriatric rehabilitation programs are other models of hospital-based geriatric care that are evolving to address the unique needs of older people.

■ LONG-TERM CARE

Long-term care refers to a continuum of care that ranges from informal assistance provided by family and friends, to formal medical and supportive services provided in the home, to specialty facilities for rehabilitation, to care in a nursing home (see Chapter 8). Long-term care services assist those with chronic disabilities and decreasing health status to maintain their physical, social, and psychologic functioning. Traditionally, nursing home care has been synonymous with long-term care, but this is misleading. Many older persons with disabilities are as likely to receive long-term care at home as in a nursing home. Long-term care accounts for 25% of all health care expenditures for older persons.[10]

Specialty Facility

Rehabilitation centers are specialty facilities that provide intensive inpatient care to rehabilitate functional disabilities. The older individual must be able to tolerate 3 to 5 hours of intensive rehabilitation daily. The usual length of stay is 2 to 4 weeks, depending on evaluations. Medicare pays 80% of the costs.

Nursing Home Care

The close association between nursing home and long-term care arises from the late 1970s, when nursing homes were the primary (and usually the only) resource for people who needed long-term care. Nursing homes are licensed by the state, and most are certified for Medicare or Medicaid reimbursement. Round-the-clock care averages $38,000 annually for basic nursing home care. About 5% of the population 65 years and older are in nursing homes at any given time.[28]

People in this age group have a 50% chance of being in a nursing home at some point in their lives.[22] Typical nursing home populations are as follows[27, 37]:

- Average age is 82 years
- There is no living spouse
- Women outnumber men by a ratio of 3:1
- More than half have a progressive dementia or arthritis, cardiovascular disorder, or both
- One third have impaired vision or impaired hearing
- Most require assistance in several or all ADL
- Twenty per cent return home, and 70% stay for longer than 1 year

Two levels of care are provided in nursing homes, with many facilities offering both. Residents needing highly *skilled* nursing care may have feeding tubes, tracheotomies, extensive wounds, or infections or may need medications that require round-the-clock supervision and treatment by a registered nurse under the direction of a physician. The length of stay is variable. Medicare Part A generally pays 100% for the first 20 days, then 80% after a co-payment. After 100 days, Part A pays nothing. Medicare Part B pays a portion of the cost after 100 days.

Intermediate care is suitable for clients who need supervision and moderate assistance with ADL and medications. Generally, nurse's aides give primary care. The average length of stay varies. Medicare does not pay for this type of care.

Subacute Care

Many hospitals and nursing homes have added subacute care units to their facilities. The typical subacute unit looks much like a medical-surgical hospital unit; however, in contrast to a hospital, it is more family-focused and flexible, with a relaxed and adaptable atmosphere.[10] Medicare Part A pays for subacute care in a manner similar to that for skilled nursing home care.

Clients in subacute units typically have short-term stays. They frequently need skilled nursing care, rehabilitation, and other services, but they may no longer meet the criteria for hospitalization. Often because of their age and frailty, they cannot tolerate the daily amount of rehabilitation mandated in inpatient rehabilitation facilities; thus, they transfer to a subacute unit to complete rehabilitation before returning home.

The goal of subacute care is to discharge the client back to home or to an appropriate living environment.

The picture of the "typical" nursing home resident mentioned earlier would accurately depict a long-term resident, but it does not apply to the many who are in nursing homes for subacute, short-term care.

Home Care

Home health care is skilled care consisting of rehabilitation services that can be received in the home if the person is homebound, has a physician's referral, needs intermittent skilled care, is making progress, and receives rehabilitation three to five times a week. The average length of stay is six weeks. Medicare Part A pays the full, approved cost for five visits a week. Home health care can provide a wide variety of services, such as social services, nutritional counseling, provision of some medical supplies and equipment, and personal care assistance (see Chapter 7). Medicare may cover some of these services for a limited time for clients who meet specific criteria.

Outpatient Rehabilitation

Outpatient rehabilitation is for the older client who has a physician's prescription for therapy. The client is responsible for a deductible and noncovered amounts. Medicare pays 80% of the fee up to a specified limit but does not pay for services by independent speech pathologists.

Hospice

Hospice is a program of care for the terminally ill, either on an inpatient basis or at home. The emphasis is on alleviation of pain, terminal care, and support for the individual and family (see Chapter 22). Physicians must certify that the client has less than 6 months to live. Medicare covers hospice care, and there is no deductible. Medicare also covers nursing, physicians, drugs, rehabilitation, homemaker, social services, short-term care, counseling, and *respite care* (short-term relief for family members who care for an older person at home).

Respite Care

The elderly client may receive respite care at home or at such locations as day care centers and health care facilities. Trained individuals care for the older person while the family member is away. Medicare generally does not pay for respite care unless the client is in a hospice program.

Adult Day Care

Day care refers to daily supervised programmed activities for moderately to minimally impaired elders. Community-based adult day care centers focus on maintaining or improving the functional abilities of the impaired older person. Typically, participants need safety supervision or assistance in several areas of functioning. Centers usually emphasize either rehabilitation or social activities and provide a variety of services ranging from health care to social programs. Most participants cannot be left at home alone during the day when family members are at work

or are unavailable. This arrangement allows the family caregiver to work outside the home. Medicare does not cover the cost of day care.

Case Management

Nursing case management provides comprehensive, individualized, and economic care for older clients with complex chronic health needs. The goal is to meet client and support caregiver needs while coordinating access to cost-effective services. The nurse case manager functions as the primary care representative and coordinates with others to form a team of acute, long-term, and community care services as needed. The nurse case manager serves as a client advocate, has a holistic view of the situation, and can help solve problems as they arise in a cost-efficient, high-quality manner. Nursing case management can become involved through a health provider referral, social service intervention, or family contact with independent case management services.

LEGISLATION AFFECTING THE ELDERLY POPULATION

Federal and state laws govern legal issues that affect the elderly and the services provided. Table 3–6 lists the major laws that affect the older population. Three of the most significant acts are Title XVIII–Medicare of 1965, the Older Americans Act of 1965, and the Omnibus Budget Reconciliation Act (OBRA) of 1987.

The Nursing Home Reform Act, part of OBRA 1987, mandated the most comprehensive legislative requirements ever to affect nursing homes and the delivery of long-term care. The intent was to improve quality of care by establishing a set of conditions for certification and regulations for resident care, rights, behaviors, quality of life, interdisciplinary evaluation, staffing requirements, and facility practices. Important changes resulted from this act. These changes include the Minimum Data Set (MDS), a standardized resident assessment that provides a nationwide research data base; (2) improved resident rights with emphasis on resident-driven rather than provider-driven care; (3) a more "humane" environment with a focus on quality of life rather than custodial care; and (4) movement toward a restraint-free environment that has reduced the use of physical and chemical restraints.

ETHICAL ISSUES THAT AFFECT THE ELDERLY

Whatever the setting, there are daily challenges to be advocated for the older client. An advocate represents the interests of others by acting in their behalf or influencing policies that affect them.[10] Issues of autonomy and self-determination arise frequently. Know the issues in order to serve as a client advocate and to ensure that both the client and family are informed.

■ AUTONOMY

Autonomy is the personal freedom and independence to direct one's own life and make decisions for and about

TABLE 3-6	LEGISLATION AND EVENTS AFFECTING THE ELDERLY
Legislation	**Content and Concerns**
1935, Social Security Act (SSA)	Provides income after retirement, based on individual's average earnings paid into social security over a defined period of years before retirement
1961, First White House Conference on Aging (WHCOA) 1971, 1981, 1995 subsequent WHCOA	Each conference focused on different concerns of the aging. Outcomes included establishment of Senate Special Committee on Aging (1961), Cabinet-level Domestic Council Committee on Aging (1971), revision of mandatory retirement laws (1981), and preservation of Medicare, Medicaid, and Older Americans Act (1995)
1965, Amendment to SSA: Title XVIII—Medicare	Provides health insurance for all eligible individuals over age 65 and some younger disabled individuals. Part A: Hospital insurance, covers important hospital care, skilled nursing home care, and some home health care. Part B: Supplemental medical insurance, covers physician services; in some outpatient services, there is an additional monthly charge
1965, Amendment to SSA: Title XIX·—Medicaid	Health assistance program for low-income individuals (<21 years and >64 years of age), frequent source of long-term care payment for elderly
1965, Older Americans Act; amended 1975, 1976, 1992	Provides federal funds to states for services, training, and research to help older persons. Amended objectives focus on health care, housing, residential repair, in-home services, transportation, senior centers, nutrition and ombudsman program, legal services, crime prevention, job counseling, and case management
1973, Area Agencies on Aging (AAA)	Coordinates plans for comprehensive Aging Service delivery at the local level
1974, Amendments to SSA: Title XV—Supplemental Security Income (SSI)	Income maintenance program for low-income people who are aged, blind, or disabled; guarantees a minimum income level
1976 Tax Reform Act	Provides income tax break on post-retirement income, sale of residence, and estate and gifts
1981 Omnibus Budget Reconciliation Act; amended 1987, 1990	Standardized assessment and process of care planning and provision in all long-term care facilities receiving federal funds; includes right to self-determination, freedom from restraints, and ombudsman advocacy
1983, Diagnosis-Related Groups (DRGs)	Instituted by Health Care Financing Administration in attempts to limit and control Medicare health costs
1990 Patient Self-Determination Act	Requires all health care facilities to provide written information concerning right to make health care decisions
1996, Managed care and Medicare	Medicare changes move most older clients into managed care systems

oneself. Autonomous people are capable of rational thought and problem-solving. They can identify problems, understand the situation, search for alternatives, and select solutions that allow continued personal freedom.

Loss of autonomy, and therefore independence, is a real fear among the elderly. No autonomous adult wishes to give up the right to decide when to get up, when to go to bed, what to eat, or what interests and activities to pursue. In many institutional settings, autonomy becomes scarce when schedules must be met and the older person moves slowly, when decreases in hearing and processing slow decision-making, and when the person's decision does not coincide with the health care provider's ideas.

Encourage the older person's autonomy in any way possible, supervise and educate staff to listen and allow the person time to make choices, and discuss with family members what is occurring and how they can enhance the older person's autonomy.

■ COMPETENCE

The term competence is used to describe a person's decision-making abilities. Competence is the ability to adequately fulfill one's role and handle one's affairs.[27] Increasingly, nurses encounter clients who are confused or mentally impaired. Are these individuals competent to give consent for tests and procedures? Can they decide whether to proceed with, stop, or refuse treatment? Can they make end-of-life decisions?

Competence usually describes a status—the ability to make all or no decisions for oneself. Competence is a legal determination made by a judge. Adults are presumed to be legally competent unless there is evidence of an inability to care for oneself or to manage affairs or both. The court generally appoints a guardian for the individual judged to be incompetent.

In recent years, the notion of capacity to make health care decisions has become an alternative to the traditional concept of competence. Determining capacity is a criteria-based judgment similar to that made by an informed lay person.[26] The criteria include that the client (1) understand there is the right to make a choice; (2) understand the medical situation, prognosis, and risks, benefits, and consequences of treatment; (3) have the ability to communicate the decision; and (4) make a decision that is stable and consistent over time. Capacity is not absolute; it recognizes that a person may be able to make some decisions and not others or may have decisional capacity only at certain times and that some decisions require a higher level of capacity than others. Health care professionals must be sensitive to the fact that some residents are lucid during certain hours of the day and disoriented or confused at others. At the appropriate time, discuss treatment options and matters that require a decision.

■ SELF-DETERMINATION

The Patient Self-Determination Act (PSDA) reaffirmed the common law right of self-determination as guaranteed by the Fourteenth Amendment.[20] This act requires all health care facilities receiving Medicare and Medicaid reimbursement to recognize *advance directives*. Self-determination encourages individuals to be active partners in guiding their medical treatment and to claim their rights in treatment decisions. Self-determination, competency, and autonomy are closely related in decision-making associated with future treatment and end-of-life decisions.

Advance Directives

"Advance directive" is an umbrella term for any document used to protect the individual's wishes for and interests in decisions about life-sustaining measures. If used, advance directives can minimize potential conflict within the family once the person loses decision-making capacity and alleviate the burden of guilt that family members may feel about decisions to withdraw or withhold treatment. These documents include the *living will* and the *durable power of attorney* for health care or health care *proxy*.

Advance directives are valuable planning tools for all adults. However, the documents have special relevance for older people because a significant percentage of them will lose decision-making capacity at some time before death.[32] Discussion of advance directives does not come easily. Many clients want to talk about advance directives with their physician but are reluctant to initiate discussion because of a belief that it is the physician's role. Only about 15% of elderly patients have advance directives.[30] Studies have shown that most older people expect and anticipate that "someone" will know what to do when the time comes,[20, 25, 32] and they prefer family members, rather than health care providers, to be surrogate decision makers.

Many factors influence a person's decisions about advance directives including religion, education, knowledge of these instruments, and cultural and ethnic values.[24] Blacks rarely execute advance directives, Hispanics use them 25% of the time, and about half of older whites and Asians have them. Elders older than 80 years of age are more likely to have recorded health care wishes. Cultural importance of family ties, religion, and death may explain some of these differences.

Living Will

A living will affirms a person's right and desire to refuse a life-prolonging intervention and becomes effective when the person is determined to be terminally ill or near death. A living will, sometimes called a *treatment directive,* is typically a series of instructions regarding the withholding, withdrawing, or implementing of life-sustaining medical care in the event of terminal illness. It is limited to the instructions in the document. A living will can be used only for terminal illness or when death is imminent.[27] It is often less flexible, covers fewer medical decisions, and can lead to disagreement about whether a condition is terminal or not. Such disagreement affects implementation of the living will. Relatives who disagree with the stated terms have been known to override the individual's wishes and not honor the living will. In most states, a living will is in effect until the writer revokes it, creates a new one, or destroys the document.

Durable Power of Attorney for Health Care or Health Care Proxy

Durable power of attorney for health care is assigned to a trusted person, often called the proxy, designated to make decisions regarding medical care for the older person in the event of future mental incapacity rather than in situations of terminal illness. A health care proxy can make all treatment decisions, not just decisions about life-sustaining measures. The proxy can guide the overall course of the elder's treatment by consenting to treatment as well as by refusing care. The proxy can clarify a living will or make decisions independently according to the client's values in situations that a living will might not address. Use of a proxy is a recommended procedure for clients with dementia and other disorders in which capacity is anticipated to decline. Older people generally name a spouse or an adult child as proxy. The proxy designee must be able to seek and understand medical information, communicate with health care professionals, and advocate effectively on the elder's behalf. The proxy must be faithful to the elder's wishes and well-being and must be willing to assume the burden of difficult decisions to honor the client's wishes.

An advance directive, although a legal document, can be disregarded or overridden. Situations in which advance directives have been disregarded include (1) family opposition; (2) caregiver disregard for, or lack of knowledge about an advance directive; and (3) state laws that mandate responding Emergency Medical Technicians (EMTs) and paramedics to resuscitate before transporting to a hospital. To guard against these occurrences, families should discuss end-of-life decisions before their occurrence, especially if the condition is one of terminal illness. All parties should understand the decisions that are made.

To educate the public about advance directives, nurses must know the different types and must have a sensitivity to individual cultural and ethnic values. Once an advance directive is available and placed on the client's chart, all caregivers should be made aware of its existence and every effort should be made to honor the individual's wishes (see Chapter 22).

Prehospital Advance Directive for Emergency Medical Services

Depending on state or local law, an advance directive may or may not be honored when an emergency medical service (EMS) system (9-1-1) is activated. California, Texas, and New Jersey have legislation that requires special forms to be prepared in order that EMTs not resuscitate a person. It is important to let families know the laws that EMTs must uphold when advance directives are involved.

CONCLUSIONS

Opportunities to care for elders exist in all settings. The number of elderly people requiring health care is considerable. The proportion of all hospital patient days accounted for by people over 65 years of age was 38% in 1980 and is expected to rise to 58% by 2000.[39] Many of these hospitalized clients will be discharged to their homes with continued care needs. The role of the nurse in acute care and community settings—to act as an advocate and to promote the physical and mental well-being of older people—will be extremely important.

Given that the elderly are the fastest growing segment of the population in the United States, every nurse involved with adult health care will undoubtedly at some point be challenged to meet the unique needs of these clients. A holistic perspective is necessary, and the physiologic, psychological, sociologic, and spiritual needs of older people must be considered.

BIBLIOGRAPHY

1. American Nurses' Association. (1995). *Scope and standards of gerontological nursing practice*. Washington, DC: Author.
1a. American Psychiatric Association. (1994). *Diagnostic and statistical manual of mental disorders* (4th ed.). Washington, DC: Author.
2. Anetzberger, G. J. (1990). Abuse, neglect and self-neglect: Issues of vulnerability. In Z. Hanel, P. Ehrlich, & R. Hubbard (Eds.), *The vulnerable aged: People, services, and policies* (pp. 140–148). New York: Springer.
3. Batt, L. (1989). Managing delirium; Implications for geropsychiatric nurses. *Journal of Psychosocial Nursing and Mental Health Services, 27*(5), 22–25.
4. Beare, P. G., & Graveley, E. (1995). Health teaching and compliance. In M. Stanley & P. Beare (Eds.), *Gerontological nursing* (pp. 63–96). Philadelphia: F. A. Davis.
5. Besdine, R. W. (1983). The educational utility of comprehensive functional assessment in the elderly. *Journal of the American Geriatrics Society, 31*, 651–656.
6. Binder, E., & Robins, L. (1990). Cognitive impairment and length of hospital stay in older persons. *Journal of the American Geriatrics Society, 38*, 759–766.
7. Burnside, I. (1988). *Nursing and the aged*. New York: McGraw-Hill.
8. Carnaveli, D., & Patrick, H. (Eds.). (1993). *Nursing management for the elderly* (3rd ed.). Philadelphia: J. B. Lippincott.
9. Darnell, J. C., et al. (1986). Medication use by ambulatory elderly: An in-home survey. *Journal of the American Geriatrics Society, 34*(1), 1–4.
9a. Davies, H. (1999). Delirium and dementia. In J. K. Stone, et al. (Eds.), *Clinical Gerontological Nursing* (2nd ed., pp. 413–443). Philadelphia: W. B. Saunders.
10. Ebersole, P., & Hess, P. (Eds.). (1998). *Toward healthy aging* (5th ed., pp. 1–29). St. Louis: Mosby–Year Book.
11. Eliopoulos, C. (1987). *Gerontological nursing*. Philadelphia: J. B. Lippincott.
12. Folstein, M. F., Folstein, S., & McHugh, P. R. (1975). Mini mental state: A practical method for grading the cognitive states of patients for the clinician. *Journal of Psychiatric Research, 12*, 189–198.
13. Foreman, M. (1989). Confusion in the hospitalized elderly: Incidence, onset, and associated factors. *Research in Nursing and Health, 12*, 21.

14. Hogstel, M. O. (Ed.). (1992). *Clinical manual of gerontological nursing*. St. Louis: Mosby–Year Book.
15. Johnson, J., Sullivan, E., & Gottlieb, G. (1987). Delirium in elderly patients on internal medicine services. *Journal of the American Geriatrics Society, 35*, 972.
16. Kane, R. A., & Kane, R. (1981). *Assessing the elderly* (pp. 59–64). Lexington, MA: Lexington Books.
17. Katz, S., et al. (1963). Studies of illness in the aged. The index of ADL: A standardized measure of biological and psychosocial functions. *Journal of the American Medical Association, 185*, 915–919.
18. King, K., Diamond, M., & McCanie, K. (1987). Coping with relocation. *Geriatric Nursing, 8*(5), 258–261.
19. Levkoff, S., Besdine, R., & Wetle, T. (1986). Acute confusional states (delirium) in the hospitalized elderly. In C. Eisdorfer (Ed.), *Annual review of gerontology and geriatrics* (Vol. 6, pp. 1–26). New York: Springer.
19a. Lipowski, A. (1983). Transient cognitive disorders (delirium, acute confusional states) in the elderly. *American Journal of Psychiatry, 140*, 1426–1436.
20. Madson, S. K. (1993). Patient self-determination act: Implications for long-term care. *Journal of Gerontological Nursing, 19*(2), 15–18.
21. Mahoney, F. I., & Barthel, D. W. (1965). Functional evaluation: The Barthel index. *Maryland State Medical Journal, 14*, 61–65.
22. McConnel, C. E. (1984). A note on the lifetime risk of nursing home residency. *The Gerontologist, 24*, 193–198.
23. McCurren, C. (1991). *Hospitalized elders: Attention deficits and confusion*. Doctoral dissertation. Lexington KY: University of Kentucky.
24. McKenna, W. A. (1995). Transcultural perspectives in nursing care of the elderly. In M. M. Andrews & J. S. Bole (Eds.), *Transcultural concepts in nursing care* (pp. 203–234). Philadelphia: J. B. Lippincott.
25. Meyer, C. (1993). "End-of-life" care: Patients' choices, nurses' challenges. *American Journal of Nursing, 93*(2), 40–47.
26. Mikulencak, M. (1993). The "graying of America": Changing what nurses need to know. *The American Nurse, 25*(7), 1, 12.
27. Miller, C. A. (1995). *Nursing care of older adults: Theory and practice* (2nd ed.). Philadelphia: J. B. Lippincott.
28. Program Resource Development, American Association of Retired Persons. (1998). *A profile of older Americans (1997)* [brochure]. Washington, DC: Author.
29. Ramsdell, J., et al. (1990). Evaluation of cognitive impairment in the elderly. *Journal of General Internal Medicine, 5*, 55–64.
30. Shawler, E., et al. (1992). Clinical considerations: Surrogate decision making for hospitalized elders. *Journal of Gerontological Nursing, 18*(6), 5–11.
31. Shugars, D. A., O'Neil, E. H., & Bader, J. D. (Eds.). (1994). *Healthy America: Practitioners for 2005*. Durham, NC: The Pew Health Professions Commission.
32. Stanley, M., & Bare, P. (Eds.). (1995). *Gerontological nursing*. Philadelphia: F. A. Davis.
33. Stewart, R. B., et al. (1991). Changing patterns of therapeutic agents in the elderly: A ten-year overview. *Age and Aging, 20*(3), 182–188.
34. Stone, J. K., Wyman, J. F., & Salisbury, S. A. (1999). *Clinical gerontological nursing: A guide to advanced practice* (2nd ed.). Philadelphia: W. B. Saunders.
35. Tideiksaar, R. (1997). *Falling in old age* (2nd ed.). New York: Springer.
36. U.S. Bureau of the Census. (1991). *Statistical abstracts of the U.S.* (111th ed.). Washington, DC: U.S. Government Printing Office.
37. U.S. House Select Committee on Aging. (1986). *The rights of America's institutionalized aged: Lost in confinement* (Committee Publication No. 99-543). Washington, DC: U.S. Government Printing Office.
38. U.S. House Select Committee on Aging. (1990). *Elder abuse: A decade of shame and inaction*. Washington, DC: U.S. Government Printing Office.
39. U.S. Senate Special Committee on Aging. (1989). *Developments in aging: 1988* (Committee Publication No. 101-4). Washington, DC: U.S. Government Printing Office.
40. Valanis, R., Yeaworth, R., & Mullis, M. (1987). Alcohol use among bereaved and nonbereaved older persons. *Journal of Gerontological Nursing, 13*(5), 26–32.

The Trait and Process of Resilience

QUESTIONS
What is meant by resilience?
How does it affect responses to illness and adversity?

CITATION
Jacelon, C. S. (1997). The trait and process of resilience. *Journal of Advanced Nursing, 25,* 123–129.

STUDIES

The author of this review selected studies to demonstrate the breadth and diversity of ideas about resilience and diversity in the behavioral science and clinical literature. Other than these goals, the method of locating and choosing the studies for inclusion was not described. The studies were conducted by researchers from social, psychological, and health care disciplines. Studies about adults are emphasized in this synopsis.

Summary of Findings

"Resilience as a Trait" (p. 123)

Resilience can be defined either as a personal trait or as a process by which people "spring back" from adversity and continue with their lives.[5] *Vulnerability* may be an opposite trait, referring to how people are easily "beaten down" by adversity and succumb to dysfunction in their lives.[9]

Resilience is manifested differently in children and adults. Studies of children in poverty,[5] of children who have parents with major affective disorders,[2] of children whose parents are divorced,[7] and of children with attention deficit disorder[6] suggest a constellation of characteristics that constitute resilience. Important contributors include:

- Personal disposition to high activity levels, self-understanding, intelligence, and positive responsiveness to others
- The presence of a caring adult or a warm cohesive family
- Strong community support and role models[5]

Adult homosexual men who are long-term survivors of acquired immunodeficiency syndrome (AIDS) were also found to have extraordinary personal resources: intelligence, education, wide-ranging interests, a positive outlook, and goals.[8] Most of them also had a confidant, access to community resources, and adequate housing.

The personality traits and responses of adults with cancer have also been studied. A correlational study examined the relationship between personality traits and the degree of atypical neoplastic growth on the cervix of 75 women who had abnormal Papanicolaou (Pap) smears.[1] An interview was conducted and a health inventory questionnaire was administered before the examination results were reported to the women. Several associations were revealed between personality variables and the degree of neoplastic growth. Women with cancer had significantly higher scores in pessimism, future despair, life-threat reactivity, and somatic anxiety than women with a very low level of or no neoplastic growth. Thus, we might infer that a positive life outlook affords resistance to development of cancer.

As part of a qualitative study, in-depth interviews were conducted with 24 older women who had adjusted well after a major loss. The themes that emerged from the interview data were:[10]

- A balanced perspective of their life experiences
- Persistence in the face of adversity
- A belief in their own abilities
- The realization that life has purpose and that one can always make a contribution
- A belief that each person's life path is unique

An experimental instrument to measure the trait of resilience has been tested on 810 older adults.[11] Resilience was found to be positively correlated with life satisfaction, morale, and physical health and negatively correlated with depression. The instrument was found to measure two main factors: personal competence and acceptance of life and self.

"Resilience as a Process" (p. 126)

The process of resilience has been described as the complex interaction of intrapsychic and social responses with demands and stresses that occur over time.[4, 9] Two stages have been delineated: (1) the *disruption* phase, "during which energy is directed at minimizing the impact of the stress or stressor"; and (2) the *reorganization* phase, "during which a new reality is accepted in part or in whole."[3] The literature suggests that resilience as a process can be learned at any point in life.[3]

Overall, studies of resilience as a *process* are fewer than studies of resilience as a personal *trait*. One investigator working with the physically disabled concluded that personal perceptions and responses to major life events are "crucial elements of survival, recovery, and rehabilitation."[3]

Limitations/Reservations. We as health care workers seem to be intrigued by the ability of children, adolescents, adults, couples, and families to bounce back from adversity and persevere. We understand the personal traits that serve as protective factors to the hurts, losses, and difficulties of adverse experiences, but we do not know why some people have these resources while other people lack them. We also do not understand how people acquire resilience and remain resilient over a long time.

The concept of resilience has been defined in various ways and is not well differentiated from other similar concepts such as hardiness, thriving, self-efficacy, and coping. Perhaps most lacking from a nursing perspective is that it is not clear whether or not interventions can promote and support resilience during difficult times.

Continued on following page

The Trait and Process of Resilience *Continued*

Research-Based Practice

Resilient people have a constellation of traits, including (1) the ability to form and maintain meaningful relationships with others, (2) a balanced perspective of life's joys and difficulties, and (3) a belief that we can determine our own future. The review author envisions that if an instrument for measuring resilience existed, "Nurses in practice could then better focus resources by capitalizing on the resilient person's strengths and by providing assistance to people who are not inherently resilient" (p. 128). This is an intriguing idea, but further development is needed to specify what should be done differently for the two groups of people; the proposed interventions would need to be tested to ensure that they work and to specify the people with whom they work. Another issue to be addressed would be how one helps people whose trait score is in the mid-range.

Attempts have been made to teach coping and problem-solving skills to clients with chronic health problems, but the extent to which the learning of these skills results in resilience has not been examined. Similarly, conducting personal resource inventories with clients who face chronic illness may help them realize what protective resources they do have and then tap into them.

Promoting support groups is another intervention that may foster resiliency. Support groups seem to benefit people who already have resiliency traits in place. It is not known whether people with tentative resiliency traits are bolstered by support groups. For older adults and clients with life-threatening illness, a life review may build resilience by helping them realize how strong they have been over their lifetime and by helping them place the current adversity into perspective.

In summary, some of the interventions already used to "support" people during difficult times may succeed by bolstering, tapping into, or bringing into conscious awareness a client's resiliency traits that were developed earlier in life.

Cited References

1. Antoni, M. H., & Goodkin, K. (1988). Host moderator variable in the promotion of cervical neoplasia. I. Personal facets. *Journal of Psychosomatic Research, 32,* 327–338.
2. Beardslee, W. R., & Poderefsky, D. (1988). Resilient adolescents whose parents have serious affective and other psychiatric disorders: Importance of self-understanding and relationships. *American Journal of Psychiatry, 145,* 63–69.
3. Fine, S. B. (1991). Resilience and human adaptability: Who rises above adversity? *American Journal of Occupational Therapy, 45,* 493–503.
4. Fonagy, P., et al. (1993). The Emanuel Miller memorial lecture 1992: The theory and practice of resilience. *Journal of Child Psychology and Psychiatry, 35,* 231–257.
5. Garmezy, N. (1993). Children in poverty: Resilience despite risk. *Psychiatry, 56,* 127–136.
6. Hechtman, L. (1991). Resilience and vulnerability in long term outcome of attention deficit hyperactive disorder. *Canadian Journal of Psychiatry, 36,* 415–421.
7. Mulholland, D. J., et al. (1991). Academic performance in children of divorce: Psychological resilience and vulnerability. *Psychiatry, 54,* 268–280.
8. Rabkin, J. G., et al. (1993). Resilience in adversity among long-term survivors of AIDS. *Hospital and Community Psychiatry, 44,* 162–167.
9. Rutter, M. (1985). Psychosocial resilience and protective mechanisms. *American Journal of Orthopsychiatry, 57,* 316–331.
10. Wagnild, G., & Young, H. M. (1990). Resilience among older women. *Image: Journal of Nursing Scholarship, 22,* 252–255.
11. Wagnild, G., & Young, H. M. (1993). Development and psychometric evaluation of the resilience scale. *Journal of Nursing Measurement, 1,* 165–178.

Sarah Jo Brown, PhD, RN, *Principal and Consultant, Practice-Research Integrations, Norwich, Vermont*

UNIT 2

Health Care Delivery Systems

4   Overview of Health Care Delivery

5   Ambulatory Health Care

6   Acute Health Care

7   Home Health Care

8   Long-Term Care

CHAPTER 4

Overview of Health Care Delivery

Mary L. Fisher

Nurses in the United States practice within a diverse and complex health care system. During the 1980s and 1990s, the system experienced a dramatic growth in scientific knowledge, coupled with an explosion of technology. This also was a period of increased competition and regulation. Additionally, the financing of health care was revolutionized in 1983, when prospective payment was introduced, and later, as managed care began to dominate the market. These events have had a profound impact on the practice of nursing. Understanding who the major stakeholders are within the field of health care and understanding recent health care history are crucial to the practice of professional nurses. This chapter strives to inform beginning practitioners of these changes and trends to prepare them for active roles in shaping the health care system for the new millennium.

MAJOR STAKEHOLDERS IN THE HEALTH CARE SYSTEM

■ GOVERNMENT

The role of government in the administration of health care in the United States cannot be overestimated. Health care expenditures accounted for 20% of the federal government's budget in 1995; by 1997, expenditures amounted to $485 billion.[16, 20] In 1997, 46.4% of health care dollars spent were funded by government programs, especially Medicare (a federal program funded at $214 billion for 1997) and Medicaid (a joint federal-state initiative funded at $160 billion for 1997).[14, 16] Other important sources of federal government funding are the Department of Veterans Affairs (VA), funded at $16.6 billion for 1997, which oversees the VA health care system, and the Department of Defense, funded at 13.4 billion for 1997, which funds health care for members of the armed forces and their dependents.[14] Workers' compensation, a joint federal and state program, was funded at $14.1 billion for 1997.[14] In addition, state and local governments support local indigent care through various mechanisms.

As the major payer, the federal government has been

active in regulating the health care industry. Approximately 40% of hospital beds are occupied on any given day by Medicare recipients. Therefore, hospitals have great incentive to comply with regulations promulgated by the federal government, because they can be fined or "decertified" as a provider of care to Medicare clients if they do not. Noncompliance can result in the loss of millions of dollars of income for the hospital.

Government regulation is frequently opposed by the health care industry because it often affects the health care practitioner's autonomy. In 1991, for example, the U.S. Supreme Court upheld the right of the federal government to restrict health care providers in family planning clinics that receive federal funds from informing pregnant women about abortion options (*Rust v. Sullivan*). Since the Supreme Court ruling, health care workers in the clinics had to alter their practice or be subject to penalty. Strong condemnation of this restriction was voiced by the American Nurses' Association (ANA) and the American Medical Association (AMA), among others. Legislation to modify the regulation was eventually passed.

The federal government is the biggest source of funding for biomedical research. The Agency for Health Care Policy and Research (AHCPR), established in 1989, conducts research on costs, quality, and medical effectiveness of health care. It received $171 billion in 1999, two thirds of which was awarded in grants and contracts.[2] The National Institutes of Health (NIH), the principal biomedical research agency of the government through its 17 institutes, received $15.6 billion for fiscal year 1999, 82% of which supports research and training.[21] The House of Representatives passed $17.9 billion for fiscal year 2000.[8] The government also directs public health programs through the Centers for Disease Control and Prevention (CDC), which received $3.1 billion for fiscal year 2000.[9] The growth of scientific knowledge related to health care is highly dependent on government funding. Nurse researchers are recipients of research grants through various government agencies, most notably the National Institute for Nursing Research at NIH. Its budget for 1999 was $70 million.[22] Research funds are an important source of revenue for major medical centers and university-affiliated hospitals.

This chapter includes material from the fifth edition written by Bonita Ann Pilon.

DIVERSITY IN HEALTH CARE

Health Care Practitioners

Americans have been socialized to believe that the United States has the best health care system in the world. This ethnocentric attitude interferes with nurses' recognition and acceptance of the value and use of traditional healers. Terms used for traditional healers include folk practitioners, indigenous healers, native healers, primitive healers, and witch doctors. Whatever the terms, they generally are given a negative connotation, and it is implied that they are not as good as Western practitioners. Health care needs to reflect an understanding of the values of diverse populations.[2]

The table identifies culture and folk practitioners, their preparation, and scope of practice.

Culture/Folk Practitioners

Practitioner	Preparation	Scope of Practice
Hispanic		
Family member	Possesses knowledge of folk medicine.	Common illnesses of a mild nature that may or may not be recognized by modern medicine.
Curandero	May receive training in an apprenticeship. May receive a "gift from God" that enables her or him to cure. Knowledgeable in use of herbs, diet, massage, and rituals.	Some may not treat illness caused by witchcraft for fear of being accused of possessing evil powers. Usually admired by community. Treats almost all of the traditional illnesses.
Espiritualista or spiritualist	Born with the special gifts of being able to analyze dreams and foretell future events. May serve apprenticeship with an older practitioner.	Emphasizes prevention of illness or bewitchment through use of medals, prayers, and amulets. May also be sought for cure of existing illnesses.
Yerbero	No formal training. Knowledgeable in growing and prescribing herbs.	Consulted for preventive and curative use of herbs for traditional and Western illnesses.
Sabador	Knowledgeable in massage and manipulation of bones and muscles.	Treats many traditional illnesses, particularly those affecting the musculoskeletal system. May also treat nontraditional illnesses.
Black		
"Old Lady"	Usually an older woman who has successfully raised her own family. Knowledgeable in child care and folk remedies.	Consulted about common ailments and advice for child care.
Spiritualist	Called by God to help others. No formal training. Usually associated with a fundamentalist Christian church.	Assists with financial, personal, spiritual, or physical problems. Predominantly found in urban communities.
Voodoo priest or priestess or *Hougan*	May be trained by another priest or priestess. In the United States, the oldest son of a priest becomes a priest. A daughter of a priest or priestess becomes a priestess if she is born with a veil (amniotic sac) over her face.	Knowledgeable about properties of herbs and interpretation of signs and omens. Can cure illness caused by voodoo. Uses communication to establish a therapeutic milieu (like a psychiatrist). Treats African Americans, Mexican Americans, and Native Americans.
Chinese		
Herbalist	Knowledgeable in diagnosis of illness and herbal remedies.	Both diagnostic and therapeutic. Diagnostic techniques include interviewing, inspection, auscultation, and assessment of pulses.
Acupuncturist	3½ to 4½ years (1500 to 1800 hours) of courses on acupuncture, Western anatomy and physiology, and Chinese herbs. Usually requires a period of apprenticeship under someone who is licensed or certified. Licensure required in North America.	Diagnosis and treatment of *Yin* and *Yang* disorders by inserting needles into meridians (pathways through which life energy flows). Heat may be applied to the acupuncture needle (moxibustion). May combine acupuncture with herbal remedies and/or dietary recommendations. Acupuncture is sometimes used as an anesthetic in surgery.

DIVERSITY IN HEALTH CARE *Continued*

Amish

Braucher or *baruch-doktor*	Apprenticeship.	Men or women use a combination of modalities, including physical manipulation, massage, herbs, teas, reflexology, and *brauche,* folk-healing art with origins in 18th and 19th century Europe. Especially effective in the treatment of bed-wetting.
Lay midwives	Apprenticeship.	Cares for women before, during, and after delivery.

Greek

Magissa "magician"	Apprenticeship.	Woman who cures *matiasma* (evil eye). May be referred to as a doctor.
Bone setters	Apprenticeship.	Specializes in treating uncomplicated fractures.
Priest (Orthodox)	Ordained clergy. Formal theological study.	May be called on for advice, blessings, exorcisms, or direct healing.

Native American

Shaman	Spiritually chosen. Apprenticeship.	Uses incantations, prayers, and herbs to cure physical, psychological, and spiritual illnesses.
Crystal gazer, hand trembler (Navajo)		Diviner diagnostician who can identify the cause of a problem by using crystals or by placing a hand over the sick person. Does not implement treatment.

Traditional healers existed long before modern nursing or medicine. It is only recently that health care professionals are becoming aware of their value. Ideally, traditional healers will soon be an integral part of the health care team.[1]

References

1. Leininger, M. (1997). Founders focus alternative to what? Generic vs. professional caring, treatments and healing modes. *Journal of Transcultural Nursing, 9*(1), 37.
2. Purnell, L., & Paulanka, B. (1998). *Transcultural health care: A culturally competent approach.* Philadelphia: F. A. Davis.

Modified from Andrews, M., & Herberg, P. (1999). Transcultural nursing care. In M. Andrews & J. Boyle (Eds.), *Transcultural concepts in nursing care* (pp. 42–43). Philadelphia: J. B. Lippincott.

Joyce Larson-Presswalla, PhD, RN, *President, "Culture Counts," Marketing Coordinator, James A. Haley Veterans Hospital, Tampa, Florida*

■ PHYSICIANS

The role of physicians in the health care system in the United States is an important one. Physicians provide direct medical services to clients in a variety of settings, including offices, clinics, hospitals, and freestanding centers. In addition, physicians control 60% to 80% of hospital costs through their decisions about the use of resources. As gatekeepers to inpatient care, physicians decide which clients to admit, where to admit clients, the length of stay, the quantity of ancillary services, whether to perform surgery, when to initiate and to discontinue treatment regimens, and which medications to prescribe.

Because physicians strongly influence health care use, health care agencies and clients are often dependent on physicians. Agencies such as hospitals rely on their medical staffs to admit clients who generate income for the hospital. Therefore, physicians are customers of the hospital, just as clients are. As a result, physicians and their lobby groups, such as the AMA, usually have strong political influence within hospital organizations, the health care system, legislatures, and government-regulating agencies.

Many physicians perceived a decline in their dominance and control of health care during the 1980s and 1990s. These perceived and real losses have created anxiety and defensive tactics among some members of the profession toward a restructured health care system. The traditions that define medical practice, such as autonomy, professional control, solo medical practice, and fee-for-service entrepreneurialism, are being questioned and reformed. Some contend that physicians will enjoy less control in a restructured health care environment than they did before. In keeping with this trend toward the loss of physician power, the AMA took the unprecedented step in 1999 of forming a collective bargaining arm to assist physicians in seeking input into practice changes.

While Western practitioners are the main group sanctioned by American society to treat disease, traditional cultural and folk practitioners are a presence in ethnic segments of our society. Providers must recognize the place of traditional healers for an ethnically diverse population (see Diversity in Health Care).

■ HOSPITAL ADMINISTRATORS AND GOVERNING BOARDS

The chief executive, chief financial officer, chief nursing officer, and governing boards of hospitals strongly influence health care delivery in their institutions. In addition, most hospitals are members of the American Hospital Association (AHA), which represents the industry's efforts to influence legislation, regulation, judicial decisions, and health policy. The AHA filed a suit in the early 1990s to stop the National Labor Relations Board from implementing new collective bargaining rules. The suit went to the Supreme Court, where the rules were upheld, but they have had little impact in fostering collective bargaining, as the AHA has feared.[7] The AHA also worked to block regulations from the Health Care Financing Administration (HCFA), which effectively decreased reimbursement for capital costs to hospitals from Medicare.[30]

■ BUSINESS AND INDUSTRY

By the year 2000, health care costs were projected to represent 19% of the gross national product (GNP), or $1.6 trillion.[17, 26] These costs are the highest of any industrialized nation, making American products less competitive in the world economy. For example, health care costs for automobile workers add $1100 to the cost of every car made in America.[13] This continuing trend is best illustrated by comparing the cost of prescription drugs in the United States with that of other wealthy nations: Great Britain's cost is 33% less; Canada's, 37% less; and France's and Italy's, 47% less.[1]

One can understand why American industries have a big stake in controlling these costs. As health care costs rose in the mid-1990s (~5% per year),[15] the influence of business and industry increased as well. Health insurance programs, such as Blue Cross/Blue Shield and commercial insurance, are purchased mainly through employee benefit programs. As the cost of health care rises, insurance costs rise as well, forcing businesses to assume greater financial burdens to insure employees and their dependents. Costs for products increase accordingly.

One major reason for the increase is the health care industry's practice of cost shifting by increasing charges to individuals and small payers to offset underpayment by Medicare, Medicaid, and other contracted payers. The result is that the private sector, insured clients, and employers pay more for care. During the past decade, business and industry leaders protested the increased costs and began to take collective action to drive costs down. Some strategies have included:

- Increased deductibles
- Larger and more frequent co-payments
- Reduced benefits and services
- Initiation of managed care programs
- Mandatory second opinions
- Precertification of admission
- Increased contracting of care to health maintenance organizations (HMOs) and preferred provider organizations (PPOs)

By 1997, 85% of the enrolled work force was in some type of managed care plan.[14]

In some areas of the United States, industry leaders have formed coalition groups that lobby their state government for laws to restrict health care spending, limit malpractice liability, and provide major reform for the health care system. Increasingly, large businesses have contracted for health care services directly with hospitals and physician groups, demanding — and receiving — significant discounts for care. The influence of large employers is expected to remain strong within the health care industry.

■ THE PUBLIC

Despite decades of public policy designed to reduce health costs, U.S. health care spending is estimated to exceed $1.6 trillion or $5700 per capita annually by 2000.[13] The American public has a stake in health care from several perspectives. First, as consumers of health care services, the public is concerned with the quality, cost, and access to care. Many Americans believe that health care is a right and should be universally available to all citizens ragardless of the cost. Paradoxically, however, most do not want to pay these costs in the form of increased taxes.

People who are uninsured (approx. 44 million, 86% of whom are employed workers and their families) or underinsured (Medicare recipients have no prescription medication coverage) do not have equal access to health care services that income and insurance provide.[13] This uninsured figure represents 16% of the non-elderly population.[15] Women and children are among those who suffer the most, since 25% of the uninsured are children.[15] Because people have not agreed on the model for health care reform or the role of government, several ideas are being explored by various interest groups.

The public also is composed of voters who can elect representatives to enact laws protecting their health care interests. Often, citizens band together to influence the passage of health-related legislation. In 1990, activist groups concerned about acquired immunodeficiency syndrome (AIDS) strongly lobbied Congress to ensure passage of the Ryan White bill (Public Law 101-381), which provided funds for AIDS education, service, and research. The American Association of Retired Persons (AARP) is another prominent group that actively supports health care legislation targeted to older people. Although many other consumer groups are concerned with health care issues, AIDS and breast cancer activist groups and the AARP represent some of the larger and more vocal constituencies that currently influence the health care industry.

Overall, public values regarding health care are changing. People are interested in receiving quality health care at a reasonable cost. In addition, the public has a more positive view of health promotion and illness prevention than in the past. Health care resources remain focused on illness, however, with only 1% of health care expenditures going to public health.[30]

■ NURSES

Nurses outnumber physicians, dentists, pharmacists, and every other single group of health care providers in the United States. As of 1996, there were 2.6 million Licensed Professional Nurses (LPNs), 1.93 million of whom were employed in nursing.[19] Among those 1.93 million

Registered Nurses (RNs), slightly fewer than two thirds worked in hospitals—a distribution that has remained constant since the mid-1980s. The supply of RNs has increased by 40% since 1980. During that time, the percentage employed in hospitals had been stable at 67% through the mid 1990s. The percentage dipped to 60% in 1996, reflecting trends toward community and outpatient care and nurses' growing concern with health maintenance, health promotion, and health education.[11, 19]

The average age of nurses has risen steadily since the 1980s. The median age for RNs neared 40 in 1996.[19] Racial and ethnic minorities except Asians are underrepresented.[23] The U.S. Bureau of Census in 1996 estimated that 72% of Americans were white, in contrast to 90% of nurses being white.[29]

Although the influence of such a large group of health care providers should be noticed, the greatest impact—and the most frequently discussed aspect of nursing—has been the recurring shortage of RNs. The voice of nursing has been heard lately, as thousands protest downsizing of hospitals, replacement of RNs by less skilled workers, and layoffs. However, the collective expertise and leadership of nurses has not yet been fully utilized to shape the reform era. Nursing's response to rapid market changes has been largely reactionary.

In 1991, the ANA, in collaboration with the National League for Nursing, the American Organization of Nurse Executives, the American Association of Colleges of Nursing, and other organized nursing groups, introduced *Nursing's Agenda for Health Care Reform.* The authors[3] stated that

Nurses provide a unique perspective on the health care system. Our constant presence in a variety of settings places us in contact with individuals who reap the benefits of the system's most sophisticated services, as well as those individuals seriously compromised by the system's inefficiencies. . . . America's health care system is . . . very costly, its quality inconsistent, and its benefits unequally distributed. . . . In short, health care is neither fairly nor equitably delivered to all segments of the population.

Nursing's health care reform proposal attempted to address the cost, quality, and access dilemmas facing the nation. This endeavor was a proactive attempt by the nursing profession to significantly alter existing health policy. A 1999 publication by ANA, *Legislative and Regulatory Initiatives for the 106th Congress* proposed mobilizing nurses politically to enact continuing influence on health care policy.[4]

FINANCING OF HEALTH CARE SERVICES

■ FUNDING MECHANISMS

Health care is paid for in various ways. The major funding programs are defined in Box 4–1.

The health care industry has evolved through significant phases since the 1920s with regard to quality, cost, and access. To understand current issues, it is useful for nurses to understand the past, which was characterized by two major periods: (1) the *period of expansion* and (2) the *period of regulation and cost containment.* The current climate is known as the *period of reform.*

■ PERIOD OF EXPANSION

During the late 1920s, a congressional committee studied various facets of health care organization and financing. It was found that the cost of health care per illness had substantially increased with the emergence of hospitalization as the appropriate method of treating illness.[24] These rising costs, coupled with the financial problems created by the Depression of 1929, led to financial difficulties for community general hospitals. Consequently, the need to spread financial risk across the community was recognized. Prepayment plans for hospital care spread slowly during the 1930s and evolved into the Blue Cross system.

PRIVATE HEALTH INSURANCE

Blue Cross plans had two goals: (1) to provide a stronger financial base for community hospitals and (2) to move the risk of economic loss caused by hospitalization away from single individuals to larger groups of people. Because these objectives were considered socially desirable, Blue Cross, and later Blue Shield organizations, benefited from favorable legislation exempting them from some of the more stringent requirements for commercial insurance companies.

The evolution of Blue Cross/Blue Shield plans and their availability to the average worker signaled the beginning of an era in which the actual cost of health care became separated from the person who purchased the care (the insurance effect). Such a separation causes the cost of health care to appear artificially low to the client, who in turn, can afford to buy more services.

Demand for health care services, as a result of insurance, grew rapidly in the 1940s and 1950s. Because of economic wage and price controls during and after World War II, salary increases to workers were limited. Fringe benefits came into vogue as a means of attracting and retaining workers. Unions began bargaining for fringe benefits in lieu of unobtainable salary increases. As a consequence, health insurance became widely available to American workers and their families. The consumption of health care services, in turn, increased.

Another important event was the passage of the Social Security Act of 1935. This legislation established as social policy the right of older people to financial security. Although health care was not affected by this law at the time of its passage, the Social Security Act would later become the vehicle through which health care needs of older people and the poor would be addressed.

HILL-BURTON ACT

After World War II, it was apparent that the nation's hospitals were obsolete and poorly distributed to meet the population's needs. There had been great shifts from rural to urban areas during the War. Immediately after the War, the baby boom began. The private sector had difficulty meeting the need for improved health care facilities.[6] Congress responded by passing the Hospital Survey and Construction Act of 1946 (the Hill-Burton Act).

The overt purpose of the Hill-Burton Act was to eliminate shortages of hospitals, especially in rural and economically depressed areas. Ratios of beds-to-population were used to measure shortage. Funds generated by the Act were dispersed over 28 years (1946 to 1974). The Act was amended during that time to include not only

BOX 4-1   Major Health Care Funding Programs in the United States

Medicare

A federally funded and administered national health insurance program for citizens age 65 years and older and for certain other clients, such as those with end-stage renal disease, regardless of age. Medicare began in 1966 and is paid for through payroll taxes of all workers (a portion of Social Security deductions) and through monthly premiums paid by recipients. The program covers both hospitalization and physician costs, but deductibles and restrictions apply. Medicare determines the maximum allowable fee for service. Health care providers receive 80% of this fee from Medicare and can bill only for the balance of the allowable fee. The maximum allowable fee is often much less than the true value of the service.

In 1983, the federal government instituted major changes in the way hospitals were reimbursed for Medicare clients. Previously, hospitals had been reimbursed costs plus an additional amount. Since 1983, hospitals have received compensation on a *prospective* basis. Hospitals are paid one predetermined sum for a given diagnosis. Similar types of diagnoses and conditions are grouped together, weighted for severity or intensity of illness, and assigned a dollar value for compensation; these are called diagnosis-related groups (DRGs). If the client's care (e.g., acute myocardial infarction) costs the hospital *more* than Medicare's payment, the hospital *loses* money. If the costs are less than the reimbursement amount, the hospital keeps the profit. This system has caused dramatic changes as hospitals struggle to survive financially. Congress is now debating whether Medicare should fund prescription coverage for recipients.

Medicaid

A joint federal and state program administered by the state governments. This insurance program provides limited funding for hospital and medical care costs of low-income citizens. Each state sets the income levels that determine eligibility. As a result, some states provide more services than others can afford. The state must budget money from its own revenues for the program matched by the government. The federal portion is always larger than the state portion.

Blue Cross and Blue Shield

Private not-for-profit health insurance companies set up through special legislation in the 1930s. The "blues" are the largest single insurer outside the federal government from which businesses and industry can purchase health insurance for employees. Both hospital and medical care insurance are available.

Commercial Insurance Companies

For-profit businesses (e.g., Traveler's, Metropolitan Life). These agencies usually sell a host of insurance packages. Businesses or individuals may buy health insurance from a commercial carrier.

Self-Insurance

Businesses that develop their own insurance programs for employees. More companies are setting aside funds (which can be millions of dollars) to cover the risk of their self-insurance program. The company may hire Blue Cross and Blue Shield or a commercial insurer to administer the program, including receiving, reviewing, and paying claims.

HMO

A health maintenance organization representing a system of bundled services. Clients pay a monthly premium to the HMO, which entitles them to checkups and preventive care, medical care, prescriptions, and hospitalization if needed. The HMO employs its own physicians and other health care providers and may own or manage its own hospitals. Some HMOs charge the clients a co-payment for some services, such as prescriptions and office visits. Clients are restricted to using only HMO facilities and physicians. If clients go outside the system, they must pay for past or all of their expenses (except in emergencies or during travel).

PPO

A preferred provider organization is a group consisting of physicians, usually at least one hospital, as well as ancillary providers that coalesces to form a system of care. This system is marketed and sold, contractually, to employers. The physicians, hospital, and others remain independent agents who agree to treat certain clients (those who join the PPO) at discounted prices.

Workers' Compensation

A federally mandated, state-funded and state-administered insurance program available to workers injured on the job. Each employer is assessed a payroll tax, which funds the plan. Clients file claims through the employer to secure funds for treatment.

Private Pay

A term used to describe clients who have no insurance and who must pay the entire health care bill.

Uncompensated Care

Health care delivered that is not paid for by an insurance program or by clients themselves. Many private pay clients contribute to the amount of uncompensated care when they cannot pay the high costs of health care. Other sources of uncompensated care include the differences between what the care costs and what Medicare or Medicaid pays the provider. By law, providers cannot bill anyone for the difference and must absorb the loss of revenue.

Capitation

A form of payment between the purchaser of health care and the provider. Capitation is often used when a large organization contracts for health services from a provider, such as a hospital or home health agency. The provider is paid in one of two ways: (1) a flat fee is paid per incident of care (no care, no payment) or (2) the provider receives a flat fee per person enrolled in the health plan for a defined level of care whether or not the enrollee seeks care. If few enrollees use the service, the provider does well financially. If not, the provider must care for every enrollee who seeks care regardless of whether the total money received covers the cost of the care provided.

construction of new facilities but also modernization of existing facilities and, later, construction of emergency departments and neighborhood health centers.[6]

Implicit within this legislation was the social policy of ensuring access to health care for all. The solution to the social problem of inadequate access was to construct more health care facilities. To ensure that people with limited ability to pay were actually served by the agencies receiving Hill-Burton Act money, the legislation stipulated a unique payback scheme. Each facility had to provide care to indigent clients, on an annual basis, that was equal in dollar value to the amount of money received by the hospital, prorated over a specified time period, usually 20 years. Much like a mortgage payment, the hospital provided free care each year equal to its annual repayment amount. These health services were provided, in lieu of payment, to people with limited access because of poverty.

The Hill-Burton Act's approach to indigent care was a noble one but did not succeed in providing access for all indigent clients. During the long payback period, the cost of health care increased dramatically as a result of new technology and inflation. Many hospitals began meeting their obligations for free care in a few weeks' time each year. After those obligations were met, hospitals were not legally bound to treat indigent clients. By the early 1970s, the bed shortage addressed by Hill-Burton legislation had reversed itself and an oversupply appeared to exist. In 1974, the Act was allowed to expire.

MEDICARE/MEDICAID ENACTED

The early 1950s featured continued wage and price controls, growth of health insurance coverage among workers, and increased discussion of a national health insurance program. National health insurance was viewed as a means of insuring every American citizen against economic loss caused by the high cost of illness, regardless of employment status, age, or health status. This concern repeatedly asserted itself during President Truman's administration. The medical and hospital lobby successfully fought such legislation as late as 1952.[25]

By the middle of the 1960s, a new social problem was identified as the nation's priority: poverty. The War on Poverty during the Johnson Administration (1963 to 1968) provided the impetus for passage of the first national health insurance plans, for which the federal government was both the insurance carrier and the payer of a large portion of the premium. These insurance programs, known as Medicare and Medicaid, were passed as amendments to the Social Security Act in 1965. The social problem of poverty was translated more specifically into limited access to health care services by the elderly and the non-elderly poor as the result of inability to pay. The social policy expressed by both pieces of legislation implied that access to health care for all citizens was a right. Government had an obligation to ensure that right.

Funding for the Medicare hospitalization plan (Part A) is provided by a payroll tax collected from every worker who pays Social Security taxes. The medical payment component (Part B) for physician care is paid by the enrollee through monthly premiums. The Medicare program is administered by the federal government through the Department of Health and Human Services (DHHS) Health Care Financing Administration.

Administration of Medicaid is delegated to the states, which must provide certain core services but are free to tailor other services to meet specific population needs. The states also determine eligibility requirements, which vary considerably from state to state. Funding for Medicaid is provided by a matching formula specific to each state. The federal funds are always the greatest portion of each Medicaid dollar spent. States receive differing amounts of federal money—and thus, provide different ranges of care—because some states can match more federal dollars than others through larger state tax revenues.

Implementation of Medicare and Medicaid substantially increased the federal government's (and, to a lesser extent, the state governments') role in the health care market. The federal government became the single largest purchaser of health care services. Subsequently, it played a growing role in regulating the health care industry in both cost and quality.

■ PERIOD OF REGULATION AND COST CONTAINMENT

In 1974, Congress passed the National Health Planning and Resources Act (Public Law 93-641), which required states to develop a statewide health plan for the use of resources. States were also required to review providers' requests to initiate or expand health services.[18] This review process, known as *certificate of need* (CON) review, required providers to demonstrate sufficient need for the service before the request was approved. This legislation represented the first federal government effort to combine health planning and regulation in one program. It was also the first significant attempt to control health care costs through the elimination of duplicate services and facilities. It was designed to curb the oversupply and increasing technology of facilities that arose during the period of expansion.

Because the CON regulation did nothing to change incentives to hospitals in the competitive health care market, it could not control costs and by the late 1970s was curtailed as a federal effort.[18] Results of CON studies support this evaluation. Steinwald and Sloan[27] suggested that "certificate-of-need controls, initiated by the states and mandated by PL 93-641, may be regarded as a classic example of regulatory failure."

During the 1970s, some state governments undertook their own regulatory programs. Rate controls were in place in at least eight states by the end of the decade. According to Steinwald and Sloan,[27] such programs "all respond to the evils of cost-based reimbursement—they seek to counteract the unrestrained nature of hospital reimbursement by superimposing constraints that the market cannot provide."

States with mandatory rate-setting programs represented the most stringent group of prospective reimbursement programs operating during the late 1970s. The rates of increase in total hospital expenses in the eight mandatory states were 9.7% and 8.6% for the years of 1976 to 1977 and 1977 to 1978, respectively, versus 15.8% and 14% for the other states and the District of Columbia.[27]

These data and other studies clearly indicated that prospective rate-setting was more effective in controlling health care costs than the CON controls were. Reimbursement for Medicaid patients also had moved to a prospective system in many states, whether or not the state had mandatory rate-setting.

FEDERAL PROSPECTIVE PAYMENT SYSTEMS

The federal government, very aware of the rising cost of health care and continuing as the nation's largest purchaser of care, began to look at methods of prospective reimbursement that could be used by the Medicare program. Research studies were under way at Yale University and other centers to develop a system of prospective payment. These studies were closely followed and sometimes funded by DHHS, previously called the Department of Health, Education, and Welfare (DHEW).

The hospital industry adopted its own form of regulation in December 1977. Known as the Voluntary Effort (VE), it consisted of "joint activities at the state level by the American Hospital Association, the American Medical Association, and the Federation of American Hospitals (the for-profit hospitals' trade organization) to control the rate of growth of hospital costs."[27] Results of the Voluntary Effort were mixed. A study by the Congressional Budget Office indicated a small, nonsignificant negative effect on hospital expenditures. A second study found a significant negative effect on the cost per admission and cost per patient day. However, the second study indicated that the cost savings were not passed on to the consumers because hospital profits increased during the same period (1978 to 1980).[27]

The inability of various regulatory programs to control the rising cost of health care (from 9% of the gross national product in 1978 to 13% by 1992) became a primary issue with Congress. The nation was trying to recover from economic recession, and inflation in all sectors of the economy was of grave concern. In addition, the population was aging and the ratio of workers (who paid Medicare taxes for hospitalization insurance) to older people (who spent the dollars paid in by using hospital services) was shrinking. Projections that the Medicare Trust Fund would be bankrupt began in the mid-1980s and continue to this day, with Congress taking only intermediate steps to bail out the program instead of overhauling the entire health care system.

For example, the Tax Equity and Fiscal Responsibility Act (TEFRA), passed by Congress in July 1982, contained temporary limits on Medicare payments and directed the Secretary of DHHS to develop a *prospective payment system* (PPS) for Medicare. The Secretary was instructed to report back to Congress by December 1982 on the status of such a system.

In December 1982, Secretary Richard Schweiker recommended to Congress that a PPS based on *diagnosis-related groups* (DRGs), developed by researchers at Yale University, be used for all Medicare patients. In March 1983, Congress passed amendments to the Social Security Act authorizing such a system. This system was to replace the *cost-based retrospective payment system* used to determine Medicare payments to hospitals. All hospitals serving Medicare clients were to switch to PPS except for certain sole community providers, specialty hospitals, and some psychiatric units within general hospitals.

The program became operational on October 1, 1983. Hospitals were phased into the system over the next 11 months, when their fiscal year began. A formula was calculated for each hospital to determine its initial reimbursement rate under DRGs. Data were gathered from the hospital's own cost history (using a base year) and from a cost history by geographical region; a national rate was also established. These rates were weighted and blended to determine the exact rate of reimbursement per DRG. Since the PPS was initiated, several adjustments have been made in blending. The goal is still to move all hospitals toward one national rate.

PRIVATE SECTOR RESPONSE

Government was not the only entity involved with rising health care costs during the early 1980s; business and industry were also concerned because they paid the majority of the health insurance premium costs for employees. Local and regional business leaders come together to discuss and try to remedy the worsening situation. With the implementation of PPS for Medicare clients, these business coalitions were joined by Blue Cross organizations and other commercial insurers. These new groups held a common fear: that hospitals would shift uncompensated costs generated by Medicare clients to clients who were still reimbursed retrospectively on a cost-plus basis. As a result of that fear, Blue Cross and other insurers have begun to restructure their payment systems to protect themselves from potential or actual cost shifting. These fears were warranted, because cost shifting became and remains a reality.

PPS has yielded other results as well. Hospitals and other health care providers increasingly compete for non-Medicare clients who are more favorably reimbursed. Hospitals also compete for certain Medicare clients whose DRG rate has been profitable for the hospital. Much traditional inpatient care has been shifted to the outpatient system or to the client's home, where the cost of care is less. Insurers and providers have teamed up in creative arrangements designed to hold down costs and yet remain competitive. Such arrangements have created alternative delivery systems based on greater efficiency and decreased costs. Among these are HMOs, PPOs, and independent practice associations (IPAs). The number of outpatient surgical centers (freestanding and hospital-based) and freestanding emergency clinics has increased rapidly.

Providers have been marketing health services to businesses and the public. HMOs and PPOs, for example, seek to contract with employers to be the sole insurer for employee groups. *Capitation* has emerged as a popular form of PPS within these arrangements. Capitation is a per-member per-month fee paid in advance for a specified set of health care services. This money is given to providers up front, whether or not clients use services. The health care provider must provide care even if all of the up front fees have been used.

Medicare also is interested in capitation as a means of payment for its enrollees. In some regions, Medicare enrollees already receive care through an HMO that receives capitation payments from the federal government. The American Hospital Association projected that most Medicare clients would be covered by capitation by the early 1990s.[12] This prediction has yet to become a reality, with many HMO providers threatening to pull out of the Medicare sector because of reimbursement concerns.

Complex *oversight systems* within managed care limited the rate of cost growth through the 1990s, but this restraint did not come without costs. The public grew wary of roadblocks to receiving needed services and applied growing pressure on Congress to control HMO gatekeeping abuses. Perhaps heralding a new trend, United Health Care, (UHC) the nation's second largest health insurer, began dismantling the costly oversight structure in late 1999.[5] Physicians in UHC plans no longer need permission for client tests and admissions. Citing studies indicating the oversight cost more than it saved and disrupted coordination of care, the insurer led the way for the next phase of managed care reform.[5]

■ PERIOD OF REFORM

By 1992, the United States began to reform its health care financing system. With the election of President Clinton, a Democrat, and with continued control of Congress by the same party, passage of national health care reform legislation seemed inevitable. President Clinton introduced the Health Security Act in early 1994, after almost a year of deliberation by economists, business people, and health care providers. First Lady Hillary Rodham Clinton chaired the panel, which attempted to examine the current system's problems (access, cost, quality) to identify the national priorities, including a new emphasis on illness prevention.[23] Much controversy surrounded this ad hoc group. No representation was allowed from organized medicine or other provider organizations. Testimony was sought from these groups, but the actual crafting of the reform plan and ensuing legislation was carried out by the task force. The plan that emerged was so complex that it contained more than 100 pages in published form. The legislation that was sent to Congress was more than 1000 pages.

President Clinton's plan met opposition from within his own party as well as from outside. Everyone publicly agreed that the system needed to be reformed, but no one could agree about how much reform was needed or could be afforded. At one point in 1994, at least six different pieces of health care reform legislation were being considered by Congress. The main points of contention centered on (1) universal access and how to pay for it and (2) employer mandates, which require all employees to be covered by insurance provided by the employer. As a result of these issues and of a general lack of political support by Congress for the President, federal health care reform initiatives did not pass. In fact, no bill was moved out of committee for a vote.

The support for reform, however, did not die in Washington. A number of states passed legislation and policy directives to halt the escalation of costs and to provide increased access to services for citizens regardless of ability to pay. Tennessee led the way in 1994, when it moved all Medicaid recipients into a managed care plan, with capitation paid to managed care companies, which in turn provided a full range of health care services to recipients. Today, Tennessee is still in the forefront of state managed care reform, with 1.3 million Medicaid eligible and uninsured and uninsurable people covered.[28]

By 1996, more than one third of all Medicaid recipients nationwide were enrolled in some form of managed care. The Balanced Budget Act (BBA) of 1997 enabled states to convert to managed care without the need for a federal Medicaid waiver.[10] The law established minimum standards for Medicaid managed care contracts, added qualifying conditions for companies to participate in the program, and ensured better access and coverage for recipients.[10]

Reform also is being driven by the health care industry itself. During 1994, Columbia Health Care System, based in Dallas, acquired Hospital Corporation of America and Health Trust (HCA), both based in Nashville, to form the largest for-profit health care delivery system in the world. In addition to owning 220 hospitals, this corporation aggressively acquired primary care practices of physicians in both rural and urban areas. Using such a strategy, Columbia is creating a network of integrated delivery systems that focuses on primary care as the most desirable and least costly level of care, with secondary and tertiary care available when needed. With such a network in place in numerous markets across the United States, Columbia actively seeks managed care contracts from large employers, generally paid on a capitation basis, although discounted reimbursement mechanisms are still mixed with fee-for-service in most markets.

The response by the not-for-profit sector has varied. In some competitive markets, the not-for-profit hospitals have banded together to form their own integrated delivery systems to compete for managed care contracts. In other areas, some not-for-profits have entered into joint venture arrangements with the for-profit sector or have been purchased by large for-profit systems. This consolidation trend continued throughout the 1990s.

Since the early 1980s, the health care system has undergone rapid change. The system is still evolving, however, and the end product is difficult to foresee. Scarcity of and competition for human and financial resources are the dominant forces operating. This situation creates a dilemma with regard to social values of the past: health care as a right versus scarcity. Nurses must recognize and grapple with these forces and the dilemmas involved in shaping the nation's future health care system.

CONCLUSIONS

Our health care system is large and complex, with many stakeholders. It is also a system under considerable pressure to change as a direct result of rising costs and lower accessibility to basic care for many citizens. This is the environment in which nursing practice takes place. Nurses are in the mainstream of service to both advantaged and disadvantaged clients. Nurses play a crucial role in delivering health care. Many believe that nurses may be the key to revamping the health care system to one that provides access to basic primary care for all citizens. The contribution of the nursing profession to the nation's health has never been more important as we move into the 21st century.

BIBLIOGRAPHY

1. Abundis, J., & Rechin, K. (1999, November 18). Drug prices cheaper abroad. *USA Today*, p. 1.

2. Agency for Health Care Policy and Research. (1999). *AHCPR at a glance.* Agency for Health Care Policy and Research, U.S. Department of Health and Human Services [On-line]. Available: *http://www.ahcpr.gov/news/glance/htm.*

3. American Nurses' Association. (1991). *Agenda for health care reform.* Kansas City, MO: Author.

4. American Nurses' Association. (1999). *Legislative and regulatory initiatives for the 106th Congress.* Kansas City, MO: Author.

5. Appleby, J. (1999, November 9). Health plan eases doctor oversight. *USA Today,* p. 1.

6. Bice, T. W. (1980). Health services planning and regulation. In S. J. Williams & P. R. Torrens (Eds.), *Introduction to health services* (pp. 267–321). New York: John Wiley.

7. Blouin, A. S., & Brent, N. J. (1994). Revisiting collective bargaining. *Journal of Nursing Administration, 24*(9), 9–10, 36.

8. Campbell, P. W., & Healy, P. (1999 November, 5). House approves 15% budget increase for the NIH—but with a hitch. *Chronicle of Higher Education,* A36, 38.

9. Centers for Disease Control and Prevention. (1999). *2000 budget.* Centers for Disease Control and Prevention, U.S. Department of Health and Human Services [On-line]. Available: *http://www.cdc.gov/2000bdg/cdcbud.pdf*

10. Center for Health Policy Research. (1999). *A nationwide study of Medicaid managed care contracts* (2nd ed.). The George Washington University Medical Center [On-line]. Available: *http://www.chcs.org/oview.htm*

11. Clemen-Stone, S., Eigsti, D. G., & McGuire, S. L. (1998). Clients with long-term care needs: Home health, hospice, and other services. In S. Clemon-Stone (Ed.), *Comprehensive community health nursing* (5th ed., pp. 630–663). St. Louis: Mosby–Year Book.

12. Clemen-Stone, S., Eigsti, D. G., & McGuire, S. L. (1998). Occupational health nursing. In S. Clemon-Stone (Ed.), *Comprehensive community health nursing* (5th ed., pp. 537–566). St. Louis: Mosby–Year Book.

13. Clemen-Stone, S., Eigsti, D. G., & McGuire, S. L. (1998). U.S. health and welfare legislation and services. In S. Clemon-Stone (Ed.), *Comprehensive community health nursing* (5th ed., pp. 67–98). St. Louis: Mosby–Year Book.

14. Health Care Financing Administration. (1999). *Expenditures for health services and supplies under public programs by type of expenditure and program: Calendar year 1997.* Health Care Financing Administration, U.S. Department of Health and Human Services [On-line]. Available: *http://www.hcfa.gov/stats/nhe-oact/tables/t18.htm*

15. Health Care Financing Administration. (1999). *Highlights of the national health expenditure projections: 1997–2007.* Health Care Financing Administration, U.S. Department of Health and Human Services [On-line]. Available: *http://www.hcfa.gov/stats/nheproj/hilites/htm*

16. Health Care Financing Administration. (1999) *Highlights: National health expenditures, 1997.* Health Care Financing Administration, U.S. Department of Health and Human Services [On-line]. Available:*http://www.hcfa.gov/stats/nhe-oact/hilites/htm*

17. Huber, D. (1996). *Leadership and nursing care management.* Philadelphia: W. B. Saunders.

18. Jacobs, P. (1995). Economics of healthcare. In G. L. Deloughery (Ed.), *Issues and Trends in Nursing* (pp. 97–128). St. Louis: Mosby–Year Book.

19. Moses, E. B. (1997). *The registered nurse population: Findings from the national sample survey of RNs.* Rockville, MD: Division of Nursing, Bureau of Health Professions, Health Resources and Services Administration, Public Health Service, U.S. Department of Health and Human Services.

20. National Center for Health Statistics. (1995). *Health, United States, 1994.* Hyattsville, MD: Public Health Service, U.S. Department of Health and Human Services.

21. National Institutes of Health. (1999). *Welcome.* National Institutes of Health, U.S. Department of Health and Human Services. [On-line]. Available: *http://www.nih.gov/welcome/nihnew.htm*

22. National Institute for Nursing Research (1999). National Institute for Nursing Research, U.S. Department of Health and Human Services. [On-line]. Available: *http://www.nih.gov/ninr/openingstatement99.htm*

23. O'Neil, E., & Coffman, J. (Eds.). (1998). *Strategies for the future of nursing.* San Francisco: Jossey-Bass.

24. Pilon, B. A., & Davis, S. (1988). Healthcare delivery cost containment practices: History, current status, future directions. In N. Sanders (Director), *Cost management education for nurses* (Contact No. 240-86-0064) Washington, DC: Division of Nursing, Bureau of Health Professions, Health Resources and Services Administration, U.S. Department of Health and Human Services.

25. Poen, M. (1979). Politics, then health: The medicare compromise. In *Harry S. Truman versus the medical lobby* (pp. 174–209). Columbia, MO: University of Missouri Press.

26. Shortell, S. M., & Kaluzny, A. D. (1997). *Essentials of health care management.* Albany, NY: Delmar.

27. Steinwald, B., & Sloan, F. (1981). Regulatory approaches to hospital cost containment: A synthesis of the empirical evidence. In M. Olsen (Ed.), *A new approach to the economics of health care* (pp. 272–307). Washington, DC: American Enterprise Institute.

28. TennCare. (1999). *TennCare fact sheet* [On-line]. Available: *http//www.state.tn.us/health/tenncare/*

29. U.S. Bureau of Health Professions. (1996). *National sample survey of registered nurses.* Washington, DC: Government Printing Office.

30. Williams, C. A. (1996). Community-based population-focused practice: The foundation of public health nursing. In M. Stanhope & J. Lancaster (Eds.), *Community health nursing: Process and practice for promoting health* (4th ed., pp. 21–33). St. Louis: Mosby–Year Book.

CHAPTER

5

Ambulatory Health Care

Sheila A. Haas
Diana P. Hackbarth

In any given year, most Americans are not hospitalized, but the average person makes 3.6 visits to ambulatory care per year.[23] This makes ambulatory settings the major site for health care delivery in the United States. Ambulatory care visits have increased for several reasons:

1. The number of hours or days people stay in hospitals for illness, surgery, or complex treatments has decreased. More clients are seen in ambulatory settings for post-hospital visits and follow-up care.
2. New technology has made ambulatory settings the site for people to undergo many surgical and complex procedures that previously required hospitalization.
3. Advances in the treatment of chronic health problems have made it possible to treat and monitor a client's progress in ambulatory care settings and to avoid costly hospitalization. As a result, both the numbers and the acuity of people cared for in ambulatory settings have increased.

There are numerous advantages to providing health care in ambulatory settings. Clients often feel less stress because they are not separated from their family, significant others, and community. Care in the community decreases exposure to nosocomial infections and other hazards of hospitalization. Ambulatory care is often less costly than hospitalization, saving money for clients, insurance companies, employers, and the government.

Socioeconomic factors have also encouraged the growth of ambulatory care. The growth of managed care organizations has increased the demand for primary care services and ambulatory facilities. Clients who are insured through a managed care plan often must see a primary care provider before obtaining referrals to specialty or hospital care. The variety of care modalities offered in ambulatory care has escalated, and the demand for professional nurses to work in ambulatory care has never been greater. The opportunities for professional nurses to work in ambulatory care settings are expected to increase in the years to come.

■ DEFINITION AND CHARACTERISTICS OF AMBULATORY CARE NURSING

Nurses have worked in ambulatory care settings for many years. Ambulatory care nurses take care of people in all age groups and with all diagnoses, both those who are healthy and those with acute, chronic, or life-threatening health problems. The definition of ambulatory nursing was developed by a panel of expert ambulatory care nurses who participated in focus groups of ambulatory care nurses across the United States.[3] The following themes arose consistently in discussions about the unique characteristics of ambulatory care nursing[3]:

- Nursing autonomy
- Client advocacy
- Skillful, rapid assessment
- Holistic nursing care
- Client teaching
- Wellness and health promotion
- Coordination and continuity of care
- Long-term relationships with clients and families
- Telephone triage, instruction, and advice
- Client and family control as major caregivers, users of the health care system, and decision-makers regarding compliance with care regimen
- Collaboration with other health care providers
- Case management

Based on these themes, the American Academy of Ambulatory Care Nursing (AAACN)[1, 3] defined ambulatory care nursing as follows:

Professional ambulatory care nursing includes those clinical, management, educational, and research activities provided by registered nurses for and with individuals who seek care for health-related problems or concerns or seek assistance with health maintenance and/or health promotion. These individuals engage predominantly in self-care and self-managed health activities or receive care from family and significant others outside an institutional setting.

Ambulatory care nursing services are episodic, less than 24 hours in duration, and occur as a single encounter or a series of encounters over days, weeks, months, or years. Ambulatory nurse-patient encounters take place in health care facilities as well as in community-based settings, including schools, workplaces, or homes.

They occur as personal visits or as encounters using the telephone and other communication devices. Ambulatory care nursing services focus on cost-effective ways to maximize wellness; prevent illness, disability, and disease; minimize symptoms of acute minor aliments; and support patients in the management of chronic disease to affect more positive health states throughout the life span up to and including a peaceful death.

Challenges are an inherent characteristic of ambulatory care nursing:

1. *Visit encounters are short,* the number of client visits per day is great, and the assessment time is compressed. In contrast to the hospital nurse, who can return to a client confined to bed to retrieve data that may have been missed, the ambulatory care nurse who misses collecting data may not be able to obtain it until the next visit. Because visits are short, the ambulatory care nurse cannot do an extensive assessment on every client but must do a focused assessment. This aspect is often a difficult transition for nurses who have worked in hospital settings.

2. Control of care and treatment modalities is in the hands of the *client and family,* not the *health care provider.* In the hospital, the nurse administers medications, administers the treatments, or supervises others providing care to the client. In ambulatory care, however, the client chooses to schedule a visit, keep an appointment, take prescribed medications, or undergo treatments as he or she sees fit. The nurse must become a teacher, coach, and advocate as well as a treatment provider because clients and families must follow through with the treatment plan on their own between visits.

3. In ambulatory care, many members of the health care team work together, and their roles always do not have clear boundaries. Nurses must be strong communicators and collaborators, often functioning as a team leader or team facilitator.

4. In ambulatory care, contacts with the nurse are often maintained through *communication devices* such as the telephone and computer. Ambulatory care nurses need highly developed assessment and communication skills, as well as critical thinking and judgment, in order to interpret data and to refer the client for appropriate follow-up.

Finally, there is *constant pressure* to increase efficiency and effectiveness of care. Nurses are working to standardize care so that health promotion, disease prevention, and early detection and treatment of health problems will be integral to the ambulatory care client encounter.[3]

CONCEPTUAL MODELS THAT INFLUENCE AMBULATORY CARE NURSING PRACTICE

■ THE CLINICAL MODEL

The organization of ambulatory care services in the United States is based on a complex mix of historical, philosophical, political, and economic factors. The way in which policy-makers, health care providers, and ordinary citizens conceptualize health and disease has a profound effect on how health care is delivered.

Most health policy experts agree that our current health care system is based on the clinical or medical model.[6, 22, 24] In this model, health is conceptualized as the absence of the signs or symptoms of disease.[25] It is assumed that the body is a machine and that modern medical technology can employ physical and chemical interventions to "fix the machine" whenever it is broken.[22]

This has led to great emphasis on expensive, acute care with high-technology treatments and relatively little attention to prevention, public health, environmental measures, or personal responsibility for health.

Most ambulatory care services, except for certain public health programs in the community, are outgrowths of this clinical model. Services were traditionally organized around physicians' delivery of reimbursable clinical model care to people who sought care only when they were ill. The traditional nursing role in ambulatory care supported physician control and the clinical model of care delivery. Although the clinical model has led to great advances in scientific medicine and technology, the focus on body parts rather than the whole and the lack of emphasis on prevention have been problematic.

Many nurse theorists, primary care providers, and public health advocates look at health in a *holistic* way. Nurses are educated to (1) consider the whole person, family, and environment; (2) to address both actual and potential health problems; and (3) to emphasize health teaching, prevention, and self-care as well as care of the sick. Newer, more holistic conceptual models are becoming increasingly important in ambulatory care. These models have been delineated by health care scholars, national and international health advocacy organizations, and ambulatory care nurses themselves.

■ LEVELS OF PREVENTION MODEL

The Levels of Prevention Model, advocated by Leavell and Clark in 1965,[20] has influenced both public health practice and ambulatory care delivery worldwide. This model suggests that the natural history of any disease exists on a continuum, with health at one end and advanced disease at the other. The model delineates three levels of the application of preventive measures that can be used to arrest the disease process at different points along the continuum.[20] The goal is to maintain a healthy state and to prevent disease or injury.

People experiencing acute or chronic disease, as well as healthy populations, are all candidates for primary prevention measures. The Levels of Prevention Model is appropriate in all health care settings and in any population group. The *Healthy People 2010 Objectives for the Nation* includes objectives at all three levels of prevention.[29] Most of these objectives can be implemented in ambulatory settings.

PRIMARY PREVENTION. Primary prevention encompasses both health promotion and specific protection.[20] Health promotion includes interventions such as health education, information on growth and development, nutrition, and exercise as well as the provision of adequate housing, safe working conditions, and other services. For example, an ambulatory care nurse might provide telephone consultation and teaching to a new mother concerned about well baby care.

Specific protection interventions are targeted at specific health risks, injuries, or diseases. For example, immunizations protect against particular infectious diseases; seat belts reduce injuries in auto crashes; smoking cessation reduces the risk of cancers and heart disease; reducing air pollution prevents exacerbations of asthma and bronchitis; encouraging a high-calcium diet with over-the-counter calcium supplements and weight-bearing exercise helps menopausal women prevent osteoporosis. Primary prevention interventions may be targeted at individual clients, families, groups, communities or populations.

SECONDARY PREVENTION. Secondary preventive measures include early diagnosis and prompt treatment as well as disability limitation.[20] Case finding, screening, and treatment of disease by medical or surgical interventions to arrest the disease process and prevent further complications are all part of secondary prevention. An ambulatory care nurse carrying out a multiphasic health screening for hypertension, diabetes, and hypercholesterolemia would be practicing secondary prevention. Other examples are administering chemotherapy to a client with cancer and positioning a client in the recovery room after outpatient surgery to ensure proper alignment of the extremities.

TERTIARY PREVENTION. Tertiary prevention is the provision of measures to rehabilitate a person or groups so they can maximize their remaining capacities.[20] Cardiac rehabilitation nurses, physical and occupational therapists, and many home care nurses focus on tertiary prevention. An example in the ambulatory surgery recovery room would be teaching crutch walking to a client after foot surgery.

■ PRIMARY HEALTH CARE, PRIMARY CARE, AND MANAGED CARE MODELS

Primary health care focuses on the universal right to basic health care. *Primary care* focuses on integrated care coordinated by one primary provider. *Managed care* approaches the use of health care services from a cost-containment perspective. *Primary prevention* is often confused with the concepts of primary health care and primary care.[14] In addition, many managed care organizations use primary care providers, such as family practice physicians and nurse practitioners, in a "gatekeeper" function, causing further confusion. Box 5–1 compares and contrasts these conceptual models. They, as well as the clinical model and the ambulatory care nursing conceptual framework, have influenced the organization of practice in ambulatory care settings.

AMBULATORY CARE NURSING CONCEPTUAL FRAMEWORK

The Ambulatory Care Nursing Conceptual Framework was developed by a think tank of experts who are also members of the AAACN.[7] The AAACN member experts

---

BOX 5–1 Prevention and Health Care Models

Primary Prevention

- Includes health promotion and specific protection
- May be directed at individuals, groups, or populations
- May be targeted at well or ill populations
- Goal: to prevent disease or injury and to reduce risk factors
- Includes individual lifestyle changes as well as healthy environments and positive social change

  - Education
  - Legislation
  - Regulation
  - Taxation
  - Health policy
  - Risk reduction and lifestyle change

- *Healthy People 2010* goals: primary prevention

Primary Care

- IOM definition (1994)[17]: "provision of integrated accessible health care services by clinicians who are accountable for addressing a large majority of personal health care needs, developing a sustained partnership with patients, and practicing in the context of family and community.
- IOM definition (1978)[18]: personal health care services that are accessible, comprehensive, coordinated, and continuous. Care delivered by accountable providers of personal health services.
- Starfield definition (1992)[26]:

  - First contact—source of care available in a timely manner
  - Longitudinal—not episodic, focused on person not episode of disease; client sees provider as regular source of care
  - Comprehensive—includes services for common problems
  - Coordinated—provider coordinates care when client is sent elsewhere for referrals, procedures, and therapies

Primary Health Care

- WHO definition (1978)[31]: "essential health care—made universally accessible to individuals and families in the community through their full participation and at a cost the community and country can afford"

  - Assumes community involvement
  - Includes both personal health care services and population-based public health services
  - Aimed at prevention as well as treatment of disease
  - Aimed at improving health status of the population or community

Managed Care

- Enthoven definition (1993)[5]:

  - Integrated financing and delivery systems with per capita prepayment and with providers placed at risk for cost and quality of care
  - First contact—ensure access to basic services; restrict access to specialized services through "gatekeeper" function of primary provider

- Starfield definition (1992)[26]:

  - Longitudinal—not addressed
  - Comprehensive—not addressed
  - Coordinated—gatekeeper as coordinator; goal is to eliminate unnecessary and inappropriate care; may also restrict access to appropriate care
  - Reduction in cost; cost containment
  - Health status of population—not addressed; in HMO organizations, goal is to keep enrolled population healthy in order to reduce utilization cost

---

IOM, Institute of Medicine; WHO, World Health Organization.

work in ambulatory care settings, perform research, and write about ambulatory care nursing. A conceptual framework is a diagram that:

- Specifies major concepts, skills, and responsibilities in an area of practice
- Reflects values and beliefs as well as the experiential knowledge of a practice discipline
- Delineates the relationships between major concepts and skills
- Acts as a model to help organize practice, guide the development of educational materials, create test items for certification examinations, and develop orientation programs
- Forms the basis of performance appraisal instruments for ambulatory care

The conceptual framework shown in Figure 5–1 delineates three roles for ambulatory care nurses: (1) the Clinical Nursing Role, (2) the Organizational/Systems Role, and (3) the Professional Role.[7] Each role has several dimensions that vary, depending on the size of the ambulatory care setting. For example, staff nurses working in larger settings, where there are multiple nurses and nurse managers, do not need to do many of the more managerial dimensions under the Organizational/Systems Role. In smaller settings, they would likely practice in all three roles. The Ambulatory Care Nursing Conceptual Framework was used to structure the Ambulatory Care Nursing Core Curriculum written for nurses to use in preparation for certification in ambulatory care.

As seen in Figure 5–1, client populations may be healthy, acutely ill, chronically ill, or terminally ill. Role dimensions highly valued by nurses are all included in this conceptual framework:

- Primary, secondary, and tertiary prevention
- Teaching and client advocacy
- Care management, a feature of primary care
- Evidence-based practice

AMBULATORY CARE PRACTICE SETTINGS

Historically, health services in the United States were delivered to people in their homes by itinerant physicians,

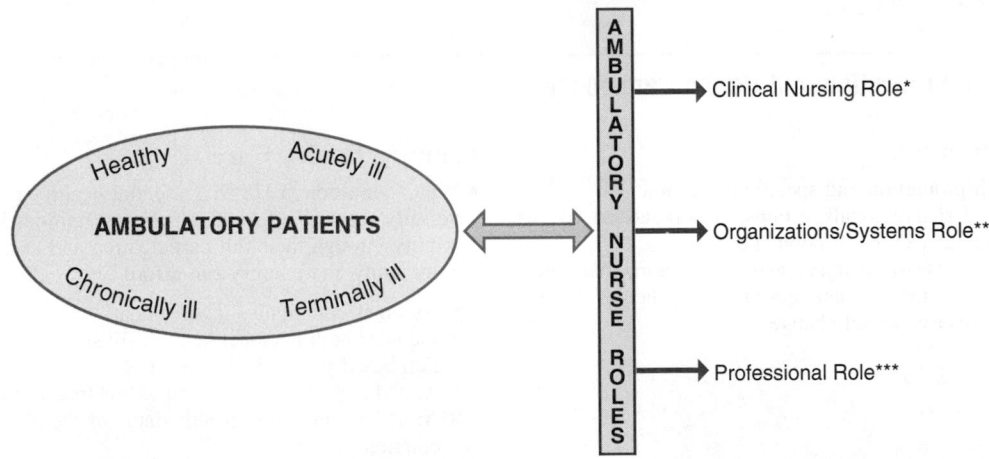

*Clinical Nursing Role
Patient Education
Advocacy (compassion, caring, emotional support)
Care Management
Assessment, Screening, Triage
Telephone Practice
Collaboration/Resource Identification and Referral
Clinical Procedures, Independent/Interdependent/Dependent
Primary, Secondary, and Tertiary Prevention
Communication/Documentation
Outcome Management
Protocol Development/Usage

**Organizations/Systems Role
Practice/Office Support
Healthcare Fiscal Management (reimbursement and coding)
Collaboration/Conflict Management
Informatics
Context of Care Delivery/Models
Care of the Caregiver
Priority Management/Delegation/Supervision
Ambulatory Culture/Cross Cultural Competencies
Ongoing Political/Entrepreneurial Skills
Structuring Customer-focused Systems
Workplace Regulatory Compliance (EEOC, OSHA)
Advocacy Inter-organizational and in Community
Legal Issues

***Professional Role
Evidence-based Practice
Leadership Inquiry and Research Utilization
Clinical Quality improvement
Staff Development
Regulatory Compliance (risk management)
Provider Self-Care

FIGURE 5–1 Ambulatory Care Nursing Conceptual Framework. (Modified from Haas, S. [1998]. Ambulatory care nursing conceptual framework. *AAACN Viewpoint, 20*[3], 16–17.) Reprinted with permission of publisher.

midwives, barbers, nurses, and "medicine men," who learned their trade through an unregulated apprentice system. In some urban areas, freestanding dispensaries were established as charity for the poor and a place for would-be physicians to learn their trade.[27] These dispensaries dissolved into outpatient departments once a system of voluntary hospitals was developed and nursing and medical education was upgraded and standardized in the beginning of the 20th century.[27]

For the purposes of data collection, the National Center for Health Statistics classifies ambulatory care settings into three main groups: physician offices, hospital outpatient departments, and hospital emergency departments.[23] Each of these may sponsor many types of ambulatory care programs, both on-site and geographically dispersed in communities. With the advent of managed care insurance plans, health maintenance organizations (HMOs) and preferred provider organizations (PPOs) have grown in importance as both sites and financiers of ambulatory care delivery.

PHYSICIAN GROUP PRACTICES. Almost 82% of all ambulatory care visits occur in physicians' offices.[23] Physician group practices arose out of the perceived need to enhance services offered to clients and to provide for more equal distribution of work among physicians. Increasingly, physicians are abandoning solo practice and aligning themselves in group practices in order to consolidate resources to meet the challenges of managed care contracting. In the past, many group practices consisted of groups of specialists, such as cardiologists or oncologists; today, larger group practices now seek to add primary care physicians.

Physician group practices usually operate on a for-profit basis and seek fee-for-service payment. In a *fee-for-service* system, providers generate more revenue the more services they provide. *Integrated* delivery systems have been developed in which hospitals align with several physician group practices to increase the hospital referral rate and provide increased coordination of care. Many physician group practices also contract with HMOs and PPOs and offer either reduced rate fee-for-service or *capitated* (prepaid at a fixed rate) services along with their traditional fee-for-service practices.

The predominant way of viewing health and disease in most physician group practices is the *clinical model*. However, family practice physicians may adhere to the *primary care model*. In the past, nurses in physician offices often served a clerical as well as an assistive function. The role of the ambulatory care nurse in physician group practices is evolving to meet the need for increasingly skilled technical services, especially in specialty practices such as oncology, freestanding birthing centers, and surgical centers.

COMMUNITY HOSPITAL OUTPATIENT DEPARTMENTS. Community hospital clinic services began in the latter part of the 19th century and took over the functions of the freestanding dispensaries.[27] Clinic services were consistent with the mission of the religious and ethnic groups that organized voluntary community hospitals. This mission included both a charitable function for the community and a place for local physicians to practice.[6] Physicians were often assigned to staff hospital clinics as a duty, in return for the privilege of hospitalizing their clients.[19, 24] Nurses trained in diploma schools staffed both the hospital and clinics.

Today, nonprofit community hospitals still provide varying amounts of uncompensated care in their outpatient departments as part of their obligation to provide "community benefits" as not-for-profit corporations. However, their goal is to maximize revenues by attracting individuals or employee groups who have insurance coverage. Thus, outpatient services constitute a key source of revenue for hospitals.

Both primary care and specialized care in a clinical model may be offered. Ambulatory services may be housed adjacent to the hospital or be freestanding in the community. Services may include outpatient surgery, emergency centers, cardiac rehabilitation centers, drug and alcohol treatment programs, mobile vans, women's health or breast centers, work site health promotion, oncology centers, home care, hospice, and community health promotion.[24] Many integrated health care systems have freestanding satellite ambulatory care sites that offer primary care services for managed care enrollees. Specialized clinics and health promotion programs staffed by nurses also exist in community hospital outpatient settings. Some of these programs are organized around the ambulatory care nursing conceptual framework.

TEACHING HOSPITAL OUTPATIENT DEPARTMENTS. Outpatient departments of teaching hospitals were developed to fulfill the mission of academic health centers: to provide medical and other health professional education, biomedical research, and client care services.[4] University hospital outpatient departments and most large hospitals run by local governments provide learning experiences for medical, nursing, and other health science students as well as opportunities for clinical research on populations of patients with highly specialized needs. Veterans Administration ambulatory care departments serve a similar function.

Clinical services are often organized around medical specialty areas for the convenience of providers. Some are regional referral centers, whereas others, especially those that are tax-supported, may provide a full range of services, including primary care for the poor.[24] Most teaching hospitals maintain a nonprofit status and provide care for those with public or private insurance as well as uncompensated care for uninsured clients (whose diseases may provide good learning experiences). Many hospitals have satellite ambulatory care centers. With the growth of managed care, increased competition, and decreased reimbursement from Medicaid and Medicare, teaching hospitals are increasingly concerned with maximizing revenue from insured clients and ensuring a flow of paying clients to make up for empty inpatient beds.

University hospital outpatient departments have traditionally espoused the clinical model and have been driven and controlled by physicians. There are, however, some nurse-managed hospital clinics that deal with specific client populations, such as clients with chronic leg ulcers or those who need monitoring of warfarin (Coumadin) therapy. Nurses play a major role in patient and family teaching and as case managers for clients with catastrophic and chronic illnesses. For example, nurses case manage the care of heart transplant clients, trauma victims, oncology clients, and high-risk mothers and infants.

HEALTH MAINTENANCE ORGANIZATIONS. HMOs began more than 50 years ago and proliferated during the 1990s in response to both federal enabling legislation and market forces. HMOs provide a defined population with a stated range of services through the prepayment of an annual or monthly capitation fee. With *capitation,* providers receive the same amount of money per patient per month, no matter how many or how few services a client uses that month or year. Thus, there is no incentive to provide expensive tests or treatments that the client may not need. HMOs are systems of care that integrate the insurance and payment mechanisms and the actual delivery of health care services.

HMOs began as nonprofit organizations but increasingly have been purchased by the for-profit sector. Philosophically, the concept of an HMO differs from traditional ambulatory services, in that value is placed on prevention and maintaining health in order to avoid more costly specialist or inpatient services. Care is coordinated by a primary care provider who acts as a gatekeeper. The goal is to lower costs through the provision of primary care, coordination of services, utilization management, and elimination of the "incentives" of the fee-for-service payment system.

Many HMOs employ nurse practitioners, nurse-midwives, and physician assistants as primary care providers. In addition to the clinical model, HMOs espouse wellness, health maintenance, and primary care. Nursing, with its more holistic approach to client care, can play an influential role in managed care settings.

EMERGENCY DEPARTMENTS. Almost 10% of ambulatory care visits are provided in emergency departments (EDs).[23] Although some of these visits are for true emergency conditions, more than half of ED visits in the United States are for non-urgent care.[21] Uninsured people and those on Medicare and Medicaid use disproportionately more ED services for non-urgent care than those who have private insurance.[23] In the United States, there are 45 million uninsured and underinsured people who lack access to appropriate primary care services in their communities.[24] Because EDs are organized according to the clinical model and are set up to meet acute care needs, they are far from the ideal place to provide primary care services.

OTHER AMBULATORY CARE SETTINGS. Many other settings provide a wide array of ambulatory care services. One unique type of ambulatory care organization is a Nurse-Managed Center or Nursing Center. These nurse-staffed community centers may provide primary health care services, home care, hospice, college health services, work site health promotion, school nursing, or wellness services. Many Nursing Centers were developed by schools of nursing as faculty practice sites and clinical sites for undergraduate and graduate students. Others were federally funded demonstration projects. Most Nurse-Managed Centers employ Advanced Practice Nurses (APNs) and are organized around a nursing or primary health care model.

Other settings in which ambulatory care nurses practice include government-funded public health clinics, migrant and community health centers, homeless shelters, school-based health centers, Native American Health Service clinics, and other community-based organizations that serve special population groups. These are either tax-supported or private nonprofit organizations and are organized around a primary health care or public health model. Most include population-based preventive services as well as personal health care.

■ CHARACTERISTICS OF AMBULATORY CARE CLIENT POPULATION

Each year in the United States, people make more than 960 million ambulatory visits. Women make more visits than men, and older adults make an average 7.5 visits a year, compared with about three visits a year for children.[23] The overall visit rate for whites is not significantly different than that for African Americans.[23] Figure 5–2 shows the distribution of ambulatory care visits, categorized by clients' expressed reasons for the visit. Figure 5–3 depicts the distribution of ambulatory care visits by primary diagnosis in the United States in 1997. Difficulty breathing, a manifestation of many problems including lung, heart, and allergic conditions, is a common reason for visits.

Ambulatory clients are often classified by their *health status.* A client may be essentially healthy but acutely ill at the time of the visit, such as a client with otitis media or appendicitis. The client can be expected to return to wellness once the acute problem is cured. Another client may be chronically ill but managing the chronic illness well. A young asthmatic person with peak flow readings within normal limits is an example. A client may be chronically ill and have an acute episode, such as an elderly diabetic client with influenza. Finally, a client may be terminally ill with end-stage renal disease or liver failure and require supportive care.

Ambulatory clients may also be classified by a major *illness,* body system, and typical *treatment* needed. For example, teaching hospital outpatient settings often have specific clinics for people with diabetes or heart failure; some have ear, nose, and throat (ENT) clinics or urology clinics for people with maladies of certain body systems; and others have programs such as a "Coumadin clinic" and "cast clinic," which classify clients according to the type of treatment to be administered.

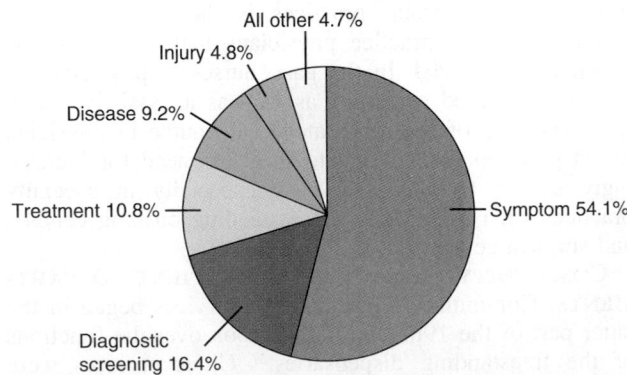

FIGURE 5–2 Per cent distribution of ambulatory care visits by patients' expressed reason for visit: United States, 1997. (From National Center for Health Statistics. [1999]. *Ambulatory care statistics: United States, 1997.* Hyattsville, MD: Centers for Disease Control and Prevention, National Center for Health Statistics.)

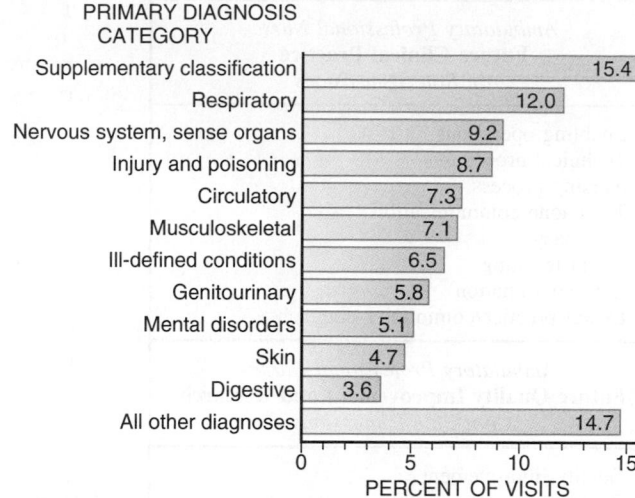

PRIMARY DIAGNOSIS
CATEGORY

Category	Percent
Supplementary classification	15.4
Respiratory	12.0
Nervous system, sense organs	9.2
Injury and poisoning	8.7
Circulatory	7.3
Musculoskeletal	7.1
Ill-defined conditions	6.5
Genitourinary	5.8
Mental disorders	5.1
Skin	4.7
Digestive	3.6
All other diagnoses	14.7

PERCENT OF VISITS

FIGURE 5–3 Per cent distribution of ambulatory care visits by primary diagnosis category: United States, 1997. The category "supplementary classification" is used for diagnoses not related to illness or injury, such as general medical examinations and normal prenatal care. (From National Center for Health Statistics. [1999]. *Ambulatory care statistics: United States, 1997.* Hyattsville, MD: Centers for Disease Control and Prevention, National Center for Health Statistics.)

Ambulatory clients may also be classified in terms of *age,* such as pediatric, adolescent, and geriatric.

Another means of categorizing clients is by the type or source of *reimbursement* for the care provided; (e.g., private insurance, Medicare, Medicaid, worker's compensation, or self-pay). Ambulatory care clients also may be defined by the type of *service,* such as primary care, which includes pediatrics, obstetrics and gynecology, family practice, and internal medicine.

As mentioned previously, in ambulatory care it is the client, client's family, or significant other who initiates an encounter or visit, travels to and from the ambulatory care setting, and chooses to collaborate with the ambulatory interdisciplinary team regarding wellness behaviors and the treatment regimen. Thus, the ambulatory care team must know, understand, and respect the client's culture, traditions, and perspective on health and illness. Cultural competence is essential, because the client, family, or significant other manages and provides health care during visits and during the interval between visits and the client controls health care decisions. Respectful communication facilitates the long-term relationships that clients often have with ambulatory care nurses and other providers.

RESEARCH IN AMBULATORY CARE NURSING

Although nurses have been working in ambulatory settings for many years, little research on the work and role of ambulatory care nurses has been done. Such research is needed for many reasons[15]:

- To help develop new models of nursing care delivery
- To delineate position descriptions for nurses working in ambulatory care
- To develop standards of client care and professional nursing practice

- To create both performance improvement programs and nursing intensity systems to determine the number and types of nursing personnel needed.[15]

One of the earliest studies, done by Hooks and colleagues in 1980,[16] delineated barriers to ambulatory nursing practice. Verran, in 1981,[30] developed seven areas of nursing responsibility in ambulatory care using a Delphi method and the opinion of expert ambulatory care nurses. Tighe and associates,[28] in 1985, further refined Verran's areas of responsibility by adding planning. In 1995, Hackbarth and co-workers[15] and Haas and colleagues[10–13] conducted a national survey of ambulatory care nurses working in many types of ambulatory care settings. An analysis of these data provided insight into the dimensions of the current staff nurse role and the dimensions of the future staff nurse role in ambulatory care.

In current practice, Hackbarth and co-workers[15] found that ambulatory care nurses spent much of their time performing activities in dimensions named Enabling Operations and Technical Procedures. These activities include locating records, ordering supplies, taking vital signs, setting up rooms, assisting with procedures, and administering oral or intramuscular (IM) medications. Some of these activities could have been done by clerks or nursing assistants. Relatively less of the staff nurses' time was spent on more professional activities in the dimensions named Telephone Communication, Advocacy, Teaching, and Care Coordination.

When nurses surveyed by Haas and Hackbarth[12] were asked what they would like to be doing in the future, they indicated that they would prefer to accomplish more activities in higher-level professional dimensions such as Teaching, Care Coordination, and Expert Practice. They even foresaw another dimension, labeled High Tech Procedures (Fig. 5–4). The implications of this research are clear. Nurses in many ambulatory settings need to have sufficient numbers of competent assistive personnel to whom they can delegate Enabling and Technical procedures if they are to have sufficient time to perform activities in higher-level dimensions such as Teaching, Advocacy, Care Coordination, High Tech Procedures, and Expert Practice.

DIMENSIONS UNIQUE TO NURSING PRACTICE IN AMBULATORY CARE

TELEPHONE NURSING PRACTICE. One dimension of the professional nurse's role that is unique in ambulatory care settings is Telephone Communication, or Telephone Nursing Practice. Telephone Nursing Practice is defined as "nursing practice using the nursing process to provide care for individual patients or defined patient populations over the telephone."[2] Defined criteria include:

- Using protocols, algorithms, or guidelines to assess and address client needs systematically
- Prioritizing the urgency of client needs
- Developing a collaborative plan of care with clients and their support systems, including wellness promotion, prevention education, advice, care counseling, disease state management, and care coordination
- Evaluating outcomes of practice and care

Ambulatory Professional Nurse **Current Clinical Practice** Core Role Dimensions	Ambulatory Professional Nurse **Future Clinical Practice** Core Role Dimensions
Enabling operations Technical procedures Nursing process Telephone communication Advocacy Teaching Care coordination Expert practice within setting	Enabling operations Technical procedures Nursing process Telephone communication Advocacy Client teaching Care coordination Expert practice/community outreach
Ambulatory Professional Nurse **Current Quality Improvement and Research** Core Role Dimensions	Ambulatory Professional Nurse **Future Quality Improvement and Research** Core Role Dimensions
Quality improvement Research Continuing education	Quality improvement Research Continuing education

FIGURE 5–4 Current and future ambulatory professional nurse role dimensions. (Data from Haas, S. A., & Hackbarth, D. P. [1995]. *Nursing Economics, 13*[4], 230–241; and Hackbarth, D. P., et al. [1995]. *Nursing Economics, 13*[2], 89–98.)

Telephone Nursing Practice is not new and has been described in the literature since the 1960s. Communication by telephone for health guidance is common in pediatric practices, obstetrics and gynecology practices, primary care, and the ED. Clients often call ambulatory care settings to report symptoms of illness and to seek advice. A 1997 document published by the AAACN identifies standards that define the responsibilities of both clinical nurses and managers when providing care via the telephone.[3]

The *Nursing Intervention Classification* (NIC) lists four telephone nursing practices:

- Telephone consultation
- Telephone follow-up
- Telephone triage
- Telephone surveillance

Each of these interventions was proposed by Haas and Androwich in 1999.[8]

1. *Telephone consultation.* The nurse assesses the client's need and readiness to learn, teaches clients, and provides advice based on protocols approved for use with telephone nursing practice. Assessing a client by telephone is far more difficult for the nurse than a face-to-face meeting with a client. The nurse must have expert communication skills to elicit information when no visual or physical assessment cues are available. The nurse must listen for nuances in the client's communication, such as inflection, pitch, volume, and rate of speech. The telephone encounter time is very limited. There is no time to reflect or have second thoughts. Although telephone assessment has some pitfalls, there are some benefits too (see later).

2. *Telephone follow-up* is used for clients who have had ambulatory surgery or complex treatments. The nurse calls the client within a specified period to assess how well the client is recovering and to provide guidance for any problems. Especially when the nurse is calling the client, the nurse must protect the confidentiality of the client and should speak with family members or significant others only if the client has given permission. Many clients appreciate telephone follow-up. It connotes caring and concern on the part of the nurse and the ambulatory care organization, and it gives the client ready access to a health professional.

3. With *telephone triage,* clients are sorted by telephone encounter based on the immediacy of the need and the type of problem. In ambulatory care, a nurse talks with a client calling from home and assesses the type of problem, how the problem should be resolved, how soon, whether the client should be seen in person, and who should resolve the problem.

4. Nurses use *telephone surveillance* to work with data coming into a central ambulatory site from monitoring equipment used by clients at home. For example, cardiac monitoring or high-risk obstetric monitoring can be accomplished by connecting the monitoring equipment to a computer or telephone in the client's home.

Telephone triage and telephone consultation by nurses has increased with the growth of managed care health insurance plans. Nurses use commercially available protocols or protocols that have been developed by physicians and nurses in their own ambulatory care organization to assess the client over the telephone and to recommend approved interventions. Nurse telephone consultation and telephone triage have some advantages. They make nurses and expert health advice readily available; they may save a trip to the ambulatory care site; and for many clients, they provide a knowledgeable and caring person to ask about a problem.

Professional nurses have stated strongly that Telephone Nursing Practice should be part of the professional nurse role.[3] It should not be done by Licensed Practical Nurses (LPNs) or assistive personnel such as receptionists or schedulers. It requires critical thinking and judgment as well as assessment and evaluation skills. Nurses need to attend educational programs designed to help them develop the knowledge and skills needed to practice these techniques effectively. Every telephone encounter should be documented on the client's medical record, including assessment data, analysis, recommendations made to the client, and the client's level of understanding of instructions, (e.g., when to come in or to call back).

EXPERT PRACTICE WITHIN THE SETTING. Another unique dimension of the current clinical nurse role in ambulatory care is Expert Practice Within the Setting. Ambulatory care nurses who develop expertise with specific client populations often are in charge of nurse-run clinics such as incontinence clinics, Coumadin clinics, or wound care clinics. In a nurse-run clinic, a nurse with at least a Bachelor's Degree in Nursing, plus experience and continuing education, works with physicians to develop protocols. Nurses monitor clients during ambulatory visits and suggest interventions for common problems that clients experience.

Nurses and clients express high levels of satisfaction with nurse-run ambulatory programs. Clients have a nurse they can call who knows them and their problems and who has insight into what works for them. The nurse often acts as their advocate in the health care system. Nurses find this type of work rewarding because they have long-term relationships with clients and families and can see the results of their teaching, advocacy, and nursing interventions.

■ AMBULATORY CARE INTERDISCIPLINARY TEAM

Nurses working in ambulatory settings are members of an interdisciplinary team. They work collaboratively with physicians; midlevel providers, such as Nurse-Practitioners (NPs), nurse-midwives, or Physician Assistants (PAs); LPNs or Licensed Vocational Nurses (LVNs); medical assistants (MAs); Nurse Assistants (NAs); and clerks, receptionists, and schedulers.

The challenges in working with a large team are numerous. Roles often are blurred, especially when people have worked together in the same clinic for many years. Sometimes team members may be asked to perform beyond their legal scope of practice; at other times, nurses may do assistive or clerical work. Both situations can prevent clients from receiving care from the best prepared provider. Nurses must continually negotiate and advocate for clients within and beyond the team.

Nurses must also delegate appropriately to assistive workers. Nurses must be aware of the specifications of their state Nurse Practice Act and delegate to LPNs or LVNs only what is legally within their scope of practice. For example, MAs in some states may administer immunizations when they have the requisite training and when they are supervised by licensed professional nurses or physicians; in other states, this might be illegal. Supervision in ambulatory care is challenging.[9] State Nurse Practice Acts often legally define both the delegation and the supervision to be done by professional nurses.

PROFESSIONAL AND LEGAL CONSIDERATIONS

STANDARDS OF CARE

Standards are written authoritative statements developed and disseminated by a professional organizational or governmental or regulatory agency by which the quality of practice, services, research, or education can be judged.[1] In 1987, the AAACN developed Ambulatory Care Nursing Administration and Practice Standards. These have been revised and updated periodically, most recently in 2000.[1] There are nine standards: Structure and Organization of Ambulatory Care Nursing, Staffing in Ambulatory Care, Competency, Ambulatory Nursing Practice, Continuity of Care, Ethics and Patient's Rights, Environment, Research, and Quality Management. AAACN also developed and published the Telephone Nursing Practice Administration and Practice Standards in 1997.[2]

Ambulatory care nurses are also guided by other sets of standards. To provide services, an ambulatory care setting must be in compliance with each state's Department of Health rules and regulations and must operate in compliance with Occupational Safety and Health Administration (OSHA) standards. Evidence-based practice standards are available through the Agency for Health Care Research and Quality (AHRQ), which has standards for many common health problems such as chronic pain, incontinence care, depression, and sickle cell anemia. These are available on the World Wide Web at *http://www.ahcpr.gov*. Professional nursing organizations, such as the American Nurses' Association (ANA) and Oncology Nurses Society (ONS), also have specific patient population standards.

COMPETENCE

Competence is the "demonstrated knowledge, skills, and ability to effectively carry out the requirements of a given role. Nurse competence is circumscribed by the individual nurse's education, knowledge, certification, experience and abilities."[3] Ambulatory care nurses demonstrate competence in core clinical practice dimensions, such as client teaching. They also have competencies that reflect the unique clinical dimensions of ambulatory care nursing, such as telephone nursing, and that correspond to the needs of the particular client populations served and the nursing interventions commonly required by such populations. For example, ambulatory oncology clients are a specific population for whom competence with chemotherapy administration is a requisite nursing intervention competence. Ambulatory care nurses who work in smaller ambulatory settings may also be required to exhibit competencies in dimensions within the leadership role, such as regulatory compliance and risk management. Any nurse who works with assistive personnel must be competent in delegation and supervision.

CERTIFICATION

Holding certification in a specialty practice area such as ambulatory care nursing is a way of demonstrating competence to consumers and colleagues. To obtain certification, practicing nurses prepare for and take an examination that is developed by a panel of experts and administered by a recognized certification agency. With increasing numbers of nurses practicing in ambulatory care and the evolution of the Ambulatory Care Nursing Conceptual Framework,[7] the AAACN and the American Nurses Credentialing Center (ANCC) service have developed a certification examination for nurses working in staff nursing positions in ambulatory care. The examination was administered for the first time in the fall of 1999.

To qualify for the examination, ambulatory care nurses must have a Baccalaureate degree in nursing and meet the requirement for hours of experience in ambulatory care nursing. To maintain certification, ambulatory nurses must continue to practice in the clinical area for the specified number of hours per year and attend a specified number of hours of sanctioned continuing education. Ambulatory care nurses are often certified in more than one area of specialty nursing practice. A nurse working with oncology clients might be certified in oncology nursing as well as ambulatory care nursing. AAACN has led the development of the Ambulatory Care Nursing Conceptual Framework, core curriculum, and ambulatory certification. AAACN Web site address is *http://www.inurse.com* and the e-mail address is *aaacn@ajj.com*.

REGULATORY COMPLIANCE

Ambulatory settings must be licensed in the state in which they are located; they may earn and maintain credentials, such as accreditation by a national association like the Joint Commission on Accreditation of Healthcare Organizations (JCAHO). Accreditation offers the opportunity for an organization to be evaluated by an external group that assesses the quality of care provided. Accreditation demonstrates compliance with a uniform set of standards; it allows comparisons with other organizations and enhances the organization's competitive edge.

Three accreditation agencies publish standards and offer external validation of quality of care for ambulatory care organizations:

1. JCAHO serves hospital-affiliated ambulatory care organizations as well as freestanding ambulatory care settings.
2. The National Committee for Quality Assurance (NCQA) serves managed care organizations and uses the Health Plan Employer Data and Information Set (HEDIS) Report Cards.
3. The Accreditation Association for Ambulatory Health Care (AAAHC) serves freestanding ambulatory surgery centers, medical group practices, student health centers, and office-based surgeons' practices.

All accreditation organizations use standards developed by the accreditation organization and on-site surveys done by teams of experts.

MULTI-STATE LICENSURE

Multi-state licensure is an issue that has emerged because (1) there are increasing numbers of national health care systems, (2) telephone nursing practice is more common, and (3) people are more mobile in seeking care. The legal authority for practice is a concern for any professional nurse who provides care for people located in a state in which the nurse is not licensed. Examples of nurses who must be concerned about multi-state licensure are (1) nurses working in integrated delivery systems and regional referral health care systems in which people come in for care from other states; (2) flight nurses; and (3) telephone practice nurses. If a nurse cares for a client by telephone, computer, or monitoring device and the client is located in a state where the nurse is not licensed, the nurse faces the risk of being cited for practicing without a license in the client's home state.

The *Mutual Recognition Model,* implemented through an *Interstate Compact,* has been recognized as the preferred model of nurse licensure. The National Council of State Boards of Nursing (NCSBN) has been working to educate nurses about the Interstate Compact. Information is available on their Web site at *http://www.ncsbn.org.* The Interstate Compact is a legal document that must be adopted by each state legislature. After adoption, nurses would obtain a license in their home state but would be able to communicate with clients in other states without violating the Nurse Practice Act in the client's home state if that state has also passed Compact legislation. The advantages of the Interstate Compact or "the one license concept" are reduced barriers to interstate practice, improved tracking for disciplinary purposes, cost-effectiveness, unduplicated counts of nurses, maintenance of a state-based system of licensure, and expanded consumer access to qualified nurses. Only a few states have adopted the Interstate Compact thus far. It will take several years for all states to sign on. Until all states have adopted the Interstate Compact, nurses need to be aware of the implications of practicing across state lines.

TRENDS AND DIRECTIONS FOR THE FUTURE

Demographic and socioeconomic trends in the United States are expected to continue to challenge ambulatory care nurses. Among these are (1) rapid changes in technology; (2) increased emphasis on demonstrated outcomes; (3) aging of the population; (4) reduced revenue to health care organizations from managed care contracts; and (5) the large number of uninsured people. A unified system ensuring access to health care for all Americans does not seem imminent. In addition, a nursing shortage is on the horizon.

Many believe, however, that the nation is experiencing a fundamental shift in emphasis on the concept of health itself, with the focus changing from the old clinical model to a wellness orientation. According to Shi and Singh,[24] health care is changing (1) from an *illness* orientation to a *wellness* orientation; (2) from an *acute* care emphasis to *primary* care; (3) from *inpatient* to *outpatient* services; (4) from *individual* health to *community* well-being; (5) from *fragmented* care to *managed* care; (6) from *independent* institutions to *integrated* systems; and (7) from service *duplication* to a *continuum* of services. If these predictions are correct, the well-educated ambulatory care nurse will be at the forefront of the health care delivery system in the new millennium.

CONCLUSIONS

Ambulatory care nursing is one of the fastest-growing areas of nursing specialty practice. Ambulatory care nurses are not only expert clinicians but also expert communicators. They play key roles in facilitating clients' successful progress through our integrated delivery systems. Ambulatory nurses make quality health care accessible for clients calling and coming into our health care delivery systems.

BIBLIOGRAPHY

1. American Academy of Ambulatory Care Nursing. (2000). *Ambulatory care nursing administration and practice standards.* Pitman, NJ: Anthony J. Jannetti, Inc.
2. American Academy of Ambulatory Care Nursing. (1997). *Telephone nursing practice administration and practice standards.* Pitman, NJ: Anthony J. Jannetti, Inc.
3. American Academy of Ambulatory Care Nursing and American Nurses Association. (1997). *Nursing in ambulatory care: The future is here.* Washington, DC: American Nurses Publishing.
4. Bentley, J., et al. (1991). Faculty practice plans: The organization and characteristics of academic medical practice. *Academic Medicine, 66*(8), 433–439.
5. Enthoven, A. (1993). The history and principles of managed competition. *Health Affairs* (suppl.), 24–28.
6. Ginzberg, E. (1994). *The road to reform.* New York: The Free Press.
7. Haas, S. (1998). Ambulatory care nursing conceptual framework. *AAACN Viewpoint, 20*(3), 16–17.
8. Haas, S., & Androwich, I. (1999). Telephone consultation. In G. Bulecheck & J. McCloskey (Eds.), *Nursing interventions: Effective nursing treatments.* Philadelphia: W. B. Saunders.
9. Haas, S., & Gold, C. (1997). Perspectives in ambulatory care: Supervision of unlicensed assistive workers in ambulatory settings. *Nursing Economics, 15*(1), 57–59.
10. Haas, S. A., & Hackbarth, D. P. (1995). Dimensions of the staff nurse role in ambulatory care: Part IV: Developing nursing intensity measures, standards, clinical ladders, and QI programs. *Nursing Economics, 13*(5), 285–294.
11. Haas, S. A., & Hackbarth, D. P. (1997). The role of the nurse manager in ambulatory care: Results of a national survey. *Nursing Economics, 15*(4), 191–203.
12. Haas, S. A., & Hackbarth, D. P. (1995). Dimensions of the staff nurse role in ambulatory care: Part III: Using research data to design new models of nursing care delivery. *Nursing Economics, 13*(4), 230–241.
13. Haas, S. A., et al. (1995). Dimensions of the staff nurse role in ambulatory care: Part II: Comparison of role dimensions in four ambulatory settings. *Nursing Economics, 13*(3), 152–165.
14. Hackbarth, D. (1995). Institute of Medicine revised definition of ambulatory care. *Viewpoint, 17*(4), 1–4.
15. Hackbarth, D. P., et al. (1995). Dimensions of the staff nurse role in ambulatory care: Part I: Methodology and analysis of data on current staff nurse practice. *Nursing Economics, 13*(2), 89–98.
16. Hooks, M., Dewitz-Arnold, D., & Westbrook, L. (1980). The role of the professional nurse in the ambulatory care setting. *Nursing Administration Quarterly, 4*(4), 12–17.
17. Institute of Medicine. (1994). *Defining primary care: An interim report.* Committee on the future of primary care. Washington, DC: National Academy Press.
18. Institute of Medicine. (1978). Primary care medicine: A definition. In *A manpower policy for primary health care: Report of a study.* Washington, DC: National Academy Press.
19. Kovner, A. (1996). *Health care delivery in the United States* (6th ed.). New York: Springer.
20. Leavell, H. R, & Clark, E. (1965). *Preventive medicine for the doctor in his community: An epidemiologic approach.* New York: McGraw-Hill.
21. McCaig, L. F. (1994). *National hospital ambulatory medical care survey: 1992 emergency department summary.* Atlanta: Centers for Disease Control and Prevention, National Center for Health Statistics.
22. McKeown, T. (1978). Determinants of health. *Human Nature, 1*(4), 60–67.
23. National Center for Health Statistics. (1999). *Ambulatory care statistics: United States, 1997.* Hyattsville, MD: Centers for Disease Control and Prevention, National Center for Health Statistics.
24. Shi, L., & Singh, D. (1998). *Delivering health care in America.* Gaithersburg, MD: Aspen.
25. Smith, J. (1983). *The idea of health: Implications for the nursing professional.* New York: Teachers College Press.
26. Starfield, B. (1992). *Primary care: Concept, evaluation and policy.* New York: Oxford University Press.
27. Starr, P. (1982). *The social transformation of American medicine.* Cambridge, MA: Basic Books.
28. Tighe, M. G., et al. (1985). A study of the oncology nurse role in ambulatory care. *Oncology Nursing Forum, 12*(6), 23–27.
29. U.S. Department of Health and Human Services, Office of Public Health and Science (1998). *Healthy people 2010 objectives: Draft for public review and comment.* Hyattsville, MD: Author.
30. Verran, J. A. (1981). Delineation of ambulatory care nursing practice. *Journal of Ambulatory Care Management, 4*(2), 1–13.
31. World Health Organization. (1978). *Primary health care: Report of the international conference on primary health care.* Alma-Ata, USSR. Geneva: Author.

CHAPTER

6

Acute Health Care

Cindy Ludwig

If you talk to a nurse who has worked in a hospital setting for the past 15 to 20 years, you are likely to hear about how much hospitals have changed. It is true. Today's hospitalized clients are sicker than they were years ago, in part because of advances in health care technology that have enabled them to survive disease and serious medical conditions longer. In the past, some of the nurse's case load included clients who were nearly well. Today, clients who are not acutely ill are discharged from the hospital and are treated in outpatient settings and by their families or significant others at home. Therefore, the case load for hospital nurses today consists of very ill clients. Chapter 4 discusses the many reasons for this change. This chapter addresses what it is like to work in a hospital today.

HISTORY OF HOSPITAL NURSING

Professional nursing in the United States is only about 100 years old. Although nursing is a young profession, it is an indispensable one. The need for nursing care is the major reason for hospitalization.

At the beginning of the 20th century, most nurses were employed by affluent clients in the client's home. Nurses worked on a fee-for-service basis and were paid by the client or the client's family. A nurse worked with only one client all day long. This early form of nursing care was called *private duty nursing.* Private duty nurses became well versed in the total care of a person because they provided physical, psychological, and social care. When care of the ill moved into the hospitals, many nurses moved into a hospital setting.

During the Great Depression, many nurses could no longer find employment in the client's home. They were forced to work in hospitals, and in many instances they worked for room and board rather than for a salary. The Blue Cross plan, developed in 1929, offered a form of prepayment of insurance to help people pay their hospital bills. During the 1930s and 1940s, more and more people purchased such insurance to protect themselves against hospital costs. The fact that hospitals could be more assured of payment put them on a sounder financial footing, and the demand for hospital-based nurses rose dramatically. Private duty nurses also moved into the hospital and provided one-to-one care for the hospitalized client at the client's request. Home-based private duty nursing care dwindled.

Today, private duty nurses can still be employed by hospitalized clients, but they are commonly employed elsewhere and are usually hired on a short-term basis. Hospitals contract with agencies, which provide a list (called a *registry*) of nurses who will work as private duty nurses.

In the 1970s and 1980s, the demand for hospital nurses continued to soar. Many schools of nursing met the demand by increasing the number of students they enrolled and graduated. History reveals cycles of nursing shortages. Nursing programs and hospitals must develop strong alliances to match the demand. There has been, and continues to be a nursing shortage. Hospital-based nurses are in shortest supply. Those who formerly chose nursing as a profession have broader career options available to them today, in home health care and other settings.

As health care costs have risen, third-party payers have begun to try to control hospital costs and soaring debts. Early discharge and the use of outpatient treatments now place clients back home quickly, even though they are still very ill. Not surprisingly, home health care nursing is increasing. Nurses still work in hospitals, but a rising percentage of nurses are caring for people in their homes.

ACUTE CARE HOSPITALS

The American Hospital Association defines a hospital as an institution with the primary function of providing diagnostic and therapeutic patient services for a variety of medical conditions, both surgical and nonsurgical. Hospitals are of three types: government-owned, voluntary, and for-profit.

GOVERNMENT-OWNED HOSPITALS. Government-owned hospitals are official agencies designed to provide care for people who receive local, state, or federal government support. Their services are often provided at no cost or at a reduced cost to the client. Many of the clients have no health care benefits. The clients may be employed, but the employer does not provide health care insurance programs.

Government-owned hospitals can be federally, state, or locally funded. Examples include the Army, Navy, Veterans Affairs, Public Health Service, and Department of Justice prison hospitals. State-supported facilities include psychiatric hospitals, state university hospitals, and state prison hospitals. Locally supported institutions include county and city hospitals.

VOLUNTARY HEALTH AGENCIES. Voluntary health agencies are nonprofit, tax-exempt organizations designed to meet the health care needs of the general public. Despite their name, nonprofit organizations still need to be concerned with their financial status. Although no stockholders are interested in profit, the hospital must have adequate resources to meet its expenses, plan for expansion, and be sustainable during economic depressions. Examples include church-affiliated, community, union, and Kaiser-Permanente hospitals. This category also includes hospitals owned by special interest groups, such as the Shriners, and hospitals for treatment of cancer or other chronic disorders.

FOR-PROFIT HOSPITALS. For-profit (*proprietary*) hospitals have the same goal as businesses: to generate profit. Like voluntary hospitals, they serve the general public. The hospitals are privately owned by large corporations, are parts of chains of hospitals, or are owned by single owners. These hospitals have stockholders. An advantage to the larger chains of hospitals is that they can purchase medical supplies in greater volume and, therefore, at less cost. They also have a slight advantage when contracting for third-party payment because of their ability to reduce costs.

Magnet hospitals are medium-sized to large urban medical for-profit centers that have a reputation for providing excellent nursing care and for having good medical outcomes. These hospitals often provide medical services for complex problems that require a team of health care providers who would be too expensive to replicate in multiple sites. For example, clients who require organ transplantation or care after a serious injury are commonly cared for in these institutions. The hospitals have a high retention rate of their staff because of their high morale and good payment systems. Most magnet hospitals employ very competent, experienced nurses who need little direct supervision.

Client Admissions

Clients in acute care hospitals include those who are acutely ill, are victims of trauma, have a potentially critical condition, need intensive monitoring, need complex diagnostic studies, need surgery or complex treatments, or have an exacerbation of a chronic disorder.

Clients can be admitted to a hospital in several ways (Box 6–1). Once the client is admitted, a primary physician (also called the *attending physician*) oversees the client's care. Consultants may be used to diagnose problems outside the physician's speciality. *Acute care* is a costly service that relies on technology and the expertise of the health care team to arrive at a diagnosis, begin treatment, stabilize the condition, and prepare for a transition to a less costly level of health care. Many people are involved in a client's care (Box 6–2).

Efficiency Measures

Hospitals continuously assess their outcomes and financial health by reviewing cost-benefit and clinical analysis data from their service lines. *Service lines* can be defined as care given to groups of clients with similar problems. For example, care of clients with heart disease or heart sur-

---

BOX 6–1   **How Clients Are Admitted to a Hospital**

Direct

A client is seen in a physician's office, and it is determined that the client needs nursing care and specialized monitoring.

Emergency

A client is seen in the emergency department, and it is determined that the client needs surgery, nursing care, and/or specialized monitoring. The disease that has been diagnosed or is considered likely cannot be managed on an outpatient or self-care basis.

Scheduled

A client has elected to undergo surgery or special diagnostic testing that requires specialized monitoring or nursing care during recovery.

---

gery would make up one service line. Many communities with two or more hospitals collaborate and then delineate service lines for each institution. For example, one hospital might provide all psychiatric services, another might provide acute service, and another might provide rehabilitation service. This is a cost-effective and a resource-effective method of providing care because duplication of effort is eliminated. Clinical outcomes are generally improved when the volume of cases increases because the staff become familiar with typical responses of clients and can detect complications earlier. In addition, equipment used to provide care can be purchased at lower costs when purchased in larger quantities.

During the late 1990s, many hospitals merged with others in efforts to reduce cost, combine services, and attract third-party payment contracts. Some of the mergers are collaborative, in which both parties are served by the merger. Some mergers are done to rescue ailing hospitals; other mergers are contested or surprise mergers. The environment of the hospital during a merger can be very volatile. Many employees realize that jobs might be lost in an effort to redesign the work environment and delivery systems, and morale often falls. Nurses should keep client care foremost in their minds and continue to provide high-quality care during the turmoil.

Subacute Care

Subacute care is designed to fill the gap between acute care hospitals and long-term care. Clients may follow a continuum from acute care to a transitional care unit (usually located within the acute care hospital but defined as a separate area) and a skilled nursing facility. If the client can provide his or her own care at home, discharge to home is appropriate. If some nursing care is still required, home health care may be used to assist the client.

Subacute care is more intensive than traditional nursing home care and less acute than acute care hospitals. For example, a client may have many complex conditions that require a lower level of care than would be given in an acute care setting but higher than could be pro-

---

BOX 6-2   Personnel and Departments in a Hospital

Professional Services

Medical staff. Consists of private practice or group practice physicians who have their own offices and use the hospital services for care of specific problems. Also made up of physicians who may work for the hospital in such departments as surgery, laboratory, radiology, and emergency.

Nursing Service. Largest group of client care providers in the hospital. Nurses are employed by the nursing service department and provide client care on one unit or ward in the hospital; in areas where no direct client care is given (such as administration and hospital-based education programs); and by the "patient care" department.

Pharmacy. Consists of pharmacists and assistants who dispense medications prescribed by physicians. Pharmacy staff also monitor the use of regulated medications, such as narcotics. Many pharmacists also teach clients about their medications.

Rehabilitation Services. Physical therapists treat diseases and injuries by restoring, improving, or maintaining the client's functional ability or status to increase musculoskeletal strength to prevent further problems. Occupational therapists teach clients ways to overcome or reduce the problems in activities of daily living resulting from their disabilities.

Support Services

Administration. Hospital staff who are accountable for the operation of the entire hospital or institution. May include the hospital president, vice-presidents, and nurse-managers who supervise client care on a given nursing unit.

Biomedical Engineering Department. Maintains the elaborate equipment in the hospital to ensure safe and proper functioning and adherence to government regulations.

Business Departments. Several departments manage the business of the hospital based on both client income and outgoing expenses (salaries, purchasing, operation of the building). The admitting office collects information on insurance and assigns a room to the client. The business office lists all client charges, prepares the hospital bill, submits it to insurance companies, and records payments received. Payroll departments monitor hours worked, disperse salaries to the employees, and keep records. Purchasing departments disperse money for purchase of new supplies.

Central Service/Material Management Department. Maintains supplies needed for client care. Provides stock supplies of routinely used items on the nursing units. Cleans and resterilizes reusable supplies.

Dietary. Prepares food for client and staff daily. Dietitians assess and manage nutritional needs of hospitalized clients.

Environmental Services. Clean the hospital, including client rooms.

Foundation. Volunteers and professional staff who often raise funds for various hospital projects (e.g., building projects). May be combined with the marketing department.

Information Technology. Computer support staff is growing in most hospitals because of the increasing use of computers. Staff members focus on design and support mechanisms for electronic data retrieval and storage.

Laboratory. Conducts diagnostic tests to help identify illness. Technicians commonly work in radiology and the various laboratories. Laboratory technicians usually collect blood samples from clients; nurses often collect all other specimens and may collect blood.

Laundry. Launders, sorts, and presses several hundred pounds of linen each day. New linen is delivered to each nursing unit daily. These services may be contracted out ("outsourced") to local providers.

Medical Records. Stores medical records for all clients. If a client is rehospitalized, former medical records are often important in diagnosis of new problems. Also compiles data for retrieval for reimbursement, service trending, and outcomes research.

Personnel/Human Resources Department. Hires new employees and concentrates on employee relations. Human resources departments may serve in public relations roles to inform the hospital staff, clients, media, and the public about the hospital and its operations. Public relations services may also be provided by the marketing department.

Volunteer Services. Operates coffee shops and gift shops, delivers mail to clients, and often raises funds for various hospital projects.

---

vided by nurses in a traditional transitional care unit in a skilled nursing facility. The requirements as outlined by the Department of Health Services are shown in Box 6-3.

Several factors have made subacute care facilities one of the fastest-growing segments of health care through the mid-1990s. Subacute care provides health care for clients with complex problems at a fraction of the cost, or at about 30% of the cost of the acute care general hospital. At one time, reimbursement was more lucrative for these care settings, and many hospitals augmented their physical structure to add subacute care units. This financial incentive changed when legislation was enacted to slow down early discharge from acute to subacute care. In some hospitals today, nursing units or beds on a given unit or actual beds can serve a dual purpose. These *swing beds* can be used either for acute care or for subacute care, depending on the circumstances.

Subacute care areas are designed for clients who are out of the fragile phase of their illness and need routine monitoring and rehabilitation. Typical candidates are clients with diagnoses of stroke, cancer, acquired immunodeficiency syndrome (AIDS), head injury, total hip replacement, vascular diseases, chronic obstructive pulmonary disease, renal failure, and wounds needing care. These clients do not need surgery or other invasive procedures, but they do require frequent assessment and longer stays. Subacute care provides coordinated services to clients by a team of nurses, nursing assistants, physicians, specialized therapists, social workers, and dietitians. Outcomes after subacute care stays are the same as, or better than, those after hospital stays.

Subacute care areas have attracted nurses from the hospital setting, because nurses feel they have more time, less pressure, and a more interdisciplinary approach to client care. Another attractive feature of most subacute

---

BOX 6–3   Nursing Hours per Day in Various Levels of Care

- *Skilled nursing:* LPN or RN + CNA = 2.5 hours/day
- *Transitional care unit:* LPN or RN + CNA = 4.9 hours/day
- *Subacute care* (distinct portion of acute care hospital) = LPN or RN + CNA = 6.0 hours/day
- *Subacute care* (freestanding) = LPN or RN + CNA = 5.8 hours/day

CNA, Certified Nursing Assistant; LPN, Licensed Practical Nurse; RN, Registered Nurse.

---

units is that the environment seems more like home to the client and family.

The four categories of subacute care units are (1) transitional, (2) general, (3) chronic, and (4) long-term transitional.

TRANSITIONAL. Transitional subacute care provides for short stays (10 days) with high levels of nursing care. It serves as a hospital step-down unit, an alternative to continued hospitalization in an acute care setting. Typical clients in transitional subacute care include those recovering from myocardial infarction (heart attack) or open heart surgery; those who must be weaned from a ventilator; those who need wound management after burn injury or for multiple pressure ulcers; those who require more rehabilitation after stroke or orthopedic surgery; or those who have complex medical conditions such as diabetes or digestive or renal problems.

GENERAL. General subacute units have some overlap with transitional units; the key difference is the *acuity level* (severity of illness) of the clients. Many clients in these units are Medicare beneficiaries, whose younger counterparts with the same level of disability would receive home care. General subacute units are used for clients who require about 3.5 hours of nursing care and 1 to 3 hours of therapy daily. Typical clients are the same as those in transitional units, although the stay is longer (10 to 40 days). The goal of care is to send clients home or to a less expensive level of care, such as to long-term care or assisted-living centers.

CHRONIC. Chronic subacute units manage clients with little hope of ultimate recovery and functional independence. Typical clients include those who cannot be successfully weaned from a ventilator, are in a long-term comatose state, or have progressive neurologic disorders. Nursing intensity is similar to that in general subacute care units. The goal of care is to stabilize the client's condition so that he or she can be transferred to home or to a long-term care center. The average length of stay is 60 to 90 days.

LONG-TERM. Long-term transitional subacute facilities provide care for clients with medically complex problems or those who are ventilator-dependent. The average length of stay is about 25 days, but it can be more. The units are staffed primarily by Registered Nurses (RNs), and each client requires about 6 to 9 hours of care per day.

ROLES OF NURSES IN HOSPITALS

Nursing is a service provided both to individual clients and to aggregates of people (e.g., families, groups, communities, populations). To fulfill nursing's commitment to contribute to the health care of people, professional nurses assume multiple roles and responsibilities. Although these roles tend to overlap, they are important to distinguish. Nurses are providers of direct care, educators, and managers.

Provider of Direct Care

Most people are familiar with nurses as providers of *direct care*. Nurses assess, care for, educate, and comfort clients. Nurses provide direct care in all settings and along all dimensions of the health-illness continuum, from health promotion to critical care and death.

Indirect care consists of processes that go on in support of the actual bedside nursing care given. Sometimes this level of care is labeled *interdependent.* The nurse interprets physicians' orders, administers medication, and provides treatment for the client when performing interdependent care.

Educator

Professional nurses provide formal and informal education to their clients, individually and in groups. Informal education goes on almost continually, as clients are taught about medications while the medications are being administered, about the importance of eating a balanced diet when they choose their menu selections, and so on. The importance of informal education should not be underestimated.

Formal education is usually provided to groups of clients and their families. The nurse may use a classroom or bring videotapes or audio tapes into the client's room. Advantages to formal education are that the client is usually prepared for learning, significant others are included, and the material presented is consistent from client to client. Many hospitals have formal educators on their staff for clients with complex learning needs. Certified diabetes educators, certified lactation specialists, oncology nurse specialists, and enterostomal therapists are examples of nurses who teach clients in the hospital and often follow up with clients when they are back in the community.

Finally, some nurses specialize in education and rehabilitation. These nurses often work in cardiac and pulmonary rehabilitation and may have a subspecialty in physical therapy or exercise physiology. Their role is to assist in the rehabilitation of clients after myocardial infarction, heart failure, or chronic obstructive pulmonary disease.

Manager

The term *manager* in this discussion means the person who coordinates human and material resources in providing care to clients. *Human resources* include (1) the client, (2) the nurse, (3) the family or significant others, (4) professional colleagues, (5) support groups (e.g., the American Cancer Society), and (6) resource groups (e.g., Vocational Rehabilitation). *Material resources* include equipment and supplies. Time is also an important resource. Finally, outcome is an important consideration in health care management. Outcomes are detailed in the next section.

The first episode of client management that you encounter as a nurse is your provision of timely care to one client. Effective time management of only one client is difficult at first because of interruptions and lack of familiarity with equipment and procedures. Even while you are caring for only one client, stay on time with assessments, medications, and treatments. Most of these aspects of nursing care are scheduled more than once every 24 hours; if you are late, the next treatment or medication may have to be delayed. As you gain experience, care of one client becomes efficient. When caring for more than one client, time management becomes even more important.

Nursing Care Delivery Systems

How client care is delivered on any nursing unit is very important. Several techniques are in use today, and each has its advantages and disadvantages.

Total Care Nursing

Total care nursing is the oldest of the care delivery systems. One nurse is assigned to one client and provides all care. The one-to-one pattern is common in critical care, with student nurses, and with private duty nurses. The advantage is that the client needs to work with only one nurse and that one nurse can focus on meeting all the biopsychosocial needs of the client and family. The disadvantage is that any given nurse must be proficient in all nursing tasks and problem-solving areas.

Functional Nursing

Functional nursing is a system of care borrowed from industry, which concentrates on duties. It can be seen as an "assembly line" of care. Functional nursing began during World War II, when the demand for patient care outstripped the supply of nurses. The RN would coordinate care for an entire unit or team. Other nurses might be assigned to pass medications and perform treatments. Personnel with less training would be assigned to provide more basic care (e.g., giving baths, making beds).

An advantage of this system is that care can be provided at a lower cost. Disadvantages are that the client interacts with several people, psychosocial needs are seldom met, and the RN seldom cares for the client and must rely on other people's assessments of the client's problems. Each member of the working group is highly dependent on the other members, and the nurse is in an autocratic position. Functional nursing is still commonly used in skilled nursing and long-term care facilities.

Team Nursing

In team nursing, the RN leads a group of health care personnel in providing care for 10 to 20 clients. Team nursing was developed in the 1950s because of social and technological changes. World War II had drawn many nurses from hospitals, causing gaps in the nursing population. In addition, several technological advances required specialized knowledge. Team nursing was felt to be one approach to using people's skills more effectively.

Advantages are that an experienced RN is head of the team and generally knows the clients. In addition, the team leader can provide guidance to new or inexperienced nurses. As in functional nursing, the talents and abilities of each member of the health care team are used. Disadvantages are that (1) it is fairly expensive (because care is fragmented), (2) a lack of delegation skills by RNs may reduce efficiency, and (3) some redundancy may occur if each team leader must perform several managerial tasks, such as making assignments.

Primary Nursing

Primary nursing is a model of care delivery and a model of organizing care to achieve high-quality care outcomes. This style of care delivery emerged during the 1980s to meet the increasingly complex needs of clients. The goal is for each client's care to be comprehensive and coordinated, from admission to discharge. Each client is assigned an RN as the primary nurse, and that nurse always provides care for that client when he or she is working. In addition, associate nurses provide care when the primary nurse is absent.

Advantages are obvious: (1) the client has the same nurse, (2) the client's psychosocial needs can be met, (3) communication with the physician is improved, and (4) the nurse feels autonomous. Disadvantages are (1) the increased cost in hiring a large RN staff, (2) possible role confusion between primary and associate nurses, and (3) many calls to physicians from one nursing unit. (When a charge nurse system is used, the charge nurse makes telephone calls and often handles several issues in one telephone call.)

Case Management

The nurse can serve a pivotal role in coordinating all of the events required for a timely recovery. Many hospitals have developed sophisticated guides, called *care pathways* or case management plans, to direct client care and recovery from predictable problems. Case management is a care delivery mode that incorporates concepts of continuity and efficiency in addressing long-term physical, psychological, and social needs of clients. The primary goals of case management are promoting self-care, upgrading the quality of life, and using resources efficiently. Case managers are nurses who coordinate care of a group of clients, monitor the implementation of interdisciplinary care plans, and maintain communication with third-party payers and referral sources.

A key distinction in the nurse's role in the case management system is that it transcends nursing unit and physician service (e.g, cardiology) boundaries. The nurse follows the client through the entire stay in the health care system and back into the community. Case managers must have a thorough knowledge of third-party reimbursement patterns and rules, community resources, and discharge planning techniques. Several care pathways are presented in this book with a discussion of how to use them.

MANAGEMENT AND DELEGATION

Today, in an effort to control costs, almost all hospitals have hired *unlicensed assistive personnel* to provide care. Other than on-the-job training, these personnel receive little formal training. The use of less trained and educated personnel to perform nursing duties is changing the face of nurse staffing in hospitals. The use of unlicensed assistive personnel is increasing despite the inconclusive amount of research demonstrating their effectiveness on client outcomes.

Different terms are used for "nurse extenders" (which may include unlicensed assistive personnel), such as *unit assistants, primary practice partners,* and *unit hostesses.* Nurse extenders with more advanced skills might be called *clinical technicians.* Assistive personnel may help with clinical duties, nonclinical duties, or both. Some of the duties that may be delegated include giving baths, taking vital signs, serving food and collecting trays, performing unit-based laboratory tests (e.g., finger sticks for blood glucose assessment), 12-lead electrocardiograms (ECGs), and skin care.

Nurses need to learn when to delegate. For example, the nurse may delegate a bed bath and linen change for a client who is stable and may give the bath herself to an unstable or new client. This book offers many examples of appropriate delegation to unlicensed assistive personnel (see, for example, the Management and Delegation features in Chapters 27 and 46).

In planning the use of nurse extenders, nurse managers and their staff must consider many key questions (Box

---

BOX 6–4   Critical Considerations for Delegating Care to Unlicensed Assistive Personnel

- What are the appropriate core duties of a Registered Nurse?
- Who should perform which tasks?
- What can be delegated?
- What is an appropriate and cost-effective staff mix?
- What is the risk management and liability at each level of caregiver?
- Who can substitute for whom?
- Who is the least expensive worker to do each task?
- How much management or supervision is needed?
- What is the philosophical commitment to the provision of total patient care by the RN here?
- Will lowering the qualification of staff add further stress and frustration to our staff?
- How will this affect recruitment?
- What is the impact on collective bargaining?

From Gardner, D. L. (1991). Issues related to the use of nurse extenders. *Journal of Nursing Administration, 21*(10), 40–45.

6–4). Two issues that demand particular attention are the functions that only an RN can perform and the minimum level of RN staffing required to provide safe client care. Nurses may have been taught that only RNs can or should perform certain clinical duties, and they may therefore have difficulty delegating them to less qualified personnel. As the pressure mounts to delegate tasks to lower-paid workers, nurses will need to develop managerial skills, especially those of leadership, delegation, and supervision. Nurses will remain professionally accountable for client outcomes whether or not the specific tasks that contribute to those outcomes have been performed by nurses or by nurse extenders. Each nurse must clearly understand what the agency defines as the role and duties of the RN, the Licensed Practical Nurse or Vocational Nurse, and the various nurse extenders.

ENSURING QUALITY HEALTH CARE DELIVERY

Amid the fast-paced changes occurring in health care delivery, health care professionals remain responsible for ensuring quality client care. Quality client care is the outcome of the integrated health care team approach that involves the corporate and hospital or agency administration, medical staff, board of trustees, employees, community, and client. Contract services, community resources, transfer agreements, and expertise of social workers or case managers enable client transitions to alternate levels of care to occur in a continuous, coordinated, and almost seamless fashion.

Through work-redesign and skill-mix reallocation, institutions are focusing goals on achieving efficient client outcomes. *Work-redesign* involves studying a job over a fixed period to discover if and how a certain job function might be made more efficient. *Skill-mix* is determined by studying the ratio of RNs to Licensed Practical Nurses or Vocational Nurses and nursing assistants on a unit. The best skill-mix delivers quality care while also controlling costs.

The "one-level-of-care" philosophy ensures that clients receive optimal care in all areas of an institution. For example, the same monitoring pertains when intravenous (IV) conscious sedation is administered in the endoscopy unit as when general anesthesia is administered in the operating room or emergency department.

The Client's Rights to Quality Care

Clients have an increased awareness of the quality-of-care issue. They are demanding and receiving more information before the initiation of treatments. Increasingly, clients' requests for information about costs, risks, benefits, and alternatives to suggested therapies are being honored. No longer automatically submissive to the suggested care, the client is becoming a participant and partner in health care, with the expectation of receiving quality care from all health care professionals.

Client rights have also reached a new level of importance for the health care consumer. Regulating agencies, insurance carriers, third-party payers, and providers are responding to ensure that these fundamental rights are maintained and that clients receive quality services.

Providing Quality Client Care

Any plan for providing client care involves the following aspects:

- Budgeting process, to assist the institution in studying, spending, and using the information to reduce costs or maintain them at the present rate
- Strategic planning, to serve as a guideline for the continued or expanded services provided by the health care agency
- Performance improvement plan, to show the steps taken to improve performance based on monitoring and evaluation of staff performance
- Risk management input, to identify and eliminate potential injuries to staff and clients
- Utilization review data, to explore items such as acuity levels (a degree of severity of illness that affects the amount and complexity of care the client requires), outcomes, and costs, and to discover what is and is not effective care
- Client satisfaction survey results, which gather data from clients at various stages of their stay in the agency (e.g., preprocedure, admission procedure, discharge)
- Physician input, to incorporate professional input into client care planning
- Census data, to plot current and future trends of health care in the organization
- Acuity levels, as designated by the health care organization, to plan an appropriate skill-mix for staffing

Changes in client population, diagnoses, programs, or staffing that would necessitate changes in the type, level, or amount of care are reviewed on an ongoing basis. Other factors contributing to quality care include (1) the adherence to, monitoring of, and evaluation of care given according to professional standards; (2) Joint Commission on the Accreditation of Healthcare Organizations (JCAHO) and Department of Health criteria; and (3) input from other regulatory agencies. In addition, clinical pathways, clinical practice guidelines, standards of practice and care, and competence standards serve as models for professional delivery of client care.

Staffing for Quality Care

Health care institutions use a combination of methods to ensure a staff of caregivers who can deliver quality care to clients. Two methods include (1) daily collection of census data (a count of the number of clients occupying beds on any given day); and (2) determination of acuity levels.

Staff are assigned or reassigned to units that have the greatest need for their expertise and experience. Staffing adjustments caused by the fluctuation of census data and acuity levels are accomplished by using per diem (daily) staff and other creative measures to ensure safe client care.

Although staffing adjustment decisions in the past were typically made at higher levels of administration, today service line leaders and empowered directors and managers are instrumental in adjusting strategies based on the many shifting variables that affect client care. These personnel are closer to the actual care setting (clients and staff) and can use their expertise to make informed decisions about staffing for quality care.

Input from the employees who actually provide care is helpful in redesigning and improving the quality of care. Because caregivers are directly involved with client care, they can contribute in important ways by reporting problems that can be addressed in a timely fashion. Such input, especially when acted on by management, helps staff members feel valued.

Unfortunately, adequate staffing is not always ensured. In 1995, nurses marched on Washington, D.C., to protest clinical staffing shortages that had already endangered and might further endanger client care. Today, RNs are still in short supply.

In an attempt to make the most effective use of available nursing staff, *cross-training* has evolved in hospitals. Whereas in the past nurses were typically assigned to one unit where they could become familiar with the other personnel and the unit routine, today's hospital nurses may be cross-trained to work effectively in two or more units (e.g., a surgical unit and a cardiac intensive care unit). Nurses are assigned to the unit where they are most needed and may arrive for work not knowing in advance the work assignment for that day. Nurses may also be assigned to similar areas (e.g., orthopedics) but at different hospitals within the larger system as a result of mergers and acquisitions. This new scenario is often stressful for nurses and other staff members.

NURSING INTENSITY CLASSIFICATION

To ensure that staffing is adequate, one must understand how ill any given group of clients is and how much nursing care they will require. Hospitalized clients are classified according to several systems in an attempt to determine *nursing intensity,* a combination of the amount of care and the skill level at which care is provided. Usually, physical care and psychosocial or teaching skills are included. For example, a stable comatose client might require a large amount of low-complexity care that could be provided by unlicensed assistive personnel. In contrast, a newly diagnosed diabetic teenager with several personal and family problems may require less time for care, but the care should be provided by an RN.

Any patient classification system has several purposes, such as:

1. *Providing staffing.* The system will establish a unit of measure for nursing time. The unit of measure will be used to determine the number and kinds of health care providers needed for any given shift.
2. *Reducing cost.* The system can be used to determine the cost of nursing care. Profits and losses can then be calculated.
3. *Tracking changes.* The acuity of care needed may change as the case mix changes or during certain times of the year.

Two methods are generally used to determine acuity.

1. *Factor evaluation method.* Each client is rated on independent elements of care; each element is scored (weighted); scores are summarized, and the client is placed in a category based on the total numerical value obtained.

2. *Prototype evaluation method.* Each client is categorized according to a broad description of care requirements. The prototypes usually have four categories that describe (a) the client's ability to perform activities of daily living (ADL), (b) general health, (c) emotional support, and (d) treatment modalities (Table 6–1).

■ MONITORING HEALTH CARE OUTCOMES

New ideas are coming into play about health care outcomes. The shift in health care originally focused on cost reduction. Fortunately, it has become recognized that cost reduction may equate to losses in quality of care. New ideas are addressing the *value* of health care (cost of care for procedure or health problem as well as outcome of care). This is a needed change in the direction of quality health care. Third-party payers in the future will probably consider the value of health care provided at various institutions before signing contracts. Some of the ways health care outcomes are monitored in an effort to track outcomes and value are now presented.

Patient Satisfaction Surveys

As in business, health care providers have learned that it is easier to keep customers than to find new ones. Patient satisfaction surveys are commonly given to the client on discharge or sent to the client's home shortly after discharge. The basic question is, "Would you return to our institution for health care in the future?" Clients are often asked about their perception of medical care, nursing care, ancillary care, the environment, and follow-up care.

Sometimes patient satisfaction surveys are discounted because of the fact that the patient has limited knowledge of what would constitute "reasonable" care. To overcome this feeling of helplessness by the client, some hospitals inform clients of the services they can reasonably expect while hospitalized. For example, clients are told that they can reasonably expect adequate pain relief. Then clients are asked to evaluate whether the outcome was met during the stay. This excellent change reminds all health care providers that the client's opinion should always be one indicator of quality of care.

Measurement of Functional Status

Functional status is a composite measurement of many components of physical health and psychosocial well-being. Because it is a composite, several instruments can be used to measure functional status; these include:

- General perception of health
- Limitations in physical ability because of health problems
- Ability to engage in social activities (including work)
- General mental health
- Pain
- Energy
- Fatigue
- Depression

Some hospitals are using these measures to monitor how interventions affect functional status. For example, it is expected that functional status will improve after coronary bypass surgery. Valid data to show improvement in a group of clients served by the hospital provides excellent evidence of health care value.

Accessibility

Because people are mobile, the location of the hospital and access to the agency are important factors. Hospitals are concerned about convenience, location, wait time, and lead time needed to find a primary care provider, to arrange an outpatient procedure, or to schedule a diagnostic procedure.

■ REGULATORY REQUIREMENTS AND ISSUES

Regulatory agencies have the primary goal of enhancing the public's ability to secure adequate health care. Health care agencies are surveyed periodically to ensure that they comply with specific rules and regulations. A survey is an in-depth study of a health care institution (e.g., a hospital or a long-term care facility) according to specific criteria set forth by the regulating agencies involved. All aspects of the institution's services are inspected. Important performance areas include client assessment, medication administration, use of restraints, client and family education, staff training, information management, and organizational performance. After the survey is completed, a report of findings is compiled and the institution is notified of its status. If a criterion is not met satisfactorily, the institution is notified, given time to correct the deficiency, and reevaluated at a later date. Sometimes the reevaluation is unannounced.

Public disclosure of survey findings has begun. Hospital surveys completed after 1994 are made available to the public, media sources, insurance companies, third-party payers, clients, and competing institutions. Other health care delivery services function under the same disclosure rules for compliance with regulations of the inspecting agencies.

Regulatory Agencies and Statutes

Several regulatory agencies have statutes that must be met by hospitals. These laws govern hiring and employment, quality controls, and conditions of the work site to reduce hazards. A full description of these laws is beyond the scope of this book; we will only look at a few of them. Employment laws include the equal employment opportunity laws that ensure equal rights in the workplace for racial and ethnic minorities, women, the elderly, and the handicapped. Contemporary changes in workplace rights for everyone would probably be incomprehensible to a worker from the 1920s.

The *Civil Rights Act* of 1964 laid the foundation for equal employment in the United States. The thrust of Title VII of the Civil Rights Act is two-fold: (1) it prohibits discrimination based on factors unrelated to job qualifications, and (2) it promotes employment based on ability and merit. The areas of discrimination specifically mentioned are race, color, religion, sex, and national origin. The Equal Employment Opportunity Commission (EEOC) is responsible for enforcing Title VII of the Civil

TABLE 6-1	PATIENT CARE CLASSIFICATION USING FOUR LEVELS OF NURSING CARE INTENSITY			
Area of Care	**Category 1**	**Category 2**	**Category 3**	**Category 4**
Eating	Feeds self or needs little food	Needs some help in preparing; may need encouragement	Cannot feed self but is able to chew and swallow	Cannot feed self and may have difficulty swallowing
Grooming	Almost entirely self-sufficient	Needs some help in bathing, oral hygiene, hair combing, and so forth	Unable to do much for self	Completely dependent
Excretion	Up and to bathroom alone or almost alone	Needs some help in getting up to bathroom or using urinal	In bed, needs bedpan or urinal placed; may be able to partially turn or lift self	Completely dependent
Comfort	Self-sufficient	Needs some help with adjusting position or bed (e.g., tubes, IV lines)	Cannot turn without help, get drink, adjust position of extremities, and so forth	Completely dependent
General health	Good—in for diagnostic procedure, simple treatment, or surgical procedure (D & C, biopsy, minor fracture)	Mild symptoms—more than one mild illness, mild debility, mild emotional reaction, mild incontinence (not more than once per shift)	Acute symptoms—severe emotional reaction to illness or surgery, more than one acute illness, medical or surgical problem, severe or frequent incontinence	Critically ill—may have severe emotional reaction
Treatments	Simple—supervised ambulation, dangle, simple dressing, test procedure preparation not requiring medication, reinforcement of surgical dressing, change pad, vital signs once per shift	Any category 1 treatment more than once per shift, Foley catheter, care, I & O, bladder irrigations, sitz bath, compresses, test procedures requiring medications or follow-ups, simple enema for evacuation, vital signs every 4 hr	Any treatment more than twice per shift, medicated IV lines, complicated dressings, sterile procedures, care of tracheotomy, Harris flush, suctioning, tube feeding, vital signs more than every 4 hr	Any elaborate or delicate procedure requiring two nurses, vital signs more often than every 2 hr
Medications	Simple, routine, not needing preevaluation or postevaluation; medications no more than once per shift	Diabetic, cardiac, hypotensive, hypertensive, diuretic, anticoagulant medications, prn medications, more than once per shift, medications needing preevaluation or postevaluation	Unusual amount of category 2 medications; control of refractory diabetics (need to be monitored more than every 4 hr)	More intensive category 3 medications; IV lines with frequent, close observation and regulation
Teaching and emotional support	Routine follow-up teaching; clients with no unusual or adverse emotional reactions	Initial teaching of care of ostomies, new diabetics, tubes that will be in place for periods of time; conditions requiring major change in eating, living, or excretory practices; clients with mild adverse reactions to their illness (e.g., depression, being overly demanding)	More intensive category 2 items; teaching of apprehensive or mildly resistive clients; care of moderately upset or apprehensive clients; confused or disoriented clients	Teaching of resistive clients, care and support of clients with severe emotional reaction

D & C, dilatation and curettage; I & O, input and output; IV, intravenous.
Modified from Marquis, B. L., & Huston, C. J. (1996). *Leadership roles and management functions in nursing* (p. 266). Philadelphia: J. B. Lippincott.

Rights Act. When a charge of discrimination is proven, the agency attempts to mediate the problem through persuasion and conciliation.

In 1967, Congress enacted the *Age Discrimination and Employment Act* (ADEA). Its purpose was to promote employment of older people based on their ability rather than their age. In early 1978, the ADEA was amended to increase the protected age to 70 years. Although people feared that this act would have serious consequences for labor-intensive occupations, such as nursing, many people are opting for earlier retirement and problems have not been reported.

The *Rehabilitation Act* of 1973 required all employers with government contracts of more than $25,000 to take affirmative action to recruit, hire, and advance handicapped people who are qualified. In 1990, Congress passed the *Americans with Disabilities Act* to eliminate discrimination against Americans with physical or mental disabilities in the workplace and in social life. Disability is defined as "any physical or mental impairment that limits any major life activity." This includes not only all individuals with obvious physical disabilities, but also individuals with cancer, diabetes, human immunodeficiency virus (HIV) infection, AIDS, and recovering alcoholics and drug users. The act not only prohibits discrimination but also delineates clear, enforceable standards.

The *Occupational Safety and Health Act* (OSHA) is broadly written legislation that requires a place of employment to be free from recognized hazards and to develop environmental safety laws for the safety of the employees. The Department of Labor enforces this act. Since the inception of OSHA, many companies have vehemently criticized the act, specifically its administration. Companies have charged that the costs of meeting OSHA standards have excessively burdened American business. However, unions have asserted that the federal government has never adequately staffed or funded the Occupational and Health Administration. They have charged that OSHA has been negligent in setting standards for toxic substances, carcinogens, and other disease-producing agents.

Finally, quality assurance standards must be met by several areas of the hospital. Laboratories must test control solutions of known substances routinely to ensure that test results are accurate. Equipment used for sterilization of instruments and other supplies must be tested daily. These precautions are critical to safe care.

Ethical Issues

Ethical issues in acute care commonly occur when the nurse is caught in the middle between clients, physicians, administrators, and other nurses and feels powerless to change the situation. Ethical distress can lead to negative consequences for everyone involved. Nurses are often called on to assist families in making informed decisions about client care, and they must be familiar with ethical, legal, economic, and emotional factors that affect the family's decision.

Legal Issues

Nurses have more responsibility today than in the past. These expanded roles open the doors to greater legal risk.

The nurse's employer is obligated to carry malpractice insurance for its employees. You should know what is covered in the policy. In addition, you should carry individual malpractice insurance.

Proper documentation is crucial to serve as evidence of the quality of nursing care provided. The court still assumes that if something was not noted in a chart, it was not done. Be specific, and document nursing actions taken and the client's response (e.g., pain relief). If unusual events occur, complete an incident report. The benefit of incident reports is that they allow the analysis of adverse client events. They should not be treated as a punitive activity but rather as a method of promoting quality care and risk management. Errors are examined to determine whether the error was due to a system problem (e.g., a faulty electrical outlet that leads to a fire or an improperly mounted side rail that allows a client to fall). If a lawsuit is filed, incident reports are usually not revealed; instead, the court system relies on the information in the medical record.

Cultural Issues

Nurses who practice in the 21st century will be interacting with an increasingly multicultural American society. It is projected that most of the American population will include groups of minorities from other cultures. Areas of the United States that seldom had immigrants now see people from all over the world. This diverse population requires that nurses be able to recognize differences and be sensitive to those differences in perceptions of health and illness, in communication styles, and in nontraditional approaches to health care. Culturally competent care in its broadest sense is knowing, explaining, interpreting, and predicting nursing care within the knowledge of the client's cultural and ethnic beliefs and practices, whether the client is well or sick.[14]

■ PERFORMANCE IMPROVEMENT AND GOALS

Hospitals and other health care organizations have been challenged by their goal of attaining a planned, systematic, multidisciplinary, nationwide approach to designing, measuring, assessing, and improving performance. These institutions generally seek to enhance their measurement activities as they relate to institutional quality indicators (Box 6-5). These indicators generally include:

- Results of basic clinical indicators
- Continuous quality improvement
- Access to care issues
- Consumer satisfaction and judgment input
- JCAHO indicators
- Human resource management
- Organization performance

Health care organizations are in the midst of a transition to performance improvement from traditional quality assurance. Relevant goals include:

- Enhancing clinical leaders' abilities to set expectations, develop plans, and manage processes to assess, improve, and maintain the quality of the organization's clinical and support activities
- Enhancing health care outcomes and the perception of these outcomes and expectations by all consumers

- Measuring outcomes to determine priorities for improvement
- Systematically improving performance of important functions and maintaining stability of these functions
- Implementing quality improvement activities that optimally affect client outcomes and cost of services and then measuring the ongoing effect of these changes on the services provided
- Instituting a flexible performance improvement plan so that new or changed services and clinical practices serve as triggers for new indicator development
- Enhancing reporting and communication mechanisms of performance improvement results so that the greatest benefit is realized
- Strengthening the client education component as a result of quality assurance and improvement of information
- Supporting performance by improving existing processes
- Designing improvement activities for new processes
- Supporting client advocacy and customer response functions by responding to complaints at the closest level of client care
- Using available resources to produce all-inclusive information and to minimize data collection by staff
- Exploring automated methods of improving clinical information systems

Qualities that enhance the important dimensions of performance are listed in Box 6–6.

■ RISK MANAGEMENT

Risk management follows the current trend of adapting business strategies to health care systems. Risk management is a planned program of loss prevention and liability control. Its purpose is to identify, analyze, and evaluate risks followed by a plan of reducing the frequency of accidents and injuries. The program requires a team of people from all departments in the institution. The risk manager or safety committee administers the program and serves as the liaison between the hospital administration, the risk management committee, and others as well as between insurance representatives, institution attorneys, and others. Risk managers have no typical profile and can be nurses, administrators, lawyers, or former insurance representatives.

Nursing personnel are crucial to a successful risk management program. The five areas of highest risk in the hospital are (1) medication errors, (2) complications from diagnostic or treatment procedures, (3) falls, (4) client or family dissatisfaction, and (5) refusal of treatment or refusal to sign consent for treatment. Most medication errors are omissions or transcription errors, not dosage calculation errors. Medical records and incident reports serve as documents of accountability. Incident reports are used to analyze problems within the five categories and to plan for corrective actions.

THE FUTURE OF ACUTE CARE HOSPITAL NURSING

Acute care nursing is changing, but a bright future exists. Major changes will continue in health care delivery, and it will be essential that nurses take a primary position to help ensure that client care remains a priority. With health care costs continuing to rise, cost containment will also remain a major concern. As a result of cost containment, goals for acute care health providers are to:

- Increase the efficiency of care to speed transfer to a less costly level of care
- Streamline care to ease movement into capitated services or managed care contracts
- Monitor clinical pathways for variances and then implement quality improvement strategies to correct the variances
- Enhance client understanding of the disease and its management through education and early discharge planning
- Target high-risk, problem-prone, high-volume client care activities for quality improvement endeavors
- Act on client satisfaction concerns to promote client advocacy
- Extract applicable client, physician, and employee satisfaction data to allow a realistic focus on pertinent issues
- Support institutional quality indicators and quality improvement team endeavors to increase the value of health care
- Enhance the dimensions of performance through the use of appropriateness, availability, timeliness, effectiveness, continuity, safety, efficiency, respect, and caring

CONCLUSIONS

Acute care hospital-based nursing has changed. Years ago, clients could stay in the hospital until they felt well enough to go home. Cost-containment issues have demanded that clients today spend as little time as possible in acute care and quickly move to less expensive areas for care. Professional nurses have become more pivotal providing high-quality care during these shortened stays. All health care providers are trying to maintain excellence in health care during these changing times.

BIBLIOGRAPHY

1. Alfred, C. A., et al. (1995). A cost-effectiveness analysis of acute care case management outcomes. *Nursing Economics, 13*(3), 129–136.
2. Badovinac, C. C., Wilson, S., & Woodhouse, S. (1999). The use of unlicensed assistive personnel and selected outcome indications. *Nursing Economics, 17*(4), 194–200.
3. Brazino, J. (1997). Reinventing nurse extenders: The emergence of UAP. *Nursing Spectrum, 6*(4), 4–5.
4. Buchan, J. (1999). Still attractive after all these years? Magnet hospitals in a changing health care environment. *Journal of Advanced Nursing, 30*(1), 100–108.
5. Doswell, W., & Erlen, J. (1998). Multicultural issues and ethical concerns in the delivery of nursing care interventions. *Nursing Clinics of North America, 33*(2), 353–361.
6. Douglas, L. M. (1996). *The effective nurse: Leader and manager* (5th ed.). St. Louis: Mosby–Year Book.
7. Fletcher, C. (1997). Failure mode and effects analysis: An interdisciplinary way to analyze and reduce medication errors. *Journal of Nursing Administration, 27*(12), 19–26.
8. Gardner, D. L. (1991). Issues related to the use of nurse extenders. *Journal of Nursing Administration, 21*(10), 40–45.
9. Huber, D. (1996). *Leadership and nursing care management.* Philadelphia: W. B. Saunders.
10. Huggins, D., & Lehman, K. (1997). Reducing costs through case management. *Nursing Management, 28*(12), 34–37.
11. Joint Commission on Accreditation of Healthcare Organizations. (1995). *Accreditation manual for hospitals* (Vol. I). Oak Brook Terrace, IL: Author.
12. Johnson, K. (1994). A practical approach to patient classification. *Nursing Management, 25,* 50–55.
13. Krapohl, G. L., & Larson, E. (1996). The impact of unlicensed assistive personnel on nursing care delivery. *Nursing Economics, 14*(2), 99–108, 122.
14. Leninger, M. (1996). Cultural care: Theory, research and practice. *Nursing Science Quarterly, 9*(2), 71–78.
15. Lipson, J., & Steiger, N. (1996). *Self-care nursing in a multicultural context.* Thousand Oaks, CA: Sage Publications.
16. Marquis, B. L., & Huston, C. J. (1996). *Leadership roles and management functions in nursing* (2nd ed.). Philadelphia: J. B. Lippincott.
17. Moore, B. W., et al. (1996). Patient care leadership within an emerging integrated delivery network. *Nursing Administration Quarterly, 20*(2), 54–64.
18. Nolan, M., et al. (1998). Preparing nurses for the acute care case manager role: Educational needs identified by existing case managers. *Journal of Continuing Education in Nursing, 29*(3), 130–134.
19. Prescott, P. A., et al. (1991). The patient intensity for nursing index: A validity assessment. *Research in Nursing and Health, 14*(3), 213–221.
20. Schaefer, J. A., & Moos, R. H. (1996). Effects of work stressors and work climate on long-term care staff's job morale and functioning. *Research in Nursing and Health, 19*(1), 63–73.
21. Sowell, R. L., & Meadows, T. M. (1994). An integrated case management model: Developing standards, evaluation and outcome criteria. *Nursing Administration Quarterly, 18*(2), 53–64.
23. Swansburg, R. C. (1996). *Management and leadership for nurse managers* (2nd ed.). Sudbury, MA: Jones & Bartlett.
24. Wagner, N., & Ronen, I. (1996). Ethical dilemmas experienced by hospital and community nurses: An Israeli survey. *Nursing Ethics, 3,* 294–302.
25. Wyld, D. C. (1996). The capitation revolution in health care: Implications for the field of nursing. *Nursing Administration Quarterly, 20*(2), 1–12.

CHAPTER

7

Home Health Care

Karen S. Martin

This chapter is intended to serve as a bridge for nurses making the transition from inpatient or long-term care facilities to home health care and community-focused service settings. Including a summary of the trends, general philosophy, risks, and practice of home health care, it is designed for the student or clinician whose primary or recent clinical experience has been in hospital, assisted living, nursing home, or other long-term care facilities. *Community health nursing* is defined as a synthesis of nursing and public health practice that is comprehensive and is intended to promote and preserve the health of populations.[27] In this chapter, community health nursing is used as an umbrella term to cover all the diverse types of home health care and community-focused services, settings, and providers. Community health settings in which nurses commonly practice include hospital-based home health care agencies, visiting nurse associations, tax-supported home health agencies, and privately or corporately owned agencies. Other community health settings include tax-supported public health agencies, nursing centers, schools, wellness and occupational health programs, parish nursing programs, clinics for the homeless, case management programs, and other programs that offer related nursing services.

Scattered throughout this book are features called Bridge to Home Health Care, written by nurses and other community-focused professionals to describe their practice. These features address environmental, psychosocial, physiologic, and health-related behavior concerns experienced by clients and their families. For example, in "Living with Failing Vision" in Chapter 65, Bernadette Mruz shares ideas that you might use with clients with vision problems who are leaving your facility to return to the challenges of living at home. The Bridge to Home Health Care features help you gain insight into the roles and responsibilities of the nurse in home health care as it is practiced with clients and families every day. You can use this information as you consider and make referrals for follow-up care.

The Bibliography in this chapter provides more extensive information about home care, public health, and related topics. After reading the chapter, you may discuss what community-focused opportunities you will have as a nursing student. If you are a staff nurse, you may consider making an appointment to accompany a colleague who practices in a home care, public health, clinic, or school setting to learn more about the specialty. Together, this chapter and the Bridge to Home Health Care features provide a review of or introduction to the world of home health care and community-focused practice.

TRENDS

The need for home health care and community-focused services has grown explosively as a result of consumer demand, the advent of Medicare reimbursement for home health services, the aging of the population, federal legislation that encouraged the expansion of home care, escalating health care costs, and the rise of managed care.[19, 20, 31] By 1996, more than 20,000 Medicare-certified and non-certified home health agencies were operating in the United States, a 1000% increase over 20 years.[31] Between 1967 and 1998, Medicare home health expenditures grew from $50 million to $42 billion.[6, 31]

These trends reflect a shift in the delivery of health care services from the hospital to the community. Ideally, this shift will decrease fragmentation and produce an improved health care system in which providers work together in the interest of their clients. The shift also has the potential to increase provider accountability and result in a more systematic delivery model that is driven by outcome data. A "seamless health care system" is the term being used to describe that new model, a system that includes a wide array of services and providers who collaborate as team members.

Although the recipients of home health care have diverse needs, circulatory disease is the primary medical diagnosis for more than half of home health clients admitted. Diabetes and cancer are the next most frequent diagnoses.[31] In general, the clients who receive home health care tend to be in the elderly population; this trend is likely to continue. Consider these projections[30, 40]:

- Since 1900, the percentage of people older than age 65 has tripled.
- More than 35 million people will be older than age 65 by the year 2000.
- People older than age 65 account for one third of health care consumption; they may represent half of the total health care dollars spent by the year 2040.
- Nearly half of all hospital admissions nationally involve older people.
- Up to 60% of older adults do not take their medications properly.

- The 4 million men and women older than age 85 constitute the fastest-growing subset of older adults, with a growth rate nearly three times that of the overall elderly population.

Because the growth of home health care promises to continue, community health nurses face challenges unlike any they have faced before. The number of clients and complexity of their needs are increasing dramatically, as are the numbers and types of community health staff members and agency programs. At the same time, demands from consumers and payers for comprehensive, economical services are increasing, the availability of staff and reimbursement is decreasing, and regulatory demands are increasing.

For example, during 1997, dramatic legislative and regulatory events occurred that cut home care reimbursement and reflected a growing federal opposition to the rate of home health care expansion. The *Interim Payment System,* scheduled to become the *Prospective Payment System* in 2000, required that all Medicare- and Medicaid-certified agencies, home health staff nurses, and physical therapists complete a 95-item start-of-care Outcome and Assessment Information Set (OASIS).[6, 7] Versions of the data set were to be completed soon after adult clients were admitted to service, at interim periods, and at client dismissal.[10, 22] Home health agencies throughout the United States oriented their staff to OASIS, developed new policies and procedures for collection and transmission of data, and purchased new paper forms or computer equipment. Two months after agencies implemented the federal regulation, it was announced that the regulation was delayed and agencies would not be required to collect OASIS data until further notice. Partly as a result of these changing demands, more than 3000 home health agencies closed because of financial losses, more than 500 agencies in Texas alone.[32]

Although some home care requirements are still in flux, some are not. Reimbursement is a challenge and responsibility that frequently confronts the staff nurse who practices in home health or community settings (see Bridge to Home Health Care: Finding Financial Help). A staff nurse in a hospital, nursing home, or other long-term care facility may not know the cost of service or supplies and may not need to discuss charges with clients and their families. In home health care agencies, however, it is usually nurses who collect financial data, either at intake or when providing the initial services. Data include:

- The source of payment
- Verification of eligibility for Medicare, Medicaid, or other programs providing payment
- Preauthorization approval from a managed care or other third-party payer
- Other concerns

Home health agencies bill third-party payers for most services; Medicare and managed care are the most common. Some clients pay for services themselves (private pay) or receive services that are paid for by taxes, United Way, foundations, or grants. Often, reimbursement regulations are complex and require extensive paperwork for both nurses and clients.[6, 22] Clients may ask their nurses for assistance as they try to deal with those regulations. The Bridge to Home Health Care: Medicare and Medicaid Coverage of Home Health Services feature summarizes eligibility, requirement, and coverage information that home health nurses must know.

BRIDGE TO HOME HEALTH CARE

Finding Financial Help

Finding financial help and support services for a chronically ill client requires patience and perseverance. As clients, families, and informal caregivers assume more responsibility for providing home health care, it is essential that the multidisciplinary health care team help in locating and obtaining needed services.

This process must start early. Waiting periods for federal, state, county, and local services—such as Medicare, Medicaid, Social Security Disability, and county assistance—make early referral not only helpful but necessary. Applications to these agencies can be started while the client is still hospitalized. Make a complete assessment of the client's present and future needs. Your assessment should address financial, environmental, and emotional concerns in addition to physical ones. Your evaluation should focus on the client's, family's, and community's ability to provide for the needs and to mobilize available resources. The health care team should be sensitive to the client's ethnic, cultural, privacy, and value diversities by affirming the client's choices and goals.

A stopgap approach may provide temporary relief for the client's problem, but a more permanent or long-term solution is preferable and avoids having to address the problem repeatedly. Consider, for example, a client who has no money to purchase medications. Finding a resource to help the client obtain medications for a few days may require only a phone call to a local community help group. A long-term solution will require additional time and creative problem-solving. Many managed care and Medicare supplement plans include prescription benefits that allow clients to purchase medications at a set fee. Selecting such a prescription program may be the best alternative for a client who has high monthly medication bills—even if the plan has relatively few additional services and benefits.

To provide the best service to your client, all team members must keep their resource materials updated. Include all team members when attempting to find a solution to a client's financial problem. They may know of appropriate resources, and they may know the staff members or volunteers who serve as gatekeepers for those resources. Local churches, human service agencies, clubs, community action groups, and health service organizations can provide numerous resources for supportive care.

Cindi Leo-Gofta, RN, BSN, *Operations Director, Resource and Referral/Business Development, Alegent Health Home Care & Hospice, Omaha, Nebraska*

BRIDGE TO HOME HEALTH CARE

Medicare and Medicaid Coverage of Home Health Services

Program	Eligibility	Requirement	Coverage
Medicare	Age 65 years or older and established entitlement to Social Security or Railroad Retirement benefits End-stage renal disease (waiting period applies) Younger than age 65 years and established eligibility for Social Security or Railroad Retirement disability benefits (waiting period applies)	Physician-prescribed plan of care Services "medically necessary" Intermittent skilled nursing, physical therapy, or speech-language pathology service Homebound	Skilled nursing, physical therapy, and speech-language pathology services Skilled occupational therapy service if initiated in conjunction with coverable skilled nursing, physical therapy, or speech-language pathology service Medical social and home health aide services if provided in conjunction with skilled service Medical supplies and equipment
Medicaid	Recipients of Aid to Families with Dependent Children (AFDC) Recipients of Aid to Aged, Blind, and Disabled (AABD) who meet specific income guidelines Others who meet federal or state income and categorical guidelines	Physician-prescribed plan of care Services "medically necessary" Homebound; requirements vary by category Additional requirements may be established by each state and may include case management and prior authorization for services	*Required* Intermittent nursing service Home health aide service Medical supplies and equipment *Optional* Physical therapy service Speech-language pathology service Occupational therapy service Private duty nursing service Personal care or housekeeping service Registered dietitian service

Nancy J. Scheet, RN, MSN, *Compliance Officer, Visiting Nurse Association of Omaha, Omaha, Nebraska*

PERSPECTIVES

The specialty of home health care and community-focused nursing has a long and distinguished history in the United States, even though it received little attention from the public or the nursing profession until the 1990s. In 1877, Francis Root was employed in New York City as the first home visit nurse. In 1893, Lillian Wald and Mary Brewster established the Henry Street Settlement in the same city. Their goal was to offer public health nursing and community programs to people of all ages who were at high risk of developing health problems and to those with acute and chronic health problems. Lillian Wald had the vision to:

- Initiate programs and group activities at the settlement to meet the community's health-related, educational, social, and employment needs
- Send nurses from the settlement to make home visits and provide care to new mothers, infants, and the sick
- Forge alliances with business and political leaders to obtain support for her programs

This comprehensive approach to health can be called *community health nursing* and represents a true blend of public health and home care practice. Collaboration between the Henry Street staff and the New York City Mission home visit staff followed and led to the formation of the Visiting Nurse Service of New York, the largest single provider of home health care services in the United States. Soon, organized home visit programs were established in populated areas along the East Coast. Lillian Wald's vision of preventive, curative, and social services for the entire community spread throughout New York City and the rest of the nation. By 1912, 2500 nurses were employed by 900 independent visiting nurse associations.[11]

By 1963, there were 1100 home health and home care aide organizations and hospices in the United States that employed professional registered nurses. The enactment of national Medicare legislation in 1965 accelerated the rate of agency growth. More than 20,000 Medicare and non-Medicare certified home care agencies now offer services to 8 million clients.[31] About 200,000 community health nurses are employed by home care and public health agencies, school systems, and industry. That number is expected to escalate dramatically in the next 10 years.

Agencies that provide Medicare- and Medicaid-certified services must meet minimum national standards; state standards also exist. Agencies voluntarily participate in national accreditation programs such as those sponsored by the National League for Nursing and the Joint Commission on Accreditation of Healthcare Organizations. Nurses and other professional staff are required to meet licensure requirements but not consistent competence standards. Accreditation and competence are becoming important concerns to administrators, clinicians, and the public because of the increased use of technology and high-risk procedures and medications in the home. To be competent, clinicians need adequate orientation, equipment, and supervision; they also need to repeat high-risk procedures with sufficient frequency that they maintain their skills.

Collaboration and communication among members of all disciplines are necessary in home health care and community-focused settings. Nurses make up the largest group of clinicians, although most home health agencies also employ or contract with home health aides and other paraprofessionals as well as other professionals. Physical therapists, occupational therapists, social workers, and speech pathologists are usually on staff. Registered dietitians, pharmacists, dentists, physicians, and clergy may be part of the team as well. Agency staff members also need to coordinate referrals and communicate about client services with various community providers.

Historically, Lillian Wald at Henry Street and other community-focused nurses demonstrated collaboration and communication skills as part of their practice. During the 1990s, a new role, that of case manager, has developed. Nurse case managers are employed by home health agencies, hospice programs, health maintenance organizations, physician group practices, private insurance companies, public health departments, school systems, and managed care organizations. Although their responsibilities vary, they attempt to coordinate the delivery and payment of services that target clients' needs.

COMMUNITY-FOCUSED PHILOSOPHY

The client who receives services may be an individual, a family, a group, or a community.[1, 27, 37, 38] As home health care and community-focused clinicians have had the opportunity to work with clients over time, they have espoused a number of core values that influence their practice. Multidisciplinary collaboration and a seamless health care environment have already been mentioned. In addition, community health nurses have frequently conducted prevention and health promotion programs involving immunizations, smoking cessation, breast self-examination, and similar concerns.[34, 37]

Nurses in home health care and community-focused settings refer to those they serve as clients, patients, consumers, or customers. Regardless of the term they use or whether they use the terms interchangeably, they tend to base their practice on beliefs related to the consumer movement. Included are beliefs that people have both rights and responsibilities and that they must be knowledgeable about their own health care and actively involved in decisions. These beliefs are linked to issues of access, cost, and quality as well as the concepts of primary health care applicable at a national and an international level. For international use, the World Health Organization[42] defined *health* as a state of complete physical, mental, and social well-being and not merely the absence of disease or infirmity; the definition further states that health is a fundamental human right and that attainment of the highest possible level of health is an important worldwide social goal.

The power of the client is an important core value for home health care and community-focused providers.[35, 37] When a clinician enters a client's home, it is the client, not the clinician, who is in charge. In the hospital or nursing home, the nurse gives the client medications and changes dressings. In the home, nurses assist clients in providing their own care or assist family members or informal caregivers in providing that care.[23, 35] The family and other informal caregivers are critical members of the health care team. Their beliefs about health care practice and treatment, the extent of their skills, and their availability influence or even determine whether a client can remain at home and the outcome of the client's care.

Hospice programs provide some of the most dramatic examples of the power of clients. The agency's hospice team usually consists of nurses, home health aides, social workers, pharmacists, registered dietitians, chaplains, and volunteers. Team members also work with the client's physician and other social service agencies. The role of the team is to support end-of-life decisions made by clients and their families as described in the Bridge to Home Health Care: Providing End-of-Life Care in Chapter 22.

Staff members who provide services to clients, their families, and other informal caregivers in their homes are human bridges to home health care. This is true whether the staff member is a nurse, another professional, or a paraprofessional. To maximize outcomes of care, all members of the home health and community-focused team should follow some basic principles as they practice their specialty:

- Remember that you are a guest in your client's home and neighborhood. Your behavior and your manners must convey that you recognize this role.
- Respect the client's cultural, religious, and ethnic heritage. Hesitate before contradicting that heritage. Clients are more likely to follow their heritage than your advice.
- It is possible that the client will not respect *your* cultural, religious, and ethnic heritage. If you are a male nurse, the client may expect, and even request, a female nurse. Develop interpersonal skills—and a tough skin.
- Almost every home health client has family members or significant others who will offer advice and will serve as your advocate or foe. Try to enlist them as your advocates.
- The client "owns" the health-related problem that initiated your services. That problem is just one portion of the client's past, present, and future. Thus, it is the client who experiences, learns to understand, and ultimately solves the problem. It is your goal to help clients and their families become independent as quickly as possible. Talk to your peers and supervisors if you sense that you may be losing that perspective.
- Enjoy the unique autonomy and challenges of providing highly complex care in the home and community setting. Home health practice requires integration of high-technology skills, teaching, case management, and monitoring. Remember the need for communication with other members of the health care team. The nurse is usually responsible for judging whether or not the client can safely remain at home, and other team members

need to share the information the nurse has through oral and written means.

• Maintain your sense of humor. You will need it!

■ RISKS

Home health care staff and students should consistently practice the Boy Scout motto, "Be prepared." Preparedness is essential regardless of your responsibilities, the size of your agency or organization, or its geographical location. If you work in a hospital or nursing home, colleagues, technology, supplies, and references are nearby. When you visit a home, school, clinic, or other community site, you are usually on your own. Help and information may be available via extra supplies in the trunk of your car, the telephone, a computer, a pager, or a Fax machine, but help may not be available immediately.

You must always consider your safety and that of your client. Plan carefully to minimize the risks of accidents or violence; make sure you know your agency's disaster plan.[18] If an accident or violence occurs, you must know how to intervene immediately and appropriately. For example, when selecting individuals, families, or groups for a student assignment, it is necessary to evaluate the client's needs, the student's educational and life experiences, the faculty member's skills and availability, where the clients are located, the timing of the visit, the availability of other sources of help, and the student's method of transportation to and familiarity with the neighborhood.

It is also important to establish an excellent working relationship among the students, faculty, and staff of the agency or institution to enhance safety and the quality of the experience for all. To improve communication and safety for both clients and students, strategies such as shared home visits, student learning centers, nursing centers, and homeless clinics are being used.[8, 15, 24, 39] The Nightingale Tracker, a computerized communication system, and other tools and techniques are additional strategies to link faculty and students (see later in this chapter).

■ RESOURCES

The home health care student and staff nurse have valuable resources that contribute to their ability to provide high-quality care: education, experience, and common sense. Use these resources consistently when making home visits.

Education

Regardless of the stage of your education or the length of time since graduation, faculty and materials provide valuable professional information. Formal and informal education beyond the professional program is important for practicing community health nurses; many educators are increasingly interested in partnerships with practitioners and agencies.[36] Consider courses in first aid; cardiopulmonary resuscitation; computers; the Internet; cultural awareness; community resources; current affairs; and political, legal, financial, and ethical issues. Read relevant publications, and attend relevant conferences. Remember what you learned, and keep updating your knowledge.

Experience

Your professional and life experiences contribute to your technical and interpersonal skills. Know where you are, and take action in the areas in which you need to improve.[2] Discuss your career goals and opportunities with a trusted friend. Take every opportunity to observe a colleague providing care or completing other responsibilities, such as documentation. Learn how to organize your practice and avail yourself of excellent practice pointers, such as the Bridge to Home Health Care features in this book.

Common Sense

Practice in community-focused settings is not the same as practice in the acute care setting. Develop and use your intuition, and listen to it.[18, 27] Expert home health care clinicians are known for their caring, flexibility, persistence, and ability to improvise. They use sound judgment to alter everything from their schedule to their interventions according to their circumstances and the available resources. Expert clinicians have more than a plan A as they begin to work with a client; they can move to a plan B or plan C at a moment's notice.

PROVIDING CARE

The concepts and principles involved in home health care and other community-focused practice settings are closely related to those of nursing practice in the hospital, outpatient departments, and long-term care. The assessment, problem identification (diagnosis), planning, intervention, and evaluation steps of the nursing process provide an important foundation for that practice. Specific systems that you may use in home health or community-focused care include the Omaha System and the Nightingale Tracker.

■ THE OMAHA SYSTEM

The Omaha System was developed and refined during three Visiting Nurse Association (VNA) of Omaha research projects funded by the Division of Nursing, U.S. Department of Health and Human Services, between 1975 and 1986. Research on reliability, validity, and usability was also completed.[25, 27, 28]

The Omaha System is designed to facilitate nursing practice, documentation, and information management. It is a series of cues or feedback loops that help remind the user about possible client problems and intervention options and about ways to evaluate the effect of the care provided. Structured language and codes enhance the precision of recording and ease of communication. Users can communicate their conclusions orally, through printed paper forms, or electronically.

The Omaha System provides a clinical data framework for agencies or programs that use manual or automated versions of client records. Establishing a clinical database that is reliable and valid enables a user to generate reports that contribute to program evaluation, long-range planning, complying with regulations required by accreditation organizations and third-party payers, and outcome statistics required as part of managed care contracts.

Many home health and community-focused agencies are making progress in their efforts to improve their client records and to develop integrated clinical and financial management information systems. The time and costs required for development of such information systems, however, are significant constraints.

Initial users of the Omaha System were community-focused home care, public health, and school practice professionals in the United States. Both the number and type of Omaha System users are expanding dramatically to include nursing center staff, hospital-based and managed care case managers, nursing educators and students, acute care staff, researchers, and the international community. Such expansion reflects the trends already described in this chapter and the trend among all types of health care providers to automate the handling of clinical data.[3, 4, 9, 12, 21, 29, 41] The Omaha System includes one of the vocabularies recognized and disseminated by the American Nurses Association.[16, 17]

Figure 7–1 illustrates the concepts of the nursing process as they relate to the Omaha System. The circular model shown depicts the dynamic, interactive nature of the nursing process; the nurse-client relationship; and related theories of diagnostic reasoning and clinical judgment, sometimes referred to as *analytic reasoning* or *expert knowledge*. The Omaha System is a research-based nursing diagnosis, intervention, and outcome measurement classification or taxonomy developed by practicing nurses.[21, 26, 27] The Problem Classification Scheme, the Intervention Scheme, and the Problem Rating Scale for Outcomes are components of the system. The relationships among the nursing process, the Omaha System, and home health care practice are described next.

A community health nurse begins service to a client after an intake or referral process. During a nurse's initial visit and all other visits, the vital importance of establishing and maintaining a positive nurse-client relationship must be recognized. Freeman and Heinrich[14] emphasized that a positive relationship is developed, not discovered. Such a relationship promotes quantity and quality of data and enhances the potential for success and client progress in relation to all components of the nursing process.

A nurse's initial activities include data collection, assessment, and analysis (i.e., Problem Classification Scheme). This process involves gathering, clustering, combining, summarizing, and validating diverse subjective and objective information about each family member, the family as an interacting unit, and the sociocultural and physical environment. A community health nurse uses principles of epidemiology to enhance systematic data collection and assessment and to identify patterns within client data. . . . The conclusion and logical end product of the data collection and assessment process is problem identification or diagnosis, which involves interpretation of the acquired data.

Planning and intervening are two of the most important concepts of the model to both a client and a nurse (i.e., Intervention Scheme). Campbell[5] described a broad interpretation of planning and intervention involving nurse and family collaboration to:

- Set priorities
- Identify client status and expected outcome(s) criteria or goals relative to specific nursing problems and time frames
- Delineate alternative courses of action
- Choose and take action

Identification of admission, interim, and discharge ratings quantifies the evaluation process (i.e., Problem Rating Scale for Outcomes). Each rating provides a baseline for contrast with later ratings during the period of client service. The evaluation component of the Omaha System allows a nurse to compare a client's health status at different points in time to determine the degree of nursing effectiveness. The nurse uses data from the evaluation process to revise and modify plans and interventions with an individual, family, or group. Thus, evaluation is both ongoing and terminal.[27]

The Problem Classification Scheme, the Intervention Scheme, and the Problem Rating Scale for Outcomes follow principles of taxonomy and consist of terms and codes arranged from general to specific. Terms are intended to be simple, clear, and concise.

The Problem Classification Scheme

The Problem Classification Scheme is a taxonomy of client problems or nursing diagnoses that has been developed from actual client data (Box 7–1). It consists of four levels[26, 27]:

Domains are four general areas that represent community health practice and provide organizational groupings for client problems: Environmental, Psychosocial, Physiological, and Health-Related Behaviors.

Problems are 40 nursing diagnoses that represent matters of difficulty and concern that adversely affect any aspect of the client's well-being. Examples include Caretaking/parenting, Integument, and Nutrition.

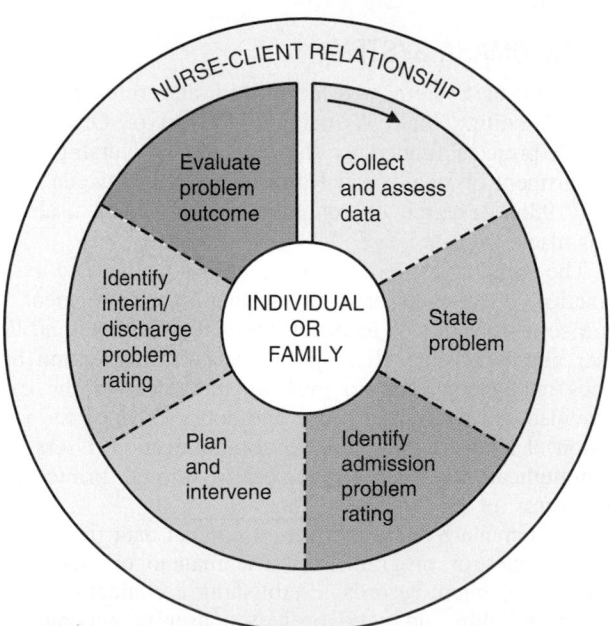

FIGURE 7–1 Steps of the nursing process as they relate to the Omaha System. (From Martin, K. S., & Scheet, N. J. [1992]. *The Omaha System: Applications for community health nursing* [p. 34]. Philadelphia: W. B. Saunders.)

BOX 7–1 Domains and Problems of the Problem Classification Scheme

Domain I. Environmental

The material resources, physical surroundings, and substances both internal and external to the client, home, neighborhood, and broader community.

1. Income
2. Sanitation
3. Residence
4. Neighborhood/workplace safety
5. Other

Domain II. Psychosocial

Patterns of behavior, communication, relationships, and development.

6. Communication with community resources
7. Social contact
8. Role change
9. Interpersonal relationship
10. Spirituality
11. Grief
12. Emotional stability
13. Human sexuality
14. Caretaking/parenting
15. Neglected child/adult
16. Abused child/adult
17. Growth and development
18. Other

Domain III. Physiological

Functional status of processes that maintain life.

19. Hearing
20. Vision

21. Speech and language
22. Dentition
23. Cognition
24. Pain
25. Consciousness
26. Integument
27. Neuromusculoskeletal function
28. Respiration
29. Circulation
30. Digestion-hydration
31. Bowel function
32. Genitourinary function
33. Antepartum/postpartum
34. Other

Domain IV. Health-Related Behaviors

Activities that maintain or promote wellness, promote recovery, or maximize rehabilitation potential.

35. Nutrition
36. Sleep and rest patterns
37. Physical activity
38. Personal hygiene
39. Substance use
40. Family planning
41. Health care supervision
42. Prescribed medication regimen
43. Technical procedure
44. Other

Data from Martin, K. S., & Scheet, N. J. (1992). *The Omaha System: A pocket guide for community health nursing.* Philadelphia: W. B. Saunders.

Modifiers are the two sets of terms used to identify ownership of the problem and degree of severity in relation to client interest, risk factors, and signs/symptoms.
Signs and symptoms are the objective and subjective evidence of a client's problem.

The Problem Classification Scheme offers a view of the wide range of client concerns that the home health or community-focused provider addresses. These include physical, emotional, social, spiritual, and economic concerns. Thus, this tool is used as a framework for assessment during a home or clinic visit and for documentation of the service provided. In that way, it constantly reminds the provider that the client needs to be viewed holistically and not as a "colostomy case" or a drug user, for example. The OASIS data set was not designed to be an assessment framework, but OASIS items can be integrated into the agency's assessment form, such as a form based on the Problem Classification Scheme.[41]

Caretaking/parenting, a problem from the Psychosocial domain, appears in Box 7–2. It has nine signs/symptoms, including difficulty providing physical care/safety and expectations incongruent with stage of growth and development. For example, you visit a 14-year-old mother and

her newborn to provide information about infant growth, development, and care. You may record:

1. The problem, Caretaking/parenting.
2. Signs/symptoms, difficulty providing physical care/safety and expectations incongruent with stage of growth and development.
3. More specific descriptive and quantitative clinical data on the client's manual or automated record.

Integument, a problem from the Physiological domain, also appears in Box 7–2. Integument has 10 signs/symptoms, including lesion and drainage. If you care for a client whose infected wound requires cleaning and a dressing change, you may record[26]:

1. The problem, Integument.
2. Signs/symptoms, lesion and drainage.
3. More specific descriptive and quantitative clinical data on the client's form or automated record.

Table 7–1 illustrates these two examples of assessment and nursing diagnosis documentation as well as terms and codes from the other two Omaha System schemes. Note that it depicts only part of the documenta-

BOX 7–2 Problems, Modifiers, and Signs/Symptoms from the Problem Classification Scheme

14. Caretaking/parenting:
  - Health promotion
  - Potential impairment
  - Impairment
  - 01. difficulty providing physical care/safety
  - 02. difficulty providing emotional nurturance
  - 03. difficulty providing cognitive learning experiences and activities
  - 04. difficulty providing preventive and therapeutic health care
  - 05. expectations incongruent with stage of growth and development
  - 06. dissatisfaction/difficulty with responsibilities
  - 07. neglectful
  - 08. abusive
  - 09. other
26. Integument:
  - Health promotion
  - Potential impairment
  - Impairment
  - 01. lesion
  - 02. rash
  - 03. excessively dry
  - 04. excessively oily
  - 05. inflammation
  - 06. pruritus
  - 07. drainage
  - 08. ecchymosis
  - 09. hypertrophy of nails
  - 10. other

Data from Martin, K. S., & Scheet, N. J. (1992). *The Omaha System: A pocket guide for community health nursing.* Philadelphia: W. B. Saunders.

tion for two nurse-client visits, not complete record entries.

The Intervention Scheme

The Intervention Scheme is a systematic arrangement of nursing actions or activities designed to help users identify and document plans and interventions in relation to specific client problems and other concepts of the nursing process (Box 7–3). It represents a research-based effort to link the effectiveness of interventions with diagnoses.[26]

The first level consists of four categories:

- Health Teaching, Guidance, and Counseling
- Treatments and Procedures
- Case Management
- Surveillance

Categories are broad areas that provide a structure for describing actions or activities. One or more categories are used to develop a plan or document an intervention specific to a client problem.

The second level is an alphabetical listing of 62 targets. *Targets* are objects of nursing intervention or nursing activities that further describe problem-specific intervention categories. For the problem Integument and the category Treatments and Procedures, useful targets include dressing change/wound care and signs/symptoms—physical. For Caretaking/parenting and the category Health Teaching, Guidance, and Counseling, possible targets are anatomy/physiology, bonding, and growth/development.

The third level is designed for client-specific information. Users generate pertinent, concise words or phrases as they develop plans or document care provided to a specific client. Although it was not part of the research

TABLE 7–1 APPLICATION OF OMAHA SYSTEM

Client Data	Problems and Signs/Symptoms	Problem Rating Scale for Outcomes	Intervention Categories	Intervention Targets
PSYCHOSOCIAL DOMAIN Jane Doe: 14-year-old new mother with 2-day-old infant boy. Says she is "scared." Has not cared for infants; asking how to hold and feed. Wants son to sleep at least 6 hr. No family in area.	14. Caretaking/parenting: actual/family 01. difficulty providing physical care/safety 05. expectations incongruent with stage of growth and development	Knowledge = 2 Behavior = 3 Status = 2	I. Health teaching, Guidance, and Counseling III. Case Management	01. Anatomy/physiology 04. Bonding 08. Caretaking/parenting skills 59. Support group
PHYSIOLOGICAL DOMAIN John Brown: 82-year-old just discharged after hemicolectomy. Has infected incision. Recalls some of discharge instructions.	26. Integument: actual/individual 01. lesion 07. drainage	Knowledge = 4 Behavior = 3 Status = 3	I. Health teaching, Guidance, and Counseling II. Treatments and Procedures	14. Dressing change/wound care 50. Signs/symptoms—physical 14. Dressing change/wound care 50. Signs/symptoms—physical

BOX 7-3   Intervention Scheme

Categories

I Health Teaching, Guidance, and Counseling

Health teaching, guidance, and counseling are nursing activities that range from giving information, anticipating client problems, encouraging client action and responsibility for self-care and coping, to assisting with decision-making and problem-solving. The overlapping concepts occur on a continuum with the variation due to the client's self-direction capabilities.

II Treatments and Procedures

Treatments and procedures are technical nursing activities directed toward preventing signs and symptoms, identifying risk factors and early signs and symptoms, and decreasing or alleviating signs and symptoms.

III Case Management

Case management includes nursing activities of coordination, advocacy, and referral. These activities involve facilitating service delivery on behalf of the client, communicating with health and human services providers, promoting assertive client communication, and guiding the client toward use of appropriate community resources.

IV Surveillance

Surveillance includes nursing activities of detection, measurement, critical analysis, and monitoring to indicate client status in relation to a given condition or phenomenon.

Targets

1. Anatomy/physiology	22. Finances	43. Rehabilitation
2. Behavior modification	23. Food	44. Relaxation/breathing techniques
3. Bladder care	24. Gait training	45. Rest/sleep
4. Bonding	25. Growth/development	46. Safety
5. Bowel care	26. Homemaking	47. Screening
6. Bronchial hygiene	27. Housing	48. Sickness/injury care
7. Cardiac care	28. Interaction	49. Signs/symptoms—mental/emotional
8. Caretaking/parenting skills	29. Laboratory findings	50. Signs/symptoms—physical
9. Cast care	30. Legal system	51. Skin care
10. Communication	31. Medical/dental care	52. Social work/counseling
11. Coping skills	32. Medication action/side effects	53. Specimen collection
12. Day care/respite care	33. Medication administration	54. Spiritual care
13. Discipline	34. Medication set-up	55. Stimulation/nurturance
14. Dressing change/wound care	35. Mobility/transfers	56. Stress management
15. Durable medical equipment	36. Nursing care, supplementary	57. Substance use
16. Education	37. Nutrition	58. Supplies
17. Employment	38. Nutritionist	59. Support group
18. Environment	39. Ostomy care	60. Support system
19. Exercises	40. Other community resource	61. Transportation
20. Family planning	41. Personal care	62. Wellness
21. Feeding procedures	42. Positioning	63. Other

Data from Martin, K. S., & Scheet, N. J. (1992). *The Omaha System: A pocket guide for community health nursing.* Philadelphia: W. B. Saunders.

projects, VNA of Omaha staff organized their suggestions into care planning guides.[26]

Table 7-1 presents the use of intervention categories, targets, and client-specific information to describe and document a plan or intervention category specific to a client problem such as Integument or Caretaking/parenting. Again, note the definitions and diversity of community-focused interventions. Nurses and other providers who practice in the community must be generalists and must develop competence in providing "hands-on" bedside care and technical skills as well as educational, referral, monitoring, and motivational skills. Recall the previous comments about the client's owning the health-related problem and being the only one who ultimately solves the problem.

Problem Rating Scale for Outcomes

The Problem Rating Scale for Outcomes is a framework for measuring a client's problem-specific Knowledge, Behavior, and Status. The scale is intended to measure the client's progress and provide both a guide for practice and a method of documentation. The scale was designed for use throughout the time of client service. When establishing the initial ratings for client problems, the user creates an independent data baseline, capturing the condition and circumstances of the client at a given point in time. This admission baseline is used to compare and contrast the client's condition and circumstances with those at the ratings completed at later intervals and at client discharge. The comparison or change in ratings over time can be used to identify the client's progress in relation to interventions and the effectiveness of the plan of care.[25-27]

The Problem Rating Scale for Outcomes is a five-point, ordinal scale comprising three subscales, or concepts (Table 7-2). *Concepts* are three major areas that represent the basic client issues of knowing (Knowledge), doing (Behavior), and being (Status):

TABLE 7-2	PROBLEM RATING SCALE FOR OUTCOMES				
Concept	1	2	3	4	5
Knowledge: the ability of the client to remember and interpret information	No knowledge	Minimal knowledge	Basic knowledge	Adequate knowledge	Superior knowledge
Behavior: the observable responses, actions, or activities of the client fitting the occasion or purpose	Not appropriate	Rarely appropriate	Inconsistently appropriate	Usually appropriate	Consistently appropriate
Status: the condition of the client in relation to objective and subjective defining characteristics	Extreme signs/symptoms	Severe signs/symptoms	Moderate signs/symptoms	Minimal signs/symptoms	No signs/symptoms

Data from Martin, K. S., & Scheet, N. J. (1992). The *Omaha System: A pocket guide for community health nursing.* Philadelphia: W. B. Saunders.

Knowledge refers to the ability of the client to remember and interpret information.

Behavior consists of the observable responses, actions, or activities of the client fitting the occasion or purpose.

Status is the condition of the client in relation to objective and subjective defining characteristics.

The scale for each of the concepts has five categories or degrees for response. For example, for the problems Integument and Caretaking/parenting, the nurse would identify baseline Knowledge, Behavior, and Status ratings during the first home or clinic visit.

■ AUTOMATION AND THE NIGHTINGALE TRACKER

The Omaha System has been described as a model for practice, documentation, and information management. The critical need to generate, store, analyze, and distribute clinical data with the help of automated information systems exists in all health care settings. For a few years early in the 1980s, the VNA developed and sold computer software. Soon other groups and agencies developed their own Omaha System software. Early in the 1990s, software companies started to develop commercially available software for home health agencies, public health departments, nursing centers, and colleges and schools of nursing.[12, 13, 21, 33, 41]

The presence of faculty and nursing students in service settings, especially students who are just beginning their nursing education, introduces additional challenges related to practice, documentation, and information management. Unlike hospital practice, community health practice may involve faculty remaining at the college or service setting while their eight or more students make independent visits and see clients at homes, clinics, schools, or other sites. These faculty and students, especially students in their early semesters of education, need to maintain communication while traveling and providing client care. Students may need to communicate with faculty quickly and often for the safety of both clients and students. These needs can be met by using reliable and efficient automated point-of-care information systems.

To help nursing students and faculty, the Helene Fuld Trust provided a 3-year (1994 to 1997) research and development grant to FITNE (formerly the Fuld Institute for Technology in Nursing Education). Staff members at FITNE developed the Nightingale Tracker, a computerized communication system using portable hand-held computers. Students use the Nightingale Tracker to document the services they provide, send and receive Fax and e-mail messages, and browse the Internet. They can also use it as a speaker phone.[12, 13]

The Omaha System terminology was selected as the clinical vocabulary for the Nightingale Tracker and is used by students as they complete clinical assignment activities. Such activities include assignment generation, preplanning, postclinical documentation, and evaluation follow-up. When the Nightingale Tracker was released in 1998, the first users were students and faculty in seven colleges and schools of nursing. These schools were selected for diversity in geographical location, size, and educational programs and included associate degree, baccalaureate degree, registered nurse completion, and graduate nurse programs.[9, 12, 33] Since 1998, the number and types of students who use the Nightingale Tracker and the Omaha System have increased to include schools and colleges that base their curriculum on the Omaha System.[29]

CONCLUSIONS

Home health care and community-focused service settings are experiencing both unprecedented growth and financial constraints. Decreased agency revenue can lead to layoffs, decreased salary and benefits, increased workloads, and a sense of insecurity. Increases in client caseloads and services, staff, and budget can be exciting. At the same time, when the internal systems of agencies experience extra pressure and become overloaded, employees are more likely to become frustrated and stressed and to make errors. Teamwork and development and improvement of systems are critical. Clinicians, administrators, students, and faculty need to use a variety of methods to communicate efficiently and work together to provide effective, high-quality services.

BIBLIOGRAPHY

1. Anderson, E. T., & McFarlane, J. M. (1996). *The community as partner* (2nd ed.). Philadelphia: J. B. Lippincott.
2. Benner, P. (1984). *From novice to expert*. Menlo Park, CA: Addison-Wesley.
3. Bowles, K. H. (1999). The Omaha System: Bridging hospital and home care. *On-line Journal of Nursing Informatics* [On-line], *3*(1). Available: *http://cac.psu.edu/~dxml/ojni.html*.
4. Button, P., et al. (1998). Challenges and issues related to implementation of nursing vocabularies in computer-based systems. *Journal of the American Medical Informatics Association, 5*(4), 332–334.
5. Campbell, C. (1984). *Nursing diagnosis and intervention in nursing practice* (2nd ed.). New York: John Wiley & Sons.
6. *Caring.* (1998). XVII(2).
7. *Caring.* (1998). XVII(10).
8. Coenen, A., Marek, K. D., & Lundeen, S. P. (1996). Using nursing diagnoses to explain utilization in a community nursing center. *Research in Nursing and Health, 19*(5), 441–445.
9. Connolly, P. M., Huynh, M. T., & Gorney-Moreno, M. J. (1999). Cutting edge or over the edge? Implementing the Nightingale Tracker. *On-line Journal of Nursing Informatics* [On-line], *3*(1). Available: *http://cac.psu.edu/~dxm12/ojni.html*.
10. Crisler, K. S., Campbell, B. M., & Shaughnessy, P. W. (1997). *OASIS basics: Beginning to use the Outcome and Assessment Information Set.* Denver: Center for Health Services and Policy Research.
11. Dolan, J. A., Fitzpatrick, M. L., & Herrmann, E. K. (1983). *Nursing in society: A historical perspective* (15th ed.). Philadelphia: W. B. Saunders.
12. Elfrink, V. L. (1999). The Omaha System: Bridging nursing education and information technology. *On-line Journal of Nursing Informatics* [On-line], *3*(1). Available: *http://cac:psu.edu/~dxm12/ojni.html*.
13. Elfrink, V. L., & Martin, K. S. (1996). Educating for community nursing practice: Point of care technology. *Healthcare Information Management, 10*(2), 81–89.
14. Freeman, R., & Heinrich, J. (1981). *Community health nursing practice* (2nd ed.). Philadelphia: W. B. Saunders.
15. Frenn, M., et al. (1996). Symposium on nursing centers: Past, present, and future. *Journal of Nursing Education, 35*(2), 54–62.
16. Helmlinger, C. (1998). New classification system recognized. *American Journal of Nursing, 98*(12), 63.
17. Lang, N. M. (Ed.). (1995). *Nursing data systems: The emerging framework.* Washington, DC: American Nurses Publishing.
18. Leahy, L. (1997). Decrease violence—increase safety. *Home Health FOCUS, 4*(1), 1, 4.
19. Martin, K. S. (1998). Economics, home health style. *Home Health FOCUS, 4*(11), 82.
20. Martin, K. S. (1998). Economics: Wishes, magic wands, and reality. *Home Health FOCUS, 4*(12), 90.
21. Martin, K. S. (1999). The Omaha System: Past, present, and future. *On-line Journal of Nursing Informatics* [On-line], *3*(1). Available: *http://cac.psu.edu/~dxm12/ojni.html*.
22. Martin, K. S. (2000). Home health care, outcomes management, and the Land of Oz. *Outcomes Management for Nursing Practice, 4*(1), 7–12.
23. Martin, K. S., & Gorski, L. A. (1998). Managed care: Effects on home health providers and stroke survivors. *Topics in Stroke Rehabilitation, 5*(3), 11–24.
24. Martin, K. S., & Norris, J. (1996). The Omaha System: A model for describing practice. *Holistic Nursing Practice, 11*(1), 75–83.
25. Martin, K. S., Norris, J., & Leak, G. K. (1999). Psychometric analysis of the Problem Rating Scale for Outcomes. *Outcomes Management for Nursing Practice, 3*(1), 20–25.
26. Martin, K. S., & Scheet, N. J. (1992). *The Omaha System: A pocket guide for community health nursing.* Philadelphia: W. B. Saunders.
27. Martin, K. S., & Scheet, N. J. (1992). *The Omaha System: Applications for community health nursing.* Philadelphia: W. B. Saunders.
28. Martin, K. S., Scheet, N. J., & Stegman, M. R. (1993). Home health clients: Characteristics, outcomes of care, and nursing interventions. *American Journal of Public Health, 83*(12), 1730–1734.
29. Merrill, A. S., et al. (1998). Curriculum restructuring using the practice-based Omaha System. *Nurse Educator, 23*(3), 41–44.
30. Mikulencak, M. (1993, July–August). Facts you should know. *American Nurse, 25*(7), 13.
31. National Association for Home Care. (1999). *Basic statistics about home care 1999.* Washington, DC: Author.
32. National Association for Home Care. (1999, March 19). *Home health agency closures rise* (NAHC Report. No. 802:1). Washington, DC: Author.
33. Nightingale Tracker Field Test Nurse Team. (1999). Designing an information technology application for use in community-focused nursing curriculum. *Computers in Nursing, 17*(2), 73–81.
34. Pender, N. J. (1996). *Health promotion in nursing practice* (3rd ed.). Norwalk, CT: Appleton & Lange.
35. Reif, L. J., & Martin, K. S. (1996). *Nurses and consumers: Partners in assuring quality in the home.* Washington, DC: American Nurses Publishing.
36. Rothert, M. L., Talarczyk, G. L., & Awbrey, S. M. (1997). Distance learning: An integral part of transforming the university and nursing education. In J. C. McCloskey & H. K. Grace (Eds.), *Current issues in nursing* (5th ed., pp. 180–184). St. Louis: Mosby–Year Book.
37. Stanhope, M., & Lancaster, J. (Eds.). (2000). *Community and public health nursing: Promoting health of aggregates, families, and individuals* (5th ed.). St. Louis: Mosby.
38. Swanson, J. M., & Neis, M. (1997). *Community health nursing: Promoting the health of aggregates* (2nd ed.). Philadelphia: W. B. Saunders.
39. Tully, M., & Bennett, K. (1992, March). Extending community health nursing services: The student learning center. *Journal of Nursing Administration, 22*, 38–42.
40. U.S. Bureau of the Census. (1996 & 1998). Resident population of the United States: Estimates and projections. Available: *http://www.census.gov/population*. Accessed: April 1, 1999.
41. Westra, B. L., & Solomon, D. A. (1999). The Omaha System: Bridging home care and technology. *On-line Journal of Nursing Informatics* [On-line], *3*(1). Available: *http://cac.psu.edu/~dxm12/ojni.html*.
42. World Health Organization/UNICEF. (1978). *Primary health care: Alma-Ata Conference.* Geneva: Author.

CHAPTER

8

Long-Term Care

Charlotte Eliopoulos

Of all the types of health care settings, long-term care facilities (LTCFs) are perhaps the most misunderstood and criticized. The media give prime coverage to the small minority of facilities that have substandard conditions while ignoring the majority that provide compassionate, competent care on a daily basis. Some professionals who have never worked in an LTCF believe that this setting is a simple, nonchallenging environment in which to work. Many families assume that nursing home staff are untrustworthy, uncaring, and lazy.

In reality, residents of LTCFs receive proper care and enjoy a good quality of life. Despite significantly fewer resources available to them, compared with those found in hospitals and other care settings, LTCFs provide adequate care for highly dependent residents. The wide range of physical and mental conditions of residents, combined with their advanced age, make them a complex population for whom to care. Because physicians typically are not on the premises at all times, nurses must be highly competent in assessing residents, recognizing changes in status, and communicating needs to physicians. It is not unusual to find very special relationships between residents and their caregivers, who often assume a family surrogate role. Why is there such a discrepancy between the reality and perception of the LTCF? Much of this is the result of the manner in which these facilities have developed. A brief review of the growth of LTCF may offer some insight into the current challenges confronting this care setting.

GROWTH OF LONG-TERM CARE FACILITIES

By the end of the 17th century, most European countries had created institutions to care for the mentally ill, aged, developmentally disabled, orphaned, poor, criminals, and people with contagious diseases. It was not unusual for a single institution to house all of these various types of people together. The interest was not to provide highly specialized and individualized care but to segregate these people from the rest of society. Not surprisingly, low public interest and limited funds caused conditions to become severe in these institutions.

Until the 19th century, the United States had few institutions. People who were sick, old, or disabled were expected to receive care at home, from private help or family. As the population grew, however, so did the number of people without the financial or family resources to provide care, and hospitals and other forms of inpatient care were needed. Hospitals, staffed by physicians who at that time were from society's elite, were less than enthusiastic about having poor people with long-term care needs remaining in their beds for extended periods. Pressure grew to create facilities that could house and care for persons over the long term. In response, communities developed institutions that were given names such as almshouse hospital, asylum, homes for the incurable, and chronic disease hospital. Most often, these institutions were located on the outskirts of town so that the average citizen would not have to have contact with the residents.

Because these early facilities relied on charities and meager public funds for their existence, needless to say, conditions were quite poor. A physician from that era, writing about those early institutions, described conditions such as grossly inadequate supplies, food so insufficient that many residents experienced recurrent incidents of scurvy, and residents forced to sleep on the floor because of overcrowding, rampant theft, open drunkenness, and sex between residents and their caregivers.[7] Residents were expected to work for their keep, and recovered residents who had no family or home in the community, remained in the institution and cooked, cleaned, or cared for other residents in exchange for room, board, and a small salary. In this environment, high quality of life, rehabilitation, residents' rights, and individuality were foreign concepts. With these conditions, most people did not view institutions that provided long-term care as highly desirable options.

The enactment of Social Security in 1935 afforded older adults the means to purchase care privately and not rely on charitable or public institutions. An informal long-term care system began to grow as people rented rooms of their homes to elders who needed room, board, and perhaps some basic personal care assistance. Many of these homes were operated by nurses, or women who called themselves nurses, thus, the term *nursing home* began to be more widely used. Small nursing homes began to appear, often developed by religious or public agencies (e.g., Jewish homes for the aged, county rest homes) and sometimes by private individuals. At this time, the government had little involvement in nursing home operations; there were no government regulations pertaining to nursing home care and no government reimbursement for long-term care services.

In 1946, the federal government took a noticeable step in promoting nursing home growth through the Hill-Burton Hospital Survey and Construction Act. This Act provided funds for hospital construction, but other institutions, such as nursing homes, could obtain funds if they met the conditions required by the Act. Since the construction requirements were developed from hospitals, the nursing homes who obtained these funds constructed facilities that were very similar to hospitals. Rather than an environment designed for the unique needs of chronically ill individuals who would reside in the setting for an extended period of time, nursing homes resembled acute hospitals in appearance and style of operation (e.g., white uniforms, rigid schedules, limited visitation schedules, subservient role of residents).

By the 1960s, the graying of the population was being realized. As the numbers of elders grew, so did their need for health services. During the Kennedy-Johnson era, federal programs proliferated to assist the disabled, the aged, and other special groups. In 1965, Medicare and Medicaid were developed to ensure a minimum level of health care for the aged and poor. There was considerable interest in the existing health care system in providing nursing home reimbursement through Medicare and Medicaid. The American Medical Association lobbied to have reimbursement for extended care facilities to ease the problems acute hospitals were experiencing in having people who no longer needed acute care services remaining in their beds because of the lack of means to pay for nursing home care. The owners of LTCFs also lobbied Congress to provide government funding for care in their facilities. Congress responded by including provisions for reimbursement for nursing home care in Medicare and Medicaid.

Along with funding came regulations—the standards or conditions that facilities had to meet in order to qualify for funds. Initially, the regulations included requirements for 24-hour licensed nursing coverage, individualized care plans, provisions for special diets, and other good standards of practice. Unfortunately, only a small minority of the existing LTCFs could meet the standards at the time and protested that it would not be possible for them to participate in the Medicare and Medicaid programs. Again, with strong lobbying efforts, these conditions were waived, and facilities were able to take advantage of government reimbursement for long-term care without having to meet what were good, basic standards. (It is interesting that there was no noticeable voice from nurses, even though these facilities were called *nursing* homes.)

With eased standards and an influx of government reimbursement, the number of nursing homes grew (Table 8-1). This rapid and unregulated growth led to problems, some of which made front page headlines. Short staffing, substandard care, and abuse were among the conditions that the media exposed and that helped to generate the negative image of LTCFs that continues to shadow this care setting. The public was outraged and demanded action. In response, the Department of Health and Human Services (DHHS) commissioned the Institute of Medicine (IOM) to study these facilities and recommend changes. The IOM study confirmed the widespread poor quality of care that existed in LTCFs and emphasized the need to develop stricter regulations.[5] In response, highly stringent

TABLE 8-1	GROWTH OF NURSING HOMES AND NURSING HOME RESIDENTS IN THE 20TH CENTURY	
Year	No. of Nursing Homes	Residents (in Thousands)
1940	1,200	25
1960	9,582	290
1970	22,004	1,076
1980	30,111	1,396
1990	14,744	1,558
1996	16,800	1,700

From U.S. Department of Commerce, Table 204: Nursing and Related Care Facilities. *Statistical Abstract of the United States: 1996* (116th ed., p. 136). Washington, DC: Bureau of the Census.

regulations were enacted under legislation called the *Omnibus Budget Reconciliation Act of 1987* (OBRA) which produced profound reforms in nursing home care. Some of the conditions that LTCFs must meet are described in Box 8-1. Both the conditions and enforcement provisions are more stringent. Facilities that do not meet the conditions described in regulations can receive sanctions that include termination of Medicare and Medicaid reimbursement. As a result of the new regulations and strict enforcement of them, conditions in LTCFs have improved.

This history can help you to understand some of the reasons for the persistent negative image of LTCFs. Further, it demonstrates that the importance of an active role for nursing in developing new services and defining nursing services that contribute to high-quality care. Nursing leadership was sorely lacking as nursing homes grew and as non-nurses determined nursing's function, role, and staffing requirements, and the results speak for themselves.

RESIDENTS OF LONG-TERM CARE FACILITIES

Residents of LTCFs can be of any age, although most are old. The risk of being in an LTCF increases with each decade of life; the average age of residents is 82 years. Women outnumber men by a ratio of 3 to 1, and 90% are single or widowed.

Most residents have conditions that impair their self-care capacity or require interventions that they cannot perform independently. About one half have a progressive cognitive impairment, such as Alzheimer's disease, arthritis, cardiovascular disease, or a combination. One third have impaired vision, and another third have impaired hearing. Most residents need assistance with at least several activities of daily living (ADL). Although most residents will spend the remainder of their lives in the facility, an increasing number will recover, have restored function, and return to the community. In the past, some who might have remained in the hospital during recovery are now convalescing in nursing homes as a result of changes in reimbursement policies. The quality and quantity of caregiver support available, rather than the medical diagnosis, determine one's risk of being admitted to an LTCF. For every resident in a nursing home, at least two

BOX 8-1   Protections Afforded to Residents of Long-Term Care Facilities as Described in Regulations*

Resident Rights

- to have rights as citizen and resident protected
- to be informed of rights, rules, regulations and responsibilities
- to inspect and obtain copies of records
- to be informed of health status
- to refuse treatment or participation in research
- to be informed of charges
- to be informed of eligibility for Medicaid
- to be informed of process for filing a complaint with the state agency
- to choose and know physician and method of contacting physician
- to be informed of changes in status, room, roommate, or rights
- to proper management of personal funds
- to have privacy respected
- to voice grievances
- to examine survey results
- to perform or refuse to perform services for the facility, and to be compensated for services performed
- to send and receive mail
- to have access to stationery, postage, and writing implements
- to receive visitors
- to use telephone privately
- to retain and use personal possessions
- to share a room with a spouse
- to self-administer drugs unless determined to be unsafe

Admission, Transfer, Discharge

- to have legitimate reason for discharge
- to be free from solicitation of gifts or money as condition for admission
- to have written policies regarding services provided by facility

Resident Behavior and Facility Practices

- to be free from restraints used for purpose of discipline or staff convenience
- to be free from verbal, physical, or mental abuse, punishment or seclusion
- to have alleged and known abuse incidents investigated and reported according to state law

Quality of Life

- to have dignity maintained and promoted
- to choose activities and care
- to organize and participate in resident groups
- to participate in social, religious, and community activities
- to have program of activities directed by qualified personnel
- to have social services provided by qualified personnel
- to have clean, safe, home-like environment
- to have private closet space, adequate lighting, and comfortable room temperatures

Resident Assessment

- to have a comprehensive assessment conducted within the first 14 days of admission and at least annually thereafter
- to be reassessed whenever there is a change in status

- to have a comprehensive care plan developed within 7 days after completion of assessment
- to have a discharge plan and summary as needed

Quality of Care

- to receive necessary services and treatments to maintain or improve condition
- to be free from developing pressure ulcers, incontinence, contractures, or dehydration unnecessarily
- to be adequately nourished and hydrated
- to not receive unnecessary drugs
- to be free from significant medication errors

Nursing Services

- to have nursing personnel provided consistent with level of care and needs of residents

Dietary Services

- to have at least 3 well balanced meals provided daily, including special diets
- to have department employ qualified personnel and follow standards for safe food procurement, preparation, and storage

Physician Services

- to be under the care of a physician
- to have the physician adhere to standards of practice

Specialized Rehabilitative Services

- to have physical therapy, occupational therapy, or speech-language therapy arranged for or provided as needed

Dental Services

- to be assisted in obtaining dental services

Pharmacy Services

- to have the facility adhere to standards for prescribing, pouring, administering, and monitoring medications

Infection Control

- to have the facility establish and maintain an infection control program

Physical Environment

- to have the facility follow standards of Life Safety Code

Administration

- to have facility be licensed by state
- to have qualified administrator
- to have nursing assistants complete training program and competency evaluation
- to have a designated medical director
- to provide or arrange for laboratory and diagnostic services
- to have clinical records safeguarded and maintained as required by state law
- to have facility emergency and disaster plans
- to have facility make transfer agreements with hospitals
- to have a utilization review committee in effect
- to have facility maintain a quality assessment and assurance committee that meets at least quarterly and develops and implements corrective actions for deficiencies

*This represents a brief outline of regulations included in the Omnibus Budget Reconciliation Act (OBRA). Please consult the full set of OBRA and state regulations for a complete description of regulatory requirements.

equally disabled people are living in the community, receiving care from family or paid caregivers.[6] Often it is a change in status of the caregiver that precipitates the dependent person's admission to an LTCF. This reinforces the importance of assessing the family and assisting these caregivers in using interventions and resources that will promote and maintain their health and well-being.

STAFF OF LONG-TERM CARE FACILITIES

Of the more than 1.3 million people who work in nursing and personal care facilities in the United States, about 1 million are nursing employees. Most of these are unlicensed personnel.[13] Regulatory standards are basic, and the only specific staffing requirements in federal regulations are that (1) a Registered Nurse must be on duty at least 8 consecutive hours per day, 7 days a week and (2) a full-time director of nursing must be on staff if the facility has more than 60 beds. The proportion of other nursing staff is not stated, although it is required that "the facility provide 24-hour nursing services which are sufficient to meet total nursing care needs."[4] The fact that most direct nursing care is provided by nursing assistants presents special challenges to nurses who must supervise these caregivers.

NURSING RESPONSIBILITIES

■ ASSESSMENT

The facility is required to assess residents within the first 14 days of admission and at least annually thereafter; residents are to be reassessed whenever there is a change in their status. The Minimum Data Set (MDS) is the tool on which the assessment is to be documented, and a Registered Nurse coordinates its completion (Fig. 8–1). Problems in need of care planning are generated from the information on the MDS.

As numerous as the items are on the MDS, it is not a *comprehensive* assessment; it a *minimum* assessment. Important pieces of information are not captured, such as the client's self-concept, spirituality, sense of power, knowledge of health condition and self-care practices, sexuality, patterns of solitude, sense of purpose, immunity, stress management, use of alternative therapies, and attitudes regarding health status and death. Since these are important areas for consideration in the long-term care of residents, you may want to supplement the MDS with these additional assessment data. Although the MDS assessment tool may be formally completed periodically, high-quality care relies on the nurse's assessment of residents with every nurse-resident contact. For example, when administering a medication, you can observe the resident's coloring and respirations, note any change in mood, and ask about the status of a previous manifestation. Often residents do not have the ability to identify and report changes in their own health status, and astute nursing assessment is thus crucial. The need to be alert to changes in status is reinforced by the reality that physicians typically do not see residents on a daily basis and must rely on nurses to detect and report manifestations.

The advanced age of the residents can create challenges in assessment. Age-related changes can cause atypical manifestations in older adults. For example, clinical manifestations of pneumonia in elders, instead of high fever and coughing, may include confusion, loss of appetite, and fatigue with activities that caused no difficulties in the past. This challenges nurses to know the norms for individual residents and to identify subtle clues of illnesses so that problems can be identified early. Timely recognition and communication of manifestations to the physician can help prevent complications.

■ CARE PLANNING

Regulations require that a care plan be written for each resident within 7 days after completion of the assessment. The care plan is an *interdisciplinary* one; nurses coordinate the input offered by each discipline and ensure that the plan is written in a correct, timely manner (Box 8–2). To the extent possible, the resident and the family should actively participate in the development of the care plan.

A care plan is not merely a paperwork requirement but a working tool to guide nursing actions; it is a blueprint for nursing actions. Goals and actions that are no longer relevant need to be revised. All members of the team, particularly nursing assistants who will perform most direct care activities, must be familiar with the care plan.

■ CAREGIVING

The direct caregiving role of nurses varies from facility to facility. In some LTCFs, nurses perform selected roles, such as administering medications and treatments; in others, they may be involved in total care activities. During the pre-employment interview, nurses should review the job descriptions for their specific positions to ensure that they have a realistic view of their role.

In addition to caregiving activities that might be performed in any setting (e.g., medication administration, treatments), special nursing support is required by residents and their families as they adjust to the LTCF. Few individuals have had experiences that prepared them for living in or having a loved one in a nursing home. Residents face many adjustments.

Environment

Many people have lived in the same home for several decades before admission and could probably locate ob-

---

BOX 8–2 **Characteristics of an Effective Care Plan**

- Is based on needs as identified in the Minimum Data Set assessment tool
- Contains goals and actions to address current needs and to prevent new problems
- States goals that are realistic, clear, specific, and measurable
- Lists actions that are related to each goal that include discipline responsible for implementation and specific directions
- Is accessible and utilized by all caregivers
- Is evaluated at least quarterly and revised as necessary

Resident _____ Numeric Identifier _____

MINIMUM DATA SET (MDS) — *VERSION 2.0*
FOR NURSING HOME RESIDENT ASSESSMENT AND CARE SCREENING
FULL ASSESSMENT FORM
(Status in last 7 days, unless other time frame indicated)

SECTION A. IDENTIFICATION AND BACKGROUND INFORMATION

1. RESIDENT NAME
a. (First)   b. (Middle Initial)   c. (Last)   d. (Jr./Sr.)

2. ROOM NUMBER

3. ASSESSMENT REFERENCE DATE
a. Last day of MDS observation period
Month — Day — Year
b. Original (0) or corrected copy of form (enter number of correction)

4a. DATE OF REENTRY
Date of reentry from most recent temporary discharge to a hospital in last 90 days (or since last assessment or admission if less than 90 days)
Month — Day — Year

5. MARITAL STATUS
1. Never married   3. Widowed   5. Divorced
2. Married   4. Separated

6. MEDICAL RECORD NO.

7. CURRENT PAYMENT SOURCES FOR N.H. STAY
(Billing Office to indicate; **check all that apply in last 30 days)**
Medicaid per diem — a.
Medicare per diem — b.
Medicare ancillary part A — c.
Medicare ancillary part B — d.
CHAMPUS per diem — e.
VA per diem — f.
Self or family pays for full per diem — g.
Medicaid resident liability or Medicare co-payment — h.
Private insurance per diem (including co-payment) — i.
Other per diem — j.

8. REASONS FOR ASSESSMENT
[Note—If this is a discharge or reentry assessment, only a limited subset of MDS items need be completed]
a. Primary reason for assessment
1. Admission assessment (required by day 14)
2. Annual assessment
3. Significant change in status assessment
4. Significant correction of prior full assessment
5. Quarterly review assessment
6. Discharged—return not anticipated
7. Discharged—return anticipated
8. Discharged prior to completing initial assessment
9. Reentry
10. Significant correction of prior quarterly assessment
0. NONE OF ABOVE
b. Codes for assessments required for Medicare PPS or the State
1. Medicare 5 day assessment
2. Medicare 30 day assessment
3. Medicare 60 day assessment
4. Medicare 90 day assessment
5. Medicare readmission/return assessment
6. Other state required assessment
7. Medicare 14 day assessment
8. Other Medicare required assessment

9. RESPONSIBILITY/ LEGAL GUARDIAN
(Check all that apply)
Legal guardian — a.
Other legal oversight — b.
Durable power of attorney/health care — c.
Durable power of attorney/financial — d.
Family member responsible — e.
Patient responsible for self — f.
NONE OF ABOVE — g.

10. ADVANCED DIRECTIVES
(For those items with supporting documentation in the medical record, **check all that apply)**
Living will — a.
Do not resuscitate — b.
Do not hospitalize — c.
Organ donation — d.
Autopsy request — e.
Feeding restrictions — f.
Medication restrictions — g.
Other treatment restrictions — h.
NONE OF ABOVE — i.

SECTION B. COGNITIVE PATTERNS

1. COMATOSE
(Persistent vegetative state/no discernible consciousness)
0. No   1. Yes (If yes, skip to Section G)

2. MEMORY
(Recall of what was learned or known)
a. Short-term memory OK—seems/appears to recall after 5 minutes
0. Memory OK   1. Memory problem **2**
b. Long-term memory OK—seems/appears to recall long past
0. Memory OK   1. Memory problem **2**

☐ = When box blank, must enter number or letter.
a. = When letter in box, check if condition applies
Code "—" if information unavailable or unknown

Form 1728RHH   © 1997 Briggs Corporation, Des Moines, IA 50306 (800) 247-2343   PRINTED IN U.S.A.
Copyright limited to addition of trigger system.
3 of 9

3. MEMORY/ RECALL ABILITY
(Check all that resident was **normally able to recall during last 7 days)**
Current season — a.
Location of own room — b.
Staff names/faces — c.
That he/she is in a nursing home — d.
NONE OF ABOVE are recalled — e.

4. COGNITIVE SKILLS FOR DAILY DECISION-MAKING
(Made decisions regarding tasks of daily life)
0. INDEPENDENT—decisions consistent/reasonable
1. MODIFIED INDEPENDENCE—some difficulty in new situations only **2**
2. MODERATELY IMPAIRED—decisions poor; cues/ supervision required **2**
3. SEVERELY IMPAIRED—never/rarely made decisions **2, 5B**

5. INDICATORS OF DELIRIUM— PERIODIC DISORDERED THINKING/ AWARENESS
(Code for behavior in the **last 7 days.)** [Note: Accurate assessment requires conversations with staff and family who have direct knowledge of resident's behavior over this time.]
0. Behavior not present
1. Behavior present, not of recent onset
2. Behavior present, over last 7 days appears different from resident's usual functioning (e.g., new onset or worsening)
a. EASILY DISTRACTED—(e.g., difficulty paying attention; gets sidetracked) 2 = **1, 17***
b. PERIODS OF ALTERED PERCEPTION OR AWARENESS OF SURROUNDINGS—(e.g., moves lips or talks to someone not present; believes he/she is somewhere else; confuses night and day) 2 = **1, 17***
c. EPISODES OF DISORGANIZED SPEECH—(e.g., speech is incoherent, nonsensical, irrelevant, or rambling from subject to subject; loses train of thought) 2 = **1, 17***
d. PERIODS OF RESTLESSNESS—(e.g., fidgeting or picking at skin, clothing, napkins, etc.; frequent position changes; repetitive physical movements or calling out) 2 = **1, 17***
e. PERIODS OF LETHARGY—(e.g., sluggishness; staring into space; difficult to arouse; little body movement) 2 = **1, 17***
f. MENTAL FUNCTION VARIES OVER THE COURSE OF THE DAY—(e.g., sometimes better, sometimes worse; behaviors sometimes present, sometimes not) 2 = **1, 17***

6. CHANGE IN COGNITIVE STATUS
Resident's cognitive status, skills, or abilities have changed as compared to status of **90 days ago** (or since assessment if less than 90 days)
0. No change   1. Improved   2. Deteriorated **1, 17***

SECTION C. COMMUNICATION/HEARING PATTERNS

1. HEARING
(With hearing appliance, if used)
0. HEARS ADEQUATELY—normal talk, TV, phone
1. MINIMAL DIFFICULTY when not in quiet setting **4**
2. HEARS IN SPECIAL SITUATIONS ONLY—speaker has to adjust tonal quality and speak distinctly **4**
3. HIGHLY IMPAIRED/absence of useful hearing **4**

2. COMMUNICATION DEVICES/ TECHNIQUES
(Check all that apply during last 7 days)
Hearing aid, present and used — a.
Hearing aid, present and not used regularly — b.
Other receptive comm. techniques used (e.g., lip reading) — c.
NONE OF ABOVE — d.

3. MODES OF EXPRESSION
(Check all used by resident to make needs known)
Speech — a.
Writing messages to express or clarify needs — b.
American sign language or Braille — c.
Signs/gestures/sounds — d.
Communication board — e.
Other — f.
NONE OF ABOVE — g.

4. MAKING SELF UNDERSTOOD
(Expressing information content—however able)
0. UNDERSTOOD
1. USUALLY UNDERSTOOD—difficulty finding words or finishing thoughts **4**
2. SOMETIMES UNDERSTOOD—ability is limited to making concrete requests **4**
3. RARELY/NEVER UNDERSTOOD **4**

5. SPEECH CLARITY
(Code for speech in the **last 7 days)**
0. CLEAR SPEECH—distinct, intelligible words
1. UNCLEAR SPEECH—slurred, mumbled words
2. NO SPEECH—absence of spoken words

6. ABILITY TO UNDERSTAND OTHERS
(Understanding verbal information content—however able)
0. UNDERSTANDS
1. USUALLY UNDERSTANDS—may miss some part/ intent of message **2, 4**
2. SOMETIMES UNDERSTANDS—responds adequately to simple, direct communication **2, 4**
3. RARELY/NEVER UNDERSTANDS **2, 4**

7. CHANGE IN COMMUNICATION/ HEARING
Resident's ability to express, understand, or hear information has changed as compared to status of **90 days ago** (or since last assessment if less than 90 days)
0. No change   1. Improved   2. Deteriorated **17***

TRIGGER LEGEND
1 - Delirium
2 - Cognitive Loss/Dementia
4 - Communication
5B - ADL Maintenance
17* - Psychotropic Drugs
(For this to trigger, O4a, b, or c must = 1-7)

MDS 2.0   1/30/98

FIGURE 8–1 Sample section of the Minimum Data Set (MDS) assessment tool for nursing home resident assessment and care screening. Other sections would include Vision Patterns, Mood and Behavior Patterns, Psychosocial Well-Being, Physical Functioning and Structural Problems, and Continence in Last 14 Days. (© 1997, Briggs Corporation, West Des Moines, IA.)

jects in their homes blindfolded. Now they are faced with adapting to the layout of a new setting, paging systems, new odors, and sounds, and other new components of their environment. They no longer have ready access to their own refrigerator if they are hungry or a spare bedroom where a grandchild can spend the night. Their personal space has shrunk to a bed, a few chairs, a closet, and several drawers. People can enter their space and invade their privacy at any hour of the day or night.

Routines

New residents soon learn that they must adjust to routines and schedules. They may now have to take a morning shower, although they may have taken a bedtime bath for more than 70 years. They may have a full breakfast placed before them at 8 AM when they seldom ate a bite of food before noon. After decades of staying awake and listening to the radio until 2 AM, they now are told that "lights out" is 9 PM.

People

After years of being on a first-name basis with neighbors, store clerks, the mail carrier, and auto repairman, residents must learn a cast of new players. In addition to other residents, they will meet at least three nurses and three nursing assistants who will care for them over a 24-hour period, the facility's medical director, administrator, social worker, housekeeper, dietitian, activities therapist, clergy, and several therapists. They must learn not only the names but also the roles of these people and how to communicate with them.

Independence

Despite a staff's best efforts to afford residents the right to make decisions, there is a loss of independence when people become residents of a nursing home. They cannot scramble an egg in the middle of the night, have a friend stay over for a few days, or paint the walls the color of their choice. They must report their whereabouts and needs to staff, and depend on others for the basics of bringing them food and taking them to the toilet.

These adjustments also affect family members at the same time that they are facing their own changing roles and responsibilities in regard to their relationship with the resident. Both residents and their families can experience such reactions as anxiety, depression, anger, helplessness, withdrawal, grief, and inattention to self-care practices. You can protect the health of residents and their families and facilitate a positive adjustment to the LTCF by taking some of the actions described in Box 8–3.

During caregiving activities, make sure that *holistic care* is provided; such care implies that every aspect—body, mind, spirit—is being addressed. This integration of body, mind, and spirit results in more powerful and meaningful care than if each aspect were addressed separately. Some ways in which holistic nursing is demonstrated are offered in Box 8–4.

■ COMMUNICATION

As mentioned earlier, the LTCF nurse carries significant responsibility for identifying and obtaining timely treatment of complications and new health problems. Because of their regular and close contact with residents, nursing assistants may be the first and only caregivers to detect changes in health status (e.g., a developing pressure ulcer or a change in eating pattern); therefore, effective channels of communication are crucial in reporting these findings. Conducting rounds, reading what has been documented, and asking specific questions are among the measures you can use to learn about a resident's condition.

You also must make sure that physicians learn of changes in a resident's condition in a timely manner. Documenting in a resident's record is not necessarily sufficient, particularly since most attending physicians do not visit LTCF residents on a daily basis. You must promptly communicate any changes and relevant information (e.g., abnormal laboratory results, family complaints) to physicians.

In between their scheduled visits to the facility, physicians may generate new orders, and most of the time these are communicated by telephone. Facilities may differ in regard to the personnel who can accept telephone orders; therefore, it is best to check with the individual facility's policy. To promote safety in telephone orders:

1. Provide the physician with complete information that can aid in medical decision-making (e.g., clinical manifestations, current and usual vital signs, prescribed medications, unusual incidents, and other relevant facts).
2. Avoid making a medical diagnosis.
3. Take the order directly from the prescribing physician, not office staff.
4. Repeat the order; if possible, have the physician fax a copy of the written order.
5. Have the order signed within 24 hours.

■ MANAGEMENT

Nurses hold a variety of administrative and managerial positions in LTCFs, such as director of nursing, assistant director of nursing, supervisor, unit manager or head nurse, charge nurse, and staffing coordinator. Even if they do not hold these formal titles, most LTCF nurses must perform some management functions, such as:

- Delegating assignments
- Supervising other staff
- Evaluating performance
- Implementing disciplinary actions
- Completing reports
- Reviewing and auditing records
- Communicating needs to other departments
- Investigating, reporting, and recording incidents and accidents
- Handling complaints
- Ordering supplies
- Communicating with insurers, regulatory agencies, and other parties

To manage effectively, your knowledge and skills must exceed those used in clinical nursing activities. You must be knowledgeable of regulations, reimbursement programs, and legal aspects of nursing practice and employee-employer relations. You must also be skillful in

BOX 8-3   Helping New Residents and Families

1. *Learn about the unique characteristics of each resident.*
   a. Find out not only about the health conditions residents have but also who they are as people and the lives they have lived.
   b. Engage residents and families in conversations about residents' histories.

c. Complete a *Profile Poster* similar to the one shown below to help staff and other residents learn about the unique backgrounds of residents and who they are as individuals.

Profile Poster

Name: *Mary Auchmeyer Luggi*
Recent home: *New York City*
Childhood home: *Frankfurt, Germany*
Schools attended: *New York City College*
Spouse's name: *Gus Luggi (deceased)*
Occupation: *High school home economics teacher*
Children: *Son: Gus Luggi Jr, Daughter: Emily Smythe*
Grandchildren: *Tom 21, Amelia 19, Gus 15, Ginny 14, Sammie 13*
Hobbies, interests: *Quilting, baseball, singing*
Other tidbits: *Travelled on several missionary trips to India, speaks German, Italian, and French*

Photos of resident and family can be added

---

2. *Identify residents' needs, preferences, and level of physical and mental function.*
   a. Assess how well residents can meet their activities of daily living and the assistance they need.
   b. Ask about their preferences in regard to food likes and dislikes, sleep and nap habits, bathing, and other activities.
   c. Incorporate findings into their plan of care.
3. *Explain and educate.*
   a. Orient residents and families to the layout of the facility, staff, routines, and activities.
   b. Explain procedures before doing them.
   c. Be available to discuss residents' and families' concerns and to answer questions.
4. *Promote maximum independence.*
   a. Encourage residents to do as much for themselves as possible.
   b. Explain to residents and families the value of residents being independent.

c. Give residents opportunities to make decisions regarding their care and activities.
5. *Make residents and families feel comfortable.*
   a. Be courteous and patient; understand that the stress associated with admission can cause residents and family members to make demands, complain, ask many questions, and forget what has been told to them.
   b. Provide privacy during visitation.
   c. Inform families of the location of visitor lounges, cafeteria, and vending machines.
6. *Be holistic.*
   a. Being holistic means that we are concerned with the whole person: body, mind, and spirit.
   b. Try to help residents meet physical, emotional, social, and spiritual needs to promote their physical, emotional, social, and spiritual health.

From Eliopoulos, C. (1997). Helping new residents and families. *Long-Term Care Educator, 8*(12), 6.

BOX 8-4   Holistic Nursing in Long-Term Care Facilities

Nurses can promote holistic care in long-term care facilities by:

- Assisting residents to achieve a higher potential of functioning
- Supporting residents in their efforts to promote health and prevent complications
- Learning about the unique life stories of residents
- Ensuring that residents receive care that is consistent with their values and beliefs and respecting cultural differences
- Aiding residents and families in discovering meaning in health status and in life and death
- Strengthening residents' abilities to live in harmony with their health condition

- Assisting residents in maintaining their connections with family, friends, and the community within and outside the facility
- Helping residents boost their natural healing abilities
- Facilitating hope and a sense of purpose in residents' lives
- Supporting residents as they respond to their spiritual identity or relate to a higher power
- Providing a nurturing, healing caregiving environment
- Offering opportunities for residents to experience joy and satisfaction
- Protecting residents from threats to their health or well-being, and promoting highest quality of life
- Adhering to accepted standards of nursing practice

From Eliopoulos, C. (1999). *Nursing administration of long-term care facilities* (3rd ed). Glen Arm, MD: Health Education Network.

assertiveness, coaching, counseling, accurate documentation, organization, time management, and communication.

OTHER FORMS OF LONG-TERM CARE

So far this chapter has focused on the role of nurses in the LTCF. However, the LTCF is only one part of the long-term care system, and other forms of long-term care are available. Box 8–5 presents additional resources.

1. *Subacute or transitional care.* For people who require ongoing care or recovery for an acute condition but do not need to receive the services on an acute hospital unit. The subacute care unit can be separate parts of a hospital or nursing home, or it can be an entire facility dedicated to this purpose.
2. *Assisted living facility.* A form of housing that provides 24-hour staffing, meals, supervision of medications, and personal care assistance.
3. *Adult day care.* A daytime program for people who typically have the same level of impairments as nursing home residents but who receive care in the community, usually by family members. The client is transported to the center and receives structured activities, meals, personal care assistance, and health care supervision.

4. *Home care.* For community-based people who are homebound and who need caregiving assistance or special treatments.
5. *Hospice.* For people who are terminally ill and in need of care. This care can be provided in the home or in a day hospital setting.

Each of these types of care have unique regulations and conditions for reimbursement.

CONCLUSIONS

The roles and responsibilities of nurses in LTCFs are varied and complex. Residents possess a wide range of physical and mental conditions that require expert assessment, interventions, and monitoring. The inability of many residents to accurately express their needs and age-related alterations in the presentation of clinical manifestations presents special challenges in detecting changes in status. The absence of physicians in the facility on a daily basis places a greater burden on nurses to identify and seek treatment of residents' problems. The high proportion of unlicensed staff demands that nurses be effective managers. An abundance of regulatory and reimbursement requirements demand that nurses be knowledgeable of these topics.

The reality that most residents will not only receive

BOX 8–5   Resources to Learn More About Long-Term Care

Adult Day Care

National Institute on Adult Day Care
600 Maryland Ave., S.W.
Washington, DC 20024
(202) 479-1200

Home Health and Community Services

American Public Health Association
Section on Gerontological Health
1015 18th St., N.W.
Washington, DC 20036

International Senior Citizens Association, Inc.
11753 Wilshire Blvd.
Los Angeles, CA 90025

National Association of Home Care
205 C St., N.E.
Washington, DC 20002

National Association of Home Health Agencies
426 C St., N.E., Suite 200
Washington, DC 20002

(202) 547-1717

National Home Caring Council
235 Park Ave. South
New York, NY 10003

Visiting Nurse Associations of America
3801 E. Florida Ave., Suite 900
Denver, CO 80210

(800) 426-2547

Long-Term Care Facilities

American Association of Homes for the Aging
901 E St., N.W., Suite 500
Washington, DC 20036
(202) 783-2242

American Health Care Association
1200 15th St., N.W.
Washington, DC 20005
(202) 833-2050

American Nurses Association, Inc.
Council on Nursing Home Nurses
600 Maryland, Ave., S.W., Suite 100 West
Washington, DC 20024
(800) 274-4262
www.nursingworld.org

National Association of Directors of Nursing Administration
   in Long Term Care
10999 Reed Hartman Hwy, Suite 234
Cincinnati, OH 45242
(800) 222-0539

National Citizens Coalition for Nursing Home Reform
1424 16th St., N.W.
Washington, DC 20036
(202) 332-2275

National Gerontological Nursing Association
7250 Parkway Drive, Suite 510
Hanover, MD 21076
(800) 723-0560
www.nursingcenter.com/people/nrsorgs/ngna

care, but will *live* in the facility for the remainder of their lives causes nurses often to serve as surrogate family. Very few practice settings offer nurses the opportunity to fill such a wide and varied range of roles. Rather than a simple, nonchallenging practice setting, LTCFs challenge nurses to use a wide range of knowledge and skills as they establish meaningful long-term relationships with residents and their families. To fill the roles and responsibilities competently, LTCF nurses must be among their profession's best.

BIBLIOGRAPHY

1. Eliopoulos, C. (1998). *Transforming nursing homes into healing centers: A holistic model for long-term care* (p. 48). Glen Arm, MD: Health Education Network.
2. Eliopoulos, C. (1999). *Integrating alternative and conventional therapies: Holistic care for chronic conditions.* St. Louis: Mosby.
3. Eliopoulos, C. (1999). *Nursing administration of long-term care facilities* (3rd ed.). Glen Arm, MD: Health Education Network.
4. *Federal Register.* (1989). Rules and Regulations (Vol. 54, No. 21). Section 483.26(c), February 2, 1989.
5. Institute of Medicine, Committee on Implications of For-Profit Enterprise in Health Care. (1986). Profits and health care: An introduction to the issues. In B. H. Gray (Ed.), *For-profit enterprise in health care* (pp. 3–18). Washington, DC: National Academy Press.
6. Kane, R. L., & Kane, R. A. (1997). Long-term care. In C. K. Cassel, et al. (Eds.), *Geriatric medicine* (3rd ed., pp. 81–96). New York: Springer.
7. Lawrence, C. (1905). *History of the Philadelphia almshouses and hospitals* (pp. 52, 123). Privately printed.
8. Muder, R. R., Brennen C., & Swenson, D. L. (1996). Pneumonia in the long-term care facility. *Archives of Internal Medicine, 156,* 2365–2370.
9. National Committee to Preserve Social Security and Medicare. (1997). *Nurse staffing in nursing homes: Viewpoint.* Legislative Agenda for the 105th Congress, April 1997.
10. Rice, V. H. (1997). Ethical issues relative to autonomy and personal control in independent and cognitively impaired elders. *Nursing Outlook, 45,* 27–34.
11. Rosenberg, C. E. (1987). *The care of strangers: The rise of America's hospital system.* New York: Basic Books.
12. Thomas, W. H. (1996). *Life worth living. How someone you love can still enjoy life in a nursing home.* The Eden Alternative in action. Acton, MA: VanderWyk & Burnham.
13. U.S. Department of Commerce. (1996). Table 654: Nonfarm industries: Employees and earnings. *Statistical Abstract of the United States: 1996* (116th ed., p. 421). Washington, DC: Bureau of the Census.

Health Assessment

9 Health History

10 Physical Assessment

11 Diagnostic Assessment

UNIT

3

CHAPTER 9

Health History

Annabelle M. Keene

The nursing process hinges on assessment of the client to provide baseline data. Assessment enhances identification of physical and psychosocial needs. The amount, depth, and level of assessment skills vary with the nurse's knowledge and expertise. Some assessment skills are basic, such as taking a temperature. Advanced assessment skills are learned and practiced in order to provide interventions and to evaluate health maintenance and promotion practices.

Familiarity with the parameters of human behavior and physiology is necessary in order to recognize abnormal situations. Normal ranges for psychosocial behavior may vary, whereas many physiologic manifestations have narrowly defined limits. For example, cell death occurs if body temperature is either too high or too low; the defined parameters are a matter of a few degrees. In contrast, depression in survivors following the death of a loved one is expected, but prolonged depression may signal mental illness. Skillful assessment requires careful observation along with the ability to decide whether an observation is normal. Consider the client's unique circumstances when comparing assessment findings to standardized norms.

Evaluate the client's reaction to the assessment process as well as the possible implications of the findings. Nursing diagnoses common to clients experiencing health assessment include *Anxiety, Fear, Knowledge Deficit, Pain, Powerlessness,* and *Situational Low Self Esteem.* Each nursing diagnosis is followed by a related factor identifying the specific cause leading to the problem. For example, a woman having a breast examination may be anxious because she never has had such an examination before or she may fear that a lump will be found.

Assessment requires skill and judgment. Chapters 9 and 10 provide information to begin developing expertise in health assessment. Proficiency requires extensive practice. Seek guidance from a skilled, competent practitioner. A broad knowledge base, repeated practice, and access to a mentor foster the ability to discriminate between findings.

Health assessment focuses on the client and is divided into two portions. The health history contains subjective information, whereas the physical examination is objective information about a client's health status. The client is a unique person with complex physical and psychosocial interactions. Keep the health history interview free from bias, prejudice, and stereotyping. For example, an

elderly client with several chronic health problems may or may not have immediate health care needs, yet the potential for complex health problems exists. Conversely, a young adult may appear "healthy" when in fact he or she may have overwhelming psychosocial problems or needs affecting both current and future health status. An individualized approach to health assessment provides a valid database for nursing care.

THE HEALTH HISTORY

■ ACCURACY

Assess the accuracy and completeness of the data throughout the health history interview. Validation allows formulation of accurate nursing diagnoses. Determine whether the client is a reliable historian, able and willing to provide information. The client may be (1) unconscious or disoriented and, therefore, may be unable to cooperate; (2) willing to cooperate but hindered by circumstances, such as a language barrier, or anxiety; (3) unwilling and mistrustful about cooperating because of anger or depression.

If the client cannot provide information, seek secondary sources, such as significant others or an interpreter. Information content and accuracy may be influenced by the perceptions and biases of the secondary sources as well as by their knowledge of the problem and recall ability.

Stereotyping jeopardizes collection of accurate data. False assumptions and generalizations may lead to questions that alienate the client and that interfere with development of trust. A mistrustful client is reluctant to divulge sensitive information, perhaps fearing rejection or ridicule, resulting in inaccurate or missed nursing diagnoses.

Similarities among people result in their being grouped according to age, sex, ethnic background, common occupation, recreational activity, health risk behavior, or type of health problem. Each person is also unique. Reliable research findings concerning group characteristics or similarities may be applied to a specific client who belongs to that group. For example, the incidence of hypertension is higher in blacks than in whites, and regular blood pressure screening should be included at every health care visit. Generalizations, particularly those grounded in assumptions or prejudice or based on limited experience, are potentially harmful.

Physical appearance or presenting manifestations may bias one's perception of a client. Similar manifestations may have different origins. For example, a client with an uneven, lurching gait and garbled speech may appear to be intoxicated or under influence of a controlled substance. In fact, the client might have residual neurologic deficits from a head injury. Initial inaccurate judgment may be costly in wasted time and effort and may result in a strained nurse-client relationship. Box 9–1 includes guidelines that may reduce stereotyping during health assessment.

Computerized health history assessment is available in clinical settings, particularly ambulatory care. Computer programs for history taking result in accurate, legible databases when data are entered correctly. Either the client or the nurse, using interactive programs, records the data directly. Data also may be entered from a client-completed questionnaire, which is reviewed and validated by a nurse skilled in health assessment. Computerized health histories tend to be complete because pertinent assessment areas are included in the programs. Branching programs direct collection of additional data when the client responds with significant information.

■ DEPTH

Many factors influence the level of assessment. Ideally, data are collected at one time and in sufficient depth to allow problem identification; however, this may not always be practical. The interview setting may be less than ideal (e.g., the scene of a motor vehicle accident). The client's reason for seeking health care may preclude in-depth interviewing (e.g., if the client has a ruptured appendix). The client's attention span, energy, and comfort level may affect ability to participate (e.g., if pain is present).

In an acute situation:

1. Collect data pertinent to the immediate problem, and assess the client's present health status.
2. Tailor the health history interview to include pertinent data while striving to be thorough.
3. Update and enlarge the database as indicated by the client's condition.

In clinical practice, many agencies provide specific health history formats. These formats are designed to meet agency purposes and may vary considerably in depth and level. Tailor the health history interview to the needs of the client and the agency. For example, you might arrange to meet several brief times with clients who have limited abilities or special needs (e.g., impaired

---

BOX 9–1 Guidelines That May Reduce Stereotyping During Health Assessment

- Do not manipulate a client's information to make it congruent with a cultural image.
- Do not assume that all of a client's reported symptoms stem from the identified medical diagnosis.
- Do not classify a client on the basis of appearance or behavior.
- Do not ignore any aspect of the client's presentation.

---

hearing or limited intellectual capacity), or an interpreter may be required when a language barrier exists.

Long Format

The health history model presented in this chapter is an *exhaustive,* or long format (Box 9–2). This holistic approach, although time-consuming, elicits a wealth of data and allows thorough assessment of how the client functions within multiple aspects. The exhaustive approach may be impractical in an acute care setting, especially in one sitting. However, to make accurate nursing diagnoses and to identify etiology, you must know each component of the history and should learn how to collect a complete database, over time if necessary. Students often learn history-taking skills in a laboratory setting using the exhaustive model. They must also learn to modify the technique to an actual setting and to a client's ability.

Short Format

An *episodic* health history assessment often suffices when a client presents with an uncomplicated, short-term health problem, such as an earache. Use a systematic approach to collect data significant to the problem (Box 9–3). Proficiency in all areas of health history assessment, which are discussed in this chapter, is necessary to conduct an accurate episodic assessment.

GUIDELINES FOR THE HEALTH HISTORY INTERVIEW

External (environmental and interpersonal) and *internal* (intrapersonal and physiologic) factors affect the health history interview. Data quality and quantity are enhanced by sensitivity to the client and by one's skill level with the interview process.

■ PREPARATION OF THE ENVIRONMENT

The following guidelines apply:

1. When possible, conduct the interview in a comfortable setting. A quiet room with a closed door decreases interruptions. If the client cannot leave a setting (e.g., a multibed room or an emergency department cubicle), screen the area by drawing the privacy drapes.
2. Reduce or eliminate distractions (e.g., turn off the television) and inform colleagues to avoid interruptions.
3. Use facing comfortable chairs to help establish rapport. Adjust their distance to the client's preference and sense of personal space.
4. Ensure a moderate room temperature to promote comfort.
5. Provide indirect lighting to prevent glare and strong shadows that may distort observation of nonverbal cues.

■ PREPARATION OF THE CLIENT

The following guidelines apply:

1. After introductions, explain the nature and purpose of the health history interview.

Text continued on page 135

BOX 9-2   An Exhaustive Health History Format

Interview date (included as a baseline for later reference)

Biographical and Demographic Data

Full name (include aliases, if applicable)
Age
Sex
Race
Nationality or ethnic background
Primary language
Date and place of birth
Significant others and relationship to client
Home address (and alternate contact address, if applicable)
Phone number(s)
Occupation (usual and current)
Social Security number
Religion
Emergency contact or next of kin
Legal guardian (if necessary)
Source of information and reliability as a historian (note use of an interpreter, if needed)
Source of referral to agency and/or usual primary health care provider
Health insurance information
Advance directive information

Current Health

Reason for seeking health care, or chief complaint (recorded in client's own words)
Symptom analysis (in-depth analysis of manifestations):

- Last time client was well (discriminate between onset of symptom and when client became concerned about it)
- Date and time of onset, including time period during which symptom evolved (slow? abrupt?)
- Setting (what was client doing and where was the client when symptom began?)
- How was client feeling before problem's onset?
- Duration or how long symptom lasts (minutes? hours? days? intermittent? constant? goes away completely?)
- Frequency or how often symptom occurs (daily? weekly? monthly?)
- Location (localized? diffuse? radiating?)
- Quality (description) of symptom's characteristics (burning? piercing? stabbing? dull? aching? throbbing?)
- Quantity or severity rated by client using an analog scale such as 1 to 10, with 1 being the least and 10 being the most or worst)
- Does symptom interfere with client's usual daily activities? Do interferences cause problems for the client? What types of problems? (sleeping? eating? activity tolerance?)
- Factors that seem to precipitate (bring on) the symptom
- Factors that seem to worsen (aggravate) the symptom (activity? weather? eating? medication? position? fatigue? time of year or day?)
- Factors that relieve symptom (rest? sleep? medication [name, strength, amount taken, and frequency]? heat? cold?)
- Associated factors or symptoms in other body systems that seem concurrent—review the associated body system at this time instead of later

Past Health History

Developmental (may not be appropriate for all adults)

- Any known problems with growth and development including prenatal or birth history (e.g., premature delivery or low birth weight) or delay in language, speech, motor skills, and so forth

Immunizations

- Record childhood immunizations and whether kept up to date (tetanus, diphtheria, pertussis, measles, mumps, rubella, chickenpox, polio, *Haemophilus influenzae* b conjugate, hepatitis B)
- Note last dates of tetanus booster and influenza vaccination
- Note whether client has received pneumococcal vaccination if age 65 or over or if there is a history of chronic illness

Past illnesses (childhood and adulthood)

- Ask about measles (rubeola), mumps, rubella, chickenpox (collectively called "usual childhood diseases"), whooping cough (pertussis), scarlet fever, strep throat, rheumatic fever, poliomyelitis, asthma, tuberculosis, pneumonia, and any sequelae or residual effects

Serious or chronic illnesses

- Note the presence of diabetes mellitus, heart disease, hypertension, kidney problems, ulcers, thyroid problems, migraine headaches, seizure disorders, stroke (cerebral vascular accident), arthritis, Lyme disease, cancer, anemia, sickle cell anemia, bleeding tendencies, or human immunodeficiency virus (HIV) infection

Hospitalizations

- Date and reason for each admission
- Summary of treatment, length of hospitalization
- Name of primary care physician
- Reaction to these events and their outcomes

Surgeries

- Date and type of procedures performed
- Name of surgeon
- Note whether procedure was performed on inpatient or outpatient basis
- Client's reaction to each procedure and its outcome

Serious injuries or accidents

- Date and type of injury or accident
- Ask specifically about head injuries, fractures, burns, or other trauma
- Note client's reaction to each and their outcomes

Obstetric history (if applicable)

- For completed pregnancies: number; course of each pregnancy, labor, delivery, and postpartum period; delivery date; birth weight, sex, and health of infant
- For incomplete pregnancies: number; duration of pregnancy; date and circumstances of termination (spontaneous or induced abortion, stillbirth)
- Complications (describe)

Last visit to health care provider

- Record most recent dates for dental, physical, vision, and hearing examinations. Identify provider if different from primary care provider
- Date and results of screening or diagnostic tests performed such as electrocardiogram (ECG), radiology studies, laboratory tests, Papanicolaou (Pap) smear, purified protein derivative (PPD) test, or tuberculosis tine test

Allergies

- Describe allergens and reactions (rash, urticaria, pruritus, watery or itching eyes, nasal congestion, running nose, breathing difficulty including asthma, pulse irregularity, convulsions, collapse)

Box continued on following page

BOX 9-2 An Exhaustive Health History Format *Continued*

- Include medications (true allergic reactions only and not side effects), food, contact agents (fabric, nickel), and environmental agents (dust, dander, pollens, cigarette smoke)

Medications currently taken, including prescriptive, nonprescriptive over-the-counter, and recreational (street) drug use

- Ask about common over-the-counter medications by name (such as aspirin, vitamins, herbals, antacids, birth control pills, cold and allergy preparations, topical creams and lotions—many people do not think of these as medications)
- For all medications, ask for: name; dose; route; frequency and time of day taken; reason for taking; any problems with drug regimen; who prescribed each drug and when

Family Health History

- Include ages, cause of death, and age at death of family members
- Ask specifically about heart disease, hypertension (high blood pressure), cerebrovascular accidents (stroke), epilepsy (seizures), migraines or headaches, mental illness, Alzheimer's disease, Huntington's chorea, alcoholism, tuberculosis, asthma, allergies, diabetes mellitus, thyroid problems, eating disorders (overeating, undereating, self-induced vomiting), obesity, kidney disease, arthritis, cancer (type), sickle cell anemia, anemia, hemophilia, HIV infection, developmental delay
- Data may be displayed in a diagram of the family tree (see Fig. 9-1)

Psychosocial History

Explore history of psychosocial problems

- Personal history
- Family history

Assess psychologic components

- General appearance

  Dress
  Hygiene and grooming
  Posture
  Motor activity
  Facial expression

- Behavior

  Verbal
  Nonverbal
  Reaction to interview

- Recent level of stress

  Current perceived level of stress
  Adjustment to past stressors
  Signs of response to stress
  Usual coping pattern

- Mental status and level of understanding

  Level of consciousness
  Orientation
  Mood and affect
  Speech and communication (language)
  Thought process and content
  Attention span
  Memory
  General fund of knowledge
  Calculation ability
  Ability to reason and think abstractly
  Perception
  Judgment
  Insight

- Personality style
- Motivation
- Personal strengths
- Values and beliefs

  Self-concept, self-esteem
  Body image
  Locus of control

- Spirituality
- Psychosocial risk factors (including coping ability, suicidal ideation)

Assess sociologic components

- Psychosocial level of development
- Social network and support systems (including pets)
- Socioeconomic status
- Lifestyle (including habits, recent travel within and outside of country)
- Sexuality

Assess cultural components (see Table 9-1)

Review of Systems

General

Do the following symptoms occur: fever, chills, sweats, night sweats, weakness, weight loss or gain (in past 6 months), fatigue, malaise, nausea or vomiting, headaches, mood changes?

Nutrition

Describe the kinds of food usually eaten, including likes and dislikes. Describe everything eaten during the last 24 hours. How much of each food was eaten? Is the client on a special type of diet, such as avoiding salt, sugar, fats, or caffeine? Does the client take vitamin or mineral pills, or anything else believed necessary in the diet? Does the client have an appetite? Has it changed recently (describe)? Has the client ever had an eating problem or disorder such as anorexia or bulimia nervosa (describe)? What is the client's usual weight? Does the weight vary (ask client to describe maximum and minimum weights)? Has the client gained or lost weight recently? (How much? Over how long a time period did this happen?) Who does the food shopping in the household? Who usually prepares meals? Does the client usually have someone to share meals with? Does the person who plans and prepares food use a system such as the Food Guide Pyramid? Does food have a special meaning for the client? Are there foods that the client looks forward to eating on special occasions (such as a religious holiday)? Are there any foods that cannot be eaten because of allergies or for other reasons? Are there any problems with following a special diet (describe)? Are there any problems with being able to swallow or chew food (describe)?

Integument

- Skin

Inquire about past skin problems (e.g., scars; birthmarks; moles; burns). Ask if the following problems occur: dryness; pruritus (itching); rashes or other skin eruptions; odor; a change in skin color, texture, or temperature; a change in any skin lesion; growths; easy bruising; psoriasis; eczema. Has the client had any skin lesions removed (describe)? Does the client have any tattoos or pierced body parts? Ask the client to describe skin care habits (e.g., use of soap, lotions, skin oils, etc.) that may affect skin texture and moisture. How much sun exposure has the client had (e.g., sunbathing, tanning salon, severe sunburns)?

BOX 9-2   An Exhaustive Health History Format *Continued*

- Hair

Are there any problems with alopecia (hair loss), dryness, brittleness, or dandruff? Does the client use hair dyes or have a permanent wave? Ask the client to describe hair care habits (e.g., frequency of shampooing, use of conditioner, combing versus brushing) that may affect hair texture.

- Nails

Are there any problems with brittleness, cracking, or splitting? Has there been a change in nail texture? Does the client bite his or her nails? Does the client wear nail polish? Have artificial nails?

Hematopoietic

Are there any problems with fatigue, unusual bleeding, easy bruising, ecchymoses (bruises), anemia, or leukemia? Has the client ever been exposed to radiation or toxic agents (describe)? Has the client ever had a transfusion of blood or a blood product (were there any problems?)? Does the client know his or her blood type (if a female is Rh-negative and has been pregnant, does she recall receiving Rho-GAM)? Does the client know if he or she has any unusual type of antibodies (describe)?

Endocrine

Have there been past problems with diabetes, goiter or thyroid, or growth and development? Has the client ever been treated with hormones (describe)? Has the client ever had neck surgery (describe)? Are there problems with polydipsia, polyuria, or polyphagia (increased thirst, urination, or hunger); heat or cold intolerance; weakness; tremors; nervousness; dry skin or hair; excessive sweating; change in hair distribution or hirsutism (excess hair growth in unusual places); impotence or a change in sexual activity or libido?

Head

Has the client ever had a blow, trauma, or injury to the head? Ask about problems with headaches (unusual or severe), dizziness or lightheadedness, syncope (fainting or loss of consciousness), vertigo, seizures.

Eyes

Has the client had past problems with eye infections (conjunctivitis or pink eye), chalazion (eyelid cyst), hordeolum (stye), glaucoma, cataracts, amblyopia (lazy eye), detached retina, or strabismus? Has the client ever received a blow to the eye? Has the client ever had eye surgery (describe)? Does the client wear an eye prosthesis (ask the client to describe how he or she cares for it)? Are there problems with a change in vision (either in general or in part of the visual field, or in night vision), failing vision or blindness, blurred vision, diplopia (double vision), spots or floaters, redness, pain, itching, lacrimation (excess tearing), dryness, discharge or drainage, swelling around the eyes, unusual sensations or twitching, photophobia (light sensitivity)? Is there difficulty reading or seeing distant objects? Do vision problems interfere with daily activities? Does the client wear eyeglasses or contact lenses (when was the last prescription change)? When was the last eye examination (results)? Last glaucoma check (results)?

Ears

Inquire about past problems with ear infections or earaches; diminution of or loss of hearing. Are there problems with difficulty hearing; deafness; increased sensitivity to sound; tinnitus (ringing), crackling, buzzing, or other sounds in the ears; feeling of fullness in the ear; ear pain; discharge or drainage (describe); vertigo? Does the client have problems with excess cerumen (ear wax)? Ask how the client cleans his or her ears (is a cotton-tipped swab, hairpin, or other sharp, foreign object used that may damage the ear canal or tympanic membrane?). Does the client wear a hearing aid? When was the last ear and hearing examination performed (results)?

Nose and Sinuses

Ask if there is a history of frequent colds, sinus infections, nasal stuffiness, allergies, hay fever, or nasal trauma or fracture. Are there current problems with sneezing, postnasal drip, rhinitis (runny nose), difficulty breathing through the nose, pain over the sinuses, or epistaxis (nosebleed)? Has there been a change in the sense of smell? Does the client use a nasal spray or other cold, allergy, or sinus medication (type, amount, frequency)?

Mouth and Pharynx

Does the client have a history of sore throats or oral infection such as strep throat, herpes (cold sores), or *Candida* (thrush)? Are there problems with mouth or tongue lesions (sore, abscess, ulcer); bleeding gums; increased saliva or dry mouth; mouth pain; sore throat; hoarseness or voice change; difficulty chewing or swallowing (dysphagia); change in taste; halitosis? Does the client use tobacco products (describe type, amount, frequency, and current use patterns)? Does the client have any dentures or bridges? Do they fit well? Are they worn most of the time? Ask the client to describe dental hygiene practices (brushing, flossing, use of fluoride dentifrice). Has the client ever had oral or dental surgery (describe)? When was the last dental examination and the results (if known)? Were x-ray films obtained at that time?

Neck

Have there been past problems with neck injury, goiter, pain, limited movement, or swollen glands? Does the client currently have stiffness, tenderness, pain, swelling, or lumps in the neck?

Breasts and Axillae

Ask the client about a history of fibrocystic breast disease and cancer of the breast (is there a family history of breast cancer?). If the client is a woman with children, ask if she breast-fed her infants. Are there current problems with breast pain, tenderness, or swelling; gynecomastia (enlargement); pruritus (itching); nipple discharge; breast lumps; dimpling or change in breast skin texture or color; change in appearance of the nipples? Does the client perform breast self-examination (if so, ask for a description of when it is done and the technique used)? If the client is a woman, has she had mammograms? When? Results, if known? How often done? Does the client take any estrogen (e.g., birth control) or corticosteroid medications (describe)? Is there a history of breast surgery (describe)?

Lungs

Inquire about a history of breathing problems, such as asthma, emphysema, wheezing, pleurisy, pneumonia, or bronchitis. Has the client ever had tuberculosis (describe any treatment

Box continued on following page

BOX 9-2   An Exhaustive Health History Format *Continued*

received) or whooping cough? Has the client smoked or used tobacco products (describe type, amount, length of time used, attempts to stop)? If the client is a former smoker, ask how long it has been since quitting. Current problems might include chronic cough, sputum production (describe), hemoptysis (blood in sputum), night sweats, dyspnea (shortness of breath) with or without exertion, inability to tolerate exercise or activities of daily living without becoming short of breath, orthopnea (difficulty breathing without elevating the head when supine), pain with breathing, and cyanosis (blue-tinged nail beds or lips). Has the client ever had a chest x-ray (results)? Has the client ever had a skin test for tuberculosis (results)?

Heart

Ask the client about a history of rheumatic fever, congenital heart problems, heart murmur, myocardial infarction, coronary artery disease, cardiac surgery, hypertension, or thyroid problems. Is there a family history of hypertension or myocardial infarction before age 50? Are there current problems with chest discomfort or pain, syncope, vertigo, palpitations, paroxysmal nocturnal dyspnea (sudden awakening at night with difficulty breathing), dyspnea on exertion, orthopnea, sudden weight gain, edema of hands or feet, hyperlipidemia, or hypercholesteremia? Has the client ever had any cardiac tests, such as an electrocardiogram (ECG), stress ECG, coronary angiograms, echocardiogram, or electrophysiologic studies (results)?

Peripheral Vascular

Has the client had previous problems with varicose veins, diabetes, hypertension, pain in the extremities, injury to an extremity (describe), or edema of the hands or feet? Are there problems with lymph node swelling or tenderness, claudication (pain in legs with walking relieved by resting), numbness or coldness of an extremity, discoloration or ulceration on extremities (especially feet and ankles), hair loss over an extremity; nail changes? Has the client ever had any vascular tests, such as Doppler studies (results)? Ask what type of hose the client wears (e.g., support hose). Does the client use garters or other means of securing the hose? Does the client spend prolonged periods of time standing?

Gastrointestinal

Inquire about a history of ulcers, indigestion, heartburn, hernia, liver disease, hepatitis (type if known), gallbladder disease, pancreatic disease, appendicitis, and use of alcohol. Is there a family history of alcohol abuse or cancer of the stomach, liver, pancreas, intestines, or colorectal area? Ask the client to describe the usual bowel pattern and characteristics. Are there problems with weight loss or gain, a change in appetite or taste, food intolerance, belching, nausea or vomiting, hematemesis (blood in emesis), pain or indigestion with eating, difficulty swallowing, diarrhea or constipation, bowel incontinence, flatulence (excess gas), changes in bowel habits or stool characteristics (e.g., clay-colored or blood in stool, ribbon-like stools), hemorrhoids (is there any pain or bleeding especially with defecation), rectal pain or itching, pain in the abdomen, ascites (swelling of the abdomen) or jaundice? Does the client use digestive aids, laxatives, enemas, or suppositories (describe)? Has the client had tests of the gastrointestinal (GI) system, such as a barium swallow, upper GI series, barium enema, sigmoidoscopy or colonoscopy, Hemoccult test, gallbladder x-rays or ultrasound, or liver scan (results)?

Urinary

Does the client have a history of bladder infection, kidney problems, urinary tract stones, or sexually transmitted disease (STD)? Is there a family history of renal disease? Are there current problems with a change in the urinary patterns, hesitancy, frequency, dysuria (pain), pyuria (pus in the urine), urgency, weak stream, dribbling or incontinence, stress incontinence, nocturia, polyuria or oliguria (increased or decreased amount of urine), flank or low back pain, a change in the color of the urine, foam in the urine (proteinuria), or discharge from the urethra. Has the client ever had tests of the urinary system such as urinalysis, cystoscopy, or intravenous pyelogram (results)?

Genitoreproductive

■ General

Is there a history of genital lesions, sores, or ulcers; urethral discharge; odor; pain, burning, or pruritus; STDs (identify); infertility; problems with sexual performance? Has the client ever had surgery involving the genitoreproductive system (describe)? Does the client use a contraceptive (type)? Is the client satisfied with the type used or is a change desired? Is the client knowledgeable about STD preventive practices or is information wanted?

■ Female

Ask about a history of pelvic inflammatory disease, endometriosis, or abnormal Pap test results. Is there a personal or family history of reproductive cancer (e.g., cervix, uterus, ovary, breast)? Review the menstrual cycle history for age at menarche and menopause (if applicable), duration and amount of menstrual flow, and last menstrual period. Are there problems with premenstrual bloating, weight gain, fatigue, or mood changes; irregular menstrual periods; menorrhagia (excessive menses); dysmenorrhea (painful menses); amenorrhea (absence of menses); metrorrhagia (bleeding other than with menses); dyspareunia (painful intercourse); postcoital pain or bleeding? Ask when the woman's last pelvic examination and Pap test were done (results).

■ Male

Inquire about a history of inguinal hernia, prostate problems, or impotence. Is there a family history of reproductive cancer (e.g., penis, testis, prostate)? Does the man have current problems with testicular pain or mass, or blood in the ejaculate? Ask when the man's last examination was, including checking the prostate and for hernia (results). Does the man know how to perform testicular self-examination (How often?) Has the man had a prostate-specific antigen (PSA) test (results)?

Musculoskeletal

Ask about past problems with sprains, strains, fractures, dislocations, arthritis, gout, backache, bursitis, osteomyelitis, scoliosis, or flat feet. Is there a family history of arthritis, gout, or muscular dystrophy? Are there current problems with muscle twitches, cramps, spasms, involuntary movements, pain, or weakness; muscle atrophy; joint pain, stiffness, swelling, redness, deformity, or limited movement; crepitation (noise or grating with joint movement); backache; spinal deformity; limitation in walking, gait, running, sports activities, or activities of daily living? Has the client ever had tests involving the musculoskeletal system such as skeletal x-rays or electromyography (results)?

BOX 9–2   An Exhaustive Health History Format *Continued*

Neurologic

Is there a history of loss of consciousness, fainting, seizures, paralysis, paresthesia (numbness or tingling), trauma to the nervous system, cerebrovascular accident (CVA)? Is there a family history of CVA, seizures, or neurologic disease such as Huntington's chorea? Are there current problems with vertigo, syncope, paresthesia, paralysis, headache, loss of balance, seizures, uncoordinated or involuntary movements (e.g., tics, tremors, spasms, clumsiness), speech problems, memory problems (short or long term)? Are there interferences with the activities of daily living from neurologic problems (describe)? Has the client ever had neurologic tests, such as electroencephalography, lumbar puncture, or computed tomography of the head (results)?

Psychiatric

Ask about a history of depression, bipolar disease, schizophrenia, obsessive-compulsive tendency (does it interfere with the client's activities of daily living?); sleeping problems; eating disorders (e.g., anorexia or bulimia nervosa); memory problems; or anxiety attacks. Is there a family history of mental health problems, such as depression, bipolar disease, or schizophrenia? Has the client ever been treated for mental or emotional health problems or taken psychotropic substances (describe)? Is there a history of suicide attempts? Does the client currently have problems with mood swings; sleeping problems, such as insomnia; anxiety, especially that interferes with activities of daily living; nervousness; increased or decreased appetite; memory lapses; inability to concentrate; change in energy level or inability to complete tasks; phobias; delusions; hallucinations? Has there been a change in relationships with significant others recently (describe)? Has there been a change in living arrangements or housing recently (describe)? Has there been a change in jobs recently (describe)?

---

2. Speak in a moderate tone of voice, calmly and patiently.
3. Ask nonprobing, client-centered questions, which help put the client at ease. As the interview progresses, focused questions and therapeutic communication techniques help identify problem areas.
4. Alternate between open-ended and closed questions, depending on the data being elicited.
5. Throughout the interview, observe nonverbal communication for signs of discomfort with topics under discussion. These areas may need gentle, further exploration (with client permission), either during the interview or at a later time.
6. Respect the client's wish to decline discussing a topic.
7. Be aware of your interview style and skills. Nonverbal behavior can either facilitate or inhibit client responses and affect the quality of the historical data.

■ PREPARATION OF THE INTERVIEWER

The following guidelines apply:

1. Reduce repetitive questioning, and proceed in a structured yet flexible manner. Until you are comfortable with the format, use a pocket-sized outline of the health history as an aid.
2. Take *brief* notes, and inform the client in advance that you will be taking notes so as not to disrupt the flow of the interview. Avoid extensive note taking, because it suggests that you are not listening attentively.
3. Compile the written history after the interview.
4. Terminate the interview by summarizing highlights and allowing the client to add or clarify information.
5. Inform the client about how the physical examination will proceed.

COMPONENTS OF THE HEALTH HISTORY

The health history includes subjective data regarding:

- Biographical and demographic information
- The health history including review of systems (ROS)
- Family health history
- Psychosocial assessment
- Appraisal of the client's health maintenance and health promotion behaviors to assess health risks

Health history assessment may be organized according to a nursing theory (e.g., Orem's theory of self-care) or by health behavior patterns (e.g., Gordon's functional health patterns). A *format* is a tool for collecting comprehensive data. In this chapter, the health history format is an extended health database model (see Box 9–2). A health history format that integrates the assessment of functional health patterns is found in Appendix B.

If data are available in other forms, compile them, thereby enhancing and expediting the interview. A single complete database is preferable for reference and retrieval of information.

■ BIOGRAPHICAL AND DEMOGRAPHIC INFORMATION

The extent and type of biographical and demographic information vary, depending on agency protocol (see Box 9–2). The date of the interview is important because the information gathered constitutes the baseline assessment. Should the client's health status change, the health history and physical examination will reflect the extent of the change over time.

BOX 9–3   An Episodic Health History Format

Include these elements in an episodic (short) health history:

■ Client's statement of the problem (i.e., chief complaint)
■ Symptom analysis
■ Review of the body system to which the symptom belongs
■ Exploration of the symptom's relationship to other body systems (including a review of the associated body systems)
■ Investigation of the current problem's relationship to the client's past health and health maintenance and promotion practices

ALTERNATIVE THERAPY

Alternative and Complementary Modalities Used by Clients

A landmark study by Eisenberg and coworkers[1] found that an estimated 60 million Americans were using some form of alternative or complementary therapy. This therapy ranged from the taking of vitamins and herbs to visits to massage therapists and acupuncturists along with a number of other modalities. Visits to alternative practitioners were estimated to exceed those to primary care physicians, with more than $13 billion spent annually on alternative care and products, and perhaps most important for physicians and nurses, more than 70% of clients using alternative therapies did not inform their medical caregivers of such use.

In a follow-up study, Eisenberg and coworkers[3] reported an increase in use of at least one of 16 identified therapies in from 33.8% to 42.1% of the respondents. Again, of particular concern, the follow-up study found that nearly 20% of clients taking prescription medications were concurrent users of herbs or high-dose vitamins.

It is being increasingly recognized that this information, or the lack thereof, about clients' use of alternative methods is of great importance to health care providers. There is much of promise in many alternative therapies, and the power of many of them, especially those involving the ingestion of herbs, vitamins, and other substances, is such that they can cause problems when combined with medications. Sometimes this is true of substances that are quite commonplace and thought to be innocuous because of their common usage. For example, several herbs may interfere with warfarin anticoagulant treatment, including celery, chamomile, fenugreek, garlic, ginger, and some Chinese medicinal herbs.[4]

The chief author of the studies cited, David Eisenberg, M.D., strongly believes in the need to explore with clients their use of alternative therapies. "Undoubtedly, talking with patients about alternative therapies requires additional skills and time. Yet, is this responsibility significantly different from exploring patients' use of alcohol or drugs, exposure to abuse, or preferences for cardiopulmonary resuscitation?"[2]

The key to this process is to be nonjudgmental about what the client is using. People use alternative and complementary therapies in an effort to become healthier, and this attempt deserves respect. Many clients believe that what they are doing is helping to achieve their goals of better health. Our task is to increase both their and our understanding of what clients are using and whether there is any potential danger in such use, either intrinsically or in combination with medical treatment. If a client is taking herbs that might have an anticoagulant effect, for example, this might be a problem if surgery is scheduled.

If clients perceive disdain or ridicule from physicians and nurses about their use of these modalities, they will continue to keep knowledge of such use from their caregivers. Many practitioners of both mainstream and alternative medicine are looking toward an "integrated" approach to medicine and health care, including the proper use and appropriate combination of all therapies relevant to a client's individual needs. A forthright and open-minded approach is the best way to communicate with clients about their use of alternative and complementary methods.

As Eisenberg has written: "We as a profession must address the challenge of discussing alternative therapies with our patients and put an end to the 'don't ask, don't tell' approach that characterizes communication in this area." Such a discussion can be a fruitful learning experience for all involved.

References

1. Eisenberg, D. M., et al. (1993). Unconventional medicine in the United States: Prevalence, costs, and patterns of use. *New England Journal of Medicine, 328*:246–252.
2. Eisenberg, D. M. (1997). Advising patients who seek alternative medical therapies. *Annals of Internal Medicine, 127*:61–69.
3. Eisenberg, D. M., et al. (1998). Trends in alternative medicine use in the United States, 1990–1997: Results of a follow-up national survey. *JAMA, 280*:1569–1575.
4. Miller, L. G. (1998). Herbal medicinals, selected clinical considerations focusing on known or potential drug-herb interactions. *Archives of Internal Medicine, 158*:2200–2211.

James Higgy Lerner, RN, LAc, *Private practice of acupuncture, traditional Oriental medicine, and biofeedback*

Biographical and demographic data provide clues about personal health risk. For example, some health risk may be ascribed to age, sex, family history, and location of residence. Various health screening procedures or recommendations are made based on age, sex, or other background data. Examples of recommended procedures include periodic pelvic examinations and monthly breast self-examinations for women, periodic prostate examinations and monthly testicular self-examinations for men, and regular screening of visual acuity and testing for glaucoma as a person ages.

■ CURRENT HEALTH

Current health status describes the reason for the health care visit.

Chief Complaint

Begin with the client's subjective statement of the reason for seeking health care (the *chief complaint*). The response may indicate concerns or anxiety on the part of the client or significant others and reveals the client's perception of the health problem. The client may talk about what the problem means and how he or she is coping. Allowing the client to elaborate can assist in avoiding generalizations. When the client reports a past or current health problem, proceed with a *symptom analysis* (see Box 9–2).

Symptom Analysis

Symptom analysis is a detailed description of the health problem. In this book, the term "manifestations" is used synonymously with "symptoms." In addition to assessing the following characteristics, ask the client to provide an opinion about the cause of the symptom or problem. Clients often have insight as to the nature and the cause of their problems and sometimes express fears and concerns while discussing them. Explore fears and concerns to identify and treat client responses to health problems.

TIMING

Timing includes onset, duration, and frequency. *Onset* refers to when a symptom was first noticed (e.g., hours, days, months). *Duration* is how long the symptom lasts (e.g., minutes, hours, days, weeks). The symptom may occur continuously, intermittently, regularly, or irregularly. *Frequency* is how often a symptom occurs (e.g., daily, weekly, monthly).

QUALITY

Ask the client to discriminate symptom quality with adjectives such as sharp, stabbing, dull, aching, cramping, cold, searing, burning, numb, tingling, loose, solid, soft, hard, tight, or crushing.

QUANTITY

Assist the client in describing the size, amount, number, or extent of symptoms as well as the severity or intensity. Quantify pain severity by asking the client to rate it on a scale (e.g., 1 to 10). Assess the symptom's effect by asking how usual daily activities have been affected, for example, "Describe how the pain has interfered with what you usually do. Does it keep you awake at night? Has it affected your appetite?"

LOCATION

Ask where a symptom, such as pain, is located on the body and whether it moves or is stationary, for example, "Does the pain stay in one place, or does it move around?" Asking the client to point helps define the location.

PRECIPITATING FACTORS

Ask what the client was doing at the time the symptom was first noticed. Does the client know what may have led to the symptom's occurrence?

AGGRAVATING AND RELIEVING FACTORS

Ask the client to recall whether any factors alleviate the symptom or make it worse, for example, "Is there anything that makes the symptom go away or become less uncomfortable?" "Is there anything that makes the symptom become worse?"

ASSOCIATED MANIFESTATIONS

Inquire whether the client has noticed anything in conjunction with the symptom. For example, "Does the symptom ever occur at other times or only when _____?"

When a symptom is reported, assess all associated physiologic areas; for example, for reported epigastric pain, review gastrointestinal, endocrine, and psychological systems. The epigastric pain may be related to problems in any of these body systems. If the reported symptom is urinary incontinence, include the following:

1. Timing
2. Quality (e.g., are incontinent episodes accompanied by dysuria?)
3. Quantity (e.g., amount of urine leakage per occurrence, effect of episodes on daily activities)
4. Precipitating factors (e.g., obesity, pregnancy, vaginal delivery)
5. Aggravating factors (e.g., coughing, sneezing, straining, lifting, caffeine intake)
6. Relieving factors (e.g., frequent toileting, medication, pelvic muscle toning exercises)
7. Associated manifestations (e.g., urgency, urinary retention, constipation).

Location does not apply in this example.

The review of body systems (described later in this chapter) should include the urinary (renal), reproductive, and gastrointestinal systems as well as a careful diet history.

■ PAST HEALTH HISTORY

The past health history may be important for determining both current and future health risk status. For example, the client who has not had chickenpox may be at risk when a community outbreak occurs or when exposed to herpes zoster (shingles). Further assess risk status, and provide information about the varicella vaccination. Box 9–2 lists the data to assess for the past health history. Throughout this part of the health history interview, note areas to explore, such as use of alternative or complementary therapies (see Alternative Therapies feature).

■ FAMILY HEALTH HISTORY

The family health history helps to identify family-linked (familial) diseases that affect health status and risk for potential health problems. The nurse should:

1. Inquire about relationships of family members to the client, their ages (if living), the age at which they died, the cause of death (if known), and the presence of significant illness or health problems.
2. Diagram the data (Fig. 9–1) as a visual display to help track the client's health risk status.
3. Include a statement summarizing health problems in the family.

Box 9–2 lists important health problems in the family health history.

■ PSYCHOSOCIAL HISTORY

Psychosocial assessment is an important part of the health history. A complete psychosocial assessment, although lengthy, is essential to a client-centered approach. Integrate psychosocial assessment throughout the history interview. If in-depth assessment is indicated, do this after the physical health history assessment, once you have established rapport. Psychosocial assessment also may come earlier (see Box 9–2), after the family health history.

Psychological status affects multiple areas of human development and behavior, such as intellectual development and capability, motivation, perception and insight, decision-making, speech and communication, motor ability, sleep and rest patterns, and nutrition and elimination patterns. It is impossible to separate a human being into discrete components. Multiple dimensions (psychological, sociologic, physiologic) interact and affect each person's behavior and responses to the environment. Interrelationships among the dimensions are neither static nor always predictable. Physiologic responses to health problems are more predictable and objectively observed, whereas two people who are faced with identical problems may not react the same way emotionally. For this reason, psychosocial assessment may be less reliable than objective assessment of physical findings. However, one may be able to develop skill and expertise in psychosocial assessment by collecting both subjective and objective data.

Psychosocial assessment assists the nurse in understanding a client's response to circumstances and events, which in turn influences the client's ability to function.

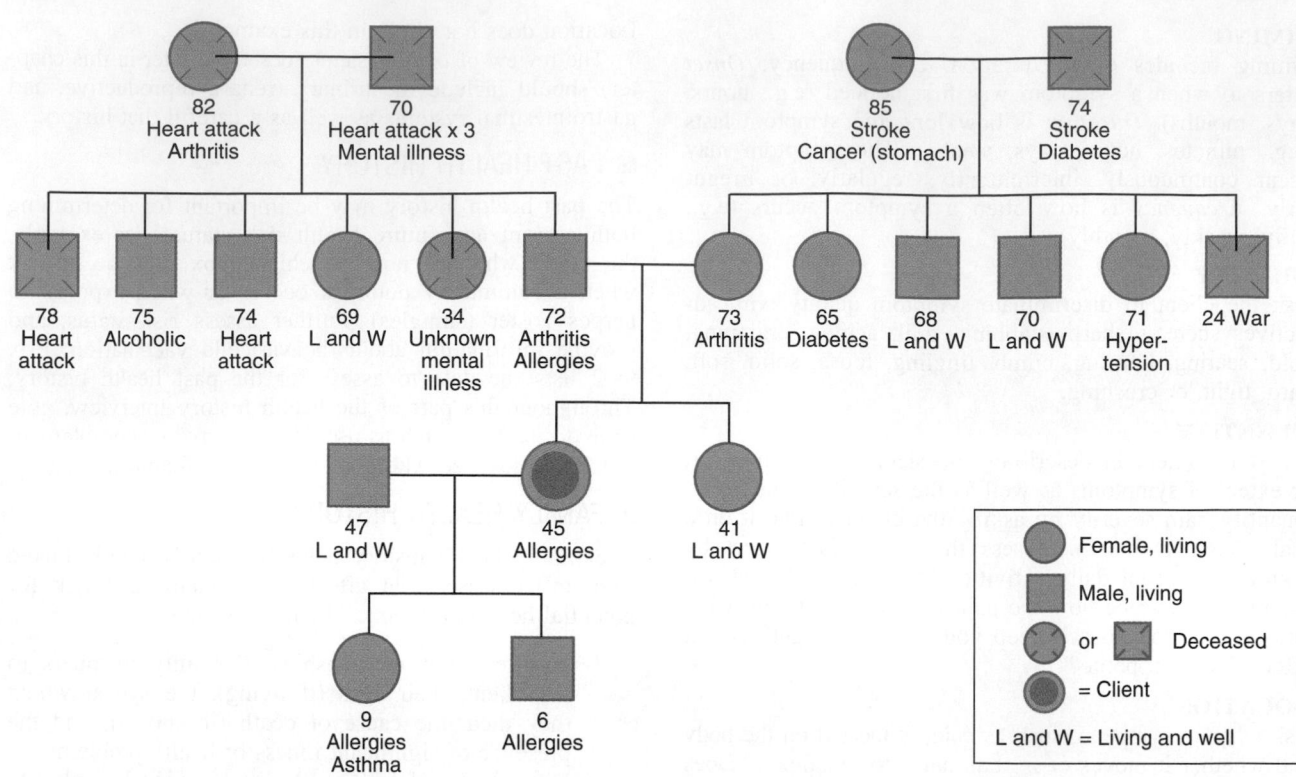

FIGURE 9-1 Family history diagram. A diagram such as this one assists in determining a client's risk for various disorders. In this case, the diagram indicates a woman with an increased inherited risk of cardiovascular disease (heart attack and stroke) and arthritis.

This understanding enables comprehensive care based on accurate nursing diagnoses. Approximately two thirds of the disorders that nurses independently identify and treat are psychosocial. Accurate assessment of responses to health problems enables the client to return to optimal levels of both physiologic and psychological functioning.

Performing the psychosocial assessment requires sensitivity and interpersonal skills. Ability to establish a therapeutic relationship directly affects the quality of the data. Because many topics are highly personal, it is imperative to be tactful and nonjudgmental and to handle confidential information professionally. An atmosphere of trust encourages the client to divulge sensitive information. Convey interest by listening attentively, making eye contact, and using skillful interview techniques. Your personal value system may influence or bias perception of a client's behavior and experiences. Self-awareness helps one to remain nonjudgmental. Free from bias, a trusting relationship promotes sharing of relevant information. Making accurate observations and sharing them allow the client opportunity to validate the nurse's perceptions and inferences.

Nature of the Psychosocial Assessment

Psychosocial assessment encompasses gathering information about *psychological patterns* (nonphysical components, such as thoughts, feelings, motivations, mental status, personal strengths, and weaknesses) and *social experiences* (parts of life that are affected by or dependent on others). The term *psychosocial* denotes the melding of the two dimensions; it is impossible to separate the effects of psychological factors from those of social factors. Similarly, the psychosocial dimension intertwines with the physiologic dimension. All dimensions interact to produce a unique individual.

Psychosocial Risk Factors

During the health history interview, assess for factors indicating risk for or an actual psychosocial problem. Box 9-4 lists guidelines for identifying psychosocial risk factors. If risk factors are present, proceed with a detailed assessment. Table 9-1 is an interview guide for in-depth assessment of selected areas of psychosocial status, including questions that may be asked during a cultural assessment.

Psychological Assessment

The psychological dimension includes perceptions about mood, thoughts, feelings, motivations, stressors, personal strengths and weaknesses, values and beliefs, and spirituality. Responses and interpretations are reflected in thought processes and in what is said and done. Observe the client's appearance and behavior throughout the interview. Observations, when validated, assist in understanding psychological status. Subjective data are recorded in the health history, and objective data are recorded in the physical examination report.

GENERAL APPEARANCE

Appearance and behavior reflect the client's mental status and comfort level with the interview. Observe the client's

BOX 9-4   Guidelines for Identifying Psychosocial Risk Factors

Social History

Social history includes information about the client's family members, social network, and lifestyle. Ask if others are available to provide emotional support to the client during stressful times. This support system may include pets.

Personal and Family History

A personal or family history of psychosocial problems increases a client's risk of having problems. A client may fear recurrence of an emotional or mental health problem or worry that he or she has inherited a family-linked illness, such as schizophrenia.

Level of Stress

Change and loss are two major influences that produce stress in individuals. Clients who have experienced stressful events within the past year are at risk for development of health problems. Assess the client's present stress level compared to the response to previous stressful events.

Usual Coping Pattern

The usual coping pattern refers to how the client copes with a serious problem or manages high levels of stress. Ask the client to describe a particularly stressful situation and how it was managed. Assess whether the client's usual coping style is adequate and appropriate for the current situation. Other coping strategies may be necessary. Psychosocial reactions to health problems are highly individual and usually occur as the client and significant others cope with the effects of illness.

Changes in Neurophysiologic Function

Neurophysiologic changes include physical manifestations of psychological stress. The stress response, regardless of its cause, results in altered levels of neurotransmitters, such as norepinephrine and serotonin, which then affect the sympathetic and parasympathetic nervous systems. The client's usual body functions, such as sleep and rest patterns, appetite, energy level, sexual function, and elimination patterns, can be affected.

Level of Understanding about Health Problem

Explore the client's level of understanding. The client may not comprehend what has happened or could happen as a result of a health problem. The client may have unrealistic expectations of the health care team. Determine how threatening a particular health problem is and whether the client has been able to prepare psychologically for its effects.

Mental Status

Mental status refers to the client's current emotional, intellectual, and perceptual functioning. If a dysfunction is evidenced, describe the problem.

Personality Style

Personality style is the way a client usually interacts with others. Examples include dependent, independent, controlled, relaxed, dramatic, suspicious, accepting, self-sacrificing, superior, inferior, uninvolved, involved, mixed (a combination of two predominant styles), or no predominant style.

Major Psychosocial Reactions

Reactions include disruption in the ability to trust, maintain self-esteem, retain feelings of control, cope with loss and guilt, and maintain intimacy.

---

posture, nonverbal behavior, facial expression, manner of dress with regard to the climate and occasion, grooming and hygiene, and attitude toward the assessment interview (e.g., cooperative, hostile, withdrawn). For example, "The client is dressed neatly, sits back in the chair, and answers questions without hesitation."

MOTOR ACTIVITY

Note motor ability, gait, coordination, reaction time, and unusual body movements (e.g., gestures, tics, tremors, foot tapping, hand wringing, grimacing, or other repetitive movements). For example, "The client drummed his fingers on the table before answering."

BEHAVIOR

Activities observed by others constitute behavior. *Verbal* behavior is what is said and includes voice tone; *nonverbal* behavior is everything done that may be observed, such as posture, movement, and facial expression. Observe and record both verbal and nonverbal behaviors.

Behavior is central to psychological assessment. Accurate assessment dictates that observed behavior be *described* rather than *interpreted*. "The client is crying" is an observed behavior, whereas "The client is depressed" is a judgmental statement. Without further assessment, the nurse does not know why the client is crying. If the client states, "I feel depressed," the recorded statement reads, "States she feels depressed."

MENTAL STATUS

Mental status assessment consists of evaluating behavior (verbal and nonverbal) and asking a series of questions. The purpose is to discover problems that may require further assessment and intervention. The level and depth of questioning vary, depending on individual circumstances. Assess a client who is alert and cooperative by listening and observing carefully during the interview. The client's responses provide information about orientation, mood, memory, attention span, general knowledge, language abilities, thought processes, judgment, and insight.

If a client demonstrates impaired cognitive function, perform a Mini-Mental State Examination (see Chapter 67). Disturbances in mood or thought processes (such as suicidality) warrant a complete, detailed mental status examination. Even though mental status data are collected during the health history, record this information with the physical examination data. The following areas are included.

LEVEL OF CONSCIOUSNESS. Level of consciousness (LOC) is the state of awareness. The client must be alert, not just awake, for a mental status assessment (see Chapter 67). The nurse should cue the client that the questions may seem "silly" but are to be answered anyway.

TABLE 9-1	INTERVIEW GUIDE FOR ASSESSMENT OF SELECTED AREAS OF A CLIENT'S PSYCHOSOCIAL STATUS

Assessment Area	Key Questions or Issues to Include*
Values and beliefs	What things in your life are important to you and help you want to live each day (e.g., health; respect for others; happiness; loving relationships with significant others; time to spend with your loved ones; friendships; religious beliefs; financial security; having a job or work to do)?
	How important is your health to you? to your family or significant others? (Ask person to rate importance on a scale of 1 to 10, with 10 being of most importance and 1 being of least.)
	What do you hope to accomplish in your lifetime (e.g., rear children successfully; become rich or famous; have a satisfying job or career)?
	Have you accomplished what you set out to do in your life? Are you satisfied/dissatisfied?
	If you were to come into a lot of money (win a lottery, receive an inheritance), what would you do with it?
	Do specific factors influence you when you have to make important decisions (e.g., being fair/ honest; getting a fair deal; examining all sides of the issue)?
	Have any of your beliefs or values been challenged recently? Are you uncomfortable that this has happened?
	Have you changed any of your values or beliefs recently? Has this change put a strain on your relationship with significant others? Are you comfortable with the change?
Self-concept, self-esteem, body image	Describe yourself as you believe others see you and as you see yourself (e.g., emotional health; usual mood and what affects it; ability to cope with daily stressors; physical appearance; stamina; intelligence).
	Describe your major strengths and areas that you would like to improve.
	What do you like about yourself? What do you wish you could change about yourself?
	Has anything happened recently to change your feelings about yourself (e.g., change in health status or physical agility; a loss of some kind; a role change)? Do you feel more positive or negative about yourself because of this change?
	Describe how you feel when you become ill or in some way incapacitated and are unable to carry on your daily activities.
Locus of control	Do you feel that you can control or manage factors that affect your state of health or illness (e.g., whether or not you smoke or exercise; what you do/do not eat; getting regular checkups)?
	Do you feel that you can control or manage factors that affect your life (e.g., your job; where you live; who your friends are)?
	Is there anything or anybody that you believe is responsible for what happens to you in your life (e.g., a supreme being; fate; luck; people who are more powerful than you)?
Spirituality	Do you have a preferred religion or religious beliefs?
	Is your religion an important influence in your life? Does it give you guidance in your daily life?
	Are there other things besides religion that are important to you as you go about your daily life?
	How often do you attend worship services? Does it bother you if you are ill or unable to attend worship services? What do you do if you cannot attend services?
	Is there someone you consider to be your spiritual advisor? Do you need to talk to this person regularly?
	Is there anything special that you do when you feel a need for spiritual support? Do you need help to practice your beliefs at this time?
	Do you have any religious or spiritual beliefs about health and illness (e.g., illness as a punishment; certain foods to eat or avoid, or practices that should be done or avoided) that the health care team should be aware of?
	Can the health care team be of spiritual help to you?
Social network and support system	Describe your family: Who are its members and what are their relationships to you?
	What roles do you and your family members have (e.g., parent, child, spouse, sibling, other relative, teacher, provider, role model, best friend, authority figure, peacemaker)?
	Who in your family do you feel closest to?
	Are there other people not related to you whom you consider important (i.e., significant others)?
	Do you and your family members (or significant others) get along with one another?
	Are there any problems within your family or with significant others that have strained your relationships with one another (e.g., change in living space; marital problems; arguments)?
	Are friendships important to you?
	Are you satisfied with the friendships that you have now?
	Whom would you identify as your best friend?
	Are your friends accepted by your family and significant others?
	Describe your relationships with your friends and coworkers.
	What types of groups, clubs, or organizations do you belong to?
	If you had a problem or were in a crisis, whom would you turn to for help? Is this person available?
	Is there someone at work whom you confide in?
	Are there other things that help you when you need support during stressful times (e.g., a pet or inanimate object)?

TABLE 9-1	INTERVIEW GUIDE FOR ASSESSMENT OF SELECTED AREAS OF A CLIENT'S PSYCHOSOCIAL STATUS *Continued*

Assessment Area	Key Questions or Issues to Include*
	Do you have a pet or animals that are important to you? Is there someone who will take care of them for you if you are unable to do so?
Sexuality	Are you satisfied with being a man (or a woman)? Have you ever wished you were of the opposite sex?
	Are you satisfied in your sexual relationships with your spouse, significant other, or other sexual partners (e.g., frequency and quality of interactions)? Has there been a change in your sexual function? If so, describe what is different and how long it has been this way. Is this change for the better or worse?
	Have you experienced any problems with sexual activity (e.g., impotence, pain, premature ejaculation, bleeding, lack of privacy, infertility, other)? Do you feel that this may be related to a health problem or some other cause? If so, have these problems affected your relationship with your sexual partner?
	How long have you been sexually active?
	How long have you been in your current relationship?
	Can you recall whether you used protection against venereal diseases with past sexual partners?
	Do you use contraceptives? If not, are you interested in information about this? Do you have any questions about the method you are using now?
	Do you use any type of protection against venereal diseases (e.g., condoms)? Have you ever been treated for a venereal disease?
	Do you have reason to believe that you have been exposed to a venereal disease such as syphilis, gonorrhea, or human immunodeficiency virus?
Cultural components	***Identification with a cultural group***
	How do you identify yourself to others when you are asked to what nationality or what ethnic group you belong?
	Describe how strongly you feel about your ethnic roots. Do you see yourself as a member of your ethnic group first, or do you think of yourself as a/an _____ (American, Canadian, or other) first?
	How do you identify yourself when you are asked about your racial background (e.g., black, white, Native American, Hispanic, Asian)?
	Where were you born? Where were your parents born?
	What countries (or regions of this country) have you lived in and when?
	Communication
	What language do you speak at home? Do you speak or read other languages? Do you prefer to speak in a language other than English? Is there someone (e.g., friend, relative) whom you want to act as an interpreter for you? Do you want a professional interpreter? Is there anyone (e.g., someone of the opposite sex; a person who is older/younger than you; a person you see as a rival or enemy) who should not act as an interpreter?
	Whom do you prefer to take care of you when you need health care (e.g., a person of the same cultural background/same sex/same age as you)?
	Values, beliefs, and attitudes
	Can you identify any special beliefs or practices of yours that are influenced by your ethnic or cultural background? For example, are there things that you or your significant others do when a baby is born? When someone dies? When you or your family members are ill?
	Is there anything special that you or your family do to stay healthy (e.g., eat or avoid certain foods; use herbs; call in someone who has special powers or gifts to help you stay well or get well)?
	Is leisure time important to you? Do you take time to relax and have fun? Describe what you do when you want to relax.
	Cultural sanctions and restrictions
	Is there anything the health care team should know about when taking care of you? For example, do you need to keep parts of your body covered to prevent others from seeing them?
	Are there certain types of procedures that are forbidden for you to have done (e.g., hysterectomy, vasectomy)?
	If you were to have a serious operation in which part of your body had to be removed (amputation) or cut out (excision), how should this body part be handled (e.g., preserved, buried, cremated, no special treatment)?
	Are there any topics or subjects that you do not wish to talk about because it is not allowed by your beliefs (e.g., discussing people who have died)?

Table continued on following page

TABLE 9-1	INTERVIEW GUIDE FOR ASSESSMENT OF SELECTED AREAS OF A CLIENT'S PSYCHOSOCIAL STATUS *Continued*
Assessment Area	**Key Questions or Issues to Include***

Health-related beliefs and practices

Is there anything in your beliefs that you feel helps you to be (or to stay) healthy? For example, do you believe certain foods, herbs, or beverages (potions) are good for you?

Is there anything special that you do or wear to help you stay healthy or bring you luck (e.g., an amulet; prayers to ancestors; praying to a saint, supreme being, or other being; certain rituals)?

Is there anything that you believe is not good for your health or that causes illness or sickness (e.g., illness is a punishment for doing something "wrong"; you are under a spell or curse; your body is not in harmony or balance with nature; there is an imbalance between good/bad [positive/negative] forces within your body such as *Yin/Yang* or hot/cold)?

Is there anything in your religious beliefs that influences what you believe about health and illness? Describe.

Do you believe in or use other types of people to help you get better or heal when you are sick (e.g., curandero; shaman; minister, priest, or other spiritual adviser)? How do you know when to contact this person?

Are there any types of healing practices or beliefs that you have or feel you need (e.g., use of herbal remedies or potions; massage or other type of special touch; wearing a special charm or talisman to ward off evil spirits; special prayers or incantations; specific healing practices or ceremonies)?

When you are ill or sick, does your family and significant others expect you to act in a certain way (e.g., to play a particular "sick role")?

Who decides when you are sick or when you are no longer sick?

Who usually helps take care of you when you are sick?

Nutritional beliefs and practices

Do you have any special beliefs that certain foods are better for you and help keep you healthy? Are there specific foods that you believe should be eaten if you have a certain kind of illness?

Identify foods that you believe are healthy for you to eat and foods that you believe you should avoid because they are unhealthy.

Describe how food is prepared in your home (e.g., frying; steaming; use of cooking oils [type]; how long foods are cooked; what types of seasonings are used or avoided; what foods may/may not be served together at the same meal; use of special cookware or dishes to serve food).

Do you have certain religious beliefs that control the type of foods you eat/should not eat (e.g., kosher diet) or how food is prepared? (Also see previous question.)

Do you fast or abstain from specific foods at certain times during the week or year because of religious beliefs?

If you believe in "fasting" for religious reasons, describe what this means to you. Do you avoid certain foods or beverages? Do you eat only at specified times during the day?

Are you ever allowed to break your religious rules of diet or fasting if you are ill? Who makes this decision and who would tell you that it is acceptable to break a dietary rule?

Socioeconomic issues

Is there anyone in your circle of family, friends, significant others, or spiritual advisers (i.e., social network) who you feel influences your health or illness status?

Are there special things that the members of your social network and support system do to help you when you are sick or to help you get better? Describe how these people would help take care of you if you were ill (e.g., stay by your side continuously; do things for you or your family; help your family).

Describe the roles that your family members play when one of the members is ill.

Do you expect your family members to help take care of you when you are sick? Describe what types of activities they might do (e.g., give you a bath; prepare your food; help to feed you; be with you).

Will your illness put a financial strain on your family? Who is the main wage earner in the family? Does anyone else help contribute to the family's income? Are there other sources for the family for financial income?

Educational background

Can you read and write in English, or do you feel more comfortable with another language?

How much education have you had in schools?

When you learn about new things, is there a special way that you prefer to learn? For example, do you like to read information first, or do you like to watch someone do a new skill and then try to repeat it? Does it help for you to talk to someone and ask questions?

TABLE 9-1	INTERVIEW GUIDE FOR ASSESSMENT OF SELECTED AREAS OF A CLIENT'S PSYCHOSOCIAL STATUS *Continued*
Assessment Area	**Key Questions or Issues to Include***
	Religious beliefs and practices
	Do your religious beliefs or practices influence you in how you feel or act when you are sick or when you are well?
	Are there special practices or healing rituals that you believe help to keep you well or to get better faster when you are ill?
	Is there someone special who performs healing rituals for you (e.g., shaman, priest)?
	Is it important to you to have a special religious person with you when you are sick or who comes to visit you (a priest or elder; imam; monk)? If so, describe how this person helps you feel better.

* The items in this guide are representative of but not inclusive for each assessment area.

ORIENTATION TO PERSON, PLACE, TIME, AND CIRCUMSTANCES. Ask the client to explain the reason for seeking health care. If the reply is unclear or if the client digresses, ask the client to state his or her name, to identify the present location, and to specify the date and time.

MOOD AND AFFECT. *Mood* is the subjective description of a personal emotion that is pervasive and sustained. Record whether the described mood matches the present situation. For example, "The client stated she was 'happy and going to celebrate' when informed that the results of her tests were normal."

Affect is the observable, outward demeanor that depicts the current emotional state, such as fear, anger, resentment, depression, anxiety, or elation. A *flat* affect is a lack of any facial expression or emotional response and is accompanied by a monotonous voice. A *blunted* affect is greatly reduced in intensity but still appropriate to the situation. Note whether the observed affect matches the immediate circumstances. For example, "When informed that discharge from the hospital was postponed because of an infection, the client first cried, then shouted at the nurse to leave the room." This indicates the client first was upset and then became angry that the discharge was delayed because of a complication. Both reactions are understandable, given the situation.

SPEECH AND COMMUNICATION (LANGUAGE). Evaluate the physical ability to speak and communicate by focusing on *how* the client talks, not the topic of speech. Observe tone of voice, pitch, rate of speech, articulation, length of responses, pauses, and pauses before the client replies to questions (latency).

THOUGHT PROCESSES AND CONTENT. Assess whether speech progresses logically and whether the stream of thought is spontaneous, natural, organized, logical, relevant, coherent, and goal-directed. What the client says should be consistent.

ATTENTION SPAN. Assess the client's ability to focus or concentrate on a task or activity over time, such as completing history forms or answering questions. If results are uncertain, further evaluate the attention span using the following tests:

1. *Digit span,* a test in which a series of five to seven numbers forward and up to five numbers backward is repeated that have been identified by the nurse.

2. *Serial 7s* and *3s,* which test attention span as well as calculation ability. Ask the client to subtract 7 (or 3) from 100 and continue to subtract by 7 (or 3) until the client cannot go any further.

MEMORY: IMMEDIATE, RECENT, AND REMOTE. Assessment of memory usually begins with recall of the past health history. Ask the client to recall information: (1) within seconds (e.g., repeat a series of numbers); (2) within several minutes to hours (e.g., recall specific words later during the interview or recall what was eaten yesterday); and (3) within hours, months, or years (e.g., identify where the client grew up). Be able to verify the client's answers.

GENERAL FUND OF KNOWLEDGE. Ask the client to identify commonly known places, events, and people. This can be done casually during conversation.

CALCULATIONS. Ask the client to perform simple arithmetic functions (addition, subtraction, multiplication, division) without using pencil or paper (see Serial 7s).

ABSTRACT REASONING AND THINKING. Answers to general questions (e.g., explaining the reason a course of action was taken for a health problem) are usually sufficient to assess abstract reasoning. If reasoning is impaired, ask the client to think beyond the concrete dimension by explaining a common proverb or by explaining similarities or differences between selected concepts. For example, "A bird in the hand is worth two in the bush." "What is the difference between a tree and a bush?"

PERCEPTUAL DISTORTION. The client should be able to discriminate reality from misperceptions. Ask the client to describe any illusions or hallucinations by asking about each of the senses. For example, "Do you ever feel that you are hearing sounds that other people do not?"

JUDGMENT. Judgment (decision-making ability) may be assessed within the context of the health history interview as the client discusses actions and decisions made in daily living. To assess further, ask about a realistic rather than a hypothetical situation. For example, "What would you do when a prescribed medication has run out?"

INSIGHT. Assess the client's insight throughout the interview as the client explains the nature of the current health problem and his or her expectations of the health care team. Evaluate whether the client demonstrates ability to perceive the self realistically and accurately.

When assessing mental status, individualize questions to the client's circumstances. Variables affecting one's ability to respond to specific questions include:

- Level of education
- Cultural background
- Degree of exposure to knowledge and information
- Familiarity with the language and vocabulary
- The client's perceived acceptance by the nurse

For example, it may be revealing to ask a teenager the name of a current popular singer but inappropriate to ask the same question of an older person. A client who has not progressed beyond a third grade level of education may be incapable of performing complicated arithmetic calculations. A proverb widely known in one culture may be meaningless to someone from a different cultural background. Finally, you must have access to correct answers for the questions asked, particularly those relating to personal circumstances, such as the location of the client's home, date and place of birth, and names of family members.

OTHER PSYCHOLOGICAL FACTORS

Assess additional psychological factors, such as personality style (see Box 9–3), motivation, and personal strengths, while interacting with the client and significant others. Although nurses do not usually participate in formal psychological testing, data from formal testing can be used to supplement psychosocial data collected in nurse-client interactions and in the health history.

MOTIVATION. Motivation is highly individual and is influenced by personal needs and desires, goals, hopes, and aspirations. Attempt to determine motivation for seeking health care. If the client is ill, ascertain the motivation for returning to an optimal level of wellness.

PERSONAL STRENGTHS. When planning care, use the client's strengths. *Resources* are personal elements that determine an individual's capability to adapt to challenges and threatening stressors. *Internal* resources are *physiologic* (e.g., immune system, nutritional state, physiologic defense systems, genetic predisposition to health, current state of each body system) and *psychological* (e.g., defense mechanisms, interpersonal style, usual coping ability, current coping ability, and spiritual state, such as the will to live). *External* resources include the social environment (e.g., usual coping style of the family, availability of social support, and the assessment skills of the health care providers) and the physical, economic, and cultural environments.

VALUES AND BELIEFS. The value system and beliefs determine whether or not the client views health care as worthwhile. The client's values and beliefs may differ from yours. Accept them as valid because they help provide insight into behavior.

SPIRITUALITY. Spiritual beliefs have implications for well-being, such as sustaining hope or assisting with coping during periods of stress. Include spirituality assessment as part of the health history, and explain the purpose for asking about it. This portion of the history is usually addressed at the end of the interview after a trusting nurse-client relationship is established. Because spirituality is very personal, respect a client's wishes not to discuss this topic. Ask whether the client prefers to consult someone else when spiritual support is needed.

Sociologic Assessment

The *sociologic dimension* includes information about social roles and functions. Assess psychosocial development, social network, socioeconomic status, lifestyle, and sexuality. View the client both as an individual and as a member of a social network.

PSYCHOSOCIAL DEVELOPMENT

Psychosocial development refers to a person's level of growth and development, including the life developmental processes and phases of growth and maturation. Psychosocial development occurs across the life span and includes physical, emotional, psychological, social, and cognitive components. These components are not distinct from one another, nor is progress through life's stages and phases always predictable or inflexible. An understanding of human growth and development provides a foundation from which to assess the client.

SOCIAL NETWORK

A *social network* is the group of people that surrounds, interacts with, and sustains a person with intimacy, social integration, nurturing, reassurance, and assistance. The nurse becomes part of a client's social network when the client enters the health care system; however, the client continues to receive support from the established social network.

Collect social network data by observing the client during interactions with family and visitors; ask questions about interpersonal relationships, and determine whether there are certain individuals with whom the client prefers to maintain contact. Do not assume that only family members are the most important people. When planning care, include the significant others who may be experiencing stress along with the client.

SOCIOECONOMIC STATUS

An individual's economic position within society is referred to as *socioeconomic status*. Ask about factors that affect financial and social well-being because they have implications for planning individualized health care, such as (1) occupation, (2) current employment status, (3) work-related concerns, (4) financial concerns, (5) effect of the client's health status on the ability to work and on finances, (6) perceived effect that the client's socioeconomic status has on access to the health care system, (7) educational background, and (8) hopes and goals for the future.

LIFESTYLE

Usual daily patterns of living are referred to as *lifestyle*. Lifestyle is closely associated with socioeconomic status but also includes relationships with others. Assess the following as they apply to the client's health:

- Usual roles and functions
- Work and study habits
- Leisure and relaxation activities
- Type and location of residence
- Living arrangements

- Usual manner of transportation
- Proximity of close friends
- Importance and influence of cultural beliefs on diet and health-seeking behavior or treatment
- Health habits (e.g., use of alcohol, medications, nicotine, recreational drugs)
- Stress level
- Coping methods used to relieve stress and their effectiveness
- Usual sleep pattern
- Degree of satisfaction with current status

SEXUALITY

Sexuality is the behavioral expression of one's sexual identity. It involves sexual relationships between people as well as the perception of one's maleness or femaleness (gender identification). Many aspects of sexuality affect health status and have significance in relation to nursing care and client outcomes. Aspects include (1) physical health problems that affect sexual behavior (e.g., mastectomy, colostomy, skin lesions, venereal diseases, paralysis, physical deformities), (2) concerns with sexual performance (e.g., impotence, premature ejaculation, inability to achieve orgasm, infertility), (3) issues of sex role function (e.g., homosexuality, bisexuality, sexual ambiguity, transsexual surgery), and (4) effects of environmental restrictions on sexual performance (e.g., residency in a long-term care facility).

Sexuality and sexual behavior are sensitive topics to discuss. Clients may want to talk about sexuality issues and may look for permission and encouragement to do so. Become comfortable with sexuality issues, and do not allow personal beliefs and values to interfere with professional care. Accept and interact with clients without judging them or their behavior.

Cultural Assessment

Cultural assessment is a systematic examination of the cultural beliefs, values, and practices as they apply to determining health care needs. These needs, and any culture-based interventions, must be viewed from the client's cultural context. Cultural assessment tends to be broad because it seeks information about group values, beliefs, and behaviors. The nurse also assesses what the larger group's tenets mean to the individual. Table 9–1 includes guidelines for assessing cultural components as part of the psychosocial assessment. Also see the Diversity in Health Care features.

A GUIDE TO PSYCHOSOCIAL ASSESSMENT

Although discussed separately, psychological and sociologic assessments are often combined (see Box 9–2). You may collect psychosocial data that indicate a psychiatric disorder. If this situation occurs, consult with other health care professionals, such as a psychiatric clinical nurse specialist and the client's physician.

■ REVIEW OF SYSTEMS

The review of systems (ROS) is a head-to-toe review of the physical health history for each body system. This review provides a focus for the physical examination.

Box 9–2 presents the information assessed. These data often are collected by having the client complete a checklist form that is then reviewed, and expanded as necessary, by a health care professional. In an episodic (short-format) health history, focus on those systems pertinent to the problem.

HEALTH PROMOTION AND HEALTH RISK APPRAISAL

Health risk appraisal examines factors that affect potential for developing a particular health problem. Risk factors are (1) *genetic* or *biologic* (e.g., race, family history, personal history), (2) *behavioral* (e.g., health habits such as smoking), or (3) *environmental* (e.g., living in a locale with smog). Determining health risk status identifies high-risk clients who may benefit from timely intervention. Explain the difference between being *at increased risk for development of* a health problem and the inevitability of *actual development of* a health problem. In health risk appraisal, assess the client's willingness and motivation to modify or reduce risk factors. For example, a client who smokes is at higher risk for pulmonary disease than a nonsmoker. You may believe that the client *should* stop smoking; however, if there is no desire to stop, your teaching will be ineffective. This client may be labeled "noncompliant" by the health care team when the client is only following a personal decision to keep smoking. Conversely, a female client at risk for osteoporosis tells you that she is concerned and desires to reduce her risk. This client is receptive to teaching about increasing dietary calcium intake and engaging in regular weight-bearing activity.

Health risk factors are categorized for assessment purposes. Some risk factors are potentially hazardous for many people (e.g., ground water pollution in a community that depends on wells for the water supply). Other risk factors may adversely affect a limited group of individuals (e.g., particle inhalation in workers who install insulation materials). Still other risk factors are significant for a family group (e.g., genetic diseases, such as Huntington's chorea). Risk categories include:

- Race and genetic or family-related factors
- Age-related factors
- Biologic factors
- Personal habits
- Lifestyle
- Environmental and occupational factors
- Socioeconomic factors

Table 9–2 summarizes examples of health risk factors, their commonly associated health problems, and suggested health promotion behaviors or screening procedures that may reduce potential risk or facilitate early detection. Awareness of health risk factors may motivate a client to seek screening procedures and to practice health promotion behaviors, particularly for health problems that are treatable or manageable through timely intervention. Environmental and occupational risk factors are linked with specific health problems and may be sus-

DIVERSITY IN HEALTH CARE

Introduction to Cultural Aspects of Health Care

Cultural knowledge is an important ingredient in health care because both health caregivers and clients interpret actions in light of their own belief systems. If clients do not respond as the nurse expects, the nurse may interpret this as unconcern or resistance. The nurse then can become anxious and frustrated. In order to incorporate cultural knowledge in care, it is important to understand some definitions and cultural components that are important in health care. Some pertinent definitions are the following:

1. *Culture:* "The learned and shared beliefs, values, and lifeways of a designated or particular group which are generally transmitted intergenerationally and influence one's thinking and action modes."[3]
2. *Ethnicity:* A characteristic of groups in which a shared social and cultural heritage is passed on to each successive generation and in which there is a sense of identity.[1]
3. *Ethnocentrism:* "The belief that one's own beliefs and ways of doing things are the best."[3]

Before we can truly appreciate and respect the belief systems of others, we must be able to recognize our own belief systems for what they are, where they originated, and how they influence perception of what others believe and do. Shaking up our own ethnocentrism is a necessary step in delivering culturally relevant care.

Another important part of delivering culturally relevant care is the use of information about the culture of the ethnic group to which the client belongs as well as the client's particular beliefs and practices. To understand the information, it is helpful to consider components of a cultural system that are pertinent to health caregivers, which are described as follows[4]:

1. *Religion:* May affect practice of health care in all phases. Religious rituals mark stages in the life cycle, influence dietary and health habits, and affect beliefs about cause of illness and effectiveness of treatment and caregiver. Religion may also influence interpreting illness as punishment from God or viewing the health professional as an instrument of God. The beliefs of some religious groups (Christian Science, Jehovah's Witnesses) have a direct influence on what is acceptable in the provision of health care (see Appendix A). Religion can also provide solace in times of stress and illness to client and family.
2. *Value Orientations*[2]
   a. *Time:* past, present, or future. All societies deal in all three but differ in their emphasis. The *past* focuses on ancestors and tradition. The *present* focuses on now; caregivers should focus on the

present value of information. The *future* is concerned with progress and change and is not concerned with present. Caregivers should focus on the long-term importance of information. All societies must deal in all three orientations.
   b. *Activity:* "doing" versus "being" versus "being-in-becoming" (self-contained; inner-controlled). *Doing* encompasses one's being valued for accomplishments. In a *being-oriented* culture, one is valued for one's existence. *Being-in-becoming* involves the value of one's striving for growth of self.
   c. *Relational:* "Collateral" versus "lineal" versus "individualistic." *Collateral* refers to the emphasis on the laterally extended group (siblings or same-age group); group goals are the primary focus. *Lineal* emphasizes kinship and continuity through time. *Individualistic* emphasizes personal autonomy and independence; individual goals dominate.
   d. *Individual-to-Nature:* "subjugated to nature" versus "dominating nature" versus "in harmony with nature." *Subjugated to nature* encompasses a fatalistic view that whatever nature causes will happen. *Dominating nature* is a major theme in the Western medical system. *In harmony with nature* concerns beliefs that balance is necessary to health.
3. *Health and illness beliefs and practices:* Involve beliefs as to causation of illness, defining of illness, toleration of pain and suffering, when to seek help, and choice of treatments and practitioners.
4. *Communication:* Differences in language or dialect, meaning, norms of social gestures, etiquette, touch, eye contact, distance zones (intimate, personal, social, public), and communication of emotions.
5. *Family and lifestyle patterns:* Includes organization and roles and relationships of family, nuclear versus extended family, gender roles, clothing, and diet.

Gathering information, both generally about the ethnic group to which the client belongs and individually about the client's beliefs and practices pertinent to these cultural components, greatly enhances nursing care and client outcomes.

References

1. Giger, J. N., & Davidhizar, R. E. (1999). *Transcultural nursing: Assessment and intervention.* (3rd ed.). St. Louis: Mosby.
2. Kluckhohn, F. (1979). Dominant and variant value orientations. In P. J. Brink (Ed.), *Transcultural nursing: A book of readings* (pp. 63–81). Englewood Cliffs, NJ: Prentice Hall.
3. Leininger, M. (1995). *Transcultural nursing: Concepts, theories, research and practices.* New York: McGraw-Hill.
4. Sharma, S. (1988). *Bridging the gap: Anthropological brokerage in nursing care.* Unpublished doctoral dissertation, University of South Florida, Tampa.

Sandra Sharma, PhD, ARNP, CS, *James A. Haley Veterans Hospital, Tampa, Florida*

ceptible to change. Socioeconomic risk factors are less easily eliminated; however, their effects may be modified through skillful case finding and risk management.

Assess the client's risk profile throughout the health history interview. A client with multiple risk factors linked to specific health problems is at greater risk for development of those problems than the client with fewer

or no risk factors. People in hazardous occupations include firefighters, police, miners, heavy equipment operators, lumber and construction workers, factory and textile workers, musicians, and workers who use chemicals or pesticides, such as farmers, landscapers, gardeners, painters, and artists. Risk for *accidental injury* or *trauma* has been linked to multiple stressors, inadequate coping abil-

DIVERSITY IN HEALTH CARE

Communicating with Culturally Diverse Clients

Nurses increasingly find themselves caring for clients from diverse cultures. In such a situation, it can be expected that the client's first language will not always be English. Most clients experience illness with some degree of anxiety. Certainly clients' anxiety is increased when language barriers do not allow them to communicate with their caregivers. The communication component of Purnell and Paulanka's Model for Culture Competence[2] describes essential variables that the nurse must assess when identifying the complexities of communication that exist when interacting with culturally diverse clients. Communication is essential to providing culturally competent care.

Certification of medical interpreters would help to ensure communication with clients who are not fluent in English.[1] Until medical interpreters are consistently available, techniques that facilitate communication can still be used.

Upon first contact with the culturally diverse client, it is essential to identify the dominant language of the client and to obtain someone who can help interpret the meaning.[2] Guidelines for communicating with clients who are not fluent in English are provided next.

Guidelines for Communicating with Clients Not Fluent in English[2]

1. Assess the client's fluency in English. Remember, clients often understand more than they can express, and they need time to think in their own language. Stress interferes with the client's ability to think and speak in English.
2. Determine whether there is a dialect that interferes with communication.
3. Given the difficulty of knowing the precise meaning of words in a language, it is best to obtain someone who can interpret the meaning and message, not just translate the individual words.
4. If there *is* an interpreter available:
   a. Use dialect-specific interpreters, not translators.
   b. Avoid using children and relatives as interpreters.
   c. Select same-age and same-gender interpreters.
   d. Give the client and interpreter time alone together.
   e. Address your questions to the client, not the interpreter.
   f. Build in time for translation and interpretation.

5. If there *is not* an interpreter available:
   a. Determine whether a third language is common to you and the client. If not, use a translator.
   b. Use pantomime for simple words and actions.
   c. Use pictures when possible (a picture is worth a thousand words).
   d. Use and also give the client paper and pencil.
   e. Avoid using technical terms.

Nonverbal Cultural Communication Patterns

Nonverbal communication is as important as verbal communication. Be attentive to both your own and the client's nonverbal messages. Nonverbal cultural communication patterns may vary from one client to another. Consequently, it is important to[2]:

1. Explore the willingness of clients to share their thoughts, feelings, and ideas.
2. Explore the practice and meaning of touch in their society: within the family, between friends, with strangers, with members of the same sex, with members of the opposite sex, and with health care providers.
3. Identify personal spatial and distancing characteristics when communicating on a one-to-one basis. Explore how distancing changes with friends versus strangers.
4. Explore the use of eye contact within this group. Does avoidance of eye contact have special meanings? How does eye contact vary among family, friends, and strangers? Does eye contact change among socioeconomic groups?
5. Explore the meaning of various facial expressions. Do specific facial expressions have special meanings? Do people tend to smile a lot? How are emotions displayed or not displayed in facial expressions?
6. Determine whether there are acceptable ways of standing.

The Challenge

It would be very convenient if there were a universal language; in reality, there is none. Cultural diversity with its accompanying many languages *is* reality. The United States has an emerging population composed of peoples from all over the world. Nurses are confronted with the challenge of communicating with and caring for these clients.

References

1. Lester, N. (1998). Cultural competence: A nursing dialogue, 1. *American Journal of Nursing, 98*(8), 26–34.
2. Purnell, L., & Paulanka, M. (1998). *Transcultural health care: A culturally competent approach.* Philadelphia: F. A. Davis.

Joyce Larson-Presswalla, PhD, RN, *President, "Culture Counts," Marketing Coordinator, James A. Haley Veterans Hospital, Tampa, Florida*

---

ity, mental and physical fatigue, decreased reaction time, and substance abuse. Stressors include strained interpersonal relationships, physical or psychological abuse, inadequate financial resources, a recent change in lifestyle, sensory stimulation overload, nutritional deficits, and hazardous environments. Lifestyle and personal habits greatly affect health status, and many are modifiable.

After assessing the risk profile, evaluate the client's health risk status. Examine each identified risk factor with the client to determine whether its effects can be modified. If the client is interested in reducing health risks

(e.g., stopping smoking or wearing seat belts), intervene either directly or indirectly. Discuss approaches to behavior changes. *Direct* interventions include teaching sessions to provide information and counseling to reinforce behavior. *Indirect* interventions include referral to an appropriate community resource or other health care professional (e.g., nutritionist, smoking-cessation program, counselor, support group for substance abusers, dieters' support programs).

The goals for the client are (1) to take responsibility for modifying factors that can affect health and (2) to

Text continued on page 155

TABLE 9–2	HEALTH PROMOTION AND RISK MANAGEMENT

| Risk Factor | Potential Health Problem | Screening and Preventive Measures | |
		Self-Care	Professional Level
RACE			
Black	Hypertension	Self-monitor BP Avoid salt in diet Maintain ideal body weight Seek professional care if systolic BP > 140 or diastolic BP > 90	Monitor if BP is elevated or client is taking antihypertensive medications
White (fair skin tones)	Skin cancer	Limit exposure to sun Wear protective clothing Use sunscreen with SPF 15 or above Perform monthly head-to-toe skin inspection Seek professional care if change noted in any moles or birthmarks, or new growths or patches do not heal	Monitor skin lesions Skin biopsy or excision and follow-up treatment
	Osteoporosis	See self-care and professional level measures listed under "Personal Habits—Inadequate calcium intake"	
Japanese	Stomach cancer	Know suspicious GI symptoms: pain, hematemesis, melena, weight loss, nausea, and so on*	Follow-up for laboratory tests and special diagnostic procedures
Hispanic	Diabetes mellitus	Regular exercise and weight control Consume balanced diet of no more than 30% fats with complex carbohydrates Know symptoms of hyperglycemia: polydipsia, polyuria, polyphagia, and delayed wound healing*	Diet counseling Follow-up for laboratory tests, diagnostic procedures, and blood glucose monitoring and control
Native American	Alcohol abuse and related diseases	Abstinence Limit alcohol intake to 1 oz/day or less if personal tendency (e.g., 1 to 2 mixed drinks or cans of beer) Know symptoms of alcoholism* Join self-help support group such as Alcoholics Anonymous (AA)	Assessment of history and physical condition Referral to a detoxification program Counseling for client and family
GENETIC OR FAMILY-RELATED			
Overweight	Obesity-related disease	Monitor weight once per week Perform regular, sustained exercise Consume balanced diet (no more than 30% fats, and calories should not exceed metabolic needs) Join self-help group such as Weight Watchers	Diet counseling Follow-up for moribund obesity (>100% of ideal body weight)
Diabetes mellitus	Diabetes mellitus or glucose intolerance	Regular exercise and weight control Consume balanced diet Know symptoms of hyperglycemia: polydipsia, polyuria, polyphagia, and delayed wound healing*	Follow-up for laboratory tests, special diagnostic procedures, and blood glucose monitoring and control
Hypertension	Cardiovascular disease Renal disease Retinopathy Cerebrovascular accident	Regular, sustained exercise Consume balanced diet Avoid excess salt intake Maintain ideal body weight Regular BP checks (self or professional) Take BP medication daily	Regular follow-up for diagnostic studies and laboratory work Monitor compliance
Heart disease (onset before age 50)	Cardiovascular disease	See "Hypertension" Know symptoms of heart disease: chest pain, dyspnea, cyanosis*	Annual physical examination, including ECG and laboratory tests

| TABLE 9–2 | HEALTH PROMOTION AND RISK MANAGEMENT *Continued* | | |

| Risk Factor | Potential Health Problem | Screening and Preventive Measures | |
		Self-Care	*Professional Level*
		Stop smoking Monitor resting pulse rate Low saturated fat diet Regular exercise	Refer to smoking cessation clinics Diet counseling
Breast cancer (in mother or sister)	Breast cancer	Learn to perform BSE Perform BSE monthly	Regular professional breast examination as indicated for age and personal history Regular mammography as indicated for age
AGE-RELATED			
Vision changes	Strabismus	Monitor for difficulty focusing, especially on near objects See ophthalmologist if symptoms occur Schedule regular eye examinations as indicated for age	Follow-up for complete eye examination and possible neurologic examination
	Visual acuity changes, cataracts, glaucoma, or macular degeneration	Monitor visual acuity See ophthalmologist if vision is "fuzzy," or seeing halos around lights Schedule regular eye examinations	Complete eye examination to screen for cataracts, glaucoma, and macular degeneration as indicated for age
	Injury or trauma	Wear protective eye gear when engaging in activity likely to result in projectiles or blunt trauma See ophthalmologist if injury should occur	Provide prompt diagnosis and treatment if injury occurs
Falls	Injury or trauma	Keep environment illuminated Remove loose scatter rugs Use a night-light Install handrails and grab bars Wipe up spills immediately	Provide prompt diagnosis and treatment if injury occurs
Self-medication errors	Overmedicating or undermedicating	Request and use prepackaged unit dose medications Prepare medicines in a well-lit area Wear corrective lenses when preparing medicines	Careful assessment of medication history; monitor for toxic response
Hearing problem	Presbycusis	Avoid exposure to loud noises Wear ear plugs when exposed to loud noise levels and limit lengths of exposure	Complete audiometric screening as appropriate for age and personal history
	Injury or trauma	Avoid putting sharp objects into ear canals Know symptoms of ear infections: pain, discharge from ear canal, vertigo, and fever*	Follow-up for prompt diagnosis and treatment if injury or infection occurs
Inadequate dental hygiene	Dental caries Periodontal disease Premature loss of teeth	Brush teeth regularly after meals and at bedtime Floss teeth daily Have damaged teeth repaired or replaced promptly Follow recommendations for fluoride treatments; use fluoridated toothpaste Schedule regular dental checkups	Provide complete dental checkups, with yearly follow-up Fluoride treatments as indicated for age and locale
Impaired immune system integrity	Community-acquired infections	Keep immunizations current as recommended for age Receive vaccinations for influenza yearly and pneumococcal infection as indicated Seek professional care if symptoms of infection occur	Provide prompt diagnosis and treatment if a contagious disease or infection is suspected

Table continued on following page

TABLE 9–2	HEALTH PROMOTION AND RISK MANAGEMENT *Continued*

| Risk Factor | Potential Health Problem | Screening and Preventive Measures | |
		Self-Care	*Professional Level*
Impaired mobility	Falls	See self-care measures listed for falls related to vision changes under Age-Related Use mobility-assistance devices (e.g., cane or walker) Avoid hazardous surfaces, such as wet floors and icy pavements	Provide prompt diagnosis and treatment if injury occurs
BIOLOGIC			
Hyperlipidemia, hypercholesteremia	Cardiovascular disease	Consume balanced diet low in saturated fats Exercise regularly Avoid or stop smoking Have blood lipid and cholesterol levels monitored periodically as recommended	Regular follow-up for monitoring serum levels
Hyperglycemia	Diabetes mellitus	Consume diet low in fats and simple carbohydrates Include complex carbohydrates Exercise regularly Have blood glucose levels monitored periodically as recommended Self-monitor blood glucose levels if diabetic and following a prescribed medical regimen	Regular follow-up for monitoring control of blood glucose levels Adjustment of medical treatment as indicated by laboratory results
Hypersensitivity reactions	Allergic reactions, including rhinitis, bronchospasm, asthma, eczema, and atopic dermatitis	Avoid known allergens Seek prompt medical treatment if self-care measures are ineffective Discuss with physician whether allergen sensitivity testing and treatment for desensitization is indicated Wear a Medic-Alert tag Learn to use and carry an emergency kit (e.g., epinephrine [Adrenalin] if indicated)	Provide prompt diagnosis and treatment if severe reactions or complications occur Initiation of desensitization therapy if indicated
PERSONAL HABITS			
Inadequate rest and sleep	Fatigue Lowered resistance to illness	Obtain sufficient sleep to feel rested on awakening (amount varies with individual need) (see Chapter 21) Avoid sedatives, caffeine, alcohol Seek professional care if chronic fatigue interferes with activities of daily living	Complete history and physical examination Evaluation in a sleep laboratory
Irregular diet habits	Obesity, diabetes, hypertension, cardiovascular disease, irritability, depression, and hyperactivity or hypoactivity	Consume meals at regular times each day Eat three balanced meals per day Limit intake of salt, caffeine, refined sugar, and fats Perform regular exercise Monitor weight weekly See self-care measures listed under obesity, diabetes, hypertension, and cardiovascular disease	Regular follow-up to monitor existing health problems Provide prompt diagnosis and treatment if a health problem arises
Inadequate calcium intake	Osteoporosis	Consume elemental calcium in recommended amount per day for age and sex. Recommended amounts range from 1000 to 1500 mg/day	Follow-up for periodic physical examination Possible estrogen hormone replacement therapy, when indicated

| TABLE 9-2 | HEALTH PROMOTION AND RISK MANAGEMENT *Continued* | | |

Risk Factor	Potential Health Problem	Screening and Preventive Measures	
		Self-Care	*Professional Level*
		Limit milk products as source of calcium; include other sources of dietary calcium, such as broccoli, carrots, green beans, spinach, collard greens, and rhubarb Consume 400–800 IU/day of vitamin D Engage in daily weight-bearing activity such as walking	Diet counseling
Excess fat intake	Colon cancer Possible breast cancer	Consume diet low in saturated fats, such as that found in beef. Substitute with fish, poultry, and beans Limit milk products and eggs Include fiber in diet such as from grains and cereals Know symptoms of colon cancer (blood in stool, change in bowel habits) and breast cancer (lump, discharge, pain)* Have stool specimen tested for occult blood Perform BSE monthly	Follow-up for laboratory tests and possible diagnostic procedures Diet counseling
Low fiber intake	Colon cancer	Consume diet high in fiber, including cereals and grains, especially bran Know symptoms of colon cancer (see earlier)* Have stool specimen tested for occult blood	Follow-up for laboratory tests and diagnostic procedures Supplemental fiber to include in diet
Alcohol abuse	Alcoholism Cancer of mouth, throat, esophagus, larynx, and liver Accidents, including those that result in death Cirrhosis Esophageal varices Pancreatitis Dementia	Abstinence, if high risk for alcoholism Limit alcohol intake to 1 oz or less per day if no personal tendency (e.g., 1 to 2 mixed drinks or cans of beer) Know the symptoms of alcoholism* Join self-help support group, such as Alcoholics Anonymous, if alcohol consumption interferes with performance of job or interpersonal relationships	Careful assessment of history and physical condition Referral to a detoxification program, if indicated Provide counseling Family counseling and support are often necessary (e.g., Al-Anon, Ala-Teen)
Drug abuse	Harmful side effects Drug interactions Allergic reactions Hepatitis HIV	Use prescribed medications only as directed Discard outdated medications Limit use of over-the-counter drugs to only those necessary Avoid recreational drug use Know symptoms of substance abuse* If using intravenous drugs, do not share needles or syringes	Careful assessment of history and physical condition Referral to a detoxification program, if indicated Provide counseling Family counseling and support are often necessary Screening for HIV infection
Tobacco use	Cancer of mouth or lung Cardiovascular disease Respiratory disease	Avoid tobacco use in any form Limit use, if unable to quit Know symptoms of tobacco-related health problems: persistent cough, oral sore that does not heal, hoarseness that persists, blood in sputum* Have regular health checkups Avoid exposing others to sidestream smoke Attend support group to help stop smoking, such as Smokers Anonymous	Follow-up for laboratory tests and special diagnostic procedures Counseling for help to stop smoking Referral of family members (if indicated) for health assessment if exposed to sidestream smoke
Safety	Unintentional injury or death	Use safety equipment as indicated (seat belts, helmet, eye shield, life vest)	Thorough teaching about medications and their side effects

Table continued on following page

TABLE 9–2	HEALTH PROMOTION AND RISK MANAGEMENT *Continued*

| Risk Factor | Potential Health Problem | Screening and Preventive Measures | |
		Self-Care	*Professional Level*
		Learn how to swim Never drink and drive. Appoint a designated driver Do not operate equipment or engage in hazardous activity if taking medication that causes drowsiness Develop safety awareness; e.g., learn to identify unsafe situations and avoid them or take corrective action	Provide prompt diagnosis and treatment if an injury occurs
Sun exposure	Sunburn Skin cancer	See self-care measures listed under skin cancer related to race	See measures listed under skin cancer related to race
LIFESTYLE			
Lack of regular exercise	Obesity Cardiovascular disease	Engage in regular aerobic exercise (brisk walking, biking, jogging, swimming) at least 3 times/week for 30 to 40 minutes each Warm up prior to exercising to increase flexibility and reduce chance of injury Do not begin an exercise program until evaluated by health care professional for a baseline health assessment Follow professional advice regarding type of exercise program and intensity of training Wear appropriate gear for activity as protection Consume a balanced diet Know warning signals of when to stop exercising (e.g., dizziness, chest pain)*	Baseline health assessment prior to beginning exercise program Provide prompt diagnosis and treatment if complications or injury occurs Periodic assessment of cardiovascular status and endurance
Stress and coping ability	Many health problems are related to high stress levels and inadequate coping	Decrease level of stress whenever possible Develop a variety of coping skills Practice relaxation techniques (e.g., biofeedback, imagery, meditation, self-hypnosis) Recognize effects of stress on self Develop a support network* Modify lifestyle to reduce stress	Provide counseling for stress management Refer to appropriate support system as indicated by the individual circumstances Teach regarding relaxation techniques Carefully assess and treat if psychosomatic health problems develop
Lack of self-care activities to promote health	Cancer of breast, testis, or prostate	Monthly practice of BSE or TSE Regular professional examination as indicated for age	Periodic, regular examination
	Cancer of the cervix	Obtain regular pelvic examination and Papanicolaou (Pap) test as indicated for age and sexual activity status	Periodic, regular examination with follow-up as necessary
	Vision and hearing problems	See self-care measures under age-related health problems	See measures listed under age-related health problems for vision and hearing
	Dental and gum disease	See self-care measures under age-related health problems	See measures listed under age-related health problems for dental hygiene
	Tetanus Influenza Pneumonia	Keep immunizations current*	Provide prompt diagnosis and treatment if an infectious disease occurs

TABLE 9-2	HEALTH PROMOTION AND RISK MANAGEMENT *Continued*		

| Risk Factor | Potential Health Problem | Screening and Preventive Measures | |
		Self-Care	*Professional Level*
	Cancer	Know the seven warning signs: change in bowel or bladder habits, a nonhealing sore, unusual bleeding or discharge, lump or thickening in breast or other area, difficulty swallowing or indigestion, change in mole or wart, and persistent cough or hoarseness* Know and follow current recommendations for prevention and early entry into the health care system	Follow-up for laboratory tests and special diagnostic procedures Provide prompt diagnosis and treatment
High-risk sexual activity	Unplanned pregnancy	Use contraceptive method acceptable to self and partner Prenatal care	Provide counseling regarding options for contraceptives Provide counseling regarding pregnancy outcome options
	Cervical cancer	Abstain from early, frequent sexual activity Limit number of sexual partners Limit number of childbirths Schedule regular Pap test as recommended for age	Regular professional pelvic examinations and Pap tests as indicated by health behavior profile
	STDs, such as HIV infection and herpes	Limit number of sexual partners Avoid anal intercourse Use condoms Avoid oral-genital intercourse Avoid oral contact with body fluids (semen, blood, feces, urine) Seek professional care for regular, periodic assessment if engaging in high-risk sexual activity Know symptoms of STDs, e.g., sore on genitals or mucous membranes, discharge from penis or vagina, abnormal bleeding, dyspareunia Refrain from sexual activity if symptoms of STDs develop	Follow-up for prompt diagnosis and treatment should STD be suspected Provide counseling regarding safe sex practices Refer to public health for contact and follow-up of possible infected partners
Travel	Diseases prevalent in locale	Obtain necessary vaccinations before departure Seek prompt treatment if illness develops while traveling or after return	Provide prompt diagnosis and treatment if illness occurs
ENVIRONMENTAL AND OCCUPATIONAL			
Sports	Fractures, sprains, and strains	Have a baseline health assessment prior to beginning a sport Wear protective gear to avoid injury (e.g., eye shield, helmet, padding)* Follow recommendations for warm-up and cool-down exercises Limit mobility of injured body part until rehabilitation begins	Provide prompt diagnosis and treatment of injuries Rehabilitation
Outdoor activity	Sunburn Skin cancer Frostbite Hypothermia or hyperthermia	Wear protective gear appropriate for the weather Use sunscreen with an SPF of 15 or above Limit exposure to extremes of heat or cold Learn survival tactics relative to activity Know early signs of hypothermia (disorientation) and hyperthermia (dry, hot skin)	Provide prompt diagnosis and treatment if a problem occurs See measures listed under skin cancer related to race

Table continued on following page

TABLE 9–2	HEALTH PROMOTION AND RISK MANAGEMENT *Continued*		
	Potential Health Problem	**Screening and Preventive Measures**	
Risk Factor		*Self-Care*	*Professional Level*
		Attempt to seek medical treatment as soon as possible if a problem arises Avoid future exposure to extremes of heat or cold because of increased vulnerability	
Loud noise	Hearing loss	Limit exposure to loud music and machinery Wear protective ear plugs Have regular screening of hearing and seek professional care if hearing loss is evident	Regular, complete audiometric screening, as appropriate
Chemical fumes, airborne particle exposure	Respiratory diseases Cancer	Provide adequate ventilation Wear protective gear (goggles, respirators) Limit exposure when possible (chemicals, dry cleaning fluid, film processing, mining, asbestos exposure, household cleaners) Evaluate occupational risks Reduce exposure by changing jobs, if necessary Know symptoms of possible disease, such as hoarseness, persistent cough, hemoptysis, chronic dyspnea* Avoid smoking	Prompt diagnosis and treatment if disease should occur
Stress-provoking activity	Many stress-related health problems may occur	See "Stress and coping ability" under Lifestyle	Provide counseling regarding stress management
High-accident-risk activity (also see "Safety" under Personal Habits)	Unintentional injury or death	Avoid high-accident-risk activities Learn safety measures Practice safety measures so they become habitual Use safety equipment such as goggles, helmets Get sufficient rest Avoid alcohol, drugs, or medications known to cause drowsiness when engaging in high-risk activity Obtain treatment if injury occurs	Provide prompt diagnosis and treatment if an accidental injury occurs
Low-level electromagnetic radiation exposure	Cancer of brain or eye Leukemia Sarcoma Possible birth defects	Limit exposure Monitor immediate environment for radiation levels Promptly seek health assessment and treatment for possible problems	Provide prompt diagnosis and treatment if a health problem occurs
SOCIOECONOMIC			
Recent immigration	Diseases common to locale of origin or where traveled	Obtain necessary immunizations before departure Seek professional care if symptoms of disease occur, especially during or after recent travel	Careful assessment of history and physical examination Provide prompt diagnosis and treatment if a health problem occurs
Lack of adequate health insurance coverage	Delayed or postponed treatment of health problems Undetected health problems	Use free walk-in health care facilities	Refer client to social services or welfare agency for assistance with applying for available health care, such as Medicaid or Medicare

*Seek professional care if symptoms are present.

BP, blood pressure; BSE, breast self-examination; ECG, electrocardiogram; GI, gastrointestinal; HIV, human immunodeficiency virus; IU, international units; SPF, sun protection factor; STDs, sexually transmitted diseases; TSE, testicular self-examination.

BOX 9-5   Example of Integrating Health Risk Appraisal into the History Interview

Biographical and Demographic Data

S. W. is a 28-year-old, single, white, female, self-employed clothing designer. Self-insured. Admitted to nursing unit after surgical repair of the right knee.

Health Maintenance Activities

Annual examinations for teeth, vision, Pap smear. No breast self-examination. Last physical examination 18 months ago.

Personal Habits

Denies smoking. Consumes one to two alcoholic drinks or glasses of wine most days. Uses own automobile frequently, wears seat belts "when [she] remembers to put them on." Uses tanning room at health spa twice a week for 30 minutes.

Diet

No restrictions, likes most foods. Prefers to limit sugar and salt intake. Typical 24-hour diet includes Food Guide Pyramid groups. Usually eats breakfast and dinner; lunch consumed "on the run." Dines out often with clients at restaurants.

Exercise

Jogs once per week for 2 to 3 miles and performs step aerobics once per week at health spa. Tripped and fell while jogging 3 weeks ago; twisted right knee.

Stress Management

Feels "moderate" pressure to succeed in business. Life becomes "hectic" when new fashion lines shown. Uses imagery for relaxation (usually effective). Denies current problems with stress management.

Sleep and Rest

Gets approximately 6 to 7 hours' sleep per night and feels rested.

Sexuality

Sexually active since age 18. Reports five or six partners in past 10 years, with one partner for past 2 years. Prescribed oral contraceptive for 6 years. Partner does not use condoms.

Past Health History

No previous illness, injury, or surgery. No allergies.

Family Health History

Mother had breast cancer at age 42; treated with surgery and is currently healthy. No other known family-linked health problems.

Health Risk Appraisal

S. W. is at risk for (1) breast cancer, (2) possible skin cancer, (3) automobile-related injury or death, (4) possible sexually transmitted diseases, including human immunodeficiency virus infection, and (5) recurrent injury to the right knee. She also is at risk for health problems related to alcohol consumption, inadequate nutrition, inadequate exercise patterns, and a stress-producing lifestyle. There may be concerns about financial security that can be explored with S. W. during further questioning.

---

strive for optimal health. Box 9-5 provides an example of how to integrate health risk appraisal into the history interview.

■ HEALTH PROMOTION ACROSS THE LIFE SPAN

Health promotion needs change with age and sex. For example, the risk for development of cancer of the bowel or breast is higher in people over age 50 years than in younger people.

Specific screening procedures are performed during health assessment to determine potential and actual health problems. For example, after age 40, glaucoma screening is recommended every 2 years. For health maintenance and prevention, specific health management behaviors are recommended based on age. For example, routine childhood vaccinations for immunization against contagious diseases are administered according to a schedule that correlates with the development of the immune system as well as with periods when exposure is most likely to occur. Adults may be deficient in routine vaccinations or may not have had previous exposure to childhood contagious diseases. These clients should have screening antibody assays and immunizations if indicated.

Recommendations for common screening procedures and health management behaviors across the life span are listed in Table 9-3. Recommendations change periodically as research and epidemiologic studies reveal information about occurrence and as newer, more easily applied or sensitive screening methods are developed. Become familiar with the most current recommendations.

Chapter 18 discusses risk factors for the common types of cancer as well as primary risk factors and secondary type of cancer prevention. The American Cancer Society Guidelines are given for early detection in asymptomatic populations.

■ SCREENING TESTS AND PROCEDURES

Screening tests and procedures are used to assess for a health problem (e.g., a skin test for tuberculosis) or for risk of future health problems (e.g., serum cholesterol screening for the risk of atherosclerosis). When inquiring whether the client has had a specific screening test or procedure, such as an eye examination or mammogram, ask when the test was last performed and what the results were. Use this information to assess health risk status and to recommend further follow-up or screening procedures.

Text continued on page 160

TABLE 9–3 RECOMMENDATIONS FOR COMMON SCREENING PROCEDURES AND HEALTH MANAGEMENT BEHAVIORS ACROSS THE LIFE SPAN*

Potential Health Problem	Recommended Preventive/Screening Examination†	Birth to 18 Months	2 to 6 Years	7 to 12 Years	13 to 18 Years	19 to 39 Years	40 to 64 Years	65 Years and over
Growth and developmental concerns	History—re: developmental disorders	Parent/family dysfunction. Physical, mental, emotional, and social growth. Behavioral and learning disorders				Relationships with significant others. Parenting behaviors. Job satisfaction.		Retirement planning; declining mental acuity
			Discipline, school readiness		Sexual practices			
	Nutrition history	Breastfeeding, iron intake	Sweets, between-meal snacks, fats (saturated), sodium, iron, calcium		Fats (saturated), cholesterol	Fats (saturated), cholesterol, complex carbohydrates, fiber, sodium, calcium		
						Iron for women until menopause		
			Caloric balance and selection of exercise program					
	Complete physical examination	Birth, 2–4 weeks, and 2, 4, 6, 9, 12, 15, and 18 months	Every year until age 5	Every 2 years	Every 2 years	Every 5 years	Every 2 years ages 40 to 50, then yearly	Every year
Vision problems	Strabismus check, amblyopia	Every visit						
	Assessment of visual acuity		Every year beginning at age 3	One time	One time	Every 2 to 4 years	Every 1 to 2 years to include glaucoma screening	
Hearing problems	Audiometry	18 months	Every year	One time	One time		Every 3 years	Every year
Dental problems	Assessment of teeth/cleaning	Every visit (baby bottle tooth decay)	Every 6 months beginning at age 3	Every 6 months to 1 year				
	Fluoride	+	+	+	+	+		
	Brushing and flossing		+	+	+	+	+	+

Table continued on following page

Infectious diseases								
Routine immunizations	DTP, OPV/IPV, MMR, Hib, HBV, VZV per protocol	DTP, OPV/IPV, MMR per protocol	MMR at age 11 to 12 if not given at 4 to 6 years					
PPD or tine test	At age 1	One time	One time	One time	One time	One time	One time	One time
Tetanus-diphtheria booster		One time between 4 and 6 years		One time between 14 and 16 years	Every 10 years	Every 10 years		
Influenza vaccine			Every year if high risk under age 65					Every year
Pneumococcal vaccine			Every 6 to 10 years if in high-risk category (e.g., asthma, cystic fibrosis, chronic pulmonary disease)					One time
Accidents and injuries								
Automobile restraints	Car seats	Car seats until age 4; seat belts	+	+	+	+	+	+
History—re: risk factors	Burns, falls, choking, poisoning, drowning	Poisoning, drowning, burns, bicycle accidents, choking	Bicycle accidents, burns, poisoning, firearms, drowning	Bicycle accidents, burns, firearms, drinking while driving, suicide	Drinking while driving, firearms, back injury, burns, suicide	Drinking while driving, burns, back injury, falls	Falls	
Substance abuse								
History—re: use of tobacco, drugs, alcohol			+	+	+	+	+	
Birth defects								
Rubella titer					Unimmunized/unexposed female			
Amniocentesis					Over age 35			
Unplanned pregnancy								
Sex education			+	+	+	+	+	
Contraceptive information			+	+	+			
Anemia								
Hemoglobin and hematocrit	One time, early infancy	Age 3 and 5 years	Ages 8, 10, and 12	Ages 15 and 18	One time	One time	Every 3 years	Every year
Bacteriuria								
Urinalysis		One time at age 3	One time	One time	Every 1 to 3 years	One time	Every year	Every year

TABLE 9–3	RECOMMENDATIONS FOR COMMON SCREENING PROCEDURES AND HEALTH MANAGEMENT BEHAVIORS ACROSS THE LIFE SPAN *Continued*							
Potential Health Problem	**Recommended Preventive/ Screening Examination†**	**Birth to 18 Months**	**2 to 6 Years**	**7 to 12 Years**	**13 to 18 Years**	**19 to 39 Years**	**40 to 64 Years**	**65 Years and over**
Bowel cancer	Rectal examination					Every year from ages 30 to 40	Every year	
	Stool examination for occult blood						Every year beginning at age 40	
	Sigmoidoscopy						Every 3 to 5 years after two negative test results 1 year apart, beginning at age 40	
Breast cancer	Breast self-examination (BSE)					Every month		
	Professional examination					Every 3 years	Every year	
	Mammogram					One time between ages 35 and 39 if high risk	Every 1 to 2 years until age 50; then every year until age 75	
Cervical cancer/ gynecologic problems	Papanicolaou (Pap) smear				Every 1 to 3 years if sexually active	Every year until 3 examination results in a row are negative; then decrease frequency		
	Pelvic examination					Every 1 to 3 years	Every year	
Heart disease	History—re: exercise program or physical activity		Every visit					
	Electrocardiogram					Every 5 years after age 50		
Hypertension	Blood pressure		Every year beginning at age 3	Every 1 to 2 years		Every 5 years after age 35; every 2 years after age 50		Every year
Hyperlipidemia	Blood cholesterol level		Age 3 if family history			Every 5 years if below 200 mg/dl		Every 3 to 5 years
Obesity	Height and weight	Every visit	+	+	+	+	+	+
Oral cancer	Professional examination					Annually	Annually	Annually

Screening/Service					
Scoliosis	Every year beginning at age 8				
Back examination					
Sexually transmitted diseases (STDs) — VDRL/RPR		One time if sexually active	One time	One time	One time
Chlamydial testing		+	+	+	+
Gonorrhea culture		+	+	+	+
HIV counseling and testing		+	+	+	+
Testicular/prostate problems — Testicular self-examination (TSE)			Every month	Every month	Every month
Professional examination			Every 5 years	Every 2 to 3 years between ages 40 and 50, then every year	Every year
Prostate cancer — Prostate-specific antigen (PSA)				Every year between ages 50 and 70 years	

*Recommendations are subject to change, based on the most current information available. Recommendations in this table are based on guidelines from the American Academy of Family Physicians, the American Academy of Ophthalmology, the American Academy of Pediatrics, the American Cancer Society, the American College of Obstetricians and Gynecologists, the American College of Physicians, the National Cancer Institute, the National Heart, Lung, and Blood Institute, Centers for Disease Control and Prevention, and the U.S. Preventive Services Task Force.

† The list of preventive/screening services is not exhaustive, nor are all services listed indicated for every client at every visit. Type and frequency of visits and services is determined by individual and family health history and personal habits.

DTP, diphtheria and tetanus toxoids combined with pertussis vaccine; HBV, hepatitis B vaccine; Hib (or HbCV [Haemophilus b conjugate vaccine]); HIV, human immunodeficiency virus; IPV, injectable polio virus; MMR, measles-mumps-rubella vaccine; OPV, oral polio vaccine; PPD, purified protein derivative; RPR, rapid plasma reagin test (for syphilis); VDRL, Venereal Disease Research Laboratory test (for syphilis); VZV, varicella-zoster virus vaccine; +, ongoing preventive behavior (these items should be assessed during each contact with the client).

ORGANIZING THE HEALTH HISTORY INTERVIEW

Organize the data collected during the health history interview by topical areas. Use a comprehensive, flexible approach while allowing for in-depth focus assessment in areas of concern. Include a head-to-toe assessment. Various formats are helpful for conducting a health history interview. Gordon's functional health patterns (FHPs) are an example.

Functional health patterns may be used to collect health history data (Box 9–6). This approach assists in identifying health patterns, deviations from these patterns, and actual or potential nursing diagnoses. Each of the 11 patterns has its own assessment criteria (see Appendix B).

RECORDING THE HEALTH HISTORY INTERVIEW

Record interview data in the health record according to agency protocol. The format is organized and may be a narrative, an outline, or a checklist with written supplementary comments. Record all pertinent data (both positive and negative findings). Data are clear, concise, comprehensive, and consistent, with no gaps or areas of ambiguity. Use approved agency abbreviations and terminology, whenever possible, to promote communication among health care team members.

APPLYING THE NURSING PROCESS TO HEALTH ASSESSMENT

In health assessment, seek to gather as much data about the client as possible, both subjective and objective. Analyze the data to determine the client's needs and responses to potential and actual health problems. Consider the client's preferences when formulating nursing diagnoses that are amenable to intervention. Establishing realistic goals and outcome criteria and planning interventions follow in logical order (Box 9–7).

CONCLUSIONS

The health history is the first component of health assessment. The history constitutes the subjective data and guides thorough assessment of specific concerns or areas identified through health risk appraisal. The history can be recorded in many ways, such as through computerized database assessments or on paper. Although a thorough history may seem time-consuming, the data provided are crucial to fully understanding the client's special needs.

BOX 9–6   Gordon's Functional Health Patterns

Health Perception and Health Management

The client's perception and understanding of the health status; this includes lifestyle and behaviors to promote, maintain, and restore health and well-being.

Nutritional-Metabolic

Food and fluid consumption in relation to the body's metabolic needs, including adequacy of nutrient supply to local tissues. Multiple factors influence behavior, such as physiologic (e.g., dehydration), pathophysiologic (e.g., peptic ulcer), psychosocial (e.g., the emotional significance of food), and socioeconomic (e.g., financial ability to purchase food).

Elimination

Patterns of excretory function, including bowel, bladder, and skin. Habits of excretory regularity and perceived difficulties are assessed.

Activity-Exercise

Activities of daily living requiring energy expenditure; these include self-care measures, physical exercise, stamina, and leisure and recreational activities.

Sleep-Rest

The usual habits of sleep, rest, relaxation, and energy level. Patterns are assessed for a 24-hour period so that circadian rhythmicity can be considered.

Cognitive-Perceptual

The ability to perceive, comprehend, and use information. The sensory functions are also involved. Pain is included in this pattern.

Self-Perception and Self-Concept

View of self, including attitudes, identity, body image, sense of self-worth, and self-esteem.

Role Relationship

The client's roles in society and interpersonal relationships.

Sexuality-Reproductive

Satisfaction or dissatisfaction with sexuality and reproductive functions; these include sex role behavior and identification, physiologic and biologic functions, and sociocultural aspects of sexual behavior.

Coping–Stress Tolerance

General coping strategies and effectiveness in managing stress, including the perception of stressors and their effect on the client.

Value-Belief

Values, beliefs (including spiritual), and goals that guide the choices and decisions, particularly in health care. Sources of strength and meaning are identified.

BOX 9-7 Applying the Nursing Process to Health Assessment: Case Example

Introduction

Mrs. L. is a 58-year-old, healthy-looking woman who visits a glaucoma screening booth at a health fair. The nurse integrates health assessment data and nursing process while talking to Mrs. L. and testing her visual acuity.

Biographical Data

Married. Works full time as a legal secretary. Has one married child who lives out of state.

Physical Health History

History negative for significant health problems. Postmenopausal. Reports seeing rings around lights and decreased side vision most noticeable when reading.

Health Risk Appraisal

Mother had cataracts. Family history positive for hypertension. Nearsighted since age 10 and wears corrective lenses. Last eye examination 5 years ago. Has smoked one pack of cigarettes per day for 40 years.

Physical Examination

Snellen chart results (with corrective lenses) are O.D. (right eye) = 20/40, O.S. (left eye) = 20/30, O.U. (both eyes) = 20/30. Visual fields to confrontation reveal superior fields less than those of the examiner. Pupils react sluggishly to accommodation. Further physical examination limited because of setting.

Nursing Diagnosis

High risk for altered health maintenance related to visual changes (decreased visual acuity and peripheral vision), family history of hypertension, and smoking history.

Expected Outcomes

Long Term

Mrs. L. will maintain present visual acuity and prevent further loss of vision.

Short Term

1. Mrs. L. will verbalize understanding of the need for an immediate, complete ophthalmologic examination.
2. Mrs. L. will identify an ophthalmologist whom she will contact no later than tomorrow for an appointment.

Interventions

1. Discuss results of visual screening with Mrs. L. and their significance.
2. Explain risk factors for glaucoma and Mrs. L.'s risk profile.
3. Assist Mrs. L. in choosing an ophthalmologist.
4. Provide Mrs. L. with pamphlets about glaucoma from the National Society to Prevent Blindness.
5. Give Mrs. L. a self-addressed, stamped postcard that is to be returned by the ophthalmologist after the first visit.

Evaluation

Long Term

Ask Mrs. L. to restate her understanding of the need to have regular visual check-ups by an ophthalmologist and to follow the recommended medical regimen for eye care.

Short Term

Ask Mrs. L. whom she plans to contact for an eye appointment and when she intends to do this.

BIBLIOGRAPHY

1. Ainslie, G., et al. (1998). Psychosocial history by automated self-report. *Federal Practitioner, 15*(3), 33–40.
2. Alfaro-LeFevere, R. (1998). *Applying nursing process: A step-by-step guide* (4th ed.). Philadelphia: J. B. Lippincott.
3. American Academy of Family Physicians (AAFP). (1996). *Summary of policy recommendations for periodic health examination.* (AAFP No. 962, reprint No. 510.) Kansas City, KS: Author.
4. American Academy of Pediatrics. (1988). *Guidelines for health supervision II* (2nd ed.). Elk Grove Village, IL: Author.
5. American Academy of Pediatrics, Committee on Infectious Diseases. (1999). Recommended childhood immunization schedule—United States, January–December 1999. *Pediatrics, 103,* 182–185.
6. Andresen, G. P. (1992). How to assess the older mind. RN, *55*(6), 34.
7. Andrews, M. M., & Boyle, J. S. (Eds.). (1995). *Transcultural concepts in nursing care* (2nd ed.). Philadelphia: J. B. Lippincott.
8. Barry, P. D. (1996). *Psychosocial nursing: Care of physically ill patients and their families.* Philadelphia: J. B. Lippincott.
9. Bozzo, J. (1999). Databases and nursing outcomes. *American Journal of Nursing, 99*(4), 22.
10. Braverman, B. G. (1990). Eliciting assessment data from the patient who is difficult to interview. *Nursing Clinics of North America, 25,* 743–750.
11. Brennan, P. F., & Romano, C. A. (1987). Computers and nursing diagnoses: Issues in implementation. *Nursing Clinics of North America, 22,* 935–941.
12. Brink, P. (1984). Value orientations as an assessment tool in cultural diversity. *Nursing Research, 35,* 198.
13. Brink, P. J. (1987). Cultural aspects of sexuality. *Holistic Nursing Practice, 1,* 12–20.
14. Buckley, G. E. (1995). Traveling healthy: A guide for counseling the international traveler. *Nurse Practitioner, 20*(10), 38–50.
15. Burnard, P. (1988). Discussing spiritual issues with clients. *Health Vision, 61*(12), 371–372.
16. Cameron, C. T., & McNeil, E. L. (1976). The importance of history. *Journal of Emergency Nursing, 2*(3), 21–22.
17. Carpenito, L. J. (1997). *Nursing diagnosis: Application to clinical practice* (8th ed.). Philadelphia: J. B. Lippincott.
18. Carson, V. B. (1999). *Spiritual dimensions of nursing practice* (2nd ed.). Philadelphia: W. B. Saunders.
19. Centers for Disease Control and Prevention. (1999). Recommended childhood immunization schedule—United States, 1999. *Morbidity and Mortality Weekly Report, 48,* 12–6.
20. Chilton, B. A. (1998). Recognizing spirituality. *Image, Journal of Nursing Scholarship, 30*(4), 400–401.
21. Clark, C. C. (1996). *Wellness practitioner: Concepts, research, and strategies* (2nd ed.). New York: Springer.
22. Diaz-Duque, O. F. (1982). Advice from an interpreter. *American Journal of Nursing, 82*(9), 1380–1382.
23. Dirckx, J. H. (1985). Talking with patients, the art of history taking. *Clinical Nurse Practitioner, 3,* 13–14.
24. Edelman, C., & Mandle, C. (Eds.). (1997). *Health promotion throughout the life span.* (4th ed.). St. Louis: Mosby–Year Book.
25. Geissler, E. M. (1994). *Pocket guide to cultural assessment.* St. Louis: C. V. Mosby.
26. Giger, J., & Davidhizar, R. (Eds.). (1995). *Transcultural nursing: Assessment and intervention* (2nd ed.). St. Louis: Mosby–Year Book.

27. Gordon, M. (1994). *Nursing diagnosis: Process and application* (3rd ed.). New York: McGraw-Hill.
28. Grasska, M. A., & McFarland, T. (1982). Overcoming the language barrier: Problems and solutions. *American Journal of Nursing, 82*(9), 1376–1379.
29. Grimes, J., & Burns, E. (1996). *Health assessment in nursing practice* (4th ed.). Boston: Little, Brown.
30. Grossman, D. (1994). Enhancing your "cultural competence." *American Journal of Nursing, 94*(7), 58–62.
31. Halloran, E. J. (1988). Computerized nurse assessments. *Nursing and Health Care, 9,* 497–499.
32. Helman, C. (1994). *Culture, health and illness* (3rd ed.). Boston: Wright.
33. Hogstel, M. O. (1996). *Practical guide to health assessment through the lifespan* (2nd ed.). Philadelphia: F. A. Davis.
34. Huff, R. M., & Kline, M. V. (Eds.). (1998). *Promoting health in multicultural populations: A handbook for practitioners.* Thousand Oaks, CA: Sage.
35. Iyer, P. W., Taptich, B. J., & Bernocchi-Losey, D. (1995). *Nursing process and nursing diagnosis* (3rd ed.). Philadelphia: W. B. Saunders.
36. Jarvis, C. (2000). *Physical examination and health assessment.* (3rd ed.). Philadelphia: W. B. Saunders.
37. Landis, B. J., & Brykczynski, K. A. (1997). Employing prevention in practice. *American Journal of Nursing, 97*(8), 40–46.
38. Lester, N. (1998). Cultural competence: A nursing dialogue. Part One. *American Journal of Nursing, 98*(8), 26–33.
39. Lester, N. (1998). Cultural competence: A nursing dialogue. Part Two. *American Journal of Nursing, 98*(9), 36–42.
40. Lipson, J. G., Dibble, S. L., & Minarik, P. A. (1996). *Culture and nursing care: A pocket guide.* San Francisco: University of California, San Francisco, Nursing Press.
41. Longo, D. C., & Williams, R. A. (1986). *Clinical practice in psychosocial nursing: Assessment and intervention* (2nd ed.). Norwalk, CT: Appleton-Century-Crofts.
42. McConnell, E. A. (1998). Communicating with a hearing-impaired patient. *Nursing, 28*(1), 32.
43. Miya, P. A., & Megel, M. E. (1997). Confidentiality and electronic medical records. *MEDSURG Nursing, 6*(4), 222–224, 212.
44. Murray, R. B., & Zentner, J. P. (1993). *Nursing assessment and health promotion: Strategies through the life span* (5th ed.). Norwalk, CT: Appleton & Lange.
45. North American Nursing Diagnosis Association (NANDA). (1999). *NANDA definitions and classification, 1999–2000.* Philadelphia: Author.
46. Pender, N. J. (1996). *Health promotion in nursing practice* (3rd ed.). Norwalk, CT: Appleton & Lange.
47. Poss, J. E., & Rangel, R. (1995). Working effectively with interpreters in the primary setting. *Nurse Practitioner, 20*(12), 43–47.
48. Purnell, L., & Paulanka, B. (1998). *Transcultural health care: A culturally competent approach.* Philadelphia: F. A. Davis.
49. *Quick reference to cultural assessment.* (1994). St. Louis: Mosby–Year Book.
50. Rahe, R. H. (1975). Life changes and near-future illness reports. In L. Levi (Ed.), *Emotions: Their parameters and measurement.* New York: Raven Press.
51. Risen, C. B. (1995). A guide to taking a sexual history. *Psychiatric Clinics of North America, 18*(1), 39–53.
52. Schneiderman, H. (1982, June). The review of systems, an important part of comprehensive examination. *Postgraduate Medicine, 71,* 151–158.
53. Spillane, R. K. (1987). Getting the patient's point of view: Early. *Nursing Manager, 18*(5), 20–28.
54. Strub, R. L., & Black, F. W. (1995). *The mental status examination in neurology* (3rd ed.). Philadelphia: F. A. Davis.
55. Tom, C. K. (1976). Nursing assessment of biological rhythms. *Nursing Clinics of North America, 11,* 621–630.
56. U.S. Department of Health and Human Services. (1998). *Clinician's handbook of preventive services* (3rd ed.). Washington, D.C.: U.S. Government Printing Office.
57. U.S. Preventive Services Task Force. (1996). *Guide to clinical preventive services* (2nd ed.). Baltimore: Williams & Wilkins.
58. VanDongen, C. J. (1998). Environmental health risks. *American Journal of Nursing, 98*(9), 16B–16F.
59. Warner, P. H., Rowe, T., & Whipple, B. (1999). Shedding light on the sexual history. *American Journal of Nursing, 99*(6), 34–40.
60. Wenger, A. F. Z. (1993). Cultural meaning of symptoms. *Holistic Nursing Practice, 7*(2), 22–35.
61. Woolf, S. H., Jonas, S., & Lawrence, R. S. (Eds.). (1996). *Health promotion and disease prevention in clinical practice.* Baltimore: Williams & Wilkins.

C H A P T E R

10

Physical Examination

Annabelle M. Keene

The physical examination is performed after the health history interview. Physical examination skills require use of the ears, eyes, and senses of touch and smell. Repeated practice reinforces integration of these skills. Learn the techniques and correct use of equipment as well as how to discriminate "normal" from "abnormal" findings.

Collect objective data systematically during the examination to supplement and validate subjective data. Evaluate both types of data to enhance holistic perception of the client. Ask the client questions about abnormal physical findings. For example, if a mass is found during palpation, ask whether the area is tender to touch. Record the client's reply in the physical examination portion of the database (e.g., "nontender") even though the data are subjective. If you are palpating a lump or mass that the client did not report initially during the history interview, ask the client whether he or she is aware of the mass's existence. If the client knows that the mass is present or reports related symptoms, proceed with a symptom analysis (see Chapter 9). Record these subjective data in the health history.

Physical examination is used in many settings. Health fairs, screening clinics, physicians' offices, independent practice clinics, home health care, and hospitals are some examples. Client health needs determine the extent and depth of examination. For example, a home health nurse visits a client who has had total hip replacement surgery. During the initial visit, the nurse performs a baseline assessment. During subsequent visits, the initial assessment findings guide evaluation of the client's progress (e.g., increased mobility and strength in the operative leg). Similarly, a coronary care nurse conducts periodic examinations of a client after a myocardial infarction to assess for life-threatening complications.

PURPOSE OF THE EXAMINATION

The purpose of physical examination is to differentiate normal from abnormal physical findings. A foundation of basic anatomy (structure) and physiology (function) is key to developing skill, expertise, and an appreciation for the wide range of findings that are considered normal. In addition to collecting baseline data, use assessment skills to make clinical judgments about health status and to evaluate the effectiveness of health care interventions. The home health care and coronary care scenarios are examples.

LEVELS OF PHYSICAL EXAMINATION

Several levels of physical examination are available, depending on client needs.

1. A *screening* physical examination is an organized, superficial check of major body systems for detecting abnormalities or possible problems.
2. If a problem is detected, the examination focuses on a *regional* or *branching* examination, which is an in-depth assessment of a specific body system. This chapter describes the screening adult physical examination. Table 10–1 shows regional examination assessments (see following unit assessment chapters for specific body systems).
3. A *complete* physical examination, which includes ancillary procedures such as x-ray studies and clinical laboratory tests, is beyond the scope of this text.

In the clinical setting, *periodic head-to-toe assessment* updates baseline data and assesses changes in health status. Individualize the depth of body system examinations according to client needs. For example, assess a client with a neurologic problem using the Glasgow Coma Scale in addition to the rest of the head-to-toe evaluation (see Chapter 68). A client with intact neurologic function would not require this depth of assessment. An example of a head-to-toe periodic assessment guide appears in Box 10–1.

ACCURACY OF PHYSICAL EXAMINATION

The physical examination helps to validate data collected during the health history interview. As with the health history, strive to collect accurate, thorough data. If you encounter difficulty with an assessment technique or question the accuracy of a finding, consult with colleagues. A second opinion or evaluation may be needed.

PHYSICAL EXAMINATION AND THE NURSING PROCESS

An accurate database is essential for formulating individualized nursing diagnoses. It may be misleading to diagnose a problem on the basis of one assessment finding. *Significant* findings (i.e., data that are either abnormal or indicate a potential risk) cue the nurse to collect addi-

Text continued on page 174

TABLE 10–1   ASSESSMENTS PERFORMED DURING REGIONAL EXAMINATIONS

Assessment Area	Client Position or Activity*	Technique†	Equipment	What to Observe
1. General survey	▪ Standing and walking during entrance (a, c) ▪ Sitting during health history interview (a, c) ▪ Changing into examining gown (a, c, f) ▪ Walking to examining table (a, b, c, d, f) ▪ Sitting on edge of examining table (a, c, e, f)	▪ Inspection (a, b, c, d, e, f) ▪ Olfaction (a)	b. Balance scale with height measure d. Snellen chart e. Thermometer; watch with second hand; sphygmomanometer; stethoscope f. Tape measure; skinfold calipers	a. General appearance and behavior; apparent age; sex; race; general state of health; signs of distress; body build; posture; gait; obvious deformity; movements and gross ROM; skin color and texture of exposed areas; dress, hygiene, and grooming; body or breath odor; mental status (expression, affect, speech, memory, eye contact); level of consciousness; level of cooperation b. Height and weight measurements c. Balance, coordination (Romberg's test, arm drift) d. Visual acuity (CN II) e. Vital signs: temperature; pulse; respirations; blood pressure, including check for auscultatory gap f. Nutritional status: body frame (wrist circumference); MAC; TSF; MAMC; IBW
2. Head and neck	▪ Sitting on edge of examining table (a, b, c, d, e, f, g)	▪ Inspection (a, b, c, d, e, f, g) ▪ Palpation (a, b, c, d, e, f, g) ▪ Percussion (e) ▪ Auscultation (a, f, g) ▪ Olfaction (a, f)	(1) Tape measure (3) Stethoscope (3) Cotton wisp; sterile safety pin (1) Snellen chart; eye cover (2) Eye cover; penlight or pen (3) Penlight or pen (4) Penlight or pen	a. *Head* (1) Inspect and palpate: skull size, shape, symmetry, contour, tenderness, lesions; measure circumference if abnormal size (2) Inspect hair and scalp: color, integrity; hair distribution and texture; presence of nits or lice; hygiene (3) Palpate temporal arteries: thickening, tenderness; auscultate for bruits if abnormality noted; rate amplitude b. *Face* (1) Inspect symmetry, skin color, hair distribution; facial movements (CN V and VII): clenched jaws, puffed cheeks, raised eyebrows, frown, eyelid strength (2) Palpate TMJ; temporal and masseter muscles (CN V); nodules (3) Test facial sensation for light touch, pressure and pain (CN V) over forehead, cheeks, and jaw c. *Eyes* (1) Visual acuity, if not performed earlier (CN II) (2) Visual fields (peripheral vision) by confrontation method (CN II) (3) EOMs through six cardinal positions of gaze (CN III, IV, VI) (4) Convergence and accommodation (CN III, IV, VI)

164

(5) Cover/uncover test (CN III, IV, VI) for movement

(6) Corneal light reflex (CN III, IV, VI) for alignment (Hirschberg's test)

(7) Inspect and palpate external eye structures:

   (a) Eyebrow symmetry, alignment

   (b) Eyelash symmetry, hair distribution, direction of growth

   (c) Eyelid position, skin characteristics, blinking

   (d) Lacrimal apparatus function

   (e) Eyeball symmetry, firmness

   (f) Conjunctiva and sclera color, texture, lesions, foreign bodies

   (g) Cornea texture, transparency; corneal reflex (CN V); omit corneal reflex testing if blinking intact

   (h) Anterior chamber transparency, depth

   (i) Iris and pupil symmetry, color, size, reaction to light and accommodation (CN III, IV, VI)

(8) Inspect internal eye structures: red reflex, retina, retinal vessels, optic disc, macula, fovea

d. *Ears*

(1) Inspect and palpate external ear structures:

   (a) Auricle symmetry, placement, skin integrity, color, mobility, tenderness over tragus

   (b) Ear canal skin integrity, cerumen, obstruction, foreign body, discharge

   (c) Tympanic membrane symmetry, color, light reflection, landmarks, scars, fluid

(2) Hearing acuity: response to normal conversation, whisper test, Weber's test for sound lateralization, Rinne's test for air and bone conduction of sound (CN VIII)

e. *Nose and sinuses*

(1) Inspect and palpate external nose alignment, symmetry; skin color, lesions, tenderness, discharge, nasal flaring, patency

(2) Inspect vestibule color, mucous membrane, septum alignment

(3) Inspect nasal mucosa for color, moisture; septum for alignment, masses, perforation; turbinates for color, exudate, inflammation

(4) Palpate and percuss frontal and maxillary sinuses for swelling and tenderness

(5) Transilluminate frontal and maxillary sinuses if client reports a problem

(6) Sense of smell (CN I) not usually tested, but if done, test with coffee grounds, cinnamon, cloves, peppermint

(5) Eye cover

(6) Penlight

(7) Penlight; cotton wisp; cotton applicator

(8) Ophthalmoscope

(1) Otoscope

(2) Tuning fork (512 Hz)

(2) Penlight

(3) Nasal speculum and penlight; or otoscope head with nasal speculum

(5) Penlight or transilluminator

(6) Various substances to smell (coffee grounds, cinnamon, cloves, peppermint)

Table continued on following page

165

Assessment Area	Client Position or Activity*	Technique†	Equipment	What to Observe
			f. Gloves; tongue blade; penlight	f. *Mouth and pharynx*
				(1) Inspect and palpate lips and oral mucosa for color, symmetry, texture, hydration, lesions, Stensen's ducts
				(2) Inspect teeth and gums and palpate gums for state of repair, hygiene, teeth alignment, missing teeth, gum bleeding, gum integrity
				(3) Inspect and palpate tongue and floor of mouth for symmetry, color, tongue position and size, texture, mobility, lesions, presence of papillae
				(4) Tongue mobility and strength (CN IX, XII)
				(5) Inspect Wharton's duct under tongue, floor of mouth, and base of tongue for lesions
				(6) Inspect roof of mouth, palates, and uvula for color, symmetry, texture, bone deformity
				(7) Test rise of uvula and soft palate with phonation (CN X)
				(8) Inspect tonsils and pillars for color, size, shape
				(9) Inspect pharynx for color, discharge on posterior wall
				(10) Test gag reflex (CN IX, X) if swallowing impairment reported or noted
				(11) Note characteristics of voice, ability to swallow (CN IX, X)
				(12) Note presence of breath odor
			(13) Various substances to taste (sugar, salt, lemon juice, bitters)	(13) Test sense of taste (CN VII, IX) only if abnormality reported with sugar, salt, lemon juice, bitters
				g. *Neck*
				(1) Inspect neck muscle symmetry, ROM, strength (CN XI); shoulder shrug
				(2) Palpate and inspect over parotid and submandibular salivary glands for swelling, tenderness
				(3) Palpate all cervical lymph nodes
				(4) Inspect and palpate trachea for symmetry and alignment
			(5) Stethoscope	(5) Inspect and palpate thyroid gland for symmetry, masses; auscultate for bruits if enlarged
			(6) Stethoscope	(6) Inspect and palpate carotid arteries; rate amplitude; auscultate for bruits
				(7) Inspect jugular venous distention

Body area	Position/Technique	Assessment	Equipment
3. Upper extremities and spine	Sitting on edge of examining table (a, b) ▪ Inspection (a, b) ▪ Palpation (a) ▪ Percussion (b)	a. *Upper extremities* (1) Inspect skin for lesions and palpate turgor (2) Inspect limbs for alignment and symmetry (3) Inspect fingernails and blanch to test capillary refill; inspect for clubbing (4) Palpate peripheral pulses: brachial, radial, ulnar; rate amplitude (5) Palpate epitrochlear lymph nodes (6) Inspect and palpate muscle groups for size, symmetry, tone; measure if they appear unequal (7) Evaluate and rate muscle strength: upper arms, forearms, wrists, fingers (8) Inspect and palpate joints for swelling and tenderness, crepitus (9) Assess ROM: shoulders, elbows, wrists, fingers; measure ROM if limitation noted b. *Spine* (1) Test DTRs and rate response: biceps, triceps, brachioradialis; test lower extremity DTRs: patellar, Achilles, and plantar cutaneous reflexes (2) Assess cerebellar functions: finger-to-finger touch; hand supination and pronation; finger-to-thumb opposition	(6) Tape measure (9) Goniometer (1) Reflex hammer
4. Posterior thorax	Sitting on edge of examining table; nurse stands behind client (a, b, c) ▪ Inspection (a, b) ▪ Palpation (a, b) ▪ Percussion (a, b, c) ▪ Auscultation (b)	a. *Spine, ribs, muscles* (1) Inspect spine for alignment; palpate spine processes for tenderness; inspect skin integrity (2) Inspect rib cage for symmetry, shape, movement with respiration (3) Measure anteroposterior-to-lateral diameter (4) Inspect and lightly palpate paravertebral muscles for tenderness, spasm (5) Assess thoracic expansion (respiratory excursion) b. *Lungs* (1) Observe respiratory pattern (2) Palpate tactile fremitus and respiratory excursion (3) Percuss posterior and lateral thorax and diaphragmatic excursion (4) Measure diaphragmatic excursion (5) Auscultate breath sounds, posterior and lateral thorax (6) Auscultate voice sounds if fremitus abnormal (bronchophony, egophony, whispered pectoriloquy) c. *Kidneys* Percuss over CVAs for kidney tenderness	(4) Ruler and pen (5) Stethoscope (6) Stethoscope

Table continued on following page

TABLE 10-1 ASSESSMENTS PERFORMED DURING REGIONAL EXAMINATIONS *Continued*

Assessment Area	Client Position or Activity*	Technique†	Equipment	What to Observe
5. Anterior thorax	▪ Sitting on edge of examining table; nurse stands on right side of client (a, b, c, d, e) ▪ Sitting up and leaning forward (b, e) ▪ Sitting with arms at sides; with hands on hips; with arms raised over head (e) ▪ Supine, arm behind head (e) ▪ Supine, head elevated 30 degrees (f, g) ▪ Left lateral recumbent (f)	▪ Inspection (a, b, c, d, e, f, g) ▪ Palpation (a, b, e, f) ▪ Percussion (a) ▪ Auscultation (a, b, c, f)	(7) Stethoscope (4) Stethoscope (5) Stethoscope (1) Stethoscope (4) Stethoscope	a. *Lungs and thorax* 　(1) Inspect skin integrity 　(2) Observe respiratory pattern 　(3) Inspect rib cage for symmetry, movement with respiration, shape, use of accessory muscles 　(4) Palpate respiratory excursion 　(5) Palpate tactile fremitus 　(6) Percuss anterior thorax 　(7) Auscultate breath sounds and voice sounds (if fremitus abnormal) b. *Heart* 　(1) Inspect precordium for lifts, heaves, apical impulse 　(2) Inspect epigastrium for aortic pulsations 　(3) Palpate precordium for thrills, apical impulse, lift, heaves 　(4) Auscultate heart sounds with client sitting up, then leaning forward 　(5) Assess heart rate and rhythm c. *Carotid vessels* 　(1) Auscultate for bruits 　(2) Rate amplitude if not done during neck examination d. *Jugular veins* 　Inspect for distention e. *Breasts and axillae* 　(1) Inspect breasts in 3 positions for size, shape, symmetry, contour, skin characteristics, lesions 　(2) Inspect areolae and nipples for size, shape, color, contour, symmetry, lesions 　(3) Inspect axillae for rashes, masses, lesions, pigmentation 　(4) Palpate axillae for lymph nodes 　(5) Palpate breasts for lumps, masses, consistency ▪ **Assist client to supine position** 　(6) Palpate breasts, areolae, and nipples with client supine and arm behind head f. *Heart* 　(1) Inspect precordium for lifts, heaves, apical impulse 　(2) Inspect epigastrium for aortic pulsations 　(3) Palpate precordium for thrills, lifts, heaves, apical impulse 　(4) Auscultate heart sounds with client supine, then in left lateral recumbent position

System	Position	Technique	Assessment	Equipment
6. Abdomen	■ Supine with arms relaxed at sides or crossed over chest; may have knees flexed slightly (a, b, c, d, e, f, i) ■ Turned to right lateral recumbent (g, h)	■ Inspection (a, i, j) ■ Auscultation (a) ■ Percussion (a, b, c, h, j) ■ Palpation (a, b, d, e, f, g, h)	*g. Jugular veins* (1) Inspect for level of venous distention with client's head elevated 30 to 45 degrees; measure level of distention between angle of Louis and angle of jaw (2) Assess for hepatojugular reflux if right ventricular failure suspected *a. Abdomen (general)* (1) Inspect skin integrity and characteristics: striae, venous pattern, hair distribution (2) Inspect contour, symmetry, umbilicus, pulsations, peristalsis, rectus muscles with straining; measure girth if distention noted (3) Auscultate all quadrants for bowel sounds (4) Auscultate major vessels for bruits: abdominal aorta; renal, iliac, and femoral arteries (5) Auscultate over epigastrium for venous hum (6) Auscultate over liver and spleen for peritoneal friction rub (7) Percuss all quadrants for masses, tenderness, gastric bubble; over bladder and spleen (8) Blunt percussion over anterior right (liver) and left (spleen) lower rib margins for tenderness (9) Lightly palpate all quadrants for masses, tenderness (10) Deep palpation for masses and tenderness, all quadrants (11) Assess rebound tenderness over RLQ and LLQ *b. Liver* (1) Percuss liver size at RMCL and MSL and mark borders (2) Measure liver span at RMCL and MSL *c. Spleen* (1) Percuss spleen size (2) Percuss for splenic enlargement if indicated *d. Aorta* Palpate for area of pulsation in epigastrium *e. Inguinal areas* (1) Palpate femoral arteries and rate amplitude (2) Palpate inguinal lymph nodes; note characteristics *f. Liver* Palpate for size, masses, nodules *g. Spleen* Palpate for size if enlargement suspected *h. Kidneys* (1) Palpate right and left kidneys for enlargement (2) Blunt percussion over CVAs (posterior thorax) for tenderness if not done earlier	(2) Tape measure (3) Stethoscope (4) Stethoscope (5) Stethoscope (6) Stethoscope (1) Pen (2) Ruler

Table continued on following page

Assessment Area	Client Position or Activity*	Technique†	Equipment	What to Observe

7. Lower extremities and spine	▪ Supine with arms relaxed (a, b)
	▪ Prone if needed to assess popliteal lymph nodes (a)
		▪ Inspection (a, b)
		▪ Palpation (a)
		▪ Percussion (b)
			i. Tongue blade
			
			(7) Tape measure
			
			(9) Tape measure
			
			(12) Goniometer
				i. *Abdominal reflexes*
				    Assess each quadrant for presence of reflex
				j. Test for ascites if indicated
				a. *Lower extremities*
				    (1) Inspect skin for lesions, hair distribution
				    (2) Inspect limbs for alignment and symmetry
				    (3) Inspect toenails and blanch to test capillary refill
				    (4) Palpate peripheral pulses: popliteal, posterior tibial, dorsalis pedis; rate amplitude
				    (5) Palpate popliteal lymph nodes
				    (6) Inspect for edema and palpate for pitting if present
				    (7) Palpate for phlebitis, varicosities; measure circumference of calves or thighs if phlebitis present
				    (8) Assess for presence of Homans' sign
				    (9) Inspect and palpate muscle groups for size, symmetry, tone; measure if appear unequal
				    (10) Evaluate and rate muscle strength: hips, hamstrings, quadriceps, ankles, toes, feet
				    (11) Inspect and palpate joints for swelling, tenderness, crepitus
				    (12) Assess ROM: hips, knees, ankles, feet, toes; measure ROM if limitation noted
				b. *Spine*
				    (1) Test DTRs if not done before at time of upper extremity evaluation; test patellar, Achilles, and plantar cutaneous reflexes
				    (2) Assess cerebellar functions: ability to slide heel down opposite shin; foot tapping

8. General neurologic and spine	▪ Supine with arms at sides, eyes closed (a)
	▪ Walking heel to toe (b)
	▪ Walking on toes, then heels (b)
	▪ Hopping on each foot (b)
	▪ Knee bends (b)
	▪ Standing with arms relaxed at sides (c)
		▪ Inspection (a, b, c)	(1) Cotton wisp
			
			(2) Sterile safety pin or needle
			
			(3) Tuning fork (128 Hz)
			
			(5) Key, coins, safety pin, paper clip
			(6) Closed pen
			(7) Two sterile safety pins
			(8) Test tubes filled with hot water and cold water
				a. *Sensory function*
				    (1) Test perception of light touch over symmetric dermatomes distally, then proximally; trunk, face, neck
				    (2) Test perception of pain vs. pressure over symmetric dermatomes distally, then proximally; trunk, face, neck
				    (3) Test perception of vibration distally on toes and fingers; progress proximally if abnormal
				    (4) Test position sense, fingers and toes
				    (5) Test object identification, both hands (stereognosis)
				
				    (6) Test graphism, both hands
				    (7) Test two-point discrimination, both index fingers
				    (8) Test temperature perception only if pain perception is impaired: distally, then proximally; trunk, face, neck

	(9) Test point localization and tactile localization (double simultaneous stimulation) only if light touch perception is impaired	(9) Finger touch		
	Help client to a standing position			
	b. *Gross motor and balance*			
	(1) Inspect gait and balance while client walks heel to toe, then on toes, then on heels			
	(2) Observe balance while client stands on one foot, then the other			
	(3) Observe balance and lower extremity strength while client hops on one foot, then the other			
	(4) Observe balance and strength while client performs shallow knee bends			
	c. *Spine*			
	(1) Inspect spine from anterior, lateral, and posterior views for kyphosis, lordosis, or scoliosis			
	(2) Assess spine ROM			
9A. Genitalia (male)	A. *Male genitalia* a. Inspect pubic hair and skin for hair distribution, rashes, lesions, parasites b. Inspect penis: shaft, prepuce, glans, urethral meatus; culture discharge if present c. Palpate penile shaft for nodules, tenderness d. Inspect scrotum for size, symmetry, shape, swelling e. Palpate scrotum for presence of testes, epididymis, vas deferens f. Transilluminate scrotum if swelling or mass palpated g. Inspect inguinal areas for hernia, first with client standing quietly, then during Valsalva's maneuver h. Palpate for direct inguinal hernia with client at rest and performing Valsalva's maneuver i. Palpate for indirect inguinal hernia with client at rest and performing Valsalva's maneuver	A. Gloves worn throughout b. Culture medium f. Transilluminator or flashlight	▪ Inspection (a, b, d, f, g) ▪ Palpation (c, e, h, i)	▪ Standing facing nurse (a, b, c, d, e, f, g, h, i) ▪ Standing and performing Valsalva's maneuver (g, h, i)
9B. Anus and rectum (male)	B. *Anus and rectum (male)* a. Inspect perianal skin for integrity, color, excoriation, rash, lesions, fissures, ulcers, hemorrhoids b. Inspect anal area for rectal prolapse, fissures, fistulas, inflammation, hemorrhoids, polyps with client performing Valsalva's maneuver c. Palpate anus, anal canal, sphincter tone, anorectal junction, rectal walls, coccyx with client at rest d. Palpate anal sphincter tone during Valsalva's maneuver e. Palpate for a descending rectal mass with client performing Valsalva's maneuver f. Palpate prostate gland: median sulcus, two lateral lobes	B. Gloves worn throughout c. Lubricant	▪ Inspection (a, b, g) ▪ Palpation (c, d, e, f)	▪ Standing and bending over examining table (a, c, f, g) ▪ Standing and bending over examining table, performing Valsalva's maneuver (b, d, e)

Table continued on following page

171

Assessment Area	Client Position or Activity*	Technique†	Equipment	What to Observe
			g. Hemoccult test; culture medium	g. Inspect gloved finger as it is withdrawn for stool and test stool for occult blood; obtain rectal culture if indicated
				■ **Female client is assisted to assume lithotomy or dorsal recumbent position**
10A. Genitalia (female)	■ Lithotomy position if both external and internal genitalia examined (a, b, c, d, e, f, g, h, i, j, k, l, m, n) ■ Dorsal recumbent if only external genitalia examined (a, b, c, d, e, f, g, h, i)	■ Inspection (a, b, c, d, e, g, j, k) ■ Palpation (f, h, i, l, m, n)	A. Gloves worn through-out	A. *Female genitalia* a. Inspect mons pubis for pubic hair distribution and texture; perineal skin for color, lesions, irritation, parasites b. Inspect labia majora for edema, symmetry c. Inspect labia for minora symmetry d. Inspect clitoris for color, presence of lesions e. Inspect introitus and hymen f. Palpate Bartholin's glands if inflamed or enlarged for size, tenderness g. Inspect urethral meatus for discharge, inflammation, swelling
			h. Culture medium; change gloves if discharge present	h. Palpate Skene's glands for discharge and obtain specimen for culture if present i. Assess integrity of pelvic floor muscles: strength, presence of cystocele or rectocele, discharge of urine
			j. Vaginal speculum; light source; wooden spatula; cotton-tipped applicator; glass slides; fixative; culture medium	j. Insert vaginal speculum and inspect cervix; adjust light as needed; note shape, position, color, lesions, discharge; obtain cervical specimens if indicated: cervical scraping, endocervical swab, vaginal pool scraping k. Inspect vagina as speculum is removed: color, rugae, mucosa

			l. Lubricant	l. Palpate vagina and cervix for nodules, masses; cervix position, mobility, consistency, tenderness
				m. Bimanually palpate pelvic structures
				  (1) Uterus (anterior wall and fundus) for masses, tenderness, position
				  (2) Ovary and adnexa for ovary size, masses, tenderness

			n. Change gloves if vaginal examination performed; lubricant	n. Rectovaginal palpation of uterus for masses, position, tenderness

	Position	Technique	Observations	Equipment
10B. Anus and rectum (female)	▪ Lithotomy position if done at same time as internal genitalia examination (a, b, c, d, e, g) ▪ Dorsal recumbent if done after external genitalia examination (a, b, c, d, e, f, g) ▪ Performing Valsalva's maneuver (b, d, e)	▪ Inspection (a, b, g) ▪ Palpation (c, d, e, f)	B. *Anus and rectum (female)* a. Inspect perianal skin for integrity, color, excoriation, rash, lesions, fissures, ulcers, hemorrhoids b. Inspect anal area for rectal prolapse, fissures, fistulas, inflammation, hemorrhoids, polyps with client performing Valsalva's maneuver c. Palpate anus, anal canal, sphincter tone, anorectal junction, rectal walls, coccyx with client at rest d. Palpate anal sphincter tone during Valsalva's maneuver e. Palpate for a descending rectal mass with client performing Valsalva's maneuver f. Palpate cervix through anterior rectal wall for shape, position, mobility, tenderness g. Inspect gloved finger as it is withdrawn for stool and test stool for occult blood; obtain rectal culture if indicated	B. Gloves worn throughout c. Lubricant g. Hemoccult; culture medium
11. Examination complete	▪ Sitting		After removal of finger, assist client in cleaning the perineum and in sitting comfortably before leaving to allow client to dress	

*Letters in parentheses after the client position or activity denote what the nurse observes.

†Letters in parentheses after technique denote the examination portions during which the nurse uses these skills to assist observations.

CN, cranial nerve; CVAs, costovertebral angles; DTRs, deep tendon reflexes; EOMs, extraocular movements; IBW, ideal body weight; LLQ, left lower quadrant; MAC, midarm circumference; MAMC, midarm muscle circumference; MSL, midsternal line; RLQ, right lower quadrant; RMCL, right midclavicular line; ROM, range of motion; TMJ, temporomandibular joint; TSF, triceps skinfold thickness.

BOX 10-1   **Head-to-Toe Periodic Assessment Guide**

1. *Vital signs:* Temperature, pulse, respirations, blood pressure
2. *Pain:* Location, type, quality, intensity
3. *Neurologic:* Orientation (person, place, time, situation), level of consciousness, gait, extremity color/movement/sensation (CMS), pupillary responses to light
4. *Pulmonary:* Respiratory pattern and effort; breath sounds; cough quality; sputum production, color, and quantity
5. *Cardiovascular:* Heart sounds and rhythm, pulses (radial, dorsalis pedis, and right and left posterior tibial), capillary refill, edema (location and amount), skin color and temperature
6. *Gastrointestinal:* Oral assessment, abdominal appearance, bowel sounds, bowel elimination pattern
7. *Genitourinary:* Bladder distention, voiding pattern
8. *Integument:* Skin integrity, wounds, dressings, drainage
9. *Psychosocial:* Sociability, affect, anxiety, attitude

Note: Perform additional assessments according to the client's specific health status and needs.

---

tional information. A complete assessment is necessary before data can be grouped and a cause determined. The initial physical assessment is the baseline for the client's functional ability. Physical assessment is also used as intervention (e.g., monitoring lung sounds) to evaluate changes in the client's physical condition and to determine whether expected outcomes have been achieved.

TECHNIQUES OF PHYSICAL EXAMINATION

Four primary techniques are used in physical assessment: *inspection, palpation, percussion,* and *auscultation.* These techniques enhance the data collected by observation of the ears, eyes, and senses of touch and smell and are used as indicated during the examination of each body region (Fig. 10-1).

■ INSPECTION

Inspection is the systematic, deliberate visual examination of the entire client or a region. Inspection yields information about size, shape, color, texture, symmetry, position, and deformities. It is the first technique of examination and begins at the outset of the client-nurse interaction. For example, inspect facial skin while collecting the history. Complete this inspection before progressing to the hands-on techniques of palpation, percussion, and auscultation.

Conduct inspection in a well-lighted setting. Uncover the body region or part sufficiently to permit complete visualization while draping the rest of the body to preserve modesty and comfort. During inspection, compare observations with the known parameters of normal findings in clients of similar age, sex, race, and ethnicity.

Inspection is enhanced with special instruments such as a penlight, oto-ophthalmoscope, and various specula (e.g., nasal and vaginal) that permit visual access to body cavities and orifices (Fig. 10-2). Other equipment includes tongue blades, a marking pen, a ruler, a tape measure, skinfold calipers, a goniometer, and eye charts.

■ PALPATION

Palpation, generally the second physical assessment technique, is the use of touch. During palpation, exert varying amounts of pressure to determine information about masses, pulsation, organ size, tenderness or pain, swelling, tissue firmness and elasticity, vibration, crepitation, temperature, texture variation, and moisture. In addition, use palpation to assess masses for position, size, shape, consistency, and mobility.

TECHNIQUE
Use the most sensitive parts of your hands and fingers to palpate specific characteristics. For example, the *fingertips* or *pads* are the most sensitive for fine touch and are used to palpate pulses, lymph nodes, and breast tissue. The *dorsum,* or back of the hand and fingers, is used to discriminate changes in skin temperature (see Fig. 48-3). Use the *palmar surface* of the hand over the metacarpophalangeal joints and the *ulnar aspect* to assess vibration of the lung with vocalization (tactile fremitus). Assess position, consistency, mobility, size, shape, and skin turgor by lightly grasping tissue between the *thumb* and *index finger.*

Facilitate palpation by positioning the client comfortably. This minimizes muscle tension and lessens the possibility of mistaking such tension for muscle rigidity. Improve client relaxation by having warm hands and short fingernails and by using a gentle approach. Encourage the client to take slow, deep breaths. Apply tactile pressure, and increase pressure gradually. Prolonged pressure decreases sensitivity in the palpating hand.

Before palpating, ask the client to indicate tender areas. Palpate tender areas last while you observe for nonverbal signs of discomfort or pain. Examine these areas, but note that this may result in client discomfort and reluctance to continue with examination.

LEVELS OF PALPATION
Palpation proceeds from light to deep (Fig. 10-3).

For *light* palpation, depress the underlying tissue approximately 1 to 2 cm (½ to ¾ inch). After light palpation, use deep palpation to determine the size and condition of underlying structures, such as abdominal organs.

For *deep* palpation, depress the underlying tissue approximately 4 to 5 cm (1½ to 2 inches), proceeding cautiously, because prolonged pressure can potentially injure internal organs. Use one or both hands (i.e., bimanual palpation).

For *bimanual* palpation, place one hand lightly on the client's skin (the sensing hand). Place the other hand (active hand) over the sensing hand to apply pressure. The sensing hand does not apply direct pressure and remains sensitive to underlying organ characteristics.

In one *variation* of bimanual palpation, one hand positions or stabilizes an organ while the other hand palpates (e.g., liver, spleen, kidney, or breast, or uterus and adnexae during gynecologic examination). Another variation involves trapping structures that move between the two hands, such as the kidney with respiration. (See also gynecologic assessment, Chapter 37.)

PRECAUTIONS
Take precautions during palpation. For example, palpate an artery so that blood flow is not obstructed. Do not

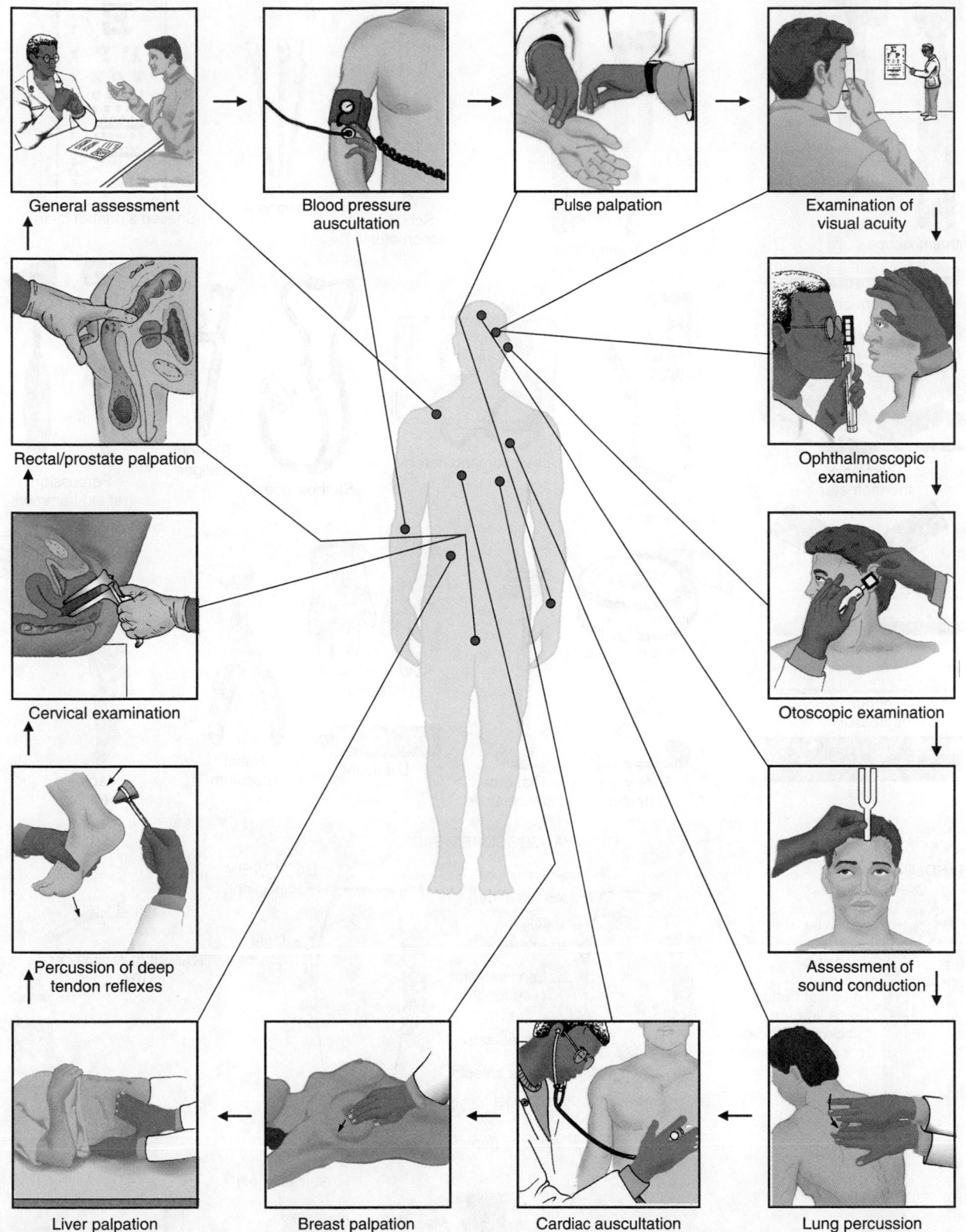

General assessment

Blood pressure auscultation

Pulse palpation

Examination of visual acuity

Rectal/prostate palpation

Ophthalmoscopic examination

Cervical examination

Otoscopic examination

Percussion of deep tendon reflexes

Assessment of sound conduction

Liver palpation

Breast palpation

Cardiac auscultation

Lung percussion

FIGURE 10–1 Common techniques of physical assessment used in a head-to-toe screening examination. The examiner wears gloves for the pelvic, rectal, and prostate examinations.

FIGURE 10–2 Instruments used in a physical examination.

176

ties. Percussion helps to confirm suspected abnormal findings from palpation and auscultation, such as a mass or consolidation in the lungs.

There are two primary methods of percussion: direct and indirect (Fig. 10–4).

Direct Percussion

Direct percussion involves striking the body surface with either one or two fingers or the fist (i.e., *blunt* percussion). Use it primarily to assess the sinuses and over the thin chest wall of a small adult or a child. Perform *blunt* percussion to elicit tenderness from an underlying structure, such as the liver or kidney, not to produce a sound. Use of a reflex hammer is another example of blunt percussion.

Indirect Percussion

TECHNIQUE

Indirect percussion involves striking an intermediary finger or hand that is placed firmly on the body's surface. Dexterity and practice are required to attain proficiency in this technique. Place the distal phalanx of the middle finger (*pleximeter*) (see Fig. 10–4) firmly on the skin surface over soft tissue. Hyperextend the remaining fingers so that only the single digit is in contact with the skin. The *plexor* must strike the pleximeter sharply and quickly; do this by relaxing the wrist, keeping the forearm stationary, and striking with the fingertip (not the pad). Errors in technique diminish (damp) the sound produced. Common errors include (1) placing the pleximeter over bone, (2) resting the palm or other fingers of the nondominant hand on the body surface, (3) losing contact between pleximeter and skin surface, (4) delivering a weak blow with the plexor, and (5) striking the pleximeter at a point other than the distal joint.

For an accurate comparison of sounds, deliver the same amount of force with each blow. A light, quick blow produces the clearest sound. The blows may be repeated rapidly two or three times to assess the sound.

TYPES OF SOUNDS

Indirect percussion results in five characteristic sounds:

1. *Flatness,* a soft, high-pitched, short sound produced by very dense tissue such as muscle. Percussion of the thigh reproduces a characteristic flat sound.
2. *Dullness,* a soft to moderately loud sound of moderate pitch and duration. It is produced by less dense, mostly fluid-filled tissue, such as the liver and spleen, and has a thudding quality.
3. *Resonance,* a moderate to loud sound of low pitch and long duration. It results from the air-filled tissue of the normal lung and has a hollow quality.
4. *Hyperresonance,* a very loud, low-pitched sound lasting longer than resonance. It is produced by the overinflated, air-filled lungs of a person with pulmonary emphysema, or it may be heard in a child's lung because of a thin chest wall. Hyperresonance has a booming quality.
5. *Tympany,* a loud, high-pitched, moderately long sound with a drum-like, musical quality. It results from enclosed, air-containing structures, such as the

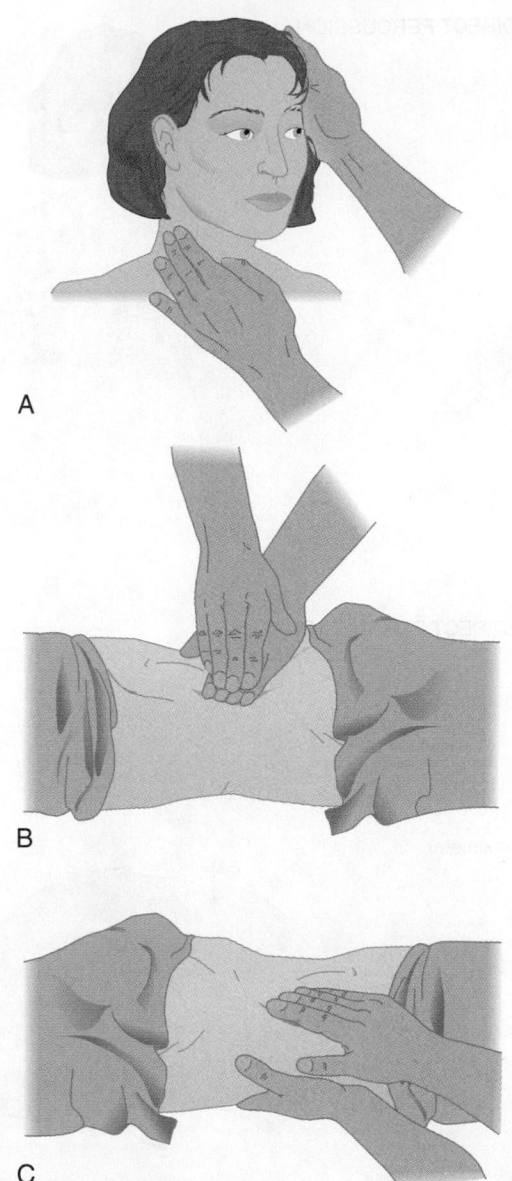

FIGURE 10–3 Palpation techniques. *A,* Light palpation employs the lightest possible pressure to assess structures under the surface of the skin, such as lymph nodes. *B,* Deep palpation is used to assess the condition of underlying organs, such as in the abdomen, using one or both hands. *C,* Bimanual palpation is used to trap and assess hard-to-palpate organs, such as the kidneys, or to stabilize an organ with one hand while the other hand palpates, as in liver palpation.

palpate the carotid arteries simultaneously because of the possibility of restricting blood flow to the brain.

■ PERCUSSION

Percussion is a technique to assess tissue density by sound produced from striking the skin. With this step, which is usually the third technique in physical assessment, 3 to 5 cm of tissue depth can be examined. Evaluate the sounds and tissue vibrations that result from percussion in relation to the underlying body structures. Percussion of body structures containing air, fluid, and solids produces various sounds, depending on their densi-

DIRECT PERCUSSION

A   B

INDIRECT PERCUSSION

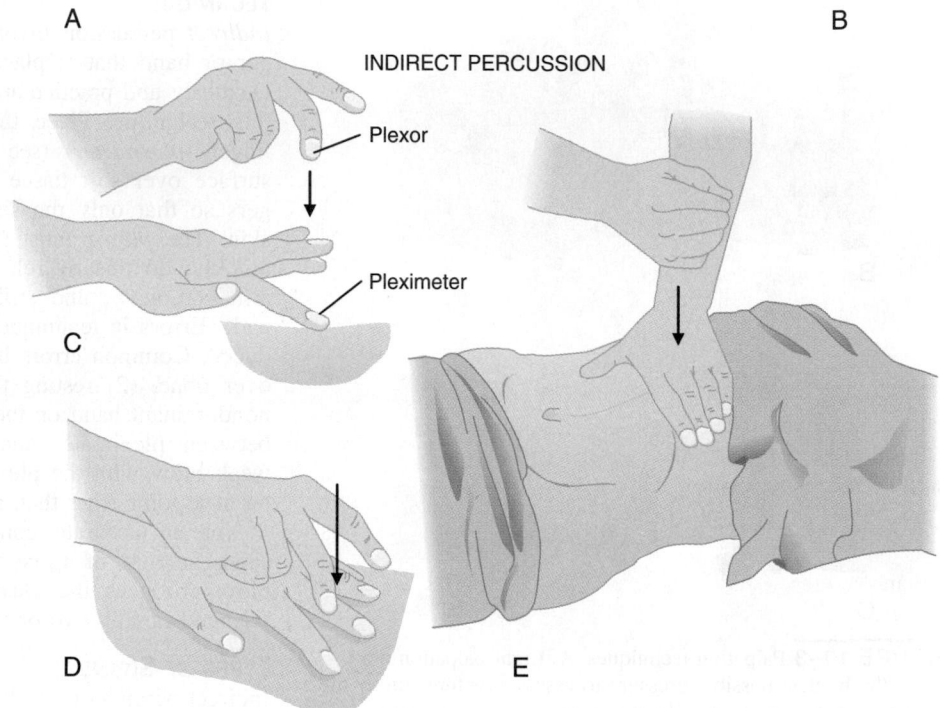

FIGURE 10–4 Techniques for the two primary types of percussion, direct and indirect. *A and B, Direct percussion. A,* Use one or two fingers to percuss directly against a body surface, such as over the sinuses, to elicit tenderness. *B,* Use the ulnar surface of your fist to gently strike the surface of the client's body over an underlying organ, such as at the costovertebral junction to assess for kidney tenderness. *C–E, Indirect percussion. C,* Place the distal phalanx of the middle finger of your nondominant hand (the pleximeter) on the client's skin over soft tissue. Bend the middle finger of your dominant hand at its distal interphalangeal joint to create a "hammer" (or plexor). *D,* Pivot the plexor down quickly in an arc to strike the pleximeter. *E,* Place the palm of your left hand over the area to be percussed. Gently strike the left hand with the ulnar surface of your right fist.

stomach (gastric bubble) and bowel. It can be reproduced by percussion over a puffed cheek.

■ AUSCULTATION

Auscultation is listening to internal body sounds to assess normal sounds and detect abnormal sounds. It is the final step in the physical examination. Use a stethoscope to enhance sounds. The sounds commonly assessed by auscultation include those produced by the heart, lungs, abdomen, and vascular system. Become proficient at auscultation by knowing which sounds are produced by each body structure and the location at which they are most readily heard. Recognizing abnormal sounds is easier once the normal sounds have been mastered.

Acute hearing ability, a reliable stethoscope, and knowing how to use the stethoscope are essential. Stethoscopes that amplify sounds are available for those who

have difficulty hearing. The basic stethoscope (Fig. 10–5) has a chestpiece with a bell and diaphragm and single or double tubing connected to double ear tubes (i.e., binaurals). A tension bar between the binaurals holds the ear pieces firmly in place and reduces kinking of the tubing.

TECHNIQUE

Hold the *diaphragm* between the index and middle fingers firmly against the skin surface; use it to hear *high-pitched* sounds, such as lung sounds, heart sounds, and blood pressure. Place the *bell* lightly in contact with the skin to hear *low-pitched* sounds, such as murmurs and bruits. Place the *chestpiece* on the skin so that it is between bones and not over them, because bone does not transmit sound. Clothing and excessive chest hair interfere with sound transmission and may introduce artifacts. Snug-fitting *earpieces* occlude the external ear canal to

FIGURE 10–5 Components of a stethoscope. The *bell* is used to listen for low-pitched sounds, such as bruits. The *diaphragm* is used to assess high-pitched sounds, such as lung sounds and sounds heard in the assessment of blood pressure.

enhance sound transmission from the chestpiece. Keep the *tubing,* no longer than 12 to 15 inches for the best sound transmission, free of contact with all surfaces to prevent extraneous noises.

A quiet environment is essential for auscultation. Close the door, and draw the cubicle curtains. If necessary, turn down the television or radio volume after informing the client about the importance of decreasing external sounds. Concentrate on the part being auscultated to determine what is causing the sounds that are heard. Once you understand the source and characteristics of normal body sounds, it is easier to recognize abnormal sounds and their origin.

TYPES OF SOUNDS

There are four characteristic auscultation sounds:

1. *Pitch,* the number or frequency of sound wave cycles per second. By varying the frequency, one may alter the pitch. For example, a high frequency results in a high-pitched sound, whereas a low frequency produces a low-pitched sound. Heart murmurs can be either high-pitched or low-pitched, depending on the structural cause. Pitch is a diagnostic clue.

2. *Intensity,* the amplitude of a sound wave. The greater the amplitude, the louder the sound; the lower the amplitude, the softer the sound.
3. *Duration,* the length of time a sound endures; it may be long, medium, or short.
4. *Quality,* a description of a sound's character, such as "gurgling," "blowing," "whistling," or "snapping."

■ OLFACTION

Olfaction is the use of the sense of smell to detect body odors. The sense of smell helps detect abnormalities not readily recognized by other means, such as inspection. For example, the smell of ammonia in urine suggests a urinary tract infection; a strong, musty odor from a casted body part suggests a wound infection under the cast; a strong, fruity breath odor indicates enhanced production of ketone by-products. Consider olfactory findings with other assessments to determine the nature of the client's health problem.

GUIDELINES FOR PHYSICAL EXAMINATION

Physical examination proceeds in a logical, orderly fashion. The approach commonly used follows a head-to-toe organization so that findings are complete. This is not an absolute rule, and the nurse who is beginning to use physical assessment skills must practice and develop a system that is comfortable to use. Once a system is developed, use it routinely to avoid inadvertently omitting portions of the examination. For a successful physical assessment, you must know both the techniques and the parameters of normal findings. Consult the following guidelines to plan and conduct a physical examination.

■ PREPARATION OF THE ENVIRONMENT

To prepare for physical examination, ensure that the environment is private, quiet, comfortable (neither too warm or too cool), and well lighted. An examination may be conducted in a special room in an office or clinic; in a client's bedroom in the home; or in the area enclosed by drawn curtains around a client's bed in a hospital room. Eliminate or control extraneous noises to enhance concentration and to encourage the client to feel free to discuss problems or concerns.

■ PREPARATION OF EQUIPMENT

Assemble all necessary equipment before beginning. Arrange equipment in order of use to facilitate examination. Practice picking up equipment, holding it in the position of use, making adjustments, assembling, and disassembling. Check equipment for adequate functioning. It is embarrassing as well as time-consuming to hunt for a replacement bulb for the oto-ophthalmoscope or to discover that the battery needs recharging in the middle of an examination.

Equipment commonly used in physical examination is shown in Figure 10–2. Additional equipment may include cotton balls, gauze sponges, a watch with a second hand, supplies for specimens, and substances to test the senses of taste and smell.

PREPARATION OF THE CLIENT

Prepare the client physically and psychologically for the physical examination. Before beginning, instruct the client to empty the bladder. If a urine specimen is needed, instruct the client in the technique for collection at this time. An empty bladder facilitates examination of the abdomen, genitalia, and rectum.

Draping

Physical preparation also includes instructing the client to dress according to the type and extent of examination to be conducted. A gown and drapes provide privacy (Fig. 10–6).

Positioning

During the examination, assist the client in assuming different positions to facilitate assessment. Figure 10–6 illustrates common positions for examination and the areas of the body that are assessed. Consider any limitations of the client that may prevent optimal positioning, such as arthritis, back injury, joint deformities, or weakness. Alternative positions may have to be assumed to complete the examination. The client may find some positions uncomfortable or embarrassing. Keep the client in these positions only as long as required and drape to prevent unnecessary exposure. Table 10–1 shows a sequence that minimizes position changes during the examination.

Psychological Preparation

Approach the client professionally and calmly. An organized, efficient approach and a relaxed tone of voice and facial expression put the client at ease and promote trust. The client may be anxious about the examination and about the possibility of finding something abnormal. Some agencies require the presence of a second staff person of the same sex as the client for examination of breasts and genitalia when the examiner is of the opposite sex. Explain what will be done before proceeding so that the client knows what to expect and cooperates to the fullest extent possible.

Explain the examination in general terms, and then provide a detailed explanation as you examine each body system. Simple terms are less confusing and less threatening than complicated explanations. Encourage the client to verbalize discomfort as the examination proceeds.

Be sensitive to the client who is uncomfortable with exposing body parts to anyone other than those who are culturally sanctioned. For example, in some cultures, a woman is restricted from revealing most of her body to a male other than her husband or immediate family. In other cultures, women are restricted from touching men other than their immediate male relatives.

Watch facial expressions and body language throughout the examination. Nonverbal communication may convey anxiety, fear, or concern. For example, the client may pull the drape closely around the body, or muscles may be tight and tense. In extreme instances, the client may wish to stop the examination and you should comply. Never coerce the client to continue. Attempt to explain the purpose of the examination and to clarify misconceptions.

PREPARATION OF THE EXAMINER

On meeting the client, begin the physical examination by focusing on appearance, movements, position, and reaction to the assessment process. Have a mental plan (assisted by an outline or checklist) so that you cover the major portions of the examination. The outline may include the general sequence, methods, equipment, and techniques needed to examine each body system.

Organization

Organization and efficiency provide a framework for a thorough physical assessment without wasting the time or energy of the nurse or client. Minimize position changes to reduce client fatigue. Use a specific piece of equipment to examine an entire region or body system. For example, use the reflex hammer to test deep tendon reflexes in quick succession, proceeding from upper to lower extremities, while the client is either seated or supine.

Sequence of Examination

The importance of organizing the physical examination systematically has already been discussed. Table 10–1 presents a suggested format for sequencing the adult general screening physical examination that integrates a head-to-toe approach incorporating regional assessments as well as each body system. Develop an individual style and approach to obtain the data necessary to diagnose the client's responses to physical problems, yet be flexible enough to accommodate individual needs.

Knowledge of Structure and Function

Anatomic landmarks are reference points for locating areas to examine and for use in recording findings. Reference to an anatomy book is recommended for the beginning practitioner in physical examination. Descriptive terms and anatomic reference points are discussed further with the examination of the respective body systems.

ADULT GENERAL SCREENING PHYSICAL EXAMINATION

GENERAL SURVEY

The general survey begins the physical examination and includes observing the overall appearance and behavior, taking vital signs, and measuring height and weight.

General Appearance and Behavior

Evaluate observations regarding general appearance and behavior in relation to the client's background (i.e., culture, educational level, socioeconomic status, current health, and illness status). Signs of problems or abnormalities direct attention to specific body areas as the examination proceeds. For example, the client who is unkempt and has obvious body odor needs thorough examination of the hair, skin, and nails for assessment of hygiene.

POSITION	AREAS EXAMINED	RATIONALE	CONTRAINDICATIONS
Sitting	Vital signs, head and neck, back, posterior and anterior thorax and lungs, breasts, axillae, heart, upper and lower extremities, reflexes	Sitting upright allows for full lung expansion and better visualization of upper body symmetry.	Elderly and weak clients may be unable to sit without support. An alternate position is supine with the head of the bed elevated.
Supine	Vital signs, head and neck, anterior thorax and lungs, breasts, axillae, heart, abdomen, extremities, peripheral pulses	This is a relaxed position for most clients. It provides access to pulse sites and prevents contracture of abdominal muscles, especially if a small pillow is placed under the knees.	Clients with cardiovascular and respiratory problems may be unable to lie flat without becoming short of breath. An alternate position is to raise the head of the bed. Clients with lower back pain may be unable to lie flat without flexing the knees.
Dorsal recumbent	Abdomen and external genitalia	Flexed knees reduce tension on lower back and abdominal muscles and increase client comfort.	Same as for supine. The client should not raise the arms over the head or clasp the hands behind the head because this increases contraction of the abdominal muscles.
Lithotomy	Female genitalia, reproductive tract, and rectum	This position maximally exposes the genitalia and facilitates the insertion of a vaginal speculum.	This position is assumed immediately before it is needed because it is embarrassing and uncomfortable. The client is kept draped. Clients with arthritis or joint deformity may be unable to assume this position. Alternate positions are dorsal recumbent and Sims'.
Sims' (posterior view)	Rectum, vagina	Flexion of the upper hip and knee improves exposure of the rectal area.	Clients with deformities of the hip or knee may be unable to assume this position. Elderly and obese clients may be uncomfortable.
Prone	Posterior thorax, hip movement, popliteal pulses	This position is used to assess hip extension. Sometimes popliteal pulse palpation is facilitated in this position.	This position is not well tolerated by the elderly or clients with cardiovascular or respiratory problems.
Knee-chest	Rectum, prostate	This position provides maximal exposure of the anal and rectal areas and facilitates insertion of instruments into the rectum.	Poorly tolerated by clients with cardiovascular or respiratory problems. Clients with difficulty flexing hips or knees may be unable to assume this position.
Standing, bent over examining table	Rectum, prostate	This is a more comfortable position than knee-chest and allows for palpation of the prostate gland.	This position is assumed immediately before it is needed because it is embarrassing. Clients with back problems may need assistance.

FIGURE 10–6 Draping and positioning the client to facilitate assessment and protect privacy.

General appearance and behavior assessments include the following.

APPARENT AGE, SEX, AND RACE. Because a client's appearance may or may not match chronologic age, direct assessment to each body system for potential problems related to aging. Other assessments are sex-specific and affect the type of procedures performed. Interpret data, and make recommendations for health teaching and further screening based on the client's health risk profile (see Chapter 9).

APPARENT STATE OF HEALTH. Assess whether the client looks "healthy," frail, or ill. Note deformities or absent body parts.

SIGNS OF DISTRESS OR DISCOMFORT. The client may display obvious signs of pain (wincing), anxiety (eyes darting around room), difficulty breathing (gasping), or other problems. Adapt the examination by including only the necessary assessments. The ideal situation is one in which the client is comfortable and in no acute distress.

BODY BUILD, HEIGHT, AND WEIGHT. Assess the client's body build for proportionate distribution of weight for height. Body build may be thin, obese, trim, or muscular, and it reflects the level of wellness, age, and lifestyle.

POSTURE. Posture may reflect mood or the presence of a physical problem. Observe the client's posture throughout the assessment process. Normal findings are an erect posture while the client is standing, with the shoulders and hips aligned over the knees and ankles. Sitting posture is with a straight back and slight rounding of the shoulders. Deviations from normal include stooping, slouching, and a curved posture. An ethnic variation may include an increased forward lumbar spine curvature (i.e., lordosis) accompanied by a forward tilt of the pelvis and abdominal protrusion.

GAIT. Observe gait as the client enters the examination room or ambulates. The gait should be smooth and coordinated as arms swing freely at the sides, in a direction opposite that of leg movement. The head and face should orient in the direction of movement. Shuffling steps and hesitancy are abnormal findings. Note devices to assist ambulation.

MOVEMENTS. Observe body movements as the examination proceeds. They are usually purposeful and controlled without tremors, tics, muscle fasciculations, signs of spasticity, or decreased muscle tone. Note immobile body parts.

DRESS. The client's manner of dress should be appropriate to the time of year, temperature, age, socioeconomic status, and current circumstances. A depressed client may wear clothing that is dull, unkempt, or mismatched. A client with a thyroid disorder may be dressed more warmly than others (hypothyroid) or may wear lightweight clothing despite a cool or cold environment (hyperthyroid).

HYGIENE AND GROOMING. Note the cleanliness of hair, nails, skin, and clothes. Does the client present a pleasant image? Consider what activity the client engaged in before the examination and whether it affects appearance.

BODY AND BREATH ODOR. Note these in relationship to activity level, such as strenuous exercise. Deficient hygiene may result in body and breath odors that are considered unpleasant or offensive. Odors include cigarette smoke, perfume, perspiration, alcohol, acetone, blood, decaying tissue, or an associated disease process.

MENTAL STATUS. Mental status includes level of consciousness, orientation, affect, speech, and thought processes. If abnormalities are noted in these areas, proceed with a full mental status assessment (see Chapters 9 and 67).

LEVEL OF COOPERATION. Assess the client's cooperation with the examination. Is the client interested, concerned, and willing to discuss information, or silent, withdrawn, hostile, angry, or suspicious? Is the client relaxed and able to engage in eye contact, or is the client tense and avoiding eye contact? Also consider cultural influences when assessing eye contact and body language. In some cultures, direct eye contact is perceived as being hostile or as dominant behavior and averted eyes are the norm when one person is talking to another person. Similarly, members of some cultural groups do not directly face a person while talking if that person is perceived as an authority figure.

Height and Weight

Measure height and weight while the client is standing. This often is done immediately after the health history interview, before the client sits on the examination table. Use a balance scale (see Fig. 10–2), which is usually very accurate. (Alternatives to the standing platform scale include bed and chair scales.) The standing scale has a telescoping ruler to measure height.

Compare height and weight with reference ranges in tables such as that developed by the Metropolitan Life Insurance Company (see Table 28–7). Weight should fall within range for sex, height, and body frame. (Determining body frame and ideal body weight is discussed in Chapter 28.) Adjust weight for clients who are missing all or part of an extremity (e.g., amputation) to account for the absent body mass using a chart or table for segmental weights.

Balance (Romberg's Test)

After measuring height and weight and before the client sits down, assess balance. Romberg's test and the test for pronation assess cerebellar function and may be done later, during the neurologic examination. Instruct the client to stand quietly with hands at the sides and feet together. Once equilibrium is attained, instruct the client to close the eyes. The client should be able to stand upright with minimal swaying and no loss of balance. Stand close by and intervene should the client begin to lose balance and fall. While standing, the client is asked to raise and extend the arms to shoulder height, then close the eyes. The client should be able to maintain the arms in extension with no downward drifting or pronation (pronation sign). (See other cerebellar assessments in Chapter 67.)

Once Romberg's test is completed, you may assess visual acuity if the eye chart is located at the correct distance from the examination table. Otherwise, test visual acuity when the eyes are examined. Instruct the cli-

MANAGEMENT AND DELEGATION

Measuring and Recording Vital Signs and Other Client Data

The measurement and recording of routine vital signs may be delegated to unlicensed assistive personnel. Delegate collection of data only when you are caring for a stable client. Emphasize the following when delegating these tasks to assistive personnel.

1. *Blood pressure.* Place the blood pressure cuff 1 to 2 inches above the antecubital fossa, with the cuff bladder overlying the brachial artery. For the leg, place the blood pressure cuff 1 to 2 inches above the popliteal space, with the cuff bladder overlying the popliteal artery. The size of the cuff should accommodate the circumference of the client's arm or leg. If the client has contraindications to blood pressure measurement on the arm or leg, inform the assistive personnel.
2. *Pulse.* Count the radial pulse for 30 seconds and multiply by 2. If the pulse seems irregular, count it for a full minute.
3. *Respiratory rate.* Count the rate of respiration without the client's being aware that it is being done. This prevents the client from consciously controlling the respiratory rate. If the respiratory rate is regular, count the rate for 30 seconds and multiply by 2. If the respiratory rate is irregular, count the rate for a full minute.
4. *Temperature.* Designate the route by which the temperature should be taken. Delay taking oral temperatures for 15 minutes if the patient has just eaten, smoked, or consumed a hot or cold liquid. If the client has dry mucous membranes and cannot hold the thermometer under the tongue with the lips closed, use the axillary, rectal, or tympanic route. If the client has contraindications to rectal temperature measurement, inform the assistive personnel.
5. *Oxygen saturation.* Designate the type of pulse oximeter sensor to be used. If a finger or toe sensor is used, you may need to remove nail polish or artificial nails. The skin at the sensor site should be clean, dry, and intact.

Findings that are immediately reportable to you, the R.N., should be described for the assistive personnel. These findings may include a blood pressure outside the range of 95/60 to 140/90 mm Hg or may be defined by the client's baseline blood pressure. For example, in a client with known controlled hypertension, a systolic reading of 140 to 170 mm Hg may be acceptable. Pulse rates less than 60 or greater than 110 beats per minute as well as any irregular pulse or inability to locate a pulse should be reported. Adult respiratory rates less than 10 or greater than 20 should be reported to you, as should any irregular respiratory rate. Temperatures outside the normal range of 97.6° to 99.4° F should be reported. An oxygen saturation level below 96% should be brought to your attention.

Even though you have delegated the collection of this information, you remain responsible for the review and interpretation of the data as well as for the full health assessment of the client. Assess cardiovascular and respiratory status daily and more frequently as the client's clinical condition warrants.

Verify the competence of the assistive personnel in performing each of these tasks during orientation and annually thereafter. Include the proper recording of the vital signs and any other client data delegated for collection.

Donna W. Markey, MSN, RN, ACNP-CS, *Clinician IV, Surgical Services, University of Virginia Health System, Charlottesville, Virginia*

ent to sit on the edge of the examination table for assessment of vital signs (see Table 10–1).

Vital Signs

Once the client is comfortably seated, measure vital signs after a brief stabilization period. Measure body temperature and blood pressure during the general survey. You may measure specific vital signs during examination of the upper extremities or heart (peripheral pulse) and thorax (respirations). A nursing fundamentals textbook would describe the techniques of vital signs measurement and equipment selection. (See Management and Delegation.)

TEMPERATURE. Oral body temperature ranges from 96.8° to 99.5° F (36° to 37.5° C), with an average of 98.6° F (37° C). Body temperatures above the normal range are *hyperthermic;* those below are *hypothermic.*

PULSE. Resting pulse rate ranges from 60 to 100 beats per minute (BPM). A rate above 100 BPM is *tachycardia;* a rate below 60 BPM is *bradycardia.* Note general characteristics of the pulse, such as rhythm (regular or irregular), amplitude (weak or bounding), and pattern. Rhythm is regular, with pulsations occurring at equal intervals, and are of similar amplitude. A slight variation in rhythm occurs with respiration and is normal. Describe *pulse amplitude* (Box 10–2) and any irregular patterns. See also Chapter 51.

RESPIRATION. Respirations range from 12 to 20 per minute. They have a regular, smooth pattern and are of consistent depth. They are quiet and effortless, without abnormal sounds such as wheezing. Respiratory depth reflects *tidal volume* (i.e., the amount of air taken in with each breath). Use the rise and fall of the chest to estimate whether respirations are shallow, moderate, or deep. Note

BOX 10–2 Pulse Amplitude

The following terms are commonly used to describe and record pulse amplitude:

Absent. The pulse is indiscernible to palpation.
Weak, thready. The pulse is difficult to palpate and easily obliterated by slight pressure.
Normal. The pulse is easily palpable and can be obliterated only with strong pressure.
Bounding. The pulse is easily palpable, forceful, and not easily obliterated by pressure.

RESPIRATORY PATTERN	DESCRIPTION

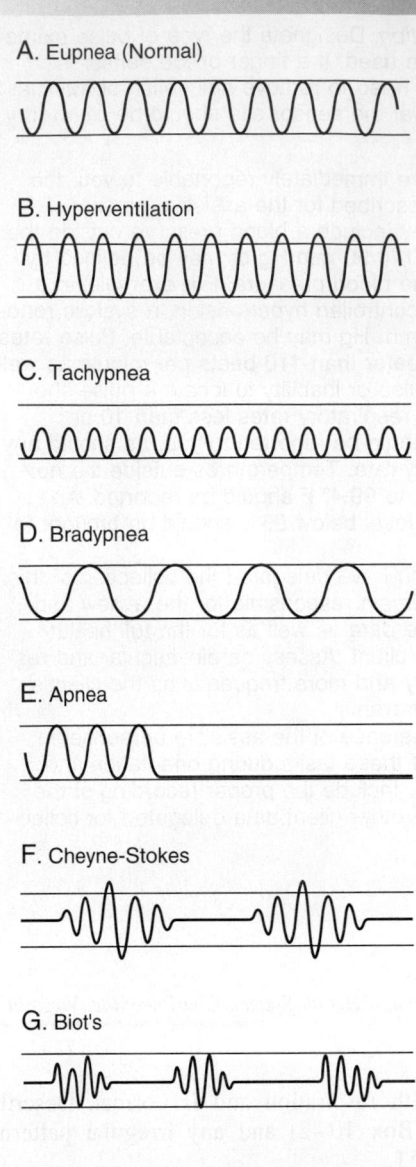

A. Eupnea (Normal)

Rate = 12 to 20 breaths per minute
Depth = Average tidal volume 350-500 mL (adults)
Rhythm = Regular, occasional sigh breath deeper
   than baseline tidal volume
I:E Ratio* = 1:2

B. Hyperventilation

Rate = May increase
Depth = Deep—large tidal volumes
Rhythm = Usually regular
I:E Ratio = Approaches 1:1
Comment = May be associated with CO_2 loss (respiratory alkalosis)

C. Tachypnea

Rate = Rapid
Depth = Shallow—small tidal volume with each breath
Rhythm = Regular
I:E Ratio = Approaches 1:1
Comment = May be associated with CO_2 retention (respiratory acidosis)

D. Bradypnea

Rate = Slow
Depth = Tidal volumes vary depending on the cause
Rhythm = Regular
I:E Ratio = 1:2

E. Apnea

Complete absence of breathing
Comment = May be temporary

F. Cheyne-Stokes

Rate = Variable
Depth = Depth of each breath varies in a cyclical pattern:
   Shallow before and after apnea, deep with hyperventilation
Rhythm = Apneic periods alternate with hyperventilation
Comment = Regular-irregular—crescendo-decrescendo pattern

G. Biot's

Rate = Variable
Depth = Depth variable—predominantly shallow
Rhythm = Unpredictable irregularity
Comment = Long periods of apnea alternate with breathing periods

H. Kussmaul's

Rate = Rapid
Depth = Deep without pauses
Rhythm = Regular
Comment = Associated with diabetic ketoacidosis

I. Apneustic

Rate = Rapid
Depth = Shallow
Comment = Prolonged inspiration followed by short,
   ineffective expiration

* Inspiration to Expiration (I:E) ratio

FIGURE 10–7 Assessing respiratory patterns.

the respiratory pattern, and record its characteristics (Fig. 10–7). See also Chapters 59 and 67.

BLOOD PRESSURE. Blood pressure varies greatly among individuals. Normal systolic pressure ranges from 100 to 140 mm Hg, and diastolic pressure ranges from 60 to 90 mm Hg. It is more accurate to evaluate consecutive blood pressure readings over time rather than make an isolated measurement for determining blood pressure abnormalities. *Hypotension* is a systolic pressure below 95 mm Hg or diastolic pressure below 60 mm Hg. *Hyper-*

tension is a systolic pressure above 140 mm Hg or diastolic pressure above 90 mm Hg. Note the difference between the systolic and diastolic pressure readings (i.e., *pulse pressure*). Report a difference of more than 40 mm Hg, which is abnormal. A slightly elevated blood pressure may be considered a normal finding in older people.

Assess blood pressure by using the bell of the stethoscope initially. Assess both arms, and compare the two readings. A pressure difference of 5 to 10 mm Hg between the two arms is insignificant. Report larger differences. Assess for an *auscultatory gap* the first time a client's blood pressure is measured. This phenomenon occurs as a period of silence between two levels of systolic pressures that may range as much as 40 mm Hg. See also Chapter 51.

Skin Color

Assess overall skin color during the health history interview, but conduct a more thorough assessment during the remainder of the examination. Observe the face and visible skin surfaces for color tones that should be congruent with the client's stated race. Abnormal findings include pallor (paleness), flushing or a ruddy complexion, cyanosis (blue cast), jaundice (yellow cast), and areas of irregular pigmentation. See also Chapter 48.

PROCESSING THE DATA

■ COMPARISON OF FINDINGS

Use the client as a "control," or self-standard, for comparison during the physical examination. Compare findings from one side of the body with those from the opposite side (*bilateral comparison*). Even though both sides of the human body are not exactly identical (i.e., symmetrical), similarities in structure and appearance are individualized and unique. Comparisons are useful and valid for findings such as a joint deformity or an extremity swelling. If a part of a limb is missing (such as from an amputation), a bilateral comparison is impractical; compare findings with a known standard.

■ COMPARISON WITH KNOWN STANDARDS

Compare physical examination findings with known parameters of "normal" for age, sex, and racial background. For example, decreased skin elasticity and loss of subcutaneous adipose tissue are expected findings for an older client but not for a 30-year-old.

■ SUSPECTED PROBLEM AREAS

Examine known or suspected problem areas carefully. Include areas identified during the health history interview as well as those predicted to be at risk based on the client's history and reactions to the physical examination. For example, thoroughly assess mouth and neck structures of the client who reports difficulty swallowing (see Chapters 28 and 42). To allay client anxiety, explain why a particular portion of the examination is more thorough.

■ HEALTH TEACHING

The physical examination process lends itself to health teaching and opportunities for providing accurate informa-

tion and correcting misconceptions. Examples include reinforcing techniques for self-examination and having the client perform a return demonstration.

TERMINATING THE HEALTH ASSESSMENT

After completing the examination, close the client's gown or allow the client to dress (assist if needed) and to assume a comfortable position. Summarize findings in understandable terms. If a serious abnormality is found, consult with the client's health care provider or refer the client to another health care professional for further assessment after explaining the general nature of the abnormality and the need for further examination.

Discard disposable, used equipment and supplies according to agency protocol. Clean or restock nondisposable equipment for future use.

RECORDING THE FINDINGS

Document physical examination findings using accurate, descriptive terms. Avoid vague, subjective terminology, such as "normal," "slight," "moderate," "healthy," or "poor," because they are easily misinterpreted. Strive to be objective, concise, clear, and thorough in the recording. However, it is better to err on the side of verbosity than to describe a significant finding vaguely or inadequately. A detailed recording is helpful as a baseline for comparison with future physical findings.

During the examination, briefly note abnormal assessment findings for later retrieval and detailed documentation. This avoids interrupting the flow of the examination to record detailed observations. After the examination, combine normal and abnormal findings in the final document.

HEALTH ASSESSMENT, NURSING DIAGNOSIS, AND NURSING PROCESS

After the collection of baseline data, which include both the health history and the physical examination results, summarize the client's health problems. Assess the client's areas of strength and health risk profile. Formalize and prioritize nursing diagnoses. Reexamine and validate the tentative diagnoses formulated after the health history interview in light of the physical examination findings.

Determine which health problems are nursing diagnoses and which are collaborative problems. Make referrals when indicated so that the client receives continuity of care and either resolution or effective management of the health problems.

CONCLUSIONS

The physical examination is the second portion of physical assessment, following the health history, in which objective data are collected through inspection, palpation, percussion, and auscultation. Once all data are collected, compare the findings with known standards and make appropriate referrals, intervene, or provide health teaching.

BIBLIOGRAPHY

1. Alfaro-LeFevre, R. (1995). *Critical thinking in nursing: A practical approach.* Philadelphia: W. B. Saunders.
2. Andrews, M. M., & Boyle, J. S. (Eds.) (1995). *Transcultural concepts in nursing care* (2nd ed.). Philadelphia: J. B. Lippincott.
3. Bates, B. (1995). *A guide to physical examination* (6th ed.). Philadelphia: J. B. Lippincott.
4. Braunwald, E. (1997). *Heart disease* (5th ed.). Philadelphia: W. B. Saunders.
5. ———— (1997). *Expert 10-minute physical examinations.* St. Louis: Mosby–Year Book.
6. Geissler, E. M. (1994). *Pocket guide to cultural assessment.* St. Louis: Mosby–Year Book.
7. Giger, J. N., & Davidhizar, R. E. (Eds.). (1995). *Transcultural nursing: Assessment and intervention* (2nd ed.). St. Louis: Mosby–Year Book.
8. Grimes, J., & Burns, E. (1996). *Health assessment in nursing practice* (4th ed.). Boston: Little, Brown.
9. Hogstel, M. O. (1996). *Practical guide to health assessment through the lifespan* (2nd ed.). Philadelphia: F. A. Davis.
10. Hurst, J. W., et al. (Eds.). (1990). *The heart* (7th ed.). New York: McGraw-Hill.
11. Iyer, P. W., Taptich, B. J., & Bernocchi-Losey, D. (1995). *Nursing process and nursing diagnosis* (3rd ed.). Philadelphia: W. B. Saunders.
12. Jacobson, N., Gift, A., & Jacox, A. (1990). Advances in physical assessment. *Nursing Clinics of North America, 25*(4), 743–833.
13. Jarvis, C. (2000). *Physical examination and health assessment* (3rd ed.). Philadelphia: W. B. Saunders.
14. Joint National Committee on Detection, Evaluation, and Treatment of High Blood Pressure. (1993). The fifth report of the Joint National Committee on detection, evaluation, and treatment of high blood pressure. *Archives of Internal Medicine, 153,* 154–188.
15. Leasia, M. S., & Monahan, F. D. (1997). *A practical guide to health assessment.* Philadelphia: W. B. Saunders.
16. Morton, P. (1994). *Quick reference to cultural assessment.* St. Louis: Mosby–Year Book.
17. Purnell, L., & Paulanka, B. (1998). *Transcultural health care: A culturally competent approach.* Philadelphia: F. A. Davis.
18. Seidel, H. M., et al. (1995). *Mosby's guide to physical examination* (3rd ed.). St. Louis: Mosby–Year Book.
19. Society of Actuaries and Association of Life Insurance Medical Directors of America. (1983). *Metropolitan Life Insurance Co. build study.* New York: Author.
20. Solomon, E. P. (1992). *Introduction to human anatomy and physiology.* Philadelphia: W. B. Saunders.
21. Strub, R. L., & Black, F. W. (1993). *The mental status examination in neurology* (3rd ed.). Philadelphia: F. A. Davis.
22. Swartz, M. H. (1997). *Textbook of physical diagnosis* (3rd ed.). Philadelphia: W. B. Saunders.
23. Thomas, C. L. (1998). *Taber's cyclopedic medical dictionary* (18th ed.). Philadelphia: F. A. Davis.
24. Weber, J. (1997). *Nurses' handbook of health assessment* (3rd ed.). Philadelphia: J. B. Lippincott.

Diagnostic Assessment

11

Annabelle M. Keene

Diagnostic assessment refers to the various tests used to detect disease and to evaluate the nature and extent of a disease, if present. During diagnostic assessment, you may have many responsibilities, ranging from preparing a client to interpreting test results to determining whether a client requires immediate medical intervention. This chapter discusses the general nursing management of clients undergoing a variety of common laboratory, imaging, endoscopic, and cytologic diagnostic tests. Specific information about individual tests is also found throughout the book.

GENERAL NURSING MANAGEMENT

■ ASSESSMENT

If your client is scheduled for a diagnostic test, you will need to assess his or her ability to participate in the test. Limitations in the client's physical condition, sensory ability, psychological condition, and functional status can all affect the successful performance of a diagnostic test. For instance, disorders of the cardiovascular or respiratory system may severely limit the client's tolerance for required position changes. Sensory limitations (such as impaired hearing or speech) or mental impairment may interfere with the client's ability to understand or carry out his or her role in accomplishing the test.

Assessment of the client's self-care ability, mobility, and nutritional status can also help you determine the client's ability to participate in diagnostic testing. Clients with impaired mobility, restricted self-care ability, or nutritional deficits may require interventions to help prepare for testing; they may need extra assistance during testing as well. If clients are agitated or unable to lie still, for instance, they may need a sedative before undergoing a lengthy imaging test. Many imaging tests require the client to lie motionless for 30 minutes or more. Similarly, for many tests, the client must have fasted for 6 to 8 hours; if the client does not follow the directions for fasting time, the test will probably need to be postponed.

■ NURSING INTERVENTIONS

Independent nursing interventions commonly needed by clients undergoing diagnostic tests include (1) preparation

---

This chapter incorporates material written by Cynthia Hromek from the fifth edition.

of the client (based in part on your assessment of the client's ability to participate), (2) collection of data, (3) collection and transport of clients and specimens, (4) monitoring of clients during diagnostic testing, and (5) supportive teaching. Naturally, it is crucial that you obtain adequate specimens (Box 11–1).

Interdependent nursing interventions commonly include (1) transcribing orders, (2) consulting with laboratory and radiology technicians, (3) sedating the client, and (4) interpreting test results to determine whether immediate action is required. Consider the underlying pathophysiologic status, current medical treatment, and laboratory result when assessing the need for immediate attention from a physician. For example, if a client's serum potassium level rises from 2.5 to 2.8 mEq/L, he has no dysrhythmias, and 80 mEq of potassium is being infused in 1 liter (L) of intravenous (IV) fluid, you may notify the physician about the potassium level during usual rounds. In contrast, if the potassium level drops from 2.5 to 2.0 mEq/L and the client has a flattened T wave and ventricular dysrhythmia, immediately notify the physician about the change in the client's status.

SPECIFICITY AND SENSITIVITY OF DIAGNOSTIC TESTS

It would be ideal if all diagnostic (or screening) tests were 100% accurate. They are not. False-positive and false-negative results occur. The concepts used to evaluate the effectiveness of a test are its specificity and its sensitivity.

Specificity is the ability of a test to correctly identify a person who is disease free. It equals the number of *true negative* results divided by the sum of true negative and false-positive results. A *false-positive* result indicates that a client has the disease or disorder being tested for when, in fact, he does not have that disease or disorder.

Sensitivity is the ability of a test to correctly identify a disease. Sensitivity equals the number of true-positive results divided by the sum of true-positive and false-negative results. A *false-negative* result indicates that a client does not have the disease or disorder being tested for when, in fact, he does have that disease or disorder.

No test is 100% specific and 100% sensitive because of (1) limitations inherent in the test and (2) various factors that can affect all tests. For example, the antinuclear antibody (ANA) test is highly sensitive for detecting systemic lupus erythematosus but is not specific because clients with rheumatoid arthritis may also have positive ANA results. The closer a test is to 100% on both counts, the more reliable its results.

MEASUREMENTS USED TO REPORT LABORATORY TEST RESULTS

■ REFERENCE VALUES

The term *reference value* (rather than "normal value") is used for reporting laboratory studies because different laboratories may produce different values. In addition, some tests (e.g., serum calcium level) have more than one accepted reference value.

Laboratory results may be influenced by several factors. The time of day, temperature, altitude, stress felt by the client, medications taken, and underlying disorder may all affect the test. When analyzing a client's laboratory test results, consider all of these influencing variables.

■ INTERNATIONAL SYSTEM OF UNITS

A comprehensive modern form of the metric system is the *International System of Units,* commonly called the *SI system* (from its French name, Système Internationale d' Unités). The SI system provides a common international language for units of measurement. The meter and kilogram are used for length and weight. Moles are used to express amounts per volume. A *mole* is the quantity of a substance in grams that is equal to its molecular weight.

Most Americans are more familiar with mass concentration units (such as milligrams) than with moles, and the United States has been slow to adopt the SI system. The rationale for changing to SI units is that biologic components react in vivo on a molar basis. Thus, moles offer a better understanding of the relative amounts of components of body fluids and of biologic processes and their interrelationships.

LABORATORY DIAGNOSTIC TESTING

Many diagnostic tests in all practice settings are performed by nurses. Some can even be delegated to assistive personnel, as discussed in the Management and Delegation feature. No matter who performs a test, its accurate outcome depends on collecting the proper specimen, in the proper manner, in the proper container, at the proper time. Anyone performing a test should:

1. Carefully follow the instructions on diagnostic test kits, and maintain the integrity of all test materials.
2. When necessary, protect the test materials from light and moisture.
3. Always check the expiration dates.

In addition to performing tests, you may be responsible for the ongoing care of portable testing equipment. Equipment requires routine maintenance, quality assurance checks, and recalibration, just as in a full-scale diagnostic laboratory. Standardized specimens should be analyzed on a routine schedule according to the agency's quality control standards and those mandated by the American Society of Pathologists and the Joint Commission on the Accreditation of Healthcare Organizations (JCAHO). The reliability of test results depends on the accuracy of procedures and equipment and the integrity of test materials.

■ MICROBIOLOGY STUDIES

Many microbiology studies can be used to identify infection-causing organisms—such as bacteria, viruses, fungi, and protozoa—and to guide treatment. Several tests can be performed to identify a specific microorganism:

1. A *smear* is a specimen that has been spread across a glass slide. It is examined under a microscope, usually after being stained.
2. A *stain* is the application of dye or a combination of dyes to help identify microorganisms. Gram's stain is a quick, commonly used method to identify general strains of bacteria by their color. Gram-positive organisms stain purple-black. Gram-negative organisms stain pink. Knowing whether a bacterium is gram-positive or gram-negative can assist in choosing an initial treatment until the specific bacterium is identified by culture.
3. A *culture* is the placement of microorganisms on culture plates to facilitate their growth. Afterward, the microorganisms can be isolated and identified. The culture process may take a few hours to several weeks, depending on the organism.

Sensitivity studies determine the type of antibiotic that will impede the growth of the organism. Small discs saturated with antibiotics are placed on the culture plate. In time, the culture is examined again. If the antibiotic stopped the growth of the microorganism, the microorganism is said to be *sensitive* to the antibiotic. If the antibiotic does not halt the growth of the microorganism, the organism is said to be *resistant* to it. Sensitivity reports typically list several antibiotics to which an organism is susceptible. The physician then chooses an appropriate treatment on the basis of cost, adverse drug effects, and so on.

Culture and sensitivity tests are commonly performed together to both identify an infecting microorganism and to determine appropriate drugs for treating it. On a physician's order, you may see these tests abbreviated as *C & S*.

Specimen collection and handling are common procedures that can raise the risk of disease transmission if they are done incorrectly. To help prevent disease transmission, wash your hands thoroughly and frequently, and wear appropriate personal protective equipment—especially gloves—whenever you could be exposed to a client's body fluids. Properly label specimens, and place in plastic containers to reduce the risk of transmission to other personnel.

Blood Cultures

Normally, blood is sterile. If bacteria enter the bloodstream, they can cause severe infections. *Bacteremia* is the term used to describe bacteria in the bloodstream. *Septicemia* is systemic disease caused by bacteria and their toxins in the blood. Blood cultures are commonly obtained for clients who have unexplained fever, a high risk of sepsis, or the appearance of being in septic shock.

To collect blood for culture, thoroughly clean the client's skin at the selected puncture site. Draw samples at specific intervals (30 minutes apart, for example) or draw a second specimen from the client's other arm. Blood samples may be examined for anaerobic or aerobic microorganisms. Ideally, blood culture specimens should be collected before antibiotic therapy begins or other blood samples are collected (if ordered at the same time).

If the client has already received an antibiotic, certain enzymes can be added to the growth medium by laboratory personnel to eliminate the activity of the antibiotic. Note on the laboratory request slip that the client is receiving an antibiotic. Once the specimen is obtained, the client should receive any prescribed antibiotics and antipyretics.

Wound Cultures

Healing is delayed in wounds that are infected. Therefore, material from inside the wound may be obtained for culture to detect and identify microorganisms in the wound. Ideally, the specimen should be collected before the client receives an antibiotic. Aseptic technique is used. Additional precautions, such as the wearing of mask, gown, and gloves, may be needed to collect specimens from draining wounds.

Culturettes (sterile, cotton-tipped applicators in special containers) are commonly used for collecting specimens for a wound culture; they should be used as follows:

1. Place the cotton tip deep into the wound without touching the surrounding skin.
2. Swab the wound where the purulent drainage is most profuse.
3. Return the applicator to the holder, and break the bottom of it to release the culture medium.

A syringe and needle can also be used to aspirate infectious material from the wound.

Note on the request slip any antibiotics the client is taking and the specific site from which the specimen was obtained. After collecting the specimen, administer any antibiotics prescribed.

Urine Cultures

Normally, urine is sterile. However, urinary tract infection (UTI) is a common disorder. Women are susceptible to UTIs because of their short urethras. In addition, nosocomial UTI is a common sequela (consequence) of indwelling catheterization. The culture test used most often to detect bacteria in the urine uses a clean-catch (or midstream) specimen. The goal of clean-catch collection is to minimize contamination of the specimen by organisms on the perineal skin. To obtain the specimen correctly, the client (1) cleans the perineum, (2) starts voiding, (3) stops voiding, (4) resumes voiding, then (5) catches the specimen in a sterile container.

As an alternative, you may need to collect a specimen

from an indwelling catheter. Urine standing in the collection bag undergoes chemical changes, may be contaminated with bacteria, and does not reflect the client's current urinary status; as a result, it should never be used as a urine specimen. Instead, obtain a specimen from the catheter or drainage tubing. Avoid opening the drainage system to air, which might introduce microorganisms. Most urinary drainage systems have a self-sealing, rubber-covered specimen collection port built into the top of the drainage tubing. Clean this area, and then aspirate the urine specimen with a sterile needle and syringe. You may need to clamp the tubing below the port for 15 to 20 minutes to allow enough urine to accumulate.

If there is no collection port and the catheter is not rubber-like silicone (Silastic), use a small 25-gauge needle and syringe to aspirate urine from the catheter itself. Using aseptic technique, insert the needle into the catheter distal to the sleeve leading to the balloon, slant the needle toward the drainage tubing, and make sure it does not enter the balloon lumen. Puncture the catheter at an angle to allow it to reseal after you withdraw the needle. This procedure cannot be performed with a Silastic catheter because it will not reseal after being punctured.

Sometimes you may need to perform a straight catheterization to obtain a urine specimen for culture. To do so, use a straight catheter of the smallest size. Insert it into the bladder under aseptic conditions, allowing urine to flow directly from the end of the catheter into the sterile specimen container. Some agencies provide special kits that include a catheter attached to a test tube. Only rarely will you obtain urine specimens by catheterization because the catheter may introduce organisms into the client's urinary tract.

■ BLOOD STUDIES

Types of blood collection methods are venipuncture, microcapillary collection, serial port sampling, and arterial blood sampling. Check your facility's laboratory procedure manual to review collection procedures, available equipment, biohazard disposal procedures, and standard precautions.

Venipuncture

The procedure for venipuncture is described in Box 11–2. Table 11–1 shows the various tubes, called Vacutainer tubes, used for drawing blood. The tubes are vacuums and fill automatically with blood. Before drawing a specimen, make sure that (1) you have the proper tube and (2) specimens from one type of tube are not mixed with those from another tube. Remember, when cells are damaged, potassium leaks and platelets migrate. A concern is that multiple venipuncture attempts or contamination with EDTA (ethylenediaminetetraacetic acid, an anticoagulant) may distort serum potassium test results. Therefore, draw specimens for potassium measurements early and consider that abnormal serum potassium readings may result from multiple punctures or contamination.

BOX 11–2 **Procedure for Venipuncture**

1. Check physician's request to verify test and time requested, client's name, and client's identification number.
2. Select materials needed: alcohol swabs, cotton or gauze swab, adhesive bandage, gloves, labels, needle, sharps container, tube holders, tourniquets, and Vacutainer tube or syringe (if using a butterfly needle).
3. Label Vacutainer tube with client's name and identification number, collection date and time, specimen source, and test.
4. Greet client, check test requested and client's name and identification number, and determine client's preparation for test. Wash your hands.
5. Place the client's arm in a position comfortable for the client and convenient for you. Support it on a firm surface. The client should be sitting or lying down.
6. Assemble the needle, needle holder, Vacutainer tube, alcohol swabs, cotton or gauze swab, and bandage. Take care not to engage the Vacutainer tube. Place any additional Vacutainer tubes in a convenient location. Use a 20- or 21-gauge, 1- to 1½-inch needle for antecubital veins.
7. Apply the tourniquet tightly enough to distend the veins but not so tightly that it cuts off circulation. Tell the client to open and close his fist several times and to keep it closed while you locate a vein. If it is difficult to locate a vein, wrap the arm in a warm compress to promote venous distention. Instead, you may use a blood pressure cuff to distend the veins; obtain a pressure between the

client's systolic and diastolic readings. Remember that a tourniquet or blood pressure cuff should never remain on the client's arm for more than 1 to 2 minutes.
8. Choose the site. Try to locate the median cubital vein. Other acceptable veins are the cephalic and basilic veins. If hand veins are selected, use a 23- or 25-gauge needle.
9. Put on gloves. Clean the venipuncture site with 70% isopropyl alcohol by making outward concentric circles. Allow the site to air-dry or wipe with sterile gauze.
10. Anchor the vein by stretching the skin below the site with your thumb. Reassure the client that any discomfort will be brief. Insert the needle bevel-up into the vein, and engage the Vacutainer tube. The needle should be at about a 15-degree angle to the client's arm and directly in line with the vein. If multiple samples are needed, remove the tube as soon as the blood flow stops and insert the next tube into the needle holder. Once good blood flow is established and before the final tube is filled, release the tourniquet.
11. Remove the last Vacutainer tube from the needle holder. Remove the needle with a swift motion, and quickly apply clean cotton or gauze over the puncture site. Apply pressure, or ask the client to apply pressure to the puncture site. Properly dispose of the needle in the sharps container. (Do not lay down or recap the needle.) Immediately label the specimen. Remove your gloves, and wash your hands. Record the client's name, the test performed, disposition of the specimen, and any condition not meeting specimen collection criteria.

Specimens for vacuum collection tubes without additives should be drawn first to prevent contamination by samples for additive-containing vacuum tubes.

A suggested sequence for blood specimen collection to prevent specimen contamination is as follows:

1. Microbiology culture specimen tubes.
2. Tubes without additives (red, speckled, or gold top).
3. Citrate-containing tubes (blue top).
4. Heparin-containing tubes (green or dark blue top).
5. EDTA-containing tubes (lavender top).
6. Oxalate/fluoride-containing tubes (gray top).

When you need to obtain blood from a superficial hand vein, use a butterfly needle (Fig. 11–1). Insert the needle and, after blood flashback is noted in the tubing, use a syringe or Vacutainer tube to withdraw blood from the vein.

Microcapillary Collection

Microcapillary blood collections may be used for a variety of purposes, including peripheral testing in clinics, for very young or very old clients, and for clients with skin disorders. The procedure for microcapillary collection is similar to that for venipuncture. The site of the skin puncture is usually the finger tip. (An ear lobe may be used for clients with edema.) No tourniquet is used.

Use the following procedure for microcapillary blood collection:

1. Hold the finger firmly.
2. Clean the area with povidone-iodine or 70% alcohol.
3. Using a microlance instead of a needle and Vacutainer tube, make a puncture perpendicular to the fingerprint lines and off the center of the finger.
4. Wipe away the first drop of blood with sterile gauze because it contains plasma, which may affect the accuracy of results.
5. Place the hand in a dependent position, and allow the next drops to flow without squeezing. A microtube or pipette may be used to collect the blood specimen.
6. After blood collection, you or the client must maintain pressure on the puncture site until the bleeding has stopped.

Serial Port Sampling

Serial port sampling refers to collection of blood specimens from an indwelling venous catheter. The advantage of this method is that it reduces client discomfort caused by multiple venipunctures. The preparation for serial port sampling is similar to that for venipuncture:

1. Stop the intravenous fluid flow.
2. After opening the stopcock or choosing the lumen, use a 10-ml syringe to aspirate 10 ml of blood from the indwelling catheter.
3. Discard the first sample.

4. Use another 10-ml syringe (or 20-ml syringe, depending on the number of tests needed) to aspirate the blood specimen needed for the study.
5. Flush the indwelling line with saline and heparin according to agency protocol.
6. Return the stopcock to the original position and adjust the intravenous fluid rate as needed.

Arterial Blood Sampling

A sample of blood is collected from an artery for blood gas analysis and, rarely, for other studies. The technique of arterial blood sampling is discussed in Chapter 59. Because this method raises a risk of bleeding and nerve injury, arterial blood sampling is performed only by staff with special training. Blood gas analysis is discussed in Chapter 14.

■ URINE STUDIES

Urinalysis

Urinalysis is one of the oldest and most common laboratory tests. It is noninvasive, the specimen is easily obtained, results are available quickly, and it is economical. It yields a large amount of information about possible disorders of the kidney and lower urinary tract as well as about systemic disorders that alter the composition of urine. Normal urinalysis results can be used to exclude a number of alternative diagnoses (Table 11–2).

Data from a urinalysis include color, specific gravity, pH, and the presence of protein, red blood cells (RBCs), white blood cells (WBCs), bacteria, leukocyte esterase, bilirubin, urobilirubin, glucose, ketones, casts, and crystals. Normal urine does not contain protein, bilirubin, urobilirubin, glucose, ketones, bacteria, or leukocyte esterase. A few RBCs, WBCs, casts, and crystals are normal (see Chapter 32).

A random-specimen urinalysis can be collected at any time. In general, an early-morning specimen gives more definitive results because the urine is concentrated and is not influenced by diet. Generally, no specific client preparation is needed. The urine should be collected in a clean container. This type of specimen cannot be used for culture and sensitivity tests because neither the container nor the collection technique is sterile.

12- or 24-Hour Urine Collection

A timed collection of urine allows for quantitative analysis of specific substances and, because the specimen is collected over time, is more accurate than a random one-time specimen. A 12- or 24-hour specimen is usually collected in one large container. The procedure may require a chemical preservative in the container and refrigeration during the collection process. If appropriate refrigeration is not available, the specimen container may be placed in ice or in insulated ice packs; in this case, make sure the cooling agent is replaced frequently to maintain the specimen at the necessary temperature. Furthermore, if the client has an indwelling catheter, the bag can be placed on ice to collect a 24-hour specimen.

TABLE 11–1	TUBES USED FOR VENIPUNCTURE			
Stopper Color	Principal Anticoagulant/Additive	Mode of Action	Commonly Used for	
Red	None Clot activator and gel separator	None Enhances clot formation	Cell/blood typing Serum blood group antibody testing Alkaline phosphatase Amylase Blood urea nitrogen (BUN) Creatine phosphokinase (CPK) Calcium Cholesterol	
Speckled			Compatibility testing Drug monitoring Glucose High-density lipoprotein (HDL) Human immunodeficiency virus (HIV) Iron profile Low-density lipoprotein (LDL)	
Gold (Hemoguard)			Liver enzymes Potassium Protein Rapid plasma reagin (RPR) Sodium Triglycerides	
Lavender	Ethylenediaminetetraacetic acid (EDTA)	Binds calcium	Complete blood count (CBC) Erythrocyte sedimentation rate (ESR) Hemoglobin electrophoresis Platelet count Reticulocyte count Sickle cell screen White blood cell differential	

When specimen collection begins, the client voids (or the urine collection bag is emptied) and this specimen is discarded. All urine voided over the next 12 or 24 hours, as appropriate, is placed in the container. After 12 or 24 hours from the time of the first voiding, instruct the client to void again (or empty the urine collection bag) and add this urine to the specimen. One of the major requirements during this collection process is careful communication among all persons involved. If any single urine specimen is inadvertently discarded, the entire procedure must begin anew. The client should also be instructed to moderately limit the amount of fluids consumed and to avoid alcohol. Other specific instructions may be needed, such as avoiding certain foods or medications.

DIAGNOSTIC IMAGING

Imaging refers to representations produced by radiography (x-rays), nuclear magnetic resonance, tomograms, ultrasound, radioisotopes, and so forth. Methods range from simple x-ray studies to very complex and expensive imaging using magnetic fields and radiowaves. Review the protocol to be followed at your facility, especially the

guidelines for preparation and follow-up care. You may need to consult with the imaging (radiology) department to obtain written guidelines for preparation and postimaging care, or to coordinate studies. For example, barium studies may make visualization for other abdominal tests impossible for up to 2 days.

Explain the procedure to the client and family and answer their questions. Many procedures may take up to an hour (follow-up x-rays are sometimes taken 30 minutes after an injection). Suggest that the client void before the procedure, unless the bladder must be full for the procedure.

■ X-RAY STUDIES
PROCEDURE
Radiography is the most widely used diagnostic procedure for the study of soft tissues and bones. A radiograph, commonly called an "x-ray," is an image of a negative on photographic film made by exposing the film to x-rays that have passed through the body. The energy of the x-rays is adjusted by varying the voltage in the x-ray tube. Because each part of the body absorbs some of the x-rays, variable amounts of exposure are needed for optimal results, depending on the body part being examined.

TABLE 11–1	TUBES USED FOR VENIPUNCTURE *Continued*		
Stopper Color	**Principal Anticoagulant/Additive**	**Mode of Action**	**Commonly Used for**
Blue	Sodium citrate	Binds calcium	Activated partial thromboplastin time (aPTT) Individual coagulation factor studies Fibrin degradation products (FDPs) Fibrinogen Prothrombin time (PT)
Green	Heparin	Inactivates thrombin and thromboplastin	Ammonia Chromosome screening Lupus erythematosus cell, preparation HLA typing
Gray	Potassium oxalate/sodium fluoride	Binds calcium Inhibits glycolysis	Glucose
Dark or royal blue	Heparin	Inactivates thrombin and thromboplastin	Trace metals (e.g., lead)

From Flynn, J. C., Jr. (1994). *Procedures in phlebotomy.* Philadelphia: W. B. Saunders.

Tissue is called *radiopaque* when transmission of x-rays is partially blocked, such as by bone. Bone appears white on x-ray film. Tissues are said to be *radiolucent* when they allow x-rays to penetrate. Lung is translucent and therefore appears dark on x-ray film. The images on x-ray films are two-dimensional, so that multiple views are often needed, such as anteroposterior (AP, front to back), posteroanterior (PA, back to front), lateral (LAT, from the side), or oblique (OBL, at an angle). It is impor-

FIGURE 11–1 A butterfly needle used for venipuncture. (From Flynn, J. C., Jr. [1994]. *Procedures in phlebotomy.* Philadelphia: W. B. Saunders.)

TABLE 11–2	NORMAL FINDINGS IN A ROUTINE URINALYSIS
Component	**Normal Values**
Color	Pale yellow to deep amber
Opacity	Clear
Specific gravity	1.002–1.035
Osmolality	275–295 mOsm/L
pH	4.5–8.0
Glucose	Negative
Ketones	Negative
Protein	Negative
Bilirubin	Negative
Red blood cells	None to 3
White blood cells	None to 4
Bacteria	None
Casts	None
Crystals	None

tant to note the position of the view of an x-ray for proper interpretation; this information is usually recorded by the x-ray technician.

X-ray examinations are important to (1) establish the presence of a mobility or structural problem, (2) follow its progress, and (3) evaluate the effectiveness of treatment. Features shown by an x-ray can help diagnose a suspected problem; for example:

- A radiopaque (rather than radiolucent) area in the lung, which may mean pulmonary edema, pneumonia, or a tumor (Fig. 11–2)
- Alterations in normal contour or density of bones, as in fractures or osteoporosis (Fig. 11–3)
- Changes in fat lines around soft tissues (e.g., with tumor or inflammation present, fat tissue is replaced by soft tissues)
- Enlargement in shadows produced by organs (e.g., an enlarged heart shadow possibly meaning an enlarged heart from heart failure or athletic activity)

Two potential risks from repeated exposure to radiation are genetic and somatic. The *genetic risk* involves changes in the chromosomes. If a developing (first-trimester) fetus is exposed to radiation, the chromosomes can mutate and the baby can be born with deformities; the eggs and sperm can be damaged by radiation, which may lead to deformities in future offspring.

Somatic changes occur in body tissues that receive excessive or repeated doses of radiation. The risks from radiation exposure are cumulative and therefore are poten-

FIGURE 11–3 An x-ray showing a hip fracture.

tially more dangerous to health care personnel than to clients. Side effects of the use of radiation for cancer treatment are discussed in Chapter 19.

Several safety measures are used to avoid exposure to x-rays. The walls in rooms in which x-ray machines are located are lined with lead. Lead-lined protection, such as aprons, eyeglasses, and thyroid shields, are used by imaging personnel. Maintaining adequate distance is also important, and x-ray rooms have a protective divider for the technician. When x-rays are taken outside the radiology department, less protection may be available. If you must remain with a client during x-ray exposure, wear a lead apron. Other personnel should step outside the room during the exposure. Clients are given lead aprons to shield their reproductive organs (gonads). Radiology personnel also wear a film badge to monitor accidental exposure.

PREPROCEDURE CARE

Before the x-ray procedure, ask the client to remove any radiopaque objects (such as jewelry, belts, or metal buttons) and to wear a gown. Additional preparation depends on the type of study. The client may be asked to move into various positions, if possible, so that x-ray films can be taken from the most useful angles.

Because various positions may be difficult or painful and x-ray tables are hard, the client may need analgesia and other pain-relieving interventions before and after the x-ray study. Nursing care for the client having diagnostic imaging studies focuses on client preparation and follow-up care.

Occasionally, you may be asked to monitor an unstable client during an imaging procedure. You will need an oximetry monitor, sphygmomanometer to measure blood pressure, stethoscope, extra intravenous fluids, and an emergency cart. Note pertinent findings—such as the presence of a pacemaker or an artificial joint—on the x-ray request.

POSTPROCEDURE CARE

Although no specific care is usually needed after an x-ray procedure, in some instances specific postprocedure care is needed. See headings corresponding to the specific x-ray procedures.

FIGURE 11–2 A chest x-ray showing right middle lobe pneumonia. The consolidation of lung tissue makes the area appear radiopaque.

Chest X-rays

Chest x-rays may be taken to detect pulmonary disease and the status of respiratory problems or trauma and to confirm the placement of an endotracheal or tracheostomy tube. Complete details are presented in Chapter 59. There is no specific follow-up care.

Plain Abdominal Films

A plain abdominal film—known as a *flat plate* or a KUB, which stands for *k*idney, *u*reter, *b*ladder—can reveal such abnormalities as tumors, obstructions, abnormal gas collections, and strictures. No follow-up care is needed for this study.

Skeletal X-rays

When fractures are suspected, x-rays are ordered for the bones in question. Generally, the procedure is not painful unless the extremity has to be moved for positioning. Examples of some x-ray projections are:

- Waters' projection, which is a posteroanterior view of the skull to show the orbits and maxillary sinuses. If the client may have a cervical spine fracture, the physician will order a lateral cervical spine x-ray instead.
- Towne's projection, which is an anteroposterior view to demonstrate the occipital bone and facial structures, such as the zygomatic arch.
- Panoramic (sometimes called Panorex, from the name of a machine used to take panoramic x-rays), a 180-degree view of the teeth and jaw.

Fluoroscopy

Fluoroscopy is a radiographic technique that permits direct observation of the body. The body part under examination is positioned between an x-ray tube and a fluorescent screen. X-rays pass through the body and project the targeted organs or bones onto the fluoroscopic screen as visual images. The benefit of fluoroscopy is that joint actions, organs, and entire body systems can be observed directly and dynamically (as they move). Radiopaque and radiolucent media enhance visualization.

Fluoroscopy can be used to monitor the progress of other diagnostic studies. For example, the progress of a radiopaque catheter can be observed as it is threaded through an artery or vein; or the progress of radiopaque barium can be seen as it is swallowed and moves through the gastrointestinal (GI) tract.

Tomography

Tomography is a radiographic technique that produces images of body tissues in a single plane or slice. Sequential images are obtained by moving the x-ray tube as it projects views at varying levels of tissue depth. Tomograms can be static body-section radiographs or can be combined with reconstruction tomography, as in computed tomography (CT) and positron emission tomography (PET), which are discussed later in this chapter.

Contrast X-rays

Contrast studies use radiopaque media to enhance visualization of an organ system or tissue under study. Contrast media include barium (a radiopaque contrast medium) and various dyes.

UPPER GASTROINTESTINAL SERIES

An upper GI series, also known as a *barium swallow,* permits radiologic visualization of the esophagus, stomach, and duodenum using fluoroscopy. It can aid in the detection of strictures, ulcers, tumors, polyps, hiatal hernias, and motility problems. A detailed discussion of the upper GI series and related client care is found in Chapter 28.

LOWER GASTROINTESTINAL SERIES

A lower GI series, which requires a barium enema, is performed to visualize the position, movements, and filling of the colon. Barium is instilled rectally, and x-rays are taken with or without fluoroscopy. This test can aid in detecting tumors, diverticula, stenoses, obstructions, inflammation, ulcerative colitis, and polyps. See Chapter 32 for a detailed discussion of this procedure and related client care.

Computed Tomography

PROCEDURE

Computed tomography scans highlight differences in bone and soft tissue. The images are generated by computerized synthesis of x-ray data obtained in many different directions in a cross-sectional plane or slice. The computed data are assembled as three-dimensional images. CT is used to identify space-occupying lesions (masses) and shifts of structures caused by neoplasms, cysts, focal inflammatory lesions, and abscesses of the head, chest, abdomen, pelvis, and extremities (Fig. 11–4). To distinguish normal tissue from abnormal masses, a contrast

FIGURE 11–4 A computed tomography scan of the head. The brain tissue is gray, and the skull is white. The mass in the left frontal lobe is blood from a head injury.

medium (dye) may be administered. The CT scan can be performed quickly, within 20 minutes, not including analysis.

PREPROCEDURE CARE

Before a CT scan, make sure that the client has given informed consent and answer any questions the client and family may have about the procedure. Explain that fasting usually is not required for a CT scan of the head, but ask whether or not the client becomes nauseated easily; if so, adjust food and fluid intake accordingly. For example, some clients prefer a light breakfast to reduce nausea and others prefer an empty stomach. Fasting is usually required for a CT scan of the abdomen. Explain that a contrast agent is commonly given. Because the contrast material is iodine-based, ask whether the client has allergies to iodine or contrast dyes (Box 11–3).

If the CT scan will be of the client's head, remove any objects from the hair (wigs, barrettes, earrings, hair pins) before the test begins. The client's hair should be combed smooth.

Explain the client's role during the scan. The client is positioned supine, and the body part to be scanned is placed into the doughnut-shaped ring of the scanner. The technician moves the table from a control room during the scan to direct the study to different areas. The client should expect to hear mechanical noises coming from the scanner. Some clients may feel claustrophobic during the test, but assure them that it is possible to communicate with the technician during the scan.

Emphasize that the client must remain still during the scan. If the client is unable to comply, sedation or even general anesthesia may be required. If sedation is needed, tell the client to (1) avoid alcohol and caffeine on the day of the scan, (2) avoid eating for 2 hours before the scan, (3) arrange for someone to drive him home after the scan, and (4) avoid driving for at least 12 hours.

POSTPROCEDURE CARE

After the test, assess the client for reactions to the contrast agent, for hematoma at the injection site, and for the quality of pulses in the limb used for injection of the contrast agent. The client may resume normal activities unless additional diagnostic tests are planned. Tell the client to expect to experience diuresis from the dye. Encourage the client to drink plenty of fluids to flush the dye and prevent nephrotoxic injury.

■ MAGNETIC RESONANCE IMAGING

PROCEDURE

Magnetic resonance imaging (MRI) is a noninvasive imaging test that uses powerful magnetic fields and radiofrequency pulses to produce the image; therefore, the client is not exposed to ionizing radiation. The magnet in the scanner is 30,000 times more powerful than the earth's magnetic field. Consequently, this test cannot be performed if clients have pacemakers, metal implants, some types of ventilators, or embedded metal fragments, such as shrapnel. The powerful magnet may move these objects inside the client's body or may interfere with their

---

BOX 11–3   Use of Contrast Agents

Certain disorders, such as tumors, are better visualized with the use of a contrast agent. Other disorders, such as bleeding and edema, can be seen better without a contrast agent. The use of contrast agents is potentially dangerous. They may irritate blood vessels, and some clients may have allergic reactions to them that, if untreated, may develop into anaphylactic shock.

Preprocedure Care

Before a test involving a contrast agent, ask the client whether he has ever had an allergic reaction to contrast dye or iodine. Note the type of allergic response on the record; for example, "Client states that he developed hives when a dye was injected for another test." Some clients report allergies, but when asked to explain the reaction, they state that they "feel warm" when given the dye. This is a normal reaction, not an allergic one.

Some clients are given contrast agents even though they report contrast allergy. To reduce the severity of the reaction, these clients are pretreated with an antihistamine or corticosteroids. Therefore, do not assure the client with a reported allergy to dye that a contrast agent will not be given. Even if the client says that he has no history of allergy, watch for symptoms of an allergic reaction after injection of contrast agent. Some anaphylactic reactions have occurred with the first dose of dye. Tell the client that it is normal to feel a hot, flushed sensation and metallic taste in the mouth when the dye is injected. Tell the client to report any difficulty breathing or itching to staff in the radiology department.

Postprocedure Care

After the procedure, the client can usually resume normal activities. Diuresis will occur shortly after the use of a contrast agent. If the client is able to do so, encourage drinking at least one glass of water or other liquid an hour after the procedure. Replacement fluid may be needed, and the client should be assessed for fluid balance. The fluid balance in clients with renal or cardiac disease should be assessed carefully after a series of tests requiring intravenous contrast agents.

Complications

Complications rarely occur with the use of contrast agents but include local and systemic allergic reactions, spasm, occlusion of the vessel by a clot, and bleeding at the injection site. Assess the affected limb for color, warmth, pulses distal to the injection site, bleeding or hematoma formation, and mobility.

Assess the client for clinical manifestations of an allergic reaction, which include pallor, tachycardia, restlessness, sneezing, coughing, erythema, tachypnea, respiratory distress, facial flushing, urticaria, pruritus, hypotension, nausea, vomiting, headache, convulsions, flank pain, hematuria, and oliguria. Assess for these reactions after the dye is injected, because clients have experienced respiratory or cardiac arrest while undergoing x-ray study. Emergency equipment should always be available.

FIGURE 11–5 Magnetic resonance imaging of the head. The eyes are evident at the top of the image. The client has a brain tumor.

function. MRIs also are not performed for pregnant clients.

When looking at an MRI, remember that the image is opposite to that of a CT scan: Bone appears black on an MRI and white on a CT scan (Fig. 11–5). A contrast agent may be used to augment the images.

PREPROCEDURE CARE
Explain to the client and family the purpose of the MRI, the sounds and sensations that the client will hear and feel during the examination, and the client's role during the test. Obtain an informed consent.

Before the test, the client should remove all metal-containing objects (brassiere, jewelry, watch, and so on). Note the presence of any internal metal objects, such as a prosthesis or pacemaker, for the physician. Intravenous fluid pumps need to be removed during the test. Special MRI-compatible monitoring devices, such as pulse oximeters and electrocardiogram (ECG) leads, can be used.

The client can eat normally and take any prescribed medication before an MRI of the head. When the scan involves the GI system, the client must fast for 6 hours before the procedure. Explain that he must lie still during the procedure, which can take from 60 to 90 minutes. Clients who are agitated or unable to remain motionless may require sedation before the scan (see instructions for CT). If the use of a contrast agent is planned, ask whether the client tends to become nauseated easily, and adjust the intake of food and fluids accordingly.

The client lies supine on a narrow padded table. Because the scanner makes loud clanging noises, the client should wear earplugs or headphones. Some clients may feel claustrophobic during the test; assure them it is possible to communicate with the technician during the scan.

POSTPROCEDURE CARE
After the test, the client may resume previous activities and diet. Tell the client to expect to experience diuresis if a contrast agent was used for the MRI (see instructions for CT).

■ POSITRON EMISSION TOMOGRAPHY
PROCEDURE
Positron emission tomography (PET) scanning produces images of metabolic and physiologic function. PET scans have diagnostic value because the function of diseased tissue commonly differs from that of normal tissues. The client is given doses of strong radioactive tracers (*radionuclides*), which emit signals to show the uptake and distribution of the traces. The images are formed by computer analysis of photons detected by annihilation of positrons emitted by the radionuclides (Fig. 11–6). PET has three primary uses:

• To determine the amount of blood flowing into specific body tissues
• To reveal how adequately tissues use blood receptors, such as medications and neurotransmitters
• To measure blood flow, glucose metabolism, and oxygen extraction

PET is used in the diagnosis of stroke, brain tumors, and epilepsy and to chart the progress of Alzheimer's disease, Parkinson's disease, head injury, schizophrenia, bipolar disorder, and cardiac hypoxemia.

PREPROCEDURE CARE
Explain to the client and family the purpose of the test, the sounds and sensations that the client will hear and feel during the examination, and the client's role during the test. Obtain an informed consent. In contrast to CT and MRI machines, the PET scanner is quiet. The client should fast for 4 hours before the scan. If the client is diabetic, it is preferred that the blood glucose be below 150 g/dl. The client must remain motionless for about 45

FIGURE 11–6 A positron emission tomographic scan showing decreased metabolic activity after a seizure (noted as green areas on the scan).

FIGURE 11–7 Coronary angiography shows stenosis, or narrowing (*arrow*), of the left anterior descending coronary artery. (From Braunwald, E. [1992]. *Heart disease: A textbook of cardiovascular medicine* [4th ed.]. Philadelphia: W. B. Saunders.)

minutes. An agitated client may require sedation. (See instructions for sedation under CT Preprocedure Care earlier.)

POSTPROCEDURE CARE
No special care is required after a PET procedure.

■ ANGIOGRAPHY
PROCEDURE
Angiography is a radiographic technique that uses a contrast agent to assess blood vessels and the blood flowing through them. A common form of angiography is coronary angiography, which is performed to determine the degree of obstruction in the myocardial circulation (Fig. 11–7). Angiography can also be used to outline veins (*venography*) or lymphatic vessels (*lymphography*). The terms *angiogram* and *arteriogram* are used interchangeably in practice.

PREPROCEDURE CARE
Before angiography, make sure the client understands the planned procedure and has given informed consent. Note any known allergies to contrast agents or iodine. Collect baseline assessment data: vital signs, quality and symmetry of pulses in the limbs, level of consciousness, speech patterns, and estimates of limb strength. The same assessments are made after the procedure. *A detailed baseline is crucial to accurate assessment of postprocedure changes.*

In most facilities, the client is given nothing by mouth for 6 to 8 hours before angiography. Some facilities allow fluids to reduce the risk of dehydration and clotting. Follow your facility's protocol. The planned puncture site may be shaved.

POSTPROCEDURE CARE
Decreased perfusion of the distal limb from hemorrhage or hematoma at the puncture site and an allergic reaction to the contrast agent are the two major complications that can develop after angiography. Assessment is crucial to their early detection. Follow your facility's protocol for

postprocedure care. Usually, it consists of the following steps:

1. If the femoral approach was used, keep the leg immobile; tell the client not to flex the hip or leg for 12 hours. If the brachial approach was used, release the pressure dressing and apply an elastic bandage to the client's arm; the arm must remain straight. Movement of the limb can dislodge the clot at the puncture site and result in bleeding.
2. Monitor the client's vital signs every 15 minutes for 2 hours, then hourly until stable. Review the signs of an allergic reaction (see Box 11–3).
3. Keep a sandbag on a femoral puncture site to maintain pressure on the site. Check puncture sites every 15 minutes for 2 hours, then hourly.
4. Monitor distal pulses every 15 minutes for 2 hours, then hourly until stable. Assess the quality of the pulses and note capillary filling time. Notify the physician if the quality of the pulse changes.
5. Expect diuresis, provide ample fluids, and keep a urinal or bedpan nearby.
6. Resume medications, if prescribed, and the client's usual diet.

■ ULTRASONOGRAPHY
PROCEDURE
Ultrasonography (also called *ultrasound* or *echography*) uses high-frequency sound waves to depict soft tissues. Ultrasonography works on the same principle as sonar and radar. When the ultrasound waves are directed into the body, they spread through the tissues. Because tissues differ in density, the sound waves are reflected (bounced back) in various ways in different tissues. The reflected waves are processed, shown as an image, and then recorded.

Ultrasound can be used to assess many structures in the body, including the heart, great vessels, liver, gallbladder, pancreas, breast, uterus and ovaries, scrotum, kidney, and thyroid gland (Fig. 11–8). It is commonly

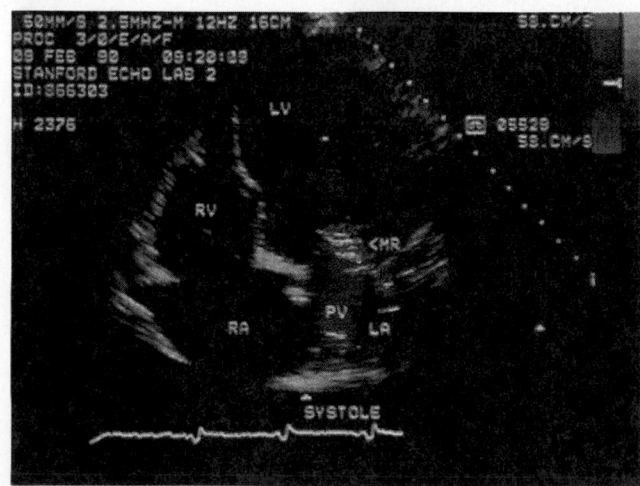

FIGURE 11–8 An ultrasound image of the heart, also known as an echocardiogram. (From Bennett, J. C., & Plum, F. [1996]. *Cecil textbook of medicine* [20th ed.]. Philadelphia: W. B. Saunders.)

used in obstetrics to determine gestational age. There is no exposure to ionizing radiation during this test, and it is noninvasive.

PREPROCEDURE CARE

No special care is required before ultrasonography. Tell the client the purpose of the test and what to expect. A gel is applied to the skin, and a transducer (a device that changes reflected high-frequency sound to electrical energy) is moved on the skin surface above the organ. The procedure is painless and fairly quick.

Sometimes a bowel preparation with laxatives is used for viewing the abdominal organs. The bladder must be very full for the uterus to be viewed. Sometimes the lighting must be dimmed for the oscilloscope to be seen.

POSTPROCEDURE CARE

No special care is required after an ultrasound study.

■ RADIONUCLIDE IMAGING

PROCEDURE

Radionuclides are radioisotopes (radioactive forms of some elements) or tracers that are used to visualize organs or regions that cannot be seen on plain films. Radioisotopes are treated the same as normal elements by living cells. Their radiation can be detected by suitable counters. Radionuclide studies may be used to diagnose disorders of the heart, thyroid, liver, brain, bone, kidney, spleen, pancreas, lung, and gallbladder.

Various isotopes are used because they concentrate in one organ or body fluid. For example, thallium concentrates in the heart, whereas iodine concentrates in the thyroid. An artificial radioactive element (technetium) is used extensively. Technetium emits gamma radiation only and therefore is safer than other isotopes that emit more damaging radiation. When combined with pyrophosphate given intravenously, technetium is taken up by bone and the entire skeleton can be surveyed. This technique is helpful in detecting bone tumors (Fig. 11–9). When combined with albumin, technetium concentrates in the lung and can be used to estimate pulmonary blood flow. It can also be used to investigate lesions in other organs and has largely replaced radioactive iodine for thyroid assessment.

Depending on the intended diagnostic purpose, a blocking agent may be administered before the radionuclide to prevent uptake by certain tissues. The blocking agent is not radioactive. For example, iodine is normally concentrated in the thyroid gland. When iodine-tagged radionuclides are used other than in thyroid studies, Lugol's solution is given to block the uptake of iodine-tagged radionuclides by the thyroid.

The radionuclide is administered orally or intravenously about 1 to 3 hours before the test to allow time for distribution. During this time, have the client drink extra fluids to clear the portion not taken up by the tissues. After the waiting period, the client is placed on a table and an imaging device records the activity of the emitted radiation.

Radioactivity may be increased or decreased in comparison with normal activity in the organ. Areas of decreased activity, called *cold-spot imaging,* usually indicate tissues that are functioning improperly. This is common when normal tissues have been replaced by tumor. Increased activity, called *hot-spot imaging,* may occur in

FIGURE 11–9 A technetium scan of the skeleton shows an area of increased radionuclide density on the right tibia that is a bone tumor. (From Walter, J. B. [1992]. *An introduction to the principles of disease* [3rd ed.]. Philadelphia: W. B. Saunders.)

tissues that are metabolically more active. For example, a diseased thyroid gland or bone infection may be detected by hot-spot imaging.

PREPROCEDURE CARE

Tell the client that the radionuclide contains very little radioactivity. If an abdominal scan is scheduled, the client may need an enema first. Make sure that the radionuclide test is scheduled before any tests that use iodinated contrast agents or barium. These substances block the exit of protons from radionuclides. This is especially important with radioactive iodine thyroid scans. The use of contrast agents for other studies can block uptake of radioactive iodine for months. Obtain an informed consent.

Obtain the following information from the client:

- Age, weight, and height to calculate the amount of radioactive substance to be used

- Menstrual history to rule out pregnancy (pregnancy is a contraindication to many radionuclide studies)
- Whether the client is breast-feeding (breast-feeding is a contraindication to many radionuclide studies)
- A history of allergy
- Recent exposure to radionuclides
- Presence of internal prostheses that could block the view of the organ
- Current treatments, such as the need for oxygen, telemetry, or timed specimen collections

POSTPROCEDURE CARE

Tell the client to drink extra fluids; otherwise, no special care is required.

FIGURE 11–10 An endoscopic view of the esophagus showing an esophageal ulcer.

ENDOSCOPY

Endoscopy is direct visualization of a body system or part by means of a lighted, flexible tube. This method is more accurate than radiologic examination because the physician can directly observe sources of bleeding and surface lesions and can determine the status of healing tissues. Arthroscopy, bronchoscopy, and gastrointestinal endoscopy are examples of this type of diagnostic technique.

Endoscopic procedures require a signed consent. Provide complete client education to enhance cooperation. Tell the client not to drive a motor vehicle for at least 12 hours after endoscopy if sedation was used during the procedure. (See earlier instructions for sedation.)

■ ARTHROSCOPY

Arthroscopy is an endoscopic examination of a joint. An arthroscope is a thin fiberoptic instrument that allows examination of various joints without need for a large incision. Biopsy specimens can be taken, articular cartilage abnormalities assessed, loose bodies removed, and cartilage trimmed. Further discussion of arthroscopy is found in Chapter 25.

■ BRONCHOSCOPY

Bronchoscopy is the passage of a lighted bronchoscope, either rigid or flexible, into the bronchial tree for diagnostic or therapeutic purposes. This procedure is covered in Chapter 59.

■ ENDOSCOPY OF THE GASTROINTESTINAL TRACT

Endoscopy of the upper GI tract consists of esophagoscopy and esophagogastroduodenoscopy (Fig. 11–10). These procedures are useful for assessing acute or chronic GI bleeding, pernicious anemia, esophageal injury, dysphagia, substernal pain, and epigastric discomfort (see Chapter 28). Endoscopy of the lower GI tract consists of proctosigmoidoscopy and colonoscopy (see Chapter 32).

CYTOLOGIC STUDIES

Cytology is the study of the anatomy, physiology, pathology, and chemistry of the cell. One of the most common cytologic studies is a staining technique developed by George Papanicolaou—the *Pap test,* which is used to detect malignant cells. Usually, this test is used to study vaginal or cervical cells. Sometimes it may be used for other tissues obtained easily by smearing or scraping, such as the mouth, genital tract, or anus.

Tissues not available for scraping must be obtained by *biopsy,* which is the removal of tissue for diagnostic study. The tissue removed must be (1) representative of the tissue in question, (2) large enough to be examined, and (3) kept intact until studied. Many times a fixative or refrigeration is used to prevent tissue decomposition. Some tissues are not placed in fixative, such as breast tissue to be analyzed for hormones.

Biopsy procedures are either closed or open.

■ CLOSED BIOPSY

In a closed biopsy, no surgical incision is used. Examples include:

- *Needle aspiration biopsy.* A trocar or needle is inserted into the tissue. The aspirated cells are then examined. This technique is common for the biopsy of breast masses.
- *Stereotactic needle aspiration biopsy.* A three-dimensional view of the abnormal tissue is created. On the basis of the imaging results, a needle is inserted into the mass. The client must be able to remain motionless for 20 to 60 minutes while the coordinates are determined. This technique is used for biopsy of certain lung lesions.
- *Core needle biopsy.* A special needle cuts a specimen from tissues not in view. This technique is common for biopsy of the kidney, prostate, liver, lung, and thyroid gland.
- *Punch biopsy.* A small specimen is removed by means of a special instrument that pierces the organ directly or through the skin. This technique is commonly used for biopsy of the skin or the cervix.
- *Brush biopsy.* Cells and tissue fragments are removed by a stiff bristle brush. The brush is advanced into the target area through an endoscope. Areas sampled in this way are the renal pelvis and bronchus.
- *Shave biopsy.* Skin lesions are shaved from the skin surface with a surgical blade or razor blade.

■ OPEN BIOPSY

A surgical incision is needed for an open biopsy. There are two types:

- *Excisional biopsy.* The entire lesion and a margin of surrounding normal tissue are removed. This is the procedure of choice in most cases.
- *Incisional biopsy.* A selected part of the lesion is removed. This form of biopsy is commonly completed during endoscopic examination.

■ SECTIONS

Two methods are used to assess for malignant cells from tissue samples:

1. *Frozen sections* are used for rapid microscopic diagnosis. A thin slice of tissue is cut from the frozen specimen and examined. The procedure requires about 10 to 15 minutes. The pathologist can determine whether malignancy is present and whether the entire tumor has been removed by looking for a margin of tumor-free tissue.
2. *Permanent sections* require about 48 hours. The tissue is placed in a fixative and then examined. It can be stained to facilitate pathologic study.

PREPROCEDURE CARE

Before a biopsy, tell the client about the purpose of the procedure and obtain informed consent. The client may express concern or anxiety about the possible results of the biopsy; be empathetic with the client and family. Some clients sign a permit that allows surgical excision of the mass if it is found to be malignant on frozen section. In these situations, perform a complete baseline assessment for postoperative comparison. Certain types of biopsy require the client's cooperation. For example, to reduce the risk of liver laceration during biopsy of the liver, the client is instructed to hold his breath.

POSTPROCEDURE CARE

Postprocedure care varies with the type of biopsy done. If organs such as the liver, lung, or kidney are sampled, the client has a risk of bleeding, peritonitis, and pneumothorax. Tailor the specific interventions to match the client's needs. Guidelines for care are offered in assessment chapters throughout this book.

CONCLUSIONS

Diagnostic testing is common in both hospital and ambulatory care settings. In all likelihood, a growing number of tests will be performed, processed, or both at the point of care rather than in a laboratory. Become familiar with the various tests on urine, blood, and other body fluids. In many settings, nurses are now required to be prepared to collect these specimens. Understanding how to collect the specimen and knowing the care needed by the client before and after the procedure are important aspects of nursing management. Diagnostic assessment of organs mandates an understanding of the test and the proper scheduling of multiple tests to avoid losing time. In addition, most laboratories call or fax results to the nurse, who is then responsible for determining whether the results warrant notification of the physician.

BIBLIOGRAPHY

1. Brunzel, N. A. (1994). *Fundamentals of urine and body fluid analysis.* Philadelphia: W. B. Saunders.
2. Chernecky, C. C., & Berger, B. J. (1997). *Laboratory tests and diagnostic procedures* (2nd ed.). Philadelphia: W. B. Saunders.
3. Cook, L. (1999). The value of lab values. *American Journal of Nursing, 99*(5), 66–75.
4. Corbett, J. (1996). *Laboratory tests and diagnostic procedures with nursing diagnosis* (4th ed.). Norwalk, CT: Appleton & Lange.
5. Edelman, R. R., & Warach, S. (1993). Magnetic resonance imaging: Part I. *New England Journal of Medicine, 328*(10), 708–716.
6. Edelman, R. R., & Warach, S. (1993). Magnetic resonance imaging: Part II. *New England Journal of Medicine, 328*(11), 785–791.
7. Fishbach, F. T. (1996). *A manual of laboratory & diagnostic tests* (5th ed.). Philadelphia: Lippincott-Raven.
8. Flynn, J. C., Jr. (1994). *Procedures in phlebotomy.* Philadelphia: W. B. Saunders.
9. Frizzell, J. (1998). Avoiding lab test pitfalls. *American Journal of Nursing, 98*(2), 34–37.
10. Greenberg, J. (1993). Physiologic imaging. *Neuroimaging, 7,* 166–174.
11. Malarky, L. M., & McMorrow, L. M. (1996). *Nurse's manual of laboratory tests and diagnostic procedures.* Philadelphia: W. B. Saunders.
12. McFarland, M. (1994). *Nursing implications of laboratory tests.* Albany, NY: Delmar.
13. Mettler, F. A. (1996). *Essentials of radiology.* Philadelphia: W. B. Saunders.
14. O'Toole, M. T. (Ed.). (1997). *Miller-Keane encyclopedia and dictionary of medicine, nursing, and allied health* (6th ed.). Philadelphia: W. B. Saunders.
15. Pagana, K. D., & Pagana, T. J. (1997). *Mosby's diagnostic and laboratory test reference* (3rd ed.). St. Louis: Mosby–Year Book.
16. Putnam, C., & Ravin, C. (1994). *Textbook of diagnostic imaging.* Philadelphia: W. B. Saunders.
17. Scheffer, K. J., & Tobin, R. S. (1997). *Better x-ray interpretation.* Springhouse, PA: Springhouse.

Patient-Centered Communication

QUESTIONS:
What is patient-centered communication?
Does patient-centered communication affect patient outcomes?
How is patient-centered communication used in clinical problem-solving?

CITATION:
Brown, S. J. (1999). Patient-centered communication. *Annual Review of Nursing Research, 17,* 85–104.

The definition of patient-centered communication (PCC) used for the review was an orientation to patient-provider discourse by which patient and provider co-produce mutual understandings and decisions.

STUDIES

The term "patient-centered communication" is used in the clinical literature quite aften, yet a comprehensive search of *CINAHL* and *MEDLINE* (1984–1998) produced only five relevant research studies. Unfortunately, the definition of PCC used in these studies was not consistent with the term's usage in the North American clinical literature. However, many studies did examine a communication behavior and then related the behavior to PCC in the conclusion. As a result, the body of studies included in the review focus more on the behavioral components of PCC than on PCC as a comprehensive health care communication style. Findings from 63 nursing and medicine studies and reviews were included.* Most studies were conducted in office settings.

Summary of Findings

What Is Patient-Centered Communication?

The following behaviors were associated with PCC:

- Allowing clients to give their accounts in their own language[9]
- A conversational style of interview[4, 13]
- Eliciting the client's thoughts, perspectives, expectations, values, and goals
- Inquiring about the client's home, work, and social lives[4]
- Responding to the client's indirect and nonverbal clues regarding emotions and problems[5]
- Providing clients with information for self-care and participation in health care decisions[7, 13]
- Creating shared understandings with clients[9]
- Collaboratively developing health care plans with clients[7]
- Expressing concern for the client's well-being[4, 13]
- Creating social connectedness with clients by humor, touch, and modest personal sharing[4, 13]

Does PCC Affect Patient Outcomes?

Contrary to what some providers think, when the behaviors of PCC are used, more accurate and more useful information about the client's illness or health status is obtained than when the provider asks a series of specific questions.[11, 14] Other outcomes associated with the behaviors of PCC include

- Increased client compliance and resolution of client concerns[6]
- Greater client satisfaction[2]
- Better physiologic outcomes[8]
- Higher overall health ratings[8]
- Increased trust in the health care provider[16]

How Is Patient-Centered Communication Used in Clinical Problem-Solving?

Three different strategies are used for incorporating PCC into clinical problem-solving discourse:

1. Some providers open the interview with a client-centered phase in which the clients take the lead and present their health problems and issues. Then the provider takes control and asks specific questions about these health problems.[10, 15]
2. Some providers allow the client's story to structure the entire interview. Interestingly, it has been found that when clients were given an uninterrupted opportunity to present their concerns, they on average took only 38 seconds to do so and never more than 2½ minutes.[1] Providers using this strategy ask questions that arise out of what the client has just said and keep the story intact as a life experience rooted in events, sequence, places, and relationships. They also avoid use of medical language and specific disease-centered questions.[4, 7, 12, 13] These providers then offer their thoughts on the underlying illness meanings of the client's experiences, carefully linking these interpretations to the client's statements.
3. In the *windows-of-opportunity approach,*[3] the provider asks an initial open-ended question, followed by specific questions that help pinpoint the health problem or diagnosis. However, the provider remains sensitive to the client's desires to talk about personal, emotional, or family issues. The provider responds to these comments by asking about them, thus allowing the client to introduce concerns and psychosocial issues into the interview.

There is no one best strategy; each has its benefits and is employed in different situations. The *integrated approach* (i.e., with the entire interview structured around the client's story) may work best when there are few health or illness problems, whereas the *phased approach* may work best when the client has an immediate concern to be addressed. The issue of when to use one strategy or another still needs to be studied.

Limitations/Reservations: We know a lot about the separate interpersonal processes that compose PCC but very little about it as a multiprocess, integrated health care communication strategy. We do not know whether or how integrated PCC affects the client's clinical outcome. In addition, most of the studies in this review focus on physicians because relatively few studies of nurses' communication processes have been conducted. The studies on communication have been performed mainly in office settings because appointments are scheduled and take place in a room, a setting that lends itself to audiotap-

---

*Not all studies for each behavior are cited.

Patient-Centered Communication *Continued*

ing or videotaping. In contrast, communication between nurses and clients in hospital is typically not scheduled and takes place as a series of short contacts, not one longer contact as in offices. Hence, we know little about how nurses and clients communicate over time (e.g. a shift or consecutive days) in hospitals.

Research-Based Practice

A wide range of communication behaviors and styles is used by health care providers in their conversations with clients. Some of the behaviors associated with PCC may help the client feel at ease (e.g., humor, touch, brief social chit-chat). Others actually help clients tell their stories (e.g., asking about home life, responding to indirect and nonverbal clues regarding emotions and psychosocial issues).

Skilled clinicians let clients tell their whole stories before asking questions. They build on what clients have said and ask focused-but-open question (not questions with yes or no answers). Then they ask a few specific questions to complete their understanding of the situation. Clients who feel that they are appreciated as unique persons and whose providers allow them to tell their stories in the sequence and manner that makes sense to them may be socially more comfortable in the health care interview. As a result, they may disclose more personal information than they would in a more traditional health care interview.

More controlling communication behaviors force clients to tell their stories in ways that impose medical or nursing language and sequences on what clients say. For example, a client may say he "gets winded." A PCC nurse might continue to listen to the rest of a story about when this happens, or might say, "Tell me more about when you get winded." In contrast, a nurse who is disease-centered may say, "Do you get this shortness of breath when you climb a short set of stairs?" This response, which changes what clients call their problem and moves it away from how clients are thinking about it, subtly "medicalizes" the description of what clients are experiencing. More relevant information will be provided by clients if nurses do not introduce specific questions at this point.

All nurses should listen to themselves and note to what extent they interrupt clients, change the language clients use to describe problems, or otherwise control the conversation. The nurse should be committed to getting in touch with the client's view of the situation and the meanings it holds for them. Each nurse should attempt to become a partner with the client, a partner who works with the client to create a true conversation. When true conversation takes place, a mutual understanding of the client's problems and mutually agreed upon ways of addressing them become possible. The plans that PCC nurses and clients make together are more likely to be realistic, to address all the important aspects of a situation, and to produce good clinical outcomes.

Cited References

1. Beckman, H. B., & Frankel, R. M. (1984). The effect of physician behavior on the collection of data. *Annals of Internal Medicine, 91*, 692–696.
2. Bertakis, K. D., Roter, D., & Putnam, S. M. (1991). The relationship of physician medical interview style to patient satisfaction. *Journal of Family Practice, 32*, 175–181.
3. Branch, W. T., & Malik, T. K. (1993). Using "windows of opportunities" in brief interviews to understand patients' concerns. *Journal of American Medical Association, 269*, 1667–1668.
4. Brown, S. J. (1994). Communication strategies used by an expert nurse. *Clinical Nursing Research, 3*, 43–56.
5. Brykcznski, K. A. (1989). An interpretive study describing the clinical judgment of nurse practitioners. *Scholarly Inquiry for Nursing Practice: An International Journal, 3*, 75–104.
6. Henbest, R. J., & Stewart, M. A. (1990). Patient-centredness in the consultation: Does it really make a difference? *Family Practice, 6*, 249–253.
7. Johnson, R. (1993). Nurse practitioner-patient discourse: Uncovering the voice of nursing in primary care practice. *Scholarly Inquiry for Nursing Practice: An International Journal, 7*, 143–157.
8. Kaplan, S. H., Greenfield, S., & Ware, J. E. (1989). Assessing the effects of physician-patient interaction on the outcomes of chronic disease. *Medical Care, 33*, 1176–1187.
9. Kristjanson, L., & Chalmers, K. (1990). Nurse-client interactions in community-based practice: Creating common ground. *Public Health Nursing, 7*, 215–223.
10. Levenstein, J. H., et al. (1986). The patient-centred clinical method. 1. A model for doctor-patient interaction in family medicine. *Family Practice, 3*, 24–30.
11. Marshall, R. S. (1988). Interpretation in doctor-patient interviews: A sociolinguistic analysis. *Culture, Medicine, and Psychiatry, 12*, 201–218.
12. Mishler, E. G. (1984). *The discourse of medicine: Dialectics of medical interviews.* Norwood, NJ: Ablex.
13. Morten, A., et al. (1991). Certified nurse midwifery care of the postpartum client: A descriptive study. *Journal of Nurse-Midwifery, 36*, 276–288.
14. Roter, D. L., & Hall, J. A. (1987). Physicians' interviewing styles and medical information obtained from patients. *Journal of General Internal Medicine, 2*, 325–329.
15. Smith, R. C. (1996). *The patient's story: Integrated patient-doctor interviewing.* Boston: Little, Brown.
16. Thom, D. H., & Campbell, B. (1997). Patient-physician trust: An exploratory study. *Journal of Family Practice, 44*, 169–176.

Sarah Jo Brown, PhD, RN, *Principal and Consultant, Practice-Research Integrations, Norwich, Vermont*

UNIT 4

Foundations of Medical-Surgical Nursing

Anatomy and Physiology Review: The Cell

12 Clients with Fluid Imbalances: Promoting Positive Outcomes

13 Clients with Electrolyte Imbalances: Promoting Positive Outcomes

14 Clients with Acid-Base Imbalances: Promoting Positive Outcomes

15 Clients Having Surgery: Promoting Positive Outcomes

16 Clients with Wounds: Promoting Positive Outcomes

17 Perspectives on Infectious Disorders

18 Perspectives in Oncology

19 Clients with Cancer: Promoting Positive Outcomes

20 Clients with Psychosocial and Mental Health Concerns: Promoting Positive Outcomes

21 Clients with Sleep and Rest Disorders and Fatigue: Promoting Positive Outcomes

22 Perspectives on End-of-Life Care

23 Clients with Pain: Promoting Positive Outcomes

24 Clients with Substance Abuse Disorders: Promoting Positive Outcomes

Anatomy and Physiology Review
The Cell

R. B. Boley
Arlene L. Polaski
David Porta

The cell is the basic unit of structure and function in biologic systems. Two fundamental types of cells are recognized on the basis of composition and organization: *prokaryotic* and *eukaryotic*. Cells found in the human body and in higher plants and animals are eukaryotic; a bacterial cell is prokaryotic. All life systems use one of these two patterns except for viruses, which are acellular and are placed in a separate kingdom: the Akaryotae.

NORMAL CELL STRUCTURE AND FUNCTION

All cells, regardless of type, have the same basic structural pattern: a cytoplasmic matrix surrounded by a plasma membrane (Fig. U4–1). Numerous *organelles* (membrane-limited structures with a complex infrastructure and unique functions) are scattered within the cytoplasm of eukaryotic cells. Their compartmentalization allows multistage metabolic and physiologic events to occur simultaneously while keeping one function separate from another. In contrast, prokaryotic cells do not have organelles and have minimal infrastructural organization. The differences between these two cell types allow clinicians to attack a prokaryotic pathogen selectively in vivo and to use drugs that do not damage eukaryotic cells.

Despite some marked differences in structure and composition, both cell types perform the same basic functions. All cells transfer energy, take up and assimilate materials from outside the cell, synthesize macromolecules, maintain a homeostatic environment, and reproduce themselves as required (Table U4–1).

Most of a cell's mass is water (60% to 95%), which aids in thermal regulation and serves as a solvent for (1) electrolytes, (2) organic molecules, and (3) chemical reactions. *Electrolytes* in the cytoplasm help maintain stable electrical and pH environments and assist with various metabolic and physiologic activities. The most common intracellular electrolytes are calcium, magnesium, phos-

Vesicles

Digestive enzymes

GOLGI COMPLEX

LYSOSOME

NUCLEAR MEMBRANE

Ribosomes

SMOOTH ENDOPLASMIC RETICULUM

ROUGH ENDOPLASMIC RETICULUM

PLASMA MEMBRANE

MITOCHONDRION

NUCLEUS

MICROTUBULES AND MICROFILAMENTS

VACUOLE

CENTRIOLE

FIGURE U4–1 A "typical" cell showing the internal organelles in the cytoplasm and the nucleus.

TABLE U4-1	CELL STRUCTURES AND THEIR FUNCTIONS	
Structure	**Description**	**Function**
Cell Nucleus		
Nucleus	Large structure surrounded by double membrane, contains nucleolus and chromosomes	DNA is transcribed using RNA to make proteins
Nucleolus	Granular body, consists of RNA and protein	Ribosomal RNA synthesis; ribosome sub-unit assembly
Chromosomes	Complexes of DNA and protein known as chromatin become visible as rod-like structures when cell divides	Contain genes that transmit hereditary information and govern cell structure and activity
Cytoplasmic Organelles		
Cell membrane	Boundary of cell	Encloses cell contents; regulates movement of materials in and out of the cell; maintains cell structure; communicates with other cells
Endoplasmic reticulum (ER)	Network of internal membranes extending throughout the cytoplasm. Two types: smooth and rough. Smooth lacks ribosomes on the outer surface; rough has ribosomes on the outer surface	Site of membrane lipids and proteins; origin of intracellular transport vesicles carrying proteins to be secreted. Smooth ER is used for lipid biosynthesis and drug detoxification; rough ER is site of protein manufacturing
Ribosomes	Granules composed of RNA and protein, some attached to ER, some free in cytoplasm	Synthesize polypeptides
Golgi complex	Stacks of flattened membrane sacs	Modifies proteins; packages secreted proteins; sorts other proteins to vacuoles and other organelles
Lysosomes	Membranous sacs	Contain enzymes to break down ingested materials, secretions, and waste
Vacuoles	Membranous sacs	Transport and store materials, waste, and water
Mitochondria	Sacs consisting of two membranes; inner membrane is folded to form cristae and encloses matrix	Site of most reactions of cellular respiration; transformation of energy originating from glucose or lipids into ATP
Microbodies (e.g., peroxisomes)	Membranous sacs containing a variety of enzymes	Sites of many diverse metabolic reactions
Cytoskeleton		
Microtubules	Hollow tubes made of tubulin protein	Provide structural support; provide for cell movement and cell division
Microfilaments	Solid, rodlike structures consisting of actin protein	Provide structural support; provide for cell movement and cell division
Centrioles	Pairs of hollow cylinders located near center of the cell	Spindles form between centrioles during mitosis; may anchor or organize microtubule formation
Cilia	Short projections extending from the surface of the cell, covered by plasma membrane	Regulate movement of material on surface of cell and some tissues
Flagella	Long projections made of microtubules, extend from surface of the cell, covered with plasma membrane	Provide for cellular locomotion by sperm cells

ATP, adenosine triphosphate; DNA, deoxyribonucleic acid; RNA, ribonucleic acid.

phate, bicarbonate, and potassium (the most abundant intracellular cation). *Molecules* within the cell consist mostly of sugars, fatty acids, amino acids, and nucleotides. These are metabolized for energy or used to synthesize macromolecules (lipids, proteins, nucleic acids, and their conjugates).

CELL DEVELOPMENT

Human life begins as an undifferentiated single cell, derived from the fusion of a male gamete (sperm) with a female gamete (ovum). By about the 7th day after fertilization, the original cell (or zygote) has already undergone several cycles of proliferation. The progeny cells begin to develop into distinctive tissues. In the embryo and fetus, these fully differentiated cells can be distinguished on the basis of both form and function.

When tissues in the developing organism reach genetically programmed size limits, the rate of cell reproduction begins to slow and finally stops or attains a steady-state replacement level. This form of growth regulation (called *contact* or *density-dependent inhibition*) is initiated by physical (contact) and chemical (nutrient and cytokine) levels. Cell replication is described later in this review.

■ CELL MEMBRANE

The cell membrane is a fluid phospholipid bilayer with a variety of proteins and conjugated proteins attached to or embedded within it (Fig. U4–2). Proteins that are weakly bound to the inner surface are called *peripheral* proteins. Those that span the lipid bilayer are called *integral;* they function as junctions or channels for the selective transport of ions and other water-soluble molecules or as receptors for various signaling molecules, including transmitters, hormones, and drugs.

The cell selectively regulates entry and exit of materials across the membrane by mechanisms that permit transport either down the concentration gradient (from

high to low concentration) or up the gradient (from low to high). In general, a mechanism is termed *passive* or *active* according to the use of energy from the hydrolysis of adenosine triphosphate (ATP). The basic transport mechanisms are summarized in Table U4–2 and are illustrated in Figure U4–3.

The fate of material after uptake in vesicles is controlled by the presence of signal sequences on molecules within the cell and by other, as yet undetermined, factors. Some substances are degraded by enzymes, and the fragments are metabolically assimilated. Viruses may be uncoated, releasing their nucleic acid component into the cytoplasm. Bacterial toxin molecules may be split and the active portion released to combine with a cytoplasmic or nuclear receptor. Other materials may be exocytosed on another side (e.g., transcytosis of substances across mucosal epithelia in the gut).

Membrane Channels

Proteins in the cell membrane provide channels into the cell. Some of the channels leak continuously, and some are gated (opened by stimuli). A *ligand-gated* channel

TABLE U4–2	MECHANISMS OF MEMBRANE TRANSPORT	
Mechanism	**Common Examples**
Passive (High to Low, No ATP)	
Osmosis	Movement of water through a lipid portion of the membrane
Diffusion	Movement of gasses and small hydrophilic molecules (oxygen, carbon dioxide, nitrogen, glycerol, urea) through the lipid portion of a membrane
Facilitated diffusion	Movement of glucose, some ions, and amino acids via specific carrier proteins
Active (Low to High, Uses ATP)	
Pumps	Hydrogen, sodium, and potassium ions moved by protein pumps
Endocytosis	Intake of substance by creating a vesicle
Pinocytosis	Random uptake of small amounts of extracellular fluid and solutes
Phagocytosis	Large-scale uptake of particles and cells, especially important in defense
Receptor-mediated	Specific uptake of molecules after binding to a ligand
Exocytosis	Secretion of products and wastes via secretory vesicles

ATP, adenosine triphosphate.

EXTERIOR OF CELL

INTERIOR OF CELL

FIGURE U4–2 The cell membrane is composed of a bimolecular layer of lipids, primarily phospholipid and cholesterol. Proteins can be attached or embedded in the membrane. Peripheral proteins are attached to the surface; integral proteins are embedded in the cell membrane.

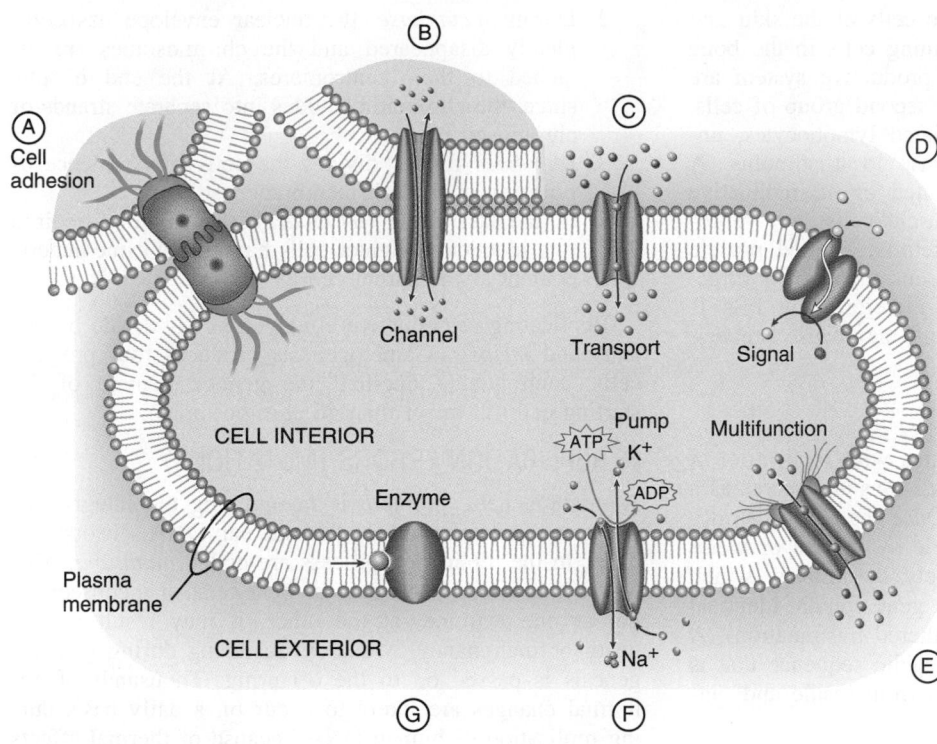

ⒶCell adhesion

Ⓑ

Channel

Ⓒ

Transport

Signal

Ⓓ

CELL INTERIOR

Enzyme

Pump
ATP   K⁺
ADP

Multifunction

Plasma membrane

CELL EXTERIOR

Na⁺

Ⓖ   Ⓕ   Ⓔ

FIGURE U4–3 The cell membrane is responsible for adhesion to adjacent cells (A) and movement of substances in and out of the cell. Several mechanisms are required: gap junctions allow communication between neighboring cells by transfer of small molecules (B); passive transport of molecules (C); signal receptor proteins that bind to surface signal molecules and transfer a message to the cell interior (D); use of integral proteins to transport specific molecules (E); ATP-driven pumps to actively transport ions from one compartment to another (F); and use of membrane bound enzymes, which have active sites on either side of the cell membrane (G). ADP, adenosine diphosphate; ATP, adenosine triphosphate.

changes shape when a protein binds to it, then opens and closes. These channels are seen in cells that respond to hormones, drugs, or neurotransmitters. A *voltage-gated* channel opens or closes when there are changes in the electrical voltage across the membrane. These channels are seen in all three types of muscle cells: skeletal, smooth and cardiac.

A *mechanically gated* channel opens in response to deforming forces, such as pressure or friction. These channels are found in blood vessels, skin, and sensory nerves. Channels that leak are important in the cardiac, nervous, and muscle tissue for the rapid transmission of electrical pacemaker messages.

Intercellular Communication

Special sites on cell membranes play a role in communication and interaction between cells, both nearby and at a distance. Membrane proteins mediate this communication, serving as ligand-binding receptors and as transducers that initiate enzymatic function in the cell. Hormones as well as an extensive group of molecules called *cytokines* are involved in intercellular signaling.

Some cell surface molecules serve as mammalian blood group isoantigens (e.g., ABO, Rh). Others act as histocompatibility antigens, which detect self and non-self in immune function and in tissue and organ transplants.

■ NUCLEUS

The nucleus is the most prominent organelle in the eukaryotic cell. It is surrounded by a porous double membrane (the *nuclear envelope*). Within the nucleus are one or more nucleoli, visible among a mass of chromosomes. The nucleus contains the genetic material of the cell in the form of chromatin threads composed of deoxyribonu-

cleic acid (DNA). Each cell, except the reproductive cells, contains a person's full genetic complement of DNA (46 chromosomes).

The DNA contains the recipes for all the proteins in the body. The DNA in the nucleus is unable to pass through the nuclear envelope into the cytoplasm; yet it is in the cytoplasm that polypeptides and proteins are synthesized. These proteins are used for structure or control of all metabolic and physiologic activities of the cell. Therefore, DNA must transfer its instructions for synthesizing proteins to molecules that can carry the information from the nucleus to the cytoplasm. It does this through a two-step process: transcription and translation.

TRANSCRIPTION. DNA serves as a template for the assembly of molecules of ribonucleic acid (RNA). The two linked chains of DNA separate from one another, exposing part of the base sequence. RNA links to the DNA template and then serves as the messenger (mRNA) and moves from the nucleus to the cytoplasm for protein synthesis.

TRANSLATION. At the ribosome, mRNA is used to assemble proteins in specific order. This step (translation) requires that the mRNA bind to the ribosome and that the ribosome "read" the RNA. Transfer RNA (tRNA) transports the amino acids in the cytoplasm to the ribosome, and the protein is assembled. In a human body, roughly 100,000 genes produce about 60,000 essential proteins. A single cell can synthesize about 20,000 different proteins (an awesome achievement).

CELL REPLICATION

Besides producing proteins, most body cells also must reproduce themselves. In the healthy adult body, somatic cells replicate at varying rates. The cells of the skin and mucous membranes, the blood-forming cells in the bone marrow, and some cells in the reproductive system are replaced at a high constant rate. A second group of cells, such as hepatocytes and differentiated lymphocytes, undergoes replication only in response to a stimulus. A third group of cells has very limited or no replicative capabilities. Individual smooth muscle cells may reproduce only once or twice in a lifetime; striated muscle cells (heart and skeleton) and neurons (except for olfactory cells) do not replicate, and therefore any loss is permanent. Thus, a spinal cord injury may cause irreversible paralysis.

■ STAGES OF REPLICATION

The process of cell replication begins with replication of the genetic information. The DNA divides and serves as a template for its own duplication. Once the DNA has duplicated, eukaryotic cells may divide by *mitosis* or *meiosis*. Somatic cells divide exclusively by mitosis, which produces two daughter cells with a gene content identical to that of the parent cell (unless altered by mutation). A cell undergoing mitosis follows a cyclic sequence that is driven by a combination of signals from inside and outside the cell (Fig. U4—4).

Mitosis involves several steps:

1. In *prophase,* two centrioles move toward opposite poles of the cell, fibers become visible, and the nucleolus disappears. The chromatin threads of DNA become visible as structures called *chromosomes.*

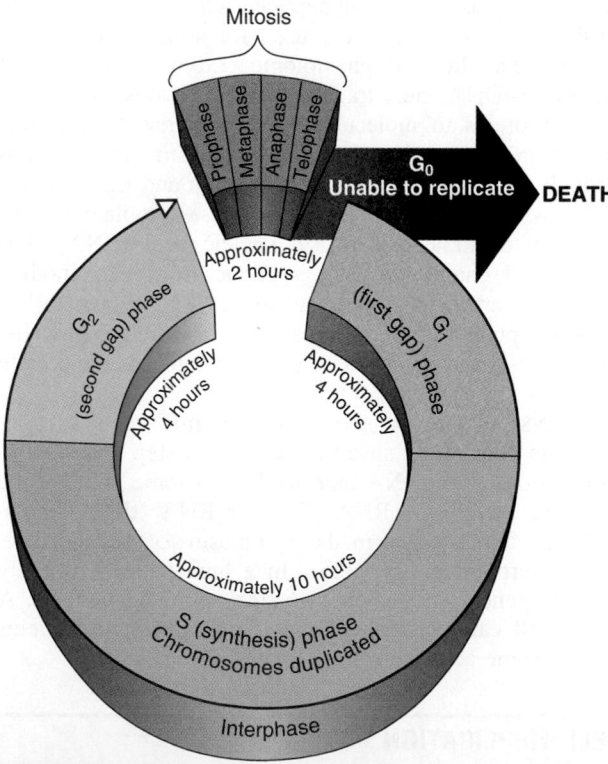

FIGURE U4—4 Phases in the life cycle of a cell. Actual times vary, depending on the type of cell.

2. During *metaphase,* the nuclear envelope has completely disappeared and the chromosomes are attached to their centromeres. At the end of this stage, the chromatin divides into separate strands of chromosomes.
3. *Anaphase* further divides the cell with evidence of pinching of the cell membrane.
4. In the last phase *(telophase),* the cell divides into two identical daughter cells having the same genetic content as the parent cell.

Replicating reproductive eukaryotic cells divide by *mitosis* and *meiosis.* Gametogenesis produces four progeny cells, each having one-half the genetic content of the starting cell (23 rather than 46 chromosomes).

■ REPLICATION ERRORS (MUTATIONS)

A major genetic problem is maintaining the integrity of the message contained in the nuclear DNA. Errors that occur in the replication process are called *mutations.* Mutation in a somatic cell may be beneficial or inconsequential at one extreme; at the other, it may result in cell death or malignancy. Mutation occurring during gametogenesis is passed on to the offspring. Thousands of abnormal changes are likely to occur on a daily basis during replication of human DNA because of thermal effects and inappropriate metabolic events. In nearly all cases, however, the DNA is restored to normal configurations by a variety of repair mechanisms. Abnormal genes that escape repair may result in diseases such as phenylketonuria or sickle cell disease.

Biotechnologists are applying recent advances in genetic engineering to the prevention and therapy of diseases. Using restriction *endonuclease* (which hydrolyzes or cuts DNA at specific sequences) and *DNA ligase* (which recombines the cut ends of DNA fragments), biotechnologists can cut selected genes out of sections of human DNA molecules, insert them into bacterial *plasmids* (extrachromosomal genetic elements in bacteria that can incorporate segments of human DNA), and produce large quantities of the gene product. Many benefits are being realized and anticipated from the use of this technology:

- Increased yields and improved antimicrobial action of antibiotics
- More effective and safer virus vaccines (prepared from gene components)
- Ability to produce mammalian proteins, including clotting factors, insulin, human growth hormone, and interferons
- Development of "magic bullets" for treating many conditions, including tumors, through precise modification of reactive sites in antibodies
- Development of transgenic plants and animals for increasing and improving nutritional sources for humans.

CELLS IN TISSUES AND ORGANS

Cells working together as a unit are called *tissues.* Tissues unite to form individual *organs.* The four major specialized types of cells that unite into larger tissue units are the following:

1. *Epithelial cells* are arranged in sheets. They cover the outside of the body (epidermis) and form the absorptive linings of the body's cavities and tubular structures (such as mucosa and glands).
2. *Nerve cells* form the highly specialized, irritable, and conductive nerve tissue. Destroyed nerve cells cannot be replaced.
3. *Muscle cells* allow mobility of body parts as well as mobility of substances (such as air, blood, and waste) within the body by contracting and relaxing.
4. *Connective tissue cells* support other cells and tissues. They include blood cells and structural cells found in bones, tendons, and ligaments. Blood cells carry oxygen to the tissues and carbon dioxide and wastes from the tissues. They also defend the body against foreign substances. Structural cells build the bony scaffolding and form the critical intercellular proteins that bind together the cells of the body. Collagen is an important extracellular connective tissue protein.

ALTERATIONS IN CELL STRUCTURE AND FUNCTION

The major causes of cellular alterations include changes in gene structure and function (either newly acquired or hereditary) and degeneration of normal tissue due to aging, excessive use, or infiltration by foreign substances (including fat, water, glycogen, and proteins).

ATROPHY

Atrophy is the wasting or decrease in size of a normally developed organ. This condition results from a decrease either in the number of cells or in the size of the cells composing it. Atrophy may follow disuse of an organ. For example, muscle atrophy may develop following denervation or prolonged immobilization. Muscular atrophy caused by aging can be greatly minimized by physical activity. Because the adrenal glands normally secrete corticosteroids, atrophy of these glands can occur when large doses of corticosteroids are administered over a prolonged period. Atrophy also accompanies the normal physiologic aging process. The thymus gland increases in size during childhood and very gradually starts to atrophy during adolescence. The ovaries atrophy after menopause.

HYPERTROPHY

Hypertrophy is an increase in the size of an organ or tissue resulting from an increase in the size of the cells. Hypertrophy sometimes represents the response of an organ to a greater workload. For example, when the heart is subjected to great strain, the left ventricle of the heart enlarges (hypertrophies) in order to handle the additional stress. Another example is the increased size of the biceps muscle in people engaged in strenuous physical activity.

PRECANCEROUS CHANGES

Hyperplasia is an increase in the number of cells. Hyperplasia can be an expected cellular response, such as increased cell regeneration in the formation of calluses. Pathologic hyperplasia can become cancerous.

Dysplasia is deranged cellular growth or a form of hyperplasia. It results from persistent severe injury or irritation.

Metaplasia is the transformation of one mature cell type or tissue into another. Usually, the new cell does not perform the functions of the cell it replaced. Metaplastic cells can transform into malignant cancer cells.

NEOPLASTIC (CANCEROUS) CHANGES

Neoplastic change is characterized by disturbances in cell differentiation and growth. When normal cells undergo transformation into cancerous cells, they fail to respond to normal regulatory forces and instead show unrestrained growth. These unregulated replicating cells *(neoplasms)* may then invade contiguous healthy tissues or become detached from the primary tumor and spread *(metastasize)* to other parts of the body where they continue to divide. This alteration in normal cell reproduction is discussed in greater detail in Chapter 18.

AGING

In a young healthy person, cells are biochemically active, have a high turnover rate (in some tissues), and have a high rate of metabolic and physiologic efficiency. In older adults, cells are less active, have a slower turnover rate, and begin to decline in efficiency. Aging cells shrink in size, protein synthesis slows, the Golgi apparatus shows signs of disintegration, and the mitochondria may undergo fragmentation. Aging affects every system of the body (Table U4–3).

Numerous theories exist regarding the aging process, but little is certain about how age-related changes occur. The age range of a cell is great. In the mature adult, an epithelial cell lining the intestinal tract lives only about 1½ days; a red blood cell can survive for 120 days. At the other extreme, nerve cells have a potential life expectancy of 100 years or more. In the immune system, immunocompetent cells appear to remain constant in numbers as people age but lose some of their interactive and regulatory properties. The resulting alteration in immune function is responsible for the increased incidence of autoimmune disease, the appearance of tumors, and the greater susceptibility to infection seen in the elderly population.

One theory of aging is that unrepaired mutations accumulate on DNA, causing changes that lead to aging. For example, highly specialized cells (such as nerve cells) do not reproduce. When these cells die from injury or disease and are not replaced, the remaining cells must assume their functions. The greater workload may stress these cells, cause them to age faster, and hasten their dying.

Another hypothesis is that each of us is born with a genetic clock that governs our life span. This theory is based on the observation that each cell type has a finite number of divisions. This concept is supported in part by similarities in life spans seen in various family groups.

TABLE U4-3	PHYSIOLOGIC CHANGES OF AGING: AN OVERVIEW
System	**Physiologic Changes**
Cardiovascular	Decreased vessel elasticity due to calcification and connective tissue (increased pulmonary vascular resistance)
	Decreased number of heart muscle fibers, with increased size of individual fibers (hypertrophy)
	Decreased filling capacity
	Decreased stroke volume
	Decreased sensitivity of baroreceptors
	Degeneration of vein valves
Respiratory	Decreased chest wall compliance due to calcification of the costal cartilage
	Decreased alveolar ventilation
	Decreased respiratory muscle strength
	Air trapping and decreased ventilation due to degeneration of lung tissue (decreased elasticity)
Renal and urinary	Decreased glomerular filtration rate due to nephron degeneration (decreased 33%–50% by age 70)
	Decreased ability to concentrate urine
	Decreased ability to regulate hydrogen (H^+)
Gastrointestinal	Decreased muscular contraction
	Decreased esophageal emptying
	Decreased bowel motility
	Decreased production of hydrochloric acid (HCl), enzymes, and intrinsic factor
	Decreased hepatic enzyme production and metabolic capacity
	Thinning of stomach mucosa
Neurologic and sensory	Degeneration and atrophy of nerve cells
	Decrease of 25% to 45% in neurons
	Decrease in neurotransmitters
	Decreased rate of conduction of nerve impulses
	Loss of taste buds
	Loss of auditory hair cells and sclerosis of the eardrum
Musculoskeletal	Decreased muscle mass
	Bone demineralization
	Joint degeneration, erosion, and calcification
Immune	Decreased inflammatory response
	Decrease in T-cell function due to involution of the thymus gland
Integumentary	Decreased subcutaneous fat
	Decreased elastin
	Atrophy of the sweat glands
	Atrophy of the epidermal arterioles, causing altered temperature regulation

From Copstead, L. C., & Banasik, J. (2000). *Pathophysiology*. Philadelphia: W. B. Saunders.

MECHANISMS OF CELL DAMAGE

When cells are injured, injured organelles no longer carry out their specific functions (e.g., mitochondria stop producing ATP). The extent of the damage depends on (1) the nature, intensity, and duration of the stressor; (2) whether the blood supply to the cells is affected; and (3) the state of differentiation or metabolic activity of the cells. Indeed, two clients exposed to the same injurious substance may not sustain the same degree of injury because of the influence of modifying factors. For example, a person's nutritional and emotional state can have a profound impact on the extent and consequences of a slight to moderate level of injury. However, there is a point after which cell death inevitably occurs. The mechanisms responsible for the transition from reversible to irreversible cellular damage are not completely understood.

■ HYPOXIA

Hypoxia (inadequate tissue oxygenation) is a leading cause of cell injury and death. Hypoxia can occur as a result of:

- Vascular disease or injury, which impedes blood flow to tissues
- Insufficient oxygenation of blood caused by conditions such as carbon monoxide poisoning

Depending on the severity of the hypoxic state, cells compensate and recover or are killed. (For example, if the femoral artery becomes stenotic, the skeletal muscles of the legs will eventually atrophy as a result of the inadequate blood flow and the consequent reduced oxygen supply. Severe or chronic hypoxia will result in cell injury or death.)

The most common cause of hypoxia is *ischemia,* or reduced blood supply. Progressive hypoxia caused by gradual narrowing of arteries (atherosclerosis) is better tolerated than sudden anoxia caused by an obstruction in the blood supply.

■ TEMPERATURE EXTREMES

Extreme heat damages cells by coagulating cytoplasmic protein. Even mild heat results in permanent cellular damage if it is applied over a prolonged period to people with impaired circulation, as seen in peripheral vascular disease. Heat in these cases increases the metabolic needs of cells and tissues and leads to insufficient oxygen levels. Coupled with a reduced capacity to dispose of waste products, this process accelerates the damage to the affected tissue.

Cold constricts the smaller blood vessels, thereby decreasing the circulation of blood and oxygen to tissues. Freezing temperatures may cause the intracellular water to crystallize, which destroys the cell's structure. Cold injury can result in frostbite, permanently injuring the tissues involved. Very low temperatures cause stasis of blood, clot formation, arterial occlusion, ischemia, and ultimately cell death and necrosis.

■ IONIZING RADIATION

Exposure to radiation causes mutations, inactivates enzymes, and interrupts cell division. The fact that radiation inhibits mitosis makes this therapy important in the treatment of cancer, a disease involving pathologic cell reproduction. Radiation affects virtually all cells, but certain cells are more susceptible than others. Reproductive cells, cells in the lymph nodes and gastrointestinal tract, and bone marrow cells are highly sensitive to damage by radiation exposure, whereas cells of cartilage, muscle, brain, and endocrine glands are relatively insensitive. People who work with radioactive materials or nuclear fission reactors or who are giving or receiving radiotherapy are most at risk for cellular trauma from radiation.

■ ELECTRICAL INJURY

Electrical energy generates heat when it passes through the body and may thus produce burns. It also interferes with neural conduction and often causes death from cardiac dysrhythmias. The extent of damage from electrical energy depends on its voltage and amperage, tissue resistance, and the pathway of the current as it passes through the body. Users of electrical equipment should be aware that exposure to 100 milliamperes (mA) can be lethal to humans. Electrical burns are discussed in Chapter 50.

■ CHEMICAL INJURY

Chemicals harm cells by destroying or altering their structure and by disrupting their metabolism. The capacity of a chemical to injure a cell depends on the strength and toxicity of the chemical as well as on the susceptibility of the cell. Many chemicals can injure cells. Highly toxic substances are called poisons. Minute amounts of poisonous substances, such as cyanide and arsenic, can cause death. Some of the most toxic substances known are bacterial exotoxins, such as diphtheria toxin and botulinum toxin.

Environmental chemicals, such as herbicides, pesticides, and air pollutants, are potential causes of cellular injury. Lead-based paint, which tastes sweet, is often eaten by children. Lead-based paint on walls and window blinds comes off in dust particles and can be inhaled. Dangerous amounts of lead may also be found in water pipes and drinking water in older homes. Ingested or inhaled lead destroys cells in the nervous system (which may lead to mental retardation in young children), affects blood cell production, and damages the kidneys.

Workers around machinery and home owners with gas appliances must guard against carbon monoxide poisoning. Carbon monoxide binds tightly and 210 times more rapidly than oxygen to hemoglobin, preventing normal exchange of oxygen and carbon dioxide.

■ BACTERIAL INJURY

Microorganisms such as bacteria injure host cells by direct attack or by the toxins they produce. Bacterial toxins are classified as (1) endotoxins or (2) exotoxins.

Endotoxins may act directly with macrophages and T lymphocytes, causing the release of cytokines. Endotoxins acting on macrophages stimulate the production of interleukin-1 (IL-1) and tumor necrosis factor (TNF), two cytokines that in large quantities cause bacterial septic shock, a condition that is often fatal. Endotoxins may also activate the complement cascade, producing disseminated intravascular coagulation (DIC), another potentially fatal condition. Successful intervention in endotoxemia is difficult and often impossible to achieve.

Exotoxins are proteins and have specific toxic effects. For example, Clostridium tetani, the organism that causes tetanus, produces a neurotoxin that blocks processes that inhibit neural transmission in the central nervous system (CNS). Preventive immunization is possible with a few exotoxins (such as C. tetani), and in some cases an exotoxemia can be successfully treated with antitoxins (e.g., diphtheria).

■ VIRAL INJURY

Viruses have been described as mobile genetic elements protected by outer layers of protein and lipoprotein. Viruses attach to specific receptors on host cell surfaces and are taken up by endocytosis. The nucleic acid core of the virus passes through the vesicular membrane into the interior of the host cell. The viral genome then subverts the host cell metabolic machinery and begins to make viral components. While inside the host cell, the virus is protected from the host's reactive cells and solutes. The assembled virions may then exit the cell either by lysing the cell remnant or by permitting the host cell to remain viable while continuously secreting virions across the cell membrane. Viruses damage host cells by killing them, depriving them of nutrients, or causing cells to transform into a tumor state.

■ MECHANICAL INJURY

Cells can be damaged by physical impact or irritation. Examples of this type of injury include blisters from tight shoes, abrasions, lacerations, and contusions (bruises). Cells can be injured in other ways as well. Light can damage cells of the cornea. Noise can damage the eardrum (tympanic membrane), the ossicle in the middle ear, and the organ of Corti in the inner ear. Prolonged contact with vibrating objects can alter muscle and bone structure as well as nerve conduction. Clients at risk for these injuries are those who work with power tools.

■ NUTRITIONAL IMBALANCE

Inadequate protein intake decreases the function of the intestinal mucosa and pancreas, which in turn reduces nutrient absorption. Plasma proteins, especially albumin, help retain fluid in blood vessels. When levels of plasma proteins decline, fluid tends to move into interstitial spaces, causing edema. Antibodies or immunoglobulins are protein; therefore, the lack of proteins adversely affects immune system function and increases the risk of infection.

Inadequate carbohydrate intake forces the body to use fats for energy. The liver becomes overwhelmed and ketone bodies are formed that accumulate in the blood, a condition known as *ketosis*. Ketosis develops because of the rapid breakdown of fatty acids stored in adipose tissue. Fatty acids are used for energy when the daily intake of carbohydrates is less than 50 g. Clients at high risk for ketosis include those with diabetes, those on starvation diets, and those on low-carbohydrate diets.

Increased fat intake often causes fat deposition in heart, liver, and muscle and may lead to obesity, coronary heart disease, stroke, or breast and colon cancer.

Growth factors include amino acids, purines and pyrimidines, and vitamins. These nutrients are required but cannot be synthesized. Insufficient quantities of these substances can seriously impair the ability of the cell to take up and metabolize nutrients or to synthesize macromolecules for structural building and reproduction.

■ CELL DEATH

Cells die as a result of being traumatized, through alteration by disease, from failure caused by genetic alterations, or through a programmed process called *apoptosis*.

Apoptosis usually does not disturb the steady-state nature of the tissue and thus gives no sign of its occurrence.

CONCLUSIONS

Cells are the basic units of life, and they serve many functions. The integrity and existence of the organism is dependent on the individual and collective ability of body cells to digest and assimilate substances, protect themselves by reacting to stimuli, replicate, metabolize, and produce energy. When cells lose their ability to function normally because of injury or attack by pathogens, the organism will show signs of distress and disease will develop.

Recent advances in molecular biology are providing the means for great improvements in the diagnosis and treatment of many human diseases. Only those professionals who keep current in the field will be able to comprehend the nature and consequences of the pathologic changes associated with disease processes and will know how to make and evaluate therapeutic decisions.

BIBLIOGRAPHY

1. Alberts, B. D., et al. (1994). *Molecular biology of the cell* (3rd ed.). New York: Garland.
2. Barnes, D. E., Lindahl, T., & Sedgwick, B. (1993). DNA repair. *Current Opinion in Cell Biology, 5,* 424.
3. Becker, W. M., Reece, J. B., & Poenie, M. F. (1995). *The world of the cell* (3rd ed.). New York: Benjamin/Cummings.
4. Berridge, M. J. (1994). The biology and medicine of calcium signalling. *Molecular and Cellular Endocrinology, 98,* 119.
5. Hartwell, L. H., & Kastan, M. B. (1994). Cell cycle control and cancer. *Science, 266,* 1821.
6. Mulligan, R. C. (1993). The basic science of gene therapy. *Science, 260,* 926.
7. Welch, W. J. (1993). How cells respond to stress. *Scientific American, 268,* 56.
8. Yeh, E. (1998, August 15). Life and death of the cell. *Hospital Practice,* 85–92.

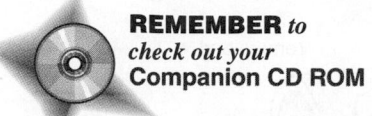
CHAPTER 12

Clients with Fluid Imbalances: Promoting Positive Outcomes

Bernadette White

Dehydration is the most common fluid and electrolyte imbalance in the United States. The Health Care Financing Administration has identified dehydration as one of the most frequent diagnoses upon hospital admission, present in more than 1 million admissions per year. Dehydration is especially common among older adults and therefore is expected to increase as our population ages. Dehydration carries a 17% to 45% morbidity and mortality rate.[36] The cost to society includes not only the cost of admission, diagnosis, and treatment of the dehydration and secondary complications but also the financial and psychological loss to the family and society of a productive contributor.

This chapter provides the basic knowledge necessary to promote positive health outcomes for clients at risk for fluid and electrolyte imbalances. Positive health outcomes are achieved through health promotion, health maintenance, and health restoration strategies. Clearly, water is not only responsible for the body's structure and function; it is also necessary for the maintenance of equilibrium and of life itself.

OVERVIEW

Fluids exist in two compartments in the body: (1) the *intracellular* fluid (ICF) compartment, inside the cells, and (2) the *extracellular* fluid (ECF) compartment, outside the cells. Two thirds of body fluid is intracellular. Although water is the predominant component in each of these compartments, the word *fluid* is used to indicate that other substances (glucose, sodium, waste products) are also found in these compartments and that they influence the water balance in and between compartments.

The ECF compartment is further divided into the *intravascular* (e.g., plasma) and *interstitial* (between cells) compartments. Cerebrospinal, lymphatic, synovial, and eye fluids are also part of the ECF compartment. Interstitial fluid compartments are also known as *tissue spaces* or *third spaces.*

Fluids move between the intracellular, intravascular, and interstitial compartments to maintain fluid balance.

Fluid in the cells is the most stable; cells are fairly resistant to major fluid shifts. Fluids in the bloodstream are the most changeable, quickly lost or gained by intake of fluids or by loss of fluids through sweat, urination, diarrhea, and so on. Fluids in the interstitial spaces are the reserve fluids, replacing fluid in the cells or the blood.

About 60% of the body's total weight is water, although this percentage varies with stature and lean body mass. Among short and obese people, 50% of body mass is water. In athletes and lean people, water comprises 70% of total body weight.

■ FLUID MOVEMENT FROM PRESSURE CHANGES

Fluids move between compartments to maintain homeostasis. Changes in pressure promote fluid movement. Most fluid movement, (i.e., water and dissolved particles in the water) takes place across the capillary wall. Forces that move fluids are constantly at work and allow the fluid taken in orally to maintain blood pressure and hydrate cells and eventually to be excreted as urine.

Figure 12–1 demonstrates *hydrostatic* and *oncotic pressures* within the capillary. Blood moves through the vascular system from areas of high pressure (arteries) to areas of low pressure (capillaries and veins) via hydrostatic pressure. *Hydrostatic pressure* is the pressure exerted against the wall of the blood vessel by the blood inside it. *Oncotic* (sometimes called *osmotic*) *pressure* results from the presence of "nondiffusible" (too large, opposing ionic charge) proteins. These proteins create a pressure that draws fluid to it. Oncotic pressures pull fluids back into the vessel on the venous end of the capillary.

As arterial blood enters the capillary, it is at higher pressure than the surrounding tissues. Fluids are pushed into the interstitial spaces from the arterial end. This passive form of fluid movement is known as *filtration.* As blood continues to flow through the capillary, the volume of blood is reduced, thereby reducing the pressure. By the time blood reaches the venous end of the capillary, pressure is higher in the interstitial space and fluid returns to

FIGURE 12-1 Pressure differences inside the capillary are responsible for movement of fluids. Fluid moves out of the capillary at the arterial end because hydrostatic pressure in the vessel exceeds pressure in the tissues. Fluids return to the vessel at the venous end because proteins (colloids) in the vessel exert a pulling pressure on them. Under normal conditions, movement of fluids is almost equal, and neither dehydration nor edema results. Fluid that remains in the interstitium is transported via the lymphatics to the vascular system. Abnormal conditions occur with the presence of too much fluid, too few proteins, changes in the capillary wall, or lymphatic obstruction.

the capillary. This form of fluid movement is known as *reabsorption.* The terms "reabsorption," "absorption," and "resorption" are clarified in Box 12-1. The movement of fluids is based on the presence of proper amounts of pressure on both sides of the capillary wall.

Proteins in the interstitial spaces and in the capillary pull fluids toward themselves. Therefore, proteins promote fluid movement both ways: into the interstitial space and into the capillary. Because these forces are due to protein, this process is often called *colloid (protein) osmotic pressure.* The most common protein in plasma is *albumin,* which is responsible for most of the fluid movement at the capillary level. Albumin comprises 50% of the plasma proteins but contributes to 80% of the osmotic force inside the capillary. The proper movement of fluids is also based on adequate amounts of protein on both sides of the capillary wall.

As blood moves through the capillary, not all of the fluid that passed into the interstitial spaces is recaptured. The remainder is returned to the central circulation by the lymphatic system. As interstitial and tissue fluid pressures

increase, one-way valves in the terminal lymphatic capillaries open and fluid enters. Pressure or skeletal muscle movement from outside of the lymphatics propels the fluid forward into larger lymphatic vessels and eventually to the thoracic duct or the right lymph duct and then into the left subclavian vein. Valves inside the lymphatic vessels prevent back flow of fluid. The lymphatics also return small proteins that have leaked into the tissues.

■ FLUID MOVEMENT BY DIFFUSION AND OSMOLALITY

Diffusion is the most important means by which substances such as nutrients and waste products move between blood and the interstitial spaces. It is the movement of fluids or substances across a membrane because of differences in concentration. Substances diffuse across the membrane to equal the concentration on each side of the membrane.

Osmolality and a related concept, *osmolarity,* refer to the concentration of solutes (electrolytes, glucose, urea, protein) in 1 liter (L) of solution. The more solute present, the higher the osmolality. Fluids of high osmolality tend to pull water across a membrane to reduce the osmolality by reducing the ratio of solute to solvent.

Osmolality is measured by the number of dissolved particles per kilogram of water. Because 1 L of water is equal to 1 kg of weight, the terms osmolality and osmolarity are frequently used interchangeably. Electrolytes, especially sodium and protein, contribute the largest number of particles to the osmolality. Urea and glucose also contribute to osmolality.

Sodium is the most abundant and easily accessible electrolyte in plasma. The concentration of sodium is used to measure osmolality. Normal plasma osmolality is 275 to 295 mOsm/kg of water. This is an *iso-osmolar* state because the fluid contains particles (*solutes*) and water (*solvent*) in approximately equal proportions. When there are *more than* 295 mOsm/kg of water, a *hyperosmolar (hypertonic)* state results. In contrast, fluid with *less than* 275 mOsm/kg of water is *hyposmolar (hypo-*

BOX 12-1   **Concepts: Absorption, Reabsorption, and Resorption**

In addition to many other concepts, three often confusing concepts are discussed in this chapter: absorption, reabsorption, and resorption.

- *Absorption* usually refers to the initial movement of substances, such as the end products of digestion or medications, into the vascular spaces from an organ, such as the gastrointestinal tract, muscle, subcutaneous or dermal tissue, or buccal or pharyngeal tissues.
- *Reabsorption* refers to the movement of water, electrolytes, vitamins, amino acids, glucose, lactate, or other essential substances from one compartment, such as the interstitium or renal tubules, back into capillaries.
- *Resorption* refers to the process of calcium salts leaving the bone and moving into the blood in an ionized form.

tonic) fluid because it has fewer particles than water. Thirst is regulated in the hypothalamus, and changes in the osmolality of circulating blood produce thirst.

■ HORMONAL REGULATION OF FLUID BALANCE

The hypothalamus regulates osmolality by producing *antidiuretic hormone* (ADH), also called vasopressin. The term *diuresis* means to produce and excrete urine; therefore, this hormone slows the production of dilute urine, thereby retaining body fluids.

ADH is stored in the posterior pituitary gland. Increasing serum osmolarity is sensed by the hypothalamus, and it signals the posterior pituitary gland to release ADH into circulation. ADH reduces urinary output by enlarging the size of the pores in the distal and collecting tubules in the nephron, returning fluids to the body rather than excreting them. ADH allows the kidneys to produce a range of urine volumes and concentrations. When body fluid levels are dangerously low, ADH also constricts arterioles to shunt blood from the peripheral areas and promote perfusion of the major organs.

ADH is released continuously in response to many conditions, not just during emergencies. These conditions include a lack of water intake (as from nothing by mouth [NPO] status), uncontrolled water loss (as from watery diarrhea), consumption of concentrated food or fluids, pain, and use of certain medications, such as narcotics, barbiturates, and anesthetics. Emotional or physiologic stress can also trigger ADH release, during surgery, trauma, severe anxiety, or prolonged exercise.

Factors that suppress ADH include hyposmolality of the ECF, increased blood volume, exposure to cold, acute alcohol ingestion, carbon dioxide inhalation, and administration of some diuretics, lithium, and some antipsychotic medications. Disorders of the pituitary gland can also lead to failure to release ADH. These situations lead to increased urine output (diuresis). Sometimes diuresis is desirable, but other times it is dangerous. Can you see potential problems with uncontrollable diuresis or with diuresis in clients who are unable to respond to thirst?

Aldosterone, another hormone that controls fluid balance, is secreted by the adrenal cortex and conserves body sodium by promoting potassium excretion from the kidneys. Sodium retains fluid, and under the action of aldosterone fluid is thus also retained.

Aldosterone secretion is a four-step process:

1. When arterial blood flow is decreased to the kidneys, renin is released by the juxtaglomerular apparatus of the kidney.
2. In the blood, renin converts angiotensinogen to angiotensin I.
3. Angiotensin I is further converted to angiotensin II by a converting enzyme from the lungs.
4. The presence of angiotensin II stimulates secretion of aldosterone from the adrenal cortex.

This process is called the *renin-angiotensin system.* Adrenocorticotropic hormone (ACTH) from the anterior pituitary is necessary for aldosterone secretion, but its effect is limited. When ACTH levels are low, the kidney is less able to respond to sodium depletion. Figure 12–2 illustrates how the kidneys interact with hormones and the thirst mechanism to maintain fluid balance.

The two most powerful stimulants for aldosterone release are (1) decreased arterial blood flow in the kidney and (2) increased plasma potassium. Conditions such as hemorrhage, dehydration, and an upright posture reduce renal blood flow. An increased plasma sodium level slightly decreases aldosterone secretion.

Atrial natriuretic peptides, prostaglandins, and *kinins* also contribute to the regulation of sodium balance. Because their major action is on sodium, and secondarily on water, they are discussed in Chapter 13.

EXTRACELLULAR FLUID VOLUME DEFICIT

Extracellular fluid volume deficit (ECFVD), commonly called *dehydration,* is a decrease in intravascular and interstitial fluids. ECFVD is a common and serious fluid imbalance that results in vascular fluid volume loss (*hypovolemia*). With *mild* ECFVD, 1 to 2 L of water or 2% of body weight is lost; with *moderate* ECFVD, 3 to 5 L of water or 5% body weight is lost; and with *severe* ECFVD, 5 to 10 L of water or 8% of body weight is lost.

Etiology

Fluid balance is maintained in the body because the intake of fluids equals the excretion of fluids. This simple concept can be used to explain common causes of fluid imbalances. A lack of fluid intake, excessive fluid output, or both can lead to dehydration. Conversely, excessive fluid intake and a lack of fluid excretion can lead to overhydration. Further, alteration in any of the regulators of fluid balance—thirst, hormones, lymphatic system, and kidneys—increases the risk for or can cause an actual fluid imbalance.

LACK OF FLUID INTAKE

Average daily fluid intake for adults is about 1500 to 2000 ml. In addition, about 800 ml of fluid is consumed through solid foods; however, cognitive and physical impairments can quickly reduce water intake. For example, clients who are hospitalized, chairbound, or bedbound may not be able to reach their glass of water or may be too confused to recognize thirst. People with dysphagia or at risk for aspiration may not be able to swallow fluids safely. Tube-fed people who are not given adequate free water, or are fed hypertonic formulas, are also at risk. Community-dwelling older adults may have decreased access to fluids because of financial or transportation barriers or debilitation. For many of these reasons, nursing home residents older than 85 years of age appear to be at greatest risk for dehydration.

Impaired thirst mechanisms can also decrease fluid intake. Thirst usually develops from low blood pressure or fluid volume depletion as small as 0.5%. Low blood pressure can be seen in people who are losing fluids because of diuresis, diarrhea, bleeding, or drainage tubes. Excessive urination can be due to the use of diuretics (e.g., furosemide), intake of hypertonic fluids (e.g., hypertonic intravenous solutions), excretion of large volumes of glucose (e.g., ketoacidosis with diabetes mellitus), or, less commonly, neurologic problems (e.g., a lack of ADH production from diabetes insipidus). The sensation of a

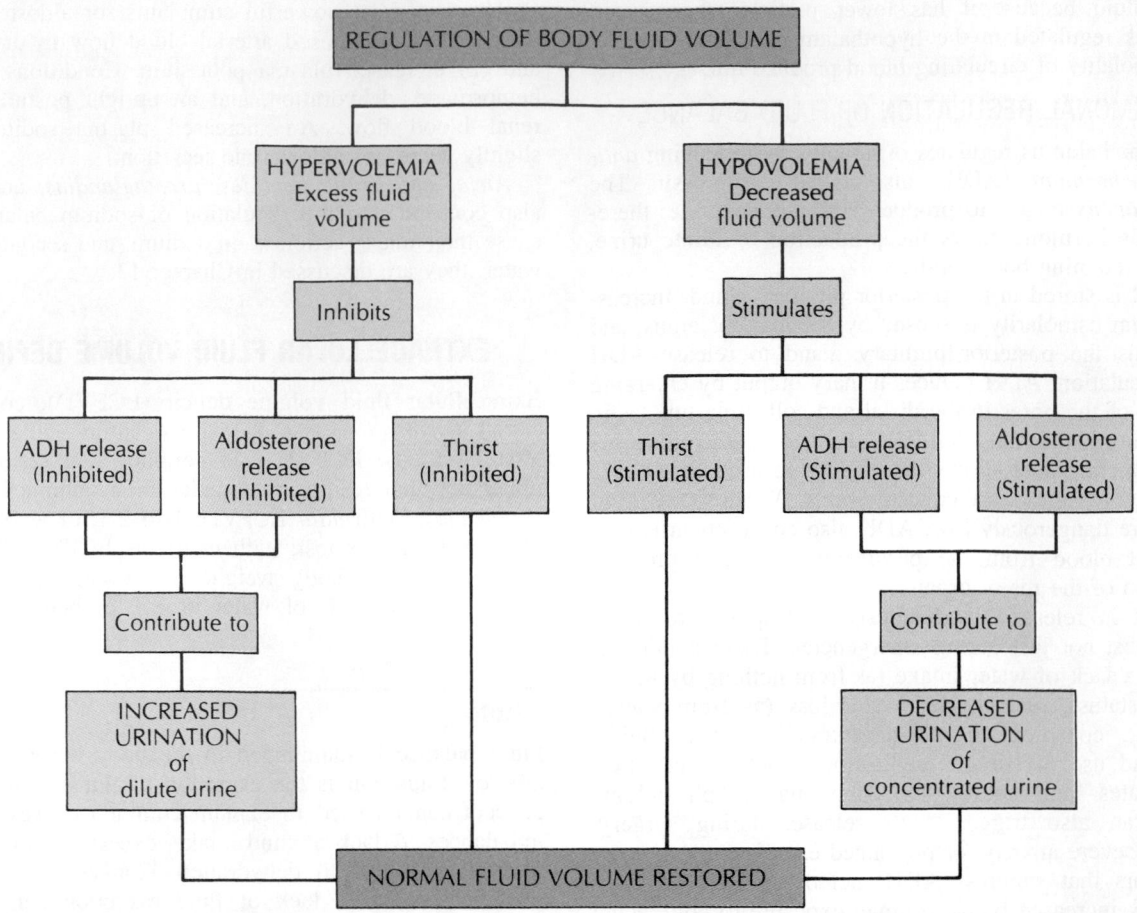

FIGURE 12–2 Regulation of body fluid volume depends on antidiuretic hormone (ADH), aldosterone, and thirst and fluid dynamics. (From White, B. [1994]. Maintaining fluid and electrolyte balance. In V. B. Bolander, [Ed.], *Sorensen and Luckmann's basic nursing: A psychophysiologic approach* [3rd ed.]. Philadelphia: W. B. Saunders.)

dry mouth also stimulates thirst. Clients may experience dry mouth from salivary gland dysfunction, head or neck radiation, smoking, mouth breathing, oxygen therapy, hyperventilation, and anticholinergic medications (such as atropine).

Most healthy people respond to decreased fluid levels by drinking fluids and thus maintain balance. However, the thirst mechanism is depressed in people with debilitating illnesses and in older adults, even the healthy elderly.[36] Several disorders also lead to inappropriate thirst mechanisms. People with excess fluids in the interstitial space, but depleted fluids in the vascular space, are commonly thirsty. Thirst is due to an increased renin-angiotensin-aldosterone response. Clients with congestive heart failure commonly experience this problem.

Osmolarity also influences thirst. Hyposmolarity inhibits the thirst response. Conversely, hyperosmolarity leads to thirst. It is common to find comatose and confused people with high plasma osmolarity, but they are unable to recognize the urge to drink.

EXCESS FLUID LOSSES

Severe vomiting and diarrhea are common causes of dehydration. These conditions are commonly associated with other clinical manifestations as well, such as changes in electrolytes. Potential causes of fluid loss include fever,

diaphoresis, hyperglycemia, gastrointestinal suction, ileostomy, fistulae, burns, blood loss, hyperventilation, hyperthyroidism, decreased ADH secretion, diabetes insipidus (nephrogenic and neurogenic),[31] Addison's disease or adrenal crisis, diuretic phase of acute renal failure, and the use of diuretics.

Again, the elderly population is at risk for excessive fluid losses for several reasons: (1) decreased renal concentration of urine, (2) an altered ADH response, and (3) an increase in body fat and thus a decrease in total quantity of body water in proportion to body weight.[14, 36] Increased drug-drug interactions and multiple chronic diseases potentiate the risk for fluid imbalances.

Third-space fluid shifts (shifting of fluid from the vascular space to interstitial space where fluid cannot be easily exchanged) can result in a fluid deficit in the vascular compartment. Spaces that are prone to third-spacing include the peritoneal, pericardial, pleural, and joint cavities. Abdominal third-spacing is called ascites.

Pathophysiology

When fluids are lost from the ECF, fluids move in from the interstitial spaces to restore vascular volume and dilute the hypernatremic state. ADH and aldosterone are secreted to retain fluids by decreasing urine output. Fluids are also recruited from fecal matter in the colon. Decreased blood volume is sensed by *baroreceptors,* which send messages to the sympathetic nervous system to increase peripheral vasoconstriction and the heart rate in an attempt to move fluids from the periphery into circulation. Low blood volume is also sensed by the osmoreceptors in the hypothalamus, which signals the thirst mechanism. These compensatory processes occur over and over again in normal healthy people. When fluid loss continues or when the compensation fails to restore blood volume, the person becomes dehydrated.

If the dehydration is not corrected, fluid is shifted from the cells because the ECF is hypertonic in relation to the ICF. The salivary glands become less active. There is less cerebrospinal fluid (CSF) and less fluid in the fat pads around the eyes. Less fluid is available for temperature regulation via sweating, and a lowered blood volume decreases the body's ability to transport core heat to the periphery for conductive loss. If cerebral cells become dehydrated, the vessels may bleed or go into spasm, and thought processes may be impaired. If sodium is lost, the muscle and nerve functions that depend on this electrolyte are slowed. A full discussion of sodium imbalances is provided in Chapter 13.

Clinical Manifestations

There are three types of extracellular fluid (ECF) volume deficits:

- *Hyperosmolar* fluid volume deficit: water loss is greater than electrolyte (sodium) loss
- *Iso-osmolar* fluid volume deficit: water and electrolyte (sodium) losses are equal
- *Hypotonic* fluid volume deficit: electrolyte loss is greater than fluid loss (rare)

LOSS OF BODY WEIGHT
Because water is a major portion of body weight, fairly rapid weight loss is an early and common result of fluid loss. A mild ECFVD exists when weight loss equals 2% of body weight. For example, in a client who weighs 150 pounds (68 kg), a 2% loss equals 1.4 L of water. Severe fluid loss exceeds 6% of body weight. In mild forms of dehydration, weight loss may not occur because it is masked by trapped fluids in the third space.

CHANGES IN INTAKE AND OUTPUT
Intake and output (I & O) measurements provide another means of assessing fluid balance. These data provide insight into the cause of the imbalance (such as decreased fluid intake or increased fluid loss). I & O measurements are not as accurate as body weight, however, because of relative risk of errors in recording.

Thirst is an early clinical manifestation of ECFVD in a conscious person. Clients often request plain, cold water rather than carbonated or caffeinated beverages. This is advantageous because caffeine is a diuretic and sweet fluids may not quench thirst.

Urine output usually decreases with ECFVD because of the effects of ADH and aldosterone. Urine is usually concentrated, with specific gravity above 1.030 and urine osmolarity above 1000 mOsm/kg. For many years, it had been thought that the kidneys had to excrete at least 30 ml of urine per hour as a mechanism for waste removal. Today, a urine output of 400 to 500 ml/day (16–20 ml/hr) is considered *oliguria* and indicates a marked compromise in kidney function. In most people (perhaps not the critically ill), urine output varies throughout the day. Normally, urine output is low and concentration is higher during the night. Thus, the view that urine should flow constantly at 30 to 40 ml/hr appears to lack justification.

Two groups of clients can become dehydrated because they do not have the ability to concentrate urine: (1) those with diabetes insipidus who do not produce ADH, and (2) those with kidney failure that prevents urine concentration.

CHANGES IN VITAL SIGNS
Inadequate fluid volume also leads to a decrease in systolic blood pressure, a weak pulse, and a decrease in central venous pressure (CVP) and pulmonary capillary wedge pressure (PCWP). For every liter of fluid lost, the cardiac output decreases by 1 L/min, the heart rate increases eight beats per minute (BPM), and the core temperature increases by 0.3° C (0.6° F).[15] Postural hypotension is a classic sign of decreased fluid volume. It is defined as a drop in systolic blood pressure of more than 25 mm Hg, a drop in diastolic pressure of more than 20 mm Hg, and a pulse increase of 30 BPM or more when the client stands up.

Sympathetic nervous system stimulation leads to vasoconstriction and increases the heart rate in an attempt to compensate for the altered tissue perfusion. Without restoring fluids, the vasoconstrictive and tachycardic (rate > 100 BPM) responses provide only a minimal and temporary solution. If these responses continue, tissue perfusion is further compromised. Serious fluid loss can lead to systolic blood pressures below 70 mm Hg. Low systolic pressure impairs tissue perfusion to vital organs that have high metabolic demands, such as cerebral, cardiac, and kidney tissues.

Flat jugular veins in a supine position and a prolonged peripheral venous filling time of more than 5 seconds are also noted. Because of the inability to cool the body core, an elevated temperature is common and can reach 105° F.

MANIFESTATIONS OF CELLULAR DEHYDRATION
The mucous membranes of the mouth and eyes become dry even though fluid is recruited from the interstitial spaces. The lips can crack, and furrows may be seen on the tongue. Swallowing can become difficult.

Tenting of the skin (decreased turgor) occurs when the skin tissues tend to stick together because of the decreased interstitial fluid. Tenting is not diagnostic of fluid deficit in older adults because tenting commonly results from loss of elastin in the skin in this population. Soft and sunken eyes may be noted. Muscle weakness from an imbalance of sodium and potassium occurs early and becomes worse as the deficit progresses. Feces become hard and decreased in number because the colon is trying to restore fluid balance.

Cerebral signs are always considered serious because it means that ICF compartmental shifting has occurred. Early signs include apprehension, restlessness, and headache. As the deficit progresses, hallucinations, maniacal behavior, and confusion occur, followed by coma.

DIAGNOSTIC FINDINGS

In hyposmolar fluid loss, more solvent is lost than solutes, which creates hemoconcentration. Plasma sodium concentration is also increased (*hypernatremia*). The following elevations are typical findings secondary to a hemoconcentrated state:

- Osmolality above 295 mOsm/kg
- Plasma sodium level above 145 mEq/L
- Blood urea nitrogen (BUN) above 25 mg/dl
- Plasma glucose above 120 mg/dl
- Hematocrit above 55%
- Urine specific gravity above 1.030

Specific gravity is a numeric value of urine concentration using solute-solvent relationships. Very concentrated urine has a high specific gravity. High specific gravity readings indicate dehydration or increased ADH. Glucose, protein, and dyes falsely elevate specific gravity. You can measure urine specific gravity by using a urinometer or by sending a urine sample to the laboratory for testing.

Hypernatremia usually indicates hyperosmolality, and hyponatremia usually indicates hyposmolality. Box 12–2 shows how to calculate plasma osmolality. Urine specific gravity may also be used as an indirect measurement of osmolality.

Outcome Management

The seriousness of a client's manifestations and the aggressiveness of treatment are related to both the *amount* and *acuteness* of the fluid loss and the client's state of health at the time of loss. Sudden loss of fluid does not give the compensatory mechanisms time to adapt; severe loss is often beyond the potential of compensatory mechanisms to adapt, resulting in vascular collapse or shock. A thorough history and physical examination, including collection of such demographic variables as age, gender, culture, presence of chronic diseases, and socioeconomic status, are critical to identifying realistic and measurable outcomes.

Medical treatment of fluid volume deficit depends on the acuteness and severity of the fluid deficit. The goals of treatment of ECFVD are to replace fluids and electrolytes (sodium primarily) that have been lost and to correct the underlying problem (such as vomiting or diarrhea).

BOX 12–2 How to Calculate Plasma Osmolality

To calculate plasma osmolality, you must know the plasma sodium (Na) level. Additionally, you should know the glucose level and blood urea nitrogen (BUN). The first formula may be used as a rough estimate of the plasma osmolality; the second formula gives a more exact plasma osmolality value.

$2 \times$ plasma Na = plasma osmolality
$2 \times$ plasma Na + (BUN/3) + (glucose/18) = plasma osmolality

---

FLUID RESTORATION

ORAL REHYDRATION. If the fluid loss is mild, the thirst mechanism is intact, and the client can drink fluid, fluids can be replaced orally. Oral glucose replacement solutions are palatable, inexpensive, and a good source of fluid, glucose, and electrolytes (Table 12–1). These solutions are quickly absorbed even if the client has diarrhea or is vomiting. Avoid cola drinks because they do not contain adequate electrolyte replacement; the sugar content also may lead to osmotic diuresis, and the caffeine may lead to diuresis.

INTRAVENOUS REHYDRATION. Whenever possible, use the oral route for replacement therapy. When the fluid loss is severe or life-threatening, intravenous (IV) fluids are used for replacement. The volume of fluid is calculated on the basis of the client's weight and the presence of any cardiac, renal, or pulmonary disorders. The type of solution used is based on the type of fluid lost from the body. Generally, isotonic ECFVD is treated with isotonic solutions, hypertonic ECFVD is treated with hypotonic solutions, and hypotonic ECFVD is treated with hypertonic solutions. Common IV fluids are listed in Table 12–2. Remember, a client with a terminal illness may have specific wishes about fluid maintenance.

MONITOR FOR COMPLICATIONS OF FLUID RESTORATION. Fluid needs must be assessed within the context of the client's overall condition. A client with severe ECFVD accompanied by severe heart, liver, or kidney disease cannot tolerate large volumes of fluid or sodium

TABLE 12–1	CONTENTS OF ORAL REHYDRATION SOLUTIONS				
Brand Name	Calories per Liter*	Sodium (mEq/L)	Potassium (mEq/L)	Chloride (mEq/L)	Citrate (mEq/L)
Gastrolyte	75	60	20	60	10
Lytren	84	50	25	45	30
Naturalyte	100	45	20	35	48
Oralyte	100	45	20	25	48
Pedialyte	100	45	20	35	30
Rapolyte	84	90	20	80	30
Rehydralyte	100	75	20	65	30
Resol	84	50	20	50	34
Ricelyte	126†	50	25	45	34

*From dextrose.
†From rice syrup.

Solution (Abbreviation)	Contents	Uses	Comments
HYPOTONIC			
5% dextrose in water (D$_5$W)	50 g dextrose No electrolytes	Replace deficits of total body water Not used alone to expand ECF volume because dilution of electrolytes can occur	Supplies 170 kcal/L and free water Distilled water cannot be given IV because it would cause hemolysis of RBCs Dextrose is metabolized on first pass through the liver, leaving a solution of water but without the hemolytic problems
ISOTONIC			
0.9% NaCl (normal saline solution, NS, 0.9% NS)	154 mEq/L of Na and Cl	ECF deficits in patients with low serum levels of Na or Cl and metabolic alkalosis Before and after the infusion of blood products	Not used for routine administration of IV fluids because it contains more sodium than ECF (140 mEq of NaCl and 103 mEq of Cl) Expands plasma and interstitial volume and does not enter cells
Lactated Ringer's solution (LR)	130 mEq/L Na 4 mEq/L K 3 mEq/L Ca 109 mEq/L Cl 28 mEq/L lactate	ECF deficits, such as fluid loss with burns and bleeding and dehydration from loss of bile or diarrhea	Solution is roughly isotonic to plasma but does not contain magnesium or phosphate Lactate is equivalent to bicarbonate, and solution can be used to treat many forms of acidosis Cannot be used in people with alkalosis; solutions of acetate Ringer's are better for these clients
HYPERTONIC			
Lactated Ringer's solution with 5% dextrose (D$_5$/LR)	50 g dextrose 130 mEq/L Na 4 mEq/L K 3 mEq/L Ca 109 mEq/L Cl 28 mEq/L lactate	ECF deficits, such as fluid loss with burns and bleeding and dehydration from loss of bile or diarrhea Provides modest calories (170 kcal)	This solution is hypertonic because it is the combination of two solutions (D$_5$W and LR) See other comments on individual solutions
5% dextrose and normal saline (D$_5$/0.9 NS)	50 g dextrose 154 mEq/L Na and Cl	ECF deficits in patients with low serum levels of Na or Cl and metabolic alkalosis Before and after the infusion of blood products Provides modest calories (170 kcal)	This solution is hypertonic because it is the combination of two solutions (D$_5$W and NS) See other comments on individual solutions
5% dextrose and 0.45% normal saline (D$_5$/0.45 NS; D$_5$/½ NS)	50 g dextrose 77 mEq/L Na and Cl	Can be used as an initial fluid for hydration because it provides more water than sodium Provides modest calories (170 kcal)	Commonly used as a maintenance fluid
5% dextrose and 0.225% normal saline (D$_5$/0.2 NS; D$_5$/¼ NS)	50 g dextrose 34 mEq/L Na and Cl	Can be used as an initial fluid for hydration because it provides more water than sodium Provides modest calories (170 kcal)	Commonly used as a maintenance fluid

Na, sodium; Cl, chloride; K, potassium; Ca, calcium; ECF, extracellular fluid; NS, normal saline; RBC, red blood cells; IV, intravenously; kcal, kilocalories.

without the risk for development of heart failure. For unstable clients, monitors to detect increasing pressures from fluids are used (e.g., measurement of CVP and pulmonary artery pressure). If the deficit has existed for more than 24 hours, it is dangerous to correct this deficit too rapidly. Sodium solutions should be infused at a rate of 0.5 to 1 mEq/L/hr. If fluid is given too rapidly, cerebral edema may result.[7]

Urine output, body weight, and laboratory values of sodium, osmolarity, BUN, and potassium are monitored closely.

CORRECTION OF UNDERLYING PROBLEM. Antiemetic and antidiarrheal drugs may be prescribed to correct problems with nausea and vomiting or diarrhea. Antibiotics may be used in clients with infectious diarrhea. Antipyretic agents may be used to reduce body temperature.

■ Nursing Management of the Medical Client

ASSESSMENT

Obtain the client's history of fluid losses. Consider whether the cause is infectious and whether isolation is warranted to reduce the spread of organisms.

Assess the client's vital signs every 2 to 4 hours, depending on the severity of the fluid loss; compare them with baseline vital signs and report marked differences. Assess for postural (orthostatic) blood pressure and pulse changes by taking blood pressure and pulse with the client lying down. Then have the client stand up; repeat the blood pressure and pulse measurements after 1 minute. Report a drop in standing systolic blood pressure of 25 mm Hg or more from the supine blood pressure; report pulse increases of more than 30 BPM. Autonomic neuropathy seen in diabetes, dysrhythmias, and some medications (e.g., antihypertensive agents) can also cause postural hypotension.

Assess the peripheral vein filling time daily. Veins with normal fluid volume should fill in 3 to 5 seconds when the arm is lowered below the level of the heart.

Monitor intake, output, and daily weights accurately in high-risk clients. Comparison of I & O data necessitates that all sources of intake (including liquids with meals and between meals, with medications, in IV lines, in tube-feedings, and in IV or tube flushes) and all sources of output (including urine, diarrhea, diaphoresis, and hyperventilation) be recorded accurately. If the ECFVD is mild, assess urine output every 8 hours and compare daily outputs. Absence of adequate renal perfusion for several hours may result in permanent renal damage. Whenever the output drops below 30 ml/hr for 2 consecutive hours, urinary output must be assessed hourly.

Teach unlicensed assistive personnel to report urine outputs of less than 30 ml/hr for 2 consecutive hours or less than 240 ml for an 8-hour period. Provide other instructions as well (see the Management and Delegation feature). Instruct the client to report fluids consumed in addition to the fluids on food trays and urine output not measured.

Monitor plasma sodium, BUN, glucose, and hematocrit levels to determine plasma osmolality. Assess the client for confusion, which is an early manifestation of ICF involvement.

Determine a history of chronic illnesses that may impair the ability to tolerate fluids at rapid speeds. Lung, renal, and heart disease reduce the body's ability to move fluids through the vascular system. Note the client's lung sounds on admission to serve as a baseline for later comparison.

Assess the client's weight and height. Do not rely on the client's stated weight because it may have decreased with fluid loss. Weigh the client daily. To increase accuracy of the measurement, weigh on the same scale, at the same time of day, with the client wearing clothing of similar weight. Help the client onto the scale; orthostatic hypotension may be present. Analyze changes in daily weights. A loss of 2.2 pounds is equivalent to 1 L of fluid. Therefore, an 8-pound weight loss equals about 3.5 L of fluid, or a moderate fluid volume deficit.

Assess the oral cavity between the gums and cheek for dryness of the mucous membranes and the tongue for dryness and longitudinal furrows.[17] A reliable method of testing for dryness of the mouth is to place your finger on the mucous membranes where the gums and cheek meet. When ECFVD is present, your finger will not glide easily because of dryness. Note any speech and swallowing difficulty. Assess closely for dried and adherent mucus on the soft palate.

Check skin turgor by gently pinching and lifting the skin (Fig. 12–3). Usually, skin returns to a normal position within 1 or 2 seconds in people younger than 60 years of age. A slower response may indicate loss of

A Assessment of skin turgor on the forearm

B Assessment of skin turgor on the sternum

FIGURE 12–3 Skin turgor assessment. This assessment can be done on the forearm (*A*) of a young to middle-aged adult. For older adults, skin turgor should be assessed over the sternum (*B*) because using a forearm yields inaccurate results because of natural loss of subcutaneous tissue.

interstitial fluids. Generalized weakness may develop because of changes in sodium levels.

DIAGNOSIS, OUTCOMES, INTERVENTIONS

Fluid Volume Deficit. Fluid volume deficit (FVD) is the state in which a person has vascular, interstitial, or intracellular dehydration. The diagnosis is *Fluid Volume Deficit related to insufficient fluid intake, vomiting, diarrhea, hemorrhage, or third-space fluid loss such as ascites or burns.*

Outcomes. The desired outcome is return of normal levels of body fluids. Indicators of adequate fluid volumes include:

- Oral intake between 1500 and 2500 ml or more in 24 hours
- Urine output greater than 600 ml in 24 hours
- Stable blood pressure and pulse in the supine and standing positions
- Increasing body weight of about 0.5 to 1.0 pound per day
- Absence of crackles (fluid in alveoli), an indicator of fluid overload from overcompensation
- Moist tongue and mucous membranes
- BUN plasma sodium hematocrit and osmolality levels approaching normal ranges over the first 48 to 72 hours

Interventions

Restore Oral Fluid Intake. Give small amounts of fluids "of choice" hourly to elderly, confused, or debilitated clients and to those who require restraints. Keep fluids fresh and within reach. Use orthotic devices as appropriate for those who can assist in their own fluid intake. Use antiemetics as needed to control nausea before drinking. When appropriate, begin with clear liquids,

such as oral replacement fluids, broth, or gelatin. Progress to full liquids and then solid foods, if tolerated without vomiting or aspiration. Encourage family members to participate in feeding.

If dysphagia (difficulty in swallowing) is present, consult the physician for swallowing studies. Once the problem has been identified, a speech pathologist can provide exercises to help the client. Reinforce the speech therapist's prescription during each feeding. You may need to give thickened fluids, elevate the headrest to 90 degrees before meals and for 1 hour after feeding, and flex the client's head slightly forward at the start of a swallow. Decrease the risk of aspiration by placing small amounts of food on the side of the mouth that has the best sensation and muscle strength. Teaching the client to chew slowly and to swallow two or three times with each mouthful and inspecting the mouth for food pocketing can also decrease the risk of aspiration. Assessing the fit of dentures is also important.

Restore Fluids by Intravenous Routes. Administer IV fluids cautiously to clients with ECFVD. Ideally, a large IV gauge (e.g., 18- to 20-gauge) should be used; however, most clients have venous collapse, and it is difficult to find a vein. A small IV site may be used initially; once fluids are reestablished, a larger needle can be inserted if fluids or an IV access is still needed. Use an IV pump or a mini-drop infusion set to regulate IV infusion and to decrease the risk of too rapid an infusion. Monitor IV solutions, IV sites, and client outcomes hourly.

Rapid fluid replacement often results in overflow diuresis without cellular replacement. Diuresis compounds dehydration and may result in hypernatremia. In elderly people or those with renal or cardiac disease, rapid fluid administration may also result in pulmonary overload.

Reduce the Risk of Fluid Volume Deficit. If your assessment indicates no fluid deficit but a risk of fluid deficit, the format for writing the problem statement is *Risk for Fluid Volume Deficit related to (risk factor).* Interventions are focused on health promotion and maintenance strategies that decrease the likelihood of a deficit. The goal of oral fluid promotion and maintenance is to maintain the level of fluid intake at 1500 ml for 24 hours.

If the client is fed by tube, give water boluses with hypertonic tube-feedings. Recommended dilution is 1 ml of water per 1 kilocalorie (kcal) of feeding formula. For example, if a can of formula has 380 kcal in 240 ml of formula, give an additional 140 ml of water, for a total of 380 ml of fluid.

Control the Underlying Problems. Diarrhea has several causes. Examine elixirs for sorbitol, which can cause abdominal distention, cramping, and osmotic diarrhea. If the onset of the diarrhea was at the same time as the new drug with sorbitol, consult the pharmacy to determine whether crushable pills rather than elixirs can be used. Consider viral infections because many have been known to result in lactose intolerance. If this is the cause, encourage the client to avoid milk-based products. Avoiding fatty or fried foods also decreases diarrhea and enhances digestion.

Give prescribed antiemetics for nausea, antipyretics for fever, and antibiotics for infection.

Monitor for Complications. When fluid balance is compromised, a person is at risk for tissue breakdown. Apply a moisturizer or skin barrier to protect the skin from the irritants, enzymes, and microorganisms found in urine and feces. Continue to assess lung sounds for manifestations of fluid overload (crackles) from overcorrection.

Altered Oral Mucous Membranes.
The nursing diagnosis of *Altered Mucous Membranes related to lack of oral intake, or other causes* is a common problem in clients with dehydration.

Outcomes. The desired outcome is that the client's mouth, gums, and teeth remain clean and free of accumulations of dried mucus.

Interventions. Give oral care with a regular toothbrush or a foam toothbrush every 2 to 4 hours, and apply lip moisturizer. Rinse the client's mouth every 1 to 2 hours. Examine the client's mouth with a penlight to make sure that it remains free of debris. Avoid mouthwashes with an alcohol base, which can dry the mucous membranes. The frequency of oral care may need to be increased to hourly if evaluation of the skin and oral assessment findings indicate lack of improvement. Artificial saliva can also be used for the client with a very dry and fissured mouth.

Risk for Injury.
If orthostatic hypotension is present, *Risk for Injury* is another problem that needs to be addressed.

Outcomes. The desired outcome is that the client will remain free of injury, as evidenced by no manifestations of falls (bruises, bumps, abrasions) or reported episodes of falls.

Interventions. Provide safety through step-progression position changes. Step-progression gives the client's body time to adapt to changes in position. First, raise the head of the bed. Next, assist the client to sit at the edge of the bed, in a "dangling" position, until the dizziness has subsided. Have the client stand, and assist the client to a chair. Do not progress to the next position until the client tolerates the preceding one (i.e., without dizziness or marked hypotension).

It is difficult to teach confused clients to remain in bed and not to get up without assistance. Use bed alarms to help identify clients who are likely to get up and fall. Restraints may be needed if all other measures to control behavior do not work.

EVALUATION

Mild to moderate fluid deficits should be corrected in 8 to 24 hours. More severe fluid losses may take several days, especially when they occur in older adults.

■ Self-Care

Client teaching is one of the primary interventions for promoting and maintaining fluid balance. Teach clients with mild fluid deficit to replace fluid with clear liquids, 30 to 60 ml or more hourly, as tolerated, to decrease nausea and replace electrolytes. Teach the importance of consulting a physician if an illness lasts longer than 24 hours or if the person is older or has a chronic illness, such as diabetes mellitus or liver, kidney, or heart disease.

Health promotion teaching is critical for those who actively exercise.[15] Teach people who exercise to:

- Understand the importance of exercise and heat acclimatization
- Avoid exercise during high heat and humidity
- Wear appropriate clothing (excess clothing decreases evaporation)
- Use more caution to prevent heat exhaustion if they are obese, because obesity impairs the sweating mechanism
- Drink cool water before exercise, 150 to 200 ml every 15 minutes during exercise, and after finishing exercise, and add 500 to 700 kcal of carbohydrates (for energy and sodium), if exercise is prolonged
- Avoid rapid fluid replacement, since this fluid only overflows to the kidneys
- Use caution when taking medications that interfere with thermoregulation, such as thyroid replacement, amphetamines, beta-blockers, haloperidol, antihistamines, anticholinergic drugs, and phenothiazines

Encourage diabetic clients who exercise to wear or carry Medic-Alert identification, to increase their protein intake, to decrease refined sugar intake, and to reduce insulin to half the usual dosage or to an amount recommended by the physician.[23] Teach people taking cortisone the importance of not missing doses, of carrying Medic-Alert identification, and of consulting a physician about increased dosage during physical or emotional stress to prevent Addison's crisis.

Reducing fluid intake as a way of decreasing urinary incontinence in older adults is inappropriate. Limited fluid intake increases bladder irritability, leading to uninhibited contractions, and alters the neurologic stimulus that controls normal bladder emptying. Emphasizing the importance of drinking even in the absence of thirst, teaching pelvic muscle exercises, and instituting a toilet schedule may help an older person overcome the problem of incontinence.

INTRACELLULAR FLUID VOLUME DEFICIT

Dehydration can become so severe that the cells become dehydrated. This condition is relatively rare in a healthy adult, but it occurs quite often in older clients and in clients with conditions that result in acute water loss. Compensatory attempts to combat the fluid deficit have the same physiologic basis as in ECFVD. Thirst and oliguria are the most common compensatory signs. Cellular manifestations are due to the dysfunction in the cerebral cells and include fever and central nervous system (CNS) changes, such as confusion, coma, and cerebral hemorrhage.

The desired outcome is restoration of fluid volume, which is initially addressed through IV replacement. Once the client becomes stable, the focus of medical management is correction or control of the underlying cause. The focus of nursing management is on prevention or early detection of complications secondary to the pathology or the treatment. Interdisciplinary communication is critical to the achievement of positive outcomes.

EXTRACELLULAR FLUID VOLUME EXCESS

ECF volume excess (ECFVE) is fluid overload or overhydration. Excess fluids can be found in the vascular system, a problem called *hypervolemia,* or in the interstitial spaces, a problem usually called *third-spacing* (see later). The water and sodium retained is in the same proportions as it exists in other ECF, and therefore is referred to as *isosmolar fluid volume excess.*

Etiology

ECF volume excess can develop from two processes: (1) simple overloading with fluids and (2) failure to excrete fluids. ECFVE often results from an increase in the total body sodium. Causes of ECFVE are shown in Table 12–3.

Pathophysiology

With a fluid volume excess, the hydrostatic pressure of the fluid is higher than usual at the arterial end of the capillary. Excess amounts are moved out into the interstitial spaces because of the pressure. The fluid is not reabsorbed at the venous end because pressure remains high in the arteriole and resists flow from the tissues. Peripheral and pulmonary edema may result (Fig. 12–4A).

As the fluid pressure increases in the interstitial area and tissues, it creates a resistance to forward blood flow and increases resistance throughout the circulatory system. A resistance to arterial flow occurs, which leads to increased pressure in the left ventricle and then in the left atrium. From the atrium, fluid is unable to be propelled forward and it backs up across the alveolocapillary membrane of the lungs, resulting in pulmonary edema. Because the lungs are low-pressure organs, they also offer little resistance to fluid accumulation. Pulmonary edema develops quickly in clients with distention of the left side of the heart muscle, and the heart cannot pump adequately. If the right side of the heart fails, peripheral edema occurs through the same retrograde process. Left-

TABLE 12–3	ETIOLOGY OF EXTRACELLULAR FLUID VOLUME EXCESS
Etiologic Factor	**Examples**
Compromised regulation of fluid movement and excretion	Cirrhosis of the liver Decreased plasma protein Heart failure Hypothyroidism Lymphatic or venous obstruction Renal disorders
Excessive ingestion of fluids or foods containing sodium	Excessive amounts of saline intravenous fluids Ingestion of high-sodium foods Excessive use of enemas with sodium (e.g., Fleet's) or medications with sodium (e.g., Alka-Seltzer)
Increased antidiuretic hormone (ADH) and aldosterone	Certain barbiturates and narcotics (e.g., morphine) Cushing's syndrome General anesthesia Glucocorticoid use Hyperaldosteronism Syndrome of inappropriate secretion of ADH

sided heart failure leads to right-sided failure and vice versa, and both pulmonary and peripheral edema may thus exist simultaneously.

When fluid overload results from renal disorders, sodium and water excretion are decreased. As fluid volume rises, the heart compensates through tachycardia and hypertrophy. When compensatory mechanisms fail, heart failure results. Uncontrolled heart failure can lead to multiple organ failure and death from massive water retention, also known as *anasarca.*

In severe liver disease, renal disease, burns, or protein malnutrition, the plasma protein and albumin levels are decreased. Therefore, oncotic pressure is decreased in the vascular fluids, resulting in less fluid reabsorption from the tissue spaces at the venous end. Peripheral edema and ascites result (see Fig. 12–4B).

When lymphatic channels are obstructed, tissue oncotic pressure rises and leads to edema (see Fig. 12–4C). Chapter 53 discusses lymphedema. Edema can also develop from conditions that increase capillary permeability, such as tissue trauma (see Fig. 12–4D). This form of edema is discussed in Chapter 27.

Clinical Manifestations

Fluid volume excess leads to respiratory and cardiovascular manifestations. The respiratory manifestations are from increasing hydrostatic pressure in the pulmonary capillaries, which results in shifting of fluid to the alveolar sacs. Fluid congestion in the alveoli manifests as coughing, dyspnea, and crackles that can be auscultated over the involved lung area. The alveolar fluid accumulation

FIGURE 12–4 Mechanisms of edema formation. *A,* Fluid overload. *B,* Decreased plasma and albumin. *C,* Lymphatic obstruction. *D,* Tissue injury.

also leads to impaired oxygen (O_2) and carbon dioxide (CO_2) transport between the capillaries and alveoli, resulting in pallor, cyanosis, decreased tissue perfusion (measured by pulse oximetry) and increased CO_2 blood gas abnormalities. If hydrostatic pressure continues to rise, fluid shifts into the pleural spaces as well; this is known as *pleural effusion.*

Cardiovascular manifestations are numerous. Delayed emptying and filling of the right ventricle leads to systemic venous engorgement, including signs of jugular venous distention, peripheral vein filling time above 5 seconds, a bounding pulse and elevated blood pressure, and increased CVP and pulmonary capillary wedge pressure (PCWP). If the delayed ventricular filling overdistends the ventricles, an extra heart sound, called S_3, can often be auscultated.

Fluid accumulates in the interstitial compartments, especially in the gravity-dependent tissues of the legs and sacrum. Edema may develop in the feet in ambulatory people and in the sacrum of bedridden clients. The continued increase in fluid pressure also causes fluid shifting into the visceral tissues. Thus, the client may exhibit signs of organ dysfunction specific to the tissues involved (e.g., anorexia and bloating from stomach involvement). Rapid weight gain is a classic sign of fluid overload regardless of the system responsible for the overload.

If any early changes in cerebral function develop, such as confusion and headache, suspect ICF shifting. As the fluid excess increases in the cerebral cells, lethargy occurs, followed by seizures and then coma.

With fluid overload, the concentration of solutes is decreased by the excess fluid volume. Typical findings include:

- Plasma osmolality less than 275 mOsm/kg
- Plasma sodium less than 135 mEq/L, depending on the type of fluid excess
- Hematocrit less than 45%
- Specific gravity less than 1.010
- BUN less than 8 mg/dl

Remember, these results must be evaluated in the context of the client's manifestations and the possibility of other pathologic processes. For example, blood loss would also cause a decreased hematocrit; a decreased protein intake would result in a decreased BUN. Chapters 56 and 63 describe heart failure and acute pulmonary edema. The plasma sodium level may appear to be within the normal range because of excess water retention, even though the actual sodium level is increased.

Outcome Management

A thorough clinical history of contributing and causative factors, medication history, manifestations of fluid overload, and laboratory findings are essential to identifying appropriate interventions. Reduction of dietary sodium, restriction of fluids, and pharmacologic interventions are the major treatments of ECFVE.

RESTRICTION OF SODIUM AND FLUIDS. According to the usual definitions, a *mildly* restricted sodium diet contains 4 to 5 g of sodium, a *moderately* restricted diet contains 2 g of sodium, and a *severely* restricted diet contains 0.5 g of sodium[1] (see Chapter 13, Box 13–2, for a list of high- and low-sodium foods). To convert milligrams of sodium to milliequivalents, divide the number of milligrams by 23 (the atomic weight of sodium). For example, 1000 mg sodium is equivalent to 43 mEq of sodium.

PROMOTING URINE OUTPUT. Mild diuretics and digitalis promote fluid loss and improve myocardial contractility. Many diuretics cause potassium and magnesium to be excreted along with the sodium and water. To counteract this, a combination of potassium-wasting and potassium-sparing diuretics may be prescribed.

Several studies have found improved myocardial contractility and decreased morbidity and mortality in clients with heart failure who, in addition to digitalis, have received angiotensin-converting enzyme (ACE) inhibitors and low-dose beta-blockers. Many of these clients showed such an improvement in their overall cardiac function that they did not need diuretics. When ACE inhibitors are used, clients should be monitored for hyperkalemia because of the potassium-sparing effect of the ACE inhibitor.[24]

▄ Nursing Management of the Medical Client

ASSESSMENT

Monitor the client's vital signs for a bounding pulse, elevated blood pressure, or both every 4 to 8 hours. Assess the apical pulse if the radial pulse is irregular or if the client is taking cardiac medication. Assess breath sounds every 4 to 8 hours for crackles, rhonchi (abnormal lung sounds indicating retention of secretions), or wheezes, noting changes in location or severity. Assess for changes in respiratory effort with activity or rest.

Each morning, palpate the sacrum and legs for pitting edema and observe the client for hand and bilateral neck vein engorgement. Jugular vein distention at or above a 45-degree headrest suggests ECFVE. Hand veins that do not flatten within 3 to 5 seconds when the hand is raised above the heart level suggest fluid overload. Assess the condition of skin on the legs. Edematous skin is very fragile and can tear easily.

Compare I & O every 4 to 8 hours. Weigh the client daily; do not rely on stated weights. Determine whether the client has had expected weight loss or unexpected weight gain. Edema does not usually occur until 3 L or more of excess fluid has accumulated. Measure extremities if edema seems pronounced.

Monitor plasma osmolality, sodium level, hematocrit, and urine specific gravity. Observe for changes in level of consciousness, which may indicate the more serious complication of ICF shifting.

DIAGNOSIS, OUTCOMES, INTERVENTIONS

Fluid Volume Excess. The diagnostic statement is written *Fluid Volume Excess* related to (specific cause, such as heart, renal, or liver failure). Be certain to specify the cause in your client's case. If your client has heart failure, also consider using the diagnosis *Decreased Cardiac Output.*

Outcomes. The desired outcome is return of normal levels of body fluids. Indicators of adequate fluid volumes include:

- Stable blood pressure and pulse
- Decreasing body weight of about 0.5 to 1.0 pound per day
- Absence of manifestations of ICFVE such as confusion
- Absence of manifestations of ECFVE such as coughing, crackles, dyspnea, jugular venous distention, peripheral edema, S_3 gallop rhythm
- BUN, plasma sodium, hematocrit, and osmolality approaching normal levels in 48 to 72 hours
- Absence of manifestations of overcorrection, such as hypotension, dry mucous membranes

Interventions

Reduce Sodium and Fluid Intake. Fluid management becomes extremely important in clients with ECFVE. Strict I & O may be crucial. Include fluids on meal trays and those given with medications as part of the total fluid intake. Collaborate with the dietitian in planning fluid restrictions. Schedule oral medications at meal times, if possible, to limit fluid intake. Use minimal amounts of water (5 to 10 ml) to dissolve crushed medications that need to be given by feeding tube. Flushing the tube with cola may decrease the need for large amounts of water and may keep the tube patent. Cold fluids decrease the sensation of thirst more than warm or hot fluids do. Give the client ice chips, if allowed, and provide frequent oral care to decrease the thirst sensation (1 cup of ice equals ½ cup of water). Instruct the client about the rationale for fluid and sodium restrictions.

Use IV pumps and/or mini-drop tubing to control IV fluid intake. Use only isotonic saline for bladder and nasogastric tube irrigations. For clients on continuous bladder irrigation, consult the physician about changing hypotonic bladder irrigations to normal saline during the postoperative period.

Sodium is a common ingredient in foods, and to many clients the low-sodium diet is bland. Suggest alternatives for seasoning to enhance the taste of foods and increase dietary compliance. Salt substitutes are available; they use potassium as the cation but taste bitter to many people. Clients who take ACE inhibitors cannot use potassium salt substitutes.

Mobilize Fluid. Instruct the client who has dependent leg edema to avoid long periods of standing and to sit with legs elevated. Bed rest alone promotes diuresis, particularly in clients with heart failure. Mobilization of edema in the supine position is probably due to diminished pooling of venous blood, a resultant increase in effective circulating blood volume and thus renal perfusion.

Reduce Complications. Elevate the head of the bed 30 to 45 degrees to decrease venous return to the heart, which decreases cardiac workload and allows for improved diaphragmatic excursion, both of which improve oxygenation. This position also promotes jugular venous drainage, which improves cerebral perfusion. If dyspnea or orthopnea is present, position the client in semi-Fowler's or Fowler's position. Give oxygen to keep oxygen saturation above 90%, according to the provider's orders.

If the client is taking diuretics and digitalis, monitor plasma electrolytes and anticipate digitalis toxic effects secondary to hypokalemia. Report the levels of plasma electrolytes, especially potassium levels.

When peripheral tissue perfusion is altered because of edema or vascular disease, provide frequent skin care, turn the client often, control moisture, and prevent friction and shear. The heel is especially at risk for decreased capillary blood flow. Therefore, it is important to keep the client's heels elevated off the mattress and to remove elastic stockings when redness is noted.

■ Modifications for Elderly Clients

In general, the interventions for each of these outcomes are the same for the older client; however, response time is usually slower and the risk for side effects is higher because of poorer renal and liver function and problems with drug interactions.[32] For instance, digitalis toxicity is much more common in the elderly. Some diagnostic studies may not be as accurate in this population. For example, a person with protein malnutrition, which is more common in the elderly, may have renal insufficiency but may have a normal BUN because of the lack of protein.

EVALUATION

Correcting ECFVE is a slow process, especially when it results from an organ disorder. Most clients are discharged without complete resolution of peripheral edema but with improvement in pulmonary edema and breathing. Self-care instructions are critical.

■ Self-Care

If the client is going home on a low-sodium diet, review allowed and restricted foods with the client and the person who prepares the meals. Canned foods should be avoided; fresh and frozen foods are usually lower in sodium. Buying these items in season and freezing them for later use save money and provide more nutrients. Encourage the food purchaser to read food labels and to avoid products with high levels of sodium or salt and food whose labels contain the word "sodium" or the symbol "Na" as a prefix. Avoid drinking or cooking with softened water, which is high in sodium. Water may need to be obtained from another source, or a water distiller may be needed.

Suggest alternatives for seasoning to enhance the taste of foods and to increase dietary compliance. Adding fresh lemon to vegetables and main dishes, condiments that come in powder form (such as garlic), or other low-sodium seasonings that can be found at health food stores can increase satiety. Remember, people taking ACE inhibitors cannot use potassium salt substitutes.

If the client is going home with fluid restriction, help the client and family plan for how fluids can be spaced. Recognize the cultural variations in fluid consumption. In Western society, offering a guest something to drink is a common practice and may influence total fluid consumption.

Instruct the client and family to notify the physician about a weight gain of more than 3 pounds per week, a marked reduction in urine output, increased shortness of breath with exertion or especially at rest, new-onset headaches, confusion, seizures, or a deterioration in level of consciousness.

INTRACELLULAR FLUID VOLUME EXCESS: WATER INTOXICATION

Although the cells are usually quite resistant to fluid shifts, certain conditions can lead to an intracellular fluid volume excess (ICFVE). Conditions that cause acute or severe fluid volume excesses have a higher incidence of ICF overload. This is because the adaptive mechanisms may be unable to compensate for large or sudden fluid excesses.

ICFVE results from either water excess or solute deficit, primarily from sodium loss. In water excess, the number of solutes is normal but they are diluted by excessive water. In solute deficit, the amount of water is normal but there are too few particles per liter of water.

The most common cause of ICFVE is the administration of excessive amounts of hyposmolar IV fluids, such as 0.45% (half-normal) saline solution or 5% dextrose in water (D_5W). ICFVE may occur in clients who receive continuous IV D_5W or in older clients who consume excessive amounts of tap water without adequate nutrient intake. Syndrome of inappropriate antidiuretic hormone (SIADH) also leads to ICFVE regardless of whether the SIADH is caused by CNS trauma, the stress of surgery, pain, or narcotic use.

People with certain psychiatric disorders, such as schizophrenia, often have compulsive water consumption behaviors. Studies have found that as many as 80% of people admitted to a hospital with a diagnosis of schizophrenia have water intoxication. You must monitor for compulsive water consumption in people with a history or current manifestations of an organic psychiatric illness.[12, 13, 35]

Hyposmolar fluids in the vessels move by osmosis to the region of higher concentration of sodium in the cells in an attempt to maintain equilibrium. Unfortunately, too much fluid accumulates in the cells, causing cellular edema. Cerebral cells absorb hyposmolar fluid more quickly than do other cells. Thus, these cell changes often present the earliest warning signs of intracellular shifting.

All neurologic manifestations are secondary to the increasing intracranial pressure (ICP). Most ICP syndromes progress cephalocaudally. Thus, the early signs are cortical and, as pressure increases, pupillary. The vital signs then change. A complete discussion of the changes caused by increasing ICP is presented in Chapter 73.

Because ICF excess is often associated with ECF excess, it is common to see a plasma sodium level of less than 125 mEq/L and a decreased hematocrit. However, there is no plasma test to reflect the cell fluid volume. Diagnostic tests, such as computed tomography (CT) and magnetic resonance imaging (MRI), are more helpful in identifying causes underlying the syndrome of ICFVE.

Neurologic cells are very vulnerable to fluid excess or deficit. The first priority is to reduce ICP with steroids and osmotic diuretics. Equally as important is identifying and addressing the cause of the fluid volume excess. Immediate surgical intervention may be critical. The interventions specific to varying causes are discussed in Chapters 68, 69, 70, and 73.

If SIADH is an impending risk, early administration of IV fluids containing some sodium chloride (NaCl) may prevent it. Saline solutions, such as $D_5/0.45\%$ NaCl, increase the osmolality of vascular fluid and prevent or help correct hyposmolality.

Because brain tissue has a very narrow margin in which life is sustained, frequent monitoring and early intervention are critical. Perform neurologic checks, including level of consciousness, vital signs, reflexes, and pupillary responses, every hour if cranial changes are present. Cerebral perfusion is altered if systolic blood pressure drops too low or rises too high. Notify the provider if the client's sensorium changes from the baseline assessment, if systolic blood pressure is less than 100 mm Hg or greater than 150 mm Hg, or if other signs persist or worsen.

Monitor IV fluids and I & O hourly, and monitor weight daily. Polyuria is a good sign and indicates that fluid has shifted to the vascular space and to the renal tubules, where it can be excreted. Administer antiemetics prophylactically, as appropriate, to promote food and fluid ingestion and retention and to decrease the risk of vomiting, which worsens the increased ICP.

Provide safety measures when the client displays behavioral changes, such as confusion or disorientation. Keep the bed in a low position with bedside rails raised. Keep suction equipment at the bedside in anticipation of seizures. If a client has a seizure, turn the client to one side to displace the tongue. Remain at the bedside until the client is safe, and document all phases of the seizure. See Chapter 69 for care of the client during a seizure.

If the manifestations of increased ICP are improving, then the client is at less risk for complications. Remember, time equals brain cell survival. The longer the manifestations of increased ICP persist and the more serious they are, the graver the prognosis.

EXTRACELLULAR FLUID VOLUME SHIFT: THIRD-SPACING

A fluid volume shift is basically a change in the location of ECF between the intravascular and the interstitial spaces. Fluid shifts are of two types: (1) *vascular* fluid shifts to interstitial spaces and (2) *interstitial* fluid shifts to vascular spaces. Fluid that shifts into the interstitial spaces and remains there is referred to as *third-space*

fluid. This abnormal fluid accumulation not only results from pathologic conditions but also reflects an inability of the lymphatic system to compensate. Common sites of third-spacing include the pleural cavity, peritoneal cavity, and pericardial sac. Third-space fluid is physiologically useless because it does not circulate to provide nutrients for cells.

Etiology

Fluids can move into interstitial spaces because of increased capillary permeability, decreased serum protein levels, obstruction of the venous portion of the capillary, or nonfunctional lymphatic drainage systems.

Any pathologic process that increases capillary permeability can cause third-spacing. Any tissue injury can lead to fluid shifting. Massive fluid shifts from the vascular to the interstitial spaces can be seen in crush injuries, major tissue trauma, major surgery, extensive burns, acid-base imbalance, bowel obstruction, and sepsis. Capillary permeability can also be altered by ischemia.

Decreased protein intake, production, or storage, as seen in protein-calorie malnutrition, leads to hypoalbuminemia. Bowel disorders that reduce protein absorption can reduce serum levels. Conditions that cause a loss of protein, such as kidney and liver disease or large draining wounds or burns, also deplete protein stores. Increased protein anabolism can occur in the healing phase of fractures or wounds; increased protein catabolism can occur with fever, infection or sepsis, and malignancy.

Lymphatic obstruction and venous thrombosis slow fluid returning through the venous system.

Pathophysiology

Tissue injury causes the release of histamine and bradykinin, resulting in increased capillary permeability, which allows more fluid, protein, and other solutes to move into the interstitial spaces than normal. This form of fluid shift is time-limited. Once the early stages of inflammation pass in about 24 to 48 hours, the capillary closes and fluid returns to the venous system.

Protein malnutrition leads to fluid shifts because protein is not present to pull fluid back into the capillary at the venous end. This form of fluid shifting is usually long term and can be seen in children who are malnourished and have large protruding abdomens and pencil-thin legs.

Two phases of fluid shift are associated with tissue injury:

1. Fluid shift from vascular to interstitial spaces, which leads to a fluid volume deficit (*hypovolemia*) (see Fig. 12–4D). Severe hypovolemia may lead to vascular collapse and death. If cellular damage is severe, a toxic response may occur from intracellular ions, such as potassium, which leak into the vascular spaces.
2. Fluid shift back from the interstitial to the vascular space, which leads to a fluid volume excess (*hypervolemia*). If the hypervolemia is severe, it may lead to heart failure. Intracellular potassium ions shift back into the cell during this phase, which increases the risk for hypokalemia.

Clinical Manifestations

Clinical manifestations of a fluid shift from the vascular to the interstitial spaces are similar to the manifestations of hypovolemic shock because the fluid is not in the vascular system. Typical clinical manifestations include pallor, cold limbs, weak and rapid pulse, hypotension, oliguria, increased skin turgor, and decreased levels of consciousness. Body weight does not change because fluid has not been lost; it has been redistributed.

If fluid collects and obstructs an organ, nerve, or vessel, other clinical manifestations may arise. For example, bowel sounds may change throughout the abdomen. Extremities may become pale, cool, and pulseless if fluid obstructs blood vessels or nerves. Laboratory results may indicate an elevated hematocrit and an elevated BUN. Urine has an elevated specific gravity.

When fluid returns to the blood vessels, the clinical manifestations are similar to those of fluid overload. Signs may include a bounding pulse, crackles, engorgement of peripheral and jugular veins, and an increase in blood pressure. Laboratory results may indicate a decrease in hematocrit and BUN. Other abnormal findings depend on the area of the body affected.

Outcome Management

As with fluid volume deficit and fluid volume excess, third-spacing is only a manifestation. It is crucial that the underlying cause be identified through a thorough history and physical examination so that interventions can be targeted to the desired outcomes.

Medical treatment begins with determining the cause of the fluid volume shift. If the third-spacing of fluid has occurred as a result of pericarditis, pericardiocentesis may have to be done to preserve organ function. If third-spacing is from a bowel obstruction, paracentesis (removal of peritoneal fluid via a large-bore needle) is the procedure of choice (see Chapters 30 and 62).

REPLACE FLUIDS

When hypovolemia results from tissue injury, such as burns or crush injuries, a large volume of isosmolar IV fluid administration is required to replace intravascular volume. When there is evidence of capillary sealing, as when urine output increases without additional fluids, albumin may be given to replace the protein lost from the trauma and to promote restoration of capillary oncotic pressures. Because third-spacing is a common occurrence after major surgery, maintaining IV fluid intake is essential to maintaining kidney perfusion. The amount of fluid infusion may be three times greater than urine output. Generally, fluids are titrated to maintain an adequate blood pressure, PCWP or PAWP, and urine output. If replacement is too aggressive, a fluid overload can occur, in part because of increased ADH.

When the capillary walls regain integrity, fluid shifts from the tissue spaces back into the vessels. If fluid replacement is too aggressive during this phase, a fluid overload can also occur.

STABILIZE OTHER PROBLEMS

The diagnosis of sepsis is confirmed by culture, and treatment is with antibiotics. Vasoactive medications may be needed to maintain blood pressure. Bowel obstructions are decompressed and surgically repaired. Inflammatory disorders are treated with massive doses of steroids to stabilize the mast cell membrane.

Nursing Management of the Medical Client

Assess vital signs often according to the client's condition. The frequency can vary from every 1 to 8 hours. If shock-like symptoms are present, assess vital signs every hour during the shock-like state. If fluid loss is a result of ascites or peripheral edema, the fluid shift is slower and changes in vital signs are usually subtle.

Monitor IV fluid replacement needs. If fluids are administered too rapidly, fluid overload or hypervolemia may occur. Assess for early signs of fluid overload, such as pulmonary crackles, difficulty in breathing, and neck vein engorgement. Notify the provider if these signs are present. Anticipate a reduction in IV fluid needs as the third-space fluid shifts back into the plasma during the capillary repair stage.

If the third-spacing is in the abdomen, as with ascites, measure the client's abdominal girth every 8 hours. If a limb is involved, measure the circumference of the limb and assess peripheral pulses every 8 hours. Use preventive measures to prevent skin breakdown of edematous areas.

Monitor urine output every hour, and report an output of less than 30 ml/hr if it persists for more than 2 hours. The client may need more fluids, not diuretics. Urine output is usually reduced after tissue injury because of decreased renal circulation and a fluid shift into the injured tissue spaces. One to 3 days after tissue injury, fluid returns to the circulation and excess fluid is excreted by the kidneys unless renal function is impaired. Monitor plasma levels of BUN and creatinine.

CONCLUSIONS

Fluid imbalances are common problems, especially in high-risk populations, such as older adults and clients with acute illnesses or multiple pathologic processes. Many health care disciplines work collaboratively toward maintaining or retoring fluid balance. The role of nursing in this collaborative effort is focused on health promotion activities, including teaching positive health behaviors, health maintenance activities (including early detection and consultation with other disciplines), and prevention and early detection of complications from the underlying diseases, coexisting conditions, or treatment. Through these interventions, you play a critical role in assisting clients and their families achieve positive health outcomes in a cost-effective manner.

THINKING CRITICALLY

1. **The admitting receptionist has just called your floor to secure a room for a 69-year-old woman with a history of 2 days of vomiting and diarrhea and a fever of 103° F secondary to suspected influenza virus. The client has a history of hypertension and heart failure. Home prescriptions include digoxin, 0.125 mg/day; furo-**

semide (Lasix), 40 mg bid; and potassium chloride, 40 mEq/day. The client has also been advised to consume a low-sodium diet. An IV line of D$_5$/NS with 30 mEq of potassium chloride was started.

Factors to Consider. What is the priority risk or problem in this scenario? What are the desired outcomes? What are the critical assessments? What medical management and nursing strategies do you anticipate?

2. **A middle-aged client is admitted to your unit with shock-like symptoms from a massive burn wound. He has pale skin, cold limbs, hypotension, and a weak, rapid pulse. Urine output via the indwelling catheter is decreased. His level of consciousness varies from an adequate response to little or no response to external stimuli.**

Factors to Consider. What is the priority risk or problem in this scenario? What are the desired outcomes? What are the critical assessments? What medical management and nursing strategies do you anticipate during this phase of fluid shifting from the vascular spaces to the interstitial spaces? How will they change when the fluid shifts back into the vascular spaces?

BIBLIOGRAPHY

1. Abraham, W., & Schrier, R. (1994). Body fluid volume regulation in health and disease. *Advances in Internal Medicine, 39,* 23–43.
2. Andrews, M., et al. (1993). Dehydration in terminally ill patients. *Postgraduate Medicine, 93*(1), 201–208.
3. Arief, I. (1999). Fatal postoperative pulmonary edema: Pathogenesis and literature review. *Chest, 115*(5), 1371–1377.
4. Banasik, J. (1995). Alterations in cardiac function. In L. Copstead (Ed.), *Perspectives on pathophysiology* (pp. 346–374). Philadelphia: W. B. Saunders.
5. Batcheller, J. (1994). Syndrome of inappropriate antidiuretic hormone secretion. *Critical Care Nursing Clinics of North America, 6*(4), 687–692.
6. Bergeron, M., Armstrong, L., & Maresh, C. (1995). Fluid and electrolyte losses during tennis in the heat. *Clinics in Sports Medicine, 14*(1), 23–32.
7. Brown, R. (1993). Disorders of water and sodium balance. *Postgraduate Medicine, 93*(4), 227–246.
8. Burge, F. (1993). Dehydration symptoms of palliative care cancer patients. *Journal of Pain and Symptom Management, 8*(7), 454–464.
9. Casa, D. J. (1999). Exercise in heat: I. Fundamentals of thermal physiology, performance implications, and dehydration. *Journal of Athletic Training, 34*(3), 246–252.
10. Carrougher, G. J. (1997). Management of fluid and electrolyte balance in thermal injuries: Implications for perioperative nursing practice. *Seminars in Perioperative Nursing, 6*(4), 201–209.
11. Corbett, J. V. (1996). *Laboratory tests and diagnostic procedures with nursing diagnoses* (4th ed.). Stamford, CT: Appleton & Lange.
12. Cosgray, R., et al. (1993). A program for water-intoxicated patients at a state hospital. *Clinical Nurse Specialist, 7*(2), 55–61.
13. Davidhizar, R., & Kriesl, R. (1993). Water intoxication: One nursing staff's response and intervention. *Journal of Advanced Nursing, 18,* 1975–1980.
14. Faull, C., Holmes, C., & Baylis, P. (1993). Water balance in elderly people: Is there a deficiency of vasopressin? *Age and Ageing, 22,* 114–120.
15. Galloway, S. D. (1999). Dehydration, rehydration, and exercise in the heat: Rehydration strategies for the athletic competition. *Canadian Journal of Applied Physiology, 24*(2), 188–200.
16. Gisolfi, C. (1996). Fluid balance for optimal performance. *Nutrition Reviews, 54*(4), S159–S166.
17. Gross, C., et al. (1992). Clinical indicators of dehydration severity in elderly patients. *Journal of Emergency Medicine, 10*(3), 267–274.
18. Hall, J. (1994). Caring for corpses or killing patients? *Nursing Management, 25*(10), 81–89.
19. Held, J. (1995). Cancer care: Correcting fluid and electrolyte imbalances. *Nursing, 95*(4), 24–28.
20. Hoot-Martin, J., & Larsen, P. (1994). Dehydration in the elderly surgical patient. *AORN Journal, 60*(4), 666–671.
21. Iggulden, H. (1999). Dehydration and electrolyte disturbance. *Elderly Care, 11*(3), 17–23.
22. Kaufmann, M. (1996). Preventing dehydration in the elderly. *Provider, 9,* 65–66.
23. Koivisto, V., et al. (1992). Fuel and fluid homeostasis during long-term exercise in healthy subjects and type I diabetic patients. *Diabetes Care, 15*(4), 1736–1742.
24. Krueger, S., et al. (1994). Treatment of heart failure: Update 1994. *Nebraska Medical Journal, 8,* 292–297.
25. Maughan, R. J. (1999). Exercise in the heat: Limitations to performance and the impact of fluid replacement strategies. *Canadian Journal of Applied Physiology, 24*(2), 149–151.
26. May D. L. (1998). The relationship between self-induced water intoxication and severity of psychiatric symptoms. *Archives of Psychiatric Nursing, 12*(6), 335–343.
27. McClousky, J., & Bulechek, G. (1996). *Nursing interventions classification (NIC): Iowa intervention project* (2nd ed.). St. Louis: Mosby–Year Book.
28. McConnell, E. (1995). What's wrong with this patient? Assessing altered level of consciousness. *Nursing, 95*(6), 66–67.
29. Miller, C. (1995). *Nursing care of older adults: Theory and practice* (2nd ed.). Philadelphia: Lippincott-Raven.
30. Miller, K. (1996). Diabetes insipidus. *Journal, 23*(3), 285–292.
31. Moseley, M. J. (1997). Perioperative problems: Nutrition and electrolytes in the elderly. *Seminars in Perioperative Nursing, 6*(1), 21–30.
32. O'Donnell, M. (1995). Assessing fluid and electrolyte balance in elders. *American Journal of Nursing, 95*(11), 41–45.
33. Oster, J., & Materson, B. (1992). Renal and electrolyte complications of congestive heart failure and effects of therapy with angiotensin-converting enzyme inhibitors. *Archives of Internal Medicine, 152,* 704–710.
34. Rehrer, N. (1994). The maintenance of fluid balance during exercise. *International Journal of Sports Medicine, 15,* 122–125.
35. Ribbe, D., & Thelander, B. (1994). Patients with disordered water balance. *Journal of Psychosocial Nursing, 32*(10), 35–42.
36. Sansevero, A. (1997). Dehydration in the elderly: Strategies for prevention and management. *Nurse Practitioner, 22*(4), 41–70.
37. Smith, S. (1995). Patient-induced dehydration: Can it ever be therapeutic? *Oncology Nursing Forum, 22*(10), 1487–1497.
38. Smith, S. (1997). Controversies in hydrating the terminally ill patient. *Journal of Intravenous Nursing, 20*(4), 193–199.
39. Spangler, A. A. (1998). Age, dependency and other factors influencing fluid intake by long term care residents. *Journal of Nutrition for the Elderly, 18*(2), 21–35.
40. Steiner, N. & Bruera, E. (1998). Methods of hydration in palliative care patients. *Journal of Palliative Care, 14*(2), 6–13.
41. Sutcliffe, J., & Holmes, S. (1994). Dehydration: Burden or benefit to the dying patient? *Journal of Advanced Nursing, 19,* 71–76.
42. Theston-Aurand, J., Olmsted R., Allen-Bridson, K., & Craig, C. (1997). Impact of dressing materials on central venous catheter infection rates. *Journal of Intravenous Nursing, 20*(4), 201–204.
43. Vonfolio, L. (1995). Back to basics: Would you hang these IV solutions? *AJN, 95*(6), 37–39.
44. Zerwekh, J. (1997). Do dying patients really need IV fluids? *AJN, 97*(3), 26–30.

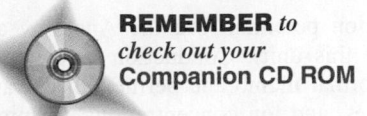

CHAPTER 13

Clients with Electrolyte Imbalances: Promoting Positive Outcomes

Bernadette White

Electrolytes are substances found in extracellular and intracellular fluid that dissociate into electrically charged particles known as ions. Ions that carry a positive charge are called *cations;* those that carry a negative charge are called *anions.* Sodium, potassium, calcium, magnesium, and hydrogen are the major cations in the body. Major anions are chloride, phosphate, bicarbonate, and protein. The principal cation in the intracellular fluid (ICF) is potassium. The principal cation in the extracellular fluid (ECF) is sodium (Fig. 13–1). Chapter 14 discusses the role of hydrogen and bicarbonate in maintaining acid-base balance. The concentrations of electrolytes in various body fluids are given in Table 13–1.

Electrolytes have several functions in the body. They regulate fluid balance and osmolality. Because of the abundance of sodium in the ECF, this ion has a major effect on fluid balance. Problems related to fluid balance are discussed in Chapter 12. The continual fluctuation of anions and cations also allows for transmission of nerve impulses and stimulation of muscle activity.[29]

ELECTROLYTE BALANCE

■ DIETARY INTAKE

Under normal circumstances, humans ingest far more electrolytes than are needed each day. Food sources for some important electrolytes are listed later in the chapter (see Boxes 13–2 to 13–5). Only when food intake is restricted does the intake of electrolytes become a concern.

■ REGULATED OUTPUT

Several hormones govern the output of electrolytes. Sodium, potassium, and chloride are closely regulated by aldosterone, antidiuretic hormone (ADH), and atrial natriuretic peptide (ANP). Calcium and phosphorus are regulated by vitamin D and calcitonin. Insulin and epinephrine promote the uptake of potassium by cells. Hormones such as gastrin, cholecystokinin, and secretin affect some degree of electrolyte absorption in the intestines. Finally,

weight-bearing and stress on bones promote calcium uptake by the bone.

ELECTROLYTE IMBALANCES

An electrolyte imbalance is present whenever there is an excess or deficit in the plasma level of a specific ion. Terms used to describe the imbalance contain the prefix *hyper-* for increased or *hypo-* for decreased, followed by the name of the electrolyte (in its Latin form for sodium and potassium) and then the suffix *-emia* to indicate presence in the blood—as measured in the plasma. For example, *hyponatremia* means low plasma sodium, and *hyperkalemia* means elevated plasma potassium. *Hypercalcemia* and *hypermagnesemia* indicate elevated calcium and magnesium levels, respectively.

Although electrolyte imbalances are very common, the literature is scant on the topic. One study found that 94% of clients coming into the emergency department with certain presenting characteristics had significant electrolyte imbalances. These variables included poor oral intake, history of vomiting or muscle weakness, use of diuretics, signs of abnormal mental status, and history of chronic hypertension, alcoholism, recent seizure or electrolyte imbalance, and age 65 years or older.

As with fluid imbalance, a client's response to electrolyte imbalance is related to several variables. The relationship of fluid status to the electrolyte level, age, health status, potential for adaptive mechanisms, and the severity and acuteness of the imbalance all influence the client's response.

To help clients achieve the most positive health outcomes, you must understand the underlying causative disorders and conditions as well as the risk factors for electrolyte imbalance and become an active participant in health promotion, health maintenance, and health restoration interventions. By increasing the emphasis on health promotion and maintenance from a community perspective, you can also decrease the need for acute care intervention, which decreases the cost of health care in addition to improving health outcomes.

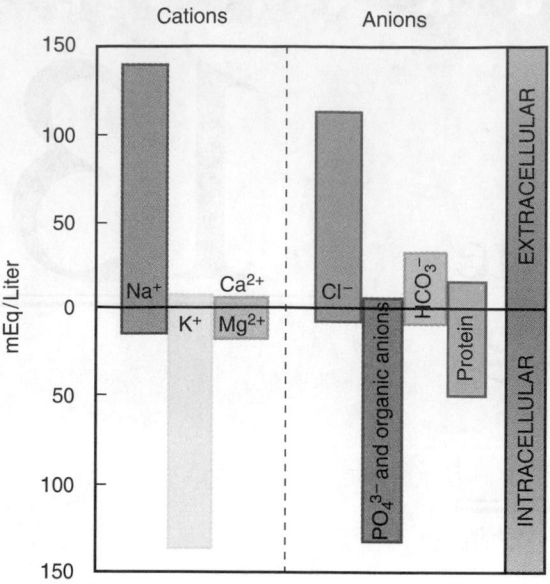

FIGURE 13–1 A comparison of electrolyte composition of the extracellular and intracellular fluid compartments. (From Guyton, A. C., & Hall, J. E. [1996]. *Textbook of medical physiology* [9th ed., p. 300]. Philadelphia: W. B. Saunders.)

Etiology and Risk Factors

Anyone who has decreased intake, decreased availability, or increased loss of electrolytes is at risk for electrolyte deficit. When body fluids are lost, the electrolytes in them are also lost. For example, the loss of gastric juice through vomiting may lead to the loss of several electrolytes. Conversely, increased intake or increased retention of an electrolyte or decreased ability to excrete certain electrolytes may increase the risk for electrolyte excess. For example, ingestion of excess sodium bicarbonate for indigestion can alter both sodium level and acid base balance.

Pathophysiology

Before you can fully understand the pathophysiology of electrolyte imbalances, you need to first understand the physiology of the action potential (see the Anatomy and Physiology section of this unit). Conduction of electrical current depends on normal membrane permeability, transportation of electrolytes, and ion concentrations. Common problems that alter the conduction of electrical current include problems with membrane permeability, ionic gradients, and concentrations.

Cells are quickly damaged by lack of blood flow or oxygen. Cardiac, nerve, and muscle cells can be damaged by lack of blood flow (as during periods of ischemia), altered by toxins (as from various medications), or directly injured (as in crush or stab injuries). Such damage typically increases the permeability of the cell membrane and increases its tendency to "fire." This phenomenon can be seen in cardiac cells after ischemia. Cells that normally do not generate action potentials begin to do so, causing abnormal heart rhythms. This same phenomenon can be the cause of seizures following brain injury.

Potassium levels can significantly influence the resting membrane potential (Fig. 13–2). When potassium levels are lower than normal, the resting membrane potential becomes more positive. It requires less stimulus to make it "fire." Cells so affected are called *hypopolarized* and respond to a weaker stimulus. Conversely, when potassium levels are higher, the resting membrane potential falls and the cell is less excitable. Such cells are called *hyperpolarized* and require a stronger-than-normal stimulus to reach threshold potential and to generate an action potential. Sodium and calcium also alter resting membrane potential.

Diagnosis

A wide range of clinical manifestations should raise suspicion about a possible electrolyte imbalance, as suggested in the Critical Monitoring feature. The diagnosis of electrolyte imbalance is made through clinical assessment and measurement of plasma levels in laboratory studies. Currently, measurement of intracellular levels of electrolytes is too costly; thus, plasma levels are used for diagnostic evaluation (Box 13–1). Plasma electrolyte studies are relatively inexpensive.

Plasma values for electrolytes can be expressed as milliequivalents per liter (mEq/L), or milligrams per deciliter

TABLE 13–1	CONCENTRATION OF ELECTROLYTES IN VARIOUS BODY FLUIDS*				
	Concentration (mEq/L)				
Fluid	*Na⁺*	*K⁺*	*Cl⁻*	*HCO₃⁻*	*H⁻*
Plasma	135–145	3.5–5.0	98–106	25–29	7.35–7.45
Gastric juice	55–100	10–15	120	5–10	90
Pancreatic juice	145–160	5	65–90	50–80	—
Bile	130–145	5–9	75–100	10–45	—
Ileum	125	10–80	55	60	—
Sweat					
Insensible	8	10	15	—	—
Sensible	10–80	6	5–85	—	—

*Levels may vary according to the physiologic state of the body.

Na⁺, sodium; K⁺, potassium; Cl⁻, chloride; HCO₃⁻, bicarbonate; H⁻, hydrogen.

From White, B. (1994). Maintaining fluid and electrolyte balance. In V. B. Bolander (Ed.), *Sorenson and Luckmann's basic nursing: A psychophysiologic approach* (3rd ed.). Philadelphia: W. B. Saunders.

FIGURE 13–2 Effects of electrolyte imbalances on the membrane potential. Conductile tissue rests at negative millivolts, called a *resting membrane potential.* When the nerve is stimulated, ion channels for sodium, potassium, and calcium open to change the firing potential. Potassium tends to lower the potential by decreasing the millivolts to more negative levels. Sodium does the opposite: It raises the action potential to more positive values (above zero). Calcium also raises the resting membrane potential to a more positive value. The closer the resting membrane potential to threshold, the more rapid the nerve firing.

(mg/dl). Values reported as mEq/L can be converted to mg/dl by multiplying by 1.2.

Using a "Collaborative Problem" Format

Currently there are no NANDA diagnoses for electrolyte imbalances. The Iowa Interventions Project approached these disorders as collaborative problems and developed a research-based list of critical and supporting activities for management of 15 fluid and electrolyte disorders. Because the nursing role primarily involves collaborating with the physician, the goal statements are also phrased differently. Note that each expected outcome is preceded by the phrase "The nurse will monitor the client for. . . ."[20] Nursing diagnoses that may apply to clients with electrolyte imbalances include *Risk for Injury, Risk for Activity Intolerance, Risk for Decreased Cardiac Output, Altered Mucous Membranes,* and *Risk for Impaired Skin Integrity.* Or you may use the appropriate collaborative problem

taxonomy to identify the problem—*hyponatremia* or *hypernatremia, hypokalemia* or *hyperkalemia, hypocalcemia* or *hypercalcemia, hypomagnesemia* or *hypermagnesemia* and *hypophosphatemia* or *hyperphosphatemia.*

SODIUM IMBALANCES

A sodium imbalance occurs when sodium concentration in plasma either decreases or increases. A sodium deficit is known as *hyponatremia.* Sodium excess is known as *hypernatremia.* Chloride is the anion that usually accompanies sodium; therefore, levels of chloride fall or rise along with levels of sodium. Manifestations of chloride imbalance are usually associated with the cation imbalance.

Sodium balance is regulated by the interaction among neural, hormonal, and vascular mechanisms. Sensing mechanisms in the atria, aorta, carotid sinus, liver, pulmonary tissue, and juxtaglomerular apparatus (JGA) in the kidneys detect changes in sodium intake and ECF volume by sensing an increase or decrease in blood pressure. Central nervous system (CNS) receptors also respond to changes in the sodium concentration in the cerebrospinal fluid (CSF).

One example of a neural-hormonal interaction is the JGA sensory mechanism in the nephron, which promotes a stimulation response of the renin-angiotensin-aldosterone hormonal system. Renin, excreted in response to hypotension, results in increased aldosterone secretion, which stimulates sodium reabsorption across the renal tubule. Prostaglandins, kallikrein, and atrial natriuretic peptide also control sodium homeostasis. Prostaglandins secreted by the kidney stimulate the production of renin to maintain renal blood flow during periods of reduced blood volume. Kallikreins are high-molecular-weight pro-

BOX 13–1	Plasma Ranges for Electrolytes*
Sodium	135–145 mEq/L
Chloride	98–106 mEq/L
Potassium	3.5–5.0 mEq/L
Calcium	4.5–5.5 mEq/L
Ionized calcium	1.18–1.30 mEq/L
Phosphorus	1.2–3.0 mEq/L
Magnesium	1.5–2.5 mEq/L

*Ranges may vary somewhat between laboratories.

CRITICAL MONITORING

Fluid and Electrolyte Imbalance Secondary to Any Disorder/Condition

- New onset of dysrhythmia
- Worsening of dysrhythmia, such as occurrence of premature ventricular contractions at a rate greater than 6 per minute, bradycardia with heart rate less than 50 BPM, tachycardia with heart rate greater than 120 BPM
- Sudden change in level of consciousness, including sudden restlessness, lethargy, and seizures
- Tetany, laryngeal spasm, or stridor
- Postural systolic blood pressure drop greater than 25 mm Hg, with a pulse increase of 30 beats/min or more
- Rapid weight loss
- Severe dryness of oral mucous membranes with tongue furrowing
- Hemorrhage
- Urinary output less than 30 ml/hr for 2 consecutive hours
- Rapid weight gain, especially with pulmonary signs of sudden onset such as crackles, dyspnea, S_3 gallop

teins produced by the distal convoluted tubule that secrete kinin. Kinin is a potent renal vasodilator that increases renal excretion of sodium. Atrial natriuretic peptide (ANP) balances the effects of ADH by promoting urinary sodium excretion (natriuresis), vasodilatation, and increased urinary output.[13] See the Nervous System review in Unit 11 and Chapter 52 for review of the influence of the baroreceptors.

The phenomenon of glomerular capillary filtration is an example of how vascular dynamics influence sodium homeostasis. The renal glomerulus filters 1000 mEq of sodium every hour, and about 99% of this is reabsorbed. Reabsorption is influenced by the pressure of the blood entering the glomeruli. Increased blood pressure promotes filtration of water and sodium and other electrolytes across the glomerular membrane. Sodium is reabsorbed in the loop of Henle, and reabsorption of the rest of the electrolytes occurs in the proximal tubule.

■ HYPONATREMIA

Hyponatremia is defined as a plasma sodium level below 135 mEq/L. It is one of the most common electrolyte disorders in adults, especially the elderly.[21, 30] Hyponatremia is usually associated with changes in fluid volume status. The four types of hyponatremic states are as follows[21]:

- Hypovolemic hyponatremia
- Euvolemic hyponatremia
- Hypervolemic hyponatremia
- Redistributive hyponatremia

When sodium loss is greater than water loss, hypovolemic hyponatremia occurs. Euvolemic hyponatremia results when the total body water (TBW) is moderately increased and the total body sodium remains at a normal level. Hypervolemic hyponatremia results when a greater increase occurs in TBW than in total body sodium. In redistributive hyponatremia, no change occurs in TBW or total body sodium; water merely shifts between the intracellular and extracellular compartments relative to the sodium concentration.

Etiology and Risk Factors

Table 13–2 lists the most common pathophysiologic causes of hyponatremia. Hyponatremia can also occur in persons who are considered healthy. For example, athletes[3, 12] and outdoor laborers are at risk for hyponatremia from excessive perspiration. Any person with an altered thirst mechanism or without access to fluids, or one who attempts to rehydrate too rapidly after excessive fluid loss, is at risk for hyponatremia. Older adults are at increased risk because of their relatively lower percentage of TBW. The preoperative use of laxatives, multiple pathologic conditions, spinal anesthesia, and noninfectious postoperative complications increase risk factors for death from hyponatremia in elderly people after surgery.

With cardiac, renal, and liver disease, the total body sodium is usually high, although the plasma sodium level may appear normal or low because of dilution from water retention. In such instances, the increase in TBW is generally greater than the sodium indicates. Renal causes of hyponatremia stem from the inability to excrete suffi-

TABLE 13–2	CLINICAL CONDITIONS AND DISORDERS THAT MAY CAUSE HYPONATREMIA
Type of Hyponatremia	**Clinical Conditions and Disorders**
Hypovolemic hyponatremia	Renal loss of sodium from diuretic use, diabetic glycosuria, aldosterone deficiency, intrinsic renal disease
	Extrarenal loss of sodium from vomiting, diarrhea, increased sweating, burns, high-volume ileostomy
Euvolemic hyponatremia	Sodium deficit resulting from SIADH or the continuous secretion of ADH due to pain, emotion, medications; many cancers; CNS disorders
Hypervolemic hyponatremia	Edematous disorders resulting in sodium deficits; congestive heart failure, cirrhosis of the liver, nephrotic syndrome, acute and chronic renal failure
Redistributive hyponatremia	Pseudohyponatremia, hyperglycemia, hyperlipidemia

ADH, antidiuretic hormone; CNS, central nervous system; SIADH, syndrome of inappropriate (secretion of) antidiuretic hormone.

ciently dilute urine.[25] Normally, when hyponatremia and hyposmolality occur, diuresis follows to promote the return of sodium and water reabsorption.

Pathophysiology

Most pathophysiologic changes caused by hyponatremia result from the decreased excitability of the membranes from a loss of sodium and changes in water volume. Recall that most sodium is outside the cell. Less sodium is available to move across the excitable membrane, resulting in delayed membrane depolarization. Excitable tissues vary in their response to decreased sodium. The cells most sensitive to change are the CNS cells.

As the concentration of sodium decreases in the ECF, the difference in gradient between the ECF and ICF compartments also decreases. When the extracellular sodium level falls, the ECF becomes hypo-osmolar. This osmotic shift can lead to intracellular edema. Water moves into the cell to the area of greater concentration to rebalance the water concentration. An increase in brain cell volume as small as 5% can cause brain herniation.[27] Brain cells attempt to compensate by reducing cerebral blood flow, shifting CSF, and decreasing the brain's intracellular osmolality. Intracellular osmolality is reduced through decreasing the amount of intracellular ions, such as sodium and potassium, and amino acids.[21, 27]

Clinical Manifestations and Diagnostic Findings

Clinical manifestations of hyponatremia vary with the cause, type, and rate of onset of sodium or fluid imbalance. A plasma sodium level of 120 mEq/L that developed slowly may be asymptomatic. The same plasma sodium level resulting from an acute loss may be life-threatening.[10]

When plasma sodium concentration is greater than 125 mEq/L, clinical manifestations may not be apparent.[10, 30] Early neurologic manifestations of headache and apprehension are from increased fluid shift into the cerebral cells. As intracranial pressure rises and plasma sodium level drops to 115 mEq/L, severe neurologic changes such as confusion, hallucinations, behavioral changes, and seizures occur. Continued shifting of water into the intracellular compartment leads to brain herniation, resulting in coma and death.[21, 27, 30]

Cardiovascular manifestations—such as a decrease in systolic and diastolic blood pressures, orthostatic hypotension, and a weak, thready pulse—are due to a decrease in vascular volume secondary to sodium and water loss. Tachycardia is a compensatory response that is the direct result of triggering of the release of sympathetic catecholamines by the baroreceptor reflex (see Unit 12 review). Chemoreceptors in the aortic arch and carotid bodies also trigger sympathetic responses if the oxygen, carbon dioxide, or hydrogen levels become affected. In severe hypovolemic hyponatremia, a shock-like state occurs, with blood pressures of 60 mm Hg and below. An exception is hypervolemic hyponatremia, in which the excess volume causes elevated blood pressure and a full, rapid pulse.

Crackles in the lungs are from fluid shifting into the pulmonary alveoli secondary to increasing fluid pressures in the pulmonary capillaries. The increasing left ventricular fluid pressure leads to a retrograde increase in pressure in the left atrium and pulmonary vasculature. The changes in respiratory rate and difficulty breathing—such as tachypnea, dyspnea, orthopnea, and feeling short of breath—are from presence of fluid in the alveoli, which alters oxygen and carbon dioxide levels. Alterations in respiratory pattern, such as with Cheyne-Stokes respirations, neurogenic hyperventilation, apneustic breathing, or ataxic breathing, are from increasing intracranial pressure.

Hyponatremia causes gastrointestinal (GI) manifestations, such as nausea, vomiting, hyperactive bowel sounds, abdominal cramping, and diarrhea, because sodium is a crucial component of normal neuromuscular activity of smooth muscle. A decrease in sodium causes increased excitability of the neurons that innervate the smooth muscle.

Although not life-threatening, the dryness of the skin, tongue, and mucous membranes that results from the decreased interstitial volume caused by a sodium deficit has other, more serious implications. There is a higher risk for altered integrity of the skin and oral mucous membranes, which increases the risk of infection and results in increased health care needs and costs.

A laboratory finding of a plasma sodium level below 135 mEq/L is diagnostic of hyponatremia. However, as noted previously, most clients are not symptomatic until levels reach 125 mEq/L or less. Because chloride is the main anion associated with sodium, a chloride level below 98 mEq/L is a very common finding. A decreased concentration of sodium is also reflected in a plasma osmolality of less than 275 mOsm/kg. The kidney attempts to compensate for the body's loss of sodium by decreasing urinary losses; thus, a typical urine sodium level is below 40 mEq/L.[36]

If the hyponatremic state and body fluid volume disorders are not corrected, potassium, calcium, chloride, and bicarbonate electrolyte imbalances may also occur.

Outcome Management

■ Medical Management

Medical management is determined by the cause of the hyponatremia, the type of hyponatremia, and the severity of the clinical manifestations. The more serious the manifestations, the more aggressive the treatment. The goal of medical intervention is correction of the body water osmolality, with restoration of cell volume, by raising the ratio of sodium to water in the ECF. The increased ECF osmolality draws water from the cells, thereby decreasing cellular edema.

RESTORING SODIUM LEVELS

If the client has hyponatremia from fluid volume excess, fluids are restricted to allow the sodium to regain balance. Intake of balanced diet is usually adequate therapy for mild hyponatremia, with sodium levels of 126 to 135 mEq/L. Fluids may be restricted to a range of 1000 to 1500 ml/day.

If the plasma sodium level declines below 125 mEq/L, sodium replacement is needed. For sodium levels of 125 mEq/L or less, intravenous (IV) therapy is the treatment of choice. Dietary supplementation may still be appropriate for a client who can ingest oral fluids or food. Foods high in sodium are listed in Box 13–2. For moderate hyponatremia, with sodium levels of 125 mEq/L, IV normal saline solution (0.9% NaCl) or lactated Ringer's solution may be ordered if the client is symptomatic. When the plasma sodium level is 115 mEq/L or less, a concentrated saline solution such as 3% NaCl may be indicated until the plasma sodium reaches 125 mEq/L. A diuretic such as furosemide (Lasix) is often given intravenously to prevent fluid overload. Demeclocycline (a tetracycline), an agent that antagonizes ADH, is the preferred agent for treatment of hyponatremia secondary to syndrome of inappropriate antidiuretic hormone (SIADH).[10, 28, 33, 77]

Rapid elevation of plasma sodium concentrations to more than 125 mEq/L increases intravascular fluid volume and may result in hypernatremia and CNS damage. Recommendations for IV replacement therapy include an infusion rate of 0.5 mEq/L/hr if the loss is chronic, not to exceed a total of 12 mEq of sodium in 48 hours, or of 1.0 mEq/L/hr if the loss is acute, not to exceed 25 mEq in 48 hours.[5] To prevent fluid shifts and exacerbation of vasospasm in persons with subarachnoid hemorrhage, normal saline is usually the IV solution of choice.[21, 37]

▪ Nursing Management of the Medical Client
ASSESSMENT

Take a complete history of risk factors and presenting manifestations. Emphasize diet and medication history, including over-the-counter medications. Older adults are especially prone to drug-drug interactions that may alter sodium balance. The client and family members should be asked about behavioral changes, headaches, increased weakness or sleepiness, dizziness, and palpitations.

Measure the client's body weight, because the stated weight may not be accurate. Calculate ideal body weight by using height, weight, and body frame; then compare measurements. Assess intake and output, peripheral vein filling time, and vital signs every 4 to 8 hours. Also, monitor plasma sodium levels and estimate the plasma osmolality. It is important to remember that in hyponatremic conditions, such as hypervolemic hyponatremia, plasma sodium levels may appear to be normal to low.

DIAGNOSIS, OUTCOMES, INTERVENTIONS

Risk of Hyponatremia. There is no specific diagnosis for hyponatremia; therefore, the collaborative problem of *Risk for Hyponatremia* can be used to label this client problem. State the problem as *Risk for Hyponatremia related to unreplaced fluid loss or limited oral intake.*

When actual hyponatremia is present, the collaborative problem is stated as *Hyponatremia related to* (e.g., *vomiting, diarrhea, gastric suctioning, burns, SIADH, surgery, or fluid overload*). The cause needs to be clear because it relates directly to the interventions.

Outcomes. The nurse will have a high index of suspicion for high-risk clients and will monitor clients who have had fluid losses or limited fluid intake for manifestations of hyponatremia. When your assessment indicates an actual sodium deficit, restoration is the primary goal. An outcome may be as follows: The nurse will monitor laboratory sodium and chloride levels and will continue to monitor for clinical manifestations of hyponatremia.

BOX 13–2 High- and Low-Sodium Foods

High-Sodium Foods (~250 mg per serving)
Breads/Cereals
Cold cereal, 1 oz
Corn chips, 14 chips
Instant hot cereal, ½ cup
Potato chips, 14 chips

Cheeses
Natural cheese, 1 oz
Processed cheese, 1 oz
Creamed cheese, ½ cup

Meats
Sausage, 1 oz
Luncheon meats, 1 oz
Frankfurters, 1 oz
Cooked bacon, 2 slices
Ham, 1 oz

Convenience Foods
Pizza, 2 to 3 slices
Pot pies, 8 oz
Ravioli, canned, 8 oz
Soups (canned/dehydrated), 1 cup

Low-Sodium Foods (<50 mg per serving)
Fruits/Vegetables
Fresh or canned, ½ cup
Fresh, frozen, ½ cup

Breads/Cereals
Unsalted pastas, ½ cup
Oatmeal, cooked, 1 cup
Popcorn (unsalted), 1 oz
Puffed rice, 1 cup
Shredded wheat, 1 biscuit

Meats
Fresh meat, 1 oz
Fresh chicken, 1 oz
Fresh fish, 1 oz

Data from Laquarta, I., & Gerlach, M. (1990). *Nutrition in clinical nursing.* Albany, NY: Delmar; and Burtis, G., et al. (1988). *Applied nutrition and diet therapy.* Philadelphia: W. B. Saunders.

Interventions
Reduce Sodium Loss in High-Risk Clients. If plasma sodium levels are above 125 mEq/L, encourage intake of 30 to 60 ml of clear liquids or more per hour as tolerated. If the client is on a low-sodium diet, do not be concerned about sodium restriction until the vomiting or diarrhea subsides and the client is taking whole foods.

To prevent sodium loss, irrigate nasogastric tubes and wounds with isotonic saline and give only minimal ice chips, even if ordered, when a nasogastric tube is connected to suction. Never give more than three tap water enemas in succession without consulting the physician about converting the enema fluid to normal saline. Treat nausea with prophylactic antiemetics. If hyponatremia is from hypervolemia, consult the dietitian for assistance in total fluid restriction. Consult the physician if (1) the sodium level is less than 125 mEq/L or sooner if client is symptomatic or (2) the client is receiving nothing by mouth (NPO status) and has no intake of electrolytes or has an increased loss of electrolytes.

Restore Sodium Balance. Encourage the intake of a well-balanced diet. Give nutrient-dense supplements between meals. If the client is receiving nutrition only through tube feedings, it is sometimes necessary to add extra salt to the feeding to achieve the desired sodium level.[29] If the hyponatremia is secondary to hypervolemia, consult with the physician and dietitian to coordinate therapeutic fluid restriction. Strict behavioral modification or psychiatric consultation may be necessary for a client who drinks water compulsively.

To decrease the thirst that accompanies fluid restriction, offer ice chips, cold fluids, and frequent oral care. Some clients feel less thirsty if they hold the fluids in their mouth first to fully moisten the oral mucous membranes before swallowing. Restricting fluids is contraindicated in persons with subarachnoid hemorrhage because it increases the risk of cerebral vasospasm and cell death.[10]

When plasma sodium levels are 125 mEq/L or less and the client is symptomatic, notify the physician immediately. Administration of hypertonic IV saline (3% saline) is the most commonly prescribed therapy. *Caution:* Hypertonic saline must be given very slowly by IV piggyback infusion in a large vein to decrease the risk of hypernatremia, pulmonary congestion, and phlebitis. If the client is confused or agitated, also initiate safety and seizure precautions.

EVALUATION

Mild to moderate deficits are usually corrected in 8 to 24 hours. More severe deficits may take several days, especially in older adults. Evaluate the client's and family members' understanding of positive health behaviors that prevent further occurrences of sodium deficit.

■ Self-Care

Teach the client to consult the physician if vomiting or diarrhea persists for more than 48 hours, or sooner if extreme weakness, dizziness, palpitations, irregular pulse of new onset, cough or dyspnea, or CNS changes (such as headache, confusion, or seizures) develop. Anyone who has a chronic disease—such as renal, liver, or heart disease or diabetes mellitus—should consult a physician if any signs or symptoms persist for more than 24 hours.

Teach clients to consult a physician before taking over-the-counter medications. Review the exercise precautions discussed in Chapter 12. Refer people with eating disorders to counseling and community support groups.

■ HYPERNATREMIA

Hypernatremia is defined as a plasma sodium level above 145 mEq/L. It occurs in about 1% of hospitalized clients and carries a high mortality rate, whether it has an acute or a chronic onset. Hypernatremia is usually associated with water loss or sodium gain. It can occur with increased, decreased, or normal total body sodium levels and decreased or increased TBW levels. The underlying cause of hypernatremia is a TBW deficit relative to the total body sodium content, which results in hyperosmolality.

Etiology and Risk Factors

Body fluid loss resulting in hypernatremia may be from renal or extrarenal causes, such as GI or skin problems. Hypernatremia can be classified as one of three types:

- Hypovolemic hypernatremia, in which TBW is greatly decreased relative to sodium (loss of hypotonic fluid)
- Euvolemic hypernatremia, in which TBW is decreased relative to the normal total body sodium
- Hypervolemic hypernatremia, in which TBW is increased but the sodium gain exceeds the water gain

Hypervolemic hypernatremia is the least common type of hypernatremia. Table 13–3 presents clinical conditions and disorders that may contribute to the development of hypernatremia.[24] Elderly and debilitated people are at highest risk for developing hypernatremia. Major risk factors include inadequate water intake in conjunction with decreased thirst (hypodipsia), lack of access to drinkable water, physical or chemical restraint, mental confusion, and NPO status. Excessive water loss and insufficient fluid replacement associated with fever, vomiting, diarrhea, excess drainage, polyuria, tube-feeding, or prolonged hyperventilation are also major risk factors.

Other factors that increase the risk for hypernatremia include increased sodium intake, such as with IV administration of hypertonic saline or hypertonic tube feedings. Retention of sodium occurs in heart, renal, or liver disease; Cushing's syndrome; hyperaldosteronism with corticosteroid therapy; and uncontrolled diabetes mellitus or insipidus. Uncontrolled diabetes mellitus results in polyuria, leading to dehydration and secondary hypernatremia. Fortunately, hypernatremia from untreated diabetes insipidus tends to be mild. Although the ADH mechanism is

TABLE 13–3	CLINICAL CONDITIONS AND DISORDERS THAT MAY CONTRIBUTE TO HYPERNATREMIA
Type of Hypernatremia	**Clinical Conditions and Disorders**
Hypovolemic hypernatremia	Renal losses; osmotic diuresis, diuretics, severe hyperglycemia Extrarenal losses: profuse diaphoresis, decreased thirst, diarrhea occurring with inadequate volume replacement or fluid replacement with hyperosmolar solutions, burns
Euvolemic hypernatremia	Excess fluid losses from the skin and lungs Hypodipsia in the elderly and infants Diabetes insipidus
Hypervolemic hypernatremia	Administration of concentrated saline solutions; hypertonic feedings, excess mineralocorticoids Accidental or intentional salt ingestion; commercially prepared soups and canned vegetables

altered, the thirst mechanism is intact and stimulates the client to drink water and fluids, which helps balance water losses and hypernatremia. See Chapter 44 for a more in-depth discussion of diabetes insipidus.

Pathophysiology

When sodium levels rise, water moves to maintain balance. However, the osmotic shift of water from the cells to the ECF in an attempt to dilute the hyperosmolar state only creates another problem: cellular dehydration. If the hypernatremia evolves slowly or is chronic, the brain develops its own osmotic particles, called *idiogenic osmoles,* to prevent fluid shifts into and out of the brain cells.[30]

The heart is sensitive to the increasing sodium levels. Calcium must move through the calcium channels for cardiac muscle contraction to occur. However, in hypernatremia, sodium molecules compete with calcium in the slow calcium channels of the heart, resulting in decreased myocardial contractility. Myocardial depolarization, however, occurs more easily with the increased sodium levels.

Generally, the body responds to increased sodium levels by suppressing the effects of aldosterone and ADH. These two substances normally act to increase renal blood flow and cause excretion of sodium and water. In hypernatremia, the magnitude of the problem overwhelms the ability of these adaptive mechanisms to compensate.

Clinical Manifestations and Diagnostic Findings

In the early stages of hypernatremia, clinical manifestations are nonspecific because two thirds of body water is intracellular; primary water losses tend to cause only modest effects on circulating blood volume. Early manifestations include polyuria followed by oliguria, anorexia, nausea, vomiting, weakness, and restlessness. The anorexia, nausea, and vomiting are related to increased fluid retention in the gastric cells. Early neurologic manifestations of restlessness, agitation, irritability, and muscle weakness are related to the sensitivity of brain cells to fluid shifting.

The response of the kidneys varies with the type of hypernatremia. In a hypervolemic state, the kidneys excrete some of the excess water. In a hypovolemic state, oliguria is the method of renal compensation. As fluid levels decrease in the interstitial compartments, the skin becomes dry and flushed, the mucous membranes become dry and sticky, and tongue furrows develop. The person experiences increasing thirst and fever. Temperature elevation is from the decreasing amount of fluid available for dissipating heat.

Cardiovascular manifestations are related to the type of hypernatremia. In hypovolemic hypernatremia, orthostatic hypotension with compensatory tachycardia (rapid heart beat) occurs. In hypervolemic hypernatremia, signs of hypertension, jugular venous distention, prolonged peripheral vein emptying, an extra heart sound (S_3 gallop), and generalized weight gain and edema are often present.

Dysrhythmia can result from the competition of sodium ions with calcium ions in the slow channels of the heart cells. Pulmonary manifestations, such as crackles, dyspnea, and pleural effusion, are also due to the increasing hydrostatic pressure seen in hypervolemic hypernatremia.

When sodium levels reach 155 mEq/L or more, cells (especially brain cells) shrink because of the increased ECF osmolality. More severe neurologic changes occur, manifested as confusion, seizures, or coma, in some cases with irreversible brain damage. Altered neuromuscular contractility and irritability lead to muscle twitching, tremor, hyperreflexia, and seizures. The development of rigid paralysis is a grave sign.

The diagnosis of hypernatremia is validated through increased plasma sodium concentration and osmolality. A plasma sodium level above 145 mEq/L and plasma osmolality above 295 mOsm/kg are diagnostic for hypernatremia. Because chloride is the major ECF ion that balances sodium, it is common to find a plasma chloride level above 106 mEq/L. Unless the sodium elevation is an acute change, many clients will not be symptomatic until plasma sodium reaches 155 mEq/L or more.

Outcome Management

Again, a thorough history and physical examination, as well as the aforementioned plasma studies, are necessary for accurate diagnosis of hypernatremia. Awareness of demographic variables is essential for choosing the appropriate interventions for restoring sodium balance.

Medical Management

Medical management is determined by the type of hypernatremia. The goal of medical intervention is correction of the body water osmolality, with restoration of cell volume, by decreasing the ratio of sodium to water in the ECF.

For a client experiencing minor manifestations from hypovolemia or euvolemic hypernatremia, the focus is on correcting the underlying disorder and giving oral fluid replacement. However, clients with cardiovascular, pulmonary, or neurologic manifestations from severe hypernatremia usually require hospitalization and the more aggressive approach of IV hypotonic saline.

To decrease total body sodium and replace fluid loss, either a hyposmolar electrolyte solution (0.2% or 0.45% NaCl) or 5% dextrose in water (D_5W) is administered. These solutions do not cause a considerable dilution of body sodium; instead, the plasma sodium level gradually decreases as excess sodium is excreted. When administered continuously, D_5W is considered to be a hyposmolar solution because the dextrose is metabolized quickly and only water remains. If the plasma sodium level is lowered too rapidly, fluid shifts from the vascular fluid into the cerebral cells, causing cerebral edema. Slow administration of IV fluids with a goal of reducing plasma sodium levels, at a rate of not more than 2 mEq/L/hr for the first 48 hours, decreases this risks.[5, 10]

Hypernatremia due to sodium excess may be treated with administration of D_5W and a diuretic, such as furosemide (Lasix).[31, 32] When hypernatremia results from diabetes insipidus, desmopressin acetate, in the form of a nasal spray, is commonly ordered to slow the rate of diuresis. It has a 20-hour duration of action compared with the 4- to 6-hour duration of vasopressin oil nasal spray.[10]

Although dietary sodium restriction is useful in preventing hypernatremia in high-risk clients, it cannot bring a high sodium level down to normal. People with renal disease may need sodium intake restricted to 500 to 2000 mg/day (see Box 13–2). In hypervolemic hypernatremia, fluids must also be restricted. Clients with diabetes insipidus who are receiving antidiuretic medications must be taught to avoid excessive water intake. Drinking excess water defeats the purpose of the medication.

■ Nursing Management of the Medical Client

ASSESSMENT

Assess for the usual clinical manifestations, especially in head-injured and other high-risk clients. Obtain a thorough diet and medication history, including the use of corticosteroids and over-the-counter medications, such as cough medicine, and food flavorings and spices (salt).

Depending on the client's condition, assess vital signs and peripheral vein filling time every 4 to 8 hours, measure intake and output every 8 hours, and monitor body weight daily. Use oral membrane and skin assessment tools to guide your interventions. Monitor for changes in plasma sodium and plasma osmolality (by estimated values). Report early signs of altered mental status, such as agitation, irritability, or confusion, to prevent the progression of hypernatremia and to detect lack of response to therapy or signs of overcorrection (resulting in hyponatremia). Monitor lung sounds every 2 to 4 hours, and notify the physician of increasing pulmonary overload.

DIAGNOSIS, OUTCOMES, INTERVENTIONS

Risk of Hypernatremia. The format for writing the collaborative problem is as follows: *Hypernatremia related to* (e.g., *decreased thirst, excessive administration of salt solutions,* or *impaired excretion of sodium and water*). The cause needs to be identified specifically, as it guides the choice of interventions.

Outcomes. The nurse will maintain a high index of suspicion for high-risk clients and will monitor plasma sodium and chloride levels and clinical manifestations of hypernatremia.

Interventions. Monitor the client for response to IV fluid replacement of hyposmolar electrolyte solutions, absence of clinical manifestations of hypernatremia, and return to normal sodium levels. Prevent osmotic diuresis from D_5W by maintaining the prescribed rate. Use IV pumps in high-risk clients. Initiate safety and seizure precautions if the client manifests weakness or cerebral changes.

Offer water and fluids hourly to clients with hypovolemic or euvolemic hypernatremia. Consult with the dietitian and the physician concerning the need for fluid and sodium restriction in those with hypervolemic hypernatremia. Teach the client and family members the food items that should be restricted as well as the rationale for these restrictions.

Give 1 ml of fluid per kilocalorie (kcal) of hypertonic feeding solution. Initiate new gastric feedings slowly. Increase the rate if the client tolerates the feeding, as evidenced by no diarrhea, with residuals less than half the amount of the feeding per hour, or up to 100 ml.

Consult the physician for signs that indicate worsening of the hypernatremia or fluid overload, such as increasing weight gain or pulmonary, cardiovascular, or neurologic manifestations.

Altered Oral Mucous Membranes. The problem statement *Altered Oral Mucous Membranes related to lack of body water secondary to hypernatremia* can be used.

Outcomes. There are several options for outcome statements, depending upon the condition of the mouth initially. If the oral membranes are simply dry, but not open or cracked, an outcome of maintaining moist oral mucous membranes is appropriate. If the oral mucous membranes are cracked or open, the outcome should state that no further deterioration will occur and that the mouth will be moist. Additional nursing diagnoses for pain from oral ulcerations or inadequate nutrition related to mouth pain should be considered.

Interventions. Provide oral care every 2 hours with a nonalcoholic mouthwash. Avoid lemon-glycerin swabs because they dry the membranes and may cause pain. Dilute saline and non-alcoholic rinses have been found to be effective. Use a soft toothbrush to prevent injury to the mucosa. Moisten the client's lips every 1 to 2 hours. Offer cool, nonacidic fluids such as apple juice. Low-acid juices provide fluid while decreasing pain and irritation. Limited ice chips may also decrease the discomfort from dry mucous membranes.

Caregivers often feel uncomfortable about giving oral care, and often the client's mouth is simply rinsed or lightly "brushed" with foam toothbrushes. This "light touch" oral care is appropriate when clients are in pain from mouth ulcers. However, lack of thorough oral care also leads to mouth ulcers, dental decay, and malnutrition. Mucus can accumulate on the roof of the mouth and impair swallowing or even breathing. Assess the mouth before and after mouth care, and be aggressive in cleaning the mouth.

EVALUATION

Even if the desired outcome of sodium maintenance has been met, continue to monitor clients at high risk. The key to evaluating health promotion strategies is evaluating not only whether the client and family members understand the health promotion activities but, more important, asking whether they have incorporated the necessary changes into their lifestyle. If change has not occurred, investigate the barriers and recommend alternatives or resources.

If the desired outcome of sodium restoration has been met or partially met, the manifestations of excess should be absent or at least lessened. Mild to moderate excesses are usually corrected in 8 to 24 hours. If the excesses are more severe or occur in very young or older clients, intervention must be more cautious, necessitating 48 hours or more before positive outcomes are noticeable. Evaluate the client with altered oral mucous membranes every nursing shift. If improvement is not seen within a few hours, increase the frequency of oral care.

■ Self-Care

Teach clients the importance of taking hourly fluids—30 to 60 ml of clear liquids or more as tolerated—and avoiding excessive caffeinated beverages (because they lead to diuresis). Impress upon family members the importance of keeping fresh foods and a variety of fluids on hand, especially for the client who lives alone. Encourage the use of community resources, such as Meals on Wheels. Instruct on reading labels and avoiding foods with high "Na" (sodium) content and over-the-counter medications unless physician-approved.

Teach the client to consult the physician if vomiting or diarrhea persists for more than 48 hours or sooner if extreme weakness, dizziness, palpitations, change in mental state, new onset of cough, or increasing restlessness occurs. Persons with a concurrent chronic disease (such as diabetes mellitus or disease of the liver, heart, or kidneys) should consult a physician if any of these manifestations persist for longer than 24 hours. Explain the importance of reporting weight gains of more than 3 pounds in 1 week.

Some clients are managed at home with IV fluids. Home health care nurses see their clients often (see Bridge to Home Health Care).

POTASSIUM IMBALANCES

Potassium helps regulate intracellular osmolality and promotes the transmission and conduction of nerve impulses and the contraction of skeletal, cardiac, and smooth muscle. It promotes enzyme action for cellular metabolism and glycogen storage in the liver. Potassium also fosters acid-base balance through cellular exchange with hydrogen.

Potassium is plentiful in cells. About 96% (150 mEq/L) of potassium is in ICF, and 4% (5 mEq/L) is in intravascular fluid. Potassium is also plentiful in the GI tract secretions. Because the greatest amount of potassium is intracellular, the plasma range is very narrow. Normal values of plasma potassium range from 3.5 to 5.0 mEq/L. Life-threatening changes occur when the plasma potassium concentration is altered; levels less than 2.5 mEq/L or greater than 7.0 mEq/L can result in cardiac arrest.

Requirements for a person with no active loss of potassium are 40 to 60 mEq/day. Because potassium is

BRIDGE TO HOME HEALTH CARE

Managing Intravenous Therapy

Intravenous (IV) therapy is commonly administered in the home setting. Some recognized advantages include increased comfort, increased client participation in care, reduced cost of services, and a reduced risk of infection compared with the hospital. However, home therapy has associated risks, including those related to the presence of an invasive device (i.e., the IV catheter) and potential adverse reactions to certain medications or with specific modalities. Thus, it is important to provide home IV therapy with a primary goal of ensuring client safety.

Clearly delineated policies and procedures and careful client selection are essential. Client selection criteria to consider in planning home IV therapy include client (1) willingness and motivation, (2) ability to learn and remember procedures, (3) visual acuity, and (4) manual dexterity.

Some degree of self-care is usually the goal of home IV therapy. Depending on the type of therapy, clients or their caregivers may assume all or part of the responsibility for administering IV therapy. This includes taking care of the IV catheter site, flushing the catheter with heparin or normal saline to maintain patency, and administering IV medications. Home IV therapies usually taught to a client or caregiver include antibiotic treatment, simple hydration, continuous chemotherapy with selected drugs, and parenteral nutrition. However, nurses administer blood transfusions and complicated chemotherapy drug regimens.

Prescribed IV medications and all necessary IV supplies (e.g., syringes, catheter valves, site dressings, IV pole) are provided and usually delivered to the client's home by the designated pharmacy. Improvisation with IV supplies is rarely needed or appropriate, although a coat hanger suspended from a curtain rod can serve as an IV pole. Home as well as inpatient-based IV therapy demands strict adherence to aseptic technique, storage of medications and IV fluids at proper temperatures, and maintenance of IV supplies and use within expiration dates.

Various methods are used to administer IV therapy in the home setting. The simple *gravity drip method* and *IV push* are cost-effective and appropriate ways to administer most antibiotics. Infusion pumps are used when rate control is necessary. Typically, home infusion pumps have computers that can be programmed, are battery-powered, and are small—about the size of a portable radio. The pump is placed in a small nylon pouch with the IV fluid container. The pouch is often worn with an over-the-shoulder strap or sometimes as a "fanny pack." IV tubing is threaded through the client's clothing to the IV catheter. The client can then ambulate while the pump is infusing the IV fluid.

Electronic home infusion pumps include complete alarm systems; the alarm sounds if a battery is low or if IV tubing is occluded. Most home infusion pumps also have "lock-out" capabilities to reduce the risk of tampering or of accidentally changing the program. The latest in home infusion pump technology allows infusion pumps to be programmed or alarms to be cleared via "telehealth" technology; a special modem can be placed in the client's home and attached to the telephone. The home care pharmacist or nurse can view the pump screen from the pharmacy and make necessary program changes without going to the client's home.

Specific client education to be addressed when an infusion pump is used includes teaching the client how to safely maneuver while the pump is in use. Client education should address bathing, dressing, checking pump function, and troubleshooting alarms.

The Intravenous Nursing Society (617-441-3008; www.INS1.org) is a national nursing organization devoted to the education of nurses practicing the specialty of IV nursing. This professional group is an excellent resource for home IV therapy; specific benefits include a professional journal, ongoing educational conferences, and local chapter meetings.

Lisa A. Gorski, RN, MS, *Clinical Nurse Specialist, Covenant Home Health and Hospice, Milwaukee, Wisconsin*

poorly stored in the body, *daily* potassium intake is necessary. A standard diet contains 50 to 100 mEq/day. Foods rich in potassium include vegetables, fruits (especially if dried), nuts, and meats.

Eighty per cent to 90% of potassium is excreted through the kidneys, and the remainder is excreted in feces. Renal excretion of potassium is influenced by plasma potassium concentration, blood flow into the kidney, acid-base status, and various hormones. An increased sodium intake promotes potassium loss.

Plasma and cellular levels of potassium are affected by acid-base imbalances. Alkalosis can cause hypokalemia. In an alkalotic state, hydrogen moves out of the cells to correct the alkalosis, and potassium moves into the cells, thus lowering the plasma potassium level. In acidosis, the reverse is true: Potassium leaves the cell, and extracellular levels rise.

Several substances can alter potassium levels. *Insulin* promotes potassium uptake by the cells by stimulating the sodium-potassium pump. Insulin-deficient clients often have hyperkalemia. *Glucagon* increases plasma levels of potassium by stimulating potassium release from the liver, and it may promote potassium movement from muscle cells. *Adrenocortical hormones,* such as cortisol and aldosterone, promote potassium excretion and sodium retention via the kidneys. During stress, cortisol and aldosterone levels are increased. Thus, hypokalemia is a risk factor in stress. *Catecholamines* and *beta-adrenergic agonists* promote cellular uptake of potassium. In response, hepatic stores of potassium are released and muscle storage is altered. Conversely, *alpha-adrenergic* agonists increase plasma potassium concentration. *Epinephrine,* which has both alpha- and beta-adrenergic properties, causes an initial transient rise in potassium. The beta-adrenergic properties subsequently become dominant, and the major effect is a reduced plasma potassium level.

■ **HYPOKALEMIA**

Hypokalemia is defined as a plasma potassium level of less than 3.5 mEq/L. It is a common electrolyte disorder, especially in the elderly population.

Etiology and Risk Factors

The body does not conserve potassium; thus, potassium deficit commonly results from inadequate potassium intake. Fortunately, potassium is found in most foods and fluids. People at high risk for hypokalemia include those who are debilitated, confused, restrained, or lacking access to dietary sources for financial or other reasons, or who are malnourished, anorexic, or bulimic.[7] Clients on potassium-restricted diets or some weight reduction diets or those receiving potassium-free IV solutions compounded by lack of dietary potassium are also at risk. Older adults are at especially high risk.

Potassium levels can also fall when the excretion or loss of potassium exceeds intake. People at high risk for loss include those with vomiting or diarrhea, nasogastric suctioning, intestinal fistulae, or ileostomy. Potassium is also lost with the osmotic diuresis that occurs with diabetic ketoacidosis. Surgical clients often develop hypokalemia secondary to the increased cortisol levels during the stress adaptation period and to the effects of general or spinal anesthesia. Some studies suggest that hypokalemia in alcoholic clients, as well as hypocalcemia, hypophosphatemia, and hypomagnesemia, is secondary to alcohol-induced nephrotoxicity. After several weeks of alcohol abstinence, electrolyte levels returned to normal.[8]

Medications that commonly cause hypokalemia include the potassium-wasting diuretics (thiazide, loop, and osmotic diuretics), cathartics, steroids, aminoglycosides, amphotericin B, digitalis preparations, beta-adrenergic drugs, cisplatin, and bicarbonate. People who ingest large amounts of natural licorice may develop hypokalemia secondary to an aldosterone-like effect.

Several conditions cause redistribution of potassium. Increased levels of insulin promote the movement of not only glucose but also potassium into the cell. In alkalosis, potassium exchanges with hydrogen across the cell wall, thus increasing the level of hydrogen but decreasing the level of potassium in the plasma. Clients who are in the healing phase after a severe tissue injury or burn also experience hypokalemia secondary to the shifting of potassium into the cell.[34]

Other factors associated with an increased risk of hypokalemia include Cushing's syndrome, the diuretic phase of renal failure, hyperaldosteronism, liver disease, cancer, wounds, and Bartter's syndrome, a chronic electrolyte-wasting syndrome.

Pathophysiology

When plasma potassium levels decrease, a decrease in potassium gradient occurs between the ICF and the plasma. The decreased gradient causes the resting membrane potential to increase, thus increasing excitability. Therefore, cell membranes are more responsive to stimuli (see Fig. 13–2). Almost all of the manifestations that occur with hypokalemia are secondary to the changes in neuronal excitability and its consequent effect on muscle function.

Clinical Manifestations and Diagnostic Findings

The clinical manifestations of hypokalemia include abnormal findings on the electrocardiogram (ECG) and GI, cardiac, renal, respiratory, and neurologic disturbances. Abnormalities may not be apparent with mild hypokalemia (3.3 to 3.4 mEq/L), especially if the decrease in the potassium concentration is gradual. Slowed smooth muscle contraction leads to early GI manifestations, which include anorexia, abdominal distention, and constipation. Slowed skeletal muscle contraction results in muscle weakness and flabbiness and leg cramps. Increased conduction of nerve impulses leads to the neurologic manifestations of fatigue, paresthesias, hyporeflexia, and irritability.

With severe hypokalemia, ECG changes (Fig. 13–3) may occur. The depressed and prolonged ST segment, depressed and inverted T wave, and prominent U wave are due to the prolongation of myocardial repolarization. Dysrhythmias are common because of increased cellular excitability. Ventricular fibrillation and cardiac arrest are the most serious consequences of impaired cellular action potentials. Hypokalemia also leads to a decrease in myo-

FIGURE 13–3 Electrocardiographic changes seen in potassium imbalances. (From McCance, K. L., & Huether, S. E. [1994]. *Pathophysiology: The biologic basis for disease in adults and children* [2nd ed.]. St. Louis: Mosby–Year Book.)

cardial contraction, which is manifested as hypotension and a slow, weakened pulse. Pulmonary manifestations of shallow respirations, shortness of breath, and apnea, culminating in respiratory arrest, are also from progressive deterioration of respiratory muscular contraction.

The progressive neurologic consequences of altered nerve conduction are manifested as dysphasia, confusion, depression, convulsions, areflexia, and coma. Extreme smooth muscle slowing leads to vomiting and an ileus as well as urinary retention. Skeletal muscle weakness may progress to paralysis. Hypokalemia also inhibits the kidney's ability to concentrate urine, which leads to polyuria, nocturia, and a decreased plasma osmolality.

Although plasma potassium levels below 3.5 mEq/L are diagnostic for hypokalemia, the ECG is the most reliable tool for identifying abnormalities in intracellular potassium level.

Outcome Management

A thorough history and physical examination with appropriate diagnostic studies are essential in accurate diagnosis and management of hypokalemia.

▮ Medical Management

Medical management is focused on identifying and correcting the cause of the imbalance. The aggressiveness of the therapy is determined by the potassium level and the clinical manifestations. Extreme hypokalemia necessitates cardiac monitoring.

RESTORE POTASSIUM LEVELS

Maintenance doses for clients not taking any source of potassium are 40 to 60 mEq/day in the IV solution. Larger amounts are needed with coexisting potassium losses.

For clients with minor potassium deficits or for those who have potassium-wasting conditions, administering foods high in potassium helps correct the deficit and offsets losses. The adult recommended allowance for potassium is 1875 to 5625 mg/day. Box 13–3 includes examples of foods that are high and low in potassium.

Mild to moderate hypokalemia is treated by correcting or controlling the cause of the loss or by supplementing potassium intake through the diet and/or with medication. Oral potassium replacement therapy is usually prescribed for mild hypokalemia (plasma potassium, 3.3 to 3.5 mEq/L) or for potassium-wasting conditions. Oral potassium (chloride or gluconate) is extremely irritating to the gastric mucosa, therefore, it must be taken with a glass of water or juice or with meals.

Severe hypokalemia requires IV intervention. A client with a plasma potassium level between 3.0 and 3.4 mEq/L needs approximately 100 to 200 mEq of IV potassium for the potassium level to rise 1 mEq/L. If the plasma potassium level is less than 3.0 mEq/L, it takes approximately 200 to 400 mEq of IV potassium to raise the level 1 mEq/L.[34] Potassium given intravenously *must always be diluted in IV fluids*. The usual concentration of IV potassium is 20 to 40 mEq/L. Potassium is *not* given intramuscularly and is *never* given as a bolus (IV push) injection. Giving potassium by IV push creates sudden, severe hyperkalemia, which may result in cardiac arrest.

For severe potassium deficits, 10 to 20 mEq of potassium can be given every hour if *diluted* in IV fluids; a cardiac monitor must be used to ensure safety. Use of saline as a diluent is recommended; avoid dextrose as a diluent, because it increases intracellular potassium shifting. Because potassium is irritating to the veins, concentrations higher than 20 to 40 mEq/L increase the risk of phlebitis, and large veins should be used for administration.

If hypokalemia is refractory to the usual treatments, assess for manifestations of hypomagnesemia. Many clients who are hypokalemic are also hypomagnesemic. Hypokalemia that does not respond to treatment is frequently associated with hypomagnesemia. Magnesium is necessary for the kidney to conserve potassium.[1]

▮ Nursing Management of the Medical Client

ASSESSMENT

Assessment focuses on identifying risk factors for hypokalemia through history-taking and a thorough physical

BOX 13–3 High- and Low-Potassium Foods

High-Potassium Foods (average: 7 mEq per serving)

Vegetables (½ cup cooked or 1 cup raw)

Artichokes
Broccoli
Brussels sprouts
Cabbage
Carrots
Celery
Collards
Cucumber
Mushrooms
Potatoes with skins
Spinach
Tomatoes

Fruits

Apricots, fresh, 4 medium
Apricots, canned, 4 halves
Apricots, dried, 7 halves
Banana, 7 inches
Cantaloupe, ¼ small
Guava, 1 medium
Honeydew melon, ⅛ medium
Nectarine, ½
Orange, 1 small
Prunes, 3 medium
Strawberries, 1¼ cups
Tangerine, 2 medium
Watermelon, 1¼ cups

Beverages

Brewed coffee
Tomato juice
Vegetable juice cocktail, unsalted

Low-Potassium Foods (average: 3 mEq per serving)

Vegetables

Corn, ⅓ cup
Sweet potato, yams, ¼ cup
Lima beans, ⅓ cup
French fried potatoes, 10 pieces

Fruit

Apple, 1 small
Apple juice, ½ cup
Applesauce, ½ cup
Blueberries, ¾ cup
Cranberries, 1¼ cups

Beverages

Coffee, instant
Cola
Cranberry juice cocktail, ⅓ cup
Ginger ale
Noncarbonated drinks
Root beer
Lemon-lime soda

Data from Mahan, K. L., & Arlin, M. (1992). *Food, nutrition & diet therapy* (8th ed.). Philadelphia: W. B. Saunders.

examination. Obtaining a diet history that focuses on intake, conditions promoting loss, and drugs such as diuretics, cortisone, and over-the-counter medications is very important. Review laboratory reports of potassium levels. Report even borderline plasma potassium levels to the physician, especially in high-risk clients, particularly those about to undergo surgery. General anesthesia not only promotes potassium loss but, in combination with lower plasma potassium levels, synergistically increases the risk of cardiac dysrhythmia. Consult the physician about the need for potassium supplementation in anyone who has been on NPO status or who has an obvious cause of potassium loss or marked decrease in potassium intake.

Ongoing assessments of the client with hypokalemia include all the body systems, because the effect of low potassium is widespread. Assess cardiac function, including apical pulses, and renal function every hour in the client with severe hypokalemia, and progress to every 8 hours as the client's condition improves. Assess neuromuscular and bowel function every 4 to 8 hours. A urine output of 30 ml/hr is necessary to prevent rebound hyperkalemia. Hypokalemia increases the risk of digitalis toxicity because low potassium levels increase the sensitivity of the myocardium to digitalis-induced dysrhythmia.[48] If the client receives digitalis, monitor for anorexia, nausea, vomiting, diarrhea, headache, weakness, blurring or visual halos, or marked change in cardiac rate or rhythm.

If the apical pulse is irregular, assess for pulse deficits. Because this procedure is impractical for self-monitoring, at least ensure that the client or a family member is able to assess a radial pulse accurately for 1 minute and is aware of the need to notify the physician if the pulse is below 60 BPM (beats/minute).

DIAGNOSIS, OUTCOMES, INTERVENTIONS

Hypokalemia. Because there is no nursing diagnosis for hypokalemia, a collaborative problem format is used. It is commonly written as *Hypokalemia related to* (specific etiology). Causative factors often include vomiting, diarrhea, Cushing's disease, prolonged or intensive diuretic use, cortisone therapy, decreased intake, and NPO status.

Outcomes. The client's potassium level will be 3.5 to 5.0 mEq/L. Because the nurse cannot treat the problem independently, the outcome can also be written: "The nurse will monitor potassium levels."

Interventions. Give oral or IV potassium as prescribed, ensuring that it is *diluted in IV fluids; it cannot be given as an IV push.* Always *agitate* IV bags before hanging them up in order to prevent giving a loading dose, which can cause cardiac arrest.[34] Monitor IV sites hourly for phlebitis, infiltration, and rate of infusion. Change IV sites every 72 hours or sooner if the vein becomes tender to palpation. Tenderness indicates damage to the intima of the vein; this is an early sign of phlebitis.

Use the smallest IV catheter possible to allow maximum plasma flow around the site at which the potassium enters the vein. This promotes dilution of the potassium, thereby decreasing the risk of phlebitis. If an IV solution containing potassium infiltrates surrounding tissue, consult the physician for advice. Potassium can cause tissue sloughing. Give IV fluids with potassium chloride by a controlled infusion pump to ensure the correct flow rate.

Notify the physician if signs of hypokalemia persist or worsen, such as dysrhythmia of increasing severity, or if signs of overcorrection occur, such as manifestations of hyperkalemia. During the administration of IV potassium, consult the physician if the client's urinary output is less than 30 ml/hr for 2 consecutive hours, if the pulse deficit is greater than 20 BPM, or if signs of impaired peripheral tissue perfusion are present. Anticipate the need for additional potassium with increased IV glucose, such as in total parenteral nutrition (TPN) resulting from the increased shift of potassium into the cell caused by the increased insulin levels.

Risk of Injury. Because potassium is needed for normal nerve conduction and muscle function, low plasma potassium levels often lead to weakness and can lead to seizures. The nursing diagnosis is stated as *Risk for Injury related to muscle weakness and hypotension or seizures secondary to hypokalemia.*

Outcomes. The client will sustain no injury, as evidenced by an absence of falls, bruises, and contusions.

Interventions. Employ safety and seizure precautions to reduce the risk of injury. Keep the bed in a low position with side rails up. Before the client walks, clear the path of obstacles and place non-slippery shoes and a gait belt on the client. Use restraints only after all other alternatives to prevent inadvertent harm to self or others have been tried. It is imperative that health care providers comply with the client's rights and follow the defined protocols for use of restraints. Refer to your agency's policy and procedure manuals for explicit guidelines for action and documentation.

Altered Nutrition: Less Than Body Requirements. If the main cause of the client's hypokalemia is inadequate consumption of foods rich in potassium, then use the nursing diagnosis *Altered Nutrition: Less than Body Requirements related to insufficient intake of foods rich in potassium.* However, this diagnosis can be used *only* if the client can eat and drink.

Outcomes. The client will demonstrate improved nutrition, as evidenced by consumption of adequate amounts of food and fluid to maintain a normal potassium level.

Interventions. Instruct the client to choose and consume foods rich in potassium, such as fruits, fruit juices, dried fruits, and vegetables, including potato skins. Fish (but not shellfish), whole grains, and nuts, such as peanuts, almonds, and walnuts, are also good sources of potassium. Some fruits have a relatively higher potassium content; bananas, cantaloupe, and honeydew melons have twice as much potassium as that in oranges. Meat and milk have moderate amounts of potassium. Instruct the client to take liquid or tablet potassium supplements with a glass or more of water or juice and food.

EVALUATION

If the desired outcome of potassium maintenance has been met, continue to monitor high-risk clients for evidence of deficit. Continue to reinforce strategies for prevention. If the outcome of potassium restoration has been met or partially met, the manifestations of deficit should be absent or at least lessened in severity. Mild to moderate deficits are usually corrected in 8 to 24 hours. Correction of more severe deficits may take several days, especially in the older adult. Continue to evaluate the client's and family members' understanding of positive health behaviors, and assess for barriers to achieving those behaviors.

■ Self-Care

Teaching is essential to the promotion and maintenance of potassium balance. Provide a copy of the list of food groups, and emphasize the importance of eating a well-balanced diet. Review alternative cooking methods, reinforcing that prolonged cooking of vegetables may result in potassium and vitamin wasting. Suggest steaming, microwaving, and, if possible, eating raw vegetables as methods to increase nutrient retention.

Teach the basic principles of sick care. These principles include ingestion of 30 to 60 ml hourly of fluids with electrolytes; for example, cola contains potassium and reduces nausea. Sick care also involves teaching clients when to consult a physician. People with chronic diseases, such as heart, liver, or kidney disease or diabetes mellitus, should consult a physician for any illness that interferes with food ingestion or causes loss of nutrients and persists for more than 24 hours. Anyone who becomes symptomatic—who develops weakness of sudden onset, irregular heartbeat, or change in mental status—should consult a physician.

Teach the importance of not taking over-the-counter medicine, especially laxatives, without physician approval. Encourage clients who are lactose-intolerant to avoid milk products or to take lactase. Reinforce the label instruction that potassium products should be taken with food to avoid GI irritation.

Encourage use of support services—first, the family or extended family and then the religious community as well as respite services, Meals on Wheels, food stamps, Alcoholics Anonymous, or other community services.

■ HYPERKALEMIA

Hyperkalemia is defined as an elevation of the potassium level above 5.0 mEq/L. Hyperkalemia is rare in clients with normal kidney function but affects more than half of people with acute renal failure.

Etiology and Risk Factors

The three major causes of hyperkalemia are as follows:

- Retention of potassium by the body because of decreased or inadequate urine output
- Excessive release of potassium from the cells during the first 24 to 72 hours after traumatic injury or burns, or from cell lysis or acidosis
- Excessive infusion of IV solutions that contain potassium or excessive oral intake, especially in a person who has renal disease

All three potential causes of hyperkalemia limit the ability of the kidneys to excrete the excess potassium. Because the kidneys are responsible for 80% to 90% of potassium excretion, the underlying cause of hyperkalemia is often related to decreased kidney function. People with as little as 5% glomerular function can maintain normal plasma potassium levels if urine output is at least 1 L/day. Shock compounds the problem because of a low volume of circulating vascular fluids and diminished kidney function. Other routes of excretion are less effective to rid the body of potassium. The GI tract and skin cannot excrete enough potassium to compensate for an acute state of hyperkalemia.

Recall that most potassium is inside the cell. Therefore, conditions that destroy cells release potassium into the circulation. People with fast-growing cancers, such as non-Hodgkin's lymphoma, acute leukemia, small cell carcinomas, and some metastatic cancers, are at risk for *tumor lysis syndrome* (TLS). TLS is the consequence of rapid destruction of tumor cells secondary to chemotherapy and/or irradiation, which results in hyperkalemia, hyperphosphatemia, hypocalcemia, and hyperuricemia. Hyperkalemia can also result from burns, crush injuries, or severe infections involving extensive cell destruction. Potassium levels can also rise after the use of stored blood, and after open-heart surgery or other surgical procedures in which a perfusion pump is used.

Therapy with potassium-sparing diuretics or concurrent use of potassium supplements and angiotensin-converting enzyme (ACE) inhibitors may also cause hyperkalemia. Disorders that decrease or inhibit secretion of aldosterone, such as adrenal insufficiency, may also cause hyperkalemia. Acidosis also increases hyperkalemia owing to the compensatory shifting of potassium out of the cell in exchange for hydrogen; the exception to this mechanism is in diabetic acidosis (see Chapter 45). See earlier discussion of hypokalemia.

Pathophysiology

Hyperkalemia increases the cell membrane's excitation threshold, causing the cell to become less excitable. Decreased irritability (excitability) of nerve and muscle results. As hyperkalemia becomes more severe, muscles become weak, flaccid, and paralyzed.

Clinical Manifestations and Diagnostic Findings

Clinical manifestations are related to the plasma potassium level and the mode of onset of the imbalance. Acute hyperkalemia may cause manifestations when the plasma level is only moderately elevated, to 6.0 mEq/L. However, if the condition developed slowly, manifestations may not be present until the plasma level reaches 7.0 mEq/L. Clinical manifestations can involve many body systems, including GI, cardiac, renal, and neurologic systems. Mild to moderate hyperkalemia (a plasma level near 6.0 mEq/L) causes nerve and muscle irritability, resulting in paresthesia (numbness, tingling), tachycardia, and intestinal colic and diarrhea.

As the plasma potassium level approaches 7.0 mEq/L, sodium channels become progressively inactivated, which causes disturbances in nerve and muscle function: impaired cardiac conduction, ventricular contraction, hypotension, cardiac arrest, convulsions, and severe neuromuscular weakness progressing to flaccid paralysis and respiratory muscle paralysis. The acidosis that occurs with hyperkalemia has a synergistic effect on the progressive

impairment of depolarization. The renal abnormalities oliguria and anuria are commonly precursors to hyperkalemia rather than consequences of the imbalance.

As noted previously, the key to the level of severity is the amount of time the body has had to adapt to the imbalance. Although a plasma potassium level above 5.0 mEq/L is diagnostic for hyperkalemia, the ECG is the most reliable tool for identifying an imbalance (see Fig. 13–3). Blood studies may yield false-positive results when hemolysis of blood specimens has occurred, when tourniquets are applied too tightly, when multiple attempts are made to obtain a sample from the same site, or when excess force is used to transfer blood into tubes or to aspirate blood into a syringe. Under these conditions, the cell ruptures and releases potassium into the sample of blood.

Other useful laboratory studies include determination of blood urea nitrogen (BUN), serum creatinine, and carbon dioxide levels. Elevated BUN and serum creatinine levels, which reflect decreased renal function, are important laboratory indicators for determining the risk of hyperkalemia. If the total carbon dioxide levels in the venous blood are low, an arterial blood gas study should be done to rule out metabolic or respiratory acidosis as a possible cause of hyperkalemia.

Outcome Management

■ Medical Management

The goals of medical management are to correct the potassium level as quickly as possible to prevent life-threatening consequences. Although a thorough history and physical examination are desirable, if the client's state is critical, intervention may preempt a thorough assessment.

RESTORE POTASSIUM BALANCE

If the plasma potassium level is less than 5.5 mEq/L, dietary restriction of potassium may be all that is needed (see Box 13–3).

If the level is higher or if the client is symptomatic, pharmacologic intervention is usually necessary. The onset of symptoms and the need for aggressive intervention are usually related to the suddenness of the development of hyperkalemia. Improving urine output by forcing fluids, giving IV saline, or giving potassium-wasting diuretics usually corrects mild hyperkalemia.

When hyperkalemia is severe, immediate action is needed to avoid lethal cardiac disturbances. Temporary corrective measures may include the following: infusion of IV calcium gluconate to decrease the antagonistic effect of the potassium excess on the myocardium; infusion of insulin and glucose or sodium bicarbonate to promote potassium uptake into the cells (useful in metabolic acidosis); and use of the beta-agonist albuterol (0.5 mg IV), which results in a decrease in plasma potassium level within 30 minutes, lasting for 6 hours.[30] These are only temporary methods for decreasing plasma potassium; repeating these methods may not be effective.[9]

As hyperkalemia persists or increases, a cation-exchange resin such as sodium polystyrene sulfonate (Kayexalate) may be given orally or rectally as a retention enema. When this medication is given, the potassium ion is exchanged for the sodium ion in the intestinal tract; the potassium ion is then excreted in the stool. To prevent the constipating effect of this drug, it is usually combined with sorbitol, and diarrhea often results. In marked renal failure, peritoneal dialysis or hemodialysis may be needed.[9]

Prevention is central to the management of TLS. Adequate hydration is the key: 3000 ml of IV fluid is given 24 hours before therapy, during therapy, and for 48 hours after therapy. Diuretics, to decrease the risk of pulmonary overload, and a uric acid blocker such as allopurinol, to increase the excretion of uric acid, are also given to prevent renal failure.

If hyperkalemia is secondary to respiratory acidosis, enhancing pulmonary function is the primary focus. If it is from metabolic acidosis, the immediate risks associated with the acidosis and hyperkalemia are addressed first, and then interventions are targeted at the system in which the acidosis originated.

■ Nursing Management of the Medical Client

Assessment

Assessment focuses on identifying risk factors for hyperkalemia through history-taking and a thorough physical examination. Obtain a history of medical conditions associated with potassium elevations. Review laboratory reports of potassium levels. Report even borderline plasma potassium levels to the physician, especially in high-risk clients, such as those who have cancer or are undergoing chemotherapy.

Ongoing assessments include checking vital signs, bowel function, urine output, lung sounds (crackles), and peripheral edema every 4 to 8 hours. Monitor plasma levels of potassium and creatinine and BUN. In severe hyperkalemia, perform hourly checks of vital signs, including apical pulses. ECG changes should be monitored continuously. In the absence of ECG monitoring, apical pulses constitute the next most valuable indicator of abnormality in intracellular potassium concentration. Monitor urine output hourly if severe hyperkalemia or a history of renal insufficiency exists or if the urine output drops to less than 30 ml/hr for 2 consecutive hours.

Monitor not only for a therapeutic response to treatment (improvement) but also for signs of overcorrection. Rapid correction places a client at risk for hypokalemia and metabolic alkalosis. In a client taking digitalis, the occurrence of hypokalemia is associated with a digitalis toxic response.

Diagnosis, Outcomes, Interventions

There is no nursing diagnosis for hyperkalemia. The problem can be written using the following collaborative problem statement: *Hyperkalemia related* to (specify etiology). Consider the contribution of renal dysfunction, shock from traumatic injuries, or burns (tissue destruction).

Outcomes. The client will have and maintain a potassium level of 3.5 to 5.0 mEq/L. Because you cannot treat the problem independently, the outcome can also specify: "The nurse will monitor potassium levels."

Interventions. Administer fluids as ordered to promote renal excretion of potassium. Report manifestations indicating the development of hypokalemia and urine outputs of less than 30 ml/hr for 2 consecutive hours, or less than 720 ml/day.

If the client is to receive a blood transfusion and is at risk for hyperkalemia, notify the blood bank so that "old" blood (more than 2 weeks old) is not supplied. Use a 19-gauge needle or 20-gauge catheter to deliver the packed cells, to prevent red blood cell (RBC) rupture with release of intracellular potassium. When obtaining blood specimens, use vacuum tubes when possible to avoid false-positive results on tests for hyperkalemia.

High potassium levels have the potential to induce life-threatening dysrhythmias. Treat them according to protocol, and report ECG changes that indicate worsening hyperkalemia or overcorrection resulting in hypokalemia.[13] Set cardiac monitor alarms with narrow limits to ensure early detection of lethal dysrhythmias. *Remember, a machine cannot replace your bedside assessment.* Cardiopulmonary resuscitation may be required, but it is seldom successful in cases of severe hyperkalemia because the heart muscle cannot respond to medications or countershock. Consult the physician for any serious change, including progression of altered tissue perfusion, especially in the heart, lungs, brain, or kidneys.

Evaluation

Evaluate the client's responses to therapy every hour if severe hyperkalemia is present or every 8 hours if mild hyperkalemia exists. Hyperkalemia must be corrected quickly because of the risk of dysrhythmia.

■ Self-Care

Teaching still remains one of the primary interventions to promote and maintain normal potassium balance for those at high risk for hyperkalemia. Explain the significance of potassium restriction. Crucial elements of teaching include dietary potassium sources and the importance of reading labels, avoiding salt substitutes, which are usually made from a potassium salt, and avoiding over-the-counter medication not approved by a physician. Clients must also understand the importance of consulting a physician if renal function worsens or if an acute illness lasts more than 24 hours. Occasionally, a person with renal insufficiency is in a state of hypokalemia secondary to an acute loss. To ensure safe administration of potassium to any client with renal insufficiency, see that a cardiac monitor is used.

Calcium Imbalances

Calcium, an extracellular and intracellular cation, has a normal plasma range of 4.5 to 5.5 mEq/L, or 9 to 11 mg/dl. About 99% of the body's calcium is in the bones and teeth. The other 1% is in the tissues and intravascular fluid. About half of the portion of calcium in the blood is bound to protein, mostly albumin, and the remaining half is free (ionized calcium). Therefore, the total plasma calcium level does not indicate the exact amount of free, active calcium in the body.

Calcium has many functions in the body:

- Acts as a catalyst in the transmission and conduction of nerve impulses

- Stimulates the contraction of skeletal, smooth, and cardiac muscle
- Maintains normal cellular permeability; increased plasma calcium levels decrease cellular permeability, and decreased plasma calcium levels increase cellular permeability
- Promotes coagulation of blood in all phases but mostly in the prothrombin to thrombin phase
- Promotes absorption and utilization of vitamin B_{12}. Promotes strong and durable bones and teeth; vitamin D is needed to absorb calcium from the GI tract

Parathyroid hormone (PTH) regulates plasma levels of calcium and phosphorus (see later discussion on phosphorus [phosphate]) by increasing resorption from bone, and reabsorption from the renal tubule or the GI tract. Thus, increased PTH increases plasma ionized calcium levels and decreases plasma phosphorus levels. Calcitonin from the thyroid gland also promotes calcium balance by opposing the action of PTH; it inhibits bone resorption.

When the level of plasma calcium falls even slightly, PTH secretion increases. Within minutes, calcium is reabsorbed from the kidney tubules; within hours, bone resorption occurs; and within days, increased absorption from the GI tract occurs (Fig. 13–4). Notice in Figure 13–4B and C how calcium and phosphate intake and output remain in balance.

■ HYPOCALCEMIA

Hypocalcemia is defined as a plasma calcium level below 4.5 mEq/L, or 8.5 mg/dl. Calcium levels are often reciprocal with phosphorus levels. Phosphate imbalances are discussed separately later on the chapter, however.

Low calcium levels are common in older adults because of inadequate intake. Hypocalcemia can also develop from an inadequate intake of vitamin D due to intentional changes in the diet or to diseases that impair absorption. Diets can be deficient in vitamin D in people with lactose intolerance, GI disease, liver disease, alcoholism, anorexia, and bulimia.[7] Decreased intake for several days, such as with NPO status, or for longer periods, as in high-protein and other weight-reduction diets, has also been linked to hypocalcemia.

Parathyroid disease decreases serum calcium levels. A deficiency of PTH results in a drop in plasma calcium levels secondary to decreased bone resorption and GI absorption and increased urinary excretion of calcium. Inadvertent (unplanned) removal of the parathyroid can occur when the thyroid is removed.

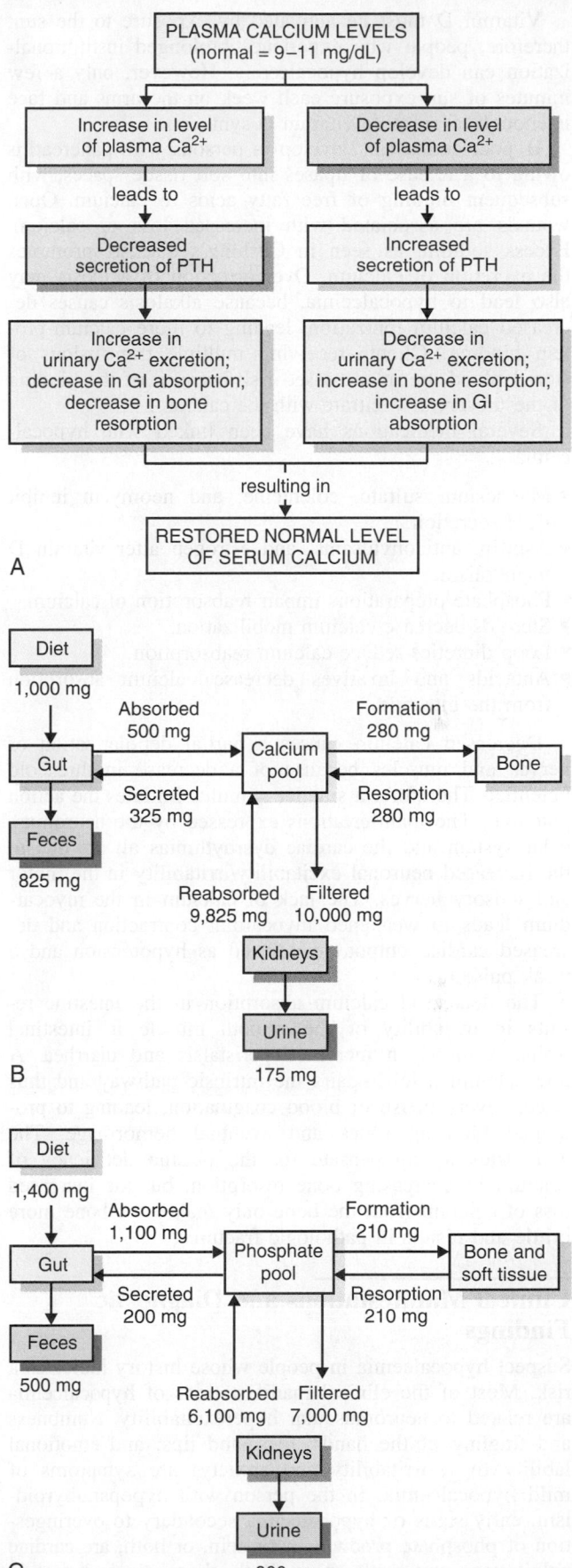

FIGURE 13–4 *A,* Parathyroid hormone (PTH) regulation of plasma calcium level. GI, gastrointestinal. *B,* Calcium homeostasis. A pool of calcium exists in the body and remains in balance by dietary intake, bowel and kidney excretion, and bone formation and resorption. *C,* Phosphate homeostasis. A pool of phosphate exists in the body and remains in balance by dietary intake, urine and bowel excretion, and bone and soft tissue formation and resorption.

Vitamin D must be activated by exposure to the sun; therefore, people who experience prolonged institutionalization can develop hypocalcemia. However, only a few minutes of sun exposure each week on the arms and face is enough to promote vitamin D synthesis.

Hypocalcemia can develop in persons with pancreatitis owing to a release of lipases into soft tissue spaces, with subsequent binding of free fatty acids to calcium. Open wounds are associated with increased loss of calcium. Excess sodium, as seen in Cushing's disease, promotes the excretion of calcium. Overcorrection of acidosis may also lead to hypocalcemia, because alkalosis causes decreased calcium ionization, leading to more calcium-protein binding. Clients receiving multiple transfusions of stored blood are at increased risk because of the binding of the preservative citrate with the calcium.

Several medications have been linked with hypocalcemia:

- Magnesium sulfate, colchicine, and neomycin inhibit PTH secretion.
- Aspirin, anticonvulsants, and estrogen alter vitamin D metabolism.
- Phosphate preparations impair reabsorption of calcium.
- Steroids decrease calcium mobilization.
- Loop diuretics reduce calcium reabsorption.
- Antacids and laxatives decrease calcium absorption from the intestine.

Decreased calcium causes a partial depolarization of nerves and muscles because of a decrease in threshold potential. Therefore, a smaller stimulus initiates the action potential. The manifestations expressed by the neuromuscular system and the cardiac dysrhythmias all are due to the increased neuronal excitability/irritability in the motor and sensory nerves. The lack of calcium in the myocardium leads to weakened myocardial contraction and decreased cardiac output, manifested as hypotension and a weak pulse.

The decreased calcium absorption in the intestine results in irritability of the smooth muscle in intestinal walls, resulting in increased peristalsis and diarrhea. A low calcium level impairs the intrinsic pathway and thus affects every phase of blood coagulation, leading to prolonged bleeding times and eventual hemorrhage. The bone tries to compensate for the plasma deficiency of calcium by increasing bone resorption, but the increased loss of calcium from the bone only makes the bone more brittle and results in pathologic fractures.

Clinical Manifestations and Diagnostic Findings

Suspect hypocalcemia in people whose history indicates a risk. Most of the clinical manifestations of hypocalcemia are related to neuromuscular hyperexcitability. Numbness and tingling of the hands, toes, and lips; and emotional lability (e.g., irritability and anxiety) are symptoms of mild hypocalcemia. In the person with hypoparathyroidism, early signs of hypocalcemia secondary to overingestion of phosphate products or protein, or both, are cardiac palpitations and restlessness. Both phosphate and protein increase calcium binding. Findings in severe hypocalcemia are cardiac insufficiency, hypotension, dysrhyth-

mias, a prolonged QT interval, carpopedal spasm (Trousseau's sign), facial twitching (Chvostek's sign), and prolonged bleeding times; these abnormalities progress to seizures, laryngeal stridor, tetany, hemorrhage, cardiac collapse, and eventual death.[38]

With prolonged hypocalcemia, cataracts may develop because of increased uptake of sodium and water by the lens. Trophic changes, such as dry, sparse hair and rough skin, may also be noted. Spontaneous fractures can occur when the bone is depleted of calcium.

A plasma calcium level below 4.5 mEq/L, or 9 mg/dl, is considered diagnostic for hypocalcemia. This measurement and the clinical manifestations are the validating data used in most situations. However, remember to interpret these findings in the context of the plasma albumin level and pH, and adjust the data if either is abnormal. Also, when clients have manifestations of hypocalcemia but have a normal plasma calcium, an ionized calcium level should be determined, as it is the only value that gives the true level of free calcium. A level below 1.18 mEq/L (<2.36 mg/dl) indicates hypocalcemia.

Also, abnormal plasma albumin and pH levels influence the interpretation of plasma calcium levels. For example, when the albumin level is low, a falsely normal plasma calcium level can be present. Conversely, when plasma albumin is high, the functional ionized calcium level is actually lower than the plasma laboratory level reveals. When albumin levels are abnormal, the total plasma calcium can be adjusted by adding or subtracting 0.8 mg/dl for every 1 g/dl decrease or increase, respectively, in plasma albumin. A basic pH causes an increase in calcium binding. The plasma level may appear normal, but the functional ionized calcium level is actually lower. The opposite is true with an acid pH. Therefore, a plasma ionized calcium (iCa) assay should be done in clients who are critically ill, those with marginal calcium imbalances, or those with an abnormal albumin level or acid-base imbalance. (See Box 13–1 for normal ranges.)

Outcome Management

The goals of medical management are to determine and correct the cause of the hypocalcemia, restore calcium levels to normal values, and determine a method to reduce recurrence.

■ Medical Management

RESTORE CALCIUM BALANCE

Asymptomatic hypocalcemia is usually corrected with oral calcium gluconate, calcium lactate, or calcium chloride. For increased absorption, the calcium supplement should be given with a glass of milk 30 minutes before meals. The vitamin D in the milk promotes calcium absorption.

Chronic or mild hypocalcemia can be treated in part by having the client consume a diet high in calcium (Box 13–4). If hypocalcemia is secondary to parathyroid deficiency, the client must avoid high-phosphate foods, such as milk products and carbonated beverages, and excess protein. Protein binds with available calcium and only exacerbates the manifestations of hypocalcemia. Maintenance needs are met through calcium and vitamin D supplements.

BOX 13–4	High- and Low-Calcium Foods

High-Calcium Foods (>100 mg per serving)

Dairy Products

Cheese, all types
Ice cream, 1 cup
Milk, 1 cup
Yogurt, low-fat with fruit, 1 cup

Other Foods

Oatmeal, instant, ¾ cup
Rhubarb, cooked, 1 cup
Spinach, frozen, ½ cup
Tofu, regular, ½ cup

Low-Calcium Foods (<25 mg per serving)

Apple, 1 medium
Banana, 1 medium
Chicken breast, baked, 3 oz
Ground beef, lean, 3 oz
Oatmeal, cooked, 1 cup
Pasta, cooked, 1 cup
Vegetable juices

Data from Laquarta, I., & Gerlach, M. (1990). *Nutrition in clinical nursing.* Albany, NY: Delmar; and Burtis, G., et al. (1988). *Applied nutrition and diet therapy.* Philadelphia: W. B. Saunders.

Tetany from acute hypocalcemia needs *immediate* attention. IV calcium chloride or calcium gluconate must be given slowly to avoid hypotension and bradycardia and other dysrhythmias. Use D_5W solutions when dilution is

necessary; avoid saline solutions, as they promote calcium loss.

Nursing Management of the Medical Client

A thorough history of the client's current and chronic illnesses, diet intake, and medications, including over-the-counter medications, assists in identifying risks for calcium deficit and guides interventions for health promotion and maintenance. If digitalis and calcium are among the medications identified, assess for digitalis toxicity as well, because hypocalcemia increases the risk of this problem.

Check for Trousseau's and Chvostek's signs in high-risk clients (Fig. 13–5). *Trousseau's sign* is the occurrence of carpopedal spasm, or contraction of the fingers and hand, when a blood pressure cuff is kept inflated on the upper arm for 5 minutes at diastolic pressure. *Chvostek's sign* is occurrence of spasm of the muscles innervated by the facial nerve when the client's face is tapped lightly below the temple. Spasm of the face, lip, or nose is also evidence of tetany. In addition, assess for paresthesias.

Assess the client's cardiac status by monitoring the ECG and vital signs, especially the apical heart rate and rhythm. Frequency of assessment varies from 1 to 4 hours, depending on the client's condition. Assess color, warmth, motion, and sensation (CWMS) and peripheral pulses to provide data for evaluation of the peripheral cardiac output.

Monitor also for bleeding in the gums and petechiae or ecchymosis in the skin. Assess for changes in the clarity of urine, as microscopic bleeding causes clear urine to become cloudy before frank bleeding is apparent. Also,

Chvostek's sign

Trousseau's sign

FIGURE 13–5 Chvostek's and Trousseau's signs. A calcium deficit (hypocalcemia) or magnesium deficit (hypomagnesemia) raises the resting potential of nerves. This rise allows nerve stimulation and firing with less stimulus. Touching the facial nerve adjacent to the ear produces twitching of the client's upper lip (Chvostek's sign). The hand and fingers can also go into spasm (Trousseau's sign or carpopedal spasm). These spasms can occur spontaneously or when blood flow is decreased (e.g., during blood pressure cuff inflation).

note black or blood-streaked stool, which may signify occult gastrointestinal bleeding. Be suspicious of an intracerebral hemorrhage when a client reports headaches of new onset. Monitor plasma calcium levels for improvement or worsening.

Monitor IV sites for infiltration or phlebitis when IV calcium is being infused. Calcium chloride is extremely irritating to the subcutaneous tissue. If infiltration occurs, notify the physician immediately, as tissue sloughing may occur. In either situation, change the IV site. Also notify the physician if the client's manifestations do not resolve or if signs of overcorrection (hypercalcemia) occur. When possible, use fresh blood for transfusions. Avoid giving calcium and bicarbonate in the same IV solution, as a precipitate will form. Use filters with TPN solutions.

To prevent pathologic fractures, use caution by obtaining adequate help to turn or move the client. Use gait belts and or extra personnel to walk or transfer the client to and from bed.

Instruct the client about foods that are rich in calcium, such as milk, cheese, yogurt, and green leafy vegetables. Encourage taking calcium supplements before meals and with vitamin D milk for better absorption. *Exception:* For persons with hypocalcemia secondary to hypoparathyroidism, phosphorus intake should be decreased by *omitting* milk, milk products, and other high-phosphorus foods (e.g., carbonated beverages). Calcium and vitamin D supplements are prescribed for this population as well. Several types of vitamin D are available. Therefore, clients with hypoparathyroidism must be advised not to take over-the-counter forms without first consulting with a physician to ensure that the right supplement is taken. These clients should also be advised to ingest protein only in amounts recommended by the American Dietetic Association (ADA). Increased intake of protein leads only to further binding of available calcium. For clients with osteoporosis, see the dietary recommendations in Chapter 26.

■ Self-Care

Reinforce intake of a well-balanced diet, avoiding high-protein diets or other non-prescribed weight-loss diets, and encourage weight-bearing exercises to prevent bone demineralization. Consult the physician about the need for mineral and vitamin supplements for clients who consume less than half of their meals (e.g., the elderly population). Tums, which contains calcium carbonate, is often recommended as an inexpensive supplement.

Older clients may have difficulty incorporating large amounts of food and fluids containing calcium into the diet. Part of the difficulty is in changing long-established eating habits. Many of today's older adults drink very little milk because of habits formed in childhood. Suggest other forms of calcium that may be more appealing, such as yogurt, cheese, milkshakes made with ice milk, or green leafy vegetables.[6]

■ HYPERCALCEMIA

Hypercalcemia is defined as a plasma level over 5.5 mEq/L, or 11 mg/dl. Hypercalcemia can occur in any age group. It is a common electrolyte disorder that can have serious physical complications.

Etiology and Risk Factors

The three most common causes of hypercalcemia arc (1) metastatic malignancy, (2) hyperparathyroidism, and (3) thiazide diuretic therapy. The most common cancers that cause hypercalcemia are malignancies of the lung, breast, ovary, prostate, bladder, bone (multiple myeloma, leukemia), kidney, head and neck, and lymph tissues. Malignancy-induced hypercalcemia is the result of either bone destruction or an increased secretion of ectopic PTH.

Other causes of hypercalcemia include an excessive intake of calcium supplements with vitamin D or of calcium-containing antacids, prolonged immobilization, metabolic acidosis, and hypophosphatemia. Prolonged immobilization causes resorption of calcium from the bone. Recall that bone density is maintained by weight-bearing stress on bone (see Chapter 26). Metabolic acidosis promotes hypercalcemia by two mechanisms: decreased binding of calcium, which increases the plasma ionized calcium levels, and inhibition of calcium excretion from the kidney. Hypophosphatemia inhibits the kidney's ability to excrete excess calcium.

Pathophysiology

Destruction of bone tissue results in an increased release of calcium into the vascular spaces. See Chapter 19 for more information related to malignancies. Excessive PTH production promotes calcium retention, which leads to hypophosphatemia. Hypophosphatemia compounds the problem by promoting more calcium retention.

When excess calcium is present, the cell membrane threshold potential becomes more positive, which results in membranes that are refractory to depolarization. This decreased cell membrane excitability requires a stronger stimulus for a response to occur. As a result, cardiac and smooth muscle activity is decreased. Excess calcium in the bloodstream also impairs renal function and precipitates as a salt, which often forms renal stones.

Clinical Manifestations and Diagnostic Findings

The clinical manifestations of hypercalcemia, which are generally nonspecific, are determined by the plasma calcium level. Mild hypercalcemia, with calcium levels near 5.5 mEq/L, or 11.5 mg/dl, is usually asymptomatic. In mild cases, the plasma calcium level may increase momentarily when the client consumes calcium-containing antacids, or a large dose of an oral calcium supplement, and the kidneys are initially unable to eliminate the excess.

In moderate hypercalcemia, with calcium levels of 6.2 mEq/L, or 13 mg/dl, manifestations usually include anorexia, nausea, vomiting, polyuria, muscle weakness, fatigue, lethargy, dehydration, and constipation. Increased calcium stimulates the release of hydrochloric acid, gastrin, and pancreatic enzymes and slows bowel transit time, which leads to the anorexia, nausea, vomiting, abdominal distention, and constipation. The weakness, fatigue, depression, and difficulty concentrating are due to neurologic depression. Hypercalcemia also causes osmotic diuresis; the polyuria leads to dehydration and thirst and further exacerbates the constipation.

Calcium precipitates tend to form ureteral or kidney stones, which results in urinary blockage and severe colicky pain. Excess calcium also impairs glomerular blood flow, which in severe cases has led to renal failure. Bone pain is often associated with cancer of the bone and is due to the pressure on nerve endings from the tumor cells. Pathologic fractures are due to the decalcification of the bony matrix and can occur with cancer of the bone or with any condition that causes resorption of calcium.[7, 14, 17]

Progressive neurologic depression from increasing hypercalcemia is manifested as extreme lethargy, a depressed sensorium, confusion, and eventually coma. Severe hypercalcemia may result in hypercalcemic crisis, which carries a 30% to 50% mortality rate. A hypercalcemic crisis occurs when calcium levels reach 7.1 mEq/L, or 15 mg/dl. The resultant increased conduction transmission, shortened repolarization, and severe cardiac depression can cause cardiac dysrhythmias, ECG changes, and cardiac arrest. Hypokalemia may occur as the body eliminates potassium rather than calcium.

A plasma calcium level above 5.5 mEq/L, or 11.5 mg/dl, is considered diagnostic for hypercalcemia. Typical ECG changes include a widened T wave and shortened QT interval.

Outcome Management

▪ Medical Management

The goals of medical management are to determine and correct the cause of the hypercalcemia, restore calcium levels to normal values, and determine a method to reduce recurrence. Prevention and early detection of complications such as renal stones and fractures are also important.

RESTORE CALCIUM BALANCE

Immediate correction of moderate and severe hypercalcemia is essential. IV normal saline, given rapidly with furosemide to prevent fluid overload, promotes urinary calcium excretion. Antitumor antibiotics such as plicamycin inhibit the action of PTH on osteoclasts in bone tissue, which reduces decalcification and the plasma calcium level. However, plicamycin has many dangerous side effects.

Calcitonin decreases the plasma calcium level by inhibiting the effects of PTH on the osteoclasts and increasing urinary calcium excretion. Corticosteroid drugs decrease calcium levels by competing with vitamin D, resulting in decreased intestinal absorption of calcium, and by inhibiting prostaglandins, resulting in decreased bone resorption. IV phosphate decreases plasma calcium; however, it is used as a last resort because it may result in severe calcification of various tissues.

Thiazide diuretics should be changed to furosemide or to another diuretic that does not cause retention of calcium. If the cause of the hypercalcemia is excessive use of calcium or vitamin D supplements or calcium-containing antacids, these agents should be either avoided or used in a reduced dosage. If the client is not nauseated, encourage oral liquids. These actions are designed to lower the calcium level in 36 to 48 hours. Etidronate disodium (Didronel) reduces plasma calcium by inhibiting

precursors to calcium mineralization and, secondarily, by reducing bone formation. The client needs to be hydrated with large volumes of normal saline before etidronate administration and must be given loop diuretics to enhance urine output and calcium excretion following drug administration.

Gallium nitrate has been effective in inhibiting bone resorption and in decreasing osteoclastic activity. The drug should be stopped if the urinary output is less than 2 L/day or if the plasma creatinine level is greater than 2.5 mg/dl.[15, 16, 22]

For client teaching, review high-calcium foods that should be restricted (see Box 13–4). Instruct the client that forcing fluids helps to lower plasma levels by flushing excess calcium through the kidney. If manifestations of renal calculi (stones) are present, teach that consumption of foods and fluids that increase urine acidity will help decrease stone formation. These include meat, cheese, eggs, whole grains, cranberry juice, and prune juice.

▪ Nursing Management of the Medical Client

Because plasma calcium levels are not routinely assessed, it is essential that you identify high-risk clients. Screening assessment includes obtaining a thorough history, focusing on risk factors, medications (including over-the-counter calcium supplements or antacids), and diet history. Assess vital signs, apical pulses, and ECG every 1 to 8 hours, depending on the severity of the client's manifestations. Bowel sounds, renal function, and hydration status should be assessed every 8 hours. Also, recall that it is important to monitor for fluid volume depletion secondary to hypercalcemia.

Early treatment may prevent a hypercalcemic crisis. Unless fluids are contraindicated (as in clients with heart failure), increase fluid intake. If flank pain or renal colic is present, strain all urine to capture renal calculi for analysis. Report urine output of less than 30 ml/hr for 2 consecutive hours. Report any manifestations that indicate worsening of the clinical status, such as an increase in severity of dysrhythmias, a decrease in sensorium, or manifestations of overcorrection (hypocalcemia).

Once the crisis is controlled, prevention of complications through teaching and safety interventions becomes the primary focus of health maintenance. Instruct the client to avoid calcium supplements. Sodium intake is increased, unless contraindicated, to promote calcium loss through the kidneys. Consumption of high-fiber foods and fluids should be increased to prevent constipation, and an acid-ash diet may be recommended to decrease the risk of stone formation. The client should also be taught to report clinical manifestations of renal calculi, such as flank pain, hematuria, or cardiac dysfunction (such as an irregular pulse or palpitations).

If the client has confusion, lethargy, or coma, institute safety precautions, including a low bed position with side rails raised. To prevent injury, turn and move the client with extreme caution and with adequate assistance. Gait belts, back braces, tripod canes, and walkers may be used to facilitate safer ambulation. Assist with resistive range of motion and weight-bearing activities to decrease calcium loss from bone. Report clinical manifestations of fractures immediately, such as bone pain or ecchymosis.

■ Surgical Management

Surgery may be used to remove an ectopic PTH-secreting tumor. Noninvasive or invasive lithotripsy or endoscopic removal of renal or ureteral calculi may be necessary. See Chapters 34 and 35 for more information related to these surgical procedures.

PHOSPHATE IMBALANCES

The normal plasma phosphorus level is 1.2 to 3.0 mEq/L. Less than 1% of phosphorus is contained in the vascular spaces; 85% is contained in the bones, and 14% is contained in the soft tissues. However, rapid shifting between cells and blood can occur, which can create a risk for severe hypophosphatemia or hyperphosphatemia.

Phosphorus promotes strong and durable bones and teeth. Phosphorus is also an integral part of the energy systems in the body—adenosine diphosphate (ADP) and adenosine triphosphate (ATP) and in the phosphate acid-base buffer system. PTH regulates plasma levels of phosphorus by the following mechanisms:

- Increasing resorption of phosphate from the bone
- Inhibiting phosphate reabsorption from the renal tubule
- Increasing phosphate absorption from the GI tract

Thus, increased PTH increases plasma ionized calcium levels and decreases plasma phosphorus levels.

■ HYPOPHOSPHATEMIA

Hypophosphatemia is defined as plasma phosphorus levels below 1.2 mEq/L. The overall major risk for hypophosphatemia is loss or long-term lack of intake. However, risk factors that are often overlooked include periods of increased growth or tissue repair and recovery from malnourished states. Each of these factors increases the demand for phosphorus.[38] Failure to meet these increased needs results in a state of phosphorus depletion.

Phosphorus depletion can occur as a result of prolonged and excessive intake of antacids. Administration of high levels of glucose via tube feeding or IV line causes phosphorus to enter the cell for glucose phosphorylation. The increased sodium found in Cushing's syndrome, the increased calcium found in hyperparathyroidism, and the decreased arterial partial pressure of carbon dioxide ($PaCO_2$) in chronic respiratory alkalosis also cause phosphorus to move into the cell. Lead poisoning leads to a decreased availability of phosphate. Phosphate loss occurs in burns, and a mild renal loss occurs with metabolic alkalosis.

Pathophysiologic changes that occur with hypophosphatemia can affect every organ system because of the effect of hypophosphatemia on optimal ATP and oxygen supply. Phosphate depletion impairs the conversion of glucose and many other intermediate substances to ATP. The ultimate result is a disruption in the sole mechanism responsible for regeneration of ATP.

Recognition of phosphate deficits is challenging because the plasma level, whether normal or low, does not always reflect the total body phosphate content. Careful review of a client's history, laboratory data, medications, and clinical manifestations, with emphasis on nutritional health in people at high risk, increases the likelihood of identifying phosphate deficiencies. The primary manifestations of hypophosphatemia are decreased cardiac and respiratory function, muscle weakness, fatigue, brittle bones, bone pain, confusion, and seizures.

Mild hypophosphatemia can be treated with diet and dietary supplementation. The major nursing roles are teaching a well-balanced diet and helping the client and family gain access to resources that alleviate barriers to positive health behaviors.

Clients who have a serious phosphate imbalance are often deficient in many other nutrients. TPN is usually the intervention of choice until the plasma levels become stable. Monitoring a client's response to IV TPN is also essential. See Chapter 29 for more information on nursing implications related to TPN.

■ HYPERPHOSPHATEMIA

Hyperphosphatemia is a rare but serious disorder. It is defined as a plasma phosphate level above 3.0 mEq/L. However, it is the total body phosphate level that determines the seriousness of the imbalance. The most common causes are excessive intake of high-phosphate foods, excess vitamin D (especially with renal insufficiency due to decreased excretion), impaired colonic motility from increased absorption, hypoparathyroidism, and Addison's disease. Clinical manifestations are related to the degree of hyperphosphatemia or to secondary hypocalcemia. Tachycardia, palpitations, and restlessness are among the earliest manifestations. Anorexia, nausea, vomiting, hyperreflexia, tetany, and more serious dysrhythmias may follow if the imbalance worsens.

In certain conditions, an increased intake or decreased excretion of phosphate or an increase in cell lysis results in high levels of phosphorus. In renal failure, the kidney is less able to excrete phosphate; the excess phosphate impairs calcium reabsorption. TLS results in a state of hyperphosphatemia from excess cell rupture. Women are at risk after menopause owing to a slight increase in phosphate secondary to a deficiency of estrogen. Exposure to lead increases the risk of phosphorus imbalances. Hyperphosphatemia leading to death has been associated with administration of Fleet Phospho-Soda enemas in the presence of altered renal or bowel function.[11] Follow manufacturer recommendations when giving Fleet Phospho-Soda enemas.

In mild or asymptomatic hyperphosphatemia, treatment focuses on limiting high-phosphate foods, especially milk, ice cream, cheeses, high amounts of meat and fish, and carbonated beverages, or giving calcium or aluminum products that promote the binding and excretion of phosphate. Dialysis is the primary treatment for renal failure that is refractory to conservative approaches (either peritoneal dialysis or hemodialysis).

For mild or moderate phosphate deficiencies, diet supplementation is usually sufficient. Sources of phosphorus include milk products, eggs, fish, whole grains, vegetables, and carbonated beverages. Hypophosphatemia, if associated with signs of total body phosphate deficit, is usually treated with IV replacement. This is most commonly given in the form of TPN if the client suffers from other electrolyte imbalances.

MAGNESIUM IMBALANCES

Magnesium is the second most abundant intracellular cation. The actions of magnesium in the body and the clinical manifestations of imbalance are similar to those for potassium. Half the body's magnesium is stored in bone, 49% is contained in the ICF, and 1% is contained in the ECF. Of the 1% in the plasma, 30% of the magnesium is bound to protein, 15% is combined with anions, and 55% is in a free, ionized form. Magnesium is absorbed from the small intestine at the same site at which calcium is absorbed. Thus, malabsorption affects both electrolytes. Magnesium is excreted in the urine and in small amounts in feces. Figure 13–6 shows how magnesium balance is maintained.

The functions of magnesium include the transmission and conduction of nerve impulses and the contraction of skeletal, smooth, and cardiac muscle. Magnesium accomplishes this through its effect on more than 300 enzyme systems. It is responsible for the transportation of sodium and potassium across the cell membrane (sodium-potassium pump) and for the synthesis and release of PTH. Therefore, a deficit can lead to hypokalemia and hypocalcemia. Magnesium is necessary for the conversion of ATP to ADP and hence the release of energy. It influences the use of potassium, sodium, calcium, and phosphate, and it activates enzymes that are necessary for the metabolism of carbohydrates, proteins, lipids, and vitamin B_{12}. Finally, magnesium promotes vasodilatation of peripheral arteries and arterioles.

Increased calcium or phosphorus intake can decrease magnesium absorption from the intestines. Conversely, a low calcium level increases magnesium absorption from the intestines.

■ HYPOMAGNESEMIA

Hypomagnesemia is defined as a plasma magnesium level below 1.5 mEq/L, or 1.8 mg/dl. Magnesium deficits are being identified more often as a result of increased knowledge about this ion. Twenty-two per cent to 42% of clients with calcium, phosphate, sodium, and potassium imbalances have been found to have a coexisting magnesium imbalance.[1] However, it is a rare imbalance in people who consume a well-balanced diet. As with other intracellular ions, plasma levels may be normal in the presence of intracellular depletion. Also, hypomagnesemia is often overlooked, because tests for plasma magnesium levels are not routinely ordered until a severe deficit has occurred. Plasma levels may be helpful in severe or acute changes, but a 24-hour urinalysis after an IV magnesium challenge, ion-selective imaging, or nuclear magnetic resonance imaging (MRI) (to determine soft tissue levels) is more predictive of total body magnesium levels, but these studies are rarely done owing to the expense.[2]

Hypomagnesemia is becoming recognized as a common cause of refractory (not responsive to treatment) hypokalemia and hypocalcemia.[1] The hypomagnesemic state inhibits potassium reabsorption; the hypomagnesemia therefore needs to be corrected before potassium and calcium imbalances respond to treatment.

Magnesium deficits are often seen in critically ill and alcoholic clients. Alcoholism decreases intestinal absorption secondary to a decrease in enzymes that are normally produced by the liver. Alcoholism also promotes magnesium wasting secondary to nephrotoxicity and leads to malnutrition. Other causes of hypomagnesemia are severe or chronic malnutrition; malabsorption syndromes, such as Crohn's or celiac disease or pancreatitis; and GI losses secondary to vomiting, GI suction, diarrhea, high-volume ileostomies, fistulas, laxative abuse, or radiation enteritis. Mechanisms for renal losses include the diuretic phase of acute renal failure and hyperphosphatemia. Prolonged IV or TPN therapy without magnesium replacement also increases the risk for hypomagnesemia. Excess calcium (as in hyperparathyroidism) and excess sodium (as in Cushing's syndrome or hyperaldosteronism) inhibit magnesium. The hyperglycemia seen in diabetic acidosis causes osmotic diuresis with loss of magnesium. Alkalosis is also associated with hypomagnesemia.

Many medications increase the risk of hypomagnesemia. Excessive amounts of phosphorus in the intestine (as from overuse of antacids) inhibit the uptake of magnesium from the intestinal villi. Some medications interfere with renal handling of magnesium as either a primary action or a side effect. The primary drugs implicated are diuretics and antibiotics. Loop, osmotic, and thiazide diuretics; aminoglycoside antibiotics (gentamicin, tobramycin); carbenicillin; amphotericin B; cisplatin; corticosteroids; and digitalis are the usual offenders. The neurologic trauma associated with cocaine abuse has also been linked to hypomagnesemia.[1]

The myocardial irritability that occurs with hypomagnesemia seems to be a result of changes in the resting membrane potential associated with the altered relationship between potassium and magnesium ions. It is thought to be secondary to the stimulation of beta$_2$-adrenergic cells; more commonly, it is associated with digitalis intake. Magnesium depletion and digitalis both promote potassium loss from myocardial cells. Digitalis uptake also seems to be increased in hypomagnesemia. GI

FIGURE 13–6 Magnesium homeostasis. A pool of magnesium exists in the body and is kept in balance by dietary intake, bowel and kidney excretion, and bone and soft tissue formation and resorption.

changes from decreased contractility, such as anorexia, nausea, and abdominal distention, can occur. Psychological disorders, such as depression, psychosis, and confusion, may also develop.[35]

Severe hypomagnesemia causes neuromuscular manifestations such as Chvostek's and Trousseau's signs, tetany, convulsions, and vasospasm leading to stroke. Cardiac abnormalities include premature ventricular contractions, atrial or ventricular fibrillation, and ECG changes (prolonged QT intervals, widened QRS complexes, and broadening of T waves). Other ECG changes are related to the concomitant low levels of potassium. Low magnesium levels have been linked with an increased incidence of ventricular dysrhythmias and decreased 1-year survival rates in clients with heart failure as well as with lethal dysrhythmias in clients who have had myocardial infarctions.[2] Studies also suggest a link between estrogen therapy in postmenopausal women and increased coagulation risk; estrogen promotes tissue uptake of magnesium and hence hypomagnesemia.[2]

Management

Treatment of hypomagnesemia includes oral magnesium replacement in the form of magnesium-containing antacids or parenteral magnesium sulfate. Increasing dietary intake of magnesium also helps ensure balance and stability.

IV magnesium reduces the tendency of the small airways to spasm and has been found useful in treating acute asthma that has been refractory to other therapy. The positive inotropic, negative chronotropic, and vasodilatory effects of magnesium have also been found to increase cardiac output and decrease oxygen consumption in people with shock and sepsis. Magnesium has also been successfully used as a mood stabilizer in clients with bipolar disease.[1]

Nursing management includes monitoring vital signs every 4 to 8 hours and reviewing ECG readings hourly. Initiate safety and seizure precautions for clients who are extremely confused or at risk for seizures. Monitor plasma magnesium, potassium, and calcium levels. Also, many experts recommend assessing the client's deep tendon reflexes. Normal reflexes suggest normal magnesium levels.

Consult a physician about the need for magnesium maintenance or replacement if the client has severe malnutrition, is on NPO status for more than 3 days (especially in the presence of coexisting losses), or has manifestations of hypokalemia or hypocalcemia even after treatment. TPN may be necessary to correct coexistent nutrient imbalances, which is common. The presence of hyperglycemia in diabetic clients increases the risk of hypomagnesemia. Therefore, maintaining glucose control in people with diabetes mellitus will decrease the risk of hypomagnesemia.

When administering magnesium intravenously, dilute it according to pharmacy recommendations. Rapid infusion of magnesium sulfate can cause a hot or flushed feeling and phlebitis. Avoid giving magnesium in saline solutions.

Instructing clients and family members about foods rich in magnesium provides information that may be essential to prevent magnesium deficiency or to correct a mild deficit (Box 13–5). Caution clients about taking mineral supplements without the advice of a dietitian or pharmacist. The calcium-to-magnesium ratio should be maintained at 4:1, because a higher ratio can lead to deposition of calcium in the soft tissues and vessels.[2] Taking magnesium without potassium causes shifting of potassium into the cell. In the alcoholic client, magnesium should be given with thiamine to promote nerve regeneration.[1]

■ HYPERMAGNESEMIA

Hypermagnesemia is defined as a plasma magnesium level greater than 2.5 mEq/L, or 3.0 mg/dl. It is a rare disorder. Hypermagnesemia may occur with renal insufficiency, excessive use of magnesium-containing antacids or laxatives, or administration of potassium-sparing diuretics. Many potassium-sparing diuretics conserve magnesium. Hypermagnesemia is also seen with severe dehydration from ketoacidosis, with decreased synthesis of aldosterone (such as in Addison's disease or after adrenalectomy), and with overuse of IV magnesium sulfate for controlling premature labor or pregnancy-induced hypertension.

Clinical manifestations are related to the blocked release of acetylcholine from the myoneural junction, which results in a decrease in muscle cell activity. With mild hypermagnesemia, peripheral vessels dilate, causing hypotension. ECG changes include prolonged PR and QT intervals. In extreme hypermagnesemia, profound sedative effects on the neuromuscular system lead to severe muscle weakness, lethargy, drowsiness, loss of deep tendon reflexes, respiratory paralysis, and loss of consciousness. Cardiac signs include delayed myocardial conduction manifested on the ECG as wide QRS complexes, elevated T wave, heart block, and premature ventricular contractions.

Management

Management of hypermagnesemia includes decreasing the use of magnesium sulfate and enhancing the elimination

---

BOX 13–5   **High- and Low-Magnesium Foods**

High-Magnesium Foods (>75 mg per serving)

Cashews, roasted, ¼ cup
Chili, with beans, 1 cup
Halibut, baked, 3 oz
Swiss chard, cooked, ½ cup
Tofu, ½ cup
Wheat germ, ¼ cup, toasted

Low-Magnesium Foods (<25 mg per serving)

Chicken breast, 3 oz
Egg, 1
Fruits
Green peas, frozen, ½ cup
Ground beef, 3 oz
White bread, 1 slice

Data from Mahan, K. L., & Arlin, M. (1992). *Food, nutrition and diet therapy* (8th ed.). Philadelphia: W. B. Saunders.

of magnesium. A saline infusion with a diuretic increases renal elimination of magnesium. However, a side effect of the treatment is a loss of calcium. Hypocalcemia may intensify the hypermagnesemia. Calcium antagonizes magnesium. Thus, IV calcium salts in solution have been used in the treatment of extreme hypermagnesemia. Albuterol has also been used to reduce magnesium levels. The presence of severe respiratory distress requires ventilatory assistance. If renal failure is present, hemodialysis may be necessary.[35]

Nursing management focuses on monitoring for early signs of hypermagnesemia in high-risk clients. Assessment includes vital signs, respiratory function, ECG recordings, urinary output, and the level of sensorium; these should be checked every 1 to 4 hours, depending on the client's condition. Safety and seizure precautions should be initiated if confusion or seizure risk is present. Changes in deep tendon reflexes should be reported. If the reflexes are normal, body levels of magnesium are normal. Keep IV calcium salts in the code cart for emergency reversal of severe hypermagnesemia.

Teach clients to avoid constant use of laxatives and antacids containing magnesium, especially if urinary output is decreased. Encourage eating foods that contain fiber and drinking adequate fluids to promote fecal elimination.

CONCLUSIONS

Electrolyte imbalances are found in all age groups in every type of health care setting. It is rare for a person to have only one electrolyte imbalance; more commonly multiple electrolyte and fluid imbalances are present, especially in high-risk populations such as the very young, older adults, and people with chronic illnesses.

Nurses play an essential role in health promotion, health maintenance, and health restoration for clients at risk for or experiencing fluid and electrolyte imbalances. Nursing management includes the following pivotal roles:

- *Teaching* clients and their families about positive health behaviors, about the importance of nutrient intake (even during non-acute illnesses), and about manifestations of fluid and electrolyte imbalance that necessitate physician consultation
- *Promoting* nutritional maintenance and replacement in clients who are at high risk for or who are experiencing fluid and/or electrolyte imbalance
- *Assisting* the physician in early detection of imbalances and of poor response to treatment or signs of overcorrection
- *Promoting* balanced nutrition in rehabilitation or extended care settings through family support, early physician referrals for supplements, dietary consultation, or management of imbalances

THINKING CRITICALLY

1. An elderly, tube-fed resident from a nursing home is admitted with recent changes in level of consciousness. Her skin and mouth are very dry, and her urine is scant and dark yellow. Laboratory assessment reveals sodium, 150 mEq/dl; chloride, 106 mEq/dl; BUN, 52; and creatine, 1.2. Her family calls and wants to know "if she will make it." How would you respond?

Factors to Consider: What do this assessment findings suggest? What interventions would you expect to be prescribed? What precautions will be needed to prevent further fluid and electrolyte shifts?

2. A 45-year-old woman was admitted with a rapid heart rate. Her past medical history is negative for cardiac disease. One week ago, she started on a new weight loss program, which included furosemide. Could her heart rate be potentially lethal?

Factors to Consider: Why would a client take furosemide in a weight-loss program? What side effects may be occurring? What laboratory studies will be ordered? Which electrolytes do you think will be abnormal?

BIBLIOGRAPHY

1. Altura, B., et al. (1994). Magnesium: Growing in clinical importance. *Patient Care, 28*(1), 130–150.
2. Altura, B., et al. (1994). Magnesium therapy: Coming of age. *Patient Care, 28*(2), 79–94.
3. Bergeron, M., Armstrong, L., & Maresh, C. (1995). Fluid and electrolyte losses during tennis in the heat. *Clinics in Sports Medicine, 14*(1), 23–32.
4. Bove, L. (1996). Restoring electrolyte balance: Sodium & chloride. *RN, 96*(1), 25–28.
5. Brown, R. (1993). Disorders of water and sodium balance. *Postgraduate Medicine, 93*(4), 227–246.
5a. Carrougher, G. J. (1997). Management of fluid and electrolyte balance in thermal injuries: Implications for perioperative nursing practice. *Seminars in Perioperative Nursing, 6*(4), 201–209.
6. Constants, T., et al. (1994). Effects of nutrition education on calcium intake in the elderly. *Journal of the American Dietetic Association, 94*(4), 447–448.
7. Crow, S., et al. (1997). Serum electrolytes as markers of vomiting in bulimia nervosa. *International Journal of Eating Disorders, 21*(1), 95–98.
8. DeAngelis, R. (1992). Hypokalemia. *Critical Care Nurse, 12*(7), 71–75.
9. DeAngelis, R., & Lessig, M. (1992). Hyperkalemia. *Critical Care Nurse, 12*(3), 55–59.
10. Diringer, M. (1992). Management of sodium abnormalities in patients with CNS disease. *Clinical Neuropharmacology, 15*(6), 427–444.
11. Fass, R., Son, D., & Hixson, L. (1993). Fatal hyperphosphatemia following Fleet Phospho-Soda in a patient with colonic ileus. *The American Journal of Gastroenterology, 88*(6), 929–932.
12. Gisolfi, C., et al. (1995). Effect of sodium concentration in a carbohydrate-electrolyte solution on intestinal absorption. *Medical Science Sports Exercise, 27*(10), 1414–1420.
13. Guyton, A., & Hall, J. (1996). *Textbook of medical physiology* (9th ed.). Philadelphia: W. B. Saunders.
14. Held, J. (1995). Cancer care: Correcting fluid and electrolyte imbalances. *Nursing, 95*(4), 24–28.
14a. Iggulden, H. (1999). Dehydration and electrolyte disturbance. *Elderly Care, 11*(3), 17–23.
15. Kaplan, M. (1994). Hypercalcemia of malignancy: A review of advances in pathophysiology. *Oncology Nursing Forum, 21*(6), 1039–1046.
16. Kaye, T. (1994). Hypercalcemia. *Postgraduate Medicine, 97*(1), 153–160.
17. King, P. (1995). Oncologic emergencies: Assessment, identification, and interventions in the emergency department. *Journal of Emergency Nursing, 21*(3), 214–217.
18. Klotz, R. (1998). The effects of intravenous solutions on fluid and electrolyte balance. *Journal of Intravenous Therapy, 21*(1), 20–26.

18a. Latzka, W. A., & Montain, S. J. (1999). Water and electrolyte requirements for exercise. *Clinics in Sports Medicine, 18*(3), 513–524.

19. McCance, K., & Huether, S. (1998). *Pathophysiology: The biologic basis for disease in adults and children* (3rd ed.). St. Louis: Mosby–Year Book.

20. McCloskey, J., & Bulechek, G. (1996). *Nursing interventions classification (NIC): Iowa intervention project* (2nd ed.). St. Louis: Mosby–Year Book.

20a. Moseley, M. J. (1997). Perioperative problems: Nutrition and electrolytes in the elderly. *Seminars in Perioperative Nursing, 6*(1), 21–30.

21. Mulloy, A., & Caruana, R. (1995). Hyponatremic emergencies. *Medical Clinics of North America, 79*(1), 155–169.

22. Mundy, G. (1994). Evaluation and treatment of hypercalcemia. *Hospital Practice, 6,* 79–86.

23. O'Donnell, M. (1995). Assessing fluid and electrolyte balance in elders. *American Journal of Nursing, 95*(11), 41–45.

24. Okun, J. (1995). Clinical pathology rounds: Severe hypernatremia. *Laboratory Medicine, 26*(8), 507–509.

25. Radke, K. (1994). The aging kidney: Structure, function, and nursing practice implications. *ANNA Journal, 21*(4), 181–190.

26. Reber, P., & Heath, H. (1995). Hypocalcemic emergencies. *Medical Clinics of North America, 79*(1), 93–107.

27. Rutecki, G. W., & Whittier, F. C. (1994). Hyponatremia: Physiologic clues to a state of disordered tonicity. *Consultant, 34*(5), 688–690, 700–702.

28. Rutecki, G. W., & Whittier, F. C. (1994). Hyponatremia: Cause of hypotonicity directs management. *Consultant, 34*(5), 705–707, 711–712.

29. Seshadri, V., & Meyer-Tettambel, O. (1993). Electrolyte and drug management in nutritional support. *Critical Care Nursing Clinics of North America, 5*(1), 31–36.

30. Sica, D. (1994). Renal disease, electrolyte abnormalities, and acid-base imbalance in the elderly. *Clinics in Geriatric Medicine, 10*(1), 197–211.

31. Simmons-Holcomb, S. (1997). Understanding the ins and outs of diuretic therapy. *RN, 97*(2), 34–40.

32. Stark, J. (1997). Dialysis choices. *RN, 97*(2), 41–46.

33. Sterns, R. (1991). The management of hyponatremic emergencies. *Critical Care Clinics, 7*(1), 127–141.

34. Terry, J. (1994). The major electrolytes: Sodium, potassium, and chloride. *Journal of Intravenous Nursing, 17*(5), 240–247.

35. Toto, K., & Yucha, C. (1994). Magnesium. *Critical Care Nursing Clinics of North America. 6*(4), 767–783.

36. Toto, K., & Yucha, C. (1996). Urine chemistry: Monitoring fluid and electrolytes. *Nursing, 96*(4), 24j, 241.

37. Vieweg, W. (1994). Treatment strategies in the polydipsia-hyponatremia syndrome. *Journal of Clinical Psychiatry, 55*(4), 154–160.

38. Yucha, C., & Toto, K. (1994). Calcium and phosphorus derangements. *Critical Care Nursing Clinics of North America, 6*(4), 747–766.

C H A P T E R 14

Acid-Base Balance

Margie Hansen

Normal function of body cells depends on regulation of the hydrogen ion (H$^+$) concentration within very narrow limits. If H$^+$ levels exceed these normal limits, acid-base imbalances result and are recognized clinically as abnormalities of serum pH. Because acid-base imbalances may be caused by disorders of any body system, their incidence in clinical settings is quite high. Along with other health care professionals, you are responsible for preventing, detecting, and intervening in acid-base imbalances.

REGULATION OF ACID-BASE BALANCE

The symbol *pH* refers to the negative logarithm of the H$^+$ concentration. It is used to express the acidity or alkalinity of a solution. A pH of 7.0 is *neutral*, having an equal number of acids and bases. An *acidic* solution has a pH less than 7.0, and an *alkaline* solution has a pH greater than 7.0. Because pH is a *negative* log (indicating a reciprocal relationship), a rise in pH reflects a drop in H$^+$. Conversely, a decline in pH indicates an increase in H$^+$.

Normal serum pH is 7.35 to 7.45. The function of cellular proteins is seriously impaired when pH falls to 7.2 or less or rises to 7.55 or more. Rapid rates of change in pH are especially detrimental. A serum pH below 6.8 or above 7.8 typically is fatal.

Three physiologic systems act interdependently to maintain a normal serum pH:

- Buffering of excess acid or base by blood buffer systems
- Excretion of acid by the lungs
- Excretion of acid or regeneration of base by the kidneys

■ MODULATION OF SERUM pH BY BLOOD BUFFER SYSTEMS

A buffer system consists of a weak acid (one that does not readily release H$^+$ into solution) and a salt of a base. For example, carbonic acid (H$_2$CO$_3$), a weak acid, and sodium bicarbonate (NaHCO$_3$), the salt of a base with which H$^+$ can combine, make up the clinically important bicarbonate buffer in the blood. The organic acids formed during cellular energy metabolism are strong acids; that is, they readily contribute free H$^+$ to body fluids, potentially producing large alterations in pH. The pH of buffered solutions tends to remain fairly stable despite the addition of strong acids or bases because buffer system components combine with added acids or bases to convert them to weaker forms. Because only free H$^+$ contributes to pH, changes in pH are minimized. Examples of buffering reactions are presented next.

Strong acid buffered:

$$HCl + (H_2CO_3/NaHCO_3) \rightarrow H_2CO_3 + NaCl$$

where HCl is hydrochloric acid and NaCl is sodium chloride.

Strong base buffered:

$$NaOH + (H_2CO_3/NaHCO_3) \rightarrow NaHCO_3 + H_2O$$

where NaOH is sodium hydroxide.

Several buffer systems are present in the blood, both within red blood cells (RBCs) and in the plasma. The numerous negative charges on proteins permit the binding of large quantities of H$^+$ cations. Accordingly, proteins such as hemoglobin in RBCs and albumin in the plasma are quantitatively (judged according to amount) the most important buffers.

In clinical settings, however, the bicarbonate buffer is monitored because of its accessibility within the plasma as well as its physiologic importance as an *open* buffer system. In an open buffer system, the end products of acid-buffering reactions are continuously eliminated from the body by the lungs and kidneys, allowing these reactions to continue without being slowed by the accumulation of end products. When bases must be buffered, the carbon dioxide (CO$_2$) consumed by carbonic acid formation is readily replenished by normal metabolism. Furthermore, the dissociation constant (p*K*a) of this system is ideal for buffering fluids such as plasma, in which the addition of acids is more prevalent than the addition of bases. The *dissociation constant* (p*K*a) of a buffer is the pH at which half its components are in the acid form and half are in the base form. At normal serum pH, the bicarbonate buffer has about 90% of its components in base form.

Since all intracellular and extracellular buffer systems operate interdependently, the status of the bicarbonate buffer is representative of acid-base homeostasis within the body as a whole. Buffer systems act instantly to minimize the impact of adding strong acids or bases to the blood; thus, these systems are the body's first line of defense against acid-base imbalance. Unlike the lungs and kidneys, however, buffers do not actually eliminate acid or base from the body.

■ REGULATION OF VOLATILE ACID BY THE LUNGS

Volatile acids are acids that can be converted to gases. During normal ventilation (breathing), the lungs exhale large quantities of "potential" acid in the form of CO_2 gas. CO_2 is continuously produced by body cells as an end product of complete oxidative metabolism of nutrients for energy. CO_2 diffuses from body cells into the blood, where it may combine with water to form H_2CO_3, which then dissociates, or separates, into its component ions: H^+ and HCO_3^- (bicarbonate). This *hydrolysis reaction*, which is reversible, is shown as

$$H_2O + CO_2 \rightleftarrows H_2CO_3 \rightleftarrows HCO_3^- + H^+$$

It is apparent from this equation that CO_2 and H_2CO_3 are directly related. As serum CO_2 levels rise, H^+ production increases and pH falls, indicating increased acidity. Conversely, lower CO_2 levels are consistent with higher (more alkaline) pH values. The hydrolysis reaction further demonstrates that some of the CO_2 entering the blood forms the base HCO_3^-. Although some hydrolysis occurs in the plasma, most takes place in the cytoplasm of RBCs, where the enzyme carbonic anhydrase (CA) catalyzes the reaction at much more rapid rates than in the plasma. The presence of CA in other cells, notably the renal tubular cells, is also important to acid-base homeostasis (discussed later).

Figure 14–1 demonstrates the hydrolysis reaction at the tissue level. Consistent with the *law of mass action*,

FIGURE 14–1 Tissue level hydrolysis. *A*, Carbon dioxide (CO_2) is formed during cellular energy metabolism. *B*, CO_2 diffuses into plasma, then into red blood cells. *C*, CO_2 enters hydrolysis catalyzed by carbonic anhydrase (CA), yielding hydrogen (H^+) and bicarbonate (HCO_3^-). *D*, HCO_3^- diffuses into plasma in exchange for Cl^- (chloride shift). *E*, H^+ is buffered by hemoglobin (Hb) and other intracellular buffers. RBC, red blood cell; ATP, adenosine triphosphate.

FIGURE 14–2 Reversal of hydrolysis in the lung. *A*, Carbon dioxide (CO_2) is exhaled, creating a gradient for diffusion of CO_2 from the blood to the alveolus. *B*, Removal of CO_2 drives reverse hydrolysis in the red blood cell (RBC). *C*, Bicarbonate (HCO_3^-) reenters the RBC in exchange for Cl^- (reverse chloride shift). *D*, Oxygen binding to hemoglobin (Hb) promotes H^+ release (reverse Haldane effect). HHb, combined hydrogen/hemoglobin.

the rate and direction of this reaction are determined by (1) the addition of substrate or (2) the removal of end product. In the tissues, the addition of CO_2 to the blood by metabolizing cells drives hydrolysis in the forward direction, forming H^+ and HCO_3^-, mostly in the RBCs. The H^+ formed by hydrolysis is buffered by hemoglobin, thereby minimizing changes in the pH of the RBC cytoplasm. The HCO_3^- formed in RBCs diffuses out into the plasma, while the chloride anion (Cl^-) moves in to maintain electroneutrality. This anion countertransport is known as the *chloride shift*. HCO_3^- formed in this way accounts for the major portion (80%) of CO_2 transported in the blood. Small amounts are transported while dissolved in plasma (8%) or are combined with hemoglobin (as carbaminohemoglobin) or other proteins (12%). The amount of carbonic acid in the blood at any time is negligible (0.0006%).

In the lungs, CO_2 diffuses along its concentration gradient from the plasma to the alveoli, from which it is exhaled. Removal of CO_2 drives the hydrolysis reaction in reverse, as shown in Figure 14–2. In a reversal of the chloride shift, HCO_3^- reenters the RBCs, and Cl^- exits. HCO_3^- combines with H^+, which has been released from its buffers, regenerating CO_2 and H_2O.

■ REGULATION OF FIXED ACIDS AND BICARBONATE BY THE KIDNEYS

Acids that cannot be converted to gases must be eliminated in the urine. These *fixed acids* include:

- Sulfuric, phosphoric, and other acids produced during protein metabolism
- Ketones produced during accelerated lipid metabolism, as in diabetic ketoacidosis

- Lactic acid produced during anaerobic glycolysis, as in shock and hypoxemia
- Occasionally, ingested toxins, such as salicylate (aspirin), drugs, and methanol

The kidneys regulate serum pH by secreting H^+ into the urine and by regenerating HCO_3^- for reabsorption into the blood. At the glomerulus, HCO_3^- is filtered from the blood into the proximal convoluted tubule. Because HCO_3^- is a large, charged particle, it is poorly reabsorbed. Any HCO_3^- filtered in excess of H^+ is excreted in the urine. H^+ is actively secreted into the renal tubules, primarily by proximal tubular cells, but also in the distal tubule and collecting duct. This system operates only until tubular pH falls to about 4.5. At lower pH values, significant amounts of H^+ leak from the tubular lumen back into the blood. Secretion of large amounts of H^+ into the renal tubules would result in a rapid fall in tubular pH and would inhibit further H^+ secretion, if not for the presence of *urinary buffer systems*. These systems permit the tubular fluid to accept large quantities of H^+ while limiting how much the urinary pH decreases.

Urinary Buffer Systems

The three principal buffer systems in renal tubules are the bicarbonate, ammonia, and phosphate (titratable acid) systems.

In the *bicarbonate buffer* (Fig. 14–3), H^+ is secreted into the tubular lumen by tubular cells in countertransport with sodium (Na^+). The combination of H^+ with filtered bicarbonate regenerates CO_2 in a reversal of the hydrolysis reaction. This CO_2 is reabsorbed into tubular cells, where hydrolysis proceeds efficiently because of the presence of CA. The HCO_3^- formed is reabsorbed with sodium into the blood. Thus, for every molecule of H^+ secreted, a molecule of HCO_3^- is returned to the blood to restore components of the plasma bicarbonate buffer system.

The *ammonia buffer* depends on the generation of ammonia (NH_3) from amino acids, such as glutamine, in renal tubular cells (Fig. 14–4). NH_3 diffuses into the tubular lumen, where it may combine with secreted H^+ to form ammonium (NH_4^+), a large, charged particle that cannot be reabsorbed. H^+ in this form is thus trapped in the tubule. NH_4^+ is excreted in the urine in combination with Cl^- from NaCl. Na^+ is actively reabsorbed, along with tubular HCO_3^-.

The *phosphate buffer* operates similarly (Fig. 14–5), resulting in the formation of weak acids that are excreted in the urine. Sodium and bicarbonate are reabsorbed.

Effects of Other Electrolytes

Although H^+ and HCO_3^- are critical determinants of acid-base balance, they are also electrolytes, subject to the *principle of electroneutrality*, which holds that total cations must equal total anions in any fluid compartment. Renal regulation of serum pH is greatly influenced by the concentrations of other electrolytes, particularly potassium (K^+), sodium (Na^+), calcium (Ca^{2+}), chloride (Cl^-), and protein (Pr^-).

When serum potassium is elevated (*hyperkalemia*), renal tubular cells secrete more K^+ but retain H^+ for electroneutrality. The opposite occurs in *hypokalemia*, which promotes renal secretion of H^+. Similarly, H^+ imbalance influences both renal regulation and cellular shifts in potassium. In cases of serum H^+ excess, more H^+ is secreted by renal tubular cells, but K^+ is retained, promoting hyperkalemia. At the tissue level, H^+ moves into cells to be buffered by intracellular proteins, and K^+ moves out into the blood to maintain electroneutrality. This shift does not represent a true K^+ excess but does contribute to clinical manifestations of hyperkalemia, which include potentially lethal cardiac dysrhythmias. Treatment of the H^+ excess causes a shift in the opposite direction, promoting hypokalemia. In response to a deficit in serum H^+, renal cells retain H^+ and secrete more K^+, and cellular proteins release H^+ to the extracellular fluid while K^+ shifts intracellularly.

FIGURE 14–3 Function of the urinary bicarbonate (HCO_3^-) buffer. *A*, Hydrogen (H^+) is actively secreted into the tubule in exchange for sodium (Na^+). *B*, HCO_3^- is filtered into the tubule at the glomerulus. *C*, H^+ and $H_2CO_3^-$ enter reverse hydrolysis, yielding water (H_2O) and carbon dioxide (CO_2). *D*, H_2O remains in the tubule as urine unless it is reabsorbed. *E*, CO_2 diffuses into tubular cells and enters hydrolysis, catalyzed by carbonic anhydrase (CA), yielding H^+ and HCO_3^-. *F*, HCO_3^- is reabsorbed, with Na^+, into the blood.

Tubular fluid   Renal tubular cells   Peritubular capillary

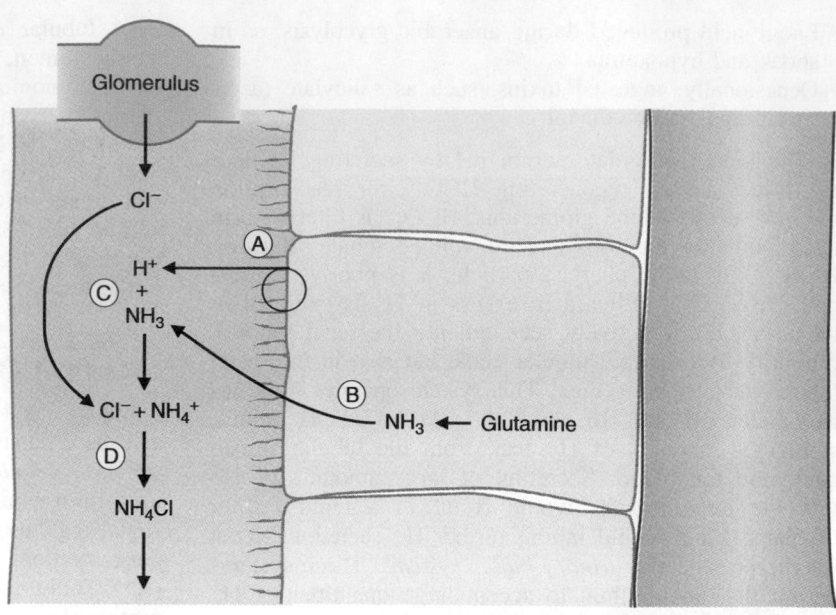

FIGURE 14–4 Function of the ammonia (NH_3) buffer. *A*, Hydrogen (H^+) is actively secreted into the tubular fluid. *B*, NH_3 is formed in the tubular cell and diffuses into the tubular lumen. *C*, Hydrogen (H^+) combines with NH_3 to form ammonium (NH_4^+), which cannot be reabsorbed. *D*, NH_4^+ combines with filtered chloride (Cl^-) for excretion in the urine. NH_4Cl, ammonium chloride.

Na^+ and Cl^- are of particular importance in maintaining fluid balance, and the kidney is the principal site of their regulation. Active reabsorption of Na^+ from the renal tubules creates gradients that drive the reabsorption of anions such as Cl^- and HCO_3^-. The juxtaglomerular cells of the renal glomeruli sense a low extracellular volume, triggering the renin-angiotensin-aldosterone system. Release of the mineralocorticoid hormone aldosterone from the adrenal cortex stimulates renal reabsorption of Na^+ from the distal tubule and proximal collecting duct. Maintenance of electroneutrality requires concurrent increases in the secretion of H^+ and K^+ as well as reabsorption of HCO_3^-. The kidney's priority in such cases is to restore volume balance, but this happens at the cost of worsening pH status. Clinical conditions that cause low serum Na^+

(*hyponatremia*) almost invariably result in low Cl^- (*hypochloremia*) as well. In Cl^- deficit, the kidney reabsorbs more HCO_3^- to maintain electroneutrality. Conversely, in conditions in which excess HCO_3^- is lost in the urine, Cl^- is retained.

Although intracellular proteins are the most important buffers in whole-body acid-base homeostasis, serum proteins such as albumin are also significant. In H^+ excess, for example, serum proteins bind circulating H^+, displacing other cations, such as calcium. The level of free (ionized) Ca^{2+} thus rises, promoting clinical manifestations of hypercalcemia. In H^+ deficit, a greater fraction of serum calcium is bound, decreasing levels of Ca^{2+}. Because H^+ excess creates a need for more urinary buffers, including ammonia (which is derived from protein), in-

FIGURE 14–5 Function of the phosphate buffer. *A*, Hydrogen (H^+) is actively secreted into the tubule. *B*, HPO_4^{2-} (hydrogen phosphate) and Na^+ are filtered into the tubule at the glomerulus. *C*, H^+ and HPO_4^{2-} combine to form dihydrogen phosphate ($H_2PO_4^-$). *D*, $H_2PO_4^-$ combines with filtered Na^+ for excretion in the urine.

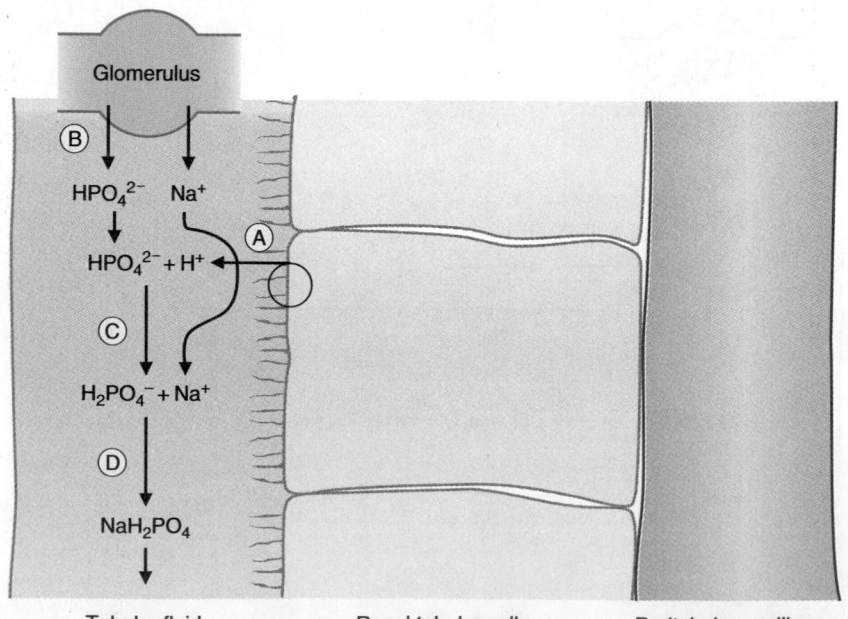

creased buffering of acid promotes depletion of protein. Similarly, deficiency of serum albumin caused by renal disease or other disorders may promote H^+ excess.

INTERACTION OF ACID-BASE REGULATORY SYSTEMS

Clinical evaluation of total acid-base homeostasis is aided by an understanding of the *Henderson-Hasselbalch equation*, which describes the relationships among pH, acid (H_2CO_3), and base (HCO_3^-):

$$pH = pKa + \log([HCO_3^-]/[H_2CO_3])$$

In this equation, pKa is a constant value (6.1). The base component is represented by serum HCO_3^- (normal value 24 mEq/L); since carbonic acid levels are negligible, the acid is represented by dissolved CO_2. Dissolved CO_2 is derived from the measurement of $PaCO_2$, the partial pressure of CO_2 in arterial blood (normal value 40 mm Hg, multiplied by a unit conversion factor of 0.03 to yield 1.2). When normal values are substituted, the equation becomes

$$7.4 = 6.1 + \log \frac{24}{1.2}$$

This equation reveals that a ratio of 20 parts base to 1 part acid must be present to yield a normal pH. An increase in the numerator (base) promotes an increase in blood pH; a decrease in base lowers pH. An increase in the denominator (acid) lowers pH; a decrease in acid raises pH (Fig. 14–6).

ACID-BASE COMPENSATION

When primary disease processes alter either the acid or the base component of the ratio, the lungs or the kidneys (whichever is unaffected by pathologic change) act to restore the 20:1 ratio and normalize pH. This process is known as *acid-base compensation*. When kidney disease impairs excretion of fixed acids, for example, the respiratory system can increase ventilation to "blow off" excess acid as CO_2. In respiratory failure, the kidneys can compensate for retention of acid (CO_2) by secreting H^+ and regenerating HCO_3^-.

As stated, blood buffers act to modulate pH changes but do not eliminate acid or base from the body. The lungs or kidneys alter the actual amounts of acid and base, but regulation by these systems is not as fast. The lungs respond within minutes, but maximal compensation takes up to 24 hours. The kidneys may require up to 72 hours to achieve optimal compensation.

In most cases, compensation does not fully restore normal pH. Respiratory compensation is limited because reducing ventilation to compensate for a renal deficit of H^+ would eventually result in hypoxemia. Because hypoxemia is a respiratory stimulant, ventilation would again increase. Similarly, renal compensation for ventilatory disorders is potentially limited by many factors, including renal blood flow, tubular flow rates, and saturability of tubular transport processes.

ACID-BASE CORRECTION

Although compensatory responses for primary acid-base disorders may nearly restore the 20:1 ratio of base to acid, the actual amounts of acid and base remain abnormal. Thus, compensation must be differentiated from *correction*, in which the ratio is restored and the absolute

FIGURE 14–6 Regulation of acid-base balance. H_2CO_3, carbonic acid; H_2O, water; CO_2, carbon dioxide; HCO_3^-, bicarbonate.

quantities of dissolved CO_2 (as derived from $PaCO_2$) and HCO_3^- are returned to the normal range. Correction occurs only with resolution of the underlying disorder.

■ ANALYSIS OF ARTERIAL BLOOD GASES

The status of acid-base homeostasis may be monitored clinically through the serial measurement of *arterial blood gases* (ABGs). Among the parameters reported are pH, $PaCO_2$, and HCO_3^-. As illustrated in Box 14–1, these values may be used to (1) determine the presence and type of acid-base imbalance and (2) evaluate the level of compensation.

DISORDERS OF ACID-BASE BALANCE

The four general classes of acid-base imbalance are (1) respiratory acidosis, (2) respiratory alkalosis, (3) metabolic acidosis, and (4) metabolic alkalosis. These disorders are not clinical diagnoses or diseases in themselves; rather, they are clinical syndromes associated with a wide variety of diseases.

Acidosis refers to any pathologic process that causes a relative excess of acid (volatile or fixed) in the body. *Acidemia* is excess acid in the blood. The presence of acidemia does not necessarily confirm an underlying pathologic process; technically, it is merely a laboratory finding.

The same distinction may be made between the terms alkalosis and alkalemia. *Alkalosis* indicates a primary condition resulting in excess base in the body, and *alkalemia* refers more narrowly to elevation of serum pH. Care must be taken not to confuse these terms conceptually, and they must not be used interchangeably in clinical practice.

The incidence of acid-base imbalances in clinical settings is high. A study of 110 consecutive admissions to a general hospital revealed an overall incidence of acid-base imbalances of 56%. The most common disorder was respiratory alkalosis (26 cases), followed by respiratory acidosis (16), metabolic alkalosis (10), and metabolic acidosis (6). Eleven clients had more than one acid-base imbalance concurrently.[11]

■ RESPIRATORY ALKALOSIS

Respiratory alkalosis is a state of relative excess of base in body fluids resulting from increased respiratory elimination of CO_2. *Acute* respiratory alkalosis lasts for 24 hours or less; *chronic* respiratory alkalosis persists for a longer period.

Etiology and Risk Factors

Respiratory alkalosis is caused by alveolar hyperventilation, in which excess CO_2 is eliminated. The most com-

---

BOX 14–1 Analysis of Arterial Blood Gases

Step 1: Classify the pH

Normal: 7.35–7.45
Acidemia: <7.35
Alkalemia: >7.45

Step 2: Assess $PaCO_2$

Normal: 35–45 mm Hg
Respiratory acidosis: >45 mm Hg
Respiratory alkalosis: <35 mm Hg

Step 3: Assess HCO_3^-*

Normal: 22–26 mEq/L
Metabolic acidosis: <22 mEq/L
Metabolic alkalosis: >26 mEq/L

Step 4: Determine Presence of Compensation

Compensation present: $PaCO_2$ and HCO_3^- are abnormal (or nearly so) in opposite directions; that is, one is acidotic and the other alkalotic.†
Compensation absent: One component ($PaCO_2$ or HCO_3^-) is abnormal, the other normal.

Step 5: Identify Primary Disorder, If Possible

If pH is clearly abnormal: The acid-base component most consistent with the pH disturbance is the primary disorder.

If pH is normal or near-normal: The more deviant component is probably primary.‡ Also, note whether pH is on acidotic or alkalotic side of 7.4. The more deviant component should be consistent with this pH.

Step 6: Classify Degree of Compensation, If Present

The limits of complete compensation are as follows:

■ *Metabolic acidosis*: The decrease in $PaCO_2$ is approximately equal to the last two digits of the pH.
■ *Metabolic alkalosis*: The $PaCO_2$ is approximately equal to 0.6 times the increase in HCO_3^-.
■ *Respiratory acidosis*: For every 10 mm Hg increase in $PaCO_2$, the HCO_3^- is increased by 1 mEq/L (in acute acidosis) or 4 mEq/L (in chronic acidosis).
■ *Respiratory alkalosis*: For every 10 mm Hg decrease in $PaCO_2$, the HCO_3^- is decreased by 2 mEq/L (in acute alkalosis) or 5 mEq/L (in chronic alkalosis).

"Compensation" beyond these limits suggests the presence of a complex disorder.

*Base excess (BE) is also reported with arterial blood gas (ABG) values and is a second index of metabolic status. Normal BE is −2 to +2. Because fluctuation in BE parallels that of bicarbonate, it is not usually necessary to classify both.

† It is possible, but less likely, that two or more opposing primary imbalances (i.e., a complex disorder) are present, resulting in the appearance of compensation. The detection of complex disorders is facilitated by the use of an acid-base map (see Fig. 14–1) and by the use of the "formulas" described in Step 6, but a complex disorder cannot always be differentiated from compensation on the basis of laboratory values.

‡ It is unlikely that the more deviant component represents compensation, because except in rare cases the body does not overcompensate for imbalance. When pH approaches the normal range, compensatory mechanisms are no longer triggered.

mon cause of respiratory alkalosis is hypoxemia from such pulmonary disorders as pneumonia, pulmonary embolism, asthma, adult respiratory distress syndrome (ARDS), and pulmonary edema. Transient respiratory alkalosis may also occur secondary to acute anxiety or as a response to respiratory stimulant drugs such as epinephrine and salicylates. Neural disorders, such as stroke and intracranial lesions, may stimulate the central respiratory drive.

The most common causes of mild, chronic respiratory alkalosis are residence in high altitudes and pregnancy. Pulmonary fibrosis and other disorders that limit ventilatory volume result in an increased ventilatory rate, with a possible net excess of CO_2 elimination.

Pathophysiology

A low partial pressure of oxygen in arterial blood (PaO_2) is sensed by peripheral chemoreceptors in the carotid bodies and aortic arch. The rate at which these receptors fire then increases, stimulating the respiratory center in the medulla and increasing the rate and depth of ventilation. Peripheral chemoreceptors are also stimulated in states of low blood flow, such as shock.

Conditions that physically impede expansion of the lungs (such as pulmonary fibrosis) stimulate activation of the respiratory center via the Hering-Breuer, or stretch reflex. The J receptors, located in the alveolar-capillary membrane, are thought to stimulate increased ventilation in disorders such as ARDS, which causes thickening of this membrane.

The central chemoreceptors and respiratory center may be stimulated excessively by chemicals or toxins. In the case of salicylate overdose, it is interesting that adults usually exhibit respiratory alkalosis and that children more often have metabolic acidosis from the acid ingestion. The reason for this difference between children and adults is unknown. In severe alkalemia, changes in the ionization of structural and regulatory proteins result in widespread organ dysfunction. Cellular shifts and increased binding of Ca^{2+} to serum proteins induce electrolyte imbalance.

The buffering response in acute respiratory alkalosis results from (1) shifting of acid from intracellular fluid into the blood and (2) movement of HCO_3^- into cells in exchange for Cl^-. An adaptive increase in lactic acid production occurs secondary to stimulation of glycolysis. Renal compensation in chronic respiratory alkalosis involves decreased H^+ secretion as well as excretion of excess filtered HCO_3^-.

Clinical Manifestations

Signs of respiratory alkalosis in a client's ABG analysis include a high pH and a low $PaCO_2$. HCO_3^- levels fall with compensation in chronic respiratory alkalosis, and serum lactate dehydrogenase levels are often elevated. Hyperventilation, the underlying cause, is clinically apparent.

Central nervous system manifestations of altered blood flow and neurotransmission are usually predominant. They include paresthesias, lightheadedness, and confusion. Musculoskeletal and cardiac manifestations of hypokalemia and hypocalcemia (such as dysrhythmias and muscle weakness) may be present.

Prognosis

The clinical outcome depends on the severity of the underlying disorder and its response to treatment. Mild alkalosis in pregnancy and at high altitudes is considered to be adaptive. Respiratory alkalosis in a critically ill client is an ominous prognostic sign, with mortality increasing proportionately with the severity of alkalosis.[2] Compensation for severe respiratory alkalosis depletes the bicarbonate buffer, increasing the client's vulnerability to later acidosis.

Outcome Management

TREATMENT OF THE UNDERLYING DISORDER
Treatment of mild, chronic respiratory alkalosis is usually not warranted because it produces little risk and few symptoms. Aggressive treatment of the underlying causes of hypoxemia is essential in cases of severe respiratory alkalosis. Electrolyte imbalances usually resolve with treatment of the underlying cause.

RESPIRATORY SUPPORT
Oxygen therapy may be used to correct underlying hypoxemia. Rebreathing of CO_2 (as from breathing into a paper bag or other closed system) provides prompt but short-term relief in anxiety-related respiratory alkalosis.

■ RESPIRATORY ACIDOSIS

Respiratory acidosis is a state of relative excess of acid in body fluids resulting from retention or excessive production of CO_2. *Acute* respiratory acidosis develops and resolves within 3 days or less; *chronic* respiratory acidosis persists over a longer period.

Etiology and Risk Factors

Respiratory acidosis nearly always results from hypoventilation. Chronic respiratory acidosis is most commonly caused by chronic obstructive pulmonary disease (COPD), also known as "chronic airflow limitation." In end-stage COPD, pathologic changes lead to airway collapse, air trapping, and disturbance of ventilation-perfusion (V/Q) relationships. Acute respiratory acidosis also occurs when respiratory infection or concurrent cardiac disease increases the work of breathing. Hypoventilation with resulting respiratory acidosis is seen in diseases of the neuromuscular junction in which diaphragmatic movement is impaired (such as Guillain-Barré syndrome) and in depression of the medullary respiratory center by drugs or lesions of the central nervous system.

Respiratory acidosis may occur iatrogenically (as a result of treatment) from inadequate mechanical ventilation or from excessive oxygen administration to clients with chronic CO_2 retention (as in COPD). In the latter case, hypoventilation results from:

• Depression of the medullary respiratory center with removal of the hypoxemic stimulus
• Worsening of V/Q relationships secondary to replacement of airway nitrogen (which helps keep airways open) with oxygen

Normally, the most important stimulus for ventilation is an increase in the acidity of cerebrospinal fluid (CSF) resulting from diffusion of CO_2 into the CSF from the blood. However, the higher level of HCO_3^- resulting from renal compensation for chronic respiratory acidosis minimizes the effect of increasing $PaCO_2$ in these clients. Oxygen therapy may worsen V/Q relationships because it displaces nitrogen, a much less soluble gas, in alveoli. As oxygen is absorbed, alveoli may collapse, contributing to hypoventilation.

The second, much less common cause of respiratory acidosis is excessive CO_2 production from hypermetabolism, or from excessive metabolism of carbohydrate fuels for energy. Clinical use of enteral feedings or parenteral nutrition formulas that are disproportionately high in carbohydrate may contribute to elevated $PaCO_2$ levels, particularly in clients who also have impaired ventilation.

Pathophysiology

CO_2 accumulates in the blood and diffuses readily into all body compartments. This *hypercapnia* drives the hydrolysis reaction forward, generating carbonic acid that dissociates into H^+ and HCO_3^-. Immediate buffering by nonbicarbonate buffers occurs. Renal compensation proceeds over 3 to 5 days, with greater secretion of H^+ and regeneration of bicarbonate. Renal ammonia production increases, enhancing the function of the ammonia urinary buffer but depleting protein stores. As serum HCO_3^- levels rise with compensation, Cl^- is excreted in greater amounts, potentially inducing hypochloremia in chronic respiratory acidosis. Renal retention of K^+ and cellular cation shifts may lead to hyperkalemia. Displacement of Ca^{2+} from albumin may result in hypercalcemia.

In acute respiratory acidosis, the rapid rise in $PaCO_2$ results in hypoxemia in clients breathing room air, as retained CO_2 displaces oxygen in alveoli. Hypoxemia poses a more serious threat to life than either acidemia or hypercapnia in severe acute respiratory acidosis. Acidemia alters the ionization of structural and regulatory proteins (enzymes, for example), resulting in widespread manifestations of organ dysfunction.

Clinical Manifestations

An arterial blood sample that has a low pH signifies that the client has acidemia, and a high $PaCO_2$ signifies hypercapnia. The client probably has hypoventilation, the usual underlying cause of respiratory acidosis; signs of hypoxemia may be present in severe cases. HCO_3^- levels are normal or, if renal compensation is occurring, elevated. Compensation is present to a greater extent in chronic respiratory acidosis than in acute respiratory acidosis.

Clinical signs of organ system dysfunction from acidemia include hypotension and cardiac dysrhythmias caused by decreased vascular tone, decreased myocardial contractility, and manifestations of electrolyte imbalance. Altered cerebral blood flow and depressed neurotransmission may manifest as tremors, seizures, lethargy, stupor, and, ultimately, coma (hypercapnic encephalopathy).

Prognosis

The clinical outcome in respiratory acidosis depends on the severity and duration of tissue hypoxia as well as on the responsiveness of the underlying disorder to treatment.

Outcome Management

TREATMENT OF THE UNDERLYING DISORDER
Treatment of respiratory acidosis is primarily focused on resolving the underlying disorder. For example, you may give an antibiotic to treat pneumonia, a narcotic antagonist to treat a drug overdose, or dialysis to clear toxins from the blood. Electrolyte imbalances usually resolve with such treatment; however, life-threatening hyperkalemia may require emergency treatment with dialysis or cation-exchange resins.

RESPIRATORY SUPPORT
Mechanical ventilation and supplemental oxygen are often employed in conditions that cause respiratory acidosis. Currently, the trend is to use ventilation at lower tidal volumes than would be required to completely restore $PaCO_2$ to the normal range. This *permissive hypercapnia* results in fewer airway injuries but comparable clinical outcomes. However, because the client's own ventilatory drive exceeds that provided by the ventilator, sedation is usually required. Administer oxygen therapy cautiously (at low flow rates or low percentages) to the client with chronic CO_2 retention to minimize the risk of worsening the client's respiratory status via nitrogen washout and blunting of the ventilatory drive.

ADMINISTRATION OF EXOGENOUS ALKALI
If the client has adequate renal function, administration of base (typically, sodium bicarbonate) to partially correct the pH is not warranted. Such treatment may actually worsen the client's condition because bicarbonate further raises CO_2 levels by driving reverse hydrolysis. An exception may be made if the client has severe bronchospasm, because alkalinization may restore the responsiveness of the airways to beta-agonist drugs.[1]

■ METABOLIC ALKALOSIS

Metabolic alkalosis is a state of relative excess of base (or H^+ deficit) in body fluids resulting from a gain of bicarbonate or a loss of fixed acids.

Etiology and Risk Factors

Metabolic alkalosis develops through a two-phase mechanism. In the *generation phase*, the imbalance is first created by (1) loss of acid (as with HCl loss during vomiting) or gain of base (as with administration of $NaHCO_3$) or (2) loss of intestinal fluids containing more Cl^- than HCO_3^-. Metabolic alkalosis associated with fluid volume loss is referred to as *contraction alkalosis*. Another common type, *posthypercapnic metabolic alkalosis*, results from too-rapid correction of chronic respiratory acidosis, in which case a compensatory increase in HCO_3^- then persists as a primary disorder.

In the *maintenance phase*, alkalosis persists because renal excretion of HCO_3^-, which would otherwise correct the disorder, is impaired. This impairment may result from hypovolemia in contraction alkalosis or, much less commonly, from aldosterone excess. In hypovolemia, greater Na⁺ reabsorption by the distal tubule (stimulated by the renin-angiotensin-aldosterone system) results in increases in both H⁺ secretion and HCO_3^- regeneration. In primary aldosteronism (or with prolonged corticosteroid administration, in which aldosterone-like effects also arise), the hormone stimulates increased Na⁺ reabsorption by the same distal tubular transport mechanism.

Metabolic alkalosis from fluid loss is referred to as "saline-sensitive," because restoration of volume with fluid containing NaCl permits the kidneys to restore acid-base homeostasis. Alkalosis in cases of aldosterone excess is not correctable with administration of a saline solution and so is termed "saline-resistant." Rarely, excessive ingestion of licorice (20 to 40 g) causes metabolic alkalosis because of its structural similarity to aldosterone.

Overcorrection of acidosis with $NaHCO_3$ may cause alkalosis, as can massive transfusion of whole blood. The citrate anticoagulant used for storing blood is metabolized to bicarbonate. Packed RBCs contain much less citrate; thus, their use in multiple transfusion is preferred. Treatment of hypovolemia with lactated Ringer's solution may also contribute, because lactate is metabolized to bicarbonate.

Loss of gastric fluid via nasogastric suction or vomiting further contributes to metabolic alkalosis because of loss of HCl. Additional HCl must be produced by gastric cells via the hydrolysis reaction. H⁺ is secreted into the stomach with Cl⁻, while the HCO_3^- produced during the reaction is reabsorbed into the blood.

Pathophysiology

Respiratory compensation for metabolic alkalosis is limited by the hypoxemia that quickly develops with hypoventilation. Most buffering occurs in the extracellular fluid, where the buffers are much less effective for base loads than for acid loads. Severe alkalemia leads to widespread organ dysfunction because of altered ionization of body proteins as well as enhanced Ca^{2+} binding to serum proteins. Neurologic and cardiovascular systems are primarily affected. Hypokalemia, which occurs from cellular shifts and renal or intestinal losses, is more prominent in metabolic alkalosis than in respiratory alkalosis.

Clinical Manifestations

Metabolic alkalosis is manifested in ABG values by a high pH and a high HCO_3^-. $PaCO_2$ rises with compensation. Adaptive hypoventilation may be apparent and may induce some hypoxemia. Signs of volume deficit are often present in association with the underlying disorder. Hypokalemia may be manifested as cardiac dysrhythmias. Central nervous system manifestations include lethargy, confusion, and seizures.

Prognosis

The outcome of metabolic alkalosis depends primarily on the severity of the underlying disorder and its responsiveness to treatment. Uncorrected metabolic alkalosis is associated with high mortality from dysrhythmias and poor tissue perfusion.

Outcome Management

TREATMENT OF THE UNDERLYING DISORDER
Prompt treatment of the underlying disease process is the primary approach. Replacement of lost fluids and electrolytes and support of renal function are often the mainstays of therapy.

ADMINISTRATION OF ACETAZOLAMIDE
Acetazolamide (Diamox) is a diuretic that inhibits carbonic anhydrase and promotes loss of bicarbonate in the urine. Losses of potassium and phosphate are also greater with the use of acetazolamide, however, and may lead to manifestations of electrolyte imbalance.

ADMINISTRATION OF EXOGENOUS ACID
In severe alkalemia, the intravenous administration of acid (HCl) or HCl precursors (ammonium chloride or arginine monohydrochloride) may be warranted to enhance physiologic compensation. Risks of acid infusion are substantial, however; they include local tissue injury (sclerosis of veins), hypervolemia, hyperosmolar imbalance (with HCl precursors), increased ammonia levels (with ammonium chloride), and hyperkalemia (with arginine monohydrochloride).

■ METABOLIC ACIDOSIS

Metabolic acidosis is a state of relative acid excess (or base deficit) in body fluids resulting from gain of fixed acids or a loss of bicarbonate.

Etiology and Risk Factors

Metabolic acidosis may be caused by either of two mechanisms: accumulation of fixed acid or loss of base. These mechanisms may be differentiated clinically by the presence or absence of a high *anion gap*. Normally, the anion gap is 6.6 ± 4 mEg/L.[13] It is calculated by subtracting the sum of the serum concentrations of the major anions, bicarbonate and chloride, from the serum concentration of sodium. The difference, or "gap," represents anions in the serum other than HCO_3^- and Cl⁻.

When acidosis results from addition of organic acid (as in lactic acidosis), bicarbonate is consumed in buffering but is not lost from the body. Unmeasured anions (primarily proteins) buffer most of the acid load, and the anion gap thus increases. Common causes of *high–anion gap acidosis* are:

- Azotemic renal failure, in which acid end products of protein metabolism cannot be effectively excreted because of impaired glomerular filtration
- Diabetic ketoacidosis, in which ketoacids accumulate because of accelerated lipid metabolism in the absence of insulin
- Lactic acidosis, a consequence of anaerobic carbohydrate metabolism
- Ingestion of toxins with acid metabolites (less common)

Non–anion gap acidosis caused by loss of base is also called *hyperchloremic metabolic acidosis*. In this case, chloride is retained by the kidneys when excess bicarbonate is lost from the body, and the anion gap remains normal. Excess bicarbonate may be lost through either the kidneys or the intestinal tract. In renal tubular acidosis, the renal tubular cells cannot reabsorb bicarbonate, which therefore is lost in the urine. Intestinal secretions, high in bicarbonate, may be lost through enteric drainage tubes (such as an ileostomy tube) or diarrhea. Drugs that inhibit carbonic anhydrase, such as acetazolamide, interfere with bicarbonate regeneration during urinary buffering. In non–anion gap acidosis caused by a gain of mineral acid (such as HCl), chloride is ingested with the acid, and bicarbonate is excreted proportionally.

Pathophysiology

Metabolic acidosis is accompanied by a compensatory increase in ventilation. Severe acidemia induces insulin resistance and depresses glycolytic enzymes, resulting in impairment of energy metabolism. The function of regulatory and structural proteins is impaired by altered ionization, leading to widespread organ dysfunction. Increased protein catabolism also occurs. Hyperkalemia occurs because K^+ shifts out of cells as excess H^+ enters. Insulin deficiency in diabetic ketoacidosis may worsen hyperkalemia because insulin normally promotes cellular uptake of K^+ along with glucose. Uptake of lactic acid by the liver is reduced, whereas hepatic lactate production is increased.

In metabolic acidosis caused by a gain of organic acids, bicarbonate stores are rapidly depleted by buffering. If renal function is not impaired, renal regeneration of HCO_3^- occurs with excretion of H^+. However, this response takes several days.

Clinical Manifestations

Metabolic acidosis is apparent in ABG values as a low pH and a low HCO_3^-. $PaCO_2$ drops as respiratory compensation occurs. Systemic signs of acidemia resulting from altered protein function and electrolyte imbalance are similar to those of respiratory acidosis, except that compensatory hyperventilation is present.

Prognosis

Clinical outcomes of metabolic acidosis depend on the severity of the underlying disorder and its responsiveness to treatment.

Outcome Management

TREATMENT OF THE UNDERLYING DISORDER
Aggressive intervention aimed at resolving the underlying disorder is the primary form of treatment. Electrolyte imbalance is treated only if life-threatening, because it normally resolves with correction of the underlying disorder.

ADMINISTRATION OF EXOGENOUS ALKALI
In severe metabolic acidosis, administration of intravenous sodium bicarbonate or other alkalinizing substances may be warranted to minimize the detrimental effects of the acidosis until the underlying disorder is resolved or until physiologic compensation is effective. Such therapy may provide a margin of safety in anticipation of continued acidifying stressors, but it is not without controversy. Fluid overload, hyperosmolar imbalance, and alkalosis

due to excessive treatment are risks of this approach. As previously mentioned, administration of bicarbonate results in increased CO_2 levels, which may be detrimental in clients with respiratory disease or advanced cardiac failure. Alternative alkalinizing agents, such as tromethamine (Tham), produce less CO_2 but have not proved more effective than $NaHCO_3$ for the treatment of severe acidemia.[1]

■ COMPLEX ACID-BASE DISORDERS

Mixed acid-base disorders, in which two primary acid-base imbalances coexist, are common. In cardiac arrest, for example, lactic acid quickly accumulates as a result of anaerobic metabolism; the carbonic acid level is elevated because of respiratory arrest. In COPD, underlying respiratory acidosis may be complicated by metabolic alkalosis secondary to diuretic or steroid therapy.

A *triple acid-base disorder* is present when metabolic acidosis and metabolic alkalosis coexist with either respiratory acidosis or respiratory alkalosis. (The two respiratory imbalances cannot coexist because they have opposite effects on ventilation.) As an example of a triple disorder, imbalances due to ingestion of methanol (an exogenous toxin that produces metabolic acidosis), vomiting (which produces metabolic alkalosis), and respiratory arrest from aspiration (which produces respiratory acidosis) may occur simultaneously.

Suspect a complex acid-base disorder when a client's $PaCO_2$ value and HCO_3^- level do not correlate with pH or when ABG evidence of compensation exceeds predicted levels (see Box 14–1). Use of an acid-base map may also facilitate detection (Fig. 14–7). If the plotted ABG values converge at a point outside the usual range for a primary imbalance, a complex disorder is likely.

■ Nursing Management of the Medical Client
ASSESSMENT
You must be alert for signs of acid-base imbalance in clients at risk for these disturbances. There is such a risk in any client who:

• Has a known disease of the pulmonary, cardiovascular, or renal system
• Is in a hypermetabolic state, such as with fever, sepsis, or burns
• Is receiving total parenteral nutrition or enteral tube feedings high in carbohydrate
• Is receiving mechanical ventilation
• Has diabetes
• Has vomiting, diarrhea, or enteric drainage
• Is elderly

Age-related decreases in respiratory and renal function may limit the client's ability to compensate for acid-base disturbances. The normal aging process results in decreased ventilatory capacity as well as loss of alveolar surface area for gas exchange; thus, older adults are susceptible to respiratory acidosis from hypoventilation and to respiratory alkalosis from hypoxemia. Older adults commonly take multiple medications for hypertension or cardiovascular disease; these drugs may contribute to hypokalemia and metabolic alkalosis. Respiratory compensa-

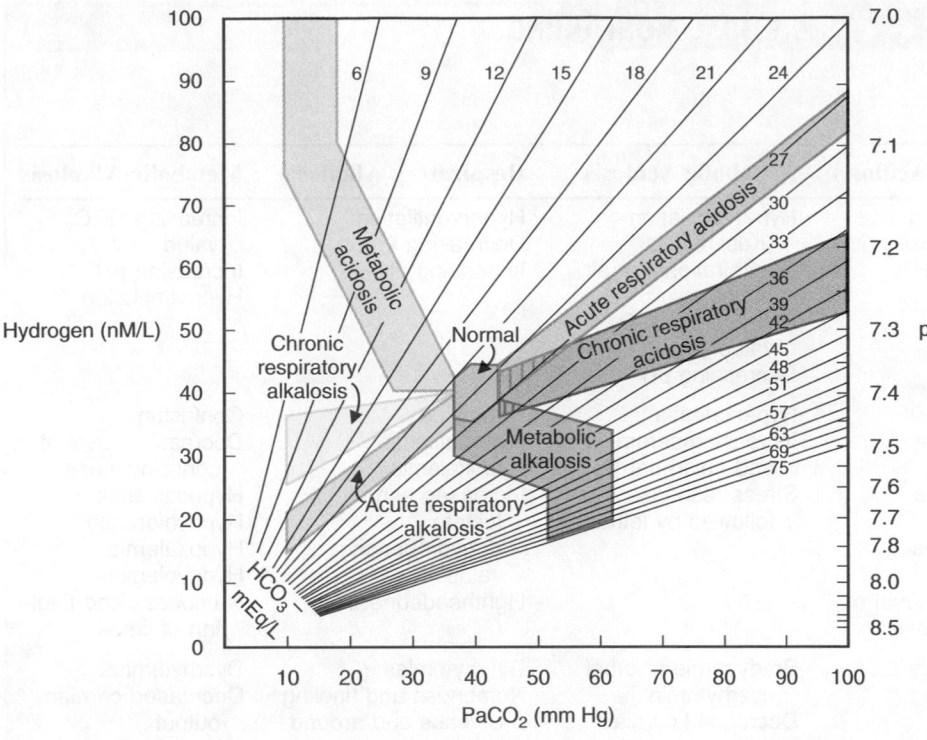

FIGURE 14–7 An acid-base map. To use the acid-base map, plot the pH on the vertical axis and the partial pressure of arterial carbon dioxide ($PaCO_2$) on the horizontal axis. Note the point at which the values intersect. If the result falls outside the normal area or the 95% confidence bands for the major primary disorders, the client probably has a complex acid-base imbalance. However, a point falling within one of the bands does not rule out a complex disorder. HCO_3^-, bicarbonate.

tion in this condition is compromised because of the structural and functional changes mentioned. Decreased cardiac output in the aging person diminishes renal perfusion and glomerular filtration. Aldosterone is less effective in older people, as is ammonia buffering. These changes limit renal compensation for respiratory imbalances and may put an elderly client at higher risk for metabolic imbalance.

To assess for acid-base imbalances, document the findings of a comprehensive physical assessment of ventilatory status, cardiovascular function, and fluid balance, as described in the Critical Monitoring chart. Carefully analyze the trends you see. Consider laboratory values as well, including ABG, electrolyte, blood urea nitrogen, creatinine, and serum lactate dehydrogenase values.

INTERPRET ARTERIAL BLOOD GAS VALUES. Your knowledgeable interpretation of ABG values is critical for timely, appropriate intervention in acid-base disturbances. Often, you are the first to see a client's ABG results. You become the communication link between respiratory therapists and physicians about potential changes in a client's status or treatment. In critical care units, many nurses are using bedside ABG analyzers to obtain these results. Systems for continuous in vivo monitoring of blood gases have recently been developed. Although ABG interpretation is essential to diagnosis and treatment of acid-base imbalance, ABG findings are helpful only when they are considered as part of the total clinical picture.

PROTECT THE CLIENT. Preventing client injury during diagnostic procedures is one of your most important responsibilities. Before a client receives a radial artery puncture for withdrawal of an arterial blood speci-

men, for example, perform Allen's test to ensure adequate circulation to the hand. Perform this test as follows:

1. Have the client tightly close the intended test hand into a fist.
2. Apply pressure over the pulse points for both radial and ulnar arteries.
3. Ask the client to open the fist; the palm has a blanched look from a lack of blood.
4. Release pressure on the ulnar artery. If the artery has adequate circulation, the client's palm reddens within 10 or 15 seconds; it is safe to use the radial artery to obtain a blood specimen.

Failure to assess collateral circulation may result in severe ischemic injury to the client's hand if the ulnar artery is compromised and the radial artery is injured by the puncture.

Critically ill clients commonly have femoral or radial arterial catheter systems from which blood specimens are drawn. Frequent sampling can result in significant blood loss if an open system is used. Nursing research has demonstrated that a minimal discard specimen of 2 ml is sufficient to clear the arterial line of heparinized solution before blood is aspirated for ABG testing.[15] Closed systems allow reinstillation of initially aspirated heparinized solution and blood. Nursing responsibilities for clients with arterial lines are discussed in Chapter 56.

ENSURE ACCURACY. You are responsible for minimizing errors in ABG analysis caused by faulty specimen collection and handling. Potential sampling errors, their consequences, and nursing implications are summarized in Table 14–1. Despite quality control procedures, erroneous blood gas data are sometimes reported. You should suspect a sampling error or transcription error

CRITICAL MONITORING

Acid-Base Imbalances

	Respiratory Acidosis	Metabolic Acidosis	Respiratory Alkalosis	Metabolic Alkalosis
Defining Signs	Hypoventilation Increasing $PaCO_2$ Decreasing pH	Hyperventilation (Kussmaul's respirations, or air hunger) Decreasing HCO_3^- value Decreasing pH	Hyperventilation Decreasing $PaCO_2$ Increasing pH	Increasing HCO_3^- value Increasing pH Hypoventilation
Commonly Seen	Dyspnea Hypercalcemia Hyperkalemia Hypochloremia Hypoxemia Stress response, followed by decreasing level of consciousness	Hyperkalemia Increasing serum Cl^- and anion gap Stress response followed by lethargy	Confusion Hypocalcemia Hypokalemia Increased serum lactate dehydrogenase value Lightheadedness	Confusion Decreasing level of consciousness Hypocalcemia Hypochloremia Hypokalemia Hypovolemia Numbness and tingling of limbs
Signs of Severe Imbalance	Hypotension Papilledema Seizures Dysrhythmias Muscle tremors	Bradycardia or other dysrhythmia Decreased cardiac output Gastrointestinal distention Hypotension Nausea and vomiting	Dysrhythmias Numbness and tingling of limbs and around mouth Muscle weakness	Dysrhythmias Decreased cardiac output Hypotension Hypoxemia Muscle cramping or tetany Muscle tremors Seizures

---

TABLE 14–1	**SOURCES OF ERROR IN SAMPLING FOR ARTERIAL BLOOD GAS ANALYSIS**	

Sampling Error	Effect	Nursing Implications
Air bubbles in syringe	↑ PaO_2 ↓ $PaCO_2$ ↑ pH	Expel all air bubbles immediately. Do not agitate syringe. Do not use any sample that appears frothy.
Inadvertent venous sample or venous contamination of arterial sample	↓ PaO_2 ↑ $PaCO_2$ ↓ pH	Avoid use of femoral artery. Use short-beveled needle. Do not overshoot artery and then withdraw to "catch" it. Watch for autofilling of syringe with arterial puncture. Verify questionable results with new sample.
Anticoagulant effects Altered pH	↓ pH	Use lithium heparin, if possible. Use 1:1000 units/ml concentration. Use minimum 2-ml discard sample with arterial line aspiration.
Dilution of sample	↑ pH ↓ all other values	Use syringe with minimal dead space. Use dried heparin if available. Use at least 3-ml sample.
Effects of metabolism of white blood cells in sample	↓ PaO_2 ↑ $PaCO_2$ ↓ pH	Place sample in ice water immediately. Have sample analyzed within 20 min. Cool sample to 5° C if it cannot be analyzed quickly. Have sample analyzed immediately if client has leukocytosis.

$PaCO_2$, partial pressure of carbon dioxide in arterial blood; PaO_2, partial pressure of oxygen in arterial blood; ↑, increase in; ↓, decrease in.
Data from Malley, W. J. (1990). *Clinical blood gases: Application and noninvasive alternatives.* Philadelphia: W. B. Saunders; and Williams, A. J. (1998). ABC of oxygen: Assessing and interpreting arterial blood gases and acid-base balance. *British Medical Journal, 317*(7167), 1213–1216.

when the reported values lack internal consistency or external congruity. *Internal consistency* means that the values make sense when considered as a whole. An alkalotic pH, for example, is inconsistent with excess $PaCO_2$ and deficient HCO_3^-. *External congruity* means that the ABG findings are consistent with other laboratory data and with clinical assessment findings. For example, a client with a pH of 7.10 should appear profoundly ill.

DIAGNOSIS, OUTCOMES, INTERVENTIONS

Nursing Diagnoses. Several nursing diagnoses may apply to the management of underlying causes and clinical manifestations of acid-base disturbances. For example, *Ineffective Breathing Pattern, Altered Tissue Perfusion,* or *Risk of Injury* may be appropriate. Acid-base imbalances are perhaps best conceptualized as collaborative problems, however, because the interventions of several health care professionals, including nurses, respiratory therapists, and physicians, are required for effective treatment.

Outcomes. When acid-base imbalances are approached as collaborative problems, the expected outcomes reflect timely resolution of underlying disorders and minimization of the detrimental effects of acidemia or alkalemia. Your role in promoting these outcomes includes implementing medical management and watching for clinical manifestations of the imbalances and the response to treatment.

Interventions. Corrective interventions address the underlying causes of acid-base imbalances and are the mainstay of treatment in such disorders. Compensatory imbalances are not treated but instead resolve spontaneously as the primary disorder is reversed. You should optimize the client's respiratory and renal function through positioning, pulmonary hygiene, and hydration. Also, help clients cope with the anxiety that often accompanies—and may contribute to—acid-base imbalance. Collaborate in the administration of drug therapy, fluid and electrolyte replacement, oxygen therapy, and mechanical ventilation when indicated.

Provide Respiratory Support. Altered ventilation is a component of all significant acid-base imbalances, whether as a contributing cause or as a result of compensation. You can help to promote optimal ventilation through such measures as repositioning, airway management, hydration, and implementation of oxygen therapy and mechanical ventilation.

Administer Exogenous Acid or Alkali. In extreme circumstances that require intravenous administration of acid or base, you must be knowledgeable about the potential risks of this therapy, and you must carefully monitor administration rates and therapeutic response. For a detailed discussion of appropriate nursing interventions for specific disorders underlying acid-base imbalances, consult the appropriate chapters of this book.

EVALUATION

Acid-base disorders can be acute and corrected quickly, with control of the underlying disorder, or they may be chronic and managed with compensation. Clients with chronic forms of acid-base imbalance must be assessed closely because they decompensate quickly.

CONCLUSIONS

In collaboration with other health care professionals, you may reduce the client's risk for adverse outcomes resulting from acid-base imbalances. Because of the narrow homeostatic range of serum pH, the client at risk must be carefully monitored in order to detect imbalance as early as possible. Nursing interventions that promote optional respiratory and renal function are particularly important in prevention and treatment of acid-base imbalances.

THINKING CRITICALLY

1. **The client is a 65-year-old widow with a long history of type 2 diabetes mellitus. She was a heavy smoker for 40 years but has not smoked in the last 5 years. She is admitted to the general medical unit because of a 1-week history of profuse diarrhea, attributed to food poisoning. She appears to be in respiratory distress. Her admission ABG values are pH, 7.26; $PaCO_2$, 13 mm Hg; HCO_3^-, 5 mEq/L. What acid-base imbalance does she have? Should you encourage her to breathe more slowly? Other than ABGs, what laboratory values should you monitor closely in this case? Why?**

Factors to Consider. What acids or bases are lost through diarrhea? Why might a respiratory change have developed if the client's primary problem is gastrointestinal (e.g., metabolic)?

2. **A 19-year-old college student is brought to the emergency department at 4:30 AM by his friends. While studying for final examinations, he grew increasingly anxious during his "cram session," frequently voicing doubts about passing a particularly difficult course. His breathing became increasingly labored, and he seemed dazed and confused. He says his "face feels numb." His pulse is rapid (165 beats per minute) and he is diaphoretic. The client was seen with bleeding duodenal ulcers 2 years ago. ABG analysis of blood samples drawn in the emergency department reveals pH, 7.58; $PaCO_2$, 21 mm Hg; HCO_3^-, 20 mEq/L. What acid-base imbalance does the client have? What caused it? What bedside assessments should you perform and why? What interventions should you consider that might prevent future episodes?**

Factors to Consider. Can rapid breathing alone alter excretion of components needed for acid-base balance?

3. **A 72-year-old retired college professor has a 55-pack-year history of cigarette smoking and advanced emphysema. He had an acute myocardial infarction 5 years ago, from which he recovered uneventfully. He sees his physician in the clinic, complaining of a "cold" that he "just can't get rid of" and "soreness" in his chest. His blood pressure is 165/90 mm Hg, and he has inspiratory crackles in both lung bases. His ankles are**

edematous. **ABG analysis of blood samples drawn during the visit revealed: pH, 7.34; PaCO$_2$, 65 mm Hg; HCO$_3^-$, 34 mEq/L. What acid-base imbalance does he have? What is the probable cause? What additional information would be helpful in planning his care? What variables should you consider in determining priorities of care?**

Factors to Consider. Consider that the client has developed heart failure. When the lungs fill with fluid, what happens to O$_2$/CO$_2$ exchange and, thereby, acid-base balance?

BIBLIOGRAPHY

1. Adrogue, H., & Madias, N. (1998). Management of life-threatening acid-base disorders: Part 1. *New England Journal of Medicine, 338*(1), 26–34.
2. Adrogue, H., & Madias, N. (1998). Management of life-threatening acid-base disorders: Part 2. *New England Journal of Medicine, 338*(2), 107–111.
3. Carpenito, L. (1995). *Nursing diagnosis: Application to clinical practice* (6th ed.). Philadelphia: J. B. Lippincott.
4. Dirks, J. (1995). Innovations in technology: Continuous intra-arterial blood gas monitoring. *Critical Care Nurse, 15*(4), 19–20, 22, 24–27.
5. Gilbert, H., & Vender, J. (1995). Arterial blood gas monitoring. *Critical Care Clinics, 11*(1), 233–248.
6. Grogono, A. (1999). *Fundamentals of acid-base balance* [Online]. Available: *http://gasnet.med.yale.edu/gta/acid-base/AB.html.*
7. Hanna, J., Scheinman, J., & Chan, J. (1995). The kidney in acid-base balance. *Pediatric Clinics of North America, 42*(6), 1365–1395.
8. Hansen, M. (1998). *Pathophysiology: Foundations of disease and clinical intervention.* Philadelphia: W. B. Saunders.
9. Laski, M., & Kurtzman, N. (1996). Acid-base disorders in medicine. *Disease-a-Month, 42*(2), 59–125.
10. Malley, W. J. (1990). *Clinical blood gases: Application and noninvasive alternatives.* Philadelphia: W. B. Saunders.
11. Palange, P., Carlone, S., Galassetti, P., et al. (1990). Incidence of acid-base and electrolyte disturbances in a general hospital: A study of 110 consecutive admissions. *Recenti Progressi in Medicina (Roma), 81*(12), 788–791.
12. Preusser, B., Lash, J., Stone, K., et al. (1989). Quantifying the minimum discard sample required for accurate blood gases. *Nursing Research, 38*(5), 276–279.
13. Rutecki, G., & Whittier, F. (1997). Acid-base interpretation: Part 1: Applying five rules in everyday cases. *Consultant, 37*(12), 3067–3070, 3073.
14. Rutecki, G., & Whittier, F. (1998). Acid-base interpretation: Part 2: Applying five rules to simplify complex cases. *Consultant, 38*(1), 131–133, 137–138, 141–142.
15. Rutecki, G., & Whittier, F. (1998). An approach to clinical acid-base problem-solving. *Comprehensive Therapy, 24*(11/12), 553–559.
16. Williams, A. J. (1998). ABC of oxygen: Assessing and interpreting arterial blood gases and acid-base balance. *British Medical Journal, 317*(7167), 1213–1216.
17. Williamson, J. C. (1995). Acid-base disorders: Classification and management strategies. *American Family Physician, 52*(2), 584–590.

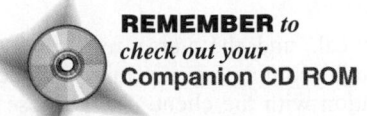

CHAPTER 15

Clients Having Surgery: Promoting Positive Outcomes

Nancy Girard

NURSING OUTCOMES CLASSIFICATION (NOC) for Nursing Diagnoses–Clients Having Surgery

Altered Thought Processes
Cognitive Ability
Cognitive Orientation
Concentration
Decision-Making
Distorted Thought Control
Identity
Information Processing
Neurologic Status: Consciousness
Anxiety
Anxiety Control
Coping
Hypothermia
Thermoregulation
Neurologic Status
Vital Signs Status
Knowledge Deficit

Concentration
Knowledge: Diet
Knowledge: Disease Process
Knowledge: Health Resources
Knowledge: Illness Care
Knowledge: Medication
Knowledge: Prescribed Activity
Knowledge: Treatment Procedure
Knowledge: Treatment Regimen
Information Processing
Pain
Comfort Lever
Pain Control
Pain: Disruptive Effects
Pain Level
Risk for Aspiration
Cognitive Ability

Endurance
Immobility Consequences: Physiologic
Infection Status
Knowledge: Treatment (Procedures)
Neurologic Status
Respiratory Status: Gas Exchange
Respiratory Status: Ventilation
Risk Control
Risk for Injury
Neurologic Status
Risk Control
Safety Behavior: Fall Prevention
Safety Behavior: Home Physical
    Environment
Safety Status: Physical Injury
Symptom Control

Having surgery is a major event in any person's life. Clients faced with surgery want to know that someone is there with them and will look out for them during a time when they may have no control or any self-protective abilities. The perioperative nurse is the member of the surgical team clients are most likely to look to for advocacy.

PERIOPERATIVE NURSING

The total surgical episode is called the *perioperative period*. This period in the health care continuum includes the time prior to surgery, or preoperative period; the time spent during the actual surgical procedure, or intraoperative period; and the period after the surgery is completed, or postoperative period. In the broadest definition of perioperative nursing practice, care can range from home, through surgery and recovery, and back to home again. A *perioperative nurse* is a Registered Nurse who uses the nursing process to design, plan, and deliver care to meet the identified needs of a client whose protective reflexes

or self-care abilities are potentially compromised because of the operative procedures to be performed. Surgery is performed in a multitude of settings, and the nurse's role as a surgical team member is partially defined by the practice setting. Thus, perioperative nursing is client-centered rather than task-oriented. The perioperative nurse must possess and apply knowledge of anatomy, physiology, psychology, and sociocultural and spiritual beliefs and practices, in addition to knowledge of all aspects of the surgical procedure to be performed. The perioperative nurse must be a good communicator, delegator, and supervisor to ensure that the needs of the patient are being met throughout the surgical experience.

BASIC CONCEPTS OF PERIOPERATIVE NURSING

Nursing care of the perioperative patient takes place before, during, and after a surgical procedure. In each of these periods, specific assessments and interventions are performed by nurses acting both as independent clinicians and as members of the health care team. The goals of perioperative nursing practice are to assist clients and their significant others through the surgical episode, to help promote positive outcomes, and to help clients achieve their optimal level of function and wellness after surgery. The management of clients' needs, both unique and predictable, may be through direct or indirect interventions. These interventions are planned to assist the client in meeting the projected outcomes in an efficient and appropriate manner. Perioperative nursing care is implemented by registered nurses who strive to assist the client by functioning in various roles.

PREOPERATIVE PERIOD

Each client responds differently to surgery. Therefore, for each client having surgery, a care plan based on the nursing process is developed. It is vital to identify potential risks and complications that may arise during the perioperative period. In addition, a care plan also identifies the need for supportive services at home or in the hospital after surgery.

■ PREOPERATIVE ASSESSMENT

Assessment is the first step in the nursing process and is designed to provide information that enables the nurse and the client to plan for optimal postoperative outcomes. A complete assessment must be done before surgery whenever possible. Generally, preoperative assessment can take place in many different places, including the physician's office before admission to a health care facility; at home during the days before the operation and on admission; the night before surgery if the client is in the hospital; and on admission on the day of surgery. In the case of emergency surgery, time may not permit complete preoperative assessment, care planning, and teaching. Nevertheless, preparation must be as thorough as possible.

Preoperative assessment includes the medical/health history, the psychosocial history, physical examination, cognitive assessment, and diagnostic testing. When surgery must be performed following a traumatic event (e.g., gunshot wound, stab wound, serious accident, or severe fall), a preoperative assessment must include details of the traumatic event described precisely as possible. If the client was injured in a fall or a motor vehicle accident, information on injury-related factors such as the position in which the injury occurred, or whether the accident appeared to cause the victim to lose consciousness, may help to assess surgical risk or to identify underlying conditions related to the injurious event. Trauma patients are usually admitted to the operating room from an emergency department. Emergency department staff provide a detailed report upon transfer.

MEDICAL/HEALTH HISTORY

Obtaining a health history allows clients to explain their understanding of impending surgery and to establish rapport with the nurse conducting the interview. Reassurance by the nurse through this process may reduce anxiety in the client and family members or significant others. In most instances, the past medical history (PMH) has been previously recorded and is found in the medical record. A complete PMH is critical, and the nurse reviews it to ensure that it is thorough, completing any missing pieces and validating information with the client. The purpose of reviewing the medical history is to determine operative risk.

The past-medical history should include, but is not limited to, the following.

PREVIOUS SURGERY AND EXPERIENCE WITH ANESTHESIA. Any untoward reactions to anesthesia (e.g., high fever, intraoperative death of family members, known malignant hyperthermia, prolonged nausea and vomiting) by the client or anyone in the family must be reported to anesthesia personnel. These problems do not preclude surgery but often require a change in the type of anesthetics used.

SERIOUS ILLNESS OR TRAUMA. This information should cover anything that might influence the surgery and recovery. An ABCDE mnemonic is often used to ascertain information:

- *A*—allergy to medications, chemicals, and other environmental products such as latex. All allergies are reported to anesthesia and surgical personnel before the beginning of surgery. If allergies exist, an allergy band must be placed on the client's arm immediately.
- *B*—bleeding tendencies or the use of medications that deter clotting, such as aspirin or products containing aspirin, heparin, or warfarin sodium. Herbal medications may also increase bleeding times or mask potential blood-related problems.
- *C*—cortisone or steroid use.
- *D*—diabetes mellitus, a condition that not only requires strict control of blood glucose levels but is also known to delay wound healing.
- *E*—emboli; previous embolic events (such as lower leg blood clots) may recur because of prolonged immobility.

Clients whose immune system is suppressed are at a much higher risk for development of a postoperative infection and have a diminished capacity to fight that infection.

ALCOHOL, RECREATIONAL DRUG OR NICOTINE USE. The use of drugs signals potential problem with the administration of anesthesia or analgesia and risk for withdrawal complications. Clients who use alcohol or drugs may experience withdrawal manifestations while the drugs are withdrawn during the postoperative course. In addition, clients addicted to alcohol often have malnutrition or unpredictable reactions to anesthetic agents. As little as two drinks per day can lead to withdrawal manifestations that may require dosage alterations in anesthesia and analgesia.

The abuse of tobacco or inhaled drugs reduces hemoglobin levels, so that less oxygen is available for tissue repair. Smokers may be more susceptible to thrombus (clot) formation because of the hypercoagulability secondary to nicotine use. Smokers are also much more likely to have damage to lung tissue. Clients are instructed to abstain from any nicotine product for at least 1 week prior to surgery. Nicotine is a potent vasoconstrictor, and the flow of blood to surgical sites is an important aspect of healing. The use of nicotine patches and nicotine gum is also inappropriate preoperatively because the body continues to receive nicotine into the bloodstream.

CURRENT DISCOMFORTS. Clients with pre-existing painful conditions may require alternate methods of pain relief while they are receiving nothing by mouth (NPO). Clients who drink a considerable amount of caffeinated beverages such as coffee often develop headaches related to their NPO status, when their caffeine intake ceases abruptly. Without appropriate preoperative assessment, the headache may be misinterpreted as a surgical problem.

CHRONIC ILLNESSES. Arthritis of the neck or back is considered in positioning the client during surgery or in extending the neck during intubation.

ADVANCED AGE. Older clients have specific perioperative needs that should be identified preoperatively and considered in developing and maintaining a plan of care.

MEDICATION HISTORY. Many clients take prescription and over-the-counter (OTC) drugs that may increase operative risks (Table 15–1). Ask if the client is taking any medications and if these have been brought to the hospital. Dosage and administration schedules for all medications should be noted on the chart.

PSYCHOLOGICAL HISTORY

Knowledge of cultural beliefs and practices is a very important component of holistic nursing care. Some cultures practice traditional health care as well as alternative

TABLE 15–1	MEDICATIONS WITH POSSIBLE EFFECTS ON THE SURGICAL CLIENT
Medication	**Possible Effects**
Antibiotics Gentamicin Penicillins	Produces mild respiratory depression; may mask infection and affect metabolism of muscle relaxants
Antiarrhythmic Agents Propranolol HCl Quinidine gluconate Procainamide HCl	Affects tolerance of anesthesia; interacts with epinephrine used in local anesthesia Depresses cardiac function Potentiates anesthetic agents that are neuromuscular blockers
Antihypertensive Agents Methyldopa Captopril	May alter response to muscle relaxants and narcotics May cause intraoperative or postoperative hypotensive crisis
Corticosteroids Dexamethasone Hydrocortisone sodium succinate Prednisone	Delays wound healing Masks infection Increases risk of hemorrhage Increases serum glucose Decreases stress response (replacement needed during surgery)
Anticoagulants Heparin sodium Warfarin sodium Aspirin NSAIDs	Increases risk of hemorrhage intraoperatively and postoperatively because of clotting abnormalities
Glaucoma Medications Pilocarpine hydrochloride	May cause respiratory or cardiovascular collapse during surgery
Antidiabetic Agents Chlorpropamide, glipizide, glyburide, insulin	Insulin needs decrease when client receives nothing by mouth; insulin levels may fluctuate because of physiologic stress Dosage alterations required, with close monitoring of blood glucose
Tricyclic Antidepressants Amitriptyline, amoxapine, doxepin	Lowers blood pressure, thus increasing the risk of shock Potentiates the effects of narcotics and barbiturates
Thiazide Diuretics Hydrochlorothiazide, Furosemide	Increased risk for dysrhythmias Can deplete potassium and cause electrolyte imbalances
Beta-adrenergic Blockers Atenolol, propranolol	Antidysrhythmics and antihypertensives, which can cause adverse effects when combined with anesthetic agents
Street Drugs Beer, whiskey, cocaine, heroin	Alcohol and narcotic abuse increase tolerance to narcotics, requiring more anesthesia and analgesia, potential for delirium tremens during surgery or immediately postoperatively; may precipitate a medical crisis

NSAIDs, nonsteroidal anti-inflammatory drugs.

and complementary practices that may include use of candles, rituals, and herbs. Certain rituals are very important to the client and should be respected by all members of the health care team. For example, in some cultures, the family may make decisions regarding health care as a unit. In other cultures, the oldest woman makes all medical decisions. The nurse must be accepting of each individual's beliefs and should play an active advocate role by supporting the client in any manner possible.

ABILITY TO TOLERATE PERIOPERATIVE STRESS

Physiologic stressors in the perioperative client include pain, tissue damage, blood loss, anesthesia, fever, and immobilization. The stressful stimuli imposed by surgery promote the physiologic stress response by combining both psychological factors (such as anxiety and fear of the unknown) and physiologic factors (including blood loss, anesthesia, pain, and immobility). The sympathetic nervous system is activated by any stressor. A person's age, physical condition, and duration of the stress determine the success of the stress response in maintaining homeostatic balance. The ability to tolerate the stress of surgery and anesthesia is decreased significantly in older and debilitated people. All body systems are affected by the stress response; therefore, this assessment is crucial throughout the perioperative experience. The nurse must be able to assess stress and to plan and implement appropriate interventions to effectively reduce or treat complications related to stress.

LIFESTYLE HABITS

Sedentary lifestyles can complicate the surgical course via poor muscle tone, limited cardiac and respiratory reserves, and decreased stress response. On the other hand, an overly active lifestyle may present postoperative compliance problems.

SOCIAL HISTORY

An important component of a social history on a preoperative patient is the support system. Identification of client occupation and physical and mental requirements for job performance also provides important information that may prove useful for care planning.

■ PHYSICAL EXAMINATION

A physical examination is performed on all clients undergoing surgery to identify the present health status and to have baseline information for comparisons during and after surgery. These data are used to determine nursing diagnoses or to identify problems and to develop pertinent outcome goals. Perform a complete physical examination whenever possible. When perioperative time is brief, such as is the case in many trauma cases, you may be required to complete the assessment in minutes. This assessment is of the utmost importance and must be accurate. Report any abnormal findings to the surgical team members immediately, as this information may affect the initiation of the surgery.

Review preoperative laboratory and diagnostic study results, and post them on the client's chart (Table 15–2). Missing laboratory data constitute a common problem in ambulatory surgery settings, especially if the client's tests were ordered days before the scheduled procedure. Missing laboratory reports could lead to cancellation of the surgery.

Examine the part of the body that will be operated on first. Next, complete a general systems assessment. Systems to be assessed include cardiovascular, pulmonary, renal, musculoskeletal, skin, and neurologic. Ask the client whether there are any particularly troublesome manifestations, and include this information in the written assessment for further investigation. Again, document all unusual findings, and communicate them to the surgical team.

The best way to organize a brief assessment in the immediate preoperative period is to develop a personal system for conducting the examination and use it consistently. Although each person will devise a particular method for gathering data, a head-to-toe examination is a common method (see Box 15–1). Assess cognition throughout the examination by noting the client's demeanor and responses to directed questioning. For example, you can assess orientation to time, place, and person in "casual" conversation with the client during the physical assessment. If possible, watch the client walk and move when he or she enters the preparation area. Include this information in the ambulatory status section of the examination.

SPECIFIC BODY SYSTEM ASSESSMENTS

Cardiovascular Assessment

Pathologic cardiac conditions or events that increase operative risk include angina pectoris, the occurrence of a myocardial infarction within the last 6 months, uncontrolled hypertension, heart failure, and peripheral vascular disease. All cardiac conditions can lead to decreased tissue perfusion with impairment of surgical wound healing. In addition to the portion of the cardiovascular assessment completed as part of the head-to-toe assessment, note specific findings that warrant further work-up. Document shortness of breath on minor exertion, hypertension, heart murmurs or S_3 gallops, and chest pain. These manifestations may be present if the client is scheduled for heart or vascular surgery, but they may make the ability to tolerate anesthesia and blood loss questionable. Laboratory studies to measure the function of the cardiovascular system include an electrocardiogram (ECG), especially for those clients over 40 years of age, and determinations of hemoglobin, hematocrit, and serum electrolytes.

Respiratory Assessment

Chronic lung conditions, such as emphysema, asthma, and bronchitis, increase operative risk because these disorders impair gas exchange in the alveoli, predisposing the client to postoperative pulmonary complications. Assessment of pulmonary conditions includes examining for the presence of shortness of breath, wheezing, clubbed fingers, chest pain, cyanosis, and coughing with expectoration of copious or purulent mucus. Question the client carefully about smoking habits. Obtain a complete history of respiratory allergies and infections. If a client demonstrates any respiratory distress at the time of the assessment, notify the surgeon before administration of anesthesia. Abnormal breath sounds may indicate the need for respiratory therapy both before and after surgery. Clients with severe respiratory disease are usually managed preoperatively with aerosol therapy, postural drainage, and antibiotics. Clients who smoke are strongly encouraged to stop smoking as early as possible before surgery. Nicotine patches

TABLE 15–2   COMMON PREOPERATIVE LABORATORY TESTS

Test	Normal Range in Serum	Conditions Often Leading to Abnormal Findings	
		Elevated in	**Decreased in**
Potassium (K⁺)	3.5–5.0 mEq/L or mmol/L	Dehydration Renal failure Acidosis Traumatic crush injury Burns Massive hemolysis of test specimen Addison's disease	NPO status when K⁺ not replaced through IV fluids Excessive use of non–K⁺-sparing diuretics Vomiting Malnutrition Diarrhea Alkalosis Aldosteronism
Sodium (Na⁺)	136–146 mEq/L or mmol/L	Dehydration Edema Cardiac failure Renal failure Excessive infusion of sodium-containing fluids Inadequate thirst Diabetic acidosis	GI fluid loss through NG tube drainage, vomiting, diarrhea Excessive use of laxatives or diuretics Excessive infusion of fluids without sodium SIADH
Chloride (Cl⁻)	98–107 mEq/L or 98–107 mmol/L	Dehydration Excessive infusion of NaCl-containing fluids Mineralocorticoid deficiency Renal failure Respiratory alkalosis	Diabetic acidosis Excessive GI losses through NG drainage, vomiting, diarrhea Excessive use of diuretics
Calcium (Ca²⁺)	8.6–10 mEq/L or 2.15–2.5 mmol/L	Excessive intake of calcium Excessive intake of vitamin D Renal failure Hyperparathyroidism Bone cancer Immobility Steroid use Adrenal insufficiency	Lack of oral intake Lactose intolerance Inadequate intake of vitamin D End-stage renal disease Low serum protein Alkalosis Acute pancreatitis Damage to parathyroid glands
Glucose (fasting)	60–100 mg/dl or mmol/L	Diabetes mellitus Gluconeogenesis with stress response Steroid use Excessive administration of glucose-containing fluids	Diabetes mellitus Excess insulin
Carbon dioxide	23–31 mEq/L or mmol/L*	Chronic airflow diseases (COPD) Intestinal obstruction Vomiting or NG suction Metabolic alkalosis	Hyperventilation Diabetic ketoacidosis Diarrhea Lactic acidosis Renal failure Salicylate toxicity
Creatinine	0.6–1.2 mg/dl or 53–106 μmol/L†	Acute or chronic renal failure End-stage renal disease Renal disease with destruction of large numbers of nephrons Renal insufficiency Shock Rhabdomyolysis	Atrophy of muscle tissue Hyperthyroidism Muscular dystrophy Paralysis
Blood urea nitrogen (BUN)	8–23 mg/dl or mmol/L*	Dehydration Renal failure Renal insufficiency Excessive dietary protein Liver failure	Overhydration Malnutrition
Albumin	3.5–5.0 g/dl	Dehydration Infection and fever	Acute burns Large open wounds Chronic liver disease Protein-calorie malnutrition

Table continued on following page

277

TABLE 15–2	COMMON PREOPERATIVE LABORATORY TESTS *Continued*

| Test | Normal Range in Serum | Conditions Often Leading to Abnormal Findings | |
		Elevated in	*Decreased in*
Prealbumin	18–40 mg/dl	Protein-calorie malnutrition	Dehydration
Hemoglobin	Females: 11.7–16 g/dl Males*: 13.1–17.2 g/dl	Dehydration Polycythemia Chronic pulmonary diseases Heart failure High altitude	Overhydration
Hematocrit	35%–47%†	Dehydration Polycythemia Chronic pulmonary diseases Heart failure	Blood loss Anemia Renal failure with loss of erythropoi- etin
White blood cell count	4500–11,000 cells/μl	Acute infection Acute inflammation Stress Lymphoma Leukemia	Bone marrow dyscrasias Use of immunosuppressant medica- tions Systemic lupus erythematosus

Differential count	Segmented neutrophils 56%	Bacterial infection, especially
		  streptococcal or staphylo-
		  coccal
		Inflammation with tissue necrosis
		Malignancy of bone marrow,
		  especially chronic myeloid
		  leukemia
			Depletion of available pool of neutro-
			phils during severe infection
			
			Bone marrow damage

	Banded neutrophils 3%	Overwhelming infection Early indicator of sepsis	
	Eosinophils 2.7%	Allergy Inflammation of skin Parasitic infection	Bacterial infections
	Basophils 0.3%	Healing phase of wounds Chronic inflammation	Acute infection Hyperthyroidism Stress

	Lymphocytes 34%	Bacterial, viral, or other causes of
		  infection
		Lymphocytic leukemia
			Lymphatic drainage
			Advanced cancers
			Bone marrow disease
			Immune deficiency that decreases T
			  lymphocytes

	Monocytes 4%	Infection (monocytes become mac- rophages) Granulomatous diseases Collagen disease	Bone marrow failure
Prothrombin time (PT)	11–15 sec	Coagulation defect Liver disease Anticoagulant use	Coagulation (clotting) disorder Extensive cancer
Partial thrombo- plastin time, acti- vated (aPTT)	35 sec	Coagulation defect Liver disease Anticoagulant use	Coagulation (clotting) disorder Extensive cancer

* Normal values vary slightly by age.
† Normal values vary slightly by age and gender.
COPD, chronic obstructive pulmonary disease; GI, gastrointestinal; IV, intravenous; NaCl, sodium chloride; NG, nasogastric; NPO, nothing by mouth; SIADH, syndrome of inappropriate antidiuretic hormone.

are usually not an appropriate alternative because of vaso-constriction caused by the nicotine.

Laboratory studies performed before surgery to diagnose respiratory conditions include chest radiography and pulse oximetry. Chest radiography (or x-rays) detect ab-normalities, if present, in the lungs, such as infections, collapsed alveoli or segments of the lung, tumors, fractures of the ribs, and size of the heart.

The pulse oximeter is used to determine gross levels of tissue oxygenation. Explain the operation and purpose

BOX 15–1   Preoperative Head-to-Toe Assessment

- Assess cognition throughout the examination by noting the client's demeanor and responses to directed questioning. For example, you can check the client's orientation to time, place, and person in the course of eliciting information during the physical assessment.
- Assess muscle strength and coordination, gait, and balance by watching the client walk and move while entering the preparation area. (This may not be possible with all clients.)
- Take a full set of vital sign measurements. Note the ease of respiration.
- Look at the client's eyes and nose, and assess the mobility of the neck.
- Listen to the heart and the lungs. Listen to the rate and rhythm of the heart. Note the character of the lung sounds, listening for any diminution of intensity or the absence of breath sounds. Shortness of breath on minor exertion should also be noted. Dyspnea, wheezing, clubbed fingers, chest pain, cyanosis, and coughing with expectoration of copious or purulent mucus should be reported to anesthesia personnel. Question the client carefully about smoking habits and recent illness with a cold or influenza. Obtain a history of respiratory allergies and infections.
- Assess range of motion of the shoulders and the strength of the arms and hand grip.
- Ask about the ability to urinate and if the client has diabetes.
- Assess the ability to flex the spine (this is important if the client is scheduled to have spinal anesthesia).
- Examine the extremities for edema, coldness to the touch, and cyanosis.

- Assess the range of motion and strength of the legs and feet.
- Assess cognition preoperatively to determine whether any postoperative changes are the effects of surgery. This is particularly important in the older adult. The effects of the operation and of associated medications frequently cause temporary cognitive deficits that can be erroneously identified as a permanent condition by the health care team. Temporary deficits in memory and recall are normal and seen in most clients, but these manifestations can persist in the older adult. Note equal movement of the face and shoulders on both sides of the body if a crude estimate of cranial nerve function is needed. Complete neurologic testing includes assessment of cranial nerve function, reflex response of the upper and lower extremities, and sensory reflexes, as well as cognitive assessment. This level of testing is performed before neurologic surgery.
- During the examination, observe the condition of the skin. Note and document lesions, pressure ulcers, necrotic tissue, skin turgor, erythema or other discoloration of the skin, and the presence of external devices. Record the approximate size, color, and location of any lesions for later comparison.
- Review the chart for results of laboratory and diagnostic tests. Commonly ordered for the client undergoing heart surgery include chest x-ray film, electrocardiogram, hemoglobin, hematocrit, serum electrolytes, and urinalysis.
- During the physical examination, pay attention to the client's verbal and nonverbal communication. Does the client complain of any pain unrelated to the impending surgical procedure?

of the oximeter to the client and why it is important to monitor oxygenation throughout the surgical experience. The definitive laboratory test for blood oxygenation is arterial blood gas (ABG) analysis. Although routine ABG analyses are not ordered preoperatively, a physician may order the test if the client has been determined to be at high risk for surgical complications. Additional pulmonary function tests may be ordered in specific situations (see Chapter 59).

Musculoskeletal Assessment

A history of fractures, contractures, joint injury, or musculoskeletal impairment is an important factor in surgical positioning and postoperative support. The physical examination should reveal any problems with joint mobility or deformities that may interfere with operative positioning as well as with the postoperative course. For example, if the preoperative assessment identifies arthritis of the neck and shoulder, the circulating nurse can incorporate this information into the care plan. Hyperextension of the arthritic neck during general anesthesia can cause postoperative pain and discomfort unrelated to the surgery. The musculoskeletal system can be assessed through passive and active range of motion and a history provided by the client or family member, or the medical record. Documentation of impairment before the surgical procedure assists in the investigation of any impairment postoperatively.

Gastrointestinal Assessment

Gastrointestinal conditions associated with poor surgical outcomes include severe malnutrition and prolonged nau-

sea and vomiting. The client's gastrointestinal system should be assessed if the planned operation is in the abdominal area or if the general physical examination reveals any abnormal data. Because narcotic analgesics increase constipation, obtain information about normal bowel patterns, so that postoperative expectations for return of function are appropriate. A client with a long history of constipation may have more difficulty postoperatively than that experienced by the client with regular bowel function.

Skin Integrity Assessment

Skin integrity must be assessed and documented preoperatively to establish a baseline for comparison postoperatively. Document and report lesions, pressure ulcers, necrotic skin tissue, skin turgor, erythema or discoloration of the skin, and the presence of external devices. Note the size, color, and location of the skin impairment to determine whether the impaired skin remains stable or worsens during and after the surgical procedure. Padding and positioning equipment should be used to maintain skin integrity and to prevent pressure ulcers. Any alterations in skin integrity that can occur intraoperatively and are not related to the actual surgical procedure are preventable by the nurse and other members of the surgical team with adequate padding and repositioning as needed during very long procedures.

Renal Assessment

Adequate renal function is necessary to eliminate protein wastes, to preserve fluid and electrolyte balance, and to remove anesthetic agents. Important renal and related disorders include advanced renal insufficiency, acute nephritis, and benign prostatic hypertrophy (BPH). If renal deficiency exists, the surgical team must be made aware of the problem. To assess renal status, ask about voiding patterns such as frequency and dysuria. Also, observe the appearance of urine if a sample is collected or an indwelling catheter is in place. Document and report abnormal urine characteristics. Monitor fluid balance by recording intake and output throughout the surgical continuum.

The most common preoperative tests to assess renal function are determination of blood urea nitrogen (BUN) and serum creatinine and urinalysis. BUN and serum creatinine levels indicate the ability of the kidney to excrete urea and protein wastes. Elevated levels may reflect dehydration, impaired cardiac output, or renal failure. Elevated creatinine is associated with renal disease. Serious renal disease and urinary infections must be treated, if possible, before surgery. Urinalysis results may indicate urinary infection, diabetes, malnutrition, renal disease, or dehydration.

Liver Function Assessment

Liver disease such as cirrhosis increases a client's surgical risk because an impaired liver cannot detoxify medications and anesthetic agents. The client may also be unable to metabolize carbohydrates, fats, and amino acids. Liver disease may be manifested by decreased albumin levels, leading to decreased immunoglobulin and fibrinogen levels. Low albumin levels predispose the client to fluid shifts, surgical wound infection, and ineffective coagulation. Clients with a history of alcoholism or other substance abuse require a careful assessment of liver function before surgery. If evidence of risk factors for liver disease is uncovered during the immediate preoperative assessment, information must be shared immediately with other members of the surgical team. Because a client with liver disease is often malnourished and debilitated and may have clotting disorders, the surgeon generally orders a high-calorie diet, or hyperalimentation during the preoperative and postoperative periods.

Cognitive and Neurologic Assessment

Serious neurologic conditions, such as uncontrolled epilepsy or severe Parkinson's disease, increase surgical risk. Important preoperative neurologic abnormalities include severe headache, frequent dizziness, light-headedness, ringing in the ears, unsteady gait, unequal pupils, and a history of seizures. Assessment of the client's orientation to time, place, and person can be accomplished by simple questioning. To determine baseline neurologic function, include testing of cranial nerves, reflex responses of the upper and lower extremities, sensory reflexes, and cerebral responses (see Chapter 67).

Assess cognition preoperatively to determine postoperative effects of surgery. This is particularly important in an older adult. The effects of the operation and of associated medications frequently lead to temporary cognitive deficiencies that can be erroneously identified as a permanent condition. Temporary deficits in memory and recall are considered normal and are seen in the majority of clients, but the older adult can experience these symptoms for a longer time.

Endocrine Assessment

Diabetes mellitus is the most common pre-existing endocrine pathophysiologic disorder. In some ethnic groups, especially Hispanic populations, diabetes is rampant. Diabetes mellitus predisposes the affected client to poor wound healing and increased risk of surgical wound infection. Corresponding cardiovascular, peripheral vascular, neurologic, visual, and renal complications may be present as well. These factors can greatly increase the surgical risk for a client with diabetes. A client who has well-controlled diabetes (i.e., blood glucose levels are consistently monitored and kept within a normal range) is less susceptible to infection. Chapter 45 describes the care of clients with diabetes mellitus.

Thyroid functioning may also need to be assessed preoperatively. Thyroid hormone replacement is usually continued throughout the perioperative period. Stopping thyroid medications may precipitate a thyroid storm or crisis, with manifestations of hypertension, tachycardia, and hyperthermia. This event can be devastating if it occurs during surgery or immediately postoperatively. In addition, the presence of hypothyroidism increases the risk of hypotension and cardiac arrest during anesthetic administration.

ADDITIONAL ASSESSMENTS

Other factors that may be considered during the planning of surgical intervention include (1) age, (2) nutrition, (3) fluid and electrolyte balance, (4) infection, and (5) hematologic conditions.

Age

Normal physiologic changes that occur with aging, along with the increased presence of disease, may adversely affect surgical outcomes. Chronic conditions commonly found in the older client that may increase surgical risk include malnutrition, anemia, dehydration, atherosclerosis, chronic obstructive pulmonary disease (COPD), diabetes mellitus, cerebrovascular changes, and peripheral vascular disease. Table 15–3 outlines major physiologic changes that occur in older adults and appropriate perioperative nursing interventions.

Pain

Pain is an important physiologic indicator that must be carefully monitored (see Chapter 23). During the preoperative nursing assessment, ask if the client is experiencing any pain. If pain is present, obtain a full assessment of the pain. Determine whether the pain is chronic and unrelated to the pathologic condition necessitating surgery or is acute and attributable to the surgical procedure. Be aware that although most operations increase pain, older adults who have undergone joint replacement surgery often state that the postoperative pain is minor compared with the chronic pain of a disintegrating joint.

Nutritional Status

Nutritional status (positive nitrogen balance) is directly related to intraoperative success and postoperative recovery. The client who is well nourished preoperatively is better prepared to handle surgical stress and to return to optimal health after surgery. Improving nutrition is usually attended to in a clinic or physician's office weeks before surgery. However, if the operation is performed on an emergency basis or has not been planned, nutritional

TABLE 15–3	INTERVENTIONS FOR PHYSIOLOGIC CHANGES IN OLDER ADULTS UNDER-GOING SURGERY

Physiologic Change	Nursing Interventions
Cardiovascular	
Decreased cardiac output	Know what anesthetic agents are being used.
Moderate increase in blood pressure	Monitor vital signs carefully.
Decreased peripheral circulation	Encourage early ambulation and leg exercises.
Dysrhythmias	Assess for hypotension or hypertension or hypothermia.
	Note changes in baseline ECG; note any changes.
Respiratory	
Decreased vital capacity	Assess for pulmonary aspiration.
Reduced oxygenation of blood	Monitor respirations carefully.
	Use vigorous pulmonary hygiene.
	Postoperatively, auscultate lung sounds.
	Monitor oxygen saturation using pulse oximeter.
Renal	
Decreased renal blood flow and glomerular filtration rate	Monitor urine output q 1–2 hr during immediate postoperative period.
Decreased ability to excrete waste products	Evaluate intake and output.
	Monitor fluid and electrolyte status.
Musculoskeletal	
Decrease in lean body mass	Assess level of mobility.
Increase in spinal compression	Position the client on operating table with padding to reduce trauma to bones and joints.
Increased incidence of osteoporosis and arthritis	Assist with early ambulation or exercises in accordance with client's ability.
	Provide adequate nutrition.
	Provide effective pain management.
Sensorimotor	
Decreased reaction time	Orient client to environment.
Decreased visual acuity	Plan individual teaching, allowing time to reinforce client learning.
Decreased auditory acuity	Maintain core body temperature.
Slowed thermoregulation	

status may be a risk factor through the perioperative period. In addition, some operations are completed to improve nutrition. For example, a client who is to undergo placement of a permanent feeding tube would be expected to have evidence of malnutrition. Likewise, a client who is to have an intestinal bypass for obesity is also malnourished (in terms of excess intake).

Assessment of nutritional status preoperatively includes obtaining a diet history, observing the general appearance of the client, laboratory diagnostic testing, and comparing current weight with ideal body weight. Laboratory tests that can assist in the assessment of nutritional status include determinations of serum albumin, hemoglobin and hemotocrit, BUN, and creatinine clearance.

Nutritional abnormalities include deficiencies and excesses. Nutritional deficiencies primarily affect clients with chronic illnesses, cancer, gastrointestinal disorders, and advanced age. Malnutrition is directly linked to delayed healing and infection.

Obesity is also associated with poorer surgical outcomes. Adipose (fatty) tissue increases the technical difficulty of surgery. Fatty tissue is less vascular and more prone to postoperative infection, incisional hernias, and wound dehiscence or evisceration. The surgeon may use an alternative closure method for a client with excess adipose tissue at or around the incision.

Obese clients frequently suffer from hypertension, heart failure, and metabolic problems. An obese client is more susceptible to postoperative pulmonary complications. Obesity decreases the efficiency of coughing and deep breathing. The pressure of the abdominal contents on the diaphragm and lungs decreases expansion, which may lead to hypoventilation. An obese client is more prone to postoperative immobility. Immobility increases the risk of venous stasis and deep vein thrombosis or pulmonary embolism. Good preoperative teaching that describes turning, coughing, deep-breathing, and moving after surgery is essential. Most complications related to obesity can be prevented, or the risk of their occurrence reduced, with appropriate interventions.

Fluid and Electrolyte Balance

Fluid volume deficits (dehydration/hypovolemia or fluid volume excess/hypervolemia) predispose a client to complications during and after surgery. Actual or potential fluid imbalance can be assessed by evaluation of skin turgor. A coated tongue can also be a manifestation of fluid volume deficit. A decrease in urine output or an increase in specific gravity is also diagnostic of decreased fluid volume. If dehydration is severe, irritability or confusion can be apparent. Dehydration results from limited fluid intake, prolonged vomiting, diarrhea, or bleeding. Fluids can be administered by the IV route if dehydration is identified.

Electrolyte imbalances also increase operative risk. Preoperative laboratory results should be checked to see whether serum sodium, potassium, calcium, and magnesium concentrations are within the normal range. In-depth assessment and management of fluid and electrolyte imbalances are discussed in Chapters 12 and 13, respectively.

Infection and Immunity

Any pre-existing infection can adversely affect surgical outcomes because bacteria may be released into the bloodstream during surgery. Their release may lead to infection elsewhere in the body. When the surgical site is near a lymph node or lymphatic vessel that is draining infectious material, the likelihood of surgical infection increases. During the preoperative assessment, documentation of any possible exposure to communicable diseases, presence of skin lesions, or manifestations of an infection (such as coughing, sore throat, or elevated body temperature) is vital. An elevated white blood cell (WBC) count also suggests an infection and should be communicated immediately to the surgical team. Because infection greatly increases surgical risk, it may be necessary to reschedule elective surgery.

A low WBC count is also a danger sign and may indicate that the client is at risk for infection. A low WBC count may be a manifestation of immunosuppression. People with diabetes mellitus, those who are undergoing radiation therapy or chemotherapy, and those with chronic medical conditions are at high risk of immunosuppression. Steroid use also decreases the client's ability to fight infection; therefore, the client taking steroids should be assessed and monitored for immunosuppression.

Hematologic Function

Clients with blood coagulation disorders are at risk for hemorrhage and hypovolemic shock during and after surgery. Five factors that should be assessed preoperatively to identify potential hematologic problems are:

- A history of bleeding or a diagnosis of a pathologic condition such as hemophilia or sickle cell anemia
- Manifestations such as easy bruising, excessive bleeding following dental extractions and razor nicks, and severe nosebleeds
- Hepatic or renal disease
- Use of anticoagulants, aspirin, or other nonsteroidal anti-inflammatory drugs (NSAIDs)
- Abnormal bleeding time, prothrombin time, or platelet count.

Remember that many clients take aspirin and other OTC medications that may increase the risk of bleeding. The client may not consider nonprescription medications important and often may not include them in a medication history. Ask specific questions regarding all prescription and nonprescription medications. Specifically ask about the use of herbal preparations. Ginkgo biloba, garlic, ginger, and ginseng may prevent blood clot formation and may lead to excess blood loss in surgery. Two other popular herbs—St. John's wort, an antidepressant, and kava-kava, a relaxant—may prolong the sedative effect of anesthesia. Advise clients to stop taking herbal products at least 2 weeks before elective surgery. Ask how often the client takes the OTC medications and when the last dose of any of those drugs was taken.

For a variety of reasons, blood transfusions are used less frequently than in past years. Many clients fear the transmission of human immunodeficiency virus (HIV) and hepatitis B. If possible, clients are encouraged to donate their own blood for use during or after surgery (autologous transfusion). Blood substitutes or fluid volume expanders can also be used in some cases to replace lost blood until the body can produce new blood cells. Blood transfusions are discussed in Chapter 75.

■ EDUCATIONAL ASSESSMENT

The client's experience with previous surgery and level of anxiety are noted. The client's education level, sensory impairments (e.g., loss of vision), expectations regarding the operation, and availability of support systems are used to guide plans for teaching. In general, clients who have undergone multiple operations need less educational preparation. However, do not assume that such clients need no reinforcement of preoperative and postoperative assessments and interventions.

The client undergoing elective surgery and planning to go home the same day requires some additional planning. See the Case Management feature.

PREOPERATIVE NURSING DIAGNOSES

Common nursing diagnoses during the preoperative period include *Knowledge Deficit related to unfamiliar surgical experience* and *Anxiety related to fear of pain, fear of death, fear of disfigurement,* or *fear of the unknown.* The outcomes for these problems must be achievable in a short preoperative time frame.

ESTIMATING MEDICAL RISK FOR SURGERY

Each surgeon determines the relative risk versus benefit from the operation for the specific client. In addition, the outcomes for many surgical procedures have been researched, and these figures can be presented to the client and family. The natural history of the condition requiring surgery (that is, the outcome if it goes untreated) is also presented. This information can then be considered by the client and family members before consenting to surgery. The surgeon presents a frank but optimistic discussion of risks of the procedure. Well-intentioned friends and family may wish to shield the client from unpleasant facts. Although medical facts may be unpleasant, it is imperative that the client have full and complete information before consenting. Some clients (such as those with malnutrition or anemia) benefit from waiting for surgery.

The type of surgery to be performed also has some inherent risk. The types of operations by category are presented in Table 15–4.

ANESTHESIA AND ANESTHETIC RISK

The anesthesia care provider visits the client before surgery to perform a complete respiratory, cardiovascular, and neurologic examination. The client's general surgical risk (the ability of the client to withstand the surgery) is expressed according to the American Society of Anesthesia (ASA) grading system (see Box 15–2). Generally, the topics discussed with the client during this examination include the type of anesthesia planned and the sensations the client may experience when undergoing anesthesia. Fears the client has concerning anesthesia are also addressed. The client's risk of side effects and complications is assessed at this time.

The pharmacologic preparation for anesthesia is based on many variables, including the client's age and physical and psychological condition, the type of surgery, and the type of anesthesia to be used. The preoperative and anesthetic medications are discussed later in the chapter.

IMMEDIATE PREOPERATIVE CARE

■ PHYSICAL CARE

PREPARE THE SKIN

Explain shower and bathing protocols for the night before a planned surgical procedure. Usually the operative area is cleaned the night before surgery with soap and water to reduce the number of microbes on the skin. Allergies to chemicals (e.g., iodine) necessitate use of other cleansing agents. If the skin assessment has identified fragile and delicate skin in an older client, nursing care must involve a gentle method for cleansing skin and hair and for any needed hair removal. Additional considerations may include use of padding over pressure points and tape that will not irritate or rip the skin, as well as lifting—rather than pulling or sliding—the client from bed to bed, to prevent traumatizing the skin.

CASE MANAGEMENT

The Elective Surgery Client

The elective surgical client presents some unique opportunities. Unlike a client arriving from the emergency department, the client undergoing elective surgery has already agreed to an operation and has had some preoperative assessment and preparation; this client will know what to expect in the perioperative period. This preparation serves as an excellent basis for case management. Case management practices become increasingly important as more procedures are being performed in ambulatory surgery settings or even in offices rather than inpatient areas. Almost all clients present the day of surgery, having undergone outpatient testing and preparation. The length of surgical stays is decreasing, especially as more laparoscopic procedures are developed. The emphasis on one-day surgery and on decreasing inpatient stays requires astute nursing assessment and intervention to prevent surgical complications and readmission.

Assess

Ideally, assessment should be initiated when the client is an outpatient. What do the client and family know about the surgical procedure, the consequences of surgery, and postoperative care needs? What other conditions might affect the client's ability to successfully undergo surgery? For instance, a client with chronic obstructive pulmonary disease having a cholecystectomy may have difficulty performing deep-breathing exercises; a client with diabetes may need to modify the insulin dose. Overlooking these situations can result in unwanted complications and increased length of stay.

How long does the client expect to be hospitalized? What plans are in place for postsurgical care? If short-term rehabilitation is planned, clients can tour facilities and can be helped to make arrangements for care even before the procedure. What is the purpose of surgery—curative, cosmetic, palliative?

Advocate

This is an ideal time to answer questions and to make sure that clients have a health care proxy and advance directives noted on their chart. If a different living situation is planned or required because of the surgery, discuss this situation with the client and family. Even if such planning is temporary, this can be viewed negatively. Be sensitive to the client's feelings about surgery as it relates to body image, especially if it may cause disfigurement or result in changes in normal body function. Many support groups are available for referral.

Prevent Readmission

Helping the client to return to optimal function in activities of daily living is an important outcome. Although simple nursing interventions such as getting the client out of bed, ambulating, and watching for return of bowel function are often dismissed as unimportant, these interventions can help clients return home safely in a shorter time. Consider hospital discharge when (1) the complete blood count and electrolyte levels are within normal range, (2) the client can be hydrated and fed, (3) voiding has occurred, and bowel function returns, and (4) mobility and ambulation are at baseline or improved levels. Especially in short-stay surgical procedures, and with older clients, watch for physical or mental effects of anesthesia. Make sure that clients and families (1) know how to perform wound care or other treatments, (2) recognize manifestations of infection or other complications, and (3) receive clear directions for follow-up.

Help clients to obtain pain medication. Referrals for nursing care, outpatient phlebotomy, physical therapy, or other home services can ensure continued improvement after surgery.

Cheryl Noetscher, RN, MS, *Director of Case Management, Crouse Hospital and Community–General Hospital, Syracuse, New York*

PREPARE THE GASTROINTESTINAL TRACT

The gastrointestinal tract needs special preparation on the evening before surgery to (1) reduce the possibility of vomiting and aspiration, (2) to reduce the risk of possible bowel obstruction, (3) to allow visualization of the intestine during bowel surgery, and (4) to prevent contamination from fecal material in the intestinal tract during bowel or abdominal surgery. Preparation involves restrict-

TABLE 15–4	CATEGORIES OF SURGICAL PROCEDURES	
Category	**Purpose**	**Example**
Aesthetic	Improvement of physical features that are within the "normal" range	Breast augmentation
Constructive	Repair of a congenitally defective body part	Cleft palate and cleft lip repair
Curative	Removal or repair of damaged or diseased tissue or organs	Hysterectomy
Diagnostic	Discovery or confirmation of a diagnosis	Breast biopsy
Exploratory	Estimation of the extent of disease or confirmation of a diagnosis	Exploratory laparotomy
Emergent	Life-saving	Repair of traumatic punctured lung
Palliative	Relief of symptoms but without cure of underlying disease	Colostomy
Reconstructive	Partial or complete restoration of a body part	Total joint replacement
Urgent	Performed as soon as client is stable and infection is under control	Appendectomy

ing food and fluid, administering enemas as needed, and inserting a gastric or intestinal tube when appropriate. Gastrointestinal tubes are usually inserted during surgery for drainage. This procedure is usually performed for clients undergoing major abdominal or intestinal tract surgery.

If a client undergoing surgery is to receive a general anesthetic, foods and fluids are restricted for 8 to 10 hours before the operation. This restriction significantly reduces the possibility of aspiration of gastric contents, which may lead to pneumonia. Because solid food must be withheld for 8 to 10 hours before surgery, clients who are to undergo anesthetic procedures must be instructed not to eat or drink anything after midnight. Therefore, clients are assigned NPO status after midnight the night before surgery is scheduled. If a client scheduled for surgery has eaten or had something to drink after midnight, the surgery may be delayed or postponed. Preoperative care for hospitalized clients also includes the restriction of food and water if anesthesia is to be used.

When a client is on NPO status, perform the following:

- Explain the reason for the fluid and food restriction.
- Remove food and water from the bedside at midnight.
- Place "NPO" signs on the door and on the bed.
- Mark the care plan or Kardex with "NPO."
- Inform the diet and nutrition department about the client's NPO status.
- Inform other caretakers and family members that the client is on NPO status.

If the client has been instructed to take important medications orally, small sips of water are permitted. For example, a client with cardiovascular disease may need to take heart medications such as digoxin on the morning of surgery. However, the client may have heard preoperative instructions not to eat or drink anything. Make sure that the medication is taken with a sip of water and inform the client that this exception is permissible. Record this medication and the amount of fluid taken on the client care record.

Enemas are not routinely ordered during the preoperative period except for surgical procedures involving the gastrointestinal tract, perianal or perineal areas, and the pelvic cavity. The client may perform the enema at home, or the nurse may complete it at the hospital. Some clients may require further bowel cleansing on the morning of surgery. Clients who are to be admitted for same-day surgery are instructed before the surgical date about the need for enemas and whether they will be self-administered. If bowel cleansing is done by the client, ensure that directions are completely understood.

■ NUTRITIONAL CARE

Nursing interventions for clients who are malnourished preoperatively include encouragement of high carbohydrate intake to increase energy, high protein intake to assist in wound healing, and supplementing the diet with vitamins to encourage healing. Vitamin C is beneficial in wound healing, whereas vitamin K will increase blood clotting times. Total parenteral nutrition (TPN) can be used preoperatively to bolster the client's nutritional status.

TPN solutions that contain lipids (fats) supply total nutritional replacement including vitamin and mineral supplements. Tube feeding (enteral nutrition) can be administered via a tube placed in the stomach or small intestine. The tube is placed through the nose or directly into the stomach through a skin incision. Both enteral and parenteral feeding can improve a client's nutritional status; either may be continued postoperatively until satisfactory swallowing or gastrointestinal functioning returns (see Chapter 29).

Treatment of obesity before surgery calls for a reducing diet, mild exercise if possible, and assessing for and controlling conditions such as hypertension and diabetes mellitus. Obese clients are not placed on a weight-reduction diet after surgery while they are healing. Wound healing is delayed when protein intake is inadequate.

■ PREOPERATIVE TEACHING

Preoperative teaching is very important to ensure a positive surgical experience for the client. Numerous research studies have supported the value of preoperative instructions in reducing both the incidence of postoperative complications and the length of stay in the hospital. The client's learning needs, level of anxiety, and fears about surgery are assessed individually so that an individualized teaching plan can be formulated.

The timing of preoperative teaching is highly individualized. Ideally, there would be enough time for the client to be given instructions and time to answer questions. If teaching is done too far in advance, the client may forget important components of the education. On the other hand, a client who is taught immediately before surgery may be too anxious to comprehend what is being taught. In many cases, the client is admitted on the day of surgery. It is imperative that the client has received written or oral instructions before this time, so that the nurse can simply reinforce these instructions and answer individual questions from the client and family members. Many ambulatory surgery or "same-day surgery" centers conduct telephone interviews before admission to educate and allow the client to ask questions.

Being aware of the effects of surgery on cognition, determine learning needs preoperatively and teach both client and family before surgery if at all possible. Only essential activities should be taught in the immediate preoperative period because of the client's total concentration on surviving the surgery. Assess the client's ability to see, hear, and understand verbal communication. Glasses and hearing aids can be worn up until the actual surgical procedure to promote learning of necessary information and to reduce apprehension and fear. As the client moves into surgery, these important items must be carefully stored or given to an accompanying adult. Add careful documentation of the location of items, such as hearing aids and glasses, to the client record to ensure retrieval after surgery. If any items are lost, the institution is responsible for replacing them.

The client should understand what the preoperative, intraoperative, and postoperative course entails. Consult with the physician before speaking to the client about specific or technical details so that you can clarify if needed. Explain all nursing care and any possible discomfort that may result as a consequence of nursing interventions. Tell the client what you will do to minimize any discomfort. If the client is scheduled to go to the surgical intensive care unit (SICU) after the operation, ask what the client and family members already know or have heard about intensive care. Take time to address any misconceptions or incorrect information.

PREOPERATIVE ANXIETY

All people are fearful of surgery. The extent to which a client fears surgery depends on many factors, such as (1) how serious the operation is, (2) individual coping abilities, (3) cultural expectations, and (4) experiences with previous surgery. Well-meaning family members and friends often contribute to the fear level unintentionally. Fear of the unknown is one of the most prevalent causes of preoperative anxiety. During the preoperative phase, clients also fear postoperative pain, the discovery of cancer, the loss of an organ or limb, anesthesia, vulnerability while unconscious, the threat of loss of job or financial security, loss of social and familial roles, disruption of lifestyle, separation from significant others, and death.

Clients respond differently to fear. Some respond by becoming silent and withdrawn, childish, belligerent, evasive, tearful, or clinging. Most clients feel helpless to some extent when admitted to a health care facility. Although surgery may be commonplace for the health care professional, it is a frightening experience for clients and their families. Report extreme anxiety and fear to the anesthesia personnel so that a sedative can be administered. A surgical procedure can be canceled if fear is overwhelming.

Allow the client to take the lead in asking questions concerning surgery and the postoperative period. Provide only as much additional information as the client wants to know. Emphasize that a nurse will be with the client throughout the total surgical experience. Stand close to the client when taking him or her into the operating room. If touch is culturally appropriate, use touch to reassure the client.

If the surgical procedure to be performed has potential long-term effects, support groups may be contacted to offer support preoperatively. Cancer organizations, amputation support groups, and enterostomal therapist associations are examples of large national organizations that offer peer support for surgical and nonsurgical patients.

■ COMPONENTS OF PREOPERATIVE TEACHING

Information provided to the client before surgery should be geared to individual needs. This information can be (1) sensory, (2) psychosocial, or (3) procedural.

Sensory information addresses the sights, sounds, and "feel" of the operating room. Instruct the client that the operating room and skin preparation fluids will be cold but that warm blankets are available. Many surgery suites are now incorporating music into their preoperative and intraoperative areas. Clients may be given headphones and can choose from a variety of music types to help them relax and to reduce external noxious sounds in the operating room environment. If the client wears a hearing aid and music is used, check with the anesthesia personnel to determine whether the hearing aid can remain in place during surgery.

Psychosocial information involves coping abilities and worries about family and similar concerns. Typical questions the client may have are the following: "What if I die?" "Who is going to care for the children?" "What if I become an invalid?" "Who is going to earn enough money to care for my family?" You can provide answers if this information is available, or you can arrange for others, such as a social worker or a member of the clergy, to talk to the client.

Procedural information details activities during the preoperative period and postoperative care. It includes information that the client needs to know and wants to know about what is going to happen. For example, you can state as appropriate: "Your family can be in the presurgical area before you are taken into the operating room," or "There will always be a nurse with you during this time, and I will remain by your side throughout the entire operation." Provide explanations and printed information about the health care facility routines, visiting hours, mealtimes, the location of the chapel and waiting room, and so on. If you find that the client is unclear about what the operation entails, the physician must be notified (see Informed Consent, p. 287). You can elaborate on or clarify information regarding surgery.

The client's role in postoperative care is taught before surgery. The nurse provides instructions on (1) deep breathing, (2) coughing, (3) turning, (4) ambulating, and (5) pain control, and the client's learning of some of these procedures is validated by return demonstration.

DEEP-BREATHING EXERCISES. To help prevent postoperative surgical complications, careful preoperative instructions and practice in deep-breathing and coughing exercises should be completed and reinforced.

Breathing and coughing exercises help to expand collapsed alveoli in the lungs and to prevent postoperative pneumonia and atelectasis. Demonstration of correct deep breathing can be done by inhaling slowly through the nose, distending the abdomen, and exhaling slowly through pursed lips. After demonstrating this method, ask the client to provide a return demonstration to ensure understanding (Fig. 15–1). The client is instructed to use this breathing method as often as possible, preferably 5 to 10 times every hour during the postoperative period of immobilization.

COUGHING EXERCISES. Coughing removes retained secretions from the bronchi and larger airways. Coughing may be painful, and analgesia may be required.

For coughing exercise, the client may remain in a sitting or supine position. Teach the client how to splint the surgical incision, to minimize pressure, and to control pain during coughing. Splinting is accomplished by lacing the fingers and holding them tightly across the incision before coughing. A small pillow or folded towel held over the incision also facilitates splinting. The client is instructed to take three deep breaths, exhaling through the mouth, before coughing from deep in the lungs. Encouragement to perform deep-breathing exercises before coughing is important because the deep breathing assists in stimulating the cough reflex and mobilizing retained secretions. Many clients simply clear their throats when coughing hurts. Encourage true coughing, and use aggressive measures to control pain, with reteaching of the procedure as intended.

Incentive spirometers are often used to promote expansion of the alveoli postoperatively by guiding the client to reach a predetermined level of lung inflation. Use of a spirometer promotes alveolar inflation and strengthens respiratory muscles that were weakened during anesthesia administration. Clients should have the opportunity to practice use of the incentive spirometer before surgery so that they can use it appropriately after surgery. Most facilities teach clients to use the incentive spirometer about 10 times an hour after surgery.

TURNING EXERCISES. Preoperative clients also need to practice turning from side to side, using the bedside rails to assist movements. Turning helps to prevent venous stasis, thrombophlebitis, pressure ulcer formation, and respiratory complications. The client should be instructed to turn and reposition in bed every 1 to 2 hours during the postoperative period.

EXTREMITY EXERCISE. Postoperative extremity exercise helps to prevent circulatory problems, such as thrombophlebitis, by facilitating venous return to the heart. The client is taught to flex and extend each joint, particularly the hip, knee, and ankle joints, while lying supine; the lower back is kept flat as the leg is lowered and straightened. The feet can be moved in circular motions while the client is lying down or sitting. The client should be encouraged to practice these exercises before surgery to gain familiarity with the appropriate exercises to be used postoperatively.

Antiembolism stockings may be used on the lower extremities perioperatively. These stockings use a low compression gradient to encourage venous blood flow. Sequential pressure stockings use compression that is applied sequentially up and down the lower extremities to massage the legs rhythmically, for even more effective prevention of clot formation.

AMBULATION. Ambulation should be encouraged whenever appropriate, as it helps to prevent many postoperative complications. Clients are taught an appropriate ambulation schedule preoperatively so that they have an idea of when they are allowed to get out of bed after surgery. Teaching of proper methods of arising from bed to prevent pain and to minimize orthostatic hypotension is important. The client is instructed to sit up slowly and pause before attempting to stand. Teach the client to use the same splinting method for providing support to the incision that is used during coughing and deep-breathing exercises in order to decrease pain on arising and sitting.

PAIN CONTROL. Uncontrolled pain is a common concern among preoperative clients. It is important to reassure clients that their pain will and can be controlled after surgery. Undertreatment of postoperative pain is unacceptable (see Chapter 23). Fears of addiction are unfounded, and clients have suffered needlessly. Preoperatively, explain the type of pain relief that will be used postoperatively. For example, some surgeons inject the surgical site with a long-acting local anesthetic before closing the wound so that the client will not feel any pain in the site until the medication wears off. The ambulatory surgery client probably will be home when the local anesthetic wears off. Because the stress of surgery or side effects of anesthesia can affect memory temporarily, give instructions on taking the postoperative pain medication before surgery to both the client and accompanying family members.

If the client is to be hospitalized after surgery, explain the type of pain medication used. During the immediate postoperative period, clients can receive medications by an IV, intramuscular, or epidural route. Clients on a demand schedule (intramuscular) ask for pain medications when they are beginning to feel uncomfortable. Clients

1. Have the client sit upright at the side of the bed or supported in bed in semi-Fowler's position (at right).

2. Instruct the client to place his or her hands on the abdomen to feel whether the chest rises to indicate that the lungs are expanding.

3. Have the client inhale through the nose until the abdomen distends.

4. Instruct the client to exhale through pursed lips while contracting the abdominal muscles.

5. Have the client repeat this exercise every hour during the first postoperative day.

FIGURE 15–1 Deep (diaphragmatic) breathing after surgery.

frequently believe that they should be stoic, and they may and hesitate to ask for relief. All clients need to be assured that they will not get addicted to pain medications in the short time for which the pain medication is required. In addition, anticipate pain when the client will be moving for the first time or when the analgesia has worn off. At such times, pain medication should be offered. If the client is to have a patient-controlled analgesia (PCA) pump after surgery, demonstrate how the machine operates, and emphasize that safety features on the equipment prevent overdosing. Without preoperative teaching about these procedures, postoperatively the client will be a groggy, sore client who may not understand how to treat the pain.

Pain can also be controlled through continuous infusion of analgesic agents through an epidural or IV route. Explain the method of planned pain control and how adjustments can be made for comfort.

EQUIPMENT. Whenever possible, explain about the equipment that will be used during the perioperative period. Depending on the type of surgery to be performed, various tubes, drains, and IV lines may be used. Discussion should focus on the purpose of specific pieces of equipment and how their use is related to the surgery.

Tubes. The most common type of tube used during the intraoperative period is an indwelling urinary catheter. Another tube commonly used is a nasogastric (NG) tube, which is used to decompress the stomach and upper bowel or to drain the stomach contents. These tubes are often inserted in the operating room.

Drains. Drains are inserted to promote evacuation of fluid from the dead space (tissue planes created during the operation) in the operative site. Many different types of drains are used. The Penrose drain works by wicking away fluid within the operative site, which then moves through the drain via gravity to an outside dressing or collection container. Drains are frequently attached to mild suction. Hemovac and Jackson-Pratt drains are commonly used suction devices.

Intravenous Infusion Devices. IV infusions are usually started before surgery. The purpose of the infusion is to administer medication, fluids, and nutrition solutions. The surgeon may request IV access for use in case of emergency even if the client is not expected to need IV medications.

■ PREOPERATIVE TEACHING FOR OLDER ADULTS

Older clients usually desire the same basic operative information as that provided for young patients. You must attend to this need in a sensitive and effective way. Preoperative teaching for older clients should include consideration of possible decreased sensory ability. Sit close to the client when teaching. Speak slowly and in a manner that results in a lower tone of voice. High-pitched sounds are frequently hard for an older people to discern. Glare from lights may bother the older client's eyes. Avoid bright lights while preparing the client preoperatively. Because the older client is more prone to hypothermia, apply blankets in the preoperative area and plan an appropriate method of warming for use in the operating room, where temperatures are usually cool.

■ INFORMED CONSENT

Anyone undergoing any invasive procedure must give informed consent for that procedure to be performed. A *consent form* is the legal document that signifies that the client has been told about and understands all aspects of a specific invasive procedure. This document guards the client against unwanted invasive procedures. It also protects the health care facility and health care professionals when a client denies understanding the procedure that was, or is planned to be, performed. Once the operative permit—indicating the client's *informed consent*—is signed, it becomes a permanent part of the client's record. This document accompanies the record to the operating room (Fig. 15–2).

Formal consent is necessary for each invasive procedure. The client or the client's legal surrogate must receive a full explanation of the operation before giving verbal and written consent. Pictures and diagrams may be necessary for a complete understanding of the surgical procedure. Moreover, the client or the surrogate must be told about who will perform the surgery; anesthesia and anesthetic choices; potential risks, complications, and risk of disfigurement or death; and whether organs or body parts may be removed. The client or the surrogate is also informed about alternative treatments. The surgeon must explain the procedure in terms the client or the surrogate readily understands. You are responsible for ensuring that the client or the surrogate receives an honest, accurate, and fair statement of what to expect during and after surgery and that the client understands it before informed consent is given.

The procedure for obtaining an informed consent varies from state to state and according to the individual policy for each health care facility. Generally, the surgeon explains the surgical procedure, the possible risks and complications, and the alternatives. The nurse may obtain and witness the client's signature on the consent form and may help to reinforce what the client has been told by the surgeon. It is not appropriate for the nurse to explain the surgical procedure, risks, complications, and alternatives unless this is done for reinforcement or clarification. The consent must be signed before the client receives any medication that may alter consciousness.

Adults sign their own operative permit unless they are unconscious or mentally incompetent. In such cases a surrogate, such as a relative or a legal guardian, is responsible for consent. If the relative or the guardian is out of state, consent can be secured via the telephone in the presence of one or two witnesses. If no relative or guardian can be found, one can be appointed by court order.

Children under legal age who are not emancipated minors must have consent given by the child's parent or legal guardian. Emancipated minors are considered to be those who are under the legal age of emancipation but because of marriage or other circumstances are independent of the parents. If the child's parent or guardian cannot be present to sign the permit, consent can be obtained from an appropriate person by telephone, Fax, or letter. When a minor's relatives cannot be located, the state in which the surgery is to be performed provides written procedures to follow in order to obtain consent via a court order.

619271 (CH Rev. 7-96)

I, _____, hereby consent to the procedures outlined below, to be performed by

_____, and his/her associates, assistants and appropriate hospital personnel.

The procedure proposed is _____

_____

_____

for diagnosis/treatment of _____ .

This procedure has been explained in terms understandable to me, which include the following:

1. The nature and extent of the procedure to be performed and risks involved, including those which, even though unlikely to occur, involve serious consequences.

2. Alternative procedures and methods of treatment.

3. The dangers and probable consequences of such alternatives (including no procedures or treatment).

4. The estimated period of hospitalization and/or incapacity and the estimated period of convalescence (assuming there are no complications).

5. The expected consequences of the procedure upon my future health.

6. I understand that there are other risks, such as the risks of infection and other serious complications, in the pre-operative and post-operative stages of my care, which can result in serious consequences such as loss of the use of parts of my body and life.

7. I have asked all of the questions which I thought were important in deciding whether or not to undergo treatment or diagnosis. Those questions have been answered to my satisfaction.

8. I understand that no assurance can be given that the procedure will be successful and no guarantee or warranty of success or cure has been given to me.

9. I have been advised that I may have anesthesia, which in rare instances has serious and even fatal complications.

10. I further authorize and request my physician and his/her associates, assistants and appropriate hospital personnel to perform such additional procedures which in their judgement are incidentally necessary or appropriate to carry out my diagnosis/treatment.

11. I have been afforded the opportunity to consult with other physicians to my complete satisfaction before signing this form and I understand that I have the right to refuse any medical and surgical procedures and treatment.

12. I authorize the hospital to dispose of or use for research any tissue or body parts which may be necessary to remove in a manner consistent with state and federal regulations for such disposal.

I certify that I have read and fully understand the above consent statement, that the explanations are understood by me, that all blanks or statements requiring insertion or completion were filled in prior to the time of my signature, that this consent was given freely, voluntarily and without reservation.

Patient's Signature:	Date:	Time:

In the event patient is a minor, unconscious or otherwise not competent to give consent: I, _____

the (relationship to patient) _____ , of _____ hereby give consent on his/her behalf.

Witness to Signature:	Date:	Time:

Clarkson Hospital
4350 Dewey Avenue
Omaha, Nebraska 68105

CONSENT FOR SURGERY OR DIAGNOSTIC/THERAPEUTIC PROCEDURES

FIGURE 15–2 Consent form for blood transfusion. (Courtesy of the Nebraska Health System, Omaha, NE.)

■ PREPARING THE CLIENT ON THE DAY OF SURGERY

Many clients are admitted into the hospital or surgical center the morning of surgery. These clients can be admitted to the hospital after the procedure if their condition requires specialized observation or nursing care. For so-called ambulatory surgery or same-day surgery, clients come to the hospital or surgery suite the morning of surgery but go home the same day to the care of family members or significant others. The ambulatory surgery approach presents a dilemma in providing preoperative instruction to the client, because time is very limited during the admission period prior to the actual surgical event. Often, the nurse will telephone the night before the procedure to remind the client of any preoperative instructions. Instructions are reinforced about starting NPO status after midnight, wearing washable clothing that is easily removed and put back on, wearing flat shoes, not wearing pantyhose, and securing a ride home after the procedure. Other instructions may be reinforced during this contact with the client. The nurse conducting the telephone educational session should convey a positive attitude about the planned surgical procedure and assist in allaying doubts or fears related to the surgery.

PREOPERATIVE PREPARATION IMMEDIATELY BEFORE SURGERY

Final preoperative preparation begins 1 to 2 hours before surgery for clients in the hospital, and upon admission for clients to have outpatient surgery. The client is asked whether there are any unanswered questions or concerns. Make sure that the client understands the operative procedure to be performed, and continue to assess for manifestations of anxiety. Delays in performing the surgery should be communicated to the client and family.

To prevent omissions in preoperative nursing interventions, most facilities supply nurses with a preoperative checklist. As each intervention on the list is completed, initial it on the form. An example of a preoperative checklist is provided in Box 15–3. Individual surgical centers may include various other actions on this form. You may need to give medications ordered preoperatively to the client before going to the operating room. You must know the approximate time the surgical procedure is scheduled for and must begin the preoperative activities early enough to have them completed when the operating room is ready.

PREOPERATIVE MEDICATIONS

Preoperative medications are given to allay anxiety, to decrease pharyngeal secretions, to reduce side effects of anesthetic agents, and to induce amnesia. Table 15–5 presents an overview of common preoperative medications. Specific drug choices are based on individual client variables, the goals of sedation, and the potential for undesirable side effects. Preoperative medications may be given in the preoperative holding area or on the nursing unit. Before administering preoperative medications, ensure that the operative permit is correctly signed because legal consent cannot be given by a medicated adult. If the preoperative medication is given on the unit, the side rails of the bed must be raised. Once medication is administered, the window shades should be lowered and bright lights turned off to avoid glare. The client is instructed not to get up without assistance because the medications are likely to cause drowsiness or dizziness. Once the client is calm and drowsy, disruptions should take place only when necessary and then be brief. Observe the client for side effects (e.g., hypotension and respiratory distress).

TRANSPORTING THE CLIENT TO SURGERY

When surgical personnel call for the client, the client is gently transferred to a stretcher. Adequate assistance for transfer must be obtained to reduce the possibility of injury to the client and staff. Appropriate covering is provided for the client, and side rails are raised. The medical record

BOX 15–3 Immediate Preoperative Activities

Before the client enters the operating room, check to determine that:

- All known allergies are recorded and allergy wristband is present if indicated.
- Vital signs are checked and recorded. Report marked differences from baseline to the surgeon or anesthesia personnel.
- The identification band is present and correct.
- The consent form is signed and the surgical procedure is listed correctly.
- Skin preparation is completed if ordered preoperatively.
- Any special orders, such as administering enemas or starting an intravenous line, are completed.
- The client has not eaten or had fluids by mouth for the last 8 hours.
- The client has just voided; measure and record the amount of urine (if indicated).
- Oral hygiene or other physical care is completed.
- The presence of dentures, bridgework, or other prostheses is noted, and the anesthesia personnel knows about it.
- Storage is arranged and documented for valuables according to health care facility policy or is given to family members.
- The client has removed jewelry. (Many facilities allow the client to keep the wedding band on as long as it is taped securely.) If jewelry is removed, it should be stored according to policy or given to the family. Assist with the removal of hairpins, wigs, and so on.
- The perioperative nurse is notified about the presence of a hearing aid. Leave it in place so that operating room personnel can communicate with the client.
- The client has a hospital gown and protective cap on. Elastic bandaging or antiembolic hose has been applied, if ordered.
- Colored nail polish has been removed from at least one fingernail for the application of the pulse oximeter (although the device can accurately read oxygen saturation levels through light-colored polish).
- Make-up is removed so that skin color can be observed.

accompanies the client to the operating room. The trip to surgery should be as smooth as possible so that the sedated client does not experience nausea and dizziness.

PREPARING THE CLIENT'S ROOM FOR POSTOPERATIVE CARE

The client's room should be prepared so that the initial care of the client on return from surgery can be orderly. Furniture should be arranged so that the stretcher can easily be brought to the bedside. The bed should be placed in high position and made with clean linen in an open position. Bed rails should be down on receiving side, up on other side. An emesis basin should be located close to the bed. Blood pressure monitoring equipment, IV setup, suction, and oxygen should be nearby. All equipment should be tested to ensure it is in working condition before the client returns.

CARING FOR SIGNIFICANT OTHERS

A designated area is usually provided for family members to wait in during surgery. If family members plan on

TABLE 15-5	COMMONLY USED PREOPERATIVE MEDICATIONS	
Medication	**Desired Effect**	**Undesired Effect(s)**
Tranquilizers		
Diazepam (Valium)	Decreases anxiety	May cause dizziness, clumsiness, or confusion
Droperidol (Inapsine)	Decreases anxiety Produces an antiemetic effect	Anxiety/hypotension during and after surgery
Sedatives		
Midazolam HCl	Induces desired sleepiness Decreases anxiety	Hypotension, undesired respiratory depression
Promethazine HCl (Phenergan)	Same as for droperidol	Hypotension during and after surgery
Secobarbital sodium (Seconal Sodium)	Decreases anxiety Promotes sedation	Disorientation, especially in elderly clients
Pentobarbital sodium (Nembutal Sodium)	Same as for secobarbital sodium	Same as for secobarbital sodium
Analgesics		
Morphine sulfate	Relieves pain Decreases anxiety Sedation	Respiratory depression Hypotension Circulatory depression Decreased gastric motility causing potential for vomiting
Fentanyl citrate (Sublimaze)	Is a short-acting analgesic for minor or outpatient surgery; adjunct to general anesthesia	Same as for morphine sulfate
Meperidine HCl (Demerol)	Same as for morphine sulfate	Same as for morphine sulfate
Anticholinergics		
Atropine sulfate	Controls secretions	Excessive dryness of mouth, tachycardia
Glycopyrrolate (Robinul)	Same as for atropine sulfate	Same as for atropine sulfate
Histamine H$_2$-Receptor Antagonists		
Cimetidine (Tagamet) (see Table 31-2 for other H$_2$ antagonists)	Inhibits gastric acid production	Mild dizziness, diarrhea, somnolence, and rash

leaving the facility during the procedure, ensure that there is a way to contact them and supply them with a phone number to the nurses' station and client's room.

When discussing the surgical procedure with the client's significant others, be sure to provide answers congruent with the information that the surgeon has already provided. Family members should also be prepared for any equipment that may accompany the client postoperatively. A preoperative explanation will assist the family in understanding what equipment is attached to their loved one, and why. Significant others need to be informed when surgery is completed or if there are any delays. The surgeon should speak with family members as soon as possible after completion of the procedure.

INTRAOPERATIVE PERIOD

Nursing care during the intraoperative phase focuses on the client's emotional well-being as well as on physical factors such as safety, positioning, maintaining asepsis, and controlling the surgical environment. The preoperative assessment assists the nurse in planning appropriate interventions for this phase of the surgical experience. The nurse remains the client's advocate during this pe-

riod, anticipating and guarding against potential complications. Whereas the surgeon concentrates on performing the surgical procedure and the anesthesia provider concentrates on the client's breathing and on maintenance of the client's physiologic stability, the circulating nurse is responsible for all other activities that take place in the operating room.

■ MEMBERS OF THE SURGICAL TEAM

The surgical team is a group of highly trained and educated professionals who coordinate their efforts to assure the welfare and safety of the client. Although the specifics of each type of surgical procedure may vary, certain key players must always be present, such as the surgeon, the anesthesiologist, the circulating nurse, and scrub personnel (see Box 15-4).

The surgeon heads the surgical team and makes decisions concerning the surgical procedure. Depending on the surgical procedure to be performed, a second surgeon or a specially trained nurse may serve as an assistant. The anesthesiologist alleviates pain and promotes relaxation with medications. The anesthesia provider maintains the airway, ensures adequate gas exchange, monitors circulation and respiration, estimates blood and fluid loss, in-

BOX 15–4   Roles of the Perioperative Nurse

Many roles are available to the perioperative nurse. The ongoing shift from tertiary care practice to community-focused practice is continuing to create even more new roles. The role these nurses play in the perioperative environment depends on their academic preparation, extended specialty education, experience, career plan, and needs of the employer. The roles of the perioperative nurse include, but are not limited to, the following:

- Circulating nurse
- Scrub nurse
- Registered Nurse First Assistant (RNFA)
- Certified Registered Nurse Anesthetist (CRNA)
- Manager
- Educator
- Case Manager, and Clinical Nurse Specialist (CNS)

Circulating Nurse

The circulating role is a major one for perioperative nurses. A nurse functioning as a circulator should be a Registered Nurse (RN). He or she assesses the client preoperatively, planning for optimal care during the surgical intervention, coordinating all personnel within the operating room, delegating and monitoring unlicensed personnel, and monitoring responsible cost compliance associated with operating room procedures. The circulator does not wear sterile clothing and can go in and out of the operating room. In addition to caring directly for the client, the circulator has very defined activities during surgery. These include:

- Ensuring all equipment is working properly
- Guaranteeing sterility of instruments and supplies
- Assisting with positioning
- Performing surgical skin preparation
- Monitoring the room and team members for breaks in sterile technique
- Assisting anesthesia personnel with induction and physiological monitoring
- Handling specimens
- Coordinating activities with other departments, such as radiology and pathology
- Documenting care provided
- Minimizing conversation and traffic within the operating room suite

Scrub Nurse

An RN or Surgical Technician (ST) can perform the role of scrub person. The duties include gathering all equipment for the procedure, preparing all supplies and instruments using sterile technique, maintaining sterility within the sterile field during surgery, handling instruments and supplies during surgery, and cleaning up after the case. During surgery, the scrub person maintains an accurate count of sponges, sharps, and instruments on the sterile field and counts the same materials with the circulating nurse before and after the surgery.

Registered Nurse First Assistant

The RNFA role is relatively new. In 1980, the American College of Surgeons supported the use of qualified RNs as first assistants in place of second or assisting physicians during surgical procedures. The Association of Operating Room Nurses (AORN) published its official statement on the role of the RNFA in 1984. The RNFA is an experienced perioperative nurse who has had additional specialized education to perform this role. The RNFA works with the primary surgeon during the surgery. This is a role separate from that of the scrub person. Some of the activities of an RNFA include providing exposure of the surgical area, using instruments to hold and cut, retracting and handling tissue, providing hemostasis, and suturing. RNFAs must work with a surgeon and are not independent practitioners.[29]

Certified Registered Nurse Anesthetist

The CRNA is a nurse who has a minimum of 2 years of additional education specializing in the administration of anesthesia. Entry into a CRNA program usually requires a Bachelor of Science degree in nursing or other appropriate field plus one year of acute or intensive care nursing experience. These nurses work under the direction of an anesthesiologist.

Manager

The role of manager of the operating room has extensive experience and has had additional education in management. It can be any Registered Nurse, but hospitals today prefer candidates with a Bachelor of Science in Nursing (BSN). Many large hospitals now require a master's degree, with a major in acute care or management. This nurse has many names, depending on the institution, such as head nurse, clinical nursing director, operating room manager, and others.

Educator

The role of educator can be played by any RN, but usually nurses with a BSN or Master's (MSN) degree who are experienced perioperative nurses are best qualified. They are responsible for staff continuing education, orientation of new staff, and working with staff to learn how to be preceptors to students. These nurses may also fulfill the role of circulator or Clinical Nurse Specialist outside their teaching responsibilities.

Case Manager

The perioperative case manager is also a new role for RNs. The role calls for extensive experience, ability to communicate, and a knowledge of the total surgical episode from home before surgery to home care needs after surgery. These nurses may have different functions within their place of work, depending on the need of the institution or employing agency. As with any role, the role of case manager should be investigated before nurses accept a position of employment.[25]

Clinical Nurse Specialist

The Clinical Nurse Specialist is an Advanced Practice Nurse.[21] These nurses must hold a MSN with a major reflecting their specialty. The major roles (depending on institutional needs) vary but incorporate direct client care; education of staff, clients, family members, people of other disciplines; consultation; and research.[21] A perioperative or surgical Clinical Nurse Specialist may not always be in the operating room but may go on rounds with physicians, interact with clients in homes, clinics, or other sites; and monitor clients in hospital surgical units. These nurses have specialized skills in heart, transplantation, renal, and cancer fields.

Perioperative nursing is performed preoperatively, intraoperatively, and postoperatively. Each of these periods is characterized by specific actions required by nurses, who participate both independently and as part of a health care team.

fuses blood and fluids, administers medications to maintain hemodynamic stability, and alerts the surgeon immediately to any complications. The circulating nurse is a core member of the surgical team and maintains the coordination of all team members while always remaining the client's advocate. Scrub personnel organize the surgical equipment and hand the surgeon appropriate instruments required for the operative procedure. Depending on the specific surgical procedure, the surgical team may include other members—for instance, a pathologist may be called in to identify tissue, an x-ray technician may be needed to perform various radiologic procedures, or a perfusionist may be required when cardiac bypass is necessary. The circulating nurse must control the traffic within the operating suite and know the designated responsibilities of each team member.

■ ANESTHESIA

Anesthesia is an artificially induced state of partial or total loss of sensation with or without loss of consciousness. Anesthestic agents can produce muscle relaxation, block transmission of pain nerve impulses, and suppress reflexes. It can also temporarily decrease memory retrieval and recall. The depth and effects of anesthesia are monitored by observing changes in respiration, oxygen saturation and end-tidal carbon dioxide (CO_2) levels, heart rate, urine output, and blood pressure.

Most clients are anxious about the anesthesia. Some are concerned about the adequacy of the pain-blocking effects, whereas others are concerned about being "put to sleep" with a drug. Some clients wonder whether they will talk during anesthesia or will experience nausea and vomiting postoperatively. Nurses must respond to these concerns by providing reassurance about the capability of the anesthesiologist, and about the availability of other drugs to reduce any unpleasant side effects of the anesthesia. The client needs frequent reminders to let the nurse or the physician know immediately about any side effects experienced from the anesthesia, and the nurse

must remain diligent in assessing for any possible complications. Bring any side effects noted to the immediate attention of the anesthesiologist.

The decision about the type of anesthesia to be used is made by the anesthesia provider in consultation with the surgeon and the client. The choice of anesthetic agent for a surgical procedure depends on many variables. The two major techniques in anesthesia are general and regional.

Agents for *general anesthesia* (general anesthetics) block pain stimulus at the cerebral cortex and induce depression of the central nervous system (CNS) that is reversed either by metabolic change and elimination from the body or by pharmacologic means. General anesthetic agents produce analgesia, amnesia, unconsciousness, and loss of reflexes and muscle tone. The neurologic, respiratory, and cardiovascular systems are affected by these agents. General anesthesia is best suited for surgery on the head, neck, upper torso, and back; for prolonged surgical procedures; or for use in clients who are unable to lie quietly for a long period of time. General anesthetic agents affect all tissues in the body to some degree.

In *regional anesthesia,* drugs are given to block the pain stimulus at its origin, along afferent neurons, or along the spinal cord. Unlike general anesthesia, regional anesthesia produces a loss of painful sensation in only one region of the body and does not result in unconsciousness. In addition to the regional anesthetic agent, the client also may receive sedative agents that produce drowsiness. The client can also receive epidural narcotics, which have a systemic effect and produce some drowsiness.

GENERAL ANESTHESIA
Stages of General Anesthesia

There are four stages of general anesthesia (Table 15–6). Surgery is performed in stage III. These stages were identified many years ago when ether was the most common drug used for anesthesia. The effects of ether allowed these distinct stages to be easily differentiated. The stages were used to guide the surgeon in determining when

TABLE 15–6	THE FOUR STAGES OF ANESTHESIA			
Stage	**Start-Point**	**End-Point**	**Physical Reactions**	**Nursing Interventions**
I: Onset	Anesthetic administration	Loss of consciousness	Client may be drowsy or dizzy. Possible auditory or visual hallucinations	Close operating room doors; keep room quiet; stand by to assist client
II: Excitement	Loss of consciousness	Loss of eyelid reflexes	Increase in autonomic activity Irregular breathing Client may struggle	Remain quietly at client's side; assist anesthetist, if needed
III: Surgical anesthesia	Loss of eyelid reflexes	Loss of most reflexes Depression of vital functions	Client is unconscious Muscles are relaxed No blink or gag reflex	Begin preparation (if indicated) only when anesthetist indicates stage III has been reached and client is breathing well, with stable vital signs
IV: Danger (death)	Functions excessively depressed	Respiratory and circulatory failure	Client is not breathing A heartbeat may or may not be present	If arrest occurs, respond immediately to assist in establishing airway; provide cardiac arrest tray, drugs, syringes, long needles; assist surgeon with closed or open cardiac massage

surgery could begin. Ether, which is no longer used because of its explosive nature, has been replaced with greatly improved anesthetic agents that provide rapid induction of anesthesia. With the rapid action of these new drugs, the stages of anesthesia are not readily apparent; however, they still occur. Some signs may be noted if the anesthetic drug is given slowly as the nurse holds the hand of the client during induction. Mild tremors of the hand may be felt as the client moves through stages I and II to stage III.

Because the last sense to be depressed during induction is hearing, remember to maintain a quiet atmosphere during this time. The client can hear and may remember conversations upon awakening. The nurse, always remaining the client's advocate, ensures that all conversation during induction and throughout the case is appropriate. Clients emerge into consciousness backward through all three stages of anesthesia after the anesthetic agents are discontinued. Therefore, hearing is the first sense to return.

Administration of General Anesthesia

General anesthesia can be administered in a variety of ways. The most common method of administering anesthesia is to use a combination of agents based on the client's need with consideration of the type of surgery to be performed. This type of anesthesia is called *neuroleptic* or *balanced anesthesia*. Balanced anesthesia is typically achieved with a combination of an inhalation agent, oxygen, a narcotic, and a neuromuscular blocking agent. Inhalation and the IV route are the most common routes of administration. Table 15–7 describes the most common general anesthetic agents used and the implications for the delivery of nursing care associated with the use of each.

Neuromuscular Blocking Agents. Neuromuscular blocking agents are classified as *depolarizing* and *nondepolarizing*. These agents block the transmission of nerve impulses to the muscle fibers. Neuromuscular blocking agents (Table 15–8) are administered via the IV route and are given mainly to facilitate intubation by easing laryngospasm, and relaxing muscles for controlled ventilation. When general anesthetics are given with neuromuscular blocking agents, the latter can be given in smaller and thus safer doses. Common muscle relaxants are succinylcholine, tubocurarine, pancuronium, and vecuronium.

Types of General Anesthesia

INTRAVENOUS ANESTHESIA. When general anesthesia is administered intravenously the client experiences an extremely rapid induction. Unconsciousness generally occurs about 30 seconds after the medication is administered. This process promotes a rapid transition from the conscious stage to the surgical anesthesia stage. It also prepares the client for a smooth transition to the surgical stage of anesthesia, as the IV anesthetic can act as a calming agent. IV anesthesia is sufficiently potent to be used alone in such minor procedures as dental extractions and pelvic examinations. Examples of IV anesthetics are thiopental sodium and ketamine.

INHALATION ANESTHESIA. For inhalation anesthesia, a mixture of volatile liquids or gas and oxygen is used. These anesthetics are advantageous because of their ease

of administration and elimination through the respiratory system. These are usually used to maintain the client in stage III anesthesia following induction. The mixture is given through a mask or through an endotracheal tube (Fig. 15–3), which is inserted once the patient is paralyzed and unconscious. Anesthesia intubation is often more difficult in an obese client because of the typically thickened neck and in the client with arthritis or a neck fracture.

When inhalation anesthetic agents are administered by mask, the gases generally flow into the mask via a finely calibrated vaporizer that is controlled by a machine. When an endotracheal tube is used to give the anesthetic, the gases flow directly into the client's tracheobronchial tree, resulting in a very quick response. Many different liquids and gases are used in inhalation anesthesia. Two commonly employed inhalation anesthetics are halothane and isoflurane. A commonly used gas anesthetic is nitrous oxide.

REGIONAL ANESTHESIA

Regional anesthetics are useful in many clinical situations. Local anesthetic agents, which are used to obtain local anesthesia, can also be administered to function as a central, peripheral, IV, regional, retrobulbar, or transbronchial nerve block. Table 15–10 (see later on) describes agents commonly used for local anesthesia. These anesthetic agents block the conduction of impulses in the nerve fibers without depolarizing the cell membrane.

Epinephrine can be added to many of the local anesthetics in an effort to prolong the anesthetic effect. Epinephrine also causes local blood vessels to constrict, thus delaying absorption of the anesthetic agent. This factor also can reduce bleeding via vasoconstriction. Epinephrine should be used with caution in older adults with cardiovascular or liver disease. Traditionally, epinephrine is not used in hand or foot surgery because of the small blood vessels in the area. Because the effect is vasoconstriction, use of epinephrine could compromise tissue perfusion, leading to adverse outcomes such as poor circulatory response. Recently, the use of epinephrine in hand and foot surgery has been reevaluated.

Types of Regional Anesthesia

Regional anesthesia can be administered in a variety of different ways: spinal, epidural, caudal, topical, local infiltration, field block, peripheral nerve block, and IV regional block.

SPINAL ANESTHESIA. Spinal anesthesia offers many advantages for clients undergoing surgical procedures involving the lower half of the body. It is often the anesthetic technique of choice for older adults because of its overall favorable profile. Benefits of spinal anesthesia include its relative safety, excellent lower body muscle relaxation, and absence of effect on consciousness; furthermore, its use does not require empty stomach. Spinal anesthesia is achieved by injecting local anesthetics into the subarachnoid space (Fig. 15–4). Autonomic nerve fibers are affected first and are also the last to recover. After blockade of the autonomic nervous system, spinal anesthesia blocks the following fibers in this order: (1) touch, (2) pain, (3) motor, (4) pressure, and (5) proprioceptive fibers—these fibers alert the brain of physical orientation. Recovery is in the reverse order.

TABLE 15–7	GENERAL ANESTHETIC AGENTS		
Drug	**Action**	**Side Effects**	**Nursing Implications**
Inhalation Agents			
Nitrous oxide	Gas has very low anesthetic potency, so it must be used with other agents; highest analgesic effect of all agents; little or no effect on BP or P; no muscle relaxant properties	Minimal side effects; little or no hypotension or respiratory depression; low incidence of malignant hypothermia	Monitor vital signs, especially BP and P; monitor effects of CNS depressants for 24 hours after administration
Halothane (Fluothane)	Volatile liquid with high anesthetic potency, so it could be used alone; has weak analgesic effect; causes moderate decrease in BP and large decrease in respirations; only a mild muscle relaxant	Hypotension, depression of myocardium with decreased cardiac output, bradycardia, respiratory depression; sensitizes heart to catecholamines; malignant hyperthermia, hepatitis, postoperative mild nausea and vomiting, decreased urine output	Monitor all vital signs closely; monitor body temperature for signs of malignant hyperthermia; keep client warm during recovery, and watch for severe shivering; avoid use of catecholamines (epinephrine or norepinephrine); monitor liver function after surgery; monitor urine output closely
Enflurane (Ethrane)	Volatile liquid with fairly high anesthetic potential; has weak analgesic effect; causes moderate decrease in BP and large decrease in respirations; is a moderate muscle relaxant	Hypotension, respiratory depression; blocks labor; minimal sensitization of heart to catecholamines; seizures with high doses	Do not give to clients with history of seizures; monitor vital signs, especially BP, P, and respirations; not for use during labor
Isoflurane (Forane)	Volatile liquid with high anesthetic potential; has weak analgesic effect; causes moderate decrease in BP and large decrease in respirations; is a moderate muscle relaxant; produces profound vasodilatation	Hypotension related to vasodilating effect; respiratory depression; suppresses uterine contractions	Does not sensitize heart to catecholamines, so it can be used with epinephrine and norepinephrine; monitor vital signs; and avoid rapid position changes because it may lead to hypotension as a result of vasodilatation
Intravenous Drugs			
Thiopental sodium (Pentothal)	Short-acting barbiturate that produces rapid unconsciousness; a weak analgesic and muscle relaxant	Respiratory depression with momentary apnea after injection, retrograde amnesia, myocardial depression, hypotension, headache, and shivering	Monitor for allergic reactions; monitor respiratory function closely, especially during induction; monitor vital signs; cannot be mixed with solutions containing atropine, tubocurarine, or succinylcholine; avoid extravasation
Fentanyl citrate– droperidol (Innovar)	A potent opioid (fentanyl) combined with a neuroleptic (droperidol); produces indifference to surroundings and insensitivity to pain; CNS depressant, which produces calming, analgesia, and reduced motor activity	Emergence delirium with hallucinations, hypotension, vasodilatation, nausea and vomiting, laryngospasm, respiratory depression, shivering, and apnea	Use with caution in clients with head injuries, increased intracranial pressure, COPD, hepatic or renal dysfunction, or bradyarrhythmias, or in elderly clients; monitor vital signs; maintain patent airway; reduce narcotic doses to one fourth or one third for first 24 hr postoperatively; when Innovar is used for induction, fentanyl citrate (Sublimaze) alone is used for maintenance of anesthesia
Ketamine HCl (Ketalar)	Produces state of dissociative anesthesia; causes sedation, immobility, analgesia, amnesia, and unresponsiveness to pain; short-acting (no antagonist)	Delirium, hallucinations, disturbing dreams, tonic and clonic movements, respiratory depression, hypotension or hypertension, decreased or increased pulse, nystagmus, increased salivation, laryngospasms, and mild nausea and vomiting	Contraindicated in clients with history of CVA and severe hypertension; use with caution in clients with alcoholism or elevated CSF; maintain airway; do not give in same syringe as for barbiturates; minimize stimulation as client emerges from anesthesia; use diazepam if hallucinations occur or delusions are severe; excellent for anesthesia in young and elderly; pad side rails of gurney; place client in quiet dark area; do not stimulate client inadvertently; any sudden moves elicit hallucinations

BP, blood pressure; CNS, central nervous system; COPD, chronic obstructive pulmonary disease; CVA, cardiovascular accident; CSF, cerebrospinal fluid; P, pulse.

TABLE 15–8	NEUROMUSCULAR BLOCKING AGENTS		
Drug	**Action**	**Side Effects**	**Nursing Implications**
Pancuronium bromide (Pavulon)	Nondepolarizing agent; prevents acetylcholine from binding to receptors on muscle end-plate, blocking depolarization	Tachycardia, hypertension, prolonged dose-related apnea, allergic reaction, and excessive sweating and salivation	Use carefully in older or debilitated clients or in clients with renal, hepatic, or pulmonary disease, myasthenia gravis, or thyroid disease; measure intake and output carefully; have resuscitation equipment available; do not mix in syringe or solution with barbiturates; neostigmine reverses effect
Vecuronium bromide (Norcuron)	Nondepolarizing agent; prevents acetylcholine from binding to receptors on muscle end-plate, blocking depolarization	Transient tachycardia; prolonged dose-related apnea, redness, itching, and induration	Has no effect on cardiovascular system; use with caution in clients with hepatic disease, obesity, or neuromuscular disease; tolerated well in renal disease; reversed with anticholinesterase and neostigmine; have emergency resuscitation equipment available
Succinylcholine chloride (Anectine)	Nondepolarizing agent that prolongs depolarization of muscle end-plate	Increased or decreased pulse rate and blood pressure, dysrhythmias, increased intraocular pressure, prolonged respiratory depression, malignant hyperthermia, postoperative muscle pain, excessive salivation, and hypersensitivity	Monitor vital signs; maintain patent airway; postoperative stiffness is normal; drug of choice for short procedures; keep emergency resuscitation equipment on hand; repeat infusions can prolong apnea; neostigmine reverses effect

Spinal anesthesia can be used for almost any type of major procedure performed below the level of the diaphragm, such as a hysterectomy or appendectomy. Figure 15–5 illustrates proper positioning for injection of drugs for spinal anesthesia. Within minutes of administration the client experiences a loss of sensation and paralysis of the toes, feet, legs, and then abdomen. Most clients exhibit a slight hypotension initially due to the vasodilatation that occurs with administration of the spinal anesthetic. The complications of spinal anesthesia are listed and described in Table 15–9, along with prevention and intervention suggestions for nurses. As with any anesthesia, the client who has undergone spinal anesthesia is at risk for neurologic, respiratory, or cardiovascular complications. However, the risk of spinal anesthesia in general is no higher than with general anesthesia.

EPIDURAL ANESTHESIA. An epidural block is achieved by introduction of an anesthetic agent into the epidural space (see Fig. 15–4). The epidural space is generally entered by a needle at a thoracic, lumbar, sacral, or caudal interspace. The needle is carefully positioned in the epidural space without penetrating the dura and without entering the subarachnoid space. When the needle is properly positioned, the cerebrospinal fluid

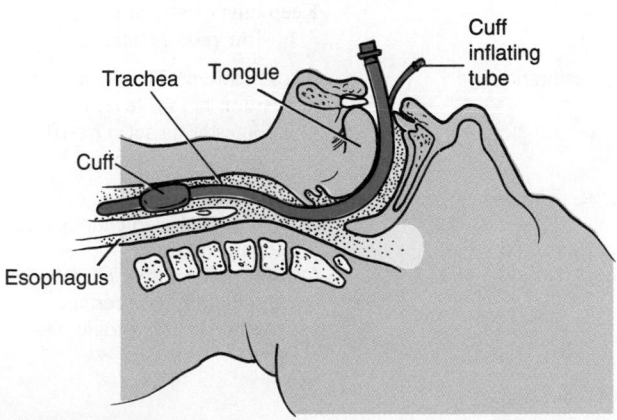

FIGURE 15–3 Correct placement of the endotracheal tube for anesthesia administration.

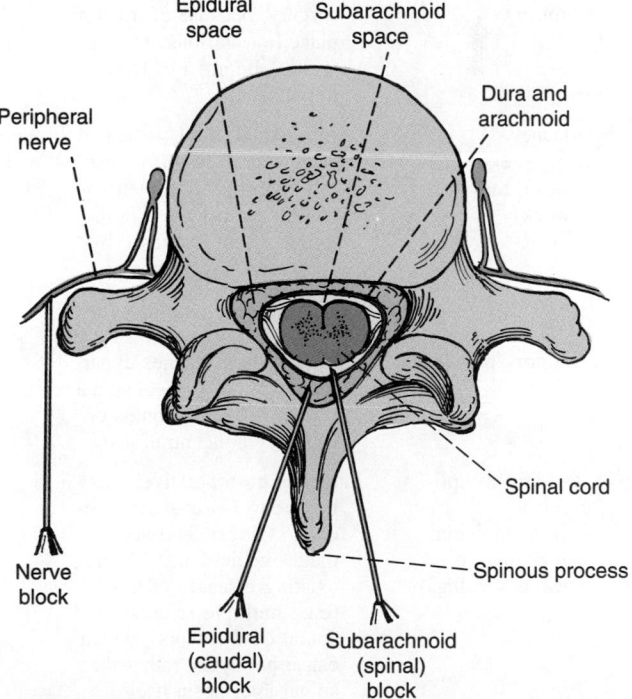

FIGURE 15–4 Cross-section of a lumbar vertebra showing injection sites for anesthesia.

FIGURE 15–5 Proper positioning for spinal anesthesia administration flexes the client's torso to expand the space between the lumbar vertebrae.

(CSF) cannot be aspirated. An epidural block, like spinal anesthesia, produces a blockade of the autonomic nerves and hypotension can result. If the level of the block is too high and the respiratory muscles are affected, then respiratory depression or paralysis may occur.

Caudal Anesthesia. Caudal anesthesia is produced by injection of the local anesthetic into the caudal or sacral canal. Caudal anesthesia is a variation of epidural anesthesia. This method is commonly used with obstetric clients.

TOPICAL ANESTHESIA. Topical anesthetic agents may be directly applied onto the area to be desensitized. The

TABLE 15–9	COMPLICATIONS AND DISCOMFORTS OF SPINAL ANESTHESIA		
Complications and Discomforts	**Causes**	**Intervention**	**Prevention**
Hypotension	Paralysis of vasomotor nerves; usually occurs shortly after induction of anesthesia	Administer oxygen by inhalation Vasoactive drugs Trendelenburg's position if level of anesthesia is fixed, 10–20 min after induction	In clients not prone to heart failure, 500–800 ml of IV fluids, administered rapidly before block
Nausea and vomiting	Occurs mainly from abdominal surgery, because of traction placed on various structures within abdomen or from hypotension	Ephedrine Antiemetics Oxygen Fluids	
Headache (can be extremely painful, may last a week)	Cerebrospinal fluid (which cushions the brain) is lost through dural hole; leakage of fluid with loss of cushioning effect increased by (1) use of a large spinal needle or (2) poor hydration	Apply tight abdominal binder Fluids Analgesics In severe cases, inject 10 ml of client's blood to plug hole (blood patch)	Use of very small spinal needle reduces incidence of spinal headache to 0.9% Administer IV and oral fluids before and after induction of spinal anesthesia Keep client flat and quiet 6–8 hr postoperatively
Respiratory paralysis	Occurs if drug reaches upper thoracic and cervical spinal levels in large amounts or in heavy concentrations	Artificial respiration	Avoid extreme Trendelenburg's position before level of spinal anesthesia set, i.e., 10–20 min after induction
Neurologic complications (e.g., paraplegia, severe muscle weakness in legs)	Paralysis postoperatively may be due to (1) unsterile needles, syringes, and anesthetic medications; (2) preexisting diseases of CNS (e.g., multiple sclerosis and spinal cord tumors), which cause paralysis, rather than spinal anesthesia itself	See Chapter 73	Strict sterile technique Heat-sterilized medications and instruments Careful preoperative neurologic examination to ascertain presence of neurologic disease

IV, intravenous; CNS, central nervous system.

TABLE 15-10	LOCAL AND TOPICAL ANESTHETIC AGENTS		
Drug	**Action**	**Side Effects**	**Nursing Implications**
Local Agents			
Bupivacaine HCl (Marcaine HCl)	Amide-type local anesthetic that blocks depolarization, preventing generation and conduction of nerve impulses; combined with epinephrine, it has prolonged action	Edema, anaphylaxis; rarely, anxiety, convulsions, respiratory arrest, cardiac arrest, blurred vision, and shivering	Contraindicated in children under 12 years of age, or for spinal or paracervical block or topical anesthesia; use with caution in older clients, or clients with hepatic disease or allergies; onset 4–15 min, duration 3–6 hr; keep resuscitative equipment available
Chloroprocaine HCl (Nesacaine)	Ester-type local anesthetic that blocks depolarization, preventing generation and condition of nerve impulses	Anaphylaxis, edema; rarely, anxiety, convulsions, respiratory arrest, cardiac arrest, blurred vision, and shivering	Contraindicated in clients with allergies to "caines," CNS disease; use cautiously in older adults; check solution for particles or discoloration; keep resuscitative equipment available; do not use solution with preservative for caudal or epidural blocks
Lidocaine HCl (Xylocaine)	Amide-type local anesthetic that blocks depolarization, preventing generation and conduction of nerve impulses; combined with epinephrine, it has prolonged action	Edema, anaphylaxis, dysrhythmias; rarely, anxiety, respiratory arrest, cardiac arrest, and tinnitus	Contraindicated in clients with hypersensitivity, severe hypertension, septicemia, spinal deformities, or neurologic disorders; use cautiously in older clients and those with heart block or general drug allergies or in severe shock; use solutions with epinephrine only in body areas with good blood supply; use preservative-free solution for spinal, epidural, and caudal blocks
Topical Agents			
Benzocaine (Americaine)	Blocks conduction of impulses at sensory nerve endings	Sensitization rash, possible tolerance	Contraindicated in clients with history of hypersensitivity to "caines"; discontinue if rash develops; avoid contact with eyes; avoid inhalation of spray; has short duration of action; do not use over infected area; if used rectally, clean area well first
Ethyl chloride spray	Produces local anesthesia by producing sensation of cold	Frostbite, tissue necrosis from prolonged use, muscle spasms, and increased pain	Do not apply over broken skin; protect adjacent skin; avoid contact with eyes; avoid inhalation; highly flammable, do not use near open flame; very short duration
Tetracaine HCl (Pontocaine HCl)	Blocks conduction of impulses at sensory nerve endings	Local sensitization and rash	Do not use in hypersensitive clients; clean rectal area well before applying; do not use if rash develops
Cocaine	Ester-type topical anesthetic that blocks uptake of norepinephrine by adrenergic neurons	CNS stimulation, euphoria, decreased fatigue, tachycardia, vasoconstriction, and hypertension	For topical use only; produces psychological dependence with prolonged or repeated use; schedule II narcotic; use cautiously in clients with history of severe hypertension or heart disease; combined with epinephrine, it can lead to cardiovascular toxicity; monitor vital signs closely

CNS, central nervous system.

anesthetic may be a solution, an ointment, a gel, a cream, or a powder. This short-acting form of anesthesia can block peripheral nerve endings in the mucous membranes of the vagina, rectum, nasopharynx, and mouth. Topical anesthesia is used in minor procedures such as a rectal examination when painful hemorrhoids are present or before a bronchoscopic examination to desensitize the bronchi. Medications used for local and topical anesthesia are listed in Table 15-10.

One drug commonly used for topical anesthesia is a 4% to 10% solution of cocaine. This agent is for topical use only and is primarily used to anesthetize the eye and the mucous membranes of the nose, mouth, and urethra. Cocaine is highly toxic. If accidentally injected, it may cause severe excitement or seizures, followed by shock, respiratory failure, and cardiac arrest. Emergency resuscitation equipment must be available when cocaine is used. Other agents commonly used for topical anesthesia include tetracaine, procaine, mepivacaine, bupivacaine, and lidocaine. To avoid anaphylactic reactions from previous sensitization to anesthetic agents, check the client's drug allergies before application of any topical anesthetic agent.

LOCAL INFILTRATION ANESTHESIA. Local infiltration anesthesia involves injection of an anesthetic agent such as lidocaine (Xylocaine) into the skin and subcutaneous tissue of the area to be anesthetized. Local anesthesia blocks only the peripheral nerves around the area of the incision. When local anesthetic is administered, the person injecting the drug must aspirate before injection to ensure the needle is not in a blood vessel. If a local anesthetic agent is inadvertently injected into the bloodstream, it becomes systemic, and cardiovascular collapse or convulsions could result.

FIELD BLOCK ANESTHESIA. The area proximal to a planned incision can be injected and infiltrated with local anesthetic agents to produce what is known as a *field block.* This block forms a barrier between the incision and the nervous system. This procedure differs from simple injection of local anesthesia, in which only the area of the incision is injected. A field block actually walls in the area around the incision and prevents transmission of sensory impulses to the brain from that area. The anesthesia provider must take precautions when performing a field block to avoid injection of the agent into a blood vessel.

PERIPHERAL NERVE BLOCK ANESTHESIA. A *nerve block* anesthetizes individual nerves or nerve plexuses rather than all the local nerves anesthetized by a field block. Nerve blocks can be obtained in a finger (digital nerve block), the entire upper arm (brachial plexus nerve block), or the chest or abdominal wall (intercostal nerve block). Nerves most commonly blocked are those within the brachial plexus and the intercostal, sciatic, and femoral nerves. Drugs commonly used as nerve block agents are lidocaine, bupivacaine, and mepivacaine. The anesthesia provider injects the anesthetic along the nerve rather than into the nerve in an effort to decrease the risk of nerve damage. Once the drug has been injected, it takes several minutes for onset of the anesthesia.

Nerve blocks, like local infiltration blocks, can produce severe systemic response if the drug is accidentally injected into a blood vessel. Because epinephrine causes vasoconstriction, particularly in the extremities, anesthetic procedures for surgery performed below the wrist or ankle typically use agents that do not contain epinephrine.

INTRAVENOUS REGIONAL EXTREMITY BLOCK ANESTHESIA (BIER BLOCK). Regional anesthesia of a limb can be achieved with an agent such as lidocaine when it is injected into a vein of the limb to be anesthetized. A pneumatic dual-cuff tourniquet applied to the anesthetized area prevents the lidocaine from circulating beyond the area undergoing the procedure. This type of anesthesia is used most commonly for procedures of the extremities that are of short duration. The tourniquet can be inflated only for 2-hour increments.

MONITORED ANESTHESIA. Monitored anesthesia is used during an operation in which the surgeon infiltrates the surgical site with a local anesthetic and the anesthesia provider supplements the local anesthetic with IV drugs to provide sedation and systemic analgesia. The anesthesia care provider monitors the client's blood pressure, heart rate, and respiration while the local anesthesia and IV support are being provided. *Local standby* and *anesthesia standby* also refer to monitored anesthesia.

Other Methods of Anesthesia and Analgesia

ACUPUNCTURE. Acupuncture is an ancient Chinese pain-killing technique that works by the insertion of long, thin needles into specific acupuncture points located on lines called *meridians* that connect anatomic sites on the body. Practitioners of acupuncture have named and numbered approximately 1000 acupuncture points, each about 0.25 cm in diameter. When performing major surgery, Chinese doctors use acupuncture as a form of anesthesia. Some advantages of acupuncture include (1) decreased anesthesia-related side effects during or after surgery, (2) less blood loss during surgery, and (3) reduced need for postoperative analgesia, because acupuncture's pain-killing effects persist for several hours.

There are several Western hypotheses to explain why acupuncture works. One hypothesis is based on the outdated gate control theory of pain control and contends that the technique stimulates the larger sensory nerve fibers that carry non-pain impulses. Another theory suggests that acupuncture triggers the release of endorphins, endogenous polypeptides with analgesic properties. Some Western physicians remain skeptical about the technique's pain-killing capabilities.

CRYOTHERMIA. Cryothermia is the use of cold to induce anesthesia. Because a very low surface temperature reduces pain, the surgical site is treated with ice preoperatively. Although there are many acceptable alternatives to cryothermia, this technique can be used in extreme conditions that threaten life and when the client cannot tolerate conventional forms of anesthesia.

■ INTRAOPERATIVE NURSING CARE

Intraoperative nursing care is the second component of perioperative nursing. It is often called "operating room nursing." Intraoperative nurses see the client immediately before surgery, either in a holding area or in an admission unit. An initial, brief assessment is completed by the intraoperative nurse. The care plans that were developed and planned preoperatively, along with the findings on the extensive admission examination, are used in this phase. Intraoperative nursing care plans incorporate safety, monitoring of the client, and control of operative resources along with considerations of the individual needs of each client.

MAINTAIN SAFETY AND PREVENT INJURY

Safety is a major consideration in the perioperative nursing. Using data gathered from the preoperative assessment, the nurse implements care individually designed for each client. This care includes positioning, controlling equipment and supplies, maintaining surgical asepsis, monitoring the physiologic status, and monitoring for potential emergencies.

Position the Client

Procedures vary among institutions, but after admission to the operating room the client is identified and then moved to the operating room bed. At this time, the client is anesthetized and positioned, and the skin is prepared and any other procedures that must be completed before draping and creating the sterile field (such as catheterization or shaving) are done. The perioperative nurse understands the various operative positions as well as the physiologic changes that occur when a client is placed in a specific position. Table 15–11 reviews these positions and the changes that may occur. Essential factors to consider in positioning a client on the operating table are (1) the site of the operation, (2) the age and size of the client, (3) the type of anesthetic used, and (4) pain normally experienced by the client on movement, such as that due to arthritis. The position must not hinder respiration or circulation, must not apply excessive pressure to skin surfaces, and must not limit surgical exposure. The following surgical positions are shown in Figure 15–6:

- *Dorsal recumbent (supine).* Commonly used for coronary artery bypass grafting hernia repair, mastectomy, or bowel resection
- *Trendelenburg.* Permits displacement of the intestines into the upper abdomen and is often used during surgery of the lower abdomen or pelvis
- *Lithotomy.* Exposes the perineal and rectal areas and is ideal for vaginal repairs, dilation and curettage, and most types of rectal surgery
- *Lateral.* Used for clients undergoing kidney, chest, or hip surgery

Many other positions can be used, depending on the type of surgery and the visualization of the site required by the surgeon. Laser techniques, endoscopy, or biopsy all may require different client positioning. Interventions may include gathering special supplies that can accommodate an obese client, arranging for an appropriate operating table to withstand excess weight, and providing extra padding to assist in skin integrity maintenance. Additional padding is applied to the operating table for the very thin client or the client with kyphosis.

Whatever the client's position on the operating table, there are general guidelines to promote safety. Most clients feel stiff and sore after a long surgical procedure and may actually complain of the effects of positioning.

Provide Equipment Safety

Almost everything in the operating room can be a source of injury if careful control is not exercised. Every action is designated to prevent accidents. These procedures include counting surgical supplies and equipment that could inadvertently be left inside the surgical incision, such as needles, sponges, and instruments. Counts are performed by two people, usually the circulating nurse and the scrub person, at three different times before the initial incision, during the surgery, and immediately before the incision is closed. A final correct count is announced to the surgeon and charted on the intraoperative chart.

Electrical safety is also controlled during surgery. All plugs and wires are inspected for correct attachment; all equipment is checked to ensure that it is in working order; and measures are taken to prevent electrical burns

TABLE 15–11	GUIDELINES FOR POSITIONING THE CLIENT DURING SURGERY
Nursing Action	**Rationale**
Explain to the client, in simple, understandable terms, why the positions and restraints are necessary.	Some clients feel that restraining straps are punitive. Some positions can be difficult or embarrassing.
Preserve the client's dignity and avoid undue exposure.	To promote a positive feeling that will encourage healing.
Place restraining straps 2 inches above the knees.	Most secure position on operating bed. Avoids pressure injury from strap on bony prominences.
Nerves, muscles, pressure points and bony prominences are padded.	To prevent nerve and tissue damage; decrease pressure that will impair or slow circulation; prevent pressure sores during long surgical procedures.
Position the client to obtain or maintain adequate respiratory exchange and vascular circulation.	To ensure tissue perfusion, oxygenation, and minimize the pooling of blood. Slow blood flow predisposes to thrombus formation.
Avoid pressure on the chest and on body parts such as the female breast and male genitalia.	Prevent injury and minimize discomfort after surgery.
Do not allow the client's extremities to dangle over the sides of the table.	Hands or feet can be inadvertently compressed against the operating room bed by surgery team personnel as they lean over the client's body. Impairment of circulation or nerve and muscle damage may result.
When using an armboard, do not abduct the upper extremity more than 90 degrees.	Hyperextension can result in permanent nerve damage caused by stretching or crushing the brachial plexus between the first rib and scapula.
Avoid excessive strain on the client's muscles.	Postoperative strain and discomfort may result.
Be certain that the client's ankles are not crossed when in the prone position.	Circulation may be occluded.
Always move both lower extremities at the same time when putting them up in stirrups and when lowering.	Hip joint could be dislocated or the muscles strained when extremities are positioned one at a time.
Monitor the total position throughout surgery.	Remember, the client may remain in one position for hours.

A. Dorsal recumbent

B. Trendelenburg

C. Lithotomy

D. Laminectomy

E. Lateral

FIGURE 15–6 *A–E,* Five surgical positions.

to the client. An *electrosurgical unit* (ESU) is used to sear the ends of capillaries and blood vessels to control bleeding during surgery. When unipolar cautery is used, place a grounding pad on a large body surface area (thigh or back) to "ground" the client and to prevent sparking and burns. Grounding pads must be placed over intact skin, away from any bony prominences and not over scars or fragile tissue. Many ESUs have a safety feature that does not allow the unit to work if the grounding pad is placed inappropriately. Bipolar cautery does not require a grounding pad.

Maintain Surgical Asepsis

The perioperative nurse ensures the sterility of supplies and equipment. All members of the health care team use sterile technique. If a suspected or actual break in the sterile field occurs, the contaminated instruments and clothing are removed and replaced with new, sterile items. Members of the surgical team who are in the "sterile area" are those actively performing or assisting in the surgical procedure. They include the surgeon and the assistants and the scrub personnel. The circulating nurse is not sterile and monitors the sterile field to maintain sterility of supplies and personnel. Surgical asepsis may be broken but must be immediately rectified. The nurse is the advocate of the client in maintaining a sterile surgical environment.

Assist with Wound Closure

After final counts are completed, the nurse anticipates the type of wound closure needed and obtains the supplies for the surgical team. The surgical wound may be closed with sutures, staples, or other materials or may be left open to heal by secondary intention. Common skin closures are illustrated in Figure 15–7. A drain is placed in a separate small incision parallel to the operative incisions to drain blood or serum from the operative site. The use of a surgical drain promotes wound healing and decreases the potential for infection. There are many types of surgical drains. The drain is chosen by surgeon preference and is based on the size of the wound and the type of drainage expected. Drains may be free-draining, attached to suction apparatus, or self-contained with suction. The intraoperative nurse and the postoperative nurse are responsible for assessing that the drainage is flowing freely through the system. When the client is transferred out of the operative area, the responsible nurse continues to monitor the patency of the drain and the characteristics of the drainage.

MONITORING
Monitor Body Temperature

Hypothermia can occur easily in the operating room. The operating room temperature is maintained at a standard cool level of 60° to 75° F. Humidity is regulated at 50%

to 60%. Temperature control is set to allow optimal performance of the surgical team members, who must wear layers of clothing, and to inhibit bacterial growth. The client can become cold in the operating room if appropriate covering is not provided. Heat is lost from the skin and from the area open for surgery. When tissues that are not covered with skin are exposed to the air, heat loss is greater than normal. The client should be kept as warm as possible to minimize heat loss without causing vasodilatation, which may cause more bleeding. Most operating rooms have a cabinet that warms blankets, and unless the surgical procedure requires cooling, the nurse should offer the client a blanket immediately upon transfer to the operating room bed. Some surgery centers allow the client to wear booties or socks during the operation to provide as much comfort as possible. The intraoperative nurse reports the lowest core body temperature to the postoperative nurse when transferring the client after surgery. Thermia blankets can also be used; these blow warm air over the client's body during the procedure. IV solutions can be warmed to assist in maintaining a warm body temperature during the operative procedure as well.

Certain operations require a hypothermic patient. Cooling of the body reduces the metabolic rate, which protects the brain and other organs during the surgical procedures.

Constant monitoring of the core body temperature is needed, and the nurse assists the anesthesia provider in this activity.

At other times a warm operating room is needed. A warm room is preferred for surgery for large body burns, for replantation, or for surgery in infants. Because of immature internal temperature controls, the infant's body temperature quickly equilibrates with the temperature of the room. Thus, room temperatures can be in the 90s. Hyperthermia can be a problem for the surgical team member who has adapted to the cool temperatures over time. If weakness, faintness, or nausea develops, the team member must leave the room at once.

Monitor for Emergencies

The perioperative nurse must be alert for potential emergencies. When these occur, knowledge, instant decision-making, and critical thinking are essential, as is speed in performing needed skills. Although almost any imaginable emergency can occur during an operation, the most common are malignant hyperthermia, cardiac or respiratory arrest, uncontrollable hemorrhage, and drug or allergic reactions.

MALIGNANT HYPERTHERMIA. Malignant hyperthermia is a genetic disorder characterized by uncontrolled skeletal muscle contraction leading to potentially fatal hyperthermia. It occurs in predisposed clients when they

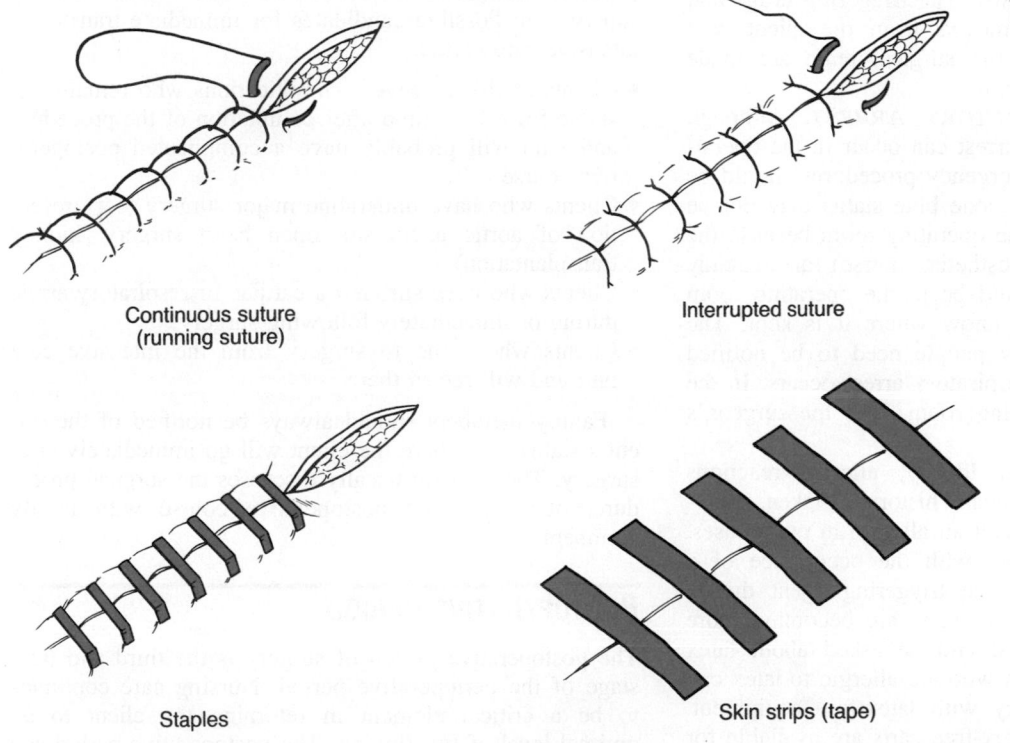

FIGURE 15–7 Skin closures.

Continuous suture
(running suture)

Interrupted suture

Staples

Skin strips (tape)

Retention suture

receive a combination of succinylcholine and inhalation agents (especially halothane). Unless the triggering event is stopped and the body is cooled, death is the result. This condition can occur within 30 minutes of anesthesia induction or several hours after surgery. The initial manifestation is increased end-tidal carbon dioxide, masseter muscle rigidity, cardiac dysrhythmias, and a hypermetabolic state. The client's fever can rise to as high as 109° F (43° C).

Everyone in the operating room must know the protocol for treatment of malignant hyperthermia. Medications for the emergency treatment of malignant hyperthermia cart should be in the operating room suite. Nurses must know where the cart is and the procedure to follow if this event occurs. Datrolene, a skeletal muscle relaxant, is used to decrease skeletal muscle rigidity. The nurse must know how to reconstitute this drug, supplied as a powder, and must be capable of assisting the surgeon or anesthesia personnel with its administration and with any other treatments needed to save the client's life.

There is a screening test for malignant hyperthermia. A muscle biopsy specimen must be taken from the vastus lateralis or abdominal rectus muscle and sent to a malignant hyperthermia laboratory for testing. This test is very expensive. A diagnosis of malignant hyperthermia can be made if there is any personal or family history of anesthesia problems. High-risk clients or those with a history of malignant hyperthermia can successfully undergo surgery if the condition is known. The triggering drugs and conditions are carefully removed from the client care plan, and all members of the surgical team are made aware of the potential problem.

CARDIAC AND RESPIRATORY ARREST. Although rare, cardiac or respiratory arrest can occur in the operating room, and the same emergency procedures should be carried out as elsewhere. A code blue status may not be called when a client is in the operating room because the key people (physician, anesthetist, nurse) are already present. The crash cart should be in the operating room suite, and everyone should know where it is kept. The nurse manager and any key people need to be notified immediately if cardiac or respiratory arrest occurs. In the case of death in the operating room, it is the surgeon's duty to talk to the family.

ALLERGIC REACTIONS. Ideally, allergic reactions should not occur if an adequate history is taken. However, some clients do not recall an allergy; in other cases, the allergy is identified only with the occurrence of a second allergic reaction to the triggering agent during surgery. For example, latex allergies are becoming more frequent, and every client should be asked about latex sensitivity or allergy. Clients who are allergic to latex can successfully undergo surgery with latex-free equipment. In many surgery centers, latex-free carts are available for such situations.

DOCUMENTATION OF INTRAOPERATIVE CARE
The intraoperative nurse documents every event and action in the operating room. Information concerning any drains, tubes, or other devices remaining in the client on completion of the surgical procedure, as well as the type of closure and dressing used, is given to the postoperative care nurse upon transfer.

MOVING AND TRANSPORTING THE CLIENT
On completion of the operation, a member of the surgical team wipes off any excess blood, skin preparation, and debris from the client's skin and puts a clean gown and blanket on the client. There should always be enough personnel for moving or transferring a client postoperatively to prevent injuries. Avoid rapid movements when changing the client's position because it can predispose the development of hypotension. In particular, move the client gradually from whatever surgical position was used onto the transportation cart. During emergence (revival) from anesthesia, the client is prone to nausea, confusion, and hypotension. Care must be taken not to catch, kink, or dislodge IV or catheter tubing, drains, or other equipment during the transfer. During transfer to the bed or stretcher, the client's modesty must be maintained. Avoid rough handling, which may damage fragile skin.

After being placed on the stretcher, the client is covered with warm blankets and secured with a safety belt. Make sure that the side rails of the stretcher are up to ensure the client's safety in case the client becomes agitated during transport from the operating room. The anesthesia care provider, as well as another member of the operating room professional staff, and sometimes the surgeon or the assistant accompany the client to the postoperative care unit.

In some hospitals, certain clients are transferred directly from the operating room to the intensive care unit (ICU) for continued specialized care and constant nursing supervision. Possible candidates for immediate transfer to intensive care include:

- Clients at risk of severe complications who remain unstable for a long time after completion of the procedure and who will probably have a complicated postoperative course
- Clients who have undergone major surgery (e.g., resection of aortic aneurysm, open heart surgery, kidney transplantation)
- Clients who have suffered a cardiac or respiratory arrest during or immediately following surgery
- Clients who came to surgery from the intensive care unit and will return there

Family members should always be notified of the client's status and where the client will go immediately after surgery. The surgeon usually discusses the surgical procedure, outcomes, and postoperative course with family members.

POSTOPERATIVE PERIOD

The postoperative period of surgery is the third and final stage of the perioperative period. Nursing care continues to be a critical element in returning the client to an optimal level of functioning. The postoperative period can be divided into three phases.

- The initial period of time for recovery from anesthesia, during which the client is monitored closely by post-anesthesia nurses
- The time from discharge from the post-anesthesia care unit (PACU) to the first day or so after surgery while the client is recovering from the effects of the surgery and is beginning to eat and ambulate

- The postoperative phase, the time of healing, which may last for weeks, months, or even years after surgery

There is certainly an overlap of these phases, but in the following discussion they are dealt with separately.

■ POST-ANESTHESIA CARE UNIT NURSING

The goal of post-anesthesia nursing is to assist a noncomplicated return to safe physiologic function after an anesthetic procedure by providing safe, knowledgeable, individualized nursing care for clients and their family members in the immediate post-anesthesia phase. The immediate post-anesthesia period is a critical time for the client. Close and constant observation is essential. The client's vital physiologic functions must be supported until the effects of the anesthetic agents abate. Until then, the client is dependent and drowsy and may be unable to call for assistance. Equipment commonly used in PACU nursing care is listed in Box 15–5.

The client is received in the PACU on a bed or a stretcher, where he or she remains, or is transferred to another bed or to a recovery chair. Proper positioning of a sedated, unconscious, or semiconscious client must ensure airway patency. For an unconscious adult patient, extend the neck and thrust the jaw forward (Fig. 15–8). The position may depend on the surgery performed. The preferred position is the lateral Sims position, because side-lying allows the client's tongue to fall forward and mucus or vomitus to drain from the mouth. Regardless of the position used, carefully monitor the client's respiratory status. Suction equipment must be ready to suction vomit or oral secretions.

FIGURE 15–8 So that the jaw can be moved forward after anesthesia, the operator's fingers are placed behind the angle of the jaw. As the jaw is moved, the tongue comes forward, opening the airway.

After the client has been positioned safely and has been determined to be stable, the nurse receives a verbal, detailed report of events from members of the operating room team (Box 15–6). The PACU nurse reviews the client's record with the anesthesia provider present, noting specifically (1) the anesthesia record for IV medications and blood received during surgery and (2) the length of time the client was in surgery. Ideally, a preoperative nursing assessment and nursing history are available in the record for comparison with the postoperative assessment.

IMMEDIATE ASSESSMENTS IN THE POST-ANESTHESIA CARE UNIT

After the transfer report from the operating room, the PACU nurse performs an assessment. The ABCs (airway, breathing, and circulation) are critical and must be assessed first. Included in the assessment are the following:

Airway: Patency; presence of tubes and respiratory assistance devices.
Breathing: Respiration rate and depth; presence of bilateral breath sounds, stridor, wheezes, hoarseness, or decreased breath sounds. Stay at the bedside until the client's gag reflex returns.

BOX 15–5   Equipment Used in the Post-Anesthesia Care Unit (PACU)

The PACU nurse prepares and checks the function of the following equipment:

- Sphygmomanometer or automatic blood pressure monitor
- Pulse oximeter—a noninvasive device that measures oxygen saturation of arterial blood and the pulse rate; provides warning of hypoxemia
- Stethoscope—to auscultate breath sounds and blood pressure
- Cardiac monitor and electrodes
- Intravenous equipment (e.g., insertion equipment, fluids, tubing, infusion pumps)
- Suction equipment (e.g., catheters, sterile saline, sterile gloves)
- Supplies to support respiration (e.g., artificial airways, oxygen, tongue depressors, oxygen tubing with masks and cannulas, intubation equipment, and anesthesia machine)
- Medications (e.g., narcotics, narcotic antagonists, hypnotics, antihypertensives, neuromuscular blocking agents)
- Emesis basin, mouth wipes, urinals, bedpans
- Thermometers—oral, rectal, and tympanic membrane types
- Warmed blankets or electric warming units to maintain body temperature
- Emergency cart containing appropriate equipment and medications—drugs including cardiotonics, vasotonics, and respiratory agents; a tracheostomy tray; endotracheal tubes; a defibrillator; a cutdown tray; a ventilator; gastric suction equipment; and chest tube insertion equipment

---

BOX 15–6   Information Given to the Post-Anesthesia Care Unit Nurse by the Perioperative Team

- Operative procedure performed
- Medical diagnosis, pertinent medical history, and daily medications
- Vital signs
- Blood loss, fluid replacements
- Urine output and presence of bladder catheters
- Anything eventful or complications during surgery
- Anesthetic agents, narcotics, neuromuscular blocking agents, or antibiotics
- Drains inserted and their locations and purpose
- Physician orders to be carried out immediately

Circulation: Pulse, blood pressure, skin color, pulse oximeter, ECG tracing if attached, wound status and dressings (this may include checking underneath the client's body for oozing or frank bleeding). A slight increase in a client's heart rate after surgery, due to stress response, may be normal. A cardiac monitor is also recommended for postoperative patients who have been under general anesthesia so that heart rhythm abnormalities can be diagnosed and treatment can be started immediately. Causes of postoperative cardiac dysrhythmias include hypovolemia, pain, electrolyte imbalances, hypoxemia, and acidosis. When dysrhythmias develop, the PACU nurse follows facility protocols if the disturbances are life-threatening and monitors the client's blood pressure, oxygen saturation, and ventilation.

Other: Level of consciousness, muscle strength, ability to follow commands, IV infusions, dressings, drains, and special equipment, tubes, and drains that must be immediately attached to containers or suction, reddened or bruised areas on skin unrelated to surgery (inspect pressure points and tape and skin preparation sites; look for signs of cautery or thermal burns), temperature (assist client to regain normal core body temperature or anticipate complications).

After receiving the admission report and review of the client's record, the PACU nurse documents all observations. Most PACUs use a flow-type method of charting, which includes a numerical rating scale measuring clients' respirations, level of consciousness, ability to move, body temperature or skin color, and blood pressure (see Fig. 15–9). As the client recovers from the anesthesia, the rating improves to a top score of 10.

NURSING DIAGNOSES

Nursing diagnoses most common during this period of care are *Risk for Injury, Hypothermia, Risk for Aspiration, Pain,* and *Altered Thought Processes.* Most common potential complications are respiratory problems, hypovolemia or hypervolemia, hemorrhage, and cardiac problems.

NURSING CARE IN THE POST-ANESTHESIA CARE UNIT

Protect the Airway

One major complication that occurs in the PACU is airway obstruction or hypoventilation. The primary nursing intervention to protect the airway is positioning the head of a minimally responsive client turned to the side with the chin extended forward to prevent respiratory obstruction. The client who is unable to clear mucus or vomitus from the throat requires suctioning immediately.

An oral or nasal airway may be in place to help maintain patency and control the tongue. The airway is a hollow rubber or plastic tube. It is inserted through the nose or mouth and passes over the base of the tongue to keep the tongue from falling back into the throat and obstructing the anatomic airway (Fig. 15–10). Airways should not be taped in place. When clients awaken and the gag reflex returns, they may spit out the airway. The PACU nurse may also remove the airway for the responsive client who is unable to remove it unassisted. Left in place too long, it can irritate the tissue, stimulate vomiting, or cause laryngospasm.

When the client is extubated, observe for the development of crowing respirations. The client may be experiencing laryngospasm. If this problem develops, the client could progress to respiratory arrest. Immediately try to ventilate the client using a face mask oxygen delivery system, securing a tight fit over the mouth and nose. The use of positive pressure sometimes alleviates the laryngospasm. If the spasm does not abate, succinylcholine is given to temporarily paralyze the voluntary muscles, including the muscles that control respiration. Respiration must be supported by mechanical means (i.e., a ventilator) when muscle relaxants are used. Respiration in clients who have received muscle relaxants must be closely monitored for at least 1 hour after the relaxants appear to have worn off because of the possibility of paralysis reoccurrence. Some clients remain intubated and ventilated, such as those who have undergone open heart surgery. They require close monitoring and intermittent suctioning.

The nurse also consults with the surgeon and the anesthesia provider and administers prescribed medications as needed. Interventions may also include the continued administration of oxygen, positive-pressure airway support, and use of reversal medications. Reversal agents such as naloxone (Narcan) are administered to reverse the respiratory depression from narcotics. Neostigmine with glycopyrrolate (Robinul) is given to reverse the effect of some neuromuscular blocking agents. Most clients receive oxygen. The rate flow of oxygen should be closely checked against physician orders. This may be administered by a respiratory therapist, but the nurse is responsible for assessment and monitoring of treatment. Oxygen levels will vary, depending on the method of delivery, such as nasal canula, simple face masks, or more controlled methods. Flow rates vary from 2 to 15 L/min with a positive pressure mask. Clients with COPD receive no more than 20%/2 L.

Maintain Normal Blood Pressure

Postoperative hypotension can have numerous causes, including inadequate ventilation, side effects of anesthetic agents or preoperative medications, rapid position change, pain, fluid or blood loss, and peripheral pooling of blood after regional anesthesia. A drop in blood pressure slightly below a client's preoperative baseline reading is common after surgery. However, a significant drop in blood pressure, accompanied by an increased heart rate, may indicate hemorrhage, circulatory failure, or fluid shifts. Do not diagnose impending hypovolemic shock on the basis of one low blood pressure reading. If you are concerned about a dropping blood pressure, measure pressure, every 5 minutes for 15 minutes to determine the variability. Decreased blood pressure can also mean that the anesthesia is wearing off or that the client is experiencing severe pain.

In addition to hypotension, manifestations of shock include tachycardia, restlessness and apprehension, and cold, moist, pale or cyanotic skin. When a client appears to be going into shock, the PACU nurse intervenes as follows: (1) administering oxygen or increasing its rate of delivery, (2) raising the client's legs above the level of the heart, (3) increasing the rate of IV fluids (unless contraindicated because of fluid excretion problems), (4) notifying the anesthesia provider and the surgeon, (5)

NHS **NEBRASKA**
HEALTH SYSTEM
CLARKSON HOSPITAL • UNIVERSITY HOSPITAL
A Partner with University of Nebraska Medical Center

NURSING NOTES:

Patient Identification (Stamp)

NAME

REG. NO.

LOCATION

DATE

Nurse Signatures	Nurse Initials

ALDRETE SCORE▲	Baseline	Post Recovery
Time		
ACTIVITY		
Able to move four extremities voluntarily or on command. 2		
Able to move two extremities voluntarily or on command. 1		
Unable to move extremities voluntarily or on command. 0		
RESPIRATION		
Able to deep breathe and cough freely. 2		
Dyspnea or limited breathing. 1		
Apneic. 0		
CIRCULATION		
Baseline BP		
Systolic BP +/- 20% of preanesthetic level. 2		
Systolic BP +/- 20-49% of preanesthetic level. 1		
Systolic BP +/- 50% of preanesthetic level. 0		
CONSCIOUSNESS		
Fully awake. 2		
Arousable on calling. 1		
Unresponsive. 0		
OXYGENATION		
Able to maintain O2 saturation > 92% on room air. 2		
Needs O2 inhalation to maintain saturation > 90%. 1		
O2 saturation < 90% even with O2 supplement. 0		
	TOTAL	

▲Aldrete, J.A. & Kroulik, D.J., *Clinical Anesthesia*, Vol. 7, Feb. 1995
and *Anesthesia & Analgesia*, Vol. 49, No. 6, 1970

Potential for Knowledge Deficit: Expected Outcome: Patient or Significant Other will Verbalize Understanding of Instructions.

DISCHARGE CRITERIA	N/A
☐ RX GIVEN AND EXPLAINED.	☐
☐ VITAL SIGNS STABLE_____	☐
☐ NAUSEA, VOMITING, DIZZINESS MINIMAL	☐
☐ POST ANESTHESIA RECOVERY SCORE 9-10	☐
☐ SWALLOW, COUGH AND GAG REFLEX PRESENT	☐
☐ ABSENCE OF RESPIRATORY DISTRESS	☐
☐ DRESSING CHECKED c̄ MINIMAL DRAINAGE	☐
☐ RESPONSIBLE ADULT PRESENT TO ESCORT HOME	☐
☐ ALERT AND ORIENTED	☐
☐ PAIN CONTROLLED	☐

Time discharged _____ per _____

Accompanied by _____

NHS-914 (6/99)

Potential alteration in fluid volume and/or urinary elimination
Expected outcome: Maintains fluid levels

INTAKE

IV			On	Off
Oral		Sequential Stockings		
		Support hose		
TOTAL:		Ice		

OUTPUT

Urine	
Drain	
TOTAL:	

☐ See extended Outpatient Flowsheet

IV DC'd at _____

CATHETER TIP INTACT? ☐ YES ☐ NO

Narcotic Waste____ mgs of _____ #1 _____ #2

Postoperative Phone Call:

Phone Number: _____   Date: _____ Time: _____

	Yes	No	☐ message left
Drsg dry/intact	☐	☐	Unsuccessful Attempts: _____
Nausea/Vomiting	☐	☐	Spoke With: _____
Pain	☐	☐	
Swelling	☐	☐	
Fever	☐	☐	
Voiding easily	☐	☐	☐ Unable to reach, chart
Surgeon/Anes. Contacted	☐	☐	returned to MR

Completed by _____ RN

OUTPATIENT PACU FLOWSHEET   PROCEDURES TAB

FIGURE 15−9 Post-Anesthesia care unit (PACU) documentation. (Courtesy of Nebraska Health Systems, Omaha, NE.)

providing medications as ordered, and (6) continuing to assess the client and response to interventions.

Hypertension may also develop. Older adults with a history of hypertension may exhibit hypertensive episodes after the stress of surgery. If the blood pressure rises above the baseline, the PACU nurse should consult with the anesthesia provider or the surgeon and administer antihypertensive medication as ordered.

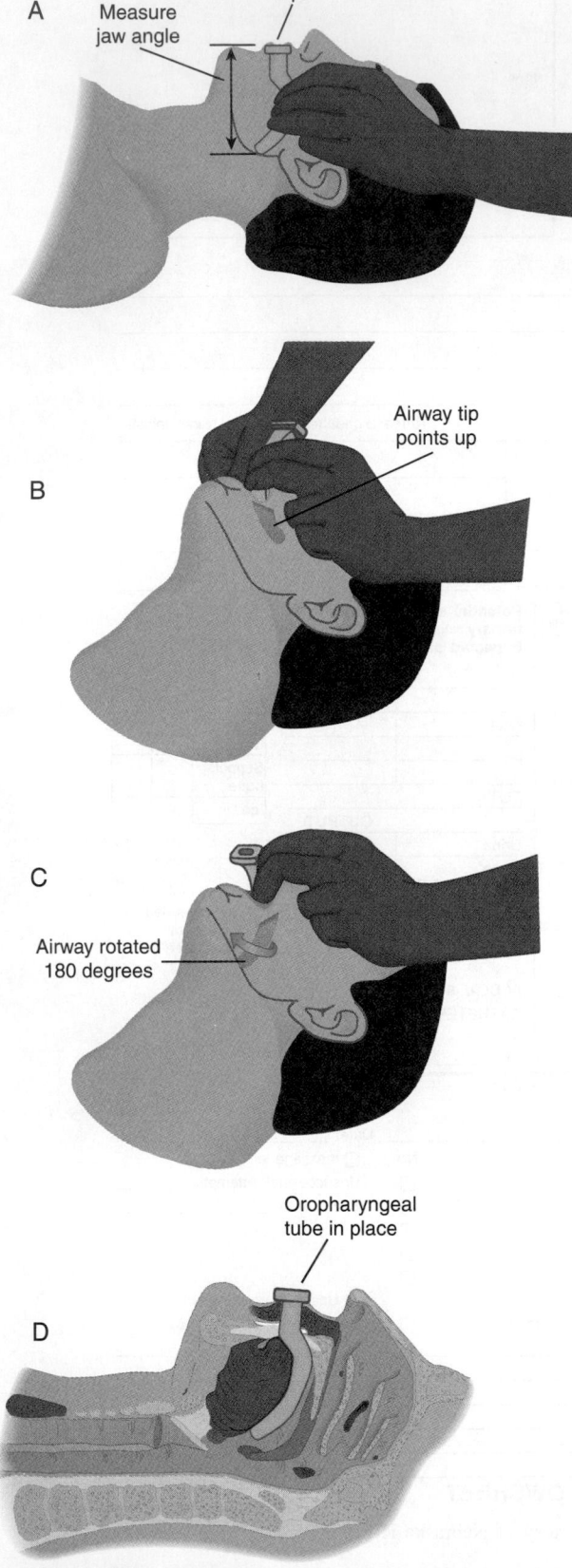

FIGURE 15–10 Artificial airway. The flattened, hollow tube prevents the tongue from falling back and occluding the natural airway.

Monitor for Return of Consciousness

The PACU nurse monitors the level of consciousness. Orientation to person is the first cognitive response to return after anesthesia. Level of orientation is assessed by noting whether the client responds to his or her name. Be certain that a client who normally wears hearing aids has them in place and turned on before you attempt to talk to the client. Orientation to place is also an important indication of postoperative return of cognitive function. Because of confusion from anesthesia and analgesia medications, the client is usually not oriented to time until after the nurse provides this information. Assessment of returning cognitive functioning includes the ability to remember facts after being told. Older adults and clients with liver or kidney impairment may take longer to regain orientation. Postoperative delirium may occur with some procedures, such as open heart surgery; therefore, do not assume that aberrations are due to age-related "senility." Rather, check the present cognitive status against that noted in the preoperative assessment to gain a truer picture of the client's level of consciousness and cognition.

Assess for Return of Sensation and Motion

In the PACU, the client is monitored carefully for return of sensation as the anesthetic agent wears off. Check return of motion to the extremities by asking clients to wiggle their toes. However, the ability to move the toes may not indicate complete recovery if client had spinal anesthesia. In such cases, the toe movement signifies that the motor blockade is wearing off, but blockade of the autonomic nervous system may still be present. Clients who are still experiencing autonomic blockade are prone to hypotension despite the presence of ability to move their toes and extremities.

Assess for Normothermia

The client in the PACU is monitored for temperature and vital signs every 15 minutes until vital signs are stable, or more often if they are unstable. The frequency of monitoring and length of time over which monitoring must be done are dictated by facility PACU policy. Clients are monitored until they are discharged from the PACU. This is usually at least 1 hour. Clients must have a minimum temperature of greater than 96.8° F (36° C) before they are discharged from the PACU. The heat loss that occurs in the operating room can continue in the PACU if the client is not warmed sufficiently. Warming requires the maintenance of temperature without overwarming and causing excessive vasodilatation, which can cause fluid shifts and a decrease in blood pressure. The PACU nurse must also realize that malignant hyperthermia can also occur in the PACU and should repeatedly assess for manifestations of this condition.

Assess Perfusion

Assessment of skin color, warmth, and turgor provides evidence of tissue perfusion. Verify skin color in clients with dark or brown skin with another nurse to avoid making incorrect assumptions. Dusky, pale, cold, moist skin is an important assessment finding that may be a manifestation of shock. Because it is not possible to detect systemic conditions by skin color alone, assessment should include other pertinent data. For example, when impending shock is suspected, check the client's blood pressure, and inspect the lips and nails as well as the skin to detect pallor or cyanosis. Consider these findings in relation to oxygen saturation and hemoglobin before assuming a diagnosis of shock.

Assess the Surgical Site
Check the dressing over the surgical incision frequently. If it is soiled, note the color, type, and amount of drainage. Reinforce the dressing, but do not change it or open it without a physician's order. If seepage is noted, draw an outline of the fluid on the dressing and note the date and time. If oozing continues, the estimation of the amount can be more easily determined by areas outside the previously marked borders. Sometimes bleeding is present but not visible on dressings. If bleeding is suspected, look for blood under the operated leg, or under the back, that may have leaked downward out of sight.

Promote Fluid and Electrolyte Balance
Assess intake and output hourly. Monitor all parenteral fluids to ensure that the proper amount and type of fluids are being infused. Intake can include solutions of IV fluids, medications, blood products, nutritional support, and colloid infusions. Check the amount of solution in the IV bottle on admission of the client to the PACU along with the rate of infusion. All types of delivery systems and lines must be considered: pumps, infusion machines, monitoring machines, IV lines, central venous lines, and arterial lines. Check the insertion sites for redness, soreness, and swelling, as these may be indications of infiltration. Note medications that have been added to solutions, so that when the next dose is ready to be infused a new bag of dilution fluid is present. This procedure ensures that there is no lapse in administration of ordered fluids or medications.

Changes in renal function and fluid and electrolyte balance may develop soon after surgery. The stress response to surgery stimulates the secretion of antidiuretic hormone (ADH) and aldosterone, which cause fluid retention. Until the stress subsides, urine volume decreases regardless of fluid intake. Avoid fluid overload while maintaining the client's blood pressure, cardiac output, and urinary output. If an indwelling bladder catheter is present, document the amount of output and compare it with the amount of input via IV fluids.

Manage Drainage Systems
Drainage tubes, such as a T-tube, gastric tube, urinary catheter, or wound drains, must be constantly monitored. For example, urinary catheters and T-tubes are unclamped and attached to gravity drainage systems. Gastric, chest, and intestinal tubes are attached to wall suction. Wound drainage systems are attached to self-contained suction devices. The PACU nurse must ensure that tubes are patent and draining freely. Check that there are no kinks in the tubes and that they are not occluded. Document the amount and characters of drainage on a regular schedule. Compare the type and amount of drainage with those expected for the surgical procedure.

Promote Comfort
Pain is an expected outcome postoperatively, yet one of the most frequent postoperative problems is inadequate analgesic administration. You must carefully and regularly assess the client's level of pain. Pain may be caused by a factor unrelated to the surgical procedure, such as

poor positioning. The discomfort of a full bladder can imitate abdominal pain even when appropriate doses of pain medication have been administered. Provide appropriate pain relief while not overmedicating. If there is any problem in making the postoperative client comfortable, call the anesthesia provider or surgeon to minimize the time the client is in pain.

Maintain Safety
Continue to be the client's advocate, and protect the client from injury that may be caused by equipment, medication, and postoperative risks. Side rails must remain in the up position to protect the client from falling out of the bed. Proper body alignment and frequent repositioning assist in maintaining circulation and relieve skin pressure. Postoperative equipment is checked to ensure that it is working properly before the client is received in the PACU. Place equipment in a safe location and electrical cords or lines out of the way so that they do not present a danger to the client or staff members.

DISCHARGE FROM THE POST-ANESTHESIA CARE UNIT
Common criteria for evaluating the client's readiness for discharge from the PACU are based on a general scoring system. The criteria that are scored include activity, respiration, circulation, consciousness, and skin color. A typical scoring system is shown in Box 15-7.

When the client is considered ready for discharge from the PACU, a report (via telephone or verbal) must be relayed to the receiving unit. The report must include the client's condition along with a summary of details of the operative procedure and events that may affect client care. Thorough documentation of the client's progress in the PACU is included in the client's permanent medical record and is an important source of information for use in providing appropriate care. If for some reason the client is to have an extended stay in the PACU, notify the family immediately, and explain the reasons for the prolonged stay.

"Same-day surgery" clients cannot be discharged until they are able to tolerate fluids by mouth, can ambulate with a steady gait and no orthostatic hypotension, and have voided. A responsible adult must accompany the client being discharged from the ambulatory care center. Taxi cabs are not an appropriate means of transportation after a surgical procedure. Discharge instructions include written and oral information. It is best if this information has been reviewed both preoperatively and postopera-

---

BOX 15-7   Criteria for Discharge from the Post-Anesthesia Care Unit (PACU)

The vital signs must be stable or at near-preoperative levels.
    Each numbered entity is scored from 0 to 3. A score of 9 or 10 usually indicates that the client is ready for transfer out of the PACU.

1. There is only moderate or light drainage from any operative site.
2. All essential postoperative care has been completed.
3. Urine output is at least 30/ml/hr for an adult.

tively. The instructions usually include information about medications, how to care for the surgical wound, the amount and type of activity that is appropriate, when and how to seek help for any problems that may arise, and when and where follow-up appointments are scheduled. The client who has had a same-day procedure is telephoned by a Registered Nurse the day after surgery to ensure that there are no complications or further questions.

■ POSTOPERATIVE NURSING CARE

After the client has been released from the PACU, the nursing assessments and interventions are similar to those performed in the PACU. The most common immediate postoperative complications are those related to spinal anesthesia and those affecting the respiratory, cardiovascular, and renal systems and fluid and electrolyte balance.

ESTABLISHMENT OF POSTOPERATIVE GOALS

At this point, the postoperative care plan is expanded and revised. The plan should include an assessment of the client's needs and goals as well as nursing interventions. Nursing diagnoses are used to specify and define postoperative problems and to guide the plan of nursing care. Findings on the preoperative assessment constitute a very important body of information at this time because the findings can be used as baseline values for comparison with those obtained in postoperative assessments. A general nursing care plan is presented. Specific assessment and care measures are often based upon the surgical procedure performed and the preoperative condition of the client.

ASSESSMENT OF THE POSTOPERATIVE CLIENT
Assess Respiratory Status

Assess for a patent airway. Observe the client and assess the breathing pattern at rest. Listen to sounds; breath respirations should be unlabored and quiet. As a result of effects of general anesthetic agents and narcotics, respiratory drive and depth may be reduced, leading to hypoxia. Clinical manifestations of hypoxia include restlessness, pale skin, pulse oximetry readings below 90%, and cool skin temperature. Although restlessness is an early sign of hypoxia, there may be other causes such as pain. Cyanosis is a very late manifestation of hypoxia.

A major complication following surgery may be decreased lung expansion, atelectasis (collapse of alveolar sacs), or aspiration of retained secretions. Lung assessment should include auscultation in all lobes as well as assessment of rate and rhythm of respirations. For many clients, incentive spirometry (Fig. 15–11) is prescribed to increase respiratory expansion and to open the alveoli. A body temperature of greater than 100° F (37.7 C) in the first 24 hours after surgery is frequently due to atelectasis.

Assess Circulation

Assess vital signs, skin color, and temperature according to facility protocols. Vital signs are assessed frequently (e.g., every 30 minutes). Reassure the client that this pattern of assessment is a matter of routine and does not indicate anything is wrong. Because the client has been immobile during the operation and may have experienced pressure on body parts that diminished circulation, extremities must be evaluated for weakness, circulation, and numbness. Bony prominences should be assessed for

stage I pressure ulcers (see Chapter 49). Although all clients must be encouraged to get out of bed and walk as soon as possible after surgery to prevent the formation of thrombus and devastating emboli, early ambulation is especially important after surgery of the abdominal area. The aorta and femoral arteries may have been manipulated during the procedure. In addition, the client may find that the dorsal recumbent position (as in a recliner chair) is most comfortable because it reduces strain on the incision. However, this position slows venous return in the pelvis and can foster thrombus formation.

Thrombus can form in any blood vessel, and you should be especially alert to any complaints of extremity pain, unilateral edema, or warmth in the calf. If the thrombus dislodges and travels via the bloodstream, it can lodge anywhere in the body, producing emergency conditions that need to be treated immediately. It is obvious when a clot suddenly lodges in the lung, heart, or brain, but embolism in other body sites may be less apparent. Walking can nullify much of the threat of thrombus formation. However, most clients do not want to move after surgery. Leg exercises should have been taught preoperatively, and you should emphasize their importance in the prevention of thrombus formation to promote an optimal postsurgical outcome.

Assess Neurologic Status

Assess the client for level of consciousness, orientation, and lingering effects of anesthesia in the first 24 hours. In older adults, cognitive deficits may remain for days or even weeks after surgery. Compare present mental status with preoperative ability to clearly define the client's neurologic status. Medications are slower to clear through aging kidneys, and hypothermia and pain can also affect

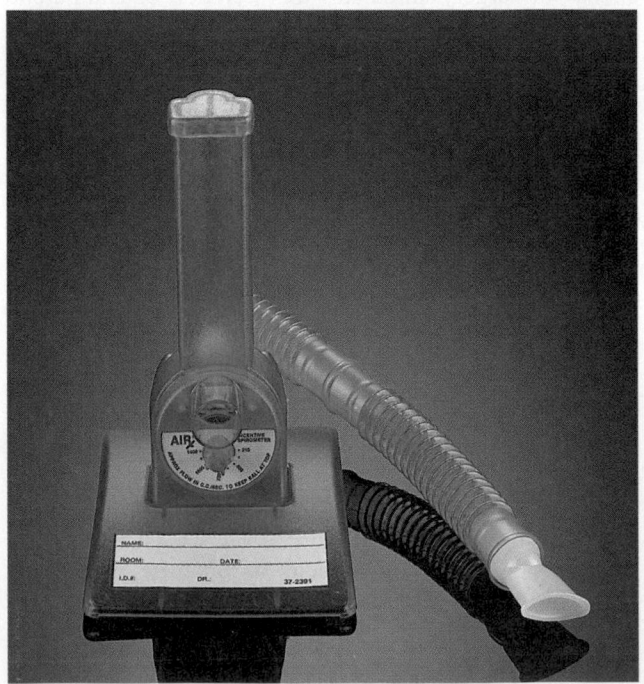

FIGURE 15–11 Use of an incentive deep-breathing exerciser promotes alveolar inflation, restores and maintains lung capacity, and strengthens the respiratory muscles. (Courtesy of Baxter Healthcare Corporation, Roond Lake, IL.)

cognition. Clients need to know that impaired cognition is to be expected—especially older clients, in whom the fear of dementia may be marked. If they are not aware that the condition is temporary, clients may believe that they have had a stroke during surgery from which they will never recover. This in turn can lead to depression with decreased coping ability. Nurses can facilitate recovery by promoting cognitive activity, repeating instructions often if needed, having patience with clients slow in recovery, and fostering hope. Document changes every shift. If a decrease in cognition appears, notify the physician immediately. Most common is the slow steady progress in return to preoperative status.

Obese clients also have a delayed return of consciousness after anesthetic procedures. Greater amounts of anesthetic agents are required for these clients. Anesthetic agents are fat-soluble, and much of the drug dose is deposited from the blood into fatty tissue. In obesity, therefore, excretion of anesthetic agents is slower because of the increased amounts of drug retained before excretion.

Monitor the Wound

Assess the dressing and the amount and character of any drainage that is present. Be alert to the method of care that the surgeon prefers. Most surgeons prefer to do the first dressing change. Some surgeons leave the original surgical dressing intact for 24 to 48 hours. Others request that the dressing be changed as it becomes soiled. If the wound is closed and left to heal by first intention, dressings on the wound may be minimal, and the client may be allowed to shower after 24 hours. If the wound healing is to be by second or third intention, then it is left open to heal from the fascia to the skin, and special wound handling must occur. Measures can include wound packing, dressings, drains, ostomy bags, and so on, depending on wound size, and location and drainage from the wound. Measure and record the amount of drainage for comparison with later assessments to guide future care plan changes (see Chapter 16).

Each client must have an individualized care plan to facilitate the most effective healing. Document the wound's appearance, drainage, and client's reports of discomfort at least every shift. If you are in doubt of how to describe the wound, it is suggested that two nurses compare observations at each change of shift.

Although it is commonplace for nurses to look at wounds, the appearance of the surgical wound is frightening to many clients. It sometimes takes days before a client can even look at the wound. Assess the client's willingness to look at the wound. Do not force the client to look at the wound until he or she is ready. Look for subtle cues—for example, the client may continue to look away from the wound while dressings are being changed. Body image is altered in response to surgery, even surgery on internal organs. Body image reintegration or restoration requires weeks or months to occur. Show acceptance of the client's appearance, and assist the client in verbalizing feelings about the postoperative appearance and the reaction of others.

If wound infection develops, the clinical manifestations appear in the wound 3 to 4 days postoperatively. Clinical manifestations include redness beyond the incision line, edema that remains after the initial swelling, increasing pain, and increased drainage. Sometimes drainage becomes purulent or foul-smelling. The client may also have fever, malaise, anorexia, and leukocytosis (increased WBC count with increased numbers of band WBCs). Notify the surgeon of any suspected wound infection. Wound cultures may be ordered to verify that organisms in the wound are sensitive to the antibiotics taken.

If collagen fibers are not mature enough to hold the incision closed without suture, the wound may open. An opening of a skin wound is called *dehiscence*. Wounds in which dehiscence has occurred are treated as open wounds—that is, they are kept clean, with application of packing or dressings and allowed to heal by secondary or tertiary intention (see Chapter 16).

If abdominal wounds become infected and the abdominal incision opens, the fascia or internal organs may be visible (Fig. 15–12). This condition is called *evisceration* and constitutes an emergency. Return the client to bed. Do not attempt to replace the organs. Cover the wound with sterile dressings moistened with normal saline. Monitor the client's vital signs, keep the client as calm as possible, and notify the surgeon immediately for emergency surgery. In many clients, evisceration is preceded by a gush of serosanguineous drainage about 48 hours earlier. Notify the surgeon of this sudden increase in drainage, and plan to put an abdominal binder on the client's body for support.

Clients must learn to care for any dressing before discharge, so education must be a written intervention in the care plan on admission to the nursing unit. Training should proceed daily until the client or a family member feels comfortable with the wound care skills necessary to promote healing.

Routine care of drains and dressings can be delegated to trained unlicensed assistive personnel. See the Management and Delegation feature.

Monitor Intravenous Lines

All IV lines must be checked for patency, type of fluid to be infused, and rate. For any client with an IV line, intake and output monitoring must be completed. This is a nursing decision; although there may be a physician's routine order, none is required to monitor the client. If

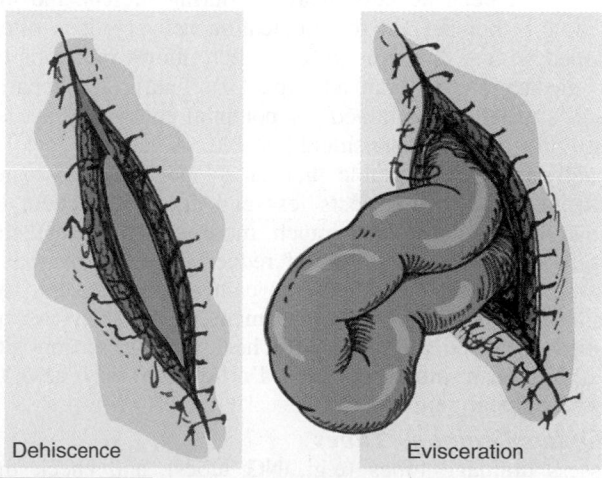

Dehiscence   Evisceration

FIGURE 15–12 Clients with wound dehiscence and evisceration after surgery require immediate attention (see text).

MANAGEMENT AND DELEGATION

Postoperative Care: Dressings and Drains

The assessment and care of postoperative wounds, including drain management and dressing changes, are your responsibility. The emptying, measurement, and recording of drainage from a postoperative wound may be delegated to unlicensed assistive personnel who have demonstrated competence in performing this task; the removal and application of some dressings may also be delegated to such personnel with special training competence.

Before delegating the care of postoperative dressings and drains, consider the type of surgical procedure performed, the extent of the wound and dressing care requirements, and the nature of the drainage and type of drain present.

Drains

1. Initially, assess the quality, character, and volume of the drainage expressed via the drain. At this time, note the patency of the drain and any leakage of fluid at the drain insertion site.
2. Ensure that the drain is secured and labeled properly. Your documentation should reflect the appropriate labeling. For example, for a client having two abdominal drains (one a right upper quadrant drain and the second a midline drain) list these as such on the output record. The drains may be labeled by name or location, at the time of placement by the physician.
3. Record the volume of drainage from each drain separately unless otherwise noted by the physician.
4. Perform the irrigation of any drain as ordered.
5. Specify the frequency with which the drain is to be emptied for the assistive personnel. A frequency of every 4 hours or once per shift may be delegated, whereas you may choose to perform more frequent measurement and recording of drainage as appropriate. For example, you might best perform hourly drain emptying with subsequent intravenous (IV) fluid re-

placement of the volume measured, which requires an hourly adjustment in the IV infusion rate.

6. Perform the assessment for air leak at intervals throughout your shift. Chest tube drainage may be measured and recorded by assistive personnel.

Dressings

1. In many institutions, the physician changes the initial postoperative dressing.
2. Assistive personnel may perform subsequent dressing changes if the wound is closed and does not require special intervention. The physician orders the type and frequency of dressing changes.
3. Delegate the dressing change to assistive personnel after your assessment of the wound. It may also be appropriate to have the assistive personnel remove the dressing in preparation for your assessment and then reapply the dressing after you examine the wound. (*Note:* A Registered Nurse should assess any wound at least once per day, more frequently as guided by the type of wound and required intervention.)
4. Specify the type of dressing (clean or sterile) for assistive personnel.

Describe findings immediately reportable to you for the assistive personnel, including changes in the color, character, and quantity of the drainage from a drain or around a drain site. Additionally, any sign of redness, swelling, tenderness, warmth, pain, bleeding, discharge, or separation of wound edges is reportable. The finding of new drainage or blood on a postoperative dressing is immediately reportable to the Registered Nurse.

In summary, even though you have delegated the completion of these tasks, you remain responsible for assessment and evaluation of the client's postoperative wound and drains. Verify the competency of the assistive personnel in performing each of these tasks during orientation and annually thereafter.

Donna W. Markey, MSN, RN, ACNP-CS, *Clinician IV, Surgical Services, University of Virginia Health System, Charlottesville, Virginia*

there have been no complications during surgery and the IV line is not needed for medication delivery, it is often capped with a "heparin lock," which allows infusions of IV medications without additional IV fluids. The heparin lock is usually maintained for potential emergency access until the client is considered stable. A heparin lock is usually more comfortable than an IV port attached to an infusion line. It also costs less and allows the client to move around and walk much more easily. Assess the insertion site for any signs of redness, swelling, or pain. If any problems are noted, the catheter may have to be removed from the vein; replacement may or may not be indicated. Application of mild heat to an insertion site that has been infiltrated with IV solution may help to decrease local pain.

Monitor Drainage Tubes

Assess drainage tubes (e.g., NG tubes), and check the client's postoperative physician's instructions to determine

whether to attach the tubes to suction or to use gravity drainage. Note the amount, color, and consistency of drainage, and document the findings. If the client has a low-suction NG tube, it must remain patent. Irrigate the tube with normal saline according to the surgeon's orders; some tubes cannot be irrigated because of increased risk of injuring internal sutures. Make sure the tube is connected to suction if ordered.

If the tube has a dual lumen and if one side is for air, do not insert medication through the air vent. Medication can easily occlude this port. If the port gurgles, do not plug the port to quiet the system. By plugging up the air vent, the suction system becomes a closed system, thereby increasing the suction on the wall of the stomach, which can cause trauma and bleeding. NG tubes inserted for decompression and removal of intestinal secretions remain in place until peristalsis begins. The removal of an NG tube requires an order by the surgeon. Assess for oral pain medication is administered. IV medications should control pain within 5 to 10 minutes. It is usually the nurse who determines whether the client is obtaining a sufficient dose of medication, whether pain is being controlled, or whether it is causing side effects such as nausea and vomiting. Communicating these details to the physician allows for a change to best suit the client's needs, leading to a positive outcome for pain relief. It is vital that pain be managed if the client is to comply with instructions for coughing, deep breathing, and ambulation. Chapter 23 addresses pain and pain management.

Reduce Nausea and Vomiting

Postoperative nausea and vomiting (PONV) do not occur frequently; however, the surgical experience for those clients with PONV will remain uniquely unpleasant. Vomiting is a reflex, and the reflex is stimulated in many ways. Stimuli can arise from gastrointestinal tract distention on irritation, vagal stimulation, centers in the cerebrum, the chemoreceptor trigger zone (CTZ) located in the floor of the fourth ventricle in the brain, rotation or disequilibrium of the vestibular labyrinths of the ear, increased intracranial pressure, pain, or sensory perceptions (such as the sight of blood or an odor or a taste). Several medications stimulate the CTZ, including morphine, meperidine, cardiac glycosides, and amphetamines.

Risk factors are shown in Table 15–12. PONV can be prevented by reducing movement, controlling pain, and early intervention with antiemetics. Several categories of medications are used to control PONV and include (1) anticholinergics and histamine type 1 (H_1) receptor an-

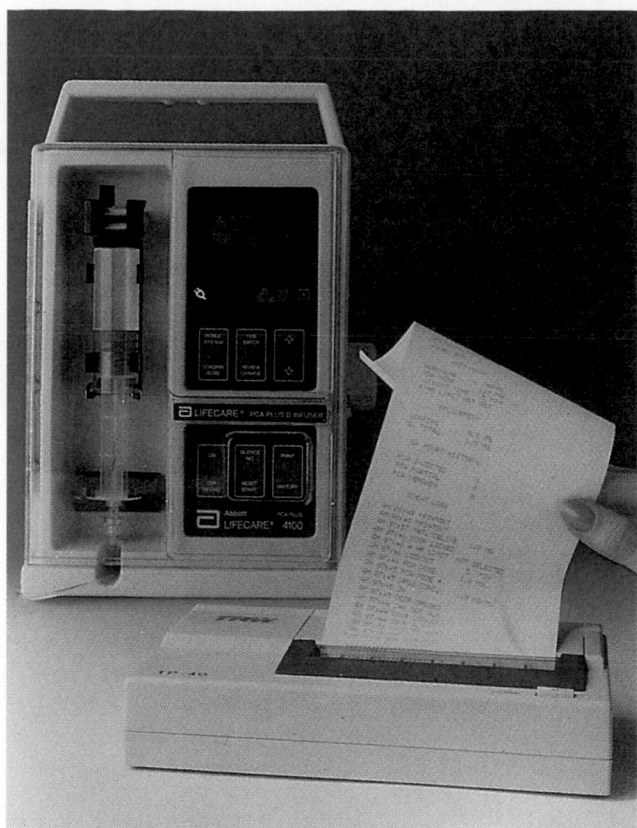

FIGURE 15–13 A patient-controlled anesthesia (PCA) device allows clients to control their own pain relief postoperatively. The printout allows the nurse to assess and record the amount of opioid analgesia. (Courtesy of Abbott Laboratories, Hospital Products Division, North Chicago, IL.)

bowel sounds, passage of flatus, and hunger as signs of peristalsis as long as the tube is in place. When peristalsis returns, the physician will probably order the NG tube to be clamped initially and then removed if the clamping was tolerated without nausea or vomiting.

Promote Comfort

All clients who have just had surgery will experience pain. Pain medication should be given when needed and before the pain becomes severe. When the "demand approach" (prn meds) is used for analgesia, it is crucial to medicate the client at the onset of the pain. When pain becomes too severe, more medication and a longer time are needed for the medication to take effect. Clients may return to the surgical unit with a patient-controlled analgesia (PCA) device for pain medication administration (Fig. 15–13). Repeat instructions on how to use the device, and assure the client that a "lock-out" function prevents inadvertent overdosing.

Document the date and time of the medication, the amount given, and the route of administration. Also include a description of the pain the client is experiencing and the effectiveness of the pain medication in controlling it. Consider the time to onset of medication effect in determining when evaluation of pain control should be assessed. For example, reassess the client 30 minutes after

TABLE 15–12	RISK FACTORS FOR POSTOPERATIVE NAUSEA AND VOMITING

Client Factors
  Ambulation
  Bowel obstruction/ileus
  Female gender
  History of motion sickness
  History of vomiting with previous anesthetic procedure
  Hypoglycemia
  Hypotension
  Obesity
  Swallowed blood
  Uncontrolled pain
  Young age

Type of Surgery
  Eye
  Intra-abdominal
  Intracranial
  Laparoscopic
  Middle ear
  Testicular

Medications
  Anticholinesterases
  Etomidate
  Isoflurane
  Nitrous oxide?
  Pentothal
  Propofol
  Regional anesthetics above T5 spinal level

tagonists, which reduce excitability of the labyrinth receptors; (2) antidopaminergic drugs, which depress the CTZ; and (3) gastrointestinal antispasmodics, which promote forward peristaltic movement. PONV has also been controlled with acupuncture.

DISCHARGE INSTRUCTIONS AND CARE

Regardless of the length of stay in the hospital or surgical center, when the client is ready to go home, ensure that the client and a family member as appropriate have the information and skills needed to continue a successful recovery. Teach skills over a period of days, with ample time for questions and "hands-on" practice. Give all information in writing to the client or family members. Most institutions provide a printed form filled out with specific postoperative information, such as instructions on medications and wound care, an appointment for a postoperative clinic visit, and names and telephone numbers in case there are further questions or an emergency arises. Drug prescriptions are also provided if medications are to be continued at home.

If the client has further health care needs after discharge, collaborate with other health care workers such as those in social services, home nursing (see Bridge to Home Health Care: Recovering from Surgery), or rehabilitation services. Many resources are available in the community for clients, and most institutions have a list for the local area. Determine the resources available in your community for the clients that you care for, what each provides, and how they are contacted. A partial listing of the most common resources follows:

- Child Protection Services
- Emergency social services or hospital social services
- Emergency legal assistance
- Hospice
- Local chapters of organizations offering help (e.g., American Cancer Society, American Heart Association, American Diabetes Association)
- Local mastectomy, laryngectomy, or colostomy support groups
- Local senior citizens assistance program
- Medic Alert Foundation
- Local sexual assault center (by law, suspected sexual abuse of minors must be reported)
- Malignant Hyperthermia Hotline
- Substance abuse treatment programs or groups
- Visiting Nurse Association or home health care services

BRIDGE TO HOME HEALTH CARE

Recovering from Surgery

An 80-year-old man is discharged from 1-day surgery in stable condition after an inguinal hernia repair. Before discharge, he is given postoperative instructions. Because he is elderly and lives alone, his physician orders a home care consultation.

On your initial visit to the client's home, you perform an assessment that includes physical, environmental, and psychosocial status. As you review the client's discharge instructions, you realize that his vision is impaired. He cannot read the instructions without help. Although he was told to take his temperature twice daily, he cannot read the thermometer. The client is on a regular diet but has little food in his house. He tells you that he recently stopped driving because of poor vision and depends on neighbors for transportation, including trips to the grocery store. He was instructed to see his physician in 1 week but is not sure how he will get to the office. The client says the doctor told him to call if there was drainage from his surgical incision; he is not sure what that means.

Before you leave, you review all of the postoperative instructions with the client to be sure that he understands them. You change his dressing and note serosanguineous drainage at the surgical site. You show him the drainage and explain that he should call you if it increases or changes color. You contact a neighbor, who agrees to take his temperature every morning and record it. You also telephone Meals-on-Wheels to have food delivered to the client's home. Most important, you tell the client that you will be back to see him tomorrow and you leave a phone number for him to call if he needs a nurse.

This client's case reflects the variety of issues that can arise during recovery from surgery at home and also illustrates the benefits of home care services in this setting. For the client to qualify for home care, certain guidelines must be followed. Medicare guidelines have required that clients be homebound and require skilled, intermittent care. Payer sources require medical orders for home care; most third-party payers require preauthorization for services.

The primary goals for the home care nurse are:

- To assess and prevent postoperative complications
- To instruct the client or the caregiver
- To assist the client in achieving an optimal level of wellness and functioning

In assessing the postoperative client, ascertain the following:

- Does the client understand the postoperative instructions?
- Does the client need specific equipment, such as a walker or dressings?
- Does the client have prescribed medications and know how to use them?
- If a special diet is ordered, can the client get the food needed for the diet?
- Does the client have needs for skilled care such as wound care or intravenous administration? Can the client or the caregiver be taught to perform this care?
- Does the client understand the prescribed level of activity?

You can help the client learn and cope during the postoperative recovery period.

Deborah L. Bayliss, RN, MS, *Community Nurse Case Manager, Poudre Valley Health System, Fort Collins, Colorado*

CONCLUSIONS

The nurse plays a critical role in the perioperative care of the client. Today, surgery ranges from outpatient procedures to complex inpatient procedures. No matter what type of surgery is performed, however, the client needs expert nursing care. The quality of nursing care can determine whether the client has a successful perioperative experience.

THINKING CRITICALLY

1. **A young adult client in the emergency department has acute appendicitis. Surgery is scheduled in 30 minutes. What teaching should be completed before the client has the surgery? What interventions must be completed before the client is taken to the operating area?**

Factors to Consider. What important client teaching is completed before any surgery in which general anesthesia is used? Are possible complications discussed at the time? What measures usually appear on a preoperative checklist?

2. **An elderly client has undergone major abdominal surgery under general anesthesia. At age 80 years, she is in relatively good health following a cerebrovascular accident about 8 years ago. Her only medication is a 325-mg aspirin tablet taken once a day. What complications are most likely in an 80-year-old client? How can these complications be prevented? How is pain tolerated by the older client?**

Factors to Consider. What complications are associated with general anesthesia? How do a thorough history and assessment help you in your plan to prevent complications after surgery? What age-related considerations must be made? Does the use of aspirin increase the risk of any complications?

BIBLIOGRAPHY

1. Acute Pain Management Guideline Panel. (1992). *Acute pain management in adults. Operative procedures.* AHCPR Pub. No. 92-0019. Rockville, MD: Agency for Health Care Policy and Research, Public Health Service, U.S. Department of Health and Human Services.
2. *AORN standards, recommended practices, and guidelines.* (2000). Denver: Association of Perioperative Nurses, Int.
3. Alves, S. L., & Deisering, L. F. (1996). Cardiovascular changes associated with aging: The anesthetic implications. *CRNA: The Clinical Forum for Nurse Anesthetists, 7*(1), 2–8.
4. Badgwell, J. M. (1996). The postanesthesia care unit: A high-risk environment for bloodborne and infectious respiratory pathogens. *Journal of Post Anesthesia Nursing, 11*(2), 66–70.
5. Beerman, C. M. (1997). The nurse's role in bioethics. *AORN Journal, 65*(5), 923–926.
6. Bogart, J. (1998). *Legal nurse consulting: Principles and practice.* American Association of Legal Nursing Consultants. Boca Raton, FL: CRC Press.
7. Britt, B., Joy, N., & Mackay, M. (1998). Anesthesia related trauma caused by patient malpositioning. In N. Gravenstein & R. Kirby,
(Eds.), *Complications of anesthesiology* (2nd ed., pp. 3654–3689). Philadelphia, W.B. Saunders,
8. Carpenito, L. J. (1999). *Nursing care plans and documentation: Nursing diagnosis and collaborative problems* (3rd ed.). Philadelphia: Lippincott.
9. Cericola, S. A. (1998). Management. Understanding informed consent. *Plastic Surgical Nursing, 18*(4), 249–251.
10. Chiarella, M. (1998). Legal and ethical issues in perioperative nursing. The nurse's responsibility for the swab and instrument count. *AORN Journal, 11*(1), 39–41.
11. Davila, Y. (1999). Cultural considerations in perioperative nursing. *Seminars in Perioperative Nursing, 8*(3), 128–136.
12. Davidhizar, R., Bechtel, G., & Giger, J. N. (1998). When your client in the surgical suite is Mexican American. *Today's Surgical Nurse, 20*(6), 29–35.
13. Dodd, F. (1996). Under pressure . . . pressure area care in theatre. *British Journal of Theatre Nursing, 6*(9), 33–35.
14. Dunn, D. (1997). Malignant hyperthermia. *AORN Journal, 65*(4), 767–776.
15. Fairchild, S. (1996). *Perioperative nursing: Principles and practice* (2nd ed). Boston: Little, Brown.
16. Fortner, P. (1998). Preoperative patient preparation: Psychological and educational aspects. *Seminars in Perioperative Nursing, 7*(1), 3–9.
17. Girard, N. (2000). Care of the geriatric patient. In M. L. Phippen & M. P. Wells (Eds.), *Patient care during operative and invasive procedures* (pp. 675–695). Philadelphia: W. B. Saunders.
18. Girard, N. (1997). Gerontological nursing in acute care settings. In M. A. Matteson, E. S. McConnell, & A. D. Linton (Eds.), *Gerontological nursing: Concepts and practice* (2nd ed., pp. 855–895). Philadephia: W. B. Saunders.
19. Girard, N. (1997). Preoperative assessment. *Nurse Practitioner Forum, 8*(4), 140–146.
20. Groah, L. K. (1996). *Perioperative nursing* (3rd ed.). Norwalk, CT: Appleton & Lange.
21. Hodson, D. M. (1998). The evolving role of advanced practice nurses in surgery. *AORN Journal, 67*(5), 998–1006, 1008–1009.
22. Ibarra, V., et al. (1997). Clinical pathways in the perioperative setting. *Nursing Case Management, 2*(3), 97–106.
23. Keller, C. (1999). The obese patient as surgical risk. *Seminars in Perioperative Nursing, 8*(3), 109–117.
24. Keller, K. (1997). The role of advanced practice nurses in surgical services. *AORN Journal, 67*(1), 16.
25. Klein, J. N. (1996). Future gazing. Perioperative case management—2001. *Surgical Services Management, 2*(1) 51.
26. McLeskey, S. W., & Korniewicz, D. M. (1998). Understanding latex allergy. *Seminars in Perioperative Nursing, 7*(4), 206–215.
27. Meeker, M. H., & Rothrock, J. C. (1995). *Alexander's care of the client in surgery* (10th ed.). St. Louis: Mosby–Year Book.
28. Murphy, J. M. (1999). Preoperative considerations with herbal medicines. *AORN Journal, 69*(1), 173, 175, 177–178.
29. Poe, D., et al. (1997). Implementation of the RN first assistant role. *AORN Journal, 65*(1), 32–44.
30. Pryor, F. (1997). Practical innovations. Key concepts in informed consent for perioperative nurses. *AORN Journal, 65*(6), 1105–1107, 1109–1110.
31. Ronk, L. (1998). Monitored anesthesia care is not synonymous with low risk. *Seminars in Perioperative Nursing, 7*(1), 54–57.
32. Rothrock, J. C. (1996). *Perioperative nursing care planning* (2nd ed.). St. Louis: Mosby–Year Book.
33. Ruzicka, S. (1997). The impact of normal aging processes and chronic illness on perioperative care of the elderly. *Seminars in Perioperative Nursing, 6*(1) 3–13.
34. Sabiston, D. C. (1997). *Textbook of surgery: The biological basis of modern surgical practice* (15th ed.). Philadelphia: W. B. Saunders.
35. Thompson, H. J. (1999). The management of postoperative nausea and vomiting. *Journal of Advanced Nursing, 29*(5), 1130–1136.
36. Vermette, E. (1998). Emergency! Malignant hyperthermia. *American Journal of Nursing, 98*, 45.
37. Williams, G. D. (1997). Preoperative assessment and health history interview. *Nursing Clinics of North America, 32*(2), 395–416.
38. Williams, H., & Reeves, F. (1998) Anesthetic techniques and positioning: Implications for perioperative nurses. *Seminars in Perioperative Nursing, 7*(1), 14–20.

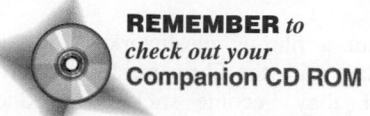

CHAPTER 16

Clients with Wounds: Promoting Positive Outcomes

Joyce M. Black

NURSING OUTCOMES CLASSIFICATION (NOC) for Nursing Diagnoses—Clients with Wounds

Impaired Skin Integrity
Tissue Integrity: Skin and Mucous Membranes
Wound Healing: Primary Intention
Wound Healing: Secondary Intention

Healing is a fundamental property of living tissue. If healing did not occur, all species would eventually become extinct. Unfortunately, many health care practices seem to lack respect for this critical attribute of healing and accept the process as passive, inevitable, and unimprovable. Popular literature assumes that if people survive, they heal, and if people are healthy, they heal.

Healing activities have always formed the basis of nursing practice. Florence Nightingale defined the nursing role as preparing the patient for the most favorable conditions for healing. Nurses today still serve as a crucial link in the process of wound healing. Nurses educate clients about disease management and wound care and support them through the physical and psychological processes of healing.

This chapter focuses on tissue injury and repair. Tissue injury is common and is seen in clients who sustain trauma as well as those who have undergone surgery. Because tissue injury is common, the body is well equipped with mechanisms of defense and healing. Defense mechanisms include intact skin and mucous membranes, phagocytes, and the immune and inflammatory responses (see Unit 16 review). In this chapter, the discussion is limited to wound healing in general. Specific information on types of wounds can be found in other chapters: diabetic foot ulcers, in Chapter 45, pressure ulcers, in Chapter 49; and venous stasis ulcers, in Chapter 53.

NORMAL WOUND HEALING

Wound healing has been defined as "a complex and dynamic process that results in the restoration of anatomic continuity and function."[12] Wound healing is a continuous sequence of signals and responses during which several cells come together outside of their usual domains, interact, perform their tasks, and having done so, resume their normal functions. Healing, specifically wound healing, is a process.

Healed wounds constitute a spectrum of repair. An *ideally healed* wound is one that has returned to normal anatomic structure, function, and appearance. In humans, this degree of healing can occur only in epidermal tissue or mucous membrane. Once there is injury through the dermis, normal appearance cannot return because scar tissue replaces missing dermis and epidermis. On the other end of the spectrum, a *minimally healed* wound has anatomic continuity (the wound has closed) but does not have sustained functional result. Hence, the wound may recur. Between these two extremes of healing, an *acceptably healed* wound is characterized by restoration of sustained function and anatomic continuity.[12] The type of wound and the intrinsic and extrinsic environments determine the timeliness of wound healing.

The type of injury has considerable influence on the form of repair. Clean approximated incisions heal with minimal synthesis of new tissue and barely test a client's resources. In sharp contrast, major burn wounds require complete regeneration of tissue and stimulate massive responses from all body systems to sustain life. The location of the wound also influences healing. Perineal wounds are likely to become infected, wounds over joints are subject to motion and therefore increased scarring, and wounds in peripheral areas or those that do not receive adequate blood supply heal slowly.

Wound healing is most apparent on the skin but occurs in all areas of the body. Bones, tendons, organs, and tissues all heal by regenerating cells to restore function. The most favorable outcome of healing is the complete return to normal structure and function. Such an outcome is possible if tissue damage is minor, no complications occur, and the destroyed tissues can regenerate. Body tissues have varying capabilities for regeneration. For example, mucous membrane is completely regenerated. Deep skin injury regenerates with a scar, which restores only a barrier. It has been thought that the central nervous system (CNS) cannot regenerate its damaged cells. Although new information is challenging that belief, today the knowledge does not exist to promote CNS tissue regeneration. It is still assumed that damaged tissues in the CNS are repaired with scar tissue, but they cannot be regenerated to regain their original function.

■ PHASES OF WOUND HEALING

Regardless of the cause of the wound, healing follows a predictable course. Events can be described in four phases:

- Vascular response
- Inflammation
- Proliferation or resolution
- Maturation, or reconstruction

At the time of injury, many actions occur simultaneously. The course is depicted in Figure 16–1.

VASCULAR RESPONSE PHASE

Within seconds after an injury, regardless of the type, blood vessels constrict to stop bleeding and reduce exposure to bacteria. Smooth muscle in the arterial walls contracts to reduce blood flow. The clotting process begins. Platelets, activated by the injury, aggregate to form a clot and stop bleeding. At the same time, the plasma protein

system begins to form a fibrous meshwork. When the platelets come in contact with the fibrin meshwork across the open vessel wall, they become sticky and adhere (aggregate) to the fibers, forming a plug. This meshwork of clotted blood and serum covers the wound while it heals and prevents further loss of blood and plasma. Platelets also release chemicals that promote clotting, such as adenosine diphosphate (ADP), to attract other platelets and a type of prostaglandin that activates other platelets. Platelets also release growth factors to stimulate healing (see later discussion).

Capillaries dilate 10 to 30 minutes after injury and remain dilated for some time because of serotonin released by the platelets. Capillary dilation allows the ingress of plasma. Plasma dilutes toxins secreted by the organisms, brings nutrients necessary for tissue repair, and carries phagocytes into the area. In addition, when the vessels dilate, the flow of blood slows and extra blood and oxygen are brought into the injured area. The capillary dilation causes the classic signs of warmth and redness seen with inflammation.

INFLAMMATION PHASE

Inflammation, the second phase of wound healing, involves a series of physiologic responses to tissue injury induced by trauma or a foreign object. It is nonspecific and occurs after every injury. The inflammatory response is essential for the repair and restoration of the structure and function of damaged tissues. The mustering of the inflammatory response is so necessary to healing that it is commonly said, "no inflammation, no healing."

The inflammatory response occurs *whenever* injury has occurred. Cellular injury can occur from trauma, oxygen or nutrient deprivation, chemical agents, microorganism invasion, temperature extremes, or ionizing radiation. Inflammation also occurs when dead cells are present. Inflammation begins at the moment of injury and may ex-

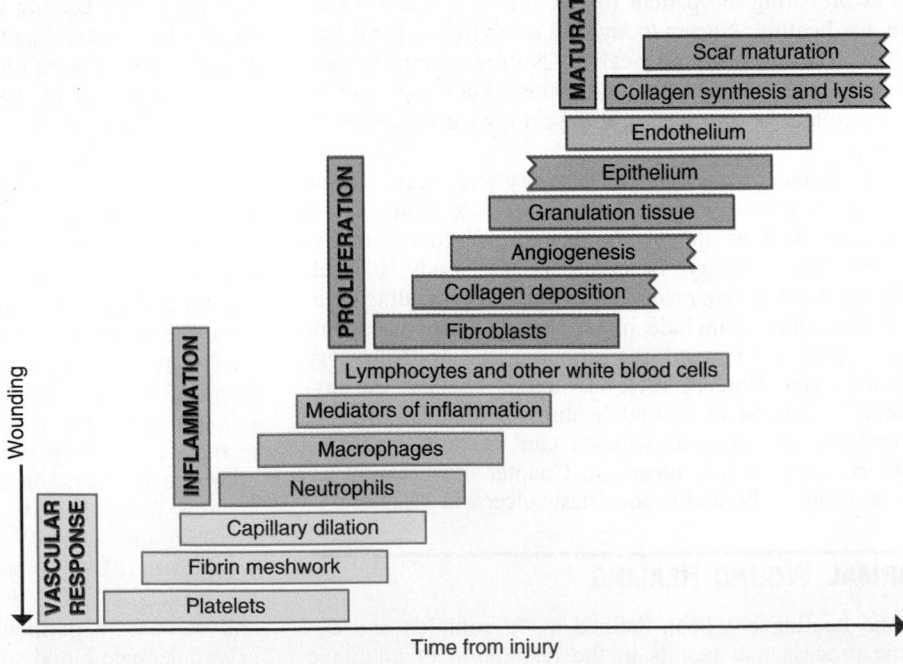

FIGURE 16–1 Normal wound healing. Wound healing proceeds through four phases: (1) the vascular response, (2) inflammation, (3) proliferation of cells to heal the wound, and (4) maturation of the wound. There are many components of each step. The jagged edge depicts an ongoing process. (Adapted from Cohen, I., et al. (Eds.). [1992]. *Wound healing.* Philadelphia: W. B. Saunders.)

tend for 4 to 6 days, depending on the extent of the injury. Inflammation is prolonged in infected wounds or wounds with necrotic tissues.

Thus, inflammation is important for healing. Unfortunately, health care terminology uses the word *inflamed* to describe the wound that is not healing normally. Do not be confused between the normal process of inflammation and the term "inflamed" to mean exaggerated inflammation. Recognize inflammation as an expected response to tissue injury, not necessarily a pathologic process.

Although inflammation can cause additional tissue injury, it is an adaptation to injury. The purpose of inflammation is to limit the effects of harmful bacteria or injury by destroying or neutralizing the organism and by limiting its spread throughout the body. The inflammatory response thereby sets up proper conditions to promote tissue repair. Unlike the *immune response,* which is slow and deliberate, using a system of specific antibodies, the effects of inflammation are immediate.

During the inflammation phase, the white blood cells (WBCs) become active to clean up the wound and initiate further healing processes. We now look closely at these WBCs and the process of phagocytosis (see Understanding Inflammation and Its Treatment).

Role of White Blood Cells

NEUTROPHILS. Neutrophils are vital defense mechanisms because they are both the first and most numerous cell types to arrive at any area of disease or injury. Within 6 hours after release from bone marrow, neutrophils migrate into tissues, where they survive for 4 to 5 days. Their role, along with tissue macrophages, is to

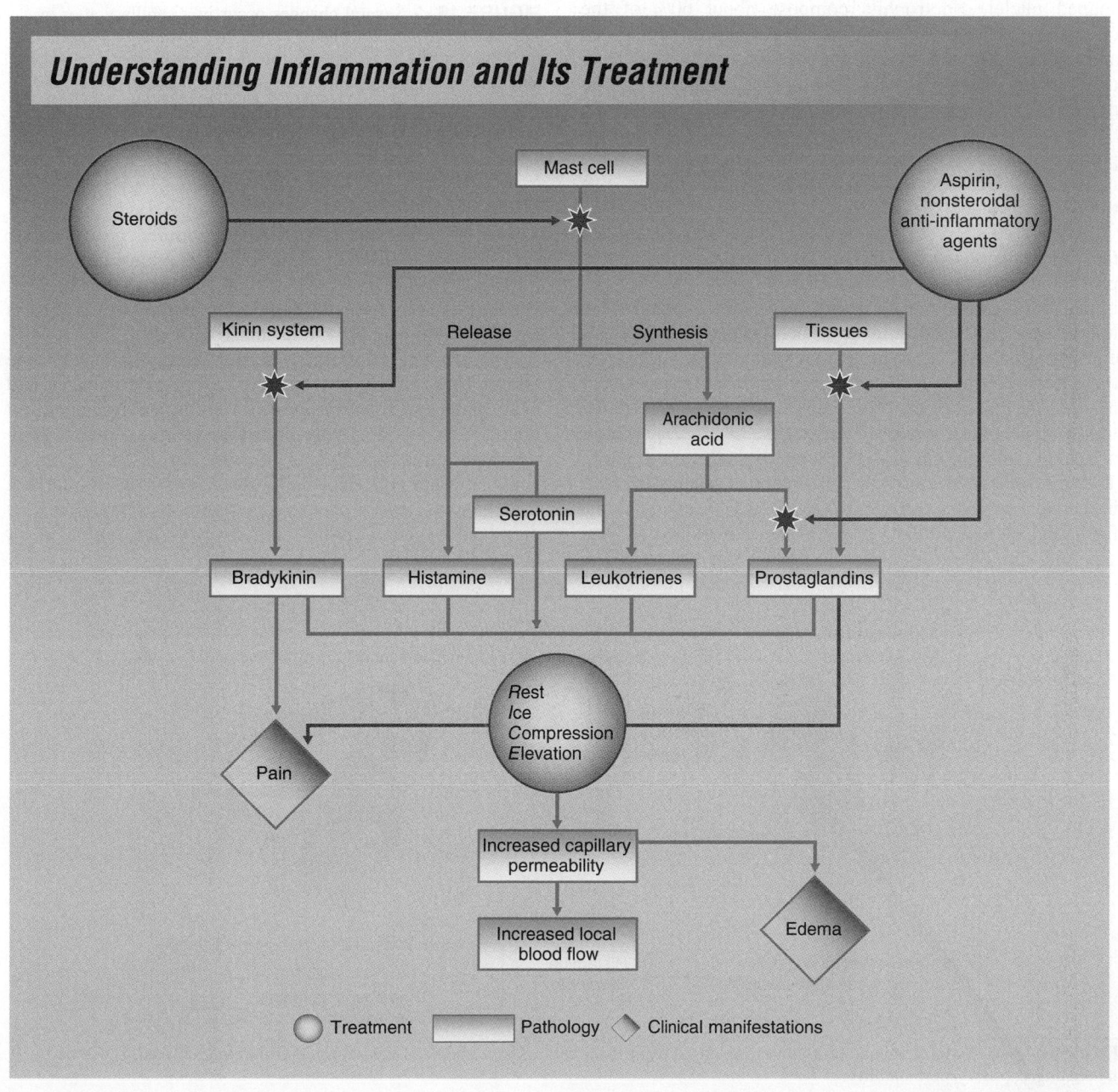

Understanding Inflammation and Its Treatment

Treatment ( )   Pathology ( )   Clinical manifestations ( )

phagocytose (ingest) injurious agents, thereby protecting against bacterial invasion.

Neutrophils are attracted to the injury site by chemotaxis. The slowed flow of blood allows the neutrophil to leave the center of the bloodstream and line the walls of the capillaries, a process called *pavementing,* or *marginating,* because the cells line up like bricks on a sidewalk. Histamine stimulates the cells that line the capillary to constrict, creating spaces in the wall. Neutrophils, which are normally too large to squeeze through the lining, can pass through the capillary wall and enter the site of tissue injury to begin phagocytosis, through a process called *diapedesis* (Figs. 16–2 and 16–3). Neutrophils phagocytose bacteria, dead cells, and cellular debris. These cells are short-lived, but they are effective in clearing a wound of debris if bacteria are not excessive in number (>100,000 per gram of tissue).

Neutrophils are sometimes called *polymorphonuclear neutrophils* (PMNs), or polys, because of their irregularly shaped nuclei. Neutrophils compose about 60% of the circulating WBCs. Mature neutrophils appear segmented and are called "segs." Immature cells are "banded" and called bands. Bands are not effective in phagocytosis. The presence of an increase in segmented WBCs indicates a bacterial invasion. The presence of increased band neutrophils indicates more severe infection because the bone marrow has released immature cells. Leukocytes are also the major producers of interferon.

MONOCYTES AND MACROPHAGES. Monocytes are the next phagocytes on the scene, stimulated by neutrophils and lymphokines. They arrive about 4 days after injury. Monocytes can phagocytose foreign material for a longer time. In addition, a large percentage of monocytes enter the tissues and become macrophages. In the tissue, these cells continue to phagocytose large numbers of bacteria. If the need arises, these cells can reenter the circulation and become mobile macrophages. Macrophages have a greater role in chronic inflammation (discussed later). The macrophage is a critical cell in wound healing because it secretes *angiogenesis factor* (AGF). AGF stimulates the formation of new blood vessels at the end of injured vessels and stimulates fibroblasts to spew forth collagen. The

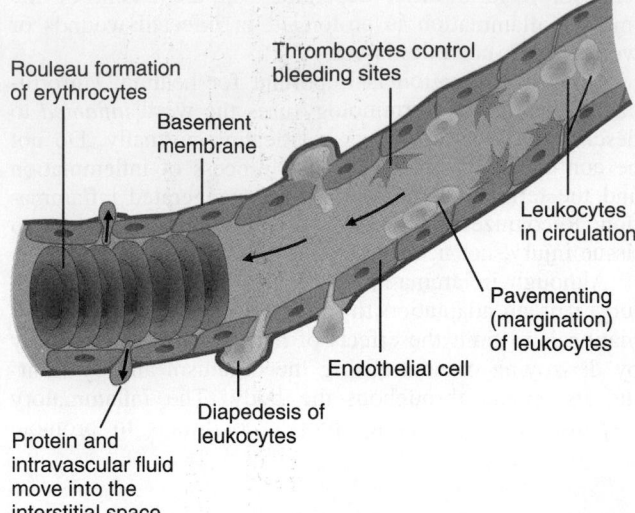

FIGURE 16–2 Several changes occur in a capillary after injury. Neutrophils are attracted to the site of injury by chemotactic factors at the site. The neutrophil leaves the blood vessel by sliding through holes in the vessel wall (diapedesis). The leukocytes also line the vessel wall, and the erythrocytes stack like coins (rouleau formation) to slow blood flow.

macrophage also secretes other cytokines such as platelet-derived growth factor (PDGF), transforming growth factor (TGF), interleukin-1 (IL-1) and basic fibroblast growth factor (bFGF). This cell has a major role in wound healing. Wounds can heal without leukocytes, but wound healing is significantly impaired without macrophages.

The amount of oxygen in the wound influences the effectiveness of phagocytic cells. Both macrophages and neutrophils can function in an anaerobic environment, but their ability to effectively digest bacteria is slowed. Macrophages are inactivated when tissue levels of oxygen are below 30 mm Hg. (Normal tissue oxygen levels are not the same as levels of oxygen bound to hemoglobin or dissolved oxygen. Tissue oxygen levels are normal at or above 30 mm Hg.)

FIGURE 16–3 Histamine and serotonin are released from mast cells. These chemical mediators of inflammation lead to edema by increasing capillary permeability.

LYMPHOCYTES AND OTHER WHITE BLOOD CELLS.
Two other forms of WBCs have much less importance in wound healing and are addressed only briefly. The lymphocytes are formed in the lymphoid tissues of the tonsils, intestines, and bone marrow, and they mature in the lymph nodes, thymus, and spleen. Lymphokines are sensitized lymphocytes. Lymphokines help the macrophages to become more effective at the site of local injury through a number of processes. Lymphocytes are controlled by the adrenocortical hormones. Therefore, clients receiving steroid therapy have reduced numbers of lymphocytes. This change places the steroid-dependent client at increased risk for infection and delayed healing.

Eosinophils and basophils may also migrate to the injured area. Eosinophils help control the inflammatory response by secreting antihistamine. Basophils secrete histamine.

"WALLING-OFF" EFFECT. A walling-off effect occurs in the damaged area to prevent the spread of injurious agents to other body tissues. Fibrinogen clots block the lymphatic channels and spaces in the tissues so that fluid barely flows through the area. The process of walling off the area partly depends on the invading agent. For example, staphylococci invade and destroy nearby tissues quickly, and therefore the process of walling off also develops quickly to control the spread. In contrast, streptococci did not cause an intense reaction in the tissues and can digest the walls. This allows the streptococci to multiply and spread. As a result, streptococcal infections have a much greater tendency to invade other organs (such as the heart valves) and are associated with a higher mortality rate.

Mediators of the Inflammation Phase
The specific mediators of inflammation are not shown in Figure 16–1. They are important, and their activity occurs throughout the healing phases. The chemicals that guide inflammation are shown in the feature called Understanding Inflammation and Its Treatment.

MAST CELLS. Several substances mediate (control) inflammation. Mast cells are found in the tissue. Mast cells are filled with histamine and neutrophil chemotactic factors, substances called vasoactive amines. Histamine and serotonin cause capillary dilation (see Fig. 16–2). The mast cell is stimulated by many factors, such as physical injury (wounds, burns, x-ray exposure), chemical injury (toxins, snake and bee venom), or immunologic means (the trigger of hypersensitivity reactions seen in allergies).

Mast cells also synthesize leukotrienes and prostaglandins. These two chemicals cause the same responses as histamine, but the response they generate lasts longer. Prostaglandins also cause pain and tend to appear in the later stages of inflammation. Leukotrienes and prostaglandins are produced from the arachidonic acid released from the mast cell membrane. Aspirin and other nonsteroidal anti-inflammatory drugs (NSAIDs) block the production of prostaglandins and can assist in reducing inflammation and pain (see Understanding Inflammation and Its Treatment). Leukotrienes and prostaglandins increase vascular permeability and enhance the action of neutrophils. The increase in blood flow brings in more nutrients and WBCs. Bradykinin, (see next section) also causes vasodilation, induces pain, and facilitates the action of the leukocyte.

KININ SYSTEM. Kinins are plasma proteins involved in inflammation. Early in injury, kinins increase vascular permeability and allow the leukocytes to enter the tissue. Later in the inflammatory process, kinins act with prostaglandin to cause pain and smooth muscle contraction and to increase leukocyte chemotaxis. Kinins increase vascular permeability, fluid in the wound, and the number of leukocytes available to assist with phagocytosis. The primary kinin is bradykinin.

OXYGEN FREE RADICALS. Free radicals are commonly regarded as the cause of some diseases. During metabolism, an unstable form of oxygen is produced. This is a single oxygen atom, derived from molecular oxygen (O_2), having an unpaired electron. This form of oxygen is called an *oxygen free radical* or a *superoxide radical*. The molecule tries to become stable again by attaching to hydrogen, lipids, or vitamin E. If the molecule attaches to hydrogen, the product is hydrogen peroxide, which is toxic to the cell. If it attaches to lipids, it can enter the cell or organelles and produce damage. When attached to vitamin E, it is stabilized and does not produce damage. Other vitamins support vitamin E; vitamin C restores vitamin E to the cell membrane. Vitamin A (beta-carotene) is present in high-density lipoproteins and is presumed to serve some role as an antioxidant, but that role is not fully understood.

Unrestrained free radicals can injure tissues and induce breaks in both single-stranded and double-stranded deoxyribonucleic acid (DNA), leading to mutations. In wound healing, free radicals serve as mediators of both acute and chronic inflammation, being stimulated by PMNs and the mast cell. They damage vascular endothelium (the inside lining of blood vessels). The exact role of free radicals in wound healing is still under investigation. The use of vitamin E as an antioxidant is becoming popular.

THE COMPLEMENT SYSTEM. The complement system is composed of a group of plasma proteins that normally lie dormant in the blood, interstitial fluid, and mucosal surfaces. Microorganisms (or antigen-antibody complexes) activate the complement system. Complement activation promotes inflammation and induces movement of leukocytes into the area of injury in a process is called *chemotaxis*. The final aspect of complement activation is the coating of microbes to make them vulnerable to phagocytosis. Many bacteria have an outer capsule that resists phagocytosis. (Complement is fully discussed in the Unit 16 review.)

PROLIFERATIVE PHASE
The third phase of wound healing, the proliferative or resolution phase, contains overlapping processes of collagen deposition, angiogenesis (formation of new blood vessels), granulation tissue development, and wound contraction. This phase ends about 2 weeks after injury, but the processes of healing are not complete and continue for 1 to 2 years.

Mediators of the Proliferative Phase
CYTOKINES. Cytokines regulate the mobility, differentiation, and growth of leukocytes. Among the best understood cytokines are interleukins and interferon. *Interleukins* promote the growth and function of several cells. Interleukin can account for many of the clinical manifestations of both acute and chronic inflammation, such as

fever, anorexia, cachexia, and movement of PMNs to the site of injury. Interferons augment immunity through several processes, especially the promotion of B-cell maturation and moderating of suppressor T-cell function.

GROWTH FACTORS. Catalysts for wound healing are growth factors released by platelets and macrophages. They can prime other cells to enter a growth phase, or they can move a cell from a growth phase to a DNA production phase. Several types of growth factors have been identified. Only major families of wound healing growth factors are described.

Platelet-derived growth factor (PDGF) is named for the platelet from which it originated. PDGF regulates the synthesis of fibronectin and fibroblasts in the matrix of the wound healing bed. Epidermal growth factor (EGF), named for the target cell, stimulates fibroblasts and endothelial cells. FGF stimulates collagen synthesis and angiogenesis. TGF-α stimulates epithelial cells and macrophages and controls cell growth and synthesis of the components of the matrix. TGF-β increases synthesis of the matrix components. Colony-stimulating factors (CSFs) are secreted by the bone marrow, monocytes, fibroblasts, and keratinocytes. Their major function appears to be enhancing the function of WBCs.

Components of Healing

COLLAGEN. Fibroblasts, normally found in connective tissue, are brought into the wound by various cellular mediators. They are the most important cells in this phase of healing because they synthesize and secrete collagen, elastin, and proteoglycans. These substances reconstruct connective tissue. Initially, collagen is gel-like, but within several weeks to months, it re-forms along lines of mechanical stress, which adds strength to the wound. Several substances are needed for normal collagen deposition, including vitamin C, zinc, oxygen, and iron.

ANGIOGENESIS. Microscopically, the development of new blood vessels (angiogenesis) begins within hours of injury. Over a period of time, the new blood vessels in the wound bed can be identified through clinical assessment. Initially, the skin edges of a wound are bright red and bleed easily. Within hours, the ends of the vessels seal and the wound drainage changes from bright red to dark red.

GRANULATION TISSUE. A matrix of collagen, capillaries, and cells begins to fill the wound space with new connective tissue, forming a scar. This tissue grows from the wound edges and the base of the wound. Granulation tissue is filled with new capillary buds, which give it a red, bumpy, or granular appearance. Fibroblasts and macrophages also surround it. The fibroblasts secrete collagen. The macrophages continue to debride the wound and stimulate fibroblasts and the process of angiogenesis. As granulation tissue is being formed, the process of *epithelialization* begins.

WOUND CONTRACTION. Wound contraction is the mechanism by which the edges of a wound are drawn together as a result of forces within the wound. Contraction is due to the action of myofibroblasts. Myofibroblasts bridge across a wound and then contract to pull the wound closed. The process of wound contraction is crucial for survival. If a wound from an acute injury did not contract, infections would be lethal complications in all acute injuries. Contraction is undesirable in some wounds

because of the cosmetic deformities that result from *contracture.*

CONTRACTURE. In large open wounds, such as burns, wound contraction can go on to become the more severe form of contracture. Contracture of the scar can produce profound deformities; contracture of the scar at the neck can pull the chin onto the chest. Wounds over joints can also contract severely. Contracture also occurs in internal organs, such as the intestine, breast, and liver.

EPITHELIALIZATION. Epithelialization is the migration of epithelial cells from surrounding skin. Epithelial buds also line hair follicles in the dermis of shallow wounds or wounds that are healing by secondary intention (discussed later). When epithelium covers a wound, the wound is considered to be closed, or healed. Large wounds or full-thickness wounds may require skin grafting because epidermal migration is normally limited to about 3 cm.

Epithelial buds can be seen in a clean granulating wound. The epithelial cells divide, and eventually the migrating epithelial cells contact similar cells from the other edges and stop migrating. At this point, they begin to differentiate into the various layers of epidermis. Epithelialization can be hastened if a wound is kept moist.

MATURATION PHASE

The final phase of wound healing (maturation or reconstruction) is marked by remodeling of the scar. This phase occurs for a year or more after the wound is closed. Collagen has been deposited, tissue is repaired, and the wound has begun to contract during the proliferative phase. During the maturation phase, the scar is remodeled, capillaries disappear, and the scar tissue regains about two thirds of its original strength. The remodeling is the process of collagen synthesis and lysis. Remodeling provides tensile strength to the wound.

Scar tissue is never as strong or durable as normal tissue. Tensile strength never reaches over 80% in scar tissue. Over the 12 months after injury, the scar becomes mature and appears thin and white instead of the red, raised appearance seen with granulation tissue. Scarring is a normal part of wound healing. Some scars are barely visible, whereas others remain very visible throughout the client's lifetime. Factors that affect scarring are discussed in Chapter 49.

■ WOUND HEALING INTENTION

Wound healing intention refers to the probable process of healing for any wound. Wounds can heal by (1) primary, (2) secondary, or (3) tertiary (delayed primary) intention (Fig. 16–4.)

PRIMARY INTENTION

Primary intention is the use of suture or other wound closures to approximate (place close together) the edges of an incision or clean laceration. Healing is primarily through collagen synthesis, and little scarring or contraction is needed. The risk of infection and tissue defects is minimal. The eventual scar is usually thin and flat.

SECONDARY INTENTION

Wounds healing by secondary intention are left open rather than closed with sutures (stitches) and heal by the generation of connective tissue. Consider open wounds like pressure ulcers or abrasions. Open wounds require

Figure 16–4 Wound healing by primary, secondary, and tertiary intention (delayed primary closure).

the regeneration of much more tissue than does the wound healing by primary intention, and there is also increased risk of infection. Wounds healing by secondary intention have a prolonged phase of inflammation because more time is required for phagocytosis of necrotic tissue. In chronic inflammation, macrophages and lymphocytes are the predominant cells. The ability of epithelial cells to migrate is limited, and epithelialization may not heal the wound. Therefore, the wound is characterized by longer phases of proliferation and maturation, leading to healing by contraction and the formation of scar tissue. Sometimes healing of is hastened by the application of skin grafts or musculocutaneous (myocutaneous) flaps (see Chapter 49).

TERTIARY INTENTION
Certain wounds may be contaminated, and although they can be closed by primary intention (e.g., by suture), they are not. Because of the increased risk of infection, these wounds are closed later, when they are free of debris. This type of wound closure is called healing by tertiary intention, or delayed primary closure.

■ NUTRITION AND WOUND HEALING
Protein and calories are needed for wound healing, and vitamins and minerals are also important components in this process (Table 16–1). Malnutrition leads to impaired collagen synthesis and an increased risk of infection. Protein-calorie malnutrition is an all too common problem in older people, especially those in institutions.

CLIENTS WITH ACUTE INFLAMMATION

Inflammation occurs in all clients who have sustained any form of tissue trauma. The trauma can be due to surgery, injury, changes in oxygen delivery to various tissues, and so on. Therefore, the information herein can be applied to many clinical settings. There are both local and systemic manifestations of inflammation. Because the response to inflammation is the same, regardless of the cause, the manifestations of inflammation are relatively consistent.

There are three systemic reactions to inflammation:

- Fever
- Leukocytosis (a rise in the number of WBCs)
- An increase in the number of plasma proteins.

Fever is caused by a pyrogen (fever-causing chemical) released from leukocytes, macrophages, and tumor necrosis factor (TNF). Prostaglandins also act on the hypothalamus to reset the internal thermostat. Fever is usually adaptive because bacterial reproduction is sensitive to even slight increases in temperature.

Outcome Management

■ Medical Management
Goals of medical management of a client with acute inflammation include (1) minimizing complications of the edema accompanying inflammation, (2) reducing the inflammatory response, and (3) monitoring systemic responses. Because the inflammatory response is a desired

TABLE 16–1	NUTRITION AND WOUND HEALING
Nutrient	**Impairments Related to Nutrient Deficiency**
Protein	Decreased collagen production, angiogenesis, and neutrophil and lymphocyte immune response; increased risk of dehiscence and infection
Calories	Too little glucose impairs immune response because energy needs of white blood cells cannot be met
Fats	Impaired inflammation
Vitamin A	Impaired monocyte and macrophage activity; delayed inflammatory response, including macrophage activity; increased risk of infection
Vitamin B complex	Not well understood; lack of B vitamins interferes with enzyme production
Vitamin C	Decreased collagen production, angiogenesis, and contraction; weakness in healed wound; increased risk of infection
Vitamin E	Delayed healing when given in excess
Zinc	Possibly impaired action of vitamin A; phagocytosis; increased risk of infection; decreased protein synthesis
Iron	Impaired oxygenation and secondary healing at very low levels

response to promote wound healing, the client with inflammation often requires only supportive care.

CONTROL THE EFFECTS OF EDEMA

Rest, Ice, Compression, and Elevation (RICE) is a mnemonic that can be used to guide care to reduce the effect of edema. If an extremity is inflamed, it is elevated and wrapped to reduce edema. Most practitioners advocate using ice to control the inflammatory response in the extremities, especially when edema and pain are present. Some physicians order ice for 24 to 72 hours to control inflammation and then apply heat to remove the accumulated waste products. When ice is ordered, be certain that the cold reaches the wound and that it is not rendered ineffective by bulky dressings. Assess for signs of skin damage if ice is applied directly to unprotected skin.

If edema is causing a detrimental alteration of tissue perfusion, anti-inflammatory agents may be required. In certain areas of the body, such as the brain and extremities, the edema that accompanies inflammation can be detrimental to tissue perfusion. These clients may require surgery to release pressure in the area or restore blood flow. Fasciotomy and bur holes are examples of these operations (see Chapters 27 and 73, respectively).

The degree of inflammation is monitored to determine whether it is leading to healing. Analgesics may be required for pain control. Temperature is monitored, and fever is treated with antipyretics when it reaches detrimental levels (e.g., >38.3° C or 101° F). If the inflammation is in response to a probable invasion by organisms, antibiotics may be prescribed.

REDUCE INFLAMMATION

Anti-inflammatory agents may be prescribed to stabilize the mast cell and reduce edema in the area. Medications in this category range from NSAIDs to corticosteroids.

MONITOR SYSTEMIC RESPONSES

Low-grade fever should not be treated with antipyretics (e.g., acetaminophen) because the high temperature retards bacterial growth. However, fever can be detrimental if it is extreme or prolonged. Therefore, the client's temperature is monitored closely to prevent harm. The client with a fever may also experience malaise, nausea, anorexia, weight loss, tachypnea, and tachycardia. The diet of the client with inflammation should be high in vitamin C, protein, calories, and fluids. Vitamin C supports WBC function, production of collagen, and angiogenesis. Protein aids in the formation of blood cells and tissue. Carbohydrates supply needed energy for fuel for healing. Additional fluids are needed to remove metabolic waste and rehydrate the client, especially if the client has been febrile.

Leukocytosis is due to the increase in the number of leukocytes in circulation to combat infection. Sometimes, in an effort to combat infection, the bone marrow releases immature leukocytes (banded neutrophils or bands). When the number of immature neutrophils is high, the client is said to have a "left shift." At times, the release of immature cells means that the body is having difficulty combating the infection with mature cells. Interpretation of the WBC differential is shown in Table 16-2.

The erythrocyte sedimentation rate (ESR) also rises

TABLE 16-2	INTERPRETATION OF DIFFERENTIAL COUNTS WITHIN A COMPLETE BLOOD COUNT			
Cell Type	**Function**	**Normal Value**	**Significance of Change**
Segmented neutrophils (segs)*	Mature neutrophils act as phagocytes	50%–60%	Elevated with infection; a "left shift" means that many band (immature) cells are present as the body fights infection; "right stuff" is the presence of more mature cells, seen with liver disease and pernicious anemia
Band neutrophils	Immature neutrophils	3%–8%	Elevated in acute stages of infection
Lymphocytes	Produced by lymphoid tissue, participate in humoral response	25%–40%	Elevated in infectious mononucleosis, cytomegalovirus infection, and infectious hepatitis; decreased in acquired immunodeficiency syndrome (AIDS), Cushing's syndrome, chronic uremia, and following trauma (e.g., burn injury)
Monocytes	A second line of defense, increasing in chronic infections	2%–8%	Elevated in chronic bacterial infection, viral disease, Hodgkin's disease, multiple myeloma, and some forms of leukemia
Eosinophils	Phagocytic, destroy antigen-antibody complexes before they can harm the body	1%–4%	Elevated in allergic disorders and parasitic infections; decreased in infectious mononucleosis, congestive heart failure, pernicious anemia, and during the use of steroids, epinephrine, and thyroxine

*To calculate the absolute neutrophil count (also called an absolute granulocyte count):

$$\text{absolute neutrophil count} = \frac{\text{total \% of neutrophils (segs + bands) WBC count (cells/mm}^3)}{100}$$

When the absolute neutrophil count falls below 1000/mm³, the client is said to be "neutropenic" and precautions must be taken to prevent infection.

with inflammation. The ESR rate ("sed rate") is the rate at which cells settle to the bottom of a glass test tube. Increased levels of fibrinogen cause the red blood cells to stack (like coins) and therefore settle more quickly. Additionally, plasma proteins rise during inflammation (e.g., fibrinogen, C-reactive protein). Most are released by the liver, and they are collectively called *acute phase reactants*. They provide components of coagulation, transportation, and complement production.

■ Nursing Assessment of the Medical Client

ASSESSMENT

The clinical manifestations of inflammation include redness, swelling, heat, pain, and loss of function. Tissues are red, warm, painful, and swollen and have limited mobility. In addition, an inflammatory exudate is formed. The exudate dilutes the toxins released by bacteria, brings certain nutrients to the wound, and carries phagocytes for defense. Various types of exudate are present, depending on the stage of inflammation and its cause.

Serous exudate is seen in early inflammation and is composed of water with a small amount of colloids, ions, and phagocytic cells. A *blister* is a common example of serous exudate. Hemorrhagic or sanguineous exudate is composed of blood. Drainage is bright red or dark red. Serosanguineous exudate is drainage composed of both serous fluid and blood. It is pink and usually fairly thin. Purulent exudate is filled with more leukocytes (pus) and is common in chronic inflammation from walled-off lesions.

The type of drainage present in the wound is indicative of the phase of healing. For example, a surgical wound initially presents with sanguineous drainage. As hemostasis progresses, the drainage becomes serosanguineous and finally advances to serous drainage (Table 16–3).

Monitor the level of WBCs, differential counts, and fever as indicators of infection. Expect the WBC level to rise in clients with known infections and after acute injury, such as a surgical incision (report elevations in WBC and clinical manifestations of infection to the physician). Monitor also the elderly, who often have infection but not necessarily elevated WBC counts.

DIAGNOSIS, OUTCOMES, INTERVENTIONS

Altered Tissue Perfusion. Edema from the inflammatory response may restrict blood vessels and entrap nerves in the traumatized area. The nursing diagnosis *Altered Tissue Perfusion related to edema* is an important problem.

Outcomes. Tissues will be perfused, as evidenced by the usual skin color, presence of pulses in areas distal to the edema, skin warmth, lack of paresthesias, and lack of escalating pain.

Interventions. Assess clients with visible injury causing inflammation for resolution of bleeding in the area, adequate blood flow, and nerve conduction distal to the affected site. Frequent assessments (every 2 hours) of the edematous area are needed. Measurement of the circumference of the area also enables the examiner to determine whether the area is becoming markedly edematous. To measure the same site, mark the area on the client with a pen to ensure appropriate location of serial measurements.

In addition to assessing the circumference, assess pulses, skin temperature, capillary refill, sensation, and movement in areas distal to the inflammation. Dressings or casts over the affected area can also form a constriction. This response can be called *compartment syndrome*. Clients who have been injured or are undergoing orthopedic surgery are at highest risk for compartment syndrome (see also Chapter 27).

Objects that may become entrapped in edematous tissues, such as rings, should be removed because they can cause serious damage. The inflamed area should be elevated. Application of cold compresses causes vasoconstriction and decreases the amount of edema. Prolonged use of cold compresses may lead to rebound vasodilation and increase the risk of tissue injury. Vasoconstriction can also decrease the inflow of new blood and thereby slow the removal of toxins and waste from the site of injury.

If the extremity is edematous, it should be elevated and assessed for the presence of distal circulation and neurologic response. Factors that impede venous flow should be controlled. For example, rolled stockings that constrict venous return should not be worn. Compression bandages may be used to reduce edema by promoting lymphatic and venous drainage. Explain the appropriate way to apply these bandages and when to rewrap them to maintain compression.

EVALUATION

The outcome of the inflammatory response is usually time-dependent. Most edema subsides over 72 hours with

TABLE 16–3	INFLAMMATORY EXUDATES	
Type	**Appearance**	**Significance**
Hemorrhagic, sanguineous	Bright red or bloody	Small amounts expected after surgery or trauma; large amounts may indicate hemorrhage; sudden large amounts of dark-red blood may indicate a draining hematoma
Serosanguineous	Blood-tinged yellow or pink	Expected for 48–72 hr after injury or trauma; a sudden increase may precede wound dehiscence
Serous	Thin, clear, yellow	Expected for up to 1 wk after trauma or surgery; a sudden increase may indicate a draining seroma
Purulent	Thin, cloudy, foul-smelling; may be thick if filled with dead cells	Usually indicates infection; may drain suddenly from an abscess (boil)
Catarrhal	Thin, clear mucus	Seen with upper respiratory infection

appropriate RICE measures. If the edema has not subsided in that time frame, consider another cause of the edematous process, such as infection.

Self-Care

Clients capable of caring for a wound or area that is likely to become inflamed need instructions on how to elevate the extremity, how to use heat or ice, how to follow the medication regimen, and how to change dressings. Clinical manifestations of edema and infection must be reported, such as changes in color, pulse, and pain.

CLIENTS WITH CHRONIC INFLAMMATION

Chronic inflammation is differentiated from acute inflammation by its duration and the cells that mediate the response. Acute inflammation is accompanied by altered capillary permeability, release of chemical mediators, and infiltration of leukocytes that engulf and destroy injured tissue and pathogens. If these elements succeed in cleaning the wound, healing begins. If the area is not cleaned, monocytes continue to perpetuate the inflammatory response, but this time the accumulation of inflammatory mediators may actually cause tissue destruction. The lymphocyte and tissue macrophages are the major phagocytes in chronic inflammation.

When the immune system is unable to eliminate the invading organisms during the acute stage of inflammation, it attempts to protect surrounding tissues from further invasion by building a wall around the infected site called a *granuloma*. Some forms of infection, such as fungi, parasites, and perhaps antibody-antigen reactions (autoimmune disease), result in granuloma formation. Tuberculosis is a good example. When tuberculosis develops, a thick wall forms around the mycobacteria. The bacteria continue to live in the walled-off area, and it is soon filled with dead tissue. As the tissue dies, the cellular enzymes are released and the fluid leaves the granuloma. The empty sac remains.

Outcome Management

The chronically inflamed wound has purulent drainage (*suppuration*) and does not heal completely. A common example of chronic inflammation is seen when foreign objects are not removed from tissues (e.g., splinter, glass, and dirt). Chronic inflammation can also occur when certain forms of bacteria cannot be killed by phagocytes. For example, the organisms that cause tuberculosis, syphilis, and leprosy have cell walls with a very high lipid and wax content, which makes them impermeable to the phagocyte.

Care of the client with chronic infection is focused on determining the source of the problem. Wounds may be *debrided* (cleaned and freed of dead tissue), and the client may be given antibiotics or anti-inflammatory agents.

CLIENTS WITH INCISIONS

Outcome Management

Wounds made intentionally with a scalpel and closed with sutures, staples, or strips of tape are called *incisions.*

Incisions are the most common example of wounds healing by primary intention. An incision should be assessed every 8 hours. If the incision is not visible, check the dressings or assess for increased girth. The incision normally appears somewhat pink and swollen; small areas of induration around the suture marks are common. However, erythema should not extend beyond a ½ inch from the incision. If the wound was closed primarily, you should be able to palpate the presence of newly synthesized collagen just under an intact suture line. This internal scar is known as a "healing ridge." When this ridge is not present 5 to 7 days after suturing, suspect slowed collagen synthesis. The client may need additional protection of the nonhealing area to prevent infection.

A wound that is healing by primary intention should be protected from further trauma, including external pressure. Keep the wound free of pulling forces that stretch the sutured skin. Keep the wound clean, but do not wash the suture line because water carries microorganisms into the wound along the sutures. Protect it from the external environment and drainage with dressings.

Apply dressings using an aseptic or sterile technique. Sterile gloves are usually not required. Hold the side of the dressing that will not touch the client's incision by the clean or gloved hands and tape it in place. The type of dressing used changes as the wound responds to treatment. Use dressings that best suit the wound. Gauze dressings are used most often on a wound healing by primary intention. Dressings for open wounds are discussed in the following section.

Wound drainage tubes can be placed in the dead space created during exposure of the operative area. Drainage of a wound is indicated when actual or potential fluid accumulation threatens the healing process. The drain facilitates removal of blood and bacteria from the wound. Assess the volume and type of fluid hourly immediately after surgery. If a reservoir is attached to the drain, measure the volume of drainage by markings on the reservoir. If the drainage is emptied from the reservoir, follow universal precautions for its disposal. In addition, if the drainage is caustic (e.g., bile), the skin around the site must be protected with skin barriers.

Teach the client how to care for the incision, the clinical manifestations of wound infection, how to care for and empty the drain reservoir, and when to return for suture removal. Sutures in areas where scarring must be controlled (e.g., on the face) are usually removed in 4 to 7 days; in other areas, sutures are usually removed in 7 to 10 days. Sutures in the hand and foot are removed in 1 to 2 weeks or more.

CLIENTS WITH OPEN WOUNDS

Outcome Management

Medical Management

The goal of medical management of an open wound is to prepare the client and the wound for the quickest and most durable form of healing. The treatment of a wound includes the removal of its cause, the correction of underlying problems that are delaying healing, and the initiation of topical (or systemic) treatments to facilitate healing.

Clients with open wounds often have other problems, such as venous insufficiency or diabetes. These disorders decrease blood flow (and thereby oxygen) into the wound and delay healing. Protein-calorie malnutrition may be present and delays healing because the protein needed to manufacture new cells is not available. If the client is immobile or incontinent, adequate prevention must be given to reduce the incidence of new areas of skin breakdown. If wound healing is delayed because of lack of venous return, the extremity requires elevation. If the cause of the wound is lack of arterial flow, the extremity should be positioned flat. If pressure is a causative or contributing factor, repositioning and proper support surfaces must be considered.

The client's diet should be high in carbohydrates, protein, iron, and vitamins. In addition, the client may remain at risk of further skin breakdown, such as pressure ulcers. Medical management may include antibiotics to reduce infection.

REMOVE DEVITALIZED TISSUE FROM THE WOUND: DEBRIDEMENT

Wound healing is optimized and the risk of infection is reduced when all necrotic (dead) tissue, exudate, and metabolic wastes are removed from the wound. Moist, devitalized tissue supports bacterial growth. Various forms of debridement are used to remove these tissues (see later). Systemic and topical antibiotics seldom stop infection because they cannot penetrate the avascular tissues.

Before a wound can heal, necrotic tissues must be removed. Debridement can be accomplished by means of a variety of techniques: (1) sharp, (2) mechanical, (3) enzymatic, and (4) autolytic (these last three are described later). Timely debridement is necessary to remove the devitalized tissue and reduce the risk of infection and the physical obstacles dead tissue places on the process of granulation. In addition, the true size of the wound cannot be known until the necrotic tissue is removed.

Sharp Debridement

Wounds covered with dead tissue, called *eschar* or *slough,* need to be cleaned to promote healing and reduce infection. *Sharp debridement* is performed by the physician and is the quickest method. The technique allows immediate treatment of the wound bed after the devitalized tissue is removed. The eschar or slough is removed to the level of red, bleeding tissues. The wound must then be protected to begin healing. The wound size, depth of the wound, contamination, and the client's status influence whether the client is in satisfactory condition to tolerate sharp debridement, which may call for general anesthesia or sedation. Pain medications should be used for clients undergoing sharp debridement.

Sharp debridement is carried out under sterile conditions, usually in an operating room, a treatment room, or an outpatient surgical setting. Risks associated with general anesthesia, blood loss, and infection are a major concern. This procedure is used for a large wound, a wound that involves a thick eschar that would not be permeated by any topical agent, and a wound that is acutely infected.

After sharp debridement, the client is monitored for signs of bleeding and bacteremia (sepsis.) Sepsis is suspected if unexplained fever, tachycardia, hypotension, or deterioration in mental status develops. The physician should be notified of these changes. Sepsis can be fatal if it is not recognized early and treated aggressively (see septic shock in Chapter 81.) Other forms of debridement commonly used by nurses are discussed later.

Once the wound is clean, surgery may be used to speed healing and to reduce the risk of infection and contracture. Skin grafts are commonly used to replace the epidermis. The partial-thickness burn wound is the best example of a wound that could heal by secondary intention but is often grafted to speed healing and reduce infection and scarring. Cutaneous or musculocutaneous flaps can also be used to close a large wound (see Chapter 49).

▉ Nursing Management of the Medical Client

ASSESSMENT

The client's history must be taken, including a history of the wound itself. The wound history includes causative and contributing factors, duration of the wound, and current and previous methods of treatment and their corresponding success. Sometimes wound treatments are used that actually impair healing, such as hydrogen peroxide or Dakin's solution, or that do not match the type of wound. This information is important when one is obtaining a complete wound history.

The history obtained by the nurse should include information about the following:

- Medical history
- Previous surgery
- Current and past medications, especially steroids and over the counter (OTC) and herbal preparations
- Nutritional state (type of diet, eats and any supplements)
- Serum glucose level if client is diabetic
- Smoking
- Degree of immobility
- Bowel and bladder continence
- Circulatory status
- Presence of infection

Many factors can lead to impaired wound healing. Assessments should be thorough and should focus on the whole client, not just the wound.

Psychosocial assessment should include the client's age, occupation, living situation, financial status, health care benefits, roles and responsibilities, cultural and spiritual beliefs, body image and self-esteem, and ability to learn self-care and comply with the treatment plan. Also note compliance with treatment of underlying disorders, such as diabetes and collagen diseases.

A complete physical assessment should be performed. Focus the data collection on height and weight; degree of range of motion; muscle wasting and level of activity; circulation, such as peripheral pulses, color, edema, and the temperature of extremities; lung sounds; and level of pain. A complete assessment is needed (Box 16-1). Clearly document data about the wound to allow for an objective evaluation at a later date. Describe the actual size of the ulcer by measuring the length (head to toe) and width (shoulder to shoulder). Describe the depth, color, type of drainage, presence of undermining, and

BOX 16-1   Wound Assessment

When assessing an open wound, obtain the following information:

1. What is the size of the wound? Use objective measures to indicate the length and width (such as centimeters or millimeters). Avoid terms such as "the size of a grape." Use a sterile gloved finger or cotton swab to measure depth. Consider using photographs to provide a baseline and serial evaluations.
2. Where is the wound located anatomically?
3. What is the color of the wound? Estimate the percentage of each color when more than one color is noted.
4. Is there granulation tissue or epithelial tissue? Granulation tissue is red, shiny, and bumpy; epithelial tissue looks like pale skin.
5. Are there sinus tracts, or are the edges undermined? Use a gloved hand or swab to measure the extent. Indicate the location and direction of tunneling.
6. Are there signs of infection in the wound? Look for erythema extending beyond the edges of the wound as well as warmth, edema, odor, and purulent exudate. (Also consider systemic signs.)
7. Is there any drainage? Note the color, odor, consistency, and approximate amount by the number of dressings saturated.
8. What is the condition of the surrounding skin? Is it intact, red, indurated, or macerated?
9. Is the wound painful?

condition of periwound skin in the assessment data for later comparison. A photograph is an excellent means of documentation and determination of the progress in healing. Obtain consent before photographs are taken. Photographs should be taken with a consistent method that includes reproducible distance, color, and grid film.

Examine laboratory values for hemoglobin, hematocrit, albumin, and WBCs, specifically lymphocytes. These values indicate the degree of nutritional impairment that may be contributing to the wound's lack of healing. Generally, the risk of delayed healing correlates with low serum albumin levels. However, albumin levels are a slow-to-change indicator of nutritional state. A pre-albumin level is more indicative of current nutritional status.

DIAGNOSIS, PLANNING, INTERVENTIONS

Impaired Skin Integrity. The nursing diagnosis should be used to indicate an actual loss of skin. The actual statement might be phrased *Impaired Skin Integrity related to delayed wound healing secondary to impaired circulation, to infection, or to malnutrition.*

Outcomes. The client will experience improved skin integrity, as evidenced by a cleaner wound within 1 week and no signs of infection in the wound. A long-term goal might be a smaller wound in 3 weeks.

Interventions. Many agencies have wound care nurses who should be contacted for up-to-date information and for assistance with complex wounds. However, every nurse must properly identify basic concepts of wound assessment and treatment.

Keep the Wound Moist. Wound healing is optimized in a moist environment. When the environment is moist,

collagen synthesis and granulation tissue formation are enhanced, cell migration and epithelial resurfacing occur more rapidly, and scab, crust, and eschar cannot form. This moist environment, however, can create a medium conducive to infection, and a clean technique must be used for wound care. Heat lamps or treatments that dry the wound must be avoided.

Wet-to-moist or continuously moist dressings are used in clean and granulating wounds. Insert dressings into the wound or place them on the wound while they are moist, again making certain to protect normal intact skin. Remove the dressings while they are still moist to avoid disrupting the granular bed. Bleeding should not occur when the dressing is removed. If the dressing is too dry to pull off, moisten it with sterile normal saline before attempting to remove it.

Prevent Injury to Healing Tissues. Avoid applying solutions on and in the clean wound that may impair healing. For example, iodine, hydrogen peroxide, and Dakin's solution were once commonly used for wound care; however, these solutions damage the wound. They are toxic to the fibroblast and therefore delay healing. In addition, use of large volumes of iodine in wounds can lead to toxicity from excess iodine absorption.

Normal saline is the only solution for wound care recommended by the Agency for Health Care Policy and Research (AHCPR). Normal saline is physiologic, does not harm tissues, and adequately cleans most wounds. Pressure may be applied to the irrigant for enhanced cleaning. If the wound is covered with adherent material, some solutions contain surfactants that aid in cleaning. Some of these chemicals can harm wound-healing cells (Table 16-4). If used, it is important to limit their use to as short a time as possible.

Protect the Periwound Skin. Moisture on normal, intact skin makes the skin more prone to breakdown. The cardinal rule is to keep the wound bed moist and surrounding skin dry. Figure 16-5 shows wound healing cascade in a dry and moist environment. Note that there is faster migration of epithelial cells on a moist wound bed.

Fill Dead Space. Dead space is empty space within a wound. In an ulcer, it is the space between the base of the ulcer and the underside of the dressing around its perimeter. If this space is closed, empty pockets may develop anaerobic infection. Long-acting normal saline gel and wound packing are good media to fill a clean wound and the pockets of empty space before a topical dressing is applied.

Perform Wound Packing. Deep wounds with channels are at high risk of infection. These wounds can also heal with "false floors," which trap bacteria and lead to further infection. It is important that an open wound heal from the inside out. Deep wounds are often packed with saline or gauze strips soaked in an antibiotic solution to debride the wound or prevent abnormal healing. Strips of gauze must be used to avoid having soiled dressings lost in the wound. The gauze is packed into the wound with enough force to hold the edges of the wound open, but not so much force that the wound is under tension. Wounds packed too tightly compromise blood flow and delay healing. The outer edge of the dressing is covered with dry dressings.

TABLE 16-4	TOPICAL AGENTS USED IN TREATMENT OF OPEN WOUNDS	
Agent	**Indications**	**Impact on Wound Healing**
ANTISEPTIC SOLUTIONS		
Normal saline	Used to moisten dry eschar; keep a clean wound healing by secondary intention	Speeds healing because solution is iso-osmolar, and it keeps the wound bed moist
Hydrogen peroxide	Used to dissolve clotted blood in a wound	Retards healing; do not use as a dressing on an open wound
Providone-iodine (Betadine)	Used for preparation of intact skin; may be used to clean very contaminated wounds	Retards healing; does not penetrate eschar
Dakin's solution	Used 3 to 2 strength to clean contaminated wounds	Retards wound healing
Acetic acid	Used to treat wounds contaminated with *Pseudomonas*	Retards wound healing slightly
ANTIBIOTIC SOLUTIONS AND OINTMENTS		
Neomycin-bacitracin-polymyxin B (Neosporin)	Used to clean wounds contaminated with gram-negative and gram-positive bacteria	Increases epidermal healing but may sensitize tissues; high incidence of allergy
Polymyxin B-bacitracin (Polysporin)	Treatment of gram-negative organisms	None known
Silver sulfadiazine	Used in wounds with eschar (e.g., burns): effective against gram-negative and gram-positive organisms	Enhances epidermal healing; penetrates eschar
Gentamicin	Most effective against gram-negative organisms, but its use may promote resistance in hospital flora	None known
Bacitracin	Effective against gram-positive and gram-negative organisms	May enhance epidermal healing

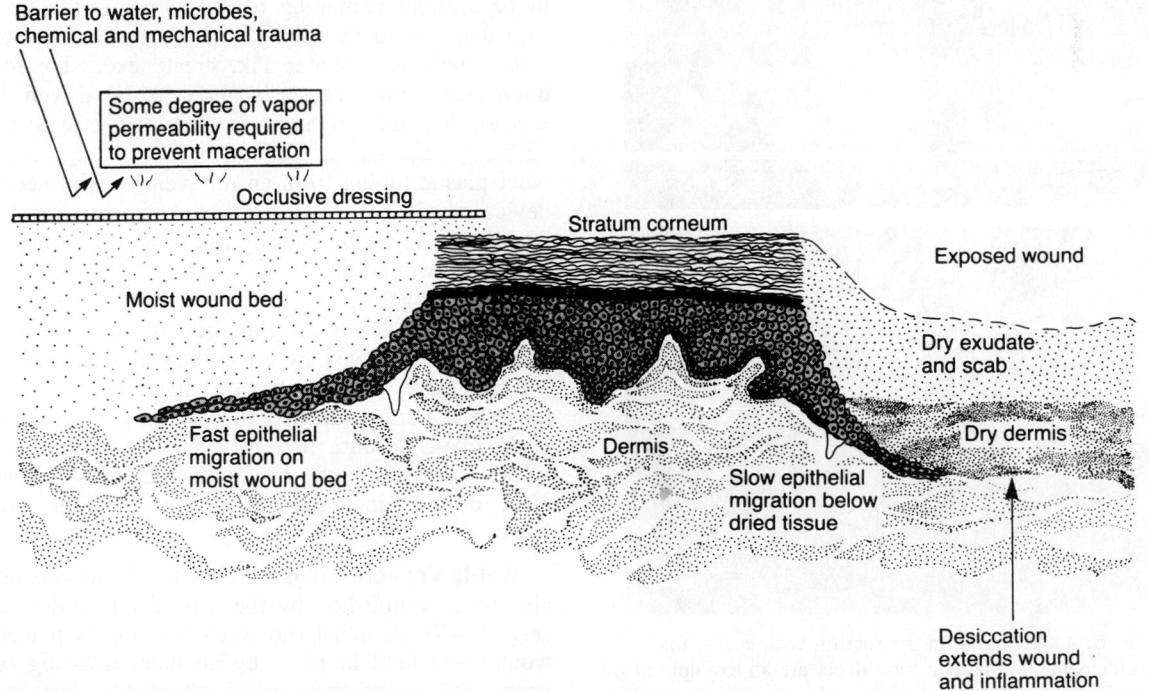

Figure 16–5 Wound healing under an occlusive dressing. (Adapted from Winter, G. D., & Scales, J. T. [1963]. Effect of air drying and dressings on the surface of a wound. *Nature, 197,* 91–92. Copyright 1963 Macmillan Magazines Limited.)

Packing is usually changed every 4 to 6 hours. Some gel packing strips are changed less often. Skin surrounding the wound should be assessed for breakdown from frequent tape removal, and dressings should be secured with other methods if needed (e.g., Montgomery straps).

Select Dressings. Red wound bases need protection to promote healing (Fig. 16–6). Red wounds are filled with granulation tissue and are beginning to heal. These wounds should not be treated with lotions, ointments, or soaps, which generally irritate or infect the area. Topical vasodilators can be used to stimulate capillary flow to the wound, but a physician's order is required. If the wound is shallow, a thin layer of antibiotic ointment and non-adhering dressing (or synthetic dressing) may be used to cover it. If the wound is deep, saline-moistened gauze can be used to pack the wound, but the dressing should not be allowed to dry out before it is changed. When an-

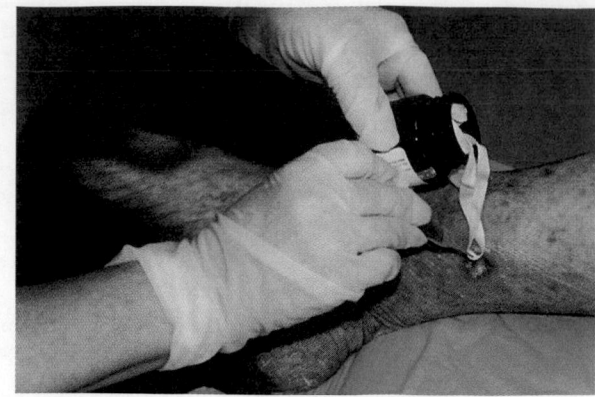

Figure 16–7 Wet-to-dry dressings are placed into a wound with the use of strip gauze.

Figure 16–6. *A,* A wound on the sacrum with eschar that needs debridement. *B,* Diabetic foot ulcers are an example of a wound with yellow, soft, slough that needs cleaning. *C,* Healing venous stasis ulcers have a clean wound filled with granulation tissue that needs protection.

adherent dressing is being changed, granulation tissue and new epithelium are also removed. If a wound is healing, the wound should be kept moist to facilitate healing.

A wound that presents with black, leathery material in the wound base is necrotic. This black, nonviable tissue is known as eschar. Yellow material in the wound base is a sloughy, necrotic substance. Black and yellow tissues present in the wound bed can be appropriately classified as devitalized, necrotic, or dead. The risk of infection rises in proportion to the amount of necrotic tissue present. Debridement techniques for removing necrotic tissue include those described in the sections that follow. (Sharp debridement was discussed earlier.)

Perform Mechanical Debridement. Mechanical debridement includes treatments with irrigation and dressings.

Irrigation. Irrigation between 4 and 15 pounds per square inch (psi), removes debris, bacteria, and necrotic tissue without damaging tissues; 8 psi is the most pressure that should be used on a wound. High-pressure devices, such as a Water Pik, create excessive force and trauma and may cause bacteria to be driven into the wound. Wound irrigation is safe and effective with a 35-ml syringe and a 19 French (19Fr.) angiocatheter, or outer plastic tubing from an intravenous (IV) needle. This device provides 8 psi of force and removes most devitalized tissue. Hydrotherapy by use of a whirlpool is also an option for wound cleaning.

When irrigating around a wound, take barrier precautions with masks or goggles, gowns, and gloves because you may be sprayed by contaminated solutions. The client may also need protection. Irrigation with pulsating devices is contraindicated in clients with wounds of the neck, eyes, or dura and in clients with exposed blood vessels. To prevent further contamination of adjacent tissues, do not increase pressure beyond the prescribed level.

Wet-to-dry dressings. Mechanical debridement can also be accomplished by the use of wet-to-dry dressings (Fig. 16–7). A moist (not wet) dressing is placed in the wound and held in place by an outer dressing or gauze wrap. The inner dressing is allowed to dry and then removed. As the dressing dries, debris, necrotic tissue, exudate, and drainage adhere to it. The wound is debrided as the dressing is gently removed. The wet dressing is obtained by saturating an all-gauze dressing with the prescribed solution and wringing the dressing out until it is just moist. The moist dressing should be placed in the wound and left long enough to begin to dry (4 to 6 hours). Use caution so that the dressing does not cause normal (or high-risk) tissues on the edges of the wound to become moist. Topical skin protectants can be used to protect surrounding intact skin. Once the dressing is dry, it is removed along with adherent tissues. The dressings are not remoistened to make removal easier because this practice defeats the purpose of the dressing, which is to debride the wound. The process is often painful, and clients should have adequate analgesia before the dressing is changed. Wet-to-dry dressings are a nonselective form of debridement and can inadvertently remove new granulation tissues as well as necrotic tissue, creating an environment that retards healing. Therefore, they are used only until the wound is clean and granulating.

Perform Enzymatic Debridement. To avoid the risk of damaging new tissue growth, which is often experienced with wet-to-dry dressings, consider chemical agents, such as enzymes, as a nonsurgical option. Enzymatic agents are expensive, requiring diligent care. Some enzymatic agents work by converting denatured proteins to peptides and amino acids. Other enzymatic preparations cause fibrin lysis. These agents cannot be used on wounds com-

municating with major body cavities, wounds with exposed nerves, or neoplastic ulcers. They must be used with caution around the eyes.

A dry eschar should be *scored* (should have small cuts made into it) before the enzymatic ointment is applied. Scoring enhances penetration. For the agent to work, the wound surface must be kept moist. The ointment is used until the eschar separates from the wound surface. Use of agents necessitates frequent dressing changes, and they should be used only on necrotic tissue. They are usually applied to only about 2 to 4 square inches of necrotic tissue at one time. Medicate clients prior to the use of enzymatic agents, which cause burning. Enzymatic agents should not be placed on viable tissue, as they cause tissue necrosis.

Perform Autolytic Debridement. With this method, a synthetic dressing is placed over the ulcer and the eschar or devitalized tissue is allowed to self-digest through the action of enzymes normally present in the wound fluid. Although not as rapid than other methods, autolytic debridement may be appropriate for clients who cannot tolerate other methods and are not susceptible to infection. Autolytic debridement is contraindicated for most infected wounds.

Select Dressings. Gauze still remains the most commonly used material for a dressing. Gauze is used as a dry cover for surgical wounds or wounds that heal by

TABLE 16–5	WOUND DRESSINGS		
Type	Product	Indications for Use	Nursing Implications
Nonadhering, nonimpregnated	Telfa	Shallow, open wounds	Second dressing or tape needed it is nonadhesive
Impregnated	Adaptic gauze, Vaseline gauze, Xeroform	Moist wounds	Nonabsorbent, occlusive, not traumatic to remove
Gauze	Adaptic gauze, Kling gauze, Nu-gauze, Primapore	Wet-to-dry debridement, wound packing	Moderately absorbent; can be used as wound packing for shallow wounds; use long strips of gauze to pack deep wounds; gauze does not provide a bacterial barrier; if allowed to dry on a wound, it may remove viable tissue when removed
Transparent films	Bio-occlusive, Op-Site, Tegaderm	Coverage of shallow wounds, intravenous sites, blisters, abrasions	Adhesive; therefore, no secondary dressing is needed; retain moisture, semipermeable, water-resistant; facilitate autolytic debridement
Hydrocolloids	Comfeel, Duoderm, Intrasite, Restore, Tegasorb, Intact, ulcer dressing	Shallow ulcers, donor sites, second-degree (partial-thickness) burns; do not use on infected wounds	Retain moisture, occlusive or semipermeable, water-resistant, adhesive; require replacement because the dressing melts; reduce pain
Hydrogels	Elastogel, wound gel, Spenco, Vigilon	Pressure ulcers, dermal ulcers, partial-thickness burns, abrasions, blisters	Hydrogels having cooling effect: maintain moist environment, relieve pain, permit autolytic debridement; easily removed unless they dry out
Exudate absorbers	Bard absorption dressing, Envisan	Deep wounds with eschar	Retain moisture, absorbent, promote autolytic debridement
Calcium alginates	Sorbsan, Kaltistat, Algiderm	Clean wounds with profuse drainage	Retain moisture, absorbent, left intact for several days
Foams	Reston, Flexan Lyofoam, Polymen	Full-thickness wounds with moderate to heavy drainage, skin tears	Moisture, absorbent, nonadherent, left intact for several days

primary intention (Table 16–5). Wet-to-dry gauze dressings can be used for nonselective debridement of wounds. More absorbent dressings should be used with exudative wounds. Only mesh gauze dressings should be used in a wound because cotton dressings are likely to leave fibers behind. Use cotton-filled gauze as an outer dressing. If the wound edges are friable or if the wound will be disrupted when the dressing is removed, a nonadherent dressing can be used. The nonadherent dressing can be impregnated or nonimpregnated. This nonadherent dressing is often chosen because when it is removed, disruption of the wound bed is minimal.

Clean granulating wounds do not require daily dressing changes. Apply hydrocolloid dressings for 3 to 5 days. Continue to observe for infection. If purulent drainage develops, do not apply occlusive dressings. Allow the wound to drain by using gauze or alginates.

Excessive exudate can delay healing. If the wound produces exudate, several absorption dressing products can be used. Absorptive dressings, calcium alginates, and hypertonic saline dressings are appropriate choices for moderate or highly exudating wounds. Foams can also be used for absorption and autolytic debridement. Table 16–5 describes the actions, indications, and nursing implications for various categories of wound dressings.

The selection of dressing type changes as the wound responds to treatment. Careful assessment and reassessment will indicate progress, or lack of progress, in wound healing. As the wound changes, variations in the dressing materials are made so that healing is maximized. No single dressing provides the optimal atmosphere required during all healing stages of the wound.

Providing Nutritional Support. In addition to local wound care, the client must be provided with a diet that is high in protein, fat, carbohydrates, vitamins, and minerals to facilitate healing. Regardless of the client's actual body weight (e.g., obesity), this is not the time to begin a weight loss diet. The wound must be healed first. If the client cannot or will not eat, the use of tube feeding or hyperalimentation should be considered.

Reducing Interface Pressure. If the client has pressure ulcers, pressure reduction is key to management and prevention. If venous stasis ulcers or lymphedema is present, use graded pressure wraps. Details on the management of these ulcers may be found in Chapter 53.

EVALUATION

Wound healing should be assessed every 24 hours, especially if the risk of infection remains high. If the wound shows no signs of healing after 2 weeks, the AHCPR suggests a 2-week trial of topical antibiotics. If no healing occurs after another 2 weeks, the AHCPR advises quantitative bacterial cultures to evaluate for infection and a bone scan to assess for osteomyelitis.

■ Self-Care

The client with open wounds often requires long-term care or community resources for safe self-care. Planning for discharge should begin several days before the client is released so that the home situation can be appraised and the necessary support, supplies, and equipment obtained. Appropriate referral to the home health agency or wound healing clinic should be made before discharge.

Social services, home health care, or a discharge planner should be involved in the plan of care. The client's financial status, home environment, and support systems must be evaluated. Third-party reimbursement may cover supplies, equipment, and nursing care.

Several areas of client education are needed. The client or family should demonstrate dressing removal, wound cleaning, and dressing application before discharge. Detailed written instructions on wound care should be provided to the client, family, and home health care nurse. Explain what changes should be expected and what changes should be reported to the health care provider. Fever, a change in drainage, or the development of an odorous drainage should be instructed as a reportable change. If the client has a pressure ulcer, provide the client or caregiver with a copy of *Treatment of Pressure Ulcers*[2] (Pub. No. 95-B0652 from the AHCPR, at 800-358-9295).

The average cost of skilled nursing services for treating wounds in the home is $1600 per healed wound. Some cost-cutting measures for saline and gloves have been designed, and it is now possible to make normal saline for home use on wounds. Use to 1 gal of distilled water or 1 gallon of tap water boiled for 5 minutes; do not use well water or sea water. Add 8 teaspoons of table salt. Mix the solution well and cool to room temperature before use. This solution can be stored for up to 1 week.

In the home, rather than purchasing gloves for dressing changes, soiled dressings can be removed with a plastic sandwich bag (Fig. 16–8). The inside of the bag is used as a glove to remove the dressing, and the dressing is disposed of in the same bag. Methods of obtaining needed wound care supplies should also be discussed with the client and family.

Alert the client to signs of complications, such as infection, and give directions on when and how to contact the health care provider. A balanced diet with frequent high-protein snacks should continue until the wound and contributing factors have been resolved. A vitamin and mineral supplement should be taken as directed. The client is often required to incorporate lifestyle changes into activities of daily living (ADL) in an effort to promote healing.

DISORDERS OF WOUND HEALING

DELAYED WOUND HEALING

Become aware of the factors that affect wound healing in order to maximize the positive factors and to minimize the negative effects of the factors that may delay healing. If the effects of unfavorable conditions in the wound or systemically within the client are compromised, these may delay healing. This not only causes the client distress but also increases the cost of wound care. Consider both the wound surface and the client's general physical condition when assessing the client, the wound, and the environment in which care will be carried out. The factors affecting wound healing are usually *intrinsic* and *extrinsic,* although some factors may fall into both categories.

Awareness of the intrinsic and extrinsic factors that

Place a small, clean bag over your hand like a mitten.

Carefully lift the dressing off the sore.

Turn the bag inside out to enclose the dressing.

Seal the bag before throwing it away.

Figure 16–8 Plastic bags used as gloves to remove a dressing in the home. (Adapted from Agency for Health Care Policy and Research. (1994). *Treating pressure sores.* Bethesda, MD, U.S. Department of Health and Human Services, AHCPR Publ. No. 95-B0654.)

can affect wound healing is required by staff who are assessing wounds, prescribing wound care products, and evaluating the care. The factors mentioned here are just a small number of conditions that can impede wound healing. As your experience grows, you will become more aware of the intrinsic and extrinsic factors that affect your clients. This knowledge is required to enable the caregiver to enhance the positive factors and to address and reduce the negative effects of intrinsic and extrinsic factors on a wound.

■ INTRINSIC FACTORS

Intrinsic factors can be divided into eight general categories: (1) health status and concurrent systemic illness, (2) age and body build, (3) nutritional status, (4) infection, (5) decreased circulation, (6) diabetes mellitus, (7) smoking, and (8) steroid use.

HEALTH STATUS AND CONCURRENT SYSTEMIC MELLITUS ILLNESS. Any systemic illness (e.g., chronic obstructive pulmonary disease, diabetes mellitus, peripheral vascular disease) may result in a reduced amount of oxygen and nutrients reaching the wound bed. Hypoxia at the tissues reduces collagen synthesis that is required for wound repair. This results in a longer time required for healing. The resulting scar has a reduced tensile strength and may be more vulnerable to reinjury.

AGE AND BODY BUILD. With age, the dermis and epidermis are not as firmly interlocked as before because the junction between them is flattened. The skin also thins and becomes less elastic, muscle tone is lost, and blood flow is reduced. There is slower healing, and the inflammatory response is diminished. Cell migration and division are slower, and all the phases of healing are lengthened. This leads to wounds remaining open for longer periods, which increases the risk of infection and thus further delays wound healing. The elderly population is more likely to have systemic disease, which also takes its toll and has a detrimental effect on wound healing.

Obese clients have increased adipose tissue, which is poorly supplied by the peripheral circulation, and therefore less oxygenated blood and nutrients are delivered to the tissues by the blood. In underweight clients, there may be inadequate storage of suitable energy, which can lead to impaired collagen synthesis and delayed healing. Both obese and underweight clients are at greater risk for pressure sore formation.

NUTRITION. Malnutrition can be present in both obese and underweight clients. Malnutrition results from a diet that is deficient in one or more of the nutrients that are essential for cells to repair damaged tissue and to help prevent damage. An adequate nutritional diet and the body's ability to effectively utilize the energy and deliver the nutrients to the cells are essential for tissue repair and for prevention and elimination of infection. Protein, vitamins, carbohydrates, fats, trace elements, and fluids are necessary and play an essential role in the wound-healing process.

INFECTION. Infection can develop when defense mechanisms are weakened, thus allowing a normal bacterial load to become overwhelming. Alternatively, the bacterial load can be greater than the body's defenses can handle. In healthy clients, the critical number is 100,000 bacteria per gram of tissue. This number is expressed as 10^5 on laboratory cultures of wounds (and other body fluids or tissues). This threshold number for bacteria holds true for all kinds of bacteria except group B streptococci, which can cause infection in lesser quantities. When bacteria are present above 10^5, the body loses control over bacterial proliferation and invasion and infection is present.

The diagnosis of infection is made through quantitative wound biopsy specimen cultures. Results take 24 to 48 hours, and the client receives a broad-spectrum antibiotic while awaiting results. Sometimes, foreign bodies within the wound are a source of infection. Examples include soil, hematoma (accumulations of blood), and bone fragments.

DECREASED CIRCULATION. An adequate blood supply is essential for all aspects of wound healing. The blood supply can be restricted through disorders of the heart, vessels, or lungs. Hypoxia impairs delivery of oxygen and nutrients to the wound and the action of various defensive cells. Neutrophils require oxygen to generate hydrogen peroxide to kill the pathogens. Likewise, fibroblast and collagen proliferation is slowed. The only aspect of wound healing that can proceed in hypoxic states is angiogenesis.

DIABETES MELLITUS. Diabetes predisposes many clients to difficulty in wound healing because of impaired collagen synthesis, angiogenesis, and phagocytosis. Elevated glucose levels interfere with the cellular transport of ascorbic acid into various cells, including fibroblasts and leukocytes. Hyperglycemia also decreases leukocyte chemotaxis. Atherosclerosis, especially of small vessels, is also common in clients with diabetes and impairs tissue oxygen delivery. Diabetic neuropathy further impairs healing by interrupting the neurologic components of healing (e.g., reducing vasodilation and the protective sensation of pain). Control of glucose levels after surgery facilitates normal wound healing.

SMOKING. Smoking causes vasoconstriction and hypoxia because of the carbon monoxide in the smoke. In addition to limiting oxygen supply, smoking increases atherosclerosis and platelet aggregation. These conditions further restrict the amount of oxygen in the wound.

STEROIDS. The use of steroids slows healing by inhibiting collagen synthesis. Clients who are taking steroids have decreased wound strength, inhibited contraction, and impeded epithelialization. Fortunately, vitamin A reverses some of the healing impairments caused by steroids.

■ EXTRINSIC FACTORS

Extrinsic factors are often the initial cause influencing the failure for wounds to respond favorably to local wound management or systemic therapy of chronic disease. Awareness of the extrinsic factors and their effects on the wound is an important component of good, consistent wound care.

Extrinsic factors of delayed wound healing include (1) mechanical stresses, (2) debris, (3) environmental temperature, (4) maceration, and (5) chemical assaults.

MECHANICAL STRESSES. Mechanical stresses that impede wound healing include friction and shear. Friction is the force that occurs when skin is dragged across a coarse surface, such as bed linens. Shearing forces occur when a mechanical force acts on an area of skin in a direction parallel to the body's surface. Shear is affected by the amount of pressure exerted, the coefficient of friction between the materials contacting each other, and the extent to which the body makes contact with the support surface. Shearing force often occurs when clients sit for a long period of time. When sitting, their skin remains stuck to the support surface while the underlying structures slide down because of gravity. This internal pressure can deter wound healing or cause new wounds.

DEBRIS. When foreign material is left in the wound it

prolongs the inflammatory response and may increase the potential for infection. Foreign material in wounds may include cotton fibers, loose grit, or necrotic or sloughy tissue. Appropriate debridement must be used to remove the foreign material.

ENVIRONMENTAL TEMPERATURE. Extreme temperatures can be devastating to a wound. Frostbite or burns can delay or prevent healing and cause extensive damage. The caregiver must be cautious when using heat or cold to treat the symptoms of the wound. Cold causes vasoconstriction and heat brings about vasodilation. The effects of these changes in circulation must be considered when temperature is used in wound care.

MACERATION. Continuous exposure of wounds and the surrounding skin to moisture from the outside or poor management of wound exudate can lead to maceration and break down the skin surrounding the wound, causing enlargement of the wounded tissues. Protection of the skin and the wound surface with appropriate wound dressings and care of the skin by careful skin hygiene help to reduce the effects of urine, feces, and sweating or excessive wound exudate.

CHEMICALS. The use of chemical substances on wounds can no longer be advocated. Topical antiseptics do not significantly reduce the numbers of bacteria in wounds and are toxic to the cells within the body attempting to repair the defect. If cleaning of a wound is required, normal saline is recommended.

WOUND INFECTION

Wound infection is a serious consequence and delays wound healing. Infection is often due to lack of blood supply, lack of oxygen, or exposure to environmental pathogens. Clinical manifestations of wound infection include increased drainage, erythema around the entire wound (not just the edges), and development of purulent drainage, pain, fever, leukocytosis, and general malaise. The infected wound is slow to heal and may open (see text on evisceration and dehiscence later).

Cultures can be used in the diagnosis of wound infection. A swab culture of wound drainage can be obtained. A quantitative culture (an actual sample of tissue) is usually needed to study open wounds. All open wounds are colonized, and using a swab culture does not reveal the true offending organisms, only organisms growing on the wound's surface.

Outcome Management

Topical antimicrobial agents can be used as the primary treatment. The ideal antimicrobial is a broad-spectrum agent and preserves the regenerating tissues. All antimicrobials compromise wound healing to some degree by having low efficacy against a particular organism or by interfering with healing. A variety of topical agents can be used to either clean or disinfect the wound (see Table 16–4).

Hydrogen peroxide breaks down into water and oxygen. When hydrogen peroxide is used in a wound, H_2O_2 must be rinsed off the wound bed with normal saline to remove any trapped oxygen before the tissues can absorb it. Povidone-iodine, acetic acid, and sodium hypochlorite are used only in debris-contaminated, infected, and malodorous wounds. These agents are cytotoxic and inhibit granular tissue growth and damage endothelial cells and fibroblasts. Therefore, their use is usually short term.

Medical Management

The goal of medical management of clients with wound infection is to promote healing. The extrinsic and intrinsic factors that lead to nonhealing are examined. Not all of these factors can be eliminated, however. Clients cannot be made younger, and some clients refuse to stop smoking, even though their nonhealing is due to inadequate circulation. At times, bypass surgery may be required to restore adequate blood flow. Cultured epithelial grafts and hyperbaric oxygen are relatively new treatments in the care of nonhealing wounds. Wound healing accelerators, such as topically applied growth factors, electric currents, and negative pressure, are being studied. Most chronic nonhealing wounds are managed by a team of health care providers that may include a wound care physician, vascular or orthopedic surgeons, a wound care nurse, a nutritionist, a physical therapist, hyperbaric medicine specialists, and social workers and psychologists. Even for these teams, chronic nonhealing wounds are a challenge.

Chronic wounds commonly affect several groups of clients. Clients with diabetes, venous or arterial disease of the legs, and collagen diseases (such as scleroderma) often do not heal quickly or completely. Several forms of adjunctive treatment are discussed briefly next.

ADJUNCTIVE WOUND HEALING TREATMENTS

ELECTRIC STIMULATION. Pulsed galvanic stimulation (Diapulse) is a form of electricity applied to the skin's surface. The electric currents stimulate DNA synthesis, increase blood flow, enhance fibroblast proliferation, and promote cell migration across the wound. This modality appears to be effective in promoting healing in wounds that have been refractory to other forms of treatment. Clients who are considering the use of electrotherapy should seek centers that have proper equipment and trained personnel.

HYPERBARIC OXYGEN THERAPY. Hyperbaric oxygen (HBO) is the administration of oxygen at greater than atmospheric pressure. When oxygen is inhaled under pressure, the level of tissue oxygen is greatly increased. The high levels of oxygen promote the action of phagocytes and promote healing of the wound by increasing the action of fibroblasts. HBO is effective in clients with complex wounds, especially clients with osteomyelitis and other types of infection. HBO is becoming more available in the United States. As with electric stimulation, a properly trained staff is critical. Clients who have inner ear problems and claustrophobia require pretreatment care.

TOPICAL APPLICATION OF GROWTH FACTORS. The same growth factors that are found in the wound bed naturally can be grown in a laboratory and applied to the wound bed. Research is ongoing to determine the biologic activity and the potential benefits of topical application of these growth factors. The efficacy of these treatments is still being studied. At the present time, only becaplermin (Regranex), a PDGF for use in diabetic foot ulcers, has gained approval for use by the Food and Drug Administration.

NEGATIVE PRESSURE WOUND THERAPY. The application of controlled negative pressure in a clean wound bed can assist and accelerate wound healing. A black sterile, reticulated foam sponge is placed in the wound bed. A connecting evacuation tube is attached to external suction and removes excess fluid in the wound and peripheral edema. The foam and tube are secured with transparent adhesive dressing. A small electrical unit controls pressure, and drainage is collected in a canister attached to the unit and to the sponge. Negative pressure wound therapy increases healing rates by up to 40%.

Nursing Management of the Medical Client

Your role in the care of the client with a nonhealing wound is to provide ample information for self-care, including how to change dressings, the disease process underlying the wound, and how to return to work or activities without increasing the risk of nonhealing. For example, a woman with venous stasis ulcers may need to return to work but can do so safely only when the ulcer is healed. She also needs to know how to apply bandages, how long to elevate her legs while at work, and how to move her legs while working (e.g., walking rather than standing). You serve a vital role in determining whether these requirements are feasible for the client and employer.

WOUND DISRUPTION

Dehiscence is the interruption of a previously intact suture line (see Chapter 16). A sharp pain in the suture line or a cough and increased serosanguineous drainage from the wound frequently precede dehiscence. *Evisceration* is the opening of a wound with exposure of internal organs. It is obviously more serious than dehiscence. If a client experiences evisceration, cover the exposed organs with sterile wet dressings, notify the physician, and prepare the client for surgery. Also notify the physician about dehiscence, although it is not an emergency.

ALTERED COLLAGEN SYNTHESIS

Hypertrophic scars are scars that are raised above the suture line. They may be painful and itch. In general, hypertrophic scars tend to regress over time. Keloids are scars that extend well beyond the suture line (Fig. 16–9). These scars tend to occur in African Americans and clients of Mediterranean descent. The scars can be excised from a wound but, unfortunately, tend to recur. Newer treatments include the use of topical forms of heat.

CONCLUSIONS

Wound healing is a complex process but often goes on with little effort on the part of the client. Only when the wound does not heal or pressure ulcers develop are the many steps in wound healing evident. Wound care follows some basic principles: debride the wound of nonviable tissues, keep the wound bed moist, protect the surrounding skin, apply the proper dressings, use safe topical agents, and fill dead space.

Figure 16—9 Keloid formation. Keloids are overgrowths of scar tissue above and beyond the normal boundaries of the scar. They are fairly resistant to treatment.

THINKING CRITICALLY

1. **You are caring for a man with large venous stasis ulcers on his lower legs. When he was admitted, the ulcers were covered with soft yellow devitalized tissue. He has been treated with wet-to-dry dressings for the past 7 days. Today, you notice that the ulcers are red and wet with a lumpy appearance. What should be done?**

Factors to Consider. Is the appearance of red and lumpy tissue in a wound good or bad? What might be happening? What type of dressing is best used on this red and lumpy tissue?

2. **You are caring for an older homeless man after emergency abdominal surgery. He has had a nasogastric tube in place for 3 days for ileus and is receiving 1 L of IV fluids of 5% dextrose with 0.45 normal saline with 20 mEq of potassium every 8 hours. Prior to surgery, serum albumin was 3.2 g/dl, hemoglobin was 9.6 g/dl, and WBCs were 17,000/mm³. His weight was 104 pounds and height 5 feet 5 inches. What are this client's chances of recovery? What interventions should be considered?**

Factors to Consider. Does this client have evidence of malnutrition? If so, what effect does malnutrition have on wound healing? What short-term and long-term interventions may need to be initiated? Does this client have a risk of fluid or electrolyte imbalance? If so, which ones, and what can be done (or is being done) to reduce the risk?

BIBLIOGRAPHY

1. Baranoski, S. (1995). Wound assessment and dressing selection. *Ostomy and Wound Management, 41* (suppl. 7A), 7S–12S.
2. Bergstrom, N., et al. (1994). *Treatment of pressure ulcers.* Clinical Practice Guideline, No. 15. Rockville, MD, U.S. Department of Health and Human Services, Public Health Service, Agency for Health Care Policy and Research. AHCPR Pub. No. 95-B0652.
3. Black, S. (1995). Venous stasis ulcers. *Ostomy and Wound Management, 41*(8), 20–32.
4. Brylinsky, C. M. (1995). Nutrition and wound healing: An overview. *Ostomy and Wound Management, 41,* 14–16.
5. Cooper, D. (1995). Indices to include in wound assessment. *Advances in Wound Care, 8*(4), 18–25.
6. Eastman, S. (1997). Negative pressure wound therapy. *Plastic Surgical Nursing, 18*(1), 27–37.
6a. Falanga, V., et al. (1995). Experimental approaches to chronic wounds. *Wound Repair and Regeneration, 3*(2), 132–140.
7. Gentzkow, G. D. (1992). Electrical stimulation for dermal wound healing. *Wounds: A Compendium of Clinical Research and Practice, 4*(6), 227–235.
8. Kerstein, M. (1997). The scientific basis of healing. *Advances in Wound Care, 10*(3), 30–36.
9. Kerstein, M., & Polasky, S. (1995). Wounds associated with decreased sensibility. *Wounds: A Compendium of Clinical Research and Practice, 7*(1), 30–34.
10. Kiy, A. M. (1997). Nutrition and wound healing: A bio-psychosocial perspective. *Nursing Clinics of North America, 32,* 849–862.
11. Ladin, D. A. (1998). Understanding dressings. *Clinics in Plastic Surgery, 25,* 433–441.
12. Lazarus, G., et al. (1994). Definitions and guidelines for assessment of wounds and evaluating healing. *Archives of Dermatology, 130,* 489–493.
13. Netscher, D., & Clamon, J. (1994). Smoking: Adverse effects on outcomes for plastic surgical patients. *Plastic Surgical Nursing, 14*(4), 205–210.
14. Stotts, N., & Hunt, T. (1997). Managing bacterial colonization and infection. *Clinics in Geriatric Medicine, 13*(3), 565–573

CHAPTER 17

Perspectives on Infectious Disorders

Carol Sharkey

For one brief moment in human history (circa 1950 to 1980), management of infectious disease did not dominate health care practice. By the close of that era, sickness and death caused by infectious diseases had plummeted as a result of multifaceted social, public health, and medical control efforts. Environmental sanitation had curbed such killers as yellow fever, cholera, typhus, malaria, typhoid fever, and plague.

International vaccination programs had eradicated smallpox. Organized efforts to vaccinate all children lowered the occurrence of vaccine-preventable diseases, particularly measles, mumps, rubella, diphtheria, tetanus, and poliomyelitis. Improved living conditions and personal hygiene had diminished parasitic diseases and gastrointestinal (GI) infections. The widespread availability of antibiotics quelled the fear of deadly tuberculosis, syphilis, gonorrhea, bacterial meningitis, scarlet fever, and rheumatic fever. Nosocomial (hospital-acquired) infections, which had already responded to medical asepsis, responded further to antibiotics, and medical technology continued to produce anti-infective agents to match the newly developing antibiotic-resistant organisms. As a result, health professionals could focus on prevention and management of chronic disease.

This brief moment in history did not last. The 1980s and 1990s brought new infectious agents, such as *Legionella,* the human immunodeficiency virus (HIV), and the Ebola virus (which actually first appeared in 1976), all reminders of human vulnerability to infectious disease. Hepatitis, tuberculosis, sexually transmitted diseases, and many vaccine-preventable diseases persist, spread, and continue to kill. Nonpathogenic organisms continue to create devastating disease in immunocompromised people and in those with chronic diseases or malnutrition. Antibiotic-resistant organisms have developed with chronic misuse and improper prescription of antibiotics. In addition, many of the major killers of the past, such as cholera and yellow fever, continue to cause death and destruction in parts of the world where poor sanitation, poor hygiene, and poverty are endemic.

All people, particularly health care professionals, must maintain vigilance to infectious diseases—to prevention rather than simply treatment. Prevention requires an understanding of the infectious process and the control measures needed. This chapter describes the process of infection and selected aspects of prevention and control. Other chapters explain the nursing care of clients with specific infectious diseases.

THE PROCESS OF INFECTION

Infection is a process by which an organism establishes a parasitic relationship with its host. The process begins with transmission of an infectious organism. Infection may end in infectious disease, a condition that depends on the response of the host to the invader. The entire process and its outcome hinge on a complex interaction of (1) the *infectious agent,* (2) an *environment* conducive to transmission of the organism, and (3) a susceptible *host.* The agent, the host, and their environmental interaction are prerequisites to infectious disease.

■ AGENT

Humans coexist with many microorganisms in complex, mutually beneficial relationships. Many organisms establish residence on or in the host and usually cause no harm. Other organisms are parasitic, maintaining themselves at the expense of their host. Some parasites arouse a pathologic response in the host and are called *pathogens* or *pathogenic agents.* In one sense, pathogens are ineffective parasites because they stimulate an inflammatory response, leading to a disease that may harm the host and eventually kill the pathogen.

All microorganisms can be distinguished by certain intrinsic properties. These properties provide the basis for identifying and classifying bacteria, viruses, fungi, and helminths. An organism's properties include its shape, size, structure, chemical composition, antigenic make-up, growth requirements, viability under adverse environmental conditions, and ability to produce toxins. Viability is a particularly important property to health care professionals because it determines the pathogen's ability to survive outside its host. Organisms that can survive drying, sunlight, heat, or other adverse environmental conditions require more aggressive tactics to prevent transmission.

■ ENVIRONMENT

Transmission of an infectious agent from a source to a susceptible host occurs within an environment. Organisms live and multiply in a *reservoir,* which can be a person, animal, plant, soil, food, or other organic substance or combination of substances. The reservoir provides what the organism needs for survival at specific stages in its life cycle. Infected people are the reservoirs for most bacteria and viruses that affect humans.

Both human and animal reservoirs may be infected and, therefore, may also be hosts. An infected host may be asymptomatic—a *carrier* of the pathogen. A carrier maintains an environment that promotes growth, multiplication, and shedding of the parasite without exhibiting manifestations of disease.

Organisms can have one or more than one *route of transmission* from the reservoir to a new host. In fact, transmission can occur through five mechanisms:

1. *Contact transmission.* Through *direct* transmission, an organism moves from an infected person (or carrier) to an uninfected person via direct contact between their body surfaces. Through *indirect* transmission, an uninfected person picks up an infectious organism from an intermediate object, such as contaminated gloves, a used needle, or a dirty dressing.
2. *Droplet transmission.* An uninfected person picks up an infectious organism when an infected person coughs, sneezes, or talks. These activities propel droplets a short distance through the air, and they may land on an uninfected person's conjunctivae, nasal mucosa, or oral mucosa. Certain procedures, such as suctioning and bronchoscopy, can generate droplets as well.
3. *Airborne transmission.* Droplets can evaporate into airborne nuclei, or microbes can become attached to floating dust particles. Unlike droplets, dry nuclei and dust particles can float a long way in the air. Relatively few organisms remain viable as airborne nuclei, but those that do can be transmitted in the air and breathed into the lungs.
4. *Common vehicle transmission.* Many uninfected people can pick up an infectious organism from the same contaminated source, such as food, water, a medication, or a device.
5. *Vector transmission,* An infected creature, such as a mosquito, fly, rat, or flea, transmits an infectious organism by biting an uninfected host.

The *portal of exit* is the place whence the parasite escapes the reservoir. Generally, this site corresponds to the *portal of entry* into the next host. For example, the portal of exit for GI parasites is generally the feces and the portal of entry into a new host is the mouth. As is the case with other links in the transmission chain, variability exists. Hookworm eggs, for example, are shed in the feces, but hookworm larvae enter through the skin of a person walking barefoot in soil containing hatched eggs. Common portals of exit include secretions and fluids (respiratory and vaginal secretions, blood, tears, semen, breast milk), excretions (urine and feces), open lesions, and exudates. Some organisms, such as HIV, have more than one portal of exit. Knowledge of the portal of exit is essential for preventing transmission of a pathogen.

A pathogen may enter a new host by ingestion, inhalation, contact with mucous membranes, percutaneously, or transplacentally. Infectious diseases vary as to the number of organisms and the duration of the exposure required to start the infectious process in a new host.

■ HOST

Some humans are more susceptible to infectious disease than others. A susceptible host has characteristics and behaviors that increase the probability of infectious disease. Factors such as age, sex, ethnicity, heredity, altitude, and temperature influence the likelihood of infection. For example, the ethnic custom of eating raw fish may increase the risk of exposure to pathogens. General health and nutritional status, hormonal balance, and the presence of concurrent disease also play a role. Living conditions and personal behaviors—such as drug use, diet, hygiene, and sexual practices—also influence the risk of exposure to pathogens and resistance once exposure has occurred. Susceptibility is also influenced by anatomic and physiologic defenses, sometimes called *lines of defense.* Even though an infectious disease is said to be caused by an etiologic (causal) agent, infection results from interactions among a variety of factors related to agent, host, and environment (Table 17–1).

The host's first-line defenses are external and act to bar invasion by pathogens. These defenses are nonspecific, in that they act against any invading pathogen. First-line defenses include (1) *physical* and *chemical barriers* and (2) the body's own natural flora.

Physical barriers include intact skin and mucous membranes; oil and perspiration on skin; cilia in respiratory passages; gag and cough reflexes; peristalsis in the GI tract; and the flushing action of tears, saliva, and mucus. All act to remove organisms before they have an opportunity to infect. The chemical composition of body secretions such as tears and sweat, together with the pH of saliva, vaginal secretions, urine, and digestive juices, further prevents or inhibits the growth of organisms. Compromise of any of these natural defenses increases host susceptibility to pathogen invasion.

Another important first-line defense is the *normal flora* of microorganisms that inhabit the skin and mucous membranes of the oral cavity, GI tract, and vagina. These microorganisms are indigenous to (occur naturally in) specific tissue. They typically coexist with their host in a mutually beneficial relationship as long as they do not migrate from the specific site. Through a mechanism called *microbial antagonism,* they control the replication of potential pathogens. The importance of this mechanism is evident when the mechanism is disturbed. An example of disturbance is the overgrowth of *Candida albicans* (thrush) that results from extensive antibiotic therapy that destroys normal flora in the GI tract or vagina.

Some normal flora can become pathogenic under specific conditions, such as immunosuppression or displacement of the pathogen to another area of the body. The opportunistic infections experienced by clients with symptomatic HIV infection are an example of immunosuppression. Displacement is seen when *Escherichia coli,* normally found in the GI tract, invades the urogenital tract

TABLE 17–1	AGENTS AND SITES OF SELECTED INFECTIOUS DISEASES			
Disease	**Infectious Agent**	**Site of Infection**	**Reservoir**	**Mode of Transmission**
BACTERIA				
Cholera	*Vibrio cholerae*	Gastrointestinal tract	Humans	Ingestion of water contaminated with feces
Diarrhea	*Escherichia coli*	Gastrointestinal tract	Humans	Ingestion of contaminated food or water
Giardiasis	*Giardia lamblia*	Gastrointestinal tract	Water, humans, wild animals	Ingestion of cysts in fecally contaminated water and food
Gonorrhea	*Neisseria gonorrhoeae*	Genitourinary tract	Humans	Sexual contact
Lyme disease	*Borrelia burgdorferi*	Skin, joints, systemic	Wild rodents and deer	Tick bite
Malaria	*Plasmodium* spp.	Red blood cells, liver	Mosquito	Bite from infected mosquito
Meningitis	*Neisseria meningitidis*	Meninges	Humans	Direct contact with droplets from respiratory passages
Pneumonia	*Streptococcus pyogenes*	Lung	Humans	Inhalation; aspiration of gastric contents
Rocky mountain spotted fever	*Rickettsia rickettsii*	Vascular endothelium	Ticks	Tick bite
Toxoplasmosis	*Toxoplasma gondii*	Eye, lung, brain	Cats	Ingestion of cysts on fecally contaminated fingers or in food; transplacental
Tuberculosis	*Mycobacterium tuberculosis*	Lung	Humans	Inhalation of droplet nuclei
Wound infection	*Staphylococcus aureus*	Connective tissue	Humans	Contaminated hands, surgical instruments
FUNGI				
Candidiasis	*Candida albicans*	Skin, mucous membranes, genital tract	Humans	Overgrowth associated with damaged skin or mucosa or use of antibiotics
Histoplasmosis	*Histoplasma capsulatum*	Lung	Bat or bird feces	Inhalation of spores
HELMINTHS				
Trichinosis	*Trichinella spiralis*	Gastrointestinal tract, muscle	Animals	Ingestion of raw or undercooked meat
VIRUSES				
Acquired immunodeficiency syndrome (AIDS)	Human immunodeficiency virus	Helper T lymphocyte	Humans	Contaminated needles, blood transfusions, sexual contact, transplacental
Hepatitis B	Hepatitis B virus	Liver	Humans	Contaminated needles, blood transfusions, sexual contact, perinatal
Influenza A	Influenza A virus	Respiratory tract	Humans	Direct contact by aerosol droplets; airborne spread
Measles (rubeola)	Paramyxoviridae	Skin, respiratory tract, systemic	Humans	Direct contact with nasal or throat secretions; airborne spread
Rabies	*Lyssavirus*	Systemic	Dogs, wild animals	Animal bite

and becomes pathogenic. Displacement of normal flora is a common cause of nosocomial infections. Invasive procedures increase the risk of displacing these organisms. For this reason, it is essential to maintain meticulous hand-washing and asepsis.

The *second line of defense* (the inflammatory process) and the *third line* (the immune response) share several physiologic components. These include the lymphatic system, leukocytes, and a multitude of proteins and enzymes.

Even after successful transmission of a pathogen, there may be more than one possible outcome. The pathogen may merely contaminate the body surface. The process ends there if the host's first-line defenses, such as intact skin or mucous membranes, block the pathogen from further invasion. Successful invasion with replication of a pathogen that does not lead to clinical manifestations or a detectable immune response is referred to as *colonization.*

When microorganisms in or on the host cause an immune response, an infection is said to be present. The period of time during which the pathogen is replicating but before it is shed from the host is called the *latent period.* During latency, host inflammatory and immune responses may ward off the organism or its by-products, thus preventing tissue damage, or the pathogen or its products may begin to destroy undefended or poorly defended tissue, producing infectious disease. Disease manifestations herald the end of the *incubation period,* which is defined as the time from invasion of the disease to the appearance of manifestations. By definition, *infectious disease* is the pathophysiologic response of a host to the destructive action of the pathogen, to its toxic products, or to the host immune responses to fight the pathogen. This pathophysiologic response is generally symptomatic. An asymptomatic pathologic response is called a *subclinical infection.*

An important point is that an asymptomatic host can still transmit a pathogen. The host may harbor the pathogen in sufficient quantities to shed it at any time after latency and toward the end of the incubation period. The time during which an organism can be shed is called the *period of communicability.* It usually precedes manifestations and coincides with part or all of the clinical disease, sometimes extending to convalescence. The communicable period, like the incubation period, varies with the pathogen and the disease.

RISKS OF HOSPITALIZATION

Nosocomial infections (which arise in a hospital or other health care facility) are a leading cause of death in the United States and are associated with significant morbidity.[18, 27] Infections present or incubating at the time of admission are referred to as *community-acquired.* From 5% to 10% of hospitalized clients acquire a nosocomial infection.[18] Occupationally acquired infections among the staff of a hospital are also considered nosocomial.

The source of nosocomial pathogens in health care facilities varies, but both health care workers and clients are reservoirs in most instances. For example, *Staphylococcus aureus* is often carried on the skin and in the nasopharynx. Respiratory secretions, feces, urine, and blood are reservoirs for some nosocomial organisms. Liquids and inanimate objects in the hospital environment may also serve as sources of nosocomial infections. The most important means of transmission is via the hands of health care workers. Hand-washing, combined with principles of asepsis and proper use of gloves, is the best method of preventing nosocomial infections.

The most common sites of nosocomial infections in clients are the urinary tract, lower respiratory tract, surgical wounds, and the bloodstream.[11] Various pathogens can cause nosocomial infections in multiple sites. For example, *Pseudomonas aeruginosa* is the organism that causes most cases of nosocomial pneumonia, but it also causes urinary tract and surgical site infections. *S. aureus* is a common cause of surgical site infection, pneumonia, and bloodstream infection. Table 17–2 lists common nosocomial pathogens.

TABLE 17–2	THE MOST COMMON CAUSES OF NOSOCOMIAL INFECTION*
Site of Infection	**Pathogen**
Bloodstream	Coagulase-negative staphylococci *Staphylococcus aureus* *Enterococcus* spp. *Candida albicans* *Enterobacter* spp.
Lung	*Pseudomonas aeruginosa* *Staphylococcus aureus* *Enterobacter* spp. *Klebsiella pneumoniae* *Haemophilus influenzae*
Surgical wound	*Enterococcus* spp. Coagulase-negative staphylococci *Staphylococcus aureus* *Pseudomonas aeruginosa* *Enterobacter* spp.
Urinary tract	*Escherichia coli* *Candida albicans* *Enterococcus* spp. *Pseudomonas aeruginosa* *Klebsiella pneumoniae*

* Organisms are listed by major site and order of importance.
Data from Centers for Disease Control and Prevention. (1997). National Nosocomial Infections Surveillance Report, data summary from October 1986–April 1997, issued May 1997. *American Journal of Infection Control, 25,* 477–487.

■ URINARY TRACT INFECTIONS

Urinary tract infections (UTIs) are the most common nosocomial infections, and about 80% stem from urethral catheterization.[18, 29] Major risk factors for catheter-related UTIs include female sex, increased duration of catheterization, breaks in the closed catheter system, and lack of administration of systemic antimicrobial agents.[27]

In most catheter-related infections in women, bacteria enter the bladder by the periurethral route. Organisms originating primarily from the fecal flora and found at the meatal and perineal areas may be introduced into the bladder during insertion of the catheter or may migrate along the external surface of the catheter into the bladder. In men, catheter-related infections usually result from *cross-infection* (transmission between clients), with bacteria introduced into the collection system at the junction of the catheter and drainage tube or at the outflow spigot; they then migrate to the bladder in 24 to 48 hours. Most nosocomial UTIs are easily managed, but bacteremia develops in 1% to 4% of affected clients. Of these, up to 15% of clients die.[29]

■ PNEUMONIA

Pneumonia is the second most common nosocomial infection and is associated with more deaths than any other nosocomial infection.[29] Most nosocomial pneumonias are caused by gram-negative bacteria. Aspiration of oropharyngeal or stomach organisms is the predominant mechanism by which nosocomial pneumonia develops.[18] Airborne transmission is usually not the cause.

Stasis (stoppage) of respiratory secretions caused by immobility and a decreased cough also contributes to nosocomial pneumonia. Postoperative clients, particularly those who have had thoracic and upper abdominal surgery, and clients who require ventilatory support are at high risk of aspiration. Clients with diminished consciousness, impaired gag reflex, intubation, or tracheostomy are also at increased risk for aspiration of oral secretions. Other risk factors include old age, decreased mobility, and severe disease, such as chronic lung disease, cardiovascular disease, renal insufficiency, and malignancies.

Nosocomial pneumonia is difficult to prevent because in most cases the microorganisms are derived from the client's own flora. Soon after hospitalization, the oropharynx of many clients becomes colonized with gram-negative bacteria that may be aspirated into the lungs. The use of histamine H_2-blockers, antimicrobial therapy, and enteral nutritional therapy have been found to promote colonization of the oropharynx with gram-negative bacteria.[18, 29] Contaminated respiratory therapy equipment can serve as a source of pathogens as well.

■ SURGICAL WOUND INFECTIONS

Surgical wound infections are a major source of hospital morbidity and account for nearly 60% of extra hospital days.[18] These infections usually result from *endogenous* (inside the host) or *exogenous* (outside the host) microorganisms that enter the wound at the time of an operation. The most common source of infecting bacteria is the client's own flora. Although the physical environment of the operating room is an uncommon source of infection, operating room personnel may shed bacteria-laden skin particles that travel through the air to the open wound.

Factors that influence the development of surgical wound infections include (1) number and types of organisms present in the wound, (2) type of operation, (3) surgeon's technique, and (4) duration of the operation. Surgical wound infection rates almost double for each hour of surgery.[18] Old age, obesity, malnutrition, and underlying immunocompromise are client-related factors that increase the risk of postoperative wound infection.

The risk of surgical wound infection also increases with the length of the client's preoperative hospital stay.[18, 29] Shortening the preoperative stay tends to reduce the risk of infection by decreasing the opportunity for colonization with nosocomial bacteria.[18, 29] Proper preparation of the surgical site is also important. Shaving the operative site—once a common practice—is now known to damage the epithelium, impair the skin's defense mechanism, and raise the risk of infection.

■ DEVICE-RELATED INFECTIONS AND BACTEREMIAS

Rates of nosocomial infection of the bloodstream are increasing, particularly in clients admitted to intensive care units.[29] The increase is partly due to the increased use of intravascular devices in this setting. Intravascular devices may include intravenous (IV) lines, intra-arterial infusion lines, and devices used for diagnostic, therapeutic, and hemodynamic monitoring. The risk of infection is influenced by factors related to the device itself, the site of insertion, and the technique used to place the device. Stiff catheters are associated with higher rates of infection than flexible catheters. Partially implantable catheters and totally implanted injection ports are associated with lower infection rates.[18]

Device-related infections and bacteremias are usually caused by microorganisms found on the client's skin that invade disrupted tissue and migrate around the site of insertion and along the device into the intravascular space. The use of semipermeable membrane dressings over the insertion site facilitates the growth of skin flora. Dressing changes following institution-specific protocols must be done at regularly scheduled intervals under aseptic conditions. Colonization of skin flora can also occur around the hub of the device, the tubing-device junction, or other connectors attached to the system. Although liquids given through the device may become contaminated, infusion-related infection is relatively uncommon.

Client factors that contribute to the risk of device-related infections include age, nutritional status, type and severity of underlying illness, skin condition, and immunosuppressive therapy. Bacteremia is especially common in clients with chronic diseases, malnutrition, and cancer.

■ ANTIBIOTIC-RESISTANT MICROORGANISMS

S. aureus is one of the pathogens most frequently reported to cause nosocomial infections because of its remarkable ability to develop resistance to antibiotics. Before the advent of penicillin in the early 1940s, the fatality rate for bacteremia caused by *S. aureus* was about 90%.[22] The use of penicillin dramatically reduced that rate, but within a few years resistant strains of *S. aureus* evolved that produced a penicillin inactivator. New antibiotics, such as methicillin, were effective in the 1960s, but they provided only a temporary solution to the problem. In the 1980s, epidemics of infections with methicillin-resistant *S. aureus* (commonly called MRSA) forced operating rooms and intensive care units to close. Once introduced into a hospital, MRSA is difficult to eliminate.[22] It spreads via nasopharyngeal secretions and via the hands of health care workers and clients.

Prior to the introduction of linezolid (Zyvox) in 2000 and the combination of quinupristin and dalfopristin (Synercid) in 1999, vancomycin was the antimicrobial agent of choice for MRSA[14, 14a]. The action of Zyvox differs from other antibimicrobials in that it blocks bacterial growth by disrupting initiation of the process that microorganisms use to make proteins. Zyvox is administered via intravenous and oral routes and is effective against gram-positive bacteria such as *S. aureus,* streptococci, and enterococci.

Strains of vancomycin-resistant *Enterococcus* (VRE) began to appear in the mid-1980s, and these organisms are now important nosocomial pathogens. Treatment of VRE infections poses a major challenge because these organisms are resistant to a wide variety of antimicrobials. Synercid and Zyvox are the only drugs currently available for treatment of VRE. Environmental cultures in hospital rooms have identified VRE-contaminated client gowns, bed rails, floors, door handles, blood pressure cuffs, stethoscopes, glucose meters, and telephones.

Person-to-person spread, probably by the hands of health care workers, may be a significant mode of transmission.

■ OTHER NOSOCOMIAL INFECTIONS

Effective screening and processing of donated blood and blood products have greatly reduced the risk of HIV transmission to clients in health care settings. The risk of provider-to-client transmission of HIV is remote,[18] although the matter has created much public anxiety. The risk of occupational exposure to HIV in the health care setting has been associated primarily with parenteral exposures to blood from clients infected with HIV. Infection after exposure of mucous membranes to infected blood is much less common.

Nosocomial infection with *hepatitis B virus* (HBV) is another concern in hospitals because the source of a typical nosocomial HBV infection is never identified. Provider-to-client transmission of HBV does not occur with routine client contact. Client-to-provider transmission is a much larger problem and is why health care workers must be vaccinated against HBV.

The resurgence of *tuberculosis* is another major concern in health care facilities. Two factors responsible for this resurgence are (1) poor compliance with therapeutic drug regimens and (2) the emergence of drug-resistant strains of *Mycobacterium tuberculosis*. When clients infected with susceptible strains of the pathogen receive appropriate therapy, sputum smears begin to clear by the third week of treatment. Clients with resistant strains, however, continue to cough up large numbers of viable organisms, exposing many health care workers. Respiratory isolation must be closely followed with high-risk clients until adequate treatment has been given.

Nosocomial infections tend to occur more frequently and with more severity in ill, debilitated, malnourished, immunocompromised, and older clients (Box 17–1). Susceptibility to infection increases when invasive procedures and indwelling devices are used. With the expanding use of invasive devices, more exposure to antimicrobial therapy, and more severely ill hospitalized clients, the risk of nosocomial infections will probably increase. Furthermore, the emergence of resistant organisms is likely to continue, resulting in infections that are more difficult to treat. Although resistance to infection may be enhanced by vaccines and immune globulin, it must be supplemented by manipulation of the physical environment to reduce the risk. This means that nurses must be ever more vigilant in administering care and in supervising those providing care.

PREVENTING AND CONTROLLING INFECTION

To be effective, strategies to prevent and control infection must be based on knowledge of agent-host-environment interactions. The goal in developing and implementing interventions is to prevent the spread of an infectious agent from its reservoir or source to susceptible hosts.

Methods for controlling transmission of infectious disease vary with the characteristics of the organism, its reservoirs, the type of pathologic response it produces, and technology available for control. In general, the aim is to intervene at the point where the greatest number of people can be protected, using the least amount of resources.

BOX 17–1   Infectious Disease in the Elderly

More than any other population, elderly clients are at risk of infection. In fact, studies show that older clients contract about three times as many nosocomial infections as younger clients. Infection frequently leads to hospitalization for nursing home residents, and it is one of the top 10 causes of death in the elderly. Many common infectious diseases, such as pneumonia, urinary tract infection (UTI), sepsis, skin and soft tissue infection, tuberculosis, and herpes zoster, become more common with advancing age.

Elderly clients have an increased risk of infection partly as a normal consequence of growing older. With aging, mechanical barriers—such as skin and mucosa—undergo structural and functional decline. The physiologic reserve capacity of organ systems dwindles, and the immune system falters. When these defense mechanisms are compromised, infection can progress locally and even spread systemically.

Many older adults have chronic diseases that further jeopardize their host defenses. Conditions associated with aging, such as diabetes mellitus and malnutrition, probably exert more influence on immunity than age itself.

Not only do older people contract more infections; they tend to experience more complications of those infections. For example, an older client with pneumonia or a UTI is more likely to develop bacteremia than a younger client with the same infection.

To make matters worse, infection can be more difficult to detect and diagnose in the older client. Older people often do not manifest typical signs and symptoms of infectious diseases. Instead, they may have worsening cognition, an abnormal mental status, lethargy, agitation, loss of appetite, incontinence, or an increased tendency to fall.

Fever—the cardinal sign of infection—may be absent in infected elderly clients, even those who have bacteremia or pneumonia. Many older people have a low baseline temperature. Suspect infection in any elderly client with an oral temperature of 100° F or higher or an increase in baseline temperature of 1.4° F or more. Coexisting diseases may mask the signs of infection even further.

Even drugs used to treat infections are less successful when given to older clients. The drugs produce a weaker response in the older person's body while producing even more adverse reactions. Age-related changes in gastrointestinal, cardiac, and renal function alter the way in which antimicrobial agents are absorbed, distributed, and excreted.

Researchers are looking for better ways to detect and better drugs to treat infections in the elderly. While these agents are being investigated in the elderly population, you can help already infected clients by encouraging individualized dosage regimens and monitoring these clients carefully.

Data from Yoshikawa, T. T., & Normal, D. C. (Eds.). (1994). *Antimicrobial therapy in the elderly client.* New York: Marcel Dekker.

The simplest and most effective way to prevent transmission is meticulous *hand-washing.* Hand-washing is an absolute necessity, even when gloves are worn. Wash your hands before donning gloves and after removing them, before and after each client contact. Teach this procedure to all personnel and continually monitor for compliance. This simple, inexpensive technique, used appropriately, is one of the most potent weapons against the spread of infection. The hygienic hand rub is also effective. This technique involves rubbing 3 to 5 ml of a fast-acting antiseptic preparation onto the hands until dry.[29]

Another method to prevent and control infectious disease involves environmental measures. Some pathogens, such as *S. aureus,* can be controlled by disinfection, sterilization, or anti-infective drugs. Other pathogens can be controlled best by eradicating their non-human reservoirs via environmental sanitation measures, such as water treatment, food safety programs, and control of animals, vectors, sewage, and solid wastes.

Transmission from the portal of exit can often be prevented by detecting and treating clients who are shedding pathogens, such as gonococci. Antimicrobials are among the drugs most frequently prescribed in the United States to treat infections. The use of antibiotics is not without problems, as shown in Box 17–2. Another example of prevention is the use of prophylactic antitubercular medications for clients who are exposed to tuberculosis and whose skin test result is positive.

■ IMMUNIZATION PROGRAMS

Several infectious diseases have been dramatically reduced by maximizing host defenses through active and passive vaccinations that stimulate the immune system to counteract the infectious agent:

Active vaccination refers to the deliberate administration of a modified infecting agent, called a *vaccine,* or a modified toxin, called a *toxoid,* to stimulate an immune response. Protection is not immediate: a period of time is needed to achieve protective antibody levels. However, induced active immunity usually results in long-lived protection against disease.
Passive vaccination refers to the administration of antibodies to a nonimmune person to provide temporary protection against a pathogenic agent or toxin. Passive immunity provides immediate but short-lived protection that lasts a few weeks.

Vaccination programs in the United States have resulted in a significant reduction in childhood infectious diseases. However, a major resurgence of measles occurred from 1989 to 1991, signaling a major problem with childhood vaccination programs.[15] Baseline data from 1989 indicated that the immunization level of preschool children was approximately 70% to 80%, with some segments of the population having levels below 50%.[28] Urban minority populations, particularly African American and Hispanic American children, had much lower immunization levels than those in the general population.[15] The goal of the Department of Health and Human Services is to vaccinate at least 90% of all children in the United States by age 2 years.[28]

An entire population does not have to be immune for prevention of a disease epidemic. When a large propor-

BOX 17–2   The Problem of Resistance to Antibiotics

Among researchers and health care professionals, there is growing concern over the frequent, widespread use of antimicrobial drugs in hospitals and long-term care facilities. Nursing home studies have revealed frequent orders for antibiotics, often without adequate evidence of underlying infection. Worse, many of these drugs were prescribed for infections not responsive to antibiotic therapy, such as viral respiratory tract infections.

Studies in hospitals have found antimicrobial drugs used routinely as prophylaxis for invasive and even noninvasive surgical procedures.[30] Although prophylaxis may be helpful when applied wisely, more than half the drugs studied were used inappropriately. Sometimes the wrong drug was ordered. Some were prescribed for unjustifiable reasons. Others were administered in the wrong dose or for the wrong duration of therapy.

Misuse of antimicrobial drugs may alter a client's normal flora and encourage resistance of pathogenic organisms. To help avoid growing resistance to antimicrobial drugs, obtain appropriate specimens for culture before starting antibiotic therapy. Also check sensitivity reports to ensure that the client receives an appropriate antibiotic.

Controlling the spread of antimicrobial resistance is difficult and requires appropriate selection and administration of antimicrobials, use of antibiotic combinations, and strict asepsis and infection control efforts. Finally, although infection control practices—such as hand-washing, aseptic techniques, and barrier precautions—do not directly limit the emergence of resistant strains, they do prevent transmission of resistant organisms from one client to another.

tion of individual members of a community becomes immune to a disease, the chance of contact between susceptible persons and infected persons decreases. This type of immunity is called *herd immunity.* For example, epidemics of measles are less likely to occur when herd immunity increases and the number of susceptible people in the community decreases.

Vaccination schedules and recommendations are established by the Committee on Infectious Diseases of the American Academy of Pediatrics (AAP) and the Advisory Committee on Immunization Practices (ACIP) of the Centers for Disease Control and Prevention (CDC). The AAP and ACIP recommend that all children be vaccinated against measles, mumps, rubella, diphtheria, pertussis, tetanus, poliomyelitis, *Haemophilus influenzae* type b, HBV, and varicella virus.[8] Hepatitis A (HAV) vaccines are recommended for high-risk children.

Vaccinations are as important for adolescents and adults as they are for children (Table 17–3). Infections seen primarily in children are now occurring in adolescents and adults who never developed active immunity. Adolescents and adults who escaped natural infection or who were not adequately immunized as children are at risk for childhood diseases and their complications. In 1996, the ACIP recommended establishing a routine vaccination visit to a health care provider for adolescents 11 to 12 years old to review their vaccination status and to administer needed vaccines for measles, mumps, rubella,

TABLE 17–3	CDC RECOMMENDATIONS FOR VACCINATION OF OLDER ADOLESCENTS AND ADULTS IN THE UNITED STATES
Disease	**Recommendation**
Polio	Primary series of oral poliovirus vaccine in childhood is sufficient. If no childhood series, vaccine need not be given except to persons at risk because of health care occupation or foreign travel.
Tetanus, diphtheria	Booster dose of tetanus and diphtheria toxoids (Td) every 10 years after primary series of Td; tetanus toxoid may be repeated in 5 years if a dirty wound is sustained. If no childhood series, initiate series of three doses within 1 year.
Pertussis	Primary series of pertussis vaccine is given in childhood only.
Measles	Documented immunity or two doses of MMR* vaccine at least 1 month apart. People who have received only one dose of vaccine since their first birthday should receive a second dose, particularly on enrolling in college, traveling to a foreign country, or entering a health care field.
Mumps	Documented immunity or two doses of MMR vaccine at least 1 month apart.
Rubella	Documented immunity or two doses of MMR vaccine at least 1 month apart. Vaccine particularly recommended for previously unimmunized women of childbearing age and susceptible health care providers.
Hepatitis A	Two doses of vaccine at least 6 months apart for persons who reside in a community that has a high rate of hepatitis A virus infection, who are at risk because of foreign travel, or who have chronic liver disease.
Hepatitis B	Complete series of three doses within 6 months for high-risk individuals including health care providers, susceptible dialysis clients, people with hemophilia, intravenous drug abusers, sexual and household contacts of hepatitis B virus carriers.
Varicella	Documented immunity or two doses of vaccine separated by 4 to 8 weeks. Recommended for health care providers, teachers of young children, day-care employees, and others at high risk for exposure and for transmitting disease.
Influenza	Annually for people older than 65; residents of nursing homes and other chronic care facilities; people with chronic cardiac or pulmonary disease, diabetes or other metabolic disorders, renal disease, severe anemia, or immunosuppression; health care providers and others in close contact with people in high-risk groups.
Pneumococcal	Single dose of vaccine for people older than 65; those with chronic cardiac or pulmonary disease, cirrhosis, alcoholism, diabetes, Hodgkin's disease, nephrosis, renal failure, cerebrovascular fluid leaks, immunosuppression, sickle cell anemia, and asplenism. Revaccination should be considered after 5 years for people at highest risk.

*MMR, measles-mumps-rubella vaccine.
Data from Centers for Disease Control and Prevention.[2, 5–7, 9, 12, 13]

HAV and HBV infections, tetanus, diphtheria, and varicella.[5]

Adolescents older than 12 years and adults through age 64 should complete a primary series of diphtheria and tetanus toxoids, plus measles-mumps-rubella vaccines if they did not receive them as children.[2] Adults 65 years and older should complete a primary series of diphtheria and tetanus toxoids but are generally considered immune to measles, mumps, and rubella. Most people born before 1957 are likely to have been infected naturally with these diseases. People who have a reliable history of varicella are considered immune; those who do not can be tested to determine their immune status or can be vaccinated without testing.[7] Vaccination for other diseases, such as influenza, pneumococcal pneumonia, HAV and HBV, is recommended for people in certain age, occupational, environmental, and lifestyle groups and for those with special health problems.

The elderly population and people with chronic diseases are at particular risk for infectious diseases because of a decline in their immune system. More than 90% of all deaths from influenza A and B viruses occur in people age 65 years and older.[12] The most effective way to reduce the impact of influenza is to vaccinate people at high risk each year before the influenza season. The ACIP recommends that influenza vaccine be administered annually to adolescents and adults at high risk and to all people age 65 and older. For people living in nursing homes and other chronic care facilities, annual vaccination can reduce the risk of influenza outbreaks by inducing herd immunity. Annual vaccination with the current vaccine is necessary because new variants of influenza continue to occur; vaccination against one strain may not confer immunity to another.

Pneumococcal pneumonia, caused by *Streptococcus pneumoniae,* is an important cause of morbidity and mortality in the very young, the elderly, and others with certain high-risk or chronic conditions. The ACIP recommends that these people receive a single dose of pneumococcal polysaccharide vaccine.

You and other nurses can be instrumental in ensuring that all children, adolescents, and adults are properly immunized. Every visit to a health care provider should be an opportunity to obtain a history of vaccination status and to provide vaccinations as needed. In addition, you and other health care providers should be concerned about improving your own resistance to infectious diseases. One important approach is to maintain your immunization status by being vaccinated against HBV infection, measles, mumps, rubella, polio, tetanus, diphtheria, varicella, and influenza.

HBV infection is a major occupational hazard for all health care providers because of the likelihood of contact with blood and blood-contaminated body fluids from infected clients. The Occupational Safety and Health Administration (OSHA) has developed regulations that require employers to offer at-risk employees the HBV vaccine at the employers' expense. Influenza vaccination is recommended yearly for health care providers in hospital, chronic care, and outpatient settings to reduce the risk of illness and to reduce the possibility of transmitting the virus to clients. The vaccinations you receive protect not only you but your clients as well.

■ INFECTION CONTROL IN HOSPITALS

Many nosocomial infections can be prevented if health care personnel adhere to infection control practices. The CDC and the Joint Commission on Accreditation of Healthcare Organizations (JCAHO) issue guidelines and establish standards for control of hospital infection. The CDC develops and updates guidelines related to the control and prevention of nosocomial infections, and JCAHO requires hospitals to establish infection control programs that meet accreditation standards. The JCAHO standards require hospital infection control committees to establish surveillance programs, implement infection control policies and procedures, and conduct continuing education for all hospital employees regarding infection control.[21] Most hospitals employ an infection control nurse or infection control practitioner (ICP) who is responsible for the coordination of a hospital-wide infection control program.

Infection control programs in hospitals address two major areas related to nosocomial infection: (1) surveillance and reporting and (2) control and prevention. The purpose of surveillance is to establish and maintain a database to track the rates of nosocomial infections. Surveillance activities include early detection of infections in clients and personnel and reporting of relevant data to designated people for appropriate action. Surveillance systems to detect both organisms and diseases are necessary components of prevention and control strategies. National data on nosocomial infections are obtained from selected hospitals in the United States by the CDC and used to estimate rates and trends.

The focus of infection control strategies is on barrier precautions to reduce infection risk for all clients and personnel and on occupational health practices to protect health care staff from infection.

Barrier Precautions

Barriers are intended to prevent the transfer of an infective organism to a susceptible host. By placing a clean layer of plastic or fabric between a susceptible site and a potential source of pathogenic organisms, we reduce likelihood of transmitting an infection. The prevented transmission can be from client to caregiver or caregiver to client. The risk for a client increases when caregivers have contact with the client's mucous membranes and non-intact skin. The risk for caregivers increases whenever they are in contact with a client's moist body substances. Protective barriers include gloves, gowns, masks, and protective eyewear.

None of the protective barriers are intended to replace hand-washing. *The most important means of preventing the spread of microorganisms is hand-washing.* Hands become soiled during client care, particularly after contact with moist body sites and substances. Soiled hands have played a major role in transferring organisms to new client hosts. Unfortunately, gloves provide a false sense of security because hands can become contaminated even when gloves are used. The use of gloves is not a substitute for hand-washing.

In the past, most barrier precautions were instituted after a client's infection was diagnosed. When an infection was suspected or recognized, a system of barrier precautions, referred to as *isolation procedures,* was instituted to prevent transmission of pathogens among hospitalized clients, health care personnel, and visitors. Depending on the diagnosis, one of several isolation strategies was used. Precautions varied, depending on the methods needed to interrupt transmission of the infection. For the isolation strategy to be effective, the diagnosis of infection had to be made or suspected early. However, most infections are communicable for some period when manifestations are absent and the infection is undetected.

In the early 1980s, unrecognized cases of HBV and HIV infection were identified as important sources of disease. Health care workers could potentially become infected through needle-sticks and body fluids contaminated with clients' blood. In response to this problem, the CDC recommended "universal precautions" as a means of preventing transmission of HIV, HBV, and other blood-borne pathogens.[1] Universal precautions focused on preventing transmission of blood-borne pathogens from infected or potentially infected clients to susceptible caregivers. Universal precautions required the use of protective barriers with all clients regardless of their presumed infection status. These precautions emphasized (1) the use of gloves and gowns to reduce contamination of skin and clothing; (2) the use of masks and goggles to reduce contamination of the mucous membranes of the mouth, nose, and eyes; and (3) prevention of needle-stick injuries. Used needles were not to be recapped by hand, and puncture-resistant containers were to be used for disposal of sharps.

In 1987, the practice of *body substance isolation* (BSI) was proposed as a system to isolate all moist and potentially infectious body substances from all clients, regardless of their presumed infection status.[20] Personnel were to use clean gloves during contact with non-intact skin and mucous membranes and when anticipating contact with blood, feces, urine, sputum, saliva, wound drainage, and other body fluids. BSI was based on the assumption that the blood and body substances of all clients might contain potentially infectious, transmissible organisms.

MANAGEMENT AND DELEGATION

Infection Control

Regulatory agencies have developed specific and complete guidelines for infection control to protect clients and staff from the transmission of infectious diseases. All health care providers must receive training and education on their role in maintaining infection control practices, including Universal Precautions. Your role in providing and delegating care of clients on isolation for known or suspected organisms includes assessment of clients and their environment. Note the level of precaution required according to your institution's system. Ensure that strict attention to isolation techniques is maintained by all who interact with the client. For the newly isolated client, you are responsible for client and family assessment and education regarding infection control measures. Unlicensed assistive personnel may then reinforce your teachings.

Some components of infection control practice may be delegated to unlicensed assistive personnel, such as room setup and maintenance of supplies and equipment. Consider delegating the following tasks:

- Stocking of gloves, gowns, and masks
- Stocking of client-specific equipment, such as thermometers, stethoscopes, and sphygmomanometers
- Cleaning of equipment after use, such as oxygen saturation machines and wheelchairs
- Removal of linen and unused equipment from the client's room

Delegation of direct care provision for clients in isolation to unlicensed assistive personnel should include reinforcement of the outlined precautions. Note: Care of a client in isolation does not change the practice parameters for what unlicensed assistive personnel may provide to the client or what you can delegate. Emphasize the ways in which the isolation status may affect delivery of care. For example, a client isolated because of methicillin-resistant *Staphylococcus aureus* (MRSA) is routinely cared for with gown, gloves, and mask. If that client is actively incontinent, you may need to give unlicensed assistive personnel additional instruction to change gloves between tasks.

Describe findings that are immediately reportable to you for the unlicensed assistive personnel. Such findings may include a disruption of isolation technique or any difficulty the unlicensed assistive personnel experience while providing care.

Kathleen Rea, BSN, RN, *Clinician III, Clinical Manager, Surgical Services, University of Virginia Health System, Charlottesville, Virginia*

In 1996, the Hospital Infection Control Practices Advisory Committee (HICPAC) of the CDC synthesized the various isolation systems into one new set of guidelines.[17] The new guidelines recommend two tiers of isolation strategies: (1) standard precautions and (2) transmission-based precautions (see inside back cover).

Standard precautions are the more important tier and are designed for the care of all clients in hospitals regardless of their diagnosis or presumed infection status. These precautions synthesize the major components of universal precautions and BSI. Standard precautions apply to non-intact skin, mucous membranes, blood, and all body fluids, secretions, and excretions except sweat.

Transmission-based precautions form the second tier and are designed only for the care of clients who have known or suspected infections or have been colonized with transmissible pathogens. These are *additional* precautions needed to interrupt transmission of a nosocomial infection and are used with standard precautions. There are three types of transmission-based precautions, and they may be combined for infections that have more than one route of transmission:

1. *Contact precautions* are designed to reduce direct and indirect contact transmission of microorganisms.
2. *Droplet precautions* are for infections transmitted by large-particle droplets such as those generated during coughing, sneezing, speaking, or suctioning.
3. *Airborne precautions* are designed to reduce the transmission of pathogens on airborne droplet nuclei.

In many cases, the risk of transmitting a nosocomial infection is highest before a diagnosis can be made. Certain clinical syndromes and conditions warrant the addition of transmission-based precautions while the definitive diagnosis is anticipated. For example, contact precautions should be implemented for incontinent or diapered clients who have acute diarrhea with a likely infectious cause such as HAV infection. Clients with infected draining skin lesions or wounds that cannot be covered warrant contact precautions because the wound may be infected with *S. aureus*. Droplet precautions should be implemented for clients with meningitis until infection with *Neisseria meningitidis* is ruled out.

Other examples include clients admitted with rashes or respiratory infections with possible etiologic agents that require additional precautions beyond standard precautions. Additional precautions should also be taken with clients who have a history of infection or colonization with multi-drug–resistant organisms or who had a recent hospital or nursing home stay in a facility where multi-drug–resistant organisms were prevalent.

Control of the spread of nosocomial infections depends on meticulous attention to infection control practices. The CDC has provided excellent institutional infection control guidelines that can be tailored to meet the needs of specific situations or environments. In addition to standard and transmission-based precautions, the CDC has issued special guidelines for preventing nosocomial transmission of tuberculosis,[3] and vancomycin-resistant *S. aureus*,[10] and VRE[4] in health care facilities. See the Management and Delegation feature on infection control.

Occupational Health Practices

The second major component of an infection prevention and control program is to protect health care workers from infection. Occupational health practices include evaluating personnel for existing infections, administering vaccinations, keeping records, managing exposures, educating employees, and developing and enforcing infection control procedures.

When it was recognized that health care workers who had contact with clients' blood were at increased risk for infection by blood-borne pathogens, infection control efforts focused on preventing employee exposure to blood. By 1989, most hospitals had implemented the universal precautions guidelines to protect employees at risk of transmission of HIV and HBV. In addition, efforts focused on HBV vaccination of employees at risk for blood exposure. New employees are screened for susceptibility to tuberculosis, HBV, measles, rubella, and chickenpox. Periodic tuberculin skin testing is recommended for employees at risk for exposure to tuberculosis.

In 1991, OSHA published guidelines—the *blood-borne pathogens standard*—to protect employees exposed to blood and other potentially infectious materials.[24] One of the most important components of the guidelines is the requirement that all health care employees at risk for exposure to blood and body fluids be offered an HBV vaccination free of charge. In addition, OSHA requires all care providers to wear protective attire when they are likely to have contact with blood and other moist body substances that may contain pathogens. Because a third of occupational exposures to HIV result from recapping needles after use, OSHA standards urge the use of needle-less or recessed needle systems. The OSHA blood-borne pathogens standard incorporates most elements of universal precautions plus barrier precautions and needle disposal systems that must be available at the point of use.

Another major area of concern has been the role and selection of respiratory protection equipment to prevent transmission of tuberculosis in hospitals. OSHA has proposed standards for respiratory protection programs to

BRIDGE TO HOME HEALTH CARE

Infection Control

Be alert for signs of high risk in every home situation, focus your teaching on clients' specific needs, and follow infection control guidelines:

1. Use a nursing bag that has a plastic liner or is made from a water-repellent material. Compartments must physically separate clean and dirty items. Store handwashing supplies in an outside pocket.
2. Hang your bag on the back of a sturdy, straight chair or place it on a hard, stable surface, not on the floor, bed, or eating surface. If environmental conditions pose a threat to the bag or its contents, place a barrier beneath the bag. Most agencies recommend clean paper towels or waxed paper and clean plastic bags if moisture is a problem. When the risk of contamination is high because of the environment, pets, children, or infectious agents such as MRSA and VRE, take only the supplies needed for the visit into the home.
3. Wash your hands using your own supplies; do not use the client's bar soap or fabric towels. Wash again after you complete care and remove your gloves. Use a rinse, gel, or foam antimicrobial product if no clean, running water is available. Wash your hands thoroughly as soon as possible after leaving. Teach and remind clients and families to use good technique.
4. Do not carry reusable equipment such as a sphygmomanometer, stethoscope, electronic thermometer, and blood glucose meter in the same compartment as for clean and sterile supplies. For general client use and in low-risk situations, it is not necessary to disinfect these items between use. Do not attempt to disinfect equipment with alcohol or a household disinfectant. If equipment becomes contaminated, follow agency protocols. Leave it in the home or place it in a plastic bag, take it to your office, and follow specific protocols

to clean and disinfect it thoroughly under controlled conditions. In high-risk situations, plan to leave a dedicated blood pressure cuff, stethoscope, or other necessary equipment in the home and teach clients and caregivers how to care for it.
5. Use designated containers to dispose of sharps and other biohazardous waste. Make certain that containers are removed from the home when they are full. Agencies should not allow their employees to transport containers because of the risk to employees and numerous regulations; nurses' vehicles are not approved to transport medical waste. Containers should be removed by a service approved to perform waste removal or mailed under strict federal guidelines to an approved waste disposal center. When neither of these plans is used, some agencies require families to make arrangements with local pharmacies or hospitals for disposal.
6. Place wound care supplies in a plastic bag, tie the bag closed, and dispose of it in the family's garbage. Use double bags only if the soiled dressings are heavily saturated or contain blood or if there is a risk that the plastic may rip or tear. Teach families to use safe disposal techniques that are consistent with local regulations.
7. If any area of the home becomes soiled with blood or body fluids, teach the family to use paper towels and then disinfect with a freshly prepared 1:10 solution of household bleach and tap water. For linens and clothing, add a cup of full-strength bleach to the laundry cycle; warn families that bleach, whether or not it is diluted, may discolor fabrics or other surfaces.
8. Encourage families to use a dishwasher with a heated drying cycle; the next best option is to wash dishes with hot soapy water, rinse thoroughly, and store in a secure, dry place.

Suzanne Shaw, RN, BSN, *Director, Walls Regional Hospital Home Health, Cleburne, Texas* protect hospital personnel from pathogens spread by the airborne route. In particular, surgical masks have not been effective in preventing inhalation of droplet nuclei, and the use of disposable particulate respirators has been recommended instead. Regulations and recommendations are continually being updated by OSHA as health care methods and techniques evolve.[25]

■ INFECTION CONTROL IN LONG-TERM CARE FACILITIES

Nosocomial infections are common among residents of long-term care facilities (LTCFs) and are a major source of morbidity and mortality. UTIs, respiratory infections (influenza, pneumonia), infected pressure ulcers, gastroenteritis, and conjunctivitis are the most common infections found in long-term care facilities.[26] Many long-term care facilities are becoming reservoirs for antimicrobial-resistant organisms, including MRSA and VRE.[23]

Many hospital-oriented infection control guidelines are relevant to long-term care facilities, but they must be adapted, depending on the acuity of residents, facility size, resources, and other factors. The long-term care facility is a home to residents, one in which they usually reside for months or years. Strict barrier approaches used in hospitals can have a negative effect on the residents and the facility's social and rehabilitative goals. Infection control programs must be designed to balance the medical and social needs of long-term care residents. The Association for Practitioners in Infection Control (APIC) has addressed this problem in its guidelines for infection control programs in long-term care facilities.[26]

■ INFECTION CONTROL IN COMMUNITY-BASED SETTINGS

Today, health care is provided to clients in their homes, in physicians' offices, in ambulatory care centers, and in outpatient specialty clinics. Intravenous infusions, hemodialysis, and mechanical ventilation are provided in the home, and nearly half of all surgical procedures are performed in outpatient settings.[29] Venipuncture, wound care, suturing, skin biopsy, bone marrow aspiration and biopsy, plastic and reconstructive surgery, and other minor surgical procedures are commonly performed in physicians' offices. Same-day surgery centers accommodate both minor and major ambulatory surgeries and procedures. Outpatient specialty clinics are available to provide hemodialysis and peritoneal dialysis.

Infections arise during the provision of care in home and outpatient settings, but identifying a break in infection control practices can be difficult. Infection control surveillance programs in community-based settings have been limited, and specific data about infections occurring in homes and outpatient settings are not readily available. Infection control guidelines from the usual resources, such as the CDC, have been written primarily for hospitals. Until setting-specific guidelines are published, commonsense adaptations of hospital infection control practices are recommended.[29] As the shift to managed care continues, it can be expected that infection surveillance and control issues will become more important as a basis for measuring the quality of care and as a requirement for agency certification.

Home care has grown to encompass services provided by family members, partners, and friends as well as health care professionals. Lay caregivers must be given simple guidelines for infection control in the home. Handwashing, use of gloves, and appropriate methods for disposal of contaminated sharps and other waste are examples of infection control practices that must be taught by the home care provider. Clients and their caregivers should be taught about safe food handling, health concerns about pets, and sanitation issues. See Bridge to Home Health Care: Infection Control.

Protecting the health care worker is a critical component of infection control in any health care setting, and the employee health plan should be similar to that used in hospitals. You should not assume that health care workers who work in outpatient settings are at lower risk for infectious diseases than those employed by hospitals. Policies should be developed that meet the requirements of OSHA and other regulating agencies and that acknowledge the unique requirements of the health care setting.

CONCLUSIONS

Infectious diseases have been killers of humans throughout recorded history. For most of this time, conquering infection has been the focus of health care. The nurse's role in preventing, detecting, and treating infectious disease is a vital one. You must be aware of agent-host-environment interactions and take appropriate steps to prevent accidental transmission in all health care settings.

BIBLIOGRAPHY

1. Centers for Disease Control. (1988). Update: Universal precautions for prevention of transmission of human immunodeficiency virus, hepatitis B virus, and other bloodborne pathogens in health-care settings. *Morbidity and Mortality Weekly Report, 37*(24), 377–387.
2. Centers for Disease Control. (1991). Update on adult immunization: Recommendations of the Immunization Practices Advisory Committee (ACIP). *Morbidity and Mortality Weekly Report, 40*(RR-12), 1–94.
3. Centers for Disease Control and Prevention. (1994). Guidelines for preventing the transmission of *Mycobacterium tuberculosis* in health-care facilities. *Morbidity and Mortality Weekly Report, 43*(RR-13), 1–132.
4. Centers for Disease Control and Prevention. (1995). Recommendations for preventing the spread of vancomycin resistance: Recommendations of the Hospital Infection Control Practices Advisory Committee (HICPAC). *Morbidity and Mortality Weekly Report, 44*(RR-12), 1–13.
5. Centers for Disease Control and Prevention. (1996). Immunization of adolescents: Recommendations of the Advisory Committee on Immunization Practices, the American Academy of Pediatrics, the American Academy of Family Physicians, and the American Medical Association. *Morbidity and Mortality Weekly Report, 45*(RR-13), 1–13.
6. Centers for Disease Control and Prevention. (1996). Prevention of hepatitis A through active or passive immunization: Recommendations of the Advisory Committee on Immunization Practices (ACIP). *Morbidity and Mortality Weekly Report, 45*(RR-15), 1–30.
7. Centers for Disease Control and Prevention. (1996). Prevention of varicella: Recommendations of the Advisory Committee on Immunization Practices (ACIP). *Morbidity and Mortality Weekly Report, 45*(RR-11), 1–36.
8. Centers for Disease Control and Prevention. (1999). Notice to readers: Recommended childhood immunization schedule: United States, 1999. *Morbidity and Mortality Weekly Report, 48*(1), 8–16.

9. Centers for Disease Control and Prevention. (1997). Immunization of health-care workers: Recommendations of the Advisory Committee on Immunization Practices (ACIP) and the Hospital Infection Control Practices Advisory Committee (HICPAC). *Morbidity and Mortality Weekly Report, 46*(RR-18), 1–42.

10. Centers for Disease Control and Prevention. (1997). Interim guidelines for prevention and control of staphylococcal infection associated with reduced susceptibility to vancomycin. *Morbidity and Mortality Weekly Report, 46*(27), 626–628, 635.

11. Centers for Disease Control and Prevention. (1997). National Nosocomial Infections Surveillance Report, data summary from October 1986–April 1997, issued May 1997. *American Journal of Infection Control, 25,* 477–487.

12. Centers for Disease Control and Prevention. (1997). Prevention and control of influenza: Recommendations of the Advisory Committee on Immunization Practices (ACIP). *Morbidity and Mortality Weekly Report, 46*(RR-9), 1–25.

13. Centers for Disease Control and Prevention. (1997). Prevention of pneumococcal disease: Recommendations of the Advisory Committee on Immunization Practices (ACIP). *Morbidity and Mortality Weekly Report, 46*(RR-8), 1–24.

14. Centers for Disease Control and Prevention. (1997). Update: *Staphylococcus aureus* with reduced susceptibility to vancomycin: United States, 1997. *Morbidity and Mortality Weekly Report, 46*(35), 813–815.

14a. Centers for Disease Control and Prevention. (2000). *Staphylococcus aureus* with reduced susceptibility to vancomycin—Illinois, 1999. *Morbidity and Mortality Weekly Report, 48*(51), 1165–1167.

15. Cochi, S. L., et al. (1994). Meeting the challenges of vaccine-preventable diseases in child day care. *Pediatrics, 94*(6, Part 2), 1021–1023.

16. Eliopoulos, G. M. (1997). Vancomycin-resistant enterococci: Mechanism and clinical relevance. *Infectious Disease Clinics of North America, 11*(4), 813–849.

17. Garner, J. S., & Hospital Infection Control Practices Advisory Committee. (1996). Guideline for isolation precautions in hospitals. *Infection Control and Hospital Epidemiology, 17,* 54–80.

18. Hoeprich, P. D., Jordan, M. C., & Ronald, A. R. (1994). *Infectious diseases: A treatise of infectious processes* (5th ed.). Philadelphia: J. B. Lippincott.

19. Institute of Medicine. (1992). *Emerging infections: Microbial threats to health in the United States.* Washington, DC: National Academy Press.

20. Jackson, M. M., & Lynch, P. (1991). An attempt to make an issue less murky: A comparison of four systems for infection precautions. *Infection Control and Hospital Epidemiology, 12,* 448–450.

21. Joint Commission on Accreditation of Healthcare Organizations. (1995). *Accreditation manual for hospitals.* Chicago: Author.

22. Maranan, M. C., et al. (1997). Antimicrobial resistance in staphylococci: Epidemiology, molecular mechanisms, and clinical relevance. *Infectious Disease Clinics of North America, 11*(4), 813–849.

23. Nicolle, L. E. (1997). Nursing home dilemmas. *Infection Control and Hospital Epidemiology, 18*(12), 806–808.

24. Occupational Safety and Health Administration. (1991). Occupational exposure to bloodborne pathogens: Final rule. *Federal Register, 56,* 64003–64182.

25. Occupational Safety and Health Administration. (1997). Occupational exposure to tuberculosis: Proposed rule. *Federal Register, 62*(201), 54159–54209.

26. Smith, P. W. & Rusnak, P. G. (1997). SHEA/APIC position paper: Infection prevention and control in the long-term-care facility. *Infection Control and Hospital Epidemiology, 18*(12), 831–849.

27. Soule, B. M., Larson, E. L., & Preston, G. A. (1995). *Infections and nursing practice: Prevention and control.* St. Louis: Mosby–Year Book.

28. U.S. Department of Health and Human Services. (1990). *Healthy people 2000.* Washington, DC: U.S. Government Printing Office.

29. Wenzel, R. P. (Ed.). (1997). *Prevention and control of nosocomial infections* (3rd ed.). Baltimore: Williams & Wilkins.

30. Yoshikawa, T. T., & Normal, D. C. (Eds.). (1994). *Antimicrobial therapy in the elderly client.* New York: Marcel Dekker.

18

Perspectives in Oncology

Patricia Meier

The face of health care, including scientific knowledge and care delivery systems, is ever changing. Likewise, the experience of cancer is changing for our clients and families. Today, a person confronted with a new diagnosis often knows someone who has survived cancer. Yet, cancer remains a frightening unknown for many. Some clients, especially older ones, still associate the word with death. Cancer nursing requires a clinical knowledge of the disease and its treatment as well as the skills to care for and support clients and their families. The pathophysiology and scientific advances discussed in this chapter provide a foundation for promoting positive outcomes for clients with cancer, discussed in the next chapter.

Approximately 1.2 to 1.3 million new cancers are diagnosed in the United States each year. Survival rates and quality of life for people living with the disease have improved. Yet, each year, approximately 552,000 Americans die of cancer. Cancer remains the second leading cause of death in the United States.[2, 20]

The National Cancer Institute (NCI) estimates that 8.4 million Americans alive today have a history of cancer. This number includes disease-free survivors who may be considered "cured," people living with cancer as a chronic disease, and those currently receiving treatment. Six of 10 clients with cancer diagnosed this year are expected to be alive 5 years after the diagnosis.[2]

TERMINOLOGY

The terms *cancer, neoplasm, malignant neoplasm,* and *tumor* are often used interchangeably by both professionals and the lay public. Strictly speaking, these words are not interchangeable. Although generally used as a synonym for cancer, the word *tumor* simply refers to a lump, mass, or swelling. That swelling can be a neoplastic mass, or it may be only an accumulation of fluid.

The word *neoplasm* (derived from the Greek *neos,* new, and *plasis,* molding) is defined as an abnormal mass of tissue that serves no useful purpose and may harm the host organism. A neoplasm can be either *benign* or *malignant.* A benign neoplasm is *usually* a harmless growth that does not spread or invade other tissues. A benign tumor does occupy space. Consequently, if it is located near a vital tube or organ, it can be fatal, as with a benign brain tumor. A malignant neoplasm is a harmful mass, capable of invasion of other tissues and *metastasis* (spread) to distant organs.

The term *cancer* is used to refer to malignant neoplasms. Cancer is a disease of the cell in which the normal mechanisms of the control of growth and proliferation have been altered. It is invasive, spreading directly to surrounding tissue as well as to new sites in the body.

The term *oncology* refers to the medical specialty that deals with the diagnosis, treatment, and study of cancer. An oncologist is a physician who specializes in cancer therapy. There are surgical, radiation, and medical oncologists. A medical oncologist is a physician with expertise in treating cancer with chemotherapy or biotherapy and in handling general medical problems related to the disease or side effects of cancer treatment. Table 18–1 lists other important terms.

EPIDEMIOLOGY

Epidemiology is the study of the distribution and determinants of diseases and health problems in specified populations. The goal of epidemiologic study is the prevention or control of the health problem. One who uses an epidemiologic approach to cancer evaluates patterns of the disease, identifies possible causes, and infers relationships between patterns of disease and determining factors. Although the causes of many cancers remain unknown, epidemiologic studies have helped to identify factors that underlie theories of causation. Nurses can utilize knowledge of the factors associated with cancer causation in promoting positive outcomes for their clients through nursing assessment and interventions.

The NCI established the Surveillance, Epidemiology, and End Results (SEER) program in 1973 as a way to report population-based data in site-specific incidences of cancer, mortality, and survival rates. This report is based on a sample of 12% of the United States population. It includes four metropolitan areas (Atlanta, Detroit, San Francisco/Oakland, and Seattle/Puget Sound). It also contains data from five states (Connecticut, Hawaii, Iowa, New Mexico, and Utah) and the Commonwealth of Puerto Rico. The SEER reporting areas reasonably represent the subsets of the population. Data are gathered from

TABLE 18-1	CANCER TERMINOLOGY
Terms	**Definitions**
Adenocarcinoma	Cancer that arises from glandular tissues. Examples include cancers of the breast, lung, thyroid, colon, and pancreas.
Anaplastic	Tumor cells that are completely undifferentiated and bear no resemblance to cells of tissues of their origin.
Aneuploid	Tumor cells that do not have the normal 46 chromosomes in a human cell. Aneuploid tumors often have a worse prognosis.
Antigens	Substances that cause activation of the immune system.
Carcinoma	A form of cancer that is composed of epithelial cells; develops in tissues covering or lining organs of the body such as the skin, uterus, or breast.
Carcinoma in situ	The earliest stage of cancer, in which the tumor is still confined to the local area, before it has grown to a significant size or has spread.
Cytokine	A substance secreted by immune system cells, usually to send messages to other immune cells.
Differentiation	The process of maturation of a cell line of cancer cells. When they are fully differentiated or well differentiated, they more closely resemble the normal cells in the tissue of origin.
Dysplasia	An alteration in the size, shape, and organization of differentiated cells. Cells lose their regularity and show variability in size and shape, usually in response to an irritant. Cells may revert to normal when the irritant is removed but may transform to a neoplasia.
Hyperplasia	An increase in the number of normal cells in a normal arrangement in a tissue or organ; usually leads to an increase in the size of the part and an increase in functional activity.
Metaplasia	The replacement of one type of fully differentiated cell by another fully differentiated cell that is not normal for that part of the body.
Oncogenes	Specific segments of cellular deoxyribonucleic acid (DNA) that, when inappropriately activated, contribute to the transformation of normal cells into malignant cells.
Sarcoma	A cancer of supporting or connective tissue such as cartilage, bone muscle, or fat.
Tumor markers	Chemicals in the blood that are produced by certain cancers.

hospital medical records. Therefore, the accuracy of the data recorded in clients' medical records by physicians, nurses, and others can affect the accuracy of the SEER data. This ongoing project provides a great deal of information about cancer incidence, prevalence, and mortality for different geographical areas and ethnic groups.

■ INCIDENCE AND PREVALENCE

The *incidence* rate for cancer reflects the number of new cases occurring in a specified population during a year, expressed as the number of cancers per 100,000 people. For the year 2000, about 1,220,100 new diagnoses of cancer were expected (Table 18-2).[20] The incidence gives perspective on the current magnitude of the problem and provides a source for establishing future priorities in cancer control programs. The *prevalence* of cancer is the total number of people alive today, whose cancer has been diagnosed in the current year (incidence) and those whose cancer has been diagnosed previously. The 8.4 million Americans living with a history of cancer (prevalence) include the 1,220,100 people whose cancer has been diagnosed in the current year (incidence).

The reported incidence of cancer appears to have increased since 1900 for several reasons. First, diagnostic methods have become more precise. Utilization of diagnostic tests, such as mammograms for breast cancer and the prostate-specific antigen (PSA) blood test for prostate cancer, has led to earlier detection than previously.

Second, data collection and analysis of cancer statistics have become more sophisticated over the years. Therefore, reported rates of incidence and mortality that are due to cancer are more accurate. Both can result in an increase in the *reported* incidence of cancer but not a true increased incidence of cancer.

Third, Americans are living longer than even a few decades ago. Most cancers take many years to develop. More people are now living long enough for cancer to develop. Therefore, the apparent rise in cancer rates can be somewhat misleading. These factors simply reflect more precise diagnostic and statistical methods combined with the trend toward a longer life span rather than a true increase in the rates of cancer. However, many lifestyle behaviors associated with cancer causation, such as smoking, alcohol intake, and multiple sex partners, are risk factors linked to true changes in cancer rates.

■ MORTALITY

The mortality rate is the number of deaths caused by cancer that occur in the specified population in a given year, expressed as the number of deaths that are due to cancer per 100,000 persons. Figures 18-1 and 18-2 show changes in the mortality rates for lung cancer for both males and females.[2] A decline in lung cancer deaths for males is a reflection of the decline in smoking by American men. Meanwhile, in the words of a long-running tobacco company advertisement, women have "come a long way baby"—all the way to increased incidence of and mortality from lung cancer. In 1987, for the first time more women died of lung cancer than of breast cancer.[27] It is predicted that neither the incidence of nor the mortality from lung cancer has yet peaked in women. The prevalence of smoking by women has begun to decline, although more recently and more gradually than in men.

■ TRENDS

In 1992, cancer rates inched down for the first time. The incidence of cancer had increased 1.2% each year between 1973 and 1992. However, from 1992 to 1995 the incidence of cancer fell 0.7% per year. Mortality rates from cancer likewise fell 2.6% (0.5% per year) from

TABLE 18-2

ESTIMATED NEW CANCER CASES AND DEATHS BY SEX FOR ALL SITES, UNITED STATES, 2000*

	Estimated New Cases			Estimated Deaths		
	Both Sexes	Male	Female	Both Sexes	Male	Female
All Sites	1,220,100	619,700	600,400	552,200	284,100	268,100
Oral cavity and pharynx	30,200	20,200	10,000	7,800	5,100	2,700
Tongue	6,900	4,500	2,400	1,700	1,100	600
Mouth	10,900	6,500	4,400	2,300	1,300	1,000
Pharynx	8,200	5,900	2,300	2,100	1,500	600
Other oral cavity	4,200	3,300	900	1,700	1,200	500
Digestive system	226,600	117,600	109,000	129,800	69,300	60,500
Esophagus	12,300	9,200	3,100	12,100	9,200	2,900
Stomach	21,500	13,400	8,100	13,000	7,600	5,400
Small intestine	4,700	2,300	2,400	1,200	600	600
Colon	93,800	43,400	50,400	47,700	23,100	24,600
Rectum	36,400	20,200	16,200	8,600	4,700	3,900
Anus, anal canal, and anorectum	3,400	1,400	2,000	500	200	300
Liver and intrahepatic bile duct	15,300	10,000	5,300	13,800	8,500	5,300
Gallbladder and other biliary	6,900	2,900	4,000	3,400	1,200	2,200
Pancreas	28,300	13,700	14,600	28,200	13,700	14,500
Other digestive organs	4,000	1,100	2,900	1,300	500	800
Respiratory system	179,400	101,500	77,900	161,900	93,100	68,800
Larynx	10,100	8,100	2,000	3,900	3,100	800
Lung and bronchus	164,100	89,500	74,600	156,900	89,300	67,600
Other respiratory organs	5,200	3,900	1,300	1,100	700	400
Bones and joints	2,500	1,500	1,000	1,400	800	600
Soft tissue (including heart)	8,100	4,300	3,800	4,600	2,200	2,400
Skin (excluding basal and squamous)	56,900	34,100	22,800	9,600	6,000	3,600
Melanoma-skin	47,700	27,300	20,400	7,700	4,800	2,900
Other non-epithelial skin	9,200	6,800	2,400	1,900	1,200	700
Breast	184,200	1,400	182,800	41,200	400	40,800
Genital system	265,900	188,400	77,500	59,000	32,500	26,500
Uterine cervix	12,800	—	12,800	4,600	—	4,600
Uterine corpus	36,100	—	36,100	6,500	—	6,500
Ovary	23,100	—	23,100	14,000	—	14,000
Vulva	3,400	—	3,400	800	—	800
Vagina and other genital, female	2,100	—	2,100	600	—	600
Prostate	180,400	180,400	—	31,900	31,900	—
Testis	6,900	6,900	—	300	300	—
Penis and other genital, male	1,100	1,100	—	300	300	—
Urinary system	86,700	58,600	28,100	24,600	15,700	8,900
Urinary bladder	53,200	38,300	14,900	12,200	8,100	4,100
Kidney and renal pelvis	31,200	18,800	12,400	11,900	7,300	4,600
Ureter and other urinary organs	2,300	1,500	800	500	300	200
Eye and orbit	2,200	1,200	1,000	200	100	100
Brain and other nervous system	16,500	9,500	7,000	13,000	7,100	5,900
Endocrine system	20,200	5,600	14,600	2,100	1,000	1,100
Thyroid	18,400	4,700	13,700	1,200	500	700
Other endocrine	1,800	900	900	900	500	400
Lymphoma	62,300	35,900	26,400	27,500	14,400	13,100
Hodgkin's disease	7,400	4,200	3,200	1,400	700	700
Non-Hodgkin's lymphoma	54,900	31,700	23,200	26,100	13,700	12,40
Multiple myeloma	13,600	7,300	6,300	11,200	5,800	5,400
Leukemia	30,800	16,900	13,900	21,700	12,100	9,600
Acute lymphocytic leukemia	3,200	1,800	1,400	1,300	700	600
Chronic lymphocytic leukemia	8,100	4,600	3,500	4,800	2,800	2,000
Acute myeloid leukemia	9,700	4,800	4,900	7,100	3,900	3,200
Chronic myeloid leukemia	4,400	2,600	1,800	2,300	1,300	1,000
Other leukemia	5,400	3,100	2,300	6,200	3,400	2,800
Other and unspecified primary sites	34,000	15,700	18,300	36,600	18,500	18,100

*Excludes basal and squamous cell skin cancers and in situ carcinomas except urinary bladder. Carcinoma in situ of the breast accounts for about 42,600 new cases annually, and melanoma carcinoma in situ accounts for about 28,600 new cases annually. Estimates of new cases are based on incidence rates from the National Cancer Institute, Surveillance, Epidemiology, and End Results program 1979–1996.

From American Cancer Society. 2000. *Cancer facts & figures 2000*. Atlanta: Author. Reprinted by permission of the American Cancer Society, Inc.

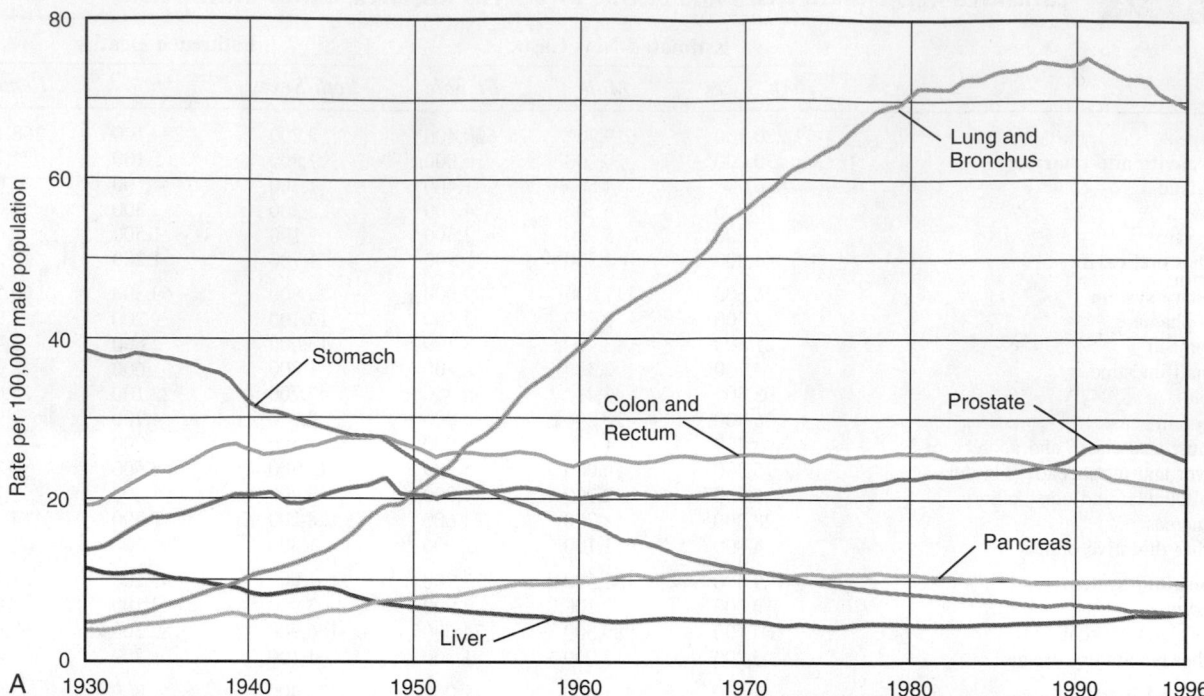

FIGURE 18–1 Cancer death rates by site in males in the United States from 1930 to 1996. Rates are per 100,000 and are age-adjusted to the 1970 U.S. standard population. (From American Cancer Society [2000]. *Cancer facts & figures 2000*. Atlanta: Author. © American Cancer Society, Inc.)

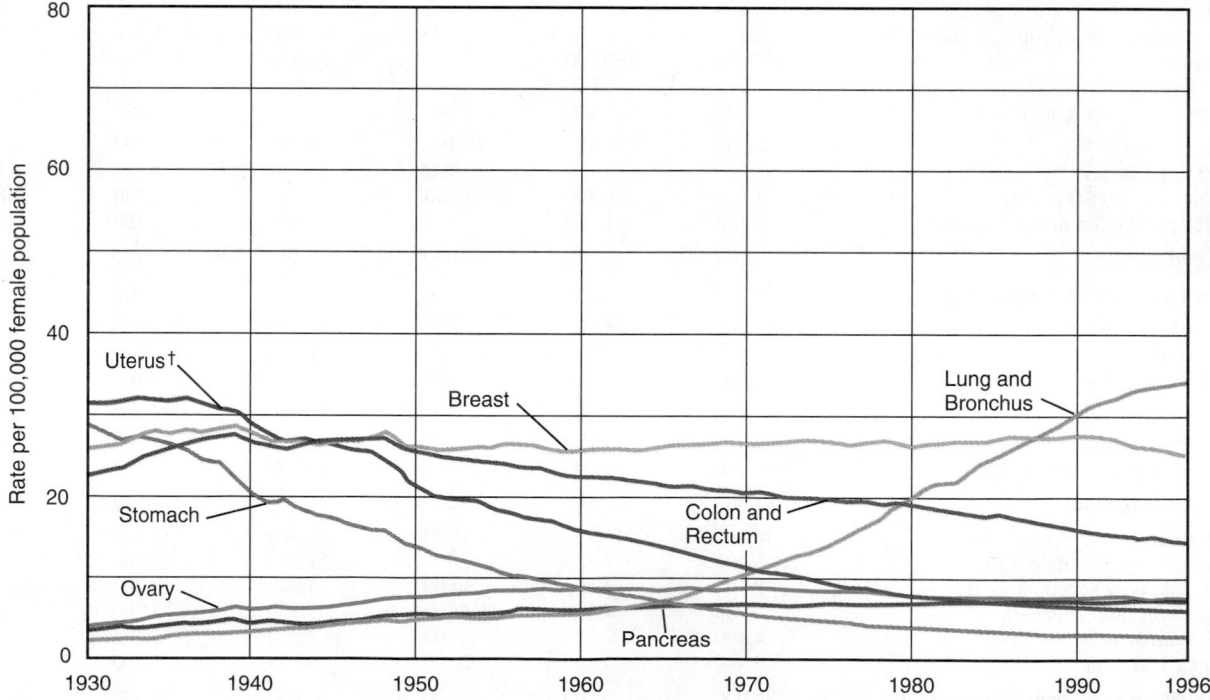

†Uterus cancer death rates are for uterine cervix and uterine corpus combined.

B

FIGURE 18–2 Cancer death rates by site in females in the United States from 1930 to 1996. Rates are per 100,000 and are age-adjusted to the 1970 U.S. standard population. (From American Cancer Society [2000]. *Cancer facts & figures 2000*. Atlanta: Author. © American Cancer Society, Inc.)

1991 to 1995. This represented about 30,000 fewer deaths than had been expected. Factors that may explain this decline include the decrease in tobacco use, better cancer research and treatment, and earlier cancer detection and prevention. Lung cancer incidence dropped 1.1% a year, mostly in men, who began quitting smoking earlier than women. Cancer is not just being treated earlier. Through cancer screening, for example, precancerous colon polyps can be removed before they become cancerous.

Although overall cancer rates inched down, declines were not seen in all areas. The incidence of deadly melanoma from chronic exposure to ultraviolet radiation is actually rising about 4% per year. Incidence rates for non-Hodgkin's lymphoma have increased nearly two-fold since the early 1970s. Although more than 25% of cancers are associated with diet, dietary patterns likely did not have an impact on the decline in overall cancer incidence. Obesity in Americans is actually increasing. Cancer rates also did not improve for some minority populations. Cancer rates increased for black males and remained level for Asian and Pacific Islander females.[2, 20, 26] Figures 18–3A and B reflect the rates of cancer incidence and mortality by race or ethnicity.[2]

Although the decline in cancer incidence is positive news, the gains are fragile. Lifestyle choices are responsible for most exposure to environmental carcinogens. The recent increase in tobacco use by teenagers may cause a rebound in cancer rates. From 1991 to 1995, the percentage of high school students who smoke frequently increased 3% to 5%. There has also been a resurgence in the use of smokeless tobacco products.[2] Lifestyle choices resulting in severe sunburn from ultraviolet radiation, especially in children, are associated with a greatly increased risk of melanoma in later life. Another concern related to melanoma is the rapid increase in the use of tanning beds. Long-term exposure to ultraviolet radiation is associated with basal cell and squamous cell skin cancers.[14] Prevention, early detection, and treatment of cancer remain significant health care concerns.

PATHOPHYSIOLOGY

Knowledge about the pathophysiology of cancer will help you better understand the significance of clinical observations and plan interventions, including client teaching, for

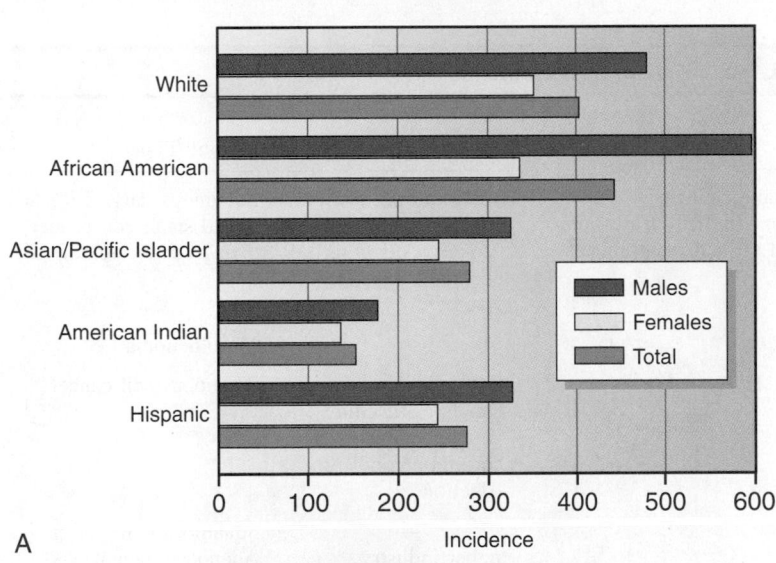

FIGURE 18–3 *A*, Cancer incidence rates (per 100,000) for all sites combined by race, ethnicity, and sex in the United States. *B*, Cancer mortality rates (per 100,000) for all sites combined by race, ethnicity, and sex in the United States. (Data from American Cancer Society. [2000]. *Cancer facts & figures 2000.* Atlanta: Author.)

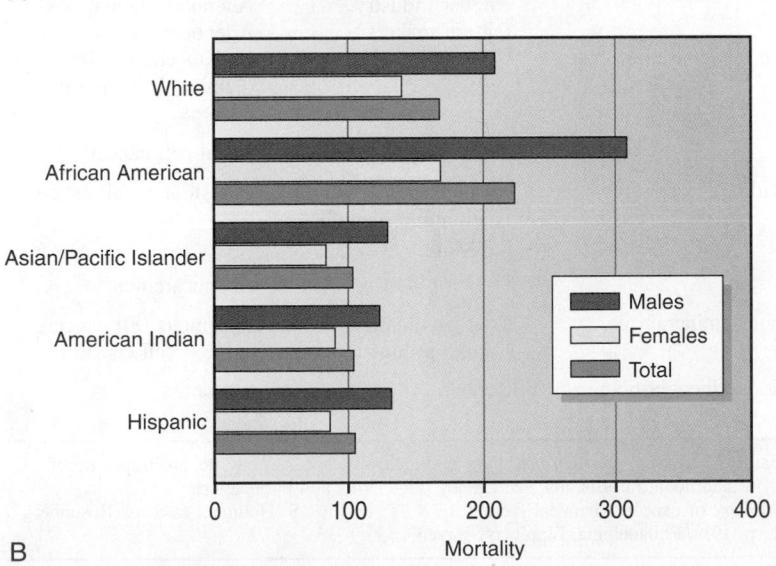

outcomes management. A common misconception is that cancer is *one* disease. Cancer is many diseases.

Cancers comprise all diseases of cells that are altered or transformed in some way but are able to multiply, grow, and spread. Cancerous cells differ from normal cells in appearance, growth, and function. The change from normal to neoplastic cells is a process, not a single event or a single alteration in cells. The development of a cancer is a series of events that generally occur over many years. Clinical manifestations are only the final stages in the natural history of a cancer.

■ CARCINOGENS

Carcinogens (factors associated with cancer causation) may be (1) radiation, (2) chemicals, (3) viruses, or (4) other physical agents (Table 18–3).[34] In addition, hormones play a significant role in the development of many cancers.[17]

Radiation

More than 80% of exposure to radiation is from natural sources.[6, 14] This includes ionizing radiation from cosmic rays and radioactive minerals, such as radon gas, radium,

and uranium. Sunlight and tanning beds are two sources of ultraviolet radiation, a complete carcinogen.

About 15% of radiation exposure comes from diagnostic or therapeutic procedures, including radiographs, radiation therapy, and radioisotopes used in diagnostic imaging. Individual doses vary widely with the numbers and types of procedures done.[14] The levels of radiation emitted by equipment for a given procedure have been falling significantly since the 1980s. Physicians commonly avoid ordering unnecessary procedures for clients. The amount of risk of a second malignancy caused by radiation therapy is still open to debate. At most, about 5% of all secondary cancers are clearly linked to radiation therapy for a previous cancer.[14]

Chemicals

Tobacco, a chemical carcinogen, remains the most important known cause of cancer in the United States, accounting for almost 30% of cancer deaths. It has been linked not only with lung cancer but also with oropharyngeal, bladder, pancreatic, cervical, and kidney cancers. Because there is a clear linear relationship between the amount and number of years of smoking and cancer risk, a nurse

TABLE 18–3	KNOWN OR SUSPECTED CHEMICAL CARCINOGENS IN HUMANS*		
Target Organ	**Agent**	**Industry**	**Tumor Type**
Lung	Tobacco smoke, arsenic, asbestos, crystalline silica, benzo[a]pyrene, beryllium, bis(chloromethyl)ether, 1,3-butadiene, chromium VI compounds, coal tar and pitch, nickel compounds, soots, mustard gas	Aluminum production, coal gasification, coke production, hematite mining, paint	Squamous, large cell, and small cell cancer and adenocarcinoma
Pleura	Asbestos	—	Mesothelioma
Oral cavity	Tobacco smoke, alcoholic beverages, nickel compounds	Boot and shoe production, furniture manufacturer, isopropyl alcohol production	Squamous cell cancer
Esophagus	Tobacco smoke, alcoholic beverages	—	Squamous cell cancer
Gastric	Smoked, salted, and pickled foods	Rubber industry	Adenocarcinoma
Colon	Heterocyclic amines, asbestos	Pattern makers	Adenocarcinoma
Liver	Aflatoxin, vinyl chloride, tobacco smoke, alcoholic beverages	—	Hepatocellular carcinoma, hemangiosarcoma
Kidney	Tobacco smoke	—	Renal cell cancer
Bladder	Tobacco smoke, 4-aminobiphenyl, benzidine, 2-naphthylamine	Magenta manufacture, auramine manufacture	Transitional cell cancer
Prostate	Cadmium	—	Adenocarcinoma
Skin	Arsenic, benzo[a]pyrene, coal tar and pitch, mineral oils, soots	Coal gasification, coke production	Squamous cell cancer, basal cell cancer
Bone marrow	Benzene, tobacco smoke, ethylene oxide, antineoplastic agents	Rubber	Leukemia

*These carcinogen designations are determined by regulatory or review agencies based on public health needs. They do not imply proof of carcinogenicity in individuals. This table is not all-inclusive. For additional information, see agency documents and publications.

Modified from Yuspa, S. H., & Shields, P. G. (1997). Etiology of cancer: Chemical factors. In V. T. DeVita, S. Hellman, & S. A. Rosenberg (Eds.), *Cancer: Principles and practices of oncology* (5th ed., p. 191). Philadelphia: Lippincott-Raven.

can often find in a physician's history the number of pack-years a client has smoked. (A "pack-year" refers to the number of packs of cigarettes smoked per day times the number of years the client has smoked. It provides a measure of the client's cigarette abuse.) Smokeless tobacco (chewing tobacco, snuff) is linked to oral cancers. Long-term users of smokeless tobacco have a nearly 50-fold increased risk of cancer of the cheek and gum.[2]

In addition to lifestyle exposure to the chemicals in tobacco products, people can be exposed to chemicals in the workplace. Occupational exposure causes 2% to 8% of all human cancers. The risk estimates are much higher among the subpopulation of people actually exposed to carcinogens in the workplace. These occupationally occurring cancers are, for the most part, preventable.[31] Health care workers wear radiation badges to ensure that they do not receive unsafe levels of exposure. Before safe handling practices were instituted, the urine of pharmacists and nurses mixing or administering chemotherapy agents was found to show mutagenic changes from cumulative exposure. Today, chemotherapeutic agents are mixed by pharmacists under laminar flow hoods. The hood draws air containing aerosolized drug away and prevents the pharmacist from breathing in the chemicals. Oncology nurses wear gowns and gloves to administer chemotherapy and use special procedures to clean up any spills to prevent absorbing the chemicals through the skin or mucous membranes.

Viruses

Some viruses are strongly associated with cancer. Table 18–4 lists biologic agents, including viruses, judged by the World Health Organization (WHO) to be involved in human cancers.[30] In the 1970s and early 1980s, many lay people thought cancer was contagious and therefore often shunned those with cancer. Occasionally, yet today, a client or family member expresses this fear. Even when there is a viral link, the cancer is not contagious. Rather, a virus at some point infected the cell, causing genetic damage to the cell's deoxyribonucleic acid (DNA), thus leading to the development of cancer.

Age, Sex, Genetics, Ethnicity

Host characteristics influencing cancer susceptibility include age, sex, genetic predisposition, and ethnicity or race. Age is a factor because the person has had more years of potential exposure to carcinogens. Females have a generally lower risk of cancer incidence. Hormonal status is associated with increased risk of neoplasia in tissues that are responsive to hormones, including breast, endometrium, prostate, ovary, thyroid, bone, and testes. In addition to biologic or genetic differences, cultural and socioeconomic factors may put an ethnic or racial group at increased or decreased risk of a specific cancer.[8, 15]

For people who do not smoke, dietary patterns and physical activities become the most important cancer risk factors that they can modify. It is estimated that at least one fourth of cancer deaths in the United States are related to diet. Research into the relationship of diet and cancer is ongoing.[6] A balanced, healthy diet that includes a high proportion of plant foods (fruits, vegetables,

TABLE 18–4	BIOLOGIC AGENTS JUDGED BY IARC (WHO) OR OTHERS AS BEING INVOLVED IN HUMAN CARCINOGENESIS
Agent	**Site of Cancer**
Aflatoxin-producing fungal strains	Liver (hepatocellular)
Hepatitis B virus	Liver (hepatocellular)
Hepatitis C virus	Liver (hepatocellular)
Helicobacter pylori	Stomach
Schistosoma haematobium	Urinary bladder
Opisthorchis viverrini	Liver (cholangiocarcinoma)
HTLV-1	Adult T-cell leukemia or lymphoma
HPV (or other sexually transmitted agent)	Uterine cervix
Epstein-Barr virus	Burkitt's lymphoma, nasopharynx, Hodgkin's disease

HPV, human papillomavirus; HTLV-1, human T-cell lymphotropic virus type I; IARC, International Agency for Research on Cancer; WHO, World Health Organization.

From Trichopoulos, D., et al. (1997). Epidemiology of cancer. In V. T. DeVita, S. Hellman, & S. A. Rosenberg (Eds.), *Cancer: Principles and practices of oncology* (5th ed., pp. 249). Philadelphia: Lippincott-Raven.

grains, and beans), limited intake of high-fat foods, a balance of caloric intake and physical activity, and limited consumption of alcoholic beverages can reduce cancer risks.[2, 30]

■ CARCINOGENESIS: TRANSFORMATION OF NORMAL CELLS INTO CANCER CELLS

The process through which normal cells are transformed into malignant or cancer cells is called carcinogenesis. Figure 18–4 depicts the multistage model of carcinogenesis.[31, 34] There are four broadly identified stages of the process of carcinogenesis:

1. *Initiation* occurs when a carcinogen damages DNA. Carcinogens cause changes in the structure and function of the cell at the genetic or molecular level. This damage may be reversible or may lead to genetic mutations if not repaired; however, the mutations may not lead immediately to cancer.
2. *Promotion* occurs with additional assaults to the cells, resulting in further genetic damage.
3. At some point, these genetic events result in a *malignant conversion*.
4. With *progression*, the cells are increasingly malignant in appearance and behavior and develop into an invasive cancer with metastases to distant body parts.

Clinicians are already using their broad understanding of this process of transformation from normal cells to malignancy. Through health promotion programs, the outcome goal of smoking cessation classes is to decrease lung cancer through prevention. Regular Papanicolaou (Pap) smears are a means of health maintenance through early detection of cervical dysplasia, a precancerous lesion. Likewise, precancerous colon polyps can be removed by colonoscopy before they progress to malig-

FIGURE 18–4 Multistage model of carcinogeneis. (Adapted from Volker, D. L. [1998]. Carcinogensis. In J. K. Itano & K. N. Taoka [Eds.], *Core curriculum for oncology nursing* [3rd ed., p. 359]. Philadelphia: W. B. Saunders; and Yupsa, S. H., & Shields, G. P. [1997]. Etiology of cancer: Chemical factors. In V. T. DeVita, S. Hellman, & S. A. Rosenberg [Eds.]: *Cancer: Principles and practices of oncology* [5th ed., p. 188]. Philadelphia: Lippincott-Raven.)

nancy. Monitoring moles for early changes can allow a potentially lethal melanoma to be removed while it is still a localized disease.

Increased knowledge of the underlying biology of the process of carcinogenesis is coming quickly. In the 1980s, the identification of oncogenes led to the recognition that cancer is largely a genetic disease. Research shifted from carcinogenesis and mutagens to oncogenes and tumor suppressor genes. In less than a decade, researchers have clarified critically important mechanisms that control cell growth and division, regulate embryologic development, and cause disease.[7] With this knowledge, scientists are developing better treatments. Powerful new chemotherapy drugs and new ways of delivering these drugs are becoming available. *Biotherapy* is now recognized as a fourth treatment modality in addition to surgery, radiation therapy, and chemotherapy. Biotherapy is moving from research to standard treatment.[11, 23]

The process of carcinogenesis transforms normal cells into cancer cells. The Anatomy and Physiology review of the cell (see beginning of Unit 4) explores the characteristics of normal cells. They differ from cancer cells in many key ways (Table 18–5). Specific concepts that help us to understand changes that occur in the neoplastic transformation of cells are (1) the cell cycle, (2) altered differentiation, (3) altered growth characteristics, and (4) metastasis.

THE CELL CYCLE

The concept of the cell cycle has increased researchers' understanding of how both normal and neoplastic cells replicate (Fig. 18–5). The cell's replication cycle is divided into the following intervals, or steps, with the letter G standing for "gap"—the interval separating cell division, or *mitosis* (M) and *synthesis* (S).

G_0 PHASE. This phase is the interval in which the cell is at rest from cell division until a trigger in the immediate environment signals the beginning of the G_1 phase. Some cells do not replicate, or they replicate so infrequently that they are said to always be in a G_0 or resting state.

G_1 PHASE. This phase is the interval in which ribonucleic acid (RNA) and protein are synthesized. The period of time the cell is in G_1 varies, depending on the type of cell and the proliferation activity of the tissue. With high activity, the G_1 interval is short. The interval lengthens when activity is low. There is a point in the G_1 phase known as the *restriction point,* after which the cell is committed to progressing into the S phase. One to 3 hours after passing the restriction point, cells initiate DNA synthesis. The acquisition of the ability to begin DNA synthesis marks the termination of the G_1 phase.

S PHASE. Synthesis of both DNA and proteins of new chromosomes occurs during the S phase. The interval of time is probably 6 to 8 hours, although it varies in certain cell populations and under different conditions. Cell proliferation can be measured in the laboratory by flow cytometry. In reading a pathology report, you may find a reference to the percentage of cells in S phase. Only a small percentage of cells should be synthesizing DNA. An increase in S phase fraction is a negative predictor of long-term survival.[22]

G_2 PHASE. Biochemical processes, including the synthesis of some RNA, occur in preparation for mitosis.

TABLE 18–5	A COMPARISON OF THE CHARACTERISTICS OF NORMAL AND CANCER CELLS	
Characteristic	**Normal Cells**	**Cancer Cells**
Mitotic cell division	Mitotic division leads to two daughter cells	Mitosis leads to multiple daughter cells that may or may not resemble the parent. Multiple mitotic spindles
Appearance	1. Cells of same type homogeneous in size, shape, and growth 2. Cells cohesive, form regular pattern of expansion 3. Uniform size to nucleus 4. Have characteristic pattern of organization 5. Mixture of stem cells (precursors) and well-differentiated cells	1. Cells larger and grow more rapidly than normal. Pleomorphic, i.e., heterogeneous in size and shape. 2. Cells not as cohesive, irregular patterns of expansion 3. Larger, more prominent nucleus 4. Lack characteristic pattern of organization of host cell 5. Anaplastic, lack of differentiated cell characteristics, specific functions
Growth pattern	1. Do not invade adjacent tissue 2. Proliferate in response to specific stimuli 3. Grow in ideal conditions (e.g., nutrients, oxygen, space, correct biochemical environment) 4. Exhibit contact inhibition 5. Cell birth equals or is less than cell death 6. Stable cell membrane 7. Constant or predictable growth rate 8. Cannot grow outside specific environment (e.g., breast cells grow only in breast)	1. Invade adjacent tissues 2. Proliferation in response to abnormal stimuli 3. Grow in adverse conditions such as lack of nutrients 4. Do not exhibit contact inhibition 5. Cell birth exceeds cell death 6. Loss of cell control a result of cell membrane changes 7. Growth rate erratic 8. Able to break off cells that migrate through bloodstream or lymphatics, or seed to distant sites and grow in other sites
Function	1. Have specific, designated purpose 2. Contribute to the overall well-being of the host 3. Cells function in specific predetermined manners (e.g., cells in the thyroid secrete thyroid hormone)	1. Serve no useful purpose 2. Do not contribute to the well-being of the host; parasitic, actually feed off host without contributing anything 3. If cells function at all, they do not function normally, or they may actually cause damage (e.g., lung cancer cells secrete ACTH and cause excessive stimulation of adrenal cortex)
Other	1. Develop specific antigens, characteristic of the particular cell formed 2. Chromosomes remain constant throughout cell division 3. Complex metabolic and enzyme pattern 4. Cannot invade, erode, or spread 5. Cannot grow in presence of necrosis or inflammation	1. Develop antigens completely different from a normal cell 2. Chromosomal aberrations occur as cell matures 3. Have more primitive and simplified metabolic and enzyme pattern 4. Invade, erode, and spread 5. Grow in presence of necrosis and inflammatory cells such as lymphocytes and macrophages 6. Exhibit periods of latency that vary from tumor to tumor 7. Have own blood supply and supporting stroma

ACTH, adrenocorticotropic hormone.

Little is known about this phase, which lasts only a few hours.

M PHASE. Actual division of the cell (mitosis) occurs during this phase, producing two daughter cells. The M phase usually ranges from less than an hour to a few hours.

In the normal mature organ, cell cycling is carefully controlled so that the organ maintains its function. Cells that die are replaced, but no extra cells are produced. Researchers are investigating the mechanisms of this control, which are not fully understood.

ALTERED CELL DIFFERENTIATION

Cells that were genetically identical in the embryo eventually assume varying structures and functions. One muscle cell looks like all the other muscle cells but not like a kidney or liver cell. In normal growth, cells become more specialized or committed to a particular cell line as they mature. This process of development is called *differentiation*. Most cells contain the entire genome. The growth and function of a particular cell line result from the expression of certain genes and the suppression of others. Transformation of a normal cell to a cancer cell can

DNA and protein synthesis

RNA synthesis

S

G_2

M Mitosis

G_1

RNA and protein synthesis

G_0 cycle: nonproliferating pool or resting state

DEATH

FIGURE 18–5 The cell cycle. Periods of deoxyribonucleic acid (DNA) synthesis (S) and mitosis (M) are divided by gaps (G) in which the cell is in a resting state (G0), producing substances in preparation for DNA synthesis (G1), or producing proteins and some ribonucleic acid (RNA) in preparation for mitosis (G2).

occur at any point in the process of differentiation. Changes in the appearance of the cell, the presence of tumor-specific antigens that are suppressed on the normal cell, and the loss of normal function can result from altered differentiation.

APPEARANCE. An obvious difference from normal cells is in the appearance of cancer cells. Normal cells have well-organized cellular components. Cancer cells have variable sizes and shapes. Nuclei may be disproportionately large, or there may be multiple nuclei. A variety of abnormal mitotic features may be present. There may be an abnormal number of chromosomes (aneuploidy) or an abnormal arrangement of chromosomes.[31] The detection of aneuploidy in a pathology report is an unfavorable prognostic factor.

A pathology report generally describes the grade of the cancer cells. When the cells are well differentiated, or low-grade, they are more mature in appearance and more like the normal cells from which they have arisen than poorly differentiated cancer cells. Anaplastic (undifferentiated) cells appear so disorganized under the microscope that they have no resemblance to the tissue of origin. Poorly differentiated and anaplastic cancers tend to be

more aggressive—an unfavorable prognostic factor. During the natural history of many malignant neoplasms, as the cancer cells grow and divide, they often lose more and more of their mature characteristics. As a result, a malignant neoplasm can be heterogeneous with more than one variation of the malignant cell line. This heterogeneity is caused by random mutations during tumor progression.[12]

At times, a neoplasm initially responds to therapy. You may read in a radiology report that the tumor has shrunk back, with a partial remission (PR) or a complete remission (CR) of all radiologic evidence of the neoplasm; then the neoplasm may come back and grow aggressively. A likely explanation is that the treatment successfully eliminated one variant of the cancer cells, causing those cells to die and the overall size of the tumor to shrink. Then other variants of the cancer cells, which were resistant to the treatment, grew and multiplied, so that the tumor increased in size.

Biochemical studies reflect differences resulting from altered cell metabolism. The cell's surface membrane is the interface between the cell and extracellular components. Cell membrane changes may result in the production of enzymes that aid in cancer spread. A loss of glycoproteins results in a loss of cell-to-cell adhesion. Loss of antigens that identify the cell as "self" or production of tumor-specific antigens can alter the immune system's ability to mount a response.[31]

Tumor cell membranes have a greater fluidity than normal cell membranes do. This may be due to changes in the lipid composition of the membrane of tumor cells. Scientists are trying to take advantage of this difference. Some chemotherapy drugs are now being delivered in *liposomes* (spheres with an outer lipid layer and internal core of drug). The tumor cells take in more of the liposomal drug than is taken in by the normal cells. The result is a better treatment effect with fewer harmful effects on the normal cells.

TUMOR-SPECIFIC ANTIGENS. Cell surfaces express antigens. Some tumors express more of an antigen than is expressed by normal cells. These tumor-specific antigens can be used as a diagnostic tool in the detection of cancer or in monitoring the effectiveness of cancer treatment. One example is the PSA test. Normally, a man's blood level of PSA is low (0 to 5 ng/ml). In the presence of prostate cancer, this antigen can be elevated. The PSA blood test is now being utilized as one early detection tool, along with the digital rectal examination, to detect prostate cancer in men who are still asymptomatic.[2] During treatment, a decline in the PSA level is an indicator of the effectiveness of the treatment. During follow-up after treatment ends, a rise in the PSA level can be an early indicator that the cancer has recurred.

FUNCTION. Unlike normal cells, cancer cells typically serve no useful purpose. The result of neoplastic growth is an abnormal tissue mass that does not contribute in any way to the well-being of the host. The mass occupies space and draws nutrition and sustenance from the host. If the cancer cells function at all, they often do not function normally and may even act in a way that causes damage to the host. For example, a functional tumor of the thyroid gland produces excess amounts of thyroid hormone, leading to a hypermetabolic state.

ALTERED GROWTH CHARACTERISTICS

Another obvious difference from normal cells is the uncontrolled growth of cancer cells. Because of changes in their cell surfaces, neoplastic cells differ from normal cells in growth patterns and mobility. Cancer cells lose the contact inhibition of normal cells, can establish metastasis, avoid normal regulation by hormones, and avoid being recognized by the immune system as altered.

CONTACT INHIBITION AND DOUBLING TIME. When normal cells are cultured in the laboratory, they exhibit a behavior known as contact inhibition. This means the cells continue to divide until they cover the bottom of the Petri dish and stop dividing when they touch the edges of the dish. Cancer cells continue to divide, piling up on the other cells. In human tissues, the growth of normal cells is carefully regulated. Cells divide to produce new cells only when needed to replace cells that have died. Cancer cells do not stop dividing and multiplying. They do not necessarily go through the cell cycle at a faster rate than the normal cells of the tissue from which they have arisen. Rather, cancer cells are almost continuously in the process of cell division, spending little time in the G_0 phase.[19]

This continuous growth results in a phenomenon referred to as *doubling time*. The doubling time of a human malignant tumor can vary from weeks to months. As depicted in Figure 18–6, it may take 10 years for a tumor to reach 1 cm in size. In only another year, that same tumor may grow to 8 cm. The smallest clinically detectable mass is about 1 g in weight or 1 cm³ in size. A *tumor burden* (amount) of 1 kg, which requires only about 10 more doublings, is potentially lethal.[31]

Clients sometimes ask whether exposing the tumor to air during surgery can cause it to grow more rapidly. More likely, if the surgeon did not see evidence of tumor in other areas, it had already spread, but the size of the tumor mass was still too small to be seen or felt. Then in a few more doubling times, without effective treatment, it became evident and proceeded to enlarge.

METASTASIS

Normal cells are adherent to the other normal cells from which they have arisen. Normal breast tissue cells, for example, are never found anywhere in the body except in the breast. Malignant or cancer cells are less adherent and more mobile than normal cells. They have the ability to spread from the original site of the tumor to distant organs. This phenomenon is called *metastasis* (from the Greek *meta*, beyond, and *stasis*, standing).

The capacity of a neoplastic tumor to metastasize to other sites is a major characteristic of malignancy—and the most frequent reason why cancer treatment fails. It is the characteristic that distinguishes malignant from benign growths. Neoplastic cells must overcome multiple barriers to successfully spread to other sites. For the purposes of study, the metastatic cascade is divided into three stages, (Fig. 18–7).

STAGE 1. Neoplastic cells from the primary tumor invade surrounding tissue and penetrate blood or lymph vessels. Increasing tumor size, leading to tissue pressure and mechanical expansion, may cause neoplastic invasion. However, the size of the primary tumor is not the sole predictor of metastasis. Tumors with identical size and histologic cell type can vary markedly in metastatic spread.[28]

Loss of tumor cell cohesiveness with increasing motility is another factor in the metastatic cascade. Tumors, even when very small, shed cells. As many as 10^7 to 10^9 cells per day may be found circulating in the bloodstream of clients with cancer.[28] Although surgery can cure most early breast cancers, some eventually recur because of these shed cells. Adjuvant chemotherapy or hormonal therapy, given when no visible tumor remains, may therefore be considered for early-stage breast cancer clients to decrease the risk of recurrence. Yet, fewer than 1% of circulating cancer cells successfully metastasize.[28] In the future, new scientific knowledge may allow oncologists to identify the clients with early-stage breast cancer who would benefit from adjuvant chemotherapy. This would allow the majority of women for whom surgery alone was curative to avoid the adverse effects of chemotherapy.

Benign neoplasms and cancer in situ do not cause destruction of the host stroma (the supporting tissues of an organ). With progression to invasive disease, the neoplasm penetrates the epithelial basement membrane and invades the interstitial stroma at multiple stages in the metastatic cascade.[28] A client's pathology report often indicates whether there was invasion of the neoplasm into surrounding tissue or into lymphatic, perineural, or vascular tissues. Such invasion may be an indication of occult (as yet undetected) metastatic disease.

Cancer cells that successfully metastasize represent a subpopulation of the primary tumor's cells. Not all cells in the primary mass share the unique genetic and biologic properties necessary for metastasis.[12]

STAGE 2. Cancer cells migrate via the lymph or blood circulation or by direct extension. The lymphatic system

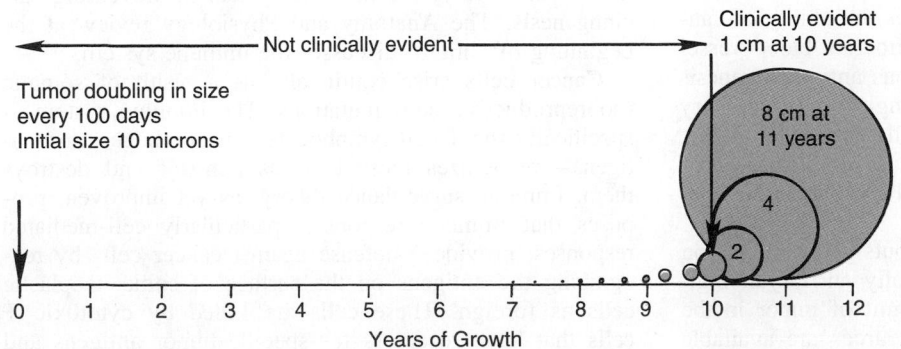

FIGURE 18–6 A depiction of tumor growth, showing doubling time related to tumor size.

STAGE 1.   Invasion of cancer cells into adjacent tissue

STAGE 2.   Spread of cancer cells

STAGE 3.   Establishment and growth at secondary site

FIGURE 18–7 The three stages of the metastatic process.

provides the most common pathway for the initial spread of malignant cancer cells. There may be spread to the lymph nodes draining the region of the primary tumor site. Lymph node involvement is seen in about 50% of all fatal cancers. The blood vessels (both veins and arteries) carry cancer cells from the primary tumor to the capillary beds of the lungs, liver, and bones. Metastatic spread to distant organs and tissues is almost always the result of cells moving through the bloodstream.

Direct extension of tumors to adjacent tissues also occurs. For example, a breast cancer may spread directly to the chest wall. In body cavities, cells may spread by gravity, resulting in new growths on other serosal surfaces. Cells shed by cancers of the ovary are often found to have fallen onto and "seeded" the entire peritoneal cavity with metastatic sites of the tumor.

STAGE 3. Cancer cells are established and proliferate at the secondary site. Researchers have observed that certain tumor cells have, for unknown reasons, an affinity for certain sites. Although the exact mechanism of metastasis is unclear, the metastatic sites of many cancers are fairly predictable. The predilection of certain malignant neoplasms for particular sites may be due to the ability of the tumor to live within only certain tissues or to some other, unknown factor. The most common site of metastasis is lymphatic tissues; the next most common sites are the liver, lungs, bones, and brain.[28]

ANGIOGENESIS. The metastatic cascade begins and ends with *angiogenesis.* A tumor cannot grow more than a few millimeters without a blood supply to transport nutrients to the tumor. Angiogenesis is the ability of cancer cells to secrete substances that stimulate blood vessel growth.[30] Scientists are studying various anti-angiogenesis strategies.[3, 12] The destruction of a single tumor capillary may be able to kill many cancer cells that rely on that vessel for nutrition. If angiogenesis is inhibited, cancer progression may be halted or slowed by preventing metastasis.[3, 12, 28]

The growth of metastatic tumors puts severe stress on the affected person, both physiologically and psychologically. As the tumor burden (the amount of tumor in the body) increases, fewer metabolic resources are available

for normal cells. As mentioned earlier, when the total burden of tumor in the body approaches 1 kg, the shear burden of the tumor is potentially lethal.

When a client's cancer metastasizes to other sites, clients and family members may erroneously believe that the client has multiple cancers; it is one cancer spread to other organs. For example, cells that have spread to the bone from a breast cancer are breast cancer cells, not malignant variants of bone tissue cells; however, a client may have two different cancers at one time. In the process of making a new diagnosis of colon cancer, for example, a clinician may also discover a previously undetected prostate cancer.

Knowing the natural history and the most likely pattern of spread can be very helpful to the clinician. If the cancer is likely to spread to the liver, bone, or brain, the clinician will want to rule out evidence of such spread in making treatment decisions and in monitoring for recurrence following treatment.

■ INABILITY OF IMMUNE SYSTEM TO RECOGNIZE CANCER CELLS

ROLE IN PREVENTING CARCINOGENESIS

The immune system usually defends against bacterial or viral invaders and plays a key role in controlling the growth of cancer cells. There are two critical components of the immune response: (1) the ability to recognize a pathogen as foreign and (2) the ability to mount a response to eliminate the pathogen.[4, 21, 25] This section addresses the role of the immune system in preventing carcinogenesis. The Anatomy and Physiology review at the beginning of Unit 16 discusses the immune system.

Cancer cells arise continually as a result of somatic (nonreproductive cell) mutations. The immune system—specifically the T-cell lymphocytes, macrophages, and antigens—recognizes these cells as non-self and destroys them. Immune surveillance theory, as yet unproven, proposes that immune responses, particularly cell-mediated responses, provide a defense against cancer cells by recognizing the antigens on the surface of some neoplastic cells as foreign. These cells are killed by cytotoxic T cells that have receptors for specific tumor antigens and by interferon-activated natural killer (NK) lymphocytes and macrophages.[4]

Macrophages, the important first line of defense, phagocytize the pathogen and present it as antigen to T and B lymphocytes. T-cell recognition of antigen stimulates proliferation of T and B cells, with B-cell production of antibodies against the pathogen and T-cell secretion of cytokines. Cytokines, hormone-like peptides or glycopeptides, regulate activation of the immune system against cancer cells. Cytokines both enhance and suppress complex immune interactions.

Antigens on cancer cells can take various forms, resulting in T-cell recognition of the cells as abnormal. The cancer cells may express antigens that are not present on normal cells. Cancer cells may have antigens that are "unmasked" and thus visible to the immune system. These same antigens when present on normal cells are masked and thus not recognized by the immune system. Cancer cells may also express antigens that are only present during oncofetal or embryonic development of normal cells. Cytotoxic T cells that have receptors for specific tumor antigens and interferon-activated NK lymphocytes and macrophages can then destroy these cancer cells.

FAILURE OF IMMUNE DEFENSES

Unfortunately, the immune defenses are not always effective. The immune system may be unable to recognize cancer cells as foreign or to mount an immune response for several reasons.

An immature, old, or weak immune system may contribute to this. People who are malnourished or chronically ill may also be immunocompromised. The tumor burden (number of cancer cells) may be too small to stimulate an immune response. Alternatively, the tumor burden may be so great as to overwhelm the immune system.

Some cancer cells may escape detection because they resemble normal cells. Other cancer cells may produce substances that shield them from recognition. Cancer cells may also escape detection by becoming coated with fibrin. Tumor invasion of the bone marrow can result in decreased production of lymphocytes needed to destroy the tumor mass.

The incidence of malignancy increases with the use of immunosuppressive drugs after organ transplantation to counteract rejection. Chemotherapeutics or radiation used to treat cancer can also induce suppression of the immune response.[4, 25, 31]

■ APOPTOSIS

With the development of molecular biology in the 1980s, scientists began to understand another important step in the process of carcinogenesis: the failure of cells to die.[1, 10, 17] In normal physiology, a damaged cell sacrifices itself for the greater good. There are two pathways to cell death:

1. *Necrosis* is cell death resulting from injury. The dead cells swell, lyse, and release their cellular contents into the intercellular spaces, causing the inflammatory response.
2. In *apoptosis* (from the Greek word for "falling off"), "cellular suicide" results in cells rapidly shrinking with loss of their intercellular contents.[17] They are quickly phagocytized and digested by macrophages and other cells in the vicinity. Inflammation is not triggered. Figure 18–8 depicts this programmed cell suicide. The morphologic changes of apoptosis can be completed in less than an hour.[10]

Most, if not all, cells manufacture a set of proteins that serve as weapons of self-destruction. As long as a cell is useful to the body, it restrains its death machinery. If the cell becomes infected or malignant or otherwise threatens the health of the organism, however, the lethal proteins are unleashed.[10]

Increasingly, scientists view cancer as both a disease of excessive cell growth and a lack of normal cell death. In the process of carcinogenesis, cells accumulate enough damage to genes that control cell growth and survival that the mutation seems irreparable. The affected cell usually kills itself rather than risk becoming deranged and potentially dangerous. If the cell does not die, it or its daughter cells may live long enough to accumulate mutations that make it possible to divide uncontrollably and to metastasize to distant sites.

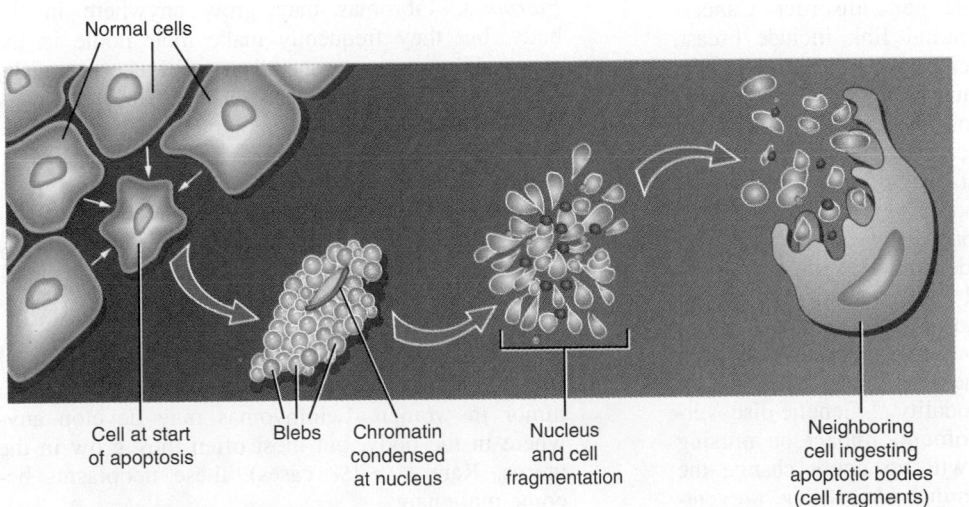

Normal cells

Cell at start of apoptosis

Blebs

Chromatin condensed at nucleus

Nucleus and cell fragmentation

Neighboring cell ingesting apoptotic bodies (cell fragments)

FIGURE 18–8 Programmed cell death resulting from apoptosis (cell "suicide"). The cell shrinks and pulls away from surrounding cells. Blebs appear on the surface of the cell. Chromatin condenses on the edge of the nucleus. The nucleus and then the cell itself breaks up. Cell fragments are ingested by other cells.

Apoptosis may not be induced in response to a cancer cell because there has also been damage to a tumor suppressor gene. In many cancers, genetic damage apparently fails to induce apoptosis because there has been damage to the gene that codes for the p53 protein. The p53 protein is a suppressor gene that can prompt activation of cell suicide. It is estimated that as many as half of solid cancers, including lung, colon, and breast cancers, have damage to the p53 protein.[10]

Still other apoptotic triggers may lead to programmed death of cancerous cells. Normal cells also tend to self-destruct when deprived of their usual growth factors or contact with other like cells. This is probably a built-in defense mechanism against metastasis. Part of the reason some cancers are resistant to the effects of radiation therapy or chemotherapy may be due to the lack of cell death through apoptosis even after cancer treatment. Researchers are investigating genetic therapies that might overcome this resistance to apoptosis.

GENETICS AND CANCER

As stated earlier, cancers comprise all diseases of cells that have been altered or transformed in some way. Throughout this chapter, genetic damage has been mentioned. The Human Genome Project, a federally funded, multibillion dollar international initiative was begun in 1990, with the goal of locating, mapping, and sequencing the more than 100,000 genes of a human's genetic composition. Approximately 60 genes have been linked to cancer. Many genes are used as molecular biologic markers of tumor prognosis, whereas others are useful markers for the screening and early detection of common cancers, including those of the breast, ovary, and colon. For example, the BRCA1 gene, isolated in 1994, is a mutation that has been linked to the susceptibility to breast, and probably ovarian, cancers in a small percentage of women.[32]

Up to 30% of rare childhood cancers result from genetic predisposition. In adults, approximately 34% of cancers have a *familial* basis; only 5% to 10% of adult cancers are *hereditary*. Some families experience a higher than normal rate of cancer that cannot be explained by environmental exposure or general risk. The cancers may be all of one type or of two or more types. There is no predictable pattern of inheritance because the cancers are probably not linked to a single gene disorder. Cancers that may have a potential familial link include breast, ovarian, colorectal, prostate, melanoma, uterine, leukemia, sarcomas, and primary brain tumors.

Hereditary cancers result from a single inherited gene disorder. Patterns of occurrence are clearly predictable. These cancers usually occur at an early age, in unusual sites, and in paired organs (both breasts, for example). There also may be multiple primary (versus metastatic) sites. Hereditary cancers include some breast, colorectal, melanoma, ovarian, and renal cell cancers as well as retinoblastoma and Wilms' tumor.[33]

Although gene therapy for cancer prevention is still futuristic, there are already some investigational studies of this treatment as a treatment modality.[33] Genetic discoveries are expected to have a profound impact on nursing practice in several areas and will no doubt change the traditional perspective on screening, identifying, preventing, and treating cancer. Precise identification of cancer-causing genetic abnormalities will significantly improve the accuracy of cancer prediction and thus the capacity to target preventive interventions to at-risk populations. As a result, the perspective of nursing will shift from symptomatic clients with cancer to counseling asymptomatic clients. Issues of confidentiality and discrimination, as well as the dilemma of predicting as yet incurable illnesses, may have an enormous negative effect on the client's and family's quality of life and psychological state.

CLASSIFICATION OF NEOPLASMS

■ BENIGN VERSUS MALIGNANT

As stated, neoplastic tumors can be either benign or malignant. The word *benign* comes from the Latin *benignus,* meaning kind. A benign tumor expands in size as it grows, but it does not infiltrate or metastasize. Because it occupies space, it may be fatal if it is located near a vital tube or organ. As a rule, though, the person with a benign neoplasm has a good prognosis because the tumor can be readily excised. Malignant neoplasms, on the other hand, represent a serious threat to the life and well-being of the host. Table 18–6 compares the characteristics of benign and malignant neoplasms.

■ TISSUE OF ORIGIN

Besides being classified as benign or malignant, neoplasms are also classified according to the tissue from which they arise. Almost all names for neoplasms end in the suffix *-oma,* meaning tumor (Table 18–7). This suffix is usually attached to a term for the parent tissue of the neoplasm. Thus, adenoma comes from the Greek *aden-,* or gland, plus *-oma.* When more than one parent tissue enters into the formation of a neoplasm, the names of the tumors are even more descriptive. For example, an adenomyoma is a benign neoplasm that contains both glandular and muscle (Greek genitive *myos*) cells.

Because epithelial tissues vary greatly, benign tumors of epithelial origin are classified according to either their *microscopic* appearance (e.g., adenoma) or their *macroscopic* appearance (e.g., polyp, from the Greek *polys* for many plus *pous* for foot).

Three of the most common benign neoplasms are:

1. *Fibromas.* Fibromas may grow anywhere in the body, but they frequently make their home in the uterus. Fibromas are generally small but occasionally grow to great size. These encapsulated, relatively harmless neoplasms cause no manifestations unless, because of their location, they press on a bone or nerve. Fibromas are easily removed surgically.
2. *Lipomas.* Lipoma, a very common benign neoplasm, arises in adipose tissue. Lipomas rarely cause manifestations, but they are poorly encapsulated and may exert pressure on surrounding tissues as they expand.
3. *Leiomyomas.* The leiomyoma, a benign neoplasm of smooth muscle origin, is the most common benign tumor in women. Leiomyomas may develop anywhere in the body, but most often they grow in the uterus. Rarely (~1% cases), these neoplasms become malignant.

TABLE 18–6   COMPARISON OF THE CHARACTERISTICS OF BENIGN AND MALIGNANT NEOPLASMS

Characteristic	Benign Neoplasm	Malignant Neoplasm
Speed of growth	Grows slowly Usually continues to grow throughout life unless surgically removed May have periods of remission	Usually grows rapidly Tends to grow relentlessly throughout life Rarely, neoplasm may regress spontaneously
Mode of growth	Grows by enlarging and expanding Always remains localized; never infiltrates surrounding tissues	Grows by infiltrating surrounding tissues May remain localized (in situ), but usually infiltrates other tissues
Capsule	Almost always contained within a fibrous capsule Capsule does not prevent expansion of neoplasm but does prevent growth by infiltration Capsule advantageous because encapsulated tumor can be removed surgically	Never contained within a capsule Absence of capsule allows neoplastic cells to invade surrounding tissues Surgical removal of tumor difficult
Cell characteristics	Usually well differentiated Mitotic figures absent or scanty Mature cells Anaplastic cells absent Cells function poorly in comparison with normal cells from which they arise If neoplasm arises in glandular tissue, cells may secrete hormones	Usually poorly differentiated Large numbers of normal and abnormal mitotic figures present Cells tend to be anaplastic, i.e., young, embryonic type Cells too abnormal to perform any physiologic functions Occasionally a malignant tumor arising in glandular tissue secretes hormones
Recurrence	Recurrence extremely unusual when surgically removed	Recurrence common following surgery because tumor cells spread into surrounding tissues
Metastasis	Metastases never occur	Metastases very common
Effect of neoplasm	Not harmful to host unless located in area where it compresses tissues or obstructs vital organs Does not produce cachexia (weight loss, debilitation, anemia, weakness, wasting)	Always harmful to host Causes death unless removed surgically or destroyed by radiation or chemotherapy Causes disfigurement, disrupted organ function, nutritional imbalances May result in ulcerations, sepsis, perforations, hemorrhage, tissue slough Almost always produces cachexia, which leaves person prone to pneumonia, anemia, etc.
Prognosis	Very good Tumor generally removed surgically	Depends on cell type and speed of diagnosis Poor prognosis if cells are poorly differentiated and evidence of metastatic spread exists Good prognosis indicated if cells still resemble normal cells and there is no evidence of metastasis

Malignant neoplasms are also categorized by tissue origin. A malignant neoplasm that arises from epithelial tissue is called a *carcinoma;* a malignant neoplasm that arises from mesenchymal origins (i.e., blood vessels, lymphatic tissue, nerve tissue) is called a *sarcoma* (from Greek *sarx,* flesh).

Three representative examples of malignant neoplasms or cancers are:

1. *Carcinoma in situ.* This is a neoplasm of epithelial tissue that remains confined to the site of origin. In situ carcinoma typically affects the cervix, and it may occur in squamous epithelium in other parts of the body. This form of cancer is, by definition, localized and thus can be removed surgically. However, in situ carcinoma can become invasive, eroding into surrounding tissues.

2. *Malignant fibrosarcomas.* These tumors are similar to benign fibromas. Fibrosarcomas tend to grow in the same sites and may originate as benign fibromas, later becoming malignant. These bulky, well-differentiated tumor masses are usually responsive to surgery. Fortunately, they rarely metastasize.

3. *Bronchogenic carcinomas.* These tumors account for 90% of all cases of lung cancer. Bronchogenic carcinomas usually develop in the lower trachea and lower bronchi. Surgical excision of the tumor is the intervention of choice. However, this type of cancer readily gives rise to metastasis; if this occurs, surgery is contraindicated.

CONCLUSIONS

Effective nursing care and client teaching to achieve outcome goals require that you understand the pathophysiol-

TABLE 18–7	CLASSIFICATION OF NEOPLASMS BY TISSUE OF ORIGIN	
Tissue of Origin	**Benign**	**Malignant**
Connective tissue		Sarcoma
Embryonic fibrous tissue	Myxoma	Myxosarcoma
Fibrous tissue	Fibroma	Fibrosarcoma
Adipose tissue	Lipoma	Liposarcoma
Cartilage	Chondroma	Chondrosarcoma
Bone	Osteoma	Osteogenic sarcoma
Epithelium		Carcinoma
Skin and mucous membrane	Papilloma	Squamous cell carcinoma
Glands		Basal cell carcinoma
		Transitional cell carcinoma
	Adenoma	Adenocarcinoma
	Cystadenoma	Cystadenocarcinoma
Pigmented cells (melanocytes)	Nevus	Malignant melanoma
Endothelium		Endothelioma
Blood vessels	Hemangioma	Hemangioendothelioma
		Hemangiosarcoma
		Kaposi's sarcoma
Lymph vessels	Lymphangioma	Lymphangiosarcoma
		Lymphangioendothelioma
Bone marrow		Multiple myeloma
		Ewing's sarcoma
		Leukemia
Lymphoid tissue		Malignant lymphoma
		Lymphosarcoma
		Reticulum cell sarcoma
Muscle tissue		
Smooth muscle	Leiomyoma	Leiomyosarcoma
Striated muscle	Rhabdomyoma	Rhabdomyosarcoma
Nerve tissue		
Nerve fibers and sheaths	Neuroma	Neurogenic sarcoma
	Neurinoma	
	(Neurilemoma)	
	Neurofibroma	(Neurofibrosarcoma)
Ganglion cells	Ganglioneuroma	Neuroblastoma
Glial cells	Glioma	Glioblastoma
Meninges	Meningioma	Malignant meningioma
Gonads	Dermoid cyst	Embryonal carcinoma
		Embryonal sarcoma
		Teratocarcinoma

ogy of the cancer. You should know the natural history of the disease, such as the normal course of disease progression, likely sites of metastasis, potential for effective treatment, and side effects and complications of both the disease and the treatments. With a basic understanding of cancer, you can build on that knowledge base by listening to the client's history, reviewing the information provided in the medical record, and consulting with colleagues, including nursing peers, nursing leaders, physicians, and oncology nurses, both locally and nationally.

BIBLIOGRAPHY

1. Ameisen, J. C. (1996). The origin of programmed cell death. *Science, 272,* 1278–1279.
2. American Cancer Society. (2000). *Cancer facts & figures—2000.* Atlanta: Author.
3. Baillie, C. T., Winslet, M. C., & Bradley, N. J. (1995). Tumour vasculature—a potential therapeutic target. *British Journal of Cancer, 72,* 257–267.
4. Brophy, L. (1998). Immunology. In J. K. Itano & K. N. Taoka (Eds.), *Core curriculum for oncology nursing* (3rd ed., pp. 383–391). Philadelphia: W. B. Saunders.
5. Calzone, K. A. (1998). Genetics. In J. K. Itano, & K. N. Taoka (Eds.), *Core curriculum for oncology nursing* (3rd ed., pp. 392–403). Philadelphia: W. B. Saunders.
6. Cartmel, B., & Reid, M. (1997). Cancer control and epidemiology. In S. L. Groenwald et al. (Eds.), *Cancer nursing: Principles and practices* (4th ed., pp. 50–74). Boston: Jones & Bartlett.
7. Caudell, K. A., Cuaron, L. J., & Gallucci, B. B. (1996). Cancer biology: Molecular and cellular aspects. In R. McCorkle et al. (Eds.), *Cancer nursing: A comprehensive textbook* (2nd ed., pp. 150–170). Philadelphia: W. B. Saunders.
8. Cortner, J., & Vande Woude, G. F. (1997). Essentials of molecular biology. In V. T. DeVita, S. Hellman, & S. A. Rosenberg (Eds.), *Cancer: Principles and practices of oncology* (5th ed., pp. 3–33). Philadelphia: Lippincott-Raven.

9. DeVita, V. T., Hellman, S., & Rosenberg, S. A. (Eds.). (1997). *Cancer: Principles and practices of oncology* (5th ed.). Philadelphia: Lippincott-Raven.

10. Duke, R. C., Ojcius, D. M., & Young, J. D. (1996). Cell suicide in health and disease. *Scientific American, 275*(6), 80–87.

11. Farrell, M. M. (1996). Biotherapy and the oncology nurse. *Seminars in Oncology Nursing, 12*(2), 82–88.

12. Fidler, I. J. (1997). Molecular biology of cancer: Invasion and metastasis. In V. T. DeVita, S. Hellman, & S. A. Rosenberg (Eds.), *Cancer: Principles and practices of oncology* (5th ed., pp. 135–148). Philadelphia: Lippincott-Raven.

13. Groenwald, S. L., et al. (1997). *Cancer nursing: Principles and practices* (4th ed.). Boston: Jones & Bartlett.

14. Hall, E. J. (1997). Etiology of cancer: Physical factors. In V. T. DeVita, S. Hellman, & S. A. Rosenberg (Eds.), *Cancer: Principles and practices of oncology* (5th ed., pp. 203–218). Philadelphia: Lippincott-Raven.

15. Henderson, B. E., Bernstein, L., & Ross, R. (1997). Etiology of cancer: Hormonal factors. In V. T. DeVita, S. Hellman, & S. A. Rosenberg (Eds.), *Cancer: Principles and practices of oncology* (5th ed., pp. 219–229). Philadelphia: Lippincott-Raven.

16. Hetts, S. W. (1998). To die or not to die. *Journal of the American Medical Association, 279*(4), 300–307.

17. Itano, J. K. & Taoka, K. N. (Eds.). (1998). *Core curriculum for oncology nursing* (3rd ed.). Philadelphia: W. B. Saunders.

18. Johnson, B. E. (1998). Tobacco and lung cancer. *Primary Care, 25*(2), 279–290.

19. Kastan, M. B. (1997). Molecular biology of cancer: The cell cycle. In V. T. DeVita, S. Hellman, & S. A. Rosenberg (Eds.), *Cancer: Principles and practices of oncology* (5th ed., pp. 121–134). Philadelphia: Lippincott-Raven.

20. Landis, S. H., et al. (1998). Cancer statistics. *CA: A Cancer Journal for Clinicians, 48*(1), 6–29.

21. Loescher, L. J. (1998). DNA testing for cancer predisposition. *Oncology Nursing Forum, 25*(8), 1317–1327.

22. Peters, J. A. (1997). Applications of genetic technologies to cancer screening, prevention, diagnosis, prognosis, and treatment. *Seminars in Oncology Nursing, 13*(2), 74–81.

23. Pitler, L. R. (1996). Hematopoietic growth factors in clinical practice. *Seminars in Oncology Nursing, 12*(2), 115–129.

24. Post-White, J. (1996). The immune system. *Seminars in Oncology Nursing, 12*(2), 89–96.

25. Post-White, J. (1996). Principles of immunology. In R. McCorkle et al. (Eds.), *Cancer nursing: A comprehensive textbook* (2nd ed., pp. 171–189). Philadelphia: W. B. Saunders.

26. Ries, L. A., et al. (Eds.). (1998). *SEER cancer statistics review, 1973–1995*. Bethesda, MD: National Cancer Institute.

27. Saenz, R. B., & Phillips, D. M. (1998). *Breast cancer. Primary care, 25*(2), 152–162.

28. Soltis, M., Hubbard, S., & Kohn, E. (1996). The biology of invasion and metastases. In R. McCorkle et al. (Eds.), *Cancer nursing: A comprehensive textbook* (2nd ed., pp. 190–212). Philadelphia: W. B. Saunders.

29. Stellman, J. M., Stellman, S. D. (1996). Cancer and the workplace. *CA: A Cancer Journal for Clinicians, 46*(70), 70–92.

30. Trichopoulos, D., et al. (1997). Epidemiology of cancer. In V. T. DeVita, S. Hellman, & S. A. Rosenberg (Eds.), *Cancer: Principles and practices of oncology* (5th ed., pp. 231–257). Philadelphia: Lippincott-Raven.

31. Volker, D. L. (1998). Carcinogenesis. In J. K. Itano & K. N. Taoka (Eds.), *Core curriculum for oncology nursing* (3rd ed., pp. 357–382). Philadelphia: W. B. Saunders.

32. Williams, J. K. (1997). Principles of genetics and cancer. *Seminars in Oncology Nursing, 13*(2), 68–73.

33. Workman, M. L. (1996). Gene therapy. In R. McCorkle et al. (Eds.), *Cancer nursing: A comprehensive textbook* (2nd ed., pp. 458–469). Philadelphia: W. B. Saunders.

34. Yuspa, S. H., & Shields, P. G. (1997). Etiology of cancer: Chemical factors. In V. T. DeVita, S. Hellman, & S. A. Rosenberg (Eds.), *Cancer: Principles and practices of oncology* (5th ed., pp. 185–202). Philadelphia: Lippincott-Raven.

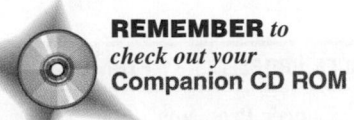

CHAPTER 19

Clients with Cancer: Promoting Positive Outcomes

Patricia Meier

NURSING OUTCOMES CLASSIFICATION (NOC)
for Nursing Diagnoses—Clients with Cancer

Altered Nutrition: Less Than Body Requirements
Nutritional Status: Food and Fluid
  Intake
Fatigue
Activity Tolerance
Endurance
Ineffective Individual Coping
Coping

Decision Making
Role Performance
Social Support
Risk for Infection
Immune Status
Risk Control
Risk Detection
Tissue Integrity: Skin and Mucous
  Membranes

Risk for Injury
Knowledge: Personal Safety
Neurologic Status
Risk Control
Risk Detection
Symptom Control

The continuum of disease progression begins with precancerous and cellular level changes discussed in the previous chapter on the pathophysiology of malignant neoplasms. The goal of health promotion is to prevent cancer or to detect it early, in its most treatable stage. After a new diagnosis of cancer, the client may experience remission, stable disease, recurrence, progressive disease, endstage or terminal disease, or long-term survivorship. Treatment modalities depend on the type and extent of the cancer but often include some combination of surgery, radiation therapy (RT), chemotherapy, and biotherapy. Bone marrow transplantation may be part of the treatment plan. Clinical trials offer the hope of new treatments for clients.

Increasingly, complementary approaches are being used in combination with other cancer treatments. The disease process and the effects of treatment on normal tissue present common complications or oncologic emergencies that require effective nursing management to achieve desired outcomes. Cancer care is not just about the disease and treatment; cancer comes in the midst of peoples' lives. Therefore, an important role of the nurse in managing outcomes is to recognize, intervene, and provide support for the human responses to living with cancer.

HEALTH PROMOTION AND MAINTENANCE

■ CANCER PREVENTION AND CONTROL

In the 1980s, the National Cancer Institute (NCI) set a goal to decrease mortality from cancer by 25% to 50% by the year 2000.[53] Cancer prevention and control were major priorities of the NCI's Year 2000 objectives. To achieve this goal, the NCI's objectives included reduction of the smoking rate in the United States to 15% or lower in order to achieve an 8% to 16% reduction in cancer mortality. Another NCI objective was to lower cancer mortality by 8% through dietary modifications. Such modifications involved decreasing fat intake to 30% of total calories and increasing dietary intake of fruits and vegetables to five or more servings daily and of grains to six or more servings daily. Another NCI objective was persuading 60% of the population to limit sun exposure, use sunscreen and protective clothing when exposed to the sun, and avoid artificial sources of ultraviolet light.

Recognizing the role of health professionals in motivating clients to alter lifestyle behaviors, the NCI also set an objective to have at least 75% of primary care providers routinely counsel clients about cessation of tobacco use, modifications of diet and exercise, and guidelines for screening.[53] These goals were difficult to achieve from the outset, given that (1) 20% to 30% of Americans smoke, (2) 90% eat too few fruits, vegetables, and grains while consuming too much fat, and (3) more than half have sedentary lifestyles.

PREVENTION, SCREENING, AND EARLY DETECTION

The three interrelated activities involved in cancer prevention and control are prevention, screening, and early detection. Primary prevention involves measures to avoid or reduce exposure to carcinogens. Screening programs help to identify high-risk populations and individuals. Early detection involves finding a precancerous lesion or a cancer at its earliest, most treatable stage.

Primary prevention activities are aimed at intervention before pathologic change has begun.[37] They can help to reduce cancer risk through alteration of lifestyle behaviors to eliminate or reduce exposure to carcinogens. Many cancers are associated with smoking, dietary habits, and alcohol consumption.[16, 37, 53] All of the cancers caused by combined tobacco and alcohol consumption could be avoided. Adapting a more healthy diet, limiting exposure to sun and other sources of ultraviolet radiation, modifying sexual practices, and decreasing exposure to environmental and occupational carcinogens would lead to further reduction in cancer incidence. Exposure to carcinogens can vary widely among population segments. In lower socioeconomic, medically underserved, and nonwhite segments of the population, the incidence of cancer is increased, and cancer is usually diagnosed at more advanced stages (Table 19–1).[69]

Secondary prevention,[37] also referred to as *early detection*, provides the opportunity to detect precancerous lesions or early-stage cancers before manifestations become readily apparent to the client and to treat them promptly. Screening efforts facilitate early detection. Methods of early detection are (1) inspection, (2) palpation, and (3) the use of tests or procedures. Inspection is useful in identifying lesions of the skin, lip, mouth, larynx, external genitalia, and cervix. Lumps or nodules in the breast, mouth, salivary glands, thyroid, subcutaneous tissue, anus, rectum, prostate, testes, ovaries, and uterus as well as enlarged lymph nodes can be detected through palpation. Mammograms, Papanicolaou (Pap) smear, occult blood testing of feces, endoscopy, and radiologic imaging studies are some of the tests or procedures that can be used. As a result of early detection, (1) premalignant lesions may be arrested, removed, or reversed or (2) cancer treatment can be started earlier, often while the cancer is in a stage more amenable to treatment.

Screening identifies high-risk groups of people more likely to have cancer or precancerous lesions. The current American Cancer Society (ACS) recommendations for screening are listed in Table 19–2. It is estimated that 75% of all cancers in the United States could be cured if all available screening tests and self-examination methods were practiced routinely.[37] Criteria for screening are as follows[30]:

- The population to be screened has a high incidence of the disease.
- The disease is detectable in its presymptomatic stage.
- Prognosis is poor if diagnosis is delayed until manifestations appear.

TABLE 19–1	CANCER PROBLEMS BY ETHNIC GROUPS
Ethnic Group	**Cancer Problems**
African American	Highest overall cancer incidence rate Highest overall mortality rate Survival 30% lower than for whites High-incidence cancers: prostate, breast, lung, colorectal, cervical, pancreatic, and esophageal
Hispanic	Gallbladder cancer among New Mexico Hispanics of Native American ancestry Liver cancer among Mexican Americans Cervical cancer among women from Central and South America Pancreatic cancer among Mexican Americans Prostate cancer
Asian/Pacific Islander	Nasopharyngeal cancer Stomach cancer
Chinese	Liver cancer Esophageal cancer
Native American	Lowest overall cancer incidence and mortality of all U.S. populations Survival rates uniformly low Important differences in tribal cancer rates

Adapted from Phillips, J., Belcher, A., & O'Neil, J. A. (1997). Special populations. In C. Varricchio et al. (Eds.), *A cancer source book for nurses* (7th ed.). Boston: Jones & Bartlett.

- An effective treatment is available for disease that is diagnosed early.
- There is an effective test for screening.
- The potential benefits of screening outweigh its potential risks and costs.

APPROACHES TO CANCER PREVENTION

Three main approaches to cancer prevention are (1) education, (2) regulation, and (3) host modification.[53] A client's health beliefs can be vital determinants of learning readiness when information is made available.

The beliefs that influence the effectiveness of *education* consist of the client's perception of susceptibility to developing cancer, beliefs about the harmful or beneficial consequences of lifestyle behaviors, and perceptions about the benefits of prevention and early detection.

Methods of *regulation* utilized in this country include prohibiting the sale of tobacco and alcohol to minors, limiting smoking in public places, imposing excise taxes, regulating the use of manufactured carcinogens such as asbestos, and prohibiting carcinogens in foods.

Host modification aims to alter the body's internal environment to decrease the risk of cancer or to reverse a carcinogenic process. Twenty per cent of cancers are associated with viruses (see Chapter 18, Table 18–4). Clinical trials of possible vaccines to immunize against some cancers have begun. Yet another avenue for host modification being studied in clinical trials is chemoprevention. This process is the use of noncytotoxic (non–cell-de-

TABLE 19–2	SUMMARY OF AMERICAN CANCER SOCIETY (ACS) RECOMMENDATIONS FOR THE EARLY DETECTION OF CANCER IN ASYMPTOMATIC PEOPLE

Site	Recommendation
Cancer-related checkup	A cancer-related checkup is recommended every 3 years for people aged 20–40 years and every year for people age 40 and older. This exam should include health counseling and, depending on a person's age, might include examinations for cancers of the thyroid, oral cavity, skin, lymph nodes, testes, and ovaries, as well as for some nonmalignant diseases.
Breast	Women 40 years and older should have an annual mammogram, an annual clinical breast exam (CBE) performed by a health care professional, and should perform monthly breast self-examination (BSE). The CBE should be conducted close to the scheduled mammogram. Women aged 20–39 should have a CBE performed by a health care professional every 3 years and should perform monthly BSE.
Colon and rectum	Men and women aged 50 years or older should follow *one* of the examination schedules below: ▪ A fecal occult blood test every year and a flexible sigmoidoscopy every 5 years. ▪ A colonoscopy every 10 years. ▪ A double-contrast barium enema every 5 to 10 years. ▪ A digital rectal exam should be done at the same time as sigmoidoscopy, colonoscopy, or double-contrast barium enema. People who are at moderate or high risk for colorectal cancer should talk with a doctor about a different testing schedule.
Prostate	The ACS recommends that both the prostate-specific antigen (PSA) blood test and the digital rectal examination be offered annually, beginning at age 50, to men who have a life expectancy of at least 10 years and to younger men who are at high risk. Men in high-risk groups, such as those with a strong familial predisposition (i.e., two or more affected first-degree relatives), or African Americans may begin at a younger age (i.e., 45 years).
Uterus	**Cervix:** All women who are or have been sexually active or who are 18 and older should have an annual Pap test and pelvic examination. After three or more consecutive satisfactory examinations with normal findings, the Pap test may be performed less frequently. Discuss the matter with your physician. **Endometrium:** Women at high risk for cancer of the uterus should have a sample of endometrial tissue examined when menopause begins.

Pap, Papanicolaou.

From American Cancer Society. (2000). *Cancer facts & figures 2000* (p. 34). Atlanta: American Cancer Society. ©American Cancer Society, Inc.

stroying) nutrients, pharmacologic agents, or both to prevent or reverse carcinogenesis.

PREVENTION AND EARLY DETECTION OF COMMON CAUSES

BREAST CANCER. Breast cancer is the most commonly diagnosed cancer, second only to lung cancer for cancer mortality, in American women. Risk factors (early menarche, late menopause, or being either nulliparous or older than 30 years at the birth of a first child) relate to their effect on circulating hormones. Incidence increases with age; more than 77% of women are older than age 50 at diagnosis. Having first-degree relatives with and a previous personal history of breast cancer also are indicators of higher risk. Many women diagnosed with breast cancer have no known risk factors.

One clinical trial has indicated the potential benefit of tamoxifen (Nolvadex), an anti-estrogen hormone, as preventive therapy for high-risk women older than 50 years. Breast cancer mortality could be reduced by 30% through early detection using routine screening mammography alone or together with an annual clinical breast examination by a primary health care provider beginning between ages 40 and 50. The ACS also recommends that women perform monthly breast self-examination (BSE) beginning at 20 years of age. The data are insufficient to determine the role of BSE in decreasing mortality; however, clients who perform BSE generally present with smaller tumors.[3, 30]

LUNG CANCER. Lung cancer is the leading cause of cancer deaths among Americans. More than 80% of lung cancers result from tobacco abuse. Other risk factors are tuberculosis (scar tumor), asbestos, exposure to radiation, and air pollution. To prevent lung cancer, clients should be counseled to not smoke. A healthy diet with at least five servings of fruits and vegetables is an added preventive step. Previous clinical trials have not found chemopreventives effective in preventing lung cancer. There is no reliable, inexpensive early detection method; therefore, screening is not of benefit.[3]

COLORECTAL CANCER. Colorectal cancer has the third highest incidence of all cancers in both men and women; the incidence is greater in men. Risk factors include familial polyposis, familial nonpolyposis syndromes, cancer family syndrome, hereditary site-specific colon cancer, and ulcerative colitis. Incidence of colorectal cancer increased with age after 50 years. A weaker risk factor associated with colorectal cancer may be a high-fat, low-fiber diet. There is no known prevention, although a healthy diet (higher in fiber and low in fat) and physical activity may be of benefit.

Early detection through routine screening is the key to decreasing mortality. The ACS recommends that people with an average risk for colon cancer be screened annually with digital rectal examinations and fecal occult blood tests beginning at age 40 and with sigmoidoscopy every 3 to 5 years beginning at age 50. For people with a high risk for colon cancer, the ACS recommendation is colonoscopy and/or double-contrast screenings beginning at age 40 (see Table 19–2).[3, 30]

PROSTATE CANCER. Age is the greatest risk factor for prostate cancer, 70 years being the median age at diagnosis. The incidence increases with each decade of life beginning at age 50. African-American men have the highest incidence of prostate cancer in the world. Another risk factor is family history; almost 25% of men with prostate cancer have two first-degree relatives with the disease. An occupationally related risk factor is exposure to cadmium. Prevention strategies include limiting exposure of workers handling cadmium batteries and keeping dietary fat intake low.

A clinical trial for prostate cancer prevention is under way with a chemopreventive agent, finasteride (Propecia). The ACS recommends that men at age 50 years and high-risk clients at age 40 years begin receiving a digital rectal examination as part of their annual physical examination as well as a prostate-specific antigen (PSA) blood test. The role of PSA findings in early detection is still unsettled. Early-stage prostate cancer is more amenable to treatment. However, the controversy centers on whether the PSA is leading to the diagnosis and treatment of prostate cancers that would never progress if not detected.[3, 30]

CERVICAL CANCER. Risk factors for cervical cancer are closely linked to sexual behavior and sexually transmitted infections. First intercourse at an early age, multiple sexual partners, or a sexual partner who has had multiple sexual partners put a woman at increased risk. The human papillomavirus and the acquired immunodeficiency syndrome (AIDS) are also risk factors, as are low socioeconomic status and cigarette smoking. Other than changing sexual behavior and avoiding tobacco use, there are no known preventive actions the client can take to avoid cervical cancer.

Routine screening for cervical cancer with the Pap smear should begin with the onset of sexual activity and should be repeated at least as often as every 3 years, annually for clients in nonmonogamous relationships. The Pap smear detects cancer in a premalignant stage, which is very amenable to treatment. With adequate screening, cervical cancer should not exist. However, there remain cultural and social barriers to prevention and early detection of this disease.[3, 30]

HEAD AND NECK CANCER. Men are at greater risk of head and neck cancer than women. A synergistic effect of alcohol and tobacco use increases the risk for cancer of the head and neck. Poor oral hygiene, long-term sun exposure, and occupational exposures (asbestos, tar, nickel, textile, wood or leather work, and machine tool operation) are additional risk factors. Southern Chinese clients are also at greater risk. All clients who smoke or combine smoking with drinking alcohol should be counseled to stop these behaviors. Retinoids have been used as a chemopreventive. The evidence does not support the value of routine screening programs, although early detection by dentists and dental hygienists can identify precancerous lesions.[3]

SKIN CANCER. Approximately 1 million new diagnoses of basal cell and squamous cell skin cancers are made each year. These highly curable cancers are not included in overall cancer statistics. The incidence of the most serious form of skin cancer, melanoma, has been increasing about 4% each year since 1973. Individuals with fair complexion, family history, multiple or atypical nevi (moles), and occupational exposure to coal tar, pitch, creosote, arsenic, or radium are at greater risk. Prevention involves avoiding ultraviolet radiation as well as limiting midday sun exposure, wearing a hat or clothing to protect the skin, using sunscreen with a sun protective factor (SPF) of 15 or higher, and avoiding severe sunburns, especially in childhood.

Early detection, especially for melanomas, is critical. Screening programs should include teaching clients how to inspect their own skin. Moles can be mapped as a baseline for future inspections. Basal and squamous cell skin cancer frequently appears as a pale, wax-like, pearly nodule or a red, scaly patch. Note should be made of any changes, such as new moles or a sore that repeatedly scabs over but fails to heal. Moles that are asymmetrical, that have irregular borders or uneven variations in color, or that change in diameter or height should be checked by a physician. A change in the color, surface appearance, or sensation of a mole should also be reported. Clients should be taught the importance of regular self-inspection and of seeking medical attention.[3]

HEALTH RESTORATION

■ MAINTAINING WELLNESS DURING TREATMENT

For clients with cancer, tertiary prevention[37] consists of limitation of disability and rehabilitation. For any client who must undergo cancer treatment, maintaining optimum wellness is important to both treatment outcome and quality of life in the midst of cancer. The nurse's role in caring for clients undergoing cancer treatment in order to maintain optimum wellness is addressed in the later discussion of outcome management during cancer treatments.

■ REHABILITATION

In addition to disease treatment, rehabilitation therapy is often important to the client's quality of life. Rehabilitation may consist of reconstructive surgery after breast cancer or surgery to reverse a temporary colostomy after colon cancer treatment. An important opportunity for rehabilitation may be an exercise program to help a client counteract chemotherapy-related fatigue.

A client whose treatment resulted in lymphedema is most grateful for the improved quality of life following a rehabilitation referral for lymphedema management. Clinicians often think of lymphedema management as benefiting only clients with breast cancer. However, professionals may overlook the possible secondary effect of lower extremity lymphedema after treatment for prostate cancer or after treatment for other cancers that affects the lymph nodes, such as surgery for melanoma or metastatic colon cancer. Additional rehabilitation strategies, such as speech therapy and prosthetic devices, are described in various chapters of the book, in discussions of specific disorders.

OUTCOME MANAGEMENT

■ DIAGNOSIS OF CANCER

Accurate diagnosis is paramount to effective cancer treatment. The vital first step in the diagnostic process is obtaining a complete history and physical examination. The history and physical assessment, together with diagnostic tests, can be highly predictive of a cancer diagnosis. Further, your careful attention to a client's history and physical status will result in accurate nursing diagnoses and interventions.

OBTAIN HISTORY

Because some cancers are linked with certain genetic and environmental factors, you will be concerned with cancer histories of blood relatives, the client's work history, and the environmental factors that may be associated with cancer causation. (See Chapters 9 and 10 for discussions of health history and physical assessment, respectively.) You should also listen for the client's previous life experiences with cancer—whether of a blood relative, the client's own history, or a friend's experience. This information will be useful in assessing both the client's previous knowledge and perceptions about cancer and the client's readiness for teaching.

ASSESS CLINICAL MANIFESTATIONS

When cancer is in its early stages, there are often few manifestations. Clinical manifestations usually appear once the cancer has grown sufficiently large to cause one or more of the following problems:

- Pressure on surrounding organs or nerves
- Distortion of surrounding tissue
- Obstruction of the lumen of vessels, intestines, ureters, and so on
- Interference with the blood supply of surrounding tissues
- Interference with organ function
- Disturbance of body metabolism
- Parasitic use of the body's nutritional supplies
- Mobilization of the body's defensive response

A localized tumor usually produces manifestations related to increased pressure or obstruction in a single region. Metastatic disease and extensive tumors of major organs may display a variety of local and systemic manifestations.

Common clinical manifestations that may arise secondary to cancer include weight loss, weakness or fatigue, central nervous system (CNS) alterations, pain, and hematologic and metabolic alterations. Close assessment of such manifestations may reveal that they are directly or indirectly related to the cancer.

Anorexia, weight loss, weakness, and fatigue are related to the body's inability to consume and use nutrients appropriately. Mechanical interference by tumors, malabsorption, paraneoplastic endocrine secretions (such as excessive secretion of thyroid hormones), and a tumor's use

of nutrients may all contribute to a process that must be interrupted to avoid general physical debility.

The client who has difficulty with vision, speech, coordination, or memory may be experiencing primary or metastatic CNS disease. Increased intracranial pressure caused by tumor growth may cause headache, lethargy, nausea, and vomiting.

Although pain is not a common manifestation of early-stage cancer, it may occur as a result of obstruction or destruction of a vital organ, pressure on sensitive tissues or bone, or involvement of nerves. Pain that is not adequately treated may become constant and progressively severe. Bone cancer is particularly painful because the rigidity of bone allows for little or no expansion as the tumor cells proliferate.[27, 57] The pain worsens when pathologic fractures produce instability and muscle spasms. Even though pain is usually a late manifestation in cancer, it may be the manifestation that brings the client to health care.

COMPLETE DIAGNOSTIC EVALUATION

In addition to the history and physical assessment, laboratory and imaging studies may provide further data to support a cancer diagnosis. Many of the diagnostic laboratory and imaging studies utilized to detect other diseases are used to detect cancer. (See Chapter 11 for a discussion of diagnostic assessment.)

A variety of blood tests can be performed to help diagnose cancer (Table 19–3). Some of the more routine tests, such as the complete blood count (CBC) and differential count, do not test for specific types of cancer but indicate the presence of nonspecific problems. These tests are also vital to monitoring the side effects of treatment. Other blood tests, such as tumor marker measurements and biochemical tests, identify the extent of a particular type of cancer. Tumor markers such as PSA can be indicators of cancer; tumor markers are often even more useful as "barometers" demonstrating the effectiveness of treatment.

Unexplained anemia often indicates a malignancy. Hematologic changes include leukopenia, leukocytosis, and bleeding disorders, which in some diseases may occur before local manifestations. Metabolic manifestations, such as Cushing's syndrome, hypercalcemia, syndrome of inappropriate antidiuretic hormone (SIADH) secretion, and carcinoid syndrome, also signify the possibility of cancer.

■ GRADING AND STAGING OF CANCER

Microscopic evidence of malignant cells from the tumor tissue, generally obtained through a surgical or needle biopsy for cytologic analysis, is the *only* definitive evidence of cancer. Once the diagnosis has been made and the microscopic cell type and grade of the tumor have been determined, the extent of spread (staging) of the tumor also needs to be identified.

Tissue may be obtained through a *biopsy*, the surgical excision of a small piece of tissue and its microscopic examination. After the excision, the pathologist prepares a frozen section or permanent paraffin section of the tissue to examine the specimen. For a frozen (or rapid) section, the tissue is immediately frozen; then the pathologist cuts the tissue into thin sections or slices and examines them

TABLE 19-3	LABORATORY BLOOD TESTS FOR CANCER

Test	Reference Values	Conditions in Which Levels May Be Altered
HEMATOLOGIC (CBC)		
Hemoglobin	M: 14–18 g/dl F: 12–16 g/dl	↓ Anemia; nonspecific; may indicate malignancy
Hematocrit	M: 40–54 ml/dl F: 37–47 ml/dl	↓ Anemia; nonspecific; may indicate malignancy
Leukocytes (WBC count)	4500–11,000/mm³	↑ Leukemia, lymphomas ↓ Leukemia, metastatic disease to bone marrow
Platelets	150,000–300,000/mm³	↑ Myeloproliferative disorders, CML, Hodgkin's disease ↓ ALL, AML, multiple myeloma, bone marrow depression
BLOOD OR SERUM		
Acid phosphatase	0.11–0.60 mU/ml	↑ Metastatic prostate cancer
ACTH	10–80 pg/ml (in AM)	↑ Lung cancer
Alkaline phosphatase	20–90 mU/ml	↑ Cancer of bone or bone metastasis, liver cancer, lymphoma, leukemia
Calcitonin	Undetectable	↑ Medullary thyroid cancer if >100 pg/ml
Calcium	9.0–11.0 mg/dl	↑ Bone metastasis, breast cancer, leukemia, lymphoma, multiple myeloma, and lung, kidney, bladder, liver, and parathyroid cancers
Gastrin	<200 pg/ml	↑ Gastric and pancreatic cancers
LDH	100–190 mU/dl	↑ Liver cancer, liver metastasis, lymphoma, acute leukemia
Parathyroid hormone	430–1860 ng/L	↑ Squamous cell lung, kidney, pancreatic, and ovarian cancers
Serotonin	50–200 ng/ml	↑ Carcinoid syndrome
SGPT (AST)	5–35 mU/ml	↑ Metastatic cancer to the liver
SGOT (ALT)	740 mU/ml	↑ Metastatic cancer to the liver
Testosterone	M: 275–875 ng/dl F: 23–75 ng/dl	↑ Adrenal and ovarian cancers
Uric acid	M: 2.5–8.0 mg/dl F: 1.4–7.0 mg/dl	↑ Leukemia, multiple myeloma ↓ Hodgkin's disease, multiple myeloma, lung cancer
TUMOR MARKERS		
AFP	<10 ng/ml	↑ Lung, nonseminomatous testicular, pancreatic, colon, and gastric cancers, choriocarcinoma
CA–125	<35 units	↑ Ovarian and pancreatic cancers
Calcitonin	<100 pg/ml	↑ Medullary thyroid, small cell lung, and breast cancers, carcinoid
CEA	0–2.5 ng/ml nonsmokers <3.0 ng/ml smokers	↑ Colorectal, breast, lung, stomach, pancreatic, and prostate cancers
Estrogen receptors	Positive >10 fmoles/mg	↑ ER + breast cancer
HCG	0–5 IU/L	↑ Choriocarcinoma, germ cell testicular cancer; ectopic production in lung, liver, gastric, pancreatic, and colon cancers
Progesterone receptor assay	Positive >10 fmoles/mg	↑ PR + breast cancer
Prostatic acid phosphatase	0.26–0.83 U/L	↑ Metastatic prostate cancer
PSA	0–4 ng/ml	↑ Prostate cancer
CA-19–9		↑ Pancreatic, colon, and gastric cancers
CA-15–3		↑ Breast cancer

ACTH, adrenocorticotropic hormone; AFP, alpha-fetoprotein; ALL, acute lymphocytic leukemia; ALT, alanine transferase; AML, acute myelogenous leukemia; AST, aspartate transaminase; CBC, complete blood count; CEA, carcinoembryonic antigen; CML, chronic myelogenous leukemia; ER, estrogen receptors; F, female; f, femto-; HCG, human chorionic gonadotropin; LDH, lactic acid dehydrogenase; M, male; mU, milliunits; PSA, prostate-specific antigen; SGOT, serum glutamic-oxalo-acetic transaminase; SGPT, serum glutamate pyruvate transaminase; U, units; WBC, white blood cell; ↑, increase; ↓, decrease.

under the microscope. The main advantage of the frozen section is the speed with which the specimen can be prepared and the diagnosis made. Only minutes are required, enabling the surgeon to receive an initial report during surgery. In contrast, the slower, more classic method of embedding the tissue in paraffin takes about 24 hours. However, the paraffin section demonstrates clearer detail than the frozen section.

The tumor *grade* is an evaluation of the extent to which tumor cells differ from their normal precursors. In low numerical grades, grades I and II, the cells are well-differentiated and deviate minimally from normal cells. High grades, grades III and IV, refer to cells that are poorly differentiated and the most aberrant compared with normal cells. A pathologist determines the grade. Tumor grading involves a histologic and anatomic description of the cancer. The pathologist also evaluates the biopsy specimen for other characteristics that help identify the cell type of the malignancy or provide important indicators of prognosis.

Basic x-rays, computed tomography (CT), magnetic resonance imaging (MRI), ultrasound, and other imaging studies are utilized in the diagnosis of cancer as well as in diagnosis of many other diseases. (See Chapter 11 for more information.) When measurable amounts of tumor remain after surgery, imaging studies such as CT scans are repeated at regular intervals to evaluate the effectiveness of chemotherapy or RT.

When a neoplastic growth is definitely diagnosed, it must be further defined in terms of its extent. This diagnostic process, called *staging*, involves a systematic search for the characteristics of the primary tumor (T), involvement of lymph nodes (N), and evidence of metastasis (M), on the basis of knowledge of the natural history of the disease. The TNM system is the accepted system for cancer staging today (Table 19–4).

According to the TNM classification, cancers may be grouped into one of four stages (I to IV) or indicated as stage 0 for carcinoma in situ (without spread). Higher stages signify more extensive disease, with stage IV consistently representing distant metastasis and the worst prognosis. Grading and staging information guides the physician in choosing the intervention and estimating the client's prognosis.

Other established classifications may be used for particular malignancies, such as Clark's classification for malignant melanomas and Dukes' classification for colorectal cancer. Clark's classification considers the level of invasion of melanomas, and Dukes' system refers to the depth of invasion of colorectal cancer. Hodgkin's disease uses the Ann Arbor classification, which refers to both the distribution of the tumor and the associated manifestations.

■ IDENTIFYING TREATMENT GOALS

The major objective of cancer therapy is to treat the client effectively with appropriate therapy for a sufficient duration so a cure (or control) of the cancer results with minimal functional and structural impairment. *Cure* is a controversial word because of the chronic nature of most cancers, so many health care providers prefer the term *control*. If a cure is not possible, important alternative goals are:

TABLE 19–4	TNM STAGING SYSTEM
Stage	**Characteristics**
Primary Tumor (T)	
TX	No primary tumor can be assessed
T0	No evidence of primary tumor
TIS	Carcinoma in situ
T1, T2, T3, T4	Increasing size and extent of the primary tumor
Regional Lymph Nodes (N)	
NX	Cannot be assessed
N0	No regional lymph node involvement
N1, N2, N3	Increasing involvement of regional lymph nodes
Distant Metastasis (M)	
MX	Presence of metastasis cannot be assessed
M0	No distant metastasis
M1	Distant metastasis

From Miaskowski, C., & Buchsel, P. (1999). Oncology nursing assessment and clinical care. St. Louis: Mosby.

- *Control* of the cancer by slowing disease progression
- *Palliation,* or alleviation of manifestations
- *Rehabilitation* to maintain a high quality of life for as long as possible or even when cure results

Decisions made at the time of first diagnosis are crucial, because early aggressive intervention usually offers the best hope of cure. Even when cure is not possible, many clients with cancer have benefited from an extended life span and an improved quality of life as a result of cancer treatment.

■ DETERMINING TREATMENT MODALITIES

Methods of treating clients with cancer are surgery, RT, chemotherapy, biotherapy, and bone marrow transplantation. The choice of method depends on the type of tumor, the extent of disease, and the client's co-morbid conditions (such as cardiac disease), performance status, and wishes.

Performance status is a way of evaluating a client's overall health status and ability to tolerate treatment. Table 19–5 describes two common performance status scales. In most cases, a client is treated with a combination of methods rather than a single therapy. This approach is called *combined modality* or *multimodal* therapy. Combined modality therapy is used in most cancer treatment regimens because it is more effective in destroying cancerous cells. For example, first surgically debulking (removing as much tumor as possible) an ovarian cancer increases the potential for the chemotherapy to be effective on the remaining tumor volume.

■ Surgical Management

Surgery plays a major role in the diagnosis, staging, and treatment of cancer. It is also an integral part of the

TABLE 19–5	PERFORMANCE STATUS SCALES

EASTERN COOPERATIVE ONCOLOGY GROUP SCALE

0	Asymptomatic
1	Symptomatic; fully ambulatory
2	Symptomatic; in bed <50% of day
3	Symptomatic; in bed >50% of day, but not bed-ridden
4	Bedridden

KARNOFSKY SCALE

100	Normal; no complaints; no evidence of disease
90	Able to carry on normal activity; minor manifestations of disease
80	Normal activity with effort; some signs or symptoms of disease
70	Can care for self; unable to do normal activity or active work
60	Needs occasional assistance; able to care for most of needs
50	Needs considerable assistance and frequent medical care
40	Disabled; needs special care and assistance
30	Severely disabled; hospitalization and death not imminent
20	Very sick; hospitalization necessary
10	Moribund; fatal processes progressing rapidly
0	Death

Adapted from Powel, L. L. (1996). *Cancer chemotherapy guidelines and recommendations for practice.* Pittsburgh: Oncology Nursing Press; and Ignatavicius, D., Workman, M. L., & Mishler, M. (1999). *Medical-surgical nursing across the health care continuum* (3rd ed.). Philadelphia: W. B. Saunders.

rehabilitation and palliation for clients with cancer. Surgery is used with less frequency as a method of cancer prevention.

Although many aspects of surgical care of the client with cancer are similar to those for all clients undergoing surgery for any reason (see Chapter 15 as well as chapters that address surgery of a specific part of the body), there are some differences. In addition to providing expert physical care, it is important that, preoperatively, you evaluate the client's understanding of the proposed procedure and the changes it involves. The emotional impact of the diagnosis may affect the client's expectations, coping, and ability to learn. Preoperatively, clients with cancer may be nutritionally compromised and may require nutritional therapy before surgery. Those who have undergone adjuvant (treatment after removal of all detected cancer) or palliative (comfort care) chemotherapy or RT may have a low red blood cell (RBC) or white blood cell (WBC) count, which needs correction before surgery. In the client undergoing a palliative surgical procedure, pain must be assessed from the perspective of normal postoperative pain in addition to pain secondary to tumor invasion.

DIAGNOSTIC SURGERY

As mentioned, the diagnosis of cancer is established by microscopic identification of malignant cells from tumor tissue. A variety of methods, most involving a surgical procedure, are used to obtain tissue for diagnostic purposes. The biology of the tumor, its size and location, and the proposed method of treatment determine which biopsy method should be used.

Cytologic specimen collection and needle biopsy are relatively simple procedures. A negative biopsy result does not prove the absence of cancer but rather may be an indication of inadequate or misplaced tissue sampling. Negative needle biopsy results generally must be followed by additional specimen collections to obtain an accurate diagnosis.

CYTOLOGIC SPECIMENS. Cytologic specimens can be obtained from tumors that tend to shed cells from their surface. Tumor cells can often be obtained from cytologic examination of fluids aspirated from effusions or ascitic fluid. The physician may obtain cytologic brushings or tissue biopsy specimens while using an endoscope to examine a questionable area. An endoscopy involves direct visualization of the gastrointestinal (GI) tract, bronchoscopy of the lungs, laryngoscopy of the larynx, colposcopy of the cervix and vagina, cystoscopy of the bladder, laparoscopy of the pelvic or abdominal cavity. During these tests, questionable areas can be examined, tissue samples and aspirates taken for biopsy, the extent of the disease staged, and pathologic processes excised.

NEEDLE BIOPSY. Needle biopsy is a simple method of obtaining tissue samples. In a *fine-needle aspiration*, tumor cells are withdrawn from the tumor with a needle and syringe. A *core-needle biopsy* is essentially the same procedure; however, the needle is larger, and a core or barrel of tissue is obtained. Core-needle biopsy allows the pathologist to examine the cells with their spatial relationships intact, whereas fine-needle aspiration provides individual cells or clumps of cells for review.

Needle biopsy is useful in obtaining samples from tumors in subcutaneous tissue, muscle, breast, pancreas, liver, and lung. Needle (aspiration) biopsy is used mainly to obtain tissue samples for identification from liver, kidney, spleen, lung, or breast. The physician aspirates a core of tissue from a questionable nodule or mass rather than excising it.

EXCISIONAL BIOPSY AND INCISIONAL BIOPSY. The size of the tumor and the purpose of the biopsy are determinants of whether an excisional or incisional biopsy is performed. If the suspected tumor is small, the entire tumor is excised for examination; this is called a *total* or *excisional* type of biopsy. It is used for small tumors (2 to 3 cm) for which the biopsy also may serve as the treatment if the tissue margins contain no tumor cells. If tumor cells remain, a wider excision is required.

If the tumor is large, only a part of the neoplasm is excised. This procedure is termed a *subtotal* or *incisional* type of biopsy. Stereotactic breast biopsy is a radiography-guided method for localizing and sampling small, nonpalpable breast lesions that are discovered on mammography and that suggest malignancy.

SURGERY FOR STAGING

Cancer staging is the process of determining the extent of disease as the basis for treatment decisions. *Clinical staging* is based on evidence acquired before treatment and obtained from physical examination, imaging, endoscopy, biopsy, laboratory tests, surgical exploration, and other diagnostic tests. It is based on all information gathered prior to the first definitive treatment used.

Pathologic staging is based on the microscopic evidence acquired before treatment, which is supplemented or modified by information obtained at surgery and from the pathologic examination of resected specimens, including the primary tumor, regional lymph nodes, and metastatic nodules. For example, the true stage of colon cancer is usually determined after surgery, when the regional lymph nodes are examined for the presence of tumor cells. Staging of ovarian cancer is based on the extent and location of disease found during surgery.

SURGERY AS TREATMENT

Surgery is performed in 55% of clients with cancer.[2] Forty per cent of clients who undergo cancer surgery are treated with surgery alone. Cancers that are localized to the organ of origin and the regional lymph nodes are potentially curable by surgery, although multimodal treatment is more likely to be used to control any submicroscopic spread.

Historically, the generally accepted concept of tumor growth was an orderly sequence of growth from the organ of origin to adjacent tissue, regional lymph nodes, and, eventually, distant sites in a systematic fashion. The logical surgical approach to this type of growth was the widest excision possible of the tumor, surrounding tissue, and regional lymph nodes. Thus, radical surgery became the standard for cancer treatment. Analysis of treatment results, however, demonstrated that despite radical excisions, tumors recurred. Current concepts of tumor biology hold that tumors probably shed cells into the systemic circulation throughout their growth and that, therefore, local therapies (surgery and radiation) must be combined with systemic therapies (biotherapy and chemotherapy) to improve client survival.

When surgery is performed with curative intent, the type of tumor determines the extent of the excision. For slow-growing tumors, such as squamous cell carcinoma and adenocarcinoma of the skin, a wide local excision may be sufficient. Tumors of the colon and breast that spread to the regional lymph nodes are removed with an en bloc excision of the tumor and regional lymph nodes. Sentinel node mapping for breast cancer is discussed in Chapter 40 (the procedure is also used for melanoma). Large tumors, such as sarcomas, which tend to spread locally without metastasis, are removed with radical excisions, such as amputations. In all surgical procedures, various operative techniques, such as glove changing, instrument cleaning, and wound irrigation with cytotoxic agents, are used to prevent dissemination of tumor cells into and beyond the operative field.

SURGERY FOR RECURRENCE AND METASTASIS

Cancer that recurs locally can be resected, resulting in occasional cure, remission, or both. Local recurrences of sarcomas as well as colon, breast, and skin cancers have been successfully excised. Solitary metastatic lesions that appear in the lungs, liver, or brain can be removed to effect a surgical cure. Excision of metastatic lesions is considered if (1) no other evidence of disease exists and (2) the metastatic lesion has appeared after a relatively long disease-free interval. The metastatic lesion must exhibit some stability and must be refractory (unresponsive) to chemotherapy and RT. Metastatic renal cell carcinomas, sarcomas, melanomas, and colon carcinomas have been removed in selected clients, resulting in cures or prolonged survival times.

PALLIATIVE SURGERY

Because surgical procedures carry an inherent potential for morbidity, use of surgery in palliative care is carefully considered and is used only if the risk-benefit ratio is favorable. Examples of palliative surgery that can benefit the client with cancer and improve quality of life include procedures that (1) reduce pain by such means as interrupting nerve pathways or implanting pain control pumps, (2) relieve airway obstructions, (3) relieve obstructions in the GI and urinary tracts, (4) relieve pressure on the brain or spinal cord, (5) prevent hemorrhage, (6) remove infected and ulcerating tumors, and (7) drain abscesses.

RECONSTRUCTIVE SURGERY

Advances in reconstructive surgery offer a different perspective on rehabilitation to the client who has experienced curative surgery. Restoration of form and function is possible to varying degrees, depending on the site and extent of surgery. Reconstructive surgery may be performed concurrently with the radical procedure or may be delayed. The major goal of reconstructive surgery is to improve the client's quality of life by restoring maximal function and appearance.

PREVENTIVE SURGERY

The client at unusually high risk for cancer may elect to undergo a preventive (prophylactic) surgical intervention. Certain conditions or diseases increase the risk of cancer occurrence so significantly that removal of the target organ is justified to prevent cancer development. Clients with familial polyposis, for example, have a 50% risk of having colon cancer by age 40 years. By the time they are 70 years old, all clients with this inherited trait have colon cancer. Clients with ulcerative colitis also have a greater risk for colon cancer. Prophylactic subtotal colectomies may be indicated for this group.

Clients with multiple high-risk factors may consider preventive surgery. Prophylactic mastectomy (breast removal) or oophorectomy (ovary removal), although uncommonly indicated, are acceptable forms of preventive therapy in certain high-risk clients.[65]

Nursing Management of the Surgical Client

Cancer operations tend to be more involved than similar procedures for benign conditions. This tendency can lead to the potential for more complications. For the most part, the postoperative care (such as wound care and prevention of infection) of the client with cancer is similar to that of any client having the same surgical procedure for a noncancer diagnosis. The difference lies in what follows. With a benign condition, although there is certainly a period of healing and perhaps rehabilitation, the surgery usually concludes the active treatment.

With cancer surgery, however, the client often has only begun one phase of multimodal treatment. Surgery is not always the first phase of treatment, because many treatment protocols begin with chemotherapy or RT to shrink the tumor mass and decrease the likelihood of micrometastasis. In the midst of the emotional impact of the diagnosis, the client and family are confronted with an often overwhelming amount of information about the diagnosis, necessary tests, treatment alternatives, and decisions to be made. The client will probably be seen or treated in multiple health care settings by many different health professionals. To effectively help the client manage outcomes, the medical-surgical nurse must not only provide excellent care during the hospitalization but also proactively assist the client with continuing care.

ASSESS DISCHARGE NEEDS

Questions you can ask as a guide to discharge planning are as follows:

- What does the client need to know, and what does the client need to be able to do?

- Does the client know how to get to the medical oncologist's office or the clinic?
- Will the client need assistance with transportation, such as an ACS Road to Recovery volunteer driver?
- Would the client benefit from initial information about chemotherapy or from talking with someone who has "been there"?
- If the client or family members have questions you cannot answer, is there a social worker, oncology nursing colleague, or chaplain who can provide assistance?

See the Case Management feature.

No one person and no one profession can meet all of the needs of the client with cancer and the family. To effectively manage outcomes requires teamwork involving the client, the family, the nurse, and other health professionals.

CASE MANAGEMENT

The Client with Cancer

A diagnosis of cancer has traditionally evoked fear of pain and death. Many clients believe that there is little to be done. However, newer therapies have made it possible for curative treatment or remission and have led to improved survival rates. As a nurse, you will be working with clients of all ages at various stages in the cancer process.

Case management for these clients involves awareness of the client's emotional, physical, and psychological state; competent clinical care; education about treatment and further options; and helping the client to use preventive measures as possible. As a good example, you should practice preventive measures—no smoking, good nutrition, weight control, screening examinations, and awareness of environmental hazards.

Assess

- Has a definitive diagnosis of cancer been made?
- What do the client and family know about the diagnosis, type of treatment, and prognosis?
- Which treatment modalities will be used—chemotherapy, surgery, radiation, or some combination?
- What does the client anticipate as a result of treatment (e.g., alopecia, nausea, leukopenia)?
- Is pain management adequate?
- Has this diagnosis affected the client's role in the family? The ability to return to work?
- Are there financial or insurance concerns? (Some insurers may not cover all treatments, especially if they are considered investigational. Loss of insurance or inability to obtain insurance or exhaustion of benefits may also be issues.)

Advocate

Clients with cancer may exhibit behavior indicative of stages in the grieving process (e.g., denial, anger). Giving support without taking the client's behavior personally can be a challenge. Always be aware of what the client

and family have been told, and make sure that all caregivers are consistent with information given. Sometimes family members will try to shield the client from knowing the extent of the disease. Honesty and knowledge of what to expect are generally more helpful and empower the client to direct treatment choices. Clients may need assistance with advanced directives or in making a will. Be aware of spiritual needs, and elicit support from the pastoral care team as the client desires.

Management of clinical manifestations is another area of advocacy. Certainly, pain management should always be considered, but other physical and psychological problems must be handled as well—nausea and vomiting, diarrhea, stomatitis, skin breakdown, anxiety, withdrawal, and self-image concerns. At some point, you may help the client to decide that palliative care is preferable to aggressive therapy.

Prevent Readmission

There are multiple reasons for readmission, depending on the type of therapy and stage of cancer. Some readmissions may be anticipated, such as a continuing course of chemotherapy or reconstructive breast surgery; others may be unexpected, such as pneumonia or another infection. Before the client leaves the hospital, consider whether the client can return to the previous living arrangement and whether caregiver support is available; also consider respite for the caregiver. Is hospice care appropriate? Many clients will have complicated care regimens, including intravenous lines or ports, total parenteral nutrition and pain medications via pump. Knowledge of treatments, medications, especially for pain and management of manifestations, can assist the client in managing successfully at home. Information and assistance in obtaining wigs, prosthetics, makeup and special clothing, as well as connecting clients with the many cancer support groups, can promote a positive outlook, leading to an improved quality of life.

Cheryl Noetscher, RN, MS, *Director of Case Management, Crouse Hospital and Community–General Hospital, Syracuse, New York*

■ RADIATION THERAPY

More than 50% of all clients with cancer receive RT at some point during the course of their disease. RT may be used as a primary, an adjuvant, or a palliative treatment. When RT is used as a *primary* modality, it is the only treatment used and aims to achieve local cure of the cancer (e.g., early-stage Hodgkin's disease, skin cancer, carcinoma of the cervix). For patients with laryngeal cancer, the potential for cure with RT is equal to the cure rate with surgery—but without the client's loss of the voice box.

As an *adjuvant* treatment, RT can be used either preoperatively or postoperatively to aid in the destruction of cancer cells (e.g., colorectal cancer, early breast cancer). In addition, it can be used in conjunction with chemotherapy to treat disease in sites not readily accessible to systemic chemotherapy, such as the brain. In some situations, chemotherapy is combined with RT and is administered before the RT dose in an attempt to enhance the effects of RT. For example, in rectal cancer, a client may receive the drug 5-fluorouracil (5-FU) by continuous infusion via an ambulatory pump while receiving RT to kill residual cancer cells left behind after the surgery. The 5-FU makes the malignant cells more sensitive to the effects of the RT.

As a *palliative* treatment modality, RT can be used to relieve pain caused by obstruction, pathologic fractures, spinal cord compression, and metastasis.

HOW RADIATION THERAPY WORKS

Radiosensitivity, the relative susceptibility of tissues to radiation, depends on the individual cells and the characteristics of the tissue itself. A highly radiosensitive tumor is greatly affected by radiation because it divides rapidly, is well vascularized, and has high oxygen content.

RT is the use of high-energy ionizing radiation to treat a variety of cancers. Ionizing radiation destroys a cell's ability to reproduce by damaging its DNA. Rapidly dividing cells are more vulnerable to radiation than more slowly dividing cells. Normal cells have a greater ability than cancer cells to repair the DNA damage from radiation. Therefore, the radiation oncologist may deliver a sufficient dose of radiation to kill the cancer cells while sparing normal cells from excessive cell death.

In addition to the DNA effects, a complex chain of chemical reactions occurs in the extracellular fluid, resulting in the formation of free radicals. Well-oxygenated tumors show a much greater response to radiation than poorly oxygenated tumors. Oxygen free radicals formed during ionization interact readily with nearby molecules, causing cellular damage. A well-vascularized tumor may therefore be more responsive to RT than the same type of tumor if it is larger and, as a result, more poorly vascularized.

TYPES OF RADIATION THERAPY

RT can be administered by a variety of methods. The RT may be delivered as external beam therapy or via a radiation source placed close to the surface of the body or inside the body.

EXTERNAL BEAM RADIATION THERAPY. External beam RT, or teletherapy, is the delivery of radiation from a source placed at some distance from the target site. It is administered in the RT department by high-energy x-ray or gamma-ray machines (e.g., linear accelerator, cobalt, betatron, or a machine containing a radioisotope). The major advantage of high-energy radiation is its skin-sparing effect; that is, the maximum effect of radiation occurs at tumor depth in the body and not on the skin surface. Neutron beam therapy delivered from a cyclotron particle accelerator is currently used to treat many types of cancers, including salivary gland tumors, sarcomas, and tumors of the prostate and lung. Therapists do not remain in the room with the client during the treatment but monitor the client via closed-circuit television and remain in voice contact via an intercom.

INTERNAL RADIATION THERAPY. Internal RT involves placement of specially prepared radioisotopes (radioactive isotopes) directly into or near the tumor itself (*brachytherapy*) or into the systemic circulation. The two major types of internal RT are (1) sealed-source RT, in which the radioactive material is enclosed in a sealed container, and (2) unsealed-source RT, in which the radioactive material is administered systemically, such as by injection or orally.

Sealed-Source Radiation Therapy. Sealed-source RT is used for both intracavity and interstitial therapy. In *intracavity* therapy, the radioisotope, usually cesium 137 or radium 226, is put in an applicator, which is then placed in the body cavity for a carefully calculated time, generally 24 to 72 hours. Intracavity RT is used to treat cancers of the uterus and cervix.

In *interstitial* therapy, the radioisotope of choice (e.g., iridium 192, iodine 125, cesium 137, gold 198, or radon 222) is placed in needles, beads, seeds, ribbons, or catheters, which are then implanted directly into the tumor. For example, clients with prostate cancer may receive implanted seeds as therapy. Implants may be left in the tumor either temporarily (when ribbons, needles, or catheters are used) or permanently (when prostatic seeds are used), depending on the half-life of the isotope.

With sealed sources of internal radiation, the radioisotope is completely enclosed by nonradioactive material. Thus, the radioisotope cannot circulate through the client's body nor can it contaminate the client's urine, sweat, blood, or vomitus. Consequently, the client's excretions are not radioactive. However, radiation exposure can result from direct contact with the sealed radioisotope, such as touching the container with bare hands or from lengthy exposure to the sealed radioisotope.

Afterloading devices have been developed in which an empty applicator (the product that holds the radiation source) is placed during an operative procedure, and the radioactive source is not loaded until the client returns to the hospital room or the radiation treatment department. The technique of remote afterloading may be used to deliver frequent, short-term, high doses of radiation directly to a selected tumor. Generally, hollow applicators are surgically placed. The radioactive source is inserted into the applicator and left in place for a specific time afterward. After a treatment, the radioactive source is removed, but the applicator is left in place if more than one treatment is planned. The client is returned to the hospital room until the next treatment. When brachytherapy is used in the hospital room, the radioactive source can be returned to the brachytherapy device while you are in the client's room providing care. Thus, the use of afterloading devices has helped to decrease radiation exposure for staff but lengthens the total time needed to deliver the dose for the client.

Unsealed-Source Radiation Therapy. Unsealed sources of internal radiation are used in systemic therapy. Unsealed sources used for internal RT are colloid suspensions that come into direct contact with body tissues. The radioisotopes may be administered intravenously, orally, or by instillation directly into a body cavity. For example, iodine 131 is given orally in very low doses to treat Graves' disease (see Chapter 43) or in high doses to treat thyroid cancer. Strontium chloride 89 (Metastron) is administered intravenously for relief of painful bony metastases.

With unsealed sources of internal radiation, the radioisotope circulates through the client's body. Therefore, the client's urine, sweat, blood, and vomitus contain the radioactive isotope.

RADIATION SAFETY STANDARDS

Three key principles you should follow to protect yourself and others from excessive radiation exposure are (1) distance, (2) time, and (3) shielding.

The greater the *distance* from the radiation source, the less the exposure dose of ionizing rays. Distance and radiation exposure are inversely related. Thus, the intensity of radiation decreases inversely with the square of the distance from the source. For example, if you stand 4 feet from a source of radiation, you are exposed to approximately one-fourth the amount of radiation you would receive at 2 feet (Fig. 19–1). When providing care to a client with a uterine implant, you will receive less radiation exposure if you stand at the head of the client's bed rather than directly beside the client.

You should aim to minimize the amount of *time* you are exposed to the radiation source, although you must still meet the client's care needs. Your exposure time should generally be limited to 30 minutes of direct care per 8-hour shift.[16] You need to plan your time in the client's room so you can spend it efficiently while providing care to the client. Time required to organize supplies should be spent outside the room. Care for the client should be rotated among available nursing staff to limit

exposure for each employee. Pregnant nurses should not be assigned to care for clients receiving RT.

The use of *shielding* devices whenever possible reduces radiation exposure. The dose of x-rays and gamma rays is reduced as the thickness of the lead shield is increased. In practice, nurses have found that lead shielding can be cumbersome to work with. When shielding is not feasible, you should maintain maximum distance from the radioactive source and limit the duration of exposure.

With sealed-source internal radioactive implants, clients require a private room and bath because of the risk of implant dislodgment and consequent exposure of other people to the radiation. Rooms at the ends of halls or stairwells may be designated for use by such clients because their location lessens the chance that others will be exposed to the radiation. Institutions with a high volume of radiation implants may have specially designed rooms with lead-shielded walls. Shields, a lead container called a *pig*, and a pair of long-handled forceps should always be present in the client's room. If the radiation source becomes dislodged, forceps are used to pick it up and place it immediately in the pig. Generally, the radiation therapist and the radiation safety officer are notified *immediately* of the situation.[21] They retrieve and secure the radiation source.

Staff caring for clients with radioactive implants are rotated to limit exposure per employee. Pregnant staff should be assigned to other clients. Staff members must wear their own film badges or dosimeters while in the client's room. Visiting policy is restricted, so the client may experience feelings of isolation. To maintain contact while keeping distance from radiation exposure, talk with the client from the doorway of the room. Encourage family and friends to telephone. Prepare the client ahead of time for limited employee contact. Before the radiation source is inserted, the client should be provided with ways to pass the time, such as reading and handwork. Such clients usually feel well but are isolated and confined to their beds as a safety measure to prevent the appliance from being dislodged when the client is to have radioactive implants inserted in the abdominal cavity. The client has a Foley (indwelling) urinary catheter and should be eating a low-fiber diet after evacuation of the colon prior to insertion of the radioactive implant. The client should not have a bowel movement before the device is removed in 2 to 3 days.

FIGURE 19–1 Inverse relationship of distance and radiation exposure.

1 meter
2 meters (1/4 of exposure)
3 meters (1/9 of exposure)
4 meters (1/16 of exposure)

The client receiving internal RT with an unsealed source also needs to have a private room and bath. Further precautions must be taken because all body secretions are radioactive. All surfaces, including the floor area the client will be walking on, are covered with Chux, paper, or other protective covering. Foods are served on disposable plates with disposable utensils. Trash and linens are kept in the client's room and are not removed until the client is ready for discharge. To further decrease the risk of radiation exposure of caregivers, bed linens are generally not changed unless they are grossly soiled. Instruct the client to flush the toilet several times after each use.

Visitor and staff contact is limited, as already described for sealed-source RT. Anyone entering the room wears a new pair of booties each time to avoid tracking the radioactive isotope out into the hallway. You must wear gloves to avoid exposure if you are handling body fluids. Any emesis (vomiting), especially that occurring shortly after the client has ingested an oral isotope, should be covered with absorbent pads, and the radiation safety officer should be called immediately. Additional precautions may be necessary, depending on the radioisotope used and the policies and procedures of the individual practice setting.

Prior to discharge, instruct the client about any precautions that should be continued at home. The radiation safety officer will scan the client to be certain that the radiation has decreased to a safe level. All precautions for the room should be continued even after the client has been discharged, until the radiation safety officer has lifted restrictions.

The U.S. Nuclear Regulatory Commission requires that radiation exposure of people be kept as low as reasonably achievable. All institutions using radioactive materials must have written policies concerning radiation protection. In addition, a radiation safety officer licensed by the U.S. Atomic Energy Commission to work with radioactive material must be available at all institutions using radioactive materials.

The law also requires monitoring devices, such as film badges, for health care workers exposed to radiation and the keeping of a record of each worker's exposure. Do not share your film badge with anyone. The film badge provides a measure of whole-body exposure. The general precautions distance, time, and shielding apply for all forms of external and internal RT. Sealed and unsealed sources of internal RT require additional precautionary measures for their safe use.

TREATMENT CONSIDERATIONS FOR RADIATION THERAPY

The goal of RT is to destroy the cancer while keeping dosages within the normal tissue tolerance to avoid harming surrounding normal tissues. Several factors determine the treatment effect and side effects of RT:

1. Tumor location in relation to surrounding normal tissue affects both treatment effect and side effects. Certain normal tissues are more sensitive to radiation and may incur permanent damage as a result of radiation. The spinal cord and the GI, integumentary, and myeloproliferative systems are at greatest

risk for damage. If the spinal cord lies in the treatment field, the maximum safe dose of RT is lower than if the RT can be delivered from directions (ports) that avoid the spinal cord. Additionally, customized shielding "blocks" may be created to protect normal tissues from ionizing rays.

2. The size of the treatment field affects the dose of RT. If a small area is treated, the client can tolerate a higher dose of radiation than if a larger area is treated. RT is a regional treatment. Widespread or metastatic disease likely extends beyond the treatment field; in such situations, RT would not be an effective curative treatment modality.

3. The client's overall health or performance status affects the ability to tolerate RT. For example, a client who already has severe chronic obstructive pulmonary disease is less able to tolerate RT to the lung.

4. The therapeutic ratio of the treatment effects on the tumor to the side effects on normal tissue is an important cost-benefit determinant in decision-making about RT.

5. The side effects a client may experience are related to the total dose of radiation. Radiation dose is prescribed in units called *grays* (Gy). This term has replaced the unit of dose known as the *rad* (radiation absorbed dose): 1 Gy equals 100 rad; 1 cGy (centigray) equals 1 rad. The RT dose is higher when the goal is curative eradication of the cancer than when the goal is pain control or palliation. A client receiving 5000 cGy for cure experiences more side effects than a client receiving 2000 cGy to the same body area for palliation.

6. In general, only the area in the treatment field is affected by the radiation. For example, hair loss occurs only in the area being treated with radiation. Therefore, a client receiving RT to the chest experiences hair loss on the chest but usually not on the scalp.

7. Administering the radiation in divided (fractionated) rather than single doses minimizes the side effects by allowing the normal cells time to recover. *Fractionation* refers to dividing the total radiation dose into small, frequent doses. A common dosage schedule for external RT is 150 to 200 cGy, 5 days per week, for a total of 4 to 5 weeks. Fractionation also increases the probability that tumor cells will be in a vulnerable phase of the cell cycle when treated; cells are more sensitive to RT during the late G_2 and early M phases. Fractionation allows normal cells time to repair themselves. At times, an RT dose is *hyperfractionated* (divided into doses given twice daily).

Nursing Management of the Client Receiving Radiation Therapy

The staff of most RT departments includes a nurse to meet the learning and manifestation management needs of the client. Yet nurses in the chemotherapy clinic, inpatient unit, or home care setting may be faced with concerns of or questions from clients and family members about the side effects of RT.

PROVIDE EDUCATION

In addition to the emotional impact of the cancer diagnosis, RT can be a source of fear and misunderstanding. Clients may experience fears of being burned or becoming radioactive. Since RT cannot be seen or felt during treatment, the client may also fear that the treatment is not effective. Education can dispel such common fears and misconceptions.

Comparing RT to the effects of the sun can be helpful. One generally does not notice the full effect of the sun immediately after coming indoors. So also, many manifestations of RT do not develop until approximately 10 to 14 days into treatment, and some do not subside until several weeks after treatment. If the cancer was not causing physical manifestations, the client may not have evidence (like seeing a suntan) of the treatment's effect. If, however, the tumor was obstructing air flow, the client may realize a few weeks into the RT that breathing is easier or coughing is diminished—even before imaging studies are performed to verify tumor shrinkage. Likewise, if RT is being delivered for painful bone metastases, the client will probably note a decrease in pain or diminished need for pain medications 1 to 2 weeks into the RT.

MINIMIZE SIDE EFFECTS

In general, skin reactions and fatigue may occur with RT to any site, whereas other side effects occur only when specific areas are involved in the treatment field. The response of normal skin to RT varies from mild erythema to moist desquamation similar in appearance to a second-degree burn. The term "burn" should not be used to describe these skin reactions, however, because doing so may frighten the client unnecessarily. Because megavoltage and cobalt deliver the maximum dose beneath the skin, skin reactions have become less significant than in years past. The accompanying Client Education Guide offers more teaching information about skin care during RT.

Site-specific manifestations of RT include mucositis, xerostomia (dry mouth), radiation caries, esophagitis, dysphagia (difficulty swallowing), nausea and vomiting, diarrhea, tenesmus (straining at stool or in urination), cystitis, urethritis, alopecia (hair loss), and bone marrow suppression. These may be the result of acute changes associated with inflammation or chronic changes associated with fibrosis. During RT, a CBC is usually performed weekly. The degree of myelosuppression varies with the amount of bone marrow within the treatment field. Areas at greatest risk are the pelvic region, sacrum, skull, lumbar and thoracic spine, ribs, shoulder region, and sternum.

In women of childbearing age, RT may cause prolonged or permanent infertility. In prostate brachytherapy, when radioactive seeds have been permanently implanted, there is a low, weakly penetrating radiation exposure for others. Therefore, the client should use a condom for sexual intercourse in the first weeks after the procedure. Also, the client should avoid close (<6 feet) contact with pregnant women and young children (younger than 3 years) for more than 5 minutes a day during the first 2 months following implantation.[1]

Many of the manifestation management strategies for side effects of RT are similar to those for side effects of chemotherapy, described later in this chapter. Information on nursing management of the general side effects of RT is included in the Oncology Nursing Society's *Manual for Radiation Oncology Nursing Practice*.[13] The NCI offers a free client education booklet, *Radiation Therapy and You: A Guide to Self-help*.[62] A nurse or therapist in the RT department is a readily accessible source of information. Furthermore, you can alert the RT staff about the client's concern and thus help the client manage outcomes of the RT side effects.

CLIENT EDUCATION GUIDE

Skin Care Within the Treatment Field

- Keep your skin dry.
- Do not wash the treatment area until you are instructed to do so. When permitted, wash the treated skin gently with mild soap, rinse well, and pat dry. Use warm or cool water, *not* hot water.
- Do not remove the lines or ink marks placed on your skin.
- Avoid using powders, lotions, creams, alcohol, and deodorants on the treated skin.
- Wear loose-fitting clothing to avoid friction over the treatment field.
- Do not apply tape to the treatment site if dressings are applied.
- Shave with an electric razor. Do not use pre-shave or after-shave lotions.
- Protect your skin from exposure to direct sunlight, chlorinated swimming pools, and temperature extremes (e.g., hot water bottles, heating pads, ice packs).
- Consult your radiation therapist or nurse about specific measures for individual skin reactions.

■ Medical Management

CHEMOTHERAPY

As with surgery and RT, the goals of chemotherapy can be cure, control, or palliation of manifestations. Chemotherapy is a systemic intervention and is appropriate when:

- Disease is widespread
- The risk of undetectable disease is high
- The tumor cannot be resected and is resistant to RT

The client who is at high risk for recurrence but shows no evidence of current disease may be a candidate for *adjuvant chemotherapy*; in this type of therapy, after initial treatment with either surgery or RT, chemotherapeutic drugs are used to eliminate any remaining submicroscopic cancer cells that are suspected to be still present. Adjuvant therapy is now well established in the treatment of breast cancer.

Neoadjuvant chemotherapy refers to the preoperative use of chemotherapy to reduce the bulk and lower the stage of a tumor, making it amenable to surgery or possibly even cure with subsequent local therapy.

The objective of chemotherapy is to destroy all malignant tumor cells without excessive destruction of normal cells. Several types of cancer are now considered curable with chemotherapy, even in advanced stages. Unfortunately, these tumors account for only about 10% of all cancers.

HOW CHEMOTHERAPY WORKS. The phases of the cell cycle are common to all cells (see Chapter 18). Normally, cells respond to the body's need for growth, repair, or regeneration in an orderly manner and cease production by entering a resting phase or slowing growth when the need is met. At any given time, normal cells may be found in all phases of growth. Cancer cells reproduce in the same manner as normal cells. However, growth occurs in an uncontrollable manner. In general, cells that are actively dividing are the most sensitive to chemotherapy.

Chemotherapy directly or indirectly disrupts reproduction of cells by altering essential biochemical processes. The desired outcome is control or eradication of all malignant cells. Experiments and clinical experience suggest that most types of chemotherapy do not kill all cancer cells during one exposure. According to the cell kill hypothesis, only a percentage of cancer cells are killed with each course of chemotherapy. Repeated doses—or cycles—of chemotherapy therefore must be used.

The use of drugs in combination, known as *combination chemotherapy*, has consistently been far superior to single-agent therapy. Drugs selected to be used in combination must each be effective against the type of cancer being treated. When combined, chemotherapeutic agents destroy more malignant cells and produce fewer side effects because each drug strikes the cancer cells at a different point in the cell cycle. Combination chemotherapy is now the standard in most situations. The regimens are complex, cyclic, and individualized for the client and the type of cancer. An example of a chemotherapy regimen for Hodgkin's disease is shown in Table 19–6.

CLASSIFICATION OF CHEMOTHERAPEUTIC AGENTS. Chemotherapeutic agents generally are classified according to their pharmacologic actions and effects on the cell generation cycle. However, the method by which cancer cells are inhibited or destroyed is not always known. A classification of common chemotherapeutic agents is shown in Box 19–1.

■ **Nursing Management of the Client Receiving Chemotherapy**

Only adequately prepared registered professional nurses who are skilled in the administration of chemotherapeutic agents should assume responsibility for performing it.[76] At a minimum, the nurse should have completed chemotherapy administration classes. Ideally, nurses providing oncology care are also Oncology Certified Nurses (OCNs), who have the specialized knowledge and skills to manage potential outcomes of cancer and its treatment. When the bedside nurse does not have the requisite knowledge, the institutional policies can ensure that a nurse with expertise in cancer care is responsible for supervising care and guiding the bedside nurse in the assessment and administration issues in order to give safe, effective care to the individual client. Recommendations

TABLE 19–6	MOPP REGIMEN FOR HODGKIN'S DISEASE
Drug	**Dosage**
M = Mechlorethamine HCl (Mustargen)	6.0 mg/m^2 IV on days 1 and 8
O = Oncovin (vincristine)	1.4 mg/m^2 IV on days 1 and 8
P = Procarbazine	100 mg/m^2 PO on days 1–14
P = Prednisone	40 mg/m^2 PO on days 1–14 during cycles 1 and 4 Repeat cycle every 28 days for at least 6 cycles or at least 2 cycles beyond the attainment of maximum response

IV, intravenously; PO, orally.
Adapted from Greco, F. A. (Ed.). (1996). *Handbook of commonly used chemotherapy regimens.* Chicago: Precept Press.

for course content, clinical practicum, and nursing practice can be found in the Oncology Nursing Society's *Cancer Chemotherapy Guidelines.*[76]

ASSESSMENT. A thorough client evaluation is necessary before cytotoxic drugs can be administered. Review the client's medical history to identify potential risk factors for chemotherapy toxicity, such as a history of impaired cardiac, pulmonary, or renal function. Carefully assess the severity and duration of side effects experienced since the previous course of therapy. Abnormal laboratory values may indicate organ-specific toxicities of chemotherapeutic agents. Before a subsequent course of chemotherapy, a CBC with differential count is vital in ensuring adequate bone marrow recovery since the last chemotherapy treatment. The differential count is used to calculate the absolute neutrophil count (ANC) (see later), a means of determining the percentage of mature white cells. Drug doses may have to be modified or delayed on the basis of these results.

The client's chart should contain either a copy of the formal drug protocol or a written summary of the planned chemotherapy regimen. Chemotherapy doses are usually based on body surface area in square meters (m^2), which is determined by the client's height and weight. Clear and complete chemotherapy prescriptions consist of (1) the name of the drug, (2) dose/m^2 and total dose, (3) route of administration, (4) administration rate for intravenous (IV) infusions, and (5) frequency of administration. Plans for antiemetic therapy, hydration, diuresis, and electrolyte supplementation are frequently included as well. It is vital that clients know what side effects to watch for and what to do when side effects arise. See the Care Plan for interventions used to manage the side effects of chemotherapy and related suggestions for client education.

Most serious side effects of the treatment do not occur in the chemotherapy clinic but develop after the client has returned home. Knowing about the expected side effects of cancer treatment and appropriate interventions increases your ability to give prompt, effective care. In a medical-surgical or home care setting, you should be able to recognize variations from normal, perform a complete

BOX 19–1   Classification of Chemotherapeutic Agents

Cell Cycle–Specific Groups

Antimetabolites

Cytarabine (Ara-C, Cytosar)
5-Fluorouracil (5-FU)
Floxuridine (FUDR)
6-Mercaptopurine (6-MP, Purinethol)
Methotrexate (Mexate)
6-Thioguanine (6-TG)
Fludarabine (Fludara)
Pentostatin (Nipent)

Vinca Alkaloids

Vinorelbine (Navelbine)
Vincristine (Oncovin)
Vinblastine (Velban)

Epipodophyllotoxins

Etoposide (VP-16)
Teniposide (VM-26, Vumon)

Taxanes

Paclitaxel (Taxol)

Miscellaneous

L-Asparaginase
Hydroxyurea (Hydrea)

Cell Cycle–Nonspecific Groups

Alkylating Agents

Busulfan (Myleran)
Carboplatin (Paraplatin)
Cisplatin (CDDP, Platinol-AQ)
Cyclophosphamide (Cytoxan)
Ifosfamide (Ifex)
Mechlorethamine HCl (Mustargen)
Thiotepa

Antitumor Antibiotics

Chlorambucil (Leukeran)
Bleomycin (Blenoxane)
Dactinomycin (Cosmegen)
Daunorubicin (Cerubidine)
Doxorubicin (Adriamycin)
Idarubicin (Idamycin)
Mitomycin C (Mitomycin)
Mitoxantrone (Novantrone)
Plicamycin (Mithracin)

Hormonal Therapy

Glucocorticoids

Prednisone (Deltasone)
Methylprednisolone (Solu-Medrol, Medrol)
Dexamethasone (Decadron)

Estrogens

Chlorotrianisene (Tace)
Diethylstilbestrol (DES)
Estradiol (Estrace)

Antiestrogens

Tamoxifen (Nolvadex)

Progestins

Depo-Provera
Megestrol acetate (Megace)
Leuprolide (Lupron)

Nitrosoureas

Carmustine (BCNU)
Lomustine (CCNU)
Streptozocin (Zanosar)

Adapted from Powel, L. L. (1996). *Cancer chemotherapy guidelines and recommendations for practice.* Pittsburgh, PA: Oncology Nursing Press.

assessment of the client's status, and then report that information in a timely manner to the client's oncology caregivers. You can therefore communicate pertinent data to the oncology professional as a basis for a medical or nursing diagnosis. Nurses in all practice settings must work together, sharing information and knowledge, to ensure continuity of care for the client undergoing chemotherapy for cancer.

ADMINISTRATION OF CHEMOTHERAPY. Before administering antineoplastic agents, consult with the pharmacist and review chemotherapy drug handbooks and investigational drug protocols for detailed information regarding drug actions, dosages, administration guidelines, and potential side effects. A critical step in the administration of chemotherapeutics is the verification of the drug, dose, and schedule.[14, 76] Chemotherapy calculations and drugs should be checked by two nurses against the written orders. Errors in chemotherapy orders may result from such factors as the misplacement of a decimal point or the dispensing of the wrong drug. An overdose of an antineoplastic agent could result in profound toxicity and death.

Educating the client and family about chemotherapy and the identification, prevention, and management of side effects is primarily a nursing function. As already mentioned, the Care Plan in this chapter offers an example of a plan for managing side effects of chemotherapy. The NCI provides an excellent booklet, *Chemotherapy and You*, free of charge for client teaching.[60] Hypersensitivity reaction and extravasation, discussed later in the chapter, can occur during the administration of chemotherapy. Other side effects are most likely to occur after the client is discharged from the outpatient clinic or inpatient unit. Potentially life-threatening side effects, such as infection during neutropenia (see later), are more likely to occur while the client is at home, when no health professionals are available.

ROUTES OF ADMINISTRATION. Two routes are discussed: intravenous and regional.

Intravenous Chemotherapy. Most chemotherapeutic agents are administered intravenously. Extravasation (escape from the vein) of some chemotherapeutic agents can cause significant harm to the surrounding tissue. There-

■ SIDE EFFECT MANAGEMENT FOR THE CLIENT RECEIVING CHEMOTHERAPY

Nursing Diagnosis. Risk for Injury related to side effects secondary to chemotherapy.

Outcomes. Client will experience minimal side effects of chemotherapy, will demonstrate knowledge of rationale for chemotherapy and treatment plan, and will demonstrate knowledge about potential side effects of drugs and related self-management strategies.

Interventions

1. Monitor client during clinic or home visits or when taking phone calls for potential side effects of the drugs—while reinforcing client education of manifestations to report.
2. Identify and monitor for known side effects of the drugs utilized in the treatment regimen, including leukopenia, nausea and vomiting, diarrhea or constipation, stomatitis, hair loss, and drug-specific side effects.
3. Perform more in-depth assessment and additional nursing interventions as indicated for the symptoms identified.

Rationales

1. Some side effects, such as drug extravasation and nausea and vomiting, may occur immediately; others are more likely to occur between treatment cycles.
2. Early detection and intervention can minimize the morbidity of adverse side effects.

3. See No. 2.

Client Education

1. Assess client's learning readiness, including previous life experience related to cancer and expectations related to chemotherapy.

2. Identify family members and other support persons whom client wished to be included in education; document this information for taking phone calls from support persons.
3. Develop a teaching plan appropriate to the client's individual needs and the specific chemotherapy regimen.
4. Verify client's understanding of the cancer diagnosis, treatment regimen, and informed consent.
5. Provide client and family caregivers with oral and written information regarding:
   a. Chemotherapy
   b. Each drug utilized in the treatment regimen.
   c. Anticipated schedule of administration.
   d. Rationale for follow-up procedures, including laboratory tests, office visits, and imaging studies.
   e. Potential side effects—when they may occur, self-care management, and manifestations to report to the physician or nurse.

Rationales

1. A family member's or friend's cancer experience—whether it has any bearing on the client's cancer experience or not—can have a major effect on the client's expectations, anxiety, and even willingness to proceed with treatment.
2. Protects client confidentiality while involving client's support persons.

3. Each client's experience will depend on the cancer, the treatment regimen utilized, co-morbid conditions, and ability to cope.
4. The information is often overwhelming to hear, the terminology and content are frequently unfamiliar.
5. Written information that reinforces teaching is vital. Recall alone is not likely to be efficient. Because most care is provided in outpatient settings, health professionals generally are not present when potentially life-threatening side effects appear.

Nursing Diagnosis. Risk for Infection related to leukopenia secondary to chemotherapy.

Outcomes. Client will remain free of infection, as evidenced by temperature remaining within normal limits. Client demonstrates knowledge related to prevention of infection.

Interventions

1. Practice good hand-washing, especially between caring for clients.

2. Keep neutropenic clients separate from others exposed to infections.
3. Care for neutropenic clients before caring for other clients.

4. Use aseptic technique in client care and treatments.
5. Check baseline vital signs.

6. Monitor hematologic laboratory results, especially complete blood count, white blood cell count, differential, and absolute neutrophil count.
7. Monitor for signs of infection, including respiratory, urinary, oral mucosa, and skin.

Rationales

1. These interventions will decrease the risk of exposure to a nosocomial infection.
   Good hand-washing is the most important means of preventing the spread of a nosocomial infection.
2. When neutropenic, a client is at greater risk for infection.
3. This helps prevent nosocomial spread of an infection to client.
4. See No. 2.
5. Provides a basis for early detection of manifestations of infection
6. See No. 5.

7. See No. 5.

Care Plan continued on following page

■

Client Education

1. Explain purpose of chemotherapy, how it works, and reason for potential side effects.

2. Explain relationship between effects of treatment on white blood cell (granulocyte) count and potential for infection.
3. Teach measures for preventing infections, including meticulous hand-washing and good oral hygiene.
4. Discuss necessity of avoiding crowds and people who have infection or have recently been vaccinated.
5. If applicable to client, note the need to avoid cleaning cat litter boxes, fish tanks, and canine or human excreta.
6. Teach the manifestations that must be reported immediately (e.g., fever, chills, sore throat, burning or pressure with voiding, purulent drainage).
7. Verify that client has, and is able to read, a thermometer.
8. Verify that client knows how to reach the health professionals after hours.

Rationales

1. Because the client is generally home when adverse side effects arise, it is vital that the client be an involved member of the health care team.
2. See No. 1.

3. Infection in the neutropenic client is potentially life-threatening.

4. See No. 3.

5. These are high-risk potential sources of infection.

6. When the client is neutropenic, an infection can become rapidly life-threatening.

7. See No. 6.
8. The consequences of not knowing how to reach professionals in an emergency can be both serious and frightening.

Nursing Diagnosis. Altered Nutrition: Less Than Body Requirements related to disease process and treatment.

Outcomes. Client will identify measures to prevent nutritional deficits and will maintain adequate nutritional status, as evidenced by body weight within preset parameters.

Interventions

1. Evaluate nutritional status:
   a. Measure height and weight.
   b. Compare with prediagnosis weight.
   c. Assess laboratory values (e.g., serum albumin, complete blood count).
   d. Obtain anthropometric measurements when indicated.
2. Monitor oral cavity for stomatitis, infection, and pain.
3. Arrange for assistance in obtaining and preparing food, if needed.

4. Refer client to the dietitian if indicators of malnutrition are present.

Rationales

1. Weight loss over time is an indicator of malnutrition. With significant decrease in weight, chemotherapy dosages must be decreased.

2. Client may avoid nutritional intake if it is painful to eat.
3. Adequate hydration and a high-protein, high-calorie diet that includes foods high in electrolytes (e.g., Gatorade, fruit juices, salty broths, soups, milk, green leafy vegetables) are vital to recovery of normal cells from the adverse effects of chemotherapy.
4. See No. 3.

Client Education

1. Discuss relationship of adequate nutrition to disease process and treatment.

2. Discuss the elements of a nutritional diet.
3. Help client identify foods that are tolerated and those that cause discomfort or have become distasteful.
4. Discuss strategies for counteracting the loss of appetite or alterations in taste and for ensuring adequate nutritional intake.
5. Emphasize good oral hygiene.

Rationales

1. The client who understands the vital role nutrition plays in the treatment is more likely to make an effort to ensure an adequate intake in spite of the loss of appetite and alterations in the sense of taste.
2. See No. 1.
3. See No. 1.

4. Suggestions specific to the client's experience (e.g., extra sweetener if foods taste bitter, popsicles for fluid intake) can be very helpful.
5. Pain and alteration of taste can impair nutritional intake.

Nursing Diagnosis. Fatigue related to cancer treatment.

Outcomes. Client will demonstrate knowledge about methods that may prevent transient tiredness states from progressing to the more intransigent states of acute or chronic fatigue and will be able to engage in a certain percentage of desired activities.

Interventions

1. Include evaluation of fatigue in nursing assessment. Obtain data on physical performance status, response to treatments over time, and impact on activities of daily living.
2. Review laboratory and other clinical data (e.g., oxygen saturation levels) for physiologic manifestations.
3. Assist client in identifying aggravating and alleviating factors.

Rationales

1. The first step in treatment is recognition of the problem. Unfortunately, cancer treatment–related fatigue is often not recognized, and its effect not appreciated, by health professionals.
2. Fatigue is multidimensional, comprising neuromuscular, attentional, and perceptual factors.
3. See No. 2.

4. Administer erythropoietin or blood transfusions as ordered.

5. Carry out treatments for dehydration or electrolyte imbalance.

6. Promote sleep and rest.

7. Assist referrals to community resources that will reduce fatigue (e.g., physical therapy, home health services, transportation services).

4. Anemia is a common cause of fatigue in clients receiving myelosuppressive therapy.

5. Dehydration and electrolyte imbalance can contribute to fatigue and weakness.

6. Clients with cancer report that sleep and rest are helpful but not completely effective in addressing cancer-related fatigue.

7. This step allows the client to conserve energy for activities that maintain quality of life.

Client Education

1. Inform client of the relationship of the therapy with fatigue.

2. Prepare client to anticipate periods during chemotherapy treatments when acute fatigue is more likely to be experienced.
3. Encourage the client to report fatigue and its effect on activities of daily living.
4. Help client identify strategies that may prevent transient tiredness from progressing to more intransigent fatigue:
   a. Vary activities.
   b. Use distraction techniques.

   c. Use relaxation techniques to dissipate the negative effects of stressors.
   d. Maintain good nutritional and fluid intake.

   e. Schedule activities to balance rest and activity in order to conserve energy.

Rationales

1. Understanding that the fatigue can result from the therapy rather than solely from the disease can alleviate undue anxiety.
2. Client can plan activities related to anticipated energy levels.

3. Professionals may be able to offer additional interventions.

4. An intervention before fatigue becomes intransigent is more effective.
   a. A variety of activities prevents boredom.
   b. Use of distraction helps the client focus on something besides fatigue.
   c. Relaxation techniques relieve fatigue by reducing effects of stressors.
   d. Nutrition provides a source of energy, and hydration promotes excretion of cell destruction end products/toxins.
   e. Results of studies of exercise programs are quite promising, whatever the exercise (bicycle ergometry, walking, or personal).

Nursing Diagnosis. Ineffective Individual Coping related to cancer diagnosis.

Outcomes. Client begins process of adapting to psychoemotional stressors. Client demonstrates functional adaptive behaviors and problem-solving capacity.

Interventions

1. Develop rapport; utilize active listening skills.

2. Assess coping by directly asking the client how he or she is coping with the cancer and the treatment.

3. Provide consistent, empathetic, and positive regard.
4. Support client's expression of feelings.
5. Guide the client to community resources such as support groups.
6. Refer client to appropriate and qualified professional for further intervention as indicated.

Rationales

1. Client will know that you are concerned about his or her well-being as a person. Listening often is the best source of data of the depth of the impact of the cancer experience.
2. When asked, the client may share fears or concerns. The professional can offer support and suggest related interventions.
3. See No. 1.
4. See No. 1.
5. Provides client opportunity to share feelings with and to learn from others who experience cancer.
6. For some clients, the emotional impact of the cancer experience—often combined with other life issues—can be overwhelming.

Client Education

1. Explain relationship between coping and the perception of stressors.
2. Help client identify problems, factors over which one has control, and coping methods that have worked for the client during previous life experiences.
3. Teach problem-solving as needed.

4. Teach client about keeping a journal for identification of events, feelings, and strategies utilized for particular problems.
5. Emphasize the importance of social network and community resources for dealing with concerns.

Rationales

1. The first step in the problem-solving process is to understand the problem.
2. Many clients experience a sense of loss of control and feelings of helplessness when confronted with a cancer diagnosis.

3. The client may not recognize that coping strategies from other life experiences can be utilized in coping with a cancer experience.
4. Keeping a journal can help the client identify specific concerns; possible solutions can then be identified.
5. A social network of support counteracts feelings of isolation.

Data from McNally, J. C., et al. (Eds.). (1991). *Guidelines for oncology nursing practice.* Philadelphia: W. B. Saunders.

fore, you must always know before administering a drug whether it is a vesicant (an agent capable of causing tissue damage).

Great care should be taken in vein selection and in venipuncture technique. Large veins in the fleshy part of the forearm are the preferred peripheral access sites. Avoid areas of impaired lymphatic drainage, phlebitis, invading neoplasm, hematoma, inflammation, sclerosis, impaired venous circulation, the lower extremities, and sites distal to a recent venipuncture site. Also avoid veins that are on the dorsal aspect of the hand or over an area of flexion, such as the wrist or elbow. When administering a vesicant drug, you must be prepared ahead of time to deal with a potential extravasation to limit tissue damage. Preparation includes having immediate availability of an antidote, if there is one.[76]

In the past, vascular access devices (VADs) were placed as a last resort in clients with poor venous access. Today, because chemotherapy regimens are complex and supportive care is extensive, VADs are being used during the initial treatment of clients requiring continuous chemotherapy, multiple access, parenteral fluids, antibiotics, and frequent blood testing.

Implanted and external vascular access catheters are usually inserted into one of the major veins of the upper chest. Centrally implanted VADs are placed by a surgeon, generally during a brief outpatient procedure. The brachial or cephalic vein in the forearm is used for peripherally inserted central catheters (PICCs), which are often placed by specially trained nurses. The distal catheter tip is advanced to the level of the superior vena cava at or above the junction of the right atrium. Proper catheter tip placement of both central and peripheral VADs is confirmed by fluoroscopy or radiography. Various types of VADs are depicted in Figure 19–2.

In addition to VADs, there are arterial, peritoneal, and intraventricular access devices that permit regional delivery of chemotherapy to the liver or peritoneal cavity or into the cerebrospinal fluid of the brain.[2] Each type of device has advantages and disadvantages, including factors such as maintenance requirements, ease of use, cost, ease of insertion, longevity, and effect on body image.

The most commonly reported complications are infection and catheter occlusion.[80] The prevention of VAD infections centers on catheter care, daily assessment for manifestations of infection, and client education. Intraluminal occlusion may occur secondary to a blood clot or precipitate. Prevention strategies include proper flushing, vigilance for drug incompatibilities, and adherence to proper drug dilutions. Other rare complications can also occur with VADs.[41] Procedures for the care and maintenance of VADs vary with each clinical setting and type of device. Nursing management strategies for VADs are extensively described elsewhere.[9, 15, 48, 54]

When the procedure for accessing a VAD is performed according to institutional policy and goes as expected, use of a VAD is relatively easy. Major, even life-threatening, problems can arise, however, if the VAD is not accessed correctly or the nurse does not know how to recognize a problem and the corrective action to take. Nurses who access VADs infrequently should review their institution's procedure before doing so. If the procedure in any way varies from the expected, obtain the advice of a nurse who is more experienced in VADs before proceeding.

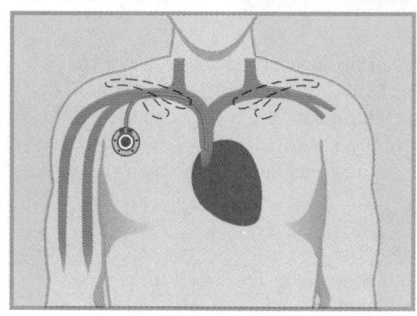

A. Implanted

Venous Access Devices

B. External

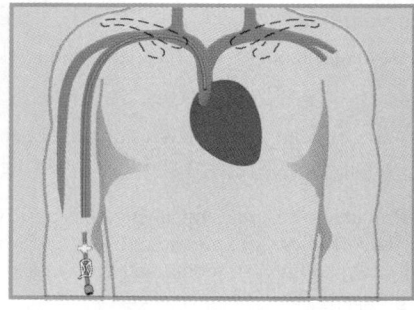

C. Peripherally inserted central catheter (PICC)

D. Implanted

Accessing Venous Access Devices

E. External

F. Peripherally inserted

FIGURE 19–2A–F, Venous access devices.

Regional Chemotherapy. Regional chemotherapy via alternative routes allows high concentrations of drugs to be directed to localized tumors. Methods are (1) topical, (2) intra-arterial, (3) intracavitary, (4) intraperitoneal, and (5) intrathecal.

Topical. Fluorouracil cream may be applied to the skin to treat actinic keratoses (sun keratoses. Squamous cell carcinoma can arise from these precancerous lesions if they are left untreated.

Intra-arterial infusions involve some risk but enable major organs or tumor sites to receive maximal exposure with limited serum levels of medications. As a result, systemic side effects are lessened.

Intracavitary therapy instills the medication directly into an area such as the abdomen, bladder, or pleural space.

Intraperitoneal chemotherapy is an option for cancer involving the intra-abdominal area, such as ovarian cancer. With this method, a high concentration of a chemotherapeutic agent is delivered to the actual tumor site with minimal exposure of healthy tissues, thereby decreasing toxic side effects.

Intrathecal. Most medications given systemically are not effective against central CNS tumors because they cannot cross the blood-brain barrier. The physician may instill chemotherapeutic agents into the CNS through a reservoir placed in the ventricle via an Ommaya reservoir (Fig. 19–3) or via a lumbar puncture. Kosier and Minkler[46] provide an excellent review of the nursing management of clients with an implanted Ommaya reservoir.

ADVERSE REACTIONS. Two potentially serious adverse reactions, the seriousness of which depends on the chemotherapeutic agents, may occur during administration: hypersensitivity reactions and extravasation.

Hypersensitivity Reaction. Hypersensitivity reaction (an exaggerated immune response to a foreign substance) to chemotherapy, although rare, can be serious and life-threatening. The antineoplastic agents most commonly implicated in the development of hypersensitivity reactions are L-asparaginase (Elspar), carboplatin (Paraplatin),

cisplatin (Platinol-AQ), paclitaxel (Taxol), bleomycin (Blenoxane), and teniposide (Vumon).[90] When administering a drug with anaphylactic potential (potential to cause a possibly fatal hypersensitivity reaction), take the following precautions to ensure client safety:

- Obtain an allergy history from the client.
- Administer a test dose if ordered by the physician.
- Stay with the client the entire time the drug is being administered.
- Have emergency equipment and drugs readily available.
- Obtain baseline vital signs.
- Establish a free-flowing IV line for the administration of fluids and emergency drugs, in case they are needed.

The manifestations of an immediate hypersensitivity reaction are (1) dyspnea, (2) chest tightness or pain, (3) pruritus (itching), (4) urticaria (wheals), (5) tachycardia, (6) dizziness, (7) anxiety, (8) agitation, (9) inability to speak, (10) abdominal pain, (11) nausea, (12) hypotension, (13) cloudy mental status, (14) flushed appearance, and (15) cyanosis. If an anaphylactic reaction is suspected, take the following actions:

- Immediately stop drug administration.
- Maintain IV access with 0.9% saline.
- Maintain the airway.
- Place the client in a supine position with the feet elevated, unless contraindicated.
- Notify the physician.
- Monitor the client's vital signs every 2 minutes until he or she is stable.
- Administer epinephrine, aminophylline, diphenhydramine (Benadryl), and corticosteroids according to the physician's orders.

Extravasation. Before administering a chemotherapeutic drug, note its vesicant potential—and its antidote, if there is one—in your review of the drug. Careful assessment of the IV site is required during and after the infusion of antineoplastic agents because some agents may cause tissue damage if extravasated (infiltrated).

Nonvesicant agents have no significant soft tissue toxicities. Vesicant chemotherapeutic agents can cause or form a blister and cause tissue destruction. Commonly utilized vesicant drugs are doxorubicin (Adriamycin) and vincristine (Oncovin). Cisplatin (Platinol-AQ) and paclitaxel (Taxol) are also vesicant drugs. Because they are commonly mixed in large volumes of fluid, the extravasation can be detected more easily before serious tissue damage occurs. Irritant drugs can produce venous pain at the site and along the vein, with or without an inflammatory reaction. Pain, erythema, swelling, and lack of a blood return indicate an extravasation.

Procedures for management of extravasation are controversial and unique to each clinical setting. Institutionally approved guidelines for the management of extravasation should be readily available. Guidelines for the management of extravasation are included in the Oncology Nursing Society's *Cancer Chemotherapy Guidelines.*[76] General recommendations are:

- Stop drug administration.
- Leave the needle in place, and attempt to aspirate any residual drug from the tubing, needle, and site.

Lateral ventricle

Reservoir implanted between scalp and skull

FIGURE 19–3 Ommaya reservoir. An Ommaya reservoir should be accessed only with a small-gauge, non-coring or butterfly needle.

- Administer an antidote, if appropriate, then remove the needle.
- Do not apply direct manual pressure to the site.
- Apply warm (for vinca alkaloid) or cold compresses as indicated.
- Observe the site regularly for pain, erythema, swelling, induration, and necrosis.
- Document the appearance of the site before and after chemotherapy.

SAFE PREPARATION, HANDLING, AND DISPOSAL. The safe administration and disposal of chemotherapeutic agents is controversial. Although evidence suggests that these agents may be carcinogenic, no valid and reliable studies have determined the risks of exposure to the health care provider. Undue exposure to antineoplastic drugs can occur from three major routes:

- Inhalation of aerosols
- Absorption through the skin
- Ingestion of contaminated materials

Several organizations, including the U.S. Occupational Safety and Health Administration (OSHA), the National Study Commission on Cytotoxic Exposure, and the Oncology Nursing Society, have prepared guidelines for the safe preparation, handling, and disposal of antineoplastics.[68, 76] These guidelines call for (1) the wearing of gloves and gowns during preparation and administration and (2) the use of a biologic safety or laminar-flow cabinet for preparation. Antineoplastic agents and their metabolites are found in the excreta and body fluids of clients undergoing chemotherapy. For this reason, you should wear gloves and disposable gowns when handling body secretions, such as blood, vomitus, or excreta, of clients who have received chemotherapy within the previous 48 hours.

BIOTHERAPY

Biotherapy is the use of agents called *biologic response modifiers* (BRMs) to affect a biologic response. The effort to understand and manipulate the human immune system has engaged scientists for decades. The observation of interactions between the immune system and malignant cells, such as spontaneous tumor remissions, continues to fuel the quest to isolate and identify effective biologic agents. Immune response remains at the core of biotherapy. Biotherapy now also includes agents that affect biologic responses in other ways. In the last decade, four major technological advances have assisted scientists in their search[37, 42, 78]:

- A greater understanding of the complex cellular nature of the immune system
- Progress in genetic engineering, enabling the development of recombinant biologic agents
- Advances in molecular biology
- Refined and improved laboratory equipment and computer systems

HEMATOPOIETIC GROWTH FACTORS. Hematopoietic growth factors are a family of glycosylated proteins that mediate hematopoiesis (formation and development of blood cells). They are used to stimulate bone marrow recovery after courses of chemotherapy. Generally, they are named for the major cell lineage they mediate: GM-CSF (granulocyte and macrophage colony-stimulating factor) affects both the granulocyte and macrophage lineage; G-CSF affects only granulocytes. GM-CSF is approved for myeloid (bone marrow) reconstitution after autologous bone marrow transplantation (BMT) and for use in clients experiencing BMT failure or engraftment delay. G-CSF and GM-CSF are approved for the treatment of chemotherapy-associated neutropenia. GM-CSF is generally well tolerated.

Side effects of these growth factors are (1) mild to moderate flu-like manifestations, such as fever, myalgia (muscular pain), bone pain, fatigue, and headache, (2) rash, (3) a transient increase in liver enzymes, and (4) thrombocytopenia (reduced platelets). The most commonly reported side effect of G-CSF is bone pain. Clients report pain in bone areas that have large marrow reserves, such as the pelvis, sternum, and long bones. This pain may be the result of the marrow expansion that occurs from the rapid increase in the neutrophil pool that G-CSF causes.

Erythropoietin, another hematopoietic growth factor, was approved by the U.S. Food and Drug Administration (FDA) in 1989 for use in treating anemia secondary to end-stage renal failure, and in 1993 to treat anemia associated with cancer chemotherapy (epoetin alfa [Procrit, Epogen]). Clients with serum erythropoietin levels greater than 200 mU/ml are unlikely to show a response to therapy. It is important to maintain adequate levels of iron, folic acid, and vitamin B_{12} because these components are essential for the development of red blood cells. The most commonly reported side effect is transient flu-like manifestations, such as arthralgias (joint pain) and myalgias.

Oprelvekin (Neumega), a hematopoietic growth factor for chemotherapy-induced thrombocytopenia, received FDA approval in November 1997. Its most common side effects are edema, dyspnea, tachycardia, and conjunctival redness. More experience with the use of this treatment is needed before broad generalizations can be made about its usefulness. It is anticipated that oprelvekin will reduce the need for platelet transfusions and allow clients to receive the desired doses of chemotherapy as scheduled.[82]

BIOLOGIC RESPONSE MODIFIERS. BRMs, which either are derived from biologic sources or affect biologic responses, are another form of biotherapy. BRMs change the relationship between the tumor and the host by altering the host's biologic response to the tumor. Many of these naturally occurring substances are hormone-like proteins or glycoproteins (proteins with a sugar attached). BRMs have multiple biologic actions, including production of immunologic or other biologic effects. They may augment, modulate, or restore the immune response; they may have direct cytotoxic effects; or they may produce other biologic effects, such as maturation of cells and interference with a tumor's ability to metastasize.[78] In addition to hematopoietic growth factors, BRM agents include interferons, interleukins, monoclonal antibodies, immunomodulators, and tumor necrosis factor.[78]

Interferons. Interferons (IFNs) are small proteins that have cellular activity in three areas: antiviral, immunomodulatory, and antiproliferative. Interferon alpha received FDA approval for use in hairy cell leukemia in 1986. The drug's clinical indications have been broadened to include AIDS-associated Kaposi's sarcoma. Clinical trials are being conducted to investigate its use in other hematologic malignancies, including chronic leukemias, multiple myeloma, cutaneous T-cell lymphoma, and low-grade non-Hodgkin's lymphoma.

Toxicities appear to be dose-related, with lower doses of IFN being associated with few side effects and high doses having side effects that may require therapy to be interrupted or stopped. A flu-like syndrome, a common side effect of IFN therapy, may consist of fever, chills, tachycardia, muscle aches, malaise, fatigue, and headaches. Continued use of IFN produces a tachyphylactic response (rapidly decreasing response after administration of a few doses) such that these manifestations decrease in intensity over time. Premedication with acetaminophen (Tylenol) and diphenhydramine (Benadryl) is helpful in reducing the client's discomfort.

Interleukins. Most interleukins (proteins that serve as regulators of the immune system) are capable of inducing multiple biologic activities. A number of interleukins have been identified. Thus far, only interleukin-2 (IL-2) has received FDA approval. It is derived from T cells, augments various T-cell activities, and enhances the function of natural killer cells. Successes have been seen in renal cell carcinoma and melanoma. Other areas of interest for its use are hematologic malignancies and bone marrow transplantation.

Major toxic responses with IL-2 therapy are due to increased capillary permeability, which may produce hypotension, ascites, pulmonary edema, fatigue, and generalized weight gain. Additionally, integumentary changes occur and may include generalized redness, rash, pruritus, and occasionally skin desquamation. Toxicity resulting from IL-2 varies greatly with the dose of drug administered. Higher doses produce greater toxicity, necessitating astute clinical management.

MONOCLONAL ANTIBODIES. Monoclonal antibodies (MoAbs) are specific antibodies directed against single antigenic determinants on the cell surface.[80] MoAbs provide high specificity lacking in other types of treatment modalities. They can be used either diagnostically or therapeutically. Diagnostic uses of these agents include the early detection of cancer by identification of surface markers on tumor cells and as a delivery agent of radioisotopes to the tumor site to aid in tumor visualization. Therapeutically, MoAbs may be used to deliver immunotoxins, such as ricin, chemotherapeutic agents, and radioisotopes, directly to the tumor site. To date, MoAbs have demonstrated limited success as a therapeutic option, and clinical trials continue for a variety of cancers.

BONE MARROW TRANSPLANTATION
BMT is discussed in Chapter 78. Although it is used as a primary treatment modality in leukemia, BMT may be used to counter the toxic effects of chemotherapy or RT in the treatment of breast cancer, lymphoma, and other cancers. BMT allows the client to receive lethal and potentially more effective doses of chemotherapy and RT without regard to hematopoietic toxicity. With BMT, the damaged bone marrow is replaced by healthy marrow.

The client's own marrow may be harvested prior to the treatment (*autologous* BMT). An *allogeneic* BMT involves the use of marrow from a matching donor. If the client's own marrow was harvested, the marrow may or may not have been chemically treated to destroy any cancer cells. It is then stored (frozen) to be reinfused after the chemotherapy or RT to "rescue" the bone marrow from the lethal effects of the treatment.

■ CLINICAL TRIALS

A *clinical trial* is a study conducted to evaluate a new treatment. New drugs or treatment modalities are first evaluated through basic research studies in the laboratory and with animals. The most promising of these treatment approaches are then further assessed in clinical trials with human subjects. There are four phases of clinical trials[64]:

- *Phase 1:* Only a small number of patients are used as subjects in phase 1 clinical trials. The purpose of the study is to determine the maximum tolerated dose of a drug or treatment. The researchers are also watching carefully for harmful side effects. Although the treatment has been tested in the laboratory and in animals, it is not yet known how humans will respond. No direct benefit in terms of disease remission can be guaranteed. Because phase 1 studies involve significant risk without any promise of benefit, participation is offered only to people with advanced disease and for whom there are no other known treatment options. Safety, comfort, and ethical considerations are primary nursing concerns during this phase of clinical drug trials.
- *Phase 2:* Phase 2 studies are developed from the information gained from the phase 1 studies. The treatment now is offered to people with types of cancer that responded to the treatment in the phase 1 studies. The purpose of a phase 2 study is to determine the effectiveness of the treatment against those cancers while continuing to learn more about the harmful effects of the treatment. As with phase 1 studies, participation in phase 2 studies is offered only to people for whom there are no known treatment alternatives.
- *Phase 3:* In a phase 3 study, a promising new treatment is compared with a standard treatment. On the basis of scientific evidence, the researchers believe that the new treatment is likely to be as good as or better than the current standard treatment. Clients who participate in clinical trials are the first people to benefit from new, more effective treatment modalities.
- *Phase 4:* In phase 4 postmarketing surveillance studies, newly introduced drugs are monitored for adverse effects. Such studies may also compare two standard treatments. For example, surgery and RT may be compared to determine whether the survival rate following RT is similar to that after surgical treatment. Clinical trials are carried out on a nationwide basis, and the pooled results of these investigations are used to determine and validate the effectiveness of treatment regimens.

Nurses have a major role to play in these research trials. Nursing responsibilities associated with caring for a client who is participating in a clinical trial are

- Client education
- Documentation of treatment benefits and side effects
- Anticipation of adverse reactions and early recognition of toxicity
- Management of side effects

Research nurses have even greater responsibilities for monitoring of clients, recruitment of participants, and dissemination of data.

Written informed consents for participation in a clinical trial are often lengthy and can be overwhelming. In most settings, nurses are responsible for reviewing the written consent and the physician's verbal teaching with the client. You can often help by highlighting key information in the consent form, such as the purpose of the study, the treatments being compared, and whom to contact for more information. An NCI pamphlet[64] describes important questions a client should ask when considering participation in a clinical trial.

▪ Self-Care

COMPLEMENTARY APPROACHES

Use by the public of alternative or complementary therapies for chronic conditions, such as back problems, depression, and cancer, is growing. Eisenberg and associates[23] estimated that in 1997, 629 million visits were made to alternative medicine practitioners, exceeding the total number of visits to all U.S. primary care physicians. These researchers found that 42.1% of the population had used at least 1 of 16 alternative therapies in the previous year.

Complementary approaches often combine one or more elements, such as (1) spiritual, psychological, nutritional, physical, pharmacologic, herbal, electromagnetic, or psychic approaches, (2) traditional medicines, (3) unconventional uses of conventional therapies, (4) unconventional instruments, and (5) humane approaches. Of these approaches, Lerner[51] points out that spiritual, psychological, nutritional, and physical approaches represent a "vital quartet of ethical approaches" that have benefited many clients with cancer. In research, prayer has been found to be a coping mechanism that correlates with perceptions of well-being.[10]

Psychological approaches that are widely recognized yet underutilized include support groups, psychotherapy, imagery, biofeedback, and hypnosis. When used with antiemetic drugs, music can be an effective diversional therapy to decrease the frequency of nausea and vomiting.[24] Guided imagery also can help control nausea and vomiting, create a relaxation response, and control pain.[10] Art therapy can be used to help an adult with cancer gain insight into his or her situation.[5]

Although diet is recognized to play a major role in cancer causation, there is no known dietary treatment that slows or cures cancer. Nevertheless, nutritional interventions can enhance a client's ability to tolerate treatment and thereby improve both the quality of life and, potentially, the treatment outcome. Physical therapy approaches, including exercises, massage therapies, and progressive relaxation, are often overlooked by health care providers.

Lerner[51] offers a framework for evaluating unconventional—and conventional—therapies. First, assess the therapy. Is there any significant scientific literature to support the therapy? Second, evaluate the practitioner. What training has the practitioner completed? What do other unconventional practitioners think of the provider? Does the practitioner share data about treatments with other practitioners? Third, assess the usefulness of the

service delivery. Do most people who have completed treatment believe that the service was reasonably related to the cost?

To date, Lerner[51] has encountered no decisive and scientifically documented cure for any type of cancer among the complementary therapies. For all their shortcomings, conventional therapies are capable of curing a number of cancers. He finds, however, that some complementary therapies, such as psychosocial support for clients with metastatic breast cancer, appear to extend life and that many complementary therapies enhance the quality of life.

HOME MANAGEMENT OF SIDE EFFECTS

Aggressive, complex, and sophisticated cancer therapies are now being delivered in the ambulatory, office, and home care settings. This shift in care settings presents additional challenges for clients, family members, and health care providers. A high level of commitment is required from the client and family caregivers for the successful management of care in the outpatient setting. Clients and family members require education regarding complex treatment regimens. They must know how to recognize manifestations of side effects or adverse events, how to prevent side effects, and what they can do to treat the manifestations. Most importantly, they must know when to report manifestations and how to reach the physician—especially after office hours. When chemotherapy is administered in the home setting, provisions must be made for the safe handling and disposal of cytotoxic drugs to minimize client, family, and nurse exposure.[76]

FINANCIAL CONCERNS

Cancer care can place a financial burden on the client and family. First are the direct costs of deductibles and coinsurance. Unless the client has a prescription card, some medications, such as the serotonin (5-HT$_3$ [5-hydroxytryptamine]) antagonist antiemetics, can be more costly than the client can afford.

In addition, cancer and its treatment often involves many hidden costs. Examples are transportation and meals for travel to clinic appointments, new clothing to accommodate weight loss or gain, medical supplies, special foods or nutritional supplements, long-distance telephone calls, and loss of income for the client or family caregiver.[58] Ten per cent, or $104 billion, of the $1 trillion spent on health care annually is utilized for cancer care; of this amount, $35 billion is utilized for direct medical care, $12 billion for lost productivity, and $57 billion for mortality costs.[11]

▪ EVALUATION OF TREATMENT RESPONSE

During and after treatment, the client is monitored for tumor response. Just as with diagnosis, listening carefully to the client's history and the physical examination are fundamental sources of data. If the client's cancer was symptomatic, the client may be able to predict that the treatment is working because the pain has lessened, breathing requires less effort, or other manifestations are subsiding.

When known disease remained after surgical intervention or diagnostic studies, repeating the imaging studies that were performed at the time of the diagnosis can be used to determine treatment effectiveness. Imaging studies are generally repeated after every two to three cycles of chemotherapy. If the tumor was associated with an elevated tumor marker at the time of diagnosis, testing for the marker again can be both a guide to the effectiveness of the chemotherapy and, later, a means of early detection of recurrence of the cancer. With ovarian cancer, a "second-look" surgical procedure may be performed after the completion of the chemotherapy to verify that no detectable disease remains.

After treatment is completed, the client continues to be monitored for manifestations of disease recurrence and for delayed or long-term after-effects of the treatment. Depending on the type of cancer, follow-up appointments may initially be at 3-month intervals, eventually extending to 6-month and then 1-year intervals.

Nursing Management of Oncologic Treatment and Emergencies

Comprehensively and successfully managing cancer-related manifestations—whether they are from the cancer itself or are side effects of treatment—is essential for achieving high-quality outcomes in cancer care. For some clinical manifestations, urgent intervention is required to prevent undue morbidity or even mortality. For example, infection, a potentially life-threatening complication in the client with neutropenia, is an oncologic emergency. When a person has few white cells, infection can quickly progress to septicemia and death unless aggressive intervention is instituted. Failure to recognize, diagnose, and intervene for new-onset back pain can result in paralysis if the pain is secondary to spinal cord compression. Uncontrolled pain, discussed in Chapter 23, is often considered an oncologic emergency in the client with cancer because it so greatly interferes with the client's relationships and activities of daily living.

Both antineoplastic medications and RT can damage and destroy not only cancer cells but also certain normal cells. Box 19–2 summarizes the side effects of antineoplastic drugs. Side effects on normal cells are evaluated or graded according to the degree of severity. Mild to moderate side effects generally do not warrant discontinuation of treatment or a decrease of the dose. More severe

---

BOX 19–2   Side Effects of Antineoplastic Drugs

Gastrointestinal

Nausea and vomiting
Constipation
Anorexia
Stomatitis
Esophagitis
Alterations in taste
Diarrhea
Weight loss
Pharyngitis

Integumentary

Dermatitis
Alopecia
Perianal ulcers
Vulvar ulcers
Hyperpigmentation
Photosensitivity
Nail changes

Hematopoietic

Anemia
Thrombocytopenia
Neutropenia

Genitourinary

Nephrotoxicity
Urine color change
Hemorrhagic cystitis
Hyperuricemic nephropathy

Hepatic

Hepatotoxicity
Cirrhosis
Hepatic fibrosis
Portal hypertension

Reproductive

Amenorrhea
Sterility
Loss of libido
Impotence
Azoospermia
Gonadal dysfunction
Menopausal manifestations
Irregular menses
Gynecomastia
Oligospermia

Cardiac

Electrocardiogram changes
Dysrhythmias
Cardiomyopathy, chronic heart failure
Tachycardia

Pulmonary

Pneumonitis
Pulmonary fibrosis

Metabolic

Tumor lysis syndrome

Neurologic, Sensory-Perceptual

Ototoxicity
Subacute meningeal irritation
Peripheral neuropathy
Cranial nerve neuropathy
Autonomic neuropathy
Cerebellar toxicity

Data from Hydzik, C. A. (1990). Late effects of chemotherapy: Implications for patient management and rehabilitation. *Nursing Clinics of North America, 25*, 423; and Ruccione, K., & Weinberg, K. (1989). Late effects in multiple body systems. *Seminars in Oncology Nursing, 5*, 4.

or unexpected toxicities require careful evaluation and dose reduction.

The onset of the side effects of chemotherapy may be acute or delayed. *Acute* toxicities (1) tend to occur in tissues composed of rapidly dividing cells (bone marrow, hair, mucosa), (2) are frequently intermittent, and (3) generally resolve with complete recovery. In contrast, *delayed* or *late* effects may produce lifelong problems. Such effects include organ-specific treatment toxicities resulting in cardiac, renal, pulmonary, hepatic, reproductive, and neurologic dysfunction.

Because many of these problems appear when the client has returned home rather than in the clinical setting, the client as well as the health care providers must be aware of, monitor for, and report side effects. When taking a telephone call from a client, you must be prepared to anticipate the potential complications related to the concern that led to the call. Telephone triage is a particularly challenging aspect of ambulatory care because you must depend almost entirely on verbal report to formulate an accurate picture of the client's situation and its urgency.

■ MYELOSUPPRESSION

NEUTROPENIA

Infection and bleeding, often resulting from diminished production of WBCs and platelets (thrombocytopenia) secondary to treatment, are two common causes of death in clients with cancer. The time after chemotherapy administration when the WBC or platelet count is at the lowest point is referred to as the *nadir*. For most chemotherapeutic agents, the nadir occurs within 7 to 14 days after drug administration. Knowledge of blood count nadirs helps the health professional predict when the client is at greatest risk for infection and bleeding. Monitoring the CBC and differential count can identify when the nadir occurs and whether the client has adequate numbers of blood cells and can demonstrate evidence of impending bone marrow recovery.

The etiology of infections associated with cancer is multifactorial. Some cancers cause specific defects in the immune response. Side effects of treatment can result in myelosuppression (decreased RBCs, WBCs, and platelets). An impaired integumentary system can increase vulnerability to infection. Corticosteroids, which are used in many treatment protocols, suppress immune functions. Neutropenia predisposes the client to infection, especially infection by opportunistic endogenous (normally resident in the client's body or surroundings) organisms. More than half of infections in clients with neutropenia are associated with organisms from the local environment. Major sources are food (raw fruits and vegetables), water, inhaled organisms, and organisms passed through direct contact. The client with neutropenia can quickly become septic; the mortality rate with septicemia can range from 30% to 80%.[98] For this reason, a CBC with differential count must be performed before administration of myelosuppressive (most chemotherapeutic) drugs and repeated periodically between treatments.

The two major types of WBCs are granulocytes (which include neutrophils) and agranulocytes. *Neutrophils* are the first and most numerous type of cell to arrive at any area of disease or tissue injury. When the number of neutrophils is substantially reduced, one of the body's prime defenses against infection is impaired. Therefore, it is important to know what proportion of WBCs are neutrophils. The absolute neutrophil count (ANC) is calculated by multiplying the WBC by the percentage of segmented and banded neutrophils in the CBC differential count:

$$ANC = WBC \times neutrophils\ (\%)$$

On a CBC laboratory report, the neutrophils are often listed as Segs (for segmented neutrophils) and as bands; the percentages of these two cells are added together to obtain the total percentage of neutrophils. For example, if the WBC count is 1200/mm^3 and the percentage of neutrophils (sum of the percentages of segmented and banded neutrophils) is 34%, the ANC is 408 (1200 × .34 = 408).

Neutropenia is commonly defined as an ANC of less than 1000/mm^3. The frequency of infection increases (1) as the ANC decreases below 500/mm^3 and (2) with duration of the neutropenia. In the client with neutropenia, the usual manifestations of infection can be absent because of the lack of neutrophils to produce an adequate inflammatory response to the infection. Therefore, fever is the cardinal, and often the only, manifestation of infection. Three oral temperature readings exceeding 38° C (100.4° F) in 24 hours or one temperature reading exceeding 38.5° C (101.3° F) is considered diagnostic of a fever.

Because infections are associated with greater morbidity and mortality, the development of fever in a client with neutropenia should be treated as an oncologic emergency that mandates prompt assessment, diagnosis, and intervention. Measures to be taken generally consist of (1) cultures, chest x-ray, and physical evaluation to attempt to identify the source, (2) broad-spectrum antibiotic therapy, and (3) monitoring of vital signs. G-CSF or GM-CSF (see earlier) may be prescribed to reduce the duration and severity of neutropenia.

Nursing management of outcomes begins with teaching clients measures to protect against infection and reinforcement of such teachings as WBC counts reach their nadir. These measures are as follows[66]:

- Practice good personal hygiene, especially handwashing.
- Perform oral care daily and frequently rinse the mouth with an alcohol-free mouthwash, such as saline and soda (1 tsp soda to 1 L of normal saline) or even just water four to six times per day.
- Maintain adequate nutrition and fluid intake.
- Do not share eating utensils with anyone.
- Avoid raw or uncooked foods during nadir period.
- Avoid crowds, people with infections, and children who have been recently vaccinated with live or attenuated vaccines.
- Avoid contact with animal excrement (e.g., bird, cat, or dog feces).
- Either avoid having cut flowers in the home, or change the water of fresh flowers daily, with 1 tsp of chlorine bleach added to the new water.
- Get adequate rest and exercise.
- Avoid indiscriminate use of antipyretics (e.g., acetaminophen, aspirin) because they can mask fever.

Clients should also be taught that even with the best precautions, infections cannot always be prevented. The importance of immediately reporting any manifestations of infection must be stressed: (1) temperature reading of more than 38° C (100° F), (2) cough, (3) sore throat, (4) chills or sweating, and (5) frequent or painful urination.

THROMBOCYTOPENIA

Thrombocytopenia due to chemotherapy may cause subtle to life-threatening bleeding. A high risk of hemorrhage exists when the platelet count is less than 20,000/mm^3. In the client with a solid (versus a hematologic) tumor, a platelet count greater than 10,000/mm^3 puts the incidence of bleeding at less than 12%; however, fatal CNS hemorrhage or massive GI hemorrhage can occur.[31] The platelet count usually recovers within 2 to 6 weeks after the recovery of the WBC count following chemotherapy. Chemotherapy is usually withheld until the platelet count rises to 100,000/mm.[3, 31]

Nursing measures to manage outcomes are utilized to prevent bleeding or detect early clinical manifestations of bleeding. Instruct the client to:

- Avoid injury, by being cautious with sharp objects and using an electric razor rather than a blade razor.
- Use lotions to prevent dryness and cracking of the skin
- Use lubrication (women) during sexual intercourse (if sexual activity is advisable during treatment).
- Maintain good oral hygiene and use either a soft toothbrush or, if the platelet count is very low, sponge oral swabs, and report excessive bleeding of gums.
- Avoid constipation; use stool softeners if needed.
- Avoid enemas or rectal suppositories, and report any rectal bleeding.
- Refrain from taking aspirin or nonsteroidal anti-inflammatory drugs (NSAIDs) without the doctor's permission.
- If nosebleeds or other external bleeding occurs, put pressure on the source of bleeding for 10 to 15 minutes.
- Avoid taking temperatures rectally at all times and orally if there is oral soreness or bleeding; take tympanic temperatures.
- Avoid intramuscular or subcutaneous injections; central lines can be used for parenteral medications.
- Notify the nurse or physician of manifestations of bleeding: petechiae (small red spots) or increased bruising, tarry stools, hypermenorrhea (heavy uterine bleeding), blood in urine or vomit, visual changes, and changes in level of consciousness (an early indication of intracranial hemorrhage).

Most oncologists use transfusions to keep a client's platelet count above 20,000/mm^3 unless the client is known to have a platelet antibody. As previously mentioned, the thrombopoietic growth factor oprelvekin (Neumega) is now available to prevent severe thrombocytopenia following myelosuppressive chemotherapy in patients with nonmyeloid malignancies.[82]

ANEMIA

Anemia in the client with cancer can have multiple causes. There may be blood loss secondary to the disease. Abnormal destruction of RBCs is commonly a secondary disorder, arising from such causes as liver or spleen disease, BMT, or drug toxicity. The most common cause of anemia in the client with cancer is inadequate production of RBCs. This can result from infiltration of the bone marrow by tumor or suppression of bone marrow production of RBCs by cancer therapy.[17] Anemia leads to an impairment of oxygen delivery that is a common and predictable sequela of many cancer therapies.[86] It may cause fatigue, headache, dizziness, fainting, pallor, dyspnea, palpitations, and tachycardia.

Anemia is an important component of cancer-related fatigue, which is one of the most common and distressing manifestations experienced by the oncology client. Fatigue is poorly understood; no one definition describes all experiences. Research on cancer-related fatigue is still in its infancy. It is difficult to predict with certainty which interventions will have therapeutic benefit for which clients.[97] As advances are made in the scientific understanding of cancer-related fatigue, recommendations for interventions will very likely be altered.

Careful evaluation of exacerbating and relieving factors, the effect of fatigue on daily life, and personal and cultural influences as well as review of laboratory data add depth to the assessment of a client's fatigue and help guide interventions.[17] Transfusions of packed RBCs may be utilized to relieve anemia that is producing manifestations. Erythropoietin may be prescribed to elevate or maintain the erythrocyte level and decrease the need for transfusions (see earlier). Other interventions can be grouped into three categories: (1) education, (2) exercise, and (3) attention-restoring activities. Clients who are taught that fatigue is expected report less fatigue than those who are not. Clients who balance exercise (such as walking) with rest report less fatigue. Engaging in activities that are interesting to the client may restore attention and the ability to think clearly.[17]

■ GASTROINTESTINAL EFFECTS

NAUSEA AND VOMITING

GI effects of chemotherapy include nausea and vomiting, anorexia, alteration in taste, weight loss, oral mucositis, diarrhea, and constipation. The vomiting center in the medulla can be stimulated by any of five different afferent pathways or by arousal of the chemotherapy trigger zone located in the fourth ventricle of the brain. The emetic potential of a particular chemotherapeutic regimen depends on the drugs given, the dose and route of administration, and the client's susceptibility to emesis. RT to the chest, abdomen, or back can stimulate afferent pathways. Radiation-related emesis is related to the area and size of the treatment field and the dose delivered.

Adequate control of nausea and vomiting is an essential factor in a client's compliance with treatment. Uncontrolled nausea and vomiting, among the most feared treatment-related side effects, is experienced by as many as 60% of people receiving chemotherapy. It can result in anorexia, malnutrition, dehydration, metabolic imbalances, psychological depression, and decreased immunity.

Three types of nausea and vomiting have been described. After the client has experienced nausea and vomiting, *anticipatory* nausea and vomiting may occur before the administration of further therapy. *Acute post-therapy* nausea and vomiting occur within minutes of the first 24 hours following therapy. *Delayed* nausea and vomiting consist of manifestations that persist or develop 24 hours after chemotherapy.[75]

Management of nausea and vomiting has greatly improved during the 1990s because of heightened interest and research. The drug armamentarium now includes premedication for chemotherapy regimens known to be highly emetogenic (causing nausea and vomiting). Newer serotonin receptor antagonists (5-HT$_3$) (e.g., ondansetron [Zofran], granisetron [Kytril], dolasetron [Anzemet]) are particularly useful for acute nausea and vomiting in the first 24 hours to control afferent pathway stimulation from the effects of the chemotherapy on the GI tract. Ongoing evaluation is essential to find the most effective dose, schedule, and combination of drugs for each client.

Nonpharmacologic interventions for nausea and vomiting related to chemotherapy include adjustment of oral and fluid intake, relaxation, exercise, hypnosis, biofeedback, guided imagery, and systemic desensitization. The client and caregivers should avoid offensive odors, such as those from flowers or foods. Food servings should be kept small and offered four to six times per day.

ANOREXIA

Anorexia and weight loss occur as a result of the disease process as well as the treatment. The client with cancer is at risk for protein-calorie malnutrition. Many variables, in addition to the effects of chemotherapy, may alter the client's ability to ingest food via the oral route. Common problems that may interfere with oral intake are anorexia, nausea and vomiting, early satiety, alterations in taste, dry mouth, stomatitis, esophagitis, viscous saliva, lactose intolerance, pain, diarrhea, and constipation.

Nursing management to prevent a compromised nutritional state is based on assessment. Weight loss of 5% or more in a 1-month period is considered significant. In assessing the client, you can begin by identifying potential interventions appropriate to the client's situation. If indicated, a referral can be made to a dietitian for a more comprehensive assessment. When medically appropriate, oral nutrition can be enhanced by relaxing dietary restrictions and emphasizing the need for a high-protein, high-calorie diet with fortification from natural food sources or commercial supplements. An excellent source of helpful tips and recipes for nutritious foods can be found in the booklet *Eating Hints*, which can be obtained free of charge from the NCI.[61] Enteral and parenteral feedings for the client with protein-calorie malnutrition are discussed in Chapter 29.

STOMATITIS

Stomatitis, or *oral mucositis*, is the term used to describe inflammation and ulceration of the mucosal lining of the mouth. The inflammation seen in the mouth is also present throughout the GI tract of a client with cancer or receiving cancer treatment. The severity of the stomatitis can affect the client's quality of life. Consequences of stomatitis include pain, decreased nutritional and fluid intake, infections, malabsorption, diarrhea, and delay of chemotherapy and radiation therapy treatments.

Nursing interventions should include teaching the client to clean and assess the mouth at least once daily and to report changes, including redness, extreme dryness, ulcers, blisters, white patches or bleeding in the mouth, difficulty swallowing, and temperature higher than 37.8° C

(100° F).[7] An oral hygiene program should start before therapy and should continue throughout treatment. Such a program consists of:

- A dental examination and treatment prior to therapy
- Thorough and gentle cleaning to avoid further trauma
- Moisturization if saliva is scanty or absent
- Avoidance of alcohol and smoking
- Culture analysis and antimicrobial therapy for infections
- Topical anesthetics and analgesics for pain or discomfort

Dietary modifications include (1) avoiding extremely hot or cold foods, spices, and citrus fruits and juices, (2) eating soft foods, and (3) taking nutritional supplements.

DIARRHEA AND CONSTIPATION

Most clinicians define *diarrhea* as an increase in stool liquid or frequency.[56] It can result from GI mucosal damage secondary to RT or chemotherapy. A low-residue or liquid diet is usually advised. Electrolytes and intake and output should be carefully monitored. Scrupulous perineal hygiene is encouraged, especially in the client with neutropenia. Antidiarrheal agents may be prescribed.

Constipation is frequently described as hard, dry stool with straining, a decrease in the number of defecations, or both. Causes include (1) a decrease in either fluid and fiber intake or mobility of clients, (2) changes in usual bowel routines, (3) mechanical changes, such as tumor pressure on the bowel, and (4) metabolic changes, such as hypokalemia or hypercalcemia.[19] The vinca alkaloid chemotherapeutic agents (vinblastine, vincristine) can slow bowel peristalsis. Other causes of constipation are narcotic use, tumor invasion of the GI tract, and depression. Preventive measures may be taken for constipation, such as increasing fluid and bulk intake, using stool softeners prophylactically, increasing physical activity, and using laxatives when necessary.

■ INTEGUMENTARY EFFECTS

ALOPECIA

Alopecia is a common side effect of many antineoplastic agents. The extent of hair loss depends on the specific drug, dosage, and method of administration. Alopecia tends to begin 2 to 3 weeks after the first treatment. It is temporary. New hair growth tends to begin 4 to 6 weeks after the completion of chemotherapy, and 8 to 9 weeks following RT. Hair color and texture may change, but the hair usually returns to its former condition within a year.[93] There can also be loss of body hair, including eyelashes, eyebrows, and pubic hair.[39]

To help the client manage this side effect, which can be a traumatic change in body image and a constant reminder of the cancer, prepare the client for its occurrence. Begin by first allowing the client to grieve for the hair loss. Having information available about where to obtain attractive wigs or turbans is helpful. Many ACS units offer a wonderful program called "Look Good, Feel Better," which involves the assistance of a volunteer beautician. Remember, hair loss bothers many men more than they may be able to acknowledge. Wigs are available for men. Many men choose to wear baseball caps to conceal the hair loss and for warmth. Hearing the experience of others with hair loss can often be helpful to both men and women.

SKIN REACTIONS

The type of skin reactions that may occur in the client receiving chemotherapy depends on the drug administered. Red patches (*erythema*) or hives (*urticaria*) may appear at the drug injection site or on other body parts. (The extravasation of vesicant drugs was discussed earlier.) These reactions generally disappear within several hours.

Darkening of the skin (*hyperpigmentation*) in the nail beds and mouth, on gums or teeth, and along the veins used for IV chemotherapy usually occurs within 2 to 3 weeks after administration of chemotherapy and continues for 10 to 12 weeks after the end of therapy. Sensitivity to sunlight (*photosensitivity*) may result in an acute sunburn after just a short exposure to the sun. The sensitivity disappears once treatment stops. Teach the client to use sunscreen or protective clothing before sun exposure.

A skin reaction called *radiation recall* may occur in clients who received RT prior to the administration of chemotherapy. When chemotherapy is given several weeks or months later, a recall reaction occurs in the previously irradiated skin area. Skin effects range from redness, shedding, or peeling to blisters and oozing. After the skin heals, it is permanently darkened. It is important to maintain meticulous hygiene to avoid a superimposed infection in the area of radiation recall. Antibiotic therapy should be initiated at the first manifestation of infection.

■ EFFECTS ON THE REPRODUCTIVE SYSTEM

Surgery, RT, and chemotherapy each can have effects on sexual health and sexual self-image. Up to 25% of women undergoing modified radical mastectomy for breast cancer report problems with sexual functioning. Surgery can affect sexual functioning through impairment of the vascular supply, removal of organs, or reduction of circulating hormone levels. Fifty-five per cent to 78% of women treated with RT for cervical cancer report sexual impairments. Body image, sexual functioning, and fertility can be affected by chemotherapy.[4, 20] Not all clients experience these effects to the same degree, however. Preliminary studies suggest that the effects of chemotherapy on gonadal function vary with respect to the client's age at the time of therapy, the drugs administered, and the total drug dosage.[42]

Administration of antineoplastic agents during the first trimester of pregnancy increases the risk of spontaneous abortion and fetal malformations. Second- and third-trimester chemotherapy exposures may result in low birth weight or prematurity.[44] A pregnancy begun after cytotoxic chemotherapy has about the same chance of a successful outcome as a normal pregnancy.[4] However, the genetic effects of chemotherapy may not be evident for several generations of offspring. Therefore, you should discuss the unpredictability of occurrence, degree, and duration of genetic damage with the client and spouse or significant other.

Although you may initially not be comfortable with sexuality issues, you can still be an important source of support by giving the client permission to express concerns about this aspect of cancer therapy. Begin simply by asking open-ended questions about how the cancer experience has changed the client's relationships. Beyond providing information yourself, offer to seek out further information or to consult with a colleague who may have additional information or suggestions to alleviate or at least ease the concern.

The PLISSIT (*p*ermission, *l*imited *i*nformation, *s*pecific *s*uggestions, *i*ntensive *t*herapy) model for evaluation of sexual function can be used for assessment purposes.[12] Pretreatment sperm banking offers the possibility of retaining reproductive capacity for some clients. Use of vaginal lubricants, methods of dilating the vagina after RT for cervical cancer (see Chapter 39), and penile prostheses (see Chapter 38) are topics you can discuss with the client. Counseling with a sexual therapist may be indicated.

■ ONCOLOGIC EMERGENCIES

Infection, pain, spinal cord compression, hypercalcemia, SIADH, cardiac tamponade, superior vena cava syndrome, tumor lysis syndrome, and disseminated intravascular coagulation (DIC) are oncologic emergencies. If not identified early and treated, oncologic emergencies can result in severe morbidity and death. Each oncologic emergency is discussed only briefly here. The focus is on your role in appreciating and urgently reporting sometimes subtle manifestations to ensure the best possible outcome for the client. Consult other cancer nursing texts for further information on oncologic emergencies.

Oncologic emergencies can be grouped as follows:

* Metabolic (infection and pain, hypercalcemia, tumor lysis syndrome, SIADH, DIC)
* Structural (spinal cord compression, superior vena cava syndrome, cardiac tamponade)

INFECTION AND PAIN

Infection, which can quickly progress as a life-threatening emergency in the client with neutropenia, was discussed in the preceding section. Although pain does not usually arise suddenly or unexpectedly, it is often regarded as an oncologic emergency because it is such a pervasive problem. As many as a third of clients in active treatment and 60% to 90% of people with advanced cancer have pain.[84] Pain can interfere with a person's ability to enjoy activities and relationships that are meaningful. When pain is uncontrolled, the goal of enabling the client to live fully cannot be met. For nursing management of pain, see Chapter 23.

HYPERCALCEMIA

After infection, hypercalcemia is the most commonly occurring oncologic emergency and can be a potentially fatal condition. Hypercalcemia is due to bone resorption (demineralization) and is defined as a serum calcium level greater than 11 mg/dl. If the client also has decreased serum albumin, a common finding with cancer, a corrected serum calcium value should be used. Eighty per cent of cases of cancer-related hypercalcemia occur with solid tumors, including breast, lung, head, neck, and renal cancers. The other 20% of cases occur in hematologic cancers, such as multiple myeloma, leukemia, and lymphoma.

If the serum calcium level rises slowly, the client may be relatively asymptomatic for a time. When it rises swiftly, renal failure, coma, cardiac arrest, and death can result. Early manifestations may be difficult to distinguish from other cancer- or treatment-related manifestations: anorexia, fatigue, nausea and vomiting, constipation, excessive thirst, polyuria, poor skin turgor, and dry mucous membranes.[25, 43] Later manifestations include severe muscle weakness, diminished deep tendon reflexes, paralytic ileus, and electrocardiogram (ECG) changes.

Nursing management begins with the recognition of clients at risk for hypercalcemia, including people with (1) cancer of the breast, lung, head, neck, or kidney, (2) multiple myeloma, (3) leukemia, (4) lymphoma, and (5) potential or actual bone metastases. Maintaining adequate hydration and mobility are important preventive measures in the client at risk. Limiting dietary intake of calcium has little or no effect. Clients and family caregivers should be instructed on manifestations to report.

Medical management of hypercalcemia is aimed at controlling the growth of the tumor causing the hypercalcemia and, possibly, administration of drugs to lower serum calcium levels, such as calcitonin (Miacalcin) and oral glucocorticoids. For the client with advanced disease, for whom other interventions are no longer effective, treatment is aimed at comfort care.

TUMOR LYSIS SYNDROME
Tumor lysis syndrome is a potentially fatal metabolic emergency that can develop as a tumor responds to treatment. When a large, bulky tumor is very responsive to treatment, especially chemotherapy, the destruction of a large number of malignant cells may rapidly release intracellular potassium, phosphorus, and nucleic acid into the circulation. Electrolyte imbalances and acute renal failure usually begin 1 to 2 days after treatment starts and end within a week following the completion of therapy. Clients with malignancies that are very responsive to treatment are at highest risk, especially if they have a very large tumor burden. Such malignancies include lymphomas, leukemias, and small cell carcinoma.

Medical management focuses on prevention in high-risk clients. Aggressive IV hydration is started before treatment begins and is continued until after treatment ends. Allopurinol (Zyloprim) is administered to decrease uric acid concentration. Sodium bicarbonate may be given in conjunction with the IV hydration to promote fecal excretion of excess phosphate.

Despite preventive measures, tumor lysis syndrome may occur. If so, the goal is to remove potassium from the extracellular fluid with medications, retention enemas, or IV 50% dextrose, which acts to increase plasma insulin and thereby forces potassium back into the intracellular fluid. When preventive and maintenance measures are not effective, the client requires renal dialysis.[43]

The most important nursing management responsibility is to recognize and report manifestations of tumor lysis syndrome immediately. Nursing management then focuses on maintenance of fluid and electrolyte balance by carrying out medical orders, including IV hydration, monitoring weight daily, and maintaining a record of intake and output. Clinical manifestations to observe for and report are (1) weakness, (2) nausea, (3) diarrhea, (4) flaccid paralysis, (5) ECG changes, (6) muscle cramps or twitching, (7) oliguria (diminished urine output), (8) hypotension, (9) edema, and (10) altered mental status. Especially when treatment is provided in the outpatient ambulatory setting, the client and family must be taught about which manifestations to report immediately.[43]

SYNDROME OF INAPPROPRIATE ANTIDIURETIC HORMONE
SIADH results from the abnormal production of antidiuretic hormone (ADH). The incidence of SIADH is relatively low, occurring in only about 1% to 2% of clients with cancer. Of clients with cancer-related SIADH, 80% have an underlying diagnosis of small cell lung cancer. Other causes of SIADH are infection, pulmonary disorders, emotional stress, CNS disorders, and some drugs, including such antineoplastic agents as cyclophosphamide (Cytoxan), vincristine (Oncovin), vinblastine (Velban), and cisplatin (Platinol-AQ). Manifestations, which are related to the rates of onset of the decrease in sodium and the increase in water retention, include (1) confusion, (2) irritability, (3) headache, (4) muscle weakness, (5) lethargy, (6) decreased urine output, (7) edema, (8) nausea and vomiting, and (9) anorexia.[26, 43]

SIADH is not a preventable complication. It is a medical emergency only when the hyponatremia is severe (<120 mEq/L) and the client experiences manifestations. Mild SIADH is treated conservatively with fluid restriction (<500 to 1000 ml/day). In about 7 to 10 days, the body should be able to normalize the serum sodium concentration and osmolality. An IV infusion of hypertonic saline (3% to 5%) is given in more severe cases to prevent pulmonary edema. Monitor intake and output. Pharmacologic agents given for SIADH include demeclocycline (Declomycin), lithium (Lithane), and urea. Beyond symptomatic treatment, the goal of medical management is to treat the underlying disease causing the SIADH.[26, 43]

DISSEMINATED INTRAVASCULAR COAGULATION
DIC involves the development of extensive, abnormal clots throughout small blood vessels. The widespread clotting consumes all circulating clotting factors and platelets, leading to excessive bleeding from several sites. The bleeding can be minimal or life-threatening. Also, clots that are blocking blood vessels decrease blood flow to major organs, which can cause pain, stroke-like manifestations, dyspnea, tachycardia, oliguria, and bowel necrosis. The mortality rate is near 70% despite appropriate treatment.

In clients with cancer, DIC is often caused by gram-negative infection or sepsis, release of thrombin or thromboplastin (clotting factors) from cancer cells, or blood transfusions. DIC is most commonly associated with leukemia and adenocarcinomas of the lung, pancreas, stomach, and prostate. Management involves treating the cancer and other measures as discussed in Chapter 75.

SPINAL CORD COMPRESSION
Even for the terminally ill client in a hospice setting, early detection of and intervention for spinal cord compression are vital. Failure to intervene in this emergency can leave the client with permanent neurologic disabilities. Spinal cord compression is caused by direct pressure on or compromise of vascular supply to the spinal cord. Back pain is often the only early presenting clinical manifestation, occurring in 95% of clients. Other early manifestations are motor weakness and decreased sensation.

Depending on the rate of tumor growth, it may take only hours or days for the spinal cord compression to progress to irreversible neurologic damage with paralysis and loss of bowel and bladder control. Late manifestations are motor loss, additional sensory loss, constipation, and urinary hesitancy.[85, 96]

In a client with known cancer, new-onset back pain should be a "red flag" signaling immediate evaluation. Pain localized over the involved area of the spine or radicular (belt-like) pain is present in more than 90% of clients with spinal cord compression. Carefully assess new-onset back pain; have the client point to the location of the pain and show you the areas of spread. Also carefully assess for any other clinical manifestations of neurologic deficit, such as numbness, tingling, constipation, and voiding hesitancy.

Data from the medical record can be helpful in determining whether the client has known bone metastasis. Give the physician a complete assessment of the pain, with a description of the location and characteristics. These data will provide the physician with the information needed to consider spinal cord compression in the differential diagnosis.

Treatment is usually with RT unless the tumor is resistant to RT or the client has already received the maximum RT dose in the involved area. A laminectomy for spinal cord decompression is an alternative. For the client in a hospice setting whose life expectancy is limited to days or weeks, administration of steroids to lessen the inflammation and swelling around the spinal cord can be a less aggressive but effective short-term alternative.

SUPERIOR VENA CAVA SYNDROME

Distressing but rarely life-threatening, superior vena cava (SVC) syndrome is a disorder resulting from internal or external obstruction of the superior vena cava. The obstruction reduces venous blood return to the heart and compromises cardiac output. SVC syndrome should be evaluated as an emergency because of concern for respiratory compromise. The onset of manifestations is usually gradual; however, if SVC syndrome was the presenting manifestation of cancer, time should be taken to accurately diagnose the underlying disease before treatment is initiated.

Typically, SVC syndrome is secondary to lung cancer, usually small cell carcinoma (65%), or lymphoma (8%). The classic presenting manifestations are dyspnea (63%) and facial swelling (50%) with jugular vein distention. The client is often sitting up and leaning forward to breathe. Other manifestations are swelling of the arms, pain in the chest, and dysphagia.

The goals of medical management are to provide rapid palliation of the distressing manifestations and to treat the underlying cancer. External-beam RT continues to be the standard of care for palliation. However, clients with small cell carcinoma of the lung or lymphoma may be palliated with the appropriate curative chemotherapy regimen with or without the addition of RT.[73]

CARDIAC TAMPONADE

With cardiac tamponade (acute compression of the heart), early detection and proper management are critical to preventing cardiovascular collapse and death. When fluid collects in the pericardial sac (pericardial effusion), it affects the heart's ability to function properly and leads to cardiac tamponade. Normally, the pericardium contains 15 to 50 ml of fluid; the pericardial sac may contain as much as 200 to 1800 ml of fluid before the heart begins to decompensate. The fluid prevents the heart from filling and contracting normally. The onset may be insidious.

The most common manifestations are tachycardia, severe dyspnea, cough, chest pain, edema, and hypotension. You may notice a narrowing of the pulse pressure (the difference between systolic and diastolic readings) or pulsus paradoxus (decreased or absent amplitude of the pulse with inspiration). Heart sounds may be muffled by the fluid. Jugular venous distention may be prominent. A chest x-ray is a cost-effective screening tool, although it cannot always visualize cardiac tamponade. An ECG shows a number of changes that could indicate tamponade.

Medical management of cardiac tamponade is individualized for the client. A pericardiocentesis (insertion of an 18-gauge needle into the chest to draw off the fluid) may be performed. Because the fluid can reaccumulate, a pericardiotomy may be performed; this surgical procedure creates a window or opening in the pericardial sac for subsequent drainage of fluid. Even then, the pericardial fluid can reaccumulate. Nursing management consists of carefully assessing clinical manifestations and teaching the client and family caregiver to watch for manifestations that may herald impending cardiac tamponade.[6]

PSYCHOSOCIAL ASPECTS OF CANCER CARE

When cancer becomes a part of life's journey, it is hard work. (See Bridge to Home Health Care: Dealing with Grief Related to a New Cancer Diagnosis.) The diagnosis of cancer affects not only the individual client but also the family. Because cancer is not just a physical disease it compels the clients—and health care professionals—to face the meaning of their lives and their relationships. Just as life experiences affect the perceptions a client brings to the cancer experience, so do your life experiences affect the perceptions you bring to the client's care. It is, therefore, valuable for you to reflect on your beliefs and values about life, death, and their meaning.

■ PROVIDING SUPPORT FOR CLIENTS

The most valuable intervention you can offer a client with cancer is your presence as a caring person. The dimensions of your presence consist of verbal expressions of empathy, positive regard, and availability of practical support.[99]

Hearing the stories of colleagues, clients, their families, and survivors can be a vehicle for a novice nurse to learn the art of cancer nursing.[89] Storytelling is becoming recognized for its value.[36, 49, 50] A story can be a means of providing comfort by offering social comparisons (helping clients know how others have fared and felt in a similar situation) or lessons from others' experiences. Using sailing as a metaphor for the teamwork that makes for a smoother journey, Janice Post-White[74] shares stories of her clients' journeys and her own family's journey with cancer. Through the stories, Post-White teaches nurses

BRIDGE TO HOME HEALTH CARE

Dealing with Grief Related to a New Cancer Diagnosis

Peoples' lives are changed forever by a new diagnosis of cancer. Grieving often begins with the news that an illness is cancer-related. When home health nurses or other nurses in the community start working with clients, they have many responsibilities in addition to meeting clients' physical needs; they also must (1) assess how the client, the family, and significant others are coping with the new diagnosis, (2) acknowledge the grief process as part of the illness, and (3) help them to express their feelings, needs, and concerns as they struggle with the process.

Consider what losses are contributing to the grief process. Losses are likely to include the sense of wellness, usual or anticipated family role, positive self-image, career, independence, and financial stability as well as the fear of loss of life. Feeling alone is not uncommon. Determine whether friends and family members are providing support for the person with cancer, or whether they need encouragement and suggestions about how to do so. Many people have difficulty knowing how to react or what to say, especially when the client is younger. Evaluate whether the client and the family feel overwhelmed as they face choices about treatment options, symptom management, and emotions that compound the reaction to the new diagnosis.

The feelings associated with a new cancer diagnosis can be very intense. Remember that feelings are not good or bad; they just are. By letting clients know that you are truly available to listen, you provide the opportunity for them to discuss various feelings that may be just under the surface. Sometimes it is easier to write about feelings rather than verbalize them. Encourage the client and others to write down questions, concerns, hopes, and fears in the form of a letter or a journal.

Teaching is an important responsibility of home health providers. Help the client, the family, and significant others learn about the disease to gain a sense of control during this time of chaos. If they know what to expect and what is "normal," they are less anxious. Provide information about the disease, treatments, management of side effects, and the dynamics of grief. The American Cancer Society is an invaluable resource for the client with a new cancer diagnosis; suggest additional resources, such as authenticated Internet sites, and support groups, such as I Can Cope and Reach to Recovery. Prepare the client and family for an information overload and for the numerous, questionable products and services that are for sale in the area.

When you help the client maintain a sense of normality, you also add to the sense of control. Work with the client to schedule daily activities and provide structure to help him or her cope with the changes that result from the illness or treatment. Encourage the client to participate in normal activities and relationships. For some clients, employment or volunteer activities are options. Planning for the future can give the client something positive to anticipate.

Remember that the grief process is very individualized. Wherever the client, family members, or significant others are in this process is the right place for them to be. Be careful to avoid a list of "shoulds" and "should nots." Validate them by acknowledging their feelings, and accept that they are real, being careful not to include bias in your acceptance. Your encouragement will help the grief process evolve in its own time and at its own pace. Teaching, listening, and offering support are critical interventions for managing the grief process.

Pamela K. Schaid, RN, MA, *Administrator, Seasons Hospice, Rochester, Minnesota*

---

that they can be the "wind behind the sails," empowering clients and their families by creating balance, uniting a team, and guiding them forward.

There is great variability in the distress, changes, and other effects of cancer in the lives of clients and their families. Responses to cancer depend on:

- The disease and the disabilities and disfigurements it may cause
- Pre-existing medical conditions that may limit treatment options
- The client's psychological make-up and spiritual well-being
- The client's family and social community
- Availability of medical and financial resources

■ PROVIDING SUPPORT FOR FAMILY

The diagnosis of cancer has an effect on the entire family as well. The daily life of the family is changed. Other family members may need to assume the role or responsibilities of the client or to serve as the family caregiver. Nursing often views the family as the context of caring for the client with cancer; the family needs to be the unit of care. A family's resources, perceptions of the cancer,

functioning patterns, coping strategies, and stressors are factors affecting their ability to respond to the crisis of cancer.[79] Much of the distress for the client and the family can be lessened with minimal assistance from the health care team. Without these services, even highly functioning families struggle.[52]

■ PROMOTING POSITIVE SELF-CONCEPT

Cancer affects all levels of functioning. Physical and psychological distress, medication, or the disease itself can cloud the client's intellectual function. The client's self-concept is affected by physical changes as well as changes in role or function. A breadwinner in the family may become dependent on others and become a consumer of family savings and resources. The young adult, striving for independence, may need to revert to an earlier level of dependency.

Body image also changes for most clients. Weight loss, hair loss, and skin changes can result from treatment. Radical surgical procedures can make devastating and permanent changes in appearance and function. Procedures such as laryngectomy, glossectomy, mastectomy, and prostatectomy may result in physical changes that humiliate and overwhelm the client.

■ PROMOTING COPING THROUGHOUT THE CANCER CONTINUUM

Although each cancer experience is unique, people with cancer have some common problems. Strategies for outcome management to help clients cope with the disease and its treatment are addressed for each phase of the *cancer continuum:* diagnosis and treatment, survivorship, recurrent disease and progression, and terminal illness.

DIAGNOSIS AND TREATMENT

Clients reach the point of cancer diagnosis in many ways. A client may have had vague manifestations, such as weight loss and fatigue, that may have been ignored or a cause of some anxiety for weeks or months. Another client may have manifestations, such as pain or abdominal bloating, that evaded diagnosis. Many times, cancer is found incidentally during a routine examination. Often the client suspects cancer, but many people are shocked when the diagnosis is made. The diagnostic period may be long and extremely stressful. This period is filled with anxiety about each test result, especially when staging procedures are performed. More than 70% of clients consider the time of diagnosis and treatment as the most stressful in the cancer experience.[95]

Most clients fear death during the first few months of the cancer experience. Weisman[95] called this stage "the existential plight." Whether clients can express their fears or not, it is an underlying cause of distress. During diagnosis, the magnitude of the client's problems becomes apparent. The client wonders: Is my disease curable? Will my disabilities be temporary or permanent? What types of physical impairment will occur? What will be the side effects of treatment? Will my manifestations be relieved? Will I be able to return to work? What adjustments have to be made in family life or work? Will finances be adequate? What plans need to be abandoned? Which changes in lifestyle will be temporary and which permanent?

Clients must deal not only with specific problems but also with the emotional distress they experience throughout this time. They may feel angry and frustrated because their lives have been changed; they may feel isolated or may worry about being abandoned by family and friends. They may be shocked and unbelieving that they are the ones with cancer. They may also feel guilty if they believe that they have contributed to their disease through behavior, such as by smoking, drinking, or putting themselves at risk for sexually transmitted diseases (see Chapter 18, Tables 18–3 and 18–4).

Clients' reactions vary greatly. Initial response to the diagnosis of cancer may be profoundly influenced by previous life experiences with the disease. When the disease is advanced at the time of diagnosis, the client and family are likely to experience more psychological distress because they are confronted with the dual stressors of a cancer diagnosis and a terminal illness.[69] Some have minimal distress, whereas others may be overwhelmed and devastated. You may sometimes feel, on the basis of your own personality and experience, that a client is responding inappropriately (i.e., too little or too much) to a cancer diagnosis. It is very important, however, to acknowledge every client's mode of response as acceptable and unique for that client.

Weisman[95] identified coping styles used by many clients with cancer (Box 19–3). *Denial,* which is a part of coping, allows a client to "repudiate what cannot be avoided, by substituting a more favorable or agreeable idea."[59] Denial can be useful as a healthy coping mechanism in the diagnostic phase, when the number of problems may be overwhelming. Denial is harmful when it prevents the client from seeking appropriate treatment. Awareness and denial can exist at the same time.

Clients who are good problem-solvers or who cope effectively tend to confront reality, avoid excessive denial, remain flexible, accept support, and remain hopeful and optimistic. Clients who cope poorly use avoidance and excessive denial; they are pessimistic and feel hopeless.[59] Box 19–4 lists factors that enable or hinder a client's ability to cope. Every client uses a variety of strategies to cope with cancer.

Families also should be assessed for their coping abilities. Use of a specific family assessment tool may not be possible, but often you will be readily able to identify "high-risk" families from your interactions with them. Unresolved past problems may affect a family's ability to cope with cancer in the present. Families who use excessive denial, exhibit strong anger and guilt, or are unreasonably demanding may be at increased risk for dysfunction. When the client is the pivotal person in the family or when the family has had a previous experience of cancer with a negative outcome, their need for ongoing psychosocial support systems may be increased.

Actively listen for remarks that describe the meaning and effect of cancer as experienced by the client. Often, time limitations may not permit you to provide support separate from physical caregiving. Consequently, while giving care, take the opportunity to initiate social interactions, such as chatting about family, sharing stories, or greeting visitors. Consider these actions a professional

---

BOX 19–3   General Coping Strategies

- Seek more information (rational inquiry).
- Share concern and talk with others (mutuality).
- Laugh it off; make light of the situation (affect reversal).
- Try to forget; put it out of your mind (suppression).
- Do other things for distraction (displacement, redirection).
- Take firm action on basis of present understanding (confrontation).
- Accept but find something favorable (redefinition, revision).
- Submit to the inevitable (fatalism, passive acceptance).
- Do something, anything, however reckless or impractical (impulsivity).
- Consider or negotiate a feasible alternative (if *x*, then *y*).
- Reduce tension with excessive drink, drugs, danger (life threats).
- Withdraw into isolation; get away (disengagement).
- Blame someone or something (externalization, projection).
- Seek direction; do what you are told (cooperative compliance).
- Blame yourself; sacrifice or atone (moral masochism).

Modified from Weisman, A. (1979). *Coping with cancer* (p. 23). New York: McGraw-Hill.

BOX 19–4 Enabling and Hindering Factors in Coping with Cancer

Enabling Factors	Hindering Factors
Social support systems	Denial
Perception of control	Avoidance
Hardiness	Helplessness
Humor	Powerlessness
Positive appraisal	Hopelessness or despair
Hopefulness	Depression
Positive comparisons	Guilt
Religiosity	Erosion of autonomy
Self-esteem	Isolation or withdrawal
Information-seeking	Wishful thinking
Open communication	Anger or hostility
Social skills	Blaming others
Problem-solving ability	Noncompliance

From Jalowiec, A., & Dudas, S. (1991). Alterations in patient coping. In S. Baird, R. McCorkle, & M. Grant (Eds.), *Cancer nursing: A comprehensive text* (pp. 806–820). Philadelphia: W. B. Saunders.

---

intervention. What did you learn about the client's perceptions of cancer? What coping mechanisms did the client or significant others use with past lifestyle changes? How will the client's and the family's life be affected? What needs for teaching or community resources did you note? Would referrals to other members of the health care team, such as the chaplain and social worker, be helpful?

Providing social support and improving the client's sense of control help reduce anxiety. Stress reduction or relaxation techniques can be taught. Speaking with cancer survivors encourages many clients. Support groups and one-to-one visitation programs such as Reach to Recovery or CanSurmount (ACS) provide this opportunity. Internet support groups offer the same opportunity for clients who are uncomfortable with the face-to-face interactions of a traditional support group.

Informational needs of the client and family are very great during the diagnostic and treatment periods. Tests, procedures, and treatments, which are often very technical and complicated, must be explained. Present consistent, accurate information in as much detail as the client wants. Be sure all health care providers are telling the client the same thing. When clients from a cancer clinic were surveyed, information and support from family, friends, and caregivers was identified as a high-priority need (Box 19–5).[32]

Address specific problems by (1) helping the client identify them, (2) providing information when necessary, and (3) referring the client to appropriate resources. Both the NCI and the ACS provide useful written materials to reinforce teaching. Site-specific information can be obtained from the NCI via the Internet *(www.nci.nih.gov* or *www.cancernet.nci.nih.gov),* Fax (301-402-5874), or telephone (1-800-4-CANCER). Other key Internet Web sites may be bookmarked on a computer in the clinical area or in a patient library.

SURVIVORSHIP

Clients who have completed successful treatment enter an indeterminate period of long-term survivorship. Survivorship has been divided into a time of acute survival fol-

lowed by a period of extended survival. Transition between these periods is not precise but evolves as time passes and the cancer does not recur.

Depending on the extent of treatment, the period of extended survival may still be one of physical fatigue and limitation. Physical rehabilitation to improve functioning may dominate the client's energy in this early period. Efforts focus on restoring the client's previous level of functioning.

The long-term physical effects of cancer treatment are now becoming apparent as data accumulate, especially from clients with pediatric cancer. The physical effects may range from minimal restriction to life-threatening complications. The effects can be organ-specific, such as cardiomyopathy or pulmonary fibrosis, or general, such as fatigue.

The potential for development of a second malignancy as a result of primary treatment is always a possibility. Although this possibility is usually rare, some studies have reported up to a 20% occurrence of another cancer after treatment of Hodgkin's disease and other cancers with alkylating agents.

Psychologically, the period of extended survival is one in which clients must take up previous roles or adjust and reorganize their lives. The possibility of recurrence may dominate their lives. Plans may be suspended. Decisions about changing jobs, buying a house, starting a family, or beginning retirement may be difficult in the face of the uncertainty of recurrence or concerns about insurance coverage.

Making sure the client carries through with routine follow-up and long-term health care with attention to prevention and early detection (health promotion) is vital to early detection of recurrent cancer and second primary sites as well as early intervention for late effects of treatment. Follow-up appointments and events such as National Cancer Survivors Day celebrations (which are held in many communities each June) are opportunities for obtaining emotional support, alleviating fears of recurrence, and enabling clients to know that they are not alone in their feelings and concerns.

BOX 19–5 Needs of Clinic Patients with Cancer

The following needs were identified and rank-ordered by a sample of clinic patients. The last three items were ranked of equal importance.

- Information about operating special equipment
- Information about radiation
- Information provided in a way that is understandable
- Ways to be active in decision-making
- Adequate preparation before discharge from hospital
- Support from family
- Support from friends
- Information about chemotherapy
- Time off from work to recuperate
- Information about what to expect in the future
- A patient caregiver
- Time off work for treatment

Modified from Gates, M. F., Lackey, N. R., & White, M. R. (1995). Needs of hospice and clinic patients with cancer. *Cancer Practice, 3*(4), 226–232.

Employment discrimination has been a problem for cancer survivors. Clients with a cancer history have proved themselves to be dependable and productive. Yet studies show that as many as 84% of blue-collar workers and 38% of white-collar workers with cancer experience some type of discrimination in employment.[34] Over the years, these issues have been partially rectified by state laws protecting the rights of the disabled.

Obtaining insurance coverage for a client with a history of cancer has also been difficult, ruinously expensive, and sometimes impossible. Legislative efforts have corrected some of these problems. Insurance discrimination can be legally appealed. Federal programs such as COBRA (Consolidated Omnibus Budget Reconciliation Act) protect the insurance coverage of an employee for 18 months following employment termination, but at an increased monthly premium. A client, spouse, or parent may be trapped in an unrewarding job to maintain the employer-funded group insurance. Direct clients who have difficulty with insurance coverage to contact the National Coalition for Cancer Survivorship (Box 19–6), the ACS, their state department of human rights, or their state insurance department. The NCI booklet *Facing Forward* provides detailed information about resources.[92]

With time, these problems usually recede and clients move into a period of extended survival. The experience of cancer is nonetheless indelibly imprinted on their lives. Amazingly, most clients cope very well and face the difficulties in their lives with courage. For many, the experience brings about a reappraisal of goals and values, making life richer and more meaningful.

RECURRENT DISEASE AND PROGRESSION

Most clients with cancer live with the threat or reality of recurrent disease. Weisman[95] describes the effect that this phase has on the client as "the hope for a cure" becoming the "struggle for existence." With recurrent cancer, therapy may once again be used to eradicate or stabilize the disease process.

Although subsequent recurrent disease may occur, it is usually the first recurrence that causes surprise, shock, and disbelief in the client. Physical impairment may be greater, and quality of life may be limited because of disease or treatment. The client who previously projected an optimistic outlook may now express a more guarded attitude. Maintain open communication and be sensitive to the informational and support needs of the client and family.

Palliative treatment and palliative care are two distinct options for the client whose cancer persists. *Palliative care* is the provision of manifestation management and psychosocial support, best offered by a multidisciplinary health care team. In the past, palliative care was linked solely to terminal care. Increasingly today, professionals are recognizing the role of palliative care for incorporating quality-of-life outcomes for clients throughout the course of their illness.[70] Surgery, RT, or chemotherapy may be used to palliate complications caused by persistent tumor growth. For example, surgery may be used to manage a malignant obstruction, or RT to prevent paralysis from spinal cord compression. Palliative treatment is not curative but, rather, is aimed at improving the quality of the remainder of the client's life, however long or short.

Communicate to the client that disease manifestations can be managed successfully and that resources are available to assist in providing supplies and support. Palliative care is effective in decreasing the stress and discomfort related to advanced cancer and offers the client and family options to help them as the disease enters the terminal phase.

TERMINAL ILLNESS

About 50% of clients with cancer still eventually die of their disease. The time from diagnosis to death ranges from weeks to years. Not all clients with cancer become terminally ill. Some clients die during the initial treatment; others die of complications of treatment. Many, however, reach an end-point at which their cancer no longer responds to treatment and progression of the disease cannot be controlled. Then, the goal of treatment is directed toward providing supportive care and minimizing distress until death occurs.

In the United States since the mid-1970s, hospice care has become the standard of care for terminally ill clients with cancer. The philosophy of hospice care emphasizes symptom control and pain management, providing comfort and dignity to enable the client to live fully until death.

In medieval times, hospices were way stations for travelers and pilgrims. Most were run by Christian religious orders. The Irish Sisters of Charity opened the first hospice specifically for the dying in the mid-19th century in London. However, it was not until 1967, when Dame Cicely Saunders opened the St. Christopher's Hospice in

---

BOX 19–6	Cancer-Related Resources

The following are a few key resources for the nurse to obtain information and share with the client with cancer.

Oncology Nursing Society (ONS)
501 Holiday Dr.
Pittsburgh, PA 15220-2749
(412) 921-7373
http://www.ons.org

Office of Cancer Communications
National Cancer Institute
Building 31, Room 11A52
Bethesda, MD 20892-4200
1-800-4-CANCER
http://www.nci.nih.gov
http://cancernet.nci.nih.gov

American Cancer Society (ACS)
1599 Clifton Rd. NE
Atlanta, GA 30333-3329
1-800-ACS-2345
http://www.cancer.org/frames/html

National Coalition for Cancer Survivorship
1010 Wayne Ave., 5th Floor
Silver Spring, MD 20910
(301) 650-8868
http://www.cansearch.org

Oncolink University of Pennsylvania
http://www.oncolink.upenn.edu

National Library of Medicine
http://www.nlm.nih.gov

London and pioneered techniques for adequate pain control, that the modern concept of hospice care emerged.[71]

The first hospice in the United States was established in 1974 in New Haven, Connecticut. Since that time, more than 1600 hospice programs have been established in the United States. A hospice can be affiliated with a hospital, community, home care agency, or skilled nursing facility. Care can be provided in the home, an inpatient hospital, or a separate facility such as a nursing home. The basic characteristics of a hospice program are:

- Control of manifestations, including pain relief
- Treatment of the client and family as a unit
- Provision of care by an interdisciplinary team
- 24-hour, 7-day-a-week services
- Coordinated home care with back-up inpatient services
- Use of trained volunteers to augment staff services
- Spiritual support
- Bereavement follow-up
- Services given on the basis of need and not ability to pay
- Structured systems of staff support

Community-based hospices also incorporate services such as nursing care, educating the family in basic nursing skills, family respite care, running errands, shopping, light housework, transportation, provision of medical equipment, and assistance to enable the client to choose to die at home. To qualify for hospice services, clients must have a life expectancy of less than 6 months and must be receiving supportive treatment only.

Clients approach death in as many ways as they approach life. Some try to remain active despite tremendous physical limitations. Others may withdraw into depression. This period is a time of suffering for both client and family as the physical loss of function and the psychological pain of anticipated and real losses in relationships and roles are intensified. See Chapter 22 for an in-depth discussion of end-of-life nursing care for the terminally ill client.

Masterful use of basic nursing skills, combined with creative management of manifestations and compassion for the client and family, is the essence of hospice nursing care. Nursing care remains the mainstay for the client and significant others. Beyond what machines and medicines and procedures can do for the client, the act of caring remains a powerful weapon in the fight against disease. It is the one thing that technology can never replace. When everything is done that can be done, compassion is the only thing that brings beauty and meaning to our lives. It is the irreplaceable gift.

CONCLUSIONS

Cancer therapy has progressed rapidly in the last half of the 20th century. Many cancers once considered incurable are now controlled with a variety of combination therapies. Even when cancer is not cured, length of life may be extended. Importantly, the quality of the extended length of life has also greatly improved. Professionals have greater knowledge of and skills in controlling pain and managing nausea and vomiting due to chemotherapy, and there are more options for helping clients cope with hair loss.

The hospice movement has demonstrated that there is still much that can be done for a client with cancer, even when cure is no longer possible. The survivorship movement has made visible the hopeful side of cancer as well as being a resource to clients in dealing with insurance, workplace, and other issues.

New treatment modalities are showing promise in clinical trials, with some already becoming standard care. The nurse in the 21st century needs to stay abreast of new developments in this rapidly expanding field.

THINKING CRITICALLY

1. **You are a nurse working in a health clinic that focuses on prevention of disease. This month, the featured goal is cancer prevention. How will you assess each client for cancer risk factors?**

Factors to Consider. How would you develop an assessment tool for the clinic nurses to use? How would you adapt teaching strategies to the cultural group being served? What teaching can help clients avoid factors that increase their risk for cancer?

2. **The client is a 22-year-old man who comes to the neighborhood health clinic with concern that his companion, who has pain and a lump in the right testicle, may have testicular cancer. The companion is at home. What teaching should be completed during this visit? What psychosocial concerns would the client and the companion have?**

Factors to Consider. What diagnostic studies should you anticipate? What care should be given to the client awaiting diagnosis after cancer testing?

3. **C. H. is a 54-year-old engineer responsible for grading, paving, and asphalting of county road surfaces. He is admitted for evaluation of chest pain and increasing shortness of breath. Because of a history of quadruple bypass surgery when he was 44, he assumes that he has additional coronary artery blockage. He has continued to smoke despite his cardiac history. Several members of his mother's family and his father died of cancer. He has lung cancer that has metastasized to the brain. He will be treated with chemotherapy and RT. What risk factors did C. H. have for lung cancer? What teaching should the nurse plan for him? What long-term plans should the nurse consider for him?**

Factors to Consider. How will this client's cardiac history affect his chemotherapy regimen? What oncologic emergencies does C. H. face? Why is he not a surgical candidate?

BIBLIOGRAPHY

1. Abel, L. J., et al. (1999). Nursing management of patients receiving brachytherapy for early stage prostate cancer. *Clinical Journal of Oncology Nursing, 3*(1), 7–15.
2. Almadrones, L., Campana, P., & Dantis, E. C. (1995). Arterial, peritoneal, and intraventricular access devices. *Seminars in Oncology Nursing, 11*(3), 194–202.

3. American Cancer Society. (2000). *Cancer facts and figures—2000*. Atlanta: Author.

4. Averette, H. D., et al. (1990). Effects of cancer chemotherapy on gonadal and reproductive capacity. *CA: A Cancer Journal for Clinicians, 40*, 199–209.

5. Bailey, S. S. (1997). The arts in spiritual care. *Seminars in Oncology Nursing, 13*(4), 242–247.

6. Beauchamp, K. A. (1998). Pericardial tamponade: An oncologic emergency. *Clinical Journal of Oncology Nursing, 2*(3), 85–95.

7. Beck, S. L. (1996). Mucositis. In S. L. Groenwald, et al. (Eds.), *Cancer symptom management* (pp. 308–324). Boston: Jones & Bartlett.

8. Berger, A., Portenoy, R. K., & Weissman, D. E. (1998). *Principles and practice of supportive oncology*. Philadelphia: Lippincott-Raven.

9. Boyle, D. M., & Engelking, C. (1995). Vesicant extravasation: Myths and realities. *Oncology Nursing Forum, 22*(1), 57–66.

10. Brown-Saltzman, K. (1997). Replenishing the spirit by meditative prayer and guided imagery. *Seminars in Oncology Nursing, 13*(4), 255–259.

11. Bruner, D. W. (1998). Cost-effectiveness and palliative care. *Seminars in Oncology Nursing, 14*(2), 164–167.

12. Bruner, D. W., & Iwamoto, R. R. (1996). Altered sexual health. In S. L. Groenwald et al. (Eds.), *Cancer symptom management* (pp. 523–551). Boston: Jones & Bartlett.

13. Bruner, D. W., et al. (1992). *Manual for radiation oncology nursing practice*. Pittsburgh, PA: Oncology Nursing Press.

14. Burke, M. B., et al. (Eds.). (1996). *Cancer chemotherapy: A nursing process approach* (2nd ed). Boston: Jones & Bartlett.

15. Camp-Sorrell, D. (1996). *Access device guidelines: Recommendations for nursing practice and education*. Pittsburgh, PA: Oncology Nursing Press.

16. Cartmel, B., & Reid, M. (1997). Cancer control and epidemiology. In S. Groenwald, et al. (Eds.), *Cancer nursing: Principles and practice* (4th ed., pp. 50–74). Boston: Jones & Bartlett.

17. Clark, P. M., & Lacasse, C. (1998). Cancer-related fatigue: Clinical practice issues. *Clinical Journal of Oncology Nursing, 2*(2), 45–53.

18. Cohen, R., & Frank-Stromberg, M. (1997). Cancer risk and assessment. In S. Groenwald, et al. (Eds.), *Cancer nursing: Principles and practice* (4th ed., pp. 108–132). Boston: Jones & Bartlett.

19. Curtiss, C. P. (1996). Constipation. In S. Groenwald, et al. (Eds.), *Cancer symptom management* (pp. 484–497). Boston: Jones & Bartlett.

20. Dockery, V. G., & Ellis, C. (1999). Sexual dysfunction. *American Journal of Nursing*, April Supplement, 28–30.

21. Dow, K. H. (1992). Principles of brachytherapy. In K. H. Dow & L. J. Hilderley (Eds.), *Nursing care in radiation oncology* (pp. 16–29). Philadelphia: W. B. Saunders.

22. Dow, K. H., & Hilderley, L. J. (Eds.) (1992). *Nursing care in radiation oncology*. Philadelphia: W. B. Saunders.

23. Eisenberg, D. M., et al. (1998). Trends in alternative medicine use in the United States, 1990–1997. *JAMA, 280*(18), 1569–1575.

24. Ezzone, S., et al. (1998). Music as an adjunct to antiemetic therapy. *Oncology Nursing Forum, 25*(9), 1551–1556.

25. Finley, J. P. (1998). Hypercalcemia. In C. R. Ziegfeld, B. G. Lubejko, & B. K. Shelton (Eds.), *Manual of cancer care* (pp. 425–430). Philadelphia: Lippincott–Williams & Wilkins.

26. Finley, J. P. (1998). Syndrome of inappropriate ADH (SIADH). In C. R. Ziegfeld, B. G. Lubejko, & B. K. Shelton (Eds.), *Manual of cancer care* (pp. 431–435). Philadelphia: Lippincott–Williams & Wilkins.

27. Fischer, B., et al. (1998). Tamoxifen for prevention of breast cancer: Report of the National Surgical Adjuvant Breast and Bowel Project P-1 study. *Journal of the National Cancer Institute, 90*, 1371–1388.

28. Fisher, G. (1997). Bone metastases: Part I—pathophysiology. *Clinical Journal of Oncology Nursing, 1*(2), 29–35.

29. Fleming, I. D., et al. (Eds.). (1997). *AJCC cancer staging manual*. (5th ed.). Philadelphia: Lippincott-Raven.

30. Frank-Stromberg, M. (1997). Cancer screening and early detection. In C. Varricchio, et al. (Eds.), *A cancer source book for nurses* (7th ed., pp. 56–66). Boston: Jones & Bartlett.

31. Fukuyama, S. N., & Itano, J. (1999). Thrombocytopenia secondary to myelosuppression. *American Journal of Nursing*, April Supplement, 5–12.

32. Gates, M. F., Lackey, N. R., & White, M. R. (1995). Needs of hospice and clinic patients with cancer. *Cancer Practice, 3*(4), 226–232.

33. Greco, F. A. (Ed.). (1996). *Handbook of commonly used chemotherapy regimens*. Chicago: Precept Press.

34. Groenwald, S., et al. (Eds.). (1997). *Cancer nursing: Principles and practice* (4th ed). Boston: Jones & Bartlett.

35. Groenwald, S. L., et al. (Eds.). (1996). *Cancer symptom management*. Boston: Jones & Bartlett.

36. Groopman, J. (1997). *The measure of our days: New beginnings at life's end*. New York: Viking.

37. Heusinkveld, K. B. (1997). Cancer prevention and risk assessment. In C. Varricchio, et al. (Eds.), *A cancer source book for nurses* (7th ed., pp. 35–42). Boston: Jones & Bartlett.

38. Hood, L. A., & Abernathy, E. (1996). Biological response modifiers. In R. McCorkle, et al. (Eds.), *Cancer nursing: A comprehensive text* (2nd ed., pp. 434–457). Philadelphia: W. B. Saunders.

39. Howser, D. M. (1996). Alopecia. In S. Groenwald, et al. (Eds.), *Cancer symptom management* (pp. 261–268). Boston: Jones & Bartlett.

40. Ignatavicius, D., Workman, M. L., & Mishler, M. (1999). *Medical-surgical nursing across the health care continuum* (3rd ed). Philadelphia: W. B. Saunders.

41. Ingle, R. (1995). Rare complications of vascular access devices. *Seminars in Oncology Nursing, 11*(3), 184–193.

42. Jassak, P. F. (1997). Biotherapy. In S. Groenwald, et al. (Eds.), *Cancer nursing: Principles and practice* (4th ed., pp. 366–392). Boston: Jones & Bartlett.

43. Jones, L. A. (1996). Electrolyte imbalances. In S. Groenwald, et al. (Eds.), *Cancer symptom management* (pp. 415–432). Boston: Jones & Bartlett.

44. Kaempfer, S. H., et al. (1985). Fertility considerations and procreative alternatives in cancer care. *Seminars in Oncology Nursing, 1*(1), 25–34.

45. Klemm, P., & Nolan, M. T. (1998). Internet cancer support groups: Legal and ethical issues for nurse researchers. *Oncology Nursing Forum, 25*(4), 673–676.

46. Kosier, M. B., & Minkler, P. (1999). Nursing management of patients with an implanted Ommaya reservoir. *Clinical Journal of Oncology Nursing, 3*(2), 63–67.

47. Kolcaba, K., & Fox, C. (1999). The effects of guided imagery on comfort of women with early stage breast cancer undergoing radiation therapy. *Oncology Nursing Forum, 26*(1), 67–72.

48. Larouere, E. (1999). The art of accessing an implanted port. *Nursing 99, 29*(5), 56–58.

49. Lehna, C. (1999). Storytelling in practice: Part one—mother's stories. *Journal of Hospice and Palliative Nursing, 1*(1), 21–25.

50. Lehna, C. (1999). Storytelling in practice: Part two—professional storytelling. *Journal of Hospice and Palliative Nursing, 1*(1), 27–30.

51. Lerner, M. (1996). *Choices in healing: Integrating the best of conventional and complementary approaches to cancer*. Cambridge: The MIT Press.

52. Lewis, F. M. (1998). Family-level service in oncology nursing: Facts, fallacies, and realities revisited. *Oncology Nursing Forum, 25*(8), 1377–1388.

53. Loescher, L. (1997). Dynamics of cancer prevention. In S. Groenwald, et al. (Eds.), *Cancer nursing: Principles and practice* (4th ed., pp. 94–107). Boston: Jones & Bartlett.

54. Lucas, A. B. (1992). A critical review of venous access devices: The nursing perspective. *Current Issues in Cancer Nursing Practice, 1*(7), 1–10.

55. McNally, J. C., et al. (Eds.). (1991). *Guidelines for oncology nursing practice*. Philadelphia: W. B. Saunders.

56. Martz, C. H. (1996). Diarrhea. In S. Groenwald, et al. (Eds.), *Cancer symptom management* (pp. 498–520). Boston: Jones & Bartlett.

57. Mayer, D. K. (1997). Bone metastases: Part II. Nursing management. *Clinical Journal of Oncology Nursing, 1*(2), 37–44.

58. Moore, K. (1998). Out-of-pocket expenditures of outpatients receiving chemotherapy. *Oncology Nursing Forum, 25*(9), 1615–1622.

59. Mullan, F. (1985). Seasons of survival: Reflections of a physician with cancer. *New England Journal of Medicine, 313*, 270–273.

60. National Cancer Institute. (1997). *Chemotherapy and you: A guide to self help during treatment*. (NIH Pub. No. 97–1136). Washington, D.C.: U.S. Government Printing Office.

61. National Cancer Institute. (1997). *Eating hints for cancer patients*. (NIH Pub. No. 97–2079). Washington, D.C.: U.S. Government Printing Office.

62. National Cancer Institute. (1997). *Radiation therapy and you: A guide to self-help during treatment.* (NIH Pub. No. 97–2227). Washington, D.C.: U.S. Government Printing Office.

63. National Cancer Institute. (1997). *Taking time: Support for people with cancer and the people who care about them.* (NIH Pub. No. 97–2059). Washington, D.C.: U.S. Government Printing Office.

64. National Cancer Institute. (1998). *Taking part in clinical trials: What cancer patients need to know.* (NIH Pub. No. 98–4250). Washington, D.C.: U.S. Government Printing Office.

65. Nelson, N. J. (1997). Studies show prophylactic surgeries seem to reduce cancer risk. *Journal of the National Cancer Institute, 89*(11), 762–763.

66. Nunez, A. M., & Liebman, M. C. (1999). Febrile neutropenia. *American Journal of Nursing,* April Supplement, 9–12.

67. Oncology Nursing Society. (1992). *Cancer chemotherapy guidelines: Recommendations for the management of vesicant extravasation, hypersensitivity, and anaphylaxis.* Pittsburgh, PA: Author.

68. Occupational Safety and Health Administration. (1995). *Workplace guidelines for personnel dealing with cytotoxic (antineoplastic) drugs.* (OSHA Instruction CPL 2–2.20B CH-4, 21-1–21-34). Washington, D.C.: U.S. Government Printing Office.

69. Pasacreta, J. V., & Pickett, M. (1998). Psychosocial aspects of palliative care. *Seminars in Oncology Nursing, 14*(2), 110–120.

70. Phillips, J., Belcher, A., & O'Neil, J. A. (1997). Special populations. In C. Varricchio, et al. (Eds.), *A cancer source book for nurses* (7th ed., pp. 56–66). Boston: Jones & Bartlett.

71. Pickett, M., Cooley, M. E., & Gordon, D. B. (1998). Palliative care: Past, present, and future perspectives. *Seminars in Oncology Nursing, 14*(2), 86–94.

72. Pickett, M., et al. (2000). Prostate cancer elder alert: Living with treatment choices and outcomes. *Journal of Gerontological Nursing, 26*(2), 22–34.

73. Pinover, W. H., & Cioa, L. R. (1998). Palliative radiation therapy. In A. M. Berger, R. K. Portenoy, & D. E. Weisman (Eds.), *Principles and practices of supportive oncology* (pp. 618–623). Philadelphia: Lippincott-Raven.

74. Post-White, J. (1998). Wind behind the sails: Empowering our patients and ourselves. *Oncology Nursing Forum, 25*(6), 1011–1017.

75. Potter, K. L., & Schafer, S. L. (1999). Nausea and vomiting: One of the most distressing chemotherapy-related symptoms. *American Journal of Nursing,* April Supplement, 2–4.

76. Powel, L. L. (1996). *Cancer chemotherapy guidelines and recommendations for practice.* Pittsburgh, PA: Oncology Nursing Press.

77. Pruett, J. (1996). Bleeding. In S. L. Groenwald, et al. (Eds.), *Cancer symptom management,* (pp. 269–288). Boston: Jones & Bartlett.

78. Rieger, P. T. (1996). Biotherapy: The fourth modality. In M. B. Burke, et al. (Eds.), *Cancer chemotherapy: A nursing process approach* (2nd ed., pp. 43–73.) Boston: Jones & Bartlett.

79. Robinson, D. (1997). Family stress theory: Implications for family health. *Journal of the American Academy of Nurse Practitioners, 9*(1), 17–23.

80. Rumsey, K. A., & Rieger, P. T. (Eds.). (1992). *Biological response modifiers: A self-instruction manual for health professionals.* Chicago: Precept Press.

81. Rumsey, K. A., & Richardson, D. K. (1995). Management of infection and occlusion associated with vascular access devices. *Seminars in Oncology Nursing, 11*(3), 174–183.

82. Rust, D. M., Wood, L. S., & Battiato, L. A. (1999). Oprelvekin: An alternative treatment for thrombocytopenia. *Clinical Journal of Oncology Nursing, 3*(2), 57–62.

83. Schulmeister, L. (1997). Preventing chemotherapy dose and schedule errors. *Clinical Journal of Oncology Nursing, 1*(3), 79–85.

84. Sheidler, V. R. (1998). Pain. In C. R. Ziegfeld, B. G. Lubejko, & B. K. Shelton (Eds.), *Manual of cancer care* (pp. 369–385). Philadelphia: Lippincott–Williams & Wilkins.

85. Shelton, B. K. (1998). Spinal cord compression. In C. R. Ziegfeld, B. G. Lubejko, & B. K. Shelton (Eds.), *Manual of cancer care* (pp. 410–419). Philadelphia: Lippincott–Williams & Wilkins.

86. Shelton, B. K. (1998). Anemia. In C. R. Ziegfeld, B. G. Lubejko, & B. K. Shelton (Eds.), *Manual of cancer care* (pp. 231–243). Philadelphia: Lippincott–Williams & Wilkins.

87. Sigley, T. (1998). Nutritional problems. In C. R. Ziegfeld, B. G. Lubejko, & B. K. Shelton (Eds.), *Manual of cancer care* (pp. 349–368). Philadelphia: Lippincott–Williams & Wilkins.

88. Somerville, E. T. (1991). Knowledge deficit related to chemotherapy. In J. C. McNally, J. Campbell Stair, & E. T. Somerville (Eds.), *Guidelines for cancer nursing practice* (2nd ed., pp. 36–39). Philadelphia: W. B. Saunders.

89. Taylor, E. J. (1997). The story behind the story: The use of storytelling in spiritual caregiving. *Seminars in Oncology Nursing, 13*(4), 252–254.

90. Tenenbaum, L., Leshin, D., & Hydzik, C. (1994). Other systems affected by chemotherapy and biotherapy. In L. Tenenbaum (Ed.), *Cancer chemotherapy and biotherapy: A reference guide* (2nd ed., pp. 371–408). Philadelphia: W. B. Saunders.

91. Tortorice, P. T. (1997). Chemotherapy: Principles of therapy. In S. Groenwald, et al. (Eds.), *Cancer nursing: Principles and practice* (4th ed., pp. 283–316). Boston: Jones & Bartlett.

92. U.S. Department of Health and Human Services. (1996). *Facing forward: A guide for cancer survivors.* (NIH Pub. No. 96–2424). Washington, D.C.: National Cancer Institute.

93. Vanderhoof, D. D., & Brant, J. M. (1999). Alopecia: The forgotten side effect? *American Journal of Nursing,* April Supplement, 17–19.

94. Varricchio, C., et al. (1997). *A cancer source book for nurses* (7th ed). Boston: Jones & Bartlett.

95. Weisman, A. (1979). *Coping with cancer.* New York: McGraw-Hill.

96. Wilkes, G. M. (1996). Neurological disturbances. In: S. Groenwald, et al. (Eds.), *Cancer symptom management* (pp. 324–363). Boston: Jones & Bartlett.

97. Winningham, M. L. (1996). Fatigue. In S. Groenwald, et al. (Eds.), *Cancer symptom management* (pp. 42–54). Boston: Jones & Bartlett.

98. Wujcik, D. (1996). Infection. In S. Groenwald, et al. (Eds.), *Cancer symptom management* (pp. 289–302). Boston: Jones & Bartlett.

99. Zewekh, J. V. (1997). The practice of presencing. *Seminars in Oncology Nursing, 13*(4), 260–262.

100. Ziegfeld, C. R., Lubejko, B. G., & Shelton, B. K. (1998). *Oncology fact finder: Manual of cancer care.* Philadelphia: Lippincott–Williams & Wilkins.

CHAPTER 20

Clients with Psychosocial and Mental Health Concerns: Promoting Positive Outcomes

Nancy Shoemaker

NURSING OUTCOMES CLASSIFICATION (NOC)
for Nursing Diagnoses—Clients with Psychosocial and Mental Health Concerns

Altered Thought Processes
Cognitive Ability
Cognitive Orientation
Communication Ability
Concentration
Decision Making
Distorted Thought Control
Identity
Information Processing
Memory
Risk Control: Alcohol Use
Risk Control: Drug Use
Safety Behavior: Personal
Anxiety
Acceptance: Health Status
Aggression Control
Anxiety Control
Coping
Impulse Control
Psychosocial Adjustment: Life Change
Self-Mutilation Restraint
Social Interaction Skills
Symptom Control
Body Image Disturbance
Acceptance: Health Status
Distorted Thought Control
Self-Esteem
Self-Mutilation Restraint
Social Involvement
Hopelessness
Comfort Level
Coping
Decision Making
Depression Control
Depression Level
Hope
Mood Equilibrium

Quality of Life
Sleep
Spiritual Well-Being
Ineffective Individual Coping
Aggression Control
Caregiver Emotional Health
Caregiver-Patient Relationship
Caregiver Well-Being
Depression Control
Depression Level
Family Coping
Family Environment: Internal
Family Normalization
Family Health Status
Knowledge Deficit
Cognitive Ability
Communication Reception: Receptive
    Ability
Concentration
Information Processing
Knowledge: Disease Process
Knowledge: Health Resources
Knowledge: Medication
Knowledge: Treatment Regimen
Memory
Risk for Self-Directed Violence
Cognitive Ability
Depression Control
Depression Level
Distorted Thought Control
Impulse Control
Loneliness
Mood Equilibrium
Quality of Life
Risk Control
Risk Control: Alcohol Use

Risk Control: Drug Use
Risk Detection
Self-Mutilation Restraint
Suicide Self-Restraint
Will to Live
Risk for Violence Directed at Others
Abuse Protection
Abusive Behavior Self-Control
Aggression Control
Cognitive Ability
Depression Control
Distorted Thought Control
Impulse Control
Quality of Life
Risk Control
Risk Control: Alcohol Use
Risk Control: Drug Use
Risk Detection
Self-Care Deficit
Self Care: Activities of Daily Living (ADL)
Self Direction of Care
Self-Esteem Disturbance
Body Image
Hope
Mood Equilibrium
Role Performance
Self-Esteem
Social Interaction Skills
Spiritual Distress
Anxiety Control
Hope
Quality of Life
Spiritual Well-Being
Suicide Self-Restraint
Well-Being
Will to Live

A sound knowledge base for responding to psychosocial and mental health concerns of clients and their families is vital in all settings where medical-surgical nursing is practiced. Psychosocial components are defined as the psychological and social aspects of the client's health status. Psychological factors include thinking, feelings, motivation, and personal strengths and weaknesses. Social issues are related to patterns of interaction with others (see also Chapter 9). For all clients seeking health care for a physical problem, there is a potential for alteration in their mental or emotional status because of the stress of illness and navigating the health care system. The North American Nursing Diagnosis Association (NANDA) currently lists 149 approved nursing diagnoses; approximately 41% are related to psychosocial functioning (see Box 20–1). To promote successful health outcomes, the nurse must address the psychosocial and mental health concerns of each client.

Some clients have a pre-existing mental disorder that may complicate or adversely affect the outcome of their medical treatment. At least 50 million Americans live with a mental illness at any given time.[23] In any one year, 23 million people suffer from anxiety disorders; 8 million more are affected by major depression; and 2.5 million are afflicted with schizophrenia.[8, 10, 25] For these clients, nursing attention to psychosocial needs makes the difference between compliance with treatment and noncompliance with resulting complications.

This chapter focuses on the psychosocial concerns of clients and families that require nursing care across various treatment settings. Basic principles regarding communication are outlined, and nursing interventions to reduce anxiety are presented. Concepts of anxiety, stress, coping mechanisms, and self-esteem are reviewed. Five clients with concurrent medical disorders and serious mental illness are discussed in order to illustrate the challenge that these individuals present for holistic nursing care. In each case, the role of the medical-surgical nurse is presented along with a suggested nursing care plan. Finally, the dimensions of culture, spirituality, and sexuality are addressed in relation to specific clients. Chapter 9 describes how to obtain a psychosocial history as part of the comprehensive nursing assessment.

Client Scenarios

Picture yourself as the nurse responsible for the clients in the following scenarios. These scenarios will help illustrate the later discussion of psychosocial and mental health issues and their application in nursing care across a variety of clinical settings.

1. You work the 3 to 11 PM shift in the emergency department (ED). You are assigned to Mrs. Barbara James, a 51-year-old black woman admitted several hours ago with acute chest pain and respiratory distress. Initial diagnostic tests to rule out myocardial infarction are negative, but final laboratory re-

---

BOX 20–1   **NANDA 1998–2000 Nursing Diagnoses Related to Adult Psychosocial Concerns**

Adjustment, Impaired
Anxiety
Body Image Disturbance
Caregiver Role Strain
Caregiver Role Strain, Risk for
Communication, Impaired Verbal
Coping, Community: Potential for Enhanced
Coping, Defensive
Coping, Family: Potential for Growth
Coping, Ineffective Community
Coping, Ineffective Family: Compromised
Coping, Ineffective Family: Disabling
Coping, Ineffective Individual
Death Anxiety
Decisional Conflict (Specify)
Denial, Ineffective
Energy Field Disturbance
Family Processes: Altered
Family Processes, Altered: Alcoholism
Fatigue
Fear
Grieving, Anticipatory
Grieving, Dysfunctional
Health Maintenance, Altered
Health Seeking Behaviors (Specify)
Home Maintenance Management, Impaired
Hopelessness
Loneliness, Risk for
Noncompliance
Parental Role Conflict
Parenting, Altered

Parenting, Risk for Altered
Personal Identity Disturbance
Post-Trauma Syndrome
Post-Trauma Syndrome, Risk for
Powerlessness
Rape-Trauma Syndrome
Rape-Trauma Syndrome: Compound Reaction
Rape-Trauma Syndrome: Silent Reaction
Relocation Stress Syndrome
Role Performance, Altered
Self Esteem Disturbance
Self Esteem, Chronic Low
Self Esteem, Situational Low
Self-Mutilation, Risk for
Sensory Perceptual Alterations (Specify: visual, auditory, kinesthetic, gustatory, tactile, olfactory)
Sexual Dysfunction
Sexuality Patterns, Altered
Social Interaction, Impaired
Social Isolation
Sorrow, Chronic
Spiritual Distress
Spiritual Distress, Risk for
Spiritual Well-Being, Potential for Enhanced
Therapeutic Regimen: Community, Ineffective Management
Therapeutic Regimen: Families, Ineffective Management
Therapeutic Regimen: Individuals, Ineffective Management
Thought Processes, Altered
Tissue Perfusion, Altered (cerebral)
Violence, Risk for: Self-Directed or Directed at Others

NANDA, North American Nursing Diagnosis Association.

sults are pending. When you introduce yourself to Mrs. James, she is crying and states, "I can't believe my heart is okay. This must be a heart attack. It can't be my nerves."

2. While on duty in a busy university medical clinic, you see a client with a recently diagnosed first-time hiatal hernia. Gregory Barnes is a 32-year-old, slightly obese black man who smiles pleasantly as you introduce yourself and shakes your hand. When you ask Mr. Barnes to describe his problem, he responds, "I don't get enough food. My stomach is connected to the elves in my basement, and they take all of my food as soon as I eat it." You notice Mr. Barnes' elderly mother sitting in the waiting room.

3. You are a staff nurse on a medical acute care unit. Returning from 2 days off, you are assigned to Mrs. Mary Conners, a 59-year-old West Indian woman admitted the previous day with diabetic ketoacidosis. Entering her room, you notice that the lights are off. She does not look up when you speak to her. When Mrs. Conners answers your second greeting, her voice is in a monotone and she quickly looks away. You observe several jars of food on her table. The admitting nurse states that Mrs. Conners had been verbal on admission and that her daughter seems very concerned about her.

4. As a home care nurse, you have recently started caring for Mr. John Moore, a 66-year-old white man who has had a second stroke. You completed his medication teaching quickly because he was familiar with most of his medicines. For the past few weeks, you have been supervising the home health aide while the physical therapist works on gait training. Today, you receive a call from the physical therapist who reports, "I don't know what to do with Mr. Moore. He has the strength to do his exercises, but he just won't try. I may have to discharge him for noncompliance."

5. You are the charge nurse in a long-term skilled nursing facility. As you are making morning rounds, one nursing assistant stops you to complain about Miss Celia Howard. She is a 75-year-old white woman who has been in your facility for 2 years because of multiple cardiac problems and the inability to care for herself. Recently hospitalized for acute dehydration, she returned 3 days ago. There has been a change in her behavior. Miss Howard is cursing and spitting at staff, and today she pushed her roommate out of the room. You remember that she was seeing the consultant psychiatrist in the past, but when you examine the chart, you note that her psychotropic medications have been discontinued.

UNIVERSAL ISSUES

Universal psychosocial concepts include anxiety, stress, coping mechanisms, and self-esteem. Additional factors that influence reactions to stress are cultural and family background, exposure to similar stressors, and repeated exposure to stressors.

■ ANXIETY

Before addressing the psychosocial concerns of clients with concurrent mental disorders, the nurse must first develop skills to manage the anxiety that is common to all clients. *Anxiety* is a universal human phenomenon, defined as a strong feeling of fear or dread with an unknown cause. All clients (and their loved ones) are vulnerable to feeling anxiety as they seek care for medical problems. Not only clients but everyone may feel anxiety at times, especially when facing an unknown situation (changing schools, starting a new job). Under normal conditions, this discomfort is short-lived and may be helpful for problem solving. Box 20–2 describes possible emotional, physical, and spiritual manifestations of anxiety.

■ STRESS

Anxiety is part of the human reaction to stress. *Stress* is defined as "a particular relationship between the person and the environment that is appraised by the person as taxing and/or exceeding his or her resources and endangering his or her well-being."[20] Resources can include one's coping skills. In the case of potential physical danger, one is mobilized for self-protection with the fight-or-flight response. Most people would experience strong reactions in the face of crisis situations such as an imminent car accident or a tornado. In addition to external stressful events, people may define stress in different ways because it is the perception of the event, not the event itself, that stimulates the response. For example, one student may feel extreme stage fright when giving a speech, whereas another may feel only mild tension. Table 20–1 describes the levels of anxiety with implications for client teaching.

BOX 20–2   **Emotional, Physical, and Spiritual Manifestations of Anxiety**

Emotional

Fearful
Helpless
Sense of impending doom
Insecure
Irritable
Fatigued
Lack of self-confidence

Physical

Increased blood pressure
Increased pulse
Increased respirations
Chest pain or tightness
Muscle tension
Excessive sweating
Dry mouth or nausea
Diarrhea or increased urination

Spiritual

Hopeless
Feeling abandoned by God
Blaming God for the suffering

TABLE 20–1	MANIFESTATIONS OF FOUR LEVELS OF ANXIETY		
Anxiety Level	Physical Manifestations	Emotional Manifestations	Cognitive Manifestations
Mild	Increased pulse and blood pressure	Positive affect	Alert, can solve a problem, prepared to learn new information
Moderate	Elevated vital signs, tense muscles, diaphoresis	Tense, fearful	Attention focused on one concern, may be able to concentrate with direction
Severe	Fight-or-flight response, dry mouth, numb extremities	Distressed	Decreased sensory perception, can focus only on details, unable to learn new information
Panic	Continued as in severe level	Totally overwhelmed	Ignores external cues, focused only on internal stimuli, unable to learn

Regardless of the source of the stressor, a person's reaction to acute stress follows a predictable course.[15] When the brain perceives a threat, the sympathetic nervous system releases epinephrine and norepinephrine within 2 or 3 seconds. The hypothalamus responds by secreting corticotropin-releasing hormone (CRH), which activates the pituitary gland to secrete adrenocorticotropic hormone (ACTH). ACTH stimulates the adrenal glands to produce the steroid hormone cortisol (the "stress hormone"). Throughout this process, various organs are affected throughout the body, creating physical effects such as elevated vital signs and dry mouth. Within 10 minutes, usually the high level of cortisol triggers the hypothalamus and pituitary to cease production of CRH and ACTH to end the acute stress response.

■ COPING MECHANISMS

Most people respond to anxiety by using *coping skills* that are learned external behaviors or internal thought processes consciously used to decrease discomfort. Coping behavior can be classified as follows[30]:

- *Emotion-focused* behaviors include thinking, saying, or doing something to make oneself feel better (crying, sharing feelings with someone)
- *Problem-focused* behaviors include seeking facts about a problem, making a plan, or studying how others have overcome similar obstacles.

Chapter 1 discusses these behaviors in more detail.

Another common response to anxiety is the use of *ego defense mechanisms,* originally defined by Freud.[31] These thought processes are not deliberate or voluntary, like coping mechanisms. Instead, they exist at an unconscious level to disguise the real threat, protecting the person from feeling anxious about the real issue. One defense mechanism frequently seen in clients with serious illness is *denial.*[29] Use of denial allows one to ignore the problematic issue and its negative consequences. For example, after hearing the diagnosis of a heart condition, a client tells the nurse that he plans to exercise as soon as he is discharged and shows no interest in learning about diet and activity limitations. Momentarily, he is protected against the distress of facing the reality of permanent changes in lifestyle. Failure to cope effectively can increase anxiety levels. See Box 20–3 for definitions and examples of selected defense mechanisms.[31]

BOX 20–3 Selected Defense Mechanisms: Definitions and Examples

Definition	Example
Denial—avoidance of a problem by ignoring or refusing to recognize it	A client with a cardiac condition tells his family that he has a "little problem" after the physician explains his diagnosis of heart attack.
Displacement—transferring feelings for a threatening topic or person to another more neutral topic or person	After a client is told that he cannot be discharged today as planned, he spends the whole shift complaining that his breakfast was cold.
Intellectualization—showing excessive thinking and logic in order to avoid uncomfortable feelings	After a leg amputation, a client shows great interest in the details of the surgery and even requests a textbook to identify the muscles and bones, but he does not watch while the nurse changes the dressing.
Projection—assigning one's own uncomfortable feelings or motivation to another person	A client tells the nurse, "Please explain about the operation again to my wife, she is so afraid that I won't wake up."
Rationalization—giving an apparently logical and acceptable explanation to cover up a feeling or motive that may not be socially acceptable	The nurse finds a client eating breakfast when he is on NPO status (nothing by mouth) for a diagnostic test. The nurse specifically told him about the procedure yesterday: when asked what happened, the client states, "Well, the aide brought me this tray so I thought it was okay."
Regression—demonstrating behavior characteristics of an earlier stage of development	An adult client insists on keeping multiple stuffed animals on her bed and bursts into tears when the nurse moves one to check her arm for intravenous access.

Assess the level of anxiety in all clients, and intervene as early as possible to try to reduce the anxiety to a manageable level. To achieve desired outcomes such as cooperation with care and compliance with discharge instructions, the client or family must be calm enough to understand the teaching. A person's anxiety level beyond the moderate range poses an emotional barrier to learning new information.[18] You can use several simple communication techniques to decrease anxiety in clients, thereby increasing the likelihood that they will benefit from health instructions. Box 20–4 lists nursing interventions that may help reduce anxiety in non-psychiatric clients.

You must also be able to recognize and support positive coping efforts by clients and their families. As noted previously, these behaviors may be emotion-focused or problem-focused, but they function to decrease anxiety. Failure to understand these behaviors may lead to nontherapeutic staff reactions. For example, a client with a new diagnosis of cancer has a wife who never leaves his bedside. She studies every action by the nurses and constantly asks questions. In addition, the client has been observed tearfully talking about his father who died of colon cancer. Several staff members have suggested that the wife have limited visiting hours because she is upsetting the client. By considering her behavior as problem-focused coping, you might involve her in teaching and allow her to participate in care as much as possible. You might also realize the client is using emotion-focused coping skills by crying and expressing his feelings of loss.

BOX 20–4   Nursing Interventions to Decrease Client Anxiety

Nonverbal Interventions	Verbal Interventions
Listen with full attention, looking at the client with unbroken eye contact.	Answer questions honestly.
Maintain a calm, unhurried approach.	Explain all procedures in simple terms.
Speak slowly in a clear, firm voice (not loud).	Give reassurance based on the data.
Offer or use touch, e.g., holding a hand or giving a back rub.	Give information about tests, medicines, and treatments as requested.
If possible, decrease the noise and bright light.	Explain the reasons for limitations on activity or other restrictions.
	Acknowledge clients' anxiety, and encourage them to explore the reasons.
	Include family members in discussions unless the client requests otherwise.
	If necessary, repeat directions patiently.

■ SELF-ESTEEM

Another universal concern that affects the client's reaction to the stress of illness is self-esteem. *Self-esteem* is defined as "the degree of worth and competence one attributes to oneself."[4] The client's pre-existing level of self-esteem strongly contributes to successful or maladaptive adjustment to illness. A person with high self-esteem shows self-confidence and positive expectations in new situations. A new medical problem may be seen as just another challenge, and the client will actively participate in learning new health behaviors. In contrast, a person with low self-esteem consistently demonstrates negative feelings about oneself and is pessimistic in new situations. The same medical diagnosis may be met with a helpless, indecisive attitude that poses a barrier to teaching and developing alternative health behaviors. Table 20–2 presents characteristics of self-esteem with implications for nursing care.

ADDITIONAL NEEDS OF CLIENTS WITH CONCURRENT MENTAL ILLNESS

After recognizing the psychosocial concerns of clients in general, you should become aware of additional needs for successful care of clients with concurrent mental illness. These needs consist of (1) comprehensive nursing assessment, (2) your self-awareness regarding communication, (3) basic mental health teaching for the client and family, and (4) referral for specialized services.

■ COMPREHENSIVE NURSING ASSESSMENT

As soon as you realize that the client is presenting with an altered mood or thought process, review the nursing database to ensure that it is complete. In many admission situations, limited data are obtained before treatment is initiated because of the severity of the manifestation or time constraints. When developing a care plan for the client with coexisting mental illness, make sure that you gather a complete psychosocial history (see Chapter 9). Significant facts concerning motor activity, mood, affect, and speech must be documented and communicated objectively. Table 20–3 lists definitions of commonly used terms to describe abnormal findings.

Psychosocial risk factors, such as a history of self-destructive, aggressive, or socially inappropriate behavior, must also be identified and documented. Secondary sources, such as family and medical records, are often helpful. Information about the client's social support system and history of mental health treatment is necessary to ensure appropriate immediate intervention and discharge planning.

In addition to the psychosocial assessment, a complete medication history provides valuable data. Some clients under treatment for anxiety or depression may not demonstrate active manifestations on admission. They usually do not volunteer that information until they are asked about the reason for taking psychotropic medications.

On the other hand, remain alert to the possibility that medication can sometimes produce psychiatric manifestations in clients without a formal diagnosis. If a client adamantly denies an emotional problem and the manifestations are of an acute onset, carefully examine prescrip-

TABLE 20–2	CHARACTERISTICS OF PEOPLE WITH HIGH AND LOW SELF-ESTEEM	
Characteristic	**High Self-Esteem**	**Low Self-Esteem**
Overall self-evaluation	Positive, "I am a good person"	Negative, "I am worthless"
Verbalization about self	Feelings of strength, pride	Feelings of weakness, shame
Perception of problem-solving ability	Self-confident, recalls past success	Insecure, dwells on past failures
Response to feedback from others	Accepts praise or criticism	Rejects praise and exaggerates criticism
Implications for nursing care	Requests active participation in care, information-seeking, makes prompt decisions	Passive involvement in care, may not ask questions, indecisive and dependent with decisions

tion and over-the-counter medication usage. Table 20–4 lists selected medicines that may cause psychiatric manifestations.[1]

■ AWARENESS OF COMMUNICATION

The second requirement in caring for psychiatric clients is to pay extra attention to all communication with them. Under ordinary circumstances, the nurse assumes that communication with clients is fairly routine and predictable, including necessary physical procedures and verbal questions, instructions, or explanations. In response, the nurse expects reactions from clients to fall within a range showing agreement, questioning, or refusing care. In es-

sence, this is the model for daily communication that many nurses take for granted.

Human communication is complex and built upon many assumptions and unspoken rules inherent in a given culture. Communication between two participants involves all of the verbal and nonverbal behavior that they perceive in each other.[38] In addition to sending words, which are carefully selected, we are simultaneously sending nonverbal signals, which are largely involuntary. Nonverbal communication includes tone and volume of voice, eye contact, facial expression, body posture, and other body language. We expect to find congruence between the words and nonverbal cues; the words match the feeling

TABLE 20–3	COMMONLY USED TERMS TO DESCRIBE ABNORMAL MENTAL STATUS FINDINGS
Term	**Mental Status Findings**
MOOD	
Depressed	Feeling sad, decreased energy and interest in usual activities
Elated	Feeling euphoric, overly optimistic, and energetic
Labile	Rapidly changing from one state to another, e.g., happy to sad or irritable
AFFECT	
Blunted	Overall decrease in emotional tone compared with a normal reaction to a situation
Flat	No expression of feelings, regardless of variation in topics
Inappropriate	Nonverbal signs of feelings do not match the verbal report of the person, e.g., person smiles when reporting sad event
MOTOR ACTIVITY	
Agitation	Physically restless, unable to sit still
Psychomotor retardation	Physically slowed down, including all movements and speech
PERCEPTION	
Hallucination	Sensory perception originating from within the brain but attributed to external sources, e.g., hearing voices
Illusion	Incorrect interpretation of external sensory input, e.g., seeing a shadow in the closet and thinking it is a person
SPEECH	
Loose association	Speech pattern where the listener cannot follow the connections between the speaker's ideas, seems illogical to listener
Pressured speech	Rapid flow of speech with intense undercurrent of feeling, may refuse to be interrupted
THOUGHT PROCESS	
Delusion	A fixed, false belief that is strongly defended by the individual, e.g., may be paranoid (suspicious) or grandiose (unrealistically wonderful)
Psychosis	Severe impairment in reality testing, with distortion in perception and analysis of external and internal stimuli

TABLE 20-4	MEDICATIONS AND SUBSTANCES THAT MAY CAUSE PSYCHIATRIC MANIFESTATIONS	
Medication	**Psychiatric Manifestations**
Anticholinergics	Disorientation, visual hallucinations, paranoia
Baclofen	Hallucinations, confusion, anxiety
Beta-adrenergic blockers	Depression, psychosis
Caffeine	Anxiety, psychosis
Calcium-channel blockers	Depression
Cephalosporins	Delusions, euphoria
Corticosteroids	Depression, mania, psychosis
DEET (diethyltoluamide [OFF])	Mania, hallucinations
Digitalis glycosides	Depression, mania, hallucinations
Fluoroquinolone antibiotics	Psychosis, agitation, depression
Histamine H_2-receptor antagonists	Confusion, aggression, psychosis
Narcotics	Dysphoria, anxiety, hallucinations
Salicylates	Agitation, confusion, paranoia
Thiazide diuretics	Depression

and tone of the body. For example, a client tells the nurse that he is in pain, and he is frowning. Another client says that she is happy about the discharge, and she is smiling. The nurse would respond to these two clients without hesitation because the verbal and nonverbal behaviors match. See Diversity in Health Care: The Significance of Cultural Assessment.

When the words and the nonverbal signs from a sender do not match, the receiving person must pause to analyze the situation. Often, this incongruent communication is the first clue that a client has a psychiatric disorder. Normal people may sometimes send a mixed message, but psychiatric clients consistently have difficulty with communicating their needs. It is generally agreed that when the verbal and the nonverbal communication are incongruent, the nonverbal communication reflects the person's true feelings.

First interactions with all clients are important. Recall Mrs. Conners' first interaction with the nurse. Looking at the words alone, the nurse greeted her and Mrs. Conners answered. The nonverbal cues—sitting in a dark room, delaying her response, and speaking in a monotone—conveyed to the nurse that this client was in an altered mental state. Conversely, Mr. Barnes' initial nonverbal communication—smiling and offering a handshake—is in stark contrast to his comment about elves in his basement.

When communicating with clients who have concurrent psychiatric problems, pay attention to the communication process for two reasons. First, thorough data must be collected to determine the nursing diagnoses and to communicate with the treatment team. Second, monitor your own nonverbal behavior to prevent sending negative nonverbal messages to the client. All clients are sensitive to the nonverbal communication of health care staff, and

psychiatric clients often expect rejection. Mental illness in our society still carries a stigma shared by clients and staff alike. Clients feel ashamed because they have an emotional problem; staff may have biases based on personal experience.[5] Recall that Mrs. James would rather believe that she has a life-threatening cardiac problem instead of an emotional problem. To communicate acceptance to these clients and to help them to overcome their self-criticism, your verbal and nonverbal communication must be congruent.

■ CLIENT AND FAMILY TEACHING

The third important requirement for all clients with concurrent psychiatric disorders is basic client and family teaching. Certainly, for the client who is receiving a new diagnosis (Mrs. James), there are many questions. Even for those who are already in treatment, their understanding about the illness and its treatment must be assessed. Basic teaching for all clients includes a definition of the illness, medications and treatment options, and relapse prevention.[26] This information is readily available in written teaching materials, which can be kept on file along with medical-surgical teaching guides. Whenever possible, include a family member in the instruction. Families often play a significant caregiver role for these clients. Repeated studies have shown that they are desperately in need of education.[40] Box 20-5 lists resources to educate and support clients and their families.

■ SPECIALIZED REFERRALS

The fourth important requirement to consider when caring for clients with concurrent mental disorders is the need for specialized referrals. Once the nursing assessment is complete, the current problems and risk factors can be analyzed. If manifestations are severe or risk factors are significant, additional evaluation is necessary. At times, this evaluation is urgent and immediate, such as when a client shows self-destructive or aggressive behavior. You are in a key position on the health care team to advocate for appropriate services. In the hospital or institutional environment, consulting psychiatric staff (nurse, social worker, psychologist, or psychiatrist) can usually be called for an in-depth assessment and disposition. Likewise, in the community setting, referrals can be made to outpatient or home care services to provide specialized care.

■ SUMMARY

The medical-surgical nurse has a clear role to play with clients who have concurrent psychiatric disorders. The four steps just outlined do not require training beyond a generalist level. They do require a professional commitment to provide holistic care to all clients and to fully utilize the multidisciplinary team available in the health care setting. There is an inherent reward in providing excellent care for clients, but the nurse is also preventing potentially serious adverse outcomes. In the managed care environment, the front-line nurse must function as the clinical manager for the client by identifying the risk for complications and coordinating efficient use of resources.[14] For example, a client with a panic disorder (such as Mrs. James) must have the diagnosis clarified on the first trip to the ED with a clear plan for follow-up. If

DIVERSITY IN HEALTH CARE

The Significance of Cultural Assessment

It is important for a nurse not only to gain adequate cultural knowledge about particular ethnic groups but also to gather information about each client's cultural background in order to provide competent care. The major focus of a cultural, or "culturalogical," assessment is to identify "culture care patterns, expressions, and meanings that reflect the client's care needs and well-being or that influence the client's patterns of illness, disabilities, or death."[5]

Nurses as well as other health caregivers must use every effort to avoid projecting onto clients their own world views and should remember that every client is a unique person who may or may not be following the beliefs and practices of his or her ethnic group. There is as much diversity within a cultural group as across cultural or ethnic groups.[3]

In performing a cultural assessment, nurses become aware of the client's beliefs and practices in health and illness and how they may enhance or interfere with an intervention or a treatment regimen. Data from a cultural assessment provide meaning to behaviors that otherwise might be judged by the caregiver as negative or confusing. Both content and process are part of a cultural assessment; the *content* covers the actual categories in which data about clients are gathered, whereas the *process* includes the techniques by which data are gathered (e.g., nonverbal and verbal communication, approach to the client, and order of elicitation of information).[1]

Various nursing authors have identified models or guides for cultural assessments.[1-3, 5-7] A helpful addition to these models is the elicitation of the client's explanatory model of his or her illness, developed by Kleinman and co-authors,[4] in which the following questions are used:

- What do you think caused your problem?
- Why do you think it started when it did?
- What do you think your sickness does to you? How does it work?
- How severe is your sickness? Will it have a short or long duration?
- What kind of treatment do you think you should receive?
- What are the most important results you hope to receive from this treatment?
- What are the chief problems your sickness has caused for you?
- What do you fear most about your sickness?

The data gathered from these questions help the nurse or other health caregiver negotiate with the client and the family about acceptable treatment and expected outcomes.

Leininger[5] noted some guidelines for an effective assessment. For instance, the nurse must maintain a role of an active listener and refrain from expressing professional opinions about the client's beliefs and practices during the assessment process. The nurse should obtain a holistic picture of the client and convey respect for beliefs. Unless the nurse can be trusted to not demean the client's beliefs, the client will not be willing to share information.

A cultural assessment, optimally, is a means to help nurses and clients communicate more effectively, to show clients that the nurse is interested and respectful of their beliefs, and to provide information that enables nursing and health care interventions to be more relevant for clients and their lifestyles. Any health teaching or treatment instructions directed toward a client must be as compatible as possible with the client's beliefs and practices if the client is expected to adhere to the treatment regimen. The client's increased adherence and satisfaction as well as the nurse's success in this endeavor are the intermediate steps desired toward the overall goal of improved client health and well-being.

References

1. Andrews, M. M., & Boyle, J. S. (1999). *Transcultural concepts in nursing care.* (3rd ed.). Philadelphia: Lippincott–Williams & Wilkins.
2. Bloch, B. (1983). Bloch's assessment guide for ethnic/cultural variations. In M. S. Orque, B. Bloch, & L. S. A. Monrroy (Eds.), *Ethnic nursing care: A multi-cultural approach* (pp. 49–75). St. Louis: C. V. Mosby.
3. Giger, J. N., & Davidhizar, R. E. (1999). *Transcultural nursing: Assessment & intervention.* (3rd ed.). St. Louis: Mosby.
4. Kleinman, A., Eisenberg, L., & Good, B. (1978). Clinical lessons from anthropological and cross-cultural research. *Annals of Internal Medicine, 88,* 251–258.
5. Leininger, M. (1995). *Transcultural nursing: Concepts, theories, research and practices* (p. 118). New York: McGraw-Hill.
6. Purnell, L. D., & Paulanka, B. (1998). *Transcultural health care: A culturally competent approach.* Philadelphia: F. A. Davis.
7. Sharma, S. (1993). Promoting cultural sensitivity in nursing practice. *Practicing Anthropology, 15*(1), 31–32.

Sandra Sharma, PhD, ARNP, CS, *James A. Haley Veterans Hospital, Tampa, Florida*

not, she is likely to return for multiple visits and even go through expensive, dangerous diagnostic tests. In the cases of Mrs. Conners and Mr. Moore, who are suffering from depression, depending on their past history of manifestations and current support systems, they may be at risk for suicide as a desperate solution to their problems.

In the sections that follow, these five psychiatric clients will be revisited in more detail. An overview of their psychiatric disorders is presented along with specific nursing care plans for management in the medical-surgical setting. For a discussion on the importance of spirituality and health, see the Alternative Therapy feature.

ANXIETY

Mrs. James presents with a classic case of panic attack. The acute manifestations can strike unexpectedly and create severe physical distress: palpitations, chest pain, elevated vital signs, dizziness, nausea, and distinct fear that one is dying. The cardiac work-up does not reveal abnormal cardiac enzymes or electrocardiogram (ECG), and the manifestations subside spontaneously. After careful diagnostic testing to rule out other medical disorders such as thyroid disease, hypoglycemia, and pheochromocytoma, panic disorder can be identified.[8]

ALTERNATIVE THERAPY

Spirituality and Health

There is a growing awareness of the importance of spirituality in health and of the need for health care providers to acknowledge this. Many clients in the health care system consider spiritual issues important and feel that such issues are too often neglected in our modern technological medical environment. A growing body of research is showing that spiritual or spiritually related activities may in fact be protective of health.[6]

For many people, spirituality may mean their particular religious practice; for others, it may be their own personal views and beliefs or the way they feel connection to something beyond themselves. In fact, connectedness may be an important component of spirituality and its positive health benefits. The social and communal aspects of many religions and spiritual practices may be a common denominator in the health benefits seen. Conversely, social isolation is considered a factor in poor health.[4]

Some authors and researchers feel that love (and the perception of being loved) is very important in health and that love may be the essence of the benefits of spirituality and connection. Author and researcher Jeff Levin states that "love indeed has everything to do with our health and well-being." Levin has researched the epidemiology of religion and found that people who were more religious or spiritual also had better health, greater well-being, and less depression.[3]

Research into the effects of intercessory prayer (prayers said on someone else's behalf), sometimes without their being aware of it consciously, is both intriguing and controversial. Preliminary data from a pilot study of a number of interventions, including intercessory prayer, in a group of clients with unstable angina and infarction showed the least adverse outcomes when they were mentioned in the prayers of others.[2] Such studies are difficult to conduct and to evaluate. Yet other research has shown that when a certain percentage of a population is engaged in Transcendental Meditation, the incidence of violence decreases in surrounding populations.[5] Such research leads some to speculate that there is a field of consciousness that we are all a part of.

Some studies have shown that clients with cancer who participate in support groups show improvement in quality of life and in survival time.[4] Perhaps this is because "all relationships are spiritual." The more intimate and loving one's relationships, the better this is for one's health.[4]

What are we, as nurses, to make of the information regarding spirituality and health? One thing we must not do is draw the wrong conclusions. As Larry Dossey points out,[1] we must not assume that being religious or spiritual is a guarantee of good health or that poor health or illness implies spiritual shortcomings in someone. "Sickly saints and healthy sinners show us that there is no invariable, linear, one-to-one relationship between one's level of spiritual attainment and the degree of one's physical health. It is obvious that one can attain immense spiritual heights and still get *very* sick." We must also not equate our own particular religion or spiritual practice as being one that others *should* follow. Each person's spirituality should be authentically his or her own, emerging "from the center of one's being."[1]

What we can do is assess each client's degree of isolation or connectedness and encourage moves toward the latter. This may mean providing information about support groups for people with various illness or putting a client in touch with a chaplain or pastoral counselor. Our interest, concern, and sharing with clients in these areas serves to deepen our relationship with them, which may in itself be healing.

References

1. Dossey L. (1993). *Healing words: The power of prayer and the practice of medicine.* San Francisco: Harper San Francisco.
2. Horrigan, B. (1999). Mitchell W. Krucoff, MD, The Mantra Project. *Alternative therapies in health and medicine.* 5(3):75–82.
3. Horrigan B. (1999). Jeff Levin, MPH, PhD, The Power of Love. *Alternative Therapies in Health and Medicine,* 5(4): 78–86.
4. Ornish D. (1998). *Love and survival.* New York: HarperCollins.
5. Sharma, H. & Clark, C. (1998). *Contemporary ayurveda.* Philadelphia: Churchill Livingstone.
6. Ziegler, J. (1998). Spirituality returns to the fold in medical practice. *Journal of the National Cancer Institute, 90,*1255–1257.

James Higgy Lerner, RN, LAc, *Private practice of acupuncture, traditional Oriental medicine, and biofeedback*

Panic disorder is one of the eight subtypes of anxiety disorders identified by the *Diagnostic and Statistical Manual of Mental Disorders,* fourth edition (*DSM-IV*).[2] Anxiety disorders as a group are the most common psychiatric disorders in the United States and affect one out of four people in a given year.[8] The eight major categories are:

- Panic Disorder
- Generalized Anxiety Disorder (GAD)
- Phobias
- Obsessive-Compulsive Disorder (OCD)
- Post-traumatic Stress Disorder (PTSD)
- Acute Stress Disorder
- Anxiety Disorder due to Medical Condition
- Anxiety Disorder Not Otherwise Specified

Manifestations may range from mild to severe. Many of these clients never request treatment because of their feelings of shame. Box 20–6 describes each diagnosis. Whereas health care professionals often joke about obsessive-compulsive traits in themselves, clients with OCD (e.g., hand-washing 50 times each day) rarely admit that they have a problem. OCD, phobias, or Generalized Anxiety Disorder may come to the attention of the nurse only accidentally while the client is being treated for another condition. However, clients with panic disorder, PTSD, or acute stress disorder frequently seek urgent care because of severe distress. One survey estimated that as many as 8% of Americans 15 to 54 years of age suffer from PTSD as a result of witnessing a tragedy, domestic violence, or sexual abuse.[11]

BOX 20-5   Resources for Mental Illness Education

Alzheimer's Disease Education and Referral
www.alzheimers.org
Web site sponsored by National Institute on Aging with educational and research information related to Alzheimer's disease.

Anxiety Disorders Association of America
301-231-9350
www.adaa.org
Information and support groups for clients with anxiety disorders.

Depression and Related Affective Disorders Association (DRADA)
Johns Hopkins Hospital
600 N. Wolfe Street
Baltimore, MD 21287-7381
410-955-4647
www.med.JHU.edu/drada
Information, support groups, and research for clients with mood disorders and their families.

National Alliance for Research on Schizophrenia and Depression (NARSAD)
60 Cutter Mill Road, Suite 404
Great Neck, NY 11021
516-829-0091
www.mhsource.com
Supports research into mental illness and offers free information and a newsletter regarding schizophrenia and mood disorders.

National Alliance for the Mentally Ill (NAMI)
200 N. Glebe Road, Suite 1015
Arlington, VA 22203-3754
800-950-NAMI (800-950-6264)
www.nami.org
Provides information, support groups, and advocacy for clients and their families.

National Depressive and Manic-Depressive Association
730 N. Franklin Street, Suite 501
Chicago, IL 60610
800-82NDMDA (800-826-3632)
Information and support for clients with bipolar illness and their families.

National Institute of Mental Health
888-8ANXIETY (888-826-94389)
www.nimh.nih.gov/anxiety
Free information and educational material on anxiety disorders.

National Mental Health Association
1021 Prince Street
Alexandria, VA 22314-2971
703-684-7722
Information and support for clients with mental illness and their families.

The WEBster
www.cyberspy.com/~webster/index.html
Web site established by a pediatric nurse to provide support to clients and their families coping with death and dying, including suicide.

■ POSSIBLE CAUSES

There is no single known cause for anxiety disorders, and research is ongoing. Three major approaches have been proposed to explain the illness: (1) biologic, (2) psychodynamic, and (3) behavioral.

BIOLOGIC VIEW

From the biologic viewpoint, there is some evidence supporting a genetic influence for Generalized Anxiety Disorder, Panic Disorder, and phobias. First-degree relatives (parents, siblings, children) of clients with these disorders have an increased risk of the same manifestations compared with normal controls.[7] Anxiety disorders often co-exist with other psychiatric problems that seem to run in families, such as depression or substance abuse.[8]

Evidence from drug studies and diagnostic imaging techniques, such as computed tomography (CT) or positron emission tomography (PET), and magnetic resonance imaging (MRI) has shown definite brain structures and neurotransmitters that are involved in the experience of anxiety. The limbic system of the brain is activated during the stress response (see the feature on anatomy and physiology of the neurologic system introducing Unit 15). The neurotransmitters epinephrine, norepinephrine, dopamine, serotonin, and gamma-aminobutyric acid (GABA) all are involved in regulating anxiety. Thus, disturbances in nerve structures or in levels of brain chemicals appear to be underlying causes of anxiety disorders.[8]

BOX 20-6   Key Features of the Anxiety Disorders

Panic Disorder—recurrent panic attacks followed by change in behavior to try and avoid another attack persisting over more than 1 month

Generalized Anxiety Disorder (GAD)—excessive anxiety for 6 or more months that is uncontrollable, often focused on health or money concern

Phobia—severe, persistent fear of an object or situation that the person recognizes as irrational but cannot overcome

Obsessive-Compulsive Disorder (OCD)—preoccupation with disturbing thoughts (obsessions) or repetitive actions (compulsions) that interferes with normal activities of daily living

Post-traumatic Stress Disorder (PTSD)—reexperiencing a real, horrifying event in nightmares or flashbacks, with a duration of manifestations more than 1 month that may be immediate or a delayed reaction

Acute Stress Disorder—similar to PTSD except that the manifestations occur within 1 month of the event and last only for approximately 1 month

Anxiety Disorder due to General Medical Condition—severe anxiety in the presence of clear physical findings of a somatic disorder, e.g., hypoglycemia

Anxiety Disorder Not Otherwise Specified—showing some anxiety or phobic manifestations but not severe enough to warrant a specific diagnosis

PSYCHODYNAMIC VIEW

Psychodynamic explanations point toward faulty psychological defenses or thinking processes. *Psychoanalytic* theory proposes that anxiety results from inability to repress (unconsciously inhibit) painful impulses, thoughts, or memories. Manifestations of anxiety are considered to be disguised forms of these repressed thoughts. *Intellectual theory* suggests that the problem is intellectual distortion; a person consistently distorts reality to see the world in a negative way. In the case of panic, the person incorrectly interprets the manifestations as impending death rather than as a reversible stress response.[31]

BEHAVIORAL VIEW

Behavioral theory views anxiety as a learned or conditioned response. A person who has experienced fear and all of its physical manifestations in a certain situation may learn to feel the same effects in a similar situation just because of past association. For example, one painful visit to the dentist as a child may condition a person to always feel anxious with a dentist even for routine, painless procedures.

■ OUTCOME MANAGEMENT

All of the anxiety disorders can be effectively treated through a combination of medication and psychotherapy. Several different classes of drugs that alter levels of neurotransmitters can be helpful. Benzodiazepines seem to increase the action of GABA. Buspirone is thought to affect serotonin receptors. Antidepressants alter the levels of serotonin or norepinephrine. Box 20–7 lists commonly prescribed anti-anxiety medications. These medicines may be prescribed for short-term or long-term use but usually are not needed permanently.

Medication may offer some immediate benefit to reduce the discomfort of anxiety, but some form of psychotherapy (individual, group, or family) is necessary to achieve lasting positive outcomes. Clients, and sometimes their loved ones, have usually tried to cope with their manifestations for a long time before seeking help. Often,

they have adopted negative patterns of thinking or avoidance behaviors that are not easily given up despite serious impairment. For example, consider the limitations of a phobic person who cannot cross bridges. This person cannot work or socialize in any location that requires going over a bridge and probably invents excuses to hide the real reason from friends or family. In the context of a therapy relationship, the client works to identify and revise dysfunctional behavior.

■ INTERVENTION

Returning to Mrs. James, the ED nurse needs to devise a care plan with a discharge plan quickly (see Care Plan). When the nurse sits down to talk with Mrs. James, she is not surprised to find that the psychosocial history is incomplete. This client had presented with potentially life-threatening manifestations, and the admitting nurse focused on selected, pertinent data such as medications and allergies. The database shows that Mrs. James has a history of hypertension and degenerative joint disease affecting her right knee, forcing her to use a cane.

COMPREHENSIVE ASSESSMENT

As the nurse explores the client's current psychological and social functioning, Mrs. James reports that this is not the first time that she has had respiratory distress. Over the past 6 months, she has had one or two episodes each month. Before this episode, they were milder and she did not have chest pain. She cannot relate the attack to any particular stressor but has learned to limit her outside activities to avoid all places where she feels anxious. Mrs. James depends on her daughter who lives with her to do all the shopping. She also describes difficulty sleeping and increased appetite. She feels she is worthless and has crying spells several times per week. She even confides that she has lost all sexual interest and that her boyfriend is starting to think that she does not love him anymore.

When asked about her past level of functioning, Mrs. James states that until 1 year ago she was working as a nurse's aide and was independent. She drove, helped to care for her mother, and enjoyed going out with friends to church and social events. After a fall resulting in a knee injury, she never recovered full ambulation and eventually applied for disability. Her daughter moved in with her to help with financial obligations. In relation to her family history for emotional problems, Mrs. James explains that her mother is alcoholic and her daughter takes antidepressants, but she has always been "too strong for that kind of problem."

COMMUNICATION AWARENESS

Throughout the interview, the nurse provides a private, supportive atmosphere. Initially, the nurse closes the curtain and moves the chair so that there is continuous eye contact. It is explained that they may have only 15 minutes before an interruption, but the nurse wants to learn as much as possible about Mrs. James. As the client talks, the nurse encourages her with nonverbal cues such as nodding her head. When the client becomes tearful at times, the nurse calmly pauses and offers her a tissue. The nurse shows no surprise or disapproval when Mrs. James mentions mental illness in her family. At the end of the assessment, the nurse tells the client that sharing this information will assist the treatment team to plan an

---

BOX 20–7   Medications for Anxiety Disorders

- Benzodiazepines
  - Alprazolam
  - Clonazepam
  - Diazepam
  - Lorazepam
  - Oxazepam
- Buspirone
- Selective serotonin reuptake inhibitors (approved for treatment of anxiety)
  - Fluoxetine
  - Paroxetine
  - Sertraline
- Tricyclic antidepressants
  - Amitriptyline
  - Clomipramine
  - Desipramine
  - Imipramine
  - Nortriptyline

■ THE CLIENT WITH DEGENERATIVE JOINT DISEASE AND CONCURRENT PANIC DISORDER: MRS. JAMES

Nursing Diagnosis. Anxiety as evidenced by panic attacks related to physical loss of independence with associated changes in social and economic functioning.

Outcomes. Mrs. James will verbalize understanding that her manifestations may be caused by an emotional disorder, will consent to evaluation by a psychiatric consultant, will accept referral to psychiatric aftercare, and will receive appropriate psychiatric treatment to resolve panic attacks and to improve her level of functioning (long-term).

Interventions	Rationales
1. Assess for other emotional problems such as depression and substance abuse and include family history.	1. Panic Disorder frequently runs in families and may coexist with other mental disorders.
2. Assess for stressors and previous level of functioning.	2. Data provide a functional baseline so that the nurse can encourage the client to set realistic goals for change.
3. Assess for family support system and acceptance of problem.	3. Family involvement increases the likelihood of follow-up with recommended treatment.
4. Demonstrate acceptance of the client's feelings and distress.	4. Manifestations of emotional illness are just as important as physical distress.
5. Educate the client and family about anxiety as a treatable illness, and explain the role of the psychiatric consultant.	5. Preparation helps the client accept mental health services.
6. Communicate the history to the social worker, including the incomplete sexual assessment.	6. Ensures continuity of care and enables the social worker to focus on the client's key issues.

Evaluation. Accomplishment of short-term outcomes should be evident before discharge from the emergency department. Accomplishment of long-term outcome may require considerable time.

effective treatment regimen; the next step is to consult with the physician for recommendations. The nurse asks Mrs. James to call a family member to come and stay with her pending her discharge.

CLIENT AND FAMILY TEACHING

The nurse reports the findings on Mrs. James' anxiety and mood to the attending physician and recommends that the psychiatric social worker or psychiatric nurse practitioner for the ED be called. The physician agrees, noting that all laboratory findings are normal. The probable diagnosis is Panic Disorder. As the physician goes to speak with the client, the nurse accesses the client education file or on-line library and obtains material on panic attack, depression, and coping skills for families. The nurse gives these pamphlets to Mrs. James and her daughter, telling them that anxiety is a common, treatable problem. The nurse also explains the role of the psychiatric consultant and asks them to wait to talk with her. The client is uncertain, but the daughter encourages her to agree.

SPECIALIZED REFERRALS

In choosing the appropriate referrals for discharge planning for Mrs. James, the nurse is aware that the medical center offers several levels of psychiatric care (see Table 20-5). Because the client is not at immediate risk to harm herself or others, referral to the inpatient unit is not indicated. Yet, the risk exists that if she is given an appointment to go to the outpatient clinic next week, she may not follow through. Mrs. James has already suffered for 6 months and is still resisting the idea that her manifestations may be due to emotional issues. Thus, the nurse selects the resource who can make an immediate, specialized assessment and disposition—namely, the ED consultant.

The psychiatric consultant (social worker, advanced practice nurse, or psychologist) will perform a full, diagnostic interview, including appropriate standardized tests for anxiety and depression. Box 20-8 lists commonly used rating scales for mental health assessment. The ED nurse shares the nursing database with the psychiatric health care worker, noting the client's report of sexual difficulties, which needs further evaluation. Box 20-9 presents the psychosocial dimension of sexuality related to the nursing assessment and intervention.

After meeting with the client and her daughter, the psychiatric consultant recommends referral to the Partial Hospital Program on the following day because of the severity of manifestations. The nurse communicates this recommendation to the physician in order to coordinate the final discharge plan for Mrs. James. In reviewing the discharge instructions, the nurse strongly recommends that the daughter accompany the client to the intake appointment, and she agrees. Upon discharge, Mrs. James is no longer crying and states, "If all of you think that I should go, then I will."

SCHIZOPHRENIA

Mr. Barnes demonstrates clear manifestations of *schizophrenia* with fixed delusions and hallucinations. He represents a generation of young, chronically mentally ill people who have been cared for primarily in the community instead of being institutionalized. Schizophrenia is an incurable, severe mental illness that usually strikes between the ages of 15 and 25.[24] *DSM-IV* lists five subtypes (Box 20-10).

In all cases, a person's thinking and communication skills are profoundly affected. Manifestations are generally classified as positive or negative.[22] *Positive* manifestations include the most obvious signs of psychosis (auditory or visual hallucinations, delusions, disorganized

TABLE 20–5	LEVELS OF PSYCHIATRIC TREATMENT SERVICES	
Level of Care	**Intensity of Psychiatric Treatment**	
Inpatient unit	Most intensive level of care for clients considered dangerous to self or others; admission may be voluntary or involuntary; brief length of stay, 1 week or less	
Partial hospitalization	One step below inpatient, to prevent hospitalization or stabilize after a brief hospital stay; voluntary admission; short length of stay, from 1 to 4 weeks, with attendance 5 to 7 days per week	
Psychosocial day program/rehabilitation	Structured daily activity for clients who need moderate, long-term supervision; voluntary admission; promotes socialization and vocational skills; indefinite length of stay	
Mobile treatment	Outreach program to follow clients who require medication and case management but refuse to attend outpatient centers; voluntary admission; intermittent visits; indefinite length of stay	
Psychiatric home care	Home visits by psychiatric nurse or social worker to treat homebound clients with an exacerbation of a *DSM-IV* diagnosis; voluntary participation; requires physician orders; length of stay 4 to 8 weeks	
Outpatient clinic or private clinician	Least intensive level of care for clients following a more intensive level of treatment or for crisis, short-term treatment; voluntary participation; length of stay indefinite	

DSM-IV, Diagnostic and Statistical Manual of Mental Disorders, 4th ed.

thinking and speech). *Negative* manifestations refer to the lack of usual emotional or social responses (blunted affect, avoidance of social contact, lack of attention to hygiene).

Schizophrenia affects at least 2.5 million people in the United States and about 1% of the world population.[24] As with other chronic illnesses such as cancer or heart disease, there are periods of exacerbation and remission. The devastating toll on clients and their families is not easily measured, but the financial cost each year in the United States for treatment, disability payment, and lost wages is approximately $48 billion.[24]

■ POSSIBLE CAUSES

In the 1960s, communication theorists and family therapists focused on disturbed patterns of communication in families with a schizophrenic member. They proposed that faulty communication and anxiety caused the illness and invented the term "schizophrenogenic mother."[32] This theory was never supported with controlled studies, but it had an unfortunate effect on therapeutic relationships with families. Many parents and family members felt blamed for their relative's illness and learned to distrust the mental health system.

Today, it is well recognized that schizophrenia is a biologic brain disorder. Repeated studies show a genetic influence, suggesting that the first-degree relatives of schizophrenics have 18.5 times the risk for the illness compared with relatives of controls.[7] CT and MRI scans have identified certain structural abnormalities in the brain, including enlargement of the ventricles and reduced size of the hippocampus.[24] The prefrontal cortex, which governs thinking and abstract mental functions, shows a decrease in the number of neurons and connections among regions.[15] It is not known whether these changes are caused by genetic, in utero, or environmental influences such as viruses, but research is ongoing.

Drug studies indicate that the neurotransmitter dopamine is implicated in schizophrenic manifestations. All of the medicines currently used for treatment are dopamine receptor blockers.[39] Dopamine is involved in mood and motivation and helps to regulate movement. Sophisticated PET scans can track the increased level of dopamine released in the brain at the same time that psychotic manifestations are observed.[34]

■ OUTCOME MANAGEMENT

The positive manifestations of schizophrenia can be controlled by antipsychotic medication, but the negative manifestations and severe social impairment require supportive psychotherapy. Antipsychotic medicines have been

BOX 20–8	Selected Standardized Tools for Assessment of Psychiatric Disorders	
Psychiatric Disorder	**Assessment Tool**	
Anxiety	Modified Spielberger State Anxiety Scale Sheehan Patient-Rated Anxiety Scale	
Cognitive status	Mini-Mental State Examination (MMSE)	
Depression	Beck Inventory Geriatric Depression Scale Hamilton's Depression Scale Zung Self-Report Inventory	
Mania	Mania Rating Scale	
Schizophrenia	Scale for Assessment of Negative Symptoms (SANS)	
General functioning	Brief Psychiatric Rating Scale (BPRS) Global Assessment of Functioning Scale (GAF)	

BOX 20–9 **Psychosocial Dimension: Sexuality and Mental Illness**

Issues related to sexuality may affect every client suffering with physical or mental illness, yet nurses often minimize or avoid this aspect of health. Human sexuality is broader than just physical sexual activity and includes gender identity, gender role, and sexual orientation. To provide holistic care, you must learn to be comfortable in promoting sexual health, "the physical and emotional state of well-being that enables us to enjoy and act on sexual feelings."*

Clients often worry about their sexual role following the effects of physical illness. There may be obvious disfigurement because of surgery or new activity restrictions resulting from compromised cardiac or respiratory status. Clients with mental illness may also suffer from altered sexual expression. In an effort to hide their feelings of anxiety or depression, some clients withdraw from intimate relationships. Loss of sexual desire is a frequent manifestation of depression, along with altered appetite and sleep. Even when clients acknowledge an emotional problem and seek treatment, they often complain of side effects from medication that alter their desire or performance.

Many clients do not volunteer their concerns but are eager to discuss questions when asked. One study showed that 76% of patients preferred the nurse to initiate discussion of sexual issues, but only 15% of the nurses included this in their assessment.[37] Common barriers that prevent nurses from exploring sexual issues include (1) not seeing the relevance to the admitting problem, (2) inadequate training, (3) embarrassment, and (4) fear of offending the client.

Sexual assessment refers to more than the client's sexual practices (see the Sexual Health Assessment tool in Chapter 37). The concepts of gender identity and gender role are important aspects. *Gender identity* refers to one's internal sense of being feminine or masculine, and *gender role* is the public expression of these beliefs. Attitudes about gender are learned in a specific sociocultural context. Learning takes place starting in early childhood in the home and in institutions such as school. By 3 years of age, children have an understanding of being male or female. Each family or community may have specific sexual values, with effects from religious and legal forces to control sexual expression.

Sexual orientation is another aspect of sexual health. About 90% of the population define themselves as *heterosexual* (preferring the opposite sex). Approximately 10% define themselves as *homosexual* (preferring the same-sex partner). A small number of people report themselves to be *bisexual* (interested in both sexes) or *transsexual* (feeling dissatisfied in their physical body because it does not match the internal view of their sexual identity).

To help the client communicate sexual concerns, the nurse must be competent in four areas: (1) knowledge about sexual function; (2) skills in assessment and intervention, including sex education and anticipatory guidance; (3) personal awareness of one's own values; and (4) awareness of the effect of one's attitude in delivering care. Becoming aware of your own values enables you to accept and respect the client's sexuality without imposing judgment. Sexual health issues should be considered part of the comprehensive nursing assessment, thus allowing clients to disclose their fears or questions in order to get resolution.

*See Edmisson (1997).[13]

---

used since the 1950s, and several classes of drugs have evolved over time in an effort to reduce unpleasant side effects (Box 20–11). These medications must be taken for a lifetime in order to control the manifestations. With medication, some clients report a total absence of hallucinations. For other clients, internal voices (auditory hallucinations) become a permanent experience. Not all voices or delusions are frightening; clients may learn to accept them as unusual but pleasant.

A major concern for most clients is the presence of side effects related to sedation and abnormal movements. Because typical antipsychotics target all dopamine receptors, including those affecting movement, muscle side effects known as *extrapyramidal symptoms* (EPS) are extremely common.[24] Manifestations of EPS may include stiffness or tremor in arms and legs, extreme restlessness with subjective discomfort, drooling, and acute muscle spasms of the tongue, neck, or face. These side effects are usually short-term and treatable with an anticholinergic agent such as benztropine or trihexyphenidyl. However, a long-term side effect of typical antipsychotics, called *tardive dyskinesia* (TD), occurs in approximately one third of clients and is usually irreversible. Common manifestations of TD are obvious, involuntary movements of the tongue, face, hands, or legs. The main benefit of the newer, atypical antipsychotics is the lower incidence of EPS and TD because the drugs are more selective in affecting neurotransmitters.

BOX 20–10 **Types of Schizophrenia and Manifestations**

Type	Manifestations
Paranoid	Presence of hallucinations and delusional thinking; fairly organized in speech and behavior, and may show some range in affect
Disorganized	Dominant manifestations of disorganized speech and behavior, with flat or inappropriate affect; may also have hallucinations and delusions
Catatonic	Presence of bizarre motor activity, either excessive and purposeless or immobilized as if in a stupor; may be mute or show incoherent speech
Undifferentiated	Presence of two or more of the following manifestations, but without a dominant feature as in the above three types: hallucinations, delusions, disorganized speech or behavior, and flat affect
Residual	Behavior does not show obvious hallucinations, delusions, or disorganization, but alterations persist in range of affect and thinking patterns

---

BOX 20-11   Medications for Schizophrenia

- Atypical antipsychotics
  - Clozapine
  - Olanzapine
  - Quetiapine
  - Risperidone
  - Ziprasidone
- Typical antipsychotics—phenothiazines
  - Chlorpromazine
  - Fluphenazine
  - Mesoridazine
  - Perphenazine
  - Thioridazine
  - Trifluoperazine
- Haloperidol
- Loxapine

One final side effect of typical antipsychotics should be noted. *Neuroleptic malignant syndrome* (NMS) is a rare but serious condition that may appear suddenly with extreme muscle rigidity, high fever, sweating, and fluctuations in consciousness. The client requires emergency hospitalization with supportive treatment to prevent seizures, coma, or even death.

Treatment of impaired social functioning involves long-term supportive therapy and psychosocial rehabilitation. Social withdrawal and lack of interest in school or work often signal the onset of the illness and may persist throughout treatment. To develop and maintain maximal level of functioning, schizophrenic clients need individual counseling and support, psychoeducation, organized rehabilitation services, and family psychoeducation.[32] Clients and families need education about the illness and coping skills to manage manifestations and prevent relapse. Rehabilitation efforts help the client complete basic schooling and learn job skills.

As with any chronic illness, the client experiences episodes of remission and exacerbation. Medication noncompliance, denial of illness, and stressful events may lead to multiple, short-term hospitalizations over a lifetime. With the consistent support of family and community resources, however, many clients can progress toward higher levels of independence and avoid long-term hospitalization.

■ INTERVENTION

Returning to the case of Mr. Barnes, the nurse immediately recognizes that the client has abnormal thinking (see Care Plan). The nurse notes that he is well groomed and shows appropriate social skills for the clinic environment; he demonstrates polite manners during the introduction. Uncertain about his reliability as a historian, the nurse asks Mr. Barnes whether his mother can be invited to join them as they complete his assessment and examination. He readily agrees.

COMPREHENSIVE ASSESSMENT

While completing the nursing assessment, the nurse evaluates the client's knowledge of his medical illness, his

psychosocial functioning, and his current level of compliance with psychiatric care. Despite his bizarre speech, Mr. Barnes offers accurate dates and descriptions of his medical manifestations and doctor appointments. He shows some awareness of his diet and casually remarks, "I have this illness called schizophrenia. It makes me talk stupid sometimes." He firmly repeats his belief in the elves in the basement that talk to him at night and cause him to feel hungry all the time.

His mother adds that Mr. Barnes' mental illness was first diagnosed in his last year of high school. Before that, she had not noticed any problems. He had been a typical child who enjoyed school and was close to his older brother. He has been hospitalized 10 times for severe paranoia and hostile threats toward his family. The most recent stay was 6 months ago. He is compliant with his medication and has been going to the same psychiatrist for 5 years. Mr. Barnes expresses satisfaction with his doctor: "He is good. He tries to give me the right medicine, but sometimes it doesn't work."

Exploration of daily activities reveals that Mr. Barnes stays home with his mother, watching television, reading, and doing chores. He does not have any contact with peers and does not work. He states, "My brother and his friends don't like me anymore." His mother comments that his brother visits him regularly and tries to take him out, but sometimes the client refuses to go. She adds that he tried to work once at a "fast food" restaurant, but people made fun of him. Now she does not allow him to go outdoors alone.

COMMUNICATION AWARENESS

Throughout the interview, the nurse takes care to include Mr. Barnes in the conversation even though his mother tends to dominate. The nurse maintains a calm facial expression when the client discusses his delusions and respectfully records his answers. No attempt is made to challenge the reality of his remarks, but the nurse does not communicate agreement with his distortions. The nurse is also careful not to invade the client's personal space, explaining all physical procedures and asking for permission before touching him.

CLIENT AND FAMILY TEACHING

Although the client and his mother seem to be familiar with the term *schizophrenia,* it is not clear how much teaching they have received about managing the illness. Neither mother nor son is involved in a community support group, and the client is socially isolated without any prospect of increased independence because of his mother's overprotective stance. Before giving them material about hiatal hernia, the nurse asks whether they would like to read more about schizophrenia. They both are interested. The nurse explains that schizophrenia is a chronic illness that can be controlled and praises the client for his knowledge of his medication and medical care. As Mr. Barnes proudly gathers up all of the teaching materials to take home, his mother smiles and says, "He always was a good reader."

SPECIALIZED REFERRALS

Before setting up the next clinic appointment, the nurse considers whether any other mental health resource is indicated. Mr. Barnes is in remission at this time, showing compliance with medications and monthly psychiatrist

■ THE CLIENT WITH HIATAL HERNIA AND CONCURRENT SCHIZOPHRENIA: MR. BARNES

Nursing Diagnosis. Altered thought processes and altered perception, as evidenced by auditory hallucinations and delusions related to paranoid schizophrenia.

Outcomes. Mr. Barnes will establish trust with the nurse and agree to return to the medical clinic, he and his mother will accept referral to the psychiatric clinical specialist to promote access to community resources, and he will remain in the community with outpatient services, which will help him develop to his maximal functioning (long term).

Interventions	Rationales
1. Assess for current compliance with psychiatric care and history of aggressive or self-destructive behavior.	1. Successful outcomes with medical condition depend on psychiatric stability; when decompensating, a schizophrenic client distorts reality and may become threatening to others or self.
2. Assess for current level of psychosocial functioning.	2. Chronic mental illness impairs social and vocational functioning even when target manifestations are under control.
3. Assess Mr. Barnes' mother's knowledge of the illness and impact on the family.	3. Families may alter their entire structure around an ill member, cutting off outside support.
4. Ask the client's permission before touching him for physical procedures.	4. A client with schizophrenia may misinterpret actions by strangers and become defensive.
5. Respond to the reality aspects of the client's speech.	5. The client is still cognitively intact and shows readiness to learn new information despite delusions.
6. Describe the role of the psychiatric nurse as just another member of the health care team.	6. The familiar environment of the medical clinic will help to reduce the client's anxiety about a new mental health provider.

Evaluation. Accomplishment of the expected outcomes will require time and a trusting relationship with the clinic nurse. Reassessment must be ongoing, with revision in the plan as necessary.

appointments; however, he feels stigmatized and has not accomplished the developmental tasks of young adulthood. He is totally dependent on his mother and experiences repeated relapses with his current living situation. To promote the best overall health outcomes for Mr. Barnes, the nurse must consider *tertiary prevention* with regard to his mental illness. (See Chapter 1 for a review of primary, secondary, and tertiary prevention.) The nurse sees that he needs additional professional support, such as participation in a structured day program, or even a part-time job to attain his maximal level of community functioning.

The nurse recommends a referral to the psychiatric clinical specialist in the outpatient clinic at the medical center. The purpose of referral is to explore community resources to support Mr. Barnes and his family. To increase the probability of their follow-up with an appointment, the nurse offers to introduce them to the psychiatric nurse at their next clinic visit. They hesitantly agree. The nurse calls the clinical specialist, who explains that one of several referrals can be made for Mr. Barnes: to a young adult supportive therapy group, a psychosocial rehabilitation program, or a mental health support group for clients and families. The clinical specialist will also call the attending psychiatrist to coordinate the treatment plan.

MOOD DISORDERS

Mrs. Conners, Mr. Moore, and Miss Howard represent clients with various mood disorders. Mood disorders are classified into three major categories: (1) Depressive Dis-

orders, (2) bipolar disorder (formerly called manic depressive illness), and (3) Mood Disorder due to General Medical Condition or Substance Use.[3] Manifestations of all depressions include a sad mood, which may be accompanied by crying spells; persistent negative thinking with hopelessness; possible suicidal thinking; decreased energy and motivation; and changes in sleep, appetite, and sexual interest.

In clients with bipolar disorder, mood can fluctuate from depression to the other extreme, mania. *Manic symptoms* include excessive cheerfulness or irritability; an unrealistic, optimistic attitude toward one's accomplishments; overabundance of energy; and decreased sleep with increased physical appetite. Box 20–12 describes mood states.[12]

The key element in mood disorders is that the person cannot control the severity of the feeling. There may or may not be a clear precipitant for the reaction. Unlike a healthy person with transient mood changes, a depressed person cannot "just get over it" and the client with mania does not wish to give up the euphoria that characterizes this mood.

Up to 15% of adults may suffer from a mood disorder at any given time, and more than 4 million Americans may have a major depressive disorder. The age of onset is usually in the 20s and 30s, and the recurrent nature of the illness impacts productivity and quality of life. Up to 70% of the people with depression experience a relapse. Women are two times more likely to have depression, but bipolar illness affects men and women equally.[28]

Mood disorders frequently co-occur with other psychiatric or medical illnesses. Clients may show depression

<table>
<tr><td>

BOX 20-12   Manifestations of Mood Disorders

Depression (major or bipolar)

Sad mood, but may be irritable
Crying spells
Negative thinking, continuously pessimistic
Feelings of guilt and hopelessness
Preoccupation with usually minor somatic complaints
Loss of pleasure in usual activities and decreased socialization
Decreased ability to concentrate and remember current events
Decreased energy level
Change in sleep, increased or decreased
Change in appetite, increased or decreased
Decreased libido and sexual activity
May feel suicidal
May develop psychosis with delusions about a negative future, e.g., fatal illness

Mania

Elated mood, not attributable to a reality event
Denial of having an emotional problem
Impulsive acts that may be dangerous or socially inappropriate, e.g., promiscuity
Increased energy level
Increased socialization to the point of becoming intrusive
Excessive, rapid speech
Change in appetite, increased or decreased
Decreased need for sleep
Increased libido

</td></tr>
</table>

with substance abuse, an anxiety disorder, or an eating disorder. Medical problems often associated with depression include stroke, diabetes, coronary artery disease, cancer, chronic fatigue syndrome, and fibromyalgia.[35] Some prescription drugs cause depressed mood as a side effect (see Table 20-4.) Whenever depressive manifestations are mixed with somatic (physical) complaints, close collaboration between a psychiatrist and primary care provider is necessary to clarify the correct diagnosis and treatment plan.

The most serious adverse outcome for mood disorders is suicide. Take all verbal expressions of suicide intent or threat seriously and act accordingly (see later in this chapter). Up to 15% of clients who are hospitalized for major depression eventually commit suicide. For clients with bipolar disorder, 10% to 15% of untreated clients commit suicide, 20 times the rate in the general population.[35] The period of greatest risk is during psychiatric hospitalization or just after release. There are known risk factors associated with suicide in the United States (see Box 20-13).[36] Older adults are at special risk; each year, more than 6300 older adults commit suicide. White men over age 80 years have the highest suicide rate. It is notable that 75% of these older suicide victims have visited their primary care physician within the month preceding their death.[9] Chapter 3 discusses depression in older people.

■ POSSIBLE CAUSES

As with anxiety and schizophrenia, there is no clear cause of mood disorders. Biologic and psychodynamic theories are offered to explain the illness, and the answer is prob-

ably a combination of both. From the biologic point of view, there are several significant findings from research. First, the genetic influence is undeniable: 25% of clients with major depression and 50% of clients with bipolar disorder have a relative with a mood disorder. Evidence from studies of families with multiple affected members indicates sections of chromosomes 6 and 11 are linked to bipolar illness.[28]

Twin and adoption studies support a genetic link.[12] Children of parents with affective (mood) illness who are adopted into families without a history of affective disorder show three times as many depressive disorders as biologic children in the same family. Twin studies reveal that genes are not the sole cause of affective illness. With identical twins, if one twin has an affective illness, the chance of a disorder developing in the other twin ranges from 50% to 90%. Thus, other biologic or environmental factors must interact with the genetic predisposition.

Data from antidepressant drug studies point to abnormalities in the level of neurotransmitters and other brain chemicals. Antidepressant drugs bring about increased levels of serotonin or norepinephrine.[17] Research with lithium for bipolar disorder indicates that it corrects an imbalance in the compound glutamate.[16] In 1998, a brain chemical called substance P was identified with mood regulation, and drug manufacturers are developing new antidepressants to block its receptors.[19]

Abnormalities in brain structure or in the endocrine system can also lead to depression. People with brain damage from Parkinson's disease, Huntington's disease, or stroke often experience depression. Similarly, people with hypothyroidism or Cushing's disease are at risk for depression.[28]

There are multiple psychodynamic explanations for depression.[31] Historically, the *psychoanalytic view* considers depression as internalized anger about the loss of a loved person or an object with symbolic meaning. It is triggered by the loss of something or someone for whom the person felt ambivalence, a mixture of positive and negative feelings. *Object loss theory* postulates that a person is predisposed to depression because of early, traumatic separation from a loved one during childhood. Thereafter, every separation in adult life recalls the initial reaction. More recently, *cognitive theory* suggests that the person has distorted thinking that defines the world in a negative way. Any disappointment or painful experience is blamed on one's own shortcomings, and life experiences reinforce a self-image of inadequacy.

<table>
<tr><td>

BOX 20-13   Risk Factors for Suicide

Depressed mood
Psychosis
Hopelessness
Serious medical disorder
Substance abuse
Male gender
Caucasian race
Family history of substance abuse
Living alone
Previous attempted suicide

</td></tr>
</table>

The behaviorists use *social learning theory* to explain depression.[31] People constantly receive feedback or reinforcement as they interact with their environment (people or events). Positive reinforcement makes a person repeat behaviors and generally feels like a reward. Lack of positive reinforcement leads a person to feel sad and starts a cycle of increasing withdrawal from social interaction. For example, lack of rewards from friendships or work decreases a person's attempts to try new social situations, further decreasing the opportunity for positive experiences. Even though medications may be needed to address altered neurotransmitters, therapists still use a theoretical model to guide their therapy to help clients examine and revise behavior that has been affected by the biochemicals.

■ OUTCOME MANAGEMENT

Mood disorders can almost always be managed effectively through a combination of medication and psychotherapy. In some cases, electroconvulsive therapy may be indicated. Antidepressant medication may be needed for up to 1 year or for a lifetime, depending on the client's potential for relapse.[36] Particularly for bipolar disorder, mood stabilizers may be needed for long-term treatment.[6] Several classes of antidepressant drugs affect neurotransmitters in different ways (see Box 20–14). If a client does not respond to the medication after a fair trial, the physician may switch to another class or try a combination. Antidepressants and mood stabilizers do not produce effects immediately, as the anti-anxiety drugs do. Thus, the depressed client often suffers for 3 to 6 more weeks when starting treatment. Hopelessness about treatment, especially if the first medication is ineffective, compounds the risk for suicide.

Several types of psychotherapy may be helpful for mood disorders. In all cases, client education is important to explain the course of the illness and the benefits of treatment despite the delay in improvement. Often, short-term therapy is beneficial with a focus on learning to manage current stressors and relationships. Marital therapy may be indicated because a mood disorder frequently causes marital discord, and conflict with loved ones often precipitates a depressive episode.[36]

Electroconvulsive therapy (ECT) is a viable treatment alternative for some clients with depression and may be provided in an inpatient or outpatient setting. An electrical shock is administered to a specific region of the brain to induce a seizure. General anesthesia is required, and the client does not remember the experience. The mechanism of action is not entirely understood but its effect on the neurotransmitter receptors may be similar to that of the tricyclic antidepressants. The client experiences short-term memory loss, but improvement is faster than with medication treatment.[28]

Although it is not usually a first-line treatment, ECT may be superior to medication under the following circumstances: psychotic manifestations with active suicidal risk; severe psychomotor retardation and vegetative symptoms; lack of response to multiple medication trials; and concurrent medical condition that poses a serious risk with psychotropic medicines.[36]

The discussion that follows illustrates the variety of manifestations found with mood disorders.

BOX 20–14 Medications for Mood Disorders

Antidepressants

Monoamine Oxidase Inhibitors (MAOIs)

Isocarboxazid
Phenelzine
Tranylcypromine

Selective Serotonin Reuptake Inhibitors (SSRIs)

Citalopram
Fluoxetine
Fluvoxamine
Paroxetine
Sertraline
Trazodone

Tricyclics

Amitriptyline
Clomipramine
Desipramine
Doxepin
Imipramine
Nortriptyline

Other

Bupropion
Methylphenidate
Mirtazapine
Nefazodone
Reboxetine
Venlafaxine

Anti-manic agents

Carbamazepine
Gabapentin
Lamotrigine
Lithium
Valproic acid

■ INTERVENTION: MAJOR DEPRESSION

After meeting Mrs. Conners (in diabetic ketoacidosis), the nurse is concerned about two major problems. First, the client's mental status appears altered and she is in distress. Second, the average length of stay for this medical diagnosis is only 1 more day, and much teaching must be done before discharge. Returning to the nursing database, the nurse notes that the psychosocial section is incomplete. It is documented that the client is a native West Indian, lives with her daughter, and has a history of major depression. She has been hospitalized three times in the past year, twice on the psychiatric unit and once for ketoacidosis (see Care Plan).

COMPREHENSIVE ASSESSMENT

The nurse decides to attempt completion of the psychosocial history, even though Mrs. Conners may not be spontaneously verbal. The assessment is explained to the client, and she is asked whether her daughter may also be contacted. Mrs. Conners agrees and states that her daughter will be visiting at lunch time. She speaks in a soft voice, with just a few words at a time, and the nurse

■ THE CLIENT WITH DIABETIC KETOACIDOSIS AND CONCURRENT DEPRESSION: MRS. CONNERS

Nursing Diagnosis. Altered thought processes with self-care deficit, as evidenced by sad mood, tearfulness, and decreased grooming and eating related to depression.

Outcomes. Mrs. Conners will cooperate with the evaluation by her psychiatrist, will agree to a safe discharge from the medical unit to an appropriate level of psychiatric care, and will be able to return to her previous level of function and remain at home with her daughter (long term).

Interventions	Rationales
1. Assess psychological and physical effects of low mood, including suicidal thoughts, and effect on diabetes management.	1. Depression causes sleep and eating disturbance, and risk of suicide must always be evaluated; irregular sleep and eating patterns affect ability to safely manage glucose levels and insulin regimen.
2. Assess the previous level of functioning and pattern of medication compliance.	2. Prior treatment history can be used to reassure the client about this episode; medication noncompliance is the major cause of relapse.
3. Accept family input regarding the client's dress and food preferences.	3. Acceptance shows respect for the client's cultural needs and promotes collaboration with the family.
4. Teach about depression and the medications, offering as a review in view of long history.	4. Teaching emphasizes that no stigma is attached to the client because of mental illness and offers hope for the current episode.
5. Explain the role of the utilization review coordinator to coordinate a safe discharge plan.	5. Contact with team members is necessary for a timely, appropriate discharge plan for complex clients.

Evaluation. Accomplishment of these expected outcomes will ensure that the client receives adequate services upon discharge from acute medical care.

---

notices a slight accent. The client says that she has had diabetes for 15 years and depression for 35 years, since the birth of her daughter. She has been going to the same psychiatrist for 20 years and asks the nurse to notify him. When asked about her medication, Mrs. Conners knows the name and dosage of all four (two antidepressant and two antipsychotic agents) and admits that she occasionally misses a dose. She does not have suicidal thoughts and has never attempted suicide.

The client describes her mood as sad, and she becomes tearful. She states that she gets along fine with her daughter and then abruptly says that she is too tired to talk to the nurse anymore. The nurse defers the rest of the interview until the daughter arrives. When the nurse returns at lunch time, she finds Mrs. Conners dressed in a long gown and wearing a colorful turban wrapped around her hair. Her daughter is coaxing her to eat some homemade soup, and she is refusing the hospital food. The daughter mentions that she suspected that her mother was depressed again but that she did not expect her to become this sick. The client has a pattern of medication noncompliance, followed by diet noncompliance with overeating, which results in rehospitalization. The daughter explains that she is aware of the client's 1800-calorie diet, but she works and the client is alone during the day. When she is well, the client enjoys cooking and dressing according to her native custom.

COMMUNICATION AWARENESS

During the interview, the nurse is careful to respect Mrs. Conners' low energy level. The nurse uses questions that require only short answers and speaks clearly and softly. When the client talks about feeling sad, the nurse does not try to cheer her up but reminds her that her depression has been successfully treated in the past.

After the input from the daughter, the nurse realizes how important the client's cultural background is for the care plan (see Box 20–15). In the West Indian culture, an older person may be uncomfortable around authority figures and may avoid eye contact. Respect and good manners are important; people expect to be greeted with "Good morning" or "Good afternoon" and are always addressed by the last name. Privacy is important, and personal issues are discussed only with family members. Mental illness is seen as a weakness and carries a strong stigma. Elderly parents are usually cared for at home by an adult daughter. Food tastes are very specific, and home-brewed teas are considered medicinal.[21] At the end of the conversation, the nurse compliments Mrs. Conners on her appearance and does not try to interrupt the daughter feeding her the homemade soup.

CLIENT AND FAMILY TEACHING

Although the client and her daughter openly discuss the diagnosis of depression, the nurse emphasizes that this is a medical illness that can be treated just like the diabetes. The fact that the client takes multiple medications suggests that this depression is probably difficult to control. Reassurance may be needed about another possible change in medication or dosage. The nurse collects information on depression, the medications, and community support groups. This information is given to the client and her daughter to review and see whether they have any questions.

SPECIALIZED REFERRALS

As soon as the nurse observes that the depression is complicating the client's medical condition, the discharge

BOX 20–15 Psychosocial Dimension: Culture and Mental Illness

Cultural background plays an important role in a person's perception of illness and participation in treatment. *Culture* is defined as the beliefs, values, patterns of behavior, customs, and language of a group of people. To provide holistic care, nurses must be sensitive to the cultural needs of clients, and must be aware of their own cultural perspective.

Nurses need to understand several concepts regarding culture. *Cultural diversity* refers to the difference between different groups of people (e.g., from different countries or even different regions of one country). *Cultural imposition* is the process of the dominant culture imposing its beliefs on a less dominant group. *Cultural sensitivity* is an awareness and acceptance of different cultures.

As you encounter clients from various cultures, it is important to be aware of both Western and non-Western health care beliefs. In American society, the following ideas are taken for granted:

- Illness is considered to have a specific cause that is discoverable and treatable.
- It is important to prevent or reduce signs of illness, and there is a focus on wellness promotion.
- Clients are seen as partly responsible for their health behavior and partly as victims of disease.
- People value cleanliness and are time-conscious, expecting immediate or rapid relief from discomfort.
- The physician is the primary practitioner who treats illness.

In non-Western cultures, illness is defined by personalistic or naturalistic viewpoints. In the *personalistic* view, illness is caused by an agent, such as a deity, ghost, or witch, and is seen as a punishment or attack. In the *naturalistic* framework, illness is due to a failure in equilibrium among opposing elements. For example, Latin Americans believe in four humors, or fluids, in the body: blood (hot and moist), phlegm (cold and moist), black bile (cold and dry), and yellow bile or choler (hot and dry). Major body organs must possess certain quantities of dry, moist, hot, and cold fluids in order to be healthy. Illness is caused by disequilibrium of these forces and is treated through foods and other means to restore balance. People seek out indigenous (local or native) healers as the primary practitioner.

In providing holistic care to clients of different cultures, be sensitive to their needs and avoid cultural imposition (see cultural assessment as part of health assessment in Chapter 9). Ask clients and their families to explain their specific needs. Whenever possible, incorporate client and family customs into the treatment plan, such as dietary preferences. If there are significant points of conflict, carefully explain the clinical rationale and convey respect for the client's choices about treatment. In addition to these nursing interventions, help link the client to community resources with similar cultural background in order to reduce feelings of isolation in our predominantly Western culture.

planner/utilization review coordinator is contacted along with the attending physician. Discharge planning for Mrs. Conners requires a coordinated effort between medical and psychiatric clinicians. The client has already asked that her psychiatrist be called, and the attending physician asks the discharge planner to arrange for a consultation.

When the discharge planner calls the psychiatrist, he states that he can visit the client this evening. He adds that he may need to transfer her to the psychiatric unit because she has a history of becoming psychotic when she relapses, refusing to eat or care for herself. The nurse introduces the discharge planner to the client and her daughter and explains the role: to ensure a timely, appropriate discharge plan that considers all of the client's needs before returning home. When Mrs. Conners hears that her psychiatrist is coming to see her, she smiles and her daughter looks relieved. The daughter states, "Maybe he will admit her to the psych unit. She always gets better there."

■ INTERVENTION: DEPRESSION

After being notified by the physical therapist about Mr. Moore's condition (second stroke), the home care nurse makes an appointment and reviews the nursing and physical therapy database. The nurse recalls that Mr. Moore quickly recovered from his first stroke with minimal residual symptoms. He had returned to his previous level of function, such as driving and doing chores (see Care Plan).

When the nurse arrives at the home, Mr. Moore is sitting in the living room with the shades drawn. As the nurse starts to say that the therapist is concerned about his status, he gruffly states, "I won't use that stupid walker. What good is it to walk like a cripple?" The nurse notes that he looks thinner, and the chart shows that he refused to allow the aide to shave him this morning. Mrs. Moore calls the nurse into the kitchen and bursts into tears, saying, "I don't know what's wrong with him. He is so negative about everything. He was never like this before."

COMPREHENSIVE ASSESSMENT

The nurse decides to repeat the entire nursing assessment. Physically, there is no improvement in Mr. Moore's walking or balance compared with 6 weeks ago. He has lost 5 pounds and blames the loss on his wife's "lousy cooking." He reports that he cannot sleep at night because the sofa is uncomfortable and he cannot go upstairs to his bedroom. He refuses to allow the therapist to order a hospital bed for downstairs.

When the nurse asks about his mood, Mr. Moore pauses and says, "What does it matter?" When the nurse persists, he finally says that he feels useless. He cannot perform any of his previous activities or household responsibilities. Knowing that he and his wife used to attend church regularly, the nurse asks whether he has tried to go out or have the minister visit. Mr. Moore snorts and says, "I'm never going back there. At first I prayed, but what good did it do?" Noting these signs of spiritual distress, the nurse further assesses his beliefs and feelings about spirituality. See Box 20–16 for a guide to spirituality and Alternative Therapy: Spirituality and Health earlier.[33]

■ THE CLIENT WITH STROKE AND CONCURRENT DEPRESSION: MR. MOORE

Nursing Diagnosis. Hopelessness with risk of self-directed violence, as evidenced by depressed mood and passive death wish related to loss of independence due to stroke.

Outcomes. Mr. Moore will agree to a no-harm contract, will accept referral for more intensive evaluation and treatment of his depression, will experience improved mood, and will cooperate with his physical therapist to attain maximal rehabilitation goals (long term).

Interventions	Rationales
1. Assess for psychological and physical signs of depression, including suicidal thoughts.	1. Depression is a common complication with stroke and can interfere with physical rehabilitation.
2. Assess risk for suicide and ability to contract for safety; inform the wife.	2. Older, white men with concurrent medical problems are at high risk for suicide, and emergency department referral may be required.
3. Listen nonjudgmentally as the client expresses anger about loss and abandonment by God.	3. Listening shows acceptance of the client's feelings of distress and may reduce the client's feelings of guilt.
4. Expect the client to make decisions and take responsibility for treatment.	4. The nurse's confidence in the client shows respect for his abilities and counteracts feelings of helplessness and powerlessness.
5. Teach that depression is a treatable illness and about the need for regular eating, sleeping, and exercise.	5. Teaching offers information and hope that the current condition can be improved with the client's active participation.
6. Explain roles of the psychiatric nurse, social worker, and physical therapist to assist in his fullest recovery.	6. Multidisciplinary services are required for this client to prevent self-harm and promote recovery.

Evaluation. Accomplishment of the expected outcomes will establish a plan for safety and offer the best opportunity for physical and emotional healing.

BOX 20–16 Psychosocial Dimension: Spirituality and Mental Illness

Spirituality is a significant aspect of humanness made up of values and beliefs about the meaning and purpose of life and may or may not include a specific religion. Suffering experienced with physical or mental illness often leads a person to question beliefs about God or a higher power; such distress can have a serious effect on recovery. As part of holistic care, assess spiritual needs in order to support the client's internal forces for healing.

Spirituality is more than religion. A religion is an organized set of practices based on specific beliefs. The human spiritual dimension is closely linked to the mind and body. When one part of the system is jeopardized, by illness for example, the other parts are also affected. When clients suffer intense, persistent pain or experience hopelessness and despair, they may begin to doubt their former spiritual support system. This state of uncertainty weakens one's resolve to improve or to survive the stressful situation.

To assist the client through this crisis, you must be able to recognize and intervene in spiritual distress. As a nursing diagnosis, Spiritual Distress is defined by expressions of anger toward a deity or questions related to the meaning of suffering. Collect the following data in a spirituality assessment.*

Subjective
- Does the client verbalize feelings about God or spiritual concerns?

- Does the client feel the illness has changed feelings about God?
- Does the client feel abandoned or separated from spiritual support?
- Does the client question the validity of faith and the religious system?
- Does the client say that the illness is a punishment from God?

Objective
- Does the client pray or read religious material?
- Does the client keep religious material nearby (e.g., rosary, medal)?
- Does the client refuse to participate in spiritual or religious rituals?

The interventions for Spiritual Distress sound simple. Provide support through active listening (i.e., giving full attention and time to accept the client's verbal and nonverbal communication). By showing patience and concern, you can encourage clients to explore their feelings and questions. At the same time, be aware of your own spiritual beliefs and be careful not to impose these on the client. Finally, encourage the client and family to seek support from the appropriate clergy person or spiritual leader of their choice.

*See Edmisson (1997).[13]

In view of his depressed mood, hopelessness, and spiritual isolation, the nurse asks whether Mr. Moore has had any thoughts about hurting himself or ending his life. Initially, he looks away and refuses to answer. But then he admits he has dreams about his death, and he thinks his wife would be better off without him.

COMMUNICATION AWARENESS

When talking with Mr. Moore, the nurse is careful not to react to his negative comments or irritable mood. The nurse asks about physical or emotional issues in a matter-of-fact tone of voice. In response to his pattern of avoiding a direct answer, the nurse rephrases the question and waits for a response. Noting that Mr. Moore may feel uncomfortable talking in front of his wife, the nurse asks her to wait in the kitchen during the interview.

When Mr. Moore states that he has thoughts of death, the nurse calmly asks specific questions to assess the risk for suicide (Box 20–17). Because the client verbally promises that he will not take action to harm himself (a verbal contract for safety), the nurse does not take emergency action.

CLIENT AND FAMILY TEACHING

Because Mr. Moore and his wife report no history of mental illness in the family, it is clear that they have no experience with mood disorders. The nurse defines the manifestations of depression and how depression can affect a person physically, emotionally, and spiritually. The nurse describes the effect on the family when one member is depressed. It is noted that depression often affects people who have suffered a stroke and that it is highly treatable. Briefly, the nurse explains medication and counseling treatment options and offers the home care resources of the psychiatric nurse and the social worker.

Mr. Moore continues to say that nothing will help, but his wife requests assistance.

SPECIALIZED REFERRALS

Before leaving the house, the nurse telephones the attending physician to report the findings and to request orders. The psychiatric nurse will further evaluate the client, offer psychoeducation, and monitor the effectiveness of medication treatment. The social worker will evaluate the need for community resources and make the necessary referrals. The physician is surprised because he had not seen the signs of depression, but he is cooperative and asks that the team members report their findings to him.

The nurse contacts the office to arrange for the referrals. Both the psychiatric nurse and the social worker are informed of Mr. Moore's passive death wish and contract for safety. The nurse also informs them of his spiritual distress at this time, since spirituality can play a significant role in physical and psychological healing. After all the arrangements are made, the nurse calls Mr. Moore to tell him of the dates for their visits. He is pessimistic but agrees to talk with them. Later, the nurse also calls the physical therapist to explain the change in treatment plan and the need to continue physical therapy despite the client's depression.

■ INTERVENTION: BIPOLAR DISORDER

Upon hearing the staff complaints about Miss Howard (dehydration with change in behavior), the nurse again reviews the medical record. It is noted that the client was admitted to the facility 2 years ago because she was unable to manage her multiple medications for heart failure. Miss Howard also has digestive problems, with a

---

BOX 20–17   Screening Assessment of Suicidal Risk

Interview Questions

1. Have you been thinking about death or hurting yourself?
2. If yes, do you have a plan?
3. Have you ever tried to hurt yourself before?
4. If yes, what did you do?
5. What would stop you from hurting yourself now?
6. Can you sign a written contract with me that you will not harm yourself for the next _____ (time period until next evaluation)?

Additional Indications of Higher Risk for Suicide

1. Has a specific plan that is available and dangerous (e.g., hanging, shooting, or jumping from a high location)
2. History of previous attempts
3. Cannot identify person or religious belief that would prevent action
4. Refusal to sign a safety contract
5. Living alone or estranged from loved ones
6. Use of alcohol or drugs
7. Presence of psychosis with command hallucinations to harm self (cannot safely contract)

Results of Screening

1. If the client shows no positive risk factors, no action is necessary except continued monitoring of behavior.

2. If the client shows positive risk factors but agrees to a written contract not to harm self, the nurse:
   a. Co-signs the contract, defining the time period from now until the next visit
   b. Notifies the attending physician (e.g., by telephone) in front of the client to report the assessment and request a psychiatric nurse evaluation; if the physician orders other actions, these are shared with the client
   c. Strongly seeks the client's permission to share the contract with a family member, if available
   d. Contacts the psychiatric nurse to give a report and schedule a visit for the following day
3. If the client shows positive risk factors but refuses to sign a "no harm contract," the nurse must take emergency action. The nurse:
   a. Instructs the client, and family if available, that this condition is a mental health emergency and requires immediate evaluation by a physician in an emergency department
   b. Calls 911 for assistance, explaining that there is a psychiatric emergency
   c. Provides brief information to the police and emergency medical team upon arrival, with a follow-up telephone report to the appropriate emergency department
   d. Notifies the attending physician of the emergency actions

■ THE CLIENT WITH DEHYDRATION AND CONCURRENT BIPOLAR DISORDER: MISS HOWARD

Nursing Diagnosis. Altered Thought Processes with risk for violence directed at others, as evidenced by agitation, verbal threats toward others related to bipolar disorder, and mania.

Outcomes. Miss Howard will not harm self or others, will eat three small meals and drink adequate fluids daily, will sleep at least 6 hours each night, will experience a stabilized mood, and will return to her previous level of functioning (long term).

Interventions	Rationales
1. Assess for mood, nutrition, sleep, and activity level.	1. Clients in a manic phase disregard sleep and food, and their hyperactivity places them at risk for physical complications.
2. Assess for safety and assign staff to observe the client; move her roommate to another room temporarily.	2. The client has decreased impulse control and the potential to hurt others or self.
3. Reduce stimuli, and assign one staff member to offer food and fluids frequently.	3. One consistent staff member reduces the opportunity for staff conflict and supports adequate nutrition.
4. Accept verbalization of anger, but set limits on cursing and aggression.	4. Letting the client "ventilate" and setting limits show acceptance of the client's feelings and maintain safety for the client and others.
5. Maintain privacy and prevent socially inappropriate behavior.	5. The client needs assistance to preserve her dignity while she has decreased control of impulses.
6. Involve the client in her plan of care, offering realistic choices in the daily schedule.	6. This step promotes the client's responsibility for self and counteracts her feelings of fear and helplessness.
7. Coordinate communication among staff and family members regarding the plan of care.	7. The client has impaired communication skills and may distort information from caregivers.

Evaluation. Accomplishment of the expected outcomes will preserve the safety of the client, peers, and staff. Reassessment must be made daily, and plan will need revision in first week if not effective.

---

family history of pancreatic cancer. Her recent hospitalization was related to uncontrolled diarrhea with dehydration. Apparently, her psychotropic medications were discontinued at the acute care hospital and she has not received them in 8 days. Her diagnosis list shows a history of bipolar disorder (see Care Plan).

The psychosocial history is sparse except to note that she lived alone before admission and has never been married. A niece is listed as the next of kin, and staff members report that she visits monthly. She received outpatient psychiatric treatment and has current orders for valproic acid and lithium. The nursing home psychiatric consultant visits monthly.

When the nurse interviews Miss Howard, the client is pacing around her room wearing only her nightgown. She has a large bruise over her right eye from falling out of bed. The chart shows that she has slept 2 to 4 hours for the past three nights. Before the nurse can greet her, Miss Howard says loudly, "I'm glad you are here. These dumb staff of yours can't even get my breakfast right. I want another roommate; that old bag snores. Call the hairdresser. I need my hair done." Her speech is rapid, and her tone of voice is insulting. This behavior is unlike that of her baseline assessment; she tends to be outgoing, with a sarcastic sense of humor, and neatly groomed.

COMPREHENSIVE ASSESSMENT
In view of the significant change in behavior, the nurse updates the nursing assessment. When the nurse tells Miss Howard that she would like to talk about her recent hospitalization, the client eagerly offers her a chair. As the nurse asks about her current mood and activities, the client talks incessantly and frequently interrupts. She does not always answer the question, but from her speech and nonverbal behavior, the nurse gathers the following information. Miss Howard says she feels scared, lonely, and misunderstood. She fears that she has pancreatic cancer and does not trust that the doctors have ordered the right tests. She starts to cry as she describes her niece, who does not visit as often as she once did. She gives numerous complaints about the staff and her roommate and threatens to hit her roommate the next time she snores.

When asked about her psychiatric history, Miss Howard is vague about her problem and complains that even the psychiatrist does not come to see her anymore. She knows that she takes two psychotropic medications but does not know their names. Seeing that the client is an unreliable historian, the nurse asks permission to call her niece for information. Miss Howard agrees and tells the nurse to order her niece to buy her five more robes.

The niece is surprised to hear about Miss Howard's behavior. She reports that her aunt has been stable for years while taking her medication for bipolar disorder. She states that the client has a history of mood swings and becomes very irritable and demanding in the manic phase. Miss Howard has received outpatient psychiatric treatment for 40 years, and the nursing home psychiatrist observes her monthly. The nurse notes that the client was hospitalized when her monthly appointment was due this month. The niece promises to visit the next day and asks the nurse to notify the psychiatrist.

Before calling the psychiatrist, the nurse informs the attending physician about the client's status. The physician agrees that her behavior is altered but refuses to order any psychotropic medication, referring her to the psychiatrist. The nurse consults with the psychiatrist, who immediately orders resumption of lithium and valproic acid, with blood levels to be assessed in 1 week. A sleeping medication is also ordered for 1 week. The psychiatrist speculates that Miss Howard suffered a manic relapse because of the stress of hospitalization and lack of medication. He asks the nurse to reduce stimuli for the client to maintain her safety and the safety of others.

COMMUNICATION AWARENESS

When communicating with Miss Howard, the nurse pays close attention to verbal and nonverbal behavior in order to avoid escalation of tension in the client. As the client talks rapidly and sometimes raises her voice, the nurse maintains a calm tone of voice and normal speed. When Miss Howard approaches the nurse too closely, the nurse moves beyond arm's reach and sets a limit on personal space. Even though the client does not seem to pose a high risk for physical harm, the nurse firmly tells her that physical aggression toward peers or staff will not be tolerated. (Miss Howard had verbally threatened her roommate.)

At the same time, the nurse acknowledges Miss Howard's fear and responds to the legitimate complaints. The nurse explains each diagnostic test and the negative results. The nurse listens seriously to the client's concerns about cold food and her roommate interfering with her sleep. The nurse suggests that part of the client's distress is due to a relapse in her mood disorder and expresses hope that she will feel better once her medications are resumed.

At the end of the interview, the nurse helps Miss Howard to put on her robe, slippers, and underwear. Together, they write a plan for the client's schedule for the rest of the day, including meals, medication, and exercise. The nurse explicitly directs Miss Howard not to threaten or hit anyone and gives her a notebook in which to write down any new complaints. The nurse promises to return at the end of the shift to reevaluate the plan.

CLIENT AND FAMILY TEACHING

The nurse believes that Miss Howard is not amenable to comprehending her illness while she is in a manic condition. Responding to the client's sleep complaint, the nurse shows her teaching materials on her medications. The nurse uses brief, simple terms to describe the desired therapeutic effects of the medication and leaves the material with the client to review.

In a 24-hour care facility, caregivers need the same information that would be given to family members in the community. Especially if physical violence is threatened, the nursing staff must have clear guidelines about communication techniques to reduce agitation. Staff members must know that the client is showing manifestations of her mental illness and that she temporarily does not have adequate impulse control. They must be cautioned not to argue with her or laugh at her behavior. It is likely that the client will recall some of her behavior and will feel guilty and embarrassed later. Efforts to preserve her dignity are just as important as attention to her safety.

SPECIALIZED REFERRALS

Knowing that time is limited for direct nursing intervention, the nurse considers the available resources of the facility. The physician, consultant psychiatrist, and family have already been called to contribute to the treatment plan. Other appropriate referrals include the facility in-service educator and social worker. The in-service instructor can present written and videotape material to the staff on how to communicate with agitated clients. In particular, the floor manager needs to know how to interact with the client so that a strong role model can be presented for the staff. The social worker can meet with the client to give her needed attention and to reassure her about her safety. If the plan does not succeed in calming the client, the nurse can recommend a referral to a partial hospital program to the psychiatrist to readjust the medication in a controlled environment.

The nurse returns to Miss Howard 3 hours later and tells her about the contacts with her niece and the staff. Miss Howard has already taken her medication and has eaten lunch. She has a new list of minor complaints but speaks with less pressure and hostility. She thanks the nurse and promises not to hit anyone.

CONCLUSIONS

The medical-surgical nurse has a vital role in caring for the psychosocial needs of all clients. Sensitivity to client and family anxiety improves the nurse's communication skills and increases the probability that clients will achieve the desired outcomes. For clients who have concurrent mental illness, the nurse must consider several additional needs in order to provide comprehensive nursing care:

- Increased attention to completing the comprehensive nursing assessment
- Heightened awareness of verbal and nonverbal communication
- Basic teaching about illness and treatment options
- Referral to appropriate specialized resources available in the health care system

To provide holistic care to clients with concurrent mental illness does not require specialized training beyond the generalist level, but nurses must learn about the range of multidisciplinary services available at the health care facility in a particular community. The nurse is in a prime position in the health care team to advocate for appropriate mental health services for clients. Recognition of mental health needs supports the accomplishment of general health outcomes while reducing the pain and suffering of preventable adverse events.

BIBLIOGRAPHY

1. Abramovitz, M. (1998). Some drugs that cause psychiatric symptoms. *Medical Letter on Drugs and Therapeutics, 40*(1020), 21–24.
2. American Psychiatric Association. (1994). *Diagnostic and statistical manual of mental disorders* (4th ed., rev.). Washington, DC: Author.
3. American Psychiatric Association. (1994). *Diagnostic criteria from DSM-IV*. Washington, DC: Author.
4. Anderson, K. N., & Anderson, L. E. (1994). *Mosby's pocket dictionary of medicine, nursing and allied health* (2nd ed.). St. Louis: Mosby–Year Book.
5. Andruzzi, E. A., & Carson, V. B. (1996). Highways for the journey: The mental health system. In V. B. Carson & E. N. Arnold

(Eds.), *Mental health nursing: The nurse-patient journey* (pp. 33–50). Philadelphia: W. B. Saunders.

6. Brightman, H. (1998). Manic and depressive recurrences: The search for mechanisms and treatments. *NARSAD Research Newsletter, 10*(2), 1–4.

7. Brown, A. (1995). Advances in genetics of psychiatric disorders. *NARSAD Research Newsletter, Fall,* 9–13.

8. Brown, A., & Lempa, M. (1996). Update on potential causes and new treatments for anxiety disorders. *NARSAD Research Newsletter, Fall/Winter,* 13–18.

9. Brown, A., & Lempa, M. (1997). Late-life depression. *NARSAD Research Newsletter, Winter Supplement,* 10–15.

10. Brown, A., & Weaver, R. (1998). Schizoaffective disorder: Just a set of symptoms or a separate disease? *NARSAD Research Newsletter, 10*(4), 25–29.

11. Clark, C. C. (1997). Posttraumatic stress disorder: How to support healing. *American Journal of Nursing, 97*(8), 27–32.

12. DePaulo, J. R., & Ablow, K. R. (1989). *How to cope with depression.* New York: Fawcett Crest.

13. Edmisson, K. W. (1997). Psychosocial dimensions of medical-surgical nursing. In J. M. Black & E. Matassarin-Jacobs (Eds.), *Medical-surgical nursing: Clinical management for continuity of care* (5th ed.). Philadelphia: W. B. Saunders.

14. Elder, K. N., et al. (1998). Managed care: The value you bring. *American Journal of Nursing, 98*(6), 34–39.

15. Fitzgerald, L. W. (1997). Explorations along the stress axis. *NARSAD Research Newsletter, 9*(2), 1–3.

16. Hall, A. (1998). A disorder yields its secrets: Breakthrough in study of manic-depression. *NARSAD Research Newsletter, 10*(3), 7–8.

17. Isaacs, A. (1998). Depression and your patient. *American Journal of Nursing, 98*(7), 26–31.

18. Katz, J. R. (1997). Providing effective patient teaching. *American Journal of Nursing, 97*(5), 33–36.

19. Langreth, R. (1998). Drug makers attack depression on a new front. *NARSAD Research Newsletter, 10*(3), 9–10.

20. Lazarus, R., & Folkman, S. (1984). *Stress, appraisal and coping.* New York: Springer.

21. Lipson, J. G., Dibble, S. L., & Minarik, P. A. (1997). *Culture and nursing care: A pocket guide.* San Francisco: University of California, San Francisco, Nursing Press.

22. Littrell, S. H., & Littrell, K. H. (1997). Recent advances in understanding negative symptoms in schizophrenia. *Journal of the American Psychiatric Nurses Association, 3*(4), 111–117.

23. ———. (1995). Mental health: Does therapy help? *Consumer Reports, 60*(11), 734–739.

24. NARSAD Research. (1997). *Understanding schizophrenia.* Great Neck, NY: Author.

25. Nemeroff, C. B. (1994). Contemporary issues in the management of depression—Introduction. *American Journal of Medicine, 97*(suppl. 6A), 15–25.

26. Rankin, E. A. D. (1996). Patient and family education. In V. B. Carson & E. N. Arnold (Eds.), *Mental health nursing: The nurse-patient journey* (pp. 503–522). Philadelphia: W. B. Saunders.

27. Reinhard, S. C. (1994). Perspectives on the family's caregiving experience in mental illness. *IMAGE: Journal of Nursing Scholarship, 26*(1), 70–73.

28. Resnick, W. M., & Carson, V. B. (1996). The journey colored by mood disorders. In V. B. Carson & E. N. Arnold (Eds.), *Mental health nursing: The nurse-patient journey* (pp. 759–792). Philadelphia: W. B. Saunders.

29. Robinson, A. W. (1999). Getting to the heart of denial. *American Journal of Nursing, 99*(5), 38–42.

30. Scherck, K. A. (1999). Recognizing coping behaviors. *American Journal of Nursing, 99*(4), 24AAA–24DDD.

31. Stuart, G. W., & Sundeen, S. J. (1991). *Principles and practice of psychiatric nursing* (4th ed.). St. Louis: Mosby–Year Book.

32. Sullivan, P. D., & Carson, V. B. (1996). Highways for the journey: The mental health system. In V. B. Carson & E. N. Arnold (Eds.), *Mental health nursing: The nurse-patient journey* (pp. 33–50). Philadelphia: W. B. Saunders.

33. Sumner, C. H. (1998). Recognizing and responding to spiritual distress. *American Journal of Nursing, 98*(1), 26–30.

34. Talan, J. (1997). Schizophrenia triggers described. *NARSAD Research Newsletter, 9*(2), 20–21.

35. U.S. Department of Health and Human Services. (1993). *Depression in primary care: Volume 1.* Rockville, MD: Agency for Health Care Policy and Research.

36. U.S. Department of Health and Human Services. (1993). *Depression in primary care: Volume 2.* Rockville, MD: Agency for Health Care Policy and Research.

37. Warner, P. H., Rowe, T., & Whipple, B. (1999). Shedding light on the sexual history. *American Journal of Nursing, 99*(6), 34–40.

38. Watzlawick, P., Beavin, J. H., & Jackson, D. D. (1967). *Pragmatics of human communication.* New York: W. W. Norton.

39. Worthington, J. F. (1995). From cause to treatment: Attacking schizophrenia from all sides. *NARSAD Research Newsletter, Summer,* 1–4.

40. Yamashita, M., & Forsyth, D. M. (1998). Family coping with mental illness: An aggregate from two studies, Canada and United States. *Journal of the American Psychiatric Nurses Association, 4*(1), 1–7.

Clients with Sleep and Rest Disorders and Fatigue: Promoting Positive Outcomes

Marlene Reimer

Nursing Outcomes Classification (NOC)
for Nursing Diagnoses—Clients with Sleep and Rest Disorders and Fatigue

Sleep Pattern Disturbance
Anxiety Control
Rest
Sleep
Well-Being
Fatigue
Activity Tolerance
Endurance
Energy Conservation
Nutritional Status: Energy
Psychomotor Energy

Most of us experience occasional problems of disturbed sleep, unwanted drowsiness, fatigue, overstimulation, or understimulation. As a nurse, you will frequently be involved with clients in whom these disturbances interfere with health, healing, and daily activities. Contributing factors may include personal lifestyle habits, environmental features, internal rhythms, and changes associated with episodic illness or chronic illness.

SLEEP AND SLEEP PATTERN DISTURBANCES

Sleep can be defined as a normal state of altered consciousness during which the body rests; it is characterized by decreased responsiveness to the environment, and a person can be aroused from it by external stimuli. Almost a third of the general population has some problems with sleep during any given year.[51] More than half of the 9000 participants in a study of sleep in elderly persons (65 years or older) reported the following as sleep pattern disturbances that they experience most of the time[29]:

- Trouble falling asleep
- Frequent awakening
- Waking too early
- Needing to nap
- Not feeling rested

These disturbances may be secondary to situational, environmental, or developmental stressors, or they may be associated with illness or with pre-existing disorders. The relationship is often reciprocal, in that the disorder decreases sleep and the decreased sleep affects the disorder. Sleep pattern disturbance also contributes to sensory disorders, such as intensive care unit psychosis.

Sleep pattern disturbance is a nursing diagnosis that is defined as a disruption of sleep time that causes discomfort or interferes with a desired lifestyle.[17, 52] A sleep pattern disturbance may be related to one of more than

80 sleep disorders identified in the International Classification of Sleep Disorders, a partial list of which is presented in Box 21–1. Intermittent sleep-related problems are also of concern for nursing diagnosis and intervention.

CHRONOBIOLOGY

Chronobiology refers to the study of biologic changes as they occur in relation to time. Knowledge of chronobiology as it relates to sleep is important to nurses in planning client care and teaching.

The *sleep-wake cycle* is one of the circadian rhythms of the body. Circadian rhythms follow an approximate 24-hour cycle through a complex process linked to light and dark. The effects of illness and hospitalization may disrupt these rhythms, particularly in older persons, who are especially vulnerable to such changes.[6] Nurses can minimize this effect by encouraging a regular schedule with appropriate environmental cues.

Ultradian cycles are circadian rhythms of less than 24 hours. The recurrent pattern of sleep stages, repeating approximately every 90 minutes in adults, is an example.

BOX 21–1   International Classification of Sleep Disorders*

I. Dyssomnias
  A. Intrinsic sleep disorders
    1. Psychophysiologic insomnia
    2. Narcolepsy
    3. Obstructive sleep apnea syndrome
    4. Central sleep apnea syndrome
    5. Periodic limb movement disorder
    6. Restless legs syndrome
  B. Extrinsic sleep disorders
    1. Inadequate sleep hygiene
    2. Environmental sleep disorder
  C. Circadian rhythm sleep disorders
II. Parasomnias
  A. Arousal disorders
    1. Sleepwalking
    2. Sleep terrors
  B. Sleep-wake transition disorders
  C. Parasomnias usually associated with REM sleep
    1. Nightmares
    2. Sleep paralysis
  D. Other parasomnias
    1. Sleep bruxism
    2. Sleep enuresis
    3. Primary snoring
III. Sleep disorders associated with medical or psychiatric disorders
  A. Associated with mental disorders
  B. Associated with neurologic disorders
  C. Associated with other medical disorders
IV. Proposed sleep disorders

* This is a partial listing of common sleep disorders.
REM, rapid eye movement.
From the Diagnostic Classification Steering Committee, Thorpy, M. J., Chairman. (1997). *International classification of sleep disorders: Diagnostic and coding manual* (Rev. ed.). Rochester, MN: American Sleep Disorders Association.

Recognizing this cycle, nurses can arrange care to avoid waking clients more frequently than is absolutely necessary.

Chronopharmacology refers to the study of how biorhythms affect the absorption, metabolism, and excretion of drugs. As an example, the blood level achieved by a continuous infusion of heparin varies throughout the day. The risk of clotting is greater in the morning, and the risk of bleeding is greater in the evening. Effectiveness of anticancer drugs varies according to the time of administration. Further, steroid medications should be administered in the morning to approximate most closely the natural elevation in cortisol levels.

PHYSIOLOGY OF SLEEP AND AROUSAL

The timing of the sleep-wake cycle and other circadian rhythms, such as body temperature, is controlled, at least in part, by the suprachiasmatic nucleus in the anterior hypothalamus. Located above the optic chiasm, this area receives input from the retina, which provides information about darkness and light. The suprachiasmatic nucleus controls the production of melatonin, which is believed to be a potent sleep inducer.[10]

Arousal from sleep, wakefulness, and the ability to respond to stimuli rely on an intact *reticular activating system* (RAS).[18] The RAS is located in the brain stem and contains projections to the thalamus and cortex. The diffuse network of neurons in the RAS is in a strategic position to monitor ascending and descending stimuli through feedback loops.[18]

Although the RAS provides the anatomic framework for arousal, it is the neurotransmitters that serve as the chemical messengers.[18] The onset of sleep and of each subsequent sleep stage is an active process involving delicate shifts in the balance of several of these neurotransmitters.

The transition from the awake state to *non–rapid eye movement* (NREM) sleep is marked by decreases in the concentrations of serotonin (5-hydroxytryptamine [5-HT]), norepinephrine, and acetylcholine. The later transition to *rapid eye movement* (REM) sleep is marked by a dramatic increase in acetylcholine and further decreases in serotonin and norepinephrine.[18, 35, 68] As REM sleep continues, the concentrations of serotonin and norepinephrine increase, eventually stopping REM sleep. Cholinergic activation with the release of acetylcholine seems to reestablish REM sleep.[35] The continuous interaction of these two systems is thought to produce the normal alterations between NREM and REM sleep.[35] Other neurotransmitters, such as gamma-aminobutyric acid (GABA) and dopamine, are also believed to have a part in the reciprocal processes involved in shifts in sleep state.

All of these neurotransmitters are actively involved in waking processes as well. For example, neurons that produce serotonin and norepinephrine play a role in the modulation of sensory input, mood, energy, and information processing, including attention, learning, and memory.[35] Thus, imbalances in these neurotransmitters induced through sleep pattern disturbances, medications, or diseases may reciprocally affect not only sleep but also aspects of sensory processing, mood, and cognition.

THE NEED FOR SLEEP

Much is known about the architecture of the sleep cycle, but much less is known about the need for sleep. It is commonly held that sleep has a restorative and protective function.[36] In sleep, sympathetic activity decreases whereas parasympathetic activity may increase. Hormonal shifts facilitate anabolic processes. Selective deprivation of "slow-wave sleep" (see later) is associated with vague physical complaints.

REM sleep may be especially important for maintaining mental activities, such as learning, reasoning, and emotional adjustment. Sleep also appears to serve as an energy-conserving measure for most of the body except the brain.[37]

SLEEP STAGES

Sleep can be defined behaviorally, functionally, and electrophysiologically. Electrophysiologic monitoring of sleep, called *polysomnography,* includes at least three parameters: (1) brain wave activity, (2) eye movements, and (3) muscle tone. Polysomnography shows that sleep can be divided into REM and NREM. NREM sleep can be further divided into stages 1 through 4. The stages vary in depth but are characterized by slow rolling eye movements, low-level and fragmented cognitive activity, maintenance of moderate muscle tone, and slower but generally rhythmic respirations and pulse rate. As a person progresses from stage 1 to stage 4 sleep, the waveforms

recorded by electroencephalography (EEG) become more synchronized, slower, and higher in amplitude (Fig. 21–1).

NREM sleep is characterized as follows:

Stage 1 is very light. Respirations begin to slow, and muscles relax. At sleep onset, some erratic breathing may occur as well as sudden myoclonic jerks (sleep starts) as the body shifts from an awake to a sleep state. Stage 1 is such a light stage of sleep that persons wakened from it often claim that they were not asleep at all.

Stage 2 is still light sleep. The brain waves are frequently mixed and low voltage in pattern, with bursts of activity called *sleep spindles* and large-amplitude waves called *K complexes.* More than 50% of sleep occurs as stages 1 and 2.

Stages 3 and 4 are known as *slow-wave sleep,* named for the characteristic high-voltage, low-frequency delta waves. Respirations become slow and even. The pulse and blood pressure fall. Oxygen consumption by muscle tissues and urine formation decrease. Dreams that occur during the NREM stages of sleep are generally thought-like ruminations about recent events and current concerns with little story line.[35]

REM sleep is characterized by low-voltage, random fast waves, as in stage 1 NREM. People in REM sleep

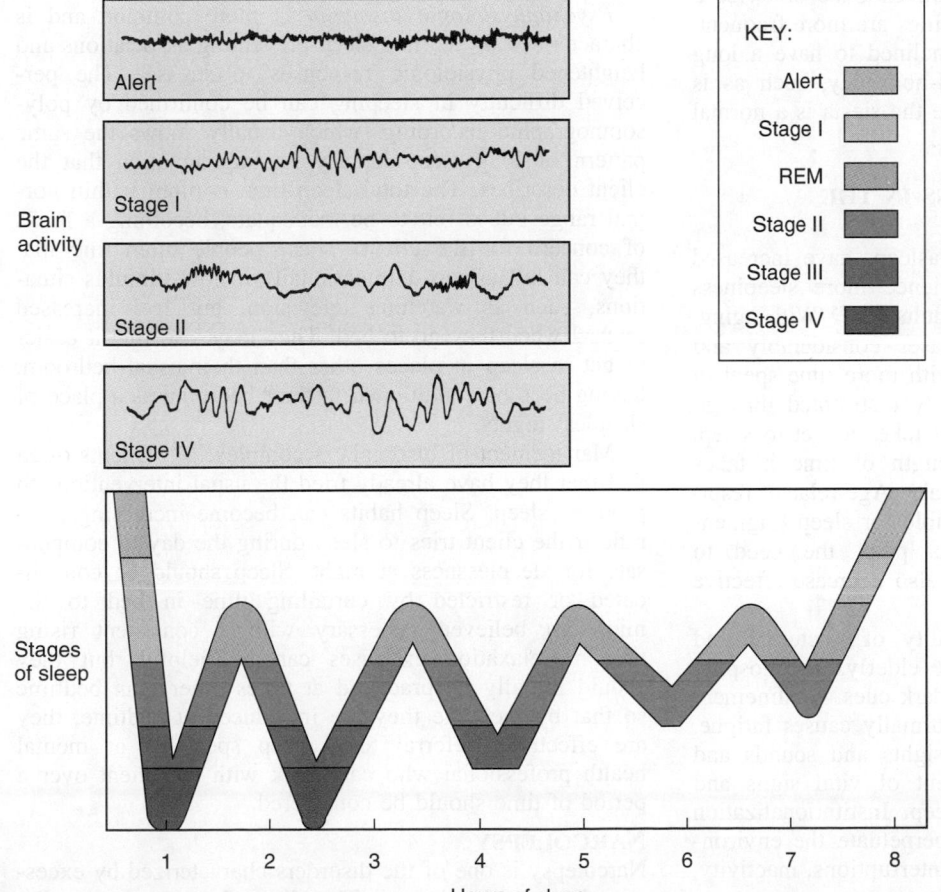

KEY:

Alert
Stage I
REM
Stage II
Stage III
Stage IV

FIGURE 21–1 The electrical activity of the brain during various stages of sleep can be shown on electroencephalograms. During the night, people go through three to five sleep cycles. Each cycle includes a sequence of sleep stages. REM, rapid eye movement. (From Solomon, E. P., Schmidt, R. R., & Adranga, P. J. [1990]. *Human anatomy and physiology* [2nd ed.]. Philadelphia: Saunders College.)

Brain activity

Alert

Stage I

Stage II

Stage IV

Stages of sleep

1   2   3   4   5   6   7   8

Hours of sleep

have characteristic rapid eye movements, erratic respirations, changes in heart rate, and very low muscle tone (see Fig. 21–1). During REM sleep, ventilation depends primarily on the movement of the diaphragm because intercostal and accessory muscle tone is markedly diminished and all postural and nonrespiratory muscles are essentially paralyzed.[61] The ventilatory response to hypoxia and hypercapnia is decreased, and thermoregulation is significantly reduced. Dreams in REM sleep are vivid, story-like, emotional, and bizarre.

Most people move through an orderly progression of NREM sleep from stages 1 to 4 and back through stages 3 to 2 before initiating a period of REM sleep (see Fig. 21–1). Although this is the typical progression, it is not essential or always seen. Atypical progressions are characteristic of some sleep disorders, such as narcolepsy, in which REM sleep is entered almost immediately after sleep onset.

In adults, each sleep cycle through the various stages lasts about 90 minutes. During the first few cycles, more time is spent in slow-wave sleep, and the percentage of REM sleep increases later in the sleep period.

Wide variations in sleep patterns exist among individuals. By explaining the range of these variations, the nurse can help clients seek a pattern that leaves them feeling reasonably refreshed and alert. Eight hours of undisturbed sleep at night with no daytime naps has become the assumed ideal pattern in North American society. However, some adults do well with 6 hours or less and other healthy adults require 10 hours or more of nighttime sleep. Even young adults often awaken once or twice a night, and, with aging, such wakenings are more frequent. Humans may be physiologically inclined to have a long and a short sleep period each 24-hour day, such as is common in warmer climates, where the siesta is a normal part of the day's schedule.[22]

CHANGES IN SLEEP PATTERNS IN THE ELDERLY

Older people take longer to fall asleep, have increased nocturnal wakefulness, and experience more sleepiness during the day than do younger adults.[6, 9, 25] With aging, the percentage of stage 4 decreases considerably and REM sleep decreases somewhat, with more time spent in stage 1. REM sleep is more evenly distributed through the night. *Sleep latency,* the time it takes to get to sleep, increases, as does the average length of time it takes to get back to sleep after arousal.[5] Age-related respiratory dysfunction may be responsible for sleep fragmentation.[4] Other problems, such as pain, the need to void, and nocturnal dyspnea, may also decrease effective sleep.

Hospitalization affects the quality of nocturnal and other sleep time, especially for the elderly. The hospital environment often lacks light and dark cues. Confinement curtails activity or exercise that normally causes fatigue. In addition, there are unfamiliar sights and sounds and frequent awakenings for assessment of vital signs and other interventions that disturb sleep. Institutionalization in a long-term care facility may perpetuate the environmental impact of noise, caregiver interruptions, inactivity, and lack of day-night cues.[63]

SLEEP DISORDERS

DYSSOMNIAS

The dyssomnias include sleep disorders characterized by difficulty initiating or maintaining sleep (insomnia) or by excessive sleepiness. These disorders may arise predominantly from within the body (*intrinsic*), from external sources (*extrinsic*), or from disruptions of circadian rhythm.[2, 21]

■ INTRINSIC SLEEP DISORDERS

INSOMNIA

Many people experience transitory periods during which they have difficulty initiating or maintaining sleep. The onset or exacerbation of illness, with or without hospitalization, may precipitate such difficulty. These sleep pattern disturbances are most often associated with disrupted or inconsistent sleep habits (*inadequate sleep hygiene*) or environmental disruptions. These disorders do not constitute insomnia, but they do predispose individuals to insomnia.

A much smaller proportion of the population has developed persistent difficulty in initiating or maintaining sleep. For them, the difficulty does not respond readily to improved sleep habits or removal of precipitating factors.[21]

Idiopathic insomnia is a rare disorder characterized by a lifelong history of inability to obtain adequate sleep. Its cause is thought to be an abnormality in the neurologic control of sleep.

Psychophysiologic insomnia is more common and is characterized by learned sleep-preventing associations and heightened physiologic responses to stress.[21] The perceived difficulty in sleeping can be confirmed by polysomnographic recording, which usually shows the same pattern of long sleep latency or fragmentation that the client describes. The total sleep time is often within normal range but is felt to be inadequate, becoming a focus of concern for the client. These people often find that they can fall asleep unintentionally in low-stimulus situations, such as watching television, but feel increased arousal when they go to bed. They may also find it easier to get to sleep in places other than their usual bedroom, having become conditioned to their bedroom as a place of sleepless nights.

Management of insomnia is complex.[27, 33] Clients often feel that they have already tried the usual interventions to promote sleep. Sleep habits can become increasingly erratic if the client tries to sleep during the day to compensate for sleeplessness at night. Sleep should be consolidated or restricted by curtailing time in bed to the minimum believed necessary with a consistent rising time.[34] Relaxation exercises can be helpful, but they should initially be practiced at times other than bedtime so that by the time they are introduced at bedtime, they are effective. Referral to a sleep specialist or mental health professional who can work with the client over a period of time should be considered.

NARCOLEPSY

Narcolepsy is one of the disorders characterized by excessive daytime sleepiness.[13] The client also experiences disturbed nocturnal sleep and repeated episodes of almost irresistible daytime drowsiness followed by brief periods of sleep, especially when engaged in monotonous activities. Many narcoleptic clients also experience *cataplexy,* a sudden loss of muscle tone at times of unexpected emotion (e.g., fright). Several other sleep-related abnormalities are commonly experienced by clients with narcolepsy. On initial wakening, they may experience *sleep paralysis* for one to several minutes, during which time they cannot move. This condition, like the other manifestations of narcolepsy, is thought to be linked to malfunctioning of the mechanism controlling REM sleep. The REM sleep that is experienced is normal, but it occurs at different times.

Another REM-like manifestation is *hypnagogic hallucinations,* hallucinatory experiences that occur at sleep onset or awakening.[13] Some people experience sleep paralysis or one of the other associated manifestations without narcolepsy. However, when these manifestations are seen together with excessive sleepiness, they constitute the narcolepsy tetrad.[21] Automatic behaviors during which there is a lapse of awareness are also frequent.

On polysomnography, the most characteristic finding is sleep-onset REM periods. A multiple sleep latency test, to measure how long it takes to fall asleep during normal waking hours, shows a sleep latency of less than 5 minutes over four or five testing periods. Occurrence of REM periods at sleep onset at least twice during the test periods is another criterion for the diagnosis.[3, 21, 32]

Narcolepsy is a genetically related condition with autosomal dominance in some cases. The prevalence is about 1 in 1000 people in the United States.[51] Genetic transmission of narcolepsy may be multifactorial and may involve a human leukocyte antigen (HLA) and another gene that is not HLA-related.[32] Environmental factors may also have a role.

The effects of the disease on lifestyle are significant, with 60% to 80% of clients reporting episodes of having fallen asleep at work, while driving, or both. The associated disruption of social and occupational roles and self-esteem may be a major factor contributing to the depression and personality disorders frequently seen in clients who have narcolepsy.[31]

Impaired release of neurotransmitters such as dopamine may also be a factor in both the narcolepsy and the associated depression.[3] Medical management of narcolepsy usually consists of low doses of stimulants to improve alertness and tricyclic antidepressants to control cataplexy.[3]

Emphasize good sleep hygiene in counseling clients who experience narcolepsy, It is important that they maintain a regular schedule with adequate nocturnal sleep. Recommend regular naps at times when clients are prone to increased sleepiness.[13] Safety is a major issue for these clients. Assistance may be needed in coping with the disruptive effects of narcolepsy on family, work, and social roles.

SLEEP APNEA SYNDROME
Sleep apnea is characterized by cessation of breathing for 10 seconds or longer occurring at least five times per hour.[21] Sleep apnea can be classified as obstructive and central nervous system (CNS) apnea. A combination of the two may be seen.

OBSTRUCTIVE SLEEP APNEA SYNDROME. In obstructive sleep apnea syndrome, respiratory efforts of the diaphragm and intercostal muscles are apparent but ineffective against a collapsed or obstructed upper airway.[28] Snoring indicates partial obstruction. Escalating snoring followed by a silent pause that ends with a gasp or snort probably indicates complete airway obstruction. As hypoxia ensues, the person eventually awakens to breathe. The frequent awakenings impair the normal sleep cycle. With sleep, the muscles of the upper airway relax and may occlude an airway that is already narrowed by enlarged soft tissue structures, jaw structure, or obesity. Partial obstruction may result in upper airway resistance syndrome with or without snoring. Repeated microarousals lead to excessive daytime sleepiness in most clients. A few, particularly older people, may present with insomnia.

Obstructive sleep apnea syndrome affects more than 1% of the adult population.[56] Prevalence may be as high as 5% in middle-aged men and much higher in people in certain occupational groups, such as truck drivers. Women are less likely than men to develop obstructive sleep apnea syndrome, particularly before menopause.[21] A much smaller percentage progress to the classic pickwickian syndrome, characterized by obesity, severe sleep apnea, daytime hypercapnia, and cor pulmonale.

Consider referral to a sleep disorders center for clients observed to have repeated periods of apnea (one a minute or more than 15 to 20 periods an hour) lasting longer than 10 seconds, whether or not these periods are associated with snoring. Because obstructive sleep apnea syndrome is particularly common among males who are obese with short, thick necks and who are heavy snorers, these clients should be observed during sleep for apneic periods. During assessment, question clients regarding the degree of daytime sleepiness experienced, and sudden nighttime awakening, with particular concern about safety in relation to driving and occupational activities.

Milder cases of obstructive sleep apnea syndrome, in which excessive daytime sleepiness is not yet a concern, may respond to weight reduction, measures to promote sleeping in positions other than supine, and avoidance of alcohol. However, once the apneic episodes are observed to occur on most nights and in all body positions, more definitive treatment is usually required.

The application of continuous positive airway pressure (CPAP) by means of a face mask covering the nose is the treatment of choice for clients with moderate to severe obstructive sleep apnea syndrome.[15] The CPAP device provides room air under increased pressure, essentially providing a pressure splint to keep the upper airway open. Bilevel positive airway pressure (BiPAP) operates by the same principle but uses lower pressure during expiration.

The CPAP mask should be applied securely over the nose and held in place by the head gear. It should be turned on whenever the client is ready to go to sleep and should be maintained throughout the sleep period. Additional humidification may be necessary, especially in dry environments. Clients may experience nasal congestion, air leaks, pressure marks on the face, or pressure intolerance. Such problems are not uncommon and may lead to discontinuation of the therapy if they are not effectively managed. It is therefore important that nurses have a working knowledge of the therapy, the importance of regularity in its use, and sources available for technical assistance (e.g., sleep disorders center, respiratory equipment supplier). CPAP units are portable and have features such as battery operation and voltage conversion to accommodate travel requirements.

People who regularly use CPAP should bring their units into the hospital with them. These clients need to be closely monitored when recovering from anesthesia and when receiving narcotics because they are at risk for ineffective breathing patterns.

A note should be made on the health record at the time of admission that the client has obstructive sleep apnea syndrome. If the client is scheduled for surgery, the anesthetist and recovery room staff must be alerted. The CPAP unit may be requested to accompany the client to the recovery room.

Question any order for benzodiazepines or other hypnotic drugs for clients with obstructive sleep apnea syndrome, chronic obstructive pulmonary disease (COPD), or loud snoring because of possible respiratory depression.[42] Teach clients with such conditions that alcohol may also worsen their manifestations because of its selective effect in relaxing the muscles of the upper airway and depression of arousal (see the Client Education Guide).

Uvulopalatopharyngoplasty (UPPP) is a common surgical procedure for reducing snoring. Resecting the uvula, the posterior portion of the soft palate, tonsils, and any excessive pharyngeal tissue, can reduce the propensity to obstruction in some clients.[24] Concern has arisen, however, that reducing or eliminating snoring may place clients at unknown risk for obstructive sleep apnea syndrome. Therefore, preoperative assessment, including respiratory pattern during sleep, is recommended before UPPP or the newer laser-assisted UPPP procedure, which is done in stages in a physician's office.[67] Somnoplasty is another surgical procedure for removal of excessive tissue through the use of high radiofrequencies that spare the mucosa. Tracheostomy may be required in severe obstructive sleep apnea syndrome.

Oral or dental appliances are being used increasingly as another treatment for sleep apnea.[62] Essentially, they act by keeping the jaw forward and the upper airway open.

CENTRAL SLEEP APNEA SYNDROME. Central sleep apnea is characterized by apneic periods during which no apparent respiratory effort occurs.[21] It may be seen with CNS lesions, such as in stroke or brain stem involvement, but it is most commonly mixed with obstructive sleep apnea. Cheyne-Stokes respirations are common with this syndrome, and CPAP is the usual treatment. As with obstructive sleep apnea, sedative-hypnotic drugs should be avoided. In severe cases with CNS involvement, use of diaphragmatic pacemakers or mechanical ventilation may be required.

PERIODIC LIMB MOVEMENT DISORDER

Periodic limb movement disorder may also contribute to daytime sleepiness and frequent nocturnal wakenings. Originally described as nocturnal myoclonus, it is characterized by periodic episodes of repetitive, stereotypic leg (or arm) movements that occur during sleep, causing partial arousals.[8, 21] The diagnosis can be confirmed during polysomnography with surface electromyography (EMG) of the anterior tibial muscles.

Periodic limb movement disorder is common in the elderly population. Clonazepam, a benzodiazepine, or baclofen, a skeletal muscle relaxant, may be ordered to diminish the magnitude of the movement and the frequency of arousals. The antiparkinsonian drug carbidopa-levodopa (Sinemet) and the tricyclic antidepressant imipramine seem to act more directly and almost eliminate the movements. Most of the other tricyclic antidepressants aggravate the condition. For some clients, the use of transcutaneous electrical nerve stimulation (TENS) before sleep has been helpful.[8]

RESTLESS LEGS SYNDROME

Restless legs syndrome involves annoying "crawling," itching, or tingling sensations of the legs while at rest and causes an almost irresistible urge to move.[8, 21] The syndrome is often most severe before sleep onset. Clients almost always have periodic limb movements during sleep. Treatment is similar to that for periodic limb movements.

■ EXTRINSIC SLEEP DISORDERS

The extrinsic sleep disorders encompass a range of factors, from environmentally to chemically induced. Some environmental factors temporarily present during hospitalization are discussed under Hospital-Acquired Sleep Disturbances.

CLIENT EDUCATION GUIDE

Living with Obstructive Sleep Apnea Syndrome

1. Avoid sleeping on your back because that is the position in which the syndrome tends to be worse. Try sleeping with pillows at your back, wearing a small backpack, or sewing a tennis ball into the back of pajamas or nightgown.
2. Aim to reduce or stabilize your weight so that body mass index (weight in kilograms divided by height in square meters) is 27 or less. Even a small weight loss may decrease the number of episodes of apnea or upper airway resistance. Increasing the amount of aerobic exercise is the most effective strategy.
3. Avoid alcohol, hypnotics, and other central nervous system depressants because of their relaxing effect on the upper airway.
4. Get adequate sleep. Chronic sleep deprivation can potentiate the effects of the syndrome.
5. Have your blood pressure checked regularly. Hypertension is often associated with this syndrome.
6. Try to limit driving to times when you feel well rested. If feeling drowsy, get someone else to drive or stop to have a nap. Snacks and caffeine drinks may provide temporary stimulation, but they cannot overcome physiologic sleepiness.
7. Carry an identification card or bracelet to alert emergency personnel to your problem.
8. If continuous positive airway pressure or an oral appliance is prescribed, use it regularly.

■ CIRCADIAN RHYTHM SLEEP DISORDERS

In the general population, the circadian rhythm sleep disorders, such as *time zone change syndrome* and *shift work sleep disorder*,[2] are not uncommon. In taking a nursing history, be alert to a history of long-time shift work.

Elderly and chronically ill clients who live alone may be vulnerable to *irregular sleep-wake patterns*. In this disorder, prolonged ignoring or absence of external cues to time, such as regular mealtimes, work periods, and daylight, leads to erratic periods of sleeping and wakefulness. Internal circadian cues may also be damped as a result of aging or diffuse brain disease.[21, 25]

Management strategies for circadian rhythm disorders include maintenance of a regular schedule (e.g., people who regularly work night shift are encouraged to maintain the same sleep schedule on nights off) and exposure to natural sunlight. Light therapy is being used to facilitate adjustments in circadian rhythms as well as in the treatment of *seasonal affective disorder* (SAD).[6, 44, 46]

SAD refers to the onset of a major depressive episode corresponding to a particular period of the year, usually late fall and early winter. Some seasonal variation in mood, activity level, and appetite is common in latitudes where climate and length of daylight change markedly.

Administration of bright light in the early morning is most effective in treating SAD or resetting habitual wakening to an earlier hour.[19, 70] Exposure to bright sunlight at those times can also be effective, but conventional indoor lighting is inadequate. Dosage of light is measured in units of illuminance (lux).[46] The usual dosage is about 5000 lux-hours, which may be taken as 2500 lux for 2 hours, 5000 lux for 1 hour, or 10,000 lux for 30 minutes. This level of illumination requires special light boxes, a variety of which are now available.

Help clients to realize that light therapy should begin only under the guidance of a clinician experienced in its use. Teaching should include appropriate positioning of the head in relation to the light source. The most common side effects are eyestrain and headache. Too much light may contribute to irritability and insomnia.[46, 70] The long-term risk of exposure of the eyes to bright light therapy is under investigation. Until more is known, the presence of retinopathy, glaucoma, or cataract is generally considered a contraindication.[46, 70]

PARASOMNIAS

The parasomnias are disorders that occur during sleep but that usually do not produce insomnia or excessive sleepiness.[21] The underlying pathologic mechanism may involve partial arousal or abnormalities in sleep-wake transition.

■ AROUSAL DISORDERS

Partial arousals typically occur during slow-wave sleep.[24] *Sleepwalking,* also known as *somnambulism,* may include semi-purposeful behavior, such as dressing. However, the behavior may be lacking in coordination and appropriateness, such as voiding in the closet. The occurrence of sleepwalking in adults is often associated with anxiety. *Sleep terrors* are sudden arousals from slow-wave sleep accompanied by screaming, tachycardia, tachypnea, diaphoresis, and other manifestations of intense fear.[21] If awakened, the person is often disoriented and has little recall of the nature of the dream image. Sleep terrors typically occur in young children but may develop in adults.

■ SLEEP-WAKE TRANSITION DISORDERS

Sleep-wake transition disorders are common in the general population, rarely causing enough disruption to be legitimately called disorders. As mentioned earlier, *sleep starts* refer to the sudden jerking movement of the legs that often occurs just as a person is falling asleep. Nocturnal leg cramps are also common. The frequency and intensity may be greater with high caffeine intake, stress, or intense physical activity before going to bed. *Sleeptalking* may also occur more frequently during times of stress.

■ PARASOMNIAS ASSOCIATED WITH RAPID EYE MOVEMENT SLEEP

Like the other parasomnias, those associated with REM sleep may be distressing but are seldom serious. *Nightmares* are frightening dreams that arise in REM sleep and are often vividly recalled on awakening. In contrast to night terrors, these dreams occur in slow-wave sleep and there is little recall. *Sleep paralysis* is one of the classic signs of narcolepsy but can occur in isolation. At sleep onset or on awakening, people experience episodes of one to several minutes during which they are unable to move.[24] This effect may be an extension of the normal state of low muscle tone during REM sleep.

■ OTHER PARASOMNIAS

Other parasomnias are not specifically associated with a particular sleep stage. *Sleep bruxism* refers to grinding of the teeth during sleep and may lead to dental damage. *Sleep enuresis,* or bed-wetting, may occur in adults in association with other disorders, such as obstructive sleep apnea syndrome.[21] *Primary snoring* is distinguished from obstructive sleep apnea syndrome by its rhythmic nature without episodes of apnea or hypoventilation.

SLEEP DISORDERS ASSOCIATED WITH MEDICAL AND PSYCHOLOGICAL DISORDERS

Secondary sleep disorders are of particular relevance in considering problems common to medical-surgical clients. Whereas some clients have a pre-existing sleep disorder of the dyssomnia or parasomnia type, others develop a sleep disorder secondary to disease or its manifestations. By remaining aware of the physiology of normal sleep, you can anticipate the risk of sleep pattern disturbances in medical-surgical clients.

■ NEUROTRANSMITTER IMBALANCES

Neurotransmitter imbalances predispose to sleep pattern disturbances.[60] These imbalances may be disease-related or drug-induced.

More than 70% of people being treated for Parkinson's disease, which results from a deficiency of the neurotransmitter dopamine, report sleep pattern disturbances.[21, 48] Insomnia is the most frequent initial concern, followed by sleep fragmentation, disturbances in the sleep-wake schedule, and visual hallucinations.

Depression is accompanied by sleep disturbance in at least 90% of people who suffer from it.[21] Milder forms of depression and those that occur in young people are often associated with sleep-onset insomnia; more severe depressions are characterized by broken sleep and early-morning wakening. Some relationship appears to exist between the pathogenesis of depression and REM sleep mechanisms in that depressed people who are deprived of REM sleep often show improved mood.[31, 40] The action of tricyclic antidepressants in suppressing REM sleep has been proposed as the primary mechanism underlying their effectiveness in treating depression.[57]

Neurotransmitter imbalances may also contribute to the sleep disturbances frequently seen with Alzheimer's disease and other dementias. The most typical pattern with dementias is frequent awakenings, with agitation progressing to loss of sleep-wake consolidation.[58] Assessing sleep patterns, minimizing caregiver-initiated awakenings (e.g., for toileting), and ensuring a regular bedtime may help to reduce nocturnal and daytime agitation.[14] The sleep-wake cycle may be completely reversed in a client with Alzheimer's disease. The client may nap during the day and be awake all night, restless, agitated, and wandering. The incidence of sleep apnea is higher in people with Alzheimer's disease, possibly as a result of associated neuronal degeneration in the brain stem. Therefore, the nocturnal respiratory patterns of these clients should be carefully assessed, with referral to a sleep disorders center if apnea is suspected.

■ HEAD INJURY

Head injury of all degrees of severity affects sleep patterns. The appearance of differentiated sleep stages on electroencephalography (EEG) in comatose clients with severe head injuries is a favorable prognostic indicator. Sleep stages indicate that connections between the brain stem, diencephalon, and telencephalon are intact and allow shifts to occur between NREM and REM sleep. Even after mild head injury, however, some degree of sleep disturbance may persist for several months.[20] Teaching clients and their families that this unsettled sleep is a typical part of *postconcussion syndrome* can allay anxiety and hasten functional recovery.

For clients in the confused, agitated stage of recovery that results from more severe head injury, use of environmental cues (e.g., light and darkness), regularity of daily schedule, and appropriate daytime exercise and activity can help to restore the sleep-wake cycle. Haloperidol (Haldol), which is often given to confused, agitated clients, blocks the activity of dopamine. This disruption of the delicate neurotransmitter balance may lead to insomnia. Thus, the health care team must balance the option of controlling agitated behavior—and its associated high consumption of energy—with the undesirable side effect of increasing sleep fragmentation through medication.[59]

■ HORMONAL IMBALANCES

Hormonal imbalances also contribute to sleep pattern disturbance. *Hyperthyroid* clients tend to have fragmented, short sleep periods with an excess of slow-wave sleep. *Hypothyroidism* is characterized by excessive sleepiness, and polysomnographic recordings show a reduction in the proportion of slow-wave sleep.

Clients with *diabetes mellitus,* particularly type 1, may experience hypoglycemic attacks during the night. Besides the usual clinical manifestations of sweating, palpitations, hunger, and anxiety, which the client may recognize as a hypoglycemic reaction, be alert to complaints of nightmares and early morning headaches. If these manifestations are present, check blood glucose levels at regular intervals during the night. Insulin dosage or timing may need to be changed. Diabetic clients who have autonomic neuropathy have a higher prevalence of breathing abnormalities during sleep because of the associated dysfunction of autonomic respiratory control; thus, their nocturnal breathing patterns should be assessed.

Sleep patterns normally vary across the menstrual cycle in response to estrogen and progesterone levels.[23] During the latter part of the cycle, when progesterone levels are higher, the first REM sleep period occurs earlier, and some studies have shown sleep disturbances to be more frequent.[45] Women with *premenstrual syndrome* tend to have less slow-wave sleep throughout the menstrual cycle than their asymptomatic peers. With *menopause,* many women experience poorer sleep quality that may result in mood changes.[7] Estrogen replacement therapy may help to reduce these symptoms. *Postmenopausal* women are also at higher risk for experiencing snoring and obstructive sleep apnea.[43]

■ RESPIRATORY DISORDERS

Nocturnal asthma attacks are common in cases of poorly managed asthma, contributing to frequent awakenings in up to 70% of people with asthma.[21] Bronchial resistance increases during the early morning hours, even in healthy people, as does sensitivity to histamine.

Chronic airway limitations, such as asthma and emphysema, contribute to difficulty initiating sleep, frequent arousals with shortness of breath or cough, and chronic fatigue. Oxygen saturation may fall, particularly during REM sleep, when ventilation depends on the diaphragm, which is often flattened and inefficient in clients with advanced chronic airflow limitation.[39, 55] In addition, ventilation and perfusion are altered. Dysrhythmias are common during sleep in clients with advanced respiratory disease, especially when oxygen saturation falls below 60%.[21] Pulmonary artery pressure increases as a result of the pulmonary vascular constriction induced by the low oxygen desaturation and the destructive processes of the underlying disease.

Ventilatory responses to hypoxia and hypercapnia are decreased during sleep, even in people with normal respiratory functioning.[4] Clients with advanced respiratory disease are even more vulnerable; therefore, hypnotics and other CNS depressants that damp arousal should be given with greater caution.

Some of the medications used in the treatment of chronic airway limitations, such as theophylline preparations, may contribute to insomnia. Anxiety and depression associated with effects of the disease may exacerbate the tendency toward fragmented sleep. Try to provide a calm, secure, and relaxed environment for clients. Stimulants such as caffeine may need to be avoided.

The recumbent posture for sleeping is problematic for many people with respiratory disorders. Encourage clients to use several pillows or to have the head of the bed elevated; during acute episodes, they may find it more comfortable to sleep in a reclining chair.

■ CARDIOVASCULAR DISORDERS

Up to 25% of people with hypertension have been found to have obstructive sleep apnea.[66] An association between snoring and hypertension has also been documented.[56] Thus, it is important that you assess clients who have hypertension or who snore while having repeated apneic periods during sleep.

In clients with severe heart failure, periodic breathing of the Cheyne-Stokes type occurs. This pattern may result in significant hypoxemia, frequent arousals, increased stage 1 sleep, and reduced total sleep time.

The variability of heart and respiratory rates during REM sleep may be a factor in nocturnal angina.[66] Clients recovering from myocardial infarction are often deprived of sleep during their stay in a critical care unit and may experience REM rebound on transfer to a step-down or standard unit. The greater cardiac demands during REM sleep may put some additional strain on the recovering heart, making continued nursing surveillance during this period particularly important.[47]

■ GASTROINTESTINAL DISORDERS

Gastric acid secretion normally decreases during sleep, but people with duodenal ulcers have higher than average levels of secretion.[66] Recurrent awakenings with epigastric pain are common, especially in the first 4 hours after sleep onset,[21] and antacids or histamine antagonists may need to be administered.

Gastroesophageal reflux (heartburn) can be more serious when it occurs during sleep, because the longer exposure of the esophagus to gastric acid can lead to esophagitis. Hypnotics should be used cautiously with such clients because the suppression of arousal makes them more vulnerable to esophagitis and pulmonary aspiration. You may suggest that these clients avoid eating within 3 hours of bedtime, consider use of antacids or histamine antagonists, and raise the head of the bed on blocks (reverse Trendelenburg position) to decrease the likelihood of reflux and subsequent aspiration.[54]

■ OTHER DISORDERS

Numerous other disorders seem to have an effect on or an association with sleep. Any condition that results in pain, discomfort, or impaired mobility has the potential to disrupt sleep.[53] Various skin conditions, such as atopic eczema, are associated with decreased REM sleep. Unrefreshing sleep, chronic fatigue, and diffuse musculoskeletal pain are among the diagnostic criteria for fibromyalgia. The EEG tracing of clients with this condition often shows a unique pattern of intrusion of alpha waves into slow-wave sleep, producing *alpha-delta activity.*[21] The clinical manifestations tend to be vague, and clients are often discouraged about the inability of health care professionals to diagnose and treat this condition. The nurse may be in a position to encourage referral to a sleep disorders center.

The effect of sleep or sleep deprivation on some disorders can be useful for diagnostic purposes. For example, the typical occurrence of erections in healthy males during REM sleep is being used as a diagnostic measure in differentiating sources of impotence.[71] REM-associated erections are also the reason that the nurse must be careful when securing an indwelling urinary catheter in a male client and allow a sufficient amount of loop to accommodate an erection.

Sleep deprivation and erratic sleep patterns reduce the seizure threshold, which you should consider in assessment and teaching of clients with seizure disorders. Seizure activity may also be a cause of sleep disturbance.[49] Partial and focal seizures can arise in all phases of sleep, including REM; generalized tonic-clonic seizures are more likely to occur during slow-wave sleep than during REM.[64] The tendency of sleep deprivation to trigger seizure activity is used diagnostically, in that clients may be required to stay awake all night before they undergo sleep-deprivation EEG. Some treatment regimens for clients susceptible to nocturnal seizures involve selective medication-induced suppression of sleep stages in which the client's seizures most frequently occur.

HOSPITAL-ACQUIRED SLEEP DISTURBANCES

Clients in the hospital may report difficulty getting to sleep, awakening frequently with difficulty getting back to sleep, or early morning awakening. The etiologic mechanism and interventions differ from each other.

■ SLEEP ONSET DIFFICULTY

Sleep onset difficulty is a common problem in hospitals because of the strange environment and the anxieties associated with illness and hospitalization. A sleep latency time of 20 to 30 minutes is within the normal range for most adults. Environmental control, such as reduction of noise and interruptions, and conservative relaxation measures, such as a back rub, should be tried before resorting to a hypnotic agent. The rapid-acting hypnotics, such as zolpidem (Ambien), are most effective with this type of insomnia.

If a hypnotic is given, monitor the client's safety in getting up at night. Most hypnotics cause some degree of antegrade amnesia, meaning that otherwise cognitively intact clients may become disoriented and forget where they are. The longer-acting hypnotics also result in some hangover effect. An increased risk of hip fractures from falls has been documented in people who are taking long-acting benzodiazepines.[59]

■ SLEEP MAINTENANCE DISTURBANCE

Sleep maintenance disturbance may be associated with sustained use of or withdrawal from a variety of medications and related substances. Alcohol hastens sleep onset but leads to awakening later in the night. In acute intoxication, REM sleep is suppressed. Abrupt withdrawal, as occurs with hospitalization, may trigger massive REM rebound. In chronic alcoholics, sleep architecture remains disturbed even several years after abstinence. Sustained use of or withdrawal from antidepressants, monoamine oxidase inhibitors, propranolol, and phenytoin can also contribute to insomnia.

Other factors that contribute to sleep fragmentation include stimuli that tend to awaken people in the middle of the night. Internal stimuli, such as pain, discomfort, and the urge to void, are frequent disturbers of sleep. Sleep disorders, such as sleep apnea and periodic limb movement, arc more frequently associated with excessive somnolence, but they do trigger awakenings, after which some people have difficulty getting back to sleep. Hospitalization provides an opportunity for nursing surveillance, which may be instrumental in detecting these disorders as distinct from disturbances triggered by natural or transitory stimuli.

External stimuli include environmental factors, such as light, noise, and temperature, as well as disruptions by other people. You can reduce nocturnal stimuli by darkening the client's room; turn lights off, except for a small night light for safety purposes, and close curtains. To reduce nocturnal stimuli, reduce as much noise as possible by avoiding unnecessary conversation, minimizing equipment noise, and closing the client's door, if possible. You can adjust the temperature by providing bed coverings according to the client's preference and by modifying room temperature (directly, by adjusting the thermostat or air conditioner, or indirectly, by closing curtains and adjusting ventilation). Remove disturbing objects to create a pleasant, tidy environment, for example, removing equipment associated with painful procedures.

You can also reduce nocturnal stimuli by spacing necessary caregiving activities (e.g., turning, taking vital signs) to allow periods of 90 minutes or more of undisturbed sleep and, when possible, synchronizing these activities with periods during which the client is already awake. Finally, coordinate the nature and timing of interruptions by other caregivers (e.g., for laboratory testing or chest physiotherapy) to preserve periods of undisturbed sleep.

■ EARLY-MORNING AWAKENING

Early-morning awakening occurs frequently among the elderly. Sensitivity to environmental disturbances increases toward morning in people of all ages but even more so in older adults. Clients who are disturbed by early-morning awakening should be screened for indications of depression.

Sleeplessness and agitation may be associated with an acute confusional state (i.e., delirium). Especially among elderly people, this transient cognitive disorder may be associated with acute illness and admission to the hospital. Unlike that of dementia, the onset is rapid and is associated with a fluctuating level of consciousness. Thinking is disorganized and fragmented, memory is impaired, and delusions and hallucinations are common. Sleep is grossly disturbed with frightening dreams, disorientation, and restlessness. Delirium is usually precipitated by a treatable systemic illness such as dehydration, infection, drug toxicity, or renal failure. It is important that you identify delirium and pursue treatment possibilities. When the cause is removed, recovery is rapid.

■ SLEEP DEPRIVATION

Sleep deprivation is of particular concern for clients in critical care units. The noise level, 24-hour lighting, and frequency of caregiver interruptions create sensory overload and sleep deprivation, which is thought to be a major factor contributing to postoperative psychosis.[5]

Clients who have had surgery are also at risk for sleep pattern disturbance because of disruptions in circadian rhythms. The cause is unclear, but the disruptions may be related to the length and type of anesthesia, postoperative analgesia, or mechanisms associated with the procedure itself. REM sleep and slow-wave sleep are suppressed. It may take 4 to 6 weeks for the client's sleep patterns to return to normal after open heart surgery with cardiopulmonary bypass. Specific assessment of sleep quality and quantity should be incorporated into the care of all surgical patients.

DIAGNOSTIC ASSESSMENT

The primary diagnostic test for sleep disorders is polysomnography (Fig. 21–2). Clients may be referred to a sleep disorders center for overnight EEG, electro-oculography (EOG), and submental EMG with surface electrodes. Clients may also have continuous recording of arterial oxygen saturation by ear or finger oximeter, air flow as detected by monitoring expired carbon dioxide, respiratory movements by means of transducers placed around the chest and abdomen, and an electrocardiogram (ECG) and heart rate determination with standard limb leads. Ambulatory monitoring systems are also available to facilitate studies in the natural home environment.

A multiple sleep latency test (MSLT) may also be performed to assess impairment of daytime alertness. The MSLT is performed the day after a standard overnight polysomnogram. The time required for clients to fall asleep when in a relaxed state is evaluated at 2-hour intervals, with each nap limited to 20 minutes. The type of sleep is also assessed, making the test particularly useful in diagnosing narcolepsy, a condition in which clients typically have sleep-onset REM periods.[13]

■ Nursing Management

ASSESSMENT

Include a brief assessment of the client's usual sleep habits and recent sleep quality as part of the initial nursing history. On the care plan, note usual bedtime and rising times as well as preferences or rituals that may enhance sleep quality. For example, clients with ineffective breathing patterns associated with conditions such as COPD and hiatal hernia may be accustomed to sleeping with several pillows or with the head of the bed elevated.

If sleep quality is reported to be poor, explore the nature of the disturbance by noting the following:

- Usual activities in the hour before retiring
- Sleep latency
- Number and perceived cause of awakenings
- Regularity of sleep pattern (e.g., shift work)
- Consistency of rising time
- Frequency and duration of naps
- Events associated with initial onset of sleep disturbance
- Ease of falling asleep in places other than the usual bedroom
- Situations in which client fights sleepiness
- Daily caffeine intake
- Use of alcohol, sleeping pills, and other medications
- Incidence of morning headache
- Frequency of snoring, apparent pauses in breathing (apneas), and kicking movements; the latter information is

TYPICAL RECORDINGS	NORMAL	LOUD SNORING	OBSTRUCTIVE APNEA	CENTRAL APNEA
TIDAL VOLUME				
PARADOXICAL BREATHING				
OXYGEN SATURATION				
HEART RATE				
BODY MOVEMENT	(MIN)	(MIN)	(MIN)	(MIN)
TYPICAL FINDINGS				
TIDAL VOLUME	SMOOTH AND REGULAR	INCREASED AND ERRATIC	REPETITIVE MAJOR FLUCTUATIONS	REPETITIVE EVENTS WITH ZERO AIRFLOW
PARADOXICAL BREATHING (INDICATION OF RESPIRATORY EFFORT)	NONE	PRESENT AND ERRATIC	OCCURS DURING EACH APNEIC EVENT	NONE
OXYGEN SATURATION	NORMAL	NORMAL	DECREASES WITH EACH APNEIC EVENT	DECREASES WITH EACH APNEIC EVENT
HEART RATE	NORMAL	NORMAL	MAJOR BRADYTACHYCARDIA	LESS PROMINENT BRADYTACHYCARDIA

FIGURE 21–2 Polysomnography is used to determine the presence of sleep disorders. These examples are taken from a screening system that may be used in a person's home (in contrast to a laboratory), where sleep patterns are more typical. Screening studies can differentiate between obstructive sleep apnea and central sleep apnea as well as between loud snoring and normal sleep patterns. When a sleep disorder is identified, further assessment is needed, including electroencephalographic and electrocardiographic readings to elucidate the cause of the problem. (Courtesy of Vitalog, Mountain View, CA.)

best obtained from the sleeping partner or from your observation while the client is in the hospital

Objective data may include visible signs of fatigue and lack of sleep, such as circles under the eyes, lack of coordination, drowsiness, and irritability.

DIAGNOSIS, OUTCOMES, INTERVENTIONS

Sleep Pattern Disturbance. Sleep pattern disturbance is a common nursing diagnosis (e.g., *Sleep Pattern Disturbance related to changes in routine due to hospitalization and pain*). It may be related to change in sleeping environment, shift work schedule, recurrent pain, or many other possibilities. Other nursing diagnoses may also be applicable (e.g., *Risk for Injury related to excessive daytime sleepiness*).

Outcomes. The client will have improved sleep patterns within three nights as evidenced by sleeping for 6 to 8 hours at one time, stated feeling of lessened fatigue, and decreased irritability.

Intervention. The client's usual bedtime routine should be followed as closely as possible. For example, if the client usually watches television before sleeping, attempt to make this possible. Schedule nursing assessments and interventions in blocks of time to allow 90 to 120 minutes of uninterrupted sleep. The environment should mimic nighttime, with lights dimmed and quiet

maintained. Offer extra blankets for external warmth. Provide a light complex carbohydrate snack, such as whole wheat crackers, if the client's condition allows.

Other techniques used to promote sleep include back massage, relaxing music, and progressive relaxation techniques. Medications to promote sleep should be used judiciously because they can alter the architecture of sleep, often reducing the REM sleep and eventually leading to REM rebound. If the client is in pain, analgesics rather than sleeping medications should be given. Clients in pain do not sleep restfully.

Sleep medications may be useful during short periods of sleep disturbance (e.g., hospitalization, bereavement, relocation). These medications are usually given at bedtime, and administration may be repeated once if they are not effective. Consider the drug's half-life and the time of night before repeating administration. To avoid prolonged drowsiness, do not repeat sleeping medications after 3 AM. In this case, you might try other measures to promote sleep, such as offering milk, analgesia, music, and back massage.

The client should be awakened with the least obtrusive stimulus possible, such as a soft touch or a soft voice. Startling the client may make it difficult for the client to go back to sleep. Many assessments and interventions can be performed without the client's being completely awake.

EVALUATION

Some sleep disturbances are temporary and related to the stress of hospitalization.[12] It is possible that temporary stress problems will be corrected only after the client's return home.

Clients with sleep disturbances may need follow-up care with repeated assessments to determine whether the problem was corrected. Clients with long-term sleep disorders may need ongoing support to maintain the effectiveness of treatment.

FATIGUE

Fatigue is a manifestation commonly associated with most acute and chronic illnesses but also experienced with normal, healthy functioning and everyday life.[1] Fatigue can be defined as a subjective state in which an individual experiences a sustained sense of exhaustion and diminished capacity for physical and mental work that is not relieved by rest.[17] It is often the first indication of an abnormal process[16, 26] and may become a chronic and debilitating condition. Fatigue differs from tiredness or sleepiness, in that sleepiness is a temporary state that results from lack of sleep, sleep disorders, improper nutrition, sedentary lifestyle, or a temporary increase in work or social responsibilities.[11]

Chronic fatigue has no recognized function and often has no apparent relation to activity or exertion.[1] The affected person perceives it as being abnormal, unusual, or excessive. It typically has an insidious onset, persists over time, and is not generally relieved by usual restorative techniques. Fatigue has a major effect on one's activities of daily living and quality of life.

Nurses have an important role in helping fatigued clients manage and cope effectively, whether they are in the hospital or in their own home. Understanding the debilitating effects of fatigue on individuals is an important component of effective nursing care.[16]

ASSESSMENT

The major defining characteristics of fatigue are as follows[17]:

- Verbalization of an unremitting and overwhelming lack of energy
- Inability to maintain usual routines
- Perceived need for additional energy to accomplish routine tasks
- Increase in physical complaints
- Emotional lability or irritability
- Impaired ability to concentrate and decreased performance
- Lethargy or listlessness
- Disinterest in surroundings
- Decreased libido
- Accident proneness

Fatigue, like pain, must be understood as multidimensional aspects that include physiologic, psychological, social, and spiritual components.[24]

Physiologic fatigue has been associated with sleep disturbances, infection, fever, pregnancy, and anemia[1]; acquired immunodeficiency syndrome (AIDS), hyperthyroidism or hypothyroidism, and menopause[17]; stroke[38]; multiple sclerosis[30]; and cancer and hepatitis.[26] Psychological fatigue has been described as a state of weariness related to diminished motivation and can be associated with stress, depression, and anxiety.[1, 17]

Chronic fatigue syndrome refers to a medical diagnosis of profound fatigue lasting at least 6 months and causing a 50% or greater reduction in physical activities not explainable by other causes.[41] Impaired concentration and generalized aching are commonly associated. It is closely related to fibromyalgia, with about 75% of people with chronic fatigue syndrome exhibiting the same characteristic tender points. They, too, frequently report sleep disturbances. As with any clients reporting manifestations of chronic fatigue, take a detailed sleep history. Coexistence of treatable sleep disorders is not uncommon, and improved sleep hygiene may reduce the overwhelming sense of fatigue.

DIAGNOSIS, OUTCOMES, INTERVENTIONS

Fatigue. Fatigue as a nursing diagnosis may be written, for example, as *Fatigue related to altered body chemistry secondary to chemotherapy.*

Outcomes. The client will report a moderate reduction in fatigue within 4 days.

Intervention. Much of the management of fatigue is based on relief of manifestations, with an emphasis on the whole person, mind, and body.[41] The goals of management are to improve the quality of sleep, reduce pain, increase neurotransmitter production, and help the person regain control of his or her life.[41]

You can support clients in understanding the causes of their fatigue and offer support in identifying energy patterns and the need for scheduling activities.[11] An understanding of the effects of conflict and stress on energy levels can help the individual learning new fatigue coping skills. Allowing the expression of feelings regarding the effects of fatigue on one's life is important. Monitor for factors contributing to fatigue on a daily basis, and intervene in a timely manner. Intervention may include carefully planning activities of daily living and daily exercise schedules with appropriate rest periods.[11] Assistance with self-care activities should be offered when needed, and attempts should be made to minimize sensory overload or sensory deprivation.

EVALUATION

Fatigue may not resolve completely, depending on the underlying factors. Thus, evaluation of outcomes and revisions to interventions should be based on mutual planning with the client and family to reduce manifestations and to improve management and quality of life. Balance is needed, so that strategies to reduce fatigue, such as avoidance of stress, do not preclude activities that are important to the client.

SENSORY DISTURBANCES

Each person has an optimal level of sensory input that facilitates a sense of well-being and optimal cognitive and motor performance. Sensory input comes from environmental and internal sources. Sensory input is received through peripheral receptors, transmitted via afferent neurons up the spinal cord, and channeled through the hypothalamus to the cerebral cortex, where it is interpreted in relation to previous patterns of experience.

People at risk for sensory overload or deprivation include those who are experiencing a new or unfamiliar environment, altered sensory input, altered cognitive processing, or impaired mobility.

It has been suggested that people with dementia have a progressively lowered stress threshold because of declining cognitive and functional abilities.[69] Other situations, such as acute illness or losses, may also reduce the ability to cope with a new or challenging environment.

CLASSIFICATION

■ SENSORY OVERLOAD

Sensory overload is a state in which the degree and nature of sensory input exceed the tolerance level of the individual, resulting in feelings of distress and hyperarousal with impaired thinking and problem-solving ability.

■ SENSORY DEPRIVATION

Sensory deprivation is a state in which the overall quantity or diversity of sensory input is decreased. People often compensate for an overall reduction in stimuli by increasing internal stimuli, such as by daydreaming or reminiscing.

DIAGNOSIS AND PREVENTION

■ DIAGNOSIS

Sensory/perceptual alterations is the nursing diagnosis relevant to sensory disturbances.[17] It is defined as a state in which the individual experiences a change in the amount or pattern of incoming stimuli accompanied by a diminished, exaggerated, distorted, or impaired response to such stimuli.

■ PREVENTION

You can minimize the risk of sensory disturbances by modifying the environment to prevent overstimulation and by enhancing orientation, meaning, and pattern. Practical interventions include reducing noise and glare and explaining not only procedures but also sights and sounds in the environment (e.g., the intercom).

Clients who have had limited prior experience with hospitalization or with health technology are at particular risk for sensory overload because they lack memories and knowledge to make sense out of much of their changed environment. In addition, clients whose sensory input is restricted or distorted are at risk for sensory deprivation in the sense that the stimuli are inappropriate to their needs. For example, a client with a spinal cord injury may be kept in a supine position initially, limiting the field of vision to the ceiling and the portions of the room that can be seen from each side.

Another major high-risk group of clients are those experiencing alterations in thought processes such as those that occur with stroke, head injury, schizophrenia, or dementia (e.g., Alzheimer's disease). Keep explanations to these clients simple and concrete. The environment should be structured and simplified, incorporating normal-izing cues (e.g., drapes open to sunlight, familiar pictures and objects). Agitation can be decreased through choice of colors, reducing television or visitor noise, and creating stability and predictability in the immediate environment.[50, 65, 69]

Associated factors that can increase the risk of sensory overload include confinement, lack of ability to control the environment, and pressures related to time, decision-making, and complex task performance.

The inability to integrate incoming stimuli may be exhibited as confusion.[58] Sensory overload caused by an excess of poorly understood environmental stimuli may be superimposed on disturbed cerebral metabolism resulting from electrolyte disturbance, drugs, organic brain disease, and cardiopulmonary problems. The nurse should monitor the client for abnormal laboratory values and possible toxic responses to drugs or drug interactions, with particular attention to implications of slower metabolic processes in elderly people.[69] (For more information on assessing the confused client, see Chapter 68.)

Modification of the environment also has the potential to enhance the client's psychological well-being. The intervention called *environmental structuring* is defined as "an assortment of nurses' actions that directly or indirectly affect environmental features or conditions."[50] As more has been learned about psychoneuroimmunology, increasing evidence suggests that environmental conditions can be modified in ways that facilitate healing. Music therapy is an example of one such intervention that you can use to reduce psychophysiologic stress and to improve breathing patterns and the ability to communicate.[72]

CONCLUSIONS

The adequacy of sleep and rest and the appropriateness of sensory stimulation are important factors to consider in caring for clients with acute or chronic illness. Disorders of sleep, fatigue, and sensory stimulation have been discussed with consideration of the reciprocity among these processes, illness, and hospitalization. The nurse can play a pivotal role in environmental modification and client teaching to minimize the impact of sleep, fatigue, and sensory disturbances.

THINKING CRITICALLY

1. **The client has just been given a prescription for zolpidem (Ambien) to treat insomnia. She confides in you that she has been using a product from a health food store, recommended by a friend. Now she asks you whether it is safe to continue taking the herbal remedy as well as her new prescription.**

Factors to Consider. What is zolpidem? Can it interact with other medications? How could you find more information about the herbal medication the client is taking?

2. **A late-middle-aged client who has had a cerebrovascular accident and is unable to move or speak is placed in a room at the end of the hall, away from the nurses' station. This client was**

assigned a window bed. He has few visitors. His roommate is a young man recovering from a mild head injury. The roommate has many visitors and uses the radio and television loudly and frequently. Which client is more likely to develop sensory deprivation? Sensory overload? What nursing assessments and interventions would help prevent sensory disturbances?

Factors to Consider. What factors (age, environmental, physical, psychological) affect sensory functioning? How do clients receive and interpret incoming stimuli? Does the room assignment contribute to the development of sensory disturbance in either client?

3. **A young adult comes to the neighborhood health clinic. She is unkempt, has circles under her eyes, and yawns frequently. She gives a history of being unable to sleep for any length of time since she gave birth recently to twin sons. She took a variety of prescription "sleeping pills" before she became pregnant and wants a new prescription to help her sleep. What might be causing her sleeplessness? What sleep assessments should be completed? What impact may lack of sleep have?**

Factors to Consider. What measures might help this young mother sleep naturally? How would her lack of sleep affect the health of her children? How normal is it for a young adult to experience difficulty with sleep and to take medications to assist with sleep?

BIBLIOGRAPHY

1. Aaronson, L. S., et al. (1999). Defining and measuring fatigue. *Image: Journal of Nursing Scholarship, 31*(1), 45–50.
2. Akerstedt, T. (1998). Shift work and disturbed sleep/wakefulness. *Sleep Medicine Reviews, 2*(2), 117–128.
3. Aldrich, M. S. (1990). Narcolepsy. *New England Journal of Medicine, 323*(6), 389–394.
4. Ancoli-Israel, S., et al. (1991). Sleep disordered breathing in community dwelling elderly. *Sleep, 14,* 486–495.
5. Ancoli-Israel, S. (1997). Sleep problems in older adults: Putting myths to bed. *Geriatrics, 52*(1), 20–30.
6. Ancoli-Israel, S., et al. (1997). Identification and treatment of sleep problems in the elderly. *Sleep Medicine Reviews, 1*(1), 3–17.
7. Baker, A., Simpson, S., & Dawson, D. (1997). Sleep disruption and mood changes associated with menopause. *Journal of Psychosomatic Research, 43*(4), 359–369.
8. Beck-Little, R., & Weinrich, S. P. (1998). Assessment and management of sleep disorders in the elderly. *Journal of Gerontological Nursing, 24*(4), 21–29.
9. Bliwise, D. L. (1994). Normal aging. In M. H. Kryger, T. Roth, & W. C. Dement (Eds.), *Principles and practice of sleep medicine* (2nd ed., pp. 26–39). Philadelphia: W. B. Saunders.
10. Cardinali, D. P., & Pevet, P. (1998). Basic aspects of melatonin action. *Sleep Medicine Reviews, 2*(4), 175–190.
11. Carpenito, L. J. (1999). *Handbook of nursing diagnosis* (8th ed). Philadelphia: J. B. Lippincott.
12. Cohen, F. L., & Merritt, S. L. (1992). Sleep promotion. In G. M. Bulechek & J. C. McCloskey (Eds.), *Nursing interventions: Essential nursing treatments* (2nd ed., pp. 109–119). Philadelphia: W. B. Saunders.
13. Cohen, F. L., Nehring, W. M., & Cloninger, L. (1996). Symptom description and management in narcolepsy. *Holistic Nursing Practice, 10*(4), 44–53.
14. Cohen-Mansfield, J., & Marx, M. S. (1990). The relationship between sleep disturbances and agitation in a nursing home. *Journal of Aging Health, 2*(1), 42–57.
15. Collard, P., et al. (1997). Compliance with nasal CPAP in obstructive sleep apnea patients. *Sleep Medicine Reviews, 1*(1), 33–44.
16. Cook, N. F., & Boore, J. R. P. (1997). Managing patients suffering from acute and chronic fatigue. *British Journal of Nursing, 6*(14), 811–815.
17. Cox, H. C., et al. (1997). *Clinical applications of nursing diagnosis* (3rd ed.). Philadelphia: F. A. Davis.
18. Curtis, S. M. & Porth, C. M. (1998). Disorders of brain function. In C. Porth (Ed.), *Pathophysiology of altered health states* (5th ed., pp. 879–920). Philadelphia: J. B. Lippincott.
19. Czeisler, C. A., & Shapiro, C. M. (1995). Circadian rhythm disorders. In C. M. Shapiro (Ed.), *Sleep solutions manual* (pp. 190–207). Pointe Claire, Quebec: Kommunicom Publications.
20. Deb, S., Lyons, I., & Koutzoukis, C. (1998). Neuropsychiatric sequelae one year after a minor head injury. *Journal of Neurology, Neurosurgery and Psychiatry, 65*(6), 889–902.
21. Diagnostic Classification Steering Committee, Thorpy, M. J., Chairman. (1997). *International classification of sleep disorders: Diagnostic and coding manual* (Rev. ed.). Rochester, MN: American Sleep Disorders Association.
22. Dinges, D. F., & Broughton, R. J. (1989). *Sleep and alertness: Chronobiological, behavioral and medical aspects of napping.* New York: Raven Press.
23. Driver, H. S., & Baker, F. C. (1998). Menstrual factors in sleep. *Sleep Medicine Reviews, 2*(4), 213–229.
24. El-Ad, B., & Korczyn, A. D. (1998). Disorders of excessive daytime sleepiness: An update. *Journal of Neurological Sciences, 153*(2), 192–202.
25. Evans, B. D., & Rogers, A. E. (1994). 24-hour sleep-wake patterns in healthy elderly persons. *Applied Nursing Research, 7*(2), 75–83.
26. Ferrell, B. R., et al. (1996). "Bone tired": The experience of fatigue and its impact on quality of life. *Oncology Nursing Forum, 23*(10) 1539–1547.
27. Fleming, J. A., & Shapiro, C. M. (1995). Insomnia management. In C. M. Shapiro (Ed.), *Sleep solutions manual* (pp. 34–49). Pointe Claire, Quebec: Kommunicom Publications.
28. Flemons, W. W., & McNicholas, W. T. (1997). Clinical prediction of the sleep apnea syndrome. *Sleep Medicine Reviews, 1*(1), 19–32.
29. Foley, D. J., et al. (1995). Sleep complaints among elderly persons: An epidemiologic study of three communities. *Sleep, 18*(6), 425–432.
30. Ford, H., Trigwell, P., & Johnson, M. (1998). The nature of fatigue in multiple sclerosis. *Journal of Psychosomatic Research, 45*(1), 33–38.
31. Fredrickson, P. A., et al. (1990). Sleep disorders in psychiatric practice. *Mayo Clinic Proceedings, 65,* 861–868.
32. Guilleminault, C. (1994). Narcolepsy syndrome. In M. H. Kryger, T. Roth, & W. C. Dement (Eds.), *Principles and practice of sleep medicine* (2nd ed., pp. 549–561). Philadelphia: W. B. Saunders.
33. Hauri, P. J. (1994). Primary insomnia. In M. H. Kryger, T. Roth, & W. C. Dement (Eds.), *Principles and practice of sleep medicine* (2nd ed., pp. 494–499). Philadelphia: W. B. Saunders.
34. Hauri, P. J., & Linde, S. (1991). *No more sleepless nights.* New York: John Wiley & Sons.
35. Hobson, J. A. (1988). *The dreaming brain.* New York: Basic Books.
36. Hodgson, L. A. (1991). Why do we need sleep? Relating theory to nursing practice. *Journal of Advances in Nursing, 16,* 1503–1510.
37. Horne, J. A. (1988). *Why we sleep.* New York: Oxford University Press.
38. Ingles, J. L., Eskes, G. A., & Phillips, S. J. (1999). Fatigue after stroke. *Archives of Physical Medicine and Rehabilitation, 80,* 173–178.
39. Johnson, M. W., & Remmers, J. E. (1984). Accessory muscle activity during sleep in chronic obstructive pulmonary disease. *Journal of Applied Physiology, 57*(4), 1011–1017.
40. Kaplan, H. I., Sadock, B. J., & Grebb, J. A. (1994). *Kaplan and Sadock's synopsis of psychiatry* (7th ed.). Baltimore: Williams & Wilkins.
41. Kenner, C. (1998). Fibromyalgia and chronic fatigue: The holistic perspective. *Holistic Nursing Practice, 12*(3), 55–63.
42. Kryger, M. H. (1994). Management of obstructive sleep apnea: An overview. In M. H. Kryger, T. Roth, & W. C. Dement (Eds.), *Principles and practice of sleep medicine* (2nd ed., pp. 736–747). Philadelphia: W. B. Saunders.
43. Krystal, A. D., et al. (1998). Sleep in peri-menopausal and postmenopausal women. *Sleep Medicine Reviews, 2*(4), 243–253.
44. Lahaie, U. (1991). Shift-workers and seasonal affective disorder. *Canadian Nurse, 87*(5), 33–34.

45. Lee, K. A., et al. (1990). Sleep patterns related to menstrual cycle phase and premenstrual affective symptoms. *Sleep, 13*(5), 403–409.

46. Levitt, A., & Shapiro, C. M. (1995). Seasonal affective disorder. In C. M. Shapiro (Ed.), *Sleep solutions manual* (pp. 126–146). Pointe Claire, Quebec: Kommunicom Publications.

47. Littrell, K. D., & Schumann, L. L. (1989). Promoting sleep for the patient with a myocardial infarction. *Critical Care Nurse, 9*(3), 44, 46–49.

48. Lowe, A. D. (1998). Sleep in Parkinson's disease. *Journal of Psychosomatic Research, 44*(6), 613–617.

49. Lugaresi, E., et al. (1988). Sleep in clinical neurology. In R. L. Williams, I. Karacan, & C. A. Moore (Eds.), *Sleep disorders: Diagnosis and treatment* (2nd ed., pp. 245–263). New York: John Wiley & Sons.

50. Mion, L. C. (1992). Environmental structuring. In G. M. Bulechek & J. C. McCloskey (Eds.), *Nursing interventions* (2nd ed., pp. 254–264). Philadelphia: W. B. Saunders.

51. National Commission on Sleep Disorders Research. (1993). *Wake up America: A national sleep alert* (Executive summary and executive report, Report of the National Commission on Sleep Disorders Research. National Institutes of Health, January, Vol. 1, pp. 1–76. DHHS Publication, Washington, DC: Supervisor of Documents, U.S. Government Printing Office).

52. North American Nursing Diagnosis Association (NANDA). (1999). *Nursing diagnoses: Definitions and classification 1999–2000.* Philadelphia: Author.

53. Ohayon, M. M., et al. (1997). How sleep and mental disorders are related to complaints of daytime sleepiness. *Archives of Internal Medicine, 157*(22), 2645–2652.

54. Orr, W. C. (1994). Gastrointestinal disorders. In M. H. Kryger, T. Roth, & W. C. Dement (Eds.), *Principles and practice of sleep medicine* (2nd ed., pp. 861–869). Philadelphia: W. B. Saunders.

55. Parkosewich, J. A. (1986). Sleep-disordered breathing: A common problem in chronic obstructive pulmonary disease. *Critical Care Nurse, 6*(6), 60–64.

56. Partinen, M. (1994). Epidemiology of sleep disorders. In M. H. Kryger, T. Roth, & W. C. Dement (Eds.), *Principles and practice of sleep medicine* (2nd ed., pp. 437–452). Philadelphia: W. B. Saunders.

57. Partonen, T. (1998). A developmental approach to severe depression. *Medical Hypotheses, 51*(2), 165–166.

58. Rasin, J. H. (1990). Confusion. *Nursing Clinics of North America, 25*(4), 909–918.

59. Ray, W., Griffen, M., & Downey, W. (1989). Benzodiazepines of long and short elimination half-life and the risk of hip fracture. *JAMA, 262*(23), 3303–3307.

60. Reimer, M. (1989). Sleep pattern disturbances related to neurological dysfunction. *Axon, 10*(3), 65–68.

61. Remmers, J. E. (1990). Sleeping and breathing. *Chest 97,* 77S–80S.

62. Schmidt-Nowara, W., et al. (1995). Oral appliances for the treatment of snoring and obstructive sleep apnea: A review. *Sleep, 18*(6), 501–510.

63. Schnelle, J. F., et al. (1998). Sleep hygiene in physically dependent nursing home residents: Behavioral and environmental intervention implications. *Sleep, 21*(5), 515–523.

64. Shouse, M. N. (1994). Epileptic seizure manifestations during sleep. In M. H. Kryger, T. Roth, & W. C. Dement (Eds.), *Principles and practice of sleep medicine* (2nd ed., pp. 801–814). Philadelphia: W. B. Saunders.

65. Sloane, P. D., & Mathew, L. J. (1990). The therapeutic environment screening scale. *American Journal of Alzheimer's Care and Related Disorders and Research, 5*(6), 22–26.

66. Smith, R. P., et al. (1998). Obstructive sleep apnea and the autonomic nervous system. *Sleep Medicine Reviews, 2*(2), 69–92.

67. Standards of Practice Committee of the American Sleep Disorders Association. (1994). Practice parameters for the use of laser-assisted uvulopalatoplasty. *Sleep, 17*(8), 744–748.

68. Steriade, M. (1994). Brain electrical activity and sensory processing during waking and sleeping states. In M. H. Kryger, T. Roth, & W. C. Dement (Eds.), *Principles and practice of sleep medicine* (2nd ed., pp. 105–124). Philadelphia: W. B. Saunders.

69. Stolley, J. M., & Buckwalter, K. C. (1992). Confusion management. In G. M. Bulechek & J. C. McCloskey (Eds.), *Nursing interventions* (2nd ed., pp. 120–134). Philadelphia: W. B. Saunders.

70. Terman, M. (1994). Light treatment. In M. H. Kryger, T. Roth, & W. C. Dement (Eds.), *Principles and practice of sleep medicine* (2nd ed., pp. 1012–1029). Philadelphia: W. B. Saunders.

71. Ware, J. C., & Hirshkowitz, M. (1994). Monitoring penile erections during sleep. In M. H. Kryger, T. Roth, & W. C. Dement (Eds.), *Principles and practice of sleep medicine* (2nd ed., pp. 967–977). Philadelphia: W. B. Saunders.

72. Wiens, M., Reimer, M., & Guyn, H. L. (1998). Music therapy as a treatment method for improving respiratory muscle strength in advanced multiple sclerosis: A pilot study. *Rehabilitation Nursing, 24*(2), 74–80.

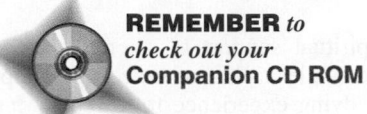

CHAPTER 22

Perspectives on End-of-Life Care

Kim K. Kuebler
Debra E. Heidrich

Nurses caring for clients with advanced diseases will ultimately witness the final stage of life—dying. The dying process is often accompanied by many different psychological, spiritual, and physical needs, and nurses are in the ideal position to identify and address them. Nurses must be knowledgeable about the normal dying process, the control of pain and other symptoms, and the role of the interdisciplinary team in order to provide optimal support and symptom management for dying clients and their families.

Note: In this chapter, *symptom* is used instead of *clinical manifestations,* the term used elsewhere in the text. The symptoms associated with dying differ from manifestations described with specific medical problems discussed in other chapters. *Symptom management* is the preferred term often used in the care of those clients with advanced illness and is the primary focus within the specialty of palliative care.

END-OF-LIFE CARE

The terms *hospice care*, *palliative care*, and *end-of-life care* sometimes are used interchangeably and at other times are used to differentiate various models of care. The following discussion briefly identifies the evolution of the hospice movement and the development of palliative care programs.

■ HOSPICE

The hospice movement began in the late 1960s in the United Kingdom. Dame Cicely Saunders established that the complex needs of dying clients were not being addressed in the traditional health care system. Her vision and understanding of the unmet needs of the dying prompted the first modern hospice, St. Christopher's Hospice in London, England.[14] Saunders believed that the dying required the multiple skills of an interdisciplinary team to provide "patient-centered care." The precepts of the hospice movement in the United States are a direct result of the work at St. Christopher's Hospice.[6, 17]

Another pioneer whose work greatly influenced the hospice movement was Elizabeth Kübler-Ross. Her theoretical framework for the death and dying process brought forth recognition of the psychological and existential needs of the dying.[24] Her life work was to help clients and society to view terminal illness not as a destructive, negative force but as one of the "windstorms" in life that can enhance inner growth.[24, 25] Kübler-Ross is most noted for identifying and defining the phases of the normal death and dying experience: (1) denial, (2) anger, (3) bargaining, (4) depression, and (5) acceptance.[24, 25] After spending many years at the bedsides of the dying, Kübler-Ross recognized the importance of the interdisciplinary team in providing support to the client and family as they experience the various phases of the dying process.[24, 25]

While Kübler-Ross was advocating for the dying and St. Christopher's Hospice was successfully caring for terminally ill clients, Florence Wald, then the dean of graduate nursing studies at Yale University, expressed interest in bringing the hospice movement to the United States. Wald recognized the tremendous need in America to improve the care of the dying. She helped integrate the British hospice movement into the first home care hospice in New Haven, Conn., in 1974.[6, 17]

At the same time, people in Canada were recognizing a need to provide better care at the end of life. Balfour Mount, the first to define *palliative care*, opened the first hospital-based palliative care service at the Royal Victoria Hospital of McGill University in Montreal in 1975.[14] The McGill model followed the interdisciplinary team approach of client-centered and family-centered care and was the first program to include research and education in the area of pain management.[6, 17]

All of these pioneers advocated for improved care of the terminally ill and their families. They believed that professionals trained to provide physical comfort through pain and symptom management as well as psychosocial and spiritual support could promote a healthy, normal dying experience.

During the 1970s, the hospice concept of care continued to grow as a grassroots movement throughout the United States. Citing the cost-effectiveness of and client and family satisfaction with this level of care, Congress approved a Medicare Hospice Benefit in 1982.[31] With a solid source of reimbursement available, the number of hospice programs grew markedly over the next several years.[6, 22, 31]

■ CONTINUED UNMET NEEDS OF THE DYING

The growth of hospices did not, however, address the needs of people dying in other health care settings. In 1995, findings of SUPPORT (Study to Understand Prognoses and Preferences for Outcomes and Risks of Treatments),[50] revealed that Americans were continuing to die in pain and without dignity. This $28 million dollar study, funded by the Robert Wood Johnson Foundation and conducted at five medical centers nationwide over 10 years, found that 80% of Americans die in institutional settings, often with unmanaged pain, in isolation, connected to mechanical ventilators, and in intensive care units. The utilization of living wills, health care proxies, and communication efforts between clients and their physicians often proved futile.[29, 35, 50]

The findings of SUPPORT stirred a massive interest in improving the care of the dying in America. Although hospice care was acknowledged as successful in addressing the concerns identified in the study, hospice care was not being accessed by the majority of dying people. Only about 17% of the American population receive hospice services.[50] There are several reasons for the underutilization of hospice services:

- Our society's being a "death-denying" one, in which many clients and health care professionals desire life-prolonging care
- Lack of knowledge regarding the availability of services
- Difficulty in determining prognoses in terms of 6 months or less

These issues, along with increasingly strict admission criteria enforced by the Health Care Financing Administration (HCFA) for Medicare clients, changed the view of hospice care from a "concept" of care to a system that pays for the care of the dying.

Thus, the benefits of hospice care for the client and family are available to only a small percentage of the population who have a limited prognosis, who elect hospice care, and who meet the highly regulated, stringent admission criteria.[53] The concept of palliative care developed from the desire to broaden the whole-person, comfort-care approach of the hospice concept and to make it available to more people in all health care settings.[14]

■ PALLIATIVE CARE

Palliative care is defined by the World Health Organization (WHO)[2] as follows:

the active total care of patients whose disease is not responsive to curative treatment. Control of pain, of other symptoms, and of psychological, social and spiritual problems, is paramount. The goal of palliative care is achievement of the best quality of life for patients and their families. Many aspects of palliative care are also applicable earlier in the course of the illness in conjunction with therapies such as anticancer treatment.

Like hospice care, palliative care recognizes that dying is a normal process that should be neither hastened nor postponed. The provision of symptom management and both emotional and spiritual support of clients and their families are considered while a plan of care is developed to promote an optimal dying experience followed by family bereavement.[14, 29, 35] Unlike clients qualifying for hospice care, clients who receive palliative care are not required to have a 6-month or shorter prognosis, making palliative care available to more people. See Bridge to Home Health Care.

DISEASE TRAJECTORY

The time from the onset of a terminal diagnosis until death is considered the *disease trajectory*. Some terminal diagnoses have a long disease trajectory with a gradual decline in functional status over time; others have a very short trajectory with a sharp decline; still others have variable trajectories with periods of remission and exacerbation.

Determining specific interventions to improve each client's quality of life is largely determined by his or her position on the disease trajectory. An example is a client who suddenly experiences spinal cord compression. If the client is not imminently dying and is considered to be active and somewhat mobile (i.e., early in the disease trajectory), it is appropriate for the client to undergo magnetic resonance imaging (MRI) with the possibility of radiation therapy. If the client is actively dying (i.e., late in the disease trajectory), he or she would not be able to tolerate a hospital admission, MRI, and radiation therapy; this client may benefit from aggressive use of corticosteroids in the home.

A comprehensive assessment is essential in determining the client's disease trajectory in order to guide identification of appropriate palliative interventions. This assessment comprises the following actions[9, 29]:

1. Define the nature of the clinical finding and symptom.
2. Perform a thorough history and physical examination, review current and tried medications, and evaluate a minimal set of diagnostic procedures to differentiate underlying pathophysiologic disorder from a reversible symptom.
3. Evaluate the problem within the context of the client's situation and allowing for prioritization. For example, the priority assigned a urinary tract infection (UTI) in a cognitively impaired, dehydrated, and bedridden client will be different from that given to a UTI in a cognitively intact client with good symptom control.
4. Define the "cost" of diagnostic and therapeutic interventions and the varying differences between clients. For example, what may be considered appropriate therapy for one client may be inappropriate for another—when evaluating the risk versus benefit of treatment and the financial burden of unnecessary interventions.
5. Discuss the various care options with the client and the family, and encourage informed decision-making.

QUALITY OF LIFE

Palliative care is offered toward the end of client's life, when a progressive illness is symptomatic and interferes with the quality of life. Many variables go into defining quality of life, including (1) socioeconomic status, (2)

BRIDGE TO HOME HEALTH CARE

Providing Hospice Care

The focus of care shifts from cure to comfort when the decision is made to use hospice and remain at home. The hospice team allows clients to maintain independence and to make informed choices about caregiving, pain control, nutrition, elimination, and skin care during frequent home visits and phone calls. The team explores and clarifies spiritual beliefs, helps clients and family members resolve estrangement and conflict, and offers information about funeral planning.

The goal of the hospice program is to achieve around-the-clock pain control by following the National Hospice Organization guidelines for scheduling, titration, and use of breakthrough pain medications. When the oral route is no longer available because of weakness or coma, rectal, transdermal, sublingual, and intravenous medications can be used effectively. Consider adjuvant medications to enhance analgesia and address different types of pain. Benzodiazepams enhance the work of analgesics. Nonsteroidal anti-inflammatory drugs help to relieve bone pain. Tricyclic antidepressants and anticonvulsants are effective for pain of neuropathic origin.

It is normal for clients to lose their appetite during the terminal stages of illness. Encourage clients to eat what they can tolerate to reduce stress and provide comfort. Prevent nausea and vomiting by giving antiemetics regularly or as needed. Schedule meals at the time of day when the client's energy is the greatest. Clients and family members need to know that dehydration will occur, but usually with few manifestations. Offer small amounts of water frequently with a spoon, syringe, eye dropper, or sponge-tipped swabs.

It is important to anticipate when equipment will be needed and to have it delivered to the home. Such preparation decreases stress, prevents injuries, and helps maintain independence. Needed equipment includes beds, wheelchairs, commodes, and walkers. Reduce oxygen hunger by using a floor fan or providing supplemental oxygen. Prevent skin breakdown with foam mats for chairs or beds. Use a draw-sheet for turning and repositioning to decrease skin tears and shearing. Save energy and prevent accidents by having the client use a commode at the bedside.

Minimize distress and discomfort by anticipating bowel and bladder changes. Schedule the administration of stool softeners and laxatives, enemas, and suppositories to increase bowel regularity and comfort. Prevent unnecessary delays by having standing orders to insert straight or Foley catheters for bladder evacuation. Keep a supply of briefs and protective pads to use when the client's condition changes quickly.

As death approaches, increase physical and emotional care to ensure dignity. Give atropine ophthalmic drops to reduce lung congestion. Use repositioning, light massage, and gentle range-of-motion exercises. Promote calmness and serenity with quiet presence, hand-holding, soft music, or prayers. Give clients permission to "go," assure them that their loved ones will be all right, and offer words of love to help clients achieve a peaceful passage. Encourage family members to do the same. It is the responsibility of nurses on the hospice team to provide details about disease progression, manifestations of approaching death, and protocols at the time of death. A nurse visits at the time of death, makes the death pronouncement, and telephones the physician, coroner, and funeral home.

The decision to use hospice is not one of giving up hope. It is one of hoping for comfort and quality of life in the moments, hours, and days that remain for a client at the end of life.

Jane Allen Austgen, RN, BSN, CRNH, *Hospice Nurse Case Manager, Alegent Health Home Care and Hospice, Omaha, Nebraska*

physical health, (3) relationships with friends and family, and (4) satisfaction with self.[12, 45] See Alternative Therapy: Spirituality and Health in Chapter 20. Quality of life is defined as "a personal statement of the positivity or negativity of attributes that characterize life."[12]

A person's quality of life is often linked to the experience of symptom distress and the meanings that the person assigns to these physical sensations.[12, 45] Nurses caring for clients who are experiencing distressing symptoms, such as pain, fatigue, constipation, and nausea, should understand that each client responds differently. The effect of a symptom on life routines varies from client to client, depending on overall functional status, coping abilities, and social supports. In palliative care, the plan of care must be based not only on the symptom itself but also on the effect of the symptom on the client's overall quality of living.

SYMPTOMS AT THE END OF LIFE

Clients with advanced diseases experience multiple symptoms, some of which are more severe than others.[18, 43, 50]

In one study, pain was found to be the most prevalent symptom among clients with advanced cancer (89% of respondents). In 87% of the clients with pain, the severity of the pain was rated to be moderate to severe. In addition to pain, the symptoms weakness, anorexia, dyspnea, constipation, early satiety, fatigue, and dry mouth were experienced by more than 40% of clients.[18, 43, 50]

Symptoms vary not only in frequency and intensity but also in the distress experienced by clients.[18, 50] Although pain may be very prevalent, it is not always identified as the most distressing symptom. Some studies have found that dyspnea, asthenia (lethargy, generalized weakness, and fatigue), dry mouth, anorexia, depression, and insomnia may actually be more distressing than pain for clients with terminal illnesses.[2, 9, 43, 50] The symptoms commonly experienced by the dying are discussed here.

■ PAIN

Pain is a multidimensional phenomenon. Not only is a person's pain experience a physical response to an underlying disorder or disease state; there are also emotional, intellectual, behavioral, sensory, and cultural dimensions.[42] When a client is nonresponsive and unable to report pain, the nurse should observe for the behavioral indicators of pain (Table 22–1). Communication within the entire health care team is essential for optimal pain management. Chapter 23 describes types of pain, subjective and objective assessment of pain, and pain management strategies.

OPIOID ANALGESICS

Opioids are the mainstay of treatment for moderate to severe pain.[1] These medications bind with opiate receptors in the central nervous system (CNS) and block the transmission of the pain impulse to the higher brain centers.[42, 43] Most opioid medications bind to the mu receptor and are called *mu agonists*. Morphine (MS Contin), hydromorphone (Dilaudid), fentanyl (Duragesic), and oxycodone (Oxycontin) are examples of mu-agonist opioids frequently used in the treatment of pain.[42] There is no ceiling to the analgesic effect of mu-agonist opioids.[18, 42] See Chapter 23 for further discussion of opioids.

In addition to modulating the transmission and perception of the pain impulse, opioids may bind with receptors in other tissues, leading to the potential for side effects. There are, for example, opioid receptors in the gastrointestinal tract. When opioids bind with these receptors, intestinal motility is decreased and gastric emptying is delayed, leading to constipation. Prophylactic treatment of constipation with both a stool softener and a stimulant is essential and should be initiated along with the first opioid dose. The clinician should not wait for the client to complain of constipation before beginning treatment. Constipation is the only side effect of opioids to which a person does not develop tolerance. A bowel protocol must be continued for the duration of treatment with opioids.

Other potential side effects of opioids are respiratory depression, nausea and vomiting, and sedation. Clinically significant respiratory depression is rare during treatment of pain if the opioid dose is increased slowly and decreased if sedation is noted. In addition, people develop tolerance to the respiratory-depressive side effects of opioids after the first several days of treatment. The client who has taken the same dose of an opioid for several weeks is not at risk for a clinically significant opioid-induced respiratory depression.[42]

Although nausea and vomiting may not be a problem for all clients, many clients do experience this as a side effect of opioids. Nausea and vomiting occur when the chemoreceptor trigger zone (CTZ) of the brain is stimulated by these medications. A client is less likely to experience nausea when opioids are administered orally than parenterally. As with respiratory depression, tolerance to this side effect of opioids develops over time. Clients who experience nausea and vomiting should be treated with antiemetics for the first 2 to 3 days after the opioid is initiated until tolerance develops. A small number of clients may experience persistent nausea from the opioids. These clients may benefit from either changing to a different opioid or continuing to use antiemetics.[42]

A client who has been in pain and receives an initial dose of an opioid may experience some degree of sedation. This is due, in part, to the direct effect of opioids on the brain. In addition to the sedative side effect of the opioid, however, the client is probably exhausted from not sleeping well when in pain. Teach the client that some sleepiness is expected and that it is probably not all due to the new medication. As with the other side effects of opioids, tolerance to the sedation develops after the first 2 to 3 days. If, however, the client is difficult to arouse or the sedation lasts more than 2 to 3 days, the opioid dose may be too high for the intensity of the pain.

Clients who are sedated from an opioid and still experiencing pain probably have pain syndromes not completely responsive to opioids. These clients require the addition of adjuvant medications in order to achieve comfort. Recognize that *there is no ceiling to the amount of opioid analgesic* required for each client to achieve a satisfactory level of analgesia. Hence, clients may require very high doses of opioids to achieve pain relief.

ADJUVANT ANALGESICS

Adjuvant medications have a primary action other than pain relief but can also serve as analgesics for some painful conditions. They are often used in combination with other analgesic medications. At each step of the WHO analgesic ladder (see Chapter 23), adjuvant medications may be added, depending on the type of pain experienced. Several classes of medications are essential to optimal management of pain (Table 22–2).

Nonsteroidal anti-inflammatory drugs (NSAIDs) can be very helpful when the inflammatory process is involved and is initiating the pain impulse, such as in bone or soft tissue damage. Clients with metastatic bone disease often require the combination of an opioid and an NSAID for comfort.

Tricyclic antidepressants (TCAs) and anticonvulsants can be effective analgesics in the management of pain syndromes that have a neurologic component.[18, 42] TCAs appear to be most helpful for pain described as burning or aching; anticonvulsants are useful in the treatment of shooting and shock-like neurologic pains. The effective analgesic dose of a TCA is much lower than the dose required for an antidepressant effect.[1, 42] Some clients are aware that these medications are used to treat depression and may be suspicious that the clinician "thinks the pain is in my head." Explain to clients that these medications are used to manage pain at low doses. Because it takes 5 to 7 days for TCAs to reach the desired plasma level, inform the client that it may take several days for this new medication to be effective.

TABLE 22–1	OBSERVATIONAL ASSESSMENT IN THE NONRESPONSIVE CLIENT
Restlessness	Agitation, frequent moving, an inability to get comfortable, fidgety, picking at things
Vocalizations	Moaning, groaning, crying out
Muscle tension	Tense muscles, not relaxed, clenched teeth, tightened fists, guarded movements
Facial expression	Frowning, grimacing, distressed
Physiologic indicators	Fast heart rate, frequent and labored breathing, sweating

TABLE 22-2	ADJUVANT ANALGESICS		
Pain Source	**Pain Character**	**Medication Class**	**Examples**
Bone or soft tissue	Tenderness over bone or joint Pain on movement	Nonsteroidal anti-inflammatory drugs	Ibuprofen Naproxen Indomethacin
Nerve damage/neuropathic	Burning, shooting, shock-like, or aching pain	Tricyclic antidepressants	Amitriptyline Doxepin
		Anticonvulsants	Carbamazepine Phenytoin Valproic acid Gabapentin
Smooth muscle spasms	Cramping or grabbing pains (intermittent)	Anticholinergics	Scopolamine Hyoscyamine Oxybutynin Dicyclomine
Anxiety	Generalized restlessness and discomfort	Benzodiazepines	Lorazepam Diazepam
		Butyrophenones	Haloperidol

People who report "colicky" pain may be experiencing the discomfort of smooth muscle spasm. This type of pain is best treated with an anticholinergic medication.

Anxiety is a complex symptom caused by physical, emotional, and spiritual concerns. People who are in pain often experience some anxiety, and it may be helpful to treat the anxiety in order to achieve comfort.[1, 11, 38] Benzodiazepine medications are frequently used for anxiety in the palliative care setting. Haloperidol, a butyrophenone, may also be used. Management of anxiety is covered in Chapter 20.

ANALGESIC DOSING

Most analgesic medication doses must be titrated up or down to achieve effectiveness, both at the beginning of therapy and during the course of treatment. For example, a client receiving morphine for bone pain may find that a lower dose of morphine is possible when an NSAID is added to the regimen. The goal is to use the smallest dose that relieves the pain so that it causes the fewest side effects.

Dose increases are usually made at the time the medication reaches its peak effect in the body. For orally administered morphine, the peak effect is generally at 60 to 90 minutes. Therefore, if a client is not comfortable 1 to 1½ hours after the last dose of the morphine, the dose can be safely increased. The peak effect of amitriptyline (Elavil) is 4 to 5 days, and dose increases should occur only every 4 or 5 days if needed.[42]

Therapeutic levels of analgesics must be maintained at all times for clients with persistent or chronic pain in order to manage the pain. Therefore, an around-the-clock (ATC) schedule (see next section) is most appropriate.[1, 18, 41] The frequency of doses to maintain therapeutic levels is determined by the route of administration and the duration of action of the medication. *Immediate-release* (short-acting) oral morphine requires dosing every 4 hours; oral hydromorphone (Dilaudid) may need to be given every 3 hours. *Sustained-release* medications offer

the benefit of more convenient dosing schedules (every 8, 12, or 24 hours).

RESCUE DOSING

The goal of ATC dosing is to keep the level of the analgesic in a range high enough to manage the pain but below the point at which a client experiences avoidable or unmanageable side effects. Unfortunately, pain does not stay at the same intensity 24 hours a day. Many clients experience pain above the normal baseline pain; this pain is often labeled "breakthrough pain." The pain may spike above (break through) the therapeutic blood level of analgesia, and additional medications are required to manage such episodes. A short-acting (or immediate-release) dose of an opioid should be administered to "cover" the spike in the client's pain.[1, 42]

For clients taking oral opioids, the recommended rescue dose is in the range of 10% to 20% of the total daily ATC dose of opioid.[1] The rescue dose should be made available every 1 to 2 hours because most immediate-release opioids reach peak effectiveness in 60 to 90 minutes. After that point, the level of the opioid in the system begins to decrease. A client experiencing pain 2 hours after a rescue dose should not be made to wait for additional medication because the level of analgesia will continue to decrease and the client will become more and more uncomfortable. As a rule, a client who requires more than two rescue doses during a 12-hour period or is awakened from sleep experiencing pain should have the pain experience reevaluated. An increase in the ATC dose is often appropriate under these circumstances.

■ DYSPNEA

Dyspnea is a subjective experience described as difficult breathing or an "uncomfortable awareness" of breathing that accounts for a high proportion of the client's inability to carry out activities of daily living (ADL) and gravely affects the perceived quality of life.[3, 15, 16] Dyspnea occurs in as many as 50% to 70% of people at the end of life.[3, 15, 16] Clients also mention labored breathing, shortness of breath, and feelings of suffocation.[1] The continuous exhaustion that accompanies breathlessness can be one of the most devastating symptoms for both the client and the observing family members.[15]

ETIOLOGY

Dyspnea generally results from a greater awareness of normal breathing, an increased workload of breathing, or abnormalities in the ventilatory system.[3, 19, 40] In a 1999 consensus statement, the American Thoracic Society[5] emphasized that many factors may contribute to the symptom of breathlessness, including pathophysiologic changes as well as clients' emotional and spiritual evaluation of the changes in their functional status and quality of living.

Disease processes commonly associated with dyspnea include (1) acute and chronic pulmonary disorders, (2) heart failure, and (3) neuromuscular disorders. In the terminally ill population, anemia and generalized weakness may also contribute to dyspnea. In addition, emotions play a major role. The fear associated with the inability to "catch one's breath" can lead to panic and worsen the sensation of dyspnea.[3, 5, 19, 40]

ASSESSMENT

Assessment of clients with dyspnea includes subjective and observational data. Clients should be asked to rate dyspnea on a scale. The scale must make sense to the client, and all people caring for that client must use the same scale. This information can help determine the severity of the symptom and provides a baseline to evaluate the effectiveness of interventions. Clients' evaluations of their own functional status and the effect of dyspnea on ADL provide helpful information about both the physical and emotional responses to dyspnea.[5, 52]

An objective assessment of the client, particularly the nonresponsive client, provides additional information about dyspnea.[26] Observe for an increased respiratory rate, use of accessory muscles, gasping or labored breathing, restlessness, and diaphoresis.

MANAGEMENT

The underlying cause of dyspnea should be treated as appropriate for the client's position in the disease trajectory. For example, pneumonia in a client who is alert and oriented and has a good quality of life (as determined by the client) should be treated. However, it may be appropriate to *not* treat pneumonia in a client who is clearly near the end of the disease trajectory if treatment of the pneumonia will not improve the quality of life. All treatment options should be reviewed with the client and family, including the option of *no* treatment.[2, 3]

Although it may not be possible to treat the underlying cause of dyspnea at the end of life, many effective interventions can be used to manage the distress and uncomfortable sensations associated with dyspnea.[3, 40] Interdisciplinary team support is essential in the management of dyspnea. The psychosocial and existential issues contributing to the symptom of dyspnea require the support of professionals trained in these areas.

OPIOIDS. Morphine is widely used for the relief of dyspnea.[3, 5, 40] Data from several clinical studies reveal that 80% to 95% of clients with terminal cancer find significant relief from the utilization of morphine. Exactly why opioids alleviate dyspnea is not known, but they are believed to blunt the perceptual response to dyspnea or to reduce the respiratory drive.[15, 16] There is no standard optimal dose of morphine for the treatment of dyspnea. Twycross[52] proposed the following recommendations based on clinical experience:

- For the client who is already taking morphine for pain and who is dyspneic, the morphine dose should be increased by 50%.
- The dyspneic client who has not been receiving morphine should be started on 2.5 to 5 mg of morphine every 4 hours as needed.

It may be appropriate to consider ATC dosing of morphine if the client is requiring frequent "as needed" doses. Sustained-release preparations may prove to be convenient and effective in this situation.[3, 15, 16]

ANTI-ANXIETY AGENTS. Both benzodiazepines and phenothiazines have been effective in the management of dyspnea. Each class of drugs has the potential to depress hypoxic or ventilator responses and to alter the emotional responses to dyspnea.[45, 50] Both classes of medications have the potential for side effects, but given the prevalence of anxiety associated with the experience of breathlessness, it is considered good palliative care to try anxiolytic therapy on an individual basis.[19]

BRONCHODILATORS. Bronchodilators help to decrease the effort of breathing, and several studies cite its effects on breathlessness. The significant decrease in dyspnea after theophylline use is believed to result from an improvement in the length-tension relationship in the diaphragm.[19, 52]

CORTICOSTEROIDS. Corticosteroids are commonly used in the palliative care setting to treat dyspnea. These medications are believed to influence the symptom of dyspnea by decreasing inflammation in the pulmonary tissue and increasing bronchodilation.[3, 19] Corticosteroid therapy is indicated when bronchodilators have been ineffective. Ahmedzai[3] states that a trial of corticosteroids is justified in almost all clients with problematic chronic airway disease, pointing out that the dose of steroid should be high enough to work efficiently but low enough not to cause potential gastric irritation or fluid retention.

OXYGEN THERAPY. Palliative care literature does not support the use of oxygen therapy for relief of dyspnea. Oxygen (O_2) therapy should only be used for clients who are hypoxic or tend to have pulmonary hypertension. If O_2 saturation is less than 90% with room air, the clinician may want to (1) consider O_2 by nasal cannula at 1 to 3 L/min, (2) recheck the client's O_2 saturation in 20 to 30 minutes, and (3) titrate the O_2 therapy up to 6 L/min by nasal cannula if necessary.[3, 26, 52]

NONPHARMACOLOGIC INTERVENTIONS. Nurses are frequently the care providers who introduce nonpharmacologic interventions to clients and families and ensure, through education and support, that the interventions are being used to maximal effectiveness. Some interventions that nurses can initiate that contribute to comfort in clients experiencing dyspnea are (1) pursed-lip breathing, (2) breathing exercises, (3) positioning, (4) having a fan blowing in the room, (5) coping techniques, (6) a calming presence, (7) relaxation therapy, (8) massage, (9) acupuncture, (10) hypnosis, and (11) visualization.[26]

■ DELIRIUM

Delirium has been found in up to 77% to 85% of terminally ill clients with cancer and in 57% of terminally ill clients with acquired immunodeficiency syndrome (AIDS).[7, 8] Some clinicians consider delirium the "hallmark" of dying. Studies have indicated, however, that 25% to 35% of episodes of delirium are reversible.[7, 11] In the palliative care setting, early detection and assessment are likely to improve outcomes.[8]

A variety of terms have been used to describe delirium, such as acute brain failure, acute confusional state, acute secondary psychosis, exogenous psychosis, sundown syndrome, and organic brain syndrome.[7, 37] According to the American Psychiatric Association's *Diagnostic and Statistical Manual of Mental Disorders (DSM-IV)* criteria,[4] *delirium* is defined as "an etiologically non-specific, global, cerebral dysfunction characterized by concurrent disturbances of level of consciousness, attention, thinking, perception, memory, psychomotor behavior, emotion, and the sleep-wake cycle." It is often identified as a sudden and significant decline in a previous level of functioning and is conceptualized as a reversible process. Delirium can also affect sleep, psychomotor activity, and emotions.[8, 21, 22, 37]

DSM-IV criteria for delirium are as follows[4]:

1. Disturbance of consciousness with reduced ability to focus, sustain, or shift attention.
2. A change in cognition (such as memory deficit, disorientation, language disturbance) or the development of a perceptual disturbance that is not better accounted for by pre-existing, established, or evolving dementia.
3. Development of the disturbance over a short time (usually hours to days) and a tendency to fluctuate over the course of the day.

ASSESSMENT

The diagnosis of delirium is based on careful observation and awareness of its key features. Because the clinical manifestations are nonspecific, the clinician must (1) look for manifestations of a disturbance in consciousness and a change in cognition, (2) identify the rapidity of onset, and (3) assess for associated medical and environmental risks that lead to a definitive diagnosis. Delirium is commonly unrecognized by clinicians and hence is misdiagnosed.[21, 22]

The most commonly used assessment instrument for identifying cognitive changes is the Mini-Mental State Examination (MMSE). The MMSE is a systematically scored method of evaluating cognitive function. The examination can indicate early changes in cognition as it relates to the cortical function of the brain.[11] The MMSE evaluates orientation, attention, recall, and language. Scores below 24, out of a maximum of 30, are indicative of cognitive changes.[11] The MMSE relies heavily on client cooperation, however, and does not account for the abrupt changes that may often occur in a client's cognitive status.[11]

MANAGEMENT

The prognosis for the client experiencing delirium is often poor. This fact, however, should not deter the clinician from looking for the underlying cause because a significant number of cases are reversible.[37, 38] Bruera and colleagues[10] were able to determine cognitive failure in 80% to 90% of clients prior to death and identified a reversible cause of delirium in 44% (29 of 66) of clients studied. Frequently cited reversible causes of delirium are (1) medications (e.g., opioids, sedatives, anticholinergics, and steroids), (2) hypoxia, (3) dehydration, (4) metabolic causes (e.g., hypercalcemia), and (5) sepsis.[21, 22] Potentially helpful interventions for these reversible causes are listed in Table 22–3.

■ DEPRESSION

The prevalence of depression in clients with cancer ranges anywhere from 10% to 25%; the prevalence appears to increase in the presence of functional losses, advancing illness, and unmanaged symptoms.[8, 49] It is believed that many cases of depression in the terminally ill go unrecognized by clinicians because many of the clinical manifestations of depression (e.g., fatigue, anorexia or weight loss, insomnia) can be attributed to the disease process itself. Key indicators of clinical depression in the terminally ill are (1) alterations in mood, (2) feelings of hopelessness, worthlessness, or excessive guilt, and (3) recurrent death wishes, including thoughts of suicide.[41]

ETIOLOGY

A terminal diagnosis potentiates both anxiety and depression. People with a family or personal history of previous depressive episodes are at even higher risk for depression than the general population. Interestingly, some cancer diagnoses, such as pancreatic cancer, have been more strongly associated with depression. It is not clear whether psychological or physiologic factors are involved in this higher risk.[4, 7]

TABLE 22–3	REVERSIBLE CAUSES OF DELIRIUM
Cause	**Intervention**
1. Medications a. Opioid metabolites may accumulate, especially in the presence of renal insufficiency.	a. Consider switching to an equianalgesic dose of a different opioid.
b. Benzodiazepine metabolites may accumulate in the presence of hepatic disease.	b. Hydration may be helpful to assist in eliminating these metabolites. If antianxiety medications are needed, consider switching the client to a butyrophenone.
2. Hypoxia	2. Intervene to improve oxygenation with bronchodilators, mucolytics, and breathing techniques. Consider oxygen therapy if O_2 saturation is <90%
3. Dehydration	3. Consider oral or parenteral hydration.
4. Hypercalemia	4. Evaluate the benefits of hydration and use of bisphosphonates.
5. Sepsis	5. Consider anti-infective therapy.

It is thought that depression is a direct result of abnormal serotonin (5-hydroxytryptamine [5-HT]) neurotransmission in the CNS. This abnormal secretion may be genetic or may be induced by some unknown mechanism. Other neurotransmitters, such as gamma-aminobutyric acid (GABA) and norepinephrine, have also been closely linked in anxiety and may be associated with depression.[48]

ASSESSMENT

Nurses play a pivotal role in identifying people with depression. An important question you can ask is "Are you depressed?" or "How has your mood been lately?" Although feeling sad and anxious at times is a normal response to a terminal diagnosis, do not ignore these symptoms. People with clinical depression should be referred to skilled health care professionals for evaluation and treatment.

MANAGEMENT

Optimal therapy is achieved with the combination of supportive psychotherapy, cognitive-behavioral techniques, and pharmaceutical management. This approach requires coordination of the interdisciplinary team.

Antidepressant medications can be very effective in treating depression. There are several classes of antidepressants. The newer selective serotonin re-uptake inhibitors (SSRIs) cause fewer side effects and are at least as effective as the TCAs.[48] A trial of antidepressant therapy is warranted in the terminally ill client because it may greatly enhance the quality of life. See Chapter 20 for further discussion of anxiety, depression, medications, and treatments.

■ FATIGUE AND WEAKNESS

Fatigue is among the most prevalent symptoms of people with advanced illnesses and is universally associated with advanced malignancy. It is a distressing, subjective experience that impedes functioning and impairs quality of life. Clients describe fatigue as tiredness, exhaustion, generalized weakness, diminished energy, increased need to rest or sleep, diminished motivation, diminished capacity to pay attention, or a disturbed mood.[39, 44]

Although the etiology of fatigue is not clearly understood, many physiologic, psycho-emotional, and spiritual factors are recognized as contributing factors to the phenomenon of fatigue.[39, 44] Fatigue may result from any one or combination of the following problems:

Disease/treatment-related: Disease process, disease treatments (surgery, radiation therapy, chemotherapy, biologic therapy), infection, anemia, malnutrition or cachexia, chronic hypoxia, metabolic or electrolyte disorders, endocrine disorders, neuromuscular disorders, medication side effects (e.g., excessive sedation from opioids).
Physiologic: Over-exertion, immobility or lack of exercise, poor sleep, pain, or other discomfort.
Psycho-emotional: Stress, anxiety, grief, depression.
Spiritual: Fear, distress.

Because of the multidimensional nature of fatigue and the potential for several contributing factors to be present at any one time, a comprehensive assessment is required. It is important to identify and treat reversible causes of fatigue. All medications should be reviewed, and any unnecessary centrally acting drugs eliminated. If the clinician suspects that opioids are contributing to fatigue, reduction of the opioid dose by 25% should be considered,

followed by evaluation of the client's cognition if pain is still controlled and fatigue is lessened.[44] If pain returns with the reduction in dose, the opioid dose should be returned to the previous level.

Note: The client who is still in pain and is sedated from opioids has an opioid-resistant pain syndrome; an adjuvant medication will be required (see Adjuvant Medications). Stress, fear, and spiritual distress may be best addressed through counseling.

Nurses can initiate many interventions to help clients cope with fatigue. Strategies to manage stress include counseling, education, relaxation, and massage. Instituting a regular exercise program can be effective in lessening fatigue in clients undergoing chemotherapy. Although no studies on the effect of an exercise program on fatigue in the palliative care setting have been published, this strategy should be considered for clients who are able to participate in some form of exercise. In addition, for clients who can eat and take in fluids, you can encourage adequate nutrition and hydration.[39, 44]

One helpful strategy is to help clients modify their activity and rest patterns. Encourage clients to (1) incorporate rest times into their daily schedules, (2) plan their most strenuous activities for the time of day when energy levels are highest, and (3) capitalize on saving energy by accepting the assistance of others, delegating tasks, and using equipment such as a bedside commode or a portable telephone.

Medications may be helpful to treat fatigue in some clients. Corticosteroids are sometimes used to treat fatigue in people with advanced cancer. The exact mechanism of action is not clear, but some researchers believe that corticosteroids may lessen fatigue by inhibiting tumor and tumor-induced substances that contribute to the symptom. Others suggest that fatigue is relieved by the central euphoric effect of these medications. If anorexia or cachexia is a contributing factor in fatigue, the appetite-stimulating effect of corticosteroids may be helpful.

Psychostimulants have also been used to treat people with fatigue (see Chapter 21). There have not been any controlled comparisons of these medications, but the largest experience in people with cancer has been with methylphenidate (Ritalin). Dextroamphetamine (Dexedrine) and pemoline (Cylert) have also been used.[39, 44]

■ SLEEP DISTURBANCES

Impaired sleep is a common, and often overlooked, problem in people with advanced illnesses. Many times, a disturbance in sleep is accepted as "part of being sick." However, it is important to recognize the importance of sleep. Sleep is associated with tissue restoration; sleep deprivation alters immune function. Although people with a terminal illness are not going to "recuperate" from their underlying disease, they can benefit from the healing and protective functions of sleep when dealing with tissue injury and infection. Excessive sleepiness is also emotionally disabling, resulting in an inability to participate in treatment, comprehend information, and share in social interactions. Furthermore, impairment of sleep may lead to depression, irritability, and withdrawal.[46]

An evaluation of the amount and quality of sleep is an important component of the overall assessment of a client in the palliative care setting.[46] This evaluation covers:

- Usual bedtime
- How long it takes to fall asleep
- Any wakefulness during the night
- Usual waking time
- Subjective feeling of being "refreshed" in the morning
- Frequency and length of daytime naps
- Use of sleep medications
- The cause of any sleep problems as identified by the client

There are many potential causes of sleep disturbances. Physiologic factors contributing to impaired sleep include pain, nausea and vomiting, respiratory problems, medications (e.g., corticosteroids, bronchodilators, antihypertensives), metabolic disturbances, and delirium. Psycho-emotional factors, such as depression and anxiety, also interfere with sleep. The client's environment definitely influences the amount and quality of sleep; unfamiliar surroundings, frequent interruptions, noise, bright lighting, and unpleasant odors can all lead to a disturbance in sleep. In addition, lack of exercise, inactivity, and boredom may lead to excessive napping during the day, resulting in poor sleep at night.

Treatable causes of sleep disturbance must be addressed with appropriate interventions and discontinuation of medications that interfere with sleep when possible. General sleep hygiene strategies include[46]:

- Establishing a regular sleep schedule
- Staying out of bed during the day
- Napping only when necessary
- Keeping active (mentally and/or physically) during the day
- Minimizing nighttime disruptions
- Avoiding stimulants at night (caffeine, nicotine)

One advantage of long-acting medications is a decreased need to awaken during the night for dose administration.

People who have difficulty falling asleep may benefit from establishing a relaxing bedtime routine. Depending on individual preferences, this relaxation routine may consist of massage, progressive muscle relaxation, imagery, music, and warm milk or herbal tea.

When other interventions are not effective in promoting or maintaining sleep, medications may be appropriate. Benzodiazepines are the main group of medications used to promote sleep. There is some controversy regarding the long-term effectiveness of the benzodiazepines, and most are recommended for short-term use. Thus, the need for sleep medications must be reevaluated on a regular basis. Benzodiazepines used for sleep disturbances include the following:

Short half-life (2 to 4 hours): Triazolam (Halcion), zolpidem (Ambien). Because of their quick onset of action, these medications are helpful for people who have difficulty falling asleep. However, they do not benefit people with sleep maintenance problems. Rebound insomnia is common if the medication is abruptly stopped. Triazolam, which is associated with adverse drug reactions, has been removed from the market in some countries.

Intermediate half-life (6 to 15 hours): Lorazepam (Ativan), oxazepam (Serax), temazepam (Restoril). These medications are helpful for promoting sleep onset and maintenance.

Long half-life (29 to 100 hours): Flurazepam (Dalmane), quazepam (Doral). Although these agents help promote sleep onset and maintenance, daytime sedation is common because of their long half-lives. Also, drug accumulation may occur in the elderly. (See Chapter 21 on sleep management.)

■ CACHEXIA-ANOREXIA SYNDROME

Cachexia is derived from the Greek words *kakos and hexis,* meaning "poor condition." The term "cachexia-anorexia syndrome" is often used loosely to define weight loss, wasting, or loss of appetite.[33] However, cachexia-anorexia syndrome is one of the most common problems afflicting clients with advanced cancer and AIDS. The incidence in clients with cancer varies with the type of primary tumor. The client who has adenocarcinoma of the breast is less likely to exhibit cachexia-anorexia syndrome than the client who has adenocarcinoma of the lung or pancreas. Wasting is not commonly observed in clients with a hematologic malignancy yet is very prevalent in clients with myelodysplastic syndromes.[33]

Several studies have identified chemical factors (due to tumor burden) that contribute to cachexia-anorexia syndrome. A number of cytokines have been identified to produce this syndrome, including tumor necrosis factor, interleukin-1 and interleukin-6, and interferon. Other causes are metabolic abnormalities, a decrease in nutritional intake, and eventual loss of appetite.[33] Correctable causes are found in clients who have obstruction of the upper or lower bowel as a result of tumor invasion. Simple starvation, which can often be corrected with parenteral or enteral nutrition (see Chapter 29), must also be considered in this client population.

Other contributing factors in cachexia-anorexia syndrome are presented in Table 22–4. Clinical manifestations commonly observed in this syndrome are (1) muscle loss, (2) impaired immunity, (3) loss of body fat, (4) glucose intolerance, (5) fluid retention, and (6) vitamin deficiencies.

Interventions are as varied as the contributing factors. Some clients may not respond favorably to the replacement of dietary supplements and require more aggressive intervention, such as a progestational (hormonal) agent. Scientific research has concluded that pharmacologic therapy alleviates cachexia-anorexia syndrome. The use of progestational agents in combination with other medications or with special diets achieves improved outcomes.

The following pharmacologic strategies are suggested for the client with cachexia-anorexia syndrome:

1. Progestational agents
2. Anabolic steroids
3. Dietary interventions involving omega-3 fatty acids and branched-chain amino acids
4. Combination approaches:
   a. Cannabinoids
   b. Dietary supplements
   c. Prokinetic agents
   d. CNS stimulants (methylphenidate)

Remember, the loss of appetite often assessed in the dying client is a normal process that should not be confused with cachexia-anorexia syndrome.

TABLE 22-4	FACTORS CONTRIBUTING TO CACHEXIA-ANOREXIA SYNDROME

Tumor involvement of gastrointestinal tract
Antitumor therapy
Infections
Taste change
Medications
Food aversions
Pain
Psychological factors
Changes in metabolism
Hormonal changes
Fatigue, weakness
Increased metabolic rate; altered fat, protein, or carbohydrate metabolism; fluid-electrolyte abnormalities; hormonal changes
Malabsorption
Tumor metabolism

INDICATORS OF IMMINENT DEATH

Certain physical, cognitive, and behavioral changes occur as a person enters the active dying process. The human body, like any other living organism, seeks survival; in doing so, it often alters normal physiology. As the body begins to die, blood is commonly shunted to the brain and the heart, the two most important organs. Thus, peripheral circulation is limited, leading to mottling and cyanosis. Because the kidneys are no longer perfused adequately, there is a decrease in urine output. Slowly, all body systems become involved in the dying process.

Tachycardia and diminished blood pressure are observed in the acute phase of decompensation (organ shutdown) of the cardiovascular system. The respiratory system works to compensate for metabolic deficiencies, causing tachypnea, dyspnea, or both. Table 22–5 highlights indicators of impending death.

COMMUNICATION

The dying process can be a time of emotional crisis for many families. You can help lead clients and families down a less threatening path to what is often termed "the unknown." In order to do so, however, you must develop a level of comfort in communicating with dying clients and their families. You will need to examine their personal feelings about death and dying before you can provide emotional support and guidance to the dying. If you are uncomfortable in this care setting, you may impede the ability of clients and families to finish their important business.

Clients and families facing the last days of life should be given the opportunity to express any or all of their concerns about issues that matter the most to them. The nurse acts as a listener, a friend, and an advocate for the client. Being available in a nonjudgmental and nonthreatening manner allows the client and family to trust the nurse. Once trust is established and the client believes that the nurse will effectively manage his or her symptoms, the client may begin to open up emotionally and discuss many concerns about the illness and death. Each client is unique, and so are the conversations that occur between nurse, client, and family. As professionals who have the most contact with clients, you are sometimes the only person with whom clients share thoughts and feelings. Emphasize to the client that the nurse is a member of a health care team and that sharing of some information with other members of the team, who can provide additional support, may be beneficial.

Communicating with dying clients and their families takes into account the multidimensional nature of people. See Diversity in Health Care: Cultural Aspects of Death and Dying. Your sensitivity to culture, spirituality, lifestyle, and emotional connections is essential for clients to feel supported.

One of the most important tasks of the bedside nurse is to empower clients and families to participate in the final act of living. Through ongoing assessment, communication, and skilled physical care, you can communicate reassurance, confidence, and support for the vulnerable client and family. The seasoned hand of a skilled professional supporting and guiding the client can change the journey through dying and death from a frightening process to one of peace and comfort.

CARE FOR THE CAREGIVERS

The families of terminally ill clients commonly serve as primary caregivers in the home care environment and are often highly involved in providing care in other palliative care settings. This "intensive caring" is physically and emotionally exhausting. In order to provide and maintain this level of care, these caregivers need education and support from all members of the interdisciplinary health care team. Coping tasks for families caring for a loved one who is dying and suggested interventions are described in Table 22–6.

Even though this intensive caring is very difficult,

TABLE 22-5	COMMON OBJECTIVE BODY SYSTEM INDICATORS OF IMMINENT DEATH
Cognition/orientation	Not always nonresponsive, may be agitated or restless, cannot subjectively respond to verbal stimuli
Cardiovascular	Tachycardia, irregular heart rate, lowered blood pressure or significant widening between systolic and diastolic, pressures, dehydration
Pulmonary	Tachypnea, dyspnea, use of accessory muscles, acetone breath, Cheyne-Stokes breathing, pooling of secretions or noisy respirations
Gastrointestinal	Diminished appetite, smaller amounts of feces (despite not eating), incontinence
Renal	Diminished urinary output, incontinence, concentrated urine
Mobility	Limited, bedbound, and requires frequent position changes

DIVERSITY IN HEALTH CARE

Cultural Aspects of Death and Dying

Death is a universal experience. Beliefs and behaviors regarding death, however, are highly personal and vary according to culture. The influx of many different cultural groups into the United States means that nurses are challenged to become knowledgeable about unique cultural beliefs and traditions related to death, dying, and bereavement.

The Problem

Nurses all too often avoid the death process because they have been educated to focus on restoring health or fostering environments in which the client returns to a previous state of health or adapts to physical, psychological, or emotional changes. Nursing education takes place within the Western view of health and illness. The U.S. health care system fosters the idea that with advanced technology, death can be controlled and postponed. Death is viewed as a medical and technological failure. This view of death as a failure of technology varies greatly from the view of cultures that perceive death as a natural part of the life cycle.[4]

"White" society is by and large viewed as a death-defying, death-denying society, whereas clients from immigrant communities may view the dying process very differently. For example, a comparison between most white and immigrant communities reveals that white society is often "I" centered; many immigrant communities are "we" centered, particularly in regard to decision-making.[6] For the client from another culture, there may be cultural conflict concerning who makes decisions about the client's impending death. Who is the decision maker—the client, the family, or the physician?

Cultural Perceptions of Death and Grieving

The way in which a family views life and death is a belief system with its core in the cultural heritage of the family. The family's basic disposition toward the meaning of life and death is expressed behaviorally.[2] For example, traditional Muslims believe that whatever happens in life is a result of destiny, or God's will. Consequently, a traditionally oriented Muslim client may believe that the time of death is predetermined and nothing can change it.[3] Such a client would not be interested in a technological intervention to prolong life. Navajos believe that speaking of the dead or expressing their emotions about the loss of a loved one can be detrimental to the living because of the power of the deceased. The Chinese view a sudden, unexpected, untimely, or violent death as a "bad" death. Such a death places shame on the family because it is thought to be caused by the transgressions of ancestors. Consequently, mourning is discouraged and grieving does not occur.[2]

Interventions

Nurses should become aware of cultural variations about grieving and perceptions of death because clients and their families are greatly in need of culturally sensitive care at this vulnerable time. Because there are many cultural variations of the perceptions about and behaviors that accompany death, dying, and bereavement, you are not expected to be knowledgeable about all of them.[4] It is important to talk with clients and families about cultural aspects of death and dying. The following guidelines to be used by the nurse for assessing death beliefs and rituals provides the structure for identifying a client's important cultural beliefs[5]:

1. Death rituals and expectations:
   a. Identify culturally specific death rituals and expectations.
   b. Explain the purpose of death rituals and mourning practices.
   c. What are specific burial practices, such as cremation?
2. Responses to death and grief:
   a. Identify cultural expectations of responses to death and grief.
   b. Explore the meaning of death, dying, and the afterlife.

Even though dying is a universal experience, its meaning varies greatly from one culture to another. Nurses are challenged to familiarize themselves with the death rituals and responses of terminally ill clients and their families. The preceding guidelines help in gathering this information. Having this knowledge enhances your ability to provide culturally competent care to clients and families when they are very vulnerable and in need of compassionate care—when they are experiencing death, dying, and bereavement.

References

1. Andrews, M. & Boyle, J. (1999). *Transcultural concepts in nursing care.* Philadelphia: Lippincott–Williams & Wilkins.
2. Esposito, L., Buckalew, P., & Chukunta, T. (1996). Cultural diversity in grief. *Home Health Care Management and Practice, 8*(4), 23–29.
3. Leininger, M. (1995). *Transcultural nursing: Concepts, theories, research and practices.* New York: McGraw-Hill.
4. O'Connell, L. (1996). Changing the culture of dying. *Health Progress, 77*(6), 16–20.
5. Purnell, L., & Paulanka, B. (1998). *Transcultural health care: A culturally competent approach.* Philadelphia: F. A. Davis.
6. Smith, J. (1996). Cultural and spiritual issues in palliative care. *Journal of Cancer Care, 5*(4), 173–178.

Joyce Larson-Presswalla, PhD, RN, *President, "Culture Counts," Marketing Coordinator, James A. Haley Veterans Hospital, Tampa, Florida*

most family caregivers are able to provide appropriate levels of care for their loved ones. Nurses play a pivotal role in assessing their educational and support needs, providing information and support, and referring caregivers to other team members and community agencies to address their needs.

SUPPORT OF THE GRIEVING FAMILY

Bereavement care is an important component of any palliative care program.[54] Providing bereavement care requires an understanding of the normal grieving process and the tasks of grief work. Grief is a normal and expected reac-

TABLE 22–6	FAMILY COPING TASKS IN TERMINAL ILLNESS
Coping Task	**Support or Interventions**
1. Acceptance versus denial	1. Provide realistic information about the illness and treatment options. Encourage open and honest communication among family members.
2. Establish a relationship with the health care team	2. Explain the roles of all interdisciplinary team members. Establish trust, maintaining open lines of communication.
3. Meet the needs of the dying person a. Physical needs	a. Provide information about pain and symptom management, use of equipment, skin care/position, rest and nutrition, infection control, safety. Reassure caregivers that they are doing a good job. Assess need for assistance, such as home health aide. Assess need for transfer to a different care setting.
b. Emotional needs	b. Encourage caregivers to take time to sit and listen to loved one and to share each other's feelings and concerns. Assess need for additional support/counseling from the interdisciplinary team.
4. Maintain functional equilibrium (i.e., the family must maintain some sense of normalcy to continue to function as a family unit)	4. Assist family to identify and prioritize activities that must be continued (e.g., going to work or school, doing laundry, buying groceries). Assist family to identify support persons to help with these tasks. Encourage caregivers to use respite care services to care for selves and to attend family events outside of direct caregiving.
5. Regulate family affect	5. Allow the caregivers the opportunity to express their feelings. Give them permission to have whatever feelings they have (i.e., "feelings just are—there's no right or wrong") Acknowledge that normally joyful times, like holidays, may not feel as joyful. Encourage formal counseling, if needed. Encourage the caregivers to address their own needs and to care for themselves, too.
6. Negotiate relationships outside the family	6. Give permission to take time to maintain friendships. Discuss options for maintaining jobs while caring for a dying loved one.
7. Cope with the post-death phase (healthy grieving)	7. Support family while they accept the finality of their loss. Discuss the functioning of the family unit without the loved one. Encourage using available bereavement supports/counseling.

Adapted from Cohen, M. S., & Cohen, E. K. (1981). Behavioral family systems interventions in terminal care. In H. J. Sokel (Ed.), *Behavioral therapy in terminal care* (pp. 177–204). Cambridge, MA: Ballinger Publishing Co.; and Ferrell, B. R. (1998). Home care. In A. Berger, R. Portenoy, & D. Weissman (Eds.), *Principles and practice of supportive oncology.* Philadelphia: Williams & Wilkins.

tion to a loss. Family members will grieve the loss of their loved ones. One role of the health care team is to reinforce the understanding that grieving is healthy, a necessary process that the family must to through to be able to move on in their lives. Nurses need to validate as normal the manifestations that the bereaved may be experiencing (Table 22–7).

In addition to knowing the normal responses to grief, it is helpful for those working with the bereaved to understand the tasks of the grieving process. Four tasks of mourning that must be accomplished in order for the bereavement to reach a satisfactory conclusion include[54]:

• Accepting the reality of the loss
• Experiencing the pain of the loss
• Adjusting to the environment in which the deceased is missing
• Finding a way to remember the deceased while moving forward with life

Most people adjust to bereavement adequately, but for some, bereavement can be complicated. It is important for health care providers to identify people with abnormal or

TABLE 22-7	MANIFESTATIONS OF GRIEF	
Psychological	**Social**	**Physiological**
1. *Avoidance phase:* Shock, denial, disbelief 2. *Confrontation phase:* Extremes emotions as person deals with the loss and its implications 3. *Reestablishment phase* Gradual decline in grief	Restlessness, inability to sit still Inability to initiate and maintain organized patterns of activity Social withdrawal	Anorexia/gastrointestinal disturbances Weight loss Sleep disturbances Crying Tendency to sigh Fatigue, lack of strength, lack of energy Heart palpitations, nervousness, tension Loss of sexual desire or hypersexuality Shortness of breath

From Rando, T. (1984). Grief, dying and death. In *Clinical interventions for caregivers.* Champaign, IL: Research Press Co.

complicated grieving and refer them for skilled counseling and support. Examples of complicated grieving are[54]:

- *Chronic grief:* prolonged grieving; the sense that person is "stuck" in the grieving process.
- *Delayed grief:* a previously insufficiently mourned loss that becomes evident at a later time.
- *Exaggerated grief:* intensification of the normal grief response to the point of dysfunction.
- *Masked grief:* grief that is hidden at the time of loss and manifests itself later as a physical or psychiatric problem.

Health care providers can assist families in their grieving process before the client dies by encouraging and supporting anticipatory grieving and by encouraging communication between client and family. As death becomes imminent, it is often helpful to encourage the family to be present with their loved one, if possible. Encouraging the family to reminisce and helping people deal with their feelings are important interventions after the death of the client.

CONCLUSIONS

The nurse caring for the dying client and family requires many skills. The nurse must possess the ability to offer compassion, assess the multitude of symptoms that occur at the end of life, and participate in symptom management. The nurse is also a member of the health care team whose focus is to help promote a healthy and positive dying experience for all involved.

THINKING CRITICALLY

1. T. S., a 57-year-old man, has stage IV squamous cell carcinoma of the right lung with metastatic bony involvement. You find that he is in excruciating pain and is so sedated that he is unable to subjectively rate his pain. He is nauseated, has not had a bowel movement in 6 days, and is anorexic and dehydrated. His current medications include sustained-release morphine 60 mg every 6 hours, a transdermal opioid of 75 μg, and immediate-release morphine 20 mg every 2 hours, which have not provided relief. What can you do to make this client more comfortable?

Factors to Consider. Besides poor pain control, what other problems need attention? Consider the addition of an adjuvant analgesic, the dosing of the opioids, and the client's hydration status.

2. F. T., a 43-year-old man, entered the emergency department with complaints of severe dyspnea. The chest x-ray revealed pleural effusion of the right lung. The results of the thoracentesis, which drained 1500 ml of fluid, were positive for adenocarcinoma. After several diagnostic studies were performed, no primary site for the tumor was identified. He was referred to an oncologist for palliative chemotherapy. You are asked to make a home visit to change the dressing on his chest tube. Your first assessment reveals a very cachectic, dehydrated, constipated, dyspneic client whose pain was well managed. The chest tube drainage totals 450 ml daily. The client and his wife are questioning the relevance of the chemotherapy, given the poor prognosis as well as his continued weight loss, loss of appetite, and weakness. He informs you that he does not want to be hospitalized and would like to remain at home and comfortable. After learning about this client's status and wishes, what actions should you take?

Factors to Consider. What actions should be taken to facilitate the client's request? Is 24-hour care needed now or in the future? What additional needs might the client or his wife have?

3. J. K. is a 38-year-old, single teacher who has diabetes mellitus and polycystic kidney disease (PKD). Her most recent kidney-pancreas transplant has been rejected, and she is undergoing hemodialysis again. She has not been compliant with her diet and fluid restrictions, and multiple dialysis access sites have become infected. She states that she does not want to continue dialysis. What should you do next? Should her parents be told of her request?

Factors to Consider. How can you be certain that the client understands the ramifications of ending the hemodialysis? What can you do to keep her comfortable once dialysis is discontinued?

BIBLIOGRAPHY

1. Agency for Health Care Policy and Research (1994). *Managing cancer pain*. Washington, DC: Department of Health and Human Services.

2. Ahmedzai, S. (1996). Making a success out of life's failure. *Progress in Palliative Care, 4*, 1–3.

3. Ahmedzai, S. (1998). Palliation of respiratory symptoms. In D. Doyle, G. Hanks, & N. MacDonald (Eds.), *Oxford textbook of palliative medicine* (2nd ed., pp. 583–616). Oxford: Oxford University Press.

4. American Psychiatric Association. (1994). *Diagnostic and statistical manual of mental disorders (DSM-IV)* (4th ed). Washington, DC: Author.

5. American Thoracic Society Standards. (1999). The diagnosis and care of patients with chronic obstructive pulmonary disease. *American Journal of Respiratory Critical Care Medicine, 159*, 321–340.

6. Bennahum, D. (1996). The historical development of hospice and palliative care. In D. Sheehan & W. Forman (Eds.), *Hospice and palliative care* (pp. 1–10). Sudbury, MA: Jones & Bartlett.

7. Brietbart, W., Chochinov, M., & Passik, S. (1998). Psychiatric aspects of palliative care. In D. Doyle, G. Hanks, & N. MacDonald (Eds.), *Oxford textbook of palliative medicine* (2nd ed., pp, 923–954). Oxford: Oxford University Press.

8. Brietbart, W., & Jacobson, P. (1996). Psychiatric symptom management in terminal care. *Clinics in Geriatric Medicine, 12*, 329–347.

9. Bruera, E., & Lawlor, P. (1998). Defining palliative care interventions. *Journal of Palliative Care, 14*, 23–24.

10. Bruera, E., et al. (1995). Frequency of alcoholism among patients with pain due to terminal cancer. *Journal of Pain and Symptom Management, 10*, 599–603.

11. Caraceni, A. (1995). Delirium in palliative medicine. *European Journal of Palliative Care, 2*, 62–67.

12. Clinch, J., Dudgeon, D., & Schipper, H. (1998). Quality of life assessment in palliative care. In D. Doyle, G. Hanks, & N. MacDonald (Eds.), *Oxford textbook of palliative medicine* (2nd ed., pp. 83–96). Oxford: Oxford University Press.

13. De Stoutz, N., & Stiefel, F. (1997). Assessment and management of reversible delirium. In R. Portenoy & E. Bruera (Eds.), *Topics in palliative care* (pp. 21–43). Oxford: Oxford University Press.

14. Doyle, D., Hanks, G., & MacDonald, N. (1998). Introduction. In D. Doyle, G. Hanks, & N. MacDonald (Eds.), *Oxford textbook of palliative medicine* (2nd ed., pp. 3–8). Oxford: Oxford University Press.

15. Dudgeon, D. (1997). Dyspnea clinical perspectives. In Symptoms in terminal illness: A research workshop treating symptoms at the end-of-life. Rockville, MD: National Institutes of Health.

16. Dudgeon, D., & Rosenthal, S. (1996). Management of dyspnea and cough in patients with cancer. *Hematology/Oncology Clinics of North America, 10*, 151–171.

17. Finn-Paradis, L. (1985). *The development of hospice in America: The hospice handbook*. Rockville, MD: Aspen.

18. Foley, K. (Ed.). (1996). Palliative medicine, pain control, and symptom assessment. In *Caring for the Dying*, pp. 11–18. Philadelphia: American Board of Internal Medicine.

19. Gift, A. (1997). Dyspnea methods perspective. In Symptoms in terminal illness: A research workshop treating symptoms at the end-of-life. Rockville, MD: National Institutes of Health.

20. Harwood, K. (1999). Dyspnea. In C. Yarbro, M. Frogge, & M. Goodman (Eds.), *Cancer symptom management* (2nd ed., pp. 45–55). Sudbury, MA: Jones & Bartlett.

21. Haskell, R., Frankel, H., & Rotondo, M. (1997). Agitation. *AACN Clinical Issues, 8*, 335–350.

22. Ingham, J., & Caraceni, A. (1998). Delirium. In A. Berger, R. Portenoy, & D. Weissman (Eds.), *Principles and practice of supportive oncology* (pp. 477–495). Philadelphia: Lippincott–Williams & Wilkins.

23. Kinzbrunner, B. (1998). Hospice: 15 years and beyond in the care of the dying. *Journal of Palliative Medicine, 1*, 127–137.

24. Kübler-Ross, E. (1969). *On death and dying*. New York: Macmillan.

25. Kübler-Ross, E. (1995). *Death is of vital importance: On life, death and life after death*. New York: Station Press.

26. Kuebler, K., et al. (1996). *Hospice and palliative care practice protocol: Dyspnea*. Pittsburgh, PA: Hospice Nurses Association.

27. Kuebler, K., & Ogle, K. (1998). Psychometric evaluation of an objective assessment instrument to measure pain, dyspnea and restlessness (Abstract). *Journal of Palliative Care, 14*, 125.

28. Leung, R., Hill, P., & Burdon, J. (1996). Effect of inhaled morphine in the development of breathlessness during exercise in patients with chronic lung disease. *Thorax, 51*, 596–600.

29. Lo, B. (1995). End-of-life care after termination of SUPPORT. *Hastings Center Report Special Supplement 25*, S6–S8.

30. Lynn, J. (1997). An 88-year-old woman facing the end-of-life. *Journal of the American Medical Association, 277*, 1633–1640.

31. Lynn, J. (1998). Complaints about hospice: Growing up or going wrong? *ABCD Exchange, 1*, 2–7.

32. Lucas, B. (1999). Coping with psychiatric emergencies in the office: Patient care for the nurse practitioner. *Clinician Reviews, 2*, 31–42.

33. MacDonald, N., Alexander, R., & Bruera, E. (1995). Cachexia-anorexia-asthenia. *Journal of Pain and Symptom Management, 10*, 151–155.

34. Mahoney, J. (1998). The Medicare hospice benefit—15 years of success. *Journal of Palliative Medicine, 1*, 139–146.

35. Marshall, P. (1995). The SUPPORT Study: Who's talking? *Hastings Center Report Special Supplement 25*, S9–S11.

36. McGuire, D. (1998). The multiple dimensions of cancer pain: A framework for assessment and management In D. McGuire, C. Yarbo, & B. Ferrell (Eds.), *Cancer pain management*. Boston, MA: Jones & Bartlett.

37. Milisen, K., et al. (1998). Delirium in the hospitalized elderly: Nursing assessment and management. *Nursing Clinics of North America, 33*, 417–439.

38. Minagawa, H., et al. (1996). Psychiatric morbidity in terminally ill cancer patients: A prospective study. *Cancer, 78*(5), 1131–1137.

39. Neuenschwander, H., & Bruera, E. (1998). Asthenia. In D. Doyle, G. Hanks, & N. MacDonald (Eds.), *Oxford textbook of palliative medicine* (2nd ed., pp. 573–581). Oxford: Oxford University Press.

40. Pereira, J., & Bruera E. (Eds.)(1997). Dyspnea. In *The Edmonton aid to palliative care*. Edmonton, Alberta, Canada: Division of Palliative Care, University of Alberta.

41. Pollack, M. (1999). New treatments for panic disorders, psychiatric illness in primary care. *Clinician Reviews, 9*(3), 4–9.

42. Portenoy, R. (1997). *Contemporary diagnosis and management of pain in oncologic and AIDS patients*. Newton, PA: Handbooks in Health Care Company.

43. Portenoy, R. (1997). Symptoms commonly experienced in terminal illness. In Symptoms in terminal illness: A research workshop treating symptoms at the end-of-life. Rockville, MD: National Institutes of Health.

44. Portenoy, R. K., & Miaskowski, C. (1998). Assessment and management of cancer-related fatigue. In A. Berger, R. Portenoy, & D. Weissman (Eds.), *Principles and practice of supportive oncology* (pp. 109–118). Philadelphia: Lippincott–Williams & Wilkins.

45. Rhodes, V., & McDaniel, R. (1999). The symptom experience and its impact on quality of life. In C. Yarbo, M. Frogge, & M. Goodman (Eds.), *Cancer symptom management* (pp. 3–8). Sudbury, MA: Jones & Bartlett.

46. Sateia, M. J., & Silberfarb, P. M.(1998). Sleep. In D. Doyle, G. Hanks, & N. MacDonald (Eds.), *Oxford textbook of palliative medicine* (2nd ed., pp. 751–767). Oxford: Oxford University Press.

47. Shepherd, S., & Geraci, S. (1999). The differential diagnosis of dyspnea: A pathophysiological approach. *Clinician Reviews, 9*(3), 52–71.

48. Sterling, L. (1999). Pharmacological review of SSRIs in panic disorder: Psychiatric illness in primary care. *Clinician Reviews, 9*(3), S10–S13.

49. Story, P. (1998). Symptom control in the dying. In A. Berger, R. Portnoy, & D. Weissman (Eds.), *Principles and practice of supportive oncology* (pp. 741–748). Philadelphia: Lippincott–Williams & Wilkins.

50. The SUPPORT Principal Investigators. (1995). A controlled trial to improve care for seriously ill hospitalized patients: The Study to Understand Prognoses and Preferences for Outcomes and Risks of Treatments (SUPPORT). *Journal of the American Medical Association, 274*, 1591–1598.

51. Trzepacz, P., et al. (1999). American Psychiatric Association Guidelines: Practice guidelines for the treatment of patients with delirium. *American Journal of Psychiatry, 156*, S1–S20.

52. Twycross, R. (Ed.) (1997). Respiratory symptoms. In *Symptom management in advanced cancer* (pp. 143–148). Abdingdon, UK: Radcliff Medical Press.

53. Walsh, D. (1998). The Medicare hospice benefit: A critique from palliative medicine. *Journal of Palliative Medicine, 1*, 147–149.

54. Weaver, S., & Eutsey, D. E. (Eds.) (1998). *Palliative care: Patient and family counseling manual*. Gaithersburg, MD: Aspen.

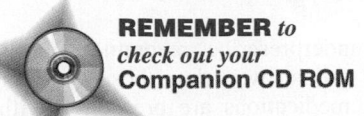

REMEMBER *to* *check out your* **Companion CD ROM**

CHAPTER

23

Clients with Pain: Promoting Positive Outcomes

Juanita Fogel Keck
Susan Baker

NURSING OUTCOMES CLASSIFICATION (NOC)
for Nursing Diagnoses—Clients with Pain

Activity Intolerance	**Ineffective Individual Coping**	Symptom Control
Endurance	Coping	Symptom Severity
Energy Conservation	Decision-Making	Well-Being
Self-Care; Activities of Daily Living	Quality of Life	**Powerlessness**
Anxiety	**Knowledge Deficit**	Health Beliefs: Perceived Control
Anxiety Control	Knowledge: Health Behaviors	**Sleep Pattern Disturbance**
Coping	Knowledge: Treatment Regimen	Comfort Level
Symptom Control Behavior	**Pain**	Pain Level
Fear	Comfort Level	Rest
Fear Control	Pain Control	Sleep
Comfort Level	Pain: Disruptive Effects	Well-Being
	Pain Level	

Pain is a complex, multifaceted phenomenon. It is an individual, unique experience that may be difficult for clients to describe or explain and often difficult for others to recognize, understand and assess. Pain often leads to debilitation, diminished quality of life, and depression. Pain management challenges every health care team member, for there is no single, universal treatment.

Nurses are probably the most important component of the team, for they are the client's primary advocate for pain relief. Listening to concerns, assessing pain intensity and distress levels, planning for care, educating the client about pain, promoting use of nonpharmacologic pain techniques, and evaluating the process for promoting positive outcomes are nursing responsibilities. An attentive nurse can identify discomfort in clients often without verbal confirmation from the client (Fig. 23–1). Nurses have the capability to relieve pain merely by acknowledging the discomfort and confirming that measures will be taken to relieve the pain. This commitment and statement of caring establish trust and rapport with the client.

This chapter summarizes what is currently known about the physiology of pain, how to assess and diagnose aspects of pain, how to implement a variety of both pharmacologic and nonpharmacologic techniques to manage the discomfort, and how to evaluate outcomes appropriately.

THE PROBLEM OF PAIN

In the natural environment, pain serves as a mechanism to warn us about the potential for physical harm. Thus, pain is the body's protective mechanism to prevent further tissue damage by providing the impetus to withdraw from the pain-producing situation. The discomfort and distress associated with pain often last far beyond the tissue-damaging experience. Pain is the primary reason people seek health care and is associated with increased length of hospital stay, longer recovery time, and poorer client outcomes.[1, 59] Pain is typically undertreated.[58, 75] In the early 1970s, researchers reported that pain was seriously undertreated after surgery.[73] Thirty years later, this situation has changed little, even though there have been immense advances in knowledge of the causes of pain and the mechanisms that contribute to pain relief. New medications and the recognition of complementary pain

FIGURE 23-1 The nurse asks the client about pain. The client is the expert regarding her pain.

management strategies have contributed to the improved ability to manage pain and to provide satisfactory pain relief. If the existing knowledge and resources were utilized to manage pain, 90% of people with pain would receive satisfactory pain relief.[75, 116] Barriers to adequate pain management may involve health care professionals, including nurses; clients, physicians, and the health care system.[35, 52, 75] These barriers are presented in Box 23-1.

BOX 23-1 Barriers to Pain Management

Problems Related to Health Care Professionals

Inadequate knowledge of pain management
Poor assessment of pain
Concern about regulation of controlled substances
Fear of client addiction
Concern about side effects of analgesics
Concern about clients becoming tolerant to analgesics

Problems Related to Clients

Reluctance to report pain
Concern about distracting physicians from treatment of underlying disease
Fear that pain means disease is worse
Concern about not being a "good" client
Reluctance to take pain medications
Fear of addiction or of being thought of as an addict
Worries about unmanageable side effects
Concern about becoming tolerant to pain medications

Problems Related to the Health Care System

Low priority given to cancer pain treatment
Inadequate reimbursement (the most appropriate treatment may not be reimbursed or may be too costly for clients and families)
Restrictive regulation of controlled substances
Problems of availability of treatment or access to it

Modified from Jacox, A., et al. (1994). *Management of cancer pain. Clinical practice guidelines No. 9.* AHCPR Pub. No. 94-1592. Rockville, MD: Agency for Health Care Policy and Research, U.S. Department of Health and Human Services, Public Health Service.

Physicians tend to underprescribe, recommending over longer periods of time doses lower than those considered therapeutic. Typically, medications are prescribed with a range of allowable doses and time periods. For example, acetaminophen with codeine may be prescribed as one or two tablets taken every 3 to 4 hours. Many nurses tend to routinely administer the smallest prescribed dose of medication over the widest time frame (e.g., one tablet every 4 hours). Health care providers need to learn more about the mechanisms of pain. A nurse's inaccurate beliefs or expectations lead to misunderstandings about the client's pain experience. Often a client's complaint of pain is ignored or not believed if that client's experience does not match the nurse's expectation.

Clients may contribute to the problem of inadequate pain management. They may be reluctant to take pain medications due to fear of addiction, they may fear being labeled a "drug user," or they may worry that taking strong medications will render them unable to be adequately medicated in the future should their pain become worse. They may believe that some degree of pain is normal and cannot be relieved. Health care providers and people in pain may believe that some degree of pain is expected and is not treatable, especially after surgery and in the presence of cancer. Pain can be totally relieved, or nearly so, with appropriate strategies.

Nurses and clients do not know enough about combination drugs for pain relief. These situations generated by nurses can lead to frustrated, angry, uncooperative clients as a result of unrelieved pain. Education is a primary action to begin to remedy the problems.

DEFINITION OF PAIN

How is *pain* defined? Does the definition include feelings of agony, distress or suffering? Is pain defined in a structural, physiologic manner only? Does the definition include individual perception of the painful stimulus? Do cultural and ethnic backgrounds, gender, or age affect pain perception?

Pain is a multidimensional phenomenon and is thus difficult to define. It is a personal and subjective experience, and no two people experience pain in exactly the same manner. You may find pain control a difficult task when caring for individual clients; however, it is one of the most important areas of care because people cannot function adequately when they are in pain. Pain is best viewed as an experience, not merely as a manifestation of a medical condition.

Health care practitioners have defined pain in many ways. It is generally related to some type of tissue damage, which serves as a warning signal, but it is much more. The International Association for the Study of Pain (IASP) offers the accepted medical definition of pain as "an unpleasant sensory and emotional experience associated with actual or potential tissue damage, or described in terms of such damage."[58]

Sternbach[115] defined pain as "an abstract concept which refers to (1) a personal, private sensation of hurt; (2) a harmful stimulus that signals current or impending tissue damage; and (3) a pattern of responses to protect the organism from harm." This definition helps the nurse's understanding of the client's pain. It focuses on pain as something that belongs to the person, because pain is both personal and private. Sternbach's definition also reminds the nurse that pain may have a protective function.

McCaffery defined pain as "whatever the experiencing person says it is and existing whenever the person says it does."[75] This definition makes each person the expert about his or her own pain. Because clinical pain is subjective, the only people who can accurately define their own pain are those who are experiencing that pain. Despite its subjective nature, the nurse is charged with accurately assessing and helping to relieve pain and McCaffery's definition helps nurses achieve this goal. Remember, all pain is real even if the cause cannot be ascertained.

PERCEPTION OF PAIN

Pain *perception,* or *interpretation,* is an important component of the pain experience. Because we perceive and interpret pain based on our own individual experience, pain is different for each person. Pain perception does not depend solely on the degree of physical damage. Both physical stimuli and psychosocial factors can influence our experience of pain. Although few agree about the specific effects of these factors, *anxiety, experience, attention, expectation,* and the *meaning of the situation* in which injury occurs affect pain perception. Cognitive functions, such as distraction, may also affect the severity and quality of the pain experience.

In the past, pain was viewed primarily as a sensation, with motivational and cognitive processes believed to influence only the reaction to pain. However, it is now apparent that mechanisms within the pain pathway can modify pain-related neural impulses before they are transmitted to the brain. Thus, pain perception is likely to be determined by a relative balance between sensory peripheral input and mechanisms of central control in the brain.

Pain perception is influenced by one's tolerance for pain. To understand tolerance, we must differentiate between *pain threshold* and *pain tolerance.* The pain threshold is defined as the lowest intensity of a painful stimulus that is perceived by a person as pain. The pain threshold may vary according to physiologic factors (such as inflammation or injury near pain receptors), but essentially it is similar for all people if the central nervous system (CNS) and peripheral nervous systems are intact.

Tolerance is defined as the amount of pain a person is willing to endure. It is different for each person who experiences pain, based on subjective factors such as the meaning of the pain and the setting. Some people have a high tolerance; that is, they can tolerate a lot of pain without distress, whereas others have a very low tolerance. Tolerance also varies for a given person, depending on a variety of factors associated with each specific pain incidence, such as nausea, fatigue, meaning of the pain, coping ability, and sensory input. Only the person, not the health care team, can determine the person's tolerance level.

Another aspect that can alter our perception of pain is our past experience with pain. Expectations regarding the new pain experience may be based on previous pain episodes. For example, when a person has had a bad experience with pain, the anticipation that future pain may be as bad can make subsequent pain episodes worse. If the person has had a good experience with pain management, future pain episodes may be more positively experienced. Therefore, it is important for nurses to facilitate adequate pain control that will result in positive client outcomes.

MISCONCEPTIONS AND MYTHS

Many misunderstandings exist about pain (Table 23–1). If nurses continue to believe these myths, adequate pain assessment and relief are hampered. For example, many health care providers believe that it is possible to predict the amount of pain people should have, based on their medical condition. However, the diagnosis or type of surgery is *not* an effective fundamental basis for determining the amount of pain the person should be experiencing or the analgesic required to relieve that pain.

Both children and older adults experience unrelieved pain because health professionals incorrectly assume that age predicts pain.[116] The fact that clients do not visibly exhibit physiologic or behavioral signs of pain often leads to the belief by the health care provider that they do not have pain. A more likely explanation is that the client has adapted to the pain. The adaptive psychological responses include:

- A shifting away from the pain
- Reporting pain only if asked directly
- Exhibiting sleepiness (which may also be due to insomnia secondary to the pain)
- Exhibiting decreased physical activity
- Showing a blank facial expression

These signs do not mean that the person is not experiencing pain but that the person is exhibiting adaptive responses to pain that continues to be present.

A major barrier to adequate pain management is concern about addiction to pain medications, particularly to opioids, which results in undermedication for clients.[116] *Addiction* is a behavioral pattern of drug use characterized by (1) overwhelming involvement with the use of a drug (compulsive use) and securing a supply of it and (2) a tendency to relapse after withdrawal from the drug (to begin taking it again whether or not pain is present). This behavior is sometimes described as the "three Cs": *c*ompulsive, *c*raving for the drug, and seeking and using the drug despite the *c*onsequences. Most people who take opioid analgesic medication for pain do not become addicted; in actuality, psychological addiction rarely occurs. (The incidence of addiction is less than 0.1%.[67]) Never use the term *addict* unless a medical diagnosis has been established, since many individuals exhibiting "drug-seeking behavior" are simply seeking better pain relief, not the medication itself (see also Chapter 24).

Education is the primary means of removing the effect of these myths on pain management. By knowing the facts about pain, pain assessment, pharmacology and pain treatment, you can provide more complete care.

■ MISINFORMATION ABOUT PAIN

One of the major blocks to accurate assessment of a person's pain is the person. If the health care team members still believe myths and have misconceptions about pain, it is likely that the client as well has been misin-

TABLE 23–1   COMMON MISCONCEPTIONS ABOUT PAIN

Myth or Misconception	Fact
• Addiction occurs with prolonged use of morphine or morphine derivatives	• The incidence of addiction is less than 0.1%
• The nurse or physician is the best judge of a client's pain	• Only the client can judge the level and distress of the pain; pain management should be a team approach that includes the client
• Pain is a result, not a cause	• Unrelieved pain can create other problems, like anger, anxiety, immobility, respiratory problems, and delay in healing
• It is better to wait until a client has pain before giving medication	• Playing "catch-up" is not an effective way to manage pain; it is better to routinely administer analgesia, thus maintaining a low pain level
• Real pain has an identifiable cause	• There is always a cause of pain, but it may be very obscure and must be assessed carefully. Pain of a psychological origin is just as real as pain of physiologic origin
• The same physical stimulus produces the same pain intensity, duration, and distress in different people	• Intensity, duration, and distress vary with each individual
• Some clients lie about the existence or severity of their pain	• Very few people lie about pain
• Very young or very old people do not have as much pain	• All clients with an intact neurological system experience pain; age is not a determinant of pain, but it may influence expression of pain
• Pain is a part of aging	• Pain does not accompany aging unless a disease process or ailment is present
• If a person is asleep, they are not in pain	• People in pain become exhausted and may truly be asleep or merely trying to sleep. Some people sleep as an escape mechanism
• If the pain is relieved by nonpharmaceutical pain relief techniques, the pain was not real anyway	• Nonpharmaceutical pain relief methods can be effective. A client's method of relief should be acknowledged as long as it does not harm
• Nurses should rely on their own definitions of pain and cultural beliefs about pain	• It is a mistake to impose one's own definitions, cultural beliefs, and values to another person's pain. Let the client tell you what the pain means

formed about pain and pain control. People sense the expectations of the health care team about their own pain. They have learned that they are expected to tolerate certain levels of pain and not to complain excessively. People have also learned to be afraid of pain medications, especially opioids. A major nursing responsibility, therefore, is to educate clients about pain and pain control. The nurse needs to help people understand that they, not the health care team, are the true experts about their pain. The nurse is also responsible for helping clients provide an accurate pain history and assessment data.

When documenting pain, avoid saying that the client "complains" of pain. This term tends to invalidate or minimize the client's experience, as if the client is fussing unnecessarily. It is more accurate and helpful simply to use the word "states" or "reports." When discussing pain (e.g., with clients) or when documenting pain, avoid using the phrase *pain attack*. Feeling that one is "under attack" may increase the feeling of powerlessness, creating the perception that the client is a victim. Use the term "episode" to promote self-control and a sense of an ability to do something to manage the episode.

TYPES OF PAIN

ACUTE PAIN

Acute pain is usually of short duration (<6 months) and has an identifiable, immediate onset, such as incisional pain after surgery. It is also regarded as having a limited and often predictable duration, such as postoperative pain, which usually disappears as the wound heals. Acute pain is often described in sensory terms, such as "sharp," "stabbing," and "shooting." It is considered a useful and limiting pain, in that it indicates injury and motivates the person to obtain relief by treatment of the cause. Acute pain is usually reversible or controllable with adequate treatment. People suffering from acute pain often come to terms with it because of the meaning or the limited nature of the pain, as in the pain of childbirth. When the pain is relieved, the person returns to the pre-pain state.

Acute pain may be accompanied by observable physical responses, including (1) increased or decreased blood pressure, (2) tachycardia, (3) diaphoresis, (4) tachypnea, (5) focusing on the pain, and (6) guarding the painful part. The cardiovascular and respiratory responses are due to stimulation of the sympathetic nervous system as part of the *fight or flight response*. These responses are often interpreted as positive evidence of a person's pain. Such interpretation is not reliable, however, because these sympathetic responses are temporary and may not be present in clients with continuing acute pain.

In 1992, the Agency for Health Care Policy and Research (AHCPR)[1] released its first set of Clinical Practice Guidelines for acute pain resulting from surgery or trauma. The guidelines were intended to serve as a resource to help health care providers and clients facilitate positive pain management outcomes. The four major pain management goals are to:

- Reduce the incidence and severity of acute postoperative or post-traumatic pain
- Encourage clients to communicate unrelieved pain so that they can receive prompt evaluation and effective treatment
- Enhance comfort and satisfaction
- Contribute to fewer postoperative complications and shorter stays after surgical procedures

These guidelines were designed to help the individual, family, and health care professionals work *together* to promote better relief of acute pain. You can obtain valuable information from these guidelines, including using them to guide pain assessment and management to improve control of acute pain for all clients. The guidelines emphasize the following[1]:

- A collaborative, interdisciplinary approach to pain control, including all members of the health care team and input from the client and client's family, when appropriate
- An individualized proactive pain control plan developed preoperatively by clients and practitioners (since pain is easier to prevent than to bring under control, once it has begun)
- Assessment and frequent reassessment of the client's pain
- Use of both drug and non-drug therapies to control or prevent pain
- A formal, institutional approach to management of acute pain, with clear lines of responsibility

■ CHRONIC PAIN

Chronic pain is a major health concern. The pain may have originally been acute in nature or may have been so obscure that the person does not know when it first developed. Chronic pain syndromes are often defined in vague terms, and many of their causes remain unknown.[120] Therefore, a diversity of treatment modalities has been used to treat the symptoms.

Chronic pain may be divided into three types:

- Chronic nonmalignant pain, such as from low back pain or rheumatoid arthritis
- Chronic, intermittent pain, such as from migraine headache
- Chronic malignant pain, from cancer

Chronic pain lasts for long periods of time and is not readily treatable.[79] A person's mental response to pain depends on its duration and, possibly, its intensity. Pain that is constant, continuous, and moderate is often described as far more difficult to bear than pain that is intense but relatively short in duration. The course of chronic pain includes months and years of pain, not minutes or hours.

Chronic pain is associated with withdrawal and despair. Anxiety may give way to depression. Some clients learn to adapt and cope with the pain, adjusting their lives. Remember, however, that absence of the expected expression of severe pain does not mean that the pain is gone; therefore the client's description of pain, not the manifestations one expects to see, is very important. Intractable, prolonged, and intense pain is very difficult to bear. Most people undergo major affective and behavioral changes when experiencing pain for prolonged periods. Such changes may be compounded, and chronic pain syndrome can develop. Characteristics of clients experiencing chronic pain syndrome include:

- Depressed mood
- Increased or decreased appetite and weight
- Drastically restricted activity level, leading to reduced work capacity, poor physical tone, and increased depression
- Social withdrawal
- Preoccupation with physical manifestations
- Poor sleep and chronic fatigue, which may result from inactivity, analgesics, and depression as well as from pain

Some clients may not exhibit any of these manifestations or may exhibit only a few. Once these changes take place, however, the pain may become more difficult to treat than the pain's original physical source.

CHRONIC NONMALIGNANT PAIN

Chronic pain is usually considered pain that lasts more than 6 months (or 1 month beyond the normal end of the condition causing the pain) and has no foreseeable end unless it is associated with very slow healing, as with burns. It is continuous or persistent and recurrent. Some disagree about whether acute recurrent pain (as in migraine and sickle cell crisis) should be classified as chronic pain, but it is usually referred to as chronic.

Chronic pain may have an identifiable cause, although the cause may be difficult to determine. It is often described in affective terms, such as "hateful," or "sickening" and it is typically much more difficult than acute pain to treat. Chronic pain is frequently associated with concomitant disability as a result of the pain experience. For example, a client immobilized by the pain of severe rheumatoid arthritis may be further compromised by the effects of the immobility.

Chronic pain is a frustrating condition, making it difficult for the person to live a normal life. Clients experiencing continuous or continually recurring chronic pain tend to become increasingly engrossed in their illness. They may seem fearful, tense, fatigued, tending to become withdrawn and isolated. Their pain is exhausting both physically and emotionally for themselves and their families. Health care providers may also feel frustrated and incompetent when their attempts to relieve chronic pain are ineffective. However, if nurses understand the anatomy, physiology, and psychosocial aspects of chronic pain, they can be very helpful to the the client and family. Professionals may be able to intervene before extreme suffering occurs.

CHRONIC INTERMITTENT PAIN

Chronic intermittent pain refers to exacerbation or recurrence of the chronic condition. The pain occurs only at specific periods; at other times, the client is free from pain. Typical, conditions include migraine and cluster headache, sickle cell crisis, and the intermittent abdominal pain associated with chronic gastrointestinal disorders, such as irritable bowel syndrome and Crohn's disease. Pain management is directed toward control of pain in much the same manner as that for individual acute pain episodes. However, chronic recurrences render the condition more difficult to control. The client anticipates continual exacerbation of the situation and is intensely influenced by psychosocial factors that are difficult to manage.

CHRONIC MALIGNANT (CANCER-RELATED) PAIN

Malignant pain is considered to have qualities of both acute and chronic pain. The category encompasses neuropathic, deep visceral, and bone pain, among others (Table 23–2). Each type of pain is best managed by strategies specific to it. Therefore, the nurse needs to carefully assess each type of pain and treat it appropriately. A diagnosis of cancer adds an additional psychological component associated with potential physical deformity and the potential for impending death, preceded by agonizing suffering. The mental anguish may intensify the perception of pain.

PHYSIOLOGY

■ PHYSIOLOGIC BASIS OF PAIN PERCEPTION

To understand the mechanisms by which pain relief might be facilitated, we must understand the neurologic contributions to pain perception. Pain is a perceptual interpretation of nerve activity that reaches consciousness. The sensation of pain depends on activation of neurons that transmit the noxious information to the CNS. Pain perception is initiated by activation of neurons along a pathway, which eventually terminates in a sensory cortex in the brain. The pathway involves both peripheral nervous system and CNS components and can be activated at any point along its path.

The typical initiation of pain producing nerve transmission begins with activation of receptors by chemical or mechanical stimuli. Receptor activation is followed by transduction of the stimulus to an electrical impulse that is transmitted from nerve cell to nerve cell along the pathway. The neuron responsible for transmitting the electrical signal is composed of three primary components: the cell body, dendrites, and an axon. Dendrites receive the signal and transmit it toward the cell body, where it is directed along the axon to activate the dendrites of the next neuron. Dendrites of the next neuron come in contact with the axon of the transmitting neuron at a synapse, a microscopic cleft at the contact area. The ends of the axons are configured with specialized structures (terminal boutons). The electrical signal is transmitted to the next neuron when specialized chemicals (*neu-*

TABLE 23–2	SOURCES OF NOXIOUS STIMULI FOR CLIENTS WITH CANCER
Source of Stimuli	**Cause**
■ Cell destruction	Cell necrosis Ulceration Tumor invasion Tissue injury
■ Inflammation	Products of cell destruction
■ Infection	Bacterial invasion
■ Nerve injury	Direct injury through incising nerve structures Tumor invasion of peripheral nerves, plexes, spinal cord, brain Chemotherapy/radiation injury
■ Ischemia/hypoxia	Edema Hematoma Occlusion of vessels by tumor
■ Noxious stretch or pressure	Distention of thoracic and abdominal viscera, fascia, periosteum Occlusion of gastrointestinal and genitourinary structures Obstruction of ducts and viscus

rotransmitters) are released by the terminal bouton. The neurotransmitter must diffuse across the synaptic cleft and attach to receptors on the dendrites of the next neuron.

Neurons involved in pain perception are A-delta (Aδ) and C fibers.[40, 44, 130] A-delta fibers transmit a signal more rapidly than C fibers do. They deliver information that allows us to recognize a pain-producing stimulus and to determine its relevant characteristics, such as location, severity, and type. A-delta fiber-mediated pain is perceived as sharp, cutting, or stabbing sensations, reflective of tissue damage. A-delta fiber activity typically results in activation of the sympathetic nervous system to prepare us to engage in fight or flight behaviors that allow us to react to the pain-producing event.[40] As a result, heart rate, respiratory rate, and blood pressure may be increased. These sympathetic reactions may or may not be observed in people with pain, since they are relatively rapidly adapting, often short-lived, responses.

C-fiber-mediated pain is conducted more slowly along the pain pathway and is characterized by dull, burning, sensations associated with suffering. C-fiber activity engages various brain stem and cerebral regions that contribute to the emotional, cognitive, and situational components of pain.

The first synapse in the pain pathway for both A-delta and C fibers occurs in the dorsal horn of the spinal cord, the area of the cord that receives all incoming sensory information[9, 40, 52] Here the nociceptive signal is transferred to the next neuron in the pain pathway and transmitted to the thalamus and brain stem structures by means of *spinal tracts*. The thalamic signal is involved in the ability to determine the location and intensity of the pain producing event. The signal is transmitted from the thalamus to the sensory cortex, where the pain as a sensation is perceived.

Secondary responses to the signal are initiated throughout the brain, including the limbic system, where the emotional response to pain is generated. Signals transmitted to brain stem structures contribute to the response we have to the pain experience and to endogenous (naturally occurring) pain modulation systems (Fig. 23–2).

RECEPTOR ACTIVATION

Pain perception depends on the generation of an electrical signal within the pain pathway. The electrical signal most often begins with activation of a receptor by high-intensity chemical, thermal, or mechanical stimuli.[40, 69, 100] Receptors associated with pain perception are found on specialized dendrites called *free nerve endings*. These receptors are categorized as *nociceptors* and are found throughout the body in the periphery in skin, fascia, bone periosteum, skeletal muscle, ligaments, and mucous membranes. In the viscera, nociceptors are found in the capsules of most organs.[40, 116]

Chemically mediated activation of nociceptors can be initiated by (1) cell wall destruction as a result of events such as tissue injury, ulceration, tumor invasion and cell necrosis, (2) inflammation, (3) infection, (4) nerve injury, and (5) extravasation of plasma from the circulatory system associated with edema, ischemia, or occlusion of vessels. Mechanically mediated activation of nociceptors is accomplished by noxious stretch or pressure due to (1) distention of viscera, fascia or periosteum, (2) occlusion of gastrointestinal or genitourinary structures, or (3) obstruction of ducts/viscus.[40, 52]

The nociceptors are at rest until they are stimulated by an event in the receptor's environment. The stimulus causes a change in the receptor membrane, which generates the electrical signal. The electrical signal is transmitted along the nerve dendrites and axon by modification of the electrical charge of the nerve cell membrane. Movement of the signal along the membrane requires that positively and negatively charged ions flow from one side of the membrane to the other.[4, 54, 75]

When at rest, the extracellular surface of the neuron membrane maintains a positive charge (the intracellular surface a negative charge). The positive charge is a result of a higher concentration of positively charged ions, primarily sodium (Na^+), in the extracellular environment, in contrast to the intracellular surface. The intracellular charge is maintained by a higher concentration of negatively charged ions, such as chloride (Cl^-), and large anions along the interior cell membrane. Potassium ions (K^+) aid in maintenance of the resting membrane charge. A change in the charge of the membrane surfaces is necessary to initiate the electrical signal. The interior must become more positive, the exterior more negative. The change is achieved by allowing Na^+ to flow into the cell and Cl^- to flow out of the cell. The addition of positively charged Na^+ inside the cell makes the inside more positive. The outward flow of Cl^- causes the extracellular surface to be less positive.

Channels in the cell membrane maintain the charge difference. The channels provide the only route for ions to move across the membrane. The nociceptive signal cannot be generated or maintained unless the channels are induced to open. When a stimulus is strong enough to initiate receptor activation, events are put into play that cause channels to open and the charged ions to move across the nerve cell membrane. This causes a change in the electrical charge of the membrane known as *depolarization* of the membrane.[4, 54, 65, 75]

Pain-producing events may initiate the nociceptive electrical signal directly, or they may sensitize the receptor, rendering it more susceptible to nociceptive activation—depending on the degree to which the ions move across the membrane. If the flow of ions is of sufficient intensity, the nerve membrane reaches threshold and "fires" initiating the electrical signal. The flow may be sufficient to change the charge of the membrane, rendering it close to threshold (partially depolarized) but not strong enough to cause the membrane to fire.[4, 44, 103] The depolarized membrane now fires in response to stimuli less intense than those originally needed.

Sensitizing chemicals are released into tissues as a result of cell wall destruction, release of plasma from the circulatory system as seen with edema, inflammation, ischemia, and infection.[114] Cells may be damaged by trauma and by the events that accompany inflammation and infection, including mast cell destruction during the release of histamine in inflammation and the effect of neutrophil activity in the presence of infection.

Chemicals sensitize receptors and nerve fiber membranes that do not typically produce pain sensations making them capable of initiating pain-producing signals. Sunburned areas produce a burning sensation when one

FIGURE 23–2 Ascending and descending nociceptive pain. (From Banasik J. *Perspectives on Pathophysiology Instructor's Manual*, 1995.)

Figure labels:
- Limbic system • Feeling and reaction to pain
- Cerebrocortex • Perception of pain
- Thalamus Axons project to other areas of brain
- Endorphin release
- Brainstem
- PAIN TRANSMISSION
- PAIN INHIBITION
- Ascending pathway • STT • SRT
- Descending pathway
- Dorsal horn • Pain inhibition
- Spinal cord
- Release of substance P
- Peripheral transmission
- Peripheral activity • Vasodilation • Edema • Hyperalgesia • Release of chemicals
- Nociceptors
- Noxious stimulus (may be chemical, thermal, or mechanical)

showers with water, which normally produces a pleasant, warm sensation. Injured areas are painful in response to touch and mild pressure that normally would not be painful. Normal peristalsis of the gut, which is typically undetectable, produces painful abdominal cramping in the presence of inflammation within the abdominal cavity.

The need for the flow of ions across the membrane provides a mechanism for pain to be intensified or decreased, depending on the activity of the membrane channels. Events or chemicals that cause channels to open and allow ions to flow across the membrane contribute to an increase in pain. Events that prevent channels from opening decrease the ability of pain-producing neurons to fire, resulting in decreased pain.

Chemicals that mediate nociception in the periphery include bradykinin, prostaglandins, substance P (sP), histamine, serotonin, leukotrienes, hydrogen ions, and nerve growth factor (NGF).[11, 55, 72, 100, 117]

Bradykinin, the most potent pain-producing chemical,[100, 135] is released into tissues when cell walls are destroyed and when plasma leaks from the vasculature.[15, 31, 69, 82] Bradykinin initiates a pain-producing signal by increasing the ability of Na^+ to flow across the membrane.

Prostaglandins result from cell wall destruction. They appear to contribute to the pain experience by sensitizing receptors, making them more responsive to other chemical, thermal, and mechanical stimuli.[24, 57, 129] They are also potent vasodilators, resulting in an increased release of bradykinin into the tissues.[24] The resulting edema may also contribute by stimulating pressure receptors. Pressure from edema typically is not painful, because the pressure is usually not strong enough to stimulate nociceptors. Prostaglandins depolarize these receptors, making them responsive to the relatively weak stimulus provided by the swelling of edema.

Substance P is released into peripheral tissues when nociceptive neurons are activated.[23, 46, 69, 129] The chemical facilitates the release of plasma by increasing vascular permeability, resulting in availability of bradykinin.[9, 69] Substance P further enhances pain responses by contributing to prostaglandin release.[23, 42, 122]

Histamine is released from mast cells when inflammation is a component of the pain-producing event. In the periphery, histamine increases vascular permeability, contributing to bradykinin activity and edema.[100] Substance P facilitates the release of histamine from mast cells.[23, 69, 129]

Serotonin is released in the periphery by platelets and mast cells.[104, 129] Therefore, any event that influences the presence of blood products in tissues or inflammation contributes to serotonin release. Serotonin causes pain directly by altering Na^+ flow in the receptive neuron membrane, causing the neuron to fire.[9, 104] Receptors are indirectly facilitated by serotonin as the chemical also sensitizes receptors to the effect of bradykinin.[15, 82]

Leukotrienes are produced by cell wall destruction during the same process that produces prostaglandins. They contribute to pain perception by attracting neutrophils to an area of injury.[65, 69] Cell wall destruction is a component of neutrophil activity to combat infection, resulting in bradykinin release. Thermal and mechanical receptors are also sensitized by leukotrienes.

Hydrogen (H^+) ions are released as a result of ischemia and hypoxia. They cause sodium channels to open, resulting in activation of neurons in the pain pathway. H^+ also facilitates calcium (Ca^{2+}) channel opening, enhancing neurotransmitter release.

Nerve growth factor is released when neurons are injured. NGF is similar to bradykinin in activating nociceptive neurons.[32, 65] NGF causes injured nerves to sprout new axons and dendrites in greater numbers than existed before the injury. As a result, the area responsive to nociceptive activation is increased in the periphery.[33] Substance P production is also increased by NGF increasing the nociceptive effect of the neurotransmitter. In addition, the number of Na^+ and K^+ channels are increased, making it easier to generate an ion flow, which will cause the neuron to "fire."

We respond to a pain-producing event with unique combinations of chemicals that modify the pain experience. For some, the combination of chemical mediators evoked may increase pain perception; for others, pain perception is limited. The multifaceted character of events that generate pain-producing signals accounts, in part, for variability in response to situations among people with similar tissue injury. Remember, we cannot predict the amount of pain a person might have in response to tissue injury or insult.

TRANSMISSION OF PAIN-PRODUCING ACTIVITY TO THE BRAIN

An electrical signal generated in the periphery must be transmitted at a synapse to the next neuron in the pathway if that signal is to result in pain perception. The first synapse occurs in the dorsal horn of the spinal cord.[30, 40, 52, 135] The neurotransmitter specific for that neuron is released into the synaptic cleft, where it flows across the cleft and engages a receptor on the postsynaptic membrane of the next neuron. Neurotransmitters associated with nociceptive transmission are substance P and glutamate. The transmitters are stored in small vesicles a short distance from the presynaptic bouton membrane. The vesicles must be moved to the membrane surface, where they can open and expel their contents into the cleft.

When enough of the vesicles have been mobilized and an adequate number of receptors on the postsynaptic membrane have been activated, the next membrane responds with opening the channels that will allow generation of the flow of ions along the next nerve fiber. Ca^{2+} initiates mobilization and emptying of presynaptic vesicles. Ca^{2+} remains in the extracellular environment until channels in the membrane open, allowing the calcium ions to flow to the neuron interior.[44, 64]

Electrical activity resulting in pain perception can be modified at the synapse by manipulating the release of neurotransmitters. An event that inhibits neurotransmitter release decreases the potential for transmission of the nociceptive signal. The inhibition may occur to an extent that extinguishes the pain-producing signal, resulting in total pain relief. Conversely, any event that facilitates release of the neurotransmitter enhances transmission of the signal. For example, an event that prohibits the opening of the Ca^{2+} channels inhibits the pain response.

INHIBITION OF PAIN-PRODUCING NEURAL ACTIVITY

Pain relief can be accomplished by (1) preventing activation of nociceptive receptors in the periphery, (2) preventing transmission of the electrical signal along the neurons in the pain pathway, and (3) preventing transfer of the signal from one neuron to the next at the synapse. Events that inhibit factors that contribute to pain (including inflammation, edema, and infection) lessen the pain experience by decreasing the availability of pain-producing chemicals.

Medications provide a primary means of modifying receptor activation. Nonsteroidal anti-inflammatory drugs (NSAIDs), for example, aspirin and ibuprofen, contribute to pain relief by preventing the production of prostaglandins and decreasing the effect of inflammation on the facilitation of pain-producing activity. Preventing unnecessary stimulation of receptors by mechanical events helps to control the pain event. Examples include controlling excess pressure on painful areas by proper positioning, avoiding pressure-producing events, and splinting an incision.

Transmission of the pain-producing signal can be inhibited by conditions that prevent opening of Na^+, Cl^-, or K^+ channels along the fiber. Some medications act directly on these channels, leading to the inability of the neuron membrane to maintain electrical activity.

A primary avenue for pain inhibition is found at the synapse in the spinal cord.[40, 42, 122] Peripheral sensory nerve cells extend from the receptor to the dorsal horn of the cord. The first synapse in the pain pathway occurs here. The dorsal horn is subdivided into layers, or *laminae*. A-delta fibers terminate in lamina I, the marginal layer, and laminae II and V. They synapse with *nociceptive-specific* (NS) neurons that transmit the signal to the thalamus. C fibers terminate primarily in laminae I, II, IV, and V.[9, 40, 130] They may activate NS neurons or *wide dynamic range* (WDR) neurons that respond to both nociceptive and non-nociceptive stimuli. These neurons extend to the brain through spinal tracts that terminate in the thalamus, the reticular formation, or the mesencephalon.

Interneurons are located in laminae II, III and IV.[40, 130] These neurons have extensively branched axons and dendrites, which may project through several laminae. They do not project beyond the dorsal horn however, suggesting that they serve a modifying function in the pain pathway. The location of the neurons, combined with their dense and extensive branching, render them capable of interacting with numerous sensory neurons. Some interactions occur with the peripheral neuron prior to the synapse. Others occur with the second neuron at postsynaptic sites. The presynaptic interactions facilitate pain relief by preventing an adequate release of nociceptive neurotransmitters. The postsynaptic interactions render the membrane less responsive to the incoming signal by modifying the electrical charge of the membrane, preventing the opening of ion channels, or by modifying the ability of receptors to receive the nociceptive neurotransmitters.[12, 55, 71]

Enkephalin and gamma-aminobutyric acid (GABA) are the primary inhibitory neurotransmitters released by dorsal horn interneurons.[3, 86, 107, 135] GABA acts to prevent "firing" of the postsynaptic membrane.[86] GABA inhibits neurotransmitter release from the presynaptic membrane by interfering with the membrane's ability to mobilize Ca^{2+}.[86] Enkephalin is one of the body's endogenous opiates. A number of opiate receptor types exist within the CNS, including mu, delta, and kappa.[3, 135] Opiates that activate mu and delta receptors initiate activity that hyperpolarizes the neuron membrane by modifying the ability of K^+ to flow across the membrane. As a result, nociceptive neurons require stronger stimuli in order to "fire." The effect occurs at both presynaptic and postsynaptic levels. When kappa receptors are engaged, Ca^{2+} channels cannot open, preventing neurotransmitter release. Enkephalin inhibits release of substance P from presynaptic terminals.

Inhibitory neurons in the dorsal horn can be activated by peripheral, mechanical and thermal stimuli, which are perceived as nonpainful. Nonpainful stimuli are transmitted to the CNS by A-beta fibers. Activation of A-beta fibers results in sensations perceived as touch, pressure, warmth, coolness, and vibration. The fibers also transmit proprioceptive information from muscle spindles and tendon insertions. These neuron fibers enter the dorsal horn and send their primary projections to the brain by means of the spinothalamic tract. Collaterals of these nerve fibers project to the dorsal horn laminae, where they terminate on enkephalin-producing interneurons. Activation of the A-beta fibers contributes to pain relief by stimulating the release of enkephalin.[3, 12, 42] One can observe the result of A-beta activity mediated by activation of peripheral skin receptors when one places a finger, mildly burned while cooking, in cold tap water. The burning sensation is extinguished while the finger is in the water. The ability of muscle contraction and joint movement to decrease pain perception is evidenced by shaking the hand when a part of the extremity has been injured.

Additional neurotransmitters are found in the dorsal horn. The cell bodies of the neurons that release these transmitters are located in areas of the brain stem. Their axons project to the spinal cord, where they synapse with the interneurons that release the inhibitory neurotransmitters. Serotonin is produced in the nucleus raphe magnus. Norepinephrine is produced by neurons in the locus ceruleus. The mechanisms by which these supraspinal nuclei contribute to pain relief are still being determined. They appear to stimulate neurons that release enkephalin, resulting in release of the inhibitory neurotransmitter.

Neurons in the raphe and ceruleus nuclei are activated by both peripheral nervous system and CNS activity. Neurons ascending to the brain in spinal tracts make connections with areas of the brain known to be involved in pain inhibition. The primary sites are the periaqueductal (PAG) and periventricular gray (PVG) areas that line the ventricles and the aqueduct of the cerebrospinal fluid (CSF) system. Enkephalin and the neurohormone endorphin are produced by PAG/PVG cell bodies. Collateral projections of the spinal tracts terminate in PAG/PVG. Nociceptive information being transmitted to the brain also activates the endogenous pain inhibition pathway by stimulating PAG/PVG neurons. Axons of these neurons project to both nucleus raphe and locus ceruleus initiating the release of serotonin and norepinephrine in the dorsal horn.[38, 42, 104, 130]

Brain areas responding to cognitive, emotional, and situational stimuli can also activate PAG/PVG, nucleus raphe magnus and locus ceruleus neurons. These nuclei receive projections from the limbic system, various cortical association areas, the hypothalamus, the basal ganglia, the auditory system, and the reticular activating system, among others.[25, 28, 38] These interconnections allow for numerous factors to contribute to pain perception through their influence on endogenous inhibitory activity. They may also serve to increase pain perception through activity that enhances the nociceptive signal or prevents the inhibitory system from operating. Figures 23–3 and 23–4 illustrate these inhibitory mechanisms.

■ GATE CONTROL THEORY OF PAIN

Historically, the gate control theory of pain has been included throughout the nursing literature as the theoretical explanation of the ability of pain management interventions to provide pain relief. Melzack and Wall posited the theory in 1965 on the basis of what was then known about the dorsal horn.[78] They proposed that pain could be inhibited by non-noxious peripheral stimuli and by brain activity associated with meaning of the experience, past pain experience, emotional arousal, cognitive activity (such as distraction), and motivational aspects of the situation. They described a gate in the dorsal horn that allowed transmission of nociceptive information when the gate was open and that prevented transmission if the gate was closed (Fig. 23–5). They suggested that interneurons in the substantia gelatinosa (SG) of the spinal cord were involved in closing the gate. When these neurons were stimulated, events occurred that rendered the transmission neuron incapable of receiving the signal. They also proposed that supraspinal activity originating in the brain and brain stem could contribute to opening or closing the gate.

The theory provided the first conceptualization of pain as a multidimensional experience. Prior to publication of the theory, the primary explanation was based on the belief that pain was a "straight through" stimulus-response phenomenon. When tissue damage occurred, specific nerve fibers were activated and the information was transmitted directly to the thalamus and then to the sensory cortex. The resulting pain perception could be accurately predicted based on the degree of tissue damage. The theory did not allow for pain inhibition by mechanisms other than interrupting the pain pathway or removing the pain-producing stimulus. The gate control theory replaced this conceptualization.

Although the theory has been helpful in bringing about a more realistic explanation of the human pain experience

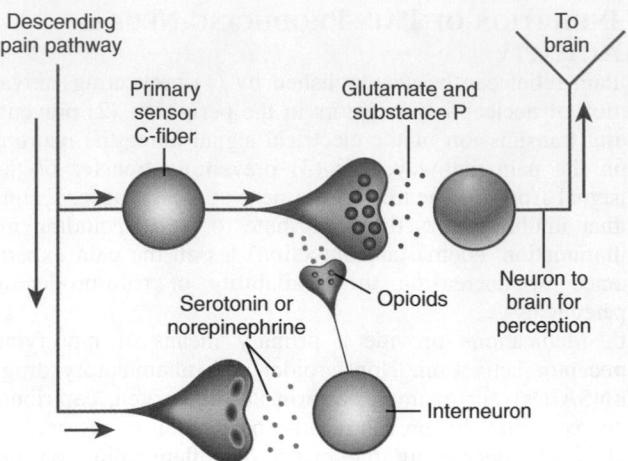

FIGURE 23–4 Endogenous inhibition in a synapse in the spinal cord. As the pain impulse enters the dorsal horn, it has the potential of being modified by interneurons in the synapse containing endogenous opioids.

FIGURE 23–3 Schematic representation of pathways involved with pain transmission and its modulation in the dorsal horn of the spinal cord. (PAG = periaqueductal gray; PVG = periventricular gray; NRM = nucleus raphe magnus; LC = locus ceruleus; WDR = wide dynamic range neuron; ENK = enkephalin releasing neuron; SG = substantia gelatinosa.

FIGURE 23–5 The gate-control theory: Mark II. The new model includes excitatory (*white circle*) and inhibitory (*black circle*) links from the substantia gelatinosa (SG) to the transmission (T) cells as well as descending inhibitory control from brain stem systems. The round knob at the end of the inhibitory link implies that its action may be presynaptic, postsynaptic, or both. All connections are excitatory, except the inhibitory link from SG to T cell. L, large-diameter fibers; S, small-diameter fibers. (From Melzack, R., & Wall, P. D. [1988]. *The challenge of pain* [2nd ed.]. New York: Penguin Books.)

at the time, it is less helpful today. Research over the past 30 years has delineated the actual mechanisms occurring in the spinal cord and has shown that the "gate" conceptualization is no longer tenable. In addition, inhibition activity is not limited to the SG. The SG is composed of dorsal horn laminae II and III. Inhibitory interneurons and their projections have been found beyond these two laminae. The theory was correct in predicting that nociceptive information was modifiable in the dorsal horn. Melzack and Wall proposed that nonpainful peripheral stimuli could initiate activation of events in the dorsal horn that would inhibit transmission of pain-producing signals beyond the spinal cord. The theory is now out of date, as subsequent research has more fully delineated the physiologic mechanisms underlying pain inhibition.

SOURCES OF PAIN

■ CLASSIFICATION

The human body is typically classified by systems. Systems involved in pain production include:

- *Superficial cutaneous* regions encompassing skin and subcutaneous tissues
- *Somatic* tissues of the body wall, including muscle, bone, periosteum, cartilage, tendons, deep fascia, ligaments, joints, blood vessels, and nerves
- *Visceral* structures, including organs and their capsules

The characteristics of a person's pain experience depends, in part, on the source of the noxious stimulation. There-fore, it is helpful to understand the typical characteristics of each pain type.

CUTANEOUS (SUPERFICIAL) PAIN

Cutaneous pain may be characterized by an abrupt onset and a sharp or stinging quality or by a slower onset and a burning quality, depending upon the type of nerve fiber involved. Cutaneous pain tends to be easily localized. The skin surface is readily divided into areas called *derma-tomes*. Each dermatome is served by one spinal nerve and dorsal root. When the skin is stimulated by a noxious stimulus, the nerve serving that dermatome is activated. The signal is transmitted to the one specific area of the sensory cortex serving the dermatome. As a result, the stimulus is perceived to occur within that dermatome. The boundaries of dermatomes may appear to be distinct in anatomic drawings, but nerve distribution actually overlaps. Excitation of one nerve may produce pain that is perceived to originate from adjacent dermatomes.

DEEP SOMATIC PAIN

Somatic structures are those of the body wall, such as muscles and bone. Table 23–3 displays a comparison of deep somatic pain with cutaneous pain. Deep somatic pain is poorly localized, may produce nausea, and may be associated with sweating and blood pressure changes. Deep somatic pain is generally diffuse and less localizable than cutaneous pain. Pain from deep structures frequently radiates from the primary site (e.g., pain from a lumbar disc is felt along the sciatic nerve).

Somatic structures vary in their sensitivity to pain. Highly sensitive structures include tendons, deep fascia, ligaments, joints, bone periosteum, blood vessels, and

TABLE 23–3	CUTANEOUS AND DEEP PAIN	
Characteristic	**Cutaneous Pain**	**Deep Pain**
Quality	Sharp, bright sensation or burning; felt superficially	Primarily dull and aching; may be described as boring, crushing, throbbing, or cramping; if less intense, described as soreness
Duration	Typically short	Often fairly long
Localization	Tends to be precise Pain is often experienced as a point, surface, or line	Often diffuse and inaccurate; seems to originate in a fairly broad area Pain frequently felt as if it were three-dimensional and occupying space
Hyperalgesia (excessive sensibility to pain)	May occur as a primary problem	May exist as secondary problem; occurring at a distance from the original noxious stimulus In referred pain, a superficial hyperalgesia may be associated with deep pain
Nausea	Rarely occurs	Sickening pain found only when deep structures are involved, as in renal and intestinal colic, gallstones, and angina
Associated symptoms	May be hyperalgesia, paresthesia, tickling, burning, or itching Also associated with brisk movements, a quick pulse, and a sense of invigoration	Resulting from autonomic responses, including pallor, sweating, nausea, vomiting, bradycardia (at times), lowering of blood pressure, syncope, faintness, and perhaps even death in shock Muscle contraction and tenderness often present Segmental spread of pain frequently noted; pain may not remain confined to original spinal segment but may spread into one or more adjacent segments

nerves. Skeletal muscle is sensitive only to stretching and ischemia. Bone and cartilage respond to extreme pressure and chemical stimulation (e.g., rheumatoid arthritis, osteomyelitis).

VISCERAL PAIN

Visceral pain refers to pain coming from body organs. It tends to be a diffuse, poorly localized, vague, dull pain. Nerve fibers innervating body organs follow the sympathetic nerves to the spinal cord. This may be the reason why autonomic manifestations (e.g., diarrhea, cramps, sweating, hypertension) frequently accompany visceral pain. Visceral pain typically includes acute appendicitis, cholecystitis, and inflammation of the biliary and pancreatic tracts, gastroduodenal disease, cardiovascular disease, pleurisy, and renal and ureteral colic. Often visceral pain is manifested as sweating, restlessness, nausea, emesis, pallor, and agitation.

Most viscera are not sensitive to stimuli that cause pain in somatic structures (such as cutting, burning, or pressure). This is understandable, because viscera are not normally exposed to such traumas, and the body thus does not "need" a response system. Although these types of stimuli do not produce pain in most viscera, other stimuli may cause severe pain, for example, violent or abnormal contractions of hollow viscera, such as the ureters and alimentary tract.

In the chest, the parietal pleura is richly supplied with pain endings through the intercostal nerves and through the phrenic nerve, on the surface of the diaphragm. The visceral pleurae in the chest, however, are insensitive to pain. The bronchi, on the other hand, are sensitive to pain. Elsewhere and throughout its serous surfaces, the visceral pericardium is insensitive to pain, except for the lower portion of the fibrous pericardium, which appears to have pain fibers from the phrenic nerve.

Pain in the gastrointestinal tract is common. It appears to arise mainly from the tract's muscular and serous lining. Gastrointestinal pain seems to occur when intestinal mucosa is inflamed, ulcerated, or otherwise abnormal or when the visceral muscles contract strongly or develop spasm. While the wall of the intestine is not sensitive to cutting, burning, or crushing, it does produce pain under other conditions, such as widespread ischemia and distention. Abdominal pain may also occur when body organs are perforated and their contents drain into the peritoneal cavity.

Visceral pain differs from cutaneous pain, in that highly localized damage to the viscera rarely causes severe pain but such damage to the body surface would cause pain. For example, a surgical cut in the gut does not cause pain but a cut in the skin would cause severe pain. If the stimulus to the viscera causes diffuse stimulation of nerve endings, the resulting pain is severe, as in ischemia (lack of oxygen) of the gut. Visceral pain is known to produce referred pain.

■ REFERRED PAIN

Referred pain is felt in an area distant from the site of the stimulus. It occurs when nerve fibers serving an area of the body distant from the site of the stimulus pass in close proximity to the stimulus. The referred pain sensation may be intense, and there may be little or no pain at the point of noxious stimuli. For example, myocardial ischemia typically is not felt as pain in the heart but most often as left arm, shoulder, or jaw pain. The fibers innervating these areas are close to those innervating the myocardium, resulting in the referred pain.

Identification of the segment of the spinal cord that is involved in transmitting referred pain is helpful diagnostically. Pain arising from a deep structure, whether a viscus or a deep somatic structure, has a referred segmental distribution, or a pattern of pain, determined according to the spinal cord segment supplying the structure. Referred pain is often baffling, warranting careful assessment. Examples of common patterns include pleural pain from the diaphragm referred to the shoulder, and the pain of cholecystitis referred to the back and in the angle of the scapula. Figure 23–6 illustrates common sites of referred pain.

■ INFLAMMATION

Inflammation is one of the most common pathologic conditions influencing pain sensitivity. Numerous harmful

FIGURE 23–6 Areas of referred pain.

substances, such as bacterial and chemical agents, can cause inflammation. Inflammatory responses may result from stressors, such as heat, cold, or trauma. Gross assessment findings associated with the inflammatory process are redness, swelling, heat, and pain. Inflammatory pain is secondary to the distention of stretch-sensitive tissue (i.e., periosteum, pleura) and the direct effect of released neuroregulators on afferent nerve endings. Principal chemical mediators of the inflammatory response are histamine, substance P, bradykinin, prostaglandins, and leukokinins.

■ NEUROPATHY

Neuropathic pain is caused by damage or injury to nerve fibers in the periphery or by damage to the CNS. Noxious electrical impulses are generated at the site of the injury. The pain is perceived to occur in the area served by the nerve. For example, an injury to a nerve that serves the hand would be perceived as pain in the hand even though the injury may be at the spinal cord level. Such pain is particularly problematic for the individual, as there is no obvious pathologic process corresponding to the pain sensation (e.g., the hand). Therefore, the person may not be believed. Neuropathic pain is also difficult to manage because it responds poorly to typical pain medications, particularly to NSAIDs[133] and opioids.[94, 133]

■ PHANTOM LIMB SENSATION

Following amputation of a body part (e.g., limb, breast), a person may continue to experience sensations in the part amputated as if that part were still present or attached. The nerve fibers that served the part continue to extend to the periphery, ending now at the incision site. The nerves have been injured by the surgery. As the cut nerve endings attempt to regenerate, they may form small neuromas at the incision cite. When nerve fibers are stimulated as a result of injury or neuroma, they continue to mediate the sensations associated with their original location. As a result, neuropathic sensations may be generated. These abnormal sensations may be perceived as presence of the limb, paresthesia, or pain.

Sensations associated with paresthesia may consist of itching, pressure, tingling, numbness, or "pins and needles." Painful sensations include throbbing, burning, stabbing, boring, and vise-like sensations experienced in the amputated area. Phantom pain also may be experienced as cramped, twisted, and abnormal posturing of a phantom limb. As a result of the nerve injury associated with the surgery, a formerly painless phantom area may gradually become painful. Phantom limb sensation is limited for most clients, resolving as the brain adapts to the loss of the amputated part. For some clients, however, the abnormal sensations persist over the long term. Fatigue, excitement, sickness, weather changes, emotional stress, or other stimuli may exacerbate the condition.

■ HEADACHE

Headache results in the most common type of pain. Many causes exist, involving both intracranial and extracranial structures. The brain itself is almost insensitive to pain, although the venous sinuses, tentorium, dura, some of the cranial nerves, and associated vasculature are pain-sensitive. Headache is discussed in Chapter 69.

■ MALIGNANCY

Pain occurs in 40% to 70% of people with solid tumors.[5, 41, 106] The Oncology Nursing Society issued a three-part position paper on cancer pain addressing the scope of nursing practice regarding cancer pain, ethical issues, practice issues, education of staff and clients, research recommendations, and sections on nursing administration, social policy, and pediatric cancer pain.[110, 111, 112] The paper also lists cancer and pain management resources and is an excellent reference for the nurse caring for clients with cancer.

Treatment of cancer pain is difficult because of its many causes. Bone pain usually responds to a combination of radiation therapy and NSAIDs, whereas other pain may require opioid analgesics, such as morphine. The client and the nurse must believe that cancer pain is controllable if correct medications are used in adequate amounts and in adequate combinations. In 1994, the AHCPR developed clinical practice guidelines with 10 goals for the management of cancer pain (Box 23–2).[59]

■ HUMAN IMMUNODEFICIENCY VIRUS INFECTION

Pain is common in clients with active human immunodeficiency virus (HIV) infection. Reports on the prevalence

---

BOX 23–2 Clinical Practice Guidelines for the Management of Cancer Pain

1. Inform clinicians and clients and their families that most cancer pain can be relieved by available methods.
2. Dispel unfounded fears that addiction results from the appropriate use of medications to control cancer pain.
3. Inform clinicians that cancer pain: (a) accompanies both disease and treatment, (b) changes over time, (c) may have multiple simultaneous causes, (d) if unrelieved, can affect the physical, psychological, social, and spiritual well-being of the client.
4. Promote prompt and effective assessment, diagnosis, and treatment of pain in clients with cancer.
5. Strengthen the ability of clients with cancer and their families to communicate new or unrelieved pain in order to secure prompt evaluation and effective treatment.
6. Provide clinicians with a synthesis of the literature and expert opinion for application to the management of cancer pain.
7. Familiarize clients and their families with options available for pain relief and to promote their active participation in selecting among these.
8. Provide a model for cancer pain management to guide therapy in selected painful, life-threatening conditions such as AIDS.
9. Provide information and guidelines on the use of controlled substances for the treatment of cancer pain that distinguishes the use of these drugs for legitimate medical purposes from their abuse as illegitimate drugs.
10. Identify health policy and research issues that affect cancer pain management.

AIDS, acquired immunodeficiency syndrome.
Modified from Jacox, A., et al. (1994). *Management of cancer pain. Clinical practice guidelines No. 9.* AHCPR Pub. No. 94-1592. Rockville, MD: Agency for Health Care Policy and Research, U.S. Department of Health and Human Services, Public Health Service.

of pain in this population range from 25% to 40% in early and ambulatory stages to 60% to almost 100% in end-stage disease.[59] The sources of pain in this population include (1) gastrointestinal or abdominal pain from colitis, esophagitis, gastritis, herpes, and cytomegalovirus (CMV); (2) peripheral neuropathy; (3) headache; (4) pleuritic pain from pneumonia; (5) oropharyngeal pain from oral candidiasis or herpes; and (6) pain from Kaposi's sarcoma lesions, which causes lymphatic obstruction. Approximately 40% of clients with HIV experience neuropathic pain, which is particularly difficult to manage pharmacologically.

Pain management is made more difficult in this population by the psychosocial correlation of the pain experience. Clients often lack the social support and resources of persons with chronic, malignant pain in other populations.[114] The multidimensional character of the pain in HIV infection and the client's personal situation requires a multidisciplinary team that can establish an open, trusting relationship in order to provide the best pain relief.[68]

Pain associated with HIV infection is usually undertreated, even in late stages.[1, 68, 114] A health care provider's opinion about the client with HIV and acquired immunodeficiency syndrome (AIDS) may be negative, resulting in lack of desire to help manage pain. The health care professional may believe that pain is an appropriate punishment for the behavior that led the person to contract HIV. Clients may be reluctant to report pain, fearing that increasing pain indicates a worsening of disease. Pain management may be complicated by a previous history of drug abuse or addiction. Prior addiction should not alter the way in which pain is treated. Clients may require higher doses of analgesics because they may have a high tolerance to opioids. Third-party payers present an additional barrier because they have considered pain management a low priority.[68]

Pain management for clients with HIV/AIDS is often difficult. It has been recommended that pharmacologic treatment be accomplished using cancer pain as a model incorporating the World Health Organization (WHO) cancer management "ladder."[59, 68] However, caution must be taken with the use of NSAIDs because of reports of cross-reaction between acetaminophen and drugs used to treat HIV infection. In addition, clients with cancer are at risk for gastrointestinal and renal diseases, which contraindicate the use of NSAIDs.[68] Recommended oral analgesics for mild to moderate pain in AIDS include aspirin and ibuprofen, choline magnesium trisalicylate (Trilisate), and weaker opioids (codeine, oxycodone, propoxyphene [Darvon]).[68] Adjuvant medications are also suggested for this population at any step in the WHO ladder.[68] It is imperative that pain of HIV/AIDS be treated vigorously, using the model of cancer pain treatment as the foundation and giving attention to the unique aspects of pain associated with this disease.

FACTORS AFFECTING PAIN

A client's reaction to pain is intensely personal and accounts for the great variability in pain experiences from person to person. Numerous factors contribute to this variability (Fig. 23–7). Some of these are discussed as examples to indicate the means by which one person's pain experience can be expected to differ from that of another person's.

■ SITUATIONAL FACTORS

The situation associated with the pain influences the person's response to it. A response to pain experienced in a formal or crowded situation may differ greatly from the response of a client who is alone or in a hospital. A woman who has had a hysterectomy for cancer may perceive her pain as more severe than that of a woman who has undergone removal of a benign cyst even though the surgical trauma is similar. Pain perception is influenced by the diagnosis in addition to the tissue trauma. A woman with a cancer diagnosis may require more aggressive pain management and additional emotional support than a woman with a benign diagnosis.

■ SOCIOCULTURAL FACTORS

Race, culture, and ethnicity are critical factors in one's response to pain.[10, 26, 36, 45, 61, 63, 89] These factors influence all sensory responses, including responses to pain. We learn how to respond to pain and other experiences from our family and ethnic group. Pain responses tend to reflect the mores of our culture. Within this framework, we

---

FIGURE 23–7 Considerations of the pain experience.

PHYSIOLOGIC FACTORS

Organic origin
Integrity of nervous system,
  including endogenous opioids
Concomitant physical influences
  (stress, fatigue)
Age
Type of pain
Location
Intensity
Duration
Frequency
Quality
Threshold
Tolerance

AFFECTIVE FACTORS

Distress of pain
Depression
Mood
Anxiety, fear, worry

I'm Unique

PSYCHOSOCIAL INFLUENCES

Family and occupational roles
Personal beliefs
Spiritual belief system
Cultural/societal influences
Sexual identity and
  stereotypes
Demographic factors

COGNITIVE

Past experience
Meaning of pain
  experience
Attention paid to
  sensation/distraction
Expectations
Coping mechanisms
Knowledge
Values/attitudes
Communication skills

learn what is appropriate and acceptable for our peer group. For example, verbally voicing pain may be considered appropriate within the Italian community and unacceptable within the German community, which values stoicism. In the Mexican culture, moaning or crying is used to help alleviate the pain rather than communicating a need for intervention.[22, 62] Cultural mores of some Hispanic groups view health as the absence of illness. If a person is not convinced that the pain is related to an illness, he or she might refuse treatment for it. The Diversity in Health Care feature discusses cultural aspects of pain response.

DIVERSITY IN HEALTH CARE

Cultural Perspectives on Pain

Anyone who has experienced severe pain understands that people are very vulnerable when they are in pain. Disease ravages the body, but pain ravages the soul. Pain is believed to be the main reason that a person initiates contact with the health care system. Nurses are responsible for evaluating clients' pain and making appropriate interventions. Consequently, nurses must realize that the meanings and expressions of pain are inextricably connected to cultural health beliefs and behaviors.[5]

Culture and Pain: Research Findings

The recognition that meanings and expressions of pain are colored by culture was first identified in the 1950s. It was reported that some patients experiencing pain were stoic and that others were expressive. For example, Americans of Northern European descent were likely to react to pain with stoicism but Italians and Jews tended to display high emotional responses to pain.[10] This research was the first to suggest that pain might be influenced by culture; however, the characterizations resemble stereotypes rather than generalizations.

Further research into how the context of culture shapes pain continues to suggest that an individual's experience of pain cannot be explained in simple physiologic terms—it is a product of culture. For example, the Navajo believe that pain is to be expected—a part of life.[2] Many Filipinos regard pain as part of life and view it as an opportunity to atone for transgressions.[6] Most Hispanics and Latinos are Catholic and consequently turn to religious practices to cope with pain. It is common for Hispanics-Latinos to believe that pain may be due to punishment and that suffering must be endured to enter heaven.[3, 4]

Another example of how culture influences the experience of pain involves African Americans, who may perceive that pain is a sign of illness or disease. This group may not take routinely prescribed medication unless pain is present (e.g., may take antihypertensive medication when they experience head or neck pain). This cultural practice interferes with effective management of hypertension.[8]

The Chinese generally believe the pain is caused from an illness that is due to a bodily imbalance. Consequently, the appropriate intervention becomes one that restores balance to the body.[8]

Mexican Americans have been shown to (1) accept pain as part of life, (2) feel obligated to "put up with" pain in the performance of their duties, (3) feel obligated to suffer stoically, and (4) feel that the type and amount of pain experienced are divinely predetermined. Their methods to alleviate pain are directed toward restoring and maintaining balance with the individual and the environment.[9]

Recognizing That Pain Is Influenced by Culture

Unfortunately, some nurses still question the importance of understanding the client's culture. Americans have been socialized to believe that the United States has the best health care system in the world. This ethnocentric attitude interferes with nurses' recognition and appreciation of culture. This is particularly troublesome because nursing supports the concept that holistic care is central to the practice of nursing. To not recognize the importance of culture is to truly miss the point of holistic care. Pain must be assessed within the context of culture.

Equally troublesome is the fact that within the subculture of nursing, it is expected that clients will be objective about the intensely subjective experience of pain. When clients are experiencing pain, they are expected to describe it in detail, but *not* to display emotional responses (i.e., to suffer in silence).[1] It has been suggested that silent suffering is probably the most valued response to pain in the United States.[7] If so, nurses are faced with the major challenge of *not* allowing their own ideas about pain to interfere with the care they give to clients in pain.

Finally, pain management is a major problem within health care. Although our communities are rich in cultural diversity, little emphasis has been devoted to pain management among culturally diverse populations. Nurses caring for clients with pain need to understand how culture influences pain. Health care providers need to be aware that their own values and perceptions may affect how they evaluate their clients' responses to pain and how they treat pain. It is important to validate the level of pain, pain intensity, and pain relief by involving the client and family. Understanding the health beliefs of different cultures regarding pain is crucial to providing culturally sensitive care.[3]

References

1. Andrews, M., & Boyle, J. (1999). *Transcultural concepts in nursing care.* Philadelphia: Lippincott.
2. Bell, R. (1994). Prominence of women in Navajo healing beliefs and values. *Nursing and Health Care, 15*(5), 232–240.
3. Juarez, G. (1997). Culture and pain. *Quality of life: A nursing challenge. 4*(4), 86–90.
4. Kumasaka, L., & Miles, A. (1996). 'My pain is God's will.' *American Journal of Nursing 96*(6), 45–47.
5. Leininger, M. (1997). Understanding cultural pain for improved health care. *Journal of Transcultural Nursing, 9*(1), 32–35.
6. Matson, S., & Lew, L. (1991). Culturally sensitive prenatal care for Southeastern Asians. *Journal of Obstetric, Gynecological, and Neonatal Nurses, 12*(1), 48–54.
7. McCaffery, P. (1979). *Nursing management of the patient with pain* (2nd ed.). Philadelphia: J. B. Lippincott.
8. Purnell, L., & Paulanka, B. (1998). *Transcultural health care: A culturally competent approach.* Philadelphia: F. A. Davis.
9. Villarruel, A., & Montellano, B. (1992). Culture and pain: A Mesoamerican experience. *Advances in Nursing Science, 15*(1), 32–38.
10. Zborowski, M. (1952). Cultural components in response to pain. *Journal of Social Issues, 8,* 16–30.

Joyce Larson-Presswalla, PhD, RN, *President, "Culture Counts," Marketing Coordinator, James A. Haley Veterans Hospital, Tampa, Florida*

Problems may also arise because of a person's view of health care team members. Members of various cultural groups may have difficulty communicating feelings to physicians and nurses who are from different backgrounds or ethnic groups.[10, 26] Health care providers may have difficulty appreciating the pain experiences of clients from unfamiliar cultural groups, because they tend to adopt white, middle-class cultural mores surrounding pain expectations and avenues for treatment.

Remember, people from different cultures may handle pain in various ways. A problem arises when the nurse does not recognize the person's way of dealing with pain or when the nurse does not accept it. Researchers found that nurses' judgments about pain their clients experienced was affected by the nurses' own beliefs and those of their culture.[22, 26] Nurses may also misinterpret expressions of pain from clients who do not speak English as a first language.[70] Health care providers must be sensitive to the contribution of cultural factors and language barriers in order to facilitate adequate pain management.

■ AGE

Age may play a significant role in perception and expression of pain. There are some variations in threshold associated with chronologic age, but no clear trends have been established.[43, 105] For example, infants perceive pain and respond to it with increasing sensitivity. Toddlers may respond to pain with crying and anger because they perceive it as a threat to security or sense that pain is a punishment. School-aged children may try to be "brave" and not cry or express much pain so that parents or nurses will not be angry with them. Adolescents may not want to report pain in front of peers, because they may perceive complaints of pain as weakness. Adults may not report pain for fear that it indicates a poor diagnosis. Pain may also mean weakness or failure for the adult.

There is controversy about pain in the elderly population. There is no reason to assume that pain perception is altered in older adults unless some damage has occurred in the CNS. The transmission and perception may be slowed with aging, but intensity of the pain is not diminished. Health care providers may underestimate the pain of older people as a result of impaired ability to express pain. Physical factors, such as paralysis and aphasia, may interfere with the ability to communicate.[115] Confused elderly clients may be unable to articulate their pain experience. Remember, altered expression does not mean absence of pain.

Age is considered an important factor in dosing of medications. Metabolic changes in the elderly affect their response to opioid analgesics. Drugs are metabolized and excreted more slowly in older people. In addition, elders frequently take combinations of medications for a variety of ailments, making them more susceptible to drug interactions.

Older people may assign different meanings to their pain. Pain may be considered a natural manifestation of aging. This may be interpreted in two ways. First, older people may think pain is simply something to be endured as a normal part of the aging process. Second, it may be seen as a sign of aging and, therefore, something to be denied because it means they are getting old. Many older people are hesitant to express pain for fear of being labeled as a "complaining" elder. These misconceptions serve to cause these people to experience pain unnecessarily. Careful assessment of the older person's pain is essential to prevent unnecessary suffering.

Few assessment instruments have been tested in the geriatric population, and visual, auditory, and motor impairments, common among elders, make typical assessment tools difficult to use.[1] Therefore, pay particular attention to verbal and nonverbal clues of pain in this population. Pain may be indicated by lack of appetite, sleeping disorders, tearing of the eyes, moaning, or splinting of a body part.

■ GENDER

Gender is an important factor in response to pain.[12, 14, 37, 123] In one study gender was a significant factor in the pain response, with men reporting less pain than women regardless of ethnicity. In some cultures in the United States, boys and men are expected to express pain less than women do. This does not mean that men feel pain less, only that they are assumed to show it less. Yet, health care providers who value bearing pain without complaint may view women as "complainers" and may ignore or devalue their pain expressions. Both men and women may experience pain unnecessarily if the nurse is not aware of gender biases in pain expression.

■ MEANING OF PAIN

The meaning of a person's pain influences his or her response to the pain.[19, 70, 128, 130] Pain caused by childbirth may be responded to differently than pain caused by surgery. If the cause of pain is known, the person may be better able to interpret meaning and to deal with the experience. If the cause is unknown, more negative psychological factors (e.g., fear, and anxiety) may be evoked, intensifying the degree of pain perceived. Pain may be perceived more intensely if the meaning of the experience is negative than pain perceived in situations with positive outcomes. For example, pain that is associated with a threat to body image may be much worse than pain that is not associated in this way. If the meaning of pain is not considered, you may make inappropriate assessments of the client's pain experience, resulting in inadequate pain control.

■ ANXIETY

The degree of anxiety experienced by the client may also influence the response to pain. Anxiety intensifies pain perception.[60] Anxiety is often related to the meaning of the pain. If the cause is unknown, anxiety is likely to be higher and the pain worse.

■ PAST EXPERIENCE WITH PAIN

Our past experience with pain affects the way we perceive our current pain. People who have had negative experiences with pain as children have reported greater difficulties with managing pain.[6, 96] The impact of past experiences, however, is not predictable. The person with a miserable experience in the past may perceive the next episode more intensely even though the medical conditions may be similar. Conversely, a person may view the next experience more positively because it is not as bad as the previous one. However, it is *not* true that the more pain we experience, the more accustomed we become to it. One might expect that the more pain we have experienced, the less anxious and more tolerant we may be. In actuality, we may be more anxious and desire rapid pain relief to avert a familiar and unpleasant painful experience.

Earlier pain experience allows us to adopt coping mechanisms that we may or may not use with subsequent episodes with pain. Discuss your clients' past experiences with pain, including how they managed the pain. In addition to methods that provided pain relief in the past, assess which measures did not have a positive outcome. Allow the client to use familiar positive intervention when possible.

■ EXPECTATION AND THE PLACEBO EFFECT

Client expectations play a major role in a person's pain experience, including perception of pain and the effectiveness of pain relief interventions.[2, 27, 119, 127] The severity of pain experienced, in addition to the emotional and cognitive overtones generated by the experience, is influenced by the client's expectations. Positive expectations engender positive outcomes; negative expectations lead to negative outcomes. Similarly, one's belief in the ability of an intervention to be effective affects the degree of pain relief attained. For example, it is not uncommon for a client to proclaim that the pain reliever Motrin is effective while Advil is not, even though the two medications are pharmaceutically identical.

You must realize that you can affect your clients' expectations by the messages you deliver regarding pain and pain management strategies. The confidence that you display regarding potential effectiveness of intervention strategies will have a significant effect on the client's ability to obtain positive pain relief outcomes.

Placebos have been administered when health care providers doubted that clients were truly in pain. Placebos are pills that look like medications but that have no medicinal properties. Historically, they have been made of sugars and inert materials. When clients are given placebos, they are told that the pills contain pain medication. It was not uncommon for these clients to obtain pain relief. It has been reported that 30% to 70% of people receiving placebos report short-lived pain relief which, in some research studies, has been reversed by naloxone (Narcan).[2, 127] The most likely explanation for the effect of placebos is the initiation of the body's endogenous opiate systems activated by the expectation of relief.[2] The response tends to be temporary, since the endogenous response is brief. A placebo response does not indicate absence of real pain; it indicates a person's ability to produce a positive pain relief outcome internally via a real physiologic mechanism.

Health care providers have incorrectly concluded that positive responses to placebos indicate that clients did not have real pain. However, a placebo response indicates that the client believes that the pill will "work" and has responded to the positive attitude portrayed by the nurse administering the pill. *Placebos should not be given.*[5, 59, 75, 134] The client's response to placebos provides no data about the nature or severity of pain. Placebo use is deceitful and unethical. It compromises the nurse-client relationship and the confidence the client has in the

nurse's ability and desire to help with pain relief. Use of placebos is costly because the client is charged for an ineffective medication, which often needs to be followed with a true pain relief preparation. Clients receiving placebos may be reluctant to report continued pain or to ask for additional pain medication, leaving them at risk for the negative physical effects of unrelieved pain.

■ Nursing Management of the Client in Pain

ASSESSMENT

The primary goals of pain assessment are to identify the cause of the pain, to understand the client's perception of the pain, and to measure the characteristics of the pain to implement pain management techniques. To assess a client's pain, obtain a pain history, a daily account of the current pain history, and a collection of subjective and objective data through use of measurement tools. Perform the assessment in an unbiased, caring manner. Assessment is a constant and ongoing task, which may occur every 15 minutes for the acute, postoperative client to every four hours for the acute, stable client with adequate pain relief. The AHCPR Clinical Guidelines for acute pain management recommend that pain be assessed every 2 hours for the first 48 hours after surgery or trauma and every 4 hours thereafter as a standard routine and more often if indicated. In addition, assessment should occur within 20 to 30 minutes after administration of any medication given for pain relief.[1]

HISTORY AND PHYSICAL EXAMINATION. A complete medical history and physical examination (H&P) focuses on basic questions about physical, behavioral, and psychological factors (Box 23-3). This H&P helps the nurse to understand the unique pain experience of the client and to formulate a plan to resolve the pain. The H&P also provides baseline data to allow assessment of the client's progression through a pain experience.

Data Collection. Data collection by use of well-tested measurement tools is essential in assessing pain for appropriate management interventions.[77, 108] Multidimensional assessment tools (e.g., McGill-Melzack Pain Questionnaire, Initial Pain Assessment Tool by McCaffery and Beebe[1]) are useful to obtain the initial H&P data and to provide information regarding the multifaceted nature of the pain experience (Figs. 23-8 and 23-9).

Single-item assessment tools include the Visual Analog Scale (VAS), numerical scales, and visual descriptor scales. These scales can be used to measure both physical pain intensity and psychological distress (Figs. 23-10 and 23-11). The tools are easy to use and provide the client and nurse with a simple means to quantify pain. They are also cost-effective when used in clinical settings because they are easily copied and can be reproduced cheaply. They do require a relatively high level of cognitive ability.

Pictorial scales measure pain in small children, such as the widely used FACES scale developed by Wong and Baker[132] (Fig. 23-12). Clients with impaired cognitive ability may be better able to report their pain with the use of pictorial scales.

Clients may experience several types of pain during one medical episode. After surgery, one may experience pain due to poor body position, incisional pain, and deep

BOX 23-3 Subjective and Objective Assessment Data

History

Age
State of consciousness
Medications currently taken/ medication for allergies
Physical state (fatigue, debility, lack of sleep, and prolonged suffering all reduce a client's ability to tolerate pain)
Emotional state (worry, fear, and anxiety reduce a person's ability to tolerate pain)
Pain expectancy (the anticipation of pain)
Pain acceptance (willingness to experience pain)
Pain apprehension (generalized desire to avoid pain)
Pain anxiety (the anxiety pain provokes because of its associated mystery, loneliness, helplessness, threat)
Effects on activities and quality of life
Methods of Pain Relief

What do you do to relieve the pain?
What has *not* worked to relieve your pain?

Physical Examination

Sympathetic Responses

Pallor
Increased blood pressure
Increased pulse
Increased respiration

Skeletal muscle tension
Dilated pupils
Diaphoresis

Parasympathetic Responses

Decreased blood pressure
Decreased pulse
Nausea, vomiting
Weakness
Pallor
Loss of consciousness

Behavioral Characteristics

Assumes a posture that minimizes pain (lying rigidly, guarding, drawing up the legs, or assuming the fetal position)
Moans, sighs, grimaces, clenches the jaws or fist, becomes quiet, or withdraws from others
Blinks rapidly
Crying, appears frightened, exhibits restlessness
Has a drawn facial expression
Has twitching muscles
Withdraws when touched
Holds or protects affected area or remains motionless

visceral pain. The client may also have a condition that produces chronic pain such as arthritis, that continues to be painful, or a secondary complication may be developing, such as pain due to myocardial infarction or pulmonary emboli. When planning interventions, learn to distinguish among the causes of pain. Each pain assessment includes location, intensity, quality, and pattern to aid in making intervention decisions.

Intensity. The single most important indicator of pain intensity is the client's self-report of the pain. Many health care facilities have incorporated *pain rating scales* for use with standard practice. These scales are used to assess current levels of pain but can be used to determine the amount of pain the client finds acceptable. This information is essential for both the client and nurse in planning and evaluating pain interventions. The AHCPR recommends the Brief Pain Inventory (Short Form) (Fig. 23–13) as a means of conducting ongoing assessments of pain intensity.[59]

You can obtain the client's self-report of pain intensity by asking clients to rate pain on a scale that they must mentally visualize or by showing the scale to the client. People in pain may have trouble concentrating on mental tasks and may find it particularly difficult to respond to a scale they must visualize. In some hospitals, it has been beneficial to provide a copy of the intensity scale in plain view of each client, typically taped to the bedside wall.

Location. Location of pain may be ascertained by verbal description or by marking the location on a drawing of the body. Use of body drawings provides an opportunity for the client to report multiple sites of pain using a self-report document that can be included in the medical record. The document is then available for use by any member of the health care team caring for that client.

Quality. Quality of the pain is typically indicated by descriptive adjectives such as "stabbing like a knife" or "throbbing" (Box 23–4). Some clients may have difficulty describing the quality of painful sensations, or they may have problems using the term "pain" to indicate their discomfort. Showing clients a list of words to describe pain may facilitate their ability to report pain quality.

Pattern. Pattern refers to the time of onset, duration, and intervals of the pain. Terms used to classify the pattern include "constant, steady, intermittent, periodic, brief, or momentary."

Distress. The psychological reactions to pain contribute to the overall pain experience. The emotional component may serve to intensify or diminish pain perception. Pain management strategies may need to be directed toward modifying the distress aspect of a pain episode.

DIAGNOSIS, OUTCOMES, INTERVENTIONS

The primary nursing diagnosis is *Pain related to tissue injury from an incision, ischemia, tumor encroachment in organs or bone.* Nurses have an impact on pain, discomfort, or suffering, no matter what the cause. In some situations, the client may be experiencing unrelieved pain. Unrelieved pain may be related to:

- Underadministration of ordered medication doses
- Administering medications in inappropriate time frames
- Not providing stronger medications when indicated
- Not providing combinations of medications when indicated
- Inadequate use of nonpharmaceutical management strategies

McGill - Melzack Pain Questionnaire

Person's Name_____ Date_____ Time_____ am/pm

Analgesic(s)_____ Dosage_____ Time Given_____ am/pm

_____ Dosage_____ Time Given_____ am/pm

Analgesic Time Difference (hours):   +4   +1   +2   +3

PRI: S _____   A _____   E _____   M(S) _____   M(AE) _____   M(T) _____   PRI(T) _____
　　　(1-10)　　　(11-15)　　　(16)　　　(17-19)　　　　(20)　　　　(17-20)　　　　(1-20)

1 FLICKERING QUIVERING PULSING THROBBING BEATING POUNDING	11 TIRING EXHAUSTING	PPI _____ COMMENTS:
	12 SICKENING SUFFOCATING	
2 JUMPING FLASHING SHOOTING	13 FEARFUL FRIGHTFUL TERRIFYING	
3 PRICKING BORING DRILLING STABBING LANCINATING	14 PUNISHING GRUELLING CRUEL VICIOUS KILLING	
4 SHARP CUTTING LACERATING	15 WRETCHED BLINDING	
5 PINCHING PRESSING GNAWING CRAMPING CRUSHING	16 ANNOYING TROUBLESOME MISERABLE INTENSE UNBEARABLE	
6 TUGGING PULLING WRENCHING	17 SPREADING RADIATING PENETRATING PIERCING	
7 HOT BURNING SCALDING SEARING	18 TIGHT NUMB DRAWING SQUEEZING TEARING	CONSTANT PERIODIC BRIEF
8 TINGLING ITCHY SMARTING STINGING	19 COOL COLD FREEZING	
9 DULL SORE HURTING ACHING HEAVY	20 NAGGING NAUSEATING AGONIZING DREADFUL TORTURING	
10 TENDER TAUT RASPING SPLITTING	PPI 0 NO PAIN 1 MILD 2 DISCOMFORTING 3 DISTRESSING 4 HORRIBLE 5 EXCRUCIATING	

ACCOMPANYING SYMPTOMS: NAUSEA HEADACHE DIZZINESS DROWSINESS CONSTIPATION DIARRHEA
COMMENTS:

SLEEP: GOOD FITFUL CAN'T SLEEP
COMMENTS:

FOOD INTAKE: GOOD SOME LITTLE NONE
COMMENTS:

ACTIVITY: GOOD SOME LITTLE NONE
COMMENTS:

FIGURE 23–8 The McGill-Melzack Pain Questionnaire, adapted for the study of narcotic drugs. The descriptors listed at left comprise four groups: 1 to 10, sensory; 11 to 15, affective; 16, evaluative; 17 to 20, miscellaneous. The rank value for each descriptor is based on its position in the words set. Total rank values comprise the pain-rating index (PRI). The present pain intensity (PPI) is based on a scale from 0 to 5. The drawings are used to designate the site of pain (From Bonica, J. J. [1980]. *Pain* [p. 145]. New York: Raven Press.)

Pain may contribute to additional diagnoses as clients respond to the pain episode. Examples of such diagnoses are presented in Table 23–4.

Outcomes. Outcomes should be determined as a team with the client, physicians, nurses, and often the extended family. A realistic outcome should be established to control or maintain the client at desired levels of pain and functioning. Desirable outcomes are that the client will (1) report freedom from pain, (2) request analgesia, and (3) perform daily activities without limitation related to pain. The goals should be those of the client, not those of the health care team.

Initial Pain Assessment Tool

Date _____

Patient's Name _____ Age _____ Room _____

Diagnosis _____ Physician _____

Nurse _____

I. Location: Patient or nurse mark drawing.

Right   Right   Left   Left   Right   Right   Left   R L L R

Left   Right   Right   Left   Right   Left   Right

II. Intensity: Patient rates the pain. Scale used _____
    Present: _____
    Worst pain gets: _____
    Best pain gets: _____
    Acceptable level of pain: _____

III. Quality: (Use patient's own words, e.g., prick, ache, burn, throb, pull, sharp) _____

IV. Onset, duration variations, rhythms: _____

V. Manner of expressing pain: _____

VI. What relieves the pain? _____

VII. What causes or increases the pain? _____

VIII. Effects of pain: (Note decreased function, decreased quality of life.) _____
    Accompanying symptoms (e.g., nausea) _____
    Sleep _____
    Appetite _____
    Physical activity _____
    Relationship with others (e.g., irritability) _____
    Emotions (e.g., anger, suicidal, crying) _____
    Concentration _____
    Other _____
IX. Other comments: _____

X. Plan: _____

FIGURE 23–9 Initial pain assessment tool. (From McCaffery M., & Beebe., A [1989]. *Pain: Clinical manual for nursing practice.* St. Louis: Mosby–Year Book.)

A widely used method of providing effective care is through use of clinical care plans or clinical pathways. Care plans and pathways provide nurses with aids to diagnose the problem, plan for expected outcomes, implement interventions, state the rationale for the interventions, and evaluate the outcome. Many health care facilities provide standard care plans or clinical pathways that are part of the department protocol. Standard plans provide the beginning basis for client care. They are then modified as indicated based on the needs of each client.

Interventions. Effective pain control is best achieved through the combination of both pharmaceutical and nonpharmaceutical therapies. Historically, pharmaceutical management has been the primary means of providing relief from pain, particularly acute pain. Although medications continue to serve as a major contributor to pain management, nonpharmaceutical techniques are being in-

creasingly used to provide pain relief. Nonpharmacologic interventions are particularly useful (1) when medications are inadequate to control pain, (2) while the client is waiting for medications to take effect, or (3) when side effects or client concerns make use of medications problematic.

ADMINISTRATION OF PAIN-RELIEVING MEDICATION. Numerous medications are used for pain relief. They are administered in a variety of ways; by mouth, rectally, topically, sublingually, by inhalation, or by injection. Medications may be injected by subcutaneous, intramuscular, or intravenous routes. Some medications may be injected spinally or paravertebrally or into selected nerves to produce nerve blocks. Physicians perform the latter types of injections, with nurses assisting with the procedures and providing aftercare. Too often nurses view the administration of pain-relieving medications as all

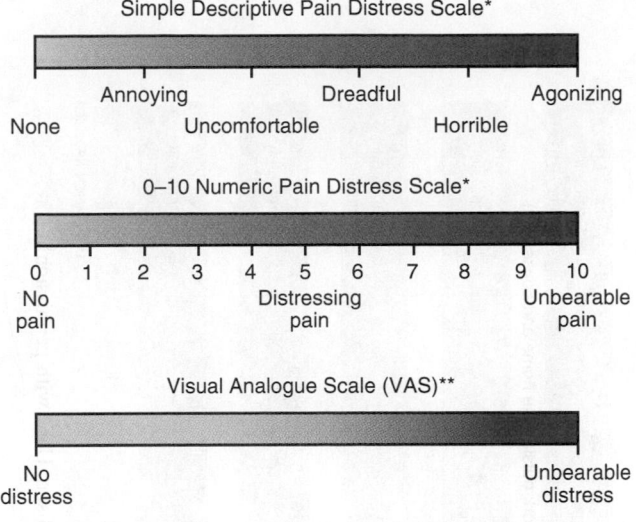

Simple Descriptive Pain Distress Scale*

Annoying   Dreadful   Agonizing
None   Uncomfortable   Horrible

0–10 Numeric Pain Distress Scale*

0   1   2   3   4   5   6   7   8   9   10
No   Distressing   Unbearable
pain   pain   pain

Visual Analogue Scale (VAS)**

No   Unbearable
distress   distress

* If used as a graphic rating scale, a 10-cm baseline is recommended.

** A 10-cm baseline is recommended for VAS scales.

FIGURE 23–10 Pain distress scales.

Simple Descriptive Pain Intensity Scale*

No   Mild   Moderate   Severe   Very   Worst
pain   pain   pain   pain   severe   possible
                                     pain   pain

0–10 Numeric Pain Intensity Scale*

0   1   2   3   4   5   6   7   8   9   10
No   Moderate   Unbearable
pain   pain   pain

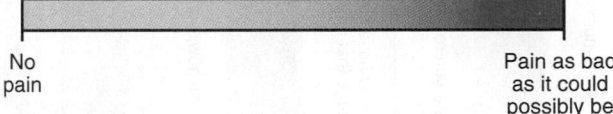

Visual Analogue Scale (VAS)**

No   Pain as bad
pain   as it could
                                            possibly be

* If used as a graphic rating scale, a 10-cm baseline is recommended.

** A 10-cm baseline is recommended for VAS scales.

FIGURE 23–11 Pain intensity scales.

they need to do for pain management. However, medication may be more effective when combined with other pain relief techniques. When you administer medication and reposition the client, give a back rub, or simply interact with a client, the effectiveness of the drug may be increased. Simply giving an injection or a pill does not replace thoughtful, comprehensive pain management.

Therapeutic interaction with someone experiencing pain may include:

- Facilitating the client's expression of feelings, which imparts a sense of being cared for
- Providing support, reassurance, and understanding, which allows the client to develop confidence in the nurse
- Teaching the client self-management strategies to relieve pain

Pain management strategies, including medications, have been found to be more effective when clients believe that

PAIN INTENSITY MEASURES

Faces:

0   1   2   3   4   5

When using the Faces, explain to the person that each face is for a person who feels happy because he has no pain (hurt for young children) or sad because he has some or a lot of pain. Face 0 is very happy because he doesn't hurt at all. Face 1 hurts just a little bit. Face 2 hurts a little more. Face 3 hurts even more. Face 4 hurts a whole lot. Face 5 hurts as much as you can imagine, although you don't have to be crying to feel this bad.

Word:

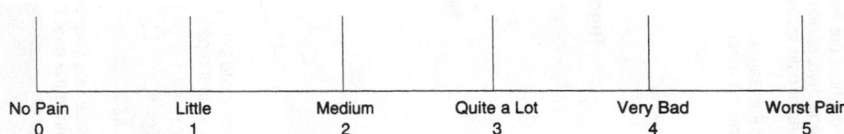

No Pain   Little   Medium   Quite a Lot   Very Bad   Worst Pain
0   1   2   3   4   5

FIGURE 23–12 Faces Pain Rating Scale. Explain to the person that each face is for a person who feels happy because he has no pain (hurt) or sad because he has some or a lot of pain. Face 0 is very happy because he doesn't hurt at all. Face 1 hurts just a little bit. Face 2 hurts a little more. Face 3 hurts even more. Face 4 hurts a whole lot. Face 5 hurts as much as you can imagine, although you don't have to be crying to feel this bad. Ask the person to choose the face that best describes how he is feeling. This rating scale is recommended for persons age 3 years and older. (From Wong, D., & Baker, C. [1988]. Pain in children: Comparison of assessment scales. *Pediatric Nursing,* *14*[1]: 9–17, 1988.)

Pain Inventory

Date: ___/___/___   Time: _____

Name: _____
        Last   First   Middle Initial

1) Throughout our lives, most of us have had pain from time to time (such as minor headaches, sprains, and toothaches). Have you had pain other than these everyday kinds of pain today?   1. Yes   2. No

2) On the diagram, shade in the areas where you feel pain. Put an X on the area that hurts the most.

Right   Left   Left   Right

3) Please rate your pain by circling the one number that best describes your pain at its **worst** in the past 24 hours.

0	1	2	3	4	5	6	7	8	9	10
No pain										Pain as bad as you can imagine

4) Please rate your pain by circling the one number that best describes your pain at its **least** in the past 24 hours.

0	1	2	3	4	5	6	7	8	9	10
No pain										Pain as bad as you can imagine

5) Please rate your pain by circling the one number that best describes your pain on the **average**.

0	1	2	3	4	5	6	7	8	9	10
No pain										Pain as bad as you can imagine

6) Please rate your pain by circling the one number that tells how much pain you have **right now.**

0	1	2	3	4	5	6	7	8	9	10
No pain										Pain as bad as you can imagine

7) What treatments or medications are you receiving for your pain?

_____

8) In the past 24 hours, how much **relief** have pain treatments or medications provided? Please circle the one percentage that most shows how much relief you have received.

0%	10%	20%	30%	40%	50%	60%	70%	80%	90%	100%
No relief										Complete relief

9) Circle the one number that describes how, during the past 24 hours, pain has **interfered** with your:

A. General activity

0	1	2	3	4	5	6	7	8	9	10
Does not interfere										Completely interferes

B. Mood

0	1	2	3	4	5	6	7	8	9	10
Does not interfere										Completely interferes

C. Walking ability

0	1	2	3	4	5	6	7	8	9	10
Does not interfere										Completely interferes

D. Normal work (includes both work outside the home and housework)

0	1	2	3	4	5	6	7	8	9	10
Does not interfere										Completely interferes

E. Relations with other people

0	1	2	3	4	5	6	7	8	9	10
Does not interfere										Completely interferes

F. Sleep

0	1	2	3	4	5	6	7	8	9	10
Does not interfere										Completely interferes

G. Enjoyment of life

0	1	2	3	4	5	6	7	8	9	10
Does not interfere										Completely interferes

UC9503409EN NP-2395EN

FIGURE 23–13 Pain Inventory, Short Form. (From Pain Research Group, Department of Neurology, University of Wisconsin-Madison. Used with permission.)

BOX 23-4   Descriptive Terms for Pain

Descriptive Word	How Pain Makes Person Feel
■ Sharp	■ Horrible
■ Piercing	■ Annoying
■ Shooting	■ Agonizing
■ Crushing	■ Killing
■ Tender	■ Miserable
■ Hurting	■ Unbearable
■ Aching	■ Frightening
■ Dull	■ Suffocating
■ Sore	■ Tortured
■ Cramping	
■ Prickly	

they are in control of the situation. A nurse who actively involves the client in the planning, intervention, and assessment of pain management strategies provides the client with enhanced potential to obtain satisfactory pain relief.

MANAGING CHRONIC INTRACTABLE PAIN. Chronic intractable pain (pain that cannot be satisfactorily relieved by typical pharmaceutical means) causes additional difficulties for those experiencing it. Clients may require a combination of nursing interventions (cognitive, behavioral, physical, pharmaceutical). Nursing and medical therapeutic regimens must be coordinated and consistent to ensure a unified approach. The client must not be promised complete pain relief, however, because this may be unrealistic.

MANAGING PROGRESSIVE PAIN. People with progressive pain, such as that seen in malignancies, may require pain-relieving medications routinely as a preventive measure, in the same way that vasodilators are regularly taken by people with ischemic heart disease. As the disease progresses, clients may require increasingly stronger drug doses. Some people hesitate to take pain-relieving medications routinely for fear of addiction. They may believe that they must avoid increasing dosages be-

TABLE 23-4   PAIN-RELATED NURSING DIAGNOSES

Diagnosis	Etiology
Activity Intolerance	related to Unrelieved pain
Ineffective Coping Strategies	related to Lack of knowledge of possible methods of coping
Powerlessness	related to Lack of participation in decision-making process
Anxiety	related to Past experiences of poor pain control
Sleep Pattern Disturbance	related to Unrelieved pain at night
Knowledge Deficit	related to Lack of exposure to informational resources
Fear	related to Anticipation of a pain experience

cause they are afraid that they will "use up" the medication's pain relief potential and will not be able to obtained adequate medication in the future. They may also be concerned that they will be labeled as drug users if they take opioids over the long term.

In reality, people experiencing pain due to widespread cancer require routine pain-relieving medications in order to function. Help is needed for clients and their significant others to understand the need for regular, often strong medications. Reassurance that adequate pain relief will be possible in the future and that routine use of the medications means only that the condition warrants it, much like a client who requires the routine use of medication for hypertension.

Many conditions associated with pain are managed at home. The treatment of acute postoperative, chronic and malignant pain is often performed by clients and family members. The Bridge to Home Health Care discusses the nurse's role in home care for pain control.

MEDICATIONS TO CONTROL PAIN

■ ANESTHETIC AGENTS

An *anesthetic* is a pharmacologic substance that, in addition to abolishing pain, generally causes loss of feeling and sensation. Many *analgesics* (pharmacologic substances that diminish or eliminate pain without producing unconsciousness), depending on their mode of action and route of administration, act as anesthetics when given in larger doses. There are many different types of anesthesia. *General anesthesia* is usually accompanied by loss of consciousness and reflexes along with amnesia regarding the experience. *Local anesthetics* produce anesthesia in a restricted area of the body without loss of consciousness.

A technique frequently used in minor surgery and other procedures is infiltration of a local anesthetic into the skin and subcutaneous tissue to produce loss of sensation, or local anesthesia. The same agent injected near a sensory nerve causes anesthesia in the distribution of the nerve (*regional anesthesia*). Nerves are often mixed in function; that is, they carry both sensory and motor fibers. Hence, a *nerve block* may cause motor weakness or paralysis, in addition to loss of sensation, in the innervated area. A nerve block is the application of a pharmacologic substance that inhibits nerve conduction (e.g., numbing the mouth for dental procedures).

Local anesthetic agents may be applied topically (on the skin or mucous membranes), infiltrated locally, used for specific nerve blocks (e.g., spinal anesthetic for surgery), or administered intravenously, depending on the reason for their use. Local anesthetic agents act by temporarily blocking nerve impulses between the peripheral structures and higher centers. Such blocks are reversible because the nerves regain their function over a period of minutes to hours.

Neurolytic agents (e.g., phenol, alcohol) produce prolonged nerve blocks, which destroy the nerves. Neurolytic blocks may not be truly permanent because nerve fibers regrow after several months. However, the growth is often disorganized. Hence, the sensation from these nerve fibers is often abnormal or painful. Consequently, neurolytic blocks are generally used only in terminally ill per-

BRIDGE TO HOME HEALTH CARE

Controlling Pain

To control the client's pain at home, you should be aware of many contributing factors. It is necessary to evaluate physical, social, emotional, and spiritual pain because each of these adds to the total pain experience. An effective plan of care should include a multidisciplinary approach to pain.

Pain control should be very individualized, and attention to age-specific needs must be considered in both assessment and treatment. A pain scale that includes pictures is effective for use with children. In addition, analgesic choices should be tailored to the age of the client, recognizing the special needs of the very young and the elderly.

Many times in the treatment of malignant pain (as with cancer), medication is given on a regular schedule to prevent exacerbations. This is in contrast to medications being taken at the time of pain or the prn (as needed) schedule used in acute care settings. This prophylactic scheduling is very effective but requires client education to ensure compliance. Scheduling may well be the single most important instruction in the use of analgesics for malignant pain. The use of adjuvant therapy, such as for pain control, should also be considered because this often increases the effectiveness of the analgesic. It is also important to consider various methods of analgesia, such as continuous, client-controlled analgesia pumps, time-released skin patches, sustained-released oral medications, and suppositories.

Fear of addiction is a major barrier for effective pain control. It is essential for the multidisciplinary team to explain that medication taken as directed will not cause addiction. For the pain of clients who are terminally ill, aggressive titration of medication is used until pain is relieved. The goal is pain control with minimal adverse reactions. When adverse reactions do occur, symptoms should be treated and the analgesic continued. Pain control is essential to quality of life and should be actively pursued. Clients should be assured that pain can and will be relieved. When the multidisciplinary team has an accurate assessment of the client's condition and home situation, the safest, most effective approach to pain management can then be determined.

Joanie J. Kush, RN, BSN, MS, *Director of Hospice, Visiting Nurse Association of Omaha, Omaha, Nebraska*

sons with a short life expectancy, such as those with cancer-related pain.

LOCAL ANESTHESIA

Chemically, local anesthetics are divided into two classes:

1. The *esters* (e.g., procaine [Novocain]) are metabolized in the plasma, are less heat-stable than the amides, and account for most of the rarely occurring allergic reactions to local anesthetics.
2. The *amides* (e.g., lidocaine [Xylocaine] and bupivacaine [Marcaine, Sensorcaine]) are metabolized in the liver.

Procaine produces analgesia in 3 to 10 minutes and lasts less than 1 hour. It is one of the least toxic of the local anesthetics, although allergies occur rarely. Procaine is not effective for topical use.

Lidocaine is one of the most commonly used local anesthetics. It acts within 5 to 10 minutes and lasts about 2 hours. It has a wide range of applications, including topical and intravascular block. Allergy to lidocaine is rare. A Bier block is an example of an intravascular block.

Bupivacaine is long-acting (4 to 8 hours) but has a slow onset. It is four times more potent than lidocaine and four to six times more toxic. Therefore, a lower concentration is used. Bupivacaine appears to block sensory nerves in preference to motor nerves when used in low concentration. Thus, effective analgesia may result without accompanying motor weakness.

Local anesthetics are usually vasodilators, increasing blood flow into the area in which they are injected. Thus, they shorten the duration of their own action by enhancing their own vascular absorption. Adding epinephrine, a vasoconstrictor, to local anesthetic solutions prolongs the anesthetic effect by decreasing the vascular uptake of the anesthetic, allowing it to stay in contact with the nerve tissue for a longer period. The recipient may sense an increased heart rate from the epinephrine.

Note: Epinephrine-containing solutions are *not* typically used for nerve blocks of the penis, fingers, or toes, where vasoconstriction could cause inadequate blood flow and necrosis of the distal extremity.

In addition to prolonging anesthesia, epinephrine-containing local anesthetic solutions offer other advantages. The supplementary use of a vasoconstrictor reduces the possibility of the anesthetic's reaching a toxic blood level. The toxicity of local analgesic medications depends on their concentration in the blood. This, in turn, depends on the speed of absorption. Vasoconstricting medications delay absorption of a local analgesic solution and thus prevent a suddenly high blood concentration, which gives the body more time to metabolize and detoxify them. Vasoconstrictors also inhibit bleeding in the area of the injection. Larger doses of epinephrine containing local anesthetic should be used cautiously in people with coronary artery disease. Care of clients who have anesthesia is discussed in Chapter 15.

TOPICAL LOCAL ANESTHESIA

Dilute solutions of local anesthetics may be applied topically in the form of pastes, sprays, or other preparations. They may reduce the severe pain of burns, abrasions, and necrosis of the mucous membranes and skin. Remember, once an area is anesthetized, it does not transmit painful sensation and the area is thus at greater risk for injury. If topical anesthetic agents are applied to burned or abraded skin or mucous membranes, absorption of the medication is almost as rapid as that following intravenous administration.

A relatively new agent, EMLA cream, is a mixture of lidocaine and prilocaine. It is useful in preventing pain from venipuncture, injections, heel sticks, and minor plastic surgery. It must be applied in advance to the area (45 minutes to 1 hour) and covered with an occlusive dressing. EMLA cream is an excellent strategy for eliminating the pain associated with penetration of the skin and should be encouraged.

■ ANALGESICS

Various factors are considered in selecting the most effective analgesic for a specific client. These factors include the cause, quality, intensity, duration, and distribution of the pain. The World Health Organization (WHO)[134] has suggested that decisions regarding pain medications may be aided by use of a "pain ladder" (Fig. 23–14). The ladder was originally designed to guide the care of persons with cancer pain, but its use has been extended to also apply to acute pain. Non-opioids, such as acetaminophen and NSAIDs, are suggested by the first ladder step. If the pain persists or increases, step 2 suggests mild opioids (such as codeine) plus non-opioid analgesics. If the pain continues to persist or increases, step 3 suggests strong opioids (such as morphine) with or without non-opioids. Adjuvant medications may be added at any step in the ladder.

Systemic analgesic medications are the most frequently used means of pain control. Analgesics are the most commonly prescribed, and thus widely used, medications. They are also purchased extensively over the counter. This is not unexpected, because pain is usually the first manifestation of injury, and most diseases begin with or include pain at some time during their course.

PHARMACEUTICAL CONSIDERATIONS

Some analgesics have a *ceiling effect,* which occurs when medications have a maximum effective dose; increasing the dose cannot increase pain relief but may increase side effects. Medications with a ceiling effect may be combined with other analgesics when additional pain relief is needed.

Tolerance

Tolerance occurs when larger doses of medications are needed to provide the same amount of pain relief as the previous smaller dose. It is common among people who require long-term pain management with opioids. The person becomes tolerant to these medications because the opiate receptors become less sensitive to them. Tolerance may be managed by continuing the dose of the opioid

and adding a non-opioid analgesic or adjuvant medication or by switching to an alternate drug.

Tolerance should not be confused with *addiction,* which is extremely rare. Concern about addiction in cases of tolerance has led health care providers to modify opioid prescriptions by ordering smaller doses over longer periods of time. Client response to the modification may lead one to conclude that addiction was the underlying problem, as these people may be forced to display behaviors often associated with psychological addiction.[5] They no longer receive adequate pain relief and may attempt to manipulate the provider into providing adequate medication. Such behavior is understandable but is often viewed as "medication-seeking," a classic definition of one psychologically addicted. Clients may "act out" their pain in the belief that if they look as if they have severe pain, their need for medication will be recognized by the health care provider. The client does not receive adequate pain relief in response to these behaviors and rationalizes that health care providers are no longer dependable. The health care provider concludes that the client's behavior is inappropriate and no longer values or believes the client. This atmosphere of mistrust creates a situation in which adequate pain relief for the client becomes increasingly unlikely. Addiction is fully discussed in Chapter 24.

Dependence

Physical dependence commonly occurs when medications are taken over a long term. Physical manifestations associated with withdrawal of the medication include anxiety, irritability, chills alternating with hot flashes, salivation, lacrimation, rhinorrhea, diaphoresis, piloerection, nausea and vomiting, abdominal cramps, and insomnia.[5] The most common example of physical dependence is seen among coffee drinkers. Their bodies become dependent on the caffeine ingested. The most common manifestation is headache when caffeine is withheld.

Physical dependence is not a problem unless opioids are to be discontinued. The effects of withdrawal can be avoided by weaning the client from the medication slowly. It is essential that health care providers, clients, and their significant others realize that physical dependence is not synonymous with psychological addiction. Client and family education regarding this matter is an expected nursing function.

TYPES OF ANALGESICS

Analgesics are medications developed to provide pain relief. The discussion is organized according to the WHO analgesic ladder,[134] which is based on the notion that pain medication decisions are based in part on the intensity and controllability of the pain. The three steps reflect mild, moderate, and severe degrees of pain intensity.

Non-opioid Analgesics

Non-opioid analgesics fall into four primary categories[5]:

- Aspirin
- Salicylate salts
- Acetaminophen
- NSAIDs

As a group, these drugs have a ceiling effect but do not cause physical dependence or tolerance. Their site of action is primarily in the periphery at the receptor site, where they serve an anti-inflammatory function and pre-

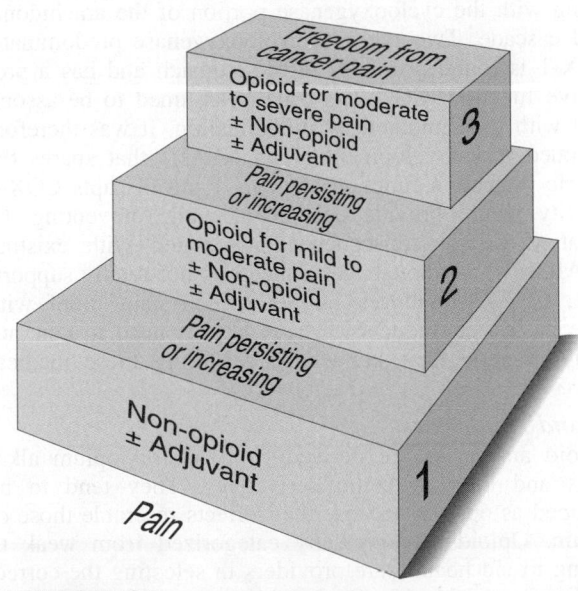

FIGURE 23–14 World Health Organization (WHO) analgesic ladder describes the steps in treating cancer pain. (From World Health Organization. [1996]. *Cancer pain relief* [2nd ed.] Geneva: Author.)

vent the production of prostaglandins. They may have a central role in pain relief, as prostaglandins inhibit the production or the release of serotonin, removing the pain relief effect of the neurotransmitter. Preventing prostaglandin production would maintain the inhibitory effect of serotonin in the dorsal horn. An exception is acetaminophen, which produces pain relief but is not an anti-inflammatory agent and does not appear to affect prostaglandins. The physical means by which acetaminophen produces pain relief is not known.[5]

The American Pain Society recommends that a non-opioid medication be included with any analgesic regimen, even when opioids are prescribed.[5] Opioids act centrally, within the brain and spinal cord. Non-opioids add peripherally mediated pain relief to the central effects of opioids when they are given in combination. Parenteral and rectal forms of non-opioids have been developed for individuals who cannot take oral medications. Refer to Table 23–5 for dosing information for non-opioid medications.

ASPIRIN. Historically, aspirin (acetylsalicylic acid, ASA) has been the primary non-opioid medication for pain. It is one of the most effective non-opioid medications available. Aspirin is available in many forms, including tablets (plain, chewable, enteric coated, sustained-release), capsules, rectal suppositories, and topical creams. As with most nonsteroidal analgesics, aspirin has an antiplatelet effect and is a gastric irritant. Side effects include bleeding associated with prolonged clotting time and gastric disturbances. Enteric-coated tablets reduce the gastric reactions because the coating remains intact until the product reaches the small intestine, where the tablet dissolves and is absorbed. Because of the association of aspirin with Reye's syndrome, a potentially fatal condition seen primarily in young children, it is not used for children under age 12 with viral illnesses. Recent cases of adults with Reye's syndrome-like symptoms and negative outcomes suggest that aspirin may pose a risk for people of any age when administered to those with viral infections.

SALICYLATE SALTS. These salts are similar to aspirin but produce fewer gastric side effects. Choline magnesium trisalicylate (Trilisate) and diflunisal (Dolobid) are typical examples. Platelet aggregation does not result when salicylate salts are used in people with normal clotting abilities.

ACETAMINOPHEN. Acetaminophen is similar to aspirin in its ability to provide pain relief, but it does not affect the gastric mucosa. It has no effect on platelet aggregation and does not affect bleeding time. Its anti-inflammatory effect is much less than that of other non-opioids. It is tolerated well by most people of any age, and it is the drug of choice when given for pain to people with viral infections.

NSAIDs. NSAIDs are nonsteroidal anti-inflammatory agents other than aspirin and acetaminophen. NSAIDs are present in numerous preparations, providing alternative medication choices. If one form is ineffective, another can be tried. NSAIDs were originally developed to treat arthritis, but they are also effective for mild to moderate pain of nonarthritic origin. NSAIDs act to decrease inflammation, but it is their ability to block prostaglandin synthesis that is credited for most of their pain-relieving properties.[21, 24, 57, 91, 102] NSAIDs are particularly helpful for clients with cancer or postoperative pain, since a major contributing factor to pain in these clients is cell destruction.

NSAIDs potentiate the effects of opiates and are often given in combination preparations that incorporate codeine or codeine derivatives. Tylenol with codeine is used widely for moderate pain. NSAIDs are particularly effective for pain resulting from bone insult, including bone metastases of malignancy and fractures. Degradation of bone tissue in these conditions produces prostaglandins. The ability of NSAIDs to prevent prostaglandin production significantly decreases pain produced by these lesions.[92] Ketoprofen and ketorolac (Toradol) also block production of leukotrienes.[57, 91]

The most common side effects associated with NSAIDs are gastrointestinal upset and possible bleeding. These agents also inhibit platelet aggregation, increasing the risk of hemorrhage. Clients taking NSAIDs must be monitored closely for the development of peptic ulcers. In clients who are taking high doses for long periods of time (as for arthritis) a histamine H_2-receptor antagonist such as ranitidine (Zantac) or misoprostol (Cytotec) may be used.

NSAIDs may also have negative effects on the renal system, particularly in clients with heart failure, chronic renal disease, lupus, blood volume depletion, diuretic use, atherosclerosis, and multiple myeloma.[5] Clients may experience sudden decreased urine output associated with water and sodium retention. These renal side effects quickly abate on discontinuance of the NSAID.

New forms of NSAIDs appear to prevent the negative side effects and to broaden the routes available for administration. For example, ketorolac was developed to provide an injectable form. The recently available cyclooxygenase (COX-2) inhibitors were developed in response to the negative gastrointestinal side effects of aspirin and NSAIDs.[51] Celecoxib (Celebrex) and meloxicam (Vioxx) disrupt the synthesis of prostaglandins by interfering with the cyclooxygenase portion of the arachidonic acid cascade. Two types of cyclooxygenase predominate. COX-1 is found primarily in the stomach and has a protective function. COX-2 is usually assumed to be associated with pain initiated by inflammation. It was therefore assumed that development of an NSAID that spares the gastric protection function of COX-1 but disrupts COX-2 activity would provide pain relief while preventing the negative gastric consequences associated with existing NSAIDs.[51, 93] Although this concept is not totally supportable, COX-2 inhibitors have provided pain relief with little gastric consequence.[46, 47, 51] Nurses need to continuously upgrade their knowledge regarding these medications.

Opioid Analgesics

Opioid analgesics are derived from natural opium alkaloids and their synthetic derivatives. They tend to be grouped as opioids because their effects resemble those of opium. Opioids are typically categorized from weak to strong to aid health care providers in selecting the correct medication (Table 23–6). Opioids are added to the medication regimen when pain is moderate to severe and non-opioids are insufficient to manage pain effectively. Tolerance and physical dependence seen in long-term

TABLE 23–5	DOSING INFORMATION FOR ACETAMINOPHEN AND NONSTEROIDAL ANTI-INFLAMMATORY DRUGS (NSAIDS)*

Chemical Class	Generic Name	Half-Life (hr)	Dosing Schedule	Recommended Oral Starting Dose (mg)	Maximum Oral Dose Recommended (mg/day)	Comments
P-Aminophenol derivatives	Acetaminophen	2	q4–6hr	650	6000	Overdosage produces hepatic toxicity. No GI or platelet toxicity. Available as liquid and for rectal administration.
Salicylates	Aspirin	3–12	q4–6hr	650	6000	Standard for comparison. May not be as well tolerated as some of the newer NSAIDs. Available for rectal administration.
	Diflunisal	8–12	q12hr	500	1500	Less GI toxicity than aspirin.
	Choline magnesium trisalicylate	9–17	q12hr	500–1000	4000	Minimal GI toxicity. No effect on platelet aggregation. Available as liquid.
	Choline salicylate	2–3	q3–6hr	870	5352	Liquid. Minimal effect on platelet function.
	Magnesium salicylate		q4–6hr	1000	4000	
	Salsalate	16	q12hr	500–1000	4000	
Proprionic acids	Ibuprofen	2	q6hr	400	3200	Available as a suspension.
	Naproxen	13	q12hr	250	1025–1375	
	Fenoprofen	2–3	q6–8hr	200	3200	
	Ketoprofen	2–3	q6–8hr	25	300	Available for rectal administration and as a topical gel.
	Flurbiprofen	5–6	q12hr	100	300	
	Oxaprozin	400	q24hr	600	1800	
Acetic acids	Indomethacin	4–5	q8hr	25	150	Higher incidence of GI and CNS side effects than proprionic acids. Available in slow-release preparations, and for rectal administration.
	Tolmetin	2–5	q8hr	200	2000	
	Sulindac	14	q12hr	150	400	Not recommended for prolonged use because of increased risk for GI toxicity.
	Diclofenac	2	q8hr	25	150	
	Ketorolac	4–7	q6hr	10	40	Use limited to 5 days. Recommended parenteral dose ≤30 mg; total daily dose ≤120 mg.
Oxicams	Piroxicam	50	q24hr	20	40	
Fenamates	Mefenamic acid	2	q6hr	250	1000	Use limited to 7 days.
	Meclofenamate	2	—	—	400	Not recommended for analgesia.
Pyranocarboxylic acids	Etodolac	7	q8hr	200	1200	
Other	Nabumetone	24	q24hr	1000	2000	Minimal effect on platelet aggregation.

*May be duplicated for use in clinical practice.
GI, gastrointestinal; CNS, central nervous system.
From McCaffery, M., & Pasero, C. (1999). *Clinical manual* (pp. 139–140). St. Louis: Mosby.

TABLE 23-6	ANALGESIC STEP PAIN LADDER	
Step One	**Step Two**	**Step Three**
NSAIDs and Others	**Opioid-Agonist Drug**	**Agonist Drugs**
Acetaminophen	Codeine	Morphine sulfate
Acetylsalicylic acid (aspirin)	Oxycodone (w/aspirin and w/acetaminophen)	Methodone
Ibuprofen	Hydrocodone	Hydromorphone
Choline magnesium trisalicylate	Meperidine	Oxymorphone
Diflunisal	Propoxyphene HCl	Levorphanol
Ketoprofen	Propoxyphene napsylate (w/aspirin and w/acetaminophen)	Fentanyl
Naproxen		
Ketorolac tromethamine	**Agonist-Antagonist Drugs**	**Agonist-Antagonist Drugs**
Piroxicam	Pentazocine HCl	Butorphanol
Sulindac		Nalbuphine
Indomethacin		Dezocine
Carbamazepine		
Celecoxib		**Partial Agonist Drugs**
Meloxicam		
Phenytoin		Buprenorphine
Amitriptyline		
Doxepin		
Imipramine		
Trazodone		
Hydroxyzine		
Lidocaine		
Mexiletine		
Tocainide		
Dexamethasone		
Dextroamphetamine		
Methylphenidate		

From the World Health Organization (1996). *Cancer pain relief* (2nd ed.). Geneva: Author.

administration are not associated with short-term opioid treatment.

Opioids bind with receptors that can be engaged by endogenous opioids, including mu (μ), kappa (κ), and delta (δ) receptor types.[94, 107] Binding with receptors in the spinal cord renders the presynaptic membrane of nociceptor fibers incapable of opening Ca^{2+} channels, inhibiting nociceptive neurotransmitter release. Opiate binding with the postsynaptic membrane hyperpolarizes the membrane by altering the ability of K^+ ions to flow across the membrane.[3, 107] Opiate receptors are found in PAG/PVG. Activation of these receptors by opioids initiates the descending effect of serotonin and norepinephrine.[28, 38, 135]

All opioids produce side effects to some degree. The side effects are determined, in part, by the receptor type engaged by the medication and by the location of the receptor. The three receptor types have very different distributions and locations with the CNS. Side effects may be managed by discontinuing one form of opiate medication with untoward side effects, and replacing it with another that binds to a different receptor type.

OPIOID AGONISTS. Opioid agonists are opiate derivatives that bring about pain relief by producing the maximum degree of receptor binding. Agonists bind fully to their corresponding receptor type and do not affect the ability of other opioid preparations to engage their specific receptor. They are typically associated with mu receptors and have no ceiling effect.

Examples of opioid agonists are displayed in Table 23-7. They include morphine-like medications, which differ from morphine in rate of onset, duration of action, route of administration, adverse side effects, and chemical configuration. The mechanisms by which they produce pain relief are similar.

OPIOID ANTAGONISTS. These agents reverse the side effects and analgesia of opioids. They have no agonist effects and thus produce no analgesia. They are used to counteract a negative effect of an opioid, typically respiratory depression. Naloxone is the most common example.

OPIOID AGONIST-ANTAGONISTS. These medications engage one receptor type while inhibiting receptor binding of another. When they are given following use of the opioid they inhibit, they precipitously reverse the medication's effects and can precipitate acute withdrawal. When the combination agents are given alone, they produce analgesia and the positive effects of opioids with fewer side effects. Respiratory depression is a less likely effect, although psychomimetic effects are more probable. Examples are displayed in Table 23-7.

METHADONE. A potent, long-acting opioid analgesic, methadone gained popularity in the management of cancer pain before the development of the long-acting forms of morphine. Unlike most morphine preparations, methadone has a long plasma half-life. This long plasma half-life, when repeated doses are given, may account for methadone's longer duration of analgesic action, but it also poses certain problems. This medication is not recommended for older people and people with compromised hepatic and renal function. The long plasma half-

TABLE 23–7	EQUIANALGESIC DOSE CHART FOR SELECTED OPIOID DRUGS

A Guide to Using Equianalgesic Dose Charts
- Equianalgesic means approximately the same pain relief.
- The equianalgesic chart is a guideline. Doses and intervals between doses are titrated according to individual's response.
- The equianalgesic chart is helpful when switching from one drug to another or switching from one route of administration to another.
- Dosages in this equianalgesic chart are not necessarily starting doses. They suggest a ratio for comparing the analgesia of one drug to another.
- The longer the client has been receiving opioids, the more conservative the starting doses of a new opioid.

Opioid	Parenteral (IM/SC/IV) (Over ~ 4 hr)	Oral (PO) (Over ~ 4 hr)	Onset (min)	Peak (min)	Duration[1] (hr)	Half-life (hr)
MU AGONISTS						
Morphine	10 mg	30 mg	30–60 (PO) 30–60 (CR)[2] 30–60 (R) 5–10 (IV) 10–20 (SC) 10–20 (IM)	60–90 (PO) 90–180 (CR)[2] 60–90 (R) 15–30 (IV) 30–60 (SC) 30–60 (IM)	3–6 (PO) 8–12 (CR)[1,3] 4–5 (R) 3–4 (IV) 3–4 (SC) 3–4 (IM)	2–4
Codeine	130 mg	200 mg NR	30–60 (PO) 10–20 (SC) 10–20 (IM)	60–90 (PO) UK (SC) 30–60 (IM)	3–4 (PO) 3–4 (SC) 3–4 (IM)	2–4
Fentanyl	100 μg/hr parenterally and transdermally ≅ 4 mg/hr morphine parenterally; 1 μg/hr transdermally ≅ morphine 2 mg/24 hr orally	—	5 (OT) 1–5 (IV) 7–15 (IM) 12–16 h (TD)	15 (OT) 3–5 (IV) 10–20 (IM) 24 h (TD)	2–5 (OT) 0.5–4 (IV) 0.5–4 (IM) 48–72 (TD)	3–4 13–24 (TD)
Hydrocodone (as in Vicodin, Lortab)	—	30 mg[5] NR	30–60 (PO)	60–90 (PO)	4–6 (PO)	4
Hydromorphone (Dilaudid)	1.5 mg[6]	7.5 mg	15–30 (PO) 15–30 (R) 5 (IV) 10–20 (SC) 10–20 (IM)	30–90 (PO) 30–90 (R) 10–20 (IV) 30–90 (SC) 30–90 (IM)	3–4 (PO) 3–4 (R) 3–4 (IV)[1,3] 3–4 (SC) 3–4 (IM)	2–3
Levorphanol (Levo-Dromoran)	2 mg	4 mg	30–60 (PO) 10 (IV) 10–20 (SC) 10–20 (IM)	60–90 (PO) 15–30 (IV) 60–90 (SC) 60–90 (IM)	4–6 (PO) 4–6 (IV)[1,3] 4–6 (SC) 4–6 (IM)	12–15
Meperidine (Demerol)	75 mg	300 mg NR	30–60 (PO) 5–10 (IV) 10–20 (SC) 10–20 (IM)	60–90 (PO) 10–15 (IV) 15–30 (SC) 15–30 (IM)	2–4 (PO) 2–4 (IV)[1,3] 2–4 (SC) 2–4 (IM)	2–3
Methadone (Dolophine)	10 mg[7]	20 mg[8]	30–60 (PO) UK (SL) 10 (IV) 10–20 (SC) 10–20 (IM)	60–120 (PO) 10 (SL) UK (IV) 60–120 (SC) 60–120 (IM)	4–8 (PO) UK (SL) 4–8 (IV)[1,3] 4–8 (SC) 4–8 (IM)	12–190
Oxycodone (as in Percocet, Tylox)	—	20 mg	30–60 (PO) 30–60 (CR)[9] 30–60 (R)	60–90 (PO) 90–180 (CR)[9] 30–60 (R)	3–4 (PO) 8–12 (CR)[9] 3–6 (R)	2–3 4.5 (CR)
Oxymorphone (Numorphan)	1 mg	(10 mg R)	15–30 (R) 5–10 (IV) 10–20 (SC) 10–20 (IM)	120 (R) 15–30 (IV) UK (SC) 30–90 (IM)	3–6 (R) 3–4 (IV)[1,3] 3–6 (SC) 3–6 (IM)	2–3
Propoxyphene[10] (Darvon)	—	—	30–60 (PO)	60–90 (PO)	4–6 (PO)	6–12

Table continued on following page

| TABLE 23–7 | EQUIANALGESIC DOSE CHART FOR SELECTED OPIOID DRUGS *Continued* |

Opioid	Parenteral (IM/SC/IV) (Over ~ 4 hr)	Oral (PO) (Over ~ 4 hr)	Onset (min)	Peak (min)	Duration[1] (hr)	Half-life (hr)
AGONIST-ANTAGONISTS						
Buprenorphine[11] (Buprenex)	0.4 mg	—	5 (SL) 5 (IV) 10–20 (IM)	30–60 (SL) 10–20 (IV) 30–60 (IM)	UK (SL) 3–4 (IV)[1, 3] 3–6 (IM)	2–3
Butorphanol[11] (Stadol)	2 mg	—	5–15 (NS)[12] 5 (IV) 10–20 (IM)	60–90 (NS) 10–20 (IV) 30–60 (IM)	3–4 (NS) 3–4 (IV)[1, 3] 3–4 (IM)	3–4
Dezocine (Dalgan)	10 mg	—	5 (IV) 10–20 (IM)	UK (IV) 30–60 (IM)	3–4 (IV)[1, 3] 3–4 (IM)	2–3
Nalbuphine[11] (Nubain)	10 mg	—	5 (IV) <15 (SC) <15 (IM)	10–20 (IV) UK (SC) 30–60 (IM)	3–4 (IV)[1, 3] 3–4 (SC) 3–4 (IM)	5
Pentazocine[11] (Talwin)	60 mg	180 mg	15–30 (PO) 5 (IV) 15–20 (SC) 15–20 (IM)	60–180 (PO) 15 (IV) 60 (SC) 60 (IM)	3–4 (PO) 3–4 (IV)[1, 3] 3–4 (SC) 3–4 (IM)	2–3

[1]Duration of analgesia is dose-dependent; the higher the dose, usually the longer the duration.

[2]As in, e.g., MS Contin.

[3]IV boluses may be used to produce analgesia that lasts approximately as long as IM or SC doses. However, of all routes of administration, IV produces the highest peak concentration of the drug, and the peak concentration is associated with the highest level of toxicity (e.g., sedation). To decrease the peak effect and lower the level of toxicity, IV boluses may be administered more slowly (e.g., 10 mg of morphine over a 15-minute period) or smaller doses may be administered more often (e.g., 5 mg of morphine every 1–1.5 hours).

[4]At steady state, slow release of fentanyl from storage in tissues can result in a prolonged half-life of up to 12 h.

[5]Equianalgesic data not available.

[6]The recommendation that 1.5 mg of parenteral hydromorphone is approximately equal to 10 mg of parenteral morphine is based on single-dose studies. With repeated dosing of hydromorphone (e.g., PCA), it is more likely that 2 to 3 mg of parenteral hydromorphone is equal to 10 mg of parenteral morphine.

[7]In opioid-tolerant clients converted from continuous IV hydromorphone to continuous IV methadone, start with 10% to 25% of the equianalgesic dose.

[8]In opioid-tolerant clients converted to methadone, start PO dosing PRN with 10% to 25% of the equianalgesic dose.

[9]As in OxyContin (oxycodone), for example.

[10]65–130 mg = approximately one-sixth of all doses listed in this chart.

[11]Used in combination with mu agonists, may reverse analgesia and precipitate withdrawal in opioid-dependent clients.

[12]In opioid-naive clients who are taking occasional mu agonists, such as codeine or oxycodone, the addition of butorphanol nasal spray may provide additive analgesia. However, in opioid-tolerant clients, such as those receiving ATC morphine, the addition of butorphanol nasal spray should be avoided because it may reverse analgesia and precipitate withdrawal.

ATC, around-the-clock; CR, oral controlled-release; h, hour; IM, intramuscular; IV, intravenous; μg, microgram; mg, milligram; min, minute; NR, not recommended; NS, nasal spray; OT, oral transmucosal; PO, oral; R, rectal; SC, subcutaneous; SL, sublingual; TD, transdermal; UK, unknown.

Modified from McCaffery M., Pasero C. (1999). *Pain: Clinical manual* (pp. 241–243). St. Louis, Mosby.

life necessitates close monitoring of any client receiving repeated doses because cumulative effects develop over 1 to 2 weeks. If the client becomes oversedated, the dosage should be reduced or the intervals between administration lengthened.

MEPERIDINE. Meperidine (Demerol) is a popular analgesic medication but has many limitations. It should not be used on a prolonged basis (more than a few doses) because of the potentially toxic breakdown product normeperidine, produced during its biotransformation. Meperidine does not provide effective pain relief with repeated doses and causes untenable CNS side effects. The metabolic by-product is toxic to the CNS and can lead to anxiety, tremors, myoclonus, and seizure activity. Nerve injury from diffusion of medication can also occur. Meperidine should not be used in clients with altered renal function.

Adverse Effects of Opioid Analgesics

Some side effects of opioid analgesics—constipation in particular—last as long as the medication is administered. Others, such as nausea and vomiting and drowsiness, decrease as the administration is continued. Other side effects (e.g., respiratory depression) are rare, and the incidence decreases precipitously with longer administration.

CONSTIPATION. Constipation is the most common side effect seen with opioid use[76, 127, 135] and results from increased smooth muscle tone and decreased motility of the gastrointestinal tract. Opioids diminish the propulsive peristaltic contractions in the small and large intestine and delay the passage of gastric contents through the duodenum. Tolerance does not develop to constipation as it does to the other side effects of opioids. Clients taking opioid analgesics need to follow a bowel regimen to prevent constipation. A diet high in fiber with plenty of fluids and stool-softening medications, such as docusate sodium (Colace) or docusate sodium casanthranol (Peri-Colace), is a common prophylactic treatment. A senna-based bulk laxative, such as Senokot-S, is also often needed.[75, 127] Constipation is treatable and is not a side effect mandating that opioid medications be discontinued.

NAUSEA AND VOMITING. Opioids may precipitate nausea and vomiting because of their action on the brain stem centers. Morphine-like medications also affect the vestibular system, which can produce these manifestations. Changing the type of opioid used may eliminate the side effect. Antiemetic agents may also be administered. Remember, this side effect decreases with analgesic use. Clients should not be denied pain relief because of this effect. Instead, they should receive treatment for the nausea and vomiting until it subsides.

RESPIRATORY DEPRESSION. Respiratory depression is caused by diminished sensitivity of the respiratory center to carbon dioxide. All opioids have the potential to produce respiratory depression, which can be rapidly reversed with an opioid antagonist, typically naloxone. The reaction is relatively rare, occurring primarily following the initial doses of opioid among those who never received the medication or whose last dose was a long time ago. It rarely occurs in awake individuals.[5]

This potential for respiratory depression should not discourage the proper use of opioids to relieve pain in people of all ages. The development of respiratory depression is not necessarily dose-related. Most clients do not respond with depressed respiratory rates regardless of dose. Another person may react with decreased respiration to relatively small doses. Rather than limit the use of opioid analgesics, carefully assess each client after giving the medication for the occurrence of respiratory depression.

Deaths that occur secondary to opioid overdose are usually due to respiratory depression and usually occur in people who have not received opioids in the past. With morphine, maximal respiratory depression usually occurs within 15 minutes of intravenous (IV) administration, within 30 minutes of intramuscular (IM) administration, within 90 minutes of subcutaneous (SC) administration, and within 4 to 12 hours of epidural administration. Remember these time ranges when assessing the respiratory status following administration of opioids. For an overdose to occur, however, doses well above the therapeutic level would have to be given. Accumulated doses, especially in clients with liver or renal failure and elderly clients, can cause an overdose.

It is also important to clearly diagnose respiratory depression. The presence of pain may result in increased respiratory rates among clients taking frequent, shallow breaths. Providing a opioid may relieve the pain allowing one's respiratory pattern to return to a more normal breathing pattern. A respiratory rate of 30 breaths per minute may be reduced to 15. This drop has been interpreted as medication-caused respiratory depression, and the pain relief achieved has been reversed by naloxone administration. Remember to assess respiratory depression in conjunction with normal functioning rather than the decrease in breaths per minute. Is the resulting respiratory rate life-threatening?

Treatment of respiratory depression includes arousing the client, establishing a patent airway, administering an opioid antagonist such as naloxone, and providing artificial ventilation as necessary.

CIRCULATORY DEPRESSION. In some clients, circulatory depression may produce hypotension.[71] In a supine client, therapeutic dosages of morphine or synthetic opioids have little effect on blood pressure and cardiac rate or rhythm. However, some people experience orthostatic hypotension when moving from a supine position to a head-up or standing position. This hypotension is secondary to a direct dilating action on the peripheral blood vessels, caused by the opioids, which reduces the capacity of the cardiovascular system to respond to gravitational shifts. Advise the client to avoid abrupt body position changes. For this reason, opioids are used very cautiously in people with reduced blood volume, since the effect is more pronounced. Increasing fluid volume decreases the orthostatic changes.

PARESTHESIAS. Paresthesias may complicate the use of intramuscular opioid analgesics. The intramuscular injection is generally not irritating to the local tissues; however, two exceptions are meperidine and methadone. SC methadone may cause local tissue irritation. Both SC and IM meperidine cause local painful tissue irritation and induration, and frequent administration can lead to severe fibrosis of muscle tissue and should be avoided when possible. If an analgesic is deposited in the region of a nerve after intramuscular injection, paresthesia and paresis may result along the course of the nerve. Proper injection techniques prevent direct nerve injury.

CUTANEOUS EFFECTS. Opioid medications may facilitate histamine release resulting in pruritus, flushing, and sweating. The client becomes tolerant to this effect with repeated administration of the opioid.[88] In the meantime, the clinical manifestations may be alleviated by ingestion of antihistamines.

URINARY RETENTION. Urinary retention may occur due to the increase in smooth muscle tone of the detrussor muscle of the bladder and the bladder sphincter.[75] The hypertoned muscle fibers resist opening preventing adequate bladder emptying. Urinary retention and urgency result. In severe cases, catheterization may be necessary.

Adjuvant Medications

Adjuvants are medications developed for other conditions but have been found to have pain reducing properties as well. Adjuvant medications may be used in combination with analgesics or may be used alone. A wide variety of medications can be classified as adjuvant analgesics.[32, 75, 87, 91, 93, 102] Tricyclic antidepressants (TCAs), such as amitriptyline (Elavil), are very effective for neuropathic pain. They can be given daily at bedtime, so that the drowsiness associated with them promotes sleep. Other effective medications for neuropathic pain are phenytoin (Dilantin), carbamazepine (Tegretol), and gabapentin (Neurontin). Nerve compression and bone pain may respond to dexamethasone (Decadron). Muscle relaxants, such as baclofen (Lioresal) and diazepam (Valium), are used to treat muscle spasm associated with pain.

Phenothiazines are not appropriate for pain relief. They are good antiemetics, but, when given for pain, phenothiazines simply increase sedation, hypotension, and respiratory depression. A phenothiazine such as promethazine (Phenergan) should never be used for pain relief. Promethazine actually increases the perception of pain.[128]

ANTIDEPRESSANTS. TCAs contribute to pain relief via the descending pain inhibitory system by blocking cellular re-uptake of serotonin and epinephrine. They may also potentiate the effect of opiates at synapses and increase their plasma bioavailability. The analgesic effect occurs with doses lower than needed to produce an antidepressant effect. TCAs are used to enhance pain relief regardless of a depression diagnosis. However, relief of depression in clinically depressed clients with pain is a positive outcome. TCAs can be given as a single daily dose at bedtime or in divided doses. Analgesic effects usually begin within a week of initiation of the TCA.

ANTI-ANXIETY AGENTS. Drugs such as diazepam and chlordiazepoxide (Librium) are believed to mediate pain by contributing to Cl^- channel opening. Movement of Cl^- ions hyperpolarizes the postsynaptic membrane, making it less receptive to incoming nociceptive stimuli. Diazepam is particularly effective for relief of painful muscle spasm.

ANTICONVULSANTS. Anticonvulsant agents are used in situations associated with nerve injury. Nerve fibers may generate electrical activity at the site of injury causing the nerve membrane to fire with a pain-producing signal. Agents such as phenytoin (Dilantin) and gabapentin (Neurontin), which stabilize the membrane, help to prevent the ectopic generation of pain-producing activity resulting in lancinating, shooting, shock-like pain.

CORTICOSTEROIDS. These drugs are used to facilitate relief for various types of pain. In the periphery, they reduce edema and inflammation, reducing the compression caused by swelling and the availability of chemical mediators of nociception. They may also inhibit the production of prostaglandins and leukotrienes. In the CNS, they function similarly to anti-anxiety agents by modifying the flow of Cl^- ions.

LOCAL ANESTHETIC AGENTS. Local anesthetics, when administered orally, are membrane stabilizers that produce analgesia by suppressing aberrant electrical activity in central neurons or peripheral axons. Membrane-stabilizing agents include mexiletine (Mexitil), lidocaine, bupivacaine, and tocainide (Tonocard). These agents appear to be effective against lancinating and continuous neuropathic pain. They operate to inactivate Na^+ or K^+ channels, preventing generation of the electrical pain-producing signal. Membrane-stabilizing agents are used primarily for their antiarrhythmic effect, and clients with heart disease must be carefully assessed before these medications are started.

MISCELLANEOUS AGENTS. *Baclofen,* a GABA antagonist, is used as an analgesic for lancinating or paroxysmal neuropathic pain. *Capsaicin* is a topical medication that depletes peptides (such as substance P) in small primary afferent neurons that mediate nociceptive transmission. It appears useful for postherpetic neuralgia and for postmastectomy pain in some clients.

FACTORS INFLUENCING THE EFFECTIVENESS OF ANALGESICS
Relative Analgesic Potency
Relative analgesic potency refers to the ratio of the doses of two analgesics required to produce the same effect. Analgesics are compared with therapeutic doses of morphine. Estimates of relative analgesic potency provide a basis for prescribing the dose when the client is being switched from one analgesic to another or from one route of administration to another. The route used to provide pain relief affects the potency of the medication.

The availability of the analgesic is determined in part by the events encountered before the drug enters the circulatory system. Orally administered medications must be dissolved in stomach contents and absorbed by the gut before the agent can contribute to pain relief. Using the IM or SC routes necessitates that the medication be absorbed from muscle or subcutaneous tissues before it becomes available. IV medications enter the circulatory system directly. Oral, IM, and SC doses must be higher than IV doses.

Duration of Action
The duration of action of an analgesic agent is the result of factors such as pain intensity, dose size, and the client's ability to absorb, biotransform, and eliminate the medication. The duration of action for the analgesics (see Table 23–7) is based on a dose that produces a peak effect equivalent to that of morphine. The time of peak effect and the duration of action of a particular opioid vary with the route of administration. For instance, the peak analgesic effect of IM morphine occurs between 30 minutes and 1 hour after administration. The peak analgesic effect of orally administered morphine occurs from 2 to 12 hours after administration. The duration of action of orally administered opioids is usually somewhat longer than that of IM analgesics. *Duration* of analgesia may not be the same as the *effect* of analgesia. Learn about peak and duration of analgesic effect so that activities that might produce pain can be planned to coincide with peak periods of action. For example, if you know that a client will be going for physical therapy at 10:00 AM, you will want to provide pain medication that will reach its peak effect around 10:00 AM.

Several new forms of morphine have been developed. An oral liquid can be given for more rapid but short-acting effects. A controlled-release form is also available. With long-acting morphine, the onset is somewhat slower but the duration ranges from 8 to 12 hours. Fentanyl is available as a patch for transdermal delivery of medication, effective for 48 to 72 hours. Fentanyl is also available for transmucosal delivery. Oral transmusocal fentanyl citrate is available in lollipop form. The medication is delivered systemically directly through the transmusocal route and partially by the amount of the medication that is swallowed.

Oral Potency
As opioids are absorbed from the intestine and pass through the liver and into the systemic circulation, they differ in the degree to which they are active. This difference in absorption accounts, in part, for the oral doses listed in Table 23–7 for various forms of oral morphine. Preparations with lower bioavailability require higher doses per pill. More recently developed forms of morphine have greater bioavailability, and therefore the dosages of these are lower than those of the older oral form. Because opioids are available in various forms, with varying onset, peak effect, duration, and half-lives, become aware of these variations. The different equianalgesic doses are based on a single dose of IV morphine (see

Table 23–7). An equianalgesic dose is expected to provide the same degree of pain relief as the single IV morphine dose. Dose requirements may decrease after the client has received a loading dose. Failure of health care providers to recognize differences in the oral and intramuscular potencies of opioids and the concept of equianalgesic doses can lead to undertreatment of a person's pain.

ADMINISTRATION OF ANALGESICS

Principles of administration of analgesics are shown in Box 23–5. The goal of analgesic administration is to provide pain relief while maintaining the ability of the client to be in control of the environment, participate in care, and reduce side effects. Assessment of the client before and after analgesic administration is necessary to ensure safe and adequate pain relief. Assess the following factors before analgesic administration:

- Medication allergies or sensitivities
- Previous response to analgesics
- Other medications being taken
- Body weight
- Individual pain experience
- Age, general state of health, mental status
- Cardiac, respiratory, renal, hepatic, and CNS

Allergies or Sensitivities to Medications

Before administering an analgesic such as morphine, ensure that the client does not have a history of untoward reactions to the medication. When possible, ask the client or significant others, and review the chart or other documentation for such information.

Concomitant Medications

Clients taking monoamine oxidase (MAO) inhibitor antidepressants should not receive meperidine. Medications that cause sedation, constipation, or orthostatic hypotension must also be considered when the client is receiving opioids.

Body Weight

The standard morphine dose is 10 mg parenterally. This dose produces satisfactory analgesia in approximately 70% of people with moderate to severe postoperative pain. The analgesic effect is dose-related. Analgesics tend to be prescribed according to a standard protocol applied to all clients with similar disease, however, rather than being based on physical characteristics, including body weight. Therefore, the standard dose may be too high for small adults and too low for obese adults. Remember, one cannot assume that the standard dose will produce adequate pain relief in all adults. You must routinely assess degree of pain relief to ensure that adequate doses are being delivered.

Individual Differences

Given the multitude of factors that contribute to any one person's pain experience, the characteristics of one client's pain may differ from those of another client. It is not possible to design a pain management regimen that will be equally effective for all people with similar pathologic processes. For example, a person's age determines, to some extent, the length of time during which an analgesic will be effective. Age may influence the amount of relief obtained from medications. While there is most likely little difference in the ability of the CNS of an older adult to respond to stimuli, decreases in muscle mass, increases in gastric pathology, and changes in circulatory characteristics may result in a decreased ability to absorb and utilize analgesics. An older person tends to receive pain relief from an opioid for a longer time compared with a younger person. This difference in duration of action may relate to the speed with which an opioid is cleared from the body. Opioid clearance is faster in younger people than in older people.

People with debilitating diseases, regardless of age, also have a heightened sensitivity to the effects of opioids. Because of individual differences in responses to

---

BOX 23–5   Principles of Pharmaceutical Pain Management

- Provide medications in adequate doses.
- Utilize a preventive approach to pain relief. Predictable and chronic pain is managed more effectively if the client maintains a therapeutic blood level of analgesics.
- Closely assess clients with particular diligence with first doses or when the medication dose or the type is changed.
- Medication doses are specific as to type and route. For example, the dose for an oral preparation is higher than that for an intravenous dose of the same medication.
- Combinations of analgesics may be more effective than those given singularly.
- Additions of adjuvant medications enhance pain relief produced by analgesics and are not intended to replace analgesics.
- Understand and be prepared to treat side effects of medications.
- Do not consider avoidance of non–life-threatening side effects (such as constipation, nausea, pruritus) more important than providing pain relief. These concomitant conditions are easily treated.
- Recognize that respiratory depression is a rare occurrence, occurring most commonly among clients who are sedated.

Respiratory depression rarely occurs after the first few doses of an opioid.
- Asking for pain medication reflects need for pain relief in 99.9% of people with pain and does not reflect an addictive personality.
- Do not use placebos for pain. The placebo response usually indicates that the responder has a effective endogenous opiate system and had obtained opiate-mediated pain relief.
- Believe the client's report of pain.
- Maintain a therapeutic relationship that facilitates mutual trust. Your attitudes and beliefs do affect the client's ability to respond to pain management strategies.
- Incorporate the goal of total pain relief into the pain management regimen for most clients.
- Operate as a team to provide the most effective pain relief outcomes. Include the client and significant others in pain interventions, allowing the client to maintain an adequate degree of personal control in the experience.
- *Only the client, and no one else, can determine the amount of pain experienced. There is no objective indicator of pain that can be observed by another.*

pain medications, you must become diligent in assessing the client's responses to the medications.

Body System Assessment

Because all analgesics have the potential to produce mild to severe side effects, it is important to assess a client's cardiac, respiratory, renal, and CNS status before administering analgesics. Hepatic function is also assessed because of the important role of the liver in detoxifying analgesics. The presence of increased intracranial pressure is cause for concern. The physician typically conducts a body system assessment prior to ordering a specific medication regimen. You will need to report changes in physical status, which may place the client at risk if given the analgesic. The physician may then determine that an alternative regimen is needed.

METHODS OF ADMINISTRATION

Nurse-Administered (Demand) Analgesia

The traditional method of treating pain is by nurse-administered pain medication on a schedule, or on a *PRN* (as needed) basis. This system has several advantages:

- It allows you to assess the pain and evaluate effectiveness of the medication
- It facilitates your ability to detect or avoid untoward reactions or side effects
- It permits dose adjustment as necessary

Unfortunately, pain is often significantly undertreated with the PRN system.

Undertreatment may occur because (1) nurses assume authority for pain management, including determination of the amount of pain experienced by the client, and (2) overconcern about possible opioid side effects and fear of inducing opioid addiction by the nurse, the client, or their significant others. The concern about negative effects of pain results in medications ordered in inadequate doses in overly long intervals. When given a range of doses over a range of times, nurses tend to give the smallest dose over the longest time.

The primary inhibitory factor is couched in the belief by the nurse that he or she is in the best position to determine pain medication needs. However, studies have shown that nurses routinely underestimate the amount of pain being experienced. Since there is no objective indicator of pain, the only one who can determine pain medication needs is the client. We as nurses have been uncomfortable with this situation because we have been taught to treat medication-seeking behavior as a sign of addiction. The problem is particularly severe when medications are ordered on a PRN basis. We have typically interpreted the order as "when the client asks for medication." When the client does ask, our fears about addictive personalities surface and the client is seen as medication-seeking and may be labeled as a potential addict. The situation is especially severe when the client is young or belongs to a social or ethnic group devalued by the nurse.

Remember, *asking for nonscheduled medications is often the only means provided clients to obtain pain medications.* In most cases, the request is based on need for pain relief and nothing else. Clients must be valued and believed in order to receive adequate pain relief. The PRN system also deprives the client of the ability to control the situation. Lack of control over pain experiences increases the pain endured during the episode. The pain may be worsened by anxiety about whether you will give the next dose in time to prevent the return of severe pain.

Intermittent dosing, such as occurs with PRN medication orders, causes wide swings in the client's blood levels of the analgesic, which may result in sedation following one dose and unacceptable pain levels preceding the next dose. PRN dosing leads to a "hill and valley" pattern of pain relief. Clients receive a dose of medication sufficient to produce adequate pain relief. They are then expected to wait until the pain is again intense before asking for the subsequent dose.

We have been encouraged by values germane to our work environment to encourage clients to hold out as long as they can so as not to risk addition and undesirable side effects. The hill and valley approach requires that each succeeding dose be maximum strength to bring the client's blood level back to a therapeutic level. Pain relief is more efficiently and effectively achieved if the valleys are avoided. If the PRN schedule is to be maintained, clients need to be encouraged to request pain medication when their pain begins to return. This problem is lessened if we can offer PRN medications on a regular, scheduled basis for clients with acute pain. If the medication is administered regularly, by the clock, pain relief is enhanced.

Patient-Controlled Analgesia

Patient-controlled analgesia (PCA) entails use of an IV or SC infusion pump that contains the analgesic and that is controlled by the client. A bolus dose may be given at the onset of PCA use to provide immediate pain relief. The client can then self-administer subsequent doses by pressing a button that releases a preset dose delivered intravenously. The pumps are programmed to deliver preset demand doses of analgesic until a maximum dose is reached. Then there is a minimal interval during which no further analgesic can be administered (i.e., a lock-out period). With this system, clients control the administration of their own pain medication within the limits prescribed by the physician.

There are many advantages to PCA:

1. The client usually reports good pain control.
2. PCA helps to relieve the client's anxiety about waiting for the nurse to administer the medication, thereby lowering the dose needed to relieve pain.
3. PCA promotes the client's independence and control over the situation.
4. Clients administer lower doses of opioids compared with traditional PRN formats.
5. Clients can adjust their analgesic doses to a near-constant blood concentration.
6. Clients report superior analgesia with a lower incidence of side effects compared with the traditional nurse-administered method.
7. As the pain lessens, clients adjust themselves to lower doses and eventually stop taking the analgesic.

Some problems are associated with PCA. Some clients complain of inadequate analgesia at night, requiring frequent wakening to redose themselves. At some institutions, a basal rate is added at night by continuous delivery at a low but constant dose through the PCA pump to avoid this situation. The success of this method depends on your understanding of the system and on how well the client is taught to use it. Failure can often be traced to a poor understanding on the part of the client, the nurse, or both.

ORAL ROUTE. Oral (PO) dosing is usually preferred. It is noninvasive, convenient, and cost-effective and allows for the greatest flexibility in medication choices. Oral preparations may be in tablet, capsule, liquid, or sublingual forms. Some tablet preparations can be crushed and added to suspensions (e.g., to applesauce) that are more easily swallowed. Oral opioids are available in immediate and sustained-release forms. Sustained-release medications are constructed to be degraded slowly in the gastrointestinal system and must not be crushed or modified. The entire dose will be released at one time if the integrity of the tablet is compromised. The peak effect of oral medications is 1½ to 2 hours for immediate-release preparations. Availability of the medication is delayed until the tablet is degraded and the medication is absorbed, passed through the liver, and made available to the circulatory system.

INTRAMUSCULAR ROUTE. IM dosing is common but is the least desirable route and should be avoided. IM injections are painful, and some people find the injections so objectionable that they are reluctant to seek relief for their pain if the medications are to be administered this way. Additional disadvantages include wide variability and unreliable absorption from muscle and subcutaneous tissues. Peak effects occur within 30 to 60 minutes and are accompanied by a rapid "fall-off" of medication effectiveness. Additional side effects of IM injections include trauma-induced fibrosis of muscle and soft tissues, nerve damage from chemical injury, and development of sterile abscesses.[4]

INTRAVENOUS ROUTE. IV dosing provides the most rapid pain relief. Medications may be provided in bolus doses or by continuous infusions. Bolus doses are given in one administration and provide the most rapid onset of pain relief. Bolus fentanyl reaches peak effect in 1 to 5 minutes, morphine in 15 to 20 minutes.[4] Continuous infusion provides a steady delivery of IV pain medication. It is usually preferred because plasma levels of the medication are maintained and the occurrence of side effects is lessened. Bolus doses may be needed is pain relief falls below acceptable levels with continuous infusion. The infusion dose may then need to be increased to maintain adequate relief.

RECTAL ROUTE. Rectal suppositories provide an alternative route to parenteral administration for people unable to take oral medications. They are provided in doses similar to those of oral preparations. Medications appropriate for the rectal route include morphine, hydromorphone (Dilaudid), oxycodone (Percocet), methadone, and oxymorphone (Numorphan).

TRANSDERMAL ROUTE. Transdermal analgesia is provided by means of a skin patch. The most common opioid administered transdermally is fentanyl, which is very potent. It is available in a variable-dosing transdermal application system that the client or family member can apply independently. The patch is designed to deliver specified amounts of medication over 48 to 72 hours. This system provides an easy means of maintaining independence and avoids the inconveniences of frequent dosing.

Analgesia from the first application may take up to 24 hours to reach an adequate blood level. During this period, supplemental analgesia is maintained. The patch is typically applied to clean, dry skin on the chest or upper back. These areas are less vulnerable to dislodgment of the patch compared with other areas. The patch may be applied to any convenient location with intact skin as long as the client can protect it. Excessive hair should be carefully clipped before application. The patch should not be applied over irritated or broken skin. The patch is left in place for up to 72 hours, when it is removed. A new patch is applied at a different site to prevent skin irritation.

TRANSMUCOSAL ANALGESIA. Transmucosal analgesia is achieved either sublingually (methadone and buprenorphine (Buprenex) or by means of a lozenge (Oralet) or a lollipop (Actiq). The transmucosal route is particularly effective for breakthrough pain in clients with scheduled opioid medications around the clock. Up to two thirds of clients with chronic or malignant pain who are treated around the clock with opioids have episodes of breakthrough pain.[95]

CONTINUOUS SUBCUTANEOUS ANALGESIA. Pain relief is achieved through an infusion setup using a pump device. A 25- or 27-gauge needle is used, or a special SC needle device can be implanted subcutaneously. The client wears a medication reservoir that can be refilled as needed. The needle site is rotated every 3 to 7 days according to the type and volume of medication administered. The volume delivered ranges from 2 to 4 ml/h.

Observe the site for redness, excessive swelling, leakage of fluid around the infusion site, or edema. If an extremity is used, carefully assess it for the presence of edema, which interferes with absorption of the medication. Closely monitor the client for adequacy of analgesic effect. If the medication is ineffective and sufficient medication is available in the reservoir, a higher concentration may be required.

INTRASPINAL ANALGESIA. Opioids are injected intrathecally or epidurally. The epidural space is outside the dura mater of the spinal cord and brain; the intrathecal space is inside the dura mater and contains the spinal fluid. The dorsal horns of the spinal cord contain receptors for endogenous opioid substances. By means of the intraspinal analgesia route, medication is delivered directly into the areas with the intended receptor sites. These receptors bind opioids and provide excellent pain relief of long duration (8 to 24 hours) without causing sympathetic and motor nerve blockade. Relatively small doses provide high opioid concentrations in the spinal fluid that bathes the dorsal columns. These concentrations are far higher than those in the spinal fluid after similar doses given by standard parenteral routes.

Repeated bolus doses, PCA, or a constant infusion via an implanted refillable infusion pump of the opioid may be given through a small catheter placed in the epidural or intrathecal space. Catheters have been left in place for days to months without adverse effects.

Possible side effects include pruritus, urinary retention, and delayed respiratory depression occurring 6 to 12 hours after a dose. Low doses of naloxone may reverse these side effects without reducing analgesia.

NERVE BLOCKS. Neuroblockade is achieved through injection of various substances (e.g., local anesthetics) close to the nerves, thereby blocking their conductivity. Blockade may be used to produce a complete, reversible interruption of nerve pathways for the following purposes:

- To eliminate a local focus of pain-producing stimulation or nervous irritation
- To interrupt the perception of pain, either at the source of the pain or anywhere along the peripheral afferent neurons
- To interrupt reflex mechanisms that are maintaining abnormal activity in blood vessels, glands, or skeletal or smooth muscle
- To eliminate reflex responses to pain (e.g., tachycardia, hypertension) by directly infiltrating skeletal muscle and other involved structures

Irreversible nerve-blocking procedures, which permanently block the pain pathway, are often used in managing pain associated with cancer. The effect of the block may be short-lived, however. The nerves may regenerate to some extent, with an associated return of sensory and motor functions.

Nerve blocks given for pain relief are called *analgesic blocks.* The analgesia is generally produced by injection of a local anesthetic agent. The anesthetic agent relieves pain and thus allows treatment that might otherwise be extremely uncomfortable, such as manipulation of a painful joint or wound debridement. Sometimes, by interrupting reflexes that are causing sustained pain, analgesic blocks can produce a beneficial effect that is prolonged beyond the effective duration of the agent injected.

Analgesic blocks are useful in various acute and chronic disorders. They often reduce the amounts of analgesic medication that might otherwise be needed. Injecting local anesthetics into tender points of muscle or skin (*trigger point injection*) causes a type of analgesic block that may modify pain and break the pain cycle, allowing manipulation and stretching of a joint. However, the pain may not be permanently eliminated unless the primary afferent impulses are either chemically or surgically terminated or until the underlying pathologic condition causing the pain is corrected.

■ NEGATIVE EFFECTS OF PAIN

A barrier to adequate pain management has been the belief that pain, while uncomfortable, has few negative physiologic effects. Unrelieved pain can affect the major organ systems—pulmonary, cardiovascular, gastrointestinal, endocrine, and immune. Unrelieved pain has resulted in untoward effects that have resulted in increased costs that affect all of society. Costs are increased because of longer hospital stays, the need to treat the negative effects of pain, and the client's loss of productivity. Pain prevents coughing, deep breathing, and sighing, leading to pulmonary complications with significant morbidity and mortality. Pain may also prevent ambulation, contributing to the development of deep vein thrombosis and potential pulmonary emboli. Pain of any type induces release of catecholamines and stress hormones. Cardiovascular complications (tachycardia, hypertension) and decreased immune activity may result.

Reflex muscle contraction may be enhanced, resulting in increased muscle tension and spasm. Abdominal wall muscle tension and spasm reduce the ability of the chest wall to expand. As a result, clients take short, shallow, frequent breaths. Oxygen and carbon dioxide exchange is less effective with this breathing pattern. Vital capacity has been reported to fall to 40% of presurgery capacity when pain was not relieved and to only 70% of presurgery values when pain was totally relieved. Although respiratory depression in response to opioids is rare, hypoventilation resulting from untreated pain is not.

Intestinal and bladder smooth muscle tone is affected such that peristalsis and bladder motility are decreased. Bowel and bladder distention may result. The decreased motility of the bowel contributes to constipation. If distention is severe enough, the abdominal contents may interfere with the ability of the diaphragm to expand. It appears as though constipation may be a complication of either opioid administration or unrelieved pain. Given the negative effects of pain, it is better to give the opioid and treat the constipation.

Catecholamine secretion in response to pain leads to increased myocardial oxygen demand and consumption. Clients with atherosclerosis may be impaired to the point of myocardial ischemia, dysrhythmias, infarction, cardiac failure, and death. Unfortunately, the elderly population—at greatest risk for atherosclerotic vascular changes—are at greatest risk for receiving inadequate pain relief. On the basis of the negative effects of pain, a reasonable goal of pain management programs is the total relief of pain.

NONPHARMACEUTICAL INTERVENTIONS

Activities such as cutaneous stimulation, acupuncture, acupressure, massage, listening to music, progressive relaxation, guided imagery, rhythmic breathing, meditation, hypnosis, humor, biofeedback, Therapeutic Touch, distraction, and magnets have been used clinically with positive results. The therapies are thought to cause physiologic changes. For example, peripheral blood vessels may be dilated, muscle tension is decreased, the immune systems is strengthened, and brain chemicals are activated or modified. Techniques such as these can be used to manage pain and to promote healthy living. It may be possible to teach clients a combination of these techniques to maximize their opportunities for self-control over manifestations of pain. Figure 23–15 presents modalities for pain relief.

■ CUTANEOUS STIMULATION

Cutaneous stimulation activates the large-diameter (A-beta) fibers, which stimulate inhibitory neurons in the spinal cord and engage the descending analgesic system. Pain relief is achieved by endogenous opiate activity.

Cutaneous stimulation can decrease the intensity of pain the client perceives and, in some instances, may eliminate it.[76, 83] It also can help in changing the sensation in a painful or noxious area to a more pleasant sensation, such as warmth. This process may also be seen as a form

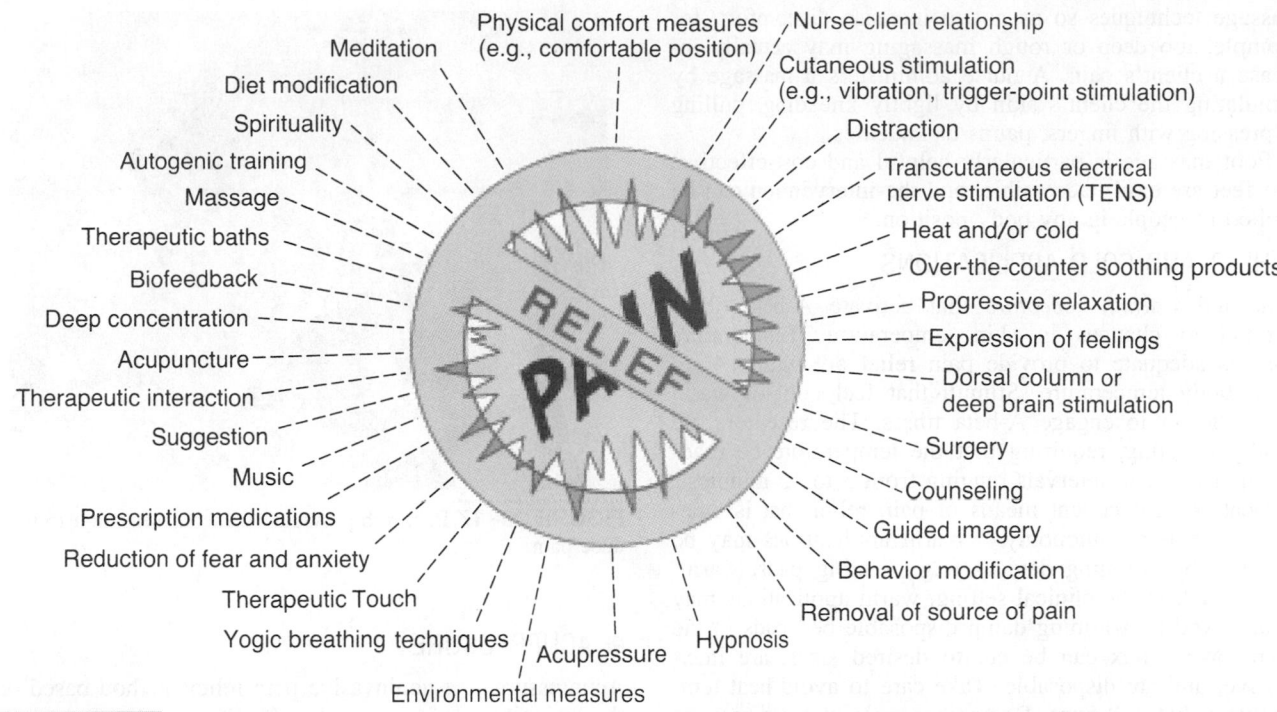

FIGURE 23–15 Pain relief measures.

of distraction because the client may focus on the sensation being created rather than the pain. Cutaneous stimulation can be applied to the unaffected side and still elicit positive benefits because the stimulated fibers cross within the spinal cord. This method is particularly useful when an area is too painful to be directly stimulated, as with burns.

■ TRANSCUTANEOUS ELECTRICAL NERVE STIMULATION (TENS)

TENS delivers electrical bursts through the skin to superficial and deep nerves. TENS is used most often for clients with chronic pain, such as muscle pain from arthritis.

TENS has been shown to relieve pain effectively in many people.[133] Success with TENS depends on the client's understanding of, interest in, and motivation to use the apparatus as well as the clinician's skillfulness in applying the device. The client needs to learn to adjust placement of the surface electrodes and the intensity and timing of the stimuli to maximize pain relief (Fig. 23–16). Involve significant others as appropriate in learning and teaching sessions. The client may need their help in applying the electrodes to areas that are difficult to reach. Electrode placement depends on the site of the pain. Positive and negative poles are usually placed within several inches of each other. Voltage and pulsation are controlled by the person wearing the device. Battery packs make the device portable.

■ MASSAGE

Massage may be effective when applied to various sites. A back rub is a good method of providing cutaneous stimulation (Fig. 23–17). It is particularly relaxing at bedtime and may block pain so as to promote more comfortable sleep. However, you should be knowledgeable in

FIGURE 23–16 Surface patches are used for transcutaneous electrical nerve stimulation (TENS) treatment.

massage techniques so as not to increase discomfort; for example, too deep or rough massaging may actually increase a client's pain. A nurse administers a massage by stimulating the client's skin by lightly kneading, pulling or pressing with fingers, palms or knuckles.

Foot massage is particularly helpful and cost-effective. The feet are easily accessible, and the intervention can be applied to people in any body position.

■ HEAT AND COLD APPLICATIONS

Cold and *warmth receptors* that activate A-beta fibers respond to changes in skin temperature. Temperature changes adequate to provide pain relief are within 4° to 5° of body temperature. Stimuli that feel cool or warm are sufficient to engage A-beta fibers. The receptors are rapidly adapting, requiring that the temperature be readjusted at frequent intervals ranging from 5 to 15 minutes.

Heat is an excellent means of pain relief that is amenable to nursing autonomy.[80] Warm applications may be achieved by warming devices (e.g., heating pads, warming towels). In the clinical setting, warm applications may be achieved by warming damp disposable bed pads in the microwave. Chux can be cut to desired sizes, are inexpensive, and are disposable. Take care to avoid heat temperatures that will burn. Remember, painful areas may be hypersensitive to skin stimuli. Heat temperatures that are typically perceived as nonpainful may become painful when applied to the sensitive area.

Cold application also brings pain relief,[81] and nurses can consider this treatment. *Ice* may also be used to provide pain relief and to prevent or reduce edema and inflammation. The effectiveness of ice applications does not depend on A-beta fiber stimulation; however, ice decreases the conduction velocity of nociceptive nerve fibers, rendering the fiber incapable of transmitting the pain signal to the spinal cord. The client perceives the application area as numb.

Thermal stimuli are most effective when applied directly to the painful area. When direct application is not possible, relief may be achieved by applying the intervention to a point proximal or distal to the painful area. A cold compress wrapped around the wrist may alleviate pain in the hand.

■ ACUPUNCTURE

Acupuncture has been practiced in Asian cultures for centuries and produces pain relief in modern health care.[39] Very thin metal needles are skillfully inserted into the body at designated locations and at various depths and angles.

Approximately 1000 known acupuncture points are widely distributed over the surface of the body in patterns known as *meridians.* Each meridian contains its own group of acupuncture points and is associated with a specific visceral organ. Meridians run bilaterally just beneath the surface of the skin and begin or terminate at the tips of the fingers or toes. "Vital energy" is believed to flow through these meridians. The acupuncture points on the surface of the body provide external access to this vital energy. Through needle insertion at specific points, various physiologic processes can be influenced or controlled and are determined by the specific pathologic condition and the desired physiologic effect.

FIGURE 23–17 Back rub provides cutaneous sensation to reduce pain.

■ ACUPRESSURE

Acupressure is a noninvasive pain relief method based on the principles of acupuncture.[66] Pressure, massage, or other cutaneous stimulation, such as heat or cold, is applied over acupuncture points.

■ MUSIC

Music has been used to relieve pain in a number of settings.[11, 48, 49, 50, 53, 118, 125] The exact physiologic mechanisms have not been determined; however, several possible theories include distraction, release of endogenous opioids, or disassociation. All three mechanisms are probably involved. Music clearly provides distraction and disassociation by focusing on the characteristics of the musical selection. The auditory pathway interacts with endogenous opiate systems at several foci within the brain, including the hypothalamus and the limbic system. These areas are known to project to PAG/PVG, providing a mechanism to contribute to pain relief through both cerebral activity and spinal cord responses mediated by descending fibers from nucleus raphe and locus ceruleus.

People in pain may find music to be relaxing. Pain relief may also be achieved through physiologic responses to relaxation. The relaxation response is mediated through the hypothalamus.

When using music for pain relief, allow clients to choose the type of music most suited to them. Some people find the use of a radio, cassette, or compact disc players with headphones a quiet way to listen to music without bothering others. This allows the client to increase the music volume or to play it softly. Encourage the family members to bring in the client's favorite selections. This also gives the family a sense of doing something to help.

■ PROGRESSIVE RELAXATION TRAINING

Progressive relaxation training is used to treat various physical and psychosocial problems, including pain.[8, 85] The client is taught to gradually tighten, then deeply relax, various muscle groups, proceeding systematically from one area of the body to the next. The deep relaxation produced by this method can decrease anxiety and excessive muscle contraction and promote the onset of sleep. Audiotape cassettes are available.

■ DEEP BREATHING FOR RELAXATION

Deep breathing for relaxation is easy to learn and contributes to pain relief by reducing muscle tension and anxiety.[75] First, the client clenches the fists while taking a deep breath. The client then holds his or her breath for a moment, and exhales while letting oneself "go limp." The cycle is followed by a slow, deep breath mimicking a yawn.

■ GUIDED IMAGERY

Guided imagery helps a client to visualize a pleasant experience. The client is coached to visualize a scene (e.g., relaxing on a beach). The coach instructs the client to imagine the sensory aspects of the scene, the sounds, sights, and emotions expressed. The more vivid the image, the more effective the intervention. Visualization may be combined with soft, lyrical, relaxing music. Audiotapes for guided imagery are available.

Imagery relieves pain through several mechanisms.[121] It is a way to help people distract themselves from their pain, which may increase their pain tolerance. Imagery may also produce a relaxation response, thus relieving pain. Last, the image can be a healing one, designed not only to relieve the pain but possibly to diminish the source of the pain,[116] (e.g., a tension headache may be alleviated).

Imagery is often combined with relaxation and biofeedback to produce a multifocal pain relief technique. The image used in this technique can be a complex scene that requires the person to think of each detail. This image would increase distraction. The image might be a relaxing scene, such as a beach or meadow, which would help with the relaxation response, or the image might consist of visualizing the pain being worn away until it is so small that it can be "blown away." When introducing an image setting, ask the client what setting is relaxing for him or her. Avoid using an image that may provoke anxiety, such as using a beach for someone who is afraid of water or a meadow for someone with severe allergies to pollen.

■ RHYTHMIC BREATHING

Rhythmic breathing is typically considered a method of both relaxation and distraction. It may also provide effective pain relief by stimulating baroreceptors in the atria and carotid sinuses. Stimulation of these receptors initiates activity in a neuropathway that sends projections to the periaqueductal and periventricular gray matter, resulting in opioid-mediated pain inhibition. This method can be combined with rhythms such as music, a ticking clock, or a metronome. Little concentration is necessary because once the individual begins the process, it takes on an automatic quality. This method focuses attention away from the pain and on the breathing and the rhythm. The Lamaze method of childbirth is a good example of a pain control method that incorporates this technique.

■ MEDITATION

Meditation focuses one's attention away from pain. It also provides energy and peace to the meditator. The client simply sits comfortably and quietly with focused attention. The focus may vary. Examples include flow of the breath, a mantra, and a picture or mental image of a great spiritual being or peaceful place. Sometimes the meditator communicates with a spiritual being. There are many meditation techniques, some with a spiritual base, such as Siddha meditation. Meditation is easily practiced anywhere, and no special equipment is required. The positive experiences available through meditation are available to anyone, including people in pain.

■ HYPNOSIS

A person's reaction to pain can be significantly altered by hypnosis. Hypnosis is based on suggestion, dissociation, and the process of focusing attention.[97, 98]

Various procedures may be used to relieve pain following induction of a hypnotic state including:

- Suggestion to alter the character of the pain or one's attitude toward it
- Body disorientation and dissociation
- Anesthesia and analgesia for superficial and deep sensation

In situations of chronic pain, a posthypnotic suggestion may be used in combination with *autohypnosis* (self-hypnosis) to provide prolonged relief. Many hypnotic subjects successfully learn to use deliberate spontaneous trance induction or autohypnosis.

Although hypnosis cannot change organic lesions that are producing pain, it can often reduce discomfort.[97, 98] The procedure itself is fairly simple and innocuous compared with the administration of many anesthetic and analgesic medications; however, take care not to probe any fears or unpleasant memories. A hypnotherapist must be skilled and informed and the client carefully selected to avoid negative effects. Increasingly nurses are being certified to provide clinical hypnotic therapies in the United States.

Hypnosis may be used as an adjunct to other pain-relieving therapies. Alteration of pain by hypnosis should be performed by those who are aware of the possible diagnostic implications of pain in the medical management of disease.

■ HUMOR

Research in the use of humor in the clinical setting has revealed that the intervention actually increases the number of NK (natural killer) cells of the immune system.[7, 17, 74] This is particularly important for implementation in clients with cancer. It has been postulated that humor elevates endogenous opioids or endorphins. Regardless of the physiologic advantages, use of humor simply makes people feel better, more relaxed, and in less pain. Clients may find some degree of pain relief by watching comedic videotapes, listening to audiotapes and compact discs they find funny or reading humorous books. You may want to suggest that hospitalized clients might bring humorous materials with them to utilize during their inpatient experience.

■ BIOFEEDBACK

Biofeedback refers to a wide variety of techniques that provide a client with information about changes in bodily functions of which the client is usually unaware, such as blood pressure. Biofeedback equipment provides immediate, continuous information. Some people learn to use this information to control previously involuntary functions. The purpose of biofeedback in pain management is to teach self-control over physiologic variables that relate to the pain, such as muscle contraction and blood flow.

Information used to reduce muscle contraction is obtained by an electromyogram (EMG) recorded from body surface electrodes. (Needle EMG electrodes are not used.) Changes in blood flow are produced by monitoring skin temperature, which increases with increased blood flow. Depending on the equipment used, clients can self-monitor their changes through *auditory displays* (decreases in muscle contractions are heard as decreases in the pitch of a tone) or *visual displays* (increases in skin temperature are seen as increases on a dial). The client tries to change the display of information in the desired direction, such as to reduce muscle contraction (relax muscle tension) and reduce blood flow. The continuous, precise information received shows the effectiveness of the effort and often helps the client learn physiologic control of these functions.[109]

Biofeedback can be performed at home with purchased or rented equipment under the guidance of a suitably prepared health care worker. Alternatively, it may be performed in an office or clinic setting with a biofeedback therapist or other specialist, such as a nurse trained in biofeedback. The equipment is expensive.

■ THERAPEUTIC TOUCH

Therapeutic Touch is a type of pain management that has been used for disorders such as tension headaches.[34, 56, 101] It is a derivative of the "laying on" of hands. The human body is believed to have energy fields that express aberrant patterns when body systems are insulted. Therapeutic Touch is thought to realign aberrant fields. Education and practice are required on the part of the nurse.

Therapeutic Touch involves three steps.

1. Become centered or focused in a meditative state. This helps you become aware of the vibrations in the surrounding energy fields.
2. Assess the client's energy field. Pass your hands over the client's body at a distance of 2 to 6 inches to sense changes in the field.
3. During the treatment step, use your hands to rearrange the client's energy field and return it to normal.

■ DISTRACTION

Cognitive strategies to modify pain perception have been effective in numerous research studies. The most effective cognitive strategy involves distraction. Attention is directed away from the painful sensation or the negative emotional arousal associated with the pain episode. The primary theoretical explanation is that a person is able to focus attention on a limited number of foci. Actively focusing attention on a cognitive task is thought to limit one's ability to attend to the noxious sensation.

To be effective, the distraction task requires considerable cognitive effort. Distraction exercises that are too easy rapidly become automatic or engage monotonous repetitive responses and are likely to be ineffective.

Interventions may be administered by a multitude of modalities that require the client to engage in highly focused interesting mental exercises. Typical techniques utilized in hospital settings include videotapes of favorite movies, audiotapes of favorite music, craft activities, and interacting with others. The distraction technique may be more effective if it involves action on the client's part. For example, listening to music and tapping one's fingers to the rhythm may be more effective than passive listening alone. Cognitive strategies need to be tailored to the client's personal preferences. Techniques used should be self-selected. People may want to bring their own tapes, videos, books, or craft items. If the items are supplied by an agency, a library of materials will be needed to allow clients to select what will be pleasing to them.

■ MAGNETS

Magnets have been used to relieve a variety of painful disorders.[90, 124] It is speculated that the pull of the magnet increases blood flow to the region, opening the Na^+ and Cl^- channels in the cells. Magnet therapy has been a mainstay in pain management in Eastern Asian countries and is gaining popularity in Western medicine.

EVALUATION AND DOCUMENTATION

■ EVALUATION

Evaluation is most effective when a formal evaluation protocol is used throughout a health care agency "across all stages of the disease and across all practice settings."[59] A formalized process within the institution provides a unified methodology that can be learned and used by every member of the health care team. According to the Clinical Practice Guidelines,[59] key items to consider include:

- Client satisfaction with pain management and its impact on their quality of life
- Satisfaction with pain management and its impact on their quality of life (particularly in chronic illness or when clients require home health care)
- The designation of who is responsible for pain management
- The systematic assessment of pain in all settings where people receive care
- The accuracy of diagnostic approaches for common pain syndromes
- The range and appropriateness of pain management options available within a particular practice setting
- The effectiveness of pain management options utilized to prevent and treat pain
- The prevalence and severity of side effects and complications associated with pain management
- The quality of pain management across points of transition in the provision of services

The effectiveness of pain management protocols needs to be evaluated frequently and throughout the course of treatment. Figure 23–18 illustrates a sample plan used to determine pain management needs for clients having sur-

FIGURE 23–18 *A* and *B,* Pain treatment flow chart.

gery.[1] The example includes the three phases of a surgical experience (preoperative, intraoperative, and postoperative).

During an evaluation, both the process used to manage pain and the outcomes achieved are assessed. Assessment and evaluation are ongoing components of the plan. Remember, there are no objective indicators of a person's pain. The only means to determine pain intensity and associated emotional discomfort accurately is to ask the person. Sometimes direct measurement of a client's report of pain is not possible, and someone else must estimate pain by observation. These assessments may or may not be accurate. Ongoing evaluation of the effectiveness of pain management interventions is essential when the client is not verbal. The pain management strategy employed for the client is based on an interpretation of need. These clients cannot provide data regarding effectiveness of the strategy. The health care provider must ascertain whether the pain was indeed relieved by the intervention they selected.

Evaluation requires the identification of a standard against which practice process and outcomes can be compared.[59] For example, the health care provider consults with the client to determine the degree of pain relief desired by the client. An evaluation criterion will consider whether the desired outcome has been achieved. If the criterion is not met, the evaluation will try to determine the reason. Modifications in the pain management program may be needed to achieve the desired outcome. These modifications should be documented to allow for evaluation of outcomes achieved by the new interventions. Some institutions have employed a standard for all clients based on the knowledge that unrelieved pain has negative physical effects. For example, a standard may mandate that medication for pain be administered if a client reports a pain intensity of 3 or greater on an 11-point numerical scale.

While the primary focus of evaluation is directed toward effectiveness of management strategies for clients, it will also be necessary to periodically evaluate the treatment protocols incorporated into hospital procedure manuals and pain management standards accepted by the clinicians. As the knowledge base underlying practice interventions increases, the standard procedures for pain management may also need to change. Conducting periodic evaluation of practice, based on research, enhances the potential for providing the best care possible. A few questions to consider are as follows:

- Is the client still in pain? If so, is progress being made to minimize or relieve the pain?
- Are the client's beliefs and values being considered?
- Are the client and family active participants in pain management planning?

- Have pain management nonpharmaceutical interventions been given ample time to be effective? Can the client try the strategy one more time?
- Are a variety of pain measures being utilized?
- Do new data indicate a new diagnosis or complication?

MM#17986

3/97

Clarian Health
Methodist · IU · Riley

F = Faces
W = Word
I = Infant Assessment Tool
A = Adult & Child Assessment Tool

PAIN MANAGEMENT FLOW SHEET

Initials	Name & Title	Initials	Name & Title

☐ In-Patient   ☐ Out-Patient

Date/Time	Scale/Rating	Resp./LOS	Location/Type	Drug Administered Dosage/Route	Other Interventions	Comments/Response	Initials

LEVEL OF SEDATION	DEGREE OF SOMNOLENCE (Patient Awakens/Responds to:)	INTERVENTIONS		COMMENTS EXAMPLES
0	Caregiver entering room	R = repositioning	M = massage	diarrhea
1	Soft verbal stimulation	F = feeding	CS = cutaneous stimulation	constipation
2	Loud Verbal Stimulation	VS = verbal support	GI = guided imagery	depressed
3	Mild Physical Contact	HR = holding/rocking	MT = music therapy	crying
4	Vigorous Physical Contact	T = toileting/diapering	HA = hot application	vomiting
		D = distraction	CA = cold application	nausea
		A = adjust environment	SO = significant other present	anxious
		E = emotional support	=	agitated
		P = play	=	itching
		S = sucking/pacifier	=	

Adapted from: Gwirtz, K.H. (1992). Single dose intrathecal opiods in the management of acute postoperative pain. In Sinatra, R., Hord, A., Ginsberg, R., & Preble, L. (Eds.). Acute Pain: Mechanisms and Management (pp.253-268). St. Louis: Mosby Publishing

19058

MEDICAL RECORDS COPY

PAIN MANAGEMENT FLOWSHEET

W-37

B-CLIN. NOTES	E-LAB	G-X-RAY	K-DIAGNOSTIC	M-SURGERY	Q-THERAPY	T-ORDERS	W-NURSING	Y-MISC.

FIGURE 23–19 Pain management flow sheet. (Courtesy of Clarian Health Partners, Indianapolis.)

■ DOCUMENTATION

Data gathered through evaluation must be documented. Documentation data are to be recorded in a manner that makes the information available to all members of the health care team. This may be best done by means of a pain document record or flow sheet (Fig. 23–19) that allows visualization of the client's pain experience throughout a hospitalization experience and that can follow the client from one health care setting to another. The flow sheet should be entered into the client's permanent hospital record.

CONCLUSIONS

The most effective pain management program may depend on use of a combination of medications and nonpharmaceutical interventions. Clients may benefit from the incorporation of several nonpharmaceutical interventions utilized simultaneously. Research has supported the efficacy of numerous nonpharmaceutical techniques. These findings plus the wide variability in the strength and types of medications makes it possible (1) to design a pain program that can be individualized and (2) to modify a pain management protocol if one finds that a component of the program is ineffective. One ineffective strategy can be replaced by another until a successful combination of treatments is determined.

The variety of potential treatments also benefits clients for whom progression of the pain experience is a component. The protocol can be modified to meet changing needs when the pain increases or abates. Box 23–2 summarizes possible interventions posited by the Clinical Practice Guidelines for Management of Cancer Pain and Pain due to Trauma, Surgery, and Painful Procedures.[59]

THINKING CRITICALLY

1. **A 33-year-old woman, Miss Brown, arrives in the emergency department with a severe headache. She has vomited twice. She states, "This is the worst headache I have ever had." The headache has lasted for about 6 hours, and two doses of acetaminophen have given no relief. Miss Brown cannot lift her head off of the pillow and cannot position herself for comfort. Her pupils are equal, and there is no diaphoresis. What further nursing history and assessments should be done? How soon can medication to alleviate the headache be administered?**

Factors to Consider. How crucial is a thorough pain assessment? How can a migraine headache mimic manifestations of a cerebral disorder? Would it be advisable to delay giving analgesia? Why? Why not?

2. **A 80-year-old client, Mrs. Parker, is terminally ill with cancer. An opiate analgesic has been prescribed for her pain. She is being cared for at home by family members who are concerned about pain control for their loved one. What should the client and family be taught about complications associated with use of opiate anal-**gesia? Who would be the ideal client to assess and coordinate the client's response to dosing of a particular opiate or combination of opiate and non-opiate medications?

Factors to Consider. What complications are associated with use of opiate analgesia? What factors contribute to the dosing schedule of a client with cancer-related pain? How much control over analgesia is given to the client? How should the caregiver and family monitor the response of the individual to the prescribed medication regimen?

BIBLIOGRAPHY

1. Acute Pain Management Guideline Panel. (1992). *Acute pain management in adults: Operative procedures. Quick reference guide for clinicians.* AHCPR Publ. No. 92-0019. Rockville, MD: Agency for Health Care Policy and Research, Public Health Service, U.S. Department of Health and Human Services.
2. Ader, R. W. (1997). The role of conditioning in pharmacotherapies: The placebo effect? *Proceedings of the American Pain Society, 16th* Annual Scientific Meeting, New Orleans, p. 53.
3. Akil, H., et al. (1998). Endogenous opioids: Overview and current issues. *Drug and Alcohol Dependence, 51*(1–2), 127–140.
4. Albers, R. W., & Siegal, G. J. (1999). Membrane transport. In G. J. Siegal, et al. (Eds.), *Basic neurochemistry: Molecular, cellular, and medical aspects* (6th ed., pp. 95–118). Philadelphia: Lippincott–Williams & Wilkins.
5. American Pain Society. (1999). *Principles of analgesic use in the treatment of acute pain and cancer pain* (4th ed.). Skokie, IL: Author.
6. Anand, K. J. S. (1998). Clinical importance of pain and stress in preterm neonates. *Biology of the Neonate, 73,* 1–9.
7. Anderson, D. L. (1997). Nurses: act now. *Journal of Practical Nursing 47*(1), 16–18.
8. Atsberger, D. B. (1995). Relaxation therapy: Its potential as an intervention for acute postoperative pain. *Journal of Post Anesthesia Nursing, 10*(1), 2–8.
9. Basbaum, A. I., & Jessell, T. (2000). The perception of pain. In E. R. Kandel, J. H. Schwartz, & T. M. Jessell (Eds.), *Principles of neural science* (4th ed., pp. 441–429). Norwalk, CT: Appleton & Lange.
10. Bates, M. S., Rankin-Hill, L., & Sanchez-Ayendez, M. (1997). The effects of the cultural context of health care on treatment of and response to chronic pain and illness. *Social Science and Medicine, 45*(9), 1433–1447.
11. Beck, S. L. (1991). The therapeutic use of music for cancer related pain. *Oncology Nursing Forum, 18,* 1327–1337.
12. Bennett, G. J. (2000). Update on the neurophysiology of pain transmission and modulation: Focus on the NMDA receptor. *Journal of Pain and Symptom Management, 19*(1 suppl), 52–56.
13. Berkley, K. J. (1997). Sex differences and pain. *Behavioral and Brain Sciences 30*(3), 371–380, 435–513.
14. Berkley, K. J., & Holdcroft, A. (1999). Sex and gender differences in pain. In P. D. Wall & R. Melzack (Eds.), *Textbook of pain* (4th ed., pp. 951–965). Edinburgh: Churchill Livingstone.
15. Bevan, S. (1999). Nociceptive peripheral neurons: Cellular properties. In P. D. Wall & R. Melzack (Eds.), *Textbook of pain* (4th ed., pp. 85–104). Edinburgh: Churchill Livingstone.
16. Bonica, J. J. (1990), *The management of pain* (Vols. 1 and 2, 2nd ed.). Philadelphia: Lea & Febiger.
17. Botterff, J., Gogag, M., & Engelberg-Lotzkar, M. (1995). Comforting: Exploring the work of cancer nursing. *Journal of Advanced Nursing, 22,* 1077–1084.
18. Brander, B., et al. (1997). Evaluation of the contribution to postoperative analgesia by local cooling of the wound. *Anesthesia, 51*(11), 1021–1025.
19. Breitbart, W., Passik, S. D., & Rosenfield, B. D. (1999). Cancer, mind and spirit. In P. D. Wall & R. Melzack (Eds.), *Textbook of pain* (4th ed., pp. 1065–1112). Edinburgh: Churchill Livingstone.
20. Breitbart, W., et al. (1996). The undertreatment of pain in ambulatory AIDS clients. *Pain, 65,* 243–249.

21. Brune, K., & Zeilhoffer, H. U. (1999). Antipyretic (non-narcotic) analgesics. In P. D. Wall & R. Melzack (Eds.), *Textbook of pain* (4th ed., pp. 1139–1153). Edinburgh: Churchill Livingstone.

22. Calvillo, E. R., & Flaskerud, J. H. (1991). Review of literature on culture and pain of adults with focus of Mexican-Americans. *Journal of Transcultural Nursing, 2,* 16–23.

23. Cao, Y. Q., et al. (1998). Primary afferent tachykinins are required to experience moderate to severe pain. *Nature, 392,* 390–394.

24. Cashman, J., & McAnulty, G. (1995). Nonsteroidal anti-inflammatory drugs in perisurgical pain management: Mechanisms of action and rationale for optimum use. *Drugs, 49,* 51–70.

25. Chapman, C. R. (1998). Psychological interventions for pain: Potential mechanisms. In R. Payne, et al. (Eds.), *Assessment and treatment of cancer pain: Progress in pain research and management* (Vol. 12, pp. 109–131). Seattle: IASP Press.

26. Cleeland, C. S., et al. (1997). Pain and treatment of pain in minority patients with cancer: The Eastern Cooperative Oncology Group minority outpatient pain study. *Annals of Internal Medicine, 127,* 813–816.

27. Cousins, M., & Power, I. (1999). Acute and postoperative pain. In P. D. Wall & R. Melzack (Eds.), *Textbook of pain* (4th ed., p. 447). Edinburgh: Churchill Livingstone.

28. Craig, A. D., & Dostrovsky, J. O. (1999). Medulla to thalamus. In P. D. Wall & R. Melzack (Eds.), *Textbook of pain* (4th ed., pp. 183–214). Edinburgh: Churchill Livingstone.

29. Craig, K. D. (1999). Emotions and psychobiology. In P. D. Wall & R. Melzack (Eds.), *Textbook of pain* (4th ed., pp. 331–343). Edinburgh: Churchill Livingstone.

30. Doubell, T. P., Mannion, R. J., & Woolf, C. J. (1999). The dorsal horn: State-dependent sensory processing, plasticity and the generation of pain. In P. D. Wall & R. Melzack (Eds.), *Textbook of pain* (4th ed., pp. 165–182). Edinburgh: Churchill Livingstone.

31. Dray, A. (1997). Kinins and their receptors in hyperalgesia. *Canadian Journal of Pharmacology, 75,* 704–712.

32. Dray, A., & Urban, L. (1996). New pharmacological strategies for pain relief. *Annual Review of Pharmacological Toxicology, 36,* 3–80.

33. Dyck, P. J., et al. (1997). Intradermal recombinant human nerve growth factor induces pressure allodynia and lowered heat-pain threshold in humans. *Neurology 48*(2), 501–505.

34. Eckes Peck, S. D. (1997). The effect of therapeutic touch for decreasing pain in elders with degenerative arthritis. *Journal of Holistic Nursing, 15,* 176–198.

35. Edwards, M. (1998, March/April). Barriers to effective pain/symptom control. *American Journal of Hospice and Palliative Care, 15*(2), 107–111.

36. Edwards, R. R., Fillingim, R. B., & Roger, B. (1999). Ethnic differences in thermal pain responses. *Psychosomatic Medicine, 61*(3), 346–354.

37. Ellermeier, W., & Westphal, W. (1995). Gender differences in pain ratings and pupil reactions to painful pressure stimuli. *Pain, 61,* 435–439.

38. Fields, H. L., & Basbaum, A. I. (1994). Central nervous system mechanisms of pain modulation. In P. Wall & R. Melzack (Eds.), *Textbook of pain* (3rd ed., pp. 243–257). New York: Churchill Livingstone.

39. Filshie, J., et al. (1996). Acupuncture for the relief of cancer-related breathlessness. *Palliative Medicine, 10*(2), 145–150.

40. Fine, P. G., & Ashburn, M. A. (1998). Functional neuroanatomy and nociception. In M. A. Ashburn and L. J. Rice (Eds.), *The Management of Pain* (pp. 1–16). New York: Churchill Livingstone.

41. Foley, K. M. (1995). Pain relief into practice: Rhetoric without reform. *Journal of Clinical Oncology, 13,* 2149–2151.

42. Furst, S. (1999). Transmitters involved in antinociception in the spinal cord. *Brain Research Bulletin, 48*(2), 129–141.

43. Gagliese, L., Katz, J., & Melzack, R. (1999). Pain in the elderly. In P. D. Wall & R. Melzack (Eds.), *Textbook of pain* (4th ed., pp. 991–1006). Edinburgh: Churchill Livingstone.

44. Gardner, E. P., & Martin, J. H. (2000). Coding of sensory information. In E. R. Kandel, J. H. Schwartz, & T. M. Jessell (Eds.), *Principles of neural science* (4th ed.). Norwalk, CT: Appleton & Lange.

45. Garro, L. C. (1990). Culture, pain and cancer. *Journal of Palliative Care, 6*(3), 34–44.

46. Geiss, G. S., et al. (1998). Safety and efficacy of celecoxib, a specific COX-2 inhibitor. *Rheumatology Europe 27(suppl 1),* 118.

47. Geis, G. S. (1999) Update on clinical developments with celecoxib, a new specific COX-2 inhibitor: What can we expect? *Journal of Rheumatology, 26*(Suppl 56), 31–36.

48. Gerdner, L. A., & Buckwalter, K. C. (1999). Music therapy. In G. M. Bulecheck & J. C. McCloskey (Eds.), *Nursing interventions: Effective nursing treatments* (3rd ed., pp. 451–468). Philadelphia: W. B. Saunders.

49. Good, M. (1995). A comparison of the effects of jaw relaxation and music on postoperative pain. *Nursing Symptom Management, 11*(4), 52–57.

50. Good, M. (1996). Effects of relaxation and music on postoperative pain: A review. *Journal of Advanced Nursing, 24,* 905–914.

51. Hawkey, C. J. (1999). COX-2 inhibitors. *The Lancet, 353,* 307–314.

52. Hawthorn, J., & Redmond, K. (1998). *Pain, causes and management.* Oxford, England, Blackwell Science.

53. Heitz, L., Symreng, T., & Scamman, F. L. (1992). Effect of music therapy in the postanesthetic care unit: A nursing intervention. *Journal of Post Anesthesia Nursing, 7,* 22–31.

54. Hille, B., & Catterall, W. A. (1999). Electrical excitability and ion channels. In G. J. Siegal, et al. (Eds.), *Basic neurochemistry: Molecular, cellular, and medical aspects,* (6th ed., pp. 119–138). Philadelphia: Lippincott–Williams & Wilkins.

55. Holz, R. W., & Fisher, S. K. (1999). Synaptic transmission and cellular signaling: An overview. In G. J. Siegal, et al. (Eds.), *Basic neurochemistry: Molecular, cellular and medical aspects* (pp. 191–212). Philadelphia: Lippincott–Williams & Wilkins.

56. Hutchison, C. P., et al. (1999). Body-mind-spirit: Healing touch: An energetic approach. *American Journal of Nursing, 99*(4), 43–48.

57. Insel, P. A. (1996). Analgesics-antipyretics and anti-inflammatory agents; Drugs employed in the treatment of gout. In J. G. Hardman & L. E. Limbird (Eds.), *The pharmacological basis of therapeutics* (9th ed., pp. 617–658), New York: Pergamon Press.

58. International Association for the Study of Pain (1986). Pain terms: A current list with definitions and notes on usage. *Pain, 3,* S216–S221.

59. Jacox, A., et al. (1994). *Management of cancer pain. Clinical practice guidelines No. 9.* AHCPR Publication No. 94-1592. Rockville, MD: Agency for Health Care Policy and Research, U.S. Department of Health and Human Services, Public Health Service.

60. Janssen, S. A., & Arntz, A. (1996). Anxiety and pain: Attentional and endorphinergic influences. *Pain, 66,* 145–150.

61. Jordan, M. S., Lumley, M. S., & Leisen, J. C. (1998). The relationships of cognitive coping and pain control beliefs to pain and adjustment among African-American and Caucasian women with rheumatoid arthritis. *Arthritis Care and Research, 11*(2), 80–88.

62. Juarez, G., Ferrell, B., & Borneman, T. (1998). Influence of culture on cancer pain management in Hispanic patients. *Cancer Practice, 6*(5), 262–269.

63. Juarez, G., Ferrell, B., & Borneman, T. (1999). Cultural considerations in education for cancer pain. *Journal of Cancer Education, 14*(3), 68–73.

64. Kandel, E. R., & Siegelbaum, S. A. (2000). Transmitter release. In E. R. Kandel, J. H. Schwartz, & T. M. Jessel (Eds.), *Principles of neural science* (4th ed., pp. 253–277). Norwalk, CT: Appleton & Lange.

65. Koester, J., & Siegelbaum, S. A. (2000). Membrane potential. In E. R. Kandel, J. H. Schwartz, & T. M. Jessel (Eds.), *Principles of neural science* (4th ed., pp. 125–139). Norwalk, CT: Appleton & Lange.

66. Kovacs, F. M., et al. (1997). Local and remote sustained trigger point therapy for exacerbations of chronic low back pain: A randomized, double-blind, controlled, multicenter trial. *Spine, 22*(7), 786–797.

67. Lander, J. (1990). Fallacies and phobias about addiction and pain. *British Journal of Addiction, 85,* 803–809.

68. Lefkowitz, M. (1998). Pain management in the HIV-positive patient. In M. A. Ashburn and L. J. Rice (Eds.), *The Management of Pain,* New York: Churchill Livingstone.

69. Levine, J. D., & Reichling, D. B. (1999). Peripheral mechanisms of inflammatory pain. In P. D. Wall and R. Melzack (Eds.), *Textbook of pain* (4th ed., pp. 59–84). Edinburgh, Churchill Livingstone.

70. Linton, S. J. (1999). Psychological factors. In I. K. Crombie, et al. (Eds.), *The epidemiology of pain.* Seattle: IASP Press (pp. 25–42).

71. Lundeberg, T. (1995). Pain physiology and principles of therapy. *Scandinavian Journal of Rehabilitation Medicine Supplement, 32,* 13–42.

72. Mains, R. E., & Epper, B. A. (1999). Peptides. In G. J. Siegal, et al. (Eds.), *Basic neurochemistry: Molecular, cellular and medical aspects.* Philadelphia: Lippincott–Williams & Wilkins.

73. Marks, R. M., & Sacher, E. J. (1973). Undertreatment of medical inpatients with narcotic analgesics. *Annals of Internal Medicine, 78,* 173–181.

74. Matz, A., & Brown, S. T. (1998). Humor and pain management. *Journal of Holistic Nursing, 16*(1), 68–75.

75. McCaffery, M., & Pasero, C. (1999). *Pain. Clinical Manual* (2nd ed). St. Louis, Mosby.

76. McCaffery, M., & Wolf, M. (1992). Pain relief using cutaneous modalities, positioning and movement. *Hospice Journal, 8,* 121–153.

77. Melzack, R., & Katz, J. (1999). Pain measurement in persons in pain. In P. D. Wall & R. Melzack (Eds.), *Textbook of pain* (4th ed., pp. 409–426). Edinburgh: Churchill Livingstone.

78. Melzack, R., & Wall, P. D. (1965). Pain mechanisms: A new theory. *Science, 150*(3699), 971–979.

79. Merskey, H., & Bogduk, N. (1994). *Classification of chronic pain: Descriptions of chronic pain syndromes and definitions of pain terms.* Seattle: IASP Press.

80. Michlovitz, S. (1996). The use of heat and cold in the management of rheumatic diseases. In S. L. Michlovitz (Ed.), *Thermal agents in rehabilitation* (2nd ed., pp. 258–274): Philadelphia: F. A. Davis.

81. Michlovitz, S. (1996). Cryotherapy: The use of cold as a therapeutic agent. In S. L. Michlovitz (Ed.), *Thermal agents in rehabilitation* (2nd ed., pp. 88–108). Philadelphia: F. A. Davis.

82. Millan, M. J. (1999). The induction of pain: An integrative review. *Progress in Neurobiology, 57*(1), 1–164.

83. Mobily, P. R., Herr, K. A., & Nicholson, A. C. (1994). Validation of cutaneous stimulation interventions for pain management. *International Journal of Nursing Studies, 31,* 533–544.

84. Moore, R., & Brodsgaard, I. (1999). Cross-cultural investigations of pain. In I. K. Crombie, et al. (Eds.), *Epidemiology of pain* (pp. 53–80). Seattle: IASP Press.

85. *NIH [National Institute of Health] Technological Assessment Statement* (1995, October 16–18). Integration of behavioral and relaxation approaches into the treatment of chronic pain and insomnia. 1–34.

86. Olsen, R. W., & DeLorey, T. M. (1999). GABA and glycine. In G. J. Siegal, et al. (Eds.), *Basic neurochemistry: Molecular, cellular and medical aspects* (pp. 335–346). Philadelphia: Lippincott–Williams & Wilkins.

87. Page, G. G., & Ben-Eliyakie, S. (1998). Pain kills: Animal models and neuroimmunological links. In R. Payne, et al. (Eds.), *Assessment and treatment of cancer pain: Progress in pain research and management* (Vol. 12, pp. 135–143). Seattle: IASP Press.

88. Paice, J. A. (1999). Pain. In C. H. Yarbo, et al. (Eds.), *Cancer symptom management* (2nd ed., pp. 118–144). Boston: Jones & Bartlett.

89. Palos, G. (1998). Culture and pain assessment in Hispanic patients. In R. Payne, et al. (Eds.), *Assessment and treatment of cancer pain: Progress in pain research and management* (Vol. 12, pp. 35–51). Seattle: IASP Press.

90. Papi, F., et al. (1995). Exposure to oscillating magnetic field influences sensitivity to electrical stimuli: II. Experiments on humans. *Bioelectromagnets, 16,* 295–300.

91. Payne R. (1998). Nonopioid analgesics for cancer pain: Update on clinical pharmacology. In R. Payne, et al. (Eds.), *Assessment and treatment of cancer pain: Progress in pain research and management* (Vol. 12, pp. 289–307). Seattle: IASP Press.

92. Payne, R., & Janjan, N. (1998). Management of metastatic bone pain. In R. Payne, et al. (Eds.), *Assessment and treatment of cancer pain: Progress in pain research and management* (Vol. 12, pp. 269–273). Seattle: IASP Press.

93. Perkins, M., & Dray, A. (1996). Novel pharmacological strategies for analgesia. *Annals of the Rheumatic Diseases, 55,* 715–722.

94. Portenoy, R. K. (1996). Opioid therapy for chronic nonmalignant pain: A review of the critical issues. *Journal of Pain and Symptom Management, 11,* 203–217.

95. Portenoy, R. K., & Lesage, P. (1999). Management of cancer pain. *The Lancet, 353,* 1695–1700.

96. Porter F. L., Grunau R. E., & Anand K. J. (1999). Long-term effects of pain in infants. *Journal of Developmental and Behavioral Pediatrics, 20*(4):253–261.

97. Price, D. D. (1996). Hypnotic analgesia: Psychological and neural mechanisms. In J. E. Berber (Ed.), *Hypnosis and suggestion in the treatment of pain: A clinical guide* (pp. 67–84). New York: W. W. Norton.

98. Price, D. D. (1999). Mechanisms of hypnotic analgesia. In *Psychological mechanisms of pain: Progress in pain research and management* (Vol. 15, pp. 183–204). Seattle: IASP Press.

99. Puntillo, K., & Weiss, S. J. (1994). Pain: Its mediators and associated morbidity in critically ill cardiovascular surgical clients. *Nursing Research, 43*(1), 31–36.

100. Raja, S. N., et al. (1999). Peripheral neural mechanisms of nociception. In P. D. Wall & R. Melzack (Eds.), *Textbook of pain* (4th ed., pp. 11–58). Edinburgh: Churchill Livingstone.

101. Ramnarine-Singh, S. (1999). The surgical significance of therapeutic touch. *AORN Journal, 69*(2), 358, 360–365, 367–369.

102. Rummans, T. A. (1994). Nonopioid agents for treatment of acute and subacute pain. *Mayo Clinic Proceedings, 69,* 481–490.

103. Shapiro, S. (1997). Neurotransmission by neurons that use serotonin, noradrenaline, glutamate, glycine and gamma-aminobutyric acid in normal and injured spinal cord. *Neurosurgery 40*(1), 168–177.

104. Siegelbaum, S. A., & Koester, J. (2000). Ion channels. In E. R. Kandel, J. H. Schwartz, & T. M. Jessell (Eds.), *Principles of neural science* (4th ed., pp. 104–124). Norwalk, CT: Appleton & Lange.

105. Simmonds, M. A. (1997). Pharmacotherapeutic management of cancer pain: Current practice. *Seminars in Oncology, 24*(5) *Suppl 16,* 516-1–516-6.

106. Simons, W., & Malabar, R. (1995). Assessing pain in elderly clients who cannot respond verbally. *Journal of Advanced Nursing, 22,* 663–669.

107. Singh, V. K., et al. (1997). Molecular biology of opioid receptors: Recent advances. *Neuroimmunomodulation, 4*(5–6), 285–297.

108. Sloan, P. A., et al. (1996). Cancer pain assessment and management by housestaff. *Pain, 67,* 475–481.

109. Spence, S. H., et al. (1995). Effects of EMG biofeedback compared to applied relaxation training with chronic, upper extremity cumulative trauma disorders. *Pain, 63*(2), 199–206.

110. Spross, J. A., McGuire, D. B., & Schmitt, R. M. (1990). Oncology Nursing Society position paper on pain: Part 1. *Oncology Nursing Forum, 17*(4), 595–614.

111. Spross, J. A., McGuire, D. B., & Schmitt, R. M. (1990). Oncology Nursing Society position paper on pain: Part 2. *Oncology Nursing Forum, 17*(5), 751–760.

112. Spross, J. A., McGuire, D. B., & Schmitt, R. M. (1990). Oncology Nursing Society position paper on pain: Part 3. *Oncology Nursing Forum, 17*(6), 943–947.

113. Staats, P. S. (1998). The pain mortality link: Unraveling the mysteries. In R. Payne, et al. (Eds.), *Assessment and treatment of cancer pain: Progress in pain research and management* (Vol. 12, pp. 145–156). Seattle: IASP Press.

114. Stephenson, J. (1996). Experts say AIDS pain 'dramatically undertreated.' *Journal of the American Medical Association, 276,* 1369–1370.

115. Sternbach, R. (1968). *Pain: A psychophysiological analysis.* New York: Academic Press.

116. Stimmel, B. (1997). *Pain and its relief without addiction: Clinical issues in the use of opioids and other analgesics.* New York, Haworth Medical Press.

117. Strand, F. L. (1999). *Neuropeptides: Regulators of physiological procedures.* Cambridge, MA: MIT Press.

118. Taylor, L. K., et al. (1998). The effect of music in the postanesthesia care unit on pain levels in women who have had abdominal hysterectomies. *Journal of Perianesthesia Nursing, 13*(2), 88–94.

119. Turk, D. C. (1999). A cognitive behavioral approach to pain management. In P. D. Wall & R. Melzack (Eds.), *Textbook of pain* (4th ed.), Edinburgh: Churchill Livingstone.

120. Turk, D. C., & Okifuji, A. (1998). Directions in prescriptive chronic pain management based on diagnostic characteristics of the client. In P. J. Vincent (Ed.), *American Pain Society Bulletin, 8*(5), 5–11.

121. Tusek, D., Church, J. M., & Fazio, V. W. (1997). Guided imagery as a coping strategy for perioperative clients. *AORN Journal, 66*(4), 644–649.

122. Urban, M. O., & Gebhart, G. F. (1999). Central mechanisms in pain. *Medical Clinics of North America, 83*(3), 585–596.

123. Vallerand, A. H. (1995). Gender differences in pain. *Image: Journal of Nursing Scholarship, 7*(3), 235–237.

124. Varcaccio-Garofalo, G., et al. (1995). Analgesic properties of electromagnetic field therapy in clients with chronic pelvic pain. *Clinical and Experimental Obstetrics and Gynecology, 22*(4), 350–354.

125. Watkins, G. R. (1997). Music therapy: Proposed physiological mechanisms and clinical implications. *Clinical Nurse Specialist, 11*(2), 43–50.

126. Watling, C. J. (1998). Management strategies for pain in the cancer patient. In M. A. Ashburn & L. J. Rice (Eds.), *The Management of Pain*. New York: Churchill Livingstone, 473–488.

127. Wall, P. (1999). Placebos. In P. D. Wall & R. Melzack (Eds.), *Textbook of pain* (4th ed., pp. 1419–1430). Edinburgh: Churchill Livingstone.

128. Weisenberg, M. (1999). Cognitive aspects of pain. In P. D. Wall & R. Melzack (Eds.), *Textbook of pain* (4th ed., pp. 345–358). Edinburgh: Churchill Livingstone.

129. Wilkie, D. J. (1995). Neural mechanisms of pain: A foundation for cancer pain assessment and management. In D. B. McGuire, C. H. Yarbro, & B. R. Ferrell (Eds.), *Cancer pain management* (2nd ed., pp. 61–87). Boston: Jones & Bartlett.

130. Williams, A. C., (1999). Measures of function and psychology. In P. D. Wall & R. Melzack (Eds.), *Textbook of pain* (4th ed., pp. 427–446). Edinburgh: Churchill Livingstone.

131. Willis, W. D., & Westlund, K. N. (1997). Neuroanatomy of the pain system and of the pathways that modulate pain. *Journal of Clinical Neurophysiology, 14*(1), 2–31.

132. Wong, D., & Baker, C. (1988). Pain in children: Comparison of assessment scales. *Pediatric Nursing, 14*(1), 9–17.

133. Woolf, C. J., & Mannion, R. J. (1999). Neuropathic pain: Aetiology, symptoms, mechanisms, and management. *The Lancet, 353,* 1959–1964.

134. World Health Organization (WHO). (1990). Cancer pain relief and palliative care. *Report of a WHO expert committee. Technical report series 804.* Geneva, Author.

135. Yaksh, T. L. (1999). Central pharmacology of nociception. In P. D. Wall & R. Melzack (Eds.), *Textbook of pain* (4th ed., pp. 253–308). Edinburgh: Churchill Livingstone.

CHAPTER 24

Clients with Substance Abuse Disorders: Promoting Positive Outcomes

Linda Carman Copel

NURSING OUTCOMES CLASSIFICATION (NOC)
for Nursing Diagnoses—Clients with Substance Abuse Disorders

Acute Confusion
Cognitive Ability
Distorted Thought Control
Information Processing
Memory
Neurologic Status: Consciousness
Altered Family Processes
Family Coping
Family Environment: Internal
Family Functioning
Family Normalization
Altered Nutrition: Less Than Body Requirements
Nutritional Status: Nutrient Intake
Altered Role Performance
Abuse Protection
Altered Sexuality Patterns
Abuse Recovery: Sexual
Body Image
Self-Esteem
Sexual Identity: Acceptance
Altered Thought Processes
Cognitive Orientation
Concentration
Decision-Making
Identity
Information Processing
Memory
Anxiety
Aggression Control
Anxiety Control
Coping
Impulse Control
Self-Mutilation Restraint
Chronic Low Self-Esteem
Self-Esteem
Body Image
Dysfunctional Grieving
Concentration
Coping

Family Coping
Grief Resolution
Psychosocial Adjustment: Life Change
Fatigue
Activity Tolerance
Endurance
Fear
Fear Control
Hopelessness
Decision-Making
Hope
Mood Equilibrium
Quality of Life
Impaired Social Interaction
Role Performance
Social Interaction Skills
Social Involvement
Impaired Verbal Communication
Communication Ability
Communication: Expressive Ability
Communication: Receptive Ability
Ineffective Denial
Fear Control
Health Beliefs: Perceived Threat
Coping
Ineffective Individual Coping
Aggression Control
Depression Control
Depression Level
Knowledge Deficit
Knowledge: Substance Abuse Control
Communication: Receptive Ability
Concentration
Noncompliance
Adherence Behavior
Compliance Behavior
Treatment Behavior: Illness or Injury
Pain
Personal Identity Disturbance
Identity

Self-Mutilation Restraint
Powerlessness
Depression Control
Depression Level
Family Participation in Professional Care
Risk for Impaired Skin Integrity
Self-Mutilation Restraint
Risk for Injury
Risk Control
Safety Behavior: Personal
Safety Status: Physical Injury
Risk for Poisoning
Risk Control: Drug Use
Risk for Trauma
Risk Control
Safety Status: Physical Injury
Risk for Violence
Abuse Protection
Abusive Behavior Self-Control
Aggression Control
Distorted Thought Control
Impulse Control
Risk Control: Alcohol Use
Risk Control: Drug Use
Risk Detection
Sensory and Perceptual Alterations
Anxiety Control
Body Image
Distorted Thought Process
Sleep Pattern Disturbance
Sleep
Social Isolation
Loneliness
Mood Equilibrium
Social Interaction Skills
Social Involvement
Social Support
Spiritual Distress
Hope

As the client passed through the hospital door, it was the beginning—the first step of many on the journey back from the world of drugs and alcohol. No longer need this person be entangled in the cycle of pain, ineffective coping with addictive substances, more pain, and more drugs. The client, struggling to think clearly, had the following thoughts: "I must be dying. My body hurts. Where am I? What is going on here? How did this happen? I can't stand it. What are they doing to me? They can't help me. I can't help me. No one can help me. My life has always been a mess. There is nothing I can do."

Clients with psychoactive substance abuse disorders struggle with an inability to solve problems. They are unable to use adaptive behaviors to handle life stresses, traumas, and demands. *Ineffective Coping, Defensive Coping, Denial, Altered Nutrition, Risk of Injury,* and *Risk for Infection* are a few of the nursing diagnoses specific to the assessment data obtained from these clients. Nurses are challenged by the myriad of physical and emotional health problems faced by clients with addiction. Their health histories and at-risk behaviors culminate in problems ranging from liver and cardiovascular disease to depression and human immunodeficiency virus (HIV). The client's physical condition is further compromised by nutritional deficits and fluid and electrolyte imbalances. In addition, many clients suffer from injuries, either self-inflicted trauma or violence at the hands of others. Often, multiple injuries in various stages of healing are evident upon examination.

Underlying the physical problems are the emotional wounds from both past and present life situations. Without effective coping skills, clients tend to repeat their self-destructive pattern of behavior over and over. The inability to perceive reality accurately and to develop and maintain supportive relationships hinders successful lifestyle changes. Accelerating bouts of depression and feelings of powerlessness continue, perpetuating a sense of incompetence. A pervasive sense of failure may be overwhelming.

Studies consistently show that substance-abusing clients need both medical and psychiatric nursing care to achieve their highest level of functioning and to maintain sobriety. Nurses have the challenge of dealing not only with the addicted client's many physiologic problems but also with the effects and withdrawal symptoms of the drugs involved. Even as you seek to assess and diagnose the physiologic effects of abused substances, clients typically offer defensiveness and may remain in denial. These clients' lack responsibility for their personal behavior. Constantly blaming and manipulating of others are typical behaviors that require your attention and intervention along with the physiologic issues. As much as any client population, this one challenges the entire health care team to provide holistic treatment for physical, emotional, and spiritual needs.

FRAMEWORKS FOR EXPLAINING ADDICTIVE BEHAVIORS

Over the past 100 years, clinicians and researchers have attempted to develop and refine the knowledge base on substance-abusing people. Early studies of alcoholism noted generational patterns of alcoholism in families. On the basis of this observation, it was suggested that alcoholism might have a genetic component. However, there is no evidence to support this supposition with other commonly abused drugs.[11, 19, 22, 31]

Various explanations of the causes of substance abuse have focused on three conceptual frameworks:

- Biologic
- Psychological
- Sociocultural

However, there is no one identifiable cause of substance use. Rather, a combination of factors typically coalesces to produce drug use patterns. A person may be at risk for substance abuse because of a complex combination of biologic, psychological, and sociocultural variables. All aspects of the client's background must be considered when treatment is initiated. In addition to what the client brings to the treatment setting, the theoretical approach used by the team to view the underlying dynamics of substance abuse influences the process of recovery.

■ BIOLOGIC FRAMEWORK

The biologic theory, or disease concept, of substance abuse views addiction as a physiologic condition that can be identified and treated. The emphasis is on a physiologic cause, such as genetic predisposition, defects in metabolism, neurobiologic abnormalities, or abnormal levels of chemicals in the body.[38] Historically, studies attempting to link genetic transmission of alcoholism have been unable to find a target gene.

Present research focuses on examining the inherited biochemical abnormalities that may predispose an individual to alcoholism.[5] It is now believed that alcohol dependence is a combination of interwoven social and psychological variables in people who are physiologically vulnerable.[30] For example, people of East Asian ancestry tend to experience a physical reaction to alcohol characterized by tachycardia, a sensation of warmth and flushing, and generalized discomfort. The response is believed to be related to the lack of activation of the enzyme aldehyde dehydrogenase, resulting in the accumulation of acetaldehyde, a toxic product of alcohol metabolism.[5, 37] This physiologic process may be the reason that Asian Americans tend to have the lowest rate of alcohol consumption and associated substance use problems compared with other racial groups.[34] Hence, an examination of biologic differences associated with the use of alcohol warrants continued investigation.

■ PSYCHOLOGICAL FRAMEWORK

Psychological theories attempt to explain the variables that may predispose someone to substance use. According to the psychoanalytic model, the person is viewed as being fixated at the oral stage of development, seeking gratification of needs through behaviors such as drinking. With the psychodynamic approach, a person experiences both interpersonal and intrapersonal difficulties that provide the foundation for the addiction.

Behavioral theories regard addiction as a learned behavior that can be unlearned in a manner similar to that of changing negative habits or dysfunctional behaviors. A *family systems approach* emphasizes that relationships, roles, and unhealthy communication patterns among family members contribute to addictive behaviors; this dysfunctional lifestyle is transmitted to future generations.[14]

For years, researchers and clinicians have sought, without success, to discover an addictive personality type. Some common characteristics noted in clients who abuse substances are low self-esteem, low frustration tolerance, inability to cope with physical and emotional pain, depression, lack of healthy relationships, and involvement in high-risk behaviors. Proponents of the psychological theories believe that people engage in substance use in an attempt to feel better about themselves and to meet their emotional needs. Thus, the use of a psychoactive substance becomes reinforced and eventually evolves into an addiction.

■ SOCIOCULTURAL FRAMEWORK

With the sociocultural theories, substance use is viewed from the perspective of cultural and social norms within various groups in society. The issues of whether to use drugs, what type of drugs to use, and how and when to use them are determined by factors in a person's background. Such factors may include values, belief systems, spiritual orientation, ethnicity, sex, family standards, or the contemporary social environment. The relationships

between these variables can contribute to a person's susceptibility to drug use and potential for addiction treatment and ongoing recovery.

DEFINITIONS AND TERMINOLOGY

According to the *Diagnostic and Statistical Manual of Mental Disorders,* fourth edition (*DSM-IV*),[2] the substance-related disorders comprise the range of substance use from taking a drug of abuse, to the adverse effects of any medication, to exposure to toxic substances. *DSM-IV* lists 11 types of substances commonly abused: alcohol, amphetamines, caffeine, cannabis, cocaine, hallucinogens, inhalants, nicotine, opioids, phencyclidine (PCP), and the group "sedatives, hypnotics, or anxiolytics."[2] Polysubstance dependence and other substance-related disorders, particularly toxins or prescribed and over-the-counter medications, are also included.[2]

To understand and assess substance abuse, you must learn the associated terminology (Table 24–1). In working with clients who are actively using substances, you must also know the types of drugs commonly used, the major routes of administration, and side effects (Table 24–2). The order and severity of manifestations are influ-

TABLE 24–1	SUBSTANCE ABUSE TERMS AND DEFINITIONS
Term	**Definition**
Psychoactive substance	A substance that affects a person's mood or behavior
Substance abuse	Continued use of a psychoactive substance despite the occurrence of physical, psychological, social, or occupational problems
Substance dependence	A range of physiologic, behavioral, and cognitive symptoms indicating that a person persists in using the substance, ignoring serious substance-related problems
Physiologic dependence	The body's physical adaptation to a drug, whereby withdrawal symptoms occur if the drug is not used
Psychological dependence	The emotional need or craving for a drug either for its effect or to prevent the occurrence of withdrawal symptoms
Addiction	A compulsion, loss of control, and progressive pattern of drug use, characterized by behavioral changes, impaired thinking, unkept promises to stop usage, obsession with the drug, neglect of personal needs, decreased tolerance, and physiologic deterioration
Polysubstance abuse	Concurrent use of multiple drugs
Intoxication	An altered physiologic state resulting from the use of a psychoactive drug
Overdose	Accidental or deliberate consumption of a drug in a dose larger than is ordinarily used, resulting in a serious toxic reaction or death
Tolerance	State resulting from metabolic changes in cell functions, whereby the tissue reaction to a drug declines and the person needs to take increasing amounts to achieve the same effect
Cross-tolerance	State whereby the effect of a drug is decreased and greater amounts are required to achieve the desired effect because the person has become tolerant to a similar drug
Predisposition	Any factor that increases the likelihood of an event occurring
Potentiation	The ability of one drug to increase the activity of another drug when taken at the same time
Drug misuse	Any use of a drug that deviates from medical or socially acceptable use
Dual diagnosis	The coexistence of a major psychiatric illness and a psychoactive substance abuse disorder
Blackout	An acute situation in which a person experiences a period of memory loss for actions as a direct result of using drugs or alcohol
Withdrawal	Discontinuation of a substance by a person who is dependent on it
Detoxification	The process of withdrawing a person from an addictive substance in a safe manner
Toxic dose	The amount of a drug that produces a poisonous effect
Recidivism	The tendency to relapse into a former pattern of substance use and associated behaviors
Recovery	Return to a normal state of health, whereby the person does not engage in problematic behavior and continues to meet life's challenges and personal goals
Sobriety	Complete abstinence from drugs while developing a satisfactory lifestyle
Abstinence	Voluntarily refraining from activities or use of substances that cause problems in the physiologic, psychological, social, intellectual, and spiritual arenas of a person's life

TABLE 24-2 CHARACTERISTIC EFFECTS OF ABUSE OF MAJOR SUBSTANCES

Drug Classification and Street Names (Route of Administration)	Effects*
Alcohol (Oral)	Relaxation and sedation Decreased inhibition Lack of coordination Unsteady gait Slurred speech Nausea and vomiting Transient visual, tactile, or auditory hallucinations Anxiety Psychomotor agitation High risk of permanent liver or brain damage
Amphetamines (Oral, injected, smoked) Dexedrine Methamphetamine "Ice" "Uppers" "Crank" "Speed"	Grandiosity Hypervigilance Hypertension or hypotension Tachycardia or bradycardia Mydriasis (dilated pupils) Euphoria Appetite suppression Personality changes Antisocial behavior Psychosis similar to paranoid schizophrenia
Caffeine (Oral)	Stimulation of senses Alertness and enhanced performance Anxiety and restlessness Flushed face Talkativeness Tremors or muscle twitching Tachycardia or cardiac arrhythmias Insomnia Irritation of the stomach
Cannabis (Smoked, oral) Marijuana "Grass" "Pot" "Hash" "Weed"	Mild intoxication Increased appetite Dry mouth Lack of coordination Impaired judgment and memory Sexual arousal Tachycardia Visual hallucinations
Cocaine (Oral, injected, inhaled) "Coke" "Crack" "Snow" "Blow" "Lady" "Powder"	Talkativeness Grandiosity Hypervigilance Anxiety Impaired judgment Tachycardia or bradycardia Hypertension or hypotension Mydriasis Muscle twitching Respiratory depression Hallucinations, paranoid delusions, or paranoia Formication (sensation of insects crawling on the skin) Personality changes Antisocial behavior Euphoria followed by depression and feeling let down
Hallucinogens (Oral, inhaled) Lysergic acid diethylamide (LSD) "Acid" Peyote Psilocybin Mescaline	Intensified perceptions and feelings Synesthesia (seeing sounds or hearing colors) Visual, auditory, or tactile hallucinations Fear of losing one's mind Mydriasis Tachycardia Palpitations Blurred vision Dizziness, weakness, and tremors Altered perceptions (flashbacks) Impaired judgment and bizarre behavior Mood swings and psychosis-like symptoms

TABLE 24–2	CHARACTERISTIC EFFECTS OF ABUSE OF MAJOR SUBSTANCES *Continued*

Drug Classification and Street Names (Route of Administration)	Effects*

Inhalants (Inhaled)
    Spray can propellants
    Paint
    Paint thinner
    Glue
    Gasoline
    Cleaning fluid
	Euphoria and giddiness
	Headache
	Dizziness, fatigue, or drowsiness
	Nystagmus (involuntary rapid eye movements)
	Unsteady gait or tremors
	Slurred speech
	Blurred vision or diplopia (double vision)
	Damage to major organs: lungs, liver, and kidneys
	Cardiac arrest

Nicotine (Inhaled, oral)	Tachycardia Vasoconstriction Irritation of oral mucosa Persistent cough Damaged alveoli and bronchioli Emphysema High risk of oral, laryngeal, or lung cancer

Opioids (Oral, injected, inhaled)
    Morphine
    Codeine
    Methadone
    Hydromorphone (Dilaudid)
    Heroin
    "Smack"
    "Horse"
	Immediate euphoria followed by dysphoria
	Psychomotor retardation or agitation
	Slurred speech
	Impaired judgment and memory
	Sedation and respiratory depression
	Constricted pupils
	Decreased sexual and aggressive drives

Phencyclidine (PCP) (Oral, injected, inhaled)
    "Angel dust"
    "Hog"
	Grandiosity and illusions of strength
	Impulsiveness
	Psychomotor agitation
	Assaultive behavior
	Decreased sensory awareness
	Hypertension and tachycardia
	Unsteady gait and lack of coordination
	Nystagmus
	Mood swings and paranoia

Sedatives, Hypnotics, and Anxiolytics (Oral, injected)
    Benzodiazepine (e.g., diazepam (Valium),
        alprazolam (Xanax), chlordiazepoxide (Librium))
    Secobarbital (Seconal)
    Pentobarbital (Nembutal)
    Methaqualone (Quaalude)
	Incoordination and unsteady gait
	Slurred speech
	Nystagmus
	Sedation
	Inappropriate sexual behavior and aggressive drives
	Impaired judgment
	Mood swings

*Drug effects are arranged in order of severity of effect, with prolonged use or a high dose of the drug associated with appearance of the later effects.

From Copel, L. C. (2000). *Nurses' clinical guide to psychiatric and mental health care.* (2nd ed.). Springhouse, PA: Springhouse.

enced by the size of the dose and the length of time the drug has been used.

GENERAL ASSESSMENT

The purposes of a drug and alcohol assessment are to:

- Determine whether substance abuse exists
- Evaluate the relationship between substance abuse and other health care problems
- Implement effective health promotion and health restoration interventions

All clients must be assessed for the use and misuse of chemical substances. Clients who struggle with addiction are found at all stages of life and therefore in all

clinical specialties. It is common for a client who abuses drugs to be hospitalized for an injury, illness, or surgical procedure. The nurse-generalist must identify clients with actual or potential substance problems (see Bridge to Home Health Care: Addressing Substance Use) and institute a collaborative team approach to provide health care.

The ability of nurses to provide care is influenced by the personal thoughts and feelings about substance abuse and the people who become addicts. Self-awareness about substance use and abuse is essential if the nurse is to establish a therapeutic relationship and provide treatment. The Seaman-Mannello Scale, a Likert-type scale that assesses nurses' attitudes toward alcohol and alcoholism, and the National Council on Alcoholism and Drug Dependence Scale can provide insight about personal values

BRIDGE TO HOME HEALTH CARE

Addressing Substance Use

Substance use is a prevalent problem, regardless of a person's age, gender, and social, economic, professional, or educational status. Nurses in community settings must collaborate with clients to prevent, screen, detect, and deal with abuse. Examples of strategies include the use of direct conversation, monitoring behavior changes, observing the environment, and providing education and referrals.

Use active listening skills consistently when you meet with clients in their homes or other informal community settings. By asking clients about their past use of substances and about substances used by their family and friends, you can gain accurate information about the client's history and current status. Often, you will be able to note changes in the client's behavior, social interactions, and lifestyle. Alcohol containers and the odor of marijuana are additional signs. When substance use is confirmed by the client and when it is suspected but denied, reassess frequently and ask questions that address the behaviors or signs observed.

It is even more critical to identify people who have substance use problems when the quality of life for others is endangered. Directly asking a pregnant woman, "How much alcohol have you consumed during the past month of your pregnancy?" allows a straightforward, honest answer. If alcohol use is detected, first give a clear message that there is no safe level of alcohol use during pregnancy, then offer assistance. When pregnant women consume alcohol, they expose their unborn children to potential birth defects, permanent brain damage, and a lifetime of physical, mental, and emotional impairments.

Provide detailed information about the effects of substances on their unborn child, such as abnormal facial features, slow growth, mental retardation, attention deficit and hyperactive disorders, learning disabilities, and problems with daily living skills. The effects of substance use are clearly seen in children growing up with *fetal alcohol syndrome* (FAS) and *fetal alcohol effects* (FAE).

School-aged children give signals that substance use is present in the home. Identify children who are often late to school or absent, whose parents miss appointments with teachers or physicians, and who may be withdrawn or show a sudden behavior change. Collaborate with the school social worker or school nurse, arrange a meeting with the parents, and assess the home situation further.

Often, adolescents use substances habitually because of peer pressure. Assist schools in writing and promoting curricula that incorporate clear and consistent messages about the dangers of drinking and driving.

The community health nurse is a source of ongoing support who can provide reassurance, education, information, and home visits for clients. When substance use is detected, offer clients appropriate resources and counseling services. Examples of resources include local inpatient or outpatient treatment programs and Alcoholics Anonymous. Suggest specific programs, such as classes for pregnant women using alcohol and support groups for families who have children with FAS. In addition, become informed about and follow mandatory reporting statutes that apply to pregnant women using substances. Such laws exist in many states.

Jill E. Timm, RN, PHN, BAN, *Public Health Nurse II, Washington County Department of Public Health and Environment, Sillwater, Minnesota*

and beliefs regarding substances.[29] Nurses can also examine their attitudes and their own use of drugs and alcohol by considering the questions of how, when, where, and under what conditions they use them.

Individual beliefs about drug and alcohol use come from the nurse's family background and previous knowledge about and experience with addicted people. This information allows nurses to anticipate their response patterns toward this group of clients. If nurses know their feelings and beliefs, they will be able to recognize a judgmental attitude, rejecting behaviors, or enabling behaviors. This knowledge can prevent the nurse from being drawn into power struggles regarding the client's manipulative behavior.

In addition to self-assessment measures for nurses some instruments allow the nurse to gain information about the client's drug and alcohol use (Box 24–1). To use a tool as part of the assessment process, the nurse must know how to score the instrument and how to correctly interpret the findings.

Interviewing the substance abuse client presents a challenge because of the client's tendency to deny or minimize the problem. A comprehensive assessment includes the client's history and physical examination. The previously mentioned screening tools can be helpful. Laboratory studies address cardiac, liver, kidney, and respiratory

functioning as well as urine toxicology. A thorough mental status assessment is a requisite part of the examination. The major components of this assessment are listed in Table 24–3.

BOX 24–1 Examples of Substance Use Screening Tools

For Use with Adults

- Michigan Alcoholism Screening Test (MAST)[33]
- Short Michigan Alcoholism Screening Test (SMAST)[34]
- Addiction Severity Index[24]
- CAGE Questions[12]
- T-ACE (a modified version of the CAGE used with pregnant women)[36]
- Alcohol Use Disorders Identification Test (AUDIT)[28]
- Alcohol Dependence Scale[35]
- Self-Administered Alcoholism Screening Test (SAAST)[39]
- Alcohol Use Inventory[18]

For Use with Adolescents

- Guided Rational Adolescent Substance Abuse Profile (GRASP)[1]
- Problem Severity Scales for Assessment of Alcohol and Drug Abuse[17]

TABLE 24–3	COMPONENTS OF THE MENTAL STATUS ASSESSMENT
General appearance	Appearance versus stated age Grooming and hygiene Posture, gait, and station Interaction during the interview Facial expressions Orientation or level of consciousness
Motor behavior	Restlessness Agitation Lethargy Tremors
Speech	Clarity and coherence of speech Rate of speech Volume and intonation Barriers to communication, such as confusion or delusions Vocabulary appropriate to socioeconomic background
Affect	Flat or labile
Mood	Euphoric, anxious, fearful
Thought processes	Thoughts presented as normal, concrete, scattered, or illogical Delusions—a false belief that is firmly maintained despite evidence to the contrary
Perception	Awareness of self and environment Illusions—misinterpretation of external stimuli Hallucinations—sensory experiences with no external stimuli present
Memory	Memory for remote, recent, and immediate past General knowledge level Ability to calculate Ability to think abstractly Insight Judgment or problem-solving ability

Attention is paid to the psychosocial evaluation, especially the components that address difficulties in family, occupational, social, or leisure functioning. Some clinicians recommend that after the history and physical examination are completed, the health care provider should take a specific drug and alcohol history that asks about drug usage for the 11 major psychoactive substances in addition to other prescription and over-the-counter substances.[10] Components of a drug and alcohol history are listed in Box 24–2.

Although all clients need to be assessed for substance abuse, of special concern are those who by virtue of lifestyle or social conditions may be at increased risk. Adolescents, women (particularly pregnant women), racial and ethnic minorities, homosexual women and men, clients with HIV infection or acquired immunodeficiency syndrome (AIDS), homeless people, older adults, and health care professionals are identified as populations requiring special prevention, treatment, and education about substance abuse.[4, 7] Extra attention must be given to clients with chronic physical or mental illnesses.

Self-medication can occur in vulnerable populations as a coping strategy to relieve physical and emotional pain associated with a chronic illness. After obtaining a comprehensive assessment, you may discover that a client struggles with polysubstance abuse. Such clients require specialized care during the withdrawal process according to the combination of drugs used.

ASSESSMENT AND MANAGEMENT OF SUBSTANCE-ABUSING CLIENTS

The immediate result of overconsumption of any psychoactive substance is acute intoxication. Nurses in an emergency department or a medical-surgical setting may care for clients suffering from trauma as a direct result of acute intoxication. In addition to treating the client's injuries, the nursing care of intoxication consists of monitoring vital signs, especially respiratory status, because respiratory depression or arrest can occur. Be vigilant for manifestations of shock, cardiac dysrhythmias, electrolyte imbalances, or subdural hematomas. Typically, intravenous (IV) fluids are given to prevent dehydration. Some people become intoxicated but do not seek medical intervention because no injuries or emergencies bring them to health care facilities.

When a person sharply reduces or stops use of a psychoactive substance, the process of *withdrawal* occurs. Depending on the drug, withdrawal may begin within 8 to 12 hours or be delayed for 1 to 3 days. Prompt recognition of withdrawal symptoms can promote client safety and prevent complications. Factors that influence the withdrawal process include (1) the specific drug used, (2) the dose taken, (3) the method of intake, (4) the time of last use, and (5) the length of time during which the drug has been used. You must also consider the client's overall health, particularly the functioning of the kidneys, lungs, and liver—the principal organs that metabolize and excrete drugs. An overview of common withdrawal symptoms for alcohol and other substances appears in Table 24–4.

■ ALCOHOL

Ethyl alcohol (ethanol), a central nervous system (CNS) depressant, is found in alcoholic beverages. The ingested alcohol is absorbed directly into the bloodstream from the

BOX 24–2	Components of a Drug and Alcohol History

- How often the drug was used (past and recent use)
- Age at first use
- Duration of use
- Age at last use
- Method of use
- Quantity used
- Initial and current reactions to the drug
- How the drug was obtained or how use of the drug was supported
- What has been done to reduce drug use
- Client's perception of use of the drug as a problem
- Use of drug related to any health problems

Drug Classification	Major Withdrawal Symptoms
Alcohol	Nausea and vomiting Tremors and weakness Sweating Tachycardia Hypertension Delusions Agitated behavior Hallucinations and nocturnal illusions
Amphetamines	Dysphoria Disorientation Fatigue and depression with suicidal potential Disturbed sleep and unpleasant dreams Hallucinations or delusions
Caffeine	Irritability and nervousness Inability to concentrate Headache Tremors Lethargy
Cannabis	No acute withdrawal symptoms; other symptoms appear over varying time periods following withdrawal Amotivational syndrome (inability to concentrate or complete tasks) Chronic respiratory problems Memory and learning difficulty Suppressed prolactin and testosterone levels
Cocaine	Severe craving for drug Severe depression ("postcoke blues") Fatigue Psychomotor agitation or retardation Anxiety Insomnia or hypersomnia Increased appetite
Hallucinogens	Symptoms appear over varying time periods following withdrawal Apprehension, fear, or panic Hyperactivity Sweating Tachycardia Altered perceptions (flashbacks) Perceptual distortions, especially hallucinations
Inhalants	Symptoms appear over varying time periods following withdrawal Central nervous system damage (cerebral atrophy or peripheral neuropathies) Acute or chronic renal failure Bone marrow depression Cardiac dysrhythmias Respiratory damage (lung or sinus damage, pneumonitis, emphysema, respiratory depression) Liver disease (hepatitis, cirrhosis)
Nicotine	Irritability and nervousness Headache Inability to concentrate Craving for cigarettes Fatigue and dizziness Tremors and palpitations
Opioids	Dysphoria Anxiety Insomnia Increased respirations and yawning Sweating Lacrimation and rhinorrhea (nasal discharge) Tremors and muscle twitching Mydriasis (dilated pupils) Piloerection (erection of the hair) Nausea, abdominal cramps, and vomiting

TABLE 24–4	COMMON WITHDRAWAL SYMPTOMS ASSOCIATED WITH PSYCHOACTIVE DRUGS *Continued*
Drug Classification	**Major Withdrawal Symptoms**
Phencyclidine (PCP)	Symptoms may appear over varying time periods following withdrawal Anxiety Withdrawn, catatonic state Hypertension Seizures Bizarre behavior and speech associated with temporary psychosis
Sedatives, hypnotics, and anxiolytics	Anxiety Sweating Tachycardia Tremors Nausea and vomiting Insomnia and disturbing dreams Transient visual, auditory, or tactile hallucinations Seizures

*See Box 24–6, Resources.
From Copel, L. C. (2000). *Nurses' clinical guide to psychiatric and mental health care.* (2nd ed.). Springhouse, PA: Springhouse.

stomach and proximal part of the small intestine. Because alcohol is water-soluble, it circulates easily throughout the body and readily passes through the blood-brain barrier. Approximately 95% of alcohol is metabolized in the liver, with the remaining 5% being excreted through the lungs, kidneys, and skin.[26] The body's mechanism for oxidizing alcohol is accomplished through the liver enzyme alcohol dehydrogenase. This process breaks down the alcohol to acetaldehyde, which is further broken down to acetic acid. Acetic acid then goes through the citric acid cycle to become carbon dioxide and water. From this chemical process, it is evident that alcohol can affect every aspect of the body. A growing number of young people may be using alcohol to enhance a drug's effect.

A blood alcohol level (BAL) test is used to measure the concentration of alcohol in the blood. The purpose of the test is to detect and estimate the level of alcohol in the brain. The legal intoxication level in most states is 100 mg/dl (0.10%); in a few states, it is 0.08%.

Although some studies suggest that small amounts of alcohol can be harmless or even healthful, large amounts produce a predictable series of deleterious effects. After drinking one or two alcoholic beverages, a person experiences a depression of the inhibitory regions of the brain that manage judgment, self-control, speech, and motor coordination. Alcohol is classified as a CNS depressant that affects all levels of the brain, starting with the reticular activating system and the cerebral cortex. Alcohol suppresses the inhibitory neurotransmitter gamma-aminobutyric acid (GABA). When the release of GABA is decreased, the initial results are an excitement or euphoric response.

With acute alcohol intoxication, alcohol continues to accumulate in the brain, resulting in depression of the cerebral cortex, cerebellum, and midbrain. In severe brain depression, disruption of the spinal reflexes, respiratory system, cardiac functioning, or temperature regulation occurs. At this point, the intoxicated person may become unconscious, and without treatment death may occur.

Early clinical manifestations of alcohol withdrawal (e.g., tremors, anorexia, anxiety, restlessness, insomnia) tend to occur within 6 to 8 hours after the last drink is ingested. During the next 2 to 3 days, the client may further experience disorientation, nightmares, abdominal pain, nausea, diaphoresis, and elevations in temperature, pulse, and blood pressure along with visual and auditory hallucinations. *Delirium tremens* (DTs) is a manifestation of severe alcohol withdrawal or its life-threatening complications. The client with DTs is at risk for cardiac dysrhythmias, hypertension, increased respirations, profuse sweating, delusions, and hallucinations.

Many clients are given medications to decrease the incidence of withdrawal manifestations and to prevent DTs. The benzodiazepines are commonly used because they cause less respiratory depression and hypertension compared with other drugs. Typically, the physician orders either a long-acting benzodiazepine (diazepam [Valium] or chlordiazepoxide [Librium]) or a short-acting benzodiazepine (lorazepam [Ativan] or oxazepam [Serax]). The long-acting benzodiazepines are often used to facilitate the withdrawal process; the short-acting benzodiazepines are used for clients with severe liver dysfunction or a high degree of cognitive impairment.

Since 1995, the drug naltrexone hydrochloride (ReVia) has been approved for the treatment of alcoholism. It has been successful in decreasing the craving for alcohol and, together with the client's participation in a recovery program, facilitates client compliance with treatment. The drug was originally intended to treat clients undergoing opioid detoxification. According to the manufacturer, the mechanisms of action for naltrexone in alcoholism are not completely known. However, because the drug is an opioid receptor antagonist, it blocks the effects of opioid drugs by its competitive site binding. The relatively few side effects of the drug are nausea, fatigue, dizziness, headache, anxiety, and insomnia. Contraindications include hepatitis, liver disease, and liver failure.[14]

Treatment with naltrexone is controversial because taking the drug conflicts with the Alcoholics Anonymous (AA) model of total abstinence from alcohol and being "drug-free." The use of any drug is seen as a "crutch" or a substitution for the alcohol. For philosophical and political reasons, some clients taking naltrexone are excluded from receiving support and the other benefits of participating in AA.

There are also nonpharmacologic approaches to treating withdrawal. The *social model,* or the nonmedicinal treatment model, incorporates the use of an extensive physical examination, followed by close medical supervision during therapy. Several studies have shown that approximately 75% of the clients enrolled in these programs improve.[27, 41]

The major nursing interventions for a client experiencing withdrawal focus on the continuous monitoring of manifestations and promoting a safe, calm, and comfortable environment. During the withdrawal period, clients need reassurance and support because they may feel that they will not survive the ordeal of detoxification. In the immediate period after the withdrawal syndrome has ceased, you can refer the client for further assessment and treatment of addiction or its complications. At this time, especially after what the client has been through, address with the client the relationship between drug use and the concomitant acute or chronic physical health problems. Common medical consequences of alcohol abuse are identified in Table 24–5.

■ AMPHETAMINES

Amphetamines have been used to treat *narcolepsy* (sudden sleep) and *attention deficit hyperactivity disorder* (ADHD). People often use amphetamines illegally to remain awake and alert, to increase their ability to perform physical tasks, or to produce a state of euphoria (a "high"). The abuse of amphetamines, according to the National Institute on Drug Abuse, is most common in the 18- to 34-year-old age group.[19] The pattern of abuse tends to be one of daily chronic use or periodic binges that end with the user overwhelmed by exhaustion ("crashing").

Amphetamines stimulate the CNS and accelerate heart and brain activity. Amphetamines block the reuptake of dopamine and norepinephrine by interfering with the transport protein, ultimately causing accumulation of dopamine and norepinephrine at the synapses.[20] Amphetamines are metabolized by the liver enzymes and excreted in the urine. In some cases, after continual drug use, half of the drug may be excreted from the body unchanged.[7]

With amphetamine intoxication, the clinical findings may include cardiac dysrhythmias, hypertension, fever, labile emotions, paranoia, delusions, panic reactions, and psychosis. For client management, perform frequent assessment of vital signs and basic body functioning and provide safe, supportive care. Closely monitor the client for changes in cardiac or neurologic status, because myocardial infarction and cerebral hemorrhage have occurred after amphetamine use. Antipsychotic agents may be used to decrease CNS stimulation, or sedatives may be given. IV amino acids may be given to speed up the detoxification process of stimulant drugs.[3]

Amphetamines commonly cause psychological dependence, often with craving behavior. Abrupt cessation of

TABLE 24–5	MEDICAL CONSEQUENCES OF ALCOHOL ABUSE
Body System	**Consequences**
Cardiac	Dysrhythmias Hypertension Cardiomyopathy Heart failure Beriberi heart disease
Gastrointestinal	Gastritis Gastric or duodenal ulcers Perforated gastrointestinal ulcers Esophageal varices Pancreatitis Interference with absorption of vitamin B$_{12}$, thiamine, and folic acid Malabsorption syndrome Alteration in nutrition, with potential for malnutrition Wernicke-Korsakoff syndrome Enlarged or fatty liver Liver enzyme changes Cirrhosis Alcoholic hepatitis Portal hypertension Ascites Hepatic encephalopathy
Hematopoietic	Anemia Thrombocytopenia Leukopenia Capillary fragility Spider nevi Palmar erythema
Neurologic	Peripheral neuropathy Brain atrophy
Musculoskeletal	Myopathy Decreased bone density with risk of fracture Fractured bones related to trauma
Immune	Depressed immune system Increased susceptibility to infections
Respiratory	Altered respirations Chronic obstructive pulmonary disease Pneumonia Tuberculosis
Endocrine	Testicular atrophy Gynecomastia Irregular menses Decreased libido Hypoglycemia Alcoholic ketoacidosis

the drug can precipitate anxiety, agitation, severe depression, hyperphagia, and hypersomnolence. An amphetamine psychosis may occur after continuous high doses. Nursing care focuses on (1) providing rest, (2) orienting the client as necessary, (3) monitoring for both physical and emotional changes, and (4) intervening to prevent complications of adverse effects or withdrawal symptoms.

■ CAFFEINE

In the United States, caffeine—a CNS stimulant—is the most commonly used psychoactive substance. Products containing caffeine include coffee, tea, chocolate, cola beverages, and prescription and nonprescription medications. People rely on caffeine to promote wakefulness, elevate their sense of well-being, decrease fatigue, and facilitate motor activity.

The mode of action within the body is stimulation of the CNS, thereby exciting the respiratory system and increasing body metabolism.[5] Caffeine is absorbed from the gastrointestinal tract, broken down in the liver, and excreted in the urine. The intake of a large quantity of caffeine can cause intoxication, manifested by cardiac dysrhythmias, sleep disturbances, mood changes, increased production of urine, gastrointestinal discomfort, and anxiety, especially panic attacks. Caffeinism and caffeine withdrawal syndrome are seen only with long-term use of caffeine, usually a documented intake of more than 500 mg/day.[19] Lack of caffeine can lead to severe headache. This problem can be seen in clients placed on NPO status (e.g., for surgery).

Nursing care begins with recognition of the clinical manifestations of excessive caffeine use and withdrawal. Monitoring the manifestations and observing for additional problems (such as whether the caffeine is exacerbating known health problems) are appropriate.

■ CANNABIS

Marijuana, a cannabis derivative, is the most widely used illegal drug in the United States, with more than 55% of young adults reporting personal use.[19] The mode of action of marijuana is not clearly understood, and researchers continue to try to identify the mechanism that accounts for its effects on the CNS and cardiovascular system.[7, 23]

Tetrahydrocannabinol (THC) is the active ingredient in marijuana and the agent responsible for the psychological effects. The amount of marijuana that crosses the blood-brain barrier depends on the method of intake used. THC is absorbed in fatty tissues, primarily the brain and testes, and is slowly released back into the bloodstream, where it is eventually excreted in urine and feces.[19]

Clients who use marijuana experience manifestations of intoxication, such as euphoria, mood changes, memory impairment, tremors, decreased body temperature, dry mouth, lack of coordination, elevated blood pressure and heart rate, and injected conjunctivae (bloodshot eyes). The CNS and cardiac, immune, and reproductive systems are affected. Long-term use also influences respiratory functioning. Marijuana residues in the lungs are considered more carcinogenic than tobacco residues.

Withdrawal from marijuana is typically an uncomfortable but not a life-threatening process. Nursing care includes monitoring the client's physical and emotional responses to the drug. It is often helpful for a nurse, family member, or friend to stay with the client, provide reassurance, and talk the client through the anxiety. Usually the client is not hospitalized unless pre-existing medical conditions or the coexistence of another psychoactive substance complicates the withdrawal process. For most clients, the initial effects of the drug dissipate within 4 to 6 hours; however, the effects of drug intoxication may last as long as 5 days.[30]

■ COCAINE

Cocaine is a narcotic obtained from the leaves of the coca plant; it was originally used by the Indians of the Andes to alleviate feelings of hunger and fatigue and to promote endurance. Today cocaine is readily available on the illicit market in the form of cocaine hydrochloride, which is soluble in water and used intravenously, inhaled (snorted), or smoked as "crack," a form of concentrated (freebase) cocaine.

Cocaine stimulates the CNS and blocks the conduction of peripheral nerve impulses. Continued use of cocaine increases the amount of dopamine in the synapses of nerve cells by preventing dopamine reuptake. Cocaine also decreases the breakdown of dopamine and other catecholamines, thereby increasing the level of catecholamine activity at the nerve cell synapses. Cocaine is metabolized in the liver and excreted in the urine. Evidence of cocaine use can be extracted from a urine sample for up to 72 hours after use.

In assessing for the effects of cocaine, remember that cocaine stimulates the CNS and the cardiovascular system. Cocaine abuse has led to myocardial infarctions in young, presumably healthy individuals. An overdose causes tremors, seizures, and delirium. Death can also result from cardiac or respiratory failure. Intervention is based on treating these identified problems and acting to prevent cardiac and respiratory complications. Cocaine intoxication may not be common in medical-surgical settings, because the half-life of cocaine is approximately 60 minutes.[3] Nursing management of a cocaine overdose focuses on preventing or handling cardiovascular collapse, respiratory distress, delirium, and hyperthermia.

Withdrawal from chronic use of cocaine ("binging") results in an exhausted state known as crashing. Clients experience a profound sense of depression, have memories of the cocaine-induced feelings of euphoria, and have cravings for the drug. Often, clients are hospitalized if there is severe depression with suicidal risk, if coexisting medical problems necessitate intense monitoring or treatment, or if there are medical problems directly related to complications of IV use. Besides providing the physical care required for the cocaine-dependent client, the nurse helps the client become aware of the need to develop effective coping skills.

■ HALLUCINOGENS

Hallucinogens, also known as *psychedelic drugs,* are both natural and synthetic substances that produce illusions, delusions, hallucinations, and alterations in thoughts, perceptions, and feelings. The effects of hallucinogens differ among individuals and are therefore unpredictable. An individual's personality may influence the reaction that occurs after hallucinogen use. Characteristic of lysergic acid diethylamide (LSD) and other psychedelic drugs are a subjective sensation of heightened awareness, an ability to look inward, and a feeling of oneness with the universe.

The mechanism of action is unknown. Hallucinogens are usually ingested and then absorbed from the gastrointestinal tract, metabolized in the liver, and excreted in the bile and feces.[7] The length of action is usually between 6 and 12 hours.[19]

The effects of hallucinogens are similar to those of other stimulants. The user experiences euphoria, dilated pupils, anxiety, and increased respirations, blood pressure, and heart rate. Panic attacks occur while the user is in a state of intoxication, accompanied by feelings of paranoia, confusion, hallucinations, possible dissociation, and loss of contact with reality. The resulting inability to perceive the environment accurately, impaired judgment, and feeling of having special powers make the person prone to dangerous activities. Suicide, homicide, and other acts of violence have been reported in people under the influence of hallucinogenic drugs. Some users also experience flashbacks. During a period of intoxication, or because of a flashback experience or the reliving of a "bad trip," a person may be brought to a health care setting.

Carefully assess the client for both physiologic and psychological problems. Nursing care focuses on attending to the panic that the client is experiencing as well as providing for client safety and creating a nonstimulating environment. Someone should stay with the client until the side effects have worn off. In the case of a severe overdose, be prepared to intervene for possible seizures, extremely high temperatures, and cardiac distress.[33] Because withdrawal symptoms may occur over a period of time, be vigilant for possible neurologic abnormalities and psychiatric manifestations.

■ INHALANTS

Inhalants are chemicals that give off fumes or vapors that readily pass through the blood-brain barrier to produce an alteration in consciousness. Commonly used inhalants are (1) solvents (glue, gasoline, nail polish remover, lighter fluid, paint thinner), (2) aerosols (hair spray, insecticides), and (3) anesthetic agents used for recreational purposes (nitrous oxide, chloroform, ether).

The probable mechanism of action is that these volatile substances alter the biologic membranes of the cells of the CNS and affect the metabolism of neurotransmitters in the brain.[19] Inhalants are metabolized in the liver and kidneys. Low doses of inhalants cause initial CNS excitement within minutes of use. Immediately after inhaling a volatile substance through the nose or mouth ("huffing"), the user experiences a "high," accompanied by feelings of giddiness and euphoria. There is a decrease in inhibitions and a slowing of the heart rate, respiratory rate, and overall mental activity. With inhalant intoxication, physical manifestations include delirium, cardiac dysrhythmias, irritation of the mucous membranes of the nose and mouth, cough, and depression of brain waves. Depending on the substance inhaled, the effects may last from a few minutes to several hours.[19]

Continuous use of volatile substances results in brain, lung, liver, kidney, and bone marrow damage. Withdrawal symptoms associated with inhalants vary with the specific substance used. Sudden death related to the use of inhalants can occur from life-threatening dysrhythmias and hypoxia.

Nursing care concentrates on prompt intervention in emergency situations (seizures, loss of consciousness, respiratory arrest). Effective management of the client's acute and chronic physiologic problems remains your primary goal.

■ NICOTINE

Nicotine is an alkaloid substance present in tobacco leaves. Using nicotine in the form of cigarettes, cigars, or chewing or pipe tobacco is an addictive habit practiced throughout the world. It is the leading cause of preventable death in the United States. Nicotine is absorbed through the lungs and within seconds crosses the blood-brain barrier and acts to stimulate the CNS. It is metabolized in the liver and excreted in the urine. Nicotine adversely affects the cardiovascular, respiratory, and gastrointestinal systems.

An overdose of nicotine is not a common occurrence. If intoxication develops, administration of oxygen and the treatment of symptoms are the nurse's priorities. Nicotine withdrawal occurs within 24 hours of smoking cessation. The withdrawal symptoms are uncomfortable, and the nurse can support the client through this process and assist with developing effective strategies for dealing with the manifestations.

■ OPIOIDS

Opioids comprise drugs produced from opium along with manufactured or semisynthetic narcotics. The human body also produces natural opiates, which facilitate feelings of well-being. Chemicals known as *endorphins* are neurotransmitters that connect with opiate receptors in the brain. When a person uses opiates or other narcotics, an interference is created in the natural opioid system and the functions of the neurotransmitters in the brain are disrupted.[16] Opioids are metabolized in the liver and excreted in the bile and urine.

An opioid overdose constitutes a life-threatening situation due to seizures, shock, respiratory depression, or cardiac dysrhythmias. The client is usually in an unconscious or lethargic state and may die without appropriate medical treatment. The nurse assesses and intervenes with the health care team to provide the required emergency care. Establishing an airway, monitoring cardiac functioning and treating dysrhythmias, maintaining hydration, and administering a narcotic antagonist such as naloxone (Narcan) are the nursing care priorities. The client should be hospitalized, with close monitoring of all body systems, for at least 24 hours.

For the client experiencing opioid withdrawal, focus on assessing and intervening for a variety of physiologic, psychological, and behavioral symptoms; these tend to occur within 72 hours of last drug use. Nursing care consists of constantly monitoring withdrawal symptoms along with providing rest, nutrition, and a comfortable environment. The initiation of a methadone program as a useful approach for treating opioid addiction is now recommended by the National Institutes of Health (NIH). Methadone therapy is useful for both detoxification and maintenance therapy. Clients often are referred to residential treatment programs to learn how to develop new, drug-free lifestyles.

■ PHENCYCLIDINE

Phencyclidine (PCP) is a synthetic drug with stimulant, depressant, and hallucinogenic properties.[7] PCP not only increases the production of dopamine but also blocks its reuptake, thus causing an increased blood pressure, heartbeat, and respiratory rates. PCP also increases acetylcholine in the CNS, thereby generating cholinergic effects manifested as diaphoresis, drooling, and pupillary constriction. Serotonin is also believed to be altered by the presence of PCP, resulting in a lack of coordination, slurred speech, and nystagmus.[19] PCP is metabolized in the liver and excreted in the urine.

Intoxication from PCP lasts up to 6 hours, and the effects of the drug are unpredictable. A person may experience euphoria, disorientation, or the racing or slowing of thoughts. In emergency departments, the client may be confused, hostile, violent, paranoid, or panicked. Nursing assessment of PCP intoxication often reveals severe cardiac or respiratory distress, which can lead to cardiac arrest. Clients under the influence of PCP can be in a psychosis-like state and can have nystagmus, abnormal muscle movements, and severe hypertension.

Nursing care concentrates on the assessment of subtle changes in vital signs and level of consciousness, gastric lavage if PCP has been ingested, and acidification of the urine.[19] In PCP withdrawal, you may see variable presentations of manifestations, particularly abnormal muscle movements. Carefully monitor the client's physical and mental condition to minimize health problems.

■ SEDATIVES, HYPNOTICS, AND ANXIOLYTICS

Sedative, hypnotic, and anxiolytic agents are considered to be CNS depressants. These medications are directly absorbed from the gastrointestinal tract into the bloodstream, where they enter the brain, are metabolized in the liver, and are eliminated via the kidneys. In cases of overdose, clients experience decreased CNS functioning along with the slowing of the cardiac and respiratory systems. Monitor vital signs and initiate emergency procedures based on the clinical manifestations presented. An overdose of any of these depressant drugs constitutes a medical emergency, with some clients requiring hospitalization in an intensive care unit (ICU).

Nursing care focuses on maintenance of adequate respiratory and cardiovascular status, hydration, and possible gastric lavage if the drugs were taken within the previous 4 to 6 hours.[33] For clients undergoing withdrawal, promote safety and rest while treating both physical and emotional manifestations. Nursing care priorities are awareness of the possibility of delirium, seizures, fever, and changes in cardiac and respiratory status as well as the interaction between adverse effects of the drug and pre-existing medical problems. Table 24–6 summarizes common health problems observed in clients who abuse drugs other than alcohol.

■ Nursing Management of Substance-Abusing Clients

The nurse plays a vital role in the care of clients experiencing intoxication and withdrawal. Nurses also meet basic needs, develop a therapeutic relationship, and teach both the client and family about addiction and its effect on the entire family. Nursing strategies for meeting actual or potential health problems are implemented for nursing diagnoses generated from assessment data. Nursing diagnoses commonly applied to the substance abuse population are listed in Box 24–3.

Education is an essential component of care to help the client understand the need for lifestyle changes. The main components of a drug education plan for clients and families are outlined in Box 24–4. Sometimes clients who abuse alcohol are referred for various treatment options and given disulfiram (Antabuse) to deter drinking. Clients receiving disulfiram must be carefully instructed about the drug. Information to include in a teaching plan is provided in Box 24–5.

Substance abuse has a major impact on family members. The family often tries to deal with a substance-abusing member by altering his or her behavior and compensating for the addict's unfilled responsibilities. Often the family inadvertently isolates itself from others as it focuses most of its energy on the addict. Personal needs of the caregiver, other adults, and children go unmet. Family members are strongly affected by the addiction and must be involved in the recovery process. A caring, supportive, and educative response from the nurse conveys that the family's concerns are understood and will be included in the treatment program. A major role of the nurse is education of client and family. The educative responsive is detailed in Box 24–4.

DRUG AND ALCOHOL INTERVENTION

■ CONFRONTATION ABOUT DRUG ABUSE

In medical-surgical settings, nurses and other members of the health care team may receive a request for assistance from family members who believe that the client needs to obtain drug and alcohol treatment. To confront the client about drug abuse, a carefully orchestrated format (a *therapeutic intervention*) can be implemented to force the client to participate in treatment.[10] The intervention must be planned in advance and executed under the guidance of a health care provider with a drug and alcohol counseling background. To prepare for the intervention, all participants compose a list of situations in which they have personal knowledge about the client's drug and alcohol behaviors.

During the therapeutic intervention, a group of family and friends gather together and bring the client face to face with the addiction problem. In an objective and nonjudgmental manner, the group states its concerns about the client, its observations about the client's substance abuse behavior, and its overall caring about the client's well-being. A plan for obtaining help from these significant people is presented to the client. This plan includes treatment recommendations and may contain a reservation for a particular treatment facility. It is believed that this loving and open confrontation can break through the abuser's denial and defensiveness. The client's family and friends must also state the consequences that will immediately ensue if help is refused.

■ TREATMENT OPTIONS

After completing a comprehensive health history and providing care for the client, you are in an optimal position to recommend a treatment modality that corresponds to

TABLE 24–6 HEALTH CONSEQUENCES OF COMMONLY ABUSED DRUGS

	Amphetamines	Caffeine	Cannabis	Cocaine	Hallucinogens	Inhalants	Nicotine	Opioids	Phencyclidine (PCP)	Sedatives, hypnotics, and anxiolytics
Abrupt withdrawal symptoms (similar to alcohol withdrawal)										X
Agitation										
Angina		X					X			
Acquired immunodeficiency syndrome (AIDS)				X				X		
Anemia								X		
Atelectasis								X		
Arthritis								X		
Aspiration				X						
Bone marrow depression						X				
Brain damage						X				
Bronchitis				X			X			
Cancer (laryngeal)							X			
Cancer (lung)							X			
Cancer (oral cavity)							X			
Cerebrovascular accident (stroke)				X			X			
Confusion									X	
Dysrhythmias	X	X			X	X		X		
Emphysema							X			
Endocarditis (bacterial)				X				X		
Excoriations (from scratching nonexistent bugs)	X									
Flashbacks					X					
Gastrointestinal distress/ulcers						X	X			
Hallucinations									X	
Hepatitis (bacterial, viral)				X		X		X		
Hypergammaglobulinemia								X		
Hypertension	X	X		X	X				X	
Immune dysfunctions									X	
Insomnia		X								
Judgment, impaired									X	
Lung abscess								X		
Lung irritation			X			X				
Lymphadenopathy								X		

TABLE 24–6   **HEALTH CONSEQUENCES OF COMMONLY ABUSED DRUGS** *Continued*

	Amphetamines	Caffeine	Cannabis	Cocaine	Hallucinogens	Inhalants	Nicotine	Opioids	Phencyclidine (PCP)	Sedatives, hypnotics, and anxiolytics
Mental slowness										X
Motor function, impaired										X
Muscle weakness						X				
Myocardial infarction				X			X			
Myositis ossificans (drug user's elbow)								X		
Nasal septal damage				X						
Nephritis								X		
Neuropathy (peripheral)						X				
Osteomyelitis								X		
Paranoid psychosis	X									
Peptic ulcers		X								
Pharyngitis (chronic)			X							
Phlebitis								X		
Pneumonia								X		
Pulmonary emboli				X						
Pulmonary fibrosis								X		
Renal failure				X		X		X		
Respiratory arrest/failure						X				
Seizures	X			X					X	X
Skin ulcers or abscesses				X						
Sinusitis (chronic)			X							
Splenomegaly								X		
Testosterone (lowered levels)			X							
Tremors		X								
Tuberculosis								X		
Visual loss (from adulterants in street drugs)								X		

BOX 24-3   Common Nursing Diagnoses for Clients Who Abuse Substances

- *Acute Confusion*
- *Anxiety*
- *Impaired Verbal Communication*
- *Ineffective Denial*
- *Altered Family Processes*
- *Fatigue*
- *Fear*
- *Dysfunctional Grieving*
- *Hopelessness*
- *Ineffective Individual Coping*
- *Risk for Infection*
- *Risk for Injury*
- *Knowledge Deficit* (specify)
- *Noncompliance* (specify)
- *Altered Nutrition: Less than Body Requirements*
- *Pain*
- *Altered Parenting*
- *Personal Identity Disturbance*
- *Risk for Poisoning*
- *Powerlessness*
- *Altered Role Performance*
- *Chronic Low Self esteem*
- *Sensory/Perceptual Alterations* (*Specify:* visual, auditory kinesthetic, gustatory, tactile, olfactory)
- *Altered Sexuality Patterns*
- *Risk for Impaired Skin Integrity*
- *Sleep Pattern Disturbance*
- *Impaired Social Interaction*
- *Social Isolation*
- *Spiritual Distress*
- *Altered Thought Processes*
- *Risk for Trauma*
- *Risk for Violence (Self-directed or directed at others)*

the needs of the client and family members. Activities that you are involved in range from primary prevention (education), to secondary prevention (outpatient services), to tertiary prevention (inpatient or outpatient detoxification and rehabilitation). The common interventions for all three levels of care are listed in Table 24–7. A list of

BOX 24-4   Components of a Client and Family Education Plan

- Concept of addiction
- Physical health problems associated with addiction
- Nutritional status
- Feelings and behaviors of all family members associated with addiction
- Areas of life affected by substance use: family, social, spiritual, sexual, occupational, financial, legal, and leisure
- Roles family members play in addiction
- Treatment options and treatment process
- Aftercare and self-help support groups or 12-step programs
- Community resources
- Skill building in the areas of communication, expression of feelings, socialization, and coping strategies
- Impact of both addiction and the recovery process on the roles and responsibilities of all family members
- Client confidentiality and right to privacy protected under the 1975 Federal Drug and Alcohol Abuse Act

BOX 24-5   Information to Include in a Teaching Plan About Disulfiram (Antabuse)

- Inform the client that disulfiram is not a cure for alcoholism; it only discourages drinking.
- Before initiating disulfiram therapy, ask whether the client has had any allergic reactions to substances such as sulfites, preservatives, or dyes.
- Ask whether the client has a history of seizures; severe mental illness, particularly psychosis; serious cardiac disease; kidney disease; diabetes mellitus; hypothyroidism; or skin allergies.
- Ask whether the client is taking anticoagulants (↑ effects), isoniazid (INH) (↑ CNS effects), metronidazole (Flagyl) (↑ toxicity), or phenytoin (Dilantin) (↑ toxicity).
- Instruct the client not to ingest any alcohol or use any products containing alcohol within 12 hours before taking disulfiram, while taking disulfiram, and for at least 14 days after discontinuing disulfiram.
- Explain to the client that it is necessary to read the labels on all products because alcohol is found in many foods, medicines, and personal hygiene products (e.g., sauces, vinegars, cough syrups, tonics, elixirs, mouthwash, colognes, after-shave lotions).
- Tell the client not to inhale chemicals that may contain alcohol (e.g., paints, varnish, shellac).
- Encourage the client not to use alcohol-containing products that are applied topically. Alcohol absorbed through the skin can cause redness, itching, headache, and nausea.
- Identify common side effects (e.g., headache, fatigue, a metallic or garlic-like aftertaste, skin rash) that may be experienced during the first 2 weeks of taking disulfiram. Inform the client that these manifestations resolve as the body adjusts to the medication.
- If the client ingests alcohol while taking disulfiram, blurred vision, chest pain, confusion, dizziness or fainting, palpitations, flushing, diaphoresis, nausea, vomiting, headache, and dyspnea may occur. These symptoms last as long as alcohol is in the body. If the client drinks a large amount of alcohol, seizures, myocardial infarction, unconsciousness, or death may result.
- Instruct the client to carry a card specifying that he or she is taking disulfiram, listing side effects of alcohol, and stating whom to contact in an emergency.

community resources that can provide education and support to substance-abusing clients and their families appears in Box 24–6.

■ PREVENTION OF RELAPSE

Clients in the recovery process may be at risk for relapse or a return to substance abuse. Anticipate the possibility of *relapse* (slipping back into substance use after a period of abstinence), and prepare clients with strategies that may prevent it. This regression can occur any time and may be defined as one-time use, brief intermittent use, or daily long-term use. Relapse should be viewed as a potential part of the illness process, much like the potential course of any other chronic illness. Seeing relapse as client failure sets the client up for defeat instead of recovery.

Physiologic, emotional, and social variables all contribute to relapse. Clients must be taught ways to assess their strengths and to identify situations that can distract them

TABLE 24–7	LEVELS OF TREATMENT STRATEGIES	
Level of Prevention	**Activities**	**Resources**
Primary prevention	Education to prevent substance abuse Risk factor identification Lifestyle guidance	School programs Community programs Health promotion activities
Secondary prevention (outpatient)	Assessment and intervention of early physical and emotional issues and problems Educational interventions Pharmacologic interventions Self-management strategies Support and self-help groups Psychotherapy	Medical facilities as appropriate Individual, family, or group therapy Psychoeducational groups Self-help groups (e.g., AA, NA, CA, Al-Anon, Alateen, Naranon, ACOA)*
Tertiary prevention (inpatient or outpatient)	Interventions to monitor withdrawal and prevent or treat complications Focusing on relapse prevention Determining plan for aftercare and methods of obtaining support Individual, family, or group therapy	Medical services, such as detoxification Aftercare, such as partial programs, supervised living, or halfway house Individual, family, or group therapy Psychoeducational groups Self-help groups (e.g., AA, NA, CA, Al-Anon, Alateen, Naranon, ACOA)*

*See Box 24–6, Resources.
AA, Alcoholics Anonymous; ACOA, Adult Children of Alcoholics; CA, Cocaine Anonymous; NA, Narcotics Anonymous.

from their recovery. Peer pressure, stress, and negative feelings may trigger a relapse. Some relapse prevention strategies to include in educational programs are listed in Box 24–7.

■ SURGERY AND SUBSTANCE ABUSE

Clients who abuse substances often experience accidents, injuries, or illnesses that require surgical intervention. In fact, many injuries seen by nurses in emergency departments are directly related to drug and alcohol use. Become skillful in observing for subtle changes, and perform frequent assessments in order to intervene immediately and prevent the escalation of manifestations. Traumatized clients usually require immediate surgery; hence, a thorough drug and alcohol assessment may not be done. It is a challenge for the nurse to distinguish medical problems, psychiatric disorders, and substance abuse disorders in a timely manner.

BOX 24–6   Resources

Alcoholics Anonymous (look in the local telephone directory, or call New York, NY: 212-686-1100 for information throughout the United States); *www.alcoholics-anonymous.org*

Al-Anon (look in the local telephone directory, or call New York, NY: 212-254-7230 for information throughout the United States); Al-Anon and Alateen Family Group Headquarters, Inc.: 888-4AL-ANON (888-425-2666); *www.al-anon.org*

Adult Children of Alcoholics (look in the local telephone directory, or call Torrance, CA: 213-534-1815 for information); *www.info@adultchildren.org*

BACCHUS (Boost Alcohol Consciousness Concerning the Health of University Students) (call Denver, CO: 303-871-3068 for information)

Children of Alcoholics Foundation, Inc. (call New York, NY: 212-351-2680 for information); 800-359-2623; *www.coaf.org*

MADD (Mothers Against Drunken Driving) (call Austin, TX: 817-268-6233 for information)

Narcotics Anonymous (look in the local telephone directory, or call Van Nuys, CA: 818-780-3951 for information); *www.na.org*

Cocaine Anonymous (call Los Angeles, CA: 800-347-8998 or 213-559-5833 for information); *www.ca.org*

Marijuana Anonymous (look in the local telephone directory, or call 800-766-6779); *www.marijuana-anonymous.org*

Dual Recovery Anonymous (look in the local telephone directory, or call 888-869-9230); *www.dualrecovery.base.org*

National Clearinghouse for Alcohol and Drug Information (call Rockville, MD: 301-468-2600 for information)

National Asian Pacific American Families Against Drug Abuse (call Bethesda, MD: 301-530-0945 for information)

Hotline Numbers

Center for Substance Abuse Treatment
   National Treatment Hotline: 800-662-HELP
   (800-662-4357)
Center for Substance Abuse Prevention Workplace
   Hotline 800-WORKPLACE 800-967-5752
National Alcohol Hotline
   HelpLine: 800-ALCOHOL (800-252-6465)
National Cocaine Hotline
   800-COCAINE (800-2622-2463)

BOX 24-7 **Strategies to Prevent Relapse**

- Assess and build on the client's coping skills.
- Take opportunities, such as role-playing, that help the client practice coping methods.
- Assist the client in identifying personal risks of relapse.
- Identify people, places, and things that can interfere with maintaining sobriety and encourage the client to minimize contact with these obstacles and develop ways to handle them.
- Change environmental variables when possible.
- Discuss the concept of craving, how to identify it, what may trigger it, and how to handle it.
- Focus on the client's physiologic feelings and sensations, and develop methods to handle them.
- Teach strategies that promote a healthy lifestyle, such as exercise, nutrition, stress management, and relaxation techniques.
- Encourage participation in support groups or self-help groups.
- Recommend group or individual therapy if the client has problems with the family of origin, struggles with daily functioning, or mental illness.

Alcoholic clients who are admitted for a surgical procedure require special attention. They are told not to drink for several days before surgery, but in reality they may have been drinking up to the night before. Postoperatively, the client begins to develop withdrawal and must be actively restrained. The challenges facing the nursing staff caring for a postoperative client with DTs are great. Client safety is a serious matter, as are wound healing and adequate nutrition. The client may be treated to reduce symptoms. In other cases, the client may be simply left to detoxify "cold turkey," a method that stops the substance abruptly. Your role as a client advocate is imperative for these clients.

If a client is addicted to CNS depressant drugs, a larger amount of an anesthetic may be needed to produce the desired effects. This situation occurs because the client has a higher tolerance to the anesthetic drug. For clients with liver impairment and overall poor health, anesthetics cannot be properly metabolized and the effect of sedation is prolonged. While undergoing surgery, the addicted client is at risk for cardiac dysrhythmias, respiratory depression, hemorrhage, and depletion of catecholamines.

In the postoperative period, these clients are susceptible to cardiac, respiratory, urinary, hemorrhagic, and wound complications. The experience of pain may be intensified because the clients often have tolerance to the pain medication. Carefully assess whether the client requires increased doses of medication for pain relief and needs to be slowly weaned from the medication during recovery. Some addicted clients may experience drug withdrawal postoperatively because withdrawal has been delayed by the use of anesthetics.

THE IMPAIRED HEALTH CARE PROFESSIONAL

Just like other people, health care professionals can become addicted to drugs and alcohol. Research on the prevalence of substance abuse among nurses has revealed no difference between nurses and other health professionals. Further, the prevalence of substance abuse among health professionals overall does not differ from that in the general population.[40] Many addicted health care professionals first started using drugs and alcohol in response to physical illness and pain, emotional difficulties, or work pressures.

The requirements of the professional nurse's role make nursing a stressful occupation. On a daily basis, the nurse is responsible for coordinating and directly providing care for clients who are in pain and crisis. The pressure of handling resources; making decisions; interfacing with medical and other personnel; working long hours, often with inadequate staff; and being responsible for the daily operation of the medical-surgical unit can be overwhelming. In addition, nurses have access to narcotics and operate on the premise that medications are a useful vehicle for relieving pain and altering states of feelings. Specialized knowledge about drugs and experience with administering them and watching their efficacy may lead health care providers to view drugs as a "pharmacologic coping method."[9, 25] It is a method that can ultimately backfire.

The signs of a chemically impaired colleague are subtle and easily overlooked by peers and supervisors. Even other health care professionals may deny and avoid the problem rather than confront the person suspected of being chemically dependent. It is essential that nurses be aware of the signs of chemical dependence in peers (Box 24-8). Document questionable or problematic incidents, and be willing to participate in an intervention if deemed appropriate. Remember, a peer who suffers from addiction cannot meet the requirements of your state nurse practice act. Some states have a law that mandates reporting of an impaired colleague.

As with clients, steps must be taken to assist an impaired nurse to obtain treatment. The use of an employee assistance program (EAP) and peer support or assistance groups from the state nurses' association can facilitate referrals to treatment and can assist with recovery. Although peer assistance programs vary from state to state,

---

BOX 24-8 **Signs of a Chemically Impaired Colleague**

- Alcohol on breath
- Mood changes or confusion
- Difficulty making judgments and impaired memory
- Red eyes with flushed face
- Unsteady gait
- Tremors or impaired eye-hand coordination
- Irritability or hyperactivity
- Lethargy or dozing on breaks
- Disheveled appearance
- Wearing long sleeves or a sweater constantly, even in hot weather
- Incorrect drug counts
- Accidents, spillages, or drugs frequently being wasted
- Frequently found in the bathroom, nurses' lounge, or off the unit
- Recurrent unfinished assignments or client care mistakes

most programs offer support, referral services, monitoring during recovery, and educational programs targeted to the health care professional.

CONCLUSIONS

Substance abuse remains a major health issue, affecting clients, families, and communities. Despite this reality many clients with substance abuse disorders are not identified and, therefore, do not obtain treatment. A lack of knowledge about addiction can perpetuate stigmatization of the client. Your challenge is to become informed about both the effects of drugs and appropriate strategies for treatment. Keen assessment skills, decision-making skills, and compassion are the prerequisites for comprehensive nursing care of the myriad physiologic and psychological needs presented by these clients.

Nurses play a vital role in developing and implementing drug and alcohol prevention strategies. Teaching how to use effective coping strategies, how to handle crises, and how to develop support systems are the primary steps that must be incorporated into the care. For you, as a nurse, it is important to spend time cultivating relationships and to allow yourself to engage in leisure activities that decrease feelings of frustration, hopelessness, and burnout.

THINKING CRITICALLY

1. **A group of young college students celebrated the end of the semester with a week-long party. Alcoholic beverages were plentiful; food was not a priority. A young couple brought their friend to the emergency department. They reported their suspicions that she might have a drinking problem (e.g., erratic behavior, presence of alcoholic beverages in the dormitory room, smell of alcohol on her breath). They were unable to awaken her for any length of time and are worried that she drank too much. She has not had a drink for about 6 hours. What assessment is required? What nursing actions are appropriate?**

Factors to Consider. How likely is it for the client to experience delirium tremens (DTs)? How will the client be treated?

2. **You are a Registered Nurse in the local "Driving Under the Influence of Alcohol" (DUI) teaching program. Your topic is "Alcohol and the Human Body." The audience is made up of clients mandated by the court to attend. After the presentation, which focuses on the complications associated with long-term drinking, the clients ask, "If alcoholism is a disease, why are we treated as criminals?" "I didn't drink so much, why did they pull me over?" What might these questions indicate?**

Factors to Consider. Is alcoholism a disease of addiction? What psychological factor is evident in such questions?

BIBLIOGRAPHY

1. Addiction Research Corporation. (1986). *GRASP: Guide's rational adolescent substance abuse profile.* Piscataway, NJ: Rutgers University Center of Alcohol Studies.
2. American Psychiatric Association. (1994). *Diagnostic and statistical manual of mental disorders* (4th ed.). Washington, DC: Author.
3. American Psychiatric Association. (1995). Practice guidelines for the treatment of patients with substance use disorders: Alcohol, cocaine, opioids. *American Journal of Psychiatry, 152*(11), Supplement 4–19.
4. Bellenir, K. (Ed.). (1996). *Substance abuse sourcebook.* Detroit, MI: Omnigraphics.
5. Blum, K., et al. (1990). Allelic association of human dopamine D2 receptor gene in alcoholism. *Journal of the American Medical Association, 15*(263), 2055–2060.
6. Bond, A., et al. (1994). Systemic absorption and abuse liability of snorted flunitrazepam. *Addiction, 89*(7), 821–830.
7. Burns, E. M., Thompson, A., & Ciccone, J. K. (1993). *An addictions curriculum for nurses and other helping professionals* (Vol. 2). New York: Springer-Verlag.
8. Clayton, L. (1997). *Tranquilizers.* Springfield, NY: Enslow.
9. Coombs, R. H. (1997). *Drug impaired professionals.* Cambridge, MA: Harvard University Press.
10. Copel, L. C. (2000). *Nurses' clinical guide to psychiatric and mental health nursing* (2nd ed.). Springhouse, PA: Springhouse.
11. Doweiko, H. (1999). *Concepts of chemical dependency.* Pacific Grove, CA: Brooks/Cole Publishing.
12. Ewing, J. A. (1984). CAGE. *Journal of the American Medical Association 252*(14):1906.
13. Freed, P. E., & York, L. N. (1997). Naltrexone: A controversial therapy for alcohol dependence. *Journal of Psychosocial Nursing and Mental Health Services, 35*(7), 24–28.
14. Freeman, E. M. (Ed.). (1993). *Substance abuse treatment: A family systems perspective.* Newbury, CA: Sage.
15. Galanter, M., & Kleber, H. D. (1994). *Textbook of substance abuse treatment.* Washington, DC: American Psychiatric Press.
16. Goldstein, A. (1994). *Addiction: From biology to drug policy.* New York: W. H. Freeman.
17. Henly, G. A., & Winters, K. C. (1988). Development of problem severity scales for the assessment of adolescent alcohol and drug abuse. *International Journal of the Addictions, 23,* 65–85.
18. Horn, J. L., Skinner, H. A., Wanberg, K. W., & Foster, F. M. (1984). *Alcohol use questionnaire (AUQ).* Toronto, Canada: Addiction Research Foundation.
19. Jaffe, J. (Ed.). (1995). *Encyclopedia of drugs and alcohol.* New York, Macmillan.
20. Jefferson, L. V. (1995). Chemically mediated responses and substance-related disorders. In G. W. Stuart & S. J. Sundeen (Eds.), *Principles and practices of psychiatric nursing* (pp. 569–605). St. Louis: Mosby–Year Book.
21. Keller, C. M. (1994). Flumazenil: A new benzodiazepine-specific antagonist. *Journal of the American Academy of Physician Assistants, 7*(8), 595–598.
22. Lowinson, J., Ruiz, P., Millman, R., & Langrod, J. (Eds.). (1997). *Substance abuse: A comprehensive textbook* (3rd ed.). Baltimore, MD: Williams & Wilkins.
23. Marx, J. (1990). Marijuana receptor gene cloned. *Science, 249,* 624–626.
24. McLellan, A. T., et al. (1992). The fifth edition of the addiction severity index. *Journal of Substance Abuse Treatment, 9*(3), 199–213.
25. Mynatt, S. (1996). A model of contributing risk factors to chemical dependency in nurses. *Journal of Psychosocial Nursing and Mental Health Services, 34*(7), 13–22.
26. Nace, E. P., & Isbell, P. I. (1991). Alcohol. In R. J. Frances & S. I. Miller (Eds.), *Clinical textbook of addictive disorders* (pp. 43–68). New York: Guilford Press.
27. Naranjo, C. A., Sellers, E. M., & Chater, M. (1983). Nonpharmacologic intervention in acute alcohol withdrawal. *Clinical Pharmacology and Therapeutics 34,* 814–819.
27a. National Consensus Development Panel. (1998). Effective medical treatment of opiate addiction. *Journal of the American Medical Association, 280*(22), 1936–1943.
28. National Institute on Alcohol Abuse and Alcoholism. (1984). *Alcohol abuse curriculum guide for nurse practitioner faculty* (DHHS

Pub. No. ADM 84-1313, Vol. 3). Rockville, MD: Health Professions Education Curriculum Resources Series.

29. National Institute on Alcohol Abuse and Alcoholism. (1990). *Seventh special report to the U.S. Congress on alcohol and health: From the secretary of health and human services* (DHHS Pub. No. ADM 90-1656). Rockville, MD: Author.

30. Ott, P. J., Tarter, R. E., & Ammerman, R. T. (1999). *Sourcebook on substance abuse: Etiology, epidemiology, assessment, and treatment.* Boston, MA: Allyn & Bacon.

31. Peele, S. (1986). The implications and limitations of genetic models of alcoholism and other addictions. *Journal of Studies on Alcohol, 47,* 63–73.

32. Pokorney, A. D., Miller, B. A., & Kaplan, H. B. (1992). The brief MAST: A shortened version of the Michigan Alcoholism Screening Test. *American Journal of Psychiatry, 129,* 342–348.

33. Selzer, M. L. (1971). The Michigan Alcoholism Screening test: The quest for a new diagnostic instrument. *American Journal of Psychiatry, 127,* 1653–1658.

34. Selzer, M., Vinokur, A., & van Roojan, L. (1975). A self-administered short alcohol screening test (SMAST). *Journal of Studies on Alcoholism, 36*(1), 86.

35. Skinner, H. A., & Horn, J. L. (1984). *Alcohol Dependence Scale (ADS): User's guide.* Toronto, Canada: Addiction Research Foundation.

35a. Smith, D. E., Wesson, D. R., & Calhoun, S. R. (1995). *Rohypnol (flunitrazepam) fact sheet.* (Available from the Haight-Ashbury Free Clinics, Inc., 409 Clayton Street, San Francisco, CA 94117.)

36. Sokol, R. J., Martier, S. S., & Ager, J. W. (1989). The T-ACE questions: Practical prenatal detection of risk-drinking. *American Journal of Obstetrics and Gynecology, 160,* 863–870.

37. Sue, D. (1987). Use and abuse of alcohol by Asian Americans. *Journal of Psychoactive Drugs, 19,* 57.

38. Sullivan, E. (1995). Nursing care of clients with substance abuse. St. Louis: Mosby–Year Book.

39. Swenson, W., & Morse, R. (1973). The use of self-administered alcoholism screening test (SAAST) in a medical center. *Mayo Clinic Proceedings, 50,* 204–208.

40. Trinkoff, A. M., Eaton, W. W., & Anthony, J. C. (1991). The prevalence of substance abuse among registered nurses. *Nursing Research, 40*(3), 172–175.

41. Whitfield, C. L., Thompson, G., & Lamb, A. (1978). Detoxication of 1,024 alcoholic patients without psychoactive drugs. *Journal of the American Medical Association, 17*(239), 1409–1411.

Decision-Making: Withholding or Withdrawing Life Support

QUESTION
What client and family factors influence decisions for or against withholding and/or withdrawing of fluids and nutrition from terminally ill adults?

CITATION
Riley, J. M., et al. (1999). Factors related to adult patient decision making about withholding or withdrawing nutrition and/or hydration. *Online Journal of Knowledge Synthesis for Nursing, 6*(3).

STUDIES

A broad search of *CINAHL, MEDLINE,* and *BIOETHICLINE* databases revealed 16 published reports that addressed the question and that were truly research studies (1977 to 1997). Some findings were embedded in more general studies about end-of-life decisions. The studies were analyzed by four collaborators, including an Advanced Practice Nurse and a nurse-ethicist.

A wide range of people and settings were studied, including 418 hospitalized clients, 1047 clinic clients, 112 residents of long-term care facilities, 2536 community-dwelling elders, and 433 family members or surrogates. Data were collected via interviews (six studies), questionnaires (seven studies), and client record audits (three studies). Four studies used hypothetical vignettes to help understand clients' and families' preferences for or against life-sustaining treatment.

Summary of Findings

Identification of Treatment Preferences

The issue of how various groups of people view life support (e.g., intravenous [IV] fluids, tube feedings, mechanical ventilation) was examined in five studies. The results showed little consensus that would be helpful in predicting how a person might feel about a particular form of life support. However, several studies suggested that in general people did not want life-sustaining measures that would prolong a diminished quality of life,[2, 5, 12] especially if they anticipated a diminished cognitive state.

Stability of Treatment Preferences

Of the four studies that examined the stability of client treatment preferences, three found that these preferences remained fairly stable in most people for 1 to 2 years.[4, 5, 12] However, in a cohort of community-based elders, the preference to forgo certain treatments was more stable than the preference to receive them.[3] For example, 75% of the people who answered "no" to tube feeding at the initial interview gave the same response 2 years later, whereas only 43% of those who answered "yes" to tube feeding did so. Some findings show that hypothetical decision-making may not predict actual choice in the event of serious illness.[5, 12]

Factors Associated with Client Decisions

An array of factors that influence end-of-life decisions has been studied, including (1) the time sequence for decision-making, (2) the presence of underlying malignancy, (3) mental status, (4) age, and (5) ethnicity. Across studies, however, none stands out as more important than the others. In one study, 74% of hospitalized clients had some interventions withdrawn or withheld before death; typically, these decisions were made near the time of death.[6] During the final episode of illness, 89% of clients decided to have limitations in their care; feeding tube limitations accounting for 11% of the interventions.[7]

Emotional state was also studied.[8, 14] When given "good" prognosis scenarios, depressed older adults wanted fewer life-saving treatments compared with older non-adults who were not depressed. With "poor" prognosis scenarios, however, preferences were similar for depressed and non-depressed elders.[8] "Increasing severity of depression explained less than 5% of the variance in decision-making in any treatment situation" (p 41).[8] Surprisingly, disease-specific factors (e.g., limitations of activity by disease, duration of illness, and clients' perceptions of the prognosis) were not significantly associated with desire for life support, nor were demographic variables (e.g., age, marital status, religion, and education).[14] However, in two studies, race did influence decisions in that African Americans and Hispanic Americans desired life support more often than whites did.[1, 14]

Client values such as not wanting to be a burden on anyone, wanting to do the most for oneself, retaining the right to choose one's own medical treatment, and viewing quality of life as more important that preservation of life influenced the preferences of many clients.[2] Previous experiences with life support were common among clinic elders (82% had at least one such experience); in one study, people with a positive experience were more likely to desire more life support than those with a negative experience.[14] In contrast, another study indicated that prior experience with life support was not a factor in a client's preference.[1]

Surrogate Decision-Making

When clients are unable to take part in the decision-making process regarding life-sustaining measures and when they have not made their wishes known, a difficult situation ensues. The research suggests that it is not clear how accurately a surrogate (i.e., the designated health care proxy) chooses what a client would choose. In one study surrogates chose life support treatments in accord with the clients' wishes about 60% of the time—a rate no better than chance guessing.[14] In contrast, another study demonstrated high agreement in the decision to accept or decline tube feedings.[9] Two studies found that many clients, including those who had written advance directives, had not conveyed their wishes to their surrogates.[2, 13] This is unfortunate, given the finding in one study that specific discussion between client and surrogate about life support was the only predictor of accurate surrogate decision-making.[14]

Many adult children–surrogates chose to continue fluid and hydration even when a parent's wishes to the contrary were known.[13] Surrogates tended to overestimate the client's preference for life-sustaining interventions, including the use of tube feedings, and often decided based on their own preferences.

Bridge continued on following page

Decision-Making: Withholding or Withdrawing
Life Support Continued

Deciding whether to withhold or withdraw tube feedings clearly makes surrogates uncomfortable, particularly if they think their decision is inconsistent with the client's decision.[10] Spouses of patients with Alzheimer's disease were more uncomfortable with decisions to forgo tube feeding than with decisions to accept it, although more of them decided to forgo it as severity of illness increased.[11]

Limitations/Reservations. The large number of studies employing hypothetical scenarios casts some doubt on how well these studies as a whole have captured clients' and families' thinking about these complex issues. The authors of the review believe that qualitative studies sensitive to the meaning of these decisions as they are anticipated, made, and lived with over time are needed (p 61). Also, little is known about the experience and sensations that accompany not receiving nutrition and hydration at the end of life; yet this is a chief source of concern for surrogates (p 63).

Research-Based Practice

There is strong societal support for a client's self-determination regarding the use of life-sustaining treatments. These studies show that such choices are highly individualized and depend on assumptions about the length and quality of life. Since these assumptions are often based on the estimations offered by physicians, surrogates often have to decide in the context of much uncertainty, which is why many people wait until a situation seems hopeless.

A person's preferences for life-sustaining interventions are relatively stable as long as his or her health state is stable but are likely to change when health status changes substantially. The likelihood that clients' preference will change as their condition worsens makes repeated discussions between clients, their surrogates, and their health care providers very important. Clients may feel one way about nutrition and another way about hydration or about cardiopulmonary resuscitation (CPR). The documented preference of many African Americans and Hispanic Americans for life support and the declining of these measures by whites should be kept in mind and respected.

The studies in this review reveal the difficulties associated with discussing end-of-life treatment decisions before illness occurs. Specific illness scenarios are a widely used tool and probably are better than discussions about options without presenting an illness context. However, the scenarios presented should be carefully chosen and carefully worded. When clients face high-risk surgery or are in a physically or mentally deteriorating state, they should discuss their treatment wishes with their surrogate or health care proxy to ensure that their wishes are known. Discussions at these times can often be more relevant in nature than when a client was well because the problems that are likely to occur and the decisions that need to be made are more predictable.

Just as clients who have a proxy should be encouraged to talk with their surrogate, surrogates should be encouraged to hold frank discussions with the client they may need to represent. Whoever begins the discussion may need guidance from a nurse. You might suggest the idea of using "what if" scenarios rather than just talking about CPR or tube feedings or IV fluids. You might also join or facilitate the discussion or request the physician to join the discussion.

You can assist patients at many points in the process of making decisions about withholding or withdrawing life-sustaining measures. As the authors of the review stated, "Nurses share in the responsibility to ensure that individual patient's personal treatment preferences are thoughtfully formulated, clearly identified, consistently communicated, and respectfully honored" (p 49).

Cited References

1. Caralis, P. V., et al. (1993). The influence of ethnicity and race on attitudes toward advance directives, life-prolonging treatments, and euthanasia. *Journal of Clinical Ethics, 4,* 155–165.
2. Cohen-Mansfield, J., et al. (1991). The decision to execute a durable power of attorney for health care and preferences regarding the utilization of life-sustaining treatments in nursing home residents. *Archives of Internal Medicine, 151,* 289–294.
3. Danis, M., et al. (1994). Stability of choices about life-sustaining treatments. *Annals of Internal Medicine, 120,* 567–573.
4. Emanuel, L. L., et al. (1994). Advance directives: Stability of patients' treatment choices. *Archives of Internal Medicine, 154,* 209–217.
5. Everhart, M. A., & Pearlman, R. A. (1990). Stability of patient preferences regarding life-sustaining treatments. *Chest, 97,* 154–164.
6. Faber-Langendoen, K., & Bartels, D. M. (1992). Process of forgoing life-sustaining treatment in a university hospital: An empirical study. *Critical Care Medicine, 20,* 570–577.
7. Fried, T. R., & Gillick, M. R. (1994). Medical decision-making in the last six months of life: Choices about limitation of care. *Journal of the American Geriatrics Society, 42,* 303–307.
8. Lee, M. A., & Ganzini, L. (1992). Depression in the elderly: Effect on patient attitudes toward life-sustaining therapy. *Journal of the American Geriatrics Society, 40,* 983–988.
9. Libbus, M. K., & Russell, C. (1995). Congruence of decisions between patients and their potential surrogates about life-sustaining therapies. *Image: Journal of Nursing Scholarship, 27,* 135–140.
10. McNabney, M. K., Beers, M. H., & Siebens, H. (1994). Surrogate decision-makers' satisfaction with the placement of feeding tubes in elderly patients. *Journal of the American Geriatrics Society, 42,* 161–168.
11. Mezey, M., et al. (1996). Life-sustaining treatment decisions by spouses of patients with Alzheimer's disease. *Journal of the American Geriatrics Society, 44,* 144–150.
12. Schneiderman, L. J., et al (1992). Relationship of general advance directive instructions to specific life-sustaining treatment preferences in patients with serious illness. *Archives of Internal Medicine, 152,* 2114–2122.
13. Sonnenblick, M., Friedlander, Y., & Steinberg, A. (1993). Dissociation between the wishes of terminally ill parents and decisions by their offspring. *Journal of the American Geriatrics Society, 41,* 599–604.
14. Suhl, J., et al. (1994). Myths of substituted judgment: Surrogate decision making regarding life support is unreliable. *Archives of Internal Medicine, 154,* 90–96.

Mobility Disorders

Anatomy and Physiology Review: The Musculoskeletal System

25 Assessment of the Musculoskeletal System

26 Management of Clients with Musculoskeletal Disorders

27 Management of Clients with Musculoskeletal Trauma and Overuse

Anatomy and Physiology Review
The Musculoskeletal System
David Porta
Joyce M. Black

Physiologically, the musculoskeletal system enables changes in movement and position. The bony skeleton provides support, protection, and movable parts. Muscles facilitate movement. Movement serves two general purposes: (1) movement is necessary to perform normal activities of daily living, and (2) movement itself is a source of pleasure. Physical activities that contribute to physical fitness and promote physical health are also enjoyable. People who participate in exercise programs describe feelings of well-being from regular physical activity.

STRUCTURE OF THE MUSCULOSKELETAL SYSTEM

MUSCLE

Muscles make up 40% to 50% of body weight. Muscles produce movement and heat by contraction. The body contains three types of muscles: (1) skeletal, (2) cardiac, and (3) smooth.

■ SKELETAL MUSCLE

Skeletal muscle attaches to bones of the skeleton. Skeletal muscles are named according to the following properties: (1) action (e.g., flexor, extensor), (2) shape (e.g., quadrilateral, pennate), (3) origin (i.e., stationary attachment of muscle to skeleton), (4) insertion (i.e., movable attachment of the muscle), (5) number of divisions, (6) location, or (7) direction of fibers (i.e., transverse). The principal muscle groups are shown in Figure U5–1.

The contraction of skeletal muscle exerts force on bones or skin and moves them (Fig. U5–2). Most skeletal muscles are under voluntary control of the nervous system, but some are controlled by the somatic division of the peripheral nervous system, such as those used to maintain balance. See detailed discussion of muscle movement on page 534.

Under microscopic examination, many nuclei of muscle cells are visible and are grouped into thread-like *myofibrils*. A close look at the myofibrils reveals alternating bands of light and dark *(striations)*. Muscle cells can be further divided into smaller segments called *sarcomeres,* delineated by Z bands. The sarcomere is the structure in the muscle where the actual contraction occurs. Two primary myofilaments are present in the sarcomere: thick myosin filaments and thin actin filaments. The filaments are proteins that briefly attach and ratchet or slide across one another to cause the muscle to contract.

Skeletal muscle is composed of many individual muscle cells called *muscle fibers.* These fibers are held together by thin sheets of fibrous connective tissue *(fascia).* Fascia also penetrates the muscle, separating it into bundles *(fasciculi).* Skeletal muscle is attached to the bones of the skeleton by very thin extensions of fascia or by tendons. *Tendons* (fibrous cords) make strong connections to bone.

■ CARDIAC MUSCLE

Cardiac muscle *(myocardium)* is involuntary and exists only in the heart. It is composed of branched, striated muscle cells having only one nucleus. Cardiac muscle is controlled by intrinsic factors (e.g., the amount of venous return to the right atrium), hormones, and signals from the autonomic nervous system. Cardiac muscle is discussed in Unit 12.

■ SMOOTH MUSCLE

"Smooth" muscle has no striations. It is involuntary and is present in the walls of hollow organs (e.g., digestive tract, blood vessels, urinary bladder) and in other areas (e.g., the eye). It is controlled by the autonomic nervous system, hormones, and intrinsic factors in the organ (e.g., stretch due to food in the intestine).

SKELETAL SYSTEM

Humans have an *endoskeleton* (i.e., it lies *within* the soft tissues of the body). It is composed of living tissue that is capable of growth, adaptation, and repair. The adult body contains 206 bones, which are divided into two major categories by position: axial and appendicular. The *axial skeleton* (80 bones) consists of the skull, vertebral column, and thorax. The *appendicular skeleton* (126 bones) includes the bones of the extremities, shoulders, and pelvis (Fig. U5–3). Bones can also be classified by their shape:

1. *Long bones* are all longer than they are wide and are found in the upper and lower extremities. The humerus, radius, ulna, femur, tibia, fibula, metatarsals, metacarpals, and phalanges are the long bones.
2. *Short bones* (e.g., carpals, tarsals) do not have a long axis; they are cubical.
3. *Flat bones* (e.g., ribs, cranium, scapula, and portions of the pelvic girdle) protect soft body parts and provide large surfaces for muscle attachments.
4. *Irregular bones* have various shapes, such as vertebrae, ear ossicles, facial bones, and pelvis. Irregular bones are similar to other bones in structure and composition.

■ GROSS ANATOMY OF BONE

A typical long bone (Fig. U5–4) has a shaft *(diaphysis)* and two ends *(proximal* and *distal epiphyses).* The diaphysis is a hollow cylinder of compact bone that surrounds a medullary cavity *(marrow).* It is lined with a thin con-

ANTERIOR

- Temporalis
- Orbicularis oculi
- Masseter
- Orbicularis oris
- Sternocleidomastoid
- Pectoralis major
- Pectoralis minor
- Serratus anterior
- Intercostals
- Biceps brachii
- Rectus abdominis
- External oblique
- Transversus abdominis
- Internal oblique
- Brachioradialis
- Sartorius
- Flexors of wrist and digits
- Rectus femoris
- Adductor muscles
- Patella
- Vastus intermedialis
- Vastus lateralis
- Vastus medialis
- Tibialis anterior
- Fibularis longus

POSTERIOR

- Splenius
- Levator scapuli
- Trapezius
- Rhomboideus
- Deltoid
- Infraspinatus
- Triceps brachii
- Serratus posterior
- Latissimus dorsi
- Intercostals
- Olecranon process
- Lumbodorsal fascia
- Extensors of wrist and digits
- Gluteus maximus
- Adductor muscles
- Iliotibial band
- Biceps femoris
- Semitendinosus
- Semimembranosus
- Soleus
- Gastrocnemius
- Achilles tendon

FIGURE U5–1 Principal muscles.

nective tissue layer called *endosteum*. In children and young adults, the epiphyses are separated from the diaphysis by *epiphyseal cartilage* or plates, where bone grows in length. When bone growth is complete, the epiphyseal cartilage is replaced with bone, which joins it to the diaphysis. Fractures of the epiphyseal plates in children can lead to slow bone growth or limb shortening.

Bones are covered with a layer of connective tissue called *periosteum*. The outer (fibrous) layer of periosteum is well supplied with blood vessels and nerves, some of which enter the bone through Volkmann's canals. This layer is very tough and can even hold fracture fragments in place with nondisplaced fractures. The inner (osteogenic) layer is anchored to the bone by bundles of collagen (*Sharpey's fibers*). There is no periosteum on articular surfaces of long bones; these areas are covered with articular cartilage.

■ MICROSCOPIC ANATOMY OF BONE

When viewed through a microscope, *compact bone* is highly organized and solid. It is organized into structural

units, called *osteons* or *haversian systems*. An osteon is essentially a cylinder of bone. Each osteon contains (1) vessels in a central canal (*haversian canal*); (2) concentric layers of bone matrix (*lamellae*); (3) tiny spaces between the lamellae (*lacunae*), which contain osteocytes; and (4) small channels (*canaliculi*). The blood vessels transport nutrients to the bone and carry wastes away from the bone.

Spongy bone does not have such an organized structure. The lamellae are not arranged in concentric circles but, rather, in directions that correspond to the lines of maximum pressure or tension placed on the bone. Spongy bone has osteocytes embedded in lacunae, and lacunae intercommunicate via canaliculi. Blood reaches the osteocytes by passing through spaces in the bone marrow.

■ COMPOSITION OF BONE

Bone's organic framework is formed from protein complexes and fibers, especially collagen (similar to the collagen found in other connective tissues). *Collagen* provides

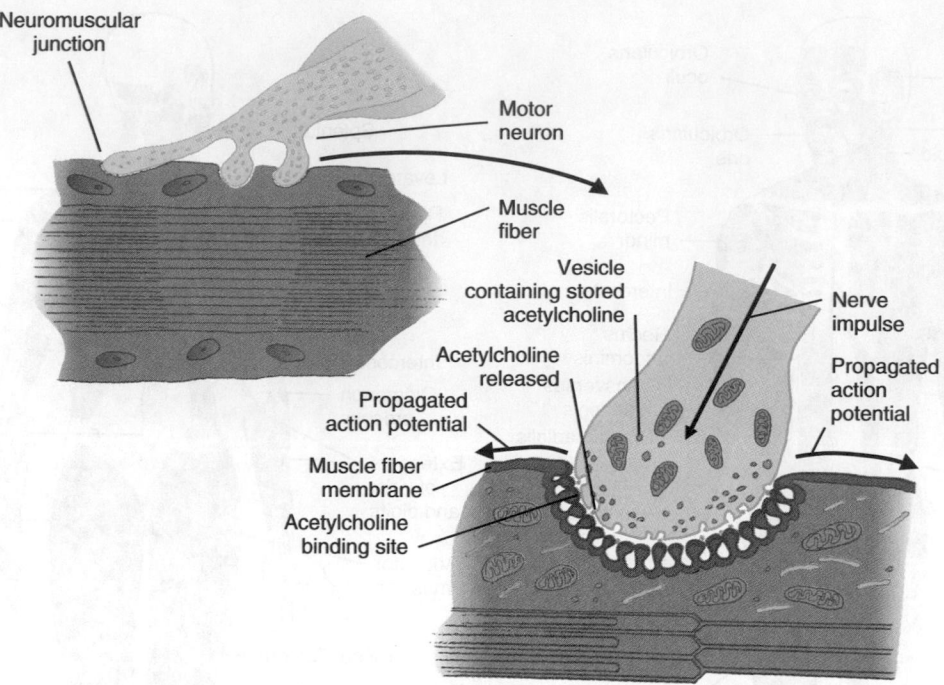

FIGURE U5–2 The neuromuscular junction. When a stimulus, such as a nerve impulse, travels to the neuromuscular junction, acetylcholine is released from storage in vesicles. The acetylcholine diffuses across the cleft and stimulates the muscle to contract.

bone with great tensile strength so that it can withstand stretching and twisting. The inorganic salts (calcium and phosphate in crystalline form, termed *hydroxyapatite*) allow bone to withstand compression. The combination of collagen and salt makes bone exceptionally strong without being brittle. The composition of bone is analogous to that of reinforced concrete, in which steel rods (the collagen) provide tensile strength, and cement, sand, and gravel (the salts) provide compression strength.

Bone contains three types of cells:

1. *Osteoblasts* are bone-forming cells; they lay down new bone by catalyzing reactions that take calcium and phosphate from the blood and form it into bone matrix in a collagen meshwork.
2. *Osteocytes* are osteoblasts that are found in the bone matrix.
3. *Osteoclasts* are cells that resorb (remove) damaged or old bone cells during periods of growth or repair. They are also critical in returning inorganic salts from bone to the bloodstream.

Bone cells allow bone to grow, repair itself, and change shape. Even mature bone constantly changes, with new cells being formed and old cells being destroyed.

ARTICULATIONS

Articulations (joints) are places of union between two or more bones. Not all joints permit movement. Joints may be synovial, fibrous, or cartilaginous.

■ SYNOVIAL JOINTS

Most of the joints in the body are synovial. They are freely movable, permitting position and motion changes. Synovial joints are capable of various movements, depending on the type of joint (see Chapter 25). Synovial joints have four characteristics:

1. Each joint is enclosed by an articular *capsule,* resulting in a joint cavity (Fig. U5–5).
2. Synovial membrane produces *synovial fluid,* which fills the cavity for lubrication and cartilage nourishment.
3. Bone surfaces in the joint are covered by *hyaline cartilage* (articular cartilage).
4. Synovial joints have additional *support* features. *Ligaments* and *tendons* reinforce the capsule and help to limit motion. *Articular discs* are located between the bones in some synovial joints to buffer forceful impact.

■ FIBROUS JOINTS

Fibrous joints are articulations in which bones are held together by fibrous connective tissue. Very little material separates the ends of the bone, and minimal movement is possible.

SUTURE JOINTS. Suture joints include the bones of the skull and sometimes the sutures between the ilium, ischium, and pubic bones. At birth, the bones of the skull are separated to facilitate birth. The bones usually fuse by 2 years. The edges of these bones have grooves (*interdigitations*) that fit firmly together and look somewhat like a suture.

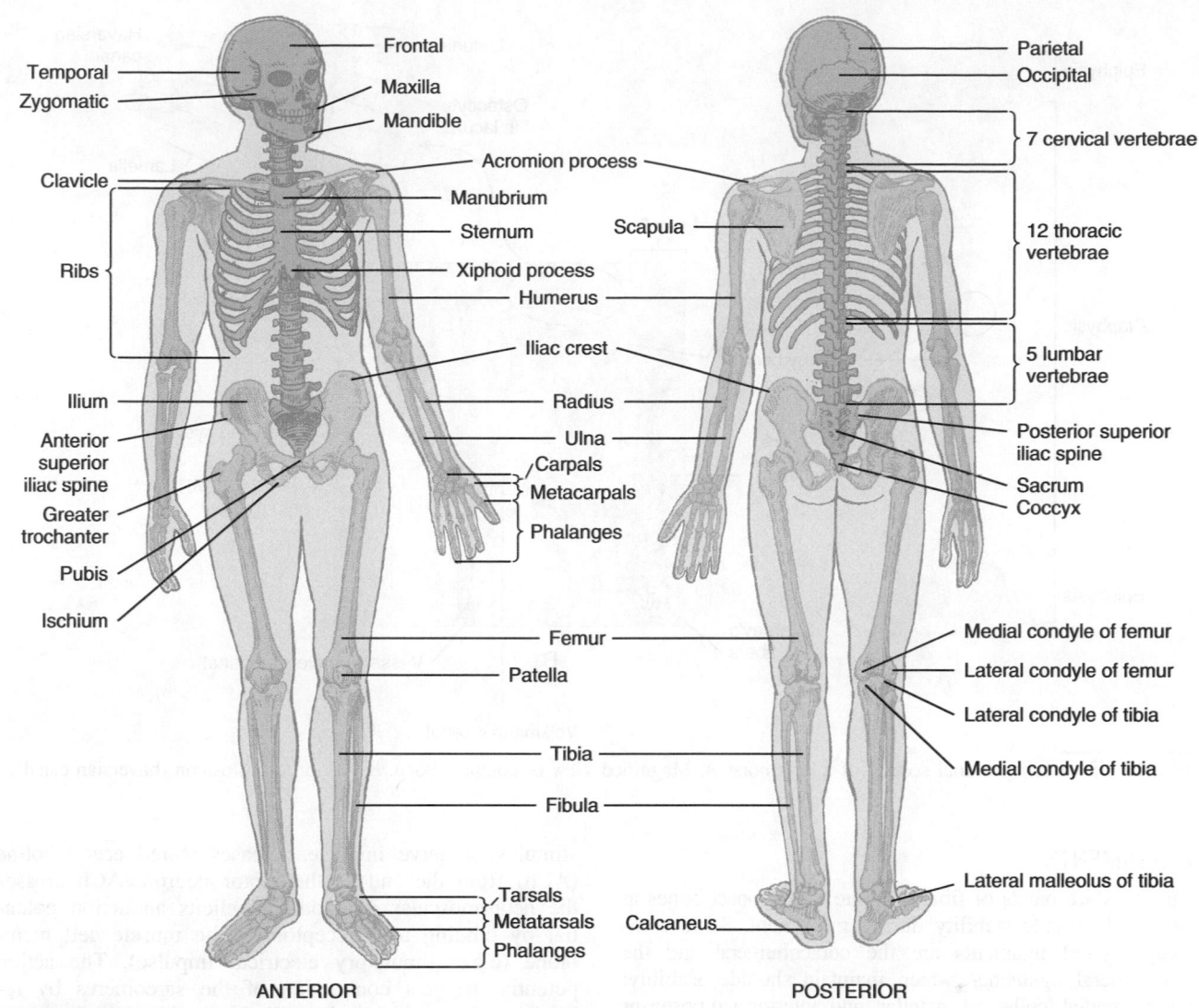

FIGURE U5–3 The adult human skeleton is composed of 206 bones. The axial skeleton is shown in blue, and the appendicular skeleton is shown in brown.

SYNDESMOSIS JOINTS. Syndesmosis (ligamentous) joints are held together by ligaments (bands of fibrous tissue) or membranes. Syndesmosis joints allow some "give." The joints at the distal end of the tibia and fibula are examples of syndesmosis joints.

■ CARTILAGINOUS JOINTS

Bones are held together by cartilage (dense connective tissue; see later). Slight movement is possible in these joints. They are of two types.

SYNCHONDROSES. Synchondroses are held together by hyaline cartilage. Joints between the epiphyses and diaphyses of long bones are replaced by bone (*ossification*) at maturity. In the ribs, this form of cartilage also is temporary and is eventually replaced by bone. In the costal cartilages, synchondroses between ribs and sternum are not usually replaced by bone.

SYMPHYSES. Symphyses are articular surfaces that have a fibrocartilaginous pad or disc connecting the artic-

ulating bones. Slight movement is allowed. Within the joint, the surfaces act as shock absorbers. The vertebrae are separated by symphyses.

CUSHIONING AND SUPPORTIVE STRUCTURES

■ BURSAE AND TENDON SHEATHS

Bursae are small sacs lined with synovial membrane and filled with synovial fluid (see Fig. U5–5). They act as cushions between structures. There are hundreds of bursae in the body. Some are subcutaneous, lying between bone and skin (e.g., the bursa between the olecranon process of the elbow and the skin).

Tendon sheaths are cylindrical synovial structures similar to bursae. They are found where tendons cross joints and may be subject to constant friction. The sheath wraps around the tendon, forming a fluid-filled cushion through which the tendon can slide.

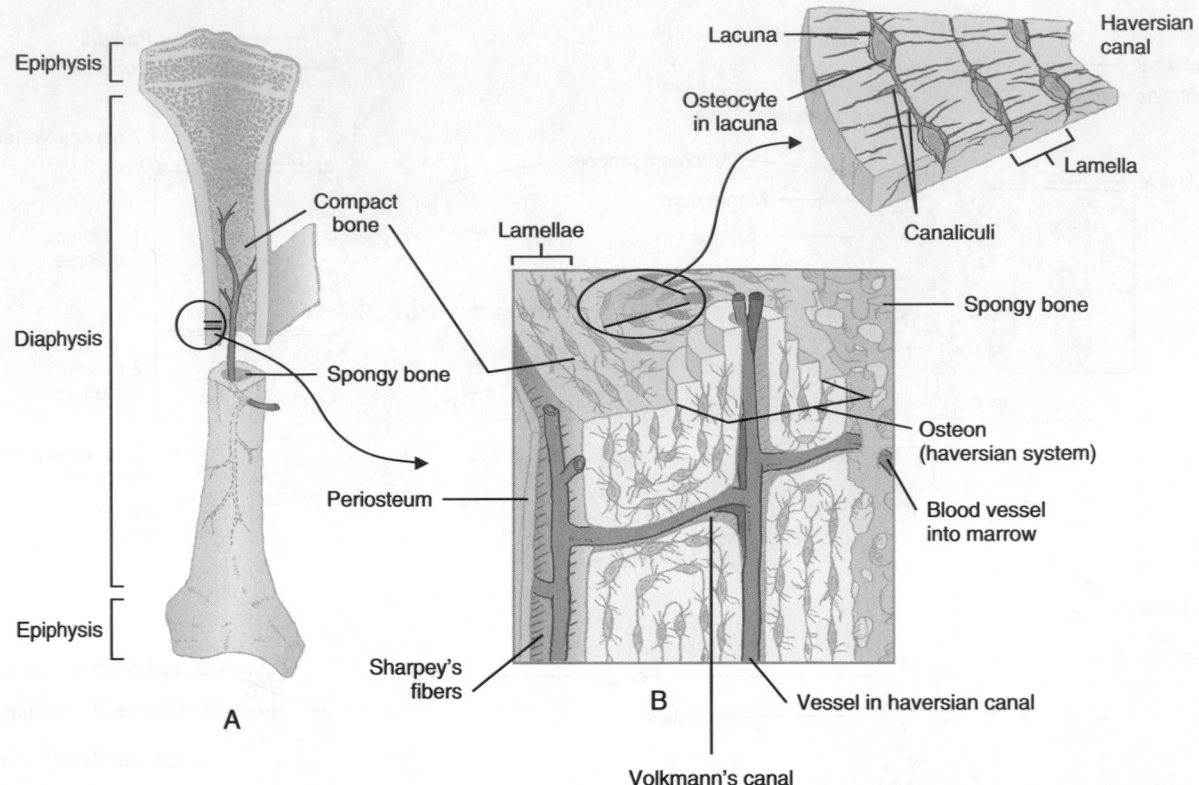

FIGURE U5—4 Longitudinal section of a long bone. *A*, Magnified view of compact bone. *B*, section of an osteon (haversian canal).

◼ LIGAMENTS

Ligaments are bands of fibrous tissue that connect bones at joints and provide stability during movement. Some commonly injured ligaments are the coracohumeral and the glenohumeral ligaments, which maintain shoulder stability; and the medial, collateral, patellar, and anterior and posterior cruciate ligaments, which support the knee (Fig. U5—6).

◼ CARTILAGE

Cartilage is a type of dense connective tissue that is prevalent throughout the musculoskeletal system. It can resist forces of tension and compression with considerable resilience. It is semi-opaque (bluish white or gray) and has limited nerve and blood supply. Most of the skeleton of an embryo is cartilage that gradually changes into bone (*ossification*).

Three types of cartilage are found in the body:

- *Hyaline cartilage,* in respiratory tract, developing bones, and ends of articulating bones
- *Fibrocartilage,* in ligaments and intervertebral discs
- *Elastin cartilage,* in the external ear

FUNCTION OF THE MUSCULOSKELETAL SYSTEM

MUSCLE

◼ MOVEMENT

Skeletal muscle contraction occurs when a stimulus excites an individual muscle fiber (see Fig. U5—2). The stimulus, a nerve impulse, releases stored acetylcholine (ACh) from the end of the motor neuron. ACh crosses the neuromuscular junction and elicits an action potential by binding to a receptor on the muscle cell membrane (e.g., stimulatory electrical impulse). The action potential triggers contraction of the sarcomeres by releasing calcium inside the cell. Nerve fibers may supply more than 100 individual skeletal muscle cells. A continuous flow of stimuli maintains muscle tone (i.e., keeps muscles partially contracted, in a state of readiness for movement).

Muscle fibers relax between contractions because calcium ions that are released during the action potential are free only for a short time. Calcium quickly returns to storage in the sarcoplasmic reticulum in the muscle. If nerve impulses arrive in rapid succession so that calcium remains free, the muscle will continue to contract (called *spasm* or *tetany*).

To generate power, muscle cells require large amounts of oxygen and glucose. Muscles thus have a rich vascular supply. An oxygen debt develops during exercise if oxygen cannot be delivered to muscles in concentrations great enough to meet the immediate metabolic needs of the cell. After exercise, increased oxygen consumption is necessary to relieve oxygen debt.

◼ PROPULSION

Smooth muscle is found in the walls of hollow conduits in the body and its contraction applies pressure that may mix, break up, or move substances forward. For example, smooth muscle of the gastrointestinal (GI) tract propels food through the tract during digestion. Smooth muscle in

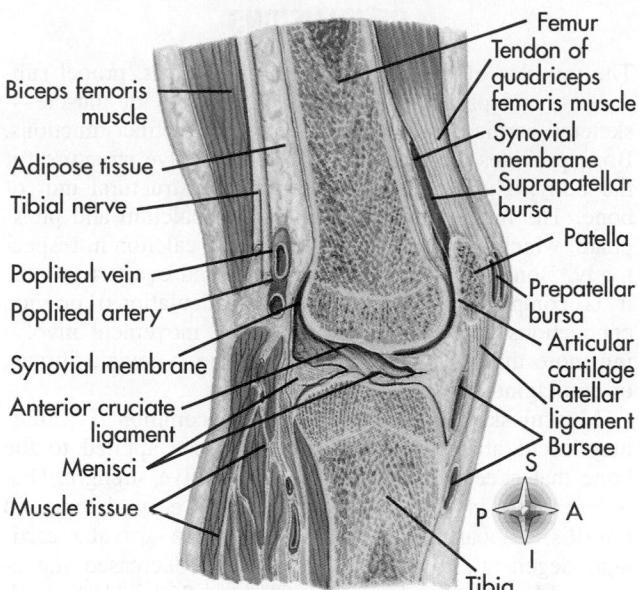

FIGURE U5–5 Anatomy of a synovial joint (knee). (From Thibodeau, G., & Patton, K. [1999]. *Anatomy and physiology* [4th ed.]. St. Louis: Mosby.)

arterioles regulates arterial blood flow by causing vasodilation and vasoconstriction. Smooth muscle in the uterus contracts during labor and smooth muscle in the airways can constrict *(bronchospasm)* or dilate to promote air movement.

■ HEAT PRODUCTION

The activity of skeletal muscle produces heat. Some of this heat can be used to maintain body temperature. During exercise, excess heat is released through sweating and vasodilation. When the body is cold, heat is generated by shivering.

SKELETAL SYSTEM

Bones give form to the body: they support various tissues and organs and permit movement by providing attachments for tendons and ligaments. The skeleton is also protective. The skull and rib cage, for example, protect the brain and special senses and the lungs, respectively.

■ HEMATOPOIETIC FUNCTION

Bone houses the hematopoietic tissues, which manufacture blood cells. In adults, blood cells form in marrow cavities in the skull, vertebrae, ribs, sternum, shoulder, and pelvis. There are two types of bone marrow: *yellow* and *red*. Some authors have noted a third type of bone marrow, brown. *Brown* marrow is generally found in older adults; it is similar to yellow marrow, in that it is inactive but lacks adipose tissue. *Yellow* marrow (connective tissue composed of fat cells) is found in the shafts of long bones and extends into the haversian systems. Yellow marrow does not produce blood cells except during times of increased blood cell need. *Red marrow* has a hematopoietic function; it manufactures red and white blood cells. It is located in the cancellous bone spaces, found in flat bones (see Unit 16).

■ ROLE OF BONE IN HOMEOSTASIS

Bones also provide a crucial portion of mineral balance; they store calcium, phosphorus, sodium, potassium, and other minerals and release them for cellular metabolism and use by other body systems. When blood levels of calcium fall, the parathyroid gland senses the decrease and releases *parathyroid hormone* (PTH). PTH increases the movement of calcium from bone into the extracellular fluids by stimulating the osteoclasts to break down bone and free calcium. PTH also decreases renal excretion of calcium, increases the excretion of phosphate, and increases the metabolic transformation of vitamin D_3 to its active form to increase calcium absorption from the intestine.

When serum calcium levels are high, *calcitonin* (a hormone from the thyroid gland) lowers plasma calcium by inhibiting calcium removal from bone (the opposite of the action of PTH).

■ BONE REMODELING

Throughout life, the bone mass continuously undergoes well-regulated processes of bone formation and bone resorption. The process of bone turnover is called *remodeling,* and it is one of the major mechanisms for maintaining calcium balance in the body. As much as 15% of the total bone mass normally turns over each year in a *three-phase process.*

Phase 1. The cycle begins when a stimulus (such as a hormone, drug, or stressor) activates the bone cell precursors to become osteoclasts.

Phase 2. Osteoclasts gradually resorb the bone. They leave behind an elongated cavity *(resorption cavity),* which matches the general structure of the haversian system or trabeculae.

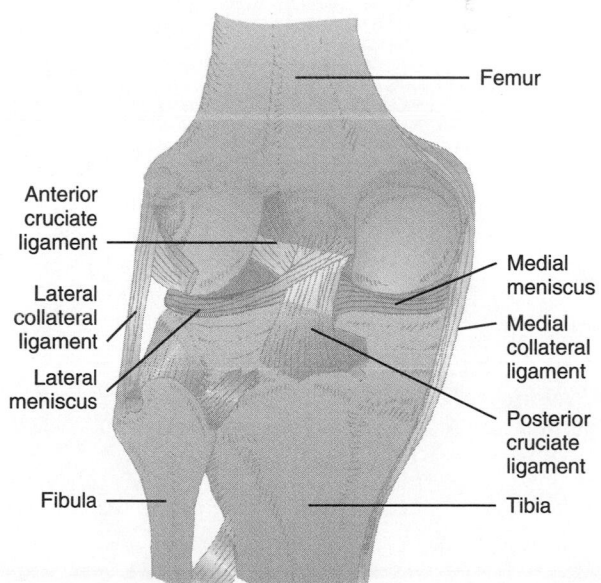

FIGURE U5–6 Posterior view of the knee. When the knee is extended, the taut anterior cruciate ligament prevents overextension. When the knee is flexed, the posterior cruciate ligament prevents the tibia from slipping posteriorly.

Phase 3. New bone is laid down by the osteoblasts. The osteoblasts follow the path of the osteoclasts to create new haversian systems and trabeculae.

The entire process takes about 4 months. Rebuilding of bone requires normal plasma concentrations of calcium and phosphate and is dependent on vitamin D.

■ BONE REPAIR

The remodeling process enables repair of small bony injuries, but breaks *(fractures)* and other wounds of bone heal in a different manner. Initially, the bone heals by forming a hematoma. The hematoma's fibrin provides a meshwork, which is the initial framework for healing. Granulation tissue *(pro-callus)* is produced, and a fibrocartilaginous callus develops prior to bony *(osseous)* depositions. Osteoblasts deposit disorganized clumps of bone matrix *(callus).* The trabeculae and haversian systems follow. Finally, the bony edges are remodeled to the size and shape of the bone before injury.

EFFECTS OF AGING

Aging affects bone, muscle, and tendons. Bone tissue is lost because the rate of loss exceeds the rate of growth. The haversian systems in compact bone erode. The lacunae enlarge, and cortical bone becomes thin and porous. *Osteoporosis,* a condition of decreased calcium in bone, leads to weak and brittle bones and increased risk of fracture.

Eventually, cartilage becomes more rigid and fragile and muscle bulk decreases. As muscle mass decreases, so does maximal strength, which can decline by 50% between the ages of 20 and 50 years. Several theories have been offered to explain these changes, including changes in activity, reduced circulation, cardiovascular disorders, and nutritional problems.

CONCLUSIONS

The muscles of the body provide movement, propel substances, and produce heat. The three types of muscle—skeletal, cardiac, and smooth—perform distinct functions. Bone provides a framework and a protective structure for the body. The haversian system is the structural unit of bone. The major minerals in bone are calcium and phosphate, which are regulated by PTH and calcitonin, respectively. Bone is constantly remodeled, and every 4 months it is completely replaced. Joints (articulations) provide connections between bones and allow movement involving more than one bone. Joints may be synovial, fibrous, or cartilaginous.

Musculoskeletal disorders are very common. Fractures may occur at any age because of forces applied to the bone that exceed its tensile or compressive strength. Disorders seen in the articular surfaces (e.g., rheumatoid arthritis, osteoarthritis) develop when the articular cartilage degenerates, leading to pain and decreased movement. Muscle disorders (see Chapter 26) include such conditions as muscular dystrophy (progressive muscle degeneration) and myasthenia gravis (loss of receptors on the muscle for acetylcholine, leading to profound muscle weakness).

BIBLIOGRAPHY

1. Berne, R., & Levy, M. (1993). *Physiology* (3rd ed.). St. Louis: Mosby–Year Book.
2. Guyton, A. (1995). *Textbook of medical physiology* (9th ed.). Philadelphia: W. B. Saunders.
3. Heveron, B., & Kaempffe, F. (1995). Tears of the rotator cuff. *Orthopaedic Nursing, 14*(6), 38–41.
4. Thibodeau, G. & Patton, K. (1999). *Anatomy and physiology* (4th ed.). St. Louis: Mosby.

CHAPTER

25

Assessment of the Musculoskeletal System

Peggy Doheny
Carol Sedlak

Assessment of the musculoskeletal system begins with a health history, which provides direction for further assessment. The musculoskeletal physical examination can be either general (as in a screening examination) or local (for a specific problem or injury). Similarly, diagnostic tests can be either general or specific. The resulting data allow you to make judgments about the client's musculoskeletal status. Musculoskeletal assessment usually also includes the client's functional status and ability to perform activities of daily living (ADL) and to meet self-care needs. This aspect of the assessment involves evaluation of the client's exercise habits and leisure activities that promote health.

HISTORY

The musculoskeletal history consists of:

- Biographical and demographic data
- Chief complaint (including symptom analysis)
- Past health history
- Family history
- Psychosocial history
- Lifestyle data
- Review of systems

Collect information to help determine the nature and extent of the client's current disorder. If the chief complaint is related to trauma, keep the history interview brief and focus on the cause of injury. You may need to defer the interview, depending on the extent of the client's injury. Once the client's condition is stable, you can obtain a more complete history.

■ BIOGRAPHICAL AND DEMOGRAPHIC DATA

Personal information enables individualized care planning. For example, knowing where the client lives and the kind of transportation the client uses helps you understand the energy required for the client to keep an appointment. Getting to know the client's significant others is essential in planning care as well.

The client's age and sex may suggest possible causes of musculoskeletal problems. For example, 85% of people older than 70 years have some osteoarthritis. Osteoporosis (porous bone) occurs most often in postmenopausal women. Reiter's syndrome is most common in men between 20 and 40 years of age. Osteogenic sarcoma is rare after age 40. Carpal tunnel syndrome occurs more often in women than in men.

■ CURRENT HEALTH

Chief Complaint

Ask the client to describe the reason for seeking health care. Common clinical manifestations related to the musculoskeletal system are pain, tenderness, muscle tightness or weakness, joint stiffness, cramps, muscle spasms, swelling, redness, deformity, reduced movement or joint range of motion (ROM), sensory changes, and other abnormal sensations. ADL may be affected. Ask the client and significant others to recount their perceptions of the problem and its cause. Their answers often provide not only information about areas for further assessment but also clues about personal fears and concerns.

Symptom Analysis

Conduct a symptom analysis for each manifestation the client reports (see Chapter 9). Examples of assessment questions for typical musculoskeletal manifestations follow.

PAIN

Ask the client to point to the exact location of the pain. Poorly localized pain usually stems from problems in blood vessels, joints, fascia, or periosteum.

Ask the client to describe the pain: Is it an ache, a sharp pain, a throbbing? Throbbing pain is usually bone-related, and aches are commonly muscular. Sharp pain may be caused by a fracture or bone infection. Ask the client to rate the pain on a scale of 0 to 10, on which 0 is no pain and 10 is the worst pain possible.

What makes the pain worse: Temperature changes? Movement? Lifting or carrying something heavy? Pain from osteoarthritis is worse in cold, damp weather. Pain that occurs with movement is typical of joint problems.

Degenerative hip conditions produce pain during weight-bearing and during and after walking. Degenerative knee problems produce pain during and after walking. Vertebral disc herniation produces pain on bending or lifting and may radiate down one leg.

Is the pain worse at a particular time of day? Does it wake the client or prevent sleeping at night? Inflammation of bursae or tendons is worse at night. Degenerative joint pain is often worse at the end of a day.

Does rest relieve the pain? Most musculoskeletal pain is helped by rest.

Which medications help to relieve the pain? Pain from inflammation is usually helped by aspirin or nonsteroidal anti-inflammatory drugs (NSAIDs). Narcotic analgesics are usually required for traumatic injury.

Have there been any recent injuries? Sometimes a client does not associate a fall or other injury with current manifestations.

Is the pain associated with chills, fever, rash, or a sore throat? Joint pain occurring 10 to 14 days after a sore throat may be from rheumatic fever.

JOINT STIFFNESS

Ask the client to point to joints that are stiff. Are they always stiff? How long does the stiffness last? Some conditions, such as ankylosing spondylitis, have remissions and exacerbations.

At what time of day is the stiffness worst? With degenerative joint disease, stiffness is often most severe in the morning after a night in bed.

What relieves the stiffness? Temperature changes? Exercise? Coldness and lack of use typically increase joint stiffness. Heat may reduce muscle spasm. Heat applied to a recently injured joint may worsen stiffness by increasing bleeding into and swelling of the joint.

Does the joint lock so it cannot move? Does the client hear or feel bones rubbing together? Bone malalignment within a joint causes locking. *Crepitus* (the sound of bone ends rubbing together) indicates fractures or joint destruction.

Does the client have pain or weakness in muscles with certain movements? Weakness in muscles may result from various neuromuscular disorders. If weakness is present, does it interfere with the client's usual activities?

SWELLING

Ask how long the client has had the swelling. Is there pain? Swelling and pain commonly accompany bone and muscle injury. With degenerative joint disease, swelling may not develop for some time, maybe weeks, after pain is present—or it may not develop at all.

Does swelling limit the client's movement? Limited movement may stem from soft tissue damage and swelling in a joint.

Does rest or elevating the part give relief? Elevation reduces swelling in acute injuries.

Ask the client whether the body part was casted recently. Removing a cast can result in temporary swelling. A casted limb also may have muscle atrophy.

Has the area been hot or red? Redness and heat indicate inflammation, infection, or recent injury and are not usually present with degenerative conditions.

DEFORMITY AND IMMOBILITY

Has the deformity developed suddenly or gradually? A gradually developing mass may be a tumor.

Is movement limited? Is this limitation always present? Is it worse after activity? Does any body position make it worse or better? Immobility from degenerative joint disease varies with the severity of the condition.

Ask how the deformity affects the client's daily activities. Does the client use any supportive equipment, such as crutches, a walker, or bandages? Use of such aids offers clues to the severity of the disability.

SENSORY CHANGES

Does the client have a history of back pain or injury? If so, where is the pain located? Does the pain travel, for example, down the back of the leg? Does the client have trouble walking? Is there a loss of feeling anywhere? If so, is the loss of feeling associated with any pain? Does the client have any tingling or burning sensation? Pressure on nerves or blood vessels can occur from swelling, tumors, or fractures, causing loss of sensation. Sensory changes may be associated with pain in an arm or hand.

■ PAST HEALTH HISTORY

Carefully assess previous trauma, accidents, or surgery involving bones or joints. The client may have sustained fractures, dislocations, strains, or sprains. Previous accidents leading to bony fracture may predispose to degenerative changes.

Question the client about a range of past health problems because many diseases can affect the musculoskeletal system. Explore both childhood and adult-onset disorders because of their possible long-term effects.

Childhood and Infectious Diseases

Health conditions may affect the musculoskeletal system directly or indirectly. For example, diabetes mellitus may predispose a client to degenerative joint disease. Blood dyscrasias, such as hemophilia, may cause bleeding in joints that produces pain, swelling, tenderness, and deformity. Psoriasis may precede psoriatic arthritis. Cartilage damage from trauma may precipitate degenerative changes in a relatively young person. Ask about a history of tuberculosis, sickle cell disease, poliomyelitis, inflammatory or degenerative arthritis, scurvy, rickets, osteomyelitis, soft tissue infection, fungus infection of bones or joints, and streptococcal and neuromuscular disorders.

Major Illnesses and Hospitalizations

Besides inquiring about diseases, such as diabetes mellitus, tuberculosis, poliomyelitis, and arthritis, ask about hospitalizations related to musculoskeletal disorders or trauma. If the client or significant others cannot remember details, ask for permission to obtain the medical records. Ask about past or present minor and major injuries, including (1) circumstances of the injury, (2) diagnosis of the injury, (3) treatment received, (4) duration of treatment, and (5) current problems resulting from the injury.

Musculoskeletal injury involves fractures, sprains, strains, and joint dislocations. Minor injuries may be treated on an ambulatory basis, whereas major injuries may require prolonged hospitalization, surgery, or rest and immobilization. Ask whether the client has residual impairment from the injury, such as a need to use an assistive device (cane, crutches, or walker). Ask whether the client has had to change or adjust ADL because of lingering limitations.

Medications

Question the client about past and present prescription and over-the-counter medications as well as herbal remedies. For each medication, find out (1) the reason for taking it, (2) the dose and frequency, (3) how long the client has taken it, and (4) any observed side effects. Ask the client about specific medications used for musculoskeletal problems, such as muscle relaxants, salicylates, NSAIDs, and steroids, because some medications affect the musculoskeletal system.

For example, corticosteroid therapy can lead to necrosis of the femur head, septic arthritis, and muscle weakness. High doses of anticoagulants can produce hemarthrosis (blood in joints). Anticonvulsants may cause osteomalacia. Phenothiazines may produce gait disturbances. Potassium-depleting diuretics may produce cramps and muscle weakness. Amphetamines and caffeine cause a generalized increase in motor activity. Hormone replacement therapy with estrogen has been shown to modify the effects of osteoporosis in postmenopausal women.

Use of NSAIDs for more than 4 weeks can lead to bleeding problems—especially in the gastrointestinal (GI) tract—because of decreased platelet aggregation. Renal and hepatic changes can also develop. Long-term use of NSAIDs requires follow-up laboratory assessments to monitor for side effects. Complete blood count and serum assays of liver enzymes, potassium, and creatinine, and urinalysis are usually assessed.

The herb cayenne (*capsicum*) or capsaicin applied externally relieves the ache and pain of arthritis. If taken internally, however, capsaicin can cause GI distress and, at high doses, may damage unmyelinated and small-diameter myelinated nerve fibers. White willow (*Salix purpurea, S. fragilis, S. daphnoides, S. alba*) has analgesic properties. It contains salicin, which may have adverse effects similar to those of salicylate.

■ FAMILY HEALTH HISTORY

Some musculoskeletal problems with a familial predisposition are arthritis, osteoporosis, ankylosing spondylitis, gout, Heberden's nodes in osteoarthritis, muscular dystrophy, and scoliosis. Thirty per cent of people with psoriatic arthritis have a family history of psoriasis.

■ PSYCHOSOCIAL HISTORY

The integrity of the musculoskeletal system enables a person to function effortlessly. However, many problems can disrupt that integrity—and the coping ability of both client and significant others. Ask about the client's daily activities and habits. When assessing a client with a chronic illness or degenerative process, ask whether the disorder has affected the client's interactions with others or view of self and others. Crippling illnesses often curtail social activity and result in lower self-esteem.

Occupation

Ask whether heavy lifting or strenuous activity is common in the client's life. Such activity can cause muscle strain, degenerative vertebral disc problems, and other trauma. Low back pain can arise from jobs involving extensive driving. Habitually carrying heavy objects, such as a mailbag, shoulder bag, attaché case, or other equipment, places uneven pressure on the spinal column. Prolonged use of computers and keyboards can cause orthopedic injuries from repetitive strain (see Chapter 27).

Activities of Daily Living

Are there everyday activities that the client finds difficult or impossible, such as (1) opening containers, pouring liquids, and cutting up food, (2) dressing, using zippers, and fastening or unfastening buttons, snaps, or hooks, (3) grooming, combing hair, and applying makeup, (4) running a bath and testing water temperature, washing hair, and shaving, (5) writing, and (6) getting out of the house, climbing stairs, or getting in and out of chairs or cars?

Ask whether physical limitations prevent the client from performing any daily activities. Also assess the client's attention to safety. Ask about safety practices used at work and at home. Does the client use recommended equipment, such as safety shoes or safety guards on power tools? There is a high incidence of accidental injury among people who pay little attention to safety practices.

Exercise

Document the details of the client's typical recreational activities and exercise pattern. Lack of exercise produces poor muscle tone, which leads to muscle strain. Sporadic exercise of poorly toned muscles is more likely to cause muscle injury and spasm. Lack of warm-up exercises increases the likelihood of injury as well.

Fractures and other trauma can arise from contact sports. Achilles tendon damage can occur from improperly landing on heels while jogging. Pain in arm joints can be caused by racket sports, such as tennis and squash, which require a strong grasp, wrist extension, and forearm rotation.

Ask about typical footwear. High-heeled shoes can shorten the Achilles tendon and pitch the center of gravity forward, leading to lordosis.

Nutrition

A dietary history can provide clues to musculoskeletal problems as well (see Chapter 28). For example, obesity stresses weight-bearing joints and predisposes to ligament instability, particularly of the lower back. Poor calcium intake can lead to bone decalcification and fractures. Ask about foods eaten on a typical day. Adequate dietary intake of vitamins A and D, calcium, and protein is important for musculoskeletal health.

Inquire about recent weight changes. Excessive weight gain can place stress on the musculoskeletal system.

Habits and Safety

Health promotion habits and a positive lifestyle can reduce the risk for development of musculoskeletal disorders. Increasing dietary calcium and weight-bearing activities, such as walking, can help prevent osteoporosis and improve strength and flexibility. Maintaining musculoskeletal health enhances a person's ability to perform ADL. Moreover, early detection of conditions such as scoliosis through screening programs can help with early intervention.

■ REVIEW OF SYSTEMS

Ask about such musculoskeletal problems as (1) muscle pain, spasm, or tenderness, (2) joint pain, stiffness, pain, swelling, or redness, (3) weakness, (4) limited movement, (5) clumsiness, (6) crepitus, (7) backache, and (8) changes in joints or bones. Investigate each reported problem. Inquire about the effect of the problem on the client's ability to perform ADL.

Assessment findings from other body systems may indicate musculoskeletal problems. Examples are:

- Pain or burning when urinating, which is associated with Reiter's syndrome
- Tachycardia and hypertension, which may accompany gout
- Chronic diarrhea, which may occur when arthritis is associated with colitis or other GI problems
- Conjunctivitis, which may indicate Reiter's syndrome, and nongranulomatous uveitis, which may occur with ankylosing spondylitis
- Skin changes, which may indicate musculoskeletal problems (dry skin over the thumb and the first two fingers suggests carpal tunnel syndrome, for example)
- Cramping leg pain with activity, which may signal intermittent claudication
- Generalized muscle cramping, which may result from electrolyte imbalances
- Joint pain with recent chills, fever, or sore throat, which may result from rheumatic fever

Detailed questions for the review of systems are found in Chapter 9.

PHYSICAL EXAMINATION

Assessment of the musculoskeletal system should proceed systematically to avoid missing hidden problems. Use an examining room big enough for the client to move around. Natural lighting is best for assessing skin color changes and swelling. Artificial light distorts some assessment findings. During the examination, have the client sit, stand, and walk unless a position is contraindicated by the client's condition.

Musculoskeletal assessment consists of inspecting and palpating (1) *muscle masses* for symmetry, involuntary movements, tenderness, tone, and strength, (2) *joints* for symmetry, crepitus, tenderness or pain, and ROM, and (3) *bones* for deformity and leg length discrepancy. As-

---

PHYSICAL ASSESSMENT FINDINGS IN THE HEALTHY ADULT

Musculoskeletal System

Inspection

Joints in alignment; posture straight; gait smooth.
Extremities symmetrical and of equal length.
Muscle groups symmetrical, without atrophy or fasciculations.
Joints without erythema, swelling, or deformities.
Full range of motion (active and passive) in all major joints.

Palpation

Muscle groups firm, symmetrical, nontender; without masses or spasms.
Joints stable and nontender; without heat, crepitus (palpable or audible), bogginess, or nodules.
Muscle strength in all major muscle groups rated 5/5.

---

sessment of muscle-stretch and deep tendon reflexes is discussed in Chapter 67.

■ GENERAL MUSCULOSKELETAL EXAMINATION

Use inspection and palpation to examine each body part. First, examine the body at rest, then assess ROM and muscle strength. Look for normal findings such as those outlined in the accompanying Physical Assessment Findings in the Healthy Adult chart.

When the client enters the examination room, assess the gait, body mobility, posture, general joint motion, and balance. While observing movement and gait, watch for (1) gait patterns associated with specific disorders (see Chapter 67), (2) objective evidence of discomfort, and (3) indications of joint stiffness or muscle weakness, lack of coordination, and deformities. Then have the client sit on the edge of the examination table. Observe the client's general appearance and body build. Examine the head, neck, shoulders, and upper extremities.

Have the client stand, and examine the chest, back, and ilium. Observe posture, body build, body contours, body alignment, and the cervical, thoracic, and lumbar spine. Observe the relationships of various body parts to one another, such as the relationship of feet to legs, legs to hips, and hips to pelvis (Fig. 25–1).

Observe the client's stance, and note any spinal deformities or other abnormalities (Fig. 25–2), such as:

- *Kyphosis*, an abnormally increased roundness of the thoracic curve or hump-back
- *Scoliosis*, a lateral deformity of the spine
- *Lordosis*, an abnormal increase in the lumbar curve, or swayback
- *Genu varum*, or bowleg
- *Genu valgum*, or knock-knee

The terms *varus (varum)* and *valgus (valgum)* refer to the direction in which the deformity lies in relationship to the midline. With a varus deformity, the de-

FIGURE 25-1 When performing a musculoskeletal assessment, have the client stand and walk if possible. Observe the client's stance, joint mobility, and posture. If you were to assess this man only while he was reclining, you might not notice his posture, the curvature of his spine, and his limited range of motion.

formity points toward the midline. With a valgus deformity, the deformity is bent or twisted away from the midline.

Last, with the client supine, examine the hips, knees, ankles, and feet for alignment, symmetry, and deformities. Determine any discrepancy between leg lengths by measuring from the anterior iliac spine to the medial malleolus. Measurements should be within 1 cm of each other. If a discrepancy is noted, determine whether it exists above or below the knee.

FIGURE 25-2 Musculoskeletal deformities observable during assessment. *A*, Kyphosis. *B*, Scoliosis. *C*, Lordosis. *D*, Genu varum. *E*, Genu valgum.

Muscles

Compare each muscle group with its contralateral side. Muscles should be free of *fasciculations* (fine muscle twitches) and smooth, without bulges or lumps. Palpate

TABLE 25-1	ASSESSING MUSCLE STRENGTH
Muscle Group	**Technique**
Deltoid	Push down client's arm while it is held up and client resists.
Biceps	Hold client's arm in extension while it is fully extended and client flexes arm.
Triceps	Keep client's arm in flexion while it is flexed and client extends arm.
Wrist and finger muscles	Push client's fingers together while client spreads them and resists.
Grip strength	Pull your own crossed index and middle fingers out from the client's grasp.
Hip muscles	Hold down client's leg while it is fully extended and while client lifts it off the table (client is supine).
Hip muscles (abduction)	Prevent client from spreading legs apart against resistance applied to the lateral surfaces of the knees (client is supine with legs extended).
Hip muscles (adduction)	Prevent client from bringing legs together against resistance applied to the medial surfaces of the knees (client is supine with legs extended).
Hamstrings	Straighten client's knees while client is supine with knees flexed and resists.
Quadriceps	Flex client's knee while client is supine with knee partially in extension and resists.
Ankle and foot muscles	Dorsiflex client's foot while client resists. Plantiflex client's foot while client resists.

muscle groups gently, from proximal to distal, feeling the *muscle tone* (the state of tension in a muscle at rest, which is felt as firmness). Muscles should feel firm and smooth and should be bilaterally equal in size and nontender. A slight increase in mass, or *hypertrophy*, on the dominant side is normal, whereas *atrophy*, or decrease in muscle mass, on either side is abnormal. If muscle groups are noticeably unequal in size, use a tape measure to assess limb circumferences. Differences of 1 cm or less between the two sides are considered within normal variation.

Assess *muscle strength* while putting joints through active ROM. If a detailed assessment is necessary, each major muscle group can be assessed separately (Table 25–1). The sternocleidomastoid and trapezius muscles are tested as part of the head and neck (cranial nerve) examination (see Chapter 67). Test muscle strength by asking the client to repeat ROM while you apply resistance. Note the strength exerted against the resistance. If you detect weakness, decrease the resistance. Because the dominant arm is usually stronger, ask whether the client is right-handed or left-handed. Rate muscle strength numerically as follows:

0 = Muscle is paralyzed with no visible or palpable contraction (zero)
1 = Contraction is palpable but muscle does not move (trace)
2 = Full ROM is present with the joint supported to eliminate gravity (poor)
3 = Full ROM is present with gravity as the only resistance (fair)
4 = Full ROM is present against moderate resistance (good)
5 = Full ROM is present against normal resistance and gravity (normal)

Include the muscle strength rating scale as part of the client's record to ensure understanding and consistency with other health care providers.

Joints and Bones

Inspect the client's joints and bones, and compare findings bilaterally. You should find symmetry without redness, swelling, enlargement, or deformity. Palpate each joint and bone for edema and tenderness, which should be absent. Palpate joints during movement for crepitus, which is abnormal. Joints should feel smooth as they move, and nodules should be absent.

ROM is the maximum range of movement attainable by a healthy joint. You can measure ROM with a goniometer, a flexible protractor-type instrument placed on a joint to measure the angles created by joint movement (Fig. 25–3). As needed, assess ROM in all the client's joints (Fig. 25–4).

Special Tests of Joint Function

Advanced practitioners may use special assessments to determine whether an injury has occurred in a joint. Some common tests are listed in Table 25–2. Two tests are shown in Figure 25–5.

FIGURE 25–3 Use of a goniometer to measure joint range of motion.

◼ NEUROVASCULAR ASSESSMENT

A neurovascular assessment is essential for clients with a past musculoskeletal injury because of the high risk of ischemia, deformity, or loss of function in the affected limb.

Components of Neurovascular Assessment

A neurovascular assessment involves checking for (1) pain, (2) pallor, (3) temperature, (4) pulses, (5) capillary refill, (6) paresthesia, and (7) mobility of affected joints.

If the client has pain, using an intensity rating scale of 0 to 10, as previously described, can help determine whether the pain is getting worse—a possible result of edema and nerve compression.

Pallor, coolness, or cyanosis can indicate circulatory compromise in the limb. Check pulses and capillary refill bilaterally to determine the adequacy of blood supply to small peripheral vessels. Capillaries should refill within 2 or 3 seconds.

Loss of sensation and motor function in a limb can signal nerve injury.

Peripheral Nerve Assessment

Test sensation and motor function in major peripheral nerves (Fig. 25–6). Check sensation with the client's eyes closed. Light touch should be perceptible if sensation is normal. If a "pins and needles" sensation is reported, assess further (see Chapter 67). The client should be able to demonstrate active motion of a specific joint upon request. Inability to move a joint and the presence of pain with passive ROM may indicate compartment syndrome.

Perform further assessments, such as of capillary refill, pulses, color, and warmth (see Chapter 27). When casts prevent full neurovascular assessment, observe for edema, capillary refill, and joint movement.

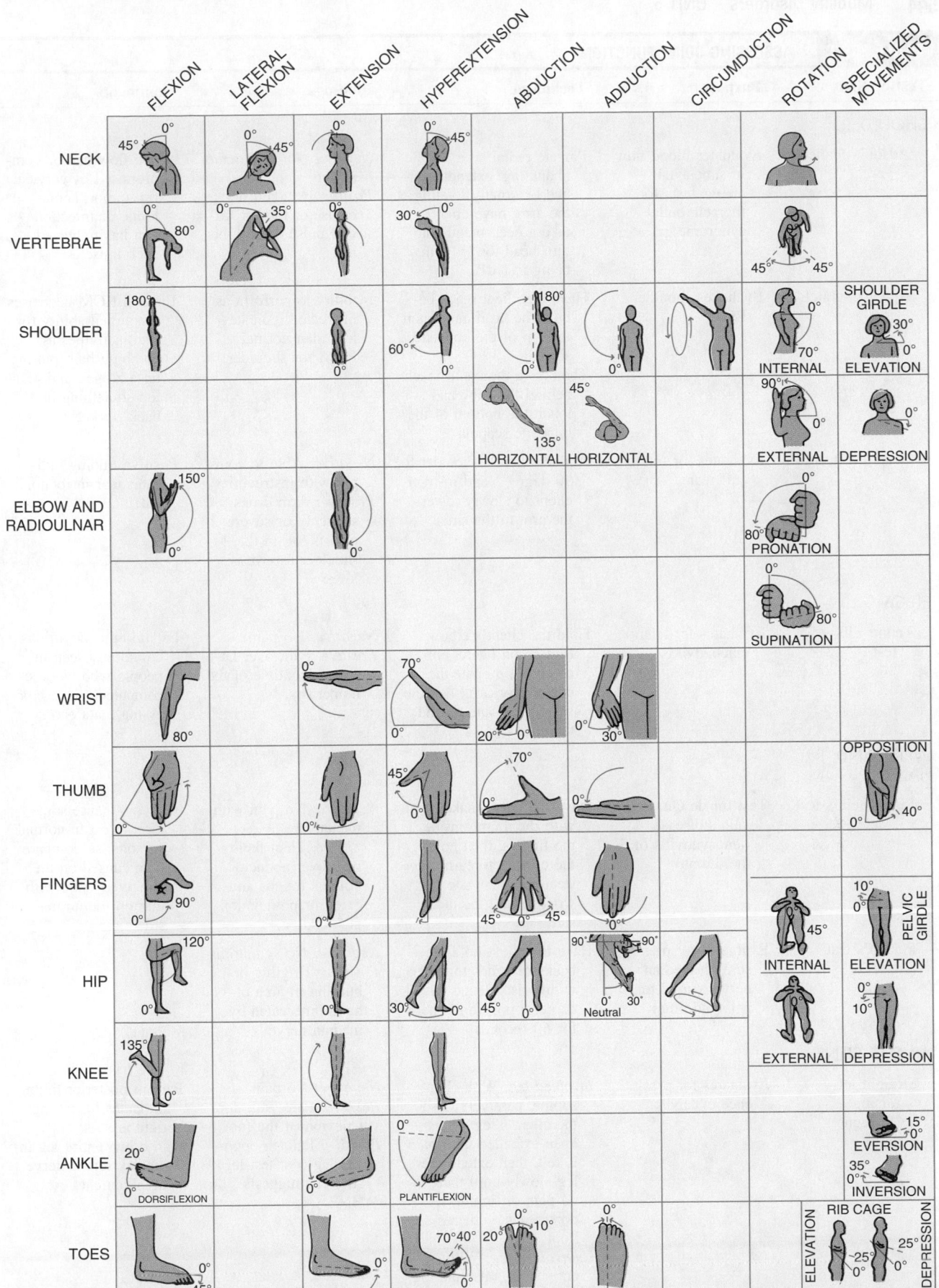

FIGURE 25–4 Joint range of motion (ROM). All joints are at 0 degrees when in anatomic position. ROM begins at 0 degrees, as shown by the *solid lines*. Attainment of average normal ROM is shown by *dotted lines* and the number of degrees in the angle formed by the two lines.

TABLE 25–2	ASSESSING JOINT FUNCTION			
Test or Sign	**Purpose**	**Technique**	**Findings**	**Comments**
SHOULDER				
Adson's maneuver	Evaluates blood flow in subclavian artery; tests for thoracic outlet syndrome	Palpate radial artery while abducting, extending, and externally rotating the arm; have client take a deep breath and turn head toward arm being tested	*Negative:* Pulse remains strong *Positive:* Marked decrease or loss of radial pulse during the test	Blood flow can be compromised by cervical rib, tumor, hematoma, or infection that has tightened neck muscles
Apley's scratch test	Evaluates shoulder ROM	Have the client reach behind the head and touch the top of the opposite scapula Then have the client reach behind the back and touch the bottom of the opposite scapula	Inability to perform as instructed indicates less than normal ROM for shoulder	Limited ROM decreases functional ability for such activities as combing hair, pulling up a zipper, and placing something in a back pocket
Drop arm test	Evaluates for rotator cuff tear	Abduct client's shoulder to 90 degrees, and instruct client to slowly lower the arm to the side	*Negative:* Able to comply with instructions *Positive:* Arm drops suddenly or severe pain is felt in the shoulder as arm is lowered	Positive finding indicates tear in rotator cuff
ELBOW				
Tennis elbow test	Evaluates for lateral epicondylitis	Hold the client's elbow (thumb on lateral epicondyle), pronate the client's forearm, flex the wrist fully, and extend the elbow	*Negative:* No pain *Positive:* Pain over lateral epicondyle of the humerus	Lateral epicondylitis is commonly seen in people who work at computers (word processing, data entry)
WRIST AND HAND				
Finkelstein's test	Test for de Quervain's disease (tenosynovitis of the thumb)	Have the client make a fist with the thumb inside the fingers, then hold the client's forearm steady and deviate the wrist toward the ulnar side	*Negative:* No pain with maneuver *Positive:* Client feels pain over abductor pollicis longus and extensor pollicis longus tendons	Test may cause some discomfort in normal persons, so compare pain caused on the "affected" side with that on the normal side
Phalen's test	Evaluates for pressure on median nerve (carpal tunnel syndrome)	Have the client hold the backs of hands together with wrists flexed 90 degrees; position is held for 60 seconds	*Negative:* No symptoms *Positive:* Tingling or burning in area of hand innervated by median nerve	
LUMBAR SPINE				
Straight leg raising (Lasègue's sign)	Evaluates for presence of HNP	*Involved leg:* With client supine, passively raise the client's leg with knee extended until pain is felt, then extend the leg slowly until there is no pain or tightness; dorsiflex the client's floot *Uninvolved leg:* With client supine, raise the leg as described for the involved leg	*Negative:* No pain *Positive:* Pain with dorsiflexion of the foot *Positive:* Pain in opposite leg (not test leg) strongly suggests HNP	Pain in posterior thigh indicates hamstring tightness Pain down entire leg indicates sciatic nerve involvement

TABLE 25-2	ASSESSING JOINT FUNCTION *Continued*			
Test or Sign	**Purpose**	**Technique**	**Findings**	**Comments**
KNEE				
Drawer test (anterior)	Evaluates stability of ACL	Have client lie on back with knee flexed to 90 degrees and hip to 45 degrees; hold the foot of the test leg in place, and then draw the tibia forward on the femur (Place your hands around the tibia with the thumbs on the medial and lateral joint lines of the knee, as shown in Fig. 25–5)	*Negative:* Movement 6 mm or less *Positive:* Movement more than 6 mm indicates tear in ACL	If PCL is injured, result may be false-positive If PCL injury is suspected, check for posterior "sag" sign (gravity and drawer test)
Drawer test (posterior)	Evaluates stability of PCL	Position client as described for anterior test and push tibia back on femur	*Negative:* Tibia does not move back *Positive:* Backward movement of tibia (felt or observed) indicates injury to PCL	
Gravity test (posterior sag sign)	Evaluates integrity of PCL	Have client lie supine with hips flexed to 45 degrees and knees to 90 degrees	*Positive:* Tibia "sagging" back on the femur indicates that PCL is torn	With minimal swelling, sag is very evident, as is obvious concavity distal to the patella
Lachman's test	Evaluates injury to the ACL	Have client lie supine with the knees between full extension and 30 degrees; then use one hand to stabilize the femur and the other hand to move the tibia forward (see Fig. 25–5*B*)	*Positive:* When tibia moves forward, the infrapatellar tendon slope disappears	This test is the best indicator of ACL injury
McMurray's test	Evaluates for medial and lateral meniscus injury	Have client lie supine with the injured leg fully flexed; then cup the heel with one hand and place your other hand on the knee (fingers on the medial joint line, thumb on the lateral joint line); first, rotate the tibia medially, changing degrees of flexion; then, rotate the tibia laterally, repeatedly changing degrees of flexion	*Positive:* If a snap or click is heard, there is probably a meniscal tear	Evaluation of meniscal injuries is difficult and requires considerable experience; because menisci have no blood or nerve supply, there may be no pain or swelling with injury

ACL, anterior cruciate ligament; HNP, herniated nucleus pulposus; PCL, posterior cruciate ligament; ROM, range of motion.
Adapted from Maher, A. B., Salmond, S. W., & Pellino, T. A. (1998). *Orthopaedic nursing* (2nd ed.). Philadelphia: W. B. Saunders.

DIAGNOSTIC TESTS

Diagnostic tests of musculoskeletal structures are grouped by whether they are invasive or noninvasive. See Chapter 11 for a more detailed discussion of many of these tests and the client preparation they require.

■ NONINVASIVE TESTS OF STRUCTURE

Radiography

Radiography (x-ray study) is the most widely used noninvasive musculoskeletal diagnostic procedure. X-ray examinations are used to:

A

B

FIGURE 25–5 Special advanced tests of joint function. *A*, The drawer test for instability of the knee ligaments. *B*, Lachman's test for anterior cruciate instability.

- Establish the presence of a musculoskeletal problem
- Follow its progress
- Evaluate the effectiveness of treatment

A plain film is obtained, usually an anteroposterior (AP) or lateral view, possibly both. Other common views include a notch (posterior or less commonly anterior) view of the knee in flexion, an oblique (45-degree angle) view, and a sunrise or patella view of the underside of the patella.

TOMOGRAPHY. *Tomograms* (body-section radiographs) show tissue at various planes through the body as though slices had been made. Tomography can be used to locate bone destruction, small cavities, foreign bodies, and lesions overshadowed by other structures and to evaluate whether a bone graft has united.

FLUOROSCOPY. Fluoroscopy may be used in conjunction with myelography to verify the location of the lumbar puncture. Fluoroscopy also can be used to monitor the progress of contrast dye injected into the subarachnoid space during myelography. See Chapter 67.

DUAL-ENERGY X-RAY ABSORPTIOMETRY. Methods to measure bone density are performed to diagnose osteoporosis because the condition is not evident in x-ray stud-

ies until 30% to 50% of bone mass is lost. One method of measuring bone mass is with dual-energy x-ray absorptiometry (commonly called a DEXA scan). An x-ray tube is used to generate dual-energy photons. DEXA causes less radiation than an x-ray exposure and takes about 10 minutes. It can detect osteoporosis in sites such as the wrist, spine, and hips. No preparation is required, although the client may require teaching about osteoporosis once the findings are known.

COMPUTED TOMOGRAPHY. Computed tomography is useful for assessing some bone and soft tissue tumors and spinal fractures.

MAGNETIC RESONANCE IMAGING. Magnetic resonance imaging, or MRI, facilitates the early diagnosis of many conditions that affect tendons, ligaments, cartilage, and bone marrow (Fig. 25–7).

■ INVASIVE TESTS OF STRUCTURE

Specialized radiographic procedures that are invasive and allow more precise visualization include arthrograms, sinography, and myelography. Other invasive tests of structure are radionuclide scanning, arthrocentesis, arthroscopy, electromyography, and biopsy. All are discussed here.

Radiography

ARTHROGRAPHY

Arthrography is a radiographic examination of soft tissue joint structures. It is used to diagnose trauma to joint capsules or supporting ligaments, especially those of the shoulder, wrist, hip, ankle, and knee. After local anesthesia has been achieved, a contrast agent or air is injected into the joint cavity with the use of aseptic precautions. A series of x-ray films is taken as the joint is moved through ROM.

Before arthrography, explain the procedure, answer any questions, and obtain the client's informed consent to the procedure. Explain that the procedure may take up to an hour (follow-up x-rays are sometimes taken 30 minutes after the injection) and that the client must remain as still as possible except when asked to reposition. Ask whether the client has any allergies, especially to local anesthetics, iodine, or contrast dyes. Suggest that the client void before the procedure. Advise that the joint may be uncomfortable for 1 to 2 days afterward and the client should thus avoid strenuous exercise for that time.

SINOGRAPHY AND MYELOGRAPHY

Sinography and myelography are similar to arthrography, in that both modalities involve injection of contrast agents and the taking of x-ray films. Sinography is used to examine sinus tracts (deep draining wounds). Myelography is discussed in Chapter 67.

Radionuclide Imaging

BONE SCANS

In bone scanning, images of the skeleton are taken after a radioisotope (usually technetium 99m) is injected intravenously and allowed to migrate to bone. The whole

Peroneal Nerve

☐ **SENSATION**
Prick the web space between the great toe and second toe

☐ **MOTION**
Have client dorsiflex ankle and extend toes at the metatarsal phalangeal joints

Tibial Nerve

☐ **SENSATION**
Prick the medial and lateral surfaces of the sole of the foot

☐ **MOTION**
Have client plantar flex ankle and toes

Radial Nerve

☐ **SENSATION**
Prick the web space between the thumb and index finger

☐ **MOTION**
Have client hyperextend thumb then wrist and hyperextend the four fingers at the MCP joints

Ulnar Nerve

☐ **SENSATION**
Prick the distal fat pad of the small finger

☐ **MOTION**
Have client abduct all fingers

Median Nerve

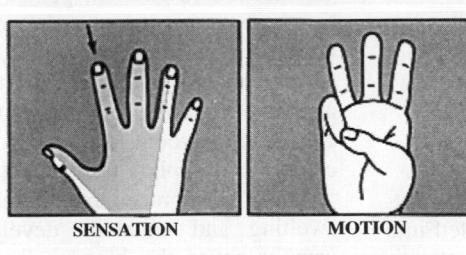

☐ **SENSATION**
Prick the distal surface of the index finger

☐ **MOTION**
Have client oppose thumb and small finger; note whether client can flex wrist

FIGURE 25–6 Neurovascular assessment of the peroneal, tibial, radial, ulnar, and median nerves. MCP, metacarpophalangeal. (Modified from Stearns, G. M., & Brunner, N. A. [1987]. *Operative care* [Vol. 1, p. 89]. Rutherford, NJ: Howmedica.)

body is usually scanned, although just a limb may be scanned (pinhole scan) if a stress fracture is suspected. Bone scanning is used to detect malignancies, osteomyelitis, osteoporosis, and some fractures, especially pathologic ones. The radioisotope concentrates in these areas, indicating abnormal bone metabolism. The radioisotope does not accumulate in poorly perfused bone.

Explain the procedure to the client and family, answer their questions, and obtain consent. The procedure takes about an hour, during which time the client lies supine. Reassure the client that the procedure is not painful and that there are no harmful effects from the isotopes. Suggest that the client void before the procedure.

After the scan, no special precautions are required ex-

FIGURE 25-7 Magnetic resonance image of the right knee.

cept that the client should drink large amounts of water for 24 to 48 hours to help eliminate the radioisotope. Because the radioisotope carries minimal radioactivity, there is no hazard to others.

GALLIUM SCANS

Gallium scans are similar to bone scans but are more specific to bone disorders. Gallium also migrates to brain, liver, and breast tissue. Because it is taken up by bone more slowly than technetium 99, gallium is given to the client by a nuclear medicine technician 2 to 3 hours before the scan. The scan takes 30 to 60 minutes to complete. Mild sedation may be needed for clients who are in pain, are restless, or are elderly. No special follow-up care is required.

INDIUM IMAGING

Indium imaging is the use of indium 111, tagged to (connected to) leukocytes to detect bone infection. The client's leukocytes are separated from a sample of blood and labeled (tagged) with indium. Then the tagged cells are reinjected. Because leukocytes naturally accumulate in areas of bone infection, the tagged leukocytes can be detected by imaging. No special preparation or follow-up care is necessary.

Other Tests

ARTHROCENTESIS

Joint aspiration, or *arthrocentesis*, is a method of aspirating synovial fluid, blood, or pus via a needle inserted into the joint cavity. It is used to diagnose rheumatoid arthritis and other inflammatory conditions or to remove fluid to relieve pain. Normal synovial fluid is clear to straw-colored and is present in minute amounts. Inflamed joints produce increased amounts. In normal joints, synovial fluid is usually thick and has a string-like appearance when expressed from a syringe.

Arthrocentesis is performed with the use of aseptic precautions after local anesthesia has been achieved and with or without fluoroscopy. Medication may be instilled into the joint, if necessary, to alleviate inflammation in septic arthritis. Apply a compression bandage after arthrocentesis, and advise the client to rest the joint for 8 to 24 hours.

ARTHROSCOPY

A fiberoptic arthroscope allows endoscopic examination of various joints (hip, knee, shoulder, elbow, wrist) without making a large incision. Arthroscopy can be used for (1) obtaining a biopsy specimen, (2) assessing articular cartilage, (3) removing loose bodies, and (4) trimming cartilage. It usually is an outpatient procedure performed with the use of local anesthesia. The client recovers more quickly than after an *arthrotomy* (opening of the joint).

Arthroscopy is contraindicated in the client whose joint flexion is less than 50% or in whom a skin or wound infection is present at the site. Complications are rare but include infection, hemarthrosis (blood in the joint), swelling, synovial rupture, joint injury, and thrombophlebitis.

Instruct the client to fast from midnight the night before. Make sure that consent forms are signed. If local anesthesia is to be used, tell the client that there may be mild discomfort as it is administered and when the endoscope is inserted.

Teach the client to watch for signs of postprocedure infection, such as temperature elevation and local inflammation at the incision site, and to report them promptly. Ensure necessary postprocedure pain relief. A normal diet may be resumed as soon as desired. Tell the client that unless a surgical incision is made and the surgeon gives specific instructions to the contrary, walking is usually permitted once sensation has returned. The client should avoid strenuous exercise for a few days.

ELECTROMYOGRAPHY

Electromyography is used to assess such problems as muscle weakness, an altered gait, or lower motor neuron lesions. Chapter 67 discusses this test in more detail because it is used for clients with neurologic disorders.

BIOPSY

Biopsy (removal and examination of a sample of tissue) is used to detect disorders such as infection, cancer of the bone, and atrophy or inflammation of the muscle. Bone or muscle biopsy specimens may be collected either during surgery or through a needle or bore not requiring a surgical incision (aspiration, punch, or needle biopsy). Aspiration biopsy sampling may be performed under radiographic control, such as for sampling of the spine. Bone biopsy specimens are collected with the use of local anesthesia and aseptic technique in either the radiology department or the operating room to prevent osteomyelitis. Bone or muscle biopsy sampling takes about 30 minutes.

After the procedure, monitor the site for bleeding, swelling, and hematoma development. Because dressings usually cover the biopsy site, analyze the client's pain level to monitor for complications. Mild to moderate discomfort is expected; more severe levels of pain may signal complications. Elevate the biopsy site for 24 hours to reduce edema. Monitor the client's vital signs every 4 hours for 24 hours. Mild analgesia is often required. Instruct the client to assess the site on a regular basis (at least daily) for signs of infection when discharged.

■ LABORATORY STUDIES

Table 25-3 lists the most common laboratory tests for clients with musculoskeletal disorders. Chapter 77 describes laboratory tests specific for rheumatic problems.

TABLE 25–3	COMMON LABORATORY STUDIES USED IN DIAGNOSIS OF MUSCULOSKELETAL CONDITIONS	
Test	**Normal Value**	**Significance of Results**
Antinuclear antibody (ANA)	Negative or at a titer ≤1:32	Positive results are associated with systemic lupus erythematosus, rheumatoid arthritis, rheumatic fever, and Raynaud's disease
C-reactive protein (CRP)	Trace amounts	Positive in acute inflammation, such as rhematoid arthritis
Erythrocyte sedimentation rate (ESR)	*Westergren method:* males, 0–15 mm/hr; females, 0–20 mm/hr *Wintrobe method:* males, 0–9 mm/hr; females, 0–15 mm/hr	Elevations common in arthritic conditions, infection, inflammation, cancer, and cell or tissue destruction
MINERAL METABOLISM		
Calcium	8.0–10.5 mg/dl or 4.5–5.5 mEq/L	Decreased levels found in osteomalacia, osteoporosis Increased levels found in bone tumors, Paget's disease, and healing fractures
Alkaline phosphatase	30–90 units/L	Elevations found in bone cancer, osteoporosis, osteomalacia, and Paget's disease
Phosphorus	2.5–4.0 mg/dl	Increased levels found in healing fractures and osteolytic metastatic tumor diseases
MUSCLE ENZYMES		
Aldolase A	1.3–8.2 units/dl	Elevations in muscular dystrophy and dermatomyositis
Aspartate aminotransferase	10–50 units/L	Found in skeletal muscle but primarily in heart and renal cells
Creatine kinase	15–150 units/L	Increased levels found in traumatic injuries, progressive muscular dystrophy, and polymyositis
Lactate dehydrogenase (LDH_4, LDH_5)	60–150 units/L	Elevations in skeletal muscle necrosis, extensive cancer, and progressive muscular dystrophy

CONCLUSIONS

Assessment of the musculoskeletal system begins with a complete history, including symptom analysis. Diagnostic studies commonly include x-rays and, in recent years, arthroscopy has evolved to allow the diagnosis and treatment of joint disorders during one procedure.

BIBLIOGRAPHY

1. Doheny, M., Linden, P., & Sedlak, C. (1995). Reducing orthopaedic hazards of the computer work environment. *Orthopaedic Nursing, 14*(1), 7–16.
2. Hunt, A. (1996). The relationship between height change and bone mineral density. *Orthopaedic Nursing, 15*(3), 57–66.
3. Jarvis, C. (2000). *Physical examination and health assessment* (3rd ed.). Philadelphia: W. B. Saunders.
4. Krowchuk, D. P. (1997). Preparticipation athletic examination (PAE): A closer look. *Pediatric Annals, 26*(1), 37–42.
5. Long, J. S. (1996). Shoulder arthroscopy. *Orthopaedic Nursing, 15*(2), 21–32.
6. Maher, A. B., Salmond, S. W., & Pellino, T. A. (1998). *Orthopaedic nursing* (2nd ed.). Philadelphia: W. B. Saunders.
7. Murray, W. J., & Gabel, T. L. (1998). *What about herbal medicine?* Unpublished Manuscript, University of Nebraska Medical Center, Omaha.
8. O'Hanlon-Nichols, T. (1998). Basic assessment series: A review of the adult musculoskeletal system. *American Journal of Nursing, 98*(6), 48–52.

CHAPTER 26

Management of Clients with Musculoskeletal Disorders

Dottie Roberts
Joan Lappe

NURSING OUTCOMES CLASSIFICATION
for Nursing Diagnoses—Clients with Musculoskeletal Disorders

Impaired Physical Mobility	**Risk for Altered Tissue Perfusion**	**Risk for Injury**
Ambulation: Walking	Tissue Perfusion: Peripheral	Risk Control
Joint Movement: Active	**Risk for Impaired Skin Integrity**	Risk Detection
Mobility Level	Immobility Consequences: Physiological	**Risk for Peripheral Neurovascular**
Transfer Performance	Tissue Perfusion: Peripheral	**Dysfunction**
Knowledge Deficit	**Risk for Infection**	Circulation Status
Knowledge: Treatment Procedures	Immobility Consequences: Physiological	Joint Movement: Active
Pain	Knowledge: Infection Control	Mobility Level
Comfort Level	Tissue Integrity: Skin and Mucous	Muscle Function
Pain Control	Membranes	Neurologic Status
Pain: Disruptive Effects	Wound Healing: Primary Intention	Tissue Perfusion: Peripheral
Pain Level		

The musculoskeletal system gives the body free movement and independent function. Bone is a vital, dynamic connective tissue that serves three major functions: (1) it provides mechanical integrity for movement and protection of internal organs, (2) it performs a major role in metabolism and mineral homeostasis, and (3) it serves as the primary site of hemopoiesis. Disorders of the musculoskeletal system cause considerable morbidity, lead to decreased quality of life, and often result in reduced life expectancy.

OSTEOARTHRITIS

Osteoarthritis (OA) is a chronic joint disease characterized by progressive degenerative changes in the articular cartilage that covers the joint surfaces. Although inflammation is not typical of OA, changes in the joint space may cause a localized inflammatory response.

Etiology and Risk Factors

OA has been classified by its cause as either primary or secondary. *Primary* OA is an idiopathic process found in

people with no history of joint injury, joint disease, or systemic illness that might be associated with the development of arthritis. The most prevalent articular disease in adults age 65 years and older, primary OA occurs more commonly in women than in men. It accounts for substantial disability in the lower extremities as a result of its effects on the large weight-bearing joints. In the past, OA was accepted as an inevitable part of the aging process. Today we know that it is not a normal part of aging.

Although OA is not considered to be a genetic disease, a strong familial disposition exists for its development. A genetic link has been found in the occurrence of Heberden's nodes associated with OA of the distal interphalangeal (DIP) joints of the hands. In addition, sex hormones and other hormonal factors are believed to play an active part in the development and progression of OA.

Secondary OA occurs more frequently in men than in women and results from trauma, other inflammatory joint disease, avascular necrosis, or neuropathic disorders—such as Legg-Calvé-Perthes disease. Traumatic arthritis can develop after fracture or open joint injury. It can also stem from repetitive injury related to the person's occupation or sport (e.g., wrist arthritis in a keyboard operator, shoulder manifestations in a baseball pitcher).

Because OA has been traditionally considered an incurable disease process, much effort has been spent on identifying modifiable risk factors. For example, studies have consistently shown that overweight people have higher rates of OA of the knee than non-overweight peers. Although overweight people also appear to be at higher risk for OA of the hip, the association is not as strong or as consistent as for OA of the knee. This risk variation is due to the different amount of force exerted across these joints when a person stands or walks. Up to six times the body's weight is exerted across the knee, whereas only three times the body's weight is exerted at the hip.

Regular exercise decreases the risk for development of OA in several ways:

- Weight-bearing exercise leads to increased joint mobility and strengthens the joint's supporting muscles, tendons, and ligaments.
- Exercise stimulates cartilage growth by driving synovial fluid through the cartilage matrix. Because articular cartilage lacks blood vessels, the mechanical process of joint movement is essential to cartilage regeneration and continued joint mobility.
- Exercise protects joints indirectly by aiding in weight control.

Pathophysiology

Healthy articular cartilage appears smooth, glistening, and white. It is characterized by unique viscoelastic and compressive properties. *Chondrocytes,* the cellular components of cartilage, constantly remodel and maintain the integrity of this slippery, shock-absorbing pad in order to protect the bone ends in a joint. Chondrocytes actually create the cartilage matrix by producing type II collagen and proteoglycans. The hydrophilic (water-attracting) properties of the proteoglycans in particular add to the ability of cartilage to resist wear with heavy joint use.

In simplest terms, OA can be described as a process of cartilage matrix degradation accompanied by the body's ineffectual attempts at repair. Early pathologic changes include a decrease in proteoglycan content in the matrix, which leads to a softening and loss of elasticity by the cartilage. As the body attempts to compensate, chondrocytes initially proliferate and increase their synthesis of proteoglycans and collagen. Progressive destruction by lysosomal enzymes eventually outweighs production, however, and the cartilage becomes increasingly susceptible to joint friction. Changes in collagen synthesis also occur, minimizing the compressibility of the cartilage. Factors that cause these changes are not clearly understood, but the effect on cartilage is the loss of its ability to resist wear with heavy use.

Fibrillation, erosion, and cracking appear in the superficial layer of cartilage as collagen fibers rupture. While cartilage becomes yellowed and worn over articular surfaces, bone growth increases at the joint margins and bony outgrowths, or osteophytes, develop (Fig. 26–1). Central loss of cartilage, accompanied by buildup of cartilage and bone peripherally, produces inequality in the joint surfaces. The normal distribution of joint stress is changed, resulting in pain and restricted motion. The synovium may also respond with excessive secretion of synovial fluid, creating an inflamed distended joint capsule.

Clinical Manifestations

The diagnosis of OA may be confirmed by radiographic changes that include the presence of osteophytes and of a narrowed joint space caused by erosion of articular cartilage. However, the American College of Rheumatology (ACR) has established classification criteria for OA that do not rely solely on radiographic findings.

Typical clinical manifestations that help in the diagnosis of OA include worsening pain and stiffness that are increased with activity and relieved by rest. Affected joints may exhibit crepitus, mild tenderness in the area of joint wear, deficits in range of motion (ROM), and possibly some joint enlargement. One or more joints may be affected, but joint discomfort is not usually symmetrical. The client may describe weight-bearing joints that "lock" or "give way" as a result of advancing disease. New bone growth in the hands may be evident in the appearance of Heberden's nodes (DIP joints) or Bouchard's nodes (proximal interphalangeal [PIP joints]) (Fig. 26–2).

Although no laboratory test has the capacity to confirm the presence of OA, specific tests may be performed to rule out other conditions such as rheumatoid arthritis (RA), infection, gout, and tendinitis or bursitis. Differentiation between OA and RA is especially important (Table 26–1). Depending on the client's clinical presentation, orders may include a test for rheumatoid factor or a serum uric acid determination. Aspiration and analysis of synovial fluid allows the practitioner to role out infection or crystal deposition. An erythrocyte sedimentation rate

A Normal   B Degenerated

FIGURE 26–1 Pathologic changes seen with osteoarthritis. *A,* Normal bony surfaces for articulation. *B,* Surfaces are altered with loss of joint space and osteophyte formation.

FIGURE 26–2 Osteoarthritis of the distal and proximal interphalageal joints. (From Moskowitz, R. W. & Bluestone, R. [1992]. General aspects of differential diagnosis. In R. W. Moskowitz et al. [Eds.], *Osteoarthritis: Diagnosis and medical/surgical treatment* [2nd ed., p. 475]. Philadelphia: W. B. Saunders.)

TABLE 26–1	DIFFERENTIATION OF OSTEOARTHRITIS AND RHEUMATOID ARTHRITIS	
	Osteoarthritis	**Rheumatoid Arthritis**
Pathology	Progressive process of cartilage degeneration and bone degeneration (spurs)	Progressive process marked by exacerbations and remissions Inflammation of synovial membrane with cartilage damage and bone destruction Ligament, tendon, and joint capsule damage
Affected joints	Weight-bearing joints (hips, knees, ankles), spine, DIP and PIP joints Asymmetric	Small joints (PIP, MCP), wrists, knees Symmetric
Joint effusions	Uncommon	Common
Clinical manifestations	Localized pain and stiffness, usually without swelling Pain with activity, improves with rest Heberden's and Bouchard's nodules	Pain, swelling, tenderness, redness, and warmth Nodules Anemia, fatigue, and muscle aches Pain at rest, especially at night Elevated ESR, frequently positive rheumatoid factor
Other affected systems	None	Lung, heart, skin
Body size	Often overweight	Usually average to below average weight for size
Age at onset	Fourth to fifth decade of life	Young to middle age
Gender	2:1 female-to-male ratio	3:1 female-to-male ratio
Heredity	One form familial	Familial tendency
Diagnostic tests	X-rays	Rheumatoid factor (80% positive); x-rays; joint fluid analysis; negative Lyme disease titer
X-ray evidence	Osteophytes, subchondral cysts	Erosions, osteoporosis
Treatment	Exercise and weight control, maintenance of activity level with joint protection Heat or cold applications Relaxation strategies Medication and/or surgery	Inflammation reduction Balanced diet and exercise program with joint protection Relaxation strategies; heat or cold applications Medication and/or surgery

DIP, distal interphalangeal; ESR, erythrocyte sedimentation rate; PIP, proximal interphalangeal; MCP, metacarpophalangeal.
Adapted from Altizer, L. L. (1998). Degenerative disorders. In A. B. Maher, S. W. Salmond, & T. A. Pellino (Eds.), *Orthopaedic nursing* (2nd ed.). Philadelphia: W. B. Saunders.

(ESR) is of use only if systemic manifestations are present. In practice, the possible diagnoses are usually narrowed greatly after completion of the history and examination.

Outcome Management

Medical Management

Goals for medical management of OA include (1) pain relief with maintenance of mobility, (2) functional independence, and (3) maintenance of quality of life. Most people with OA can be successfully treated with a conservative approach that involves the simultaneous use of several modalities.

All clients benefit from a careful balance between rest and exercise. A sedentary lifestyle can lead to weight gain, which exacerbates arthritic symptoms. Low-impact aerobic exercise, such as brisk walking, does not cause further harm to damaged joints. In fact, walking can relieve pain and improve joint mobility. It also increases muscle tone and enhances joint stability. Exercise can help in weight loss, which should be encouraged in the obese client, who faces more rapid destruction of joints in the lower extremities.

The client with OA needs to understand the importance of rest if an affected joint becomes painful. A neoprene or elastic brace may reduce pain and help stabilize the joint during activity. Joints can also be rested when the client uses a cane in the contralateral hand during episodes of severe hip or knee pain. A collar, sling, or corset may be useful for manifestations in the neck, shoulder, or back.

Some clients also obtain relief by applying heat to affected joints or by alternating applications of heat and cold (contrast baths). Diathermy (deep heat therapy), ultrasound, or microwave treatments have not proved effective in clinical trials. Cold applications have proved beneficial for some people, especially immediately after exercise or in those with muscle spasms.

Many people with OA report good results from topical application of capsaicin cream to affected joints several times a day. The cream can be used alone or with oral medication. Capsaicin is especially effective for OA of the knees and hands. About 50% of capsaicin users describe a cutaneous burning, but this reaction usually declines with continued use.

Until recently, nonsteroidal anti-inflammatory drugs (NSAIDs) were the mainstay of pharmacologic management of OA. Because OA has only a minor inflammatory component, NSAIDs may not be the best first-line choice. Furthermore, research suggests that NSAIDs actually disrupt articular cartilage metabolism. Many deaths among older adults are also attributed to NSAID use each year, usually because of gastrointestinal bleeding. ACR guidelines recommend acetaminophen as the drug of first choice for those with hip or knee OA because of its effectiveness, safety, and low cost. It is less likely than NSAIDs to cause gastrointestinal, hepatic, or renal damage. The recommended maximum dose of acetaminophen is 1 g every 6 hours, or 4 g in a 24-hour period.

According to ACR guidelines, a person with OA should be switched to an NSAID when severe pain persists despite the maximum acetaminophen dose. Acetami-

nophen use often continues on an as-needed (PRN) basis as an adjunct to the NSAID, which should be started in an over-the-counter (OTC) strength. Progression to prescriptive strengths only occurs when clinical manifestations worsen. To minimize gastrointestinal effects, the NSAID can be prescribed with a synthetic prostaglandin such as misoprostol (Cytotec). Newer NSAIDs—the COX-2 selective agents—are now in use in prescriptive strength. While their analgesic properties initially appear greater than traditional NSAIDs, their long-term side effects have not been fully investigated. Medications used for OA are listed in Table 26-2.

Other compounds are also being considered as alternative therapies in the treatment of OA. Glucosamine and chondroitin appear to provide pain relief, perhaps even slowing the disease process. Glucosamine apparently stimulates cartilage cells to manufacture proteoglycans, while chondroitin may inhibit enzymes that break down cartilage. Recent research has examined only the short-term effects of these compounds. It is difficult to determine whether clients with OA will benefit over the long term or if they will experience adverse effects.

Nursing Management of the Medical Patient

The goal of nursing management is promotion of a healthy, positive adaptation in the client with OA. Education is the key to successful treatment of the disease, and the nurse plays a major role as a client educator. Clients and their families need accurate information about the disease and about steps to take to minimize its impact. Effective education can alter behavior, empowering clients to make a positive change in their health status. Important areas in client education include (1) pain management, (2) rest-activity balance, (3) nutrition and weight loss, and (4) self-care strategies.

Teaching clients about their medications is an important part of your role in successful long-term pain management. For example, a client who is taking an NSAID must be informed of the manifestations of gastrointestinal bleeding, such as abdominal pain, tarry stools, and hematemesis. Reinforce the client's need to notify the physician immediately if these manifestations occur. Also encourage the client to keep a pain journal to help focus on manifestations and identify cues that signal the need for rest or activity. Suggest nonpharmacologic pain management strategies (e.g., relaxation techniques, guided imagery) to decrease the feelings of anxiety or powerlessness that accompany disease progression. Other modalities, such as transcutaneous electrical nerve stimulation (TENS), can also be considered to reduce pain.

To assist with self-care deficiencies related to OA, collaborate with an occupational therapist in providing assistive devices that help the client maintain independence with dressing and hygiene. Self-fastening tape (Velcro) closures, zipper pulls, or elastic shoelaces can make dressing easier. Long-handled combs or thick-barreled toothbrushes can also help clients with basic self-care tasks. The client with OA can learn to maintain affected joints in a neutral position at rest in order to avoid flexion contractures that will affect functional ability.

Also recognize the possible influence of OA on the client's sexual role functioning. Pain and stiffness, along with limited ROM, can create problems with sexual ex-

TABLE 26-2	MEDICATIONS FOR TREATMENT OF OSTEOARTHRITIS		
Category (Example)	**Indications and Contraindications**	**Adverse Effects**	**Nursing Considerations**

Analgesics (acetaminophen)	*Indications*
	  Analgesia
	Contraindications
	  Hepatic disease
		Hepatic toxicity in excess doses	Maximum dose is 4 g in 24 hr.
			Avoid use in alcohol-abusing clients.

NSAIDs (ibuprofen)	*Indications*
	  Analgesia
	  Inflammation
	Contraindications
	  Aspirin allergy
		GI bleeding
		Injury to articular cartilage
		Sodium retention and hypertension
		Renal and hepatic damage, especially with long-term use
			Administer with food.
			Observe for weight change.
			Observe for CNS changes, such as confusion, in older adults.

Prostaglandin synthesis inhibitor, or COX-2 inhibitor (rofecoxib [Vioxx])	*Indications*
	  Osteoarthritis
	  Acute postoperative pain
	  Dysmenorrhea
	Contraindications
	  Aspirin allergy
	  Rofecoxib allergy
		GI bleeding, ulceration
		Lower extremity edema
		Hypertension
		Epigastric pain
		Nausea
		Back pain
			Absorption is not slowed by food.
			Calcium products reduce bioavailability.
			Monitor for GI bleeding, skin rash, unexplained weight gain or edema.
			Avoid administration with ACE inhibitors, aspirin, furosemide, lithium, rifampin, and warfarin.

ACE, angiotensin-converting enzyme; CNS, central nervous system; COX, cyclooxygenase; GI, gastrointestinal; NSAIDs, nonsteroidal anti-inflammatory drugs

pression. Joint deformities can also negatively affect self-image, leading to reduced libido and depression. Inform the client about alternative sexual positions (e.g., side-by-side) that promote comfort during intercourse, and encourage the client to use analgesics or to take warm baths to alleviate pain and stiffness before sexual activity.

Surgical Management

OSTEOTOMY
Osteotomy is a surgical fracture, a cut across a bone with resection of a bone fragment to either correct a deformity or to alter stresses on a joint. In early hip OA, when joint congruency still exists and motion is relatively normal, proximal femoral osteotomy may be performed. A wedge of bone is removed from the region of the lesser trochanter to realign the angle of the femoral neck and shaft. Partial weight-bearing is required for at least 3 months after surgery to allow healing of the osteotomy site. Because manifestations of OA generally progress despite this procedure, as many as 75% of clients treated with osteotomy require further surgery within 10 years.[2] Osteotomy is more frequently performed on clients in their 40s, with the full expectation that total joint replacement will be needed in the future.

ARTHRODESIS
In an arthrodesis (joint fusion) procedure, the surgeon removes articular joint surfaces and holds the bone ends together so that they unite like a fracture. Initial fixation may be provided with pins, braces, or casts. Arthrodesis is indicated for irreparable joint damage or instability. The procedure produces a sound, painless limb, but the

resulting loss of movement may be a serious disadvantage in large joints such as the hip or knee.

Arthrodesis remains the operation of choice for the young client with advanced unilateral OA, severe post-traumatic arthritis, or septic arthritis. Hip fusion can result in shortening of the affected extremity by 1 to 1.5 inches, and the client commonly needs a shoe lift postoperatively to help maintain a normal gait. Knee fusion results in shortening of the affected leg by about 0.5 inch, which usually does not create significant postoperative dysfunction. Many clients resume a vigorous, active life following arthrodesis. After hip fusion in particular, they experience few of the initial limitations posed by hip replacement surgery.

TOTAL HIP REPLACEMENT (ARTHROPLASTY)
Total hip replacement (THR), or arthroplasty, is performed to restore joint motion by replacing arthritic bone with metal components. (See Chapter 77 for a discussion of shoulder, elbow, and hand arthroplasty.)

Indications
Indications for THR include (1) failure of conservative treatments, (2) severe compromise of the client's functional ability, and (3) significant pain. The client's subjective complaints frequently have a greater impact on the decision for surgery than radiologic changes do. Total hip replacement may also be performed for complications of femoral neck fractures, congenital disease or deformity, and failure of previous fixations or arthroplasties.

Both *cemented* and *noncemented* hip arthroplasties can be performed. Use of polymethyl-methacrylate (PMMA) bone cement allows immediate intraoperative fixation of femoral and acetabular components. Cemented prostheses are used for elderly clients or for those with compromised bone strength due to conditions such as osteoporosis. In younger, active, or heavier clients, cemented total hip replacements loosen at a rate of about 1% per year, usually from failure of the PMMA bone cement.[2] For these clients, use of prostheses with porous surfaces allows fixation without cement. Instead, bone grows into the porous surface as the client remains on limited weight-bearing status for a number of weeks following surgery. Although short-term outcomes of the two procedures are equivalent, long-term results must be determined in order to justify the cost of noncemented surgical technology. Many hospitals and orthopedic surgeons currently use a "demand matching" system to appropriately choose cemented or noncemented components based on client needs.

Contraindications

Contraindications to THR include (1) recent or active joint sepsis (except in joint revision due to infection), (2) neutrotrophic joints, or (3) an inability to cooperate with immediate postoperative requirements or long-term joint rehabilitation. In addition, the client's general health must allow tolerance of anesthesia, blood loss, and surgical stress. Heart, lung, liver, and metabolic disorders should be stable before surgery.

Surgical Techniques

Although a number of vendors have developed total hip prostheses, a common design currently in use is a three-component set: (1) the femoral neck and stem, (2) a slide-on femoral head, and (3) a metal acetabulum with or without fixation screw holes. Hip prostheses may be made of several different metal alloys that contribute to the relative lightness and durability of the components (Fig. 26–3).

Depending on physician preference and on the type of exposure needed for the procedure, the surgical approach may be (1) anterolateral, (2) direct lateral, (3) transtrochanteric, or (4) posterolateral. You must know the surgical approach in order to understand the leg position used to dislocate the operative hip. If that position is replicated after surgery, the client's risk for dislocating the hip prosthesis increases.

With an *anterolateral* position, the client lies supine on the table. The operative hip is externally rotated and extended, with the knee flexed. With the *posterolateral* position, the client lies on his or her side, with the operative hip internally rotated, flexed, and adducted. Many orthopedic surgeons use the posterolateral position for the anterior and posterior approaches.

Once the hip has been exposed, the surgeon performs an osteotomy of the femoral neck to expose the acetabulum. Osteophytes and cysts are removed from the acetabulum to prepare it for reaming and for the prosthesis. Trial prostheses are placed, and their fit is evaluated before final choice of appropriately sized components. If the prosthesis is to be *press-fit (noncemented)*, the bone is prepared for pegs or spikes. The surgeon presses the cup firmly into place and evaluates its apposition to the bone. If a *cemented* prosthesis is used, anchor holes are drilled

FIGURE 26–3 Hip prostheses. *A,* Coated femoral head and all-polyethylene acetabular cup for cemented total hip arthroplasty. *B,* Porous femoral and two types of acetabular components with femoral head for cementless total hip arthroplasty. (From Maher, A. B., Salmond, S. W., & Pellino, T. A. [Eds.] [1998]. *Orthopedic nursing* [2nd ed., p. 508]. Philadelphia: W. B. Saunders.)

into the iliac subchondral bone. After cleaning the bone thoroughly with pressure-pulsed lavage, the surgeon cements the cup into position.

To prepare the femur, the surgeon forms a tunnel by reaming the bone's intramedullary canal. After placement of a trial prosthesis, the hip is reduced to assess for motion, stability, and length. If results are acceptable, the surgeon removes the trial components. For a press-fit prosthesis, the femoral stem is pressed into the reamed intramedullary canal. For a cemented prosthesis, the femur is cleaned and the canal is plugged to prevent the cement from traveling too far distally. The surgeon fills the canal with cement, inserting the femoral stem and then placing the femoral head. After the hip is reduced, the surgeon evaluates the extremity for motion, stability, and length.

Before closing the incision (~10 inches long), the surgeon may place a closed wound drainage system, such as a Hemovac, to help prevent hematoma—which can increase the risk of infection. However, use of wound drainage systems has decreased in recent years as they have been found to be ineffective in preventing hematomas while possibly increasing the risk of blood loss and contamination of the surgical wound.

COMPLICATIONS

In-hospital mortality is only about 0.5%, but other postoperative complications can occur in as many as 25% of clients over 65 years of age after a THR.[2] While many complications are short-lived and reversible, others can have a great impact on the client's physical and psychological recovery from surgery. The most common and most serious complication is venous thromboembolism. Prevention of deep vein thrombosis (DVT) or pulmonary embolism (PE) requires early mobilization, often with a combination of pharmacologic and nonpharmacologic methods.

Infection following a THR is a serious concern because of the possible development of osteomyelitis. Prophylactic antibiotics are considered essential, and careful wound assessment must begin immediately after surgery. Bladder or urinary tract infection is also possible because of urinary stasis or the presence of an indwelling urinary catheter. Because any localized infection can also spread to the wound, prompt recognition and treatment of clinical manifestations is imperative.

Postoperative joint instability increases the risk for dislocation or subluxation. The risk is even greater following revision arthroplasty because of the extended surgical exposure and soft tissue deficiencies. Hip dislocation occurs in approximately 2% of clients who have undergone arthroplasty, with the greatest risk in the first 8 weeks after surgery.[2] All clients require a great deal of monitoring and education regarding the positions that should be avoided while soft tissues heal around the new joint. Positioning precautions are continued for about 6 weeks, until the surgical incision has healed and the client's periarticular muscle tone has improved.

After surgery with the commonly used posterolateral approach, the client must avoid positions of extreme hip flexion (>90 degrees), adduction, or internal rotation. Appropriate postoperative positioning requires an extended hip that is maintained in external rotation and abduction, often with a foam wedge. An anterolateral approach is used less often. The client must maintain the hip in hyperflexion, adduction, and internal rotation. After this surgical approach, the client can sit up at 90 degrees of hip flexion without increasing the risk of dislocation.

OUTCOMES

A THR commonly results in immediate reduction in the client's pain. Surgical or incisional pain is often described as substantially less than the bone-on-bone pain of OA, and it is frequently more manageable with postoperative analgesia. The client's functional status improves over the course of rehabilitation, with most clients achieving about 90% functional return by 1 year after surgery.[40] With the current emphasis on wellness, an increased number of clients now desire to resume sports activities after hip surgery. High activity levels are associated with decreased longevity for replacement components. However, low-impact activities, such as walking or hiking, swimming, bicycling, intermediate snow skiing, doubles tennis, golf, and bowling, are considered fairly safe for client participation and contribute greatly to improved quality of life after surgery.

Revision surgery may be needed for about 10% of clients because of prosthetic loosening or other complications.[2] However, improvements in component design and surgical technique help ensure that most older clients should never need revision.

▊▊ Nursing Management of the Surgical Client

TOTAL HIP REPLACEMENT

In the current managed care environment, clients who have undergone THR do not typically remain in the acute care hospital setting for more than 4 or 5 days after a THR. They may be discharged to a rehabilitation unit, extended care facility, or even home. Although there is no universally accepted rehabilitation program after THR, coordination of care in the perioperative period speeds the client's recovery and return to independent living.

PREOPERATIVE CARE
ASSESSMENT

Because most clients are admitted to the hospital on the day of surgery, the preadmission assessment of their physical and psychological readiness is currently accomplished in a variety of ways. Telephone interviews may be used, but many hospitals invite clients into a preoperative clinic for nursing assessment and for laboratory tests or x-rays. Some programs also arrange home visits to allow a physical therapist or nurse to assess the client's ambulation and to introduce assistive devices. Discharge needs can often be identified based on the home environment and the extent of support available to the client.

DIAGNOSIS, OUTCOMES, INTERVENTIONS

Knowledge Deficit. The client's previous inexperience with hospitalization and surgery in general, or with THR and its postoperative restrictions, may be described with the nursing diagnosis of knowledge deficit. The diagnosis can be written *Knowledge Deficit related to prior inexperience with surgery (total hip replacement).*

Outcomes. The client will demonstrate understanding of the proposed surgery, postoperative restrictions, and rehabilitation, as evidenced by statements and adherence to the postoperative regimen.

Interventions. A common strategy for providing information about the details of hospitalization for THR is the use of a group class or "total joint camp." Clients receive information about various topics, from preoperative strengthening exercises and nothing by mouth (NPO) requirements to postoperative pain management and dietary advances. Topics include autologous blood donation and other transfusion options. Clients also often have the opportunity to use a walker or crutches for the first time as they are coached by a nurse or physical therapist. Instructors emphasize appropriate positioning precautions to prevent postoperative hip dislocation. Because poor dentition is also a potential infection source, the client should be encouraged preoperatively to achieve and maintain good oral hygiene.

EVALUATION

Clients will provide a simple explanation of the surgery and verbalize their role in recovery. Mild anxiety may heighten the client's receptiveness to information, but severe anxiety can be a powerful barrier to learning. Provide frequent reinforcement of teaching, and encourage the client to ask questions about unclear information.

POSTOPERATIVE CARE

General care of clients following THR does not differ greatly from the usual care provided for any postoperative client. (For a review of general postoperative care, see Chapter 15.) After a THR, however, the client cannot assist with turning and repositioning. Prop the client up with pillows to maintain a side-lying position, and then return the client to a supine position on a 2-hour schedule. Do not turn the client to the operative side unless ordered by the physician. Because of the client's impaired mobility, pay careful attention to maintenance of skin integrity. A pressure reduction mattress overlay may be indicated, especially if the client is frail or malnourished.

Indwelling urinary catheters are not routinely used because of the risk of infection, but women are still likely to have a catheter because of the difficulty of positioning on a bedpan or transferring to a bedside commode in the immediate postoperative period. Perform perineal and catheter care carefully, recognizing the client's surgical pain and positioning precautions. Men are less likely to have an indwelling urinary catheter, but they need assistance to sit or stand at the bedside in order to void.

ASSESSMENT

Frequent assessment of neurovascular status is imperative after a THR. Assess both legs according to hospital protocol for color, warmth, capillary refill, pedal pulses, movement, and sensation. Report any deficits promptly to the surgeon. Ensure that the client's postoperative position is maintained in accordance with specified hip precautions.

The surgical dressing applied at the end of the procedure, used to create pressure and promote hemostasis, is often bulky. It is left in place until removed by the surgeon, usually 2 to 3 days after surgery. However, it should be regularly assessed for excessive drainage and may be reinforced according to the surgeon's order. After removal of the original dressing, the wound is covered with a light dressing or left open to air according to surgeon order. If the surgeon also orders that the wound

be kept dry, it should be covered with a transparent occlusive dressing when the client showers. Afterward, carefully examine the wound to be certain that no water has seeped through the dressing, since excessive wetness can interfere with wound healing.

In addition, a closed wound drainage system, such as a Hemovac, may be in place. Drainage is usually less than 200 ml per 8 hours (or 600 ml per 24 hours), but this amount can be increased if the client has been heavily hydrated. Measure drain output, and promptly report excessive drainage to the surgeon.

DIAGNOSIS, OUTCOMES, INTERVENTION

Pain. Acute pain is expected after any surgery, including THR. The diagnosis can be written as *Pain related to local tissue trauma from surgical incision.*

Outcomes. The client will demonstrate pain control after surgery, as evidenced by movement without grimacing, by requesting analgesics no more frequently than ordered, and by stating that the pain is tolerable and not interfering with rest or physical therapy.

Interventions. In the immediate postoperative period, the client may experience intense pain and require injected opioid analgesics to attain acceptable control. Common interventions include patient-controlled analgesia (PCA) or epidural analgesia. Within 24 to 48 hours, the client should be tolerating fluids and be able to take oral analgesics. Because pain is intensified with movement, the client may attempt to limit activity because of the expected increase in discomfort. Medicate the client before physical therapy or activities such as showering, and reinforce the importance of ambulation in decreasing the risk for postoperative complications. Although a THR can reduce pain in the operative joint, the client with arthritis in other joints continues to experience chronic pain. Use of opioid analgesics can help in reducing general discomfort.

Regularly assess for side effects of opioid analgesics. Respiratory depression is more likely with PCA or epidural analgesia than with oral opioids. Use pulse oximetry and regular assessment of vital signs to assess the client's respiratory status. Constipation, a very common problem following THR, is related to the client's impaired mobility, opioid use, and progression to a regular diet. Encourage the client's intake of fluids and dietary fiber. In addition, stool softeners or laxatives may be indicated. If the client regularly uses a bulk-forming laxative or other strategy to maintain bowel regularity at home, assist the client in continuing that program in the hospital. Regular assessment and implementation of a proactive bowel program are important to minimize client concerns about bowel elimination.

Impaired Physical Mobility. The client's degree of immobility following a THR will be affected by pain and fear of movement as well as by arthritic limitations in other joints. The diagnosis can be written as *Impaired Physical Mobility related to pain or fear of movement.*

Outcomes. The client will demonstrate improved physical mobility, as evidenced by the need for less assistance in transfers (bed to chair, bed to standing), by safe use of a walker or crutches, and by the ability to ambulate a functional distance (150 feet).

Interventions. Moving the client after a THR can create much anxiety for both the client and the nursing staff. First, be aware of any weight-bearing limitations ordered for the client before transfer. Following a THR with a cemented prosthesis, the client is often allowed to put as much weight as desired on the operative extremity. This order is written as WBAT (weight-bearing as tolerated) or FWB (full weight-bearing). Although incisional pain may keep the client from putting full body weight on the operative extremity, he can safely put weight through the leg without harming the prosthesis. If the surgery was accomplished with a noncemented prosthesis, the physician may order NWB (non–weight-bearing), TTWB (toe-touch weight-bearing), or PWB (partial weight-bearing with a percentage specified, as 25%). If the client is not allowed to bear full weight, pay careful attention to the operative extremity during transfers to be sure the client avoids passing any weight through the leg.

In addition to postoperative limitations, the client may suffer from arthritis in other joints that increases pain and affects the ability to transfer from the bed to the chair. While in-bed exercises may begin the day of surgery, the client is not usually ready to attempt transfer to a bedside chair until the morning after surgery. When the client stands and transfers for the first time, the assistance of at least two staff members will be required. Use of appropriate technique will ensure a safe transfer for the client and will minimize the risk of injury to the staff member's lower back.

Transfer the Client. All intravenous (IV) lines, urinary catheters, wound drains, and oxygen tubing should be freed for ready movement. Although you will typically determine the side of the bed for transfer, the client usually moves away from the operative side. If the bedside chair has brakes, they should be locked before client transfer is made. The client should also be wearing shoes or slippers with non-skid soles. Staff should assist the client to the edge of the bed, maintaining the operative leg position in accordance with appropriate hip precautions. Encourage the client to push off the bed with his or her arms to reach a sitting position. However, because of weakness in the hip abductors and upper arms, the client may need help to pivot in bed and to sit up.

Once the client is seated at the edge of the bed, apply a gait belt to the client's waist to help with transfer. Use of the gait belt allows you to help with standing and transfer without risking injury to yourself. If the client becomes dizzy or starts to fall, the gait belt also helps you control the client's movement to the floor or back onto the bed. Place the walker directly in front of the client, ready for use once he is standing. However, do not use it to help the client to a standing position because it will tip.

To help the client to stand, first position your foot in front of the client's foot to keep it from slipping on the floor. Standing close to the client, grasp the gait belt and encourage the client to push off the bed with his hands. Once the client is standing, he can grasp the walker and pause for a moment to take slow, deep breaths as needed.

Remain aware of the risk for falling, and ask the client about dizziness—a manifestation of orthostatic hypotension—before attempting the final transfer to the chair. To help increase awareness of surroundings, encourage the client to stand erect when using the walker rather than stooping over and looking at the floor. With coaching about weight-bearing status, the client should need no more than a few pivoting movements with the walker to reach the chair. Remind the client not to attempt to sit until he feels the chair seat against the back of his legs. Then the client should reach back to grasp the arms of the chair and lower himself slowly to a sitting position. You can assist the client by grasping the gait belt and guiding his descent into the chair. The client's legs can be elevated for comfort on a footstool or another chair, but pay close attention to maintaining flexion restrictions. For example, keeping the client's operative leg in a relaxed position, with the knee slightly lower than the hip, allows maintenance of precautions regarding hip flexion related to a posterolateral surgical approach. The gait belt can be loosened after the client is safely settled in the chair.

When the client is ready to return to the bed, coach him to slide forward to the edge of the chair and tighten the gait belt around the client's waist. Again, remind the client to keep the knee slightly lower than the hip as a positioning precaution. With the walker in position in front of the chair, the client uses the arms of the chair to push to a standing position before grasping the walker. Using the same ambulation process, return the client to bed and help him to a supine position. Maintain leg position according to individual hip precautions.

Introduce Additional Client Exercises. If the client is alert postoperatively, in-bed exercises are often begun the afternoon of surgery. Coach the client in ankle pumps and quadriceps and gluteal isometrics ("quad sets" or "glute sets"). Transfers and ambulation with a physical therapist generally begin the morning after surgery. In addition, the therapist may perform gentle active and assisted ROM exercises. The client will continue exercises that improve ROM and strengthen hip muscles, occasionally receiving physical therapy at home or on an outpatient basis after discharge from the acute hospital setting.

Because of its stability, a walker is often used by older clients to assist with ambulation. If the client has arthritis in the shoulders or hands, a special walker with arm platforms may be indicated. Walkers also necessitate less energy expenditure for the client who has respiratory disease. Crutches may be used if the client has no balance problems.

Risk for Peripheral Neurovascular Dysfunction. Surgery on any joint carries a risk for neurologic or vascular impairment. Be aware of the potential for compartment syndrome and nerve injury related to edema or extremity positioning that places pressure on the peroneal nerve. The diagnosis can be written as *Risk for Peripheral Neurovascular Dysfunction related to lower extremity edema or positioning.*

Outcomes. The client will demonstrate normal neurovascular status, as evidenced by adequate peripheral pulses with capillary refill time of less than 3 seconds and by absence of sensory impairments and motor weakness in the operative extremity.

Interventions. Assess the neurovascular status of the operative extremity at least every 4 hours or as directed by the surgeon. More frequent monitoring may be indicated by the client's condition. Assess the presence and quality of bilateral pedal pulses, skin color and temperature of the extremity, capillary refill in the toes, sensation and movement of the toes, and the client's ability to perform dorsiplantar flexion of the foot. Report any pallor or coolness, numbness or tingling, or inability to move the extremity promptly to the surgeon.

Risk for Injury. Because the hip is unstable as the surgical incision heals, the risk for dislocation of the prosthesis is a significant concern after a THR. Client education and attention to hip positioning precautions are essential. The diagnosis can be written as *Risk for Injury related to prosthesis dislocation.*

Outcomes. The client will demonstrate understanding of the risk for hip dislocation, as evidenced by an ability to verbalize positioning precautions and the use of precautions during ambulation or transfers.

Interventions. Following a THR, assess the client's position frequently to ensure that precautions related to the specific surgical approach are maintained. Remind the client of appropriate precautions through the use of instructional handouts or fliers that can be posted at the head of the bed. Performance of prescribed exercises such as gluteal isometrics also strengthens muscles surrounding the joint capsule and decreases the risk for dislocation.

If the surgeon has used a posterolateral approach, the client should not flex the hip beyond a 90-degree angle, should not bend over to tie or slip on shoes, and should not reach for sheets that are fan-folded at the bottom of the bed. Special attention should be paid to precautions when the client is getting in and out of bed or a chair. To avoid extremes of flexion, the client will need an elevated toilet seat (at least 21 inches high). The client should not cross his legs and should not inwardly rotate the operative leg.

To help maintain precautions after the posterolateral approach, the client may use a triangular foam abduction pillow placed between the legs and secured with straps (Fig. 26–4). Use of the pillow prevents adduction and flexion of the operative hip. However, you must carefully position the straps to avoid placing pressure on the client's peroneal nerve. Less commonly, balanced suspension or traction may be used to maintain the leg in abduction. If the client's leg is weak, a trochanter roll can be placed to maintain straight alignment. When using a walker, the client should be coached to point toes outward slightly. This position avoids internal rotation, particularly when the client is turning toward the operative side. Hip precautions must also be followed as the client is turned from back to side. The abductor pillow is left in place, and the client's side-lying position is maintained through the use of pillows at his back.

If the surgeon has used an anterolateral approach, precautions are almost the opposite of those for the posterolateral approach. Because the client should avoid active abduction, the legs should be maintained side by side without a pillow or wedge between them. When the client walks, he should avoid turning the toes and knee outward. The operative leg should not be extended backward. To help maintain anterolateral precautions, place the tray table and phone on the client's operative side.

To help the client maintain appropriate hip precautions, an occupational therapist may suggest several assistive devices. Long-handled shoe horns, sock donners, and

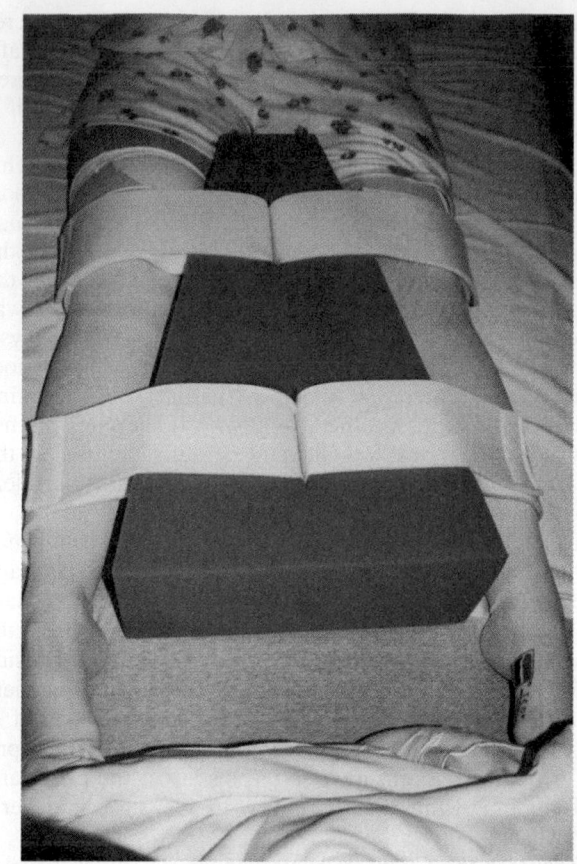

FIGURE 26–4 Abduction wedge is used to assist in maintaining the correct position of the hips after hip replacement. The main function is to prevent adduction and flexion of the hip.

reachers help the client avoid extreme hip flexion and provide more independence in dressing. The therapist or case manager can also assist the client in acquiring bathroom equipment, such as an elevated toilet seat and shower chair, for use after discharge. Reinforce the importance of using these devices to decrease the risk of hip dislocation.

Risk for Infection. Following a THR, the client is at increased risk for joint infection that may lead to the development of osteomyelitis. Although the incidence of infection is low (only 0.5% to 1%),[2] it is a great concern as a factor in possible surgical failure, leading to the removal of the prosthetic components. Joint replacements that are close to the skin surface or have poor soft tissue coverage, as in a thin patient, are more at risk for infection. *Revision* THR carries an increased infection rate compared to *primary* THR because of the longer operative time and the larger surgical exposure. The diagnosis can be written as *Risk for Infection related to surgical procedure (total hip replacement).*

Outcomes. The client will remain free from wound infection, as evidenced by normal temperature and white blood cell (WBC) count, absence of purulent drainage from the wound, and absence of redness or inflammation at the surgical site.

Interventions. Prophylactic IV antibiotics are routinely ordered immediately before surgery because of the risk of infection following a THR. The first dose is typically given 2 to 4 hours before surgery, and antibiotics are continued for 2 to 3 days postoperatively. If surgical drains are used to remove wound exudate, they should be emptied at least once a shift via aseptic technique. Because the drainage can harbor pathogens, note its color and odor and promptly report any abnormalities to the surgeon. Also routinely assess the surgical site for redness or purulent drainage. Use of staples is associated with a lower infection rate, but delays in wound healing can suggest superficial infection. Perform dressing changes using strict aseptic technique. Take the client's temperature at regular intervals, and perform careful assessments to determine the cause of any fever.

Increasing joint pain after superficial wound healing is also a possible sign of delayed, deep infection. Instruct the client to report this manifestation promptly to the physician and to inform other health care providers of the surgery.

Risk for Impaired Skin Integrity. Following a THR, the client is at high risk for pressure ulcers as a result of decreased physical mobility. Clients are often unable to change positions in bed without a great deal of assistance. Clients are also at risk for tape injury with dressing changes. This risk is due to (1) skin changes that occur in older adults, (2) intraoperative positioning and joint manipulation that lead to soft tissue edema, (3) the type of tape used to secure postoperative dressings, and (4) the method and direction of tape application. The diagnosis can be written as *Risk for Impaired Skin Integrity related to decreased physical mobility or to the application of tape with dressing changes.*

Outcomes. The client will demonstrate intact skin, as evidenced by absence of ulcers over bony prominences and absence of epidermal stripping beneath tape used to secure postoperative dressings.

Interventions. To decrease the risk of pressure ulcer development, assist the THR client with position changes on a regular schedule in the immediate postoperative period. As the client regains mobility, he will also regain independence in position changes. Carefully assess the skin over bony prominences such as the sacrum and coccyx, scapulae, elbows, and heels. In addition to using a regular turning schedule, place a pressure reducing mattress on the client's bed. Pressure on heels can be relieved using a towel roll for brief periods under the Achilles tendon. Examination gloves filled with water can also provide pressure relief under heels.

Avoid epidermal stripping by placing postoperative dressings over a skin sealant that is applied wherever the tape touches the skin. Elastic tape should be placed vertically (superior to inferior) without tension to allow for stretching related to postoperative edema. Evaluate any redness, blistering, or epidermal stripping, and consult an enterostomal nurse specialist about the client's care as appropriate.

Risk for Altered Tissue Perfusion. Venous thromboembolism, the most common complication after a THR, can be manifested as DVT. Risk factors include a surgical procedure of more than 30 minutes, advanced client age, previous history of thromboembolism, venous stasis, cardiac conditions such as heart failure or dysrhythmias, lower extremity trauma, obesity, use of oral contraceptives, sepsis, malignancy, long-term immobilization, stroke, and pregnancy. The client is most subject to development of blood clots in the thigh. The diagnosis can be written as *Risk for Altered Tissue Perfusion related to surgical procedure and immobility* (or other identified factors).

Outcomes. The client will remain free from thromboembolism, as evidenced by absence of calf or thigh pain, redness, or edema.

Interventions. Routinely assess the client for evidence of thrombophlebitis: excessive pain, unilateral edema, or a red vein track. Homans' sign is a more nonspecific indicator. The client may have thrombophlebitis but have a negative Homans' sign. Conversely, a positive Homans' sign can result from other conditions, such as shin splints. In reality, many clients have asymptomatic blood clots.

To decrease the risk of DVT, the surgeon may order various pharmacologic and nonpharmacologic interventions. Early mobilization is a key factor in decreasing DVT risk. Encourage the client to perform ankle pumps regularly because they contract the calf muscles, simulating the movements of ambulation and encouraging venous blood return. Physical agents such as pneumatic compression devices and elastic compression stockings are commonly used; they should be applied to both legs to promote adequate venous return. Compression devices or stockings should be worn until the client is fully ambulatory and should be removed only for brief periods to allow for showering or skin assessment. The pneumatic devices should be applied even when the client is sitting in a chair at the bedside because the dependent position of the lower extremities can contribute to increased venous stasis.

Pharmacologic agents used to decrease the risk of DVT include aspirin, low-dose heparin, low-molecular-weight heparin (LMWH), and warfarin sodium. These medications may be used singly or in combination, depending on surgeon preference and client risk. For example, a client may be started on both warfarin and LMWH on the evening after surgery. LMWH, which does not require laboratory monitoring, works quickly to bring about anticoagulation. Warfarin is slower to reach therapeutic blood levels but is less expensive and easier for the client to take after discharge. A prothrombin time or International Normalized Ratio (INR) is ordered to monitor the effects of warfarin, and the nurse promptly reports laboratory results to the surgeon to allow for timely ordering of the current day's dose.

Extensive education about anticoagulants is essential in order to maximize their effectiveness and to minimize the likelihood of complications. Inform the client of manifestations of internal bleeding, such as tarry stools, rust-colored or tea-colored urine, hematemesis, and abdominal or flank pain. Explain that even a minor cut will bleed for a longer period of time. Instruct the client to apply direct pressure, for example, following a shaving cut or a cut with a kitchen knife. Urge clients to seek immediate evaluation for any head injury because significant intracranial bleeding can occur in response to even minor trauma if an anticoagulant is being taken. If the client is to take warfarin, reinforce the importance of consistent intake of foods that contain vitamin K (e.g., green leafy vegetables). Many of these foods are nutritionally important and should not be totally avoided, particularly by clients with a history of heart disease who follow a low-fat diet. If the client will be discharged with a prescription for LMWH, start instruction on injection technique early enough in the hospital to allow ample time for practice and reinforcement.

If you suspect a blood clot, immediately notify the surgeon. Venography or Doppler ultrasound of the leg is commonly used in the diagnosis of DVT. If the test reveals the presence of a clot, the client will be placed on bed rest, with the leg elevated to promote venous return. A continuous heparin infusion and warfarin are often initiated at the same time, with the infusion continuing until a short time before discharge, and a warfarin prescription is written for home use. The surgeon may order calf measurements to aid in the detection of increased swelling related to DVT.

Because of the risk of pulmonary embolism, you must frequently assess the client's respiratory status. A clot in the leg can dislodge and move to the lung, typically causing dyspnea, anxiety, and a pleuritic chest pain. Because pulmonary embolism is often fatal, address suspicious manifestations promptly.

EVALUATION

Goals should be mutually established by the client and an interdisciplinary care team that includes surgeon, nurse, physical and occupational therapists, and case manager. A list of goals can be posted in the client's hospital room as a reminder of the focus for each postoperative day. Clinical pathways are commonly used to map the care of clients after a THR because of the consistent postoperative needs of this population (see Guide to Clinical Pathway: Total Hip Replacement). Pathways help providers limit the number of tasks, such as laboratory orders, that may be forgotten or overlooked. Outcomes are often also indicated on the clinical pathway to consistently track client progress. Pathways often extend from admission through acute care to client rehabilitation in another setting. They also allow for later review of discrepancies or "outliers," those clients whose experiences do not conform to the usual postoperative course.

■ Self-Care

The typical acute hospital stay after THR is 4 to 5 days. Because many clients require additional rehabilitation, they are sent from the hospital to rehabilitation centers or extended care facilities until they regain functional independence. Clients can be discharged home if they can transfer independently to and from the bed, walk alone a functional distance of 150 feet on a flat surface, and safely negotiate stairs.

Provide discharge instructions to the client and any family members or friends who will serve as support persons during the recovery period. The client must understand the hip precautions indicated by the surgical approach (anterolateral or posterolateral) in order to avoid dislocation. Precautions may continue for 6 months to a year after surgery, depending on the surgeon's assessment of soft tissue healing around the joint capsule.

Assistive devices, such as walker or crutches and bathroom equipment, should be available for immediate use at home. The client will progress from walker to crutches or

---

GUIDE TO CLINICAL PATHWAY

Total Hip Replacement

The client undergoing a total hip replacement expects to be hospitalized about 4 days and then discharged home to complete rehabilitation on an outpatient basis. During the first 24 hours, pain management is important. Without adequate pain control, the goals of ambulation will not be met. Medicate the client before any movement.

The nursing goal on the first day after surgery is to have the client sitting up in the chair in the morning and again in the afternoon. Assess the degree of assistance the client needs to move from bed to chair. The rapid mobilization of the client is an interdisciplinary process. Note that on day 1, the goals of physical and occupational therapists are to have the client stand and sit at the bedside, ambulate 5 to 10 feet with the assistance of one to two people, and move in bed with the assistance of two people. Goals for ambulation continue to progress throughout the acute care stay. By the time the client is discharged, he or she should be able to ambulate 20 feet with the assistance of one person, move in bed with minimal assistance, and dress the lower extremities with adaptive equipment (the client cannot bend forward).

Thrombus remains a serious complication of orthopedic surgery and immobility. Baseline prothrombin time is assessed on admission, and anticoagulation begins on day 2. Warfarin (Coumadin) is ordered daily on the basis of International Normalized Ratio range.

The CareMap is reprinted with permission from Bergan Mercy Medical Center.

The CareMap shown is an excerpt of one that covers PO Day 1–4.

Helen Andrews, BSN, RN, *Care Manager, Alegent Health Bergan Mercy Medical Center, Omaha, Nebraska, and* **Linda R. Haddick, MSN, RN,** *Clinical Nurse Specialist, Alegent Health Home Care & Hospice, Omaha, Nebraska*

---

cane as muscle strength increases, perhaps within 4 to 6 weeks after surgery if a cemented prosthesis was used. Clients with a noncemented prosthesis may have limited weight-bearing (e.g., TTWB) for 6 weeks, followed by WBAT with the use of a crutch for another 6 weeks.

Clients frequently have questions about driving or returning to work. Clients with sedentary occupations may be cleared by the surgeon to drive and to return to work within 6 to 8 weeks. However, they may be counseled to take regular breaks in order to avoid extended periods of sitting. It may be 3 months before a client can return to an occupation that requires lifting and bending, and activity will remain limited even after going back to work. Low-level physical activity, such as walking or swimming, is usually approved by the surgeon.

Depending on surgeon preference, the client may be allowed to shower after discharge. Safety measures, such as a nonslip mat and handrails in the shower area, are important. The client should not soak in a tub because water can enter the incision, increasing the risk of infection. Getting in or out of a tub may also violate hip precautions. The client can consume a regular diet but

Bergan Mercy Medical Center CareMap®
Total Hip Replacement

—Addressograph—

Date or Time									
Time Frame	**PO Day 1**		N	D	E	**PO Day 2**		N D E	

Assessments & Evaluations	Routine vital signs & neuro √ to affected leg
	Pt reports pain 4 or < with PCA/PCEA/IM meds:
	             Reported Level:
			__ __ __			Routine vital signs & neuro √ to affected leg
						Pt reports pain 4 or < with IM or oral meds with movement at rest
						             Reported Level:
								__ __ __	

	Check BM - laxatives prn
	Consider d/c drain
	Dry dressing to wound daily and as needed once initial
	dressing removed
	Pt demonstrates:
	  - no excessive edema > 2+(>1")
	  - no numbness
	  - able to dorsi/plantar flex without pain
	Wound/dressing clean and intact
			_____
			
			_____
			
			__ __ __
			__ __ __
			__ __ __
						Check BM
						Monitor hemovac exit site
						Dry dsg to would daily & as needed once initial dsg removed
						Pt demonstrates:
						  - no excessive edema >2+(>1")
						  - no numbness
						  - able to dorsi/plantar flex without pain
						Wound/dressing clean and intact
								__ __ __
								
								__ __ __
								__ __ __
								__ __ __	

Consults	Anesthesia if epidural Pastoral Care as appropriate for spiritual needs R.D. nutritional evaluation								
Diagnostics	CBC Protime if on Coumadin					Protime if on Coumadin			
Medications	DVT prophylaxis					DVT prophylaxis **Coumadin effective - INR range 1.8 - 2.5**		_____	
Diet/Fluid Balance	Intake and output IV & IV antibiotics Post-surgical diet - self feed Ensure a.m. and HS snacks		B__ L__ D__			IV intake and output if foley D/C IV if no foley/drains Post-surgical diet - self feed Ensure a.m. and HS snacks		B__ L__ D__ _____	

Activity/ Safety	Nsg: Encourage pt to use trapeze for repositioning
	**Nsg: Pt tolerates transfer activities with assist
	    of one or two**
	Nsg: Up in chair a.m./p.m.
	Nsg: Reinforce P.T. exercises
	P.T.: BID, transfer train/exercise at bedside/
	    department
			
			__ __
			__ __ __
			
			__ __
						Nsg: Encourage pt to use trapeze for repositioning
						**Nsg: Pt demonstrates transfer activities with assist of
						    one or two**
						Nsg: Up in chair a.m./p.m.
						Nsg: Reinforce P.T. exercises
						P.T.: BID, transfer train/exercise at bedside/department
								__ __
								
								__ __
								
								__ __	

	P.T.: Sit to stand with mod assist one or two **P.T.: Ambulated 5-10 ft with mod assist of two** **P.T.: Bed mobility with mod assist of two**		_____ _____ _____			**P.T.: Sit to stand with min assist of one** **P.T.: Ambulated 15 ft with min assist of one** **P.T.: Bed mobility with mod assist of one** O.T.: Demonstrates understanding of precautions with minimal verbal cues		_____ _____ _____ _____	
	Weight bearing to affected leg with walker or crutches ☐ as tolerated ☐ 50% ☐ 25% ☐ Touch ☐ NWB					Weight bearing to affected leg with walker or crutches ☐ as tolerated ☐ 50% ☐ 25% ☐ Touch ☐ NWB			
Education	CareMap® review Hip film - O.T. remind pt to view **O.T. & Nsg: Hip precautions teaching** Verbal home assessment if not done pre-op		_____ _____ _____						

	Have pt. view Coumadin film
	O.T.: Lower extremity dressing, bathing options,
	    adaptive equipment
			_____
			_____
						O.T. & Nsg: Hip precautions teaching
						
						O.T.: Lower extremity dressing, bathing options,
						    adaptive equipment
								_____
								
								_____	

Treatment Modalities	PCA/PCEA Foley if hip revision Cath PRN Time: ____ Time: ____ Time: ____ ↑ heels Place two pillows between legs Foot pump		__ __ __ __ __ __ __ __ __ __ __ __			D/C PCA/PCEA D/C Foley catheter ↑ heels Place two pillows between legs Foot pump		__ __ __ __ __ __ __ __ __ __ __ __	

Discharge Planning	CM/MSS to see and make arrangements for home ☐
	    or subacute rehab ☐
	Team: Assess assistance at home vs. home care
	    needs
			_____
			
			_____
						Subacute evaluation completed
						
						Obtain appropriate communication for discharge from MD			

should also continue to be aware of any bowel elimination needs. Sexual activity can typically be resumed without discomfort as long as the client observes hip precautions.

The client should understand any medications, such as anticoagulants, that will be taken after discharge, and should note follow-up laboratory and surgeon appointments. If the surgeon has ordered home care services or outpatient therapy, provide agency telephone numbers or locations for appointments. After a THR, prophylactic antibiotics are recommended whenever a transient bacteremia is expected, such as with dental work or a minor surgical procedure. The health care provider prescribes oral antibiotic coverage before the procedure.

In addition to bathroom safety features, the client may need other home modifications to aid independent recovery. Ramps, for example, may allow easier access to entrances. If the client lives in a multilevel home, encourage him to remain on a ground level until recovery is complete.

TOTAL KNEE REPLACEMENT

After the hip and the spine, the knee is the third most common site of arthritic involvement. An extremely complex joint, the knee actually demonstrates movement in three separate planes (Fig. 26–5). Biomechanical stress during normal walking allows three times a person's body weight to be transmitted through the knee. Going up and down stairs increases the force to four or five times the body weight. The force is unevenly distributed, with the medial side of the knee often receiving the larger amount of stress. OA of the knee is better tolerated than OA of the hip, however, because the knee is not usually painful at rest.

Conservative treatment of OA of the knee is similar to that for the hip. Weight loss, activity modification, use of assistive devices, and use of analgesics or anti-inflammatory medications all help to decrease disease manifestations. Physical modalities such as ice or heat may also offer some pain relief.

Indications

If conservative interventions no longer control the client's symptoms, surgery may be appropriate. Options for OA management include (1) osteotomy, (2) fusion, and (3) arthroplasty. A tibial *osteotomy* may relieve the pain of knee OA by correcting the varus deformity (bow-leg) that follows wear of the medial compartment. Knee *fusion* is indicated for young, active clients who are poor candidates for joint replacement surgery; fusion results in an immobile joint fixed in extension.

Total knee replacement (TKR), or *arthroplasty,* allows resurfacing of the arthritic joint with the use of metal and polyethylene prosthetic components. The surgeon attempts to recreate the motions of flexion, extension, rotation, abduction, and adduction that may have been lost with progressive arthritis. TKR also relieves pain and corrects deformity.

Contraindications

Clients under 65 years of age who weigh more than 200 pounds or are extremely active may be better served by

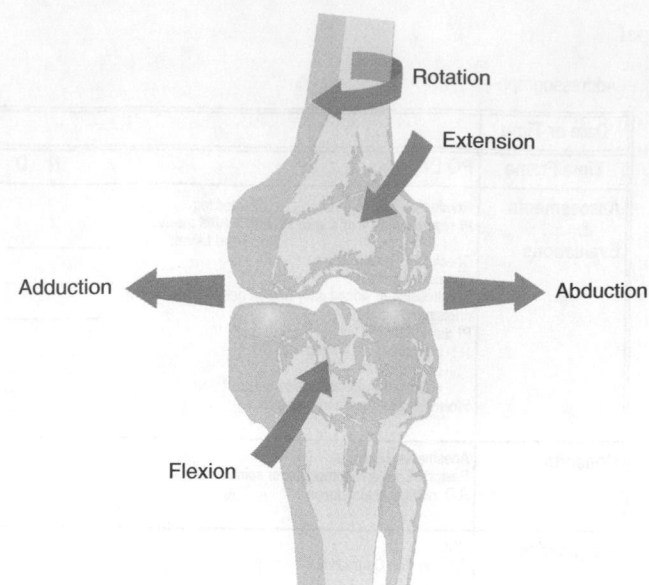

FIGURE 26–5 Movement of the knee occurs in three separate planes; the knee is not just a simple hinge joint. During normal gait, the knee moves through 70 degrees of flexion and extension, 10 degrees of abduction and adduction, and 10 to 15 degrees of internal and external rotation. (After Tooms, R. E. [1992]. Arthroplasty of the ankle and knee. In A. H. Chenshaw [Ed.], *Campbell's operative orthopaedics* [8th ed., p. 391]. St. Louis: Mosby–Year Book.)

alternatives to TKR if possible. Improved prostheses and surgical techniques, however, are slowly extending the indications for this procedure with younger clients. Conditions such as diabetes mellitus and peripheral vascular disease increase the client's risk for infection and delayed wound healing. Other contraindications are similar to those for prospective THR candidates.

Surgical Technique

Knee prostheses most commonly include three components: the femoral component, the tibial plate, and the

FIGURE 26–6 Total knee prostheses. This prosthesis consists of a femoral, a tibial, and a patellar component. *A,* A set of components for cementless arthroplasty of the knee. *B,* Components for a cemented total knee arthroplasty. (From Maher, A. B., Salmond S. W., & Pellino, T. A. [Eds.] [1998]. *Orthopedic nursing* [2nd ed., p. 521]. Philadelphia: W. B. Saunders.)

patellar button (Fig. 26–6). These tricompartmental prostheses vary in size to ensure the most accurate fit for each client. Some parts may also be specific for the right or left knee. A unicompartmental prosthesis, which is rarely used, replaces the femoral and tibial surfaces on only one side of the knee.

The surgical incision for TKR extends from 4 or 5 inches above the patella to 2 or 3 inches below it. Approach is either medial parapatellar or lateral parapatellar. Soft tissue is balanced across the joint, and the proximal tibia and distal femur are trimmed to fit the chosen prosthesis. Any flexion contractures or deformities (varus or valgus) may also be corrected. After osteotomy, the surgeon prepares the bone surfaces to accept the prosthesis based on use of cemented or press-fit (noncemented) components. The patella is resurfaced with a polyethylene button after the surgeon ensures that the patellar prosthesis will track normally during flexion and extension of the knee.

Wound drains may be placed prior to closure of the incision, and a bulky pressure dressing applied. If the client is to start *continuous passive motion* (CPM) immediately, a lighter dressing is used.

Complications

Infection, a potentially severe complication, occurs in about 2% of TKR clients.[2] Venous thromboembolism is also a serious possibility. Other complications may include patellar subluxation or dislocation, impaired wound healing, knee stiffness (inability to regain ROM), and loosening of the prosthesis.

▌ Nursing Management of the Surgical Client

Preoperative assessment and care are the same as for the client undergoing THR. Postoperative care concerns are also similar, but there is more emphasis on knee exercise because dislocation is not a significant risk. The goal of knee rehabilitation—to obtain maximal ROM with good muscle control—can be accomplished with consistent physical therapy or use of a CPM machine (Fig. 26–7). This apparatus moves the knee slowly through its arc of motion, with settings determined by physician order. The machine, which is placed in a slightly abducted position on the bed, is frequently initiated at 0 degrees of exten-

sion and 10 to 40 degrees of flexion. Settings should be gradually and regularly increased, with the client and nurse working collaboratively to achieve the goal of 90 degrees of flexion.

According to surgeon preference, the client may be placed in the machine immediately after surgery. Some physicians delay initiation of CPM until the evening of surgery or the morning after surgery. The CPM machine should be used a minimum of 6 to 8 hours a day. The client must be supine during use of the CPM machine, with the head of the bed elevated no more than 15 degrees, and should thus be removed from the machine for meals. The client may also find it uncomfortable to use the CPM machine during sleep; this concern should be discussed with the surgeon.

When the client is out of the CPM, a knee immobilizer may be ordered to promote knee extension. Make sure that the immobilizer is of the correct length for the client and it does not rub on the heel. No pillows should be placed under the client's knee when he is in bed because this promotes flexion contracture.

ROM and strengthening exercises are an important part of functional recovery following TKR. Ankle pumps decrease the risk for blood clots in the lower extremities. The physical therapist may lead the client in active ROM exercises or may perform gentle passive ROM and stretching to increase knee flexion or extension. Isometric exercises to strengthen the quadriceps, hamstrings, and gluteal muscles are an important part of the regimen. Straight-leg raises also help with muscle strengthening. A home exercise program after hospital discharge includes ROM exercises and isometrics, with weekly increases in resistance, as tolerated, without producing joint irritation. To obtain optimal knee function, the client should continue exercises for at least 6 weeks after surgery.

The client is usually allowed to transfer from bed to chair within 24 hours after TKR. Carefully supporting the operative extremity, nursing staff members help the client move to a sitting position on the side of the bed. Coach the client to push off from the bed to stand in front of the walker before gripping it. Weight-bearing status is determined by surgeon order based on the use of cemented or noncemented components. The client with a cemented prosthesis is often allowed to bear weight as tolerated, while NWB or TTWB is ordered for the client with a noncemented prosthesis. Once the client is in the chair, the operative leg can be elevated for comfort or gently flexed to the floor. When the client has regained enough muscle strength to move the operative leg without assistance, crutch-walking can begin if desired. Use of the assistive device continues until the client has sufficient quadriceps function to ambulate independently.

METABOLIC BONE DISORDERS

Inappropriate functioning of the metabolic processes results in disorders manifested by changes in both physical and chemical structure of the bone. Disorders that alter bony equilibrium and affect bone turnover can be due to estrogen deficiency, parathyroid gland abnormalities, vitamin deficiency, malabsorption, or physical inactivity.

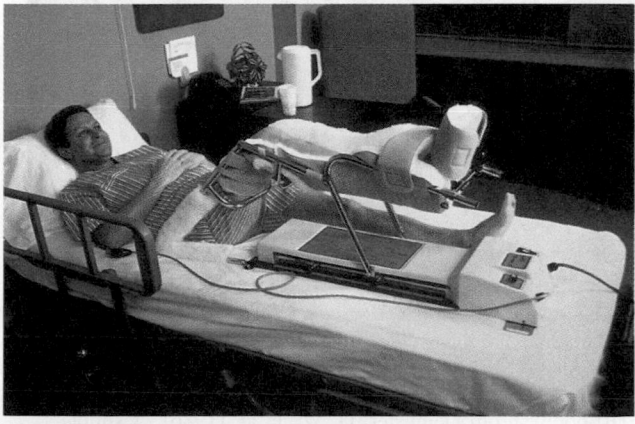

FIGURE 26–7 A continuous passive motion exerciser in use. (Courtesy of the Chattanooga Group, Inc., Hixson, TN.)

OSTEOPOROSIS

Osteoporosis is defined as a systemic skeletal disease characterized by low bone mass and microarchitectural deterioration of bone tissue that leads to increased bone fragility and susceptibility to fracture. *Fragility fractures* result from low trauma, such as bending over to pick up a newspaper, which would not cause fractures in healthy bone. Fragility fractures due to osteoporosis most commonly involve the hip, vertebrae, and radius (Colles' fracture).

The term *osteopenia* refers to a low *bone mineral density* (BMD) compared with that expected for the person's sex and age. Persons with osteopenia have a greater risk for osteoporotic fracture than persons with normal or above-average density. Osteopenia is a risk factor for fracture just as hypertension is a risk factor for stroke.

In an attempt to assess the risk of osteoporotic fracture, the World Health Organization (WHO) has developed several general categories to clarify the definition of osteoporosis. These cut-offs are commonly used with table dual-energy absorptiometry (DXA) but cannot be universally applied to BMD measurements at all sites with all devices. The categories include:

1. *Normal*—a value for BMD or *bone mineral content* (BMC) that is not more than 1 standard deviation (SD) below the young adult mean value (Fig. 26–8A).
2. *Low bone mass (osteopenia)*—a value for BMD or BMC that lies between 1.0 and 2.5 SDs below the young adult mean value.
3. *Osteoporosis*—a value for BMD or BMC that is more than 2.5 SD below the young adult mean value (Fig. 26–8B).
4. *Severe (established) osteoporosis*—a value for BMD or BMC more than 2.5 SD below the young adult mean value *and* the presence of one or more fragility fractures.

Osteoporosis is a major public health problem in many parts of the world, and its scope will increase as the population ages. It affects between 13% and 18% of post-menopausal white women in the United States, and an additional 30% to 50% have osteopenia at the hip. One of every two women will experience a fracture at some point during her life. Nonwhite women and men are also at risk for osteoporotic fractures, although their risk is lower than that for white women.

Osteoporotic fractures also create a heavy economic burden; direct medical costs in 1995 were estimated at $13.8 billion. Hip fractures incur the greatest osteoporosis-related costs, and the number of these fractures may increase three-fold by the year 2040. Thus, any reduction in hip fractures would have a large impact on health care expenditures.

Etiology and Risk Factors

Many factors, both genetic and environmental, are involved in the development of osteoporosis. Bone mass, which is measured by bone densitometry and reported as BMC or BMD, is an important risk factor in osteoporosis. To understand the relationship of bone density and risk of fracture, it is helpful to review some facts about bone mass.

Peak bone mass is the highest bone mass attained. Although longitudinal growth usually is complete by about age 20 years, consolidation of bone continues so that peak bone mass is not attained until about age 30 years in both men and women. This is noteworthy because it indicates that interventions to increase peak mass can be effective up until about age 30.

What happens to bone mass in women between age 30 and menopause is uncertain. Most likely, bone mass plateaus until menopause or else decreases slightly during this period. Bone loss in the hip probably starts as early as age 20 years. Although it is debated as to when bone loss naturally begins, during perimenopause women experience a marked acceleration in bone loss due to the loss of natural estrogen. Women start to lose bone about 1.5 to 2 years before their last menstrual period and continue rapid loss until about 1.5 years after their last menses. They may lose as much as 15% of their total mass during the perimenopausal period, after which the rate of bone

FIGURE 26–8 Electron micrographs of normal (*A*) and osteoporotic (*B*) bone. (From Dempster, D. W., et al. [1986]. A simple method for correlative light and scanning electron microscopy of human iliac crest bone biopsies: Qualitative observations in normal and osteoporotic subjects. *Journal of Bone and Mineral Research, 1,* 15–21.)

loss slows to a rate of about 1% per year. Rapid bone loss also occurs in women whose ovaries have stopped functioning, such as women being treated for prevention and treatment of ovarian and breast cancer.

Although men have larger and stronger skeletons than women, they can experience a marked loss of bone as they age, possibly resulting in fragility fractures. Bone loss in men starts later in life and progresses more slowly. Men do not experience the rapid bone loss associated with the perimenopausal decline in estrogen production seen in women. There are several reasons for loss of bone in men, including declining testosterone levels. In addition, estrogen may play a crucial role in men's bone health and changes in estrogen levels with age may be as important, if not more so, as changes in testosterone levels.

Those who have not gained their maximum peak bone mass have less bone "in the bank" to draw upon once the inevitable bone loss begins. Thus, peak bone mass as well as later bone loss is a major determinant of osteoporotic fracture. For this reason, osteoporosis has been described as a pediatric disorder. Strong adult skeletons are built during childhood.

From 60% to 80% of the risk for this disorder is inherited. A history of fracture in a first-degree relative is a risk for fragility fracture. Factors other than heredity known to influence development of osteoporosis include:

- Low body weight (<127 pounds)
- Prolonged premenopausal amenorrhea or early menopause
- Inadequate physical activity
- Low intake of dietary calcium
- Suboptimal levels of serum vitamin D
- Cigarette smoking
- Excessive consumption of alcohol

Osteoporosis can also result from underlying medical conditions, such as thyrotoxicosis, hyperparathyroidism, anorexia nervosa, and Cushing's syndrome and from long-term use of medications such as thyroid hormone, anticonvulsants, furosemide, and corticosteroids. A person who has had one osteoporotic fracture is five times more likely to suffer another fracture than a person without a fracture. Thus, history of a low-trauma fracture is an important risk factor.

Pathophysiology

Bone is a dynamic tissue that undergoes continuous *remodeling,* the process by which old bone is replaced by new (Fig. 26–9). Bone remodeling serves two principal functions:

1. Replaces old bone with new so that the biomechanical properties of the skeleton are not compromised by continuous use
2. Plays a role in mineral homeostasis by transferring calcium and other ions into and out of the skeletal reservoir.

The remodeling sequence starts with activation of *osteoclasts,* which resorb a small portion of bone over a relatively short period of time (as short as 7 to 10 days). Bone formation then takes place as *osteoblasts* form an organic matrix that is subsequently mineralized.

Peak bone mass and the subsequent rate and duration of bone loss are important determinants of whether skeletal integrity will be compromised to the degree that a fragility fracture will result. In addition, as bone tissue is lost, other alterations in the skeleton (e.g., changes in architecture, aging of the bone tissue, accumulation of microdamage) contribute to fracture risk. The supporting structures become so weak that even minimal stress can cause fractures. Spinal fractures occurring with osteoporosis are usually compression fractures that occur when one or more vertebrae collapse from carrying the weight of the upright body (see Fig. 26–8A and B).

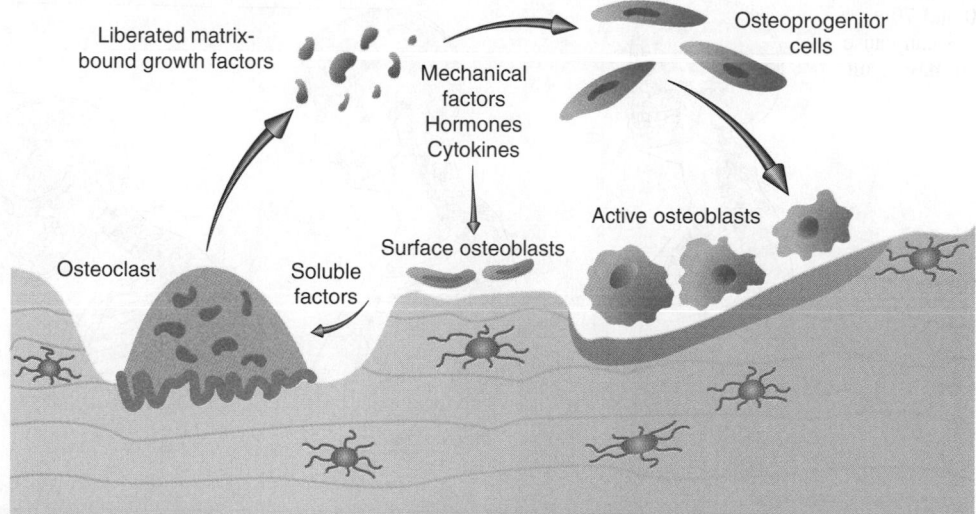

FIGURE 26–9 Bone remodeling is a process of bone resorption and bone formation. These two processes are controlled by systemic factors (the need for calcium) and local cytokines, some of which are found in the bone matrix. Cytokines are of key importance in communication between the osteoblasts and the osteoclasts. (Modified from Cotran, R. S., Kumar, V., & Robbins, S. L. [1994]. *Robbins pathologic basis of disease* [5th ed., p. 1217]. Philadelphia: W. B. Saunders.)

Clinical Manifestations

In many people, the diagnosis of osteoporosis is made after a fracture, often a vertebral compression fracture. Clinical manifestations of vertebral compression fracture include sudden onset of severe back pain that worsens on movement and is relieved by rest. This acute pain usually subsides within 2 to 6 weeks. Most compression fractures, however, are discovered accidentally on routine x-ray. Progressive vertebral deformities lead to shortened stature and progressive dorsal kyphosis (Fig. 26–10). The lower ribs eventually rest on the iliac crests, and downward pressure on viscera causes abdominal distention and bloating. Respiration may also be impaired by restricted lung expansion.

Bone loss can also occur in the mandible, which may lead to loss of teeth or poorly fitting dentures as well as changes in the appearance of the face. Unfortunately, fractures of the wrist in postmenopausal women are often not recognized as osteoporotic fractures.

The many changes in appearance and the difficulty in finding clothing that fits can have a profound negative effect on self-esteem. Quality of life may be affected by chronic pain and functional disability. Fear of subsequent fracture may cause people to reduce their activity.

The "gold standard" for measuring BMD is full-table DXA (Fig. 26–11). This technique carries low risk and takes only a few minutes. The most commonly measured sites with DXA are the spine and the hip. BMD is commonly reported as a "T-score," which is the difference between the patient's BMD and the BMD of "young normal adults" of the same gender. The difference between the patient's score and the young adult norm is expressed as SD below or above the average. (This is the basis for the WHO definition of osteoporosis discussed earlier.) Thus, a person with a T-score of −2.0 would have a BMD that is 2 SDs below the average for a young adult of the same gender. Under the WHO criteria, this person would be considered *osteopenic.*

In recent years, the number of peripheral densitometers has increased dramatically. These devices measure BMD at peripheral sites such as the heel or finger. They include *quantitative ultrasound* (QUS) devices and peripheral DXAs. These devices are smaller and less expensive than full-table DXAs, and the QUS devices involve no radiation exposure. However, criteria for interpreting results with peripheral devices are not well developed.

The National Osteoporosis Foundation (NOF) Guidelines for Treatment and Prevention of Osteoporosis recommend that the decision to test BMD should be based on a person's risk and that testing is not indicated unless the results of the testing would influence choices about treatment. According to NOF Guidelines, BMD testing should be performed for the following:

- All postmenopausal women under age 65 years who have one or more additional risk factors for osteoporosis (besides menopause)
- All women age 65 years and older regardless of additional risk factors
- Postmenopausal women who present with fractures (to confirm diagnosis and determine disease severity)
- Women who are considering therapy for osteoporosis if BMD testing would facilitate the decision
- Women who have been taking *hormone replacement therapy* (HRT) for prolonged periods of time

Laboratory tests may be performed to rule out secondary osteoporosis or other metabolic bone diseases. These

FIGURE 26–10 Osteoporotic changes: A normal spine at age 40 years and osteoporotic changes at ages 60 and 70 years. These changes can cause a loss of height and may result in dorsal kyphosis.

Height

−5'6"

−5'3"

−5'

−4'9"

−4'6"

−4'3"

40   60   70

Age

Collimated x-ray detector

X-ray source

Dual-energy
x-ray beam

FIGURE 26–11 Dual-photon absorptiometry. (Adapted from an original illustration in *Clinical Symposia,* illustrated by Frank Netter, M.D., copyright by Ciba-Geigy Corporation.)

tests include blood count, urine calcium, multichannel screen, serum alkaline phosphatase, serum 25-hydroxyvitamin D, parathyroid hormone, ionized calcium, protein electrophoresis in urine and serum, and thyroid function. Biochemical markers of bone remodeling, such as urinary collagen cross-links, are sometimes used in conjunction with DXA or QUS to monitor effectiveness of therapy. However, biochemical markers alone are not appropriate for diagnosis of osteoporosis or for predicting the risk of fracture in the future.

Outcome Management

■ Medical Management

The goal of medical management is to prevent bone loss and fragility fractures. Lifestyle changes focused on dietary intake of adequate calcium and vitamin D and weight-bearing exercise are prescribed to prevent bone loss. *Estrogen replacement therapy* (ERT) is considered for women who are postmenopausal (see later discussion). Cigarette and alcohol cessation is advised.

PREVENTING LOSS OF BONE MASS

Osteoporosis is preventable. Strategies for prevention are most effective when they are started in childhood in order to maximize peak bone mass and to establish lifelong bone-healthy behaviors. Several interventions that maximize and preserve bone mass have general health benefits, including:

- Adequate intake of calcium and vitamin D
- Regular weight-bearing exercise
- Avoidance of tobacco and alcohol abuse

Calcium and Vitamin D Intake

A well-balanced diet containing the recommended level of calcium is an important component of bone health (Table 26–3). The major sources of dietary calcium are dairy products. Calcium can also be obtained from the wide range of calcium-fortified foods that are available (Box 26–1). National surveys of dietary intake indicate that many Americans are not consuming enough calcium. Most women consume less than half of the recommended daily levels. As early as age 10, the calcium intake of

girls is considerably below that needed for optimal bone health.

People who have difficulty digesting milk due to a lack of the enzyme lactase, which breaks down the milk sugar lactose, may be able to tolerate acidophilus milk, yogurt, and hard cheeses; in addition, milk products may be tolerated if taken in small amounts. Skim milk and low-fat yogurt can be recommended for persons who are trying to maintain low-cholesterol diets. Diets high in dairy foods do not cause obesity; in fact, people who consume high amounts of dairy foods appear to have higher lean body mass.

TABLE 26–3	RECOMMENDED CALCIUM INTAKE LEVELS
Group	**Calcium Intake (mg/day)**
INFANTS	
Birth–6 mo	400
6 mo–1 yr	600
CHILDREN	
1–5 yr	800
6–10 yr	800–1200
11–24 yr	1200–1500
ADULTS	
Women 25–50 yr	1000
Postmenopausal women < 65 yr	
Taking estrogen	1000
Not taking estrogen	1500
Women > 65 yr	1500
Men < 65 yr	1000
Men > 65 yr	1500
PREGNANT WOMEN	
400 mg+ recommendation for age group	1400–1900

Data from National Institutes of Health Consensus Development Panel on Optimal Calcium Intake. (1994). Optimal calcium intake. *Journal of the American Medical Association, 272,* 1942–1948.

BOX 26–1 **Calcium Equivalents of Dietary Sources (300 mg)**

1 cup of milk
1 carton of low fat yogurt with fruit
1¼ cup frozen yogurt
1 cup vanilla pudding
1 cup baked egg custard
1 oz Swiss cheese
1 slice cheese pizza
½ cup ricotta cheese, part skim
1½ oz cheddar cheese
2¼ cup cottage cheese
11 dried figs
4 cups broccoli
7 oz baked wall-eyed pike fillet
¾ cup whole dried almonds

Prepared by Patricia T. Packard, R.D., C.N., Creighton University Osteoporosis Research Center, Omaha, NE.

Dietary calcium from a well-balanced nutritional plan is the preferred approach, but calcium supplements should be used when an adequate dietary intake cannot be achieved. All calcium supplements should be taken with food to enhance absorbability. Chewable supplements are preferred over those that are swallowed. Although a high dietary calcium intake is thought to increase the risk of renal calculi (stones), research findings suggest that high-calcium diets do not commonly result in renal calculi and may, in fact, protect against stone formation.

Vitamin D plays a major role in both calcium absorption and bone metabolism. Vitamin D is made in the skin in the presence of sunlight, or it may be obtained from food sources, primarily vitamin D–fortified milk. Although exposure to sunlight is necessary for cutaneous synthesis of vitamin D, prolonged exposure to sunlight does not necessarily increase the amount synthesized. An average of 15 minutes a day of sunlight exposure to hands, face, arms, and legs probably meets the requirements for most people. Although the use of sunscreen remains important to reduce photoaging and the risk of skin cancer, overuse of sunscreen is not advised. When sunscreen is applied so heavily that the skin receives no sunlight, vitamin D is not synthesized in the skin. Vitamin D supplementation (400 to 800 IU/day) is recommended for the institutionalized elderly, for persons living in high northern or southern latitudes, and for people who have limited sun exposure.

High dietary intake of sodium increases loss of calcium in the urine, and people who take in large amounts of sodium should increase their calcium intake accordingly. Although caffeine modestly increases calcium excretion in the urine, the loss is negligible compared with the effects of protein and sodium. The effect of caffeine can be offset by adding 40 mg of calcium to the diet for each cup of coffee. Phosphorus intake, as that in carbonated beverages, does not significantly affect calcium balance; however, people who drink a large number of carbonated beverages may not be consuming adequate calcium in the form of milk.

Low protein intake appears to play a distinct detrimental role in the causes and complications of hip fracture. Many older adults have an inadequate protein intake. The clinical outcome after hip fracture is significantly improved with the use of daily oral nutritional supplements, such as Ensure, which normalize protein intake. Protein supplementation also reduces further bone loss in elderly patients who have sustained a hip fracture.

Exercise

Weight-bearing exercise, such as walking and running, is necessary for maintaining bone mass because disuse results in bone loss. Swimming and biking have not been found effective in maintaining bone mass, probably because they do not adequately load the bones. The inactivity of older people increases the rate of bone loss and the risk of hip fracture. It has been suggested that regular exercise by the elderly would reduce the risk of hip fracture by at least half. In addition to maintaining bone mass by loading the bones, exercise leads to improved physical fitness, which is associated with improved muscle strength, stability, reaction time, balance, and coordination.

All of these factors help to decrease the risk of falling and subsequent fractures. Exercise regimens and weight training have been found to increase muscle strength even in persons older than 90 years of age. In light of the positive effects of exercise on bone and on health in general, nurses should recommend regular exercise for all clients. Previously sedentary clients who wish to start a more rigorous exercise program should undergo a physical evaluation before starting.

The American College of Sports Medicine recommends that at least 30 minutes of any physical activity be incorporated into daily schedules. Even activities such as walking, hiking, gardening, biking, and housework or yardwork increase daily energy expenditure and help promote muscular strength, flexibility, coordination, and endurance, which may ultimately decrease the number and severity of falls.

Alcohol and Tobacco

Alcohol abuse and smoking cigarettes increase the risk of osteoporosis. Current smokers have 2.1 times the risk of hip fractures as nonsmokers. If a woman quits smoking, she reduces her risk of hip fracture by 40%. Excessive alcohol intake reduces bone density and increases the risk of falls. Moderate alcohol intake has no known negative effect on BMD.

ESTROGEN REPLACEMENT AND PREVENTION OF BONE RESORPTION

Medications approved by the Food and Drug Administration (FDA) to prevent and treat osteoporosis include ERT, alendronate, raloxifene, risedronate, and calcitonin (Table 26–4). Clients receiving drug therapy for osteoporosis should be taught about the importance of calcium, vitamin D, physical activity, and avoidance of smoking and alcohol abuse as part of any treatment regimen. Treatment should not be limited to persons who have had a fragility fracture. Clients at high risk for osteoporotic fracture should be treated prophylactically. Clients receiving corticosteroid therapy are at very high risk of fracture and should always be treated prophylactically.

ERT has been effective in preventing and treating osteoporosis. In addition, it offers other health benefits, such

TABLE 26-4	MEDICATIONS FOR PREVENTION OF OSTEOPOROSIS		
Category (Example)	Indications and Contraindications	Adverse Effects	Nursing Considerations
ESTROGEN (prevents bone loss, reduces risk of fracture, provides cardioprotective effects)			
Conjugated estrogens (Premarin)	*Indications* Early menopause Osteoporosis *Contraindications* Active thrombophlebitis Known or suspected estrogen-dependent cancers Known or suspected pregnancy Undiagnosed genital bleeding	Gallbladder disease Hypertension Hypercalcemia Vaginal candidiases Melasma (dark areas on the face) Hirsutism Headache, migraine	Teach the client to monitor for breast tenderness, mood changes, fluid retention and vaginal bleeding. Teach the client to report unilateral leg pain or swelling or any shortness of breath (signs of DVT). Teach the client to have regular mammograms and PAP smears. Monitor serum calcium level.
Selective estrogen receptor modulators (raloxifene [Evista])	*Indications* Prevention of osteoporosis in early menopause *Contraindications* Active thrombophlebitis Known or suspected pregnancy	Leg cramps Hot flashes Weight gain Peripheral edema Sinusitis Sweating	Avoid administration with ampicillin, indomethacin, naproxen, diazepam and clofibrate if possible. Do not administer with cholestyramine.
BISPHOSPHONATES (inhibit osteoclasts, reduce bone resorption)			
Alendronate (Fosamax)	*Indications* Osteoporosis Paget's disease *Contraindications* Delayed esophageal emptying Hypocalcemia	Gastric irritation, heartburn, dysphagia, flatulence, diarrhea, headache	Poorly absorbed: Administer on an empty stomach and do not eat or drink for 30 min. Take medication with water (not juice) and remain upright after swallowing. Do not chew or suck on the tablet. Monitor serum calcium levels. Monitor for gastric irritation for clients taking aspirin or NSAIDs.
Calcitonin (Miacalcin)	*Indications* Osteoporotic fractures Paget's disease Hypercalcemia *Contraindications* None known	Nausea, flushing, nasal irritation, serious allergic reactions	Administered by nasal spray Has analgesic effects also

as prevention of cardiovascular disease. ERT is most effective in maintaining bone health if it is started during the perimenopausal period, before rapid bone loss begins; however, it is also beneficial when started after menopause, even in women with established osteoporosis. The skeletal effects of estrogen are obtained with both oral and transdermal preparations. Rapid bone loss occurs if and when ERT is discontinued. Estrogen in lower doses (0.3 mg/day) is effective in maintaining bone mass and has fewer side effects than conventional doses.

Estrogen is usually given in combination with progesterone in women with an intact uterus to prevent uterine cancer. Administration of estrogen and progesterone continuously eliminates monthly bleeding in many women.

Side effects of combined HRT include breast tenderness, mood changes, fluid retention, and vaginal bleeding. ERT also increases the risk of deep vein thrombosis and gallbladder disease. There is a perception that ERT causes weight gain; however, although postmenopausal weight gain may be common, women receiving ERT gain less weight than those not receiving ERT.

The major concern with prolonged ERT is the increased risk of breast cancer. After using ERT for 5 years or more, a woman's breast cancer risk has been found to increase by about 35%. However, more women in the United States die of heart disease than of all types of cancer combined. Thus, the benefits of ERT for heart and bone health may outweigh the risk of breast cancer. The decision to use ERT should be made by a woman in consultation with her primary care provider.

Marketed as Evista, raloxifene is a member of a class of drugs called *selective estrogen receptor modulators* (SERMs). SERMs provide the benefits of estrogen but avoid the risks. They prevent bone loss, reduce the incidence of osteoporotic fracture, and provide cardioprotective effects. They do not increase the risk of breast or uterine cancer. Evista increases the risk of DVT in a manner similar to that of ERT. Evista also increases hot flashes and is thus not effective in relieving menopausal symptoms.

Drugs that inhibit bone resorption are also prescribed. Alendronate and risedronate are bisphosphonates and are available as Fosamax and Actonil, respectively. Calcitonin, a hormone that slows bone resorption, is available as Miacalcin and is delivered as a single daily dose of nasal spray. Calcitonin is less effective than Evista or Fosamax in maintenance of bone mass. Interestingly, calcitonin has analgesic effects, which may help to relieve pain associated with fractures.

PROMOTION OF HEALING AFTER FRACTURE

The goals of treatment after fracture are to manage pain, regain mobility and strength, promote healing, reduce bone loss, and prevent further fracture. Furthermore, treatment is directed toward limiting the disability associated with existing fractures.

MANAGING PAIN. One of the most important interventions in the care of the client with an osteoporotic fracture is pain management. Often clients present with back pain resulting from vertebral crush fracture syndrome. Strict bed rest lasting between 5 and 7 days has been found to be most effective in relieving pain and shortening the course of pain. The client should lie supine or in a side-lying position. After 5 to 7 days of bed rest, the client is instructed to gradually increase activity.

Non-narcotic analgesics may be needed for 1 to 2 weeks to aid in relief of pain. If NSAIDs are used, protect the client from gastric ulceration by administering medications with food or antacids.

Flexible corsets with adjustable self-fastening tape (Velcro) may help to relieve back pain and fatigue. However, these corsets cannot correct the underlying problem of bone loss and spinal deformity. Corsets may be worn in bed but are most helpful if worn when the person is in the upright position.

Physical therapy is of utmost importance in the long-term treatment of back pain. Often chronic back pain is associated with decreased ROM, weakness, muscle spasm, postural change, muscle tenderness, and decreased endurance. Physical therapy should be started during the period of bed rest with ROM exercises and mild resistive exercises of the extremities in bed. Heat or ice, ultrasound, and TENS may be used for pain relief.

REGAINING MOBILITY AND STRENGTH. After acute pain subsides, clients should carry out exercises specifically prescribed for them, such as stretching and strengthening. Water aerobics may be initiated early in the treatment before the client can tolerate weight-bearing exercise. A long-term physical activity program should include weight-bearing and aerobic exercise in addition to strengthening and flexibility exercise. Since osteoporotic clients are at risk for subsequent fractures, they should be taught how to move safely while maintaining or increasing physical activity. See the Management and Delegation feature for techniques on assisting with mobility.

PROMOTING HEALING. Good general nutrition should be encouraged after fractures to promote healing. Optimal calcium and vitamin D intake continue to be important, and special attention should be given to adequate protein in the diet, especially in the elderly.

PREVENTING FURTHER FRACTURES. Medications and treatments used to prevent osteoporosis are continued after a fracture to maintain and improve bone mass in existing bone.

▨ Nursing Management of the Medical Client

Nursing management for the client with osteoporosis is detailed in the Care Plan.

▨ Self-Care

Assess clients at high risk for fracture for activity level and dietary adequacy, and perform appropriate teaching to prevent fractures. In addition, assess the risk of falling in these clients. Assessment includes visual acuity, medications that may cause dizziness or postural hypotension, and difficulties with balance or coordination as well as the home environment for potential safety hazards. Evaluation of the home setting is performed via the admission assessment, discussions with the client, consultation with a specialist in social services, and home safety evaluation by a visiting nurse.

Discussion about fall prevention strategies is imperative. Instruct clients who are prone to dizziness to get up slowly from a lying position, sitting on the side of the bed first. Their eyeglass prescription may need to be updated to improve vision. An aid to ambulation, such as a cane or walker, may also be indicated to prevent falling. Alterations to the home may be recommended. Handrails in the bathroom, removal of scatter rugs, and increased lighting are some of the modifications that may be necessary.

Specific resources in the community that may be helpful to clients with osteoporosis include support groups and exercise programs. The National Osteoporosis Foundation (*www.nof.org*) is an excellent source of educational resources.

PAGET'S DISEASE

Paget's disease (osteitis deformans) is defined as an idiopathic bone disorder characterized by abnormal and accelerated bone resorption and formation in one or more bones. The normal bone is replaced by abnormal, structurally weaker bone that is prone to fractures. Paget's disease most frequently produces painful deformities of the femur, tibia, lower spine, pelvis, and cranium.

While the cause of Paget's disease is unknown, it is thought to be of viral origin. Laboratory data suggest involvement of the measles virus, respiratory syncytial virus (RSV), or canine distemper viruses, but these findings have not been confirmed. Although no definite hereditary pattern has been established, a familial clustering has been reported. However, only 4% to 5% of patients

MANAGEMENT AND DELEGATION

Assisting with Mobility and Use of Splints

Muscle overuse, traumatic injuries, and muscle disuse associated with prolonged bed rest can each contribute to complications of immobility. An important aspect of care is the prevention of these unnecessary complications. Interventions to minimize the complications of immobility include passive and active range-of-motion (ROM) exercises as well as the use of splints to maintain normal joint alignment and position. The performance of ROM exercises and the application and removal of splints may be delegated to unlicensed assistive personnel.

Although you may delegate these tasks, as the nurse, you remain responsible for assessment of the client's baseline level of function and development of a plan to prevent the complications associated with immobility. Interdisciplinary collaboration with physical and occupational therapists is often necessary to develop a comprehensive plan of care. Additionally, you will be monitoring the client's progress and response to these interventions and adjusting the plan of care in collaboration with the other involved disciplines.

When delegating these tasks to assistive personnel, emphasize the following:

- Specify any physical limitations that clients may have that would prohibit their ability to move an extremity through its normal range of motion.
- Identify the time at which this activity is best performed with a client. Establish a schedule of which the client and assistive personnel are aware. Often ROM activities are incorporated into the morning bath routine, which limits this activity to one time per day. Most clients, confined to bed, would be better served if passive or active ROM activities were performed two to three times per day, from the onset of illness. Plan these activity periods to allow for adequate rest intervals.
- Encourage or assist the client to be as independent as possible in performing activities of daily living. Hair-combing, teeth-brushing, bathing, and eating are all

good opportunities for clients to use their extremities through the normal ROM. Care providers are often tempted to do these things for a client to get the job done, but this does not enhance the client's independence, strength, or endurance.

- Remind assistive personnel to observe and report any signs of redness or deformity overlying a joint or extremity.
- Instruct assistive personnel that a new complaint of pain on movement is cause to cease the activity and report to you for further assessment. Delegated personnel should put no joint through its full range of motion if the client complains of pain.
- During removal and application of splints, observe the skin and involved bony prominence. Any signs of redness and irritation are cause for your examination. Revision of the splint, by the appropriate practitioner, may be necessary. Splints are often fitted by occupational therapists, although this may vary.
- Allow clients to stand to transfer from a bed to a chair rather than be slid from a bed to a stretcher chair. This action preserves and promotes the function of the quadriceps and lower leg muscles; these muscles are essential to the client's ability to resume walking activities. Standing, in contrast to sliding, the client also reduces the incidence of skin shearing that can occur via the slide method. Reserve sliding from bed to chair for clients who lack the mental capacity to follow instructions for standing or clients who are deemed too weak or unsafe to stand.
- Make sure that ambulation progresses from short to long distances. Assess the client's gait and balance. Instruct assistive personnel to monitor the client's balance and the ability to walk safely.

Verify the competency of assistive personnel in performing ROM exercises, transfer techniques, and splint application and use during orientation and annually thereafter.

Donna W. Markey, MSN, RN, ACNP-CS, *Clinician IV, Surgical Services, University of Virginia Health System, Charlottesville, Virginia*

with Paget's disease have a strong family history. Most cases are probably due to environmental causes.

Paget's disease increases in frequency with age in Western countries and is more prevalent in men than in women. It is seen infrequently in Africa and Asia. Epidemiologic studies suggest that Paget's disease is decreasing in both severity at the time of diagnosis and in prevalence.

In many instances, Paget's disease is diagnosed because the client has experienced trauma and x-rays demonstrate the characteristic changes of the disease. Ten per cent to 20% of persons with the disease are asymptomatic. Before clinical manifestations occur, x-ray films show increased bone expansion and density. After clinical manifestations have developed, the bone shows a characteristic mosaic appearance (Fig. 26–12). Bone scans are the most reliable means of identifying pagetic bone. Laboratory tests include urinary hydroxyproline and serum alkaline phosphatase (AP) that may be increased in active Paget's disease.

In symptomatic Paget's disease, the most common presenting complaints include one or more of the following: deep, aching bone pain; skeletal deformity, such as a barrel-shaped chest, bowing of the tibia or femur, or kyphosis; changes in skin temperature; pathologic fractures through diseased bone; and symptoms related to nerve compression. Diseased bone pressing on the cranial nerves may result in vertigo, hearing loss with tinnitus, and blindness. Rheumatoid arthritis, ankylosing spondylitis, and gout are commonly associated with Paget's disease.

NSAIDs, such as ibuprofen, and newer COX-2 inhibitors can often control bone pain. Pain may also be relieved with heat therapy, massage, and bracing. Further

■ THE CLIENT WITH OSTEOPOROSIS

Nursing Diagnosis. Altered Nutrition: Less Than Body Requirements, related to calcium imbalance

Outcomes. The client will meet U.S. Recommended Daily Allowances (RDA) requirements for calcium and vitamin D, will describe foods high in calcium and types of calcium supplements, will use less caffeine and alcohol, and will discuss ways to avoid the effects of lactose intolerance (as needed).

Interventions	Rationales
1. Teach the importance of diet to reduce the risk of further bone loss.	1. Dietary calcium is needed to maintain serum calcium levels, to maintain bone mass.
2. Refer to the dietitian for consultation.	2. Dietitians can offer assistance with food choices.
3. Encourage the client to eat foods high in calcium, such as plain yogurt, dairy products, seafood, sardines, green vegetables, calcium-fortified orange juice, and cereals.	3. These foods are excellent sources of calcium.
4. Provide current information about calcium supplements.	4. A calcium intake of 1000 to 1500 mg each day is easier to achieve with supplements.
5. Teach the need to reduce alcohol intake.	5. Excessive alcohol use increases bone resorption.
6. Teach ways to reduce risk of lactose intolerance, such as the use of acidophilus milk and commercially prepared lactase.	6. Lactose intolerance is caused by the inability to break down milk sugar lactose.

Evaluation. Changing nutritional habits takes time. Expect that this will be an ongoing problem for many weeks. Encourage small improvements.

Nursing Diagnosis. Impaired Physical Activity related to osteoporosis

Outcomes. The client will comply with the physical mobility plan to level of independent activities of daily living (ADLs), use assistive devices to perform independent ADL, and will identify and avoid potential hazards, thereby avoiding falls and fractures resulting from minimal injury.

Interventions	Rationales
1. Consult with physical therapist to develop an exercise program of weight-bearing exercises and strengthening exercises such as walking, tennis, hiking, and ballroom dancing. Discuss the benefits of walking at least ½ mile every day. Teach the importance of exercise in prevention of osteoporosis.	1. Weight-bearing exercises decrease bone loss. Strengthening exercises increase muscle tone and circulation. The National Institutes of Health (NIH) Consensus on Osteoporosis (1984) recommends walking, tennis, hiking, and ballroom dancing.
2. Assist with ADL allowing the client to remain independent.	2. Pain may limit the client's ability to perform ADL.
3. Evaluate the need for assistive devices for ADL and home use.	3. Devices may be needed for independent ADL.
4. Establish a hazard-free hospital environment: a. Provide adequate lighting b. Adjust bed to lowest position with side rails up when client is in bed c. Place necessary articles within client's reach d. Keep client area free of spills and clutter	4. A hazard-free environment reduces the risk of falls.

Evaluation. Increasing safe and weight-bearing activities will take several weeks. The client will be pain-free and develop muscle strength and flexibility before independence can be gained.

Nursing Diagnosis. Pain related to fracture (vertebral, Colles' wrist, hip)

Outcomes. The client will experience pain reduction or relief to perform independent ADL.

Interventions	Rationales
1. Assess the client's needs for pain medication. Plan a medication schedule with the client.	1. The client may not be receiving adequate medication because of inadequate dosing, need for around-the-clock administration, or iatrogenic causes of pain.
2. Administer non-narcotic analgesics.	2. Non-narcotic analgesics block production of chemical mediators of pain.
3. Monitor the effectiveness of analgesia.	3. Monitoring allows for revisions in the Care Plan.
4. Teach alternative modalities of pain relief, such as positioning, warm compresses, application of assistive devices, distraction, imagery, biofeedback, and hypnosis.	4. Alternative modalities can be effective in reducing pain.

Evaluation. Pain relief should be accomplished within a few days when the client is immobile. Expect to revise plans to control pain once the client is mobile or exercising.

FIGURE 26–12 A pagetoid bone, demonstrating the characteristic mosaic pattern seen on x-ray. (From Merkow, R. L., & Lane, J. M. [1990]. Paget's disease of bone. *Orthopaedic Clinics of North America, 21*[1], 173.)

orthopedic treatment may be indicated for severe disabling arthritis, severe bowing deformities of the femur or tibia, and pathologic fractures.

The recent development of potent bisphosphonates, such as pamidronate (Aredia), alendronate (Fosamax), and residronate (Actonil), have greatly improved the treatment of Paget's disease. After a course of treatment, bone turnover indices such as AP return to normal in 60% to 70% of patients, reflecting suppression of abnormal bone turnover. Existing data suggest that effective disease suppression will likely reduce future disabling problems. Unfortunately, deformity and hearing loss are not corrected with these medications. Re-treatment is indicated if bone turnover markers exceed the upper limit of normal (once they had decreased to within normal limits).

OSTEOMALACIA

Etiology and Pathophysiology

Osteomalacia is a disease in which the bone becomes abnormally soft because of a disturbed calcium and phosphorus balance secondary to vitamin D deficiency. Osteomalacia is characterized by widespread decalcification and softening of bones, especially in the spine, pelvis, and lower extremities. Bones become bent and flattened as they soften. This leads to marked deformities of the weight-bearing bones and to pathologic fractures.

Osteomalacia mainly affects women, and it is endemic in Asia. It is also seen in Moslem women living in Western countries. Their style of dress prevents them from obtaining adequate vitamin D from sunlight exposure. Some causes are:

- Chronic use of anticonvulsants
- Strict vegetarianism
- Very-low-fat diets
- Renal osteodystrophy
- Hyperthyroid-induced osteopenia
- Fibrous dysplasia

Women who have had multiple pregnancies and who have breast-fed their children have a higher rates of the disease. Osteomalacia is similar to rickets, which occurs in children, and the condition is called *adult rickets.*

Clinical Manifestations

Clients generally report easy fatigability, malaise, and bone pain, which is diffuse, poorly localized, and accompanied by a general bony tenderness. Muscular weakness is often seen in severe cases. Serum calcium and phosphorus levels are reduced, and the AP level is moderately elevated. Radiographs indicate generalized demineralization with trabecular bone loss. Pseudofractures (Milkman's syndrome) and cyst formation are common. Bone biopsy is frequently necessary for diagnosis.

Outcome Management

Intervention for clients with osteomalacia includes daily vitamin D until signs of healing take place, when a daily low maintenance dose is continued. Adequate intake of calcium and phosphorus as well as protein should be ensured.

GOUT AND GOUTY ARTHRITIS

Gout is a metabolic bone disorder in which purine (protein) metabolism is altered and the by-product, uric acid, accumulates. Gout is classified as primary or secondary. *Primary* gout is caused by an inherited defect of purine metabolism, leading to increased or decreased renal excretion. Primary gout accounts for 85% of all cases, of which 95% affect males. The initial attack of gout occurs in the 30s or 40s.

Secondary gout is an acquired condition, following hematopoietic (multiple myeloma, polycythemia vera, and leukemia) or renal disorders. In hematopoietic disorders, there is an increase in cell turnover and increased uric acid production. In addition, gout may develop from the rapid induction of chemotherapy or radiation therapy when there is massive destruction of cells. Renal disorders that decrease the excretion of uric acid may lead to gout. Hyperuricemia may also result from use of aspirin, thiazide, and mercurial diuretics, and some antituberculosis medications. Alcohol intoxication and starvation increase serum urate levels by inhibiting renal excretion due to lactic acidosis and ketosis, respectively. In addition, alcohol ingestion increases urate production by stimulating purine breakdown. Prolonged use of diuretics and other medications (levodopa, nicotinic acid, low-dose salicylates) also reduce excretion of uric acid and precipitate gout.

In the body, uric acid is made by the enzymatic breakdown of tissue and dietary purines. Hyperuricemia develops because of underexcretion or overproduction of uric acid. In addition to accumulation in the blood, uric acid is concentrated in the synovial fluid, myocardium, kidneys, and ears. When uric acid levels reach a certain level, they crystallize, and the crystals (tophi) are deposited in connective tissue. Because the crystals are deposited in connective tissue, gout is classified as a form of arthritis (Fig. 26–13).

Clinical manifestations of gout develop in stages (Table 26–5). The diagnosis of gout is confirmed by the presence of persistent hyperuricemia (>7.0 mg/dl) in addition to the clinical manifestations. The presence of uric acid in an aspirated sample of synovial fluid confirms the diagnosis.

Outcome Management

The management of the client with gout has two components: (1) management of the *acute* attack and (2) *long-term* management of hyperuricemia.

Management of the acute attack includes the use of colchicine and NSAIDs to reduce pain and inflammation. Colchicine reduces the migration of leukocytes to the synovial fluids. The initial dose of colchicine is 0.6 to 1.0 mg followed by 0.5 mg/hr until pain is relieved or signs of toxicity develop. Use caution when giving colchicine because the therapeutic dose is close to the toxic dose. Signs of toxicity include nausea, vomiting, and diarrhea. Other NSAIDs can be used, such as indomethacin or naproxen. In resistant cases of gout, adrenocorticotropic hormone (ACTH) or steroids may be required. Ice over the inflamed joints may also relieve pain.

Medications to lower uric acid include allopurinol, which blocks formation of uric acid, and probenecid, which promotes resorption of uric acid deposits and excretion of uric acid. Long-term medication use is advised in clients who have more than two attacks of gout a year, secondary forms of gout, or persistent hyperuricemia. Salicylates (aspirin) antagonize the action of uricosuric agents and must not be used concurrently.

Opinions differ regarding dietary treatment for gout. In the past, a low-purine intake was used to eliminate many proteins from the diet. Some physicians have prescribed a decrease in red and organ meats; others prescribe no dietary changes at all. Encourage ample fluid intake (2000

TABLE 26–5	MANIFESTATIONS OF GOUT BY STAGE
Stage	**Manifestations**
Stage I	Asymptomatic hyperuricemia
Stage II	Asymptomatic hyperuricemia again; laboratory and x-ray findings are unchanged from stage II.
Stage III	Acute attack is accompanied by redness, swelling, and exquisite tenderness in one joint (toes, fingers, wrists, ankles, knees, or other joints). The great toe is the most common site. This first attack develops quickly, often overnight. Fever, tachycardia, malaise, and anorexia may be noted. The acute episode usually subsides within a week. As the edema subsides, pruritus and local desquamation (tissue loss) may be noted. After the initial attack the affected joint returns to normal and the client may be asymptomatic for years. Eventually, other attacks occur.
Stage IV	Permanent changes in multiple joints with restrictions in movement. Tophi may be detected on the ears, hands, elbows, feet, and knees. Renal and cardiac disorders may also develop. The client may have uric acid renal stones, renal colic, and hypertension. Atherosclerosis occurs in about 50% of all clients.

to 3000 ml/day) to promote excretion of uric acid. A moderate intake of distilled forms of alcohol does not seem to precipitate gouty attacks. Beer, ale, and wine may precipitate them. Excessive alcohol in any form should be avoided.

Gradual weight loss is encouraged after the initial attack. Weight loss alone may reduce the incidence of attacks and uric acid levels. However, a sudden loss of weight may precipitate an attack because of the destruction of cells, which release uric acid.

Clients who can recognize early manifestations of gout may be able to avert the attack by prompt use of colchicine or indomethacin. Long-term side effects (alopecia, bone marrow suppression, hepatic damage) from these agents, although rare, should be explained to the client.

Nursing management of the client with gout includes pain control. The client is usually placed at bed rest until pain subsides. Once ambulating, the client's need for crutches or a walker should be considered until gait is stable. Explain dietary restrictions, fluid requirements, and long-term self-management.

SPINAL COLUMN DEFORMITIES

The characteristic S curve of the lateral spine develops during fetal life and early childhood. Because other abnormal curves can occur due to defects in the bone, muscles, or nerves, every spinal problem must be considered from both an orthopedic and a neurologic viewpoint.

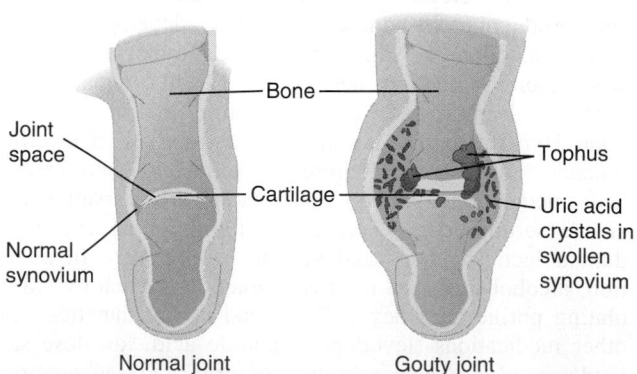

FIGURE 26–13 Comparison of a gouty joint and a normal joint.

SCOLIOSIS

In the coronal plane, the spine should appear completely straight. Scoliosis is lateral curvature of the spine in any area—cervical, thoracic, thoracolumbar, or lumbar. It is important to distinguish curvature of *structural* origin from that of *nonstructural* origin. A structural curvature does not correct itself on forced bending against the curvature, and vertebral rotation is demonstrated. A nonstructural curvature is easily corrected on forced bending or in the supine position, and rotation of the vertebral bodies is not demonstrated.

Idiopathic scoliosis is the most common form, appearing in growing children with no other apparent health problems. The incidence is less than 1%,[43] occurring most often in preadolescents and adolescents. Scoliosis was once believed to be primarily a problem in girls, but school screening studies have shown small degrees of abnormal spinal curvature in equal numbers of boys and girls. Both boys and girls should be observed until it is proved that a curve is not progressive. Continued curve progression is possible even after skeletal maturity if the curvature is greater than 40 or 45 degrees, and excessive curvature can lead to cardiopulmonary problems and pain that prompt the client to seek medical care. The client may also seek help because of cosmetic deformity and loss in height. Skeletally mature clients with a curve less than 20 degrees do not require treatment. Skeletally immature clients with a curve between 20 and 40 degrees require brace management, while clients with curves greater than 45 degrees need surgical intervention.

Etiology

The cause of scoliosis can be congenital or neuromuscular. Congenital scoliosis results from a malformation of the bony vertebral segment of the spine, either because of failure of (1) formation (absence of a portion of a vertebra) or (2) segmentation (absence of normal separations between vertebrae). Neuromuscular conditions associated with spinal deformities include cerebral palsy, syringomyelia, polio, myelomeningocele, spinal muscle atrophy, spinal cord tumors, trauma, and myopathic conditions such as muscular dystrophy.

Clinical Manifestations

Clinical manifestations and a family history of spinal deformity are significant, but diagnosis is confirmed by upright posteroanterior and lateral radiographs that reveal a curvature of 10 degrees or more (Fig. 26–14A). X-rays are the only exact tool for monitoring changes in spinal deformity, but excessive radiation exposure is inappropriate in children. Two other noninvasive stereophotogrametic techniques—Moire topography and the integrated shape-imaging system (ISIS)—produce images on the back surface shape that can be correlated to underlying spinal deformities.

FIGURE 26–14 *A,* Scoliosis. *B,* Postoperative x-ray after correction with Cotrel-Dubousset instrumentation. (From Maher, A. B., Salmond, S. W., & Pellino, T. A. [Eds.]. [1998]. *Orthopedic nursing* [2nd ed., p. 557]. Philadelphia: W. B. Saunders.)

Outcome Management

Nonsurgical treatments for clients with spinal deformity consist of observation, bracing, and exercise. Each client needs to be individually evaluated, not only for the medical problem but also for willingness to participate in any suggested therapies. One client may refuse to wear a brace under any circumstances; another may insist on treatment for even a slight curvature.

The decision to proceed with surgical treatment is based not only on failure of conservative treatments but also on additional factors, such as the client's emotional stability and readiness to undergo a major procedure. Spinal fusion is the ultimate goal in many cases, attaching adjacent vertebrae to each other with a bone graft to prohibit motion between them. The surgical approach can be posterior or anterior, depending on the location of the deformity. A combined anterior-posterior approach has become increasingly popular for adults with severe thoracolumbar scoliosis.

Various types of instruments can be used to stabilize the spine and correct deformity. The choice of instrumentation is based on the diagnosis, the magnitude of the curvature and the flexibility of the curve, the client's age and inherent bone strength, and the client's ability to wear a postoperative immobilization device. The Cotrel-Dubousset (CD), Texas Scottish Rite Hospital (TSRH), Moss-Miami, and Luque systems are commonly used for a posterior approach (see Fig. 26–14). The Harrington rod system, developed in the 1960s, is still in use because of its availability and because many surgeons are very familiar with it. The most common types of instrumentation for an anterior approach are the Zielke and Harris systems.

COMPLICATIONS

Possible complications following scoliosis surgery include neurologic compromise, infection, respiratory problems, spinal fluid leakage, phlebitis, excessive blood loss, implant problems, and pseudarthrosis. The most devastating complications are paralysis and death.

POSTOPERATIVE CARE

Postoperative nursing management focuses on:

- Assessment of blood loss and maintenance of hemodynamic stability
- Assessment of motor and sensory function in the lower extremities
- Administration of adequate analgesia and fluid replacement
- Client education for effective pulmonary hygiene
- Wound and skin care
- Progressive ambulation

(Chapter 71 also discusses nursing management after lumbar fusion.)

KYPHOSIS

Also called "humpback" or "dowager's hump," the term kyphosis describes a posterior rounding of the thoracic spine. While a certain degree of kyphosis is considered normal, curvatures greater than 45 degrees are believed to be excessive and require additional evaluation as to the cause. Kyphosis is identified as *postural* if the client can voluntarily hyperextend the spine to correct the curvature and if there is no x-ray evidence of structural change. Kyphosis is common in metabolic disorders such as osteoporosis and osteomalacia, but it can also accompany neuromuscular diseases such as cerebral palsy and muscular dystrophy. Severe curvature can affect cardiopulmonary and gastrointestinal function, making intervention essential.

Kyphosis is most often treated with bracing or corsets to straighten the spine. Exercises to strengthen muscles and ligaments may also be encouraged. Spinal fusion with or without instrumentation may be required if response to other interventions is inadequate.

LORDOSIS

Lordosis is an excessive inward curvature of the lumbar spine sometimes seen in pregnant or obese clients or in those with large abdominal tumors. Extreme lordosis may lead to *swayback,* in which the lumbosacral spine curves sharply and the thoracolumbar spine exhibits kyphosis. Lordosis is often associated with sagging shoulders, an exaggerated pelvic angle, and medial rotation of the legs. If necessary, treatment may consist of bracing, spinal fusion, or osteotomy. Hyperlordosis in young children and prepubertal girls is a self-correcting problem thought to be related to rapid skeletal growth without corresponding soft tissue growth.

BONE INFECTIONS

Musculoskeletal system contamination can result either as infection spreads from other sites in the body or from external insults (e.g., puncture, surgery). Infections are often severe and difficult to treat because the bones are relatively inaccessible to protective macrophages and antibodies. Even a small number of microorganisms can be enough to establish a serious infection that can lead to loss of function or even death. For this reason, nurses should be diligent in wound care and alert to any symptoms that suggest infection.

OSTEOMYELITIS

Pathophysiology

Osteomyelitis is a severe pyogenic infection of bone and surrounding tissues. Although generally bacterial in origin, osteomyelitis can also be caused by a virus or fungus. *Staphylococcus aureus* is the most common infecting organism, but *Escherichia coli, Pseudomonas, Klebsiella, Salmonella,* and *Proteus* may also be found. Because osteomyelitis can be extraordinarily difficult to cure even with long-term antibiotics, prompt recognition is crucial. Delayed identification or inadequate treatment can result in a chronic infection accompanied by continuing pain, chronically draining sinuses, loss of function, amputation, or death.

Osteomyelitis occurs most frequently in the femur and

tibia. Males are affected more often than females, often as a result of trauma. Susceptibility to infection increases with intravenous drug use, diabetes, immunocompromising diseases, or a history of bloodstream infections. Limiting the spread of osteomyelitis may also be more difficult in clients with a disorder such as malnutrition, alcoholism, or liver failure.

Clinical Manifestations

Clinical manifestations may vary slightly according to the site of involvement. Infection in the long bones is accompanied by acute localized pain and redness or drainage, often with a history of recent trauma or newly acquired prostheses. Fever and malaise may be present, but adults do not always appear acutely ill with other systemic signs. Infection in the vertebrae usually brings pain and mobility difficulties. The client with vertebral osteomyelitis often reports a history of genitourinary infection or drug abuse. Osteomyelitis in the foot is most commonly associated with vascular insufficiency.

Laboratory studies and x-rays or bone scans are important in the definitive diagnosis of osteomyelitis. Elevated WBC and ESR, along with clinical manifestations, usually allow initial diagnosis and early treatment while the physician waits for further evidence from blood cultures or needle aspirate analysis. Radiographic changes related to osteomyelitis are generally evident within 7 to 10 days, but in some cases the diagnosis is not confirmed on x-rays until 3 to 4 weeks after infection develops. Early acute osteomyelitis is more efficiently identified by radionuclide bone scans, which can detect lesions within 24 to 72 hours after the onset of infection. Because of its ability to distinguish between soft tissue and bone marrow, magnetic resonance imaging (MRI) is also being used increasingly for definitive diagnosis of osteomyelitis.

Outcome Management

Elimination of the infecting organism, both locally from the bone and systemically from the body, is the major treatment goal for acute osteomyelitis. Prompt treatment also prevents further bone deformity and injury, increases client comfort, and avoids complications of impaired mobility. Surgery is initially performed on the adult client with osteomyelitis to ensure effective debridement and drainage, elimination of dead space, and adequate soft tissue coverage. Antibiotics alone rarely resolve infection in adults, but they do work more effectively after surgical preparation of the treatment area. High doses of parenteral antibiotics are frequently administered for 4 to 8 weeks to achieve a bactericidal level in the bone tissue. Oral antibiotics are continued for another 4 to 8 weeks, with serial bone scans and ESR measurements performed to evaluate the effectiveness of drug therapy. Open, draining wounds are packed with gauze to promote drainage. If initial treatment is delayed or inadequate, the necrotic bone separates from the living bone to form *sequestra,* which serve as a medium for additional microorganism growth. Chronic osteomyelitis can result.

SEPTIC ARTHRITIS

Etiology and Pathophysiology

Septic arthritis (also known as pyogenic arthritis, infectious arthritis, septic joint disease, bacterial arthritis, and suppurative arthritis) is a closed-space infection caused by invasion of the synovial membrane by pus-forming bacteria or other pathogens. Joints most commonly affected in adult clients are the knee, hip, shoulder, wrist, and ankle.

A variety of microorganisms may infect the joint, but *Neisseria gonorrhoae* is the most common causative pathogen in adults under age 30 years. A significant percentage of staphylococci, the second most common causative organism in adults, is methicillin-resistant. *Staphylococcus aureus* invades the joint through hematogenous spread, as an extension of adjacent soft tissue infection, or from direct inoculation following trauma or an invasive procedure.

Hematogenous spread, in which organisms reach the joint from a remote site, is the most common etiologic mechanism. Because the synovial membrane is very vascular, any microorganism that is circulating in the blood may be easily trapped in the synovial space. Upper respiratory infection, otitis media, furuncle, or impetigo may seed a susceptible site such as a previously traumatized or diseased knee joint.

The presence of septic arthritis typically reflects the failure of multiple defense mechanisms. In the early stages of infection, the synovial membrane swells and becomes infiltrated with neutrophils. A purulent effusion distends the joint as the neutrophils release lysosomal proteolytic enzymes that destroy the articular cartilage, subchondral bone, and joint capsule. Enzymatic cartilage destruction can actually occur in 3 to 24 hours, creating a medical emergency that requires prompt treatment to avoid permanent joint damage.

Clinical Manifestations

The client often presents with complaints of pain, swelling, warmth, and tenderness in a single joint and also generally experiences an acute systemic reaction. The adult client is more likely than the child to experience only a low-grade fever and malaise. However, high temperatures and shaking chills are generally present in the client who has positive blood cultures.

Assessment focuses on the presence of factors that may predispose the client to joint infection, such as recent surgery or injury, diagnostic procedures, intravenous drug abuse, or systemic disease. Because effective treatment requires accurate identification of the causative agent, initial laboratory studies attempt to differentiate septic arthritis from autoimmune diseases with joint involvement (such as rheumatoid arthritis). CBC, ESR, the antinuclear antibody (ANA) test, and rheumatoid factor (RF) measurements are often among studies that are ordered. In addition, joint fluid is aspirated for analysis, and a synovial biopsy is performed. Radioisotope scanning techniques may also be helpful in early detection of infection.

Outcome Management

Antibiotic therapy is a critical part of effective treatment of septic arthritis and must be promptly initiated to prevent permanent joint damage. Penicillin G, a bactericidal agent, is often administered initially because many common causative organisms are susceptible to the drug. After the specific organism and its sensitivities have been identified from synovial fluid cultures, the antibiotic therapy may be altered. Treatment time varies according to duration of clinical manifestations, the causative organism, and the status of the client's immune system. For most clients, parenteral antibiotics are administered for 2 to 3 weeks and oral antibiotics continue for another 1 or 2 weeks. However, elderly clients or those with more complex presentations may require parenteral therapy lasting 4 to 6 weeks. Decompression of the infected joint is also necessary, although controversy exists about the best methods. Open synovectomy and debridement or repeated joint aspirations and irrigations may be performed. Arthroscopic drainage and debridement have also been successful.

Effective nursing management requires scrupulous attention to the client's joint position, exercise, and rehabilitation. In the acute phase of septic arthritis, the client is likely to hold the joint in slight to moderate flexion as a position of comfort. Because this can lead to flexion deformities, slings, immobilizers, or splints may be used temporarily to hold the joint in an optimal position. As inflammation begins to resolve, passive ROM exercises are initiated to preserve joint function. CPM has also been used with some success. Active motion and weight-bearing may not be initiated until clinical manifestations and inflammation have almost totally disappeared. Pain management is also important for the client with septic arthritis to provide comfort and to allow greater ease in exercise participation.

BONE TUMORS

A bone tumor (neoplasm) may be benign or malignant (Table 26–6 and Fig. 26–15). Benign bone tumors may remain undiagnosed because they often cause no pain.

TABLE 26–6	PRIMARY BONE AND CARTILAGE TUMORS
Type	**Description**
BENIGN CARTILAGE-FORMING TUMOR	
Enchondroma	Lesion in mature cartilage but lacking histologic characteristic of chondrosarcoma; found in hands and feet; age range, 20–40 yr
Osteochondroma	Most frequent bone tumor; cartilage-capped bony projection on external bone surface; metaphyses of long bone, especially proximal tibia and distal femur; age range, 0–30 yr
BENIGN BONE-FORMING TUMOR	
Osteoid osteoma	Small osteoblastic lesion (less than 1 cm) with demarcated outline and reactive bone formation; femur and tibia; age range 10–20 yr
Osteoblastoma	Similar to osteoid osteoma but larger (>2 cm); spine
Giant cell tumor (osteoclastoma)	Aggressive benign bone tumor with richly vascularized tissue consisting of plump spindle-shaped cells and numerous giant cells; distal femur, proximal tibia, distal radius, proximal humerus; age range, 20–40 yr
MALIGNANT BONE-FORMING TUMOR	
Osteosarcoma	Most common primary malignant bone tumor; formation of bone or osteoid by tumor cell; metaphyses, especially of distal femur, proximal tibia, and proximal humerus; intramedullary region involved; age range, 10–30 yr
Ewing's sarcoma	Composed of densely packed small cells with round nuclei; often confused with osteomyelitis because it presents with fever, anemia, leukocytosis, increased ESR; diaphyseal regions of long and flat bones; age range, 5–15 yr
Fibrosarcoma	Formation of interlacing bundles of collagen fibers by spindle-shaped tumor cells; absence of other types of histologic differentiation; femur, tibia; age range, 5–80 yr
MALIGNANT CARTILAGE-FORMING TUMOR	
Chondrosarcoma	Formation of cartilage by tumor cells; higher cellularity and greater pleomorphism than in chondromas; femur, pelvis, ribs, scapula; age range, 30–60 yr

Adapted from Piasecki, P. (1996). Tumors. In S. W. Salmond, N. E. Mooney, & L. A. Verdisco (Eds.), *Core curriculum for orthopaedic nursing* (3rd ed.). Pitman, NJ: National Association of Orthopaedic Nurses.

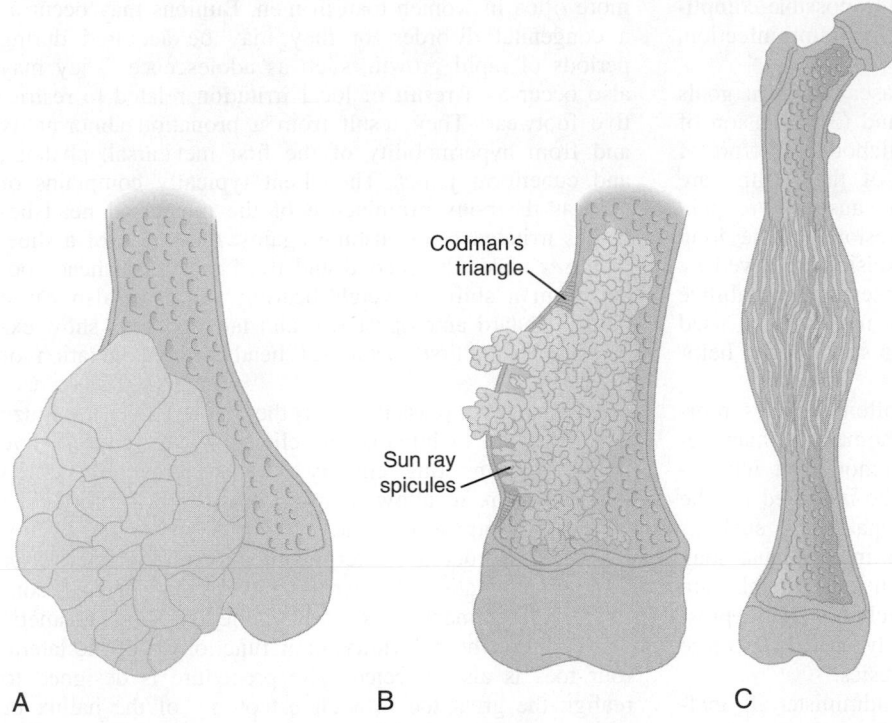

Codman's triangle

Sun ray spicules

A   B   C

FIGURE 26–15 Bone tumors. *A,* A giant cell tumor. *B,* An osteogenic sarcoma. *C,* A malignant endothelioma (Ewing's sarcoma). (After Hughes, S. [1983]. *A short textbook of orthopedics and traumatology* [3rd ed.]. New York: ARCO.)

They may be noted as an incidental x-ray finding when the client is being evaluated for another complaint, such as fracture through a bone cyst. However, benign tumors that grow aggressively can cause bone pain, weakness, and destruction. In such a case, surgery is then indicated.

MALIGNANT BONE TUMORS

Primary malignant tumors originate in bone cells or form within the bone. Each year, about 2500 new cases of primary bone tumors are diagnosed, including osteosarcoma, chondrosarcoma, and Ewing's sarcoma.[24] Clients typically present with a mass or lesion, or a pathologic fracture. They may also report weight loss, fever, chills, or pulmonary manifestations.

The exact cause of primary bone tumors remains largely unknown, but several factors are believed to play a role in their development. Past trauma has been associated with tumor development, as has exposure to carcinogens such as asbestos, dioxin, and radium. Bone tumors may also develop from benign medical conditions (enchondromatosis, neurofibromatosis) or from metabolic conditions (Paget's disease). Fewer than 5% of clients with malignancies have a hereditary predilection to cancer.[24]

Metastatic bone tumors, winch are more prevalent than sarcomas, spread to the bone from primary carcinomas in sites such as the breast, prostate, lung, and kidney. Thyroid, bladder, uterine, colorectal, and vaginal cancers can also metastasize to bone. Cancer cells may spread directly within a body cavity, or they may metastasize by hematogenous or lymphatic spread.

Laboratory studies such as CBC, blood and urine calcium levels, and ESR assist in client evaluation, but they are not diagnostic themselves. Other laboratory tests, however, are used as tumor markers. An elevated serum AP level may be noted with osteoblastic tumors, for example, and lactate dehydrogenase (LDH) may mark tumor progression for Ewing's sarcoma. A plain radiograph in anterior and posterior views may provide an initial diagnosis, but other studies—such as a CT scan, MRI, or bone scan—are also commonly performed. A bone biopsy is needed for definitive diagnosis of metastatic bone disease.

Outcome Management

The treatment goal for the client with a primary tumor is to eradicate the tumor completely and promote long-term survival. *Chemotherapy* has dramatically increased the survival of clients diagnosed with primary bone tumors. *Radiation therapy* has become safer because of increased understanding of cancer and radiobiology; it is also now better tolerated through the use of radiation machines that reduce skin sensitivity. *Surgery* may be performed to eradicate the disease, either through excision of the tumor and a wide zone of surrounding normal tissue or through amputation. If the tumor is excised, the resulting defect is repaired by using a joint prosthesis or bone graft with internal fixation. The bone graft can be taken from the client at another anatomic site, or allograft (cadaver) bone may be used.

Pain management following surgery is a major focus. Opioids are often delivered by patient-controlled analgesia (PCA) pumps or via epidural catheter. Pain should be addressed aggressively and medication effectiveness assessed regularly. Frequent position changes and stimulation of non-tumor areas through heat, cold, or massage may be beneficial. Nonpharmacologic strategies, such as music therapy, imagery, and relaxation techniques, may provide powerful adjuncts to opioid administration. Postoperative nursing care also addresses the possible complications related to orthopedic surgery, including infection, DVT, and non-union of grafted bone.

For the client with metastatic disease, treatment goals include (1) palliation, (2) remission, and (3) extension of life. Pain management requires a collaborative effort of the client, family, and all members of the health care team. Because metastatic tumors can cause severe pain and have the potential to fracture, lesions in the long bones are commonly managed with excision, followed by intramedullary rodding and cement insertion to stabilize the weakened bone. Radiation therapy may also be used to decrease tumor size, improving bone strength and helping in pain management.

Pharmacologic treatment of pain often includes morphine. Oral administration facilitates home care management for the client with metastatic tumors, but intravenous or transdermal medications may be indicated for the client with gastric problems. Other analgesics, such as acetaminophen and anti-inflammatory medications, may also be used because they act on the peripheral pain mechanism. Adjuvant medications, including antidepressants and anticonvulsants, are frequently used to increase the effectiveness of conventional analgesics.

The key to pain management is to administer all analgesics on an around-the-clock (ATC) rather than on an as-needed (PRN) basis. Nonpharmacologic measures should also be employed to maximize pain relief.

As with postoperative treatment of the client with a primary tumor, pain should be addressed aggressively and medication effectiveness assessed regularly. Attempts at pain management for the client with a metastatic bone tumor may ultimately lead to a palliative neurosurgical procedure, such as a chordotomy, in which the anterolateral spinal cord tracts are severed to provide relief in the affected areas.

DISORDERS OF THE FOOT

HALLUX VALGUS (BUNIONS)

Bunions, a common foot deformity that involves the first metatarsal and the great toe (hallux), occur nine times more often in women than in men. Bunions may occur as a congenital disorder, or they may be acquired during periods of rapid growth, such as adolescence. They may also occur as a result of local irritation related to restrictive footwear. They result from a pronation abnormality and from hypermobility of the first metatarsal, phalanx, and cuneiform joints. The client typically complains of pain as the bony prominence of the metatarsal head becomes irritated from pushing against the inside of a shoe. *Calluses* under the second and third metatarsal heads occur from a shift in weight-bearing and may also cause pain. Standard anteroposterior and lateral x-rays show exostosis of the first metatarsal head with subluxation or dislocation.

To decrease pressure over the bunion and minimize the likelihood of bursitis, the client may try conservative treatment, consisting entirely of wearing shoes with a larger toe box to allow more space for the forefoot. If a change in footwear does not provide enough relief, orthoses may be ordered or steroid injections administered for acute inflammation. Surgery may be considered if conservative treatment fails, if the client desires cosmetic correction of the deformity, or if functioning of the lateral four toes is also affected. The procedure is designed to realign the great toe through osteotomy of the hallux or through fusion of the metatarsophalangeal joint (Fig. 26–16). Kirschner wires are inserted vertically through the involved toes, remaining in place for about 3 weeks after surgery. Bits of cork are placed on the wire tips for protection. In addition to routine care, the client who has undergone bunionectomy may use wooden postoperative shoes for ambulation.

MORTON'S NEUROMA (PLANTAR NEUROMA)

Athletes commonly experience Morton's neuroma because of excessive pressure placed on the branch of the medial plantar nerve between the third and fourth toes. The pressure causes a neuroma, or swelling of the nerve, that leads the client to complain of pain in the ball of the foot. Depending on the extent of the compression, pain may radiate into the toes and be accompanied by numbness. Pain may be increased if the client wears tight-

FIGURE 26–16 Bunions and their surgical correction.

Bunion   Bunionette

Typical cuts in the bone

Typical realignment and screw fixation

fitting or high-heeled shoes. Hyperextension of the metatarsophalangeal joints or repetitive impact on the forefoot may also increase pain.

The usual treatment involves changing the type of shoe to one with a larger toe box that provides more room for the forefoot. Anti-inflammatory medications are often prescribed. If they are ineffective, steroid injections may be administered. Surgery to remove the neuroma may be considered if other treatments do not produce long-term relief.

HAMMER TOE

Hammer toe is a deformity caused by a flexion contracture of the proximal interphalangeal joint (PIP) with extension or slight hyperextension of the distal interphalangeal joint (DIP) (Fig. 26–17). This deformity often accompanies hallux valgus and may occur in clients with a family history of hammer toe, RA, and clawfeet. Hammer toe leads to improper fit of footwear, creating pain with walking and a change in gait patterns. Corns and calluses on pressure areas of the foot may need to be removed.

Treatment centers on choosing footwear with a wide toe box. Pads and inserts can help relieve pressure, but they can also cause previously unaffected areas of the foot to rub against the shoe. Osteotomy of the toe and

FIGURE 26–17 Hammer toe.

resection of the proximal phalanx may be required for symptom relief.

MUSCULAR DISORDERS

MUSCULAR DYSTROPHY

Muscular dystrophy (MD) is a term that generally designates a group of genetic disorders involving gradual degeneration of muscle fibers. The client experiences progressive weakness and skeletal muscle wasting, accompanied by disability and deformity. The various forms of MD are differentiated by the affected muscle groups, the client's age at onset of the disease, the rate of progression, and the inheritance mode (Table 26–7). *Pseudohypertrophic MD (Duchenne's MD)* is the most

TABLE 26–7	CLINICAL FEATURES IN MUSCULAR DYSTROPHY (MD)		
	Duchenne's MD	**Becker's MD**	**Limb Girdle MD**
Incidence	Most common type of MD	Less common than Duchenne's MD	Less common than Duchenne's or Becker's MD
Age at onset	Usually <3 yr	Usually 5–15 yr	Usually by second decade
Inheritance	Sex-linked recessive gene, autosomal <10%	Sex-linked recessive gene	Usually autosomal recessive
Pattern of muscle involvement	Onset: Selected symmetrical weakness of proximal pelvic muscles, 3–5 yr	Similar to Duchenne's MD	Proximal shoulder and pelvic girdle
	Later: shoulder girdle muscle involvement		
Late muscle involvement	Affects all muscles, including facial, oculopharyngeal, and respiratory	Face spared	Peripheral brachioradialis, hand, and calf
Pseudohypertrophy	Calf muscles	Calf muscles	Occurs in fewer than one third of cases
Contractural deformities	Common	Less common	Occurs in late disease; milder than Duchenne's MD
Scoliosis/kyphoscoliosis	Common in late disease	Not severe	Mild in late disease
Heart involvement	Yes	Uncommon in late disease	Rare
IQ	Decreased	Normal	Normal
Course	Steady progression	Slow progression	Slow progression, with greater variation among clients

IQ, intelligence quotient.
Adapted from Doleysh, N. (1996). Neuromuscular disorders. In S. W. Salmond, N. E. Mooney, & L. A. Verdisco (Eds.), *Core curriculum for orthopaedic nursing* (3rd ed.). Pitman, NJ: National Association of Orthopaedic Nurses.

common and severe form of the disease. A sex-linked recessive disorder that affects males almost exclusively, it has been linked to an abnormality of the Xp21 gene locus. The client experiences wheelchair dependency in early adolescence. Respiratory muscles are eventually involved, and myocardial degeneration leads to cardiomegaly and tachycardia.

Diagnosis of MD is accomplished through use of multiple modalities in an attempt to differentiate the disease from other disorders, such as myasthenia gravis and polymyositis. The most valuable laboratory test is serum creatine kinase analysis; levels are elevated in clients with MD because of an abnormality of striated muscle function. Enzyme levels do decrease, however, as muscle mass decreases. Muscle biopsy is essential to diagnosis of a neuromuscular disease such as Duchenne's MD. Muscle shows degeneration, with fibers replaced by connective tissue and fat in later stages of the disease.

Treatment is largely symptomatic and supportive because there is currently no cure for MD. Care is aimed at increasing the comfort and functional ability through corrective surgery for related deformities or use of braces for the spine or lower extremities. Breathing exercises may also be initiated for respiratory decompensation. More than 60% of clients with MD live to age 21 years, but survival beyond age 30 is unusual.[6] Death generally results from respiratory or cardiac failure.

CONCLUSIONS

The focus of this chapter has been musculoskeletal disorders, including metabolic bone diseases such as osteoporosis. Osteoarthritis is a common degenerative disorder that is often treated with joint replacement surgery. Special nursing care is required after such surgery to maximize the client's outcome. Benign and metastatic bone tumors, common foot disorders, and MD, a hereditary neuromuscular disorder, have also been discussed.

An understanding of these disorders is essential for the nurse who provides care for affected clients.

THINKING CRITICALLY

1. **You meet an older woman in the total joint class who is considering joint replacement surgery but has not yet scheduled the procedure with her orthopedist. She has osteoarthritis and, because of increasing pain in her hips, she now uses a wheelchair when she goes out in public. She tells you she also has diabetes mellitus. What would you discuss with her to help her prepare appropriately for surgery?**

Factors to Consider. What would be the benefit of increased upper arm strength for this client? Is she maintaining tight control of the diabetes? Is weight loss an issue before surgery?

2. **A middle-aged client is concerned about bone loss resulting from osteoporosis. She tells you that her mother has severe osteoporosis, and she realizes her lifestyle and family history are predisposing factors. She asks you to suggest a lifestyle program for her and her daughters. How should you proceed?**

Factors to Consider. What focused assessment should you complete? How should you complete teaching for the client and her daughters?

3. **An elderly woman tells you her physician wants her to eat a diet high in calcium. He wants her to consume 1500 mg of calcium without taking enriched antacids or calcium supplements. This woman is lactose-intolerant and has a hiatal hernia. She lives alone on a limited income. What problems might impair her compliance with the prescribed treatment regimen?**

Factors to Consider. What dietary sources of calcium are appropriate for the lactose-intolerant client? How does the presence of a hiatal hernia affect dietary intake?

BIBLIOGRAPHY

1. Altizer, L. (1995). Total hip arthroplasty. *Orthopaedic Nursing, 14*(4), 7–18, 63.
2. Altizer, L. L. (1998). Degenerative disorders. In A. B. Maher, S. W. Salmond, & T. A. Pellino (Eds.), *Orthopaedic nursing* (2nd ed.). Philadelphia: W. B. Saunders, pp. 480–544.
3. American College of Rheumatology Ad Hoc Committee on Clinical Guidelines. (1996). Guidelines for the initial evluation of the adult patient with acute musculoskeletal symptoms. *Arthritis and Rheumatology, 39,* 1–8.
4. Anderson, L. P., & Dale, K. G. (1998). Infections in total joint replacements. *Orthopaedic Nursing, 17*(1), 7–10.
5. Aubin, M., & Marks, R. (1995). The efficacy of short-term treatment with transcutaneous electrical nerve stimulation for osteo-arthritic knee pain. *Physiotherapy, 81*(11), 669–675.
6. Bender, L. H. (1998). Congenital and developmental disorders. In A. B. Maher, S. W. Salmond, & T. A. Pellino (Eds.), *Orthopaedic nursing* (2nd ed.). Philadelphia: W. B. Saunders, pp. 586–662.
7. Blaylock, B., et al. (1995). Tape injury in the patient with total hip replacement. *Orthopaedic Nursing, 14*(3), 25–28.
8. Bonatz, E. (1996). Overuse syndromes of the hand and wrist. In V. R. Masear (Ed.), *Primary care orthopaedics.* Philadelphia: W. B. Saunders, pp. 346–349.
9. Burrage, R. L., & Sutter, C. A. (1999). Arthritis. In J. T. Stone, J. F. Wyman, & S. A. Salisbury (Eds.), *Clinical gerontological nursing: A guide to advanced practice.* Philadelphia: W. B. Saunders, pp. 469–487.
10. Cerrato, P. L. (1998). Alternatives. Complementary therapies: Can these compounds curb arthritis? *RN, 6*(4), 57–58, 67.
11. Clough, J. D., Lambert, T., & Miller, D. R. (1996). The new thinking on osteoarthritis. *Patient Care, 30*(14), 110–113, 117–118, 121–124.
12. Crescimbeni, J. A. (1997). From bed to chair: Transferring the non–weight-bearing patient. *Orthopaedic Nursing, 16*(2), 47–50.
13. DiNubile, N. A. (1997). Osteoarthritis. How to make exercise part of your treatment plan. *The Physician and Sportsmedicine, 25*(7), 47–50, 52, 55–56.
14. Doleysh, N. (1996). Neuromuscular disorders. In S. W. Salmond, N. E. Mooney, & L. A. Verdisco (Eds.), *Core curriculum for orthopaedic nursing* (3rd ed.). Pitman, NJ: National Association of Orthopaedic Nurses, pp. 315–352.
15. Evans, J. A., & Madrid, C. L. (1995). High tibial osteotomy: Treatment for unicompartmental arthritis. *Operative Techniques in Sports Medicine, 3*(2), 112–116.
16. Facts and Comparisons (1998). The review of natural products: Chondroitin. St. Louis: Author.
17. Facts and Comparisons (1998). The review of natural products: Glucosamine. St. Louis: Author.
18. Felson, D.T. (1996). Weight and osteoarthritis. *American Journal of Clinical Nutrition, 63*(3S), 430S–432S.

19. Flynn, R. (1996). Arthritic disorders. In S. W. Salmond, N. E. Mooney, & L. A. Verdisco (Eds.), *Core curriculum for orthopaedic nursing* (3rd ed.). Pitman, NJ: National Association of Orthopaedic Nurses, pp. 217–263.

20. Fracaro, M. L. (1996). Infection. In S. W. Salmond, N. E. Mooney, & L. A. Verdisco (Eds.), *Core curriculum for orthopaedic nursing* (3rd ed.). Pitman, NJ: National Association of Orthopaedic Nurses, pp. 281–296.

21. Haynes, K. (1998). Neoplasms of the musculoskeletal system. In A. B. Maher, S. W. Salmond, & T. A. Pellino (Eds.), *Orthopaedic nursing* (2nd ed.). Philadelphia: W. B. Saunders, pp. 769–803.

22. Jaffe, K. (1996). Tumors of the musculoskeletal system. In V. R. Masear (Ed.), *Primary care orthopaedics*. Philadelphia: W. B. Saunders, pp. 263–288.

23. Jaffe, K., Greco, J., & Wade, J. (1996). Orthopaedic emergencies and infections. In V. R. Masear (Ed.), *Primary care orthopaedics*. Philadelphia: W. B. Saunders, pp. 35–49.

24. Kessenich, C. R. (1997). Myths & facts . . . about osteoarthritis. *Nursing97, 27*(8), 67.

25. Kettelman, K. (1998). Controlling bone pain: How to keep nausea and oversedation out of the picture. *Nursing98, 28*(11), 22.

26. Killian, J. T., & Coen, J. (1996). Developmental conditions in children. In V. R. Masear (Ed.), *Primary care orthopaedics*. Philadelphia: W. B. Saunders, pp. 289–303.

27. Kopp, M. (1997). Caring for the adult patient undergoing anterior/ posterior spinal fusion. *Orthopaedic Nursing, 16*(2), 55–59.

28. Krug, B. (1997). Rheumatoid arthritis and osteoarthritis: A basic comparison. *Orthopaedic Nursing, 16*(5), 73–75.

29. Ling, S. M., & Bathon, J. M. (1998). Osteoarthritis in older adults. *Journal of the American Geriatrics Society, 46*(2), 216–225.

30. Lotkey, P. A. (1998). Knee arthroplasty: Alternatives, techniques, and management issues. DVT prophylaxis options: Facts and fictions. *Orthopaedics, 21*(9), 1025–1026.

31. Maher, A. B. (1998). Assessment of the musculoskeletal system. In A. B. Maher, S. W. Salmond, & T. A. Pellino (Eds.), *Orthopaedic - nursing* (2nd ed.). Philadelphia: W. B. Saunders, pp. 168–189.

32. Morris, N. S. (1999). Complications associated with orthopaedic surgery. In *An introduction to orthopaedic nursing* (2nd ed.). Pitman, NJ: National Association of Orthopaedic Nurses, p. 123–145.

33. Mosher, C. M. (1999). Total hip and knee replacement. In *An introduction to orthopaedic nursing* (2nd ed.). Pitman, NJ: National Association of Orthopaedic Nurses, pp. 67–81.

34. Osteoarthritis: Old scourge, new hope (1996). *Consumer Reports on Health, 8*(1), 3–5.

35. Pemberton, C. (1995). Diagnosing and treating bone metastases. *Nursing Times, 91*(3), 33–34.

36. Piasecki, P. (1996). Nursing care of the patient with metastatic bone disease. *Orthopaedic Nursing, 15*(4), 25–33.

37. Piasecki, P. (1996). Tumors. In S. W. Salmond, N. E. Mooney, & L. A. Verdisco (Eds.), *Core curriculum for orthopaedic nursing* (3rd ed.). Pitman, NJ: National Association of Orthopaedic Nurses, pp. 451–471.

38. Rodts, M. F. (1996). Spine. In S. W. Salmond, N. E. Mooney, & L. A. Verdisco (Eds.), *Core curriculum for orthopaedic nursing* (3rd ed.). Pitman, NJ: National Association of Orthopaedic Nurses, pp. 397–414.

39. Rodts, M. F. (1998). Disorders of the spine. In A. B. Maher, S. W. Salmond, & T. A. Pellino (Eds.), *Orthopaedic nursing* (2nd ed.). Philadelphia: W. B. Saunders, pp. 545–585.

40. Salmond, W. S. (1998). Infections of the musculoskeletal system. In A. B. Maher, S. W. Salmond, & T. A. Pellino (Eds.), *Orthopaedic nursing* (2nd ed.). Philadelphia: W. B. Saunders, pp. 804–858.

41. Schultz, D. L. (1995). The role of the neuroscience nurse in lumbar fusion. *Journal of Neuroscience Nursing, 27*(2), 90–95.

42. Stein, R. R. (1999). An overview of the lumbar spine. In *An introduction to orthopaedic nursing* (2nd ed.). Pitman, NJ: National Association of Orthopaedic Nurses, pp. 83–95.

43. Stephenson, S. (1996). Arthritis and degenerative conditions. In V. R. Masear (Ed.), *Primary care orthopaedics*. Philadelphia: W. B. Saunders, pp. 329–336.

44. U.S. Department of Health and Human Services, Public Health Service. (1991). *Healthy People 2000: National health promotion and disease prevention objectives*. Washington, DC: U.S. Government Printing Office.

45. What's new in drugs: Experts recommend acetaminophen for osteoarthritis (1996). *RN, 59*(3), 70.

46. Whittington, C. F. (1998). Exercise- and sport-related disorders. In A. B. Maher, S. W. Salmond, & T. A. Pellino (Eds.), *Orthopaedic nursing* (2nd ed.). Philadelphia: W. B. Saunders, pp. 746–768.

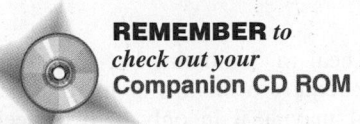

CHAPTER 27

Management of Clients with Musculoskeletal Trauma or Overuse

Dottie Roberts

NURSING OUTCOMES CLASSIFICATION
for Nursing Diagnoses—Clients with Musculoskeletal Trauma or Overuse

Impaired Physical Mobility	Medication Response	**Risk for Peripheral Neurovascular**
Ambulation: Walking	Mobility Level	**Dysfunction**
Joint Movement: Active	Self-Care: Nonparenteral Medication	Joint Movement: Active
Mobility Level	**Risk for Impaired Skin Integrity**	Mobility Level
Pain	Immobility Consequences: Physiological	Tissue Perfusion: Peripheral
Comfort Level	Tissue Integrity: Skin and Mucous	**Self-Care Deficit**
Pain Control	Membranes	Self-Care: Activities of Daily Living (ADL)
Pain: Disruptive Effects	**Risk for Infection**	Self-Care: Bathing
Risk of Constipation	Tissue Integrity: Skin and Mucous	Self-Care: Dressing
Bowel Elimination	Membranes	Self-Care: Grooming
Hydration	Treatment Behavior: Illness or Injury	Self-Care: Hygiene
Knowledge: Medication		

Anyone who has experienced a broken bone or a ligament strain can appreciate the challenges facing a client who is recovering from musculoskeletal trauma or overuse. Activity restrictions and assistive devices both complicate and facilitate the healing process. Types of fractures and their medical and nursing management as well as common soft tissue injuries are discussed in this chapter.

FRACTURES

More than 58 million Americans experience injury from accidents each year. Trauma is the leading cause of death among people aged 1 to 37 years; motor vehicle accidents and falls are the most common causes of accidental death.[31] Because 4 million injured people are treated in hospitals each year, trauma also adds over $200 billion to the cost of health care in the United States.[36] Fractures account for a high percentage of traumatic injuries. Fractures occur in all age groups, but their incidence peaks in both males and females between the ages of 6 and 16 and in elderly people. Fractures can create significant changes in a person's quality of life by causing activity restrictions, disability, and economic loss.

A fracture is any disruption in the normal continuity of a bone. When fracture occurs, surrounding soft tissue is often damaged as well. A radiograph (x-ray) may confirm the bone injury, but it does not show evidence of the torn muscles or ligaments, severed nerves, or ruptured blood vessels that can complicate the client's recovery. To care appropriately for the client with a fracture, the nurse needs a concise and accurate description of the injury.

Etiology and Risk Factors

Fracture results from mechanical overload of the bone, when more stress is placed on the bone than it can absorb. The actual amount of force necessary to cause a fracture may vary greatly, depending in part on the characteristics of the bone itself. A client with a metabolic bone disease such as osteoporosis, for example, may experience fracture with even minor trauma because the bone is weakened by the pre-existing disorder. Fracture may result from direct force, as when a moving object strikes the body area over the bone. Force may also be applied indirectly, as when a powerful muscle contraction pulls against the bone. In addition, stress or fatigue can lead to fracture because of the bone's decreased ability to withstand mechanical force.

The two types of bone also respond differently to mechanical load. *Cortical* bone, the compact outer layer, is porous and can tolerate more stress along its axis (longitudinally) than across the bone. *Cancellous,* or *spongy,* bone is the dense inner bone material. It contains web-like formations and spaces filled with red marrow that make it better able to absorb force than is cortical bone. Bony projections, called trabeculae, separate the spaces and are arranged along lines of stress, making cancellous bone even stronger.

Predisposition to fracture results from biologic conditions such as osteopenia (caused by steroid use or Cushing's syndrome) or osteogenesis imperfecta, which alters the strength and composition of the bone. Neoplasms can also increase the risk for fracture. Postmenopausal estrogen loss and protein malnutrition lead to decreased bone mass. For persons with healthy bones, fractures can result from high-risk recreation or employment-related activities (e.g., skateboarding, rock climbing). Victims of domestic violence are also among people treated for traumatic injuries.

Pathophysiology

When fracture occurs, muscles that were attached to the ends of the bone are disrupted. The muscles can undergo spasm and pull the fracture fragments out of position. Large muscle groups can create massive spasms that displace even large bones, such as the femur. Although the proximal portion of the fractured bone remains in place, the distal portion can become displaced in response to both the causative force and the spasm in the associated muscles. Fracture fragments may be displaced sideways, at an angle (angulated), or as overriding bone segments. They may also be rotated or offset.

In addition, the periosteum and blood vessels in the cortex and marrow of the fractured bone are disrupted. Soft tissue damage frequently occurs. Bleeding occurs from both the soft tissue and from the damaged ends of the bone. In the medullary canal, a hematoma forms between the fracture fragments and beneath the periosteum. Bone tissue surrounding the fracture site dies, creating an intense inflammatory response. Vasodilation, edema, pain, loss of function, exudation of plasma and leukocytes, and infiltration of other white blood cells result. These processes serve as the initial step in bone healing.

BONE HEALING

Unlike other specialized body tissues, bone healing occurs uniquely through tissue regeneration rather than scar tissue formation. Fracture repair occurs by the same mechanism as bone formation during normal growth and maintenance, with organized mineralization of newly synthesized bone matrix followed by remodeling to form mature bone. Adequate circulation to the fracture site and adequate fragment immobilization are crucial for effective bone healing. Factors such as the presence of systemic or bone diseases, the age and general health of the client, the type of fracture, and the treatment can also affect the speed and success of healing. For example, an impacted fracture may heal within several weeks but a displaced fracture may take months or even years to heal. A radial

or ulnar fracture may heal in 3 months, but fractures in the tibia or femur may require 6 months or more to heal. A fracture in an infant may heal in only 4 to 6 weeks, but the same fracture in an adolescent may require 6 to 10 weeks to heal. The rate of fracture healing is not significantly decreased in older adults unless the client also has a metabolic disorder such as osteoporosis.

Fracture healing occurs in five stages (Table 27–1). These stages do not occur independently but tend to overlap as bone healing progresses. They are sometimes combined into a three-stage process.

FACTORS AFFECTING BONE HEALING

If fracture healing is altered in any of the five stages, problems with bone union can result. Factors affecting bone healing are summarized in Box 27–1.

Most fractures heal adequately without any problems, but biologic interventions may be employed to stimulate fracture healing. For example, autogenous or allogeneic bone grafts can be used to stimulate bone growth. Injection or implantation of autogenous bone marrow is another intervention that is the subject of current research in fracture healing. A three-dimensional implant or graft can also be used as an aid to bone healing by supporting the attachment, spreading, division, and differentiation of bone cells. Osteoinduction involves the use of substances such as platelet-derived growth factor to stimulate bone healing.

Clinical Manifestations

Fracture diagnosis is based on the client's clinical manifestations and history, physical examination, and radiographic findings. Some fractures are immediately obvious; others are detected only on x-ray. Use of the correct radiologic view is essential for adequate evaluation of the suspected fracture. Two views (e.g., anteroposterior and lateral) taken at right angles are generally considered to be the minimal number needed for evaluation, and they should include the joints above and below the suspected fracture to identify additional dislocations or subluxations. Abnormal x-ray findings include soft tissue edema or displacement of air in relation to a shift of the bone after injury. Radiographs of the fractured bone show an alteration in its normal contour and a disruption of the normal joint relationship. The fracture line itself demonstrates increased radiolucency (Fig. 27–1). Radiographs are commonly taken before fracture reduction, after reduction, and then periodically during bone healing.

Physical assessment may reveal any of the following clinical manifestations:

Deformity. Swelling from local hemorrhage may cause deformity at the fracture site. Muscle spasms can cause limb shortening, a rotational deformity, or angulation. In comparison to the uninjured side, the fracture site may also have altered curves.

Swelling. Edema may appear quickly as a result of localization of serous fluid at the fracture site and extravasation of blood into surrounding tissues.

Bruising (ecchymosis). Bruising results from subcutaneous bleeding at the fracture site.

Muscle spasm. Frequently accompanying fractures, involuntary muscle spasm actually serves as a natural splint to decrease further motion of fracture fragments.

TABLE 27–1	STAGES OF BONE HEALING		
Stage	**Diagram**	**Description**	**Time**
Stage I: Hematoma stage or inflammatory stage		Immediate formation of a hematoma at the site of the fracture. The amount of damage to the bone, as well as to surrounding soft tissue and blood vessels, determines the size of the hematoma. The blood forms a clot among the fracture fragments, providing a small amount of stabilization. Necrosis of adjacent bone occurs in direct relation to the loss of blood supply to the affected region and will extend to the area where collateral circulation begins. Vascular dilatation occurs in response to the accumulation of dead cells and debris at the fracture site, and exudation of fibrin-rich plasma initiates the migration of phagocytic cells to the area of injury. If the vascular supply to the fracture site is inadequate, stage I healing will be greatly impaired.	1–3 days
Stage II: Fibrocartilage formation		Fibroblasts, osteoblasts, and chondroblasts migrate to the fracture site as a result of the acute inflammation and form fibrocartilage. Organization of the hematoma then offers the foundation for stage II bone and tissue healing. Osteoblastic activity is stimulated by periosteal trauma, and bone formation occurs quickly. The periosteum is elevated away from the bone, and within a few days, the combination of periosteal elevation and granulation tissue formation creates a collar around the end of each fracture fragment. As the collars advance, they form a bridge across the fracture site. This early formation of fibrous tissue is sometimes called the *primary callus,* and it results in gradually increasing stability for the fracture.	3 days to 2 weeks
Stage III: Callus formation		Granulation tissue matures into a provisional callus (procallus) as newly formed cartilage and bone matrix disperse through the primary callus. The procallus is large and loosely woven. It is generally wider than the normal diameter of the injured bone. The procallus secures the bone fragments, extending some distance beyond the fracture site to serve as a temporary splint, but it does not provide strength. If cells are distant from the blood supply and oxygen tensions are relatively low, cartilage is formed. When calcium is deposited in the collagen network of the granulation tissue, fibrous bone forms. Proper bone alignment is essential during stage III. This stage may be the most important in determining successful healing, and if it is slowed or interrupted, the final two stages cannot occur. Delayed union or non-union can then result.	2–6 weeks
Stage IV: Ossification		A permanent callus of rigid bone crosses the fracture gap between the periosteum and the cortex to join the fragments. In addition, medullary callus formation occurs internally to establish continuity between the marrow cavities. Trabecular bone gradually replaces the callus along stress lines. Bone union, which can be confirmed by x-ray, is said to have occurred when there is no motion with gentle stress and no tenderness with direct pressure at the fracture site. Weight-bearing in lower extremity fractures is also pain free after bone union.	3 weeks to 6 months

Table continued on following page

TABLE 27–1	STAGES OF BONE HEALING *Continued*		
Stage	**Diagram**	**Description**	**Time**
Stage V: Consolidation and remodeling		Unnecessary callus is resorbed or chiseled away from the healing bone. The process of bone resorption and deposition along stress lines allows bone to withstand the loads applied to it. The actual amount and timing of remodeling depends on the stresses imposed on the bone by muscles, weight-bearing, and age.	6 weeks to 1 year

Pain. If the client is neurologically intact, pain always accompanies fracture; the intensity and severity of the pain differ from client to client. Pain is usually continuous, increasing in severity until the fracture is immobilized. It results from muscle spasm, overriding of fracture fragments, or damage to adjacent structures.

Tenderness. Tenderness over the fracture site is caused by underlying injuries.

Loss of function. Any loss of function results either from pain caused by the fracture or from loss of the lever-arm function in the affected extremity. Paralysis may be caused by nerve damage.

Abnormal mobility and crepitus. These manifestations are caused by motion in the middle of a bone or by fracture fragments rubbing together to create grating sensations or sounds.

Neurovascular changes. Neurovascular injury results from damage to peripheral nerves or to the associated vascular structures. The client may complain of numbness.

Shock. The client who experiences blood loss or other injuries may need treatment for shock.

FRACTURE CLASSIFICATION

More than 150 types of fractures have been identified according to various classification methods. See Table 27–2 for common descriptors.

The simplest classification method is based on whether the fracture is *closed* or *open* to the environment. A closed fracture has intact skin over the site of injury, whereas the open fracture is characterized by a break in the skin over the bone injury. Tissue damage can be extensive with open fractures, which are graded according to their severity:

Grade I. The wound is smaller than 1 cm; contamination is minimal.

Grade II. The wound is larger than 1 cm; contamination is moderate.

Grade III. The wound exceeds 6 to 8 cm; there is extensive damage to soft tissue, nerve, and tendon; and there is a high degree of contamination.

Because the wound communicates with the external environment, the risk of infection must be promptly recognized and addressed.

Outcome Management

Medical Management

The goals of medical management include prompt and thorough assessment of the client to discover all injuries, reduction and stabilization of the fracture with immobilization, monitoring for complications, and eventual remobilization and rehabilitation.

THOROUGH INITIAL ASSESSMENT

Basic principles of trauma care must be followed during emergency management of fractures. Assessment and treatment are performed simultaneously as the rescuer addresses the general condition of the injured client. During primary assessment, the rescuer focuses on airway man-

---

BOX 27–1 Factors Affecting Bone Healing

Favorable

Location

- Good blood supply at bone ends
- Flat bones

Minimal damage to soft tissue
Anatomic reduction possible
Effective immobilization
Weight-bearing on long bones

Unfavorable

Fragments widely separated
Fragments distracted by traction
Severely comminuted fracture
Severe damage to soft tissue
Bone loss from injury or surgical excision
Motion/rotation at fracture site as a result of inadequate fixation
Infection
Impaired blood supply to one or more bone fragments
Location

- Decreased blood supply
- Midshaft

Health behaviors such as smoking, alcohol use

FIGURE 27-1 Fracture of the supracondylar femur. (Note radiolucency of fracture line.) Reduction of the fracture with traction. The fracture was eventually pinned.

agement, bleeding, and manifestations of shock. Any potentially life-threatening injuries must be stabilized immediately and emergency assistance summoned to transport the client to a medical facility for additional intervention. An injured client should not be moved unless the current location is not safe.

Because most fractures do not pose a serious threat to life, their management becomes a secondary priority in trauma care. Suspected injuries to extremities should be carefully splinted and moved as little as possible because multiple fractures frequently occur in the same limb. If the client complains of muscle spasm after a cervical spine or head injury, a fracture or dislocation is presumed to be present until radiographs can be performed and interpreted. The rescuer must stabilize the affected area and help the client remain still. An unconscious client should receive emergency management while the rescuer carefully notes any spontaneous movement as well as the client's position, head, and extremities. The rescuer performs a neurologic assessment that is based on the type of known or suspected injury. Any soft tissue damage must also be assessed because the injury may indicate a fracture site. Open fractures should be covered with sterile dressings and remain covered to prevent additional contamination until a thorough examination can occur in the nearest hospital.

When the client reaches the emergency department, the neurologic condition and vital signs are closely monitored, and the client is kept on *nil per os* (nothing by mouth; NPO) status in case surgery is indicated. Health care providers carefully examine the injured area and obtain the client's history. Details of the injury are very helpful in determining the probable type of fracture as well as associated injuries. If the client was in a motor vehicle accident, for example, was he or she sitting in the back or front seat? Was the client wearing a seat belt? What was the angle of impact? Was the client pulled from the car after a major collision? Or did the injury occur as a result of a fall on a hip or an outstretched arm?

Arterial damage is a possible early complication after fracture. The arteries may have been contused or lacerated, or they may have been constricted by tightly applied bandages or casts. With a displaced fracture, a hematoma may develop in the soft tissue as a result of damage to large blood vessels. Other indications of arterial damage include a variable pulse or absence of a pulse, poor capillary return, swelling, pallor or patchy cyanosis distal to the injury, pain, paresthesias, or coolness of an extremity as a result of poorly filled veins. Blood loss may be considerable, particularly with femur or pelvic fractures, and hypovolemic shock may become another complica-

Text continued on page 596

TABLE 27–2	COMMON TYPES OF FRACTURES	
Name by Fracture	**Description**	**Illustration**
APPEARANCE		
Burst	Characterized by multiple pieces of bone; often occurs at bone ends or in vertebrae	
Comminuted	More than one fracture line; more than two bone fragments; fragments may be splintered or crushed	
Complete	Break across the entire section of bone, dividing it into distinct fragments; frequently displaced	

TABLE 27-2	COMMON TYPES OF FRACTURES *Continued*	
Name by Fracture	**Description**	**Illustration**
Displaced	Fragments out of normal position at fracture site	
Incomplete	Fracture occurs through only one cortex of the bone; usually nondisplaced	
Linear	Fracture line is intact; fracture is caused by minor to moderate force applied directly to the bone	

TABLE 27-2	COMMON TYPES OF FRACTURES *Continued*	
Name by Fracture	**Description**	**Illustration**
Longitudinal	Fracture line extends in the direction of the bone's longitudinal axis	
Nondisplaced	Fragments aligned at fracture site	
Oblique	Fracture line occurs at approximately 45-degree angle across the longitudinal axis of bone	
Spiral	Fracture line results from twisting force; forms a spiral encircling the bone	

TABLE 27-2	COMMON TYPES OF FRACTURES *Continued*	
Name by Fracture	**Description**	**Illustration**
Stellate	Fracture lines radiate from one central point	
Transverse	Fracture line occurs at 90-degree angle to longitudinal axis of bone	

GENERAL DESCRIPTION

Avulsion	Bone fragments are torn away from body of the bone at site of attachment of a ligament or tendon	
Compression	Bone buckles and eventually cracks as the result of unusual loading force applied to its longitudinal axis	

TABLE 27-2	COMMON TYPES OF FRACTURES *Continued*	
Name by Fracture	**Description**	**Illustration**
Greenstick	Incomplete fracture in which one side of the cortex is broken and the other side is flexed but intact	
Impacted	Telescoped fracture, with one fragment driven into another	
ANATOMIC LOCATION		
Colles'	Fracture within the last inch of the distal radius; distal fragment is displaced in a position of dorsal and medial deviation	
Pott's	Fracture of the distal fibula, seriously disrupting the tibiofibular articulation; a piece of the medial malleolus may be chipped off as a result of rupture of the internal lateral ligament	

tion. Extensive bleeding can occur even with closed fractures, and emergency surgery may become necessary; loss of blood supply to the fracture can result in areas of bone necrosis. Soft tissue infection can easily follow open fracture, and for optimal effectiveness, antibiotic therapy should begin as soon as possible after the injury.

REDUCING FRACTURES

The first step in management of a displaced fracture is reduction: the manipulation of the fracture to restore alignment, position, and length by bringing the fragments into close approximation. Reduction, which is also called *bone setting,* alleviates compression or stretching of

nerves and blood vessels. Because reduction is generally painful, sedation or local or general anesthesia may be needed.

Not all fractures require reduction. Fragments of a nondisplaced fracture, for example, are already in proper alignment. Splinting or casting allows the alignment to be maintained as the fracture heals. A few other fractures cannot be adequately splinted and instead are treated simply by resting the affected area until healing occurs (e.g., distal phalangeal fractures).

When a fracture of an extremity divides a bone into two fragments, the fragments are referred to as *proximal* (nearer the trunk) and *distal* (farther from the trunk).

FIGURE 27-2 Closed reduction to realign a supracondylar fracture.

Because of its muscle attachment and location, the proximal fragment cannot be manipulated or moved when the fractured bone is being set. Instead, the distal fragment is moved to realign it with the proximal bone segment. Reduction methods can be used alone or in combination.

Closed Reduction

To perform closed reduction, a health care provider applies manual traction to move the fracture fragments and restore bone alignment (Fig. 27-2). Closed reduction should be performed as soon as possible after injury to decrease the client's risk for loss of function, to prevent or delay joint degeneration (traumatic arthritis), and to minimize the possible deforming effects of the injury.

Manual reduction is accomplished through four maneuvers, beginning with a longitudinal pull on the distal end of the fracture or extremity. Because it reverses the mechanism of injury, this pull overcomes any initial muscle spasm, any effects on limb length, and the overriding of bone fragments. Second, the bone ends of the fracture must be disengaged from each other. This is sometimes accomplished by rotating the distal portion of the fracture. In the third maneuver, the fracture fragments are realigned. This is a complex step because forces from various muscle groups have held the fragments in their new positions. Finally, the distraction force is released while alignment is maintained.

Because gravity, weight-bearing, and muscle contraction can again move the fragments, an immobilization device must be applied after x-ray studies have confirmed bone alignment. The immobilizer most commonly used after closed reduction is a cast, a temporary device made of plaster of Paris (anhydrous calcium sulfate) or synthetic materials such as fiberglass or thermoplastic polymer. Casts are used for several purposes in addition to immobilization: prevention or correction of deformity; maintenance, support, and protection of realigned bone; and promotion of healing in order to allow early weight-bearing for ambulation. Casts may be applied in a hospital emergency department, in the operating room, or at the client's bedside in the hospital. They are also commonly applied in a physician's office or clinic.

Synthetic materials are used to construct a strong, light-weight cast that sets in about 5 minutes. They also come in a variety of colors and patterns that can enhance self-esteem in both young and older clients after injury. Synthetic casts maintain their shape and firmness even if they become wet, but they must be dried thoroughly to prevent skin maceration. If there is no incision under the cast, synthetic materials can be dried with a hair blow dryer on a low setting; however, several hours are needed for the cast to dry thoroughly.

Plaster of Paris bandages are individual rolls of precut crinoline impregnated with plaster. They come in various sizes, and the body part to be casted determines the amount of plaster to be used. Plaster casts take at least 24 hours longer than synthetic casts to dry, and they lose their shape if they are allowed to get wet again.

Open Reduction and Internal Fixation

To perform open reduction, the surgeon makes an incision and realigns the fracture fragments under direct visualization. Open reduction is the treatment of choice for compound fractures that are comminuted or accompanied by severe neurovascular injury; it is also required if fracture fragments are widely separated or if soft tissue is interposed between pieces of bone.

Open reduction is usually performed in combination with internal fixation for femoral and joint fractures. Screws, plates, pins, wires, or nails may be used to maintain alignment of the fracture fragments (Fig. 27-3). Rods may also be placed through the fragments or fixed to the side of the bone, or they may be inserted directly

FIGURE 27-3 Examples of different types of internal fixation devices. *A,* Tension band wiring with Kirschner wires for a fracture of the phalanx. *B,* Compression plate and screws in the lateral aspect of the femur. *C,* Sliding hip screw. *D,* Intramedullary nail fixed to both the proximal and distal ends of the femur.

into the bone's medullary cavity. Internal fixation provides essential immobilization and helps prevent deformity, but it is not a substitute for bone healing. If proper healing fails to occur, the internal fixation device may actually loosen or break as a result of stress.

External Fixation

Depending on the client's condition and the physician's judgment, external fixation devices may be used for fracture fragment immobilization (Fig. 27–4). If, for example, soft tissue damage precludes the use of a cast, external fixation would be indicated for fracture immobilization. External fixation devices maintain position for unstable fractures and for weakened muscles, and they support areas with tissue or bone infection. They allow the client to use contiguous joints while the affected area remains immobilized. External fixation may also be indicated for bony non-union if fracture healing has not been successful after a certain time. Common sites for external fixation include the face and jaw, extremities, pelvis, ribs, fingers, and toes. Pins used in external fixation vary in number, length, and thickness on the basis of the treatment area.

Client selection is critical to the successful use of external fixation. Any potential problems with compliance should be thoroughly discussed with the client and family, including the effects of external fixation on the client's lifestyle. Noncompliance with the medical regimen can lead to pin loosening, loss of fracture stabilization, and infection. Specific activity orders are written after application of an external fixator, with special attention to weight-bearing status when the pelvis or a lower extremity is involved.

Traction

Traction has been used to treat fractures since prehistoric times, and its principles were well known to Hippocrates. Traction is the application of a pulling force to an injured body part or extremity while a countertraction pulls in the opposite direction. The pulling force can be achieved through the use of hands (manual traction) or, more commonly, the application of weights. The purposes of traction are shown in Box 27–2. With improved surgical technique and the development of femoral prostheses and intramedullary rods, traction is not as prevalent as it once was in the treatment of orthopedic injuries. Lower extremity traction, such as Buck or Russell traction, currently has limited application in the preoperative management of a client with a fractured hip, for example. However, skeletal traction continues to be an option for multiple trauma clients who are not immediate candidates for open reduction and internal fixation of orthopedic injuries. Various types of traction may also be treatment options before and after surgical reduction of injuries such as cervical fractures, and for chronic conditions such as low back pain.

Skin traction involves the application of a pulling force directly to the skin through the use of skin strips, boots, or foam splints. Cervical halters and pelvic belts allow traction to be applied to the neck or pelvis. Skin traction bears a low longitudinal force load (5 to 7 pounds), which gives it minimal effectiveness. Because of the risk of skin breakdown, this type of traction should be used only temporarily.

Skeletal traction uses pins to apply force to the bone. With skeletal traction, a direct force can be applied after the physician aseptically inserts stainless steel pins through the bone itself. The most common sites for pin insertion are the distal femur, the proximal tibia, and the proximal ulna. Skeletal traction can be tolerated for longer periods than can skin traction. Weights may reach 15 pounds, although 7 to 10 pounds are more commonly used.

In addition to the mode of application, traction can be categorized as *static* (continuous) or *dynamic* (intermittent). Suspension may also be running or straight (exerting a direct pull on the affected part) or balanced (exerting a pull on the affected part and also supporting the extremity in a splint). Table 27–3 describes major types of traction.

Major disadvantages include the potential need for pro-

FIGURE 27–4 External fixation to provide immobilization of a tibial fracture. (From Stryker Howmedica Osteonics.)

A

B

BOX 27–2   Purposes of Traction

- Reduce, realign, and promote healing of fractured bones
- Decrease muscle spasms that may accompany fractures or follow surgical reduction
- Prevent soft tissue damage through immobilization
- Treat deformities
- Rest an inflamed, diseased, or painful joint
- Reduce an treat dislocations and subluxations
- Prevent the development of contractures
- Reduce muscle spasms associated with low back pain or cervical whiplash
- Expand a joint space during arthroscopy or prior to major joint reconstruction

From Ceccio, C. M. (1999). Key concepts in the care of patients in traction. In *An introduction to orthopaedic nursing* (2nd ed.). Pitman, NJ: National Association of Orthopaedic Nurses.

longed bed rest and the resulting effects of extended immobility. Long-term hospitalization is not always indicated if the client in traction can qualify for home care nursing services or, depending on the type of traction, receive additional treatment as an outpatient.

COMPLICATIONS AFTER FRACTURE

Continuously assess the client with orthopedic trauma for potential complications and then intervene quickly to minimize effects. Certain client characteristics increase the likelihood of complications, particularly after surgical repair of fractures. These include age, the presence of other health problems (co-morbidities), and the client's use of medications that affect bleeding, such as warfarin, corticosteroids, and nonsteroidal anti-inflammatory drugs (NSAIDs).

Nerve Injury

Bone fragments and tissue edema associated with the injury can cause nerve damage. Be alert for pallor and coolness of the client's affected extremity, paralysis or paresthesia, complaints of increasing pain, or changes in the client's ability to move the extremity.

Compartment Syndrome

Muscle compartments in the upper and lower extremities are enclosed by tough, inelastic fascial tissue that does not expand if the muscle swells (Fig. 27–5). Edema that occurs in response to a fracture can lead to an increase in compartment pressure that reduces capillary blood perfusion. When the local blood supply is unable to meet the tissue's metabolic demands, ischemia begins. Compartment syndrome is a condition of compromised circulation related to progressively increased pressure in a confined space. It is caused by anything that decreases the compartment size, including external compression forces such as a tight cast or internal factors such as bleeding or edema. Continued ischemia results in histamine release by the affected muscles, leading to even greater edema and a further decrease in perfusion. An increase in lactic acid production causes more anaerobic metabolism and a sub-

TABLE 27–3	**MAJOR TYPES OF TRACTION**			
Traction	**Type**	**Common Conditions Treated**		**Duration**
CERVICAL				
Chin halter	Skin	Severe strains or sprains; cervical trauma nerve root compression; torticollis		Intermittent
Skeletal tongs: Gardner-Wells, Crutchfield, Vinke	Skeletal	Fractures or dislocations of cervical or high thoracic vertebrae		Continuous
Halo traction	Skeletal	Fractures or dislocations of cervical or high thoracic vertebrae		Continuous
UPPER EXTREMITY				
Side-arm	Skin or skeletal	Vertical suspension to forearm		Continuous
Overhead/90-90	Skin or skeletal	Vertical traction to humerus; horizontal suspension to forearm		Continuous
Pelvic				
Pelvic belt or sling	Skin	Low back pain		Intermittent or continuous
LOWER EXTREMITY				
Buck	Skin	Hip and knee contracture; preoperative immobilization and muscle spasm relief for hip fractures		Continuous
Balanced suspension: Thomas ring and Pearson and Brady attachment	Skeletal	Used mainly with skeletal pins for supracondylar femur fracture; hip and knee contracture; postoperative positioning and immobilization		Continuous

Adapted from Bryant, G. G. (1998). Modalities for immobilization. In A. B. Maher, S. W. Salmond, & T. A. Pellino (Eds.), *Orthopaedic nursing* (2nd ed.). Philadelphia: W. B. Saunders; and from Ceccio, C. M. (1999). Key concepts in the care of patients in traction. In *An introduction to orthopaedic nursing* (2nd ed.). Pitman, NJ: National Association of Orthopaedic Nurses.

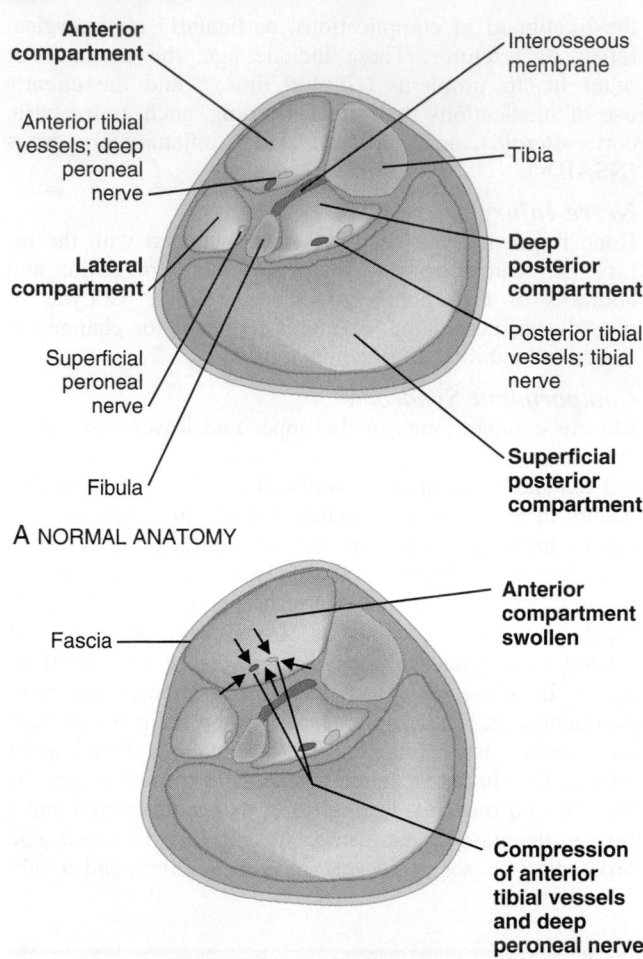

A NORMAL ANATOMY

B ANTERIOR COMPARTMENT SYNDROME

FIGURE 27–5 Compartments of the proximal third of the lower leg. The four compartments are (1) anterior, (2) lateral, (3) deep posterior, and (4) superficial posterior. As the compartment swells, it reaches its maximal size as a result of the inelastic fascia, which covers each compartment. As edema continues, pressure is exerted inward onto the nerves and vessels within the compartment.

sequent increase in blood flow that, in turn, increases the tissue pressure. This leads to a cycle of increasing compartment pressure. Compartment syndrome can occur anywhere in the body but occurs most often in the lower leg and forearm. If it goes unrecognized or untreated, the client can lose nerve and muscle function. Infection, myoglobinuria, and renal failure may follow, and amputation may be necessary.

Intracompartmental pressures can be measured by various monitors currently on the market. Normal compartment pressure is considered to be 0 to 8 mm Hg.[8] Although co-morbid conditions such as shock or compensatory hypertension can affect the client's response, compartment pressures ranging from 30 to 45 mm Hg have historically been considered high enough to cause tissue necrosis if treatment is not initiated. According to more recent medical consensus, imminent surgical intervention is not required for pressures greater than 40 mm Hg if the client's diastolic blood pressure remains high enough to perfuse the muscle compartment.[8]

The primary treatment of compartment syndrome is relief of the source of pressure. To accomplish this, the physician may order a constrictive bandage to be removed or a cast to be bivalved (to be described). The affected extremity should be kept at heart level because elevation above the heart actually decreases local arterial perfusion, further compromising blood flow. Adequate hydration is important for maintaining the client's mean arterial blood pressure. Pain should be managed to decrease the vasoconstrictive effects of the sympathetic nervous system.

If relief of external pressure is not enough to keep compartment pressures from rising, a fasciotomy may be necessary. An incision through the skin into the fascia of the muscle compartment allows for tissue expansion and restores blood flow by relieving pressure on the microcirculation. The incision is typically left open until the swelling decreases; the area is then loosely wrapped and the wrapping is left on for several days. The wound is closed by tertiary intention when edema has subsided.

Volkmann's Contracture
Volkmann's contracture is a limb deformity that results from unrelieved compartment syndrome. As prolonged pressure causes ischemia, muscle is gradually replaced by fibrous tissue that traps tendons and nerves. Tibial fractures have been linked to the development of this condition, which can lead to deformities such as cavus of the foot, equinus, and adduction of the forefoot with varus of the hindfoot. In the upper extremities, Volkmann's contracture most commonly occurs after fractures of the elbow and forearm or after crushing injuries of the forearm, or it is caused by tight bandages or casts. It can lead to a permanently stiff, claw-like deformity of the hand and arm. Contractures may be avoided through prompt recognition of manifestations of compartment syndrome, followed by limb splinting and compartment decompression as indicated.

Fat Embolism Syndrome
Fat embolism syndrome (FES) is a major cause of delayed recovery and mortality after fracture. The mechanical theory of FES origin describes the release of fat globules from the bone marrow into the venous circulation after fracture, particularly fractures of the long bones, pelvis, ribs, sternum, vertebrae, and clavicle. A biochemical or metabolic theory suggests that trauma leads to the release of fatty acids and neutral fats. Platelet aggregation and fat globule formation then occur. In reality, the pathophysiologic process of FES is unknown; it may include parts of both theories or reflect an entirely different, unknown etiology.

The deposit of embolic fat in the pulmonary circulation can lead to the rapid onset of a disorder similar to acute respiratory distress syndrome (ARDS). Perfusion pressure increases, and pulmonary vessels become engorged. As the lung becomes more rigid, the workload of the right side of the heart increases. The fat globules occluding the pulmonary circulation are hydrolyzed into free fatty acids that increase capillary permeability and activate lung surfactant. Hemorrhagic pulmonary edema and patchy alveolar collapse occur, leading to severe hypoxia. Diagnosis of FES is not made on the basis of a single manifestation, laboratory test, or radiologic study.

Instead, the client's presentation must be reviewed system by system.

While subclinical FES occurs in at least 50% of clients with pelvic or long bone fractures, the incidence of overt FES that necessitates intervention is only 1% to 5%.[32] FES varies with the number and type of fractures (open versus closed) and the treatment method. The syndrome occurs more often after closed fracture than after injury treated with external decompression. Clients who undergo open reduction with internal fixation (ORIF) within 24 to 48 hours of injury are at lower risk for FES than clients who are treated nonsurgically.

Prevention of FES begins with prudent treatment of long bone fractures, including careful handling, appropriate splinting, and avoidance of unnecessary manipulation of the injured area. In addition to prompt ORIF after injury, early aggressive resuscitation to prevent hypovolemic shock, adequate pain management, blood transfusion through a 20-μm filter, and prevention of sepsis are also considered standard preventive care.

Should FES occur, supportive treatment is directed at preserving the client's respiratory function. Oxygen is administered; intubation and continuous positive airway pressure (CPAP) are sometimes necessary. Steroids are commonly administered to decrease the inflammatory effects of the fatty acids on the alveolocapillary membrane. Hypotension is treated aggressively.

Deep Vein Thrombosis and Pulmonary Embolism

The client with orthopedic injuries is at high risk for thromboembolic conditions such as deep venous thrombosis (DVT) and pulmonary embolism (PE). DVT results from the formation of a blood clot (thrombus) in a deep vein in the lower extremity. If the thrombus travels into the pulmonary circulation, it is termed a PE.

Prevention of DVT is a primary goal. Clot prophylaxis is recommended through the use of pharmacologic agents such as subcutaneous fixed-dose low-molecular-weight (LMW) heparin or low-intensity oral anticoagulation. For appropriately selected clients, physical-mechanical measures such as intermittent pneumatic compression devices or elastic stockings may also have a role in DVT prevention. DVT is fully discussed in Chapter 53.

Infection

Infection continues to be a cause of morbidity among clients who have open or surgically repaired fractures. Pathogens can contaminate an open fracture or may be introduced at the time of surgery. Contamination during the postoperative period usually results from *Staphylococcus aureus* or *Staphylococcus epidermidis*. Osteomyelitis, a severe infection of the bone itself, can also result (see Chapter 26).

Cast Syndrome

Cast syndrome occurs when the duodenum is compressed between the superior mesenteric artery anteriorly and the aorta and vertebral bodies posteriorly (Fig. 27–6). Cast syndrome can develop weeks or even months after cast application; therefore, constant assessment of the limb is a priority. Because complete gastrointestinal obstruction can develop, immediate nursing intervention is needed. Untreated cast syndrome can be fatal because the obstruction of the superior mesenteric vein can lead to gastrointestinal hemorrhage and necrosis.

LONG-TERM COMPLICATIONS OF FRACTURES

JOINT STIFFNESS OR POST-TRAUMATIC ARTHRITIS. After injury or prolonged immobilization, joint stiffness may occur and can lead to joint contracture or muscle atrophy. Active range-of-motion exercises should be performed to the extent of client tolerance. Also perform passive range-of-motion exercises to decrease the risk for stiffness. The occurrence of post-traumatic arthritis, which can also lead to joint stiffness, is influenced by the severity of the initial injury and the success of bone reduction. Use of acetaminophen or NSAIDs may decrease joint discomfort. Exercise to tolerance may also ameliorate the symptoms of developing arthritis. However, surgical joint replacement may eventually be needed.

AVASCULAR NECROSIS. Avascular necrosis (AVN) of the femoral head occurs primarily in fractures proximal to the femoral neck. It results from local circulatory compromise. An x-ray film demonstrates collapse of the femoral head, and the client complains of pain that occurs months to years after fracture repair. Replacement of the femoral head with a prosthesis is required. The best chance for avoiding the development of AVN is prompt surgical repair after fracture diagnosis.

NONFUNCTIONAL UNION AFTER A FRACTURE. Several types of problems can result in regard to proper bony union.

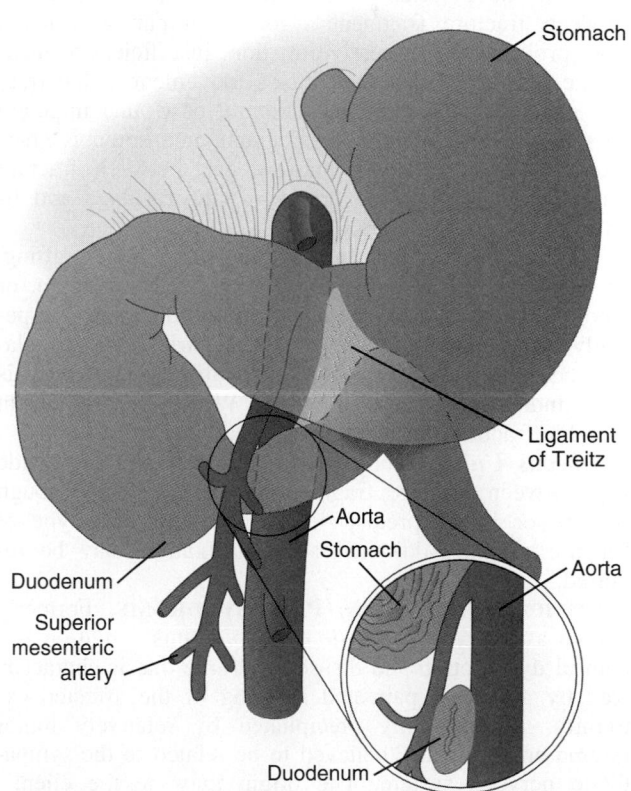

FIGURE 27–6 Cast syndrome results from the compression of the duodenum between the aorta and the superior mesenteric artery. The external compression is usually caused by a tight body cast. (After Cohen, L. B., Field, S. P., & Sachar, D. B. [1985]. The superior mesenteric artery syndrome: The disease that isn't, or is it? *Journal of Clinical Gastroenterology, 7,* 113.)

Malunion. Malunion results when fracture fragments heal in improper alignment as a result of unequal muscle pull and gravity. It can occur if the client bears weight on the affected extremity against medical advice or when an ambulatory device is applied before adequate healing has begun at the fracture site. The primary manifestation is external deformity of the involved extremity. Malunion is diagnosed by radiography. If it is identified early in the course of fracture healing, malunion can be corrected with adjustment of traction or remobilization. Malunion that is diagnosed after healing is complete must be surgically corrected. Prevention is accomplished by adequate fracture reduction and immobilization and by ensuring that the client understands the importance of any activity or position restrictions.

Delayed Union. Suspect delayed union if the client complains of continuation or increase in bone pain and tenderness beyond the healing period expected on the basis of the degree of trauma (3 months to 1 year). Healing is slowed but not completely stopped, possibly as a result of distraction of the fracture fragments or a systemic cause such as infection. If the cause can be identified and corrected early, the fracture usually heals.

Non-union. Non-union is identified when fracture healing has not occurred 4 to 6 months after the initial injury and when spontaneous healing is unlikely to occur. It is generally caused by insufficient blood supply and uncontrolled repetitive stress on the fracture site, possibly as a result of the presence of muscle, tendon, or soft tissue between fracture fragments. Non-union can also result from prolonged or excessive traction; insufficient or inadequate immobilization that allows movement at the fracture site; inadequate internal fixation; or wound infection after internal fixation. On radiograph, non-union is characterized by a relatively narrow gap between fracture fragments. A soft tissue bridge of fibrocartilage and fibrous tissue spans the gap.

Once diagnosed, non-union is treated by bone grafting, internal or external fixation, electric bone stimulation, or a combination of these methods. Client education is especially important before the use of electric bone stimulation because weight-bearing on the affected extremity is contraindicated for 6 to 8 weeks. Weight-bearing on an unstable fracture further prolongs healing time.

Fibrous Union. Fibrous tissue is interposed in a wide gap between fracture fragments. Loss of bone through surgery or injury predisposes the client to this type of fracture union. Additional surgical fixation may be required.

COMPLEX REGIONAL PAIN SYNDROME. Formerly known as *reflex sympathetic dystrophy,* this condition is a painful dysfunction and disuse syndrome that is characterized by abnormal pain and swelling of the affected extremity. It is usually precipitated by relatively minor trauma and generally believed to be related to the sympathetic nervous system. The origin may be the client's pain, fear, or anxiety. Symptoms may include disproportionate pain at the site of injury, edema, muscle spasm or vasospasm, stiffness and decreased joint mobility, increased sweating, atrophy, contractions, and loss of bone mass. Some treatment success has been experienced with sympathetic nerve blocks, especially in early stages of the syndrome. Drug therapies typically involve use of analgesics, muscle relaxants, and antidepressants. Physical therapy and transcutaneous electric nerve stimulation (TENS) may also be ordered. Psychological counseling is often suggested for the client living with this chronic condition.

■ **Nursing Management of the Medical Client**

CARE OF THE CLIENT IN A CAST

Closed reduction of fractures is followed by immobilization to relieve pain and to prevent rotation and shearing at the fracture site. Immobilization is most often accomplished through the use of a cast or splint (Fig. 27–7). Before application of a cast, the nurse's role may entail preparation of the client for casting, including a detailed explanation of the procedure. Skin preparation involves thorough cleansing and assessment of any lesions. Presence of unremovable dirt or foreign particles should be reported to the physician. After the skin preparation, padding or web-roll is applied to the extremity surrounding the fracture site. Additional padding made be indicated over bony prominences, but too much padding can actually increase pressure. Stockinette is applied over the padding and is cut several inches longer than the expected finished cast length so that excess portions can be pulled over exposed cast ends to protect the client's skin. Make sure that these coverings fit smoothly and without wrinkles, which could produce pressure areas on underlying tissues.

Rolls of casting materials, whether plaster or synthetic, are individually submerged in clean water in a bucket. Excess water is squeezed from the roll, and then the bandage is applied to encircle the injured body part. Assist during cast application by supporting the extremity from underneath, using only the palms of your hands to avoid applying pressure to any one area. Fingertips should not be pressed into the cast, and the cast should not be allowed to rest on a hard or sharp surface; these actions might cause flattening or indentations in the cast, which could create pressure. As soon as the casting procedure is complete, the client's skin must be cleansed of excess casting material. Plaster-laden water should never be emptied into an ordinary sink because the plaster sediment solidifies and plugs the plumbing. If a sink with a plaster trap is not available, wait for sediment to settle to the bottom of the bucket, and then drain off the water from the top. The remaining plaster sediment can be scraped from the bottom of the bucket and placed into the garbage container.

Drying a Cast

As the water from a newly applied cast eventually evaporates, a mature cast of full strength develops. Synthetic casts dry to the touch in a few minutes, but they take about 30 minutes to set completely and allow weight-bearing. Plaster casts set quickly but take hours to days to dry completely; a lower extremity plaster cast may not be totally dry for up to 48 hours, and larger casts can take even longer. Because both plaster and synthetic casts generate heat while drying; the client should be instructed to expect the sensation of heat. The cast should not be covered with a blanket or towel while it is drying because the retained heat can burn the client. Several towels may be placed under the cast on the pillow to absorb dampness. While the cast is still damp, the client may feel cold

Fracture of distal radius

SHORT ARM CAST

Fibular head

Lateral malleolus — Medial malleolus

SHORT LEG
WEIGHT-BEARING CAST

LONG LEG CYLINDER CAST,
WEIGHT BEARING

Fracture site

Weight

HANGING CAST WITH
WEIGHT TO PROVIDE
TRACTION ON
FRACTURE SITE

Fibular head

Lateral malleolus

NON-WEIGHT-BEARING
LONG LEG CAST

Fibular head

Fracture site

Lateral malleolus — Achilles tendon

LONG LEG CAST
FOR UNSTABLE
FRACTURE OF TIBIA

HIP SPICA CAST

FIGURE 27–7 Common types of casts.

and may experience a decrease in body temperature. Adequate covering is provided for the client while dry, warm air is allowed to circulate around the damp cast. To avoid excessive chilling for the client who is in a large cast, sections of the cast should be exposed for brief periods of time alternately. Unless it is contraindicated, the client should also be turned regularly to expose more of the new cast to air. Rapid drying through use of a blow dryer is not advised because it can burn the client's skin under the cast and crack the cast.

A wet plaster cast smells musty and is dull on percus-sion, gray, and cold to the touch. When dry, the plaster cast is odorless, resonant, and white, and it feels close to room temperature when touched. Wet fiberglass casts feel hot and sticky to the touch. A wet fiberglass cast should not be placed over drainage-containing pads, such as incontinence pads, because paper and plaster adhere and the paper will become a permanent part of the cast. Once the cast is completely dry, it can safely be placed on a hard surface (e.g., a casted arm can rest on a table), but the client is usually more comfortable in continuing to rest the casted area on pillows.

Windowing or Bivalving a Cast

Bivalving a cast means cutting the cast along both sides and then splitting it to decrease pressure on underlying tissue. Windows may also be cut into the cast to allow the physician or nurse to visualize wounds under the cast or remove drains. In addition, windows may be cut to allow pulse assessment or to prevent "cast syndrome." Bivalving also allows removal of half of the cast for wound care or x-rays. The remaining half of a bivalved cast is often used as an intermittent splint that can be removed and reapplied as the client adjusts to being without a cast. When reapplying a bivalved cast, take care not to pinch the client's skin between the cast halves. When the cast halves are properly fitted, secure them with an elastic wrap.

Neurovascular Assessment

Although casts are protective and therapeutic, they can also cause serious complications. Careful nursing assessment and prompt intervention are necessary to minimize the client's risk for detrimental effects. Be aware of the client's neurovascular status by assessing the following in a casted extremity:

- Color, warmth, pulses distal to the cast, capillary refill (circulatory function)
- Movement of distal fingers or toes, awareness of light touch distal to the cast, changes in sensation (nerve function)

The deep and superficial peroneal nerves and the tibial nerve are most at risk for injury with lower extremity fractures, whereas radial and ulnar nerve function must be assessed with upper extremity injuries. Encourage the client to report any numbness or tingling, although neither may be present even with nerve compression. Pulse, color, and warmth of the injured extremity should also be assessed by comparison with the unaffected extremity. Neurovascular assessment should be performed every 30 minutes for 4 hours after cast or splint application and then every 3 to 4 hours. Table 27–4 describes the technique used for assessment and expected findings.

Another helpful way to remember significant areas of assessment in the casted client is to use the "6 Ps" mnemonic: *p*ain, *p*allor, *p*aralysis, *p*ulselessness, *p*aresthesia, and *p*oikilothermia (skin cold to the touch).

TABLE 27–4	NEUROVASCULAR ASSESSMENTS	
Parameter Being Assessed	**Technique**	**Expected Finding**
Color of affected extremity	Inspect the color of affected leg, foot, arm, or hand; compare to opposite side	Color should be the same; it is normal to have some paleness (pallor) in injured tissues; if incisions are present, some redness (erythema) may be noted along incision lines
Temperature of affected extremity	Use dorsum (back) of your hand to assess temperature	Temperature should be the same in each extremity; report any coolness or heat in the extremity
Movement of affected extremity	Ask client to "move your toes/fingers"	Movement should be the same on each side; if decreased movement is noted, determine whether extremity normally moves (e.g., if the client has had a stroke, limited movement may have been present before); if client had surgery on toes or fingers, expect decreased movement as a result of pain and edema; look for even slight movement in the area
Sensation of affected extremity	Ask clients if they feel you touching their toes or fingers; ask specifically if they have a "pins and needles" sensation or if the extremity feels as if it is "asleep"	Sensation should be the same on each side; any alterations in sensation should be reported
Capillary refill in nail beds	Compress nail bed and measure time needed for refill (return of color)	Should be 2–4 sec; slowing to 4–6 sec should be reported
Edema	Inspect for edema in both extremities	No edema should be present; if edema is noted in affected extremity, consider whether it is caused by the trauma or surgery or thrombophlebitis; if present in both extremities, consider causes such as heart disease
Pain	Ask clients to rate pain on scale of 0–10, 0 being no pain and 10 being the worst pain they have ever felt	Pain is common in injured extremities; if no pain is reported, client may have recently had pain medication; uncontrollable pain usually signals compartment syndrome and should be reported
Pedal pulses	Palpate for pedal pulses on dorsum of foot	Pedal pulses should be present bilaterally; if absent, may be normal variation; absent pulses could also signal compression of vessels from edema

Assessment of Pain

Careful assessment of pain must be completed regularly, and the client must be encouraged to verbalize the degree of pain. Inadequate analgesic effects should be reported promptly to the surgeon because an increased dosage or change in medication may be indicated. Unrelieved pain is also a classic symptom of compartment syndrome; therefore, any complaint of pain should be given your full attention. Be especially alert to complaints of progressive pain or pain out of proportion to the injury or treatment.

Assessment of the Cast

The skin around the cast edges should be observed for damage or swelling. Also assess the cast itself. "Hot spots"—areas of the cast that feel warmer than other sections—may indicate tissue necrosis or infection under the cast. "Wet spots" may indicate drainage under the cast or a need for additional drying. Stains can indicate wound drainage or bleeding, and any stained areas should be carefully measured and documented. Also be aware of possible pressure points on underlying structures, such as the lateral malleolus under a short leg cast or the epicondyle under a short arm cast. Closely inspect areas of the cast that are known to cover wounds with the understanding that drainage on the surface of synthetic casts may not wick outward but may go to a dependent area determined by cast position (e.g., beneath the cast if it is flat, posterior and superior if the limb is elevated).

An older cast may develop a sour smell because of perspiration or normal sloughing of outer skin layers. Musty, offensive odors under the cast, however, may indicate tissue necrosis or infection. If the odor of mildew is present, the synthetic cast may have not been thoroughly dried after it became wet; notify the physician because the cast needs to be changed.

Assessment for Complications

COMPARTMENT SYNDROME Any client with an extremity fracture should be regularly assessed for compartment syndrome for the first week after injury. Traumatic injury and treatment such as closed reduction usually produces swelling, which progresses for the first 12 to 24 hours after injury. The greatest swelling is likely to be evident in the first 24 to 48 hours. Mild swelling is expected; however, moderate or severe swelling associated with pain or discoloration is abnormal. Excessive swelling constricts the enclosed soft tissues and introduces the risk for compartment syndrome.

The affected extremity should be regularly compared with the uninjured extremity, and current findings should also be compared with baseline assessment data. Manifestations of compartment syndrome can begin as early as 30 minutes after ischemic injury. The primary manifestation is increasing pain or pain that is out of proportion to the injury. Specifically, pain with passive stretching of the muscles in an affected compartment is one of the earliest indicators. Assess for the presence of tingling or paresthesia in the affected extremity; muscle strength and motion; and circulation, including the presence and quality of pulses distal to the injury, capillary refill, skin color, and temperature. Increased tenseness and erythema of the skin also suggest increasing compartment pressures. If the intracompartmental pressure increases to a level above the client's systolic blood pressure, pulses are absent, capil-

lary refill is delayed, and pallor results. Paralysis is a very late sign of compartment syndrome. If compartment syndrome goes unrecognized and tissue pressures are not relieved, muscle damage becomes irreversible after 4 to 6 hours of ischemia; nerve damage becomes irreversible after 12 to 24 hours.[8] The physician must be notified immediately of assessment findings that suggest the development of compartment syndrome (see Critical Monitoring: The Client in a Cast).

FAT EMBOLI. Be alert to manifestations of hypoxemia, such as apprehension, anxiety, agitation, or acute confusion. The client with FES also exhibits fever (>103° F), dyspnea, tachypnea, and tachycardia. Diffuse rales and rhonchi may occur as late signs of FES. In 50% to 60% of clients, petechiae are noted on the chest, axillae, flanks, abdomen, clavicular fossae, and soft palate.[34]

INFECTION. The client may describe new pain or an increased level of pain and feelings of increased warmth under a bandage or cast. Your assessment may reveal fever or chills, an odor from the area of injury, erythema and warmth around the wound, purulent drainage, and poor wound healing.

DEEP VENOUS THROMBOSIS. The typical manifestations of DVT are unilateral edema, at or below the site of thrombosis, that results from venous inflammation or obstruction. Affected clients often complain of pain and tenderness at the site, which may also be red and warm. Homans' sign (in which dorsiflexion of the foot causes discomfort in the upper calf) is present in less than one third of symptomatic clients with DVT. Because Homans' sign is present in more than 50% of symptomatic clients who do not have DVT, it is not considered specific or sensitive to the condition. Venous ultrasonography is a

---

CRITICAL MONITORING

The Client in a Cast

Compartment Syndrome

- Pulselessness: slow nail bed capillary refill (longer than 3 sec)
- Skin pallor, blanching, cyanosis, or coolness
- Increasing pain, swelling, painful edema peripheral to cast, pain on passive motion
- Paresthesias (tingling, prickling), heightened sensitivity, numbness; hypesthesia (diminished sensitivity to touch); anesthesia (numbness)
- Motor paralysis of previously functioning muscles
- Hypesthesia (diminished sensitivity); anesthesia (numbness); paresthesias (tingling, prickling, heightened sensitivity, numbness)

Infection

- Musty, unpleasant odor over cast and/or at ends of cast
- Drainage through cast or cast opening
- Sudden unexplained body temperature elevation
- "Hot spot" felt on cast over lesion

Cast Syndrome

- Bloated feeling
- Prolonged nausea; repeated vomiting
- Abdominal distention; vague abdominal pain
- Shortness of breath

sensitive, accurate, noninvasive examination that has become the standard for diagnosis of DVT.

PE results if a thromboembolism lodges in the pulmonary circulation, leading to decreased or absent blood flow distal to the clot. Because manifestations of PE can be nonspecific and vary greatly, PE is often undetected or misdiagnosed. The most common clinical manifestations are sudden unexplained dyspnea and pleuritic chest pain. In the event of a massive PE, diagnosis and successful treatment may be extremely difficult because of the extensive loss of gas exchange area and the severe strain placed on the right chambers of the heart by pulmonary hypertension. Although pulmonary angiography is still considered the standard for diagnosis with a 98% sensitivity, the ventilation/perfusion ($\dot{V}/\dot{Q}$) scan is commonly ordered because it has a high sensitivity in ruling out PE. A chest radiograph can also be helpful in ruling out other pulmonary perfusion problems. (DVT is fully discussed in chapter 53, and PE is discussed in chapter 62.)

CAST SYNDROME. If the client is in a body cast, closely attend to any complaints of nausea, abdominal pressure, vague abdominal pain, feelings of bloating or tightness, or inability to take a deep breath. These may be clinical manifestation of cast syndrome, a serious complication that can follow prolonged supine positioning, spinal surgery, or use of a body cast.

Management of suspected cast syndrome includes cutting a window or bivalving the cast to relieve pressure. Nasogastric intubation may be indicated to decompress the intestine, intravenous fluids may be ordered, and the client may be placed on NPO status. Antiemetics should be given sparingly to any client in a body cast because they can mask the manifestations of cast syndrome. The client who is discharged in a body cast should receive careful instruction about the clinical manifestations of cast syndrome and be encouraged to report any complaints promptly to the surgeon.

Interventions for Clients in Casts
To prevent or relieve swelling, the nurse typically elevates the entire casted extremity higher than the client's heart for the first 24 to 48 hours. The affected extremity may be placed on pillows. A casted arm may also be elevated in a sling attached to an intravenous (IV) pole. The entire arm, including the elbow, wrist, and hand, must be supported, and the fingers must be kept higher than the elbow to minimize swelling. Also apply ice bags around the cast, and exercise the client's fingers or toes to encourage circulation. Relieve pressure at the cast edges by petalling the cast or loosely padding an uncomfortable area. To prevent footdrop in a casted leg, splint or support the client's foot with the ankle in 90 degrees of flexion.

For the client in a hip spica or body cast, the buttocks should be exposed to prevent soiling or dampening of clothing during elimination and to provide adequate skin care. To further prevent soiling, incontinence pads can be tucked into the edge of the cast before the client uses a fracture bedpan. Slightly raising the head of the bed facilitates elimination and also prevents excrement from running under the cast; such raising is usually allowed unless the client is in shock, is hemorrhaging, or has a spinal injury. Dampness causes skin irritation and may increase the risk of infection if an open wound is present; there-

fore, thorough perineal care must be completed after elimination.

Position changes at least every 2 hours are needed to help prevent complications of immobility, and a turning schedule is useful for ensuring that the client does not remain in one position too long. Give instructions on turning to encourage client activity, but also provide assistance with bed mobility as needed. When mobility assistance is needed, always have adequate staff help to reposition a casted client. Three or four people may be needed to turn a client in a body or hip spica cast, for example. Roller boards or mechanical lifts may also be useful.

Clients in casts can often bear weight as soon as the cast is dry, depending on the nature of the injury and the physician's orders. Be aware of the client's weight-bearing status when attempting a transfer. For client safety, also use a transfer belt when getting the client out of bed. Weak, elderly, or debilitated clients may find the weight of the cast difficult to deal with and may tire rapidly with initial activity. The client should be instructed about the likelihood of increased pain when a casted leg is lowered to a dependent position with initial attempts at ambulation. Help the client lower the leg, encouraging him or her with regard to the decrease in pain as the leg becomes accustomed to the increased blood flow.

To ensure client cooperation, provide instruction on every aspect of care. Ensure that the client understands the availability of analgesics for treatment of pain and is allowed to voice any concerns about their use, such as fears of addiction. Initiate an honest discussion about any barriers to analgesic use if the client seems hesitant about taking or asking for medication. Administer analgesics as prescribed, and promptly inform the surgeon of inadequate effects. Client instruction should also include alternative methods of pain management, such as distraction, visualization, or massage, that may help the client relax.

CARE OF THE CLIENT IN EXTERNAL FIXATION
ASSESSMENT. The potential for neurovascular deficit or compartment syndrome is high when external fixation is used. The risk is increased because many clients with external fixation have extensive soft tissue injury. Even though the external fixator may be used for treatment of an open fracture, compartment syndrome can nonetheless develop in another compartment of the same extremity. Ongoing assessment of neurovascular status is critical. Current findings should be compared with baseline data, and the affected extremity should be compared with the unaffected extremity. Instruct the client to report any changes, and address any complaints promptly.

As with the client in a cast, careful assessment of pain must be completed regularly. Analgesia should be assessed, and inadequate effects should be reported promptly to the surgeon because an increased dosage or change in medication may be indicated. Unrelieved pain should raise suspicion of compartment syndrome, and any complaint of pain should be given full attention. Be especially alert to complaints of progressive pain or pain out of proportion to the injury or treatment.

Pin sites and wounds must be constantly assessed for signs of infection, and pins should be checked for loosening. A small amount of bleeding immediately after pin insertion is expected and can be controlled with small pressures dressings. However, bleeding that continues for more than 24 hours should be brought to the surgeon's attention. The progress of wound healing must be assessed, and changes must be carefully documented. The movement of adipose tissue at the pin sites may produce fatty drainage that looks a great deal like pus. Be alert to more specific signs of infection such as pin instability, drainage with odor or color, and skin tension or puckering at the insertion site (tenting). If tenting occurs, the surgeon should be notified so that the wound can be extended.

The client's nutritional status greatly affects bone and wound healing; pay attention to the adequacy of food intake as well as the client's ability to eat and swallow. Be aware of complaints of nausea or vomiting. Any abnormal laboratory values should also be assessed as possible evidence of poor nutrition.

INTERVENTIONS. Antibiotics may need to be administered prophylactically for 48 to 72 hours after application of an external fixator. Later, wound care may involve the application of wet-to-dry dressings. Because pin care methods still remain somewhat controversial, follow the surgeon's orders or institutional standards. Loose pins must be reported promptly to the surgeon; they will be removed to prevent osteomyelitis.

The client's sense of balance can be altered by the weight of a fixator frame on the lower extremity. Because the client often also has a prescribed weight-bearing status after application of a lower extremity external fixator, be scrupulous in assessing adherence to any weight-bearing restrictions and correct use of ambulatory aids. If the surgeon determines that the frame itself can be used to moved the affected extremity, the client should be instructed to move the extremity and the external fixator as a unit to avoid stress on the fracture site. The amount of support needed from the nurse is determined by the client's ability to control the extremity during movement.

Nausea or vomiting should be addressed aggressively with an antiemetic agent, as ordered, to decrease the risk for nutritional deficits or aspiration. Dietary supplements may be used, as needed. Client and family education is critical for achieving a successful outcome with use of external fixation. By the time of discharge, the client should have begun to accept the change in body image that accompanies use of external fixation. The client should also understand his or her responsibility for pin and wound care. He or she should be knowledgeable about manifestations of infection and should be aware of the significance of neurovascular or integumentary changes. The client must also receive instruction on use of analgesics and antibiotics as ordered by the surgeon. Instruction should include alternative methods of pain management, such as distraction, visualization, or massage, that may help the client relax.

Before discharge, teach the client how to meet hygiene needs and discuss any resumption of sexual activity. Clothing may need to be modified with snaps or self-fastening (Velcro) closures before discharge to fit over fixators. Advise the client with a pelvic fixator to reduce intake of gas-producing foods, which can lead to abdominal distention. Once the affected bone is healed, the fixator is removed.

CARE OF THE CLIENT IN TRACTION

ASSESSMENT. As with the other modalities for immobilization, the client in traction must be assessed for neu-

rovascular compromise, pain, skin breakdown, nutrition deficit, and signs of infection. Pin tract infection and development of osteomyelitis are risks for the client in skeletal traction. Other complications of immobility such as constipation or respiratory compromise can also occur, especially in older clients and in clients with long-term traction use.

The client's position in bed, along with the traction positioning and alignment, requires constant vigilance. Bedside rounds between shifts may be useful to ensure proper positioning and alignment, especially if the client is active, confused, or noncompliant. Traction ropes and knots must be intact and secure. Ropes should move easily over pulleys and weights, which hang freely at the end or side of the bed. Traction mechanics should be checked at the beginning of each shift and after each application or position change; all clamps on the traction frame must be tight, and ropes should be unfrayed. A photograph or sketch of the correct traction setup may be useful for nursing staff.

INTERVENTIONS. If the client's nutritional status becomes a concern, dietary supplements may be ordered. Small, frequent meals may be indicated for the client in a halo vest to avoid a feeling of excessive fullness. Bent straws and adapted utensils may be indicated for clients who have limitations on head elevation.

To provide client comfort with elimination, provide a fracture bedpan and ensure privacy when the client needs to use it. The client's diet should include ample fluids and fiber if there are no contraindications. Stool softeners are often prescribed and should be administered regularly. Also determine whether the client has regular, effective strategies for previous treatment of constipation; those methods should be used to assist with elimination.

Encourage independence in client activities within the limitations of the traction. The client should be instructed on repositioning techniques, possibly using extended horizontal bars with roller traction to allow movement to a chair at the bedside. Unaffected joints should be exercised regularly through the use of free weights, foam balls, or elastic pull bands. A record book may be used to encourage the client to cross off the exercise session when it is completed.

Immediately after traction removal, the client is often weak and unsteady as a result of muscle atrophy or orthostatic hypotension. The client should be gradually assisted to a sitting position and then to a standing position later as tolerated. Movement of a previously bedridden client to a sitting or standing position may take several days, depending on the effects of previous immobility. Ensure adequate assistance and provide careful physical support when assisting the client with these position changes. An assistive device such as a walker or crutches may be needed for temporary support of weak muscles and stiff joints.

SPECIFIC FRACTURES

HIP FRACTURES

Hip fractures have become one of the leading causes of morbidity and mortality among the older population. The estimated occurrence is as high as 300,00 fractures each year, and more than 90% of those involve adults aged 70 years or older.[21, 44] Epidemiologists predicted a six-fold increase in the number of hip fractures worldwide between 1990 and 2050.[12] Hip fractures also have a significant impact on health care costs; the annual expense of medical and nursing services is estimated to be $7 billion to $10 billion. This amount is predicted to reach $16 billion by the year 2040 and, with 5% inflation, will approximate $240 billion.[27]

The first-year postfracture mortality rate ranges from 12%[44] to 24%.[21] Among the clients who survive the first year, most do not return to their prefracture functional status. Half of the affected persons become partially dependent, often requiring the care of a spouse or adult child as they continue to live in the community. They may remain unable to walk without an assistive device. One third of those with hip fractures require placement in a long-term care facility. In fact, up to 25% of previously independent clients remain in institutions for more than a year after a hip fracture.[6]

Etiology and Risk Factors

Numerous studies have associated low bone mass and increasing age with an increased risk of hip fracture. Women begin to lose bone about 1.5 years before the last menstrual period; the bone loss continues rapidly until about 1.5 years after the last menses. The rate of bone loss then slows, matching the rate of loss in men by age 65 or 70.[32] The development of low bone mass is known to be influenced by genetic factors. For example, women tend to have lower bone mass if their mothers or fathers have experienced vertebral fractures. Additional factors that can lead to the development of low bone mass include (1) low body weight, (2) physical inactivity, (3) low dietary calcium intake, (4) inadequate levels of serum vitamin D, (5) cigarette smoking, and (6) consumption of alcohol.

More than 90% of hip fractures are caused by falling. However, attempts to decrease the risk of falling through controlled trials have generally been ineffective. Some researchers have concluded that it is the dynamic interaction between the client's physical environment and intrinsic risk factors that actually increases the person's vulnerability to fall and injury.

Other factors have been associated with occurrence of falls that lead to hip fractures. These include the client's use of barbiturates or long-acting benzodiazepines, orthostatic hypotension, impaired vision, lower limb dysfunction, and neurologic conditions. Environmental hazards may also contribute to the elderly client's tendency to fall. These include loose carpeting or rugs, slippery floors, poor lighting, a slippery tub or shower, irregular pavement, and loose clothing or footwear.

Pathophysiology

Fractures of the hip are either *intracapsular* (located within the joint capsule) or *extracapsular* (located outside the joint capsule). Fractures are also described on the basis of their location in one of the four anatomic areas of the proximal hip (Fig. 27–8). Femoral neck fractures are more common in frail older persons, especially

women, and are often associated with osteoporosis. They generally result from relatively mild trauma. Intertrochanteric fractures (between the femoral neck and the greater trochanter) and subtrochanteric fractures are more often seen in males and in vigorous older persons; they are likely to be associated with greater traumatic force.

Because blood flow to the hip is an important influence on fracture healing, delayed healing or non-union may occur in areas of the hip where circulation is impaired after injury. Healing of femoral head fractures, for example, is unlikely if AVN develops after local circulatory compromise.

Clinical Manifestations

Hip fracture is often caused by a fall at home that involves only a moderate amount of trauma, such as slipping out of a chair onto the floor. Immediately after the fall, the client is unable to bear weight on the affected leg. Objective findings include a shortened leg and an externally rotated hip. Deformity may also be evident in the lateral hip if the fracture is displaced. Ecchymosis at the hip is most likely to occur with subtrochanteric fractures. Location of pain depends on the specific fracture site (see Fig. 27–7A, C, E, G). A femoral neck fracture, for example, is characterized by groin and hip pain that increases with hip movement. Intertrochanteric fractures are accompanied by severe pain over the greater trochanter of the femur, whereas subtrochanteric fractures typically produce pain over the proximal thigh. Additional tissue trauma such as head or hand lacerations may also be evident.

Diagnosis of hip fracture is based on the client's clinical manifestations, history of trauma, and radiologic findings. The presence of a fracture is often confirmed by anteroposterior radiograph, although in some instances additional studies may be ordered. Computed tomographic (CT) scans, bone scans, fluoroscopy, myelograms, or magnetic resonance imaging (MRI) may be necessary to identify the fracture site.

Outcome Management
Medical Management

For a relatively few clients, nonoperative treatment is the best option following hip fracture. A client who cannot tolerate anesthesia or who was nonambulatory before the fracture may be treated with skeletal traction or spica casting. While the client remains in traction (approximately 8 to 12 weeks), develop a plan of care that will decrease the effects of immobility. For example, excellent skin care must be provided to reduce the risk of pressure ulcer development. Because older clients are at increased risk for skin impairment even before immobilization, a pressure-reducing mattress is essential. Perform careful daily assessment of bony prominences such as the heels, sacrum, scapulae, and vertebrae. In addition, instruct the client about leg exercises that will decrease the probability of thromboembolism; pneumatic compression devices or anticoagulant medications may also be used to lessen the likelihood of clot development. The Care Plan: The Client in Traction presents additional interventions.

Anatomic regions

A Intertrochanteric fracture

B Repair of an intertrochanteric fracture with an endoprosthesis

C Intracapsular fracture

D Repair of an intracapsular fracture with compression screws

E Femoral neck fracture

F Repair of a femoral neck fracture with compression screws

G Subtrochanteric fracture

H Repair of a subtrochanteric fracture with compression screws

FIGURE 27-8 Anatomic regions of the proximal femur and blood supply, and fracture patterns of the hip and surgical repairs.

■ THE CLIENT IN TRACTION

Nursing Diagnosis. Risk for Impaired Skin Integrity related to inability to change position secondary to skeletal traction

Outcomes. Client will retain intact skin, as evidenced by no reddened areas, no abrasions.

Interventions	Rationales
1. Assess pressure points (sacrum, heels, skin under ropes, and bones) every shift	1. These are common pressure points for clients in supine position
2. Provide skin care every shift by lifting client	2. Clients in traction cannot turn
3. Place therapeutic mattress on bed	3. Some mattresses (Geo-Matt) reduce surface pressure (egg-crate mattresses improve comfort only)

Evaluation. Expect the client's skin to remain intact with adequate pressure reduction interventions.

Nursing Diagnosis. Impaired Physical Mobility related to confinement in traction

Outcomes. The client will not experience complications of immobility, as evidenced by maintaining preinjury range of motion (ROM) in noninvolved joints, not developing thrombophlebitis, having a bowel movement every other day, and maintaining clear lung sounds.

Interventions	Rationales
1. Place all joints (except those immediately proximal and distal to fracture) through ROM every shift	1. ROM assists in maintaining muscle tone
2. Assess lung sounds every shift	2. Immobility and use of analgesia may cause hypoventilation and atelectasis
3. Teach client to deep breathe and cough every shift	3. Deep breathing and coughing cause hyperventilation and clear secretions
4. Assess for clinical manifestations of thrombophlebitis: unilateral leg edema or pain; do not rely on Homans' sign as an indicator	4. The presence of Homans' sign is not an accurate indicator of thrombophlebitis; other signs are assessed
5. Monitor bowel movements	5. Constipation is a side effect of narcotic use and immobility
6. Encourage the patient to consume fluids and food containing fiber	6. Fiber and fluids assist in adding bulk and soften stool, making its passage easier
7. Administer laxatives as needed	7. Laxatives irritate or stimulate the colon

Evaluation. After 3 to 5 days of immobility, clients may develop some of these complications. An aggressive prevention program should be effective.

Nursing Diagnosis. Risk for Injury related to traction

Outcomes. The client will sustain no injury while in traction, as evidenced by maintaining effective pulling force and desired vector of force.

Interventions	Rationales
1. Ensure that weights hang freely from pulleys	1. If weights rest on the bed or floor, traction is not effective
2. Ensure that knots in the rope do not catch in the pulleys	2. Traction is not effective when knots catch in pulleys
3. Add and remove weights slowly with physician's order	3. Slow, steady pull reduces muscle spasms
4. Assess skin at pin site daily or bid for signs of infection	4. Infection can develop in pin sites
5. Pin site care per agency policy	5. Reduces risk of infection
6. Adjust the position of the bed per physician's orders	6. Provides countertraction

Evaluation. Expect the client to maintain adequate pulling forces via traction and with adequate nursing assessment and care.

Collaborative Problem. Risk for compartment syndrome and neurovascular compromise

Outcomes. Clinical manifestations of compartment syndrome will be promptly recognized and reported.

Interventions	Rationales
1. Monitor color, warmth, movement, and sensation of extremity distal to traction every shift	1. Clinical manifestations of compartment syndrome include pallor, pulselessness, cool extremities, inability to move, loss of or change in sensation, and pain that is not relieved with usual analgesics.
2. Assess pedal radial pulse every shift	2. Distal pulses indicate peripheral blood flow.
3. Monitor reports of degree of pain and relief by analgesia	3. Pain that is increasing or beyond what is common with the injury may indicate ischemia.

4. Immediately inform physician of changes in skin color, pulses, skin temperature, motion, sensation or an increase in pain

4. Compartment syndrome mandates immediate medical intervention.

Evaluation. Risk of compartment syndrome exists until edema subsides (about 72 hours).

Nursing Diagnosis. Self Care Deficit related to inability to move in environment

Outcomes. The client will participate in self-care activities if possible, given sites of fractures.

Interventions

1. Place necessary equipment and supplies within easy reach
2. Allow client to schedule procedures, such as bath or linen changes
3. Medicate for pain before movement

Rationales

1. Facilitates maximal self-care and independence
2. Provides client some control
3. Movement increases pain and spasm in fracture site

Evaluation. The client should be able to assist with his or her own feeding, bathing, and dressing.

Nursing Diagnosis. Diversional Activity Deficit related to prolonged immobility, inadequate environmental stimulation, or lack of variation

Outcomes. The client will remain mentally and emotionally stable and will demonstrate interest in surroundings.

Interventions

1. Plan varied activities of interest to the person to fill each day, such as reading, writing, listening to the radio, and watching television
2. Be sure a telephone is convenient
3. Sit with, talk with, and touch the client as appropriate
4. Place the client's bed beside a window; keep the door open as possible
5. Provide accurate clock, current calendar and publications, clean eyeglasses and hearing aids, if worn by the client; obtain prism glasses if client is supine
6. Have the radio and television clearly tuned, but do not leave them on continuously if the client cannot control them independently

Rationales

1. Variety is a normal aspect of life
2. Telephone can be used to maintain contact with significant others
3. Provides contact with nurses outside of usual activities (medications, cares)
4. Allows passive interaction with outside
5. Normal aids to orientation; prism glasses may help a person read more easily while lying flat
6. Continuous noise can increase confusion

Evaluation. Problems with diversional activities develop after about 2 weeks, when pain is minimal and client must wait for bones to realign.

■ Surgical Management

Extensive blood loss can occur after hip fracture, particularly in older clients with other medical conditions. Additional deterioration can occur rapidly if the client is left on bed rest; therefore, prompt surgical intervention and early mobilization are keys to successful rehabilitation. The goal of surgical treatment is to achieve a stable reduction and fixation of the fracture segments internally to support early ambulation.

OPEN REDUCTION AND INTERNAL FIXATION
Postoperative treatment goals include:

- Complete union of the fracture (4 to 8 months)
- Prevention of deformity and contractures to the hip, knee, or foot
- Restoration of weight-bearing ambulation with the use of assistive devices if needed
- Relief of pain and fear; prevention of complications
- Maintenance of optimal physiologic function

Fixation may be accomplished through the use of screws, plates, intramedullary pins or implants (see Fig.

27–8B, D, F, H). The term *open reduction* indicates that a surgical incision was made to expose the bone, in contrast to a closed reduction of a fracture (see earlier). *Internal fixation* indicates that instruments were used to hold the bones in alignment during healing. It may be difficult to achieve perfect anatomic reduction and fixation if the client has decreased bone density as a result of osteoporosis. If the fracture is highly comminuted or the head of the femur has been destroyed, use of an endoprosthesis to replace the entire head of the femur may be necessary. For the client who has an accompanying acetabular fracture, total hip arthroplasty may be indicated (see Chapter 26).

■ Nursing Management of the Surgical Client
PREOPERATIVE CARE
Clients who require surgical reduction and fixation of hip fractures most often go directly from the emergency department to the operating room. Delay in repair not only places an elderly client at risk for additional effects of immobility but also increases the likelihood that AVN

will develop as a result of inadequate blood supply to the fracture fragments. Assess routine blood work, and the client's baseline weight preoperatively. A bed scale should be used to minimize client discomfort with this procedure. Do not accept a stated weight from the client or family member, because accurate comparison with postoperative changes will be impossible.

Occasionally, a client may require stabilization of medical conditions before being cleared for surgery. Underlying disorders such as heart failure or malnutrition, for example, must be evaluated and controlled. In such cases, skin traction through use of a Buck's boot is commonly applied to decrease painful muscle spasms surrounding the hip joint.

Routine preoperative assessment is performed (see Chapter 15). For the client who has experienced a hip fracture, preoperative assessment also includes determination of preinjury level of functioning. Data should clearly address usual activities, ability to walk independently, and previous falls. Under the best of circumstances, the preoperative level of functioning is the level that the client can optimistically expect to achieve after surgery. Unfortunately, some loss of function is likely after fracture repair.

One significant factor in successful rehabilitation is the client's previous social functioning. The client who was previously independent and active and who enjoyed multiple social contacts is more likely to experience a full recovery than is the client who had restricted activity before injury.

POSTOPERATIVE ASSESSMENTS

After ORIF, the same basic nursing assessments are required as for any other surgical client (see Chapter 15). Additional assessment includes a comparison of the quality of peripheral pulses in the affected extremity with that in the unaffected extremity. Prompt recognition of abnormal data allows for early intervention for any neurovascular compromise. As the client progresses into rehabilitation, collaborate with physical and occupational therapists in assessing the client's mobility and self-care needs.

Complications seen after hip fracture repair include fat emboli and infection (see section on fractures). Complications specific to or of high incidence in clients with hip fractures are discussed here.

Deep Venous Thrombosis. Prevention of DVT is a primary goal for the client after ORIF of a hip fracture. Clot prophylaxis is recommended through the use of pharmacologic agents such as subcutaneous fixed-dose LMW heparin or low-intensity oral anticoagulation. For appropriately selected clients, physical-mechanical measures such as intermittent pneumatic compression devices or elastic stockings may also have a role in DVT prevention. DVT is discussed more fully in Chapter 53.

Pressure Ulcers. A pressure ulcer is tissue damage that results from unrelieved pressure, usually over a bony prominence. Its development may have begun as the injured client lay on a hard floor at home, on hard surfaces in an ambulance or in the emergency department, on a table for radiographs or surgery, or in the bed after surgery. Pressure ulcer development is compounded because the client is unable to turn independently after injury or surgery; without assistance, the client remains

supine or in a semi-Fowler position for most of the hospitalization.

A turning schedule is essential for eliminating sustained pressure over bony prominences on the head, scapulae, vertebrae, coccyx, and heels. Other areas such as the elbows, ankles, and medial surfaces of the knee may also be affected by pressure that lasts as little as 15 minutes. Bony areas should be cushioned and supported with each position change. Heels should be elevated with calf pillows or foam boots. Prevention of ischemia can also be accomplished through the use of pressure-reduction bed overlays. An "egg-crate" mattress may contribute to client comfort in the bed, but it does not relieve pressure. Specialty mattresses or air beds are the only appropriate alternatives to assist in pressure reduction. The client who is using a specialty bed must still be turned on a regular schedule. Identification of the client's risk for skin impairment can be accomplished through use of an assessment tool such as the Braden Scale, presented in Chapter 49.

Acute Confusion. Confusion is characterized by an abrupt onset of numerous global, transient changes in a client's attention, cognition, psychomotor activity, or sleep-wake cycle or in several of these. The client may appear forgetful, inattentive, disoriented, or fearful. Daytime sleepiness and nighttime insomnia may be noticed. In the hospitalized client, confusion creates concerns about safety and dependence on others for self-care needs. It can greatly affect the emotional status of the client and family. It can also lead to prolonged hospitalization, possibly contributing to placement in a long-term care facility and definitely increasing costs. Some degree of confusion has been identified in up to 60% of hospitalized older clients.[29] The incidence of confusion after hip surgery may be as high as 42%.[29] Most affected clients have no history of confusion or mental impairment.

Consistent predictors of or risk factors for acute confusion have been difficult to identify clearly. The risk for development of confusion may in fact be a cumulative function of the client's biopsychosocial integrity, the level of illness and functional impairment, and the timing and magnitude of added stressors. Known contributors to confusion may be an unfamiliar environment; sensory overstimulation or deprivation; the client's loss of control and uncertain future; a disrupted routine, immobility and pain; and a disrupted elimination pattern. Because use of medications with anticholinergic effects has also been linked to client confusion, carefully monitor all medications.

Careful assessment of the client's attention, memory, orientation, psychomotor behavior, and sleep-wake cycle is needed. The risk for confusion may also be decreased by maintaining appropriate hydration, perfusion, and oxygenation in the client. Attention must be paid to managing pain, meeting nutritional requirements, and correcting metabolic imbalances. The client must have easy access to glasses, hearing aids, and other functional devices. Also address environmental factors by reorienting the confused client in a consistent way and minimizing disruption to the usual diurnal rhythms. Companionship of family members or volunteers is helpful, as is the use of calendars, clocks, and newspapers to provide a time reference for the client. Follow institutional guidelines for the use of restraints.

DIAGNOSIS, OUTCOMES, INTERVENTIONS

Risk for Impaired Skin Integrity. If the client has fallen while alone and experienced an extended time lying down before help arrived, even early assessment may show the development of pressure ulcers over bony prominences. After surgery, the client's mobility limitations and pain increase the risk for skin impairment. Malnutrition and dehydration, which may have existed before injury and may be exacerbated postoperatively, may also contribute. Older clients and clients receiving long-term corticosteroid therapy may have especially tissue paper–thin skin that is even more prone to breakdown and tears. Finally, the type of tape used to secure postoperative dressings and the method and direction of tape application can contribute to the development of skin blisters. An appropriate diagnostic statement may be *Risk for Impaired Skin Integrity related to mobility limitations or to the application of tape with dressing changes.*

Outcomes. The client will demonstrate intact skin, as evidenced by absence of ulcers over bony prominences and heels and absence of epidermal stripping beneath tape used to secure postoperative dressings.

Interventions. After ORIF of the hip, the client should be assisted with position changes at least every 2 hours. These clients can be turned to either side; however, they are usually most comfortable on the nonoperative side with a pillow to support the operative leg. Carefully assess the skin over bony prominences such as the sacrum, coccyx, scapulae, elbows, and heels. If areas of skin breakdown are noted, measure and describe them thoroughly. Treat the ulcer using institutional protocols or see Chapter 49.

In addition to using a regular turning schedule, place a pressure-reducing mattress on the client's bed. Pressure on heels can be relieved by placement of a towel roll for brief periods under the Achilles tendon. Examination gloves filled with water can also provide pressure relief under heels. Specific skin care products are available to be massaged gently into affected areas at the first sign of redness. Direct massage of stage I pressure ulcers is contraindicated.

Avoid epidermal stripping by placing postoperative dressings over a skin sealant that is applied wherever the tape would touch the skin. Elastic tape should be placed vertically (superior to inferior) without tension to allow for stretching that is related to postoperative edema. Any redness, blistering, or epidermal stripping should be evaluated, and an enterostomal nurse specialist should be consulted on the client's care as appropriate. Clients with thin skin should not have tape on their skin; use gauze wraps instead. Treatment of skin tears is discussed in Chapter 49.

Pain. Acute pain is expected after any surgery, including ORIF of the hip. The client may also have contusions or abrasions caused by the fall that led to hip fracture. The diagnosis can be written as *Pain related to local tissue trauma from surgical incision or other injuries.*

Outcomes. The client will demonstrate comfort after surgery, as evidenced by movement without grimacing, by requesting analgesics no more frequently than ordered, and by statements that the pain is tolerable and not interfering with rest or physical therapy.

Interventions. In the immediate postoperative period, the client may experience intense pain and require injectable analgesics to attain acceptable control. Common interventions include patient-controlled analgesia (PCA) or epidural analgesia. Ice application over the dressed surgical wound may also increase the client's comfort. See the Management and Delegation feature on safe use of ice. Within 24 to 48 hours, the client should be tolerating fluids and able to take oral analgesics. Because pain is intensified with movement, the client may attempt to limit activity because of the expected increase in discomfort. Medicate the client before physical therapy or activities such as transferring to the chair, and reinforce the importance of ambulation in decreasing the risk for postoperative complications. Use of non-narcotic analgesics can also help with acute pain management, muscle spasms, and other chronic medical problems such as arthritis.

Concerns about becoming addicted to narcotics should be addressed openly. Many older persons fear that they will become addicted quickly, and they may therefore tolerate unnecessary pain, delaying their recovery. Narcotic addiction is rare, but the fear is quite intense.

Regularly assess for side effects of narcotic analgesics. Respiratory depression is more likely to occur with PCA or epidural analgesia than with oral narcotics. Pulse oximetry and regular measurement of vital signs help you assess for hypoxemia that results from shallow or slow breathing. Most clients raise their oximetry readings with stimulation. Seldom is naloxone needed.

Constipation, a very common problem after hip fracture and repair, is related to the client's impaired mobility, narcotic use, and progression to a regular diet. Encourage the client's intake of fluids and dietary fiber. In addition, stool softeners or laxatives may be indicated. If the client uses a bulk-forming laxative or other strategy to maintain bowel regularity at home, assist in continuing that program in the hospital. Regular assessment and implementation of a proactive bowel program are important for minimizing clients' concerns about bowel elimination.

Impaired Physical Mobility. The client's degree of immobility after ORIF of the hip is affected by pain and fear of movement, as well as any limitations in other joints. If previous mobility limitations contributed to the fall, the client may have even greater problems with mobilization after surgery. The diagnosis can be written as *Impaired Physical Mobility related to pain or fear of movement.*

Outcomes. The client will demonstrate improved physical mobility, as evidenced by the need for less assistance in transfers (bed to chair, bed to standing), by safe use of a walker or crutches, and by the ability to ambulate a functional distance (150 feet). For the client with previous mobility limitations, outcomes may focus on bed mobility only.

Interventions. Moving the client after ORIF of the hip can create a great deal of anxiety for both the client and the nursing staff. First be aware of any weight-bearing limitations ordered for the client before transferring him or her (see Table 27–5 for a description of weight-bearing limitations). Non-weight-bearing orders are often received after hip fracture repair, and these must be strictly followed to avoid disruption to bone healing. If the client is not allowed to bear full weight, careful attention to the

MANAGEMENT AND DELEGATION

Application of Heat and Cold

Any equipment used to apply heat or cold may injure the client. Injury may result if the client is unable to perceive discomfort because of decreased peripheral circulation, decreased feeling, decreased sensorium, sedation, or agitation. The client may also be at risk if he or she cannot be left alone safely or if the client alters the controls of the heating pad or cooling device.

The application of heat or cold to an inflamed or painful area that is closed may be delegated to unlicensed assistive personnel. Before delegating the application of heat or cold, consider the following:

- What is the indication for the application of heat or cold? Check the physician's order. The order and indication may be sufficient to tell you whether you can delegate this task or not.
- What is the condition of the affected site? Assess for any areas of redness, swelling, breakdown, or scar tissue. It is important to know the baseline condition of the site before the application of heat or cold. There may be an indication to withhold this treatment or to confer with the physician about the order. You will also need to assess the condition of the site on completion of the treatment.
- What is the client's diagnosis? Is there any history of diabetes mellitus or impairment in sensorium or mentation? This may be an indication for you to perform this treatment yourself. If there is impairment of the client's mental or sensory status, it may be necessary for the unlicensed assistive personnel to remain with the client throughout the treatment.
- What is the competency level of the unlicensed assistive personnel who might perform this task?

Instruct the unlicensed assistive personnel providing the heat or cold application to do the following:

- Wash their hands
- Assemble the necessary equipment. Advise them as to which method of applying heat or cold is ordered.
- Check the temperature of the heat or cold device before applying it to the client's skin. A safe range for heat applications is 115° to 125° F for adults.
- Wrap any heat or cold application with a protective cover, such as a towel or a flannel sleeve.
- If using a heating pad, start with the device on the lowest setting to initiate treatment.
- Instruct the client not to adjust the heat setting.
- Check the client's response immediately. If the device is too hot or cold, an adjustment is necessary. Double the protective layer between the device and the skin or allow the temperature of the device to moderate slightly.
- Check the client's skin after 5 minutes. If it is tolerated, leave the heat or cold in place for 20 minutes. If it is not tolerated, the heat or cold should be removed immediately, and you should be made aware of this. Assess the situation and notify the physician as appropriate.
- Remove the heat or cold application at 20 minutes and to inform you that the treatment is complete.

You are responsible for examining the affected area and reassessing the client's skin at the completion of this treatment. You should document your findings and the client's response to treatment in the medical record. The unlicensed assistive personnel should immediately report any difficulty encountered during the course of treatment.

Donna W. Markey, MSN, RN, *Clinician IV, Surgical Services, University of Virginia Health System, Charlottesville, Virginia*

operative extremity is required while a transfer is made, to ensure that the client avoids passing any weight through the leg. Record the amount of assistance that the client requires for safe transfer. This information provides

TABLE 27–5	WEIGHT-BEARING STATUS
Non-weightbearing	The client does not bear weight on the affected extremity; the affected extremity should not touch the floor
Touch-down weight-bearing	The client's foot of the affected extremity may rest on the floor, but no weight is distributed through that extremity
Partial weight-bearing	The client bears 30%–50% of weight on the affected extremity
Weight-bearing as tolerated	The client bears as much weight as he or she can tolerate on the affected extremity without undue strain or pain
Full weight-bearing	The client bears weight fully on the affected extremity

Adapted from Maher, A. B., Salmond, S. W., & Pellino, T. A. (1998). *Orthopaedic nursing.* Philadelphia: W. B. Saunders.

the benchmark that will determine whether the goal for increased mobility is being met. For example, the client may have needed the assistance of two staff members on the morning after surgery; by the next afternoon, increased mobility was demonstrated when only one nurse was needed to assist with transfer.

In addition to postoperative limitations, the client may suffer from arthritis in other joints or may have residual effects from a previous stroke. These conditions can increase pain and affect the ability to transfer from the bed to the chair. When the client stands and transfers for the first time, he or she will require the assistance of at least two staff members. Use of appropriate technique ensures a safe transfer for the client and also minimizes the risk of injury to the staff member's lower back (see Chapter 26 for additional information on requirements for appropriate mobility assistance). Make sure that the devices are on the client whenever he or she is in the bed or chair, which is when the legs are dependent and venous return may be affected.

Self-Care Deficit. After hip fracture and surgical repair, the client is likely to experience some degree of self-care deficit in hygiene and dressing. Limited mobility may decrease independence in self-care, and assistive devices may be required. The diagnostic statement may read

Self-Care Deficit: Bathing/Hygiene, Dressing/Grooming related to mobility impairment following hip fracture.

Outcomes. The client will resume pre-injury level of independence in meeting self-care needs.

Interventions. After ORIF of the hip, the client will be aided in recovery by physical and occupational therapists. Physical therapists assist with ambulation and strengthening. They offer instruction on climbing stairs and on getting in and out of a car. They also provide assistive devices that help in functional independence, including an elevated toilet seat and a walker. Occupational therapists instruct the client on bathing and dressing techniques. They may suggest use of a tub bench or a long-handled sponge. They may also provide long-handled reachers or sock aids to help the client dress with minimal assistance from others. Nursing staff will reinforce the use of techniques and assistive devices to encourage the client's optimal recovery.

Risk for Infection. Bone infection is a serious threat and can lead to loss of joint function. Pre-existent poor health status also contributes to risk. State this diagnosis as *Risk for Infection related to loss of primary defenses (skin) and malnutrition.*

Outcomes. The client will remain free of manifestations of infection, as evidenced by (1) white blood cell (WBC) count within normal limits, (2) an afebrile state, (3) absence of purulent wound drainage, (4) absence of increasing pain in wound, and (5) no inflammation in wound after 72 hours.

Interventions. Clients often receive prophylactic antibiotics during surgery and in the immediate postoperative period. After ORIF, the physician may prefer to perform the initial dressing change. Use strict aseptic technique in performing subsequent dressing changes, carefully assessing the wound each time for signs of healing or infection.

Risk for Peripheral Neurovascular Dysfunction. Be aware of the risk for neurologic or vascular impairment after surgery on any joint. Edema or extremity positioning can place pressure on adjacent nerves. The diagnosis can be written as *Risk for Peripheral Neurovascular Dysfunction related to lower extremity edema or positioning.*

Outcomes. The client will demonstrate normal neurovascular status, as evidenced by adequate peripheral pulses with capillary refill time of less than 3 seconds and by absence of sensory impairments and motor weakness in the operative extremity.

Interventions. Assess the neurovascular status of the operative extremity at least every 4 hours or as directed by the surgeon, and then compare findings to the unaffected extremity. More frequent monitoring may be needed if indicated by the client's condition. Assessment includes the presence and quality of bilateral pedal pulses, skin color and temperature of the extremity, capillary refill in the toes, sensation and movement of the toes, and the client's ability to perform dorsiplantar flexion of the foot. Any pallor or coolness, numbness or tingling, or inability to move the extremity should be reported promptly to the surgeon.

Risk for Constipation. Impaired mobility and the use of narcotic analgesics can lead to constipation. The risk is increased in older clients who have a pre-existing dependence on laxatives. The diagnosis could be written as *Risk for Constipation related to impaired physical mobility and side effects of narcotics.*

Outcomes. The client will maintain a pattern of regular bowel elimination by consuming adequate fluids and high-fiber foods and by having a bowel movement at least every 2 to 3 days.

Interventions. The client's diet should include ample fluids and fiber if not contraindicated. Stool softeners are often prescribed and should be administered regularly. Also, determine whether the client has regular, effective strategies for treating constipation and, if so, use those methods to assist with elimination. The client should be assisted to transfer to a bedside commode or ambulate to the bathroom whenever possible to meet elimination needs. To assist the bedridden client with bowel elimination, offer a fracture bedpan and ensure privacy when the client needs to use it.

Risk for Nutritional Deficit. After surgery, the client may experience nausea that delays the progression to a regular diet. Decreased activity may also lead to poor appetite. If the client has experienced blood loss, a nutritional deficit may also occur. Remember that the presence of obesity does not ensure that the client is well-nourished. This diagnosis may be stated as *Risk for Nutritional Deficit related to nausea or poor appetite following hip fracture.*

Outcomes. The client will maintain adequate dietary intake, as evidenced by energy for participation in physical therapy and by appropriate wound and bone healing.

Interventions. Stress the importance of a high-carbohydrate and high-protein diet for adequate healing, and then assist the client in making food choices as necessary. If the client's appetite remains poor, offer small, frequent meals. Encourage the client to eat at least some of every food at every meal to achieve balanced intake. After blood loss, increased dietary iron or iron supplements may be required. Encourage the client to eat foods high in iron, and administer a supplement as ordered. Inform the client that stool may appear black or tarry while he or she is taking an iron supplement.

EVALUATION

Clinical pathways or care maps are now often used to determine which outcomes have been met for the client with a hip fracture; they often suggest a time frame for each goal. Pain should decrease fairly soon after surgery. Injectable narcotic analgesics are not typically required after 24 to 36 hours. The client should advance to oral analgesics as soon as nausea is controlled and liquids are being taken freely. A regular diet should be offered by the first or second day after surgery, again on the assumption that nausea is controlled. Early feeding primes the gastrointestinal tract, helping the client avoid postoperative ileus. Adequate diet also contributes greatly to the client's physical stamina and to wound healing. If an indwelling urinary catheter has been used, it should be removed as soon as the client can transfer to a bedside commode, in order to decrease any risk for urinary tract infection (see Case Management: Hip Fracture).

A clinical pathway also often describes the involvement of a case manager or social worker in planning the client's discharge. In collaboration with the bedside nurse and the physician, the case manager assesses the client's

CASE MANAGEMENT

Hip Fracture

A hip fracture is an unexpected event, usually involving an older woman who falls at home. Sometimes the client is unable to summon help and is found after having fallen hours earlier.

The best case management is prevention of the fracture. Prevention of osteoporosis through good nutrition, exercise, and monitoring of bone density are important measures. Weight reduction and maintenance of optimum range of motion can also help to prevent bone problems. Correction of visual deficits and home safety (e.g., good lighting, elimination of throw rugs, safe footwear, grab bars) can also prevent accidents.

Assess

- What events led to the hip fracture?
- How long was it before help arrived?
- Are there underlying conditions that contributed to the hip fracture (osteoporosis, cancer, arthritis, incontinence, urinary tract infection)?
- Are there other chronic conditions that might inhibit recovery or make rehabilitation more difficult, such as anemia, heart disease, or a cognitive impairment?
- Are cognitive or sensory changes apparent? What is the client's pain status?
- If surgery is anticipated, what preparations are needed? Does the client have a health care proxy or advance directives?

Advocate

Take time to explain what is happening, taking into account cognitive and sensory deficits. If the client had to wait for assistance for some time after falling, consider dehydration, weakness, or even pneumonia as a consequence. Give the client and family information to help them make decisions about surgery or other treatments. Make sure that pain is managed. Frequently, older people do not ask for pain medication and suffer needlessly as a result. Inquire about the client's home situation and care needs; some assistance or change of residence may be required.

Prevent Readmission

Explain the surgical intervention and how to prevent dislocation. Many hospitals offer educational materials showing proper positioning and exercises. Physical and occupational therapists can aid the client in learning exercises, correct weight-bearing, and transfer and ambulation techniques as well as how to make changes in activities of daily living. Often short-term rehabilitation can assist the client, especially if no caregiver is available at home.

Monitor for manifestations of infection and teach the client to continue monitoring after discharge. Make sure that pain control is adequate and that the client understands necessary medication regimens, especially anticoagulants. Prevent complications, such as thrombophlebitis and bowel problems, through early mobilization. Refer appropriately for home nursing care, social services, physical therapy, and phlebotomy. Make sure that the client knows when follow-up appointments are scheduled and what to do if an emergency, especially dislocation, occurs.

Cheryl Noetscher, RN, MS, *Director of Case Management, Crouse Hospital and Community–General Hospital, Syracuse, New York*

discharge needs on the basis of information about the home environment and social support. An extended-care facility or rehabilitation unit may be one possible destination after acute care hospitalization. If the client can move from bed to chair with minimal or no assistance, he or she may instead go directly home with possible visits from a home health aide or nurse to meet other skilled needs, such as hygiene and mobility assistance. When the client is discharged directly to the home, the nurse must ensure that the family can safely assist the client with mobility needs and activities of daily living. The case manager assists the client in obtaining any durable medical equipment that may be needed, such as a walker or crutches, and finalizes discharge transportation if necessary (see Bridge to Home Health Care).

CONDYLAR FRACTURES

The condyles are bony prominences at the distal end of the femur. Condylar fractures occur most often with high-energy injuries in young clients. They may be among several injuries sustained in a motor vehicle accident, for example, when the client's flexed knee strikes the dashboard. Less severe condylar fractures are treated with knee immobilizers or casting. For more severe injury,

ORIF is indicated. Bone grafting is used for comminuted fractures. Loss of knee mobility is a common outcome, and surgical revision may be needed to improve bony alignment. If the client develops severe pain and disability, arthrodesis (fusion) or arthroplasty (joint replacement) may be required.

PELVIC FRACTURES

The pelvis is a ring-like structure composed mostly of cancellous bone, with a thin cortex. This structure provides great strength, allowing the pelvis to offer structural support and also to serve as a shock absorber that protects the abdominal organs. Pelvic fractures have been on the rise since 1990 as a result of an increase in high-energy trauma, such as motor vehicle accidents and gunshot wounds. About two thirds of all pelvic fractures occur as a result of traffic accidents; pedestrians are injured more often than are the occupants of involved vehicles.[1]

Because fractures of the pelvic ring can vary in stability, their management depends on the severity of the injury. Most cases can be diagnosed correctly with an anteroposterior radiograph. If there is any indication of an unstable fracture, a urethrogram or intravenous pyelogram is used to assess for possible damage to the kidneys and lower urinary tract. Pelvic fractures also often result in hemorrhage, and the pelvis can hold as much as 4 L of blood. Unstable fractures have been treated aggressively since the mid-1990s with internal fixation in which plates and screws are used to achieve an intact pelvic ring. External fixation is also still used. Less severe pelvic fractures may be treated with bed rest alone. The client needs adequate pain management as well as assessment for neurovascular compromise or the development of complications such as thrombophlebitis or fat embolism.

PATELLAR FRACTURES

Fracture of the patella (kneecap) often results from a direct blow to the area. Some separation or splitting of the patella invariably occurs, and the client is unable to fully extend the knee because of pain and related damage to extensor mechanisms. Patellar fractures are usually more evident on a lateral radiograph than on other views. A stellate fracture (cracked patella without fragment displacement) can be managed conservatively by placing the client in a long leg cast for several weeks and then beginning mobilization. Indirect trauma, such as a forced flexion injury sustained in a fall, can result in a transverse fracture. ORIF is often necessary to minimize the potential for later problems with knee motion or chondromalacia. After a comminuted fracture, fragments may be difficult to reduce accurately, and removal of the patella may be best. Surgical repair of extensors such as the quadriceps tendon and the patellar tendon may also be needed.

TIBIAL AND FIBULAR FRACTURES

The fibula can be fractured alone in several ways: from direct trauma to the outer surface of the leg, producing a transverse or comminuted fracture; through twisting injuries, which produce a spiral fracture; or from repeated stress as in long-distance running, which can cause a fatigue fracture usually just above the inferior tibiofibular ligament. Fatigue fractures necessitate immobilization; for other nondisplaced fibular fractures, a cast may be needed to immobilize the ankle.

The tibia can also be broken, leaving the fibula intact. Fracture can result from direct trauma. Repeated stress can lead to a fatigue fracture at the junction of the middle and upper thirds of the tibia. This injury is commonly seen in long-distance runners, hurdlers, and ballet dancers who jump excessively. Twisting injuries rarely result in a lone tibial fracture. Tibial fractures are reduced and treated through cast immobilization, internal fixation, or external fixation. Although it may seem helpful to have the fibula intact, the undamaged bone actually holds the ends of the tibia apart and it may be necessary to cut the fibula in order to attain satisfactory alignment of the tibia.

Fractures of both the tibia and fibula are common results of motor vehicle accidents and sports injuries. Treatment concerns include possible problems with fracture union, vascular and soft tissue damage, skin loss, and the development of compartment syndrome. As with lone tibial fractures, fragments may be held in the reduced position through casting from groin to toe. Alternatively,

internal fixation would be the treatment of choice for clients with unstable or multiple fractures. External fixation would be necessary if the wound is dirty or if there is skin loss.

If the knee is struck violently on the lateral surface, a tibial plateau fracture may result. Four fracture patterns can occur: the lateral tibial plateau may be split vertically; part of the tibial plateau may be thrust downward into the tibia to produce a depressed fracture; both of these can occur together; or the whole plateau may be depressed. Because the full extent of injury may not be apparent on radiographs, CT scanning or MRI may be needed to determine the fracture anatomy. Any large fragment split off the tibia must be secured back in place with screws to restore the contour of the bone. Large depressed fragments can be elevated to reconstitute the bone's surface, but the cavity that results below the fracture must be filled with a cancellous bone graft. If only a slight depression occurred in the tibial plateau, more conservative treatment with early mobilization may be appropriate.

FOOT FRACTURES

Because it provides a contact point with the ground and protrudes forward from the body, the foot is especially susceptible to injury. Fracture is most often caused by falls or jumps from great heights, running or twisting, motor vehicle accidents, or objects dropped on the foot. As with any other injury, the client with open fractures should be taken to the operating room for surgical debridement and repair. Closed fractures of the foot, however, can generally be treated conservatively through cast or brace immobilization or through the use of walking shoes. Weight-bearing is progressively resumed as tolerated.

UPPER EXTREMITY FRACTURES

Fractures of the proximal humerus are a common traumatic injury in older persons, often caused by a fall on an outstretched arm. A fall need not be serious to produce a humeral fracture in an osteoporotic client. Injury to the dominant arm of an older client can lead to dependence and immobility. The risk of falling also increases because the sense of balance is impaired as a result of loss of use of the arm. If the fracture is nondisplaced or minimally displaced, the extremity is usually immobilized with a sling. Gentle range-of-motion exercises can be started when shoulder discomfort subsides, usually within 2 or 3 weeks after injury. A displaced fracture is treated by ORIF. Prosthetic replacement is occasionally indicated for an intra-articular fracture or one that is severely comminuted. Prompt, appropriate treatment reduces the risk that AVN of the humeral head will develop.

Fractures of the humeral shaft usually result from a direct blow to the arm, a motor vehicle accident, a gunshot injury, or a crush injury. Humeral fractures can also result from indirect injuries such as a fall on an outstretched hand or on the elbow. Most humeral shaft fractures can be treated by initial immobilization with a U-shaped splint. Once the swelling has subsided, a commercially available humeral fracture brace may be used in conjunction with an arm sling. Heavy hanging arm casts should be avoided because they may contribute to a non-union. Surgery would be indicated for debridement of an open fracture. Surgical stabilization would also be required for any fracture associated with a vascular injury.

Intra-articular injuries of the elbow include condylar, olecranon, and radial head or neck fracture. These injuries frequently result from falls on or direct blows to the elbow. Because associated injuries to the three major peripheral nerves (radial, median, and ulnar) are possible, careful neurovascular assessment is critical. A high potential for compartment syndrome also exists after intra-articular fractures of the elbow. Most nondisplaced fractures can be treated with immobilization, followed by early range-of-motion exercises once acute discomfort has diminished (usually after 1 week). A posterior long arm splint may be used with a shoulder sling. Displaced fractures, especially supracondylar fractures, often necessitate ORIF. Repair of the brachial artery may also be necessary after traumatic injury. After surgery, immobilization can be accomplished with a posterior elbow splint, a cast, or traction.

Fractures of the shafts of the radius and ulna usually result from a direct blow to the forearm, a motor vehicle accident, or a fall on an outstretched arm. Associated injuries to the nerves (median, ulnar, and radial) and arteries (radial and ulnar) are possible. A sugar-tong splint can be used to provide initial immobilization of forearm fractures. Circumferential cast immobilization is generally not recommended in early treatment because fracture swelling in association with the constriction provided by the cast may lead to a compartment syndrome. Immobilization must include the wrist and the elbow to control rotation of the forearm. In adult clients, surgical treatment may be indicated for displaced or open fractures.

As with proximal humeral fractures, fractures of the distal radius are common injuries in older persons. Many older clients have a good outcome even with a residual deformity because their routine activities may not demand full use of the limb. However, deformity and possible resulting arthritic changes in younger clients may lead to inability to perform their current jobs. Colles' fracture is a common injury in which the distal radius fragment is displaced dorsally and proximally. Fracture reduction is

---

BRIDGE TO HOME HEALTH CARE

Managing the Immobile Client

To prevent skin breakdown and manage other physical and emotional effects of immobility, the multidisciplinary team must collaborate with clients who are paralyzed or have other desensitized areas, with their family members, and with their informal caregivers. The core team members are a nurse, a physical therapist, a social worker, and an occupational therapist.

If the person is chair- or wheelchair-bound, good seat cushions can be purchased from most pharmacies and vendors. Choose a cushion to match the client's seating problems. Some cushions are designed for active paraplegics that distribute pressure onto the posterior thigh. Heavy foam (4 inches thick) provides pressure reduction for clients with wheelchairs that have sling seats. Cushions of air can be inflated to reduce pressure and prevent posture problems. Pillows or gel should not be used: A pillow allows too much hip adduction and internal rotation and becomes uncomfortable; gel is expensive and heavy, breaks down, and makes it harder to move a wheelchair.

Evaluate how clients sit and use cushions. Inspect every cushion frequently for signs of wear. Avoid folds, wrinkles, or pockets on surfaces. The proper sitting position includes 90 degrees of flexion at the hips and knees. Clients should sit erect in chairs on their buttocks, not on the sacrum. Place pillows behind a client's back to promote more erect posture.

Teach clients to protect tissue, toughen skin, and avoid massaging lotion over bony prominences; massage makes skin soft and susceptible to breakdown or shearing. Minimize friction; avoid having tissue squeezed between two hard surfaces such as bedding and bony prominences. Teach clients, especially those with paraplegia, to use a mirror to check for friction or pressure. Clients who are confined to bed need to be repositioned at least every

2 hours, and use a footboard, a thoroughly padded plastic crate, or a box to prevent feet from being forced into extreme plantar flexion. Their heels, ankles, trochanters, sacrum, scapulae, elbows, and ears need to be checked at least daily. Pillows, blanket or towel rolls, balloons, foam, or rolled-up clothing are useful for padding and positioning. Sheepskin, elbow and heel protectors, and egg-crate cushions provide little protection; thick foam is better. Even though good-quality alternating pressure pads are best, there are other options, including waterbeds, silicon bead beds, and air mattresses. When alternating pads are used watch the skin for several days to ensure that the client is getting enough lift (see Chapter 49).

Daily exercise is essential. Passive exercise only increases flexibility, whereas active exercise increases circulation and air exchange, maintains joint lubrication and mobility, and helps prevent contractures. Provide all exercise gently to avoid joint or tissue damage. Movement of any kind can trigger spasms. Keep a firm hold on the extremity, moving it through the range of motion. Wait for any spasm to subside; then continue. If the spasticity is too strong or you feel uncertain about whether to continue the exercise, request assistance from a physical therapist.

After clients progress through the acute stage, they need to consider long-term issues and dramatic lifestyle changes. Provide information about alternative housing options, transportation, yard and housekeeping services, financial assistance, recreation, and stores that deliver prescriptions. Mental health and sexuality issues are important, too. Clients also need to consider and make decisions about nutrition, clothing, informal caregivers, and health care services. Some clients may be eligible for specially trained dogs or the Helping Hands Program that supplies capuchin monkeys for aid and companion assistance.

Mary E. McQuin, BSPT, *Physical Therapist, Visiting Nurse Association of Omaha, Omaha, Nebraska*

greatly enhanced by the use of a nerve block such as the Bier block. This fracture may be treated with 2 weeks of splinting followed by 3 weeks in a short arm cast. Comminuted fractures may necessitate external fixation or ORIF with bone grafting.

Fractures of the metacarpals and phalanges account for 10% of all hand fractures.[5] More than half of those fractures are work-related. A delay in seeking evaluation and diagnosis can make fracture reduction difficult because fractures in the hand form early callus within 7 to 10 days and become difficult to manipulate. Treatment involves accurate fracture reduction, movement of the uninvolved fingers to prevent stiffness, and elevation of the extremity to decrease edema. Simple measures such as "buddy taping" or splinting are usually sufficient treatment for stable fractures. Comminuted fractures and those necessitating open reduction take longer to consolidate and are not ready as quickly for mobilization. Client motivation plays a critical role in rehabilitation after hand injury and can often be enhanced by a brief course of physical therapy. Motion can typically be started about 21 days after injury for clients with closed, nondisplaced fractures.

Neurovascular assessment is critical for all clients with upper extremity fractures. Carefully compare the color, warmth, movement, sensation, and capillary refill of the affected extremity with those of the unaffected extremity. Elevation of the injured extremity is typically indicated. At night, the client should be observed frequently to be certain the arm does not move into a dependent position. If a cast or splint has been applied, the client and family should receive careful instruction about cast care and about the clinical manifestations of compartment syndrome.

DISLOCATIONS AND SUBLUXATIONS

Dislocation and subluxation both describe changes in joint relationships. In a dislocation, the opposing joint surfaces are no longer in contact. In subluxation, the joint surfaces are in partial contact, but their relationship is abnormal. Both injuries are caused by acute deforming forces applied to ligaments or tendons from a fall, a blow, or a strong muscle contraction. For example, the client who tries to break a fall down the stairs by holding on to the handrail may dislocate a shoulder.

After dislocation, the client often complains of severe pain that increases with attempted movement. Swelling around or below the joint is likely, along with complete or nearly complete loss of function and a visible deformity that may alter the length of the extremity. Fracture of the joint surface often accompanies dislocation. Neurovascular status of the affected extremity must be carefully assessed because the displaced bone may tear blood vessels and impede circulation, damage nerves, and rupture ligaments or muscle attachments. Immediate reduction is preferred before inflammation and spasm can become significant. If immediate reduction is not possible, analgesics and muscle relaxants must be given before any later attempt to reduce the dislocation. A splint, a harness, or padding should be used for 4 to 8 weeks after acute dislocation or until pain is significantly reduced and muscle function provides adequate support in cases of recur-

rent dislocation. Like fractures, dislocations are described in terms of the relationship of the distal bone to the proximal bone. In a posterior dislocation of the knee, for example, the tibia lies posterior to the femur.

After subluxation, the client experiences variable pain and the feeling that the joint was out of position briefly. The joint typically feels weak, and pain increases with attempted movement. Because radiographs are often normal with subluxations, the physician must rule out other possible injuries such as sprain, strain, muscle tear, and fracture. Muscle-strengthening exercises can help the client avoid future subluxations. Joint restrictive supports such as a shoulder harness may also be useful.

SPORTS INJURIES

OVERUSE SYNDROMES

Overuse syndromes are common sports-related problems. They begin insidiously as the result of microtraumas that often do not completely stop the affected person's activity. The client must understand that the manifestations of pain, tenderness, and swelling result from repeated stress on musculoskeletal structures. Eventual failure is likely because of fatigue or erosion if the client continues to exercise. Nonoperative treatment of stress injuries always includes relative rest. For example, the runner may be restricted from impact-loading activities but still allowed to cycle or run in the buoyancy of a swimming pool. Ice, compression (when swelling occurs), and NSAIDs are used routinely to reduce inflammation related to the injury. A supervised, stepped rehabilitation program is also helpful if the client plans to return to the athletic activity.

People who are at greatest risk for overuse include competitive athletes, first-time athletes, "born again" athletes (those who were once very active and now seek a return to athletics after a decade or more of sedentary living), and those recovering from injury. Other factors can contribute to an increased risk for injury (Box 27–3) and should be shared with clients who exercise regularly or are considering involvement in an exercise program. The risk for developing an overuse syndrome decreases if the client avoids the following:

• Training errors, such as progressing too fast or allowing inadequate time for conditioning

---

BOX 27–3   Factors that May Increase Risk for Injury

■ Age over 40 yr
■ Current inactive lifestyle
■ Overweight by 20 lb or more
■ Family history of cardiac disease
■ Any past experience of pain or pressure in chest, arm, or throat
■ Taking medications on a regular basis
■ Documented high cholesterol level
■ Smokes or has history of pulmonary disease
■ History of diabetes or other chronic disorders
■ History of joint disease

- Improper technique based on the individual activity (e.g., elbow problems from poor tennis technique)
- Improper equipment, such as incorrect shoes for the sport
- Unsafe environment, such as exercising on a slippery surface or experiencing repeated impact on a hard surface

Prevention, the key to overuse injuries, is enhanced by pre-participation assessment and client teaching. Rather than trying to ensure that the client is in optimal health, a pre-participation assessment allows recognition of potential problems that can occur as the client progresses in a sport. Client teaching should emphasize the importance of stretching to maintain joint flexibility and range of motion. Stretching exercises should be static (i.e., holding muscles in a stretched position for a few moments rather than repeatedly stretching and relaxing them). Static stretching reduces the danger of overstretching and tissue damage, causes less muscle soreness than a bouncing stretch, and relieves muscle soreness when it occurs. Box 27–4 presents additional information about injury prevention in fitness programs.

Overuse syndromes are classified according to severity

BOX 27–4 Preventing Injuries in Fitness Programs

Lack of fitness is one of the main causes of sport injury.

Warm-up and Stretching Exercises

Always warm up and stretch before strenuous exercises. To warm up means to begin and finish exercises gradually. Stretching exercises increase muscle flexibility.

Pacing

Build up an exercise program gradually. It takes at least 6 to 8 weeks to get into strong condition. Add small, gradual increments of exercise. Proceed gradually and do not overdo. Tired muscles are prone to injury.

Intensity

When preparing for a specific event, plan training programs accordingly (e.g., a marathon demands a more intensive training program than does a 10-km race).

Capacity Level

Exercise to the capacity of physiologic limits.

Strength

Build strength gradually to gain greater endurance, speed, and power.

Motivation

Success in an exercise program depends on individual motivation.

Relaxation

Relaxation exercises relieve fatigue and tension.

Routine

Regular exercise is more valuable and less likely to lead to injury than bursts of activity followed by long periods of inactivity.

---

of injury. Intervention generally depends on the severity more than on the specific type of injury (Table 27–6).

■ LOWER EXTREMITIES

Common overuse injuries of the lower extremities include the following.

STRESS FRACTURE

The most common stress fracture occurs in the foot, in which fatigue or erosion commonly manifests as pain and swelling. Forces acting on the leg at heel contact during running are three to eight times an individual's body weight, repeated up to 2000 times.[18] Stress fractures commonly occur in the tarsal bones. Tarsal navicular stress fractures are fairly common in jumping athletes, but their recognition is frequently delayed. Once diagnosed, bone grafting and screw fixation may be necessary to obtain healing.

PLANTAR FASCIITIS

One of the most common overuse syndromes of the foot results from repetitive strain to the plantar fascia, the long ligament that attaches to the plantar surface (sole) of the calcaneus (heel bone); its fibers fan out to attach to the forefoot. At times a bone spur is seen on radiographs at the plantar origin of the fascia as new bone forms, as a result of repeated tearing of the fascia. Plantar fasciitis can be very difficult to correct. Heel cups are used routinely, and arch supports may also be useful. Other standard modalities such as ice and ultrasonography with hydrocortisone cream can at times relieve pain. Direct injections of corticosteroid preparations may be indicated in resistant cases.

SHIN SPLINTS

A medial tibial stress syndrome results from excessive strain of the posterior tibial muscle origin. Shin splints are characterized by pain with activity and residual tenderness at the muscle origins for days after running or other repetitive activity. Shin splints are best treated by strengthening the involved muscles and by using orthotics to correct misalignment of the feet and reduce strain on injured muscles.

PATELLAR TENDINITIS

Also known as "jumper's knee," patellar tendinitis results from repetitive loads placed on the knee's extensor mechanism through sports that require jumping, such as basketball and volleyball. The client complains of pain, tenderness, and sometimes swelling at either pole of the patella. The pain is aggravated by additional jumping. Patellar tendinitis is usually unilateral and rarely progresses to complete rupture. Treatment includes NSAIDs, reduction in the irritating activity, and improvement in the flexibility of the hamstrings and rectus femoris to improve efficiency of knee flexion and extension.

■ UPPER EXTREMITIES

Overuse injuries that occur in the upper extremities include:

IMPINGEMENT SYNDROME

Impingement syndrome is one of the most common problems encountered by the athlete involved in repetitive activity with arms upward over the client's head (e.g.,

TABLE 27-6	GRADES OF OVERUSE INJURIES			
	Grade I	**Grade II**	**Grade III**	**Grade IV**
ASSESSMENT				
History	Hurts after, not during, activity	Hurts after and sometimes during activity	Hurts during and after activity	Hurts all the time
Physical examination	Generalized tenderness	Generalized tenderness over area	More localized tenderness	Localized tenderness
X-rays	Negative	Negative	Usually negative	May be positive
Bone scan	Negative	Negative	May be positive	Usually positive
TYPE OF TISSUE INJURED	Soft tissue	Soft tissue	Soft, hard, or bony tissue	Hard or bony tissue
MANAGEMENT	Ice Treat underlying problem	Ice Correct underlying problem Anti-inflammatory medication, e.g., aspirin Decrease exercise 25%–33%	Ice Correct underlying problem Anti-inflammatory medication, e.g., aspirin, NSAIDs; possibly prednisone Decrease exercise 50%–75%	Ice Correct underlying problem Anti-inflammatory medication, e.g., aspirin, NSAIDs; possibly prednisone Stop exercising altogether

NSAIDs, nonsteroidal anti-inflammatory drugs.
Adapted from The athlete's leg (1985). *Emergency Medicine, 17,* 83.

painters). Manifestations include pain and weakness associated with forward flexion or lateral abduction of the shoulder above 70 degrees. The subacromial bursa, long head of the biceps muscle, and the rotator cuff are the most frequently affected structures in the "painful arc." Initial treatment involves relative rest and NSAIDs. A subacromial injection of anesthetic and cortisone is also an accepted treatment. Physical therapy represents a major portion of recovery. Return to activity should be slow and progressive.

TENNIS ELBOW

Despite the common term "tennis elbow," lateral humeral epicondylitis is seen not only in tennis players but also in anyone involved in activities that require repetitive use of the wrist extensors or flexors. Most affected clients are 30 to 45 years of age. Nonoperative treatment to reduce inflammation is followed by a careful rehabilitation program that includes gradual stretching and isometric exercises. As the client returns to full activity, a counter-force brace can be worn to inhibit full muscle expansion and decrease tension on the injured tissue.

GOLFER'S ELBOW

The etiology and treatment of medial humeral epicondylitis are similar to those of tennis elbow.

TENDINITIS

Tendinitis involving the hand and wrist is quite common but usually transitory. When it persists, tendinitis may impair the client's ability to work. People at risk include those who engage in activities that require gripping, pinching, pulling, or lifting with repetitive wrist motion. Radiographs are obtained to rule out foreign bodies, arthritis, calcification, fractures, and other abnormalities.

STRAINS

Strains result from trauma to a muscle body or to the attachment of a tendon from overstretching, overextension, or misuse. They often arise from twisting or wrenching movements and may occur in any body part that contains muscles and tendons. Strains can occur *acutely* during unaccustomed vigorous exercise. They may also be *chronic,* developing after repetitive muscle overuse.

Strains are characterized by muscle spasm and discomfort; severity of clinical manifestations is related to the degree of injury. With more severe strains, ecchymosis and edema may be evident, and range of motion may be quite limited. Radiographs are necessary to rule out the possibility of fracture.

Acute strains necessitate rest and, if possible, splinting. The injured part should be elevated and ice should be applied for the first 24 to 48 hours to decrease swelling. Heat may be prescribed for comfort after 72 hours; it also hastens reabsorption of blood and fluid and promotes healing. Surgical repair may be needed if a rupture is present at the tendon-bone interface. During healing after strain (4 to 6 weeks), movement of the injured part should be minimized. Activity should never progress to the point that symptoms such as pain or swelling result. After mature scar tissue has formed, the injured part can be gradually and progressively exercised. Overactivity must absolutely be avoided during rehabilitation.

SPRAINS

A sprain is a ligamentous injury resulting from overstress that damages ligament fibers or their attachment to a bone. The ankle is the joint most frequently injured during sports participation. An ankle sprain most often occurs when the foot is forced inward to cause stretching or tearing of the ligaments that hold the joint in place. The greater the stress and the longer it is applied to the ankle, the more severe the sprain is. The severity of the swelling depends on the extent of tissue injury. However, ecchymosis does not always reliably indicate either the severity or the site of the injury. In order to plan treatment, it is important to determine the number of ligaments affected and the severity of injury to them.

Sprains may be *mild* (first degree), *moderate* (second degree), or *severe* (third degree) (Fig. 27–9). In a first-degree sprain, only a few ligament fibers are torn, with no loss of function and no weakening of the ligament. Appropriate treatment for this level of injury includes *r*est, *i*ce, *c*ompression, and *e*levation (RICE) for 3 to 5 days. Gentle range-of-motion and strengthening exercises can then be started. In a second-degree sprain, a portion of the ligament is torn, producing some loss of function. Protection is crucial to prevent further tearing. Immobilization with a splint or brace is indicated until initial swelling has diminished, usually 1 to 2 weeks. Pain and swelling typically mandate restricted weight-bearing as well, and the client may need instruction on walking with crutches. A brace such as an airsplint can be used to prevent ankle inversion and eversion. In a third-degree sprain, a ligament is completely torn, either from its attachment or within the ligament body itself. With complete ligament rupture, surgical repair is often required. Cast or brace immobilization is needed for 4 to 6 weeks after the injury.

Once the conventional immobilizer is removed, the injured ankle can be placed in an aircast to allow dorsiflexion and plantar flexion of the foot while restricting lateral movements of the ankle. At this point, gentle range-of-motion and strengthening exercises can be initiated. When the client returns to full exercise, adequate taping and protection are needed for the next 6 months. Sprains can also lead to avulsion fractures (Fig. 27–9D).

Client education following an ankle sprain is extremely important. Explain all phases of recovery, and offer strategies to prevent future injury to the ankle.

ROTATOR CUFF TEARS

Pathophysiology

Most shoulder injuries involve the soft tissues, and many result directly from repetitive activities such as throwing or overhead motion within the shoulder girdle. The shoulder girdle includes the sternoclavicular joint, the acromioclavicular joint, the glenohumeral joint, the subacromial space, and the scapulothoracic space. Movement at all of these articulations allows for the complexity of a pitcher's throwing motion. Four muscles also contribute to the shoulder's varied movements and form the rotator cuff: (1) the subscapularis (anterior), (2) the supraspinatus, (3) the infraspinatus, and (4) the teres minor (posterior).

Normal shoulder movement is a smooth, pain-free activity of the rotator cuff muscles. However, excessive joint activity can lead to repetitive trauma, or muscles can

be injured by an external force. Careful history and appropriate examination by the physician often lead to a diagnosis of the extent of injury. If the rotator cuff is torn, the client is not able to perform abduction and external rotation. Activity at the glenohumeral joint is also painfully impaired. Confirmation can be gained through use of radiography, arthrography, CT scans, MRI, or arthroscopy.

Treatment of rotator-cuff injury often begins conservatively with rest and sling support for the shoulder. NSAIDs may relieve discomfort. Some physicians also advocate intra-articular injection of analgesics or steroids. When acute manifestations subside, the client should begin active exercises that address range of motion and strengthen the rotator cuff muscles. Any elastic graded equipment (e.g., TheraBand) can be used in a daily program of progressive gentle exercises. Exercise may be preceded by application of heat and followed by ice if discomfort occurs.

Surgery may be necessary to repair a tear in the rotator cuff. Repair may be performed on an outpatient basis, or the client may have a short hospital stay. Postoperative management includes instruction on the use of a shoulder immobilizer and introduction of a program of gentle exercises such as the pendulum shoulder movement. The neurovascular status of the affected arm should be assessed at regular intervals, and findings should be compared to

FIGURE 27–9 Various types of sprains (with the ankle as an example). *A,* Mild (first-degree) sprain is a small hematoma in a localized area. *B,* Moderate (second-degree) sprain is more severe, with more than half of the fibers torn. *C,* Severe (third-degree) sprains tear completely through the ligament.

the nonoperative arm. Pain management should also be a focus of postoperative care.

ANTERIOR CRUCIATE LIGAMENT INJURIES

One of the most common knee injuries in sports is a tear of the anterior cruciate ligament (ACL) (Fig. 27–10). For example, an estimated 80% of ski injuries involve the ACL. About 80% of the injured athletes are able to return to sports, but 50% to 65% are reinjured in 1 to 2 years; after 5 years, only 35% still participate. ACL injury also occurs in sports such as basketball, gymnastics, football, and soccer.

The ACL is usually injured as part of a complex mechanism of hyperextension, internal rotation, extremes of external rotation, and deceleration. The ligament may actually be torn from the femur or tibia. More commonly, however, the tear occurs in the midportion of the ACL. The injured client often describes hearing a loud pop. Severe swelling can occur in the first few hours after injury. The knee feels unstable ("gives way"), particularly in rotation, and full extension is difficult.

The physician may attempt to determine knee stability during examination by using the Lachman test, the most sensitive test for ACL insufficiency. The client rests in a relaxed supine position with the injured knee flexed at 15 to 30 degrees. Placing one hand around the client's distal thigh and the other around the client's proximal tibia, the physician attempts anterior-posterior translation. The test result is positive when anterior-posterior sliding occurs. Routine radiographs may also be used for diagnosis of ACL injury, but the MRI is especially sensitive and specific for difficult cases. Arthroscopy, the most important advance in the diagnosis of knee disorders, can enable the physician to confirm the degree of ACL damage and determine the extent of associated intra-articular injuries. Arthroscopy is also the surgical treatment of choice for ACL reconstruction.

Initial treatment focuses on decreasing pain and swelling and on protecting the joint from further injury by immobilization. ACL reconstruction can be accomplished within several weeks of injury and still allow a return of joint function and stability. Repair is often accomplished with the use of a portion of the client's patellar tendon. After ACL reconstruction, the surgeon often orders the use of a continuous passive motion (CPM) machine to help the client achieve rapid, satisfactory knee mobility. The CPM machine is generally applied in the recovery area and should be used at least 8 hours a day or until full range of motion is achieved. Some surgeons advocate the use of a long leg brace with fixed knee flexion, either alone or in combination with the CPM machine. After ACL reconstruction, the client receives instructions on performance of isometric exercises such as quadriceps setting, bent-knee leg exercises, and foot exercises. The exercise program is progressed over the next 4 to 6 weeks.

MENISCAL INJURIES

The meniscus is the fibrous cartilage that lies on top of the tibia, between the tibia and the femur, and acts as the

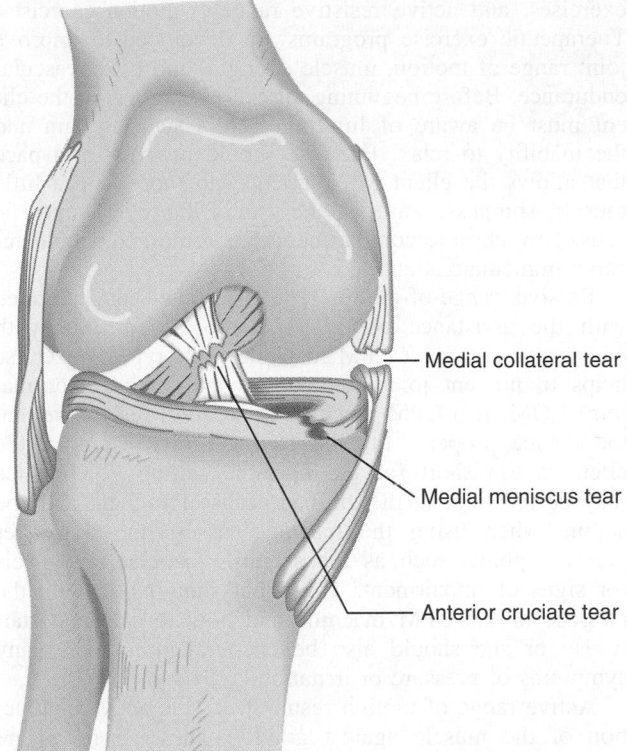

FIGURE 27–10 Common knee injuries: medial collateral tear, commonly caused by inversion and twisting. Anterior cruciate ligament injury, commonly caused by twisting a hyperextended knee. Medial meniscal injury, commonly caused by twisting an everted knee.

shock absorber of the knee. It is torn less frequently than the ACL, but most longitudinal tears of the meniscus occur in conjunction with ACL or medial collateral ligament injuries (Fig. 27–10). Because the meniscus has very little blood supply, it heals very slowly, if at all, after injury.

Meniscal injuries often result from fixed-foot rotation in weight-bearing with the knee flexed. A combination of compression and rotational forces are thus exerted on the meniscus. Mild swelling may be evident, and the client may complain of joint-line pain. Popping, slipping, catching, or buckling of the knee can also occur, particularly if a piece of the cartilage is torn and floating within the knee capsule. Routine radiographs are usually normal, although some spurring may be evident if the tear has been present for a long time. Arthrography enables the physician to diagnose posterior tears, but MRI is a more sensitive and specific procedure for reliable diagnosis. Arthroscopy has an additional advantage as both a diagnostic and treatment option. After surgery, the leg is elevated and ice is applied. Effective pain management is an initial priority. An exercise program includes quadriceps strengthening and range of motion for the knee.

REMOBILIZATION AFTER TRAUMATIC INJURY

Strategies for remobilization include therapeutic exercise, use of CPM machines, passive and active range-of-motion exercises, and active resistive range-of-motion exercises. Therapeutic exercise programs are developed to improve joint range of motion, muscle strength, and cardiovascular endurance. Before beginning an exercise program, the client must be aware of limiting factors such as pain and the inability to relax. Exercise should progress at a pace that allows the client to experience no more than a little muscle soreness. Pain in the exercising client may be caused by chronic compartment syndrome and should receive immediate attention.

Passive range-of-motion exercises can be performed with the assistance of a therapist or a nurse or with equipment such as a CPM machine. This type of exercise helps to prevent joint contractures and maintain normal joint ROM. If a CPM machine is ordered, make sure that the device properly fits the client. If, for example, the client is too short for the machine settings, the device may be too tight in the groin. Because the client must be supine when using the machine, assess the skin over pressure points such as the sacrum, scapulae, and heels for signs of impairment. The client should be taught the purpose of the CPM machine and how to stop and start it. He or she should also be encouraged to report any symptoms of pressure or irritation.

Active range of motion results from the active contraction of the muscle against gravity. These exercises are part of a program that increases muscle strength and endurance. Examples include straight-leg raises and knee flexion and extension when the client is in a sitting position. In active assistive range of motion, the therapist, a mechanical device, or the opposite extremity provides an external force to the affected extremity during joint motion. This type of exercise is often a second step in rehabilitation. It includes isotonic exercise, such as weight lifting, or isokinetic exercise through use of equipment such as Cybex machines.

Difficulties with ambulation can occur as a result of disorders of the musculoskeletal, nervous, and cardiovascular systems. Cognitive awareness, balance, and coordination are also important for safe walking. After an orthopedic injury, the client should ambulate as soon as possible. The client who has been bedridden even for brief periods may exhibit muscle atrophy and weakness, decreased endurance and cardiovascular fitness, and decreased joint flexibility. Orthostatic hypotension is also common after bed rest. A gradual progression of exercise is needed to remobilize the client. Bed exercises may be the first intervention. If the client has been on extended bed rest, a tilt table can be used to assist him or her to an upright position.

Be aware of the client's weight-bearing status before attempting to assist with ambulation. The degree of protected weight-bearing is determined by the physician on the basis of the client's injury and any surgical procedure. Ambulatory assistive devices such as canes, a walker, or crutches can be used as needed.

CONCLUSIONS

Musculoskeletal trauma ranges from simple strains or sprains to complex, life-threatening injuries. Your role is to promote early mobility, prevent possible complications, and teach the client how to prevent further injury.

THINKING CRITICALLY

1. **A young college student arrives in the emergency department holding his arm close to his body. His wrist is obviously misshapen, but swelling is minimal. He tells you he was playing basketball with friends and hit the gym wall after running toward the goal to attempt a lay-up shot. He complains of pain with attempted flexion or rotation of the wrist. A radiograph confirms a wrist fracture, and cast application is planned. What intervention should receive priority? What teaching about cast care should be completed?**

Factors to Consider. How should you relieve the client's pain? What is involved in the healing process for a fracture? What complications might the client face because of the cast?

2. **Friends of a 22-year-old woman assist her into the doctor's office. She twisted her knee on the pitcher's mound during a competitive softball game and says she heard a popping sound. Swelling over her knee is significant. The client states that her knee buckled when she attempted to walk off the field. What is your priority for care? What will be the long-range care goals?**

Factors to Consider. What is the initial treatment for this type of injury? What postoperative treatments will be ordered?

3. **An 80-year-old woman is brought to the nursing unit to await surgical repair of a femoral neck fracture. She is mildly confused. A neighbor says he found her on her kitchen floor after an apparent fall. What assessments should be performed on an ongoing basis? What will be the treatment goals after ORIF of the fracture?**

Factors to Consider. What possible complications could result after hip fracture? How can they be prevented?

BIBLIOGRAPHY

1. Alonso, J. E. (1996). Pelvic and acetabulum fractures. In V. R. Masear (Ed.), *Primary care orthopaedics* (pp. 63–71). Philadelphia: W. B. Saunders.
2. Anders, R. L., & Ornellas, E. M. (1997). Acute management of patients with hip fracture: A research literature review. *Orthopaedic Nursing, 16*(2), 21–46.
3. Bonatz, E. (1996). Bone and soft tissue injuries of the hand. In V. R. Masear (Ed.), *Primary care orthopaedics* (pp. 185–198). Philadelphia: W. B. Saunders.
4. Bonatz, E. (1996). Overuse syndromes: Overuse syndromes of the hand and wrist. In V. R. Masear (Ed.), *Primary care orthopaedics* (pp. 246–249). Philadelphia: W. B. Saunders.
5. Bryant, G. G. (1998). Modalities for immobilization. In A. B. Maher, S. W. Salmond, & T. A. Pellino (Eds.), *Orthopaedic nursing* (2nd ed., pp. 296–350). Philadelphia: W. B. Saunders.
6. Buddenberg, L. A., & Schkade, J. K. (1998). Special feature: A comparison of occupational therapy intervention approaches for older patients after hip fracture. *Topics in Geriatric Rehabilitation, 13*(4), 52–68.
7. Cailliet, R. (1996). *Soft tissue pain and disability* (3rd ed.). Philadelphia: F. A. Davis.
8. Ceccio, C. M. (1999). Key concepts in the care of patients in traction. In *An introduction to orthopaedic nursing* (2nd ed., pp. 45–60). Pitman, NJ: National Association of Orthopaedic Nurses.

9. Childs, S. G. (1998). Anatomy and physiology of the musculoskeletal system. In A. B. Maher, S. W. Salmond, & T. A. Pellino (Eds.), *Orthopaedic nursing* (2nd ed., pp. 145–267). Philadelphia: W. B. Saunders.

10. Conklin, M. J. (1996). Orthopaedic evaluation. In V. R. Masear (Ed.), *Primary care orthopaedics* (pp. 1–34). Philadelphia: W. B. Saunders.

11. Cooper, C., & Campion, G. (1992). Hip fractures in the elderly: A world-wide projection. *Osteoporosis International, 2,* 285–289.

12. Eckhouse-Ekeberg, D. R. (1999). Care of the patient with an external ambulatory device. In *An introduction to orthopaedic nursing* (2nd ed., pp. 31–43). Pitman, NJ: National Association of Orthopaedic Nurses.

13. Fisher, M., & Mowatt, M. Fractured neck of femur: The role of the nurse. (1997). *Nursing Times, 93*(24), 5–8.

14. Fisher, M., & Mowatt, M. Fractured neck of femur: Professional issues. (1997). *Nursing Times, 93*(25), 9–12.

15. Garth, W. P., Jr. (1996). Overuse syndromes: Overuse syndromes of the upper and lower extremities. In V. R. Masear (Ed.), *Primary care orthopaedics* (pp. 236–246). Philadelphia: W. B. Saunders.

16. Hager, C.A., & Brncick, N. (1998). Fat embolism syndrome: A complication of orthopaedic trauma. *Orthopaedic Nursing, 17*(2), 41–46, 58.

17. Herzberg, M. A. (1997). *Osteoporosis independent study.* Pitman, NJ: National Association of Orthopaedic Nurses.

18. Johnson, J., et al. (1995). Roller traction: Mobilizing patients with acetabular fractures. *Orthopaedic Nursing, 14*(1), 21–24.

19. Jonas, G., & Masear, V. R. (1996). Fractures and ligament injuries of the wrist. In V. R. Masear (Ed.), *Primary care orthopaedics* (pp. 169–184). Philadelphia: W. B. Saunders Company.

20. Koval, K. J., et al. (1998). Predictors of functional recovery after hip fracture in the elderly. *Clinical Orthopaedics and Related Research, 348,* 22–28.

21. Lappe, J. M. (1998). Prevention of hip fractures: A nursing imperative. *Orthopaedic Nursing, 17*(3), 15–23.

22. Lee, D. H. (1996). Fractures and dislocations of the shoulder. In V. R. Masear (Ed.), *Primary care orthopaedics* (pp. 42–155). Philadelphia: W. B. Saunders.

23. Lee, D. H. (1996). Fractures of the forearm. In V. R. Masear (Ed.), *Primary care orthopaedics* (pp. 165–168). Philadelphia: W. B. Saunders.

24. Lee, D. H. (1996). Injuries to the humerus and elbow. In V. R. Masear (Ed.), *Primary care orthopaedics* (pp. 156–164). Philadelphia: W. B. Saunders.

25. Maher, A. B. (1996). Trauma. In S. W. Salmond, N. E. Mooney, & L. A. Verdisco (Eds.), *Core curriculum for orthopaedic nursing* (3rd ed., pp. 415–449). Pitman, NJ: National Association of Orthopaedic Nurses.

26. Masear, V. R. (1996). Fractures and dislocations of the foot. In V. R. Masear (Ed.), *Primary care orthopaedics* (pp. 128–141). Philadelphia: W. B. Saunders.

27. McAndrew, M. (1996). The treatment of geriatric hip fractures. *Topics in Geriatric Rehabilitation, 12*(1), 32–37.

28. Miller, J., et al. (1996). A study of discomfort and confusion among elderly surgical patients. *Orthopaedic Nursing, 15*(6), 27–34.

29. Morris, N. S. (1999). Complications associated with orthopaedic surgery. In *An introduction to orthopaedic nursing* (2nd ed., pp. 123–145). Pitman, NJ: National Association of Orthopaedic Nurses.

30. National Association of Orthopaedic Nurses. (1993). *The impact of orthopaedic conditions on the health and economy of the United States.* Pitman, NJ: Author.

31. Nye, P. J. (1996). Complications. In S. W. Salmond, N. E. Mooney, & L. A. Verdisco (Eds.), *Core curriculum for orthopaedic nursing* (3rd ed., pp. 147–163). Pitman, NJ: National Association of Orthopaedic Nurses.

32. Orwoll, E., & Klein, R. (1995). Osteoporosis in men. *Endocrine Review, 16,* 87–166.

33. Pellino, T. A., et al. (1998). Complications of orthopaedic disorders and orthopaedic surgery. In A. B. Maher, S. W. Salmond, & T. A. Pellino (Eds.), *Orthopaedic nursing* (2nd ed., pp. 212–295). Philadelphia: W. B. Saunders.

34. Rauscher, N. A. (1996). Musculoskeletal assessment. In S. W. Salmond, N. E. Mooney, & L. A. Verdisco (Eds.), *Core curriculum for orthopaedic nursing* (3rd ed., pp. 25–57). Pitman, NJ: National Association of Orthopaedic Nurses.

35. Roberts, D. (1999). Introduction to bone: Structure and function, fractures, and osteoporosis. In *An introduction to orthopaedic nursing* (2nd ed., pp. 3–16). Pitman, NJ: National Association of Orthopedic Nurses.

36. Rockwood, C., et al. (1996). *Fractures in adults* (4th ed.). Philadelphia: Lippincott-Raven.

37. Slauenwhite, C. A., & Simpson, P. (1998). Patient and family perspectives on early discharge and care of the older adult undergoing fractured hip rehabilitation. *Orthopaedic Nursing, 17*(1), 30–36.

38. Snyder, P. E. (1998). Fractures. In A. B. Maher, S. W. Salmond, & T. A. Pellino (Eds.), *Orthopaedic nursing* (2nd ed., pp. 663–717). Philadelphia: W. B. Saunders.

39. Stephenson, S. (1996). Fractures and ligamentous injuries of the knee: Fractures about the adult knee. In V. R. Masear (Ed.), *Primary care orthopaedics* (pp. 106–109). Philadelphia: W. B. Saunders.

40. Taggart, H. M. (1999). Caring for the elderly hip fracture patient. In *An introduction to orthopaedic nursing* (2nd ed., pp. 113–122). Pitman, NJ: National Association of Orthopedic Nurses.

41. Thompson, D. (1996). Therapeutic modalities. In S.W. Salmond, N.E. Mooney, & L.A. Verdisco (Eds.), *Core curriculum for orthopaedic nursing* (3rd ed., pp. 187–209). Pitman, NJ: National Association of Orthopaedic Nurses.

42. Whittington, C. F. (1998). Exercise- and sport-related disorders. In A.B. Maher, S.W. Salmond, & T. A. Pellino (Eds.), *Orthopaedic nursing* (2nd ed., pp. 746–768). Philadelphia: W. B. Saunders.

43. Williams, M. A., et al. (1996). Family caregiving in cases of hip fracture. *Rehabilitation Nursing, 21*(3), 124–138.

44. Wolinsky, F. D., Fitzgerald, J.F., & Stump, T.E. (1997). The effect of hip fracture on mortality, hospitalization, and functional status: A prospective study. *American Journal of Public Health, 87*(3), 398–403.

45. Zuckerman, J. D., et al. (1995). Postoperative complications and mortality associated with operative delay in older patients who have a fracture of the hip. *Journal of Bone and Joint Surgery, American Volume, 77*(10), 1551–1556.

Falls Among the Elderly

QUESTIONS
What factors predict falls among older adults?
What preventive interventions do these factors support?

CITATION
Rawsky, E. (1998). Review of the literature on falls among the elderly. *Image: Journal of Nursing Scholarship, 30*, 47–52.

STUDIES

More than 100 studies published between 1979 and 1996 were included in the analysis of this review. They were identified using a *MEDLINE* search; however, how the studies came to be included or excluded from the review analysis was not explained in the report. Many of the studies consisted of retrospective chart reviews, although some prospectively compared adults who had previously fallen with those who had not (i.e., a control group). The review includes studies of falls in hospitals, homes, extended-care facilities, and nursing homes.

Summary of Findings

Intrinsic Factors

Risk factors for falls can be classified as *intrinsic* (characteristics of individuals) or *extrinsic* (contextual and environmental in nature). Cognitive impairment and sensory deficit have been implicated in a few studies. In 16 studies, cognitive impairment was found to be associated with falls; in seven studies, sensory deficit was associated. A study of specific cognitive impairments and falling implicated poor problem-solving, general anxiety, and attention deficits.[15]

Another grouping of associated factors is mobility, gait, and balance problems; in 14 studies, at least one of them was found to be associated with falling. Other associated factors include a fall history (six studies), elimination patterns (six studies), and postural hypotension (four studies). It is not clear whether increased age itself should be considered a risk factor, although "older elderly" people experience more adverse sequelae from falls compared with "younger elderly" persons.[17, 19] Men have a higher incidence of falling than women,[3, 9] although the one study with a control group revealed that gender did not make a difference.[12]

An interesting issue is the extent to which falls result in injury.[7, 17, 20] A prospective, case-controlled study of community-dwelling elders found that falls occurring while a person was turning were more likely to result in a hip fracture.[4] One study found that women are more at risk than men for hip fracture as a result of falling.[21] In turn, hip fracture often leads to death, particularly in people over age 75.

Extrinsic Factors

Changes in physiologic adaptive abilities (such as balance, proprioception, and vestibular stability) make compensation for environmental irregularities more difficult.[1, 21] Hazards include poor lighting, slippery or uneven flooring, objects in path, stairs, and steps.[20] High-gloss floors have been associated with falling, and vinyl flooring is more likely to result in injury compared with carpeted surfaces.[7] A somewhat unexpected finding is that environmental hazards may be more likely to contribute to falls in elders who are in better health than in their more frail counterparts.[2, 13]

Ironically, assistive devices can actually contribute to falls.[12, 21]; mechanical restraints do not appear to reduce the incidence of falls and may actually worsen outcomes.[5, 6, 8, 22] The extent to which staffing patterns and assignments affect the incidence of falls is uncertain, although in one hospital study a discrepancy between recommended and actual hours of staffing contributed to an increased number of falls.[24] Moreover, several studies have found that patients who had fallen had not asked for help.[26]

Interventions

"Anticipatory nursing" (e.g., routine assistance with toileting, and offering assistance for future activities rather than waiting for patients to ask for help) appears effective in reducing the frequency of falling.[3, 18] Providing appropriate footware[14] and treaded slipper socks can reduce the incidence of falls.[11] Various types of exercise programs, particularly those aimed at muscle strengthening and improving balance, have been effective in reducing the incidence of falls in older people in the community and in nursing homes.[10, 16, 23] Two studies have documented the benefits of *Tai Chi*, an ancient Chinese exercise form, in reducing falls.[16, 25]

Limitations Reservations: This review did not examine the effectiveness of assessment tools for fall risk and did not comprehensively address interventions to reduce the risk of falling or programs to prevent falls. There is considerable research on preventing falls among community-dwelling elders but much less among older people in hospitals and nursing homes. The most recent studies included in the review are from 1996.

Research-Based Practice

At the individual practice level, nurses should know how to assess clients for the presence of risk factors related to falling; these assessments should be done at the time of admission and whenever the client's condition changes. The cognitive part of this assessment should go beyond orientation to time, place, and person to include the abilities to problem-solve and to pay attention to tasks at hand; general anxiety should also serve as a "red flag" for fall risk. Assessing the person's balance, gait, vision, and hearing and identifying people with frequent or urgent urination or bowel needs are also important in identifying those at risk.

Once a person is identified as being at risk because of the presence of several of the factors just discussed, you will be able to decide on the appropriate level of intervention. Simple anticipatory actions, such as readily available call lights, assurances that you want to be called to help them get up, and uncluttered pathways to the bathroom (the most frequent destination), all help prevent falls. Wiping up liquids or urine on the

Falls Among the Elderly *Continued*

floor is another simple but effective action. Low bed positions and treaded slipper socks also help.

For higher-risk clients, bed alarms or door alarms can alert the staff that the client is getting up without assistance or is moving around. Another intervention for high-risk patients would be referral to physical therapy for gait and balance training.

At the institutional level, the physical characteristics of the environment can help lower the risk of falls and fall injuries. Good lighting, grab bars in bathrooms, handrails in halls (not blocked by equipment), and unslippery floor surfaces may help reduce adverse outcomes from falls. The maintenance of and use of wheel locks on over-bed tables and bedside cabinets also play a role because patients may lean on them, not realizing that the furniture is on wheels and will move. The choice of side rails is critical because their design can protect patients from falls or can increase the likelihood of their occurrence.

In all settings, prevention of falls is very effective when an organized fall prevention program is in place.[3, 18] Such a program can identify clients at risk and can set forth measures to be put in place. Intervention algorithms are helpful, providing quick guides to the measures that should be activated.

Some clients who have not exhibited any risk factors may fall, just as some who have several risk factors may not fall. Still, risk factors are useful in identifying those at risk for a fall. These risk factors cannot be converted to a simple formula, but you can keep in mind the many factors that are associated with falls and enact an individualized package of several interventions.

Cited References

1. Adler-Traines, J. (1994). Falls in the senior population. *Physical Therapy Forum, 9*, 14–17.
2. Baldwin, R., Craven, R., & Diamond, M. (1996). Falls: Are rural elders at greater risk? *Journal of Gerontological Nursing, 22*(8), 14–21.
3. Brady, R., et al. (1993). Geriatric Falls: Prevention strategies for the staff. *Journal of Gerontological Nursing, 19*(9), 26–32.
4. Cumming, R., & Klineberg, R. (1994). Fall frequency and characteristics and the risk of hip fractures. *Journal of American Geriatrics Society, 42*, 774–778.
5. Evans, L., & Strumpf, N. (1990). Myths about elder restraint. *Image: Journal of Nursing Scholarship, 22*, 124–128.
6. Gaebler, S. (1993). Predicting which patients will fall again . . . and again. *Journal of Advanced Nursing, 18*, 1895–1902.
7. Healey, F. (1994). Does flooring type affect risk of injury in older inpatients? *Nursing Times, 90*, 40–41.
8. Janken, J., Reynolds, B., & Swiech, K. (1986). Patient falls in the acute care setting: Identifying risk factors. *Nursing Research, 35*, 215–219.
9. Kilpack, V., Boehm, J., & Smith, N. (1991). Using research-based interventions to decrease patient falls. *Applied Nursing Research, 4*, 50–56.
10. McNeely, E., Clements, S., & Wolf, S. (1992). A program to reduce frailty in the elderly. In S. Funk, et al. (Eds.), *Key aspects of elder care* (pp. 89–96). New York: Springer.
11. Meddaugh, D., Friedenberg, D., & Knisley, R. (1996). Special socks for special people: Falls in special care units. *Geriatric Nursing, 17*, 24–26.
12. Morse, J., Tylko, S., & Dixon, H. (1987). Characteristics of the fall prone patient. *The Gerontologist, 27*, 516–522.
13. Northridge, M., et al. (1995). Home hazards and falls in the elderly: The role of health and functional status. *American Journal of Public Health, 85*, 509–515.
14. Orhon-Jech, A. (1992). Preventing falls in the elderly. *Geriatric Nursing, 34*, 43–44.
15. Persad, C., et al. (1995). Neuropsychological predictors of complex obstacle avoidance in healthy older adults. *Journal of Gerontology, Series B, Psychological Sciences & Social Sciences, 50*(5), P272–P277.
16. Province, M., et al. (1995). The effects of exercise on falls in elderly patients: A preplanned meta-analysis of the FICSIT trials. *Journal of the American Medical Association, 273*, 1341–1347.
17. Rhymes, J., & Jaeger, R. (1988). Falls: Prevention and management in the institutional setting. *Clinics in Geriatric Medicine, 4*, 613–622.
18. Ruckstuhl, M., et al. (1991). Patient falls: An outcome indicator. *Journal of Nursing Care Quality, 6*, 25–29.
19. Sattin, R. (1992). Falls among older persons: A public health perspective. *Annual Review of Public Health, 13*, 489–508.
20. Shroyer, J. (1994). Recommendations for environmental design research correlating falls and the physical environment. *Experimental Aging Research 20*, 303–309.
21. Tideiksaar, R. (1993). Falls in older persons. *Mount Sinai Journal of Medicine, 60*, 515–521.
22. Tinetti, M., Liu, W., & Ginter, S. (1992). Mechanical restraint usage and fall-related injuries among residents of skilled nursing facilities. *Annals of Internal Medicine, 116*, 369–374.
23. Tinetti, M., et al. (1994). A multifactorial intervention to reduce the risk of falling among elderly people living in the community. *New England Journal of Medicine, 331*, 821–827.
24. Whedon, M., & Shedd, P. (1989). Prediction and prevention of patient falls. *Image: Journal of Nursing Scholarship, 21*, 108–114.
25. Wolf, S. et al. (1993). The Atlanta FICSIT study: Two exercise interventions to reduce frailty in elders. *Journal of the American Geriatrics Society, 41*, 329–332.
26. Wright, B., et al. (1990). Frequent fallers: Leading groups to identify psychological factors. *Journal of Gerontological Nursing, 16*(4), 15–19.

Sarah Jo Brown, PhD, RN, *Principal and Consultant, Practice-Research Integrations, Norwich, Vermont*

UNIT
6

Nutritional Disorders

Anatomy and Physiology Review: The Nutritional (Gastrointestinal) System

28 Assessment of Nutrition and the Digestive System

29 Management of Clients with Malnutrition

30 Management of Clients with Ingestive Disorders

31 Management of Clients with Digestive Disorders

Anatomy and Physiology Review
The Nutritional (Gastrointestinal) System

Robert G. Carroll

The nutritional or gastrointestinal (GI) system is a long, hollow tube that passes through the body, providing an isolated environment for digestion and absorption of nutrients. Ingested contents pass sequentially through the following structures: mouth, esophagus, stomach, small intestine (duodenum, jejunum, and ileum), and large intestine (colon), before exiting the body at the anus.

GI tract function is regulated by a complex series of neural, hormonal, and local control systems. The *enteric nervous system* integrates motor and secretory activities along the GI tract. Ganglia have sensory neurons that respond to temperature, chemical agents, and mechanical deformation. Ganglia also have effector neurons to smooth muscle, secretory cells, endocrine cells, and autocrine cells. GI secretion and motility are enhanced by parasympathetic activity and inhibited by sympathetic activity.

GI hormones, which control and integrate both motility and secretion, are distributed in the stomach and small intestine. GI hormones are also important trophic factors, stimulating proliferation of the GI tract to enhance absorptive capacity.

Finally, the GI tract has an extensive *immune system.* Gut-associated lymphoid tissue (GALT) may account for up to 80% of the immunoglobulin-producing cells in the body. These cells are important because of the intimate association of the GI system and the "outside environment," the chyme in the lumen of the GI tract.

STRUCTURE OF THE GASTROINTESTINAL SYSTEM

In cross-section, the GI tract generally has four distinct layers (Fig. U6–1). The innermost layer is the *mucosa,* where epithelial cells contact ingested food. The mucosa often has microvilli to increase the surface area available for absorption. Beneath the mucosa is the *submucosa (lamina propria),* containing glands, blood vessels, and lymph nodules. Next is a *muscular layer,* with smooth muscle oriented either circularly or longitudinally. The outermost layer is the *connective tissue serosa layer.*

The entrance (mouth, upper esophagus) and exit (external anal sphincter) of the GI tract contain GI-associated skeletal muscle, which is partially under voluntary control. The remainder of the GI tract (Fig. U6–2) has smooth muscle, under involuntary control. GI smooth muscle is electrically connected by gap junctions, allowing a wave of depolarization and contraction to spread along the tract (see Motility).

Food is chewed (*masticated*), mixed with saliva in the mouth, and swallowed. It passes through the pharynx and into the *esophagus.* The upper third of esophagus has striated (voluntary) muscle, the middle third has both types of muscle, and the lower third has only smooth muscle. The vagus nerve innervates both the smooth and skeletal muscle of the esophagus. Sphincters isolate the esophagus from the remainder of the GI tract. The upper esophageal sphincter prevents entry of tracheal air, and the lower esophageal sphincter prevents reflux of gastric contents (*aspiration*). Acute failure of the lower esophageal sphincter causes *esophagitis* (heartburn), and chronic gastric reflux causes digestion of the esophagus. The opposite problem, *achalasia,* occurs if the lower esophageal sphincter does not relax sufficiently to allow food to pass into the stomach.

The *stomach* is divided into the *fundus, body,* and *antrum.* The fundus and body are highly distensible, and act as a reservoir for the ingested meal. Food can be stored unmixed in fundus and body for up to 1 hour. During this time, there may be a separation due to density, because fats float to the top and liquids accumulate on the bottom. Thus, liquids are the first to leave the stomach and to be absorbed through the intestine. Gastric contents empty from the antrum through the pylorus into the duodenum. The gastroduodenal junction is important in sequestering acid in the stomach and bile in the duodenum.

The *small intestine* is divided into *duodenum* (25 cm), *jejunum* (2.5 m), and *ileum* (3.6 m). The duodenum and jejunum are the major sites of digestion and absorption. Pancreatic and biliary ducts carry digestive enzymes, bicarbonate, and bile to the lumen of the duodenum. The continuous epithelial cell lining of the small intestine separates luminal contents from the body and provides a barrier across which nutrients must be absorbed. Epithelial cells reproduce rapidly and are lost (exfoliated) at the tip of the microvilli.

Chyme, the nonabsorbed component of the diet, passes through the *ileocecal valve* (a sphincter) to enter the *large intestine.* The large intestine (~1.5 m in length) includes the *cecum* (a pouch where small and large intestines join and from which the appendix projects); the *ascending, transverse, descending,* and *sigmoid colon;* and the *rectum* (anal canal). The large intestine contains mucus-secreting goblet cells and cells specialized for absorption; it lacks villi and does not produce digestive enzymes. An internal sphincter (smooth muscle) and an external sphincter (voluntary muscle) govern the expulsion of feces (defecation).

GASTROINTESTINAL BLOOD SUPPLY AND LYMPHATIC DRAINAGE

Arterial blood enters the GI tract by various branches of major arteries. Venous drainage, however, is unique in

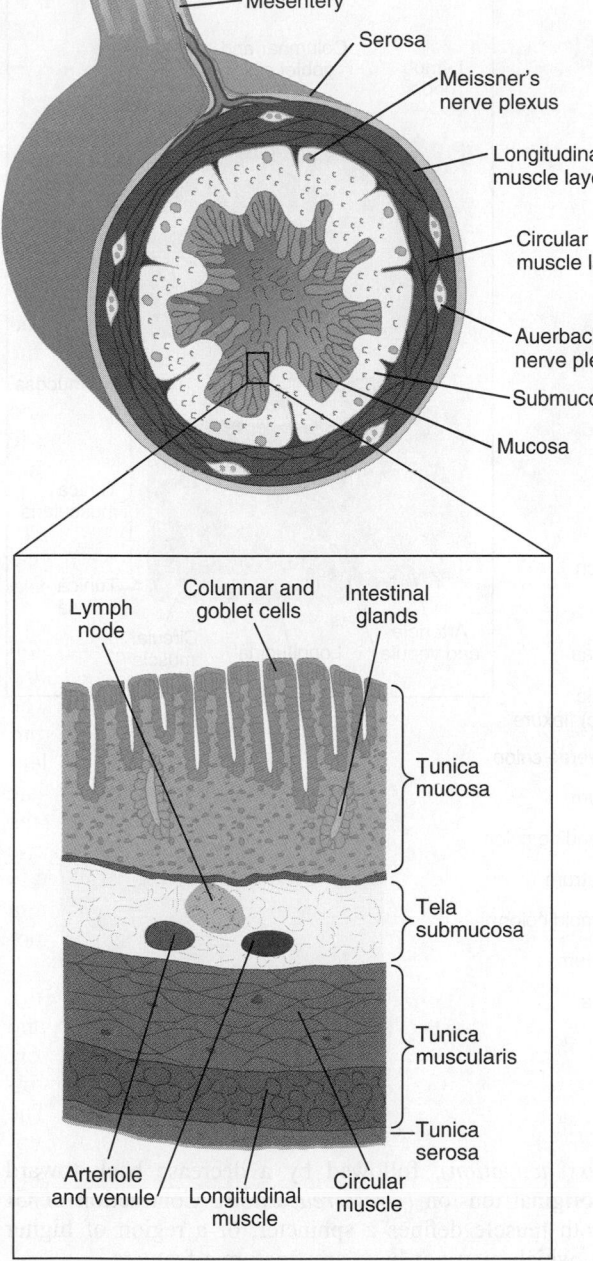

FIGURE U6–1 Typical cross-section of the gastrointestinal tract. *Inset* shows enlargement of a cross-section of the small intestine.

that the veins from the GI tract empty into the hepatic portal vein. Portal venous blood passes through the liver before entering the vena cava. This arrangement allows the liver to begin processing and detoxifying compounds absorbed across the stomach and intestines before those compounds enter the general circulation.

The esophageal arteries, the inferior thyroid artery, and the left gastric artery provide the esophagus with its arterial blood supply. The left gastric and inferior phrenic arteries supply the gastroesophageal area. Venous blood is returned via the azygos, thyroid, and left gastric veins. Lymphatic drainage from the cervical esophagus and from the tracheal and postmediastinal nodes flows to the

internal jugular vein while intercostal nodes drain the thoracic esophagus. The lymphatic drainage of the lower esophagus occurs through the diaphragmatic, intracardiac, and left gastric lymph nodes.

The arterial blood supply to the stomach is derived from the celiac artery, which branches off the lesser and greater curvatures. Gastric arteries, from the splenic artery, supply the fundus. The portal vein provides the venous drainage of the stomach. The right and left gastroepiploic veins drain the greater curvature; the right gastric and coronary veins drain the lesser curvature. Lymph nodes of the stomach arise in the submucosa and drain into the thoracic duct.

Except in the duodenum, arterial blood supply to the small intestine is derived from the superior mesenteric artery. Arterial blood from the hepatic artery supplies the duodenum. Venous drainage is via the superior mesenteric vein, which unites with the inferior mesenteric, splenic, and gastric veins and then empties into the portal system.

NEURAL REGULATION

Enteric Nervous System

The enteric system regulates motility and secretion along the entire length of the GI tract. The enteric nervous system can function independently of the central nervous system (CNS). Enteric reflexes, originating from GI sensory nerves, synapse in either the submucosal plexus or the myenteric plexus. Efferent nerves then supply the smooth muscle or secretory glands. Enteric activity can be modulated by external inputs, particularly by the sympathetic and parasympathetic nerves.

Auerbach's plexus (motor function) and *Meissner's plexus* (sensory function) provide intrinsic innervation for the stomach. Both begin in the esophageal wall and extend the length of the gut. Stimulation of Auerbach's plexus (between the longitudinal and circular muscle layers) generates gastric motility, increasing the intensity and rate of contractions and the release of gastrin from the antrum. *Meissner's plexus* (in the submucosa) functions with Auerbach's plexus to coordinate the motor and secretory activity of the gastric mucosa.

Sympathetic and Parasympathetic Nervous Systems

Sympathetic nerves supplying the GI tract originate in the celiac, superior mesenteric, inferior mesenteric, and hypogastric ganglia. In general, *sympathetics* inhibit activity in enteric plexuses, constrict GI system blood vessels, and decrease glandular secretions. GI motility is also decreased through contraction of circular muscle and certain sphincters, and indirect inhibition of peristalsis.

The vagus is the primary parasympathetic nerve supplying the GI tract, innervating all structures from the salivary glands to the transverse colon. Nerves from the hypogastric plexus innervate the remainder of colon. Parasympathetic postganglionic neurons are located in intramural plexus. In general, *parasympathetics* stimulate motor activity, secretory activity, and endocrine secretions.

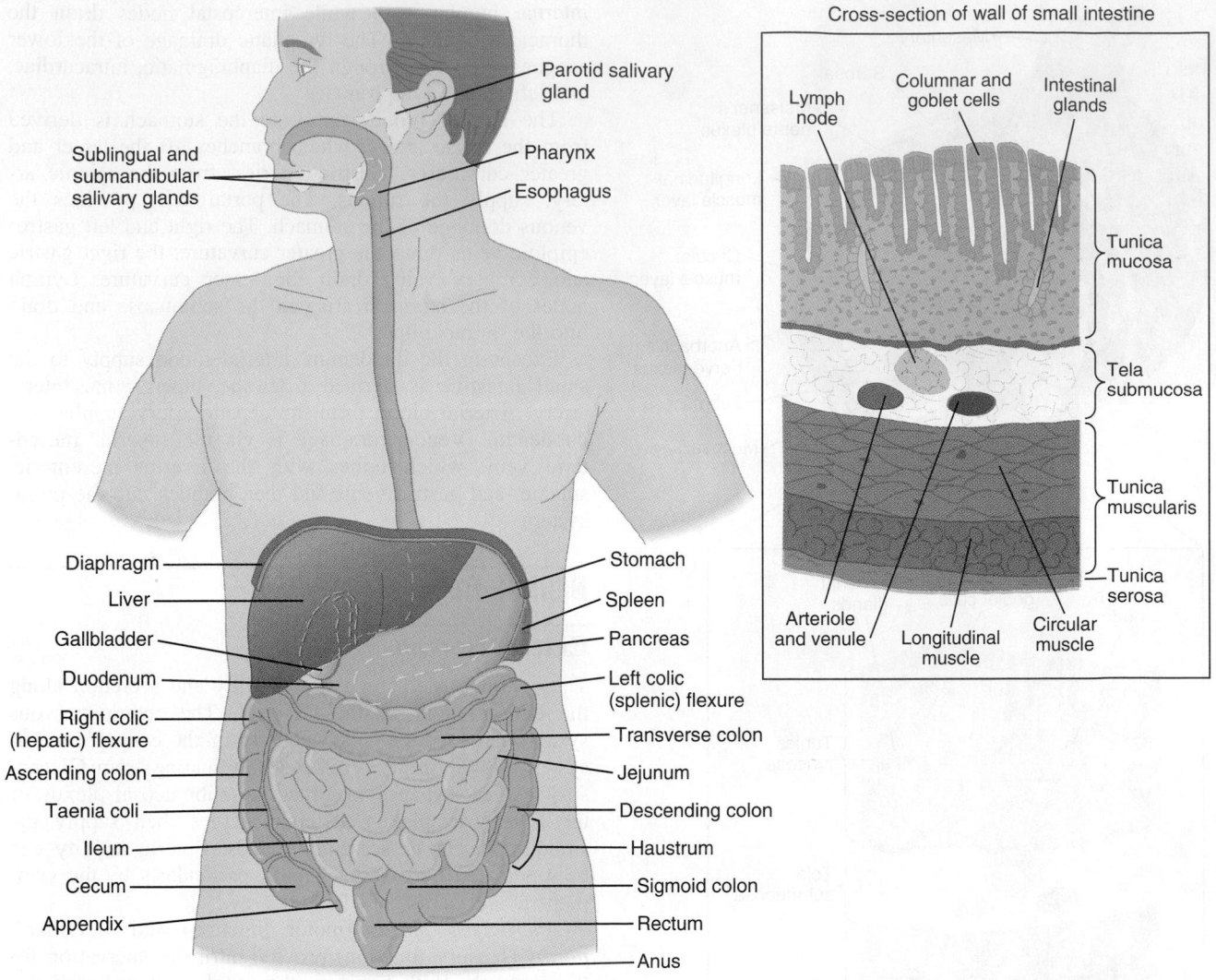

Cross-section of wall of small intestine

FIGURE U6-2 The digestive system.

FUNCTION OF THE GASTROINTESTINAL SYSTEM

The GI system isolates ingested food and provides an environment for digestion and absorption of nutrients. The major functions of the GI tract are (1) motility, (2) secretion, (3) digestion, and (4) absorption.

MOTILITY

Smooth Muscle

Smooth muscle of the GI tract is electrically connected by gap junctions, allowing a wave of depolarization and contraction to spread along the tract. Pacemakers along the length of the GI tract set the slow-wave contraction frequency. Nerves and hormones alter this rate and, therefore, GI motility.

GI smooth muscle produces long, strong contractions. Muscle basal tone provides some tension even at rest and is influenced by neurotransmitters, hormones, and drugs. Stretch of GI system increases action potential frequency

(stress activation), followed by a decrease back toward the original tension *(stress relaxation).* Contraction of GI smooth muscle defines a sphincter, or a region of higher tone, which may not have any anatomic features.

Peristalsis is an organized wave of contraction of the longitudinal muscle layer that propels contents aborally (away from the mouth). Distention of a segment of intestine elicits a reflex contraction. The smooth muscle aboral to the contraction relaxes, and the contents move. This sequence is repeated, and contents are moved for a short distance before the wave diminishes and disappears. A descending wave of peristalsis initiates sphincter relaxation, mediated by vasoactive intestinal peptide (VIP) neurotransmitter in vagal nerves. Decreased vagal cholinergic activity also contributes to relaxation.

Intrinsic motility regulation uses interneurons to coordinate activity. The enteric nervous system has neuromodulators, similar to those in the brain. Intrinsic plexuses inhibit basal activity, and action potentials are thus elicited by fewer than half of the slow waves.

Contractions of the various layers of smooth muscle propel and mix luminal contents. Peristaltic contraction of the longitudinal muscle layer accomplishes aboral movement. Contraction of circular muscle mixes luminal contents (chyme) and increases contact with microvilli.

MOUTH TO ESOPHAGUS. The process of moving food from the mouth into the esophagus is illustrated in Figure U6–3. The esophageal phase of swallowing is involuntary. Contraction of the upper esophageal sphincter isolates the pharynx from the esophagus. A primary peristaltic wave, controlled by the swallowing center,

moves food through esophagus in 10 seconds. Secondary peristalsis is initiated by esophageal distention (enteric nervous system); it propels any food still remaining in the esophagus into the stomach.

STOMACH. Gastric contractions after feeding occur at a rate of three per minute. They begin in the middle of the body, increasing in force and velocity as they approach the antrum. The antrum produces strong contractions that fragment food into smaller particles and mix it

1.

ORAL PHASE (VOLUNTARY)

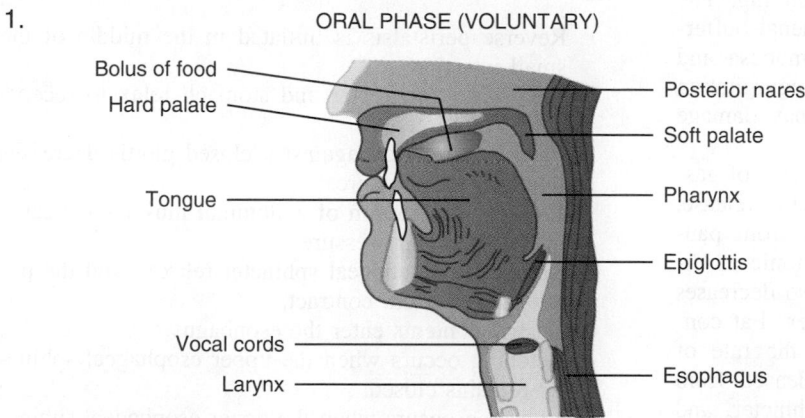

- Bolus of food
- Hard palate
- Tongue
- Vocal cords
- Larynx
- Posterior nares
- Soft palate
- Pharynx
- Epiglottis
- Esophagus

FIGURE U6–3 Swallowing occurs in three phases: (1) *Voluntary* or *oral* phase. The tongue presses food against the hard palate, forcing it toward the pharynx. (2) *Involuntary, pharyngeal* phase. *Early:* wave of peristalsis forces bolus between tonsillar pillars. *Middle:* Soft palate draws upward to close posterior nares, and respirations cease momentarily. *Late:* vocal cords approximate and larynx pulls upward, covering the airway and stretching the esophagus open. (3) *Involuntary, esophageal* phase. Relaxation of the upper esophageal (hypopharyngeal) sphincter allows a peristaltic wave to move the bolus down the esophagus.

2.

PHARYNGEAL PHASE (INVOLUNTARY)

Early   Middle   Late

3.

ESOPHAGEAL PHASE (INVOLUNTARY)

- Bolus of food in esophagus
- Contracted muscle
- Bolus of food in esophagus
- Peristalsis
- Relaxed muscle

with gastric secretions to initiate digestion. The rate of contractions is increased by gastrin and decreased by secretin. Sensory afferents from the stomach play a role in satiety. Increased intragastic pressure, gastric distention, gastric acidity, and pain all lessen the desire to ingest food.

GASTRODUODENAL JUNCTION. Gastric contents empty into the duodenal bulb at a controlled rate. The pylorus and terminal end of antrum contract almost simultaneously *(systolic contraction),* allowing only a small amount of antral content to enter duodenum. The remainder of antral contraction moves antral contents backward *(retropulsion)* and causes further mixing. The rate of gastric emptying must match the duodenal buffering ability, or acid may damage duodenal mucosa and cause duodenal ulcers. The pylorus prevents regurgitation of duodenal contents into stomach, or bile may damage stomach mucosa, causing gastric ulcers.

Duodenal acidity (pH < 3.5) decreases the rate of gastric emptying. A neural reflex causes secretin release, which increases bicarbonate buffer secretion from pancreas and liver. Chyme becomes more hypertonic as digestion progresses. Duodenal hypertonicity also decreases the rate of gastric emptying by a neural reflex. Fat content in the duodenal chyme also decreases the rate of gastric emptying. Cholecystokinin (CCK) released from duodenum and jejunum contracts pyloric sphincter, and glucose-dependent insulinotropic peptide (GIP) may also have a role. Fatty acids (especially long-chain and unsaturated) decrease the rate of gastric emptying. Monoglycerides increase contractility of pyloric sphincter. Amino acids (tryptophan) and peptides in duodenum slow gastric emptying by promoting gastrin release, which constricts the pylorus.

SMALL INTESTINE. Peristalsis moves chyme aborally an average of 10 cm per contraction, and chyme takes 2 to 4 hours to move the 6 meters. *Segmentation,* the most frequent type of intestinal contraction, can be rhythmic, with adjacent sites alternating contraction and relaxation. Eating actually slows aboral movement of chyme. The enteric nervous system controls the frequency of segmentation and peristalsis. An intrinsic rate of 11 to 13 contractions per minute exists in the duodenum, which declines to eight to nine per minute in the terminal ileum. This rate is modified by extrinsic neural and hormonal inputs.

MIGRATING MYOELECTRIC COMPLEX. The migrating myoelectric complex generates periods of intense electrical activity, followed by long quiescent periods. The resulting contractions, initiated in stomach, traverse the entire small intestine. There is evidence for both vagal and hormonal (motilin) role in initiation, and the enteric nervous system is required for propagation. This process sweeps the intestines clean and inhibits the retrograde movement of bacteria from colon into the small intestine.

LARGE INTESTINE. Although chyme may move through the small intestine in 2 to 4 hours, it takes 1 to 3 days to complete its passage through the large intestine. Here sodium and water are absorbed. Bacteria consume more nutrients and release some vitamins (e.g., vitamin K). Solid wastes (sloughed epithelial cells, bile pigments, unabsorbed food) are prepared for elimination as feces. Abnormally fast movement of chyme through the large

intestine results in diarrhea; abnormally slow movement results in constipation. Inflammation of the appendix *(appendicitis)* can lead to peritonitis and other complications.

Vomiting

Vomiting expels gastric (and sometimes duodenal) contents by mouth. Retching, an action in which gastric contents are forced into the esophagus, but not the pharynx, precedes vomiting. The vomiting reflex follows a set pattern:

1. Reverse peristalsis is initiated in the middle of the small intestine.
2. The pyloric sphincter and stomach relax to receive duodenal contents.
3. Forced inspiration against a closed glottis decreases intrathoracic pressure.
4. Forceful contraction of abdominal muscles increases intra-abdominal pressure.
5. The lower esophageal sphincter relaxes, and the pylorus and antrum contract.
6. Gastric contents enter the esophagus.
7. Retching occurs when the upper esophageal sphincter remains closed.
8. Vomiting occurs when the upper esophageal sphincter opens.
9. The trachea closes, as in normal swallowing, to prevent aspiration.

The medulla has a separate vomiting center and retching center that normally interact. Afferent inputs include stomach and duodenal distention, and pain in the genitourinary system. Dizziness or tickling the back of throat can also induce vomiting. Emetics are used to induce vomiting by stimulating receptors in the stomach and duodenum (ipecac), or by activating a chemoreceptive trigger zone (CTZ) in the area postrema (morphine).

SECRETIONS

Most ingested food cannot be absorbed directly. GI secretions digest foods into absorbable components, assist absorption, and help prevent autodigestion (Table U6–1). GI secretions are regulated by a series of hormonal and neural feedback mechanisms. Secretions include lubricants, ions, absorption facilitators, and bile.

Lubricants

Chewing of foods *(mastication)* is the initial step in digestion. Chewing mixes the food with salivary mucus, subdivides food, and exposes starches to salivary amylase. Chewing facilitates the mechanical breakdown of food, but chewing is not an essential component of digestion.

Saliva, with both watery and mucous secretions, helps lubricate food as it enters the GI tract. Mucus-secreting cells are located along the entire GI tract, but digestive secretions are limited to the prejejunal GI tract. Salivary glands contribute about 1.5 L/day into the GI tract. The stomach secretes about 2 L/day, and the pancreas secretes 1.5 L/day, helping to liquify the chyme. The small intestine secretes 1.5 L/day, and the large intestine secretes 400 ml/day. In addition, 0.25 to 1.5 L/day of hepatic secretions enter the duodenum.

Gastric secretions begin protein digestion and protect the gastric epithelium. After a meal, there are three distinct phases of gastric acid secretion.

1. The *cephalic phase* is caused by a neural reflex initiated by the sight, smell, or taste of food. The drop in antral pH acts directly on the parietal calls to attenuate the cephalic phase.
2. The *gastric phase* is due to gastric distention caused by food in the stomach.
3. The *intestinal phase* is initiated by chyme entry into duodenum.

Gastric parietal cell hydrochloric acid (HCl) secretion involves the interplay of acetylcholine, gastrin, histamine, and a second cell type, the enterochromaffin cell. A powerful synergistic interaction between these stimuli causes difficulty in diminishing acid secretion by blocking only one pathway. HCl secretion can be blocked by atropine (acetylcholine) or cimetidine (H_2 histamine), but a

blocker for gastrin is not yet available. Ranitidine is more effective, producing fewer side effects, and is used to treat duodenal ulcers. Gastric ulcers, although associated with increased HCl secretion, involve a gram-negative bacterium, *Helicobacter pylori,* which damages the gastric mucosa. Other agents, such as aspirin and nonsteroidal anti-inflammatory drugs (NSAIDs) can damage the gastric mucosa and cause gastric ulcers.

Absorption Facilitators and Ions

Pancreatic enzymes are essential for the normal absorption of lipids, proteins, and carbohydrates. Table U6–1 lists the important enzymes and ionic pancreatic secretions.

Bile and the Enterohepatic Circulation

Bile acids are secreted by liver as bile, stored in the gallbladder, and released into the duodenum after a meal. Bile acids are reabsorbed by both diffusion and active transport in the terminal ileum and returned to the liver by the he-

TABLE U6–1	GASTROINTESTINAL (GI) SYSTEM–ASSOCIATED SECRETIONS		
Class	**Location**	**Secretion**	**Role**
Lubricants	Entire GI tract	Mucus	Lubricant
	Salivary gland	Water	Lubricant, solvent
	Pancreas	Water	Lubricant
	Small intestine	Water	Lubricant
Digestive enzymes	Salivary glands	Amylase	Digestion of starch
		Lingual lipase	Digestion of triglycerides
	Stomach	Pepsin (pepsinogen)	Digest proteins
		Gastric lipase	Digest triglycerides
	Pancreas	Amylase	Digest starch
		Lipase	Digest triglycerides
		Colipase	Digest triglycerides
		Phospholipase	Digest phospholipods
		Trypsin	Digest peptides
		Chymotrypsin	Digest peptides
		Nucleases	DNA, RNA
	Intestinal epithelium	Disaccharidases	Disaccharides
		Peptidases	Peptides
Hormones and neurotransmitters	Stomach	Gastrin	Hydrochloric acid secretion
	Pancreas	Somatostatin	Inhibition of insulin, glucagon release
	Small intestine	Cholecystokinin	Pancreatic enzyme secretion
		Secretin	Pancreatic bicarbonate secretion
		Glucose-dependent insulinotropic peptide (GIP)	Pancreatic insulin release
		Motilin	GI smooth muscle contraction
		Enteroglucagons	Pancreatic insulin release
Enteric neurons		Vasoactive intestinal peptide (VIP)	GI smooth muscle relaxation Pancreatic secretion
		Bombesin	Gastrin release
Ionic secretions	Salivary glands	Sodium bicarbonate	Alkalinize ingested food
		Potassium chloride	Maintain secretion osmolality
	Stomach parietal cells	Hydrochloric acid	Activation of pepsin
	Mucus cells	Potassium bicarbonate	Protection of stomach from acid
	Pancreas	Sodium bicarbonate	Neutralization of gastric secretion
Absorption facilitators	Stomach	Intrinsic factor	Ileal absorption of vitamin B_{12}
	Liver	Bile acids	Small-intestine lipid absorption

DNA, deoxyribonucleic acid; RNA, ribonucleic acid.

patic portal vein. The liver then actively extracts bile acids from the portal venous blood and secretes the reabsorbed bile acids into bile, beginning the process anew. Only about 15% to 35% of the bile acid pool is lost in feces each day and is replaced by new synthesis of bile acids.

Bile acids are normally secreted conjugated to glycine or taurine and at neutral pH of small intestine are salts (bile salts).

With the sphincter of Oddi at the junction of the bile duct and duodenum normally contracted, bile is diverted to and stored in gallbladder between meals. The gallbladder extracts sodium ions (Na$^+$) actively, anions via electroneutrality, and water osmotically, concentrating bile. CCK is the primary stimulus for the gallbladder to contract (expel contents) into the duodenum. Vagal nerves also contract the gallbladder and relax the sphincter of Oddi, and sympathetics and VIP inhibit gallbladder emptying.

Disorders of bile secretions lead to crystal (stone) formation. Gallstones are primarily cholesterol crystals around a bilirubin crystal core. Bile pigment stones, a calcium salt of unconjugated bilirubin, can also form. If cholesterol content exceeds the dissolving capability of the micelles, cholesterol crystals form and act as a nucleus for gallstones.

DIGESTION AND ABSORPTION

Complex carbohydrates are broken down to absorbable monoglycerides. Poorly absorbed large proteins are broken down into monopeptides, dipeptides, and tripeptides. Pancreatic lipases digest lipids to components, which are absorbed primarily as bile acid micelles.

Carbohydrates
Digestion and absorption of carbohydrates occurs primarily in the duodenum and the jejunum. The ability to absorb carbohydrates greatly exceeds normal dietary intake. Occasionally, an inability to absorb dietary carbohydrates from the diet occurs because of deficiency of digestive enzymes or transport proteins. Microflora metabolize any carbohydrates that pass through to the colon, producing gas, increased motility, and diarrhea. The diagnosis of malabsorption is confirmed by exposure to a specific carbohydrate, such as an oral glucose tolerance test (GTT) or a biopsy of jejunal epithelial cells. Treatment involves dietary restriction or supplemental enzyme ingestion.

One common disorder, lactose malabsorption syndrome *(lactose intolerance),* is a genetic lactase deficiency that affects 50% of adults. This syndrome is almost universal in those of Asian ancestry, common in native Africans and those from Mediterranean areas but infrequent in those of Northern European backgrounds.

Proteins
A protein intake of 0.5 g/kg/day is necessary for normal balance, and a higher intake is required for growth. Dietary intake varies among cultures. Separately from ingestion, the body provides some protein for the intestines, mostly from digestive secretions (20 g/day) and desquamated epithelial cells (20 g/day). Fecal elimination is low and is due mostly to colonic bacteria, desquamated cells, and proteins in colonic mucous secretions.

Digestion occurs in the stomach and small intestine, and absorption occurs primarily in the duodenum and jejunum. Large proteins are poorly absorbed. L-isomers and single amino acids as well as dipeptides and tripeptides are absorbed by an Na$^+$-coupled process. Genetic malabsorption and intolerance affects intestinal and renal transport proteins. Hartnup's disease is a rare genetic defect in neutral amino acid transporter, and prolinuria is a rare defect in proline transporter.

Lipids
Triglycerides are the major component of dietary lipids; other components include sterols, sterol esters, and phospholipids. Lipids are hydrophobic and separate from the remainder of chyme as an oily phase in the stomach. In the duodenum, lipids are emulsified by bile acids and are digested to form micelles with bile acids. The micelles are absorbed at the intestinal brush border.

Some digestion occurs in the intestine and stomach, but the duodenum, as a result of pancreatic lipases, is the major site of lipid digestion.

Micelles are essential to increase contact area for absorption in the duodenum and jejunum. Lipophilic cholesterol, fatty acids, and lysophosphatides diffuse across the cell membrane. The lipids accumulate in smooth endoplasmic reticulum and are resynthesized to triglycerides, phospholipids, and cholesterol esters. They are then packaged in chylomicrons and extruded by exocytosis. After entering the lacteals, chylomicrons pass through the lymphatics to enter venous circulation at thoracic duct.

Fat lost in feces comes primarily from colonic microflora and desquamated cells. Malabsorption of lipids is tied to impaired digestion or absorption. Complete bile deficiency reduces absorption of fatty acids by 50% and impairs absorption of other lipids. Complete absence of pancreatic lipases impairs absorption of all classes of lipids. Impaired absorption can also result from epithelial cell damage, such as intestinal mucosal atrophy, tropical sprue, and gluten enteropathy. Note that the addition of nonabsorbable lipids (e.g., Olestra) and lipid absorption inhibitors impair absorption of fat-soluble vitamins (A, D, E, and K).

Water and Electrolytes
The GI tract absorbs 99% of ingested water. Absorption is greatest in the jejunum and least in the colon as a result of the tightness of the "tight junctions" on the epithelial cells. The GI tract receives 2 L/day from ingestion and 7 L/day from GI secretions and loses only 50 to 100 ml/day in feces. The colon absorbs 400 ml/day against an apparent osmotic gradient.

The jejunum is also the primary site of Na$^+$ absorption, secondary to amino acid and carbohydrate transport. The colon has an active Na$^+$ absorption. Potassium (K) is reabsorbed in jejunum and ileum, but net K balance is determined in the colon. The colon reabsorbs K$^+$ if the luminal K$^+$ concentration is high, and secretes K$^+$ if the luminal K$^+$ concentration is low. A significant K$^+$ loss accompanies water loss from diarrhea.

Intestinal chloride load is from ingestion and pancreatic secretions. Chloride is reabsorbed in jejunum, ileum, and colon. Bicarbonate intestinal load is from pancreatic secretions. It is absorbed in jejunum and may be secreted in the ileum and colon by a HCO$_3^-$/Cl$^-$ exchange. There is a net secretion if HCO_3^- levels are high (*alkalosis*) and a net reabsorption if HCO_3^- levels are low (*acidosis*).

Intestinal Ion and Water Balance

Sympathetic activity enhances water and sodium chloride (NaCl) absorption, and parasympathetic activity decreases water and NaCl absorption. Aldosterone provides the major hormonal control of absorption, causing Na^+ and water reabsorption and colonic K^+ loss. Enkephalin (opioid peptides) enhance NaCl and water absorption, and somatostatin enhances colonic NaCl and water absorption.

Excessive GI secretions are a clinically important problem. Na^+, Cl^-, and water secretion in crypts in the small intestine can exceed the absorptive capacity of the remainder of the GI tract. Cholera toxin stimulates crypt cell secretion, as do other cyclic adenosine monophosphate (cAMP) stimulators, such as VIP and prostaglandins. Pancreatic cholera results from a pancreatic tumor that secretes VIP.

Impaired nutrient absorption causes an excessive osmotic load and causes water and potassium loss in diarrhea. Carbohydrate malabsorption syndromes and fat malabsorption cause water loss in feces if colon absorptive capacity is exceeded.

Calcium absorption in the duodenum and jejunum is stimulated by vitamin D. Dietary iron is also reabsorbed primarily in the duodenum and jejunum, with about 20% of ingested heme iron absorbed. Approximately 50% of ingested magnesium is absorbed along the length of the intestine. Phosphate is also absorbed along the length of the intestine, possibly by active transport.

Flora

The flora of the small intestine are predominantly grampositive lactobacilli, streptococci, and staphylococci. *Aerobacter aerogenes*, *Bacteroides*, *Candida albicans*, *Escherichia coli*, *Proteus*, *Pseudomonas*, and *Streptococcus faecalis* are also found. Bile acids and gastric acid may inhibit bacterial proliferation in the intestine.

Vitamins

Vitamins are essential amino acids that must be absorbed from a dietary source. Water-soluble vitamins can be absorbed by membrane transport proteins. Folic acid and nicotinic acid are absorbed by diffusion or facilitated diffusion. Diffusion causes absorption of pyridoxine and riboflavin. Secondary active transport causes absorption of vitamin C in the ileum, biotin in the duodenum and ileum, and folic acid and thiamine in the jejunum. Vitamin B_{12} absorption across the ileum requires intrinsic factor, a gastric secretion. Lipid-soluble vitamins (A, D, E, K) are absorbed in micelles. Compounds that diminish or impair fat absorption also impair absorption of fat-soluble vitamins.

EFFECTS OF AGING

Physiologic changes in the GI tract occur with aging. In the mouth, teeth may become loose from loss of supporting gums and bone. Circulation in the gums is reduced, and aging teeth may darken, become uneven, and fracture. Decreased output of the salivary glands leads to dryness of mucous membranes and increased susceptibility to breakdown. This decrease can cause difficulty in swallowing and decreased stimulation of taste buds.

Secretion of digestive enzymes and bile also decreases. In the stomach, atrophy of gastric mucosa leads to a decreased secretion of HCl. A decrease in HCl causes reduction in iron and vitamin B_{12} absorption and a proliferation of bacteria. This reduction leads to the development of anemia. Increased bacteria in the gut may result in diarrhea and infection. With a decrease in bile secretion, absorption of fats and fat-soluble vitamins becomes impaired. This decreased absorption of fat can lead to weight loss, and the decrease in fat-soluble vitamins can lead to various problems, such as altered calcium metabolism and bleeding from the decrease of vitamin K, which is needed to synthesize prothrombin.

CONCLUSIONS

A thorough knowledge of the structure and function of the GI system helps the nurse to provide knowledgeable care to clients. Medical disorders are related to the four major functions of the GI system: motility, secretion, digestion, and absorption. To provide effective interventions, the nurse must understand the normal physiology and the digestive organs.

BIBLIOGRAPHY

1. Guyton, A. C., & Hall, J. (1996). *Textbook of medical physiology* (9th ed.). Philadelphia: W. B. Saunders.
2. Fauci, A. S., et al. (1998). *Harrison's principles of internal medicine* (14th ed.). New York: McGraw-Hill.
3. Johnson, L. R. (1997). *Gastrointestinal physiology* (5th ed.) St. Louis: Mosby–Year Book.
4. Silverthorn, D. (1998). *Human physiology*. Upper Saddle River, NJ: Prentice Hall.

CHAPTER

28

Assessment of Nutrition and the Digestive System

Vicki M. Ross

Adequate and appropriate nutrition underlies the success of all medical therapies. Nutritional health requires a gastrointestinal (GI) tract that can receive, transport, absorb, and metabolize nutrients. Similarly, adequate and appropriate nutrition is necessary for the GI tract to function properly. Because of this interdependence, assessment of the GI tract and nutritional status occurs simultaneously or in close succession. Systematic and thorough assessment of nutritional status and the upper GI tract can detect a wide range of actual or potential health problems.

This chapter focuses on assessment of nutritional status and the upper GI tract, which we will consider to include the mouth, esophagus, stomach, and small intestine. Assessment of the large intestine (colon), rectum, and accessory organs (liver, pancreas, and gallbladder) are discussed in Chapters 32 and 42.

SCREENING AND ASSESSMENT OF NUTRITIONAL STATUS

■ NUTRITIONAL HEALTH

Nutritional health is the result of consistently meeting the body's nutrient requirements.[4] Because of the many variables that differ from person to person—such as gender, age, size, metabolism, activity level, and more—it is difficult, if not impossible, to determine the exact nutrients required. However, we can determine average nutrient requirements by comparing individual characteristics with published standards or reference groups, such as the *Recommended Dietary Allowances* (RDAs) or the *Food Guide Pyramid*.

RDAs were developed by the Food and Nutrition Board of the National Council/National Academy of Sciences and are commonly used to determine nutritional requirements for specific groups of people.[12] The RDA system lists specific types and amounts of nutrients (e.g., protein, vitamins, minerals, and trace elements) for average, healthy people of various ages and sizes. RDAs are set at levels that may exceed actual individual nutrient requirements. Assess the adequacy of a client's diet by having the client complete a food diary (Fig. 28–1) and by comparing nutrient intake to that listed in the RDAs for people with characteristics similar to those of the client. For example, the RDA for iron is 15 mg for a 30-year-old, nonpregnant woman. If a client with these characteristics consumes on average 7 mg of iron per day, she is at risk for anemia.

RDAs should not be confused with *Reference Daily Intakes* (RDIs) for specific nutrients. RDIs are based on the amount of essential nutrients required to meet the physiologic needs of people in specific age or gender groups. Although RDIs include some micronutrients that are also included in the RDAs, the recommended amounts may be larger. An RDI may list a tolerable upper intake level and an adequate intake level, or it may list an estimated average requirement. An RDA is calculated from the estimated average requirement; otherwise, the adequate intake level is used. The adequate intake level is a goal for nutrient intake, based on the consensus of experts. Clients who consume less than the RDI amount may or may not be receiving adequate amounts of micronutrients. Consistent consumption of a nutrient above the tolerable upper intake level increases risk of adverse effects.

Another standard for assessing dietary intake is the Food Guide Pyramid published by the U.S. Department of Agriculture. It is a graphic representation of the types and proportions of foods recommended for average, healthy persons (see Chapter 2, Fig. 2–1). The Pyramid may be used to compare the client's daily food intake with recommended servings and food groups. Clients who consistently omit foods from one or more of the food groups are at nutritional risk.[10]

Because the RDA system and the Food Guide Pyramid are based on average, healthy populations, it may not be appropriate to apply these standards to clients who are ill or outside the average height or weight range. Nutritional requirements differ if clients are ill or have underlying disease. Fever, for example, increases caloric requirements 7% for each degree Fahrenheit of temperature increase. Some specialty groups publish nutritional standards or recommendations for clients with specific

Record *all* foods and drinks that you had during the day and during the night.

Day of the Week (Mon   Tues   Wed   Thurs   Fri   Sat   Sun)

Breakfast
  Foods and Drinks   Amounts (cups, tbsps)

Lunch
  Foods and Drinks   Amounts (cups, tbsps)

Dinner
  Foods and Drinks   Amounts (cups, tbsps)

Snacks
  Foods and Drinks   Amounts (cups, tbsps)

Do you take vitamin or mineral supplements?   Yes_____   No_____
Please list kind and how many per day.

FIGURE 28–1 A food diary form. (From U.S. Senate Select Committee on Nutrition and Human Needs. [1977]. *Dietary goals for the United States.* Washington, DC: U.S. Government Printing Office.)

diseases or conditions.[1, 13] In general, protein requirements decrease and nonprotein calorie requirements increase if kidney or liver function is impaired. Dietary fats are restricted if a client has pancreatic exocrine dysfunction; carbohydrates are restricted if a client has pancreatic endocrine dysfunction.

The National Health and Nutrition Examination Surveys, National Food Consumption Survey, and the Continuing Survey of Food Intakes by Individuals are examples of population-based surveys that describe dietary intake, nutritional status, or health outcomes related to nutrition. Information from these studies may be used in assessments of similar populations. For example, data from such surveys indicate that the body weight of Americans continues to increase. In addition to changes in caloric intake, sedentary lifestyles appear to contribute to this weight gain. When conducting an assessment and using information from these surveys, include questions about the client's physical activity in addition to dietary intake (see Chapters 1 and 2).

■ MALNUTRITION

When nutrient availability is inadequate or excessive over an extended period, malnutrition occurs. Malnutrition incorporates both starvation and obesity.

Starvation, or the inadequate delivery of nutrients to the body, can be primary or secondary.

- *Primary* malnutrition occurs when adequate nutrition is not delivered to the upper GI tract over an extended period (e.g., famine, anorexia, mechanical obstructions of the GI tract, fad diets)
- *Secondary* malnutrition occurs when the upper GI tract fails to absorb, metabolize, or use nutrients (e.g., ischemic bowel or Crohn's disease).

Marasmus, kwashiorkor, or mixed-type malnutrition result when inadequate amounts of protein or calories are delivered or absorbed over an extended period (Table 28–1). The development of a specific type of malnutrition depends on a number of factors that are defined by clinical presentation and laboratory values.[11, 18]

TABLE 28–1	TYPES OF MALNUTRITION ASSOCIATED WITH PROTEIN AND CALORIE DEFICITS		
Type of Malnutrition	**Clinical History**	**Clinical Manifestations**	**Laboratory Results**
Kwashiorkor	Inadequate protein intake with adequate calorie intake	Body weight at or above ideal range Edema sometimes present	Visceral proteins (albumin, prealbumin, transferrin) below normal
Marasmus	Inadequate calorie and protein intake	Cachectic appearance Body weight and anthropometric measurements below normal	Visceral proteins within normal range
Mixed	Inadequate calorie and protein intake with increased nutritional requirements	Cachectic appearance Body weight and anthropometric measurements below normal	Visceral proteins below normal

Inadequate food consumption rarely causes deficits of single nutrients. Instead, clients typically present with deficits of multiple nutrients. Micronutrient malnutrition occurs when vitamins, minerals, or trace elements are not delivered, absorbed, or used by the gut. Because vitamin, mineral, or trace element deficits occur in combination, it is difficult to identify deficits of single micronutrients. Laboratory tests designed to measure vitamin or trace element levels are rarely specific or sensitive enough to accurately determine if adequate amounts are available in the body.[14] The best method to identify actual or potential micronutrient deficits is with a thorough history and meticulous physical examination. Table 28–2 lists clinical manifestations of micronutrient deficits and foods that contain specific micronutrients.

In addition to protein or calorie malnutrition, suspect micronutrient malnutrition in clients who have had previous gastric surgery, chronic pancreatitis, short-bowel syndrome, pressure ulcers, various types of cancer, and acquired immunodeficiency syndrome (AIDS). Gastric surgery can impair absorption and use of vitamin B_{12}. Chronic pancreatitis can lead to fat malabsorption and decreased absorption of fat-soluble vitamins. Short-bowel syndrome results in decreased transit time and micronutrient absorption. Pressure ulcers can cause zinc and vitamin C deficits. Some drug therapies, especially those for cancer and AIDS, decrease the absorption or use of vitamins and minerals such as folate, potassium, and magnesium. If the client's dietary intake is inadequate or if the client presents with a clinical history such as these, suspect and assess for micronutrient malnutrition.

Although not commonly regarded as a type of malnutrition, *obesity* results from nutrient delivery that exceeds the client's nutrient requirements. In the United States, the incidence and prevalence of obesity are rising. Clients who consume recommended amounts of nutrients but have sedentary lifestyles are at risk for obesity, as are clients who consume excess calories[16] (see Chapter 2).

■ NUTRITION SCREEN OR ASSESSMENT?

Nutrition screening and nutrition assessment are not the same. Nutrition screening is a method of categorizing clients at high or low risk for malnutrition. Tools for nutrition screening usually contain a brief list of questions about changes in weight or dietary intake, any underlying disease or upper GI problems, and a comparison of the client's current weight to a standard. On the basis of the client's responses to nutrition-related questions, an assigned score determines whether the client is at low or high risk of malnutrition.[6, 9]

The Nutrition Support Screening Alert is one example of a nutrition screening tool. Developed by a multidisciplinary panel of experts, this tool is a tiered approach designed to identify older clients at risk for malnutrition (Box 28–1). Each tier, or level, of the instrument requires a more sophisticated assessment. The client or caregiver can perform the initial assessment for nutritional risk. *Level I* calls for additional information, including calculation of the client's body mass index, and *Level II* calls for information from the previous levels plus laboratory measurement of serum proteins. This instrument and all nutritional screening tools are used to identify clients at risk for malnutrition.

In general, nutritional screening takes place within the first few days of the client's encounter with the health care system and includes general questions about nutritional status and upper GI function. A client entering an inpatient setting should be assessed upon admission. When the nutritional screen indicates that a client is at risk for malnutrition, an in-depth nutrition and upper GI assessment are performed. Nutritional and upper GI assessments are client-centered and include an in-depth history, physical examination, and diagnostic testing to determine actual or potential problems involving the upper GI tract, nutritional status, or both. As needed, ask a dietitian to consult during this process.

HISTORY

Assessment of nutritional status and the upper GI tract begins with collection of history data. The historical account determines the direction and focus of the physical examination and the required diagnostic testing. Historical data include (1) biographical information, (2) chief complaint, (3) previous illness or hospitalization, (4) medications, (5) dietary supplements, (6) allergies, (7) family health, (8) psychosocial factors, and (9) a review of systems.

■ BIOGRAPHICAL AND DEMOGRAPHIC DATA

Analyze the client's demographic data (e.g., gender, age, religious affiliation, and marital status) within the context of nutritional status and upper GI function. For example, because women are more likely to experience problems related to calcium deficiency, include specific questions

TABLE 28-2	SOURCES OF MICRONUTRIENTS AND EVIDENCE OF DEFICIENCY

Micronutrient	Selected Foods with High Micronutrient Content	Evidence of Deficit
Vitamin A	Dark green, leafy or yellow-orange vegetables Milk fat Egg yolks	Loss of appetite and taste Night blindness Bumpy or scaly skin
Vitamin B_1 (thiamine)	Lean meats Egg yolks Legumes Enriched or whole grain cereals and breads	Paresthesias and peripheral neuropathies Mental confusion Heart failure Edema
Vitamin B_6 (pyridoxine)	Yeast Wheat germ Pork Liver Whole grain cereals Legumes	Sore, reddened tongue Seborrhea-like dermatitis Paresthesias
Vitamin B_{12} (cobalamin)	Beef Fish Milk Eggs Cheese	Sore, reddened mouth Atrophy of the tongue Megaloblastic anemia Paresthesias
Vitamin C (ascorbic acid)	Oranges Lemons Strawberries Tomatoes Cabbage Green peppers	Gingivitis Dry mouth Alopecia Pruritus (itching) Ecchymotic lesions on the skin
Calcium	Dairy products Sardines Salmon Dark green, leafy vegetables	Osteoporosis Osteomalacia
Copper	Organ meats Legumes Chocolate Nuts	Decreased absorption of iron Anemia Neutropenia Leukopenia
Vitamin D (calciferol)	Fish and fish oil Fortified dairy products	Softening of the bones Joint pain Fatigue Muscle tetany
Vitamin E (tocopherol)	Sunflower, corn, or soybean oil Wheat germ oils	Lipid absorption or transport abnormalities
Folate (folic acid)	Legumes Liver Dark green or leafy vegetables Lean beef Potatoes	Sore, reddened tongue and mouth Glossitis Megaloblastic anemia
Iodine	Seafood Iodized salt	Enlargement of the thyroid gland
Iron	Organ meats Shellfish Poultry Legumes Blackstrap molasses Fortified cereals	Hypochromic, microcytic anemia
Vitamin K	Broccoli Cabbage Turnip greens Green tea	Ecchymotic lesions Bruising

Table continued on following page

TABLE 28–2	SOURCES OF MICRONUTRIENTS AND EVIDENCE OF DEFICIENCY *Continued*	
Micronutrient	**Selected Foods with High Micronutrient Content**	**Evidence of Deficit**
Manganese	Whole grains Legumes Nuts Tea	Magenta tongue Dermatitis
Niacin	Organ meats Brewer's yeast Peanuts Fish Poultry Whole grains Beans	Sore, reddened mouth Atrophy of the tongue Angular stomatitis Dermatitis
Riboflavin	Liver Milk Cheddar cheese Cottage cheese Yogurt Brewer's yeast	Sore, reddened tongue and mouth Angular stomatitis Seborrhea-like dermatitis
Zinc	Oysters Wheat germ Beef Cheese	Angular stomatitis Seborrhea-like dermatitis Alopecia (hair loss)

Adapted from Mahan, L. K., & Escott-Stump, S. (Eds). (2000). *Krause's food, nutrition, and diet therapy* (10th ed.). Philadelphia: W. B. Saunders.

about calcium intake in the history. Because older people who live alone face an increased risk of inadequate food intake, question them about how and what they eat. People in their teens or 20s may be at increased risk of duodenal ulcers or gastric cancers, whereas older clients are more are at risk for gastric ulcers and colon cancers.

Women in their 20s and 30s are at risk for inadequate nutritional intake.

For clients in these age ranges, include specific questions about changes in GI function. Culture and ethnic origin also affect the type, amount, and frequency of dietary consumption (see Chapter 9).

BOX 28–1   Nutrition Support Screening Alerts

If an older person indicates that the following questions listed on the Nutrition Health Checklist, Level I and II screens are descriptive of their condition or life situation, nutrition counseling and support interventions may help them solve their nutritional problems and improve their nutrition status.

Determine Your Nutritional Health Checklist Alerts

I have an illness or condition that made me change the kind and/or amount of food I eat.
Without wanting to, I have lost or gained 10 pounds in the last 6 months.
I am not always physically able to shop for, cook for, or feed myself.

Level I Screen Alerts

Has lost or gained 10 pounds or more in the past 6 months
Body mass index < 22
Body mass index > 27
Is on a special diet

Has difficulty chewing or swallowing
Has pain in mouth, teeth, or gums
Usually or always needs assistance with preparing food or shopping for food

Level II Screen Alerts

In addition to Level I Screen Alerts:

Has pain in mouth, teeth, or gums
Midarm muscle circumference < 10th percentile
Triceps skinfold < 10th percentile
Triceps skinfold > 95th percentile
Serum albumin < 3.5 g/dl
Serum cholesterol < 160 mg/dl
Clinical evidence of mental/cognitive impairment
Clinical evidence of depressive illness
Clinical evidence of insulin-dependent diabetes, adult-onset diabetes, heart disease, high blood pressure, stroke, gastrointestinal disease, kidney disease, chronic lung disease, liver disease, osteoporosis, or osteomalacia.

Adapted from the Nutrition Screening Initiative, a project of the Amercian Academy of Family Physicians, the American Dietetic Association, and the National Council on Aging, Inc., and funded in part by a grant from Ross Products Divisions, Abbott Laboratories, Inc.

DIVERSITY IN HEALTH CARE

Cultural Influences on Nutrition

Probably no subject has intrigued human beings more universally and persistently than food. Food is more than a source of nutrition. Food has always served many functions and uses with culturally unique symbols and meanings. It is important that nurses understand their clients' food beliefs, functions, symbols and practices.[3] The nurse can obtain this knowledge by conducting a nutritional assessment. This information assists the nurse in providing nursing care that is safe and congruent with the client's culture.

The following case study provides a poignant example of the importance of understanding the client's cultural food beliefs and behaviors.

Case Study

Maria is a 17-year-old pregnant, English-speaking, Mexican American who comes for her prenatal appointment. Her blood pressure was significantly elevated, and she had a marked increase in weight. The examining physician admitted her to the hospital for tests. Maria had several consultations during her 3-day stay. It was a mystery why her hematocrit level ranged from 15 to 17 and her platelet and blood counts were dangerously low. Even a hematologist could not explain the abnormal blood levels.

The client received a pint of blood. An intern familiar with traditional health beliefs asked Maria one question: Was she eating anything other than her normal food? It was discovered that she was daily eating eight bars of Magnesia de Carbonate (chalk). She was experiencing heartburn and vomiting as well as craving dirt and ice (pica). She acknowledged that a family member had given her the chalk to cleanse her stomach. The family member also prevented her from eating ice because of the belief that eating ice would give her and the baby pneumonia and bronchitis.[2]

An assessment of the client's cultural influences on nutrition would have prevented this scenario and the resulting hospitalization.

The table identifies guidelines the nurse may use for assessing cultural influences regarding nutrition.

Guidelines for Determining Cultural Influences Regarding Nutrition

Meaning of Food

1. Explore the meaning of food to this group.

Common Foods and Food Rituals

1. Identify foods, preparation practices, and major ingredients commonly used by this cultural group.
2. Identify specific food rituals.

Dietary Practices of Health Promotion

1. Identify dietary practices used to promote health or to treat illness in this group.

Nutritional Deficiencies and Food Limitations

1. Identify enzyme deficiencies or food intolerances commonly experienced by this group.
2. Identify large-scale or significant nutritional deficiencies experienced by this group.
3. Identify native food limitations in America that may cause special health difficulties.[4]

Cultural Food Practices and Religion

Cultural food practices are often interconnected with religious practices. Most Americans have little knowledge about the cultural food practices of other religions. The following table summarizes the food-related practices of selected religious groups.

Food Restrictions for Selected Religions

Group Restrictions	Cultural Implications
Church of Jesus Christ of Latter-Day Saints (Mormonism)	
No alcoholic beverages	Avoid medicines containing alcohol (e.g., cough suppressants).
No stimulants (caffeinated beverages, such as coffee, tea, sodas)	For clients on liquid diets, substitute decaffeinated beverages for brewed and instant regular coffee, teas, cocoa, and carbonated beverages containing caffeine (e.g., colas).
	Avoid medicines containing caffeine, such as the following over-the-counter drugs: *Analgesics:* Anacin, Bromo-Seltzer, Cope, Empirin, Excedrin *Stimulants:* NōDōz, Vivarin, Caffedrine *Diet Pills:* Dexatrim, similar generic brands Many cold preparations
Observant Mormons fast on the first Sunday of each month. Fasting means refraining from food and liquids.	Fasting is not required during illness or in persons with diabetes, hypoglycemia, ulcers, or other medical condition for which fasting is contraindicated.

Chart continued on following page

DIVERSITY IN HEALTH CARE *Continued*

Group Restrictions	Cultural Implications

Judaism

Three major groups:
1. Orthodox (strict observance)
2. Conservative (basic observance)
3. Reform (less ceremonial emphasis and observance of dietary laws)

The dietary laws (Kashrut) dictate which foods are permissible under religious law:
1. Only meat from cloven-hoofed animals that chew cud (cattle, sheep, goat, ox, or deer) is allowed. These animals must be slaughtered ritually in a manner that results in minimal pain to the animal and maximal blood drainage. Two methods are used to prepare Kosher meats:
   a. The meat is soaked in cold water for 30 minutes, salted, and drained to deplete blood content. It is then washed under cold water and drained again before cooking, *or*
   b. The meat is first prepared by quickly searing or cooking over an open flame, which permits liver to be eaten.

Kosher (fit or proper to use) meals are available in hospitals and other health care settings. They usually are served on paper plates with plastic utensils that are sealed. Do not unwrap the utensils or transfer food onto another dish.

Do not bring nonkosher foods into the home of a Jewish client who follows the laws of Kashrut.

When teaching clients about special diets, be sure that sample menus are congruent with dietary laws.

Be aware that keeping a kosher kitchen requires two sets of dishes, pots, and utensils.

2. Meat and dairy products cannot be served at the same meal, and they cannot be cooked or served in the same set of dishes. Milk or milk products may be consumed just before a meal but not until 6 hours after eating a meal in which meat has been consumed. Milk may not be used in coffee if served with a meat meal. Nondairy creamers can be substituted if they do not contain sodium caseinate, which is derived from milk. Fish, eggs, vegetables, and fruits are considered neutral *(parve)* and may be eaten with dairy products or meats.

3. Fish with fins and scales are allowed. No shellfish (crab, lobster, shrimp, clam, oyster) or scavenger fish (catfish, shark, porpoise) may be eaten. Crocodile, frog, snail, snake, and tortoise also are prohibited. *Note:* Kosher foods in stores are marked with one of two symbols:
   a. The letter "K" with a circle (Kosher)
   b. The encircled letter "U" (the seal of the Union of Orthodox Jewish Congregations of America)

Additional dietary laws are followed during the week of Passover. No bread or product with yeast may be eaten; instead, matzah or unleavened bread is eaten. Products that are fermented or that can cause fermenting or souring may not be eaten.

There are a number of fast days in the Jewish calendar, with the holiest being Yom Kippur (Day of Atonement), during which Jews abstain from food and drink from sunset the evening before the holy day until after sunset the following day.

Encourage Jewish clients to consult with a rabbi if their insistence on fasting may be detrimental to health (e.g., those with insulin-dependent diabetes, hypoglycemia, or ulcers). Maintaining one's health supersedes the laws of fasting.

Islam

Pork, pork products, animal shortening, and alcohol are strictly prohibited.

Clients in hospitals and other health care settings may need assistance in identifying foods that have been prepared using animal shortenings or pork seasonings. Clients should avoid regular gelatin made with pork, marshmallow, and other confections made with pork. Avoid medicines containing alcohol, such as some cough suppressants. Avoid extracts such as vanilla or lemon that contain alcohol.

The slaughter of poultry, beef, and lamb must be done ritually by a Muslim to ensure that it is *halal* (slaughtered in a prescribed way).

Although many health care settings do not routinely provide foods that are *halal,* these products are often available at specialty grocery stores, particularly in large urban areas.

DIVERSITY IN HEALTH CARE *Continued*

Group Restrictions

Fasting is common. During the month of Ramadan, no foods or beverages are consumed until after sunset. *Note:* Recent immigrants from the Middle East may eat and pass food with the right hand. Because the left hand is used for toileting, it is considered extremely impolite to eat with the left hand.

Cultural Implications

Fasting is not required for persons who are ill.

Roman Catholicism

Abstinence from meat and meat products (gravy, soups) and fasting on Ash Wednesday and the Fridays during a 40-day period of religious observance called Lent.
Rules of fasting apply to those between the ages of 12 and 65 years. Fasting refers to eating one regular meal and two smaller meals per day.

Fish, cheese, or other meat substitutes are offered on these days.
Fasting is not required for children or the elderly or anyone who is ill.

Seventh Day Adventism

Fermented or alcoholic beverages are prohibited.

Avoid medicines containing alcohol (e.g., cough medicines). Avoid vanilla and lemon extract.

Optional vegetarianism may take three forms:
1. Strict vegetarians (e.g., vegans): Include no animal-derived products in their diet
2. Ovolactovegetarians: Use milk, milk products, and eggs but no meats.
3. Semivegetarians: Refrain from pork or pork products, shellfish, and blood
Snacking between meals is discouraged.

Strict vegetarians may need assistance in selecting a balanced diet from the hospital menu.

Some clients with diabetes, hypoglycemia, or ulcers may require between-meal snacks.

Summary

Food has many uses and meanings.
   Assess the role that food plays in keeping people well and in aiding in recovery from illness. Use the knowledge to provide safe and culturally competent care.

References

1. Andrews, M. (1999). Culture and nutrition. In M. Andrews & J. Boyle (Eds.) *Transcultural concepts in nursing care* (pp. 350–352). Philadelphia: J. B. Lippincott.
2. Cooper, T. (1996). Culturally appropriate care: Optional or imperative. *Advanced Practice Nursing Quarterly, 2*(2), 1–6.
3. Leininger, M. (1995). *Transcultural nursing: Concepts, theories, research and practices.* New York: McGraw-Hill.
4. Purnell, L., & Paulanka, B. (1998). *Transcultural health care: A culturally competent approach.* Philadelphia: F. A. Davis.

Joyce Larson-Presswalla, PhD, RN, *President, "Culture Counts," Marketing Coordinator, James A. Haley Veterans Hospital, Tampa, Florida*

■ CURRENT HEALTH

Chief Complaint

Chief complaints related to nutritional status and upper GI function include nausea and vomiting, indigestion, abdominal pain, diarrhea, and changes in weight or appetite from psychological, mechanical, or metabolic causes. When a client presents with these manifestations, conduct a symptom analysis.

Symptom Analysis

Include the following questions (see Chapter 9 for additional questions).

NAUSEA AND VOMITING. When does the nausea or vomiting occur? How long does it last? Is it related to food intake? Does food relieve or worsen the symptoms? Does the vomitus contain undigested food or bile? What does it look like? How much is vomited per episode? Is pain associated with the onset of nausea and vomiting?

INDIGESTION. Are the symptoms of indigestion related to food intake? Which foods worsen or relieve them? Does the client take any medications or antacids for the indigestion? How does the client describe the indigestion? Is it a "burping" or burning sensation?

ABDOMINAL PAIN. Did the pain begin rapidly or gradually? What is the intensity of the pain? Does the pain radiate? Does it worsen or improve with movement?

Does the client have a fever with the pain? Does food worsen or ease the pain? What specific foods alter the pain?

Abdominal pain is associated with a number of disorders, some of which are life-threatening (Table 28–3). Naturally, it is crucial to differentiate abdominal pain caused by a life-threatening condition from pain caused by a more minor condition.

WEIGHT AND APPETITE CHANGE. Ask specific questions about the client's usual appetite and weight and the amount of weight lost or gained and over what period of time. Was the weight gain or loss intentional? If so, ask about the diet. Does a specific weight loss organization or health club sanction the client's diet? Does the client take diet pills, such as appetite stimulants or suppressants?

Unintentional changes in weight may stem from psychological, physiological, or metabolic causes. Ask the following:

- Are weight changes associated with changes in mood?
- Does the client feel sad or depressed?
- Has there been a change in activity level?
- Has the client experienced early satiety, anorexia, or any changes in the taste of food?
- Does the client have trouble chewing or swallowing or problems with the teeth or gums? If the client wears dentures, ask how they fit. Ill-fitting dentures can decrease appetite and lead to weight loss.

DIARRHEA. How many stools does the client expel per day? Can the client describe the amount of stool (do feces fill the toilet or is the amount small)? Are stools liquid or solid? What color are they? Are they black or bloody? Do they sink or float? Does the client experience pain with defecation? Does abdominal bloating or cramping accompany the diarrhea? Does the diarrhea occur during the day, the night, or both day and night? Does the client experience fecal incontinence? How many days or weeks has the diarrhea persisted? Does the diarrhea decrease at certain times during the month (indicating a hormonal influence)? Does physical activity change the diarrhea symptoms?

Ask specifically about the relationship of stool output and dietary intake. Bloating and diarrhea that occur when the client consumes dairy products may signal lactose intolerance (see Allergies). High-fat diets that result in floating, greasy stools may indicate fat malabsorption. If there is copious or persistent diarrhea or vomiting, assess for fluid and electrolyte deficits (see Chapters 12 and 13).

Nonspecific GI problems, such as nausea, vomiting, and diarrhea, can result from food-borne poisoning (Table 28–4). When clients present with these manifestations, ask about the type of food consumed over the past 2 or 3 days, how the food was prepared, and whether anyone else who ate the same food also became ill.

■ PAST HEALTH HISTORY

Major Illnesses and Hospitalizations

The client's history of illnesses and hospitalizations can provide clues about nutritional status and the function of the upper GI tract. For example, a client with a history of bleeding is at increased risk for iron deficiency. A client with liver disease may have an increased risk for protein malnutrition. Has the client had or been hospitalized for peptic ulcer disease, vomiting blood (hematemesis), anemia, jaundice, gallbladder disease, pancreatitis, cancer, a change in bowel habits, tarry stools, or unexplained weight loss or gain?

Has the client had diagnostic tests of the upper GI system, such as a barium swallow, upper GI studies, endoscopic retrograde cholangiopancreatography (ERCP), or computed tomography (CT)? If the client has undergone previous diagnostic testing, the results may offer clues about current health problems in addition to providing baseline data. For example, for a client who reports having had a previous endoscopic procedure, ask about the purpose and results of the procedure.

Past surgical procedures also provide information about nutritional status and the structure and function of the upper GI tract. Ask specifically about any previous surgery of the mouth, throat, stomach, liver, pancreas, gallbladder, or abdomen. Include dates and outcomes for all tests, procedures, and operations.

Medications

Obtain detailed information about current or previous prescribed and over-the-counter medications (Table 28–5).

- Does the client use aspirin, aspirin compounds, or nonsteroidal anti-inflammatory drugs (NSAIDs) that may contribute to gastritis or bleeding?

TABLE 28–3	SOURCES AND CHARACTERISTICS OF ABDOMINAL PAIN
Source	**Characteristics**
Intestinal obstruction	Distended abdomen
	No bowel movements or flatus
	Intermittent or colicky pain
	Right upper quadrant pain radiating to shoulder associated with gallbladder
	Pain near umbilicus associated with small bowel
	Lumbar pain associated with colon
Peritoneal inflammation (perforated ulcer, ruptured spleen, ruptured appendix)	Steady, aching pain directly over area of inflammation
	Pain increasing with motion
	Intensity of pain varying with source of inflammation
	Gastric acid may produce more pain than alkaline content of small bowel
	Sometimes associated with manifestations of shock
Vascular obstruction	May be preceded by 2 to 3 days of mild to moderate pain and hyperperistalsis, followed by severe abdominal pain and manifestations of shock

TABLE 28-4	FOOD-BORNE POISONING: SOURCES AND MANIFESTATIONS	
Organism	**Associated Food**	**Clinical Manifestations**
Bacillus cereus	Fried rice	Watery diarrhea
Campylobacter jejuni	Raw or undercooked poultry, unpasteurized milk, untreated water	Fever, headache, and myalgias, followed 2 to 4 days later by abdominal pain, cramping, and watery diarrhea
Clostridium botulinum	Improper canning of fruits and vegetables. Honey used as a sweetener in infant formulas	Mild to severe manifestations occur in 18 to 36 hours; nausea and vomiting with no fever; cranial nerve involvement results in ptosis, diplopia, dysarthria, and dysphagia
Enterotoxigenic *Escherichia coli*	Fecal-oral route (contaminated water, contaminated meat, uncooked vegetables, unpasteurized apple cider)	1- to 2-day incubation period, followed by watery explosive diarrhea and abdominal cramps
Salmonella (non-typhoidal salmonellosis)	Contaminated raw eggs, unpasteurized dairy products	24- to 48-hour incubation period, followed by nausea, vomiting, and abdominal cramps
Staphylococcus aureus	Ham, poultry, potatoes, egg salad, mayonnaise, cream pastries	Nausea, vomiting, watery diarrhea within hours of consuming contaminated food
Trichinella	Undercooked pork or meat from carnivores	Mild to severe abdominal pain, nausea, vomiting, diarrhea during first week and progressing over next 3 to 4 weeks to include edema, rash, and muscle weakness
Vibrio parahaemolyticus	Shellfish	Cramping and inflammatory diarrhea more than 6 hours after ingestion of contaminated food

- Does the client take antacids? If so, note the type and the frequency. Does the client use laxatives or stool softeners?
- Does the client take any vitamin or mineral supplements? Ask specifically about supplements containing iron, because iron can cause gastric irritation and can change stool color and consistency.

Nutritional Supplements

Nutritional supplements include vitamins, minerals, herbs used for medicinal purposes, amino acids, and meal supplements or replacements. Because nutritional supplements are sold over the counter, they are often viewed as harmless. Taken in excess or in combination with certain drugs or supplements, however, nutritional supplements can be harmful.

If the client takes a vitamin supplement, determine the amount of each vitamin, mineral, and trace element contained in each dose. Multivitamins contain differing amounts of individual micronutrients. Indeed, some vitamins contain more than 100% of the RDA for specific micronutrients; others contain less than 100% of the RDA. In excessive doses, some vitamins can produce toxic side effects. Excess amounts of vitamin A, for example, may cause yellowing of the skin and abnormal liver function test results.

Does the client consume any herbs or similar products? Because herbal products contain varying amounts of active ingredients, note the amount and brand of the herbal preparation (Table 28-6).

Various forms of amino acids and hormones are also gaining notoriety as nonprescription remedies. Does the client consume such preparations as glucosamine, melatonin, or dehydroepiandrosterone (DHEA)?

Meal supplements or replacements are usually purchased in a liquid form and provide a convenient means of increasing nutritional intake. Because of the wide variation in nutritional content and the potential for consuming inadequate or excessive amounts of specific micronu-

TABLE 28-5	DRUG-NUTRIENT INTERACTIONS
Drug Class	**Possible Nutrient Interactions**
Antacids	Decreased absorption of calcium, iron, magnesium, and zinc
Anticoagulants	Vitamin K antagonist
Anticonvulsants	Decreased folate and biotin
Antituberculosis drugs	Disrupted metabolism of vitamins B_6 and B_{12}
Cathartics	Non-renal losses of calcium, potassium, water
Cholesterol-reducing drugs	Inhibited fat digestion and absorption
Diuretics	Increased renal loss of potassium, calcium, magnesium, and zinc
Histamine H_2 blockers	Decreased vitamin B_{12} absorption
Monamine oxidase inhibitors	Interactions with tyramine-containing foods (cheese, smoked fish, wine, yeast)

TABLE 28-6	COMMON HERBAL SUPPLEMENTS			
Herb	**Common Name**	**Purported Indications**	**Form**	**Side Effect**
Allium sativum	Garlic	Atherosclerosis Hypertension Anticlotting agent Increased peristalsis	Capsules, powder, liquid, bulb	Heartburn, flatulence, rare allergic reaction; caution needed if client is taking aspirin or anticoagulants
Echinacea angustifolia, E. purpurea, E. pallidus	Echinacea, purple coneflower, narrow-leaved echinacea	Immune stimulant Anti-infective Topical wound therapy	Capsules, tea, liquid	Potential for allergic reactions
Ephedra sinica Stapf, *E. equisetina* Bunge	Ephedra, *ma huang,* ephedrine (illegal in some areas)	Nasal decongestant Central nervous system stimulant Bronchodilator	Capsules, tea	Increased blood pressure, heart rate, irritability; avoid with hypertension, diabetes, and thyroid disease
Eleutherococcus senticosus Maxim, *Acanthopanax senticosus* Harms	Siberian ginseng, eleuthero	Increased mental alertness and physical endurance	Tea	Not related to Ginseng class but commonly confused with it
Ginkgo biloba Linneaus	Ginkgo	Vasodilatation Increased cerebral and/or peripheral blood flow	Leaf extracts in solid or liquid form	Headache, gastrointestinal upset, dizziness, nausea and vomiting, diarrhea, decreased clotting times
Hypericum performatum Linneaus	St. John's wort, klamath weed, amber touch-and-heel, goatweed, rosin rose	Treatment of depression, anxiety, bedwetting, diuretic, hemorrhoids, topical treatment for burns	Tea, capsules, tinctures, oil macerates	Fatigue, allergic reactions, photosensitivity
Panax ginseng C. A. Mey (Orient), *P. quinquefolium* Linneaus (American)	Ginseng	Strengthen body functions Increase vitality Aphrodisiac	Fresh dried roots, capsules, tablets, teas, gum	Nervousness, excitation, diarrhea, skin eruptions; avoid with hypertension

trients, ascertain the brand and amount of meal supplement consumed per day.

Allergies

Inquire about allergies to foods. Distinguish between actual allergic responses and food intolerances or preferences. Food allergies typically result in systemic types of responses, such as hives or dyspnea. If allergies are suspected, question the client about associated manifestations. How does the client describe an allergic reaction? What GI problems does the client have: cramping, flatulence, diarrhea?

Lactose intolerance is a common condition for many adults, because inadequate amounts of *lactase* (an enzyme in the small bowel) cannot break down large lactose molecules. As a result, fluid is drawn into the small bowel, resulting in abdominal cramping and diarrhea. If the client's manifestations result from lactose intolerance, eliminating lactose from the diet eases them. Some people benefit from taking lactase in tablet form before eating dairy products. Products such as Lact-Aid and dairy substitutes (e.g., lactose-free milk and ice cream) are also available.

■ FAMILY HEALTH HISTORY

A family history of certain GI problems may influence a client's current and past health problems. Inquire about the health status of family members. Is there a family history of cancer, ulcers, or colitis? Many diseases, such as ulcerative colitis and Crohn's disease, seem to have a familial component. Some diseases may result from genetic or environmental predisposition. Is there a family history of jaundice, alcoholism, hepatitis, pancreatitis, obesity, peptic ulcers, or irritable bowel syndrome?

■ PSYCHOSOCIAL HISTORY

Occupation

Ask about the client's occupation. Are toxic substances (e.g., arsenic, lead, mercury, carbon tetrachloride) present in the workplace? Does the client travel for work? The onset of GI problems, such as diarrhea or nausea, may be related to recent travel to foreign countries. For some travelers, invasion of the GI tract by bacteria, protozoa, helminths, or other parasites may cause nausea, vomiting, or diarrhea.

Nutrition

The type, amount, and time of food intake are heavily influenced by psychosocial factors, such as culture and ethnic origin (see the Diversity in Health Care feature). Social deprivation and institutionalization have been associated with decreased nutritional intake and malnutrition. Ask the client to describe a typical meal. Who purchases and prepares the meal? Who usually dines with the client?

Does the client consume alcohol? If so, ask how much, what type, and how frequently it is consumed?

Diet

How does the client describe her appetite (little, normal, ravenous)? Has there been any change in appetite? Ask the client to describe the usual foods and fluids (including coffee, colas, and alcohol) typically consumed in a 24-hour period. Has the client modified her usual diet and, if so, why?

Consider having the client complete a food intake record to determine dietary intake (see Fig. 28–1). Typically, a food intake record includes two weekdays and a weekend day. Because memory lapses decrease the reliability of information, instruct the client to record everything she ate immediately after she eats it. After the client completes the food intake record, consult a registered dietitian to collaborate in determining the adequacy of the diet. In general, the average, healthy person requires about 30 to 35 calories per kilogram and 0.8 to 1.2 g of protein per kilogram of body weight. For example, a woman weighing 55 kg (120 pounds) would require 1650 to 1925 calories and 44 to 46 g of protein.

■ REVIEW OF SYSTEMS

Inquire about the condition of the client's mouth, including the presence of dental caries, number and condition of teeth, condition of the gingivae, and use of dentures.

- Are there any oral lesions, halitosis, excessive salivation, or mouth dryness?
- How often does the client floss and brush?
- When was the last visit to the dentist for teeth cleaning?
- Does the client have trouble chewing or swallowing?
- If pain is reported with eating, is it related to specific foods or associated events?

Has the client had a change in bowel habits or stool characteristics? Are changes in appetite, upper GI symptoms, or bowel movements associated with menstrual cycles? Ask specifically about problems of the hepatic and biliary systems, such as jaundice, pruritus, ascites, dark-colored urine, pale stools, or bleeding problems. Detailed questions for the review of systems are found in Chapter 9.

PHYSICAL EXAMINATION

■ ANTHROPOMETRIC MEASURES

Anthropometric measures provide an assessment of body mass or body compartments. Height, weight, frame size, body mass index, midarm muscle circumference (MAMC), and waist-to-hip proportions are examples of anthropometric measures.

Height and Weight

Use a telescoping ruler and balance scale to measure height and weight. If the client cannot bear weight, consider using a calibrated sling or wheelchair scale. Describe clothing and other accessories (light clothing, shoes with or without heels, orthopedic casts, braces, and so on) worn by the client.

If the client cannot stand, use an arm span measurement to approximate height. To do so, extend the client's arms laterally and measure from the tip of the middle finger on one hand to the tip of the middle finger on the other hand.

Compare the client's current weight to her reported usual weight. Unintentional weight changes of less than 90% or more than 110% of the client's usual weight are considered significant. For example, for a client who usually weighs 100 pounds, a weight change of ±10 pounds (current weight < 90 pounds or > 110 pounds) would place the client at nutritional risk. To calculate the difference as a percentage of usual weight, divide the client's current weight by the usual weight and multiply times 100:

$$\% \text{ usual weight} = \frac{\text{current weight}}{\text{usual weight}} \times 100$$

Ideal Body Weight and Frame Size

Most methods for determining ideal or desirable body weight require an estimation of body frame size (Box 28–2). Calculate body frame size by measuring the client's wrist circumference and dividing it into the height. Compare the resulting r value with a chart to determine the client's body frame size. An alternative method for calculating body frame size is to measure the elbow breadth.

Ideal body weight may be calculated by several methods. A traditional method is to use a formula based on height, weight, and body frame size (Box 28–3). Factor the body frame size into the calculation for ideal body weight.

Another method is to compare the client's weight with the Metropolitan Life Insurance Company recommendations (Table 28–7). When using this table, adjust height and weight to account for the height of shoes and the weight of clothing. The client's weight should fall within the range for gender, height, and body frame size. A weight more than 20% above or 10% below the calculated ideal body weight indicates nutritional risk. This table is only a guideline and does not account for variations based on genetic or cultural factors.

Body Mass Index

An acceptable method of standardizing height-for-weight measurement is the body mass index (BMI). To calculate the BMI, divide the client's weight in kilograms by the height in meters squared as follows:

BOX 28–2   Calculating Body Frame Size

Wrist Circumference Method

1. Measure the client's right wrist (in centimeters) at the point of the smallest circumference, just distal to the styloid process of the radius and ulna.

2. Obtain the client's height (in centimeters) without shoes.
3. Divide the client's wrist circumference into the client's height to obtain the *r* value:

$$r = \frac{\text{height (in cm)}}{\text{wrist circumference (in cm)}}$$

4. Use the chart below to determine the client's body frame size based on the calculated *r* = value and sex:

	Men	*Women*
Small frame	*r* > 10.4	*r* > 10.9
Medium frame	*r* = 9.6–10.4	*r* = 9.9–10.9
Large frame	*r* < 9.6	*r* < 9.9

Elbow Breadth Method*

1. Instruct the client to extend his or her right arm, then bend the forearm to a 90-degree angle with the fingers pointing straight up.
2. Measure the width of the client's right elbow (in inches) across the greatest breadth of the joint between the bony prominences of the lateral and medial epicondyles of the humerus. To measure, either use calipers or place your thumb and index finger on the epicondyles and measure the distance between the thumb and finger.
3. Use the chart below to determine the client's body frame size based on the client's elbow breadth, sex, and height in 1-inch heels. The values shown are for a medium body frame. Measurements less than the values shown indicate a small frame; greater values indicate a large frame.

Height	Elbow Breadth
Men	
5′2″–5′3″	2½″–2⅞″
5′4″–5′7″	2⅝″–2⅞″
5′8″–5′11″	2¾″–3″
6′0″–6′3″	2¾″–3⅛″
6′4″	2⅞″–3¼″
Women	
4′10″–4′11″	2¼″–2½″
5′0″–5′3″	2¼″–2½″
5′4″–5′7″	2⅜″–2⅝″
5′8″–5′11″	2⅜″–2⅝″
6′0″	2½″–2¾″

*Courtesy of Metropolitan Life Insurance Company.

$$\text{BMI} = \frac{\text{wt (kg)}}{\text{ht (m}^2)} \quad or \quad \frac{\text{wt (lb)}}{\text{ht (in.}^2)} \times 703$$

For example, a 60-kg (132 pounds) client with a height of 145 cm (57 inches) has a BMI of 28.5, putting the client in the overweight range. Figure 28–2 contains normal and abnormal ranges for different BMI values.

Circumferential Measurements

Circumference measurements assess muscle mass and body fat proportions and distribution. Midarm muscle circumference and waist-to-hip ratio are examples of circumferential measurements.

To obtain a client's midarm muscle circumference, measure the triceps skinfold (TSF) thickness and midarm circumference (MAC) and calculate the MAMC. Compare these measurements and calculated results with published standards for the client's gender and age (Fig. 28–3).

Determine waist-to-hip proportions by dividing the waist measurement at its smallest circumference by the hip measurement at its largest circumference. Waist-to-hip proportions greater than 0.8 for women and 1.0 for men indicate fat distribution that is associated with negative health outcomes.

■ MOUTH

Assessment of the oral cavity includes inspection and palpation. Good illumination is essential. A headlamp

BOX 28–3 Calculating Ideal Body Weight (IBW)

Adult Male*

Take 106 lb for the first 5 ft of height; add 6 lb/inch for each additional inch over 5 ft

Adult Female*

Take 100 lb for the first 5 ft of height; add 5 lb/inch for each additional inch over 5 ft

Small Frame Calculate 10% of the amount for medium frame and subtract it from the first amount (i.e., IBW is 10% *less* for persons with small frames)

Large Frame Calculate 10% of the amount for medium frame and add it to the first amount (i.e., IBW is 10% *more* for persons with large frames)

Example An adult male is 6′1″ tall with a large body frame. His IBW is calculated as follows:
6′1″ = 5 ft plus 13 inches
First 5 ft of height = 106 lb
Additional height over 5 ft = (13) × (6)
= 78 lb
Medium frame IBW = 106 + 78 = 184 lb
Allowance for large frame = (10%) × 184
= 18.4 lb
Large frame IBW = 184 + 18.4 = 202.4 lb

*These formulas are for adults with a medium body frame. Adjust formulas for clients with small or large frames (adjustment is the same formula for both sexes).
Data from The American Dietetic Association. (1981). *Handbook of clinical dietetics.* New Haven: Yale University Press.

provides direct illumination, and a head mirror provides indirect lighting; both items keep your hands free for the physical examination. A penlight and tongue blade may also be used.

Inspection

Begin your assessment of the client's mouth by inspecting the lips for symmetry, color, hydration, lesions, or nodules. Put on clean gloves, and ask the client to remove any dentures. Note the symmetry of facial movements and the fit of the dentures as the appliance is removed. Instruct the client to open her lips while clenching her teeth. Inspect the position of the upper and lower teeth for malocclusion or missing teeth.

Next, ask the client to open her mouth wide, and inspect the structures inside (Fig. 28–4). Start at the left side of the mouth, and continue in a clockwise fashion. Note any evidence of dental caries, missing or broken teeth, or receding gums. Note the color of the mucosa and gums. Inspect for red lesions (erythroplakia), white lesions (leukoplakia), swelling, bleeding, or ulcers. Survey the pharynx for abnormalities of the tonsils, such as redness, swelling, lesions, ulcers, uvular deviations, drainage, or unusual mouth odor.

Inspect the tongue for symmetry, color, and moisture. Note any areas of atrophy, abnormal coatings, swelling, or lesions. Next, ask the client to stick out her tongue and move it from side to side, upward, and downward. Observe for symmetry of movement and voluntary or involuntary movement of the tongue. Abnormal tongue movement may be a result of infiltration of muscle by tumor or nerve entrapment.

Palpation

Palpate the client's lips, gingivae, and buccal mucosa. Check for loose teeth, masses, swellings, or areas of tenderness. If you find lesions, note the location, size, color, consistency, and presence or absence of tenderness.

Gently grasp the client's tongue with cotton gauze. Extend and lift it while inspecting and palpating the un-

TABLE 28–7 METROPOLITAN LIFE TABLE OF ADULT WEIGHT STANDARDS

Weights* for men (according to frame, ages 25–29) for greatest longevity†					Weights* for women (according to frame, ages 25–59) for greatest longevity†				
Height‡		**Small Frame**	**Medium Frame**	**Large Frame**	**Height‡**		**Small Frame**	**Medium Frame**	**Large Frame**
Feet	*Inches*				*Feet*	*Inches*			
5	2	128–134	131–141	138–150	4	10	102–111	109–121	118–131
5	3	130–136	133–143	140–153	4	11	103–113	111–123	120–134
5	4	132–138	135–145	152–156	5	0	104–115	113–126	122–137
5	5	134–140	137–148	144–160	5	1	106–118	115–129	125–140
5	6	136–142	139–151	146–164	5	2	108–121	118–132	128–143
5	7	138–145	142–154	149–168	5	3	111–124	121–135	131–147
5	8	140–148	145–157	152–172	5	4	114–127	124–138	134–151
5	9	142–151	148–160	155–176	5	5	117–130	127–141	137–155
5	10	144–154	151–163	158–180	5	6	120–133	130–144	140–159
5	11	146–157	154–166	161–184	5	7	123–136	133–147	143–163
6	0	149–160	157–170	164–188	5	8	126–139	136–150	146–167
6	1	152–164	160–174	168–192	5	9	129–142	139–153	149–170
6	2	155–168	164–178	172–197	5	10	132–145	142–156	152–173
6	3	158–172	167–182	176–202	5	11	135–148	145–159	155–176
6	4	162–176	171–187	181–207	6	0	138–151	148–162	158–179

* Weight in pounds (in indoor clothing weighing 5 lb for men, 3 lb for women).
† Metropolitan no longer labels these weights "ideal" or "desirable," because these adjectives mean different things to different people.
‡ In shoes with 1-inch heels.
Courtesy of Metropolitan Life Insurance Company, copyright 1983.

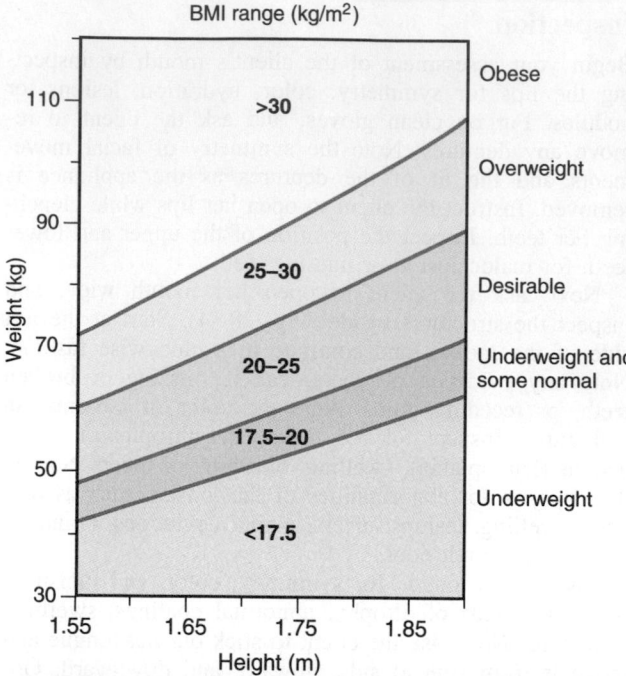

FIGURE 28-2 Weight and height for different ranges of body mass index (BMI). (From Elia, M. [1997]. Assessment of nutritional status and body composition. In G. L. Rombeau & R. H. Rolandelli [Eds.], *Clinical nutrition and enteral and tube feeding* [3rd ed.]. Philadelphia: W. B. Saunders.)

derside of the tongue and the floor of the mouth. Palpate all areas of the tongue and floor of the mouth for masses, swellings, or areas of tenderness. Note any lesions or areas of color changes. Many precancerous oral lesions are pain-free and asymptomatic. Clients with suspected lesions that do not clear within 2 to 3 weeks should be referred for further evaluation.[15]

Release the tongue, and depress it with a tongue blade. Ask the client to say "aah." Note the symmetry and movement of the uvula and soft palate. If there are no contraindications, give the client a sip of water. As the client swallows, observe for symptoms of difficulty in swallowing (*dysphagia*). Clients who exhibit difficulty with swallowing or asymmetrical movement of oral cavity structures should be evaluated for dysphagia and risk for aspiration. Oral-pharyngeal dysphagia typically presents as difficulty moving solid foods to the back of the mouth and indicates further assessment and evaluation to rule out cranial nerve involvement (see Chapter 67). Esophageal dysphagia presents as difficulty swallowing solids or liquids and indicates motor disease or obstruction of the esophagus. A speech therapist can evaluate further.

■ ABDOMEN

Because a full bladder can interfere with abdominal assessment, ask the client to void before the examination. Place the client in a supine position with her arms at her sides. Place a small pillow under the client's knees to relax the abdominal muscles. Because percussion and palpation can alter intestinal activity, assess the abdomen in

the following sequence: inspection, auscultation, percussion, and palpation. Visualize the underlying organs as you assess, and describe the abdomen by anatomic regions, or quadrants (Fig. 28-5).

Inspection

Stand at the client's right side, and begin inspecting the abdomen by noting the condition of the skin and the abdominal contour. The skin should be smooth and intact, with varying amounts of hair. The contour should be flat, concave, or rounded, depending on the client's body type. Note any areas of distention or irregular contour, which may suggest obstruction, hernia, tumor, or previous surgery. Bulging flanks and glistening, taut skin are abnormal findings and suggest ascites (see Chapters 32 and 42).

Inspect the abdomen for rashes, discoloration, scars, petechiae, striae (stretch marks), and dilated veins. Scars on the abdomen should correlate with the client's history of past surgical procedures, and striae should correlate with reported changes in weight. The umbilicus should be concave, located at the midline, and the same color as the abdominal skin, with no evidence of drainage. Note the shape, position, color, and presence of any discharge at the umbilicus.

Next, sit at eye level to the client's abdomen and observe for peristaltic movement or abdominal pulsation. Normally, peristaltic movements are not visible but abdominal pulsations may be observed in a very thin client.

Diastasis recti is a separation of the rectus muscle that results from obesity, pregnancy, or other conditions in which the abdominal muscles are subjected to sustained increased intra-abdominal pressure. This condition is not a true hernia and, for most clients, of no clinical significance. If there are no contraindications, instruct the client to bear down and perform a Valsalva maneuver or attempt a sit-up. The increased intra-abdominal pressure enhances the separation of weakened rectus muscles at the midline, where a bulge appears.

Inspect the rectal area after the abdominal examination is completed. Chapters 32 and 37 explain the rectal examination.

Auscultation

Using the diaphragm of your stethoscope, begin auscultating the client's abdomen. Press the diaphragm lightly to the abdominal wall, beginning in the right lower quadrant at the area of the ileocecal valve. Continue in a clockwise fashion, auscultating each quadrant or region. As air and fluid move through the GI tract, soft clicks and gurgles can be heard every 5 to 15 seconds. Note the frequency and character of bowel sounds. Normal bowel sounds occur irregularly at a rate of 5 to 35 per minute.[8] Loud, high-pitched bowel sounds (*borborygmi*) represent hyperactivity of the GI tract. Borborygmi may be present in clients who are hungry or who have gastroenteritis, or they may be present in early intestinal obstruction.

Hypoactive bowel sounds occur at a rate of one or fewer every minute. To determine the absence of bowel

A

Acromial process

Midpoint

Olecranon process

B

C

D Calculate the midarm muscle circumference (MAMC) using the following formula:
MAMC (in cm) = [MAC in cm] − [(0.314) × (TSF in mm)]

MEASUREMENT		STANDARD	90%	60%
Midarm circumference (MAC)	Men	29.3 cm	26.4 cm	17.6 cm
	Women	28.5 cm	25.7 cm	17.1 cm
Triceps skinfold (TSF)	Men	12.5 mm	11.3 mm	7.5 mm
	Women	16.5 mm	14.9 mm	9.9 mm
Midarm muscle circumference (MAMC)	Men	25.3 cm	22.8 cm	15.2 cm
	Women	23.2 cm	20.9 cm	13.9 cm

FIGURE 28–3 Measuring adipose and skeletal muscle tissue to estimate the client's reserves of protein and calories. *A,* Locate the *midpoint* of the client's relaxed, nondominant upper arm by palpating the acromial and olecranon processes and measuring the distance between the two points with a tape measure. Mark the posterior aspect of the arm at the midpoint with a pen. *B,* Measure *midarm circumference* (MAC) at the midpoint, keeping the tape measure level. *C,* Just above the midpoint at the posterior aspect of the arm, grasp the client's skin and subcutaneous tissue between thumb and index finger, freeing it from the underlying muscle mass. Place the calipers at the midpoint just below the fold of grasped tissue. Squeeze the calipers until they are equilibrated at the "measure" markings. Read the measurement to the nearest millimeter. Repeat the readings two more times, allowing a rest period of 3 seconds between readings. Calculate the average of the three readings for the *triceps skinfold thickness* (TSF). *D,* Compare the client's values for MAC, TSF, and *midarm muscle circumference* (MAMC) to the following standards to determine nutritional risk status. *Undernutrition* is indicated by a measurement below 90% of the standard. *Protein-calorie malnutrition* is indicated by a measurement of less than 60% of the standard, especially for MAMC. *Obesity* is indicated by a triceps skinfold measurement of 120% or more above the standard.

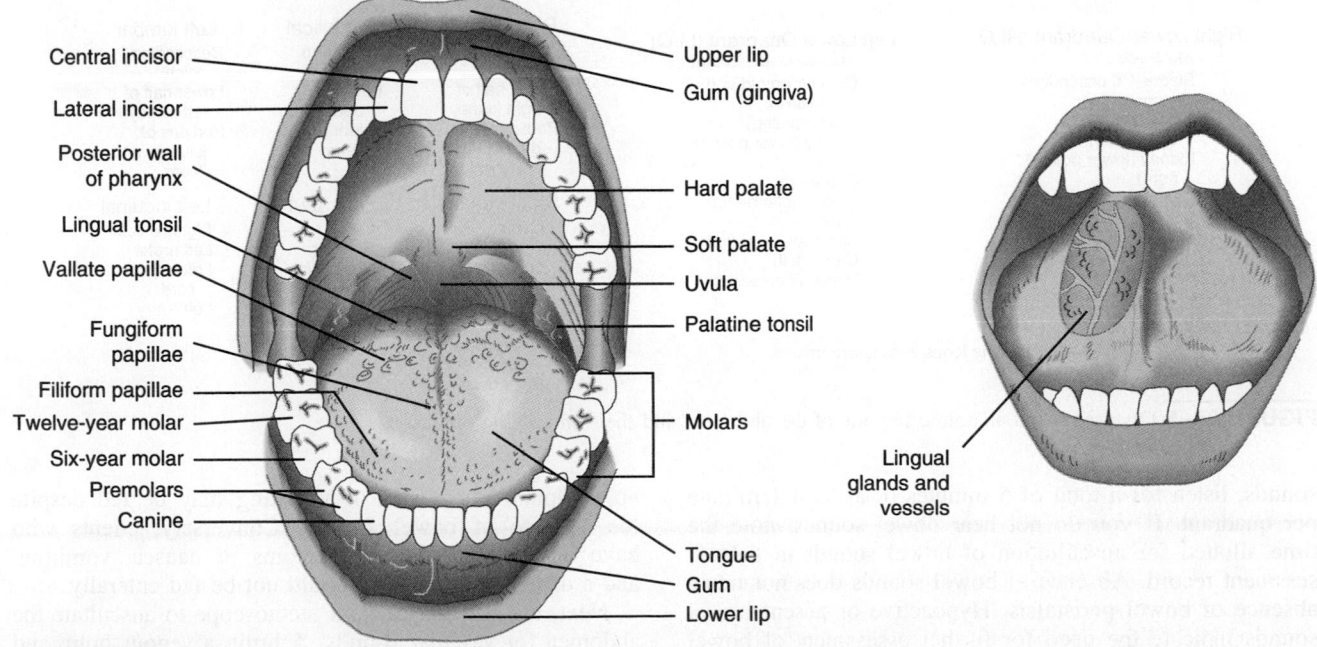

Central incisor

Lateral incisor

Posterior wall of pharynx

Lingual tonsil

Vallate papillae

Fungiform papillae

Filiform papillae

Twelve-year molar

Six-year molar

Premolars

Canine

Upper lip

Gum (gingiva)

Hard palate

Soft palate

Uvula

Palatine tonsil

Molars

Tongue

Gum

Lower lip

Lingual glands and vessels

FIGURE 28–4 Assessment of the oral cavity: terminology and normal findings.

QUADRANTS OF THE ABDOMEN
AND THEIR UNDERLYING ORGANS*

Right Upper Quadrant (RUQ)
Adrenal gland (right)
Colon (hepatic flexure
  and portions
  of ascending and
  transverse)
Duodenum
Kidney (portion of
  right)
Liver (right lobe)
Gallbladder
Pancreas (head)
Pylorus

Left Upper Quadrant (LUQ)
Adrenal gland (left)
Colon (splenic flexure
  and portions
  of transverse and
  descending)
Kidney (portion of left)
Liver (left lobe)
Pancreas (body)
Spleen
Stomach

Right Lower Quadrant (RLQ)
Appendix
Bladder (if distended)
Cecum
Colon (portion of
  ascending)
Kidney (lower pole of
  right)
Ovary (right)
Salpinx (uterine tube;
  right)
Spermatic cord (right)
Ureter (right)
Uterus (if enlarged)

Left Lower Quadrant (LLQ)
Bladder (if distended)
Colon (sigmoid and
  portion of
  descending)
Kidney (lower pole of
  left)
Ovary (left)
Salpinx (uterine tube;
  left)
Spermatic cord (left)
Ureter (left)
Uterus (if enlarged)

*Small intestine loops in all quadrants.

ANATOMIC REGIONS OF THE ABDOMEN
AND THEIR UNDERLYING ORGANS

Right hypochondriac
Right lobe of
  liver
Gallbladder
Portion of
  duodenum
Hepatic
  flexure of
  colon
Portion of right
  kidney
Adrenal gland
  (right)

Epigastric
Pyloric end of
  stomach
Duodenum
Pancreas
Portion of
  liver

Left hypochondriac
Stomach
Spleen
Tail of
  pancreas
Splenic flexure
  of colon
Upper pole of
  left kidney
Adrenal gland
  (left)

Right lumbar
Ascending
  colon
Lower half of
  right kidney
Portion of
  duodenum
  and jejunum

Umbilical
Omentum
Mesentery
Lower
  duodenum
Jejunum and
  ileum

Left lumbar
Descending
  colon
Lower half of
  left kidney
Portions of
  jejunum and
  ileum

Right inguinal
Cecum
Appendix
Ileum (lower
  end)
Right ureter
Right
  spermatic
  cord
Right ovary

Suprapubic
Ileum
Bladder
Uterus (in
  pregnancy)

Left inguinal
Sigmoid colon
Left ureter
Left spermatic
  cord
Left ovary

FIGURE 28–5 Quadrants and anatomic regions of the abdomen and their underlying organs.

sounds, listen for a total of 5 minutes or at least 1 minute per quadrant. If you do not hear bowel sounds, note the time allotted for auscultation of bowel sounds in the assessment record. Absence of bowel sounds does not mean absence of bowel peristalsis. Hypoactive or absent bowel sounds indicate the need for further assessment of bowel function. Clients who have a nondistended abdomen and

no complaint of nausea or vomiting may be fed despite the absence of bowel sounds. Conversely, clients who have bowel sounds and symptoms of nausea, vomiting, and a distended abdomen should not be fed enterally.

Next, use the bell of your stethoscope to auscultate the abdomen for vascular sounds. A bruit, a venous hum, and a friction rub are examples of abnormal sounds that may be auscultated during the abdominal examination. Bruits auscultated over major blood vessels indicate turbulent blood flow, such as an aneurysm or partial obstruction of a vessel. A continuous venous hum heard in the periumbilical area indicates engorged liver circulation. Friction rubs sound like two pieces of leather rubbing together and suggest a hepatic tumor or splenic infarction.

Percussion

Percuss the abdomen to determine the size and location of abdominal organs and to detect fluid, air, or masses. Percuss all quadrants or regions, and compare the sounds to expected findings. Normally, percussion sounds over the abdomen are high-pitched, loud, or "musical" (tympanic) over gas and dull (thud-like) over fluid or solid organs. Percussion can be used to determine the size and position of the liver and spleen (see Chapter 42) and to assess the level of a distended bladder (see Chapter 32). If you suspect an abdominal aneurysm or if the client has undergone abdominal organ transplantation, percussion is contraindicated.

Palpation

Palpate the abdomen in a systematic, quadrant-to-quadrant or region-to-region manner, beginning with nontender areas and progressing to painful ones. Start with light palpation, depressing the abdomen 1 to 2 cm. Palpate for masses or areas of tenderness. Note any areas of involuntary abdominal rigidity or guarding. McBurney's point is located in the right lower quadrant midway between the umbilicus and the anterior iliac crest. Localization of pain in this area suggests appendicitis.

After lightly palpating all areas, use deep palpation to determine the size and shape of abdominal organs and masses. Use caution when examining any tender areas. Rebound tenderness suggests peritoneal inflammation. To elicit rebound tenderness, depress the abdomen deeply over the area of tenderness and then quickly release it. If rebound tenderness is present, the client will report an increase in pain and tenderness upon release.

Palpation of organs such as the kidney, liver, and spleen is discussed in Chapters 32 and 42, and techniques are described in Chapter 10. The Physical Assessment Findings in the Healthy Adult feature is an example of a recording of a normal abdominal physical examination.

DIAGNOSTIC TESTS

Diagnostic tests provide information about the nature and severity of upper GI tract or nutritional problems. Laboratory tests, radiography, ultrasonography, endoscopy, cytology, gastric analysis, and other tests are commonly used to identify and treat nutrition and upper GI tract problems.

■ LABORATORY TESTS

Nutritional Anemias

Normal hematologic function requires adequate intake, absorption, use, and storage of nutrients, such as protein, iron, vitamin B_{12}, and copper. Assessment of red blood

---

PHYSICAL ASSESSMENT FINDINGS IN THE HEALTHY ADULT

Gastrointestinal System

Inspection

Mouth. Lips symmetrical, pink, moist, without lesions. Buccal mucosa and gingivae pink, moist, intact, without lesions. Hard and soft palates pink, intact. Tonsils behind pillars, without inflammation. Posterior pharynx pink, without exudate. Uvula rises midline with phonation. Tongue midline, mobile, without deviation or fasciculations.

Abdomen. Flat, symmetrical, with umbilicus inverted, centered, and midline. No scars, lesions, dilated veins, visible peristalsis or pulsations, or separation of rectus muscles at rest or with straining.

Anus and Rectum. Perianal area free of lesions, inflammation, fissures, bulges, or external hemorrhoids.

Auscultation

Abdomen. Bowel sounds present in all four quadrants.

Percussion*

Abdomen. General tympany throughout, with liver and splenic dullness. Liver span 10 cm at right midclavicular line.

Palpation*

Abdomen. Liver and spleen nonpalpable. Abdomen soft, nontender, no masses or rebound tenderness; muscle tone firm, relaxed.

Anus and Rectum. Anus and rectum without tenderness, masses, hemorrhoids, or prolapse. Rectal mucosa smooth. Stool negative for blood.

*In assessment of the abdomen, palpation is performed after auscultation so that the bowel is not stimulated.

---

cell function and iron stores is crucial to nutritional assessment. Chapter 74 describes assessment for hematologic disorders and anemias.

Serum Proteins

Serum proteins are important in maintaining fluid pressures and as carrier molecules. Tests for serum proteins include albumin, prealbumin, retinol-binding protein, and transferrin. Measurement of serum proteins calls for a venous blood sample to be drawn with the client in a fasting or nonfasting state. Obtaining blood samples for laboratory tests is discussed in Chapter 11.

Table 28–8 lists serum proteins, normal values, half-lives, and conditions associated with abnormal values. In general, serum proteins with long half-lives (e.g., albumin) tend to be global indicators of nutritional status. Serum proteins with shorter half-lives (e.g., prealbumin and transferrin) suggest acute changes in nutritional status.

Total Lymphocyte Count

Immune function and nutritional status are closely related. Consequently, total lymphocyte count (TLC), an indicator

TABLE 28-8	SERUM PROTEINS		
Protein	Normal Range	Half-Life	Associated Conditions
Albumin	3.5–5.0 g/dl	14–20 days	Values increased in dehydration Values decreased in malnutrition, overhydration, trauma, protein loss, and liver disease
Prealbumin	20–40 mg/dl	3–5 days	Values increased in nutrition intake and renal failure Values decreased in poor dietary intake
Retinol-binding protein	3–6 mg/L	8–12 hr	Values decreased in overhydration, liver disease, zinc and vitamin A deficiency
Transferrin	200–400 mg/dl	8–10 hr	Values increased in pregnancy and iron deficiency Values decreased in chronic infection, cirrhosis

of immune function, provides a gross measure of nutritional status as well. To determine TLC, obtain a white blood cell (WBC) count with differential from the client's venous blood sample. Next, multiply the percentage of lymphocytes by the total WBC count. For example, a client with a WBC count of 7000/mm^3 and 30% lymphocytes would have a TLC of 2100.

TLCs below 1800/mm^3 suggest malnutrition. Keep in mind, however, that this count is a gross indicator of immune function and nutritional status. Clients who are not malnourished may have a low TLC after chemotherapy. Alternatively, an elevated TLC may be found in malnourished clients with sepsis.

D-Xylose Absorption Test

D-Xylose, a monosaccharide, is absorbed in the small intestine and is used to assess malabsorption. The client receives nothing by mouth (NPO) for 10 to 12 hours before the test. A blood sample and first-voided morning urine specimen are collected. After oral administration of a known quantity of D-xylose in water, blood and urine levels of D-xylose are measured. Blood is drawn 2 hours after D-xylose is given, and all urine is collected for a specified time. Instruct the client to remain in bed during the test because activity alters the results. Decreased values of absorbed D-xylose in blood and urine indicate possible malabsorption in the small intestine.

Nitrogen Balance

Nitrogen balance is a measure of one's anabolic or catabolic state. To determine the nitrogen balance, simultaneously record the amount and type of food consumed in a 24-hour period and obtain a 24-hour urine collection. The start and stop times for the food intake record and the 24-hour urine collection must be the same. Instruct the client about the procedure and about the importance of recording all food intake and saving all urine for 24 hours.

The 24-hour urine collection begins with discarding the first voided specimen, then collecting all urine for the next 24 hours in an iced, preservative-free container. After completing the 24-hour urine collection, send the urine to the laboratory for measurement of the urine urea nitrogen (UUN). Urine creatinine, sodium, and potassium may also be measured to determine the adequacy of the urine collection. Consult a registered dietitian to calculate the client's 24-hour protein intake from the food intake record. If the client received tube feedings or parenteral nutrition during the 24-hour test period, the amount of protein from these sources must be included in the calculation.

Protein is approximately 16% nitrogen. To determine the amount of nitrogen consumed over the 24 hours, multiply the amount of protein consumed (in grams) by 0.16. UUN is the major source of nitrogen excretion. Subtract the UUN (in grams) from the amount of nitrogen consumed. Because nitrogen is also lost through the skin, stool, and the GI tract, subtract a correction factor of 3 from the nitrogen consumed, as follows:

nitrogen balance =
    nitrogen consumed (in grams) − UUN (in grams) − 3

Normal nitrogen balance is positive and ranges from 4 to 6 g. Negative values indicate catabolic states or increased nutritional requirements.

Fecal Analysis

Fecal content is an indicator of the absorptive capacity of the gut. Chapter 32 presents laboratory tests for fecal lipids and stool cultures.

■ RADIOGRAPHY

General principles for the following radiographic tests are explained in Chapter 11.

Flat Plate of the Abdomen

A flat plate of the abdomen is an x-ray (radiograph) of the abdominal organs. This test can help identify abnormalities, such as tumors, obstructions, abnormal gas, fluid collections, and strictures.

Upper Gastrointestinal Series

An upper GI series, also known as a *barium swallow*, permits radiologic visualization of the esophagus, stomach, duodenum, and jejunum. It can aid in the detection of strictures, ulcers, tumors, polyps, hiatal hernias, or motility problems. The client drinks a radiopaque contrast medium (barium) while standing in front of a fluoroscopy tube. The client may also be asked to assume other positions, such as lying on the x-ray table. This test is usually done after a barium enema or gallbladder radiographic series to prevent the swallowed barium from interfering with other diagnostic images.

PREPROCEDURE CARE

The client cannot have food or fluids for 6 to 8 hours before the test. Instruct the client about the procedure and about the barium preparation. Barium has a thick consistency and a chalky taste. It may be necessary to drink up to 16 ounces for the procedure. The test lasts about 45 minutes.

POSTPROCEDURE CARE

A laxative is usually given to help expel the barium and to prevent a fecal impaction. Assess the abdomen for distention, and observe the stool to determine whether the barium has been eliminated. Initially, the stool is white, but it should return to its normal brown color within 72 hours. A distended abdomen and constipation may indicate a barium impaction. Clients with ostomies should be closely monitored for retained barium.

Because the barium swallow is commonly performed on an outpatient basis, inform the client that the stool may be white for up to 72 hours after the procedure. Instruct the client to contact the physician immediately if constipation and abdominal distention occur.

Modified Barium Swallow

A modified barium swallow, also known as *videofluoroscopy* or an oropharyngeal motility study, is performed to assess swallowing and the risk of aspiration. While sitting in a chair equipped with videofluoroscopy, the client is given a small amount of barium to swallow in liquids and foods of various textures. During the procedure, a speech therapist or radiologist observes the client for difficulty with swallowing.

Clients are maintained on NPO status before the procedure. Maintain hydration with intravenous (IV) fluids if the client is expected to remain NPO for an extended period. After the procedure, nothing should be ingested by mouth until the speech therapist, radiologist, or physician has evaluated the test results. If diet alterations are required, consult a registered dietitian, speech therapist, or both to collaboratively develop an appropriate and adequate nutrition plan.

■ COMPUTED TOMOGRAPHY

CT scanning is used to identify masses, such as neoplasms, cysts, focal inflammatory lesions, and abscesses of the liver, pancreas, and pelvic areas (Fig. 28–6). CT also aids in evaluating local tumor spread, especially if barium studies suggest tumor growth beyond the bowel wall.[7] To distinguish normal bowel from abnormal intraperitoneal masses, dilute oral barium or other contrast media may be administered. The client is placed supine on the examination table and asked to lie still and hold her breath when instructed.

FIGURE 28–6 Normal computed tomography (CT) scan of the stomach. The CT scan is through the body of the stomach (B) at a level just below the spleen. The lateral segment of the left lobe of the liver (LS), head of the pancreas (P), and splenic flexure of the colon (C) are adjacent structures. A, aorta; D, duodenum; V, inferior vena cava. *Solid arrow* represents the superior mesenteric artery, and *open arrow* represents the vein. The rugae *(curved arrows)* are well visualized. (From Moss, A., Gamsu, G., & Genant, H. K. [1992]. *Computed tomography of the body: With magnetic resonance imaging* [Vol. 3, 2nd ed.]. Philadelphia: W. B. Saunders.)

The client receives nothing by mouth for 6 to 12 hours before the procedure. Report any client allergies to iodine to the radiologist. Non-iodine contrast medium may be used when the client is allergic to iodine. No follow-up care is needed. Chapter 11 covers the general preparation and care of the client undergoing CT scanning.

■ ULTRASONOGRAPHY

Ultrasonography of the GI system helps to identify pathophysiologic processes in the pancreas, liver, gallbladder, spleen, or retroperitoneal tissues. Ultrasound studies can be used to identify fluid, masses (such as tumors), adipose tissue, abscesses, or hematomas. Physical examination is enhanced by ultrasound techniques because palpable masses and areas of tenderness can be correlated with anatomic structures while the client is on the examining table (see Chapter 11).

Because gas may interfere with the procedure, the client may take nothing by mouth for 8 to 12 hours beforehand. Reassure the client that the test is painless and safe. There are no specific postprocedure precautions or observations related to ultrasound.

■ ENDOSCOPY

Endoscopy is the direct visualization of the GI system by means of a lighted, flexible tube. It is more accurate than radiologic examination because the physician can directly observe sources of bleeding, surface lesions, or healing tissues.

PROCEDURE

Upper GI tract endoscopy includes esophagoscopy, gastroscopy, and esophagogastroduodenoscopy (Fig. 28–7). These procedures are useful for examining clients who have acute or chronic GI bleeding, pernicious anemia, esophageal injury, masses, strictures, dysphagia, substernal pain, epigastric discomfort, or inflammatory bowel disease. Conscious sedation with a sedative, narcotic, or tranquilizer (e.g., diazepam, midazolam, or meperidine) may be given before or during the procedure. Anticholinergic medications may be given to decrease oropharyngeal secretions and to prevent reflex bradycardia.

When the client is sedated, a local anesthetic is sprayed on the posterior pharynx to ease discomfort and prevent gagging during insertion of the endoscope. The anesthetic often tastes unpleasant and makes the tongue feel swollen. To reduce the risk of aspiration, the client is placed in the left lateral decubitus (Sims) position to allow saliva to drain from the side of the mouth.

After the client is positioned, sedated, and anesthetized, a flexible fiberoptic tube is passed orally into the esophagus, stomach, pylorus, and duodenum. Some endoscopes are equipped with a camera that allows the physician to obtain color photographs. If cancer is suspected, cells or tissue can be collected for cytologic examination. Small, single polyps may be removed.

During the procedure, monitor for cardiac or respiratory complications. Assess the client's heart rate, blood pressure, respiratory rate, and pulse oximetry frequently. Specific antagonists to benzodiazepines and narcotics should be available for emergency reversal of drug effects. Upper GI endoscopy should not be performed in clients with severe cardiovascular disease.

PREPROCEDURE CARE

Clients undergoing endoscopic procedures require a signed consent. If the client will be going home within 24 hours after the procedure, someone should be available to drive her home. For clients with a history of cardiac valve disease or replacement, administer antibiotic prophylaxis. To prevent aspiration of stomach contents into the lungs, keep the client NPO for 8 to 12 hours before the procedure. Assess the oral cavity, and report any loose teeth or lesions to the gastroenterologist. Remove the client's dentures and any removable bridges.

FIGURE 28–7 Endoscopy showing normal gastric mucosa *(A)* and normal duodenal mucosa *(B)*.

Even with anesthesia, the client may experience some discomfort, nausea, or pressure. Tell her to breathe through her nose during the procedure. Explain that the room will be cool and dark and that she will not be able to talk while the endoscope is in place.

POSTPROCEDURE CARE

To prevent aspiration, place the client in the Sims position until the sedation and local anesthesia wear off. Withhold fluids and solids for 2 to 4 hours after the procedure or until the gag reflex returns. Test for return of the gag reflex by stroking the back of the client's throat with a tongue blade to see if gagging occurs. Once the gag reflex returns, the physician may order anesthetic throat lozenges or normal saline gargles to ease throat irritation or hoarseness.

Monitor for bradycardia or other dysrhythmias that may occur as a result of sedatives or anesthetics. Assess for signs of esophageal or gastric perforation. Esophageal perforation may cause crepitus (crackling) in the neck (from air leakage), fever, bleeding, or pain. Neck and throat pain, aggravated by swallowing or moving, may also occur. Mid-esophageal perforation results in referred substernal or epigastric pain. Distal esophageal perforation results in shoulder pain, dyspnea, or manifestations similar to those of perforated ulcers. If you suspect perforation, an x-ray study should be obtained to confirm the presence of free air.[2]

Endoscopic examination of the lower GI tract is discussed in Chapter 32.

■ EXFOLIATIVE CYTOLOGIC ANALYSIS

Exfoliative cytologic analysis, developed by George Papanicolaou, is a study of cells that have sloughed off from a tissue. The examination is performed in an effort to distinguish benign from malignant lesions. Malignant cells exfoliate more readily than normal cells. Specific areas of the GI tract are lavaged, and cells are collected and sent to the laboratory for analysis. Cells of the esophagus, stomach, small intestine, and colon can be examined. Stomach contents are examined for the presence of *Helicobacter pylori*, a bacterium that can cause gastritis and peptic ulcer disease. In this procedure, a nasogastric tube is placed and cells are obtained by saline lavage through the tube.

Explain the procedure to the client and, if required, obtain a written consent. Keep the client NPO before the procedure. Afterward, the client rests and may resume eating.

■ GASTRIC ANALYSIS

Gastric analysis is performed to measure secretions of hydrochloric acid (HCl) and pepsin in the stomach. Analysis of gastric contents can aid in the diagnosis of duodenal ulcer, Zollinger-Ellison syndrome, gastric carcinoma, and pernicious anemia. Gastric analysis consists of (1) the basal cell secretion test and (2) the gastric acid stimulation test.

PROCEDURE

For the *basal cell secretion test*, a nasogastric tube is inserted and attached to suction. Stomach contents are collected every 15 minutes for 1 hour. Label specimens carefully with time, volume, and client identification. The specimens are analyzed. If abnormal gastric secretion is suggested, a gastric acid stimulation test is performed.

The *gastric acid stimulation test* measures the amount of gastric acid for 1 hour after subcutaneous injection of a drug that stimulates its secretion (pentagastrin and betazole). If results are abnormal, radiographic studies or endoscopy may be done to determine the cause. A markedly increased level of gastric secretion may indicate Zollinger-Ellison syndrome, whereas a moderately increased level suggests a duodenal ulcer. Decreased levels of gastric secretion may indicate gastric ulcer or carcinoma.

PREPROCEDURE CARE

The client ingests nothing orally for 12 hours before the test. Insert a nasogastric tube, and remove any contents left in the stomach. Do not administer drugs that interfere with gastric acid levels, such as cholinergics, histamine blockers, or antacids. If a client requires coronary vasodilator therapy, change the oral form to an ointment or sublingual preparation during the procedure.

POSTPROCEDURE CARE

If the nasogastric tube is left in place, attach it to low intermittent suction. Record the amount and color of the drainage.

■ ACID PERFUSION TEST

The acid perfusion test, also known as the *Bernstein test,* determines whether a client's chest pain is related to acid perfusion across the esophageal mucosa. A nasogastric tube is inserted, and gastric contents are aspirated. Normal saline solution (0.9%) and 0.1% HCl are alternately instilled into the lower esophagus. If the client does not experience pain, the test is considered normal. If pain occurs, normal saline is administered until pain ceases. To ensure that the pain is caused by acid perfusion, 0.1% HCl is readministered. After the test, the nasogastric tube is withdrawn.

Keep the client NPO the night before the test. Instruction about the procedure includes preparing the client for insertion of the nasogastric tube. After the procedure, the client may receive an antacid.

■ ESOPHAGEAL MANOMETRY

Manometry is used to assess esophageal motor function and can be used to assess and diagnose dysphagia, esophageal reflux, spasm, motility disorders, and hiatal hernia. A special enteric tube with fused small-caliber catheters is inserted into the esophagus. The tube is designed to measure simultaneous pressures of the esophagus and lower esophageal sphincter by infusion of water into the catheters. The client is asked to swallow small amounts of water, and esophageal pressures are recorded during muscular relaxation and contraction.

Instruct the client about the procedure, and maintain NPO status for 6 to 8 hours before the procedure. The test takes about 15 to 20 minutes. After the test, remove the enteric tube. The physician may recommend medications or diet alterations based on the results.

■ AMBULATORY ESOPHAGEAL pH MONITORING

The relationship between pH changes in the esophagus and symptoms of chest pain and indigestion may be assessed by ambulatory esophageal pH monitoring. This test is used to distinguish chest pain caused by gastric acid reflux into the esophagus from chest pain caused by angina or myocardial infarction. Location of the lower esophageal sphincter (LES) is determined by esophageal manometry, and a nasoenteric tube with a pH sensor is inserted 5 cm above the LES. The enteric tube is secured to the client's face and attached to a battery-operated recorder. The client is then instructed to push a button on the recorder when she starts and ends specific activities, such as eating, sleeping, and smoking. She is told to note when chest pain or indigestion starts and ends.

Because the location of the LES must be determined, inform the client that esophageal manometry may be performed first after which a second enteric tube may be placed for the pH monitoring. You may need to stop giving the client drugs that affect the GI tract (e.g., H_2 histamine blockers and motility drugs) before the procedure. Instruct the client about the importance of recording activities and symptoms. The tube must remain securely taped. Tell the client to avoid bumping or pulling the tube when dressing or washing her face. After the procedure, remove the tube and advise the client that she may resume normal activities.

CONCLUSIONS

Nutritional health and a functional upper GI tract are basic to health. Systematic assessment of nutritional status and the upper GI tract can lead to prompt diagnosis and treatment of disorders. The diagnostic process is facilitated by performing a careful and thorough assessment and by properly preparing the client for procedures to maximize the potential for optimal health.

BIBLIOGRAPHY

1. A.S.P.E.N Board of Directors. (1993). Guidelines for the use of parenteral and enteral nutrition in adult and pediatric patients. *JPEN: J Parenteral and Enteral Nutrition, 17,* 1SA–25SA.
2. Barkin, J., & O'Phelan, C. A. (Eds.). (1994). *Advanced therapeutic endoscopy* (2nd ed.). New York: Raven Press.
3. Bartels, C. L., & Miller, S. J. (1998). Herbal and related remedies. *Nutrition and Clinical Practice, 13*(1), 5–19.
4. DeHoog, S. (1996). The assessment of nutritional status. In L. Mahan & S. Escott-Stump (Eds.). *Krause's food, nutrition, and diet therapy* (9th ed., pp. 361–386). Philadelphia: W. B. Saunders.
5. Fauci, A. S., et al. (Eds.). (1998). *Harrison's principles of internal medicine* (14th ed.). New York: McGraw-Hill.
6. Grindel, C. G., & Costello, M. C. (1996). Nutrition screening: An essential assessment parameter. *MEDSURG Nursing, 5*(3), 145–156.
7. Haubrich, W. S., Schaffner, F., & Berk, J. E. (Eds.). (1995). *Bockus gastroenterology* (5th ed.). Philadelphia: W. B. Saunders.
8. Jarvis, C. (2000). *Physical examination and health assessment* (3rd ed.). Philadelphia: W. B. Saunders.
9. Kovacevich, D. S., et al. (1997). Nutrition risk classification: A reproducible and valid tool for nurses. *Nutrition in Clinical Practice, 12*(1), 20–25.
10. Krebs-Smith, S. M., et al. (1997). Characterizing food intake patterns of American adults. *American Journal of Clinical Nutrition, 65*(suppl), 1264S–1268S.

10a. Mahan, L., & Escott-Stump, S. (Eds.). (2000). *Krause's food, nutrition, and diet therapy* (10th ed.). Philadelphia: W. B. Saunders.

11. Mitchell, M. K. (1997). *Nutrition across the life span.* Philadelphia: W. B. Saunders.

12. National Academy of Science. (1989). *Recommended dietary allowances* (10th ed.) Washington, DC: National Academy Press.

13. Schears, G., & Deutschman, C. (1997). Common nutritional issues in pediatric and adult critical care medicine. *Critical Care Clinics, 13*(3), 669–690.

14. Shenkin, A. (1997). Micronutrients and outcome. *Nutrition, 13*(9), 825–828.

14a. Shils, E., Olson, J. A., & Shike, M. (Eds.). (1999). *Modern nutrition in health and disease* (9th ed.). Baltimore: Williams & Wilkins.

15. Shugars, D. C., & Patton, L. L. (1997). Detecting, diagnosing, and preventing oral cancer. *The Nurse Practitioner, 22*(6), 105–132.

16. Solomon, C. G., & Manson, J. E. (1997). Obesity and mortality: A review of the epidemiologic data. *American Journal of Clinical Nutrition, 66*(suppl), 1044S–1050S.

17. Stone, R. (1996). Primary care diagnosis of acute abdominal pain. *The Nurse Practitioner, 21*(12), 19–41.

18. Torun, B., & Chew, F. (1994). Protein-energy malnutrition. In M. E. Shils, J. A. Olson, & M. Shike (Eds.), *Modern nutrition in health and disease* (8th ed.). (pp. 950–976). Philadelphia: Lea & Febiger.

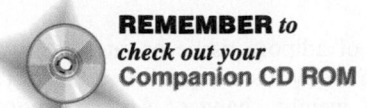

CHAPTER 29

Management of Clients with Malnutrition

Nancy Evans Stoner
Candace Cantwell

NURSING OUTCOMES CLASSIFICATION (NOC)
for Nursing Diagnoses—Clients with Malnutrition

Altered Nutrition: Less Than Body Requirements
Nutritional Status
Nutritional Status: Food and Fluid Intake
Nutritional Status: Nutrient Intake
Weight Control
Altered Nutrition: More Than Body Requirements

Nutritional Status: Food and Fluid Intake
Nutritional Status: Nutrient Intake
Weight Control
Feeding Self-Care Deficit
Nutritional Status
Nutritional Status: Food and Fluid Intake
Self-Care: Eating
Swallowing Status

Impaired Swallowing
Swallowing Status
Risk for Injury: Dysrhythmias
Cardiac Pump Effectiveness
Circulation Status
Electrolyte and Acid-Base Balance
Tissue Perfusion
Vital Signs Status

Malnutrition can develop as a result of acute or chronic diseases and treatments that affect the ability to ingest or digest foods. In turn, it can cause such problems as delayed wound healing, impaired immune function, and a decreased functional status. Obesity, anorexia nervosa, and bulimia nervosa are eating disorders that alter nutritional health. Nursing diagnoses pertinent to malnutrition include *Altered Nutrition: Less than Body Requirements,* *Altered Nutrition: More than Body Requirements,* and *Feeding Self-Care Deficit.*

PROTEIN-ENERGY MALNUTRITION

Malnutrition broadly describes *undernutrition* or *overnutrition* related to excess or deficient dietary intake. Protein-energy malnutrition (PEM) results when the body's need for protein and/or energy (glucose and fat) is not supplied by dietary intake. Prolonged deficiencies in energy and protein can result in any of these clinical syndromes of malnutrition:

• Kwashiorkor, which reflects primarily a deficiency in protein
• Marasmus, which reflects primarily an energy deficit
• Marasmic kwashiorkor, which reflects both an energy and a protein deficit

PEM can be classified as *primary* when the deficits result simply from poor food intake. *Secondary* PEM refers to malnutrition associated with acute or chronic disease that causes one or more of the following: (1) decreased food intake, (2) decreased nutrient absorption, (3) increased nutrient losses, or (4) increased nutrient requirements.[6, 17, 20]

PEM is a significant problem in adult medical-surgical clients in both hospital and home settings. Initial studies of malnutrition found PEM in up to 40% of hospitalized medical and surgical clients.[3, 4] More recent studies have found similar rates of documented malnutrition on admission to the hospital in general medical clients (46%), clients with respiratory disease (45%), and geriatric clients (43%).[9, 13, 19]

Malnutrition was documented in 10% of 441 clients who lived at home with cancer and chronic disease.[6, 9] The elderly population is at particular risk for malnutrition; in one study of nursing home residents, 85% of those assessed had significant nutritional deficits.[6, 9] Among community-dwelling elderly, the prevalence of PEM may be 5% to 10%.[6, 9] Decreases in functional capacity, mobility, and independence, which are common in older adults, can result from malnutrition or may contribute to its development. The most important changes in body composition associated with aging are a loss of lean body mass and a gain in body fat. The loss of lean body mass is an important factor in the impairment of pulmonary function, immune function, and strength.[6, 9, 18]

The cost of treating malnutrition varies greatly, depending on the level of nutritional care, for example, simply providing supplemental formulas ($4 to $5 per six-pack). More sophisticated nutritional support therapies used to treat and prevent malnutrition are more expensive; *total enteral nutrition* (TEN) costs $30 to $40 per day, and *total parenteral nutrition* (TPN) costs $250 to $350 per day. Even so, these costs are small when compared to the costs of not using therapies to prevent or treat malnutrition. The consequences can include an increased length of stay, delayed wound healing, and prolonged infection. In the Veterans Affairs TPN Cooperative Study, the use of TPN in severely malnourished clients greatly reduced the number of complications related to surgery.[21]

Etiology and Risk Factors

The etiologic mechanism of PEM is multifactorial and is usually associated with the presence of acute or chronic disease. Causes of PEM can be related to social factors, economic factors, or physiologic changes in nutrient absorption or nutrient requirements. Socioeconomic factors that have a negative effect on nutritional status include:

- Social isolation
- Limited access to food
- Emotional depression
- Substance abuse
- Poverty

Physiologic factors leading to malnutrition usually result from other diseases that can cause compromised food intake, decreased absorption of nutrients, or increased demand for nutrients. Changes in nutrient intake can result from the disease or from its treatment.

Inadequate food intake is common in hospitals and can lead to malnutrition if diminished intake is prolonged or severe. Many disease processes affect the client's swallowing function and are common reasons for decreased food intake (see Chapter 30). Inadequate absorption of nutrients is the result of various disorders of the gastrointestinal (GI) tract, such as inflammatory bowel disease (see Chapters 31 and 33). In addition, the demand for nutrients increases in response to critical, chronic, and infectious illnesses

In your role of preventing and restoring nutritional status, you should take a multidisciplinary approach. Health *promotion* interventions include activities that support the client's knowledge of normal nutrition and provide nutritional information to maintain optimal health and prevent disease. Such strategies might include diet information related to decreasing cancer risk or identifying support for an elder who cannot prepare meals independently. Health *maintenance* interventions include targeting specialized diet therapy for a client with an illness (such as diet instruction for a client with Crohn's disease). Health *restoration* activities can include retraining a client to swallow after a stroke or administering TPN to a malnourished client with severe inflammatory bowel disease.

Pathophysiology

PEM can develop gradually over weeks to months, or quickly over days to weeks, when coupled with severe stress and illness. When the total supply of nutrients is less than the body's requirement, malnutrition can occur. When the primary deficit is in energy balance, the result is, first, the depletion of adipose tissue or fat stores, with eventual loss of lean body tissue (muscle mass). This deficit is reflected in weight changes. An unintentional weight loss of 5% in 1 month or 10% in 6 months suggests that the client is at significant risk for malnutrition.[13]

When the nutrient deficit is primarily in protein intake, the result is a depletion of nonessential tissue, such as skeletal muscle. When the client is hypermetabolic from severe illness, however, there is a marked depletion of the skeletal muscle and the visceral proteins, such as albumin, transferrin, and prealbumin. This depletion results from a decrease in the synthesis of visceral proteins, such as albumin, as well as from an increase in protein breakdown.[17] Starvation related to severe stress affects organ function at the cellular level by impairing specific biochemical functions, which increases the risk of mortality and morbidity.[6, 19]

Clinical Manifestations

Table 29–1 presents the pathophysiology and related clinical manifestations of malnutrition. In addition to these, you may also notice hair loss or hair that is dull and dry. The client's skin may be dry and bruised. Nails are brittle. Saliva production decreases. Periodontal disease and bleeding gums as well as cheilosis may be present. Most malnourished clients are also anemic. The client may have decreased neurologic reflexes, weakness, edema, increased sensitivity to cold, amenorrhea, impotence, and atrophied breasts. Most clients experience delayed wound healing.

Abnormal laboratory values that may indicate malnutrition include decreased hemoglobin, blood urea nitrogen (BUN), creatinine, albumin, total protein, transferrin, prealbumin, and lymphocyte proliferation. All of these findings are related primarily to a protein deficit.

Outcome Management

▇ Medical Management

Management of PEM starts with identifying clients who are malnourished as well as clients at risk for malnutrition. Assess or screen all clients for nutritional problems. First-level screening can be done through admission forms or simple questionnaires. Nutritional screening generally focuses on a few key data points (such as a weight change, a change in dietary habits, and GI manifestations) to identify clients that require a more comprehensive nutritional assessment.

A comprehensive nutritional assessment includes a review of the medical history, weight and diet history, anthropometric measures, biochemical profiles, and physical examination (see Chapter 28 for an in-depth review of nutritional assessment).

DEFINE NUTRIENT OUTCOMES

The outcomes for weight and fat stores and protein stores define the nutrient goals for each client. Weight maintenance is appropriate for clients within 90% to 120% of a reference weight, whereas depletion of fat stores and weight loss is appropriate for obese clients (>120% of reference weight). Clients with severely depleted fat stores and more than 10% weight loss need calories sufficient to replete these stores and to gain weight.

TABLE 29-1	CONSEQUENCES OF MALNUTRITION	
Organ System	**Pathophysiology**	**Clinical Manifestations**
Cardiac	Decreased cardiac muscle mass	Postural hypotension Diminished venous return
Pulmonary	Decreased diaphragm strength Decreased respiratory strength Decreased endurance	Inability to clear secretions Decreased exercise tolerance Inability to wean from ventilator
Immune function	Decreased cell-mediated immunity Delayed cutaneous hypersensitivity	Increased incidence and severity of infection
Wound healing	Decreased collagen synthesis	Delayed wound healing
Skeletal muscle strength	Altered muscle contractions Relaxation response Decreased muscle endurance	Fatigue Inability to perform activities of daily living Risk of falling
Gastrointestinal function	Impaired intestinal absorption of lipids Decreased rate of glucose absorption Decreased gastric, pancreatic, and bile production	Diarrhea

Data from Kinney J. M., et al. (1988). *Nutrition and metabolism in patient care.* Philadelphia: W. B. Saunders.

The energy needs of most clients can be determined with formulas that estimate the basal energy expenditure (BEE). The Harris-Benedict equation is the most commonly used formula:

$$\text{BEE (men)} = 66 + (13.7 \times \text{weight in kg}) + (5 \times \text{height in cm}) - (6.8 \times \text{age})$$

$$\text{BEE (women)} = 655 + (9.6 \times \text{weight in kg}) + (1.7 \times \text{height in cm}) - (4.7 \times \text{age})$$

The BEE represents the basal metabolic rate and is multiplied by a factor that accounts for stress and activity. Table 29–2 outlines targets for daily energy requirements using predictive equations. These equations are most useful in mildly stressed clients and may overestimate or underestimate energy needs during critical illness. Indirect calorimetry can be used for severely stressed clients for a precise measurement of energy expenditure.

The protein needs of a hospitalized client are nearly twice those of normal needs. Protein repletion is necessary to maintain equilibrium when the client experiences increased protein breakdown and decreased protein synthesis. Protein requirements for the metabolically stressed client range from 1.5 g of protein per kilogram (kg) to as much as 2.5 g protein per kg of *ideal body weight* (see later discussion of obesity).

TABLE 29-2	DETERMINING DAILY ENERGY REQUIREMENTS	
Goal for Fat Stores	**kcal (in Hospital)**	**Requirement (kcal/kg/day)**
Replete	BEE × 1.5	30–35
Maintain	BEE × 1.3	25–30
Reduce	<BEE	20–25

BEE, basal energy expenditure.
From Evans Stoner, N. (1997). Nutritional assessment. *Nursing Clinics of North America, 32*(4), 648.

DETERMINE ROUTE OF FEEDING
The goals to meet nutrient needs must be translated into a practical, safe, and medically appropriate nutritional plan of care. To prevent or correct existing malnutrition through oral dietary manipulation, a registered dietitian can assist in meal planning or can recommend diet modification to increase oral intake. Supplements to boost the oral intake of calories and protein are available in a variety of forms, such as liquid milk-like drinks, clear juice-like drinks, nutrient bars, and puddings (Table 29–3).

When the client is unable to eat or when oral intake is contraindicated, an alternate means of nutritional support is necessary, such as TPN or TEN. If the GI tract is functional, TEN should be used. If the GI tract is not functional, the client is a candidate for TPN. Figure 29–1 presents an algorithm for determining the appropriate route of feeding.

Nursing Management of the Medical Client
ASSESSMENT
Nurses play a vital role in identifying clients with nutritional problems. Of all the various health care providers that clients see, you are typically the first to assess clients as they enter a health system. You also have the most constant contact during a hospitalization. You are also the last to see clients before they leave. Naturally, you are in a key position to evaluate a client's nutritional intake.

Nursing admission forms should include questions regarding weight history, weight change, diet history, and food tolerances. Daily flow sheets or nursing records must include a section on nutrition, including weight measures and tolerance to nutritional therapy. Box 29–1 is an example of an admission nutrition screening tool that can be used to determine a client's nutritional risk.

DIAGNOSIS, OUTCOMES, INTERVENTIONS
Feeding Self-Care Deficit. The nursing diagnosis most appropriate for the intervention of feeding is *Feeding Self-Care Deficit related to impaired motor function, impaired cognitive function, sensory-perceptual altera-*

TABLE 29-3	ORAL NUTRITIONAL SUPPLEMENTS		
Type of Product	Calories Per Serving	Protein (g Per Serving)	Features
MILK-BASED			
Nutra Shake (4 oz)	200	8	High-calorie/protein, lower-volume supplement
Carnation Instant Breakfast (8 oz) made with 2% milk	250	12	Widely available, economical, high-calorie/protein supplement
Ensure Pudding (5 oz)	250	6.8	Thicker consistency (dysphagia), low-volume supplement with added vitamins and minerals
LACTOSE-FREE			
Boost Plus (8 oz)	360	14.6	High-calorie/protein supplement with added vitamins and minerals
Probalance (8 oz)	300	13.5	High calorie/protein, fiber-containing supplement with added vitamins and minerals
DISEASE-SPECIFIC			
Nepro (8 oz)	475	16.6	Specialized for clients with renal failure who are receiving dialysis; low in electrolytes and volume
Resource Diabetic (8 oz)	250	15	High-calorie/protein, low-carbohydrate supplement, lactose-free
NUTRITIONAL BARS			
Boost Bar (44 g)	190	4	Candy bar appeal, convenient, with added vitamins and minerals; various flavors
Powerbar Essentials (65 g)	180	10	High-protein, low-fat supplement with added vitamins and minerals; various flavors

tions, or decreased appetite. Neuromuscular impairments, such as Parkinson's disease, muscular dystrophy, myasthenia gravis, muscular weakness, and central nervous system tumors, are contributing factors. Visual disorders can occur with glaucoma, cataracts, or a cerebrovascular accident. A situational factor may include immobility, trauma, or the placement of external fixating devices that restrict arm movement. Older clients may have decreased visual and motor abilities, increased muscle weakness, and altered taste and appetite.

Outcomes. The client will maintain an ideal body weight or will gain 1 to 2 pounds per week to return to an ideal body weight by overcoming decreased appetite or motor, sensory-perceptual, or cognitive impairments.

Interventions

Improve Nutritional Intake. General strategies to improve nutritional intake relate to choices of menu items and the accessibility of dietitians and food service personnel who can evaluate client food preferences and assist in meal planning. Clients should be able to choose from a menu in order to avoid food monotony. Dietitians should be accessible during mealtimes to help assess individual preferences. Kitchen facilities and supplies should be available at the unit level to increase client choices. Dedicated refrigeration and microwave equipment for client and family use may encourage the families to bring foods that are appealing to the client and may allow more flexible mealtimes that coincide with the client's appetite.

Increase Appetite. Appetite is often impaired in a hospital setting for a variety of reasons. Several strategies can be used to maximize or enhance a client's desire for food. First, you can create a pleasant environment during mealtime. Clear the area of unsightly bedpans, urinals, suctioning equipment, and dressing supplies. Ensure adequate pain relief before meals, and avoid invasive procedures just before a meal. Increased activity through regular exercise may also increase the client's appetite.

Appetite can be enhanced by taste, smell, and vision. Taste alterations can occur from injury after radiation to the oral cavity, surgical resection to the tongue, medications, and oral infections. Oral hygiene is important to support the optimal function of taste buds. Routine mouth care should include:

- Cleansing the mouth after each meal and at bedtime
- Using a soft-bristle toothbrush
- Rinsing with warm saltwater
- Avoiding alcohol-containing mouthwash
- Avoiding glycerin and lemon juice

The ability to smell prepared foods may also stimulate the appetite. Although clients cannot participate in food preparation, offering them a chance to smell food before a meal may be helpful. Reduce all noxious odors that might negatively affect appetite. Let the client see the food to help stimulate appetite, position the food to make it visible, and describe the different foods. Your description is especially important for clients with visual impairment.

Increase Social Interaction. Eating is ordinarily a time for social interaction, yet clients are usually given meals in their own rooms. Creating social contact by feeding clients in a central area or encouraging family and friends to visit during mealtimes may be an option. Client care assignments should be designed so that clients requiring feeding can be assigned to the same caregiver as much as possible. As the client and caregiver develop a therapeutic

FIGURE 29–1 Algorithm to determine appropriate route of feeding. (Data from Mahan, L. K., & Escott-Stump, S. E. [2000]. *Krause's food, nutrition, & diet therapy* [10th ed., p. 467]. Philadelphia: W. B. Saunders; modified and adapted from Gorman R. C., Morris, J. B. [1997]. Minimally invasive access to the gastrointestinal tract. In J. L. Rombeau & R. H. Rolandelli [Eds.], *Clinical nutrition: Enteral and tube feeding* [p. 174]. Philadelphia: W. B. Saunders.)

BOX 29–1 Features of the Admission Nutrition Screening Tool

A. Diagnosis

If the client has one or more of the following conditions, circle it, proceed to section E, and consider the client AT NUTRITIONAL RISK. If the client has none of these conditions, proceed to section B.

- Anorexia nervosa/bulimia nervosa
- Cachexia (temporal wasting, muscle wasting, cancer, cardiac disease)
- Coma
- Diabetes
- End-stage liver disease
- End-stage renal disease
- Malabsorption (celiac sprue, ulcerative colitis, Crohn's disease, short-bowel syndrome)
- Major gastrointestinal surgery within the past year
- Multiple trauma (closed-head injury, penetrating trauma, multiple fractures)
- Nonhealing wounds
- Pressure ulcers

B. Nutrition Intake History

If the client has one or more of the following manifestations, circle it, proceed to section E, and consider the client AT NUTRITIONAL RISK. If the client has none of these manifestations, proceed to section C.

- Diarrhea (>500 ml for 2 days)
- Vomiting (>5 days)
- Reduced intake (<½ normal intake for more than 5 days)

C. Ideal Body Weight Standards

Compare the client's current weight for height to a chart of ideal body weights. If the client weighs less than 80% of ideal body weight, proceed to section E and consider the client AT NUTRITIONAL RISK. If the client weighs more than 80% of ideal body weight, proceed to section D.

D. Weight History

Any recent unplanned weight loss? No _____ Yes _____
    Amount _____ (lb or kg)
If yes, within the past _____ weeks or _____ months
Current weight _____
Usual weight _____
Height _____
Find percentage of weight loss:

$$\frac{\text{usual wt} - \text{current wt}}{\text{usual wt}} \times 100 = \underline{\hspace{1cm}} \% \text{ wt loss}$$

Compare the percentage of weight lost with the values on the following chart; circle the applicable value.

Length of Time	Significant (%)	Severe (%)
1 wk	1–2	>2
2–3 wk	2–3	>3
1 mo	4–5	>5
3 mo	7–8	>8
5+ mo	10	>10

If the client has experienced a significant or severe weight loss, proceed to section E and consider the client AT NUTRITIONAL RISK.

E. Nurse Assessment

Using the above criteria, what is this client's nutritional risk? (check one)

_____ LOW NUTRITIONAL RISK
_____ AT NUTRITIONAL RISK

Adapted from Kovacevich, D., et al. (1997). Nutrition risk classification: A reproducible and valid tool for nurses. *Nutrition in Clinical Practice, 12,* 22.

---

relationship, the feeding will become a more pleasurable and successful experience for both.

Minimize Sensory-Perceptual Deficits. Clients with sensory-perceptual deficits require specific nursing actions to ensure adequate food intake. Make sure the client is wearing corrective lenses, if needed, and that they fit properly. If needed, describe the food and its location on the tray. The use of different-colored trays and dishes is helpful to clients with these deficits. Arranging the food in a clock-face pattern is an easy way to orient the client to the position of various foods on the tray. Describing the position of foods is imperative for clients with visual field disturbances. Do not place foods on the client's blind side.

Minimize Neuromuscular Impairments. Various neuromuscular impairments can make the seemingly simple task of eating difficult or impossible. The occupational therapy staff can help in planning the feeding intervention and teaching the correct use of assistive devices. For a client with physical impairment, ensure privacy, allow adequate time for eating, position the client at a 90-degree angle with the meal tray at elbow height, and provide assistive devices, such as plate guards and built-up spoons.

Minimize Cognitive Impairments. Cognitive impairments can result in the client's misunderstanding the task of eating or being unable to complete the task because of a short attention span. If so, the client will require frequent cues and close supervision. The following nursing actions are useful steps in feeding clients with cognitive impairments:

1. Create a quiet, unhurried environment.
2. Explain the procedure.
3. Orient the client to the purpose of feeding equipment.
4. Provide frequent cues to the client (e.g., "Mrs. S, pick up the toast" or "Mr. S, chew the food in your mouth").
5. Provide several small meals for clients with short attention spans.

Minimize Fatigue. Another physical factor that can affect a person's ability to feed oneself is endurance. The client may be able to start the task but becomes quickly fatigued and cannot complete it. The client's ability to maintain a level of performance is related to cardiovascular, respiratory, neurologic, and musculoskeletal function.

For a client with reduced endurance, plan rest periods before mealtimes, especially when the meal follows an activity, such as physical therapy or ambulation. Help the client conserve energy for eating by helping with meal setup, opening packages, and cutting food.

Impaired Swallowing. Chewing and swallowing dysfunction are frequent additional reasons for difficulties in eating. The client may experience malnutrition because of problems with swallowing. In this case, an appropriate nursing diagnosis is *Impaired Swallowing related to neuromuscular impairment (decreased or absent gag reflex), mechanical obstruction (edema, tracheostomy tube, tumor), fatigue, or limited awareness.*

Outcomes. The client will be able to freely swallow solids or liquids and will not experience any aspiration problems.

Interventions

Use a Team Approach. A team approach has been described in the literature in the successful management of clients with swallowing impairments.[6, 17] In addition to nurses, physicians, physical and occupational therapists, and speech pathologists can be helpful in localizing the impairment and suggesting useful strategies. You must also understand the complexity of normal swallowing mechanisms in order to plan appropriate interventions.

Assess Swallowing. Take these four steps before feeding to assess client readiness:

1. Assess level of consciousness; the client must be alert.
2. Assess the client's gag reflex by tickling the back of the throat.
3. Have the client produce an audible cough.
4. Have the client produce a voluntary swallow.

Implement Swallowing Techniques. Feeding should take place in a calm, adequately supervised environment. Place the client in a normal eating position with the feeder clearly visible. Some clients may have trouble moving the food bolus from the front to the back of the mouth. Food should be placed in the unaffected side of the mouth. If the tongue is damaged or impaired, assistive devices, such as adapted feeding syringes, can move food toward the pharynx, where the swallowing reflex (if intact) takes over.

Once the food bolus arrives at the pharynx, the client should tilt the chin down to decrease the risk of aspiration. Massaging the throat on the affected side helps stimulate the tactile areas that initiate the swallowing reflex. If the client has difficulty coordinating chewing, breathing, and swallowing, instruct the client to hold the head forward and to hold the breath before swallowing.

Watch the thyroid cartilage to see whether the client has swallowed, and inspect his or her mouth before placing more food in the oral cavity. Allowing sufficient time between each mouthful helps to ensure that the client adequately chews and swallows the food. Stay alert for signs that the client is becoming fatigued, restless, or agitated. Keep suction equipment available in case of an emergency. Also, know how to perform the Heimlich maneuver to prevent choking.

See Bridge to Home Health Care: Managing Swallowing Difficulties.

BRIDGE TO HOME HEALTH CARE

Managing Swallowing Difficulties

Swallowing difficulty (dysphagia) can vary in severity and duration. It can be mild to severe, short term (acute), or long term (chronic).

When you feed clients who have dysphagia, use good observational skills and plenty of communication and patience. Observe their responses to what you are doing. They may frown, spit, clamp their jaws together, or cough when food choices are not appealing. Try to adapt meals to their tastes. For example, if a client enjoys bananas, dice, mash, or blend them into a shake, or even freeze them to offer variety; select the consistency that your client tolerates best.

Promote use of the sense organs during mealtime. Encourage your clients to think or talk about their favorite foods before meals to stimulate saliva flow and to aid in chewing. Ask clients to close their eyes and to visualize tasting and chewing these foods. Provide mouth care before and after the client eats meals and swallows medications to keep the mouth and breath fresh and facilitate saliva production. If your clients find it pleasurable, have them watch the food being prepared, smell the food cooking, and participate in the meal preparation as much as possible. Use an activity such as folding napkins to begin involvement. Play the client's favorite music tapes during mealtime.

The home health nurse should schedule shared visits periodically with the speech or occupational therapist to promote continuity of care. Discuss strategies related to mealtime and food preparation. Work with the therapists to help clients strengthen their mouth muscles by practicing pushing their lips or "puckering," humming, or whistling. Demonstrate the techniques you are trying to teach; hold a mirror so that clients can see their own mouth.

A high Fowler's position with 90-degree flexion of the hips is usually the best position for mealtime. Position your client with shoulders back and torso erect. Slightly flexing the client's head forward may aid in swallowing. Placing a pillow at the lower back and a towel roll behind the neck can facilitate a smooth flow of food from the mouth into the stomach. Observe your clients closely to see which position makes them most comfortable. Cushions, pillows, or bedrolls are used to support any dependent limbs or "weak" sides. Increasing physical comfort decreases distraction and allows more focus on eating.

Maintaining the high Fowler's position, with at least 75- to 80-degree flexion at the hips for at least 30 minutes after a meal, helps reduce reflux and aspiration. Check your client's mouth carefully for lingering food pockets that may become dislodged and cause aspiration long after the meal. For your safety, never place your unprotected fingers in the client's mouth when teeth or dentures are in place.

Close observation, good communication, and a sense of humor will keep mealtime pleasurable for your client and you.

Bernice Christopher, RN, BSN, *Keystone Mercy Health Plan, Philadelphia, Pennsylvania*

■ **Medical Management of the Client Receiving Parenteral Nutrition**

PARENTERAL NUTRITION

TPN is indicated to maintain nutritional status and prevent malnutrition when the client cannot be fed orally or by tube feeding. TPN should not be used when the GI tract is functional. Box 29–2 outlines some common indications for the use of parenteral nutrition.

The TPN prescription is guided by the nutritional assessment and the definition of nutrient goals for calories and protein. The TPN solution contains carbohydrate and fat to meet the calorie goal and amino acids to meet the protein goal.

Carbohydrates

Glucose is the most commonly used carbohydrate to supply energy and calorie needs; it usually accounts for 50% to 70% of the nutrient prescription. At least 100 or 150 g of glucose (350 to 500 kcal) should be given daily to support the nitrogen-sparing effect of carbohydrate.

Fat Emulsions

Intravenous (IV) fat emulsions (lipids) generally provide about 10% to 30% of the daily nutrient prescription. Fat emulsions (1) provide a calorie-dense isotonic energy source and (2) supply fatty acids to prevent essential fatty acid deficiency.

Amino Acids

Crystalline amino acids of differing composition and a concentration varying from 3% to 15% are the source of protein in parenteral solutions. The standard commercially available solution is a mix of essential and nonessential amino acids. Some amino acid solutions have been developed to target specific clinical problems, such as renal failure and liver failure. However, the increase in efficacy over the general amino acid solution is not conclusive.

Fluids, Electrolytes, Vitamins, and Trace Elements

Fluids, electrolytes, vitamins, and trace elements are all equally important in the parenteral nutrient solution. The daily electrolyte regimen should be individualized and should reflect the client's clinical condition (including any ongoing losses) and the function of major organ systems. Table 29–4 outlines recommendations for daily electrolyte requirements and situations that can result in an increased or decreased need.

Vitamins and trace elements are needed to promote optimal nutritional repletion, and they support a variety of important metabolic pathways. One injectable multivitamin preparation contains both water-soluble and fat-soluble vitamins for daily use (Table 29–5). Vitamin K, a fat-soluble vitamin, is not contained in these commercial preparations and must be added to the TPN formula weekly (10 mg) or daily (1 mg). Other vitamins are sometimes added to the standard vitamin preparation, such as vitamin C, to promote wound healing, and vitamin B_{12}, thiamine, and folic acid to correct deficiencies commonly associated with alcohol abuse.

Guidelines for the administration of trace elements have been outlined by the American Medical Association's Nutritional Advisory Group (Table 29–6). Supplemental zinc may be indicated for clients with high-output fistulae, large wounds, or extreme catabolism.

BOX 29–2 Clinical Indications for Total Parenteral Nutrition

■ Malabsorptive syndromes

  ■ Severe short-bowel syndrome
  ■ Severe, prolonged radiation enteritis
  ■ High-output fistulae that cannot be bypassed with small bowel enteral feeding

■ Motility disorders

  ■ Persistent postoperative or disease-related ileus
  ■ Intestinal pseudo-obstruction
  ■ Severe persistent vomiting (as in hyperemesis gravidarum)

■ Intestinal obstruction
■ Perioperative nutrition for severe malnutrition
■ Critically ill client when enteral therapy is contraindicated
■ Low-flow state

Data adapted from Shils, M., & Brown, R. (1999). Parenteral nutrition. In M. Shils, et al. (Eds.), *Modern nutrition in health and disease* (p. 1658). Baltimore: Williams & Wilkins.

Combination Systems

A *total* nutrient admixture (TNA) is a single-bag TPN delivery system that contains glucose, lipids, amino acids, electrolytes, vitamins, and trace elements. The main advantages of the TNA are a shortened preparation and

---

TABLE 29–4 DAILY ELECTROLYTE RECOMMENDATIONS

Electrolyte	Daily Replacement	Factors Affecting Daily Requirement	Effect
Sodium	80–150 mEq	Diuretic therapy	↑
		Renal failure	↓
		Fluid overload	↓
Chloride	80–150 mEq	Gastric losses	↑
Potassium	80–100 mEq	Aggressive refeeding	↑
		Diuretic therapy	↑
		Gastrointestinal losses	↑
		Renal failure	↓
Calcium	10–20 mEq	Blood transfusions	↑
Magnesium	8–30 mEq	Aggressive refeeding	↑
		Gastrointestinal losses	↑
		Renal failure	↓
Phosphorus	15–45 mMol	Aggressive refeeding	↑
		Excessive antacid administration	↑
		Renal failure	↓
Acetate	0–60 mEq	Metabolic acidosis	↑
		Metabolic alkalosis	↓
		Sepsis	↑

↑, increased requirement; ↓, decreased requirement.
From Evans, N. (1994). The role of total parenteral nutrition in critical illness: Guidelines and recommendations. In M. Ackerman, K. Puntillo, & J. Clochesy (Eds.), *Clinical issues in critical care nursing.* Philadelphia: J. B. Lippincott.

TABLE 29-5	PARENTERAL MULTIVITAMIN SUPPLEMENTATION*
Vitamin	Amount Supplied
A	1 mg/3300 IU
D	5 μg/200 IU
E	10 mg/10 IU (as dl-α-tocopherol acetate)
B_1	3 mg
B_2	3.6 mg
B_3	40 mg
B_5	15 mg
B_6	4 mg
B_{12}	5 μg
C	100 mg
Biotin	60 μg
Folic acid	0.4 mg

*Roche and Astra products. Amounts of vitamins reflect the 1979 Nutritional Advisory Group recommendations of the American Medical Association.
From Galica, L. (1997). Parenteral nutrition. *Nursing Clinics of North America, 32*(4), 711.

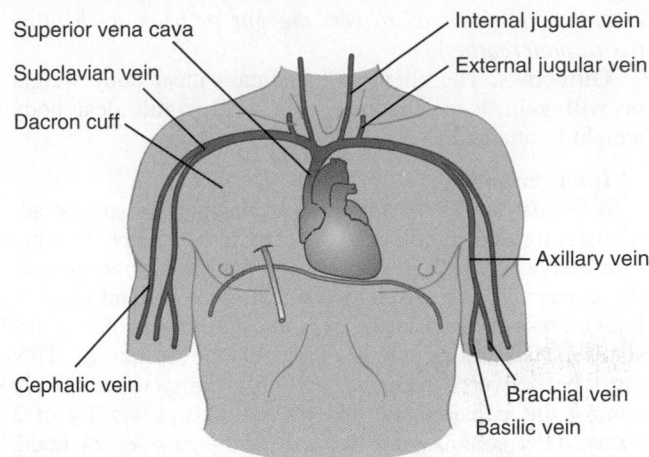

FIGURE 29-2 Insertion of catheter into superior vena cava via right subclavian vein. Once in place, this catheter may be used to administer total parenteral nutrition. (From Mahan, L. K., & Escott-Stump, S. E. [2000]. *Krause's food, nutrition, & diet therapy* [10th ed., p. 474]. Philadelphia: W. B. Saunders.)

administration time and possibly decreased contamination from fewer manipulations of the IV delivery system. The main disadvantage is that TNA supports the growth of some microorganisms better than a simple glucose–amino acid solution does.

VASCULAR ACCESS

TPN is infused into the central venous circulation. In contrast, nutrient solutions infused into a peripheral vein are known as *peripheral parenteral nutrition* (PPN). PPN generally results in underfeeding because, in order to keep the osmolarity of the solution under 1000 mOsm/L, glucose administration must be reduced. Its use should be limited to the client with adequate peripheral vascular access who needs parenteral therapy for 5 to 10 days. In the client with poor peripheral access or with severe hypermetabolism and hypercatabolism, TPN is recommended.

In central vascular access, the tip of the catheter must be positioned in a high-flow vein, such as the superior or inferior vena cava. Access to this central system can be achieved through several veins, such as a peripheral vein, the jugular vein, the subclavian vein, or the femoral vein (Figure 29–2). Temporary central venous catheters are percutaneous nontunneled catheters that are best used in an acute care setting for a short time.

More recently, the peripherally inserted central venous catheter (PICC) has offered an option for long-term use. For extended therapy (>3 months), external tunneled central venous catheters or totally implanted ports are the best option.

Nursing Management of the Client Receiving Parenteral Nutrition

ASSESSMENT

In addition to the nutritional assessment measures outlined earlier, you must check the infusion bag for correct ingredients and appearance of the solution, assess the condition of the venous access site, monitor blood glucose levels and the rate of infusion, and observe the client for untoward reactions to the solution.

DIAGNOSIS, OUTCOMES, INTERVENTIONS

Altered Nutrition: Less Than Body Requirements. The nursing diagnosis most appropriate for the client receiving TPN is *Altered Nutrition: Less Than Body Requirements related to the need for IV delivery of nutrients, fluids, and electrolytes to maintain nutritional status secondary to malabsorption problems of the GI tract, gastric cancer, cancer cachexia, anorexia nervosa, excessive metabolic needs (as in extensive burns or draining*

TABLE 29-6	DAILY PARENTERAL TRACE ELEMENT SUPPLEMENTATION			
Trace Element	AMA Guidelines	M.T.E.-4	M.T.E.-5	M.T.E.-5 Concentrate
Zinc	2.5–4.0 mg	1 mg	1 mg	5 mg
Copper	0.5–1.5 mg	0.4 mg	0.4 mg	1 mg
Manganese	0.15–0.8 mg	0.1 mg	0.1 mg	0.5 mg
Chromium	10–15 μg	4 μg	4 μg	10 μg
Selenium	20 μg	—	20 μg	60 μg

AMA, American Medical Association; M.T.E., multiple trace elements.
From Galica, L. (1997). Parenteral nutrition. *Nursing Clinics of North America., 32*, 4, p. 711.

wounds), or the need to rest the gut to promote healing (as in pancreatitis).

Outcomes. The client will maintain ideal body weight or will gain 1 to 2 pounds per week until ideal body weight is attained.

Interventions

Administer TPN. You are responsible for safely administering and monitoring the infusion of TPN. Just before delivery, check every solution for its expiration date, the correct ingredients (glucose, fat, protein, and electrolytes), leaks or tears in the bag, and the appearance of the solution (separating or cracking of the solution). TPN must be delivered using a peristaltic pump to accurately control the infusion rate and prevent the possibility of a bolus. TPN solutions are typically infused over 24 hours in the acute care setting. In the home, clients often receive TPN while sleeping.

Monitor Serum Glucose Levels. The first time TPN is administered, serum glucose levels should be monitored every 6 hours to assess the client's response to glucose. If blood glucose is within the normal range for 24 hours, monitoring can be changed to daily. Persistent elevations of blood glucose are managed by delivering regular insulin in the TPN solution after the daily requirement for insulin is determined. If the client's clinical status is unstable, the insulin dose cannot be stabilized over a 24-hour period, or both, the insulin should be delivered outside of the TPN as an insulin drip or intermittent subcutaneous injections. Most clients can tolerate an acute discontinuation of TPN and therefore do not need to be weaned from TPN gradually.

Observe for Allergy to Lipids. TPN solution that contains lipids (fats) should be introduced slowly the first time to assess for reaction to the lipid. Although rare, allergic reactions to IV lipid preparations have been reported and usually present within 30 minutes. A clinical manifestation of reactions can be any of the following: fever, shaking chills, shortness of breath, chest pain, or back pain. If the client complains of any of these manifestations, stop the TPN infusion immediately and inform the health care team of the manifestations.

Maintain Vascular Access. You play a pivotal role in ensuring the proper functioning of the vascular access system and preventing catheter-related infection. Maintain catheter patency by following a routine heparin flush protocol. Table 29-7 outlines the suggested protocols for central catheters that deliver TPN.

Prevent Infection. Prevention of catheter-related infection is key to the successful use of parenteral nutrition. Most infections that do occur result from contamination of the exit site or catheter hub.[6, 7] You must follow strict guidelines/protocols for the care of the vascular access device before, during, and after its insertion. Although

TABLE 29-7	CENTRAL VENOUS CATHETER MAINTENANCE	
Catheter Type	**Site Care**	**Flushing**
Nontunneled central venous catheter	▪ *Dressing:* Transparent or gauze ▪ Transparent dressing enhances catheter stability ▪ Performed as a sterile dressing ▪ Skin antisepsis protocols include one or a combination of the following: 70% alcohol (3 swabs), 10% povidone-iodine (3 swabs), chlorhexidine	*Internal volume:* 0.1–0.53 ml *Flush volume:* 1–2 ml *Frequency:* Usually daily
Tunneled, cuffed central venous catheter	▪ *Dressing:* Transparent or gauze until incision healed ▪ Dressing commonly discontinued when incision healed and suture removed ▪ Performed as an aseptic dressing (skin antisepsis as above) ▪ Hydrogen peroxide may be used to remove crusting at the site	*Internal volume:* 0.15–1.8 ml *Flush volume:* 3–4 ml *Frequency:* Usually daily *Groshong catheters:* 5 ml 0.9% normal saline solution weekly
Peripherally inserted central catheter	▪ *Dressing:* Transparent preferred to enhance catheter stability ▪ Performed as a sterile dressing (skin antisepsis as above) ▪ Dressings required as long as catheter is in place	*Internal volume:* 0.04–1.2 ml *Flush volume:* 2–3 ml *Frequency:* Daily
Ports	▪ *Dressing:* Transparent when port is accessed to stabilize needle ▪ Sterile gauze may be placed between needle and skin ▪ Huber needle changed at least every 7 days ▪ Sterile approach needle insertion and dressing recommended (skin antisepsis as above before needle placement) ▪ Dressing remains until healed (several days postoperatively)	*Internal volume:* 0.5–1.5 ml *Flush volume:* At least 3 ml *Frequency:* Every 4 weeks

From Krzywada, E., & Edmiston, C. (1998). Parenteral access/equipment. *The ASPEN nutrition support practice manual.* Silver Spring, MD: ASPEN Board of Directors, with permission.

catheter site care is somewhat varied and is controversial, strict adherence to hand-washing and aseptic technique is clearly the most important way to prevent infection. Dedicate (and mark) one lumen of a multilumen catheter to the infusion of TPN to minimize manipulations of the IV system. The most recent recommendations from the Centers for Disease Control and Prevention (CDC) are to change the tubing for lipid-containing TPN solutions every 24 hours.[7]

Provide Dressing Changes. The dressing change protocol for central venous access devices continues to be controversial. Various protocols exist for skin cleaning and the type and frequency of dressing change. The catheter exit site should be cleaned with an antiseptic agent, such as 70% alcohol and 10% povidone-iodine. Another product that has shown positive results in preventing catheter-related infections is chlorhexidine. Antibiotic ointments should not be applied to the catheter exit site.

The type of dressing applied over the catheter exit site should be either a sterile gauze or a transparent dressing. Frequency of dressing changes depends on client needs (e.g., more frequent changes are needed for a diaphoretic client) and the type of dressing. Gauze dressings typically are changed every 48 hours, transparent dressings every 3 to 7 days. The most important concept is that the dressing must remain adherent to be effective. Therefore, any dressing must be changed immediately if it becomes damp, soiled, or loose. Follow your agency's policy regarding dressing change protocols.

▇ Medical Management of the Client Receiving Enteral Nutrition

ENTERAL NUTRITION

"Total enteral nutrition" (TEN) refers to a method of infusing nutrient solutions or formulas directly into the GI tract through tubes that enter through the nose, mouth, or abdominal wall. Enteral nutrition is indicated when the client has impaired ingestion but normal intestinal absorption.

Some common indications for enteral nutrition are listed in Box 29–3. Enteral feeding is contraindicated in clients with complete intestinal obstruction, ileus, severe pseudo-obstruction, severe diarrhea, intestinal ischemia, severe acute pancreatitis or malabsorption syndrome. In clients with impairments of the proximal GI tract, from fistulae or tumor, enteral feeding may be used if the tip of the tube is positioned distal to the impairment.

In clients with adequate GI tract function, *enteral* rather than *parenteral* nutrition should be used. One of the most important benefits of enteral nutrition relates to the importance of utilizing the GI tract to maintain and support gut integrity and function and prevent atrophy of the gut mucosa. The protection offered by using the GI tract can result in a reduction of infectious complications.[1, 2, 6] Other factors that make enteral therapy desirable include reduced cost and safer administration.

The TEN prescription is guided by the nutritional assessment and the definition of nutrient goals for calories and protein. The selection of an enteral formula is based on the client's nutrient needs, the absorptive function of the GI tract, the fluid status, and the level of stress. More than 100 enteral formulas are available on the market

---

BOX 29–3   Indications for Enteral Feeding

Neurologic and Psychiatric

Anorexia nervosa
Cerebrovascular accident
Demyelinating disease
Failure to thrive
Inflammation
Cancer
Severe depression
Trauma

Oropharyngeal and Esophageal

Inflammation
Cancer
Trauma

Gastrointestinal

Fistula (not mid-gut)
Mild inflammatory bowel disease
Mild malabsorption
Mild pancreatitis
Preoperative bowel preparation
Short-bowel syndrome (later stages)

Miscellaneous

Acquired immunodeficiency syndrome (AIDS)
Burns
Chemotherapy
Organ transplantation
Radiation therapy

Adapted from Guenter, P., et al. (1997). Delivery systems and administration of enteral nutrition. In J. Rombeau & R. Rolandelli (Eds.), *Clinical nutrition: Enteral and tube feeding* (3rd ed., p. 240). Philadelphia: W. B. Saunders.

---

today. Most can be placed into one of the following three classifications:

- *Standard formula:* contains intact (nonhydrolyzed) protein; may be concentrated, high-protein, or fiber-enriched
- *Predigested elemental formula:* not in the "intact state"; instead, contains hydrolyzed protein in the form of dipeptides and tripeptides
- *Disease-specific formula:* contained in a standard or elemental form reported to enhance specific organ function, such as the kidneys, liver, pulmonary system, or immune system

Table 29–8 outlines the classification of enteral products and includes brief descriptions of formula characteristics. Standard formulas, which contain 1 kcal/ml, are used most often. Concentrated calorie-dense formulas, which contain 1.5 to 2.0 kcal/ml, are helpful for clients who are fluid-restricted or unable to tolerate high volumes of formula. High-protein formulas contain more than 50 g/L of protein and are useful for critically ill clients who are hypercatabolic and have a proportionally lower calorie and fluid need with high protein requirements. The addition of fiber to standard formulas can help regulate bowel function and prevent diarrhea and constipation.

Enteral formulas are designed to provide the recommended dietary allowance (RDA) of vitamins and trace

| | TABLE 29-8 | CLASSIFICATION OF ENTERAL NUTRITION PRODUCTS |

Classification	Formula Characteristics	Sample Products
Intact protein blenderized	Isotonic; nutritionally complete; containing fiber; lactose and lactose-free	Compleat Modified Formula Compleat Regular Formula, Vitaneed,
Low-residue standard protein	Isotonic; nutritionally complete; lactose-free	Entrition 1.0, Isocal, Isolan, Isosource, Osmolite, Resource
Intermediate, high-protein	Isotonic; nutritionally complete; lactose-free	Entrition 1.0, Isocal HN, Isosource HN, Osmolite HN
Concentrated	Calorically dense (1.5–2.0 cal/ml); lactose-free; nutritionally complete; hyperosmolar	Isocal HCN, Magnacal, TwoCal HN, Nutren 2.0
Fiber-supplemented	Isotonic; nutritionally complete; lactose-free; fiber range, 5–14 g/L; standard to intermediate protein	Fibersource, Jevity, Fiberlan, Ultracal
Disease-specific renal (pre-dialysis)	Low- and standard protein; low-mineral, vitamin A, and vitamin D content; lactose-free; calorically dense; hyperosmolar	Suplena
Glucose-intolerant	Low-carbohydrate, high-fat; lactose-free; isotonic; containing fiber; nutritionally complete	Glucerna
Pulmonary	Low-carbohydrate, high-fat; lactose-free; nutritionally complete; hyperosmolar; calorically dense	Nutrivent, Pulmocare, Respalor
Trauma/stress	High-protein; isotonic to hyperosmolar; lactose-free; nutritionally complete; some containing fiber, hydrolyzed protein, supplemental amino acids (BCAA, arginine, glutamine), and β-carotene; low-fat	AlitraQ, Impact, Impact w/Fiber, Immun-Aid, Isotein HN, Promote, Replete, Replete w/Fiber, TraumaCal
Hydrolyzed protein, very-low-fat	Nutritionally complete; lactose-free, fewer than 10% of calories from fat; hyperosmolar, varying in peptide length; containing amino acids	Accupep HPF, Criticare HN, Vital High Nitrogen
Low-fat	Nutritionally complete; lactose-free, 11%–30% of calories from fat; hyperosmolar; varying in peptide length; containing amino acids	Travasorb HN, Travasorb STD
Moderate-fat	Nutritionally complete; lactose-free, 30%–35% of calories from fat (high MCT); hyperosmolar, varying in peptide length; containing amino acids	Peptamen, Reabilan
Disease-specific; trauma	Nutritionally complete; lactose-free, intermediate to high in protein content; 25%–35% of calories from fat (high MCT); varying in peptide length; containing amino acids; sometimes containing supplemental arginine and β-carotene	Perative, Reabilan HN
Crystalline amino acids	Nutritionally complete; lactose-free, low-fat (1%–3% of total calories); low to standard protein content; hyperosmolar	Tolerex, Vivonex T.E.N.
Disease-specific; hepatic failure	High BCAA; nutritionally incomplete; lactose-free; low-fat	NutriHep
Renal failure (with dialysis)	Essential and nonessential amino acids: nutritionally incomplete but containing water-soluble vitamins; hyperosmolar; lactose-free; low-fat	Nepro

MCT, medium-chain triglyceride; BCAA, branched-chain amino acid; LCT, long-chain triglyceride.
Adapted from Hopkins, B. (1994). Enteral nutrition products. In G. Zaloga (Ed.), *Nutrition in critical care*. St. Louis: Mosby–Year Book, p. 447.

elements based on an intake of 1500 to 2000 calories/day. Clients receiving lower-calorie regimens may require supplemental vitamins during extended enteral nutrition.

The daily fluid needs of the client receiving enteral nutrition must be calculated to avoid overhydration or underhydration. The most vulnerable client is the one receiving a calorie-dense or concentrated formula, which contains less free water than that in a standard formula. Such a client may require additional water delivered as an intermittent flush or bolus throughout the day to meet fluid needs. A client with excessive GI losses may also require supplemental water to maintain hydration.

ENTERAL ACCESS

Enteral feeding requires the administration of a liquid solution through a tube into the GI tract. Enteral nutrients can be delivered into the stomach (intragastrically) or into the small intestine (postpylorically). Selection of the type of enteral access device depends on the functional status of the GI tract, the risk for aspiration, and the estimated length of therapy. Figure 29–3 depicts the various types of enteral access placements.

The functional status of the client's GI tract often defines the site of feeding. Resections, obstructions, motility disorders, or fistulae of the upper GI tract necessitate that the client be fed into the small bowel, distal to the impairment. A client who has aspirated or is at risk for aspiration may benefit from postpyloric feeding. The duration of enteral therapy defines the type of tube placed: temporary tubes for short-term therapy (<4 to 6 weeks) and permanent tubes for long-term therapy (>4 to 6 weeks).

For short-term feeding, nasogastric or nasoenteric tubes are the tubes of choice. Tubes varying in length and ranging in size from 5 to 16 French (Fr.) are placed into the stomach or small intestine at the bedside, and the tip position is then verified with an abdominal radiograph. If postpyloric feeding is indicated, the tip of the tube can be advanced under fluoroscopy, or via endoscopy, client positioning, or the administration of prokinetic agents (e.g., cisapride, metoclopramide, or erythromycin). Small-bore enteral feeding tubes are made of polyurethane or silicone plastic and are thus softer and more flexible than a standard nasogastric tube used for decompression.

For long-term enteral feeding, gastrostomy and jejunostomy tubes are indicated. These tubes can be placed surgically, endoscopically, or radiologically. Surgically placed devices (gastrostomy or jejunostomy tubes), are used most commonly in clients undergoing a laparotomy, and general anesthesia is required. More recently, the percutaneous endoscopic gastrostomy (PEG) or jejunostomy (PEJ) approach has become the most common method of placing a permanent long-term feeding device. This nonsurgical approach avoids the need for general anesthesia and can be performed on an outpatient basis.

Table 29–9 describes various enteral feeding devices and their indications. Various GI tubes and their placement and management are discussed in Chapters 30 and 31.

METHODS OF ADMINISTRATION

Enteral feeding can be administered by either an *intermittent* or *continuous* drip. The method of delivery is determined by (1) the location of the tube tip and (2) the client's tolerance. When the tube tip is located in the small intestine, continuous feeding is the desired choice. For gastric feedings, the type of administration can be (1) bolus, (2) intermittent, or (3) continuous.

In *intermittent* or *bolus* feedings, 300 to 500 ml of enteral formula are delivered several times per day. Bolus feedings are usually delivered via a syringe over 10 to 15 minutes.

In *intermittent* feeding, formula is placed into a gravity bag and dripped in over 30 to 60 minutes. An infusion pump may also be used. Intermittent feeding is a more common method than bolus feeding to deliver periodic feedings into the stomach in the acute care setting because of improved tolerance.

Continuous feedings are administered via an infusion pump to more closely control the rate of infusion. The feedings are generally infused over 24 hours at rates ranging from 50 ml to 150 ml. As clients are switched to cycled nocturnal feedings in preparation for discharge, they often require and can tolerate continuous rates slightly above 150 ml/hr. However, clients usually cannot tolerate continuous feeding into the small intestine at rates above 200 ml/hr.

Continuous feeding into the stomach has been associated with less gastric distention and aspiration compared with bolus or intermittent feeding into the stomach.[6, 10] In addition, continuous gastric feedings may reduce metabolic complications and protect against stress ulcers more effectively compared with intermittent gastric feedings.[6, 10]

■ Nursing Management of the Client Receiving Enteral Nutrition

ASSESSMENT

In addition to the nutritional assessment measures described earlier, you should review the type of formula being used; the time, frequency, and amount of feeding; the client's specific indications; and the placement and

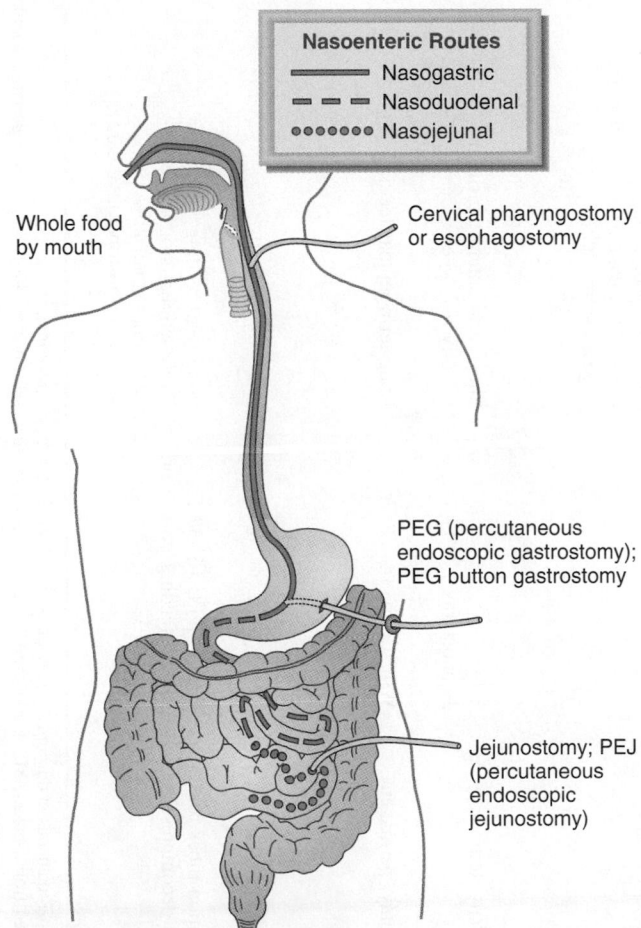

Nasoenteric Routes
— Nasogastric
- - - Nasoduodenal
•••••• Nasojejunal

Whole food by mouth

Cervical pharyngostomy or esophagostomy

PEG (percutaneous endoscopic gastrostomy); PEG button gastrostomy

Jejunostomy; PEJ (percutaneous endoscopic jejunostomy)

FIGURE 29–3 Placements for enteral access. (From Mahan, L. K., & Escott-Stump, S. E. [2000]. *Krause's food, nutrition, & diet therapy* [10th ed., p. 468]. Philadelphia: W. B. Saunders.)

TABLE 29-9 ENTERAL ACCESS DEVICES

Enteral Access	Tube Size and Length	Indications	Advantages	Disadvantages
Nasogastric (small-bore feeding tube)	8–12 Fr., 17–36 inches	Functional stomach Upper gastrointestinal tract obstruction Dysphagia to solids Not at risk for aspiration	Placed at bedside Low morbidity Easily inserted Continued use of GI tract	Client discomfort Risk of aspiration
Nasoduodenal	14–18 Fr., 35–45 inches	Gastric atony Risk of aspiration	Decreased risk of aspiration Continued use of GI tract	Client discomfort Difficult placement Easily malpositioned
Nasojejunal	14–18 Fr., 36–45 inches	High risk for pulmonary aspiration of gastric contents Functional small bowel	Decreased risk of aspiration Continued use of GI tract	Increased cost of tube and skilled professional needed to place tube Easily malpositioned
Gastrostomy, surgical	14–30 Fr.	Inability to use percutaneous placement GI surgery Long-term feeding	Continued use of GI tract Can be placed in clients with esophageal or pharyngeal cancers Used in obese clients when unable to transilluminate abdominal wall for PEG placement	General anesthesia Tube migration Easily obstructed Local stoma site complications
Gastrostomy, percutaneous	14–22 Fr.	Long-term feeding tube No history of aspiration	No surgical procedure needed Placement without general anesthesia Continued use of GI tract	Potential for aspiration Cannot be used in obese clients
Low-profile gastrostomy device (G-Button)	18–28 Fr.	Long-term feeding Ambulatory patients Disoriented patients who pull at the gastrostomy tube	Increased mobility Decreased cost over time because of device longevity Decreased nursing time compared with time needed for replacement tube change Continued use of GI tract	Skilled professional needed for placement Increased trauma to client compared with replacement tube Increased cost compared with cost of gastrostomy tube change Second procedure required after gastrostomy tube placement
Jejunostomy, temporary	5 Fr. Jejunostomy kit, 14 Fr.	Short-term enteral nutrition Usually ≤2 weeks	Continued use of GI tract	Surgical placement Tube easily obstructed Costly
Jejunostomy, permanent	Whistle tip, 14–18 Fr.	Long-term jejunal feeding	Silicone plastic Continued use of GI tract Easily replaced when fistulous tract is formed Larger-bore Location proximal jejunum, thus elemental products not required Continued use of GI tract	Continuous or slow intermittent tube feeding required via a pump
Combination tubes for gastric decompression	Gastric port, 16–30 Fr. Jejunal feeding port, 9 Fr.	Long-term feeding Dysfunctional stomach Functional small bowel Short-term postoperative care	Can decompress a dysfunctional stomach and prevent regurgitation of gastric contents during small intestine feeding Continued use of GI tract	Skilled professional needed for placement Expensive process Jejunal feeding needed Can be dislodged from original position Placed during surgery

PEG, percutaneous endoscopic gastrostomy; Fr., French; GI, gastrointestinal.
Adapted from Shuster, M., & Mancino, J. (1994). Ensuring successful home tube feeding in the geriatric population. *Geriatric Nursing, 15,* 67–82.

patency of the tube. Monitor the client for aspiration of tube feeding or GI contents.

See Bridge to Home Health Care: Managing Tube Feedings.

DIAGNOSIS, OUTCOMES, INTERVENTIONS

Altered Nutrition: Less Than Body Requirements. The nursing diagnosis most appropriate for the client receiving enteral feeding is *Altered Nutrition: Less Than Body Requirements related to difficulty swallowing, esophageal or gastric resection or obstruction, or inability to ingest adequate calories and nutrients.*

BRIDGE TO HOME HEALTH CARE

Managing Tube Feedings

Home health agency nutrition support teams usually consist of a nurse, a registered dietitian, and a pharmacist. When these professionals regularly visit a client who has a new feeding tube, the chances for successfully managing the client and the tube feedings at home are greatly increased. In addition to providing direct care, the team provides instructions to the client and family, communicates with the client's physician, prevents problems if possible, and monitors any problems that develop.

Consistently flushing the tube with water before and after each feeding enhances the longevity of the tube. Although flushing the tube with carbonated beverages has been suggested, studies indicate few or no benefits over flushing with water. Flush all types of feeding tubes with a 50-cc syringe; smaller syringes can create pressure high enough to rupture a tube.

Teach the client and family to secure a nasogastric tube firmly to the nose and to either side of the face or to another position of comfort. To secure the tube, use tape, a transparent occlusive dressing, or a commercial tube holder with a hydrocolloid backing with a self-fastening tape (Velcro) closure.

When the client has a percutaneous endoscopic gastrostomy (PEG) or a percutaneous endoscopic jejunostomy (PEJ), observe daily for tube dislodgment, leaking, skin irritation, and clinical manifestations of infection. Clean the site daily with hydrogen peroxide followed by normal saline rinse. Slide the external bridge away for cleaning, then reposition. No dressing is required. Good hand-washing technique is essential for all personnel.

Management of tube feedings varies with the type of infusion: continuous infusion with a pump, bolus infusion, or infusion by gravity. Numerous commercial products are available to meet the client's nutritional needs. The physician and the registered dietitian are responsible for assessing the type of feeding and method of infusion. However, the client may tolerate one formula better than another. Positioning clients at a 45-degree angle or greater helps them tolerate the feeding. Changing the rate and frequency of infusion may decrease or eliminate nausea, diarrhea, or tube displacement. Successful tube feeding begins in the hospital and continues at home as the client, family, home care nurse, registered dietitian, pharmacist, and physician work together as a team.

Colette H. McVaney, RN, BSN, *Lead Nurse, Geriatric Clinic, Nebraska Health System, Omaha, Nebraska*

Outcomes. The client will maintain ideal body weight or will gain 1 to 2 pounds per week until ideal body weight is attained.

Interventions

Prevent Contamination of Formula and Delivery System. You are primarily responsible for administering and monitoring enteral feeding. The care and handling of the feeding formula and equipment is a key factor in the success of enteral feeding. To prevent contamination of the enteral formula, you must adhere to strict hand-washing before handling the feeding formula and equipment. *Open delivery systems,* which use cans and syringes and bags, are the most vulnerable because of the great degree of manipulation. Formulas administered via an open system should hang for only 4 hours before being changed and the tubing flushed or rinsed. The equipment should be changed every 24 hours. *Closed delivery systems,* which use a prefilled container, minimize the amount of preparation; thus, the chance of formula contamination is reduced and the hang time is extended (24 to 48 hours).

Assess Tube Location. Before administering an enteral feeding, ensure that the tube is positioned properly. If a nasoenteric tube is being used to feed a client for the first time, make sure that an abdominal radiograph has verified that the tip is located in the GI tract.

Routinely evaluate the position of the enteral feeding device, and be alert for the possibility of tube migration or dislodgment. Nasoenteric tubes can be marked to indicate the position so that it will be evident if the tube has moved. Nasoenteric tubes can easily migrate when the client coughs or vomits, but more often the tubes are dislodged when a confused or agitated client inadvertently removes the tube.

In addition to determining whether the tube has migrated, you may need to evaluate the location of the tube tip. Is the tube tip in the stomach, small intestine, or respiratory tract? Three methods can be used to evaluate tip location:

- *Auscultation:* injecting air into the feeding tube and listening with a stethoscope for the sound
- *Aspiration:* observing the fluid that is removed through the feeding tube
- *pH paper testing:* checking the pH of the fluid removed from the feeding tube

Auscultation is the least reliable method and should not be used to evaluate the tube tip position. Observing the aspirated fluid and checking its pH are more useful. However, aspiration should not replace a radiographic evaluation after the initial placement or when tube migration is suspected.

An enterostomy (e.g., gastrostomy, jejunostomy) tube can migrate in or out if it is not properly secured at the exit site with sutures or a tube attachment device. Enteral feeding tubes that are not well secured at the exit site can pivot, causing an accumulation of granulation tissue and a widening of the tract. If the tract becomes widened, formula and digestive enzymes can come up through it and excoriate the skin on the abdomen.

Administer Feedings. Starter regimens for enteral feedings differ according to tube tip location and the client's clinical status. Continuous feedings into the small intestine are usually started at 30 to 40 ml/hr and advanced as tolerated every 12 to 24 hours until the daily goal is reached. Intermittent feedings into the stomach are initiated at 100 to 120 ml every 4 hours and advanced every 12 to 24 hours as tolerated.

Prevent Aspiration. Preventing aspiration during enteral feeding is crucial. The use of postpyloric or small bowel feeding is recommended for a client with a high risk of aspiration. Proper administration and delivery techniques are especially important during gastric feedings. The head of the bed must be elevated 45 degrees for 1 hour before and 1 hour after gastric feeding. Continuous gastric feedings require that the head of the client's bed remain elevated. Gastric residuals can be monitored every 4 hours initially and then as needed to assess gastric emptying and to prevent aspiration. A significant gastric residual is approximately 100 to 150 ml. Feeding into the jejunum theoretically reduces the risk of aspirating enteral formula. However, the head of the bed should still be elevated about 30 degrees during continuous jejunal feeding.

Maintain Enteral Access. Maintenance of enteral access consists of caring for the external site, maintaining tube patency, and maintaining the correct tube position. Nasoenteric tubes most often exit the nose and are secured to the nose or cheek with tape or an adhesive attachment device. The nasoenteric tube should exit the nose, hang straight down, and then be gently looped up and secured to the cheek. Tubes that are sharply angled as they exit the nostril can cause necrosis or obstruct the flow of enteral formula through the tube. With any method of securing, the tube should be repositioned and resecured at least every other day to prevent skin irritation.

For tubes that exit the abdominal wall (e.g., PEG, gastrostomy, and jejunostomy tubes), a dressing is required for the first 24 hours after placement. The site care consists of a daily cleaning with mild soap and rinsing with warm water. Dressings are optional for healed enterostomy sites, but a light nonocclusive dressing may help secure the tube as well as contain mucus that commonly drains from the tube tract.

Maintaining the patency of the enteral feeding tube is a critical nursing intervention for the client receiving enteral feeding. Enteral feeding tubes clog for a variety of reasons, the most common of which is the improper administration of medications through the tube. Medication administration via enteral feeding tubes is probably the most poorly understood part of working with enteral feeding devices and thus highly prone to error. Medications should be given through an enteral access device only when there is an absolute contraindication to taking them by mouth. Problems that can result from incorrect medication administration via an enteral feeding tube include tube clogging, altered drug availability, and diarrhea. Box 29-4 lists some steps to follow for safe administration of medications via an enteral feeding tube.

Tubes of any diameter will clog without strict adherence to a flushing protocol. The most effective irrigant for flushing an enteral feeding tube is water. Flush the tube with at least 30 ml of warm water every 4 hours during continuous feedings and before and after each in-

---

> **BOX 29-4** **Guidelines for the Administration of Medications via an Enteral Feeding Tube**
>
> - If possible, administer the medication by mouth.
> - Use a liquid form of the medication if available.
> - If the medication can be crushed, crush it to a fine powder and dissolve it in 30 ml of water.
> - Do not crush enteric-coated or time-released tablets or capsules.
> - Flush the tube with 30 ml of water before and after giving each medication.
> - Do not mix multiple medications or give them together.
> - Do not deliver a medication that must be absorbed in the stomach into the small intestine, such as sucralfate (Carafate) or antacids.
> - Hold feedings 1 to 2 hours before and after giving a medication that might have drug-nutrient interactions, such as phenytoin (Dilantin).

---

termittent feeding or medication. Acidic flushing solutions, such as cranberry juice, may precipitate with protein and obstruct the tube; thus, they are not recommended.[6]

See the Management and Delegation feature.

EVALUATION OF NUTRITIONAL INTERVENTIONS

When caring for a client receiving TEN or TPN, you must regularly evaluate the client's response to therapy. Assessing the client's tolerance to the nutrient regimen includes evaluation of the fluid status (intake/output data and weights) and a thorough assessment of the GI system. Evaluation also includes monitoring vital signs, reviewing laboratory tests, and assessing the function of the nutritional access device. Together with a nutritional support team, you will be collecting pertinent data, such as weight and visceral protein measures, to assess the success of the nutrient prescription.

Table 29-10 outlines common parameters used to monitor clients receiving enteral or parenteral nutrition. Comprehensive and routine monitoring can prevent complications related to nutritional support therapies.

Self-Care

Nutritional support therapies, such as TEN and TPN, are routinely administered in the home setting. Nurses play a pivotal role in determining appropriate candidates for home nutrition support by helping to determine the plan of care and providing client and family education.

The nursing assessment includes a comprehensive review of the client and family or caregivers. The physical and cognitive abilities of the client or caregiver must be evaluated so that you can be sure of their ability to carry out complex procedures. Manual dexterity and eyesight are particularly important when care involves programming pumps for infusion and drawing up medication in syringes. The client's home environment must be evaluated to ensure that it is safe for home therapy. The client or caregiver education process should ideally start in the hospital and be reinforced after discharge. Clients receiving either TPN or tube feedings need to learn a wide range of related skills (Box 29-5).

MANAGEMENT AND DELEGATION

Care of Nasogastric Tubes, Small-Bore Feeding Tubes, and Gastrostomy and Jejunostomy Tubes

Nasogastric Tubes

Decompression relieves stomach pressure by removing gas and fluids from the stomach. It can be used to prevent nausea, vomiting and gastric distention when gastrointestinal (GI) motility is delayed or absent or when the client has a distal obstruction or has had recent GI tract surgery. Nasogastric tubes may also be used to initiate enteral feedings upon resumption of bowel motility.

The detailed assessment and potential risks associated with nasogastric tube insertion, maintenance, and removal prevent delegation of these procedures to unlicensed personnel. You may delegate the gathering of equipment and the measurement, recording, and testing of nasogastric drainage to assistive personnel. Delegation of short-term disconnection of nasogastric tubes (for the purposes such as toileting or ambulation) may be appropriate under the supervision of a Registered Nurse (RN). Reconnection of the nasogastric tube to suction requires the RN to verify pressure settings. You may delegate skin care of the client's nose and comfort care for the client's mouth to unlicensed personnel.

Nasogastric Tubes: Mouth and Nose Care

Instruct assistive personnel to:

1. Wash hands and don gloves.
2. For nasal care:
   a. Gently clean and lubricate the client's external nares to prevent buildup of crusted secretions and skin breakdown.
   b. Use a clean cotton-tipped swab and a water-soluble lubricant to clean the client's nostril.
   c. Make sure that the skin on the client's nose is clean and dry.
   d. Apply tincture of benzoin or other skin adhesive on the tip of the patient's nose and allow to dry.
   e. Secure tube with hypoallergenic tape, taking care to avoid pressure on nares
3. For mouth care:
   a. Offer or administer frequent oral hygiene with non-alcohol containing solutions to remove debris, increase comfort and maintain a healthy oral cavity.
   b. Brush teeth or assist patient to do so.

Small-Bore Feeding Tubes and Gastrostomy and Jejunostomy Tubes

The most desirable and appropriate method of providing nutrition is via the oral route. For clients who are unable or unwilling to meet their nutritional needs orally, enteral tube feedings may be an option. Tube-feedings may be delivered through large-bore or small-bore gastric tubes that may be inserted by the RN with a physician's order, through gastrostomy tubes, or through jejunostomy tubes. A gastrostomy tube is large and is surgically or endoscopically placed directly into the stomach, exiting through an incision in the left upper quadrant of the abdomen. A jejunostomy tube is also placed surgically (directly into the jejunum for small bowel feedings), or endoscopically (into the gastrostomy tube and passed through to the jejunum).

A physician's order is required for placement of a small-bore nasogastric or nasointestinal feeding tube. Accuracy of feeding tube placement is confirmed by abdominal radiograph. Insertion of nasogastric tubes and verification of placement of nasogastric, gastrostomy and jejunostomy tubes require problem-solving and knowledge application unique to the professional nurse. For this reason, delegation of these skills is inappropriate. You may delegate skin care to the exit site of the tube to unlicensed personnel.

Gastrostomy and Jejunostomy Exit Site Care:

Exit site care is performed 24 hours after feeding tube insertion. Instruct assistive personnel to:

1. Wash hands and don gloves.
2. Remove the old dressing.
3. Clean around the tube insertion site with normal saline to remove exudate or dried blood.
4. Do not use hydrogen peroxide or any antiseptic cream unless specifically ordered by the physician.
5. Rinse the tube insertion site with clean water and dry thoroughly.
6. Apply a new split drain sponge dressing if needed.

Describe findings that are immediately reportable to you for assistive personnel, including redness, swelling, abnormal drainage (thick, foul-smelling, yellow or green color), or pain at the tube's insertion site. Have assistive personnel report any complaints of abdominal pain, bloating, cramping, or diarrhea. Verify the competence of assistive personnel in performing these tasks during orientation and annually thereafter.

Hilary S. Blackwood, MSN, RN, *Clinician IV, Surgical Nutrition Support Services, University of Virginia Health System, Charlottesville, Virginia*

EATING DISORDERS

OBESITY

Obesity is characterized by an excess accumulation of fat and reflects an overall imbalance between energy intake and expenditure.

Etiology and Risk Factors

The etiology of obesity is multifactorial, making effective treatment a challenge. When a positive energy balance occurs (more calories are consumed than expended), obesity or an accumulation of stored energy (fat) occurs. Causes of obesity can be related to either side of this energy equation. The most important factors[5] seem to be:

1. *Genetic tendency.* Genetic makeup determines the *basal metabolic rate* (BMR), defined as the energy required for basic maintenance of the body's cells and functions. The BMR can vary widely (as much as 30%) and is often higher in the obese client.[7] More recent studies of causes of obesity are focusing on other genetic factors, such as neurotransmitters and peptide levels, that may control and regu-

TABLE 29–10	SUGGESTED NUTRITION MONITORING PROTOCOL

Parameter	Frequency of Assessment
BIOCHEMICAL MEASURES	
Electrolytes	Daily
Magnesium, calcium, phosphorus	Daily
Glucose	Every 6 hours for 48 hours, then daily
Albumin, prealbumin, transferrin	Weekly
Triglyceride	Pre-infusion, post-infusion, then daily
Liver function tests	Pre-infusion, then weekly
Complete blood count, prothrombin time, partial thromboplastin time	Weekly
NURSING ASSESSMENT	
Weight	Daily
Intake/output	Hourly/every 8 hours
Infusion rate	Every 4 hours
Temperature	Every 8 hours
NUTRITIONAL MONITORING	
24-hour urine collection for urinary urea nitrogen	Weekly
Measured resting energy expenditure	Weekly

late food intake and affect the development of obesity.

2. *Environment.* The relationship between environmental factors and obesity is unclear. However, societal factors that may play a role include a more sedentary lifestyle, which is typical of our industrialized society. Much of our daily lifestyle no longer requires physical work. In addition, when food is plentiful, particularly high-fat alternatives, obesity can develop.

BOX 29–5	Teaching Topics for Clients Who Need Enteral or Parenteral Feedings at Home

Care of the Nutritional Access Device

- Flushing the venous access or feeding tube
- Changing the dressing
- Observing for evidence of infection

Formula Preparation

- Adding medication to the TPN formula
- Placing enteral formula in feeding bag
- Setting up enteral or parenteral feeding pump or bag
- Obtaining formula for TPN and related supplies

Monitoring for Complications

- Assessing temperature
- Monitoring weight

TPN, total parenteral nutrition.

3. *Diet.* The composition of diet is increasingly important and continues to receive public attention. The intake of a high-fat, calorie-dense diet can increase the likelihood of obesity.[16]

Pathophysiology

Obesity is a serious health risk and has been associated with increased mortality and morbidity. With obesity, the risk for cardiovascular disease is increased; with increasing weight, elevated blood pressure, blood lipids, and glucose levels have been documented.[8, 12, 15, 16]

A strong relationship between obesity and the development of type 2 diabetes mellitus has been known for some time. The cause is thought to be the increased amount of fat stores, which are associated with glucose intolerance and abnormal metabolism of insulin. Other serious health problems that occur more often in obesity include respiratory problems, gallbladder disease, and arthritis.

More recently, a relationship between obesity and cancer has been suggested. Some cancers, such as colorectal, breast, and prostate cancer, have been linked to obesity. However, whether this link between cancer and obesity is simply due to the excess weight or to specific dietary factors is unclear.

Clinical Manifestations

Obesity is a significant problem in the United States. Estimates from 1988 to 1991 indicated that approximately 33% of Americans are obese, an increase from 23% in 1971.[8] Obesity is defined as more than 45% above *ideal body weight* (IBW) for women and more than 35% above ideal body weight for men. *Body mass index* (BMI) is another way to quantify obesity. A BMI above 27 kg/m^2 is characteristic of obesity. To determine BMI, use the following formula:

$$ BMI = \frac{wt\ (kg)}{ht\ (m^2)} \quad or \quad \frac{wt\ (lb)}{ht\ (in.^2)} \times 703 $$

Outcome Management

■ Medical Management

The medical management of obesity should include a combination of diet and behavior modification, exercise, and occasionally medication. Diet instruction with a trained registered dietitian is the optimal intervention to encourage weight loss. A balanced hypocaloric diet in the range of 1100 to 1200 kcal is regarded as the most successful approach to long-term diet modifications. More severe calorie restrictions are difficult to maintain for longer periods and can result in severe vitamin and mineral deficiencies. Clients on low-calorie diets should consume about 60 g/day of protein (~25% of total calories).

An exercise program should be part of the overall care of the obese client. Exercise is an important way to increase the energy expenditure and to facilitate weight loss. Diet restriction in combination with an exercise program, compared with diet restriction alone, is a more successful way to lose weight and maintain the weight loss.

The role of medication in promoting weight loss is controversial, in part because of the known dangers of some regimens. Drugs used to treat obesity are categorized by the following three mechanisms: (1) reduction of food intake, (2) decrease in the absorption of nutrients, and (3) increase in energy expenditure.[15] Although various drugs have been effective in promoting weight loss, any prescribed drug therapy regimen should be under the strict supervision of a qualified health care team to prevent potentially life-threatening complications.

■ Surgical Management

Surgical treatment of obesity may be considered when the client has been unsuccessful after diet modification, behavioral therapy, exercise, and drug therapy. Two surgical approaches have been used.

JEJUNOILEAL BYPASS. A "shortened small bowel" is created, resulting in malabsorption of nutrients. However, severe metabolic complications—including hypokalemia, hypocalcemia, vitamin B deficiency, and hepatic toxicity—have made this procedure less than optimal.

GASTRIC STAPLING. The more favorable option is revision of the stomach to create a smaller pouch, which limits oral intake. Gastric stapling is the most common surgical approach for the morbidly obese client. This procedure involves creation of a small pouch (~50 to 60 ml) and an outlet to the small intestine. This surgical approach is associated with fewer complications than jejunoileal bypass. Diet instruction must be part of the postoperative care of these clients, focusing on the increased frequency and decreased size of meals. In addition, clients are instructed to take a multivitamin every day.

ANOREXIA NERVOSA AND BULIMIA NERVOSA

Anorexia nervosa and bulimia nervosa have become of increasing concern to nurses and other health care professionals. These abnormalities in eating behavior can result in life-threatening complications. Together, these disorders afflict about 1.2 million young women in the United States. Clients with these disorders are frequently seen by medical-surgical nurses for treatment of the nutritional problems. Mental health consultations are particularly important for these clients.

A client with anorexia nervosa intentionally imposes severe dietary restrictions, resulting in weight loss, endocrine dysfunction, and fluid and electrolyte imbalance. The client's body image is grossly distorted, and her attitude toward eating is impaired. Clients with bulimia nervosa have similar distortions in attitudes toward weight and eating; however, this disorder is characterized by frequent binge eating and purging (vomiting).

Etiology and Risk Factors

The etiology of eating disorders involves biologic, psychological, and social factors. Endocrine changes related to the onset of puberty may be the influencing biologic factor, since dramatic changes in physical appearance and weight gain are occurring. Psychological factors may play a contributing role, especially early sexual and/or physical abuse. The social aspects relate to our society's obsession

with thinness. The group most at risk for development of eating disorders is young females 15 to 24 years of age. The incidence of bulimia nervosa is twice that of anorexia nervosa.

Early recognition can lead to treatment before the client's life is in jeopardy. Although the disorders are psychological in origin and not responsive to education, health promotion activities include instruction about avoidance of fad diets, proper nutrition, and ways to build self-confidence safely.

Pathophysiology

The pathophysiologic changes associated with severe eating disorders are similar to those seen in starvation. When nutrient intake is severely limited, the body adapts by utilizing the body's fat stores and sparing protein and glucose stores. With prolonged starvation, significant shifts in fluid and electrolyte balance can occur and can be life-threatening. Alterations in the metabolism of insulin, thyroid hormone, and catecholamines explain common clinical manifestations, including decreases in pulse, respiratory rate, blood pressure, cardiac output, and gut motility.[11] The hypothalamus responds to the lack of nutrient intake with changes in pituitary function, resulting in amenorrhea and infertility.

Clinical Manifestations

Clients with anorexia nervosa are usually first introduced to the health care system when the disordered eating behavior results in obvious weight loss. Clients may limit themselves to 200 to 500 kcal/day—only 60% to 70% of the amount needed for ideal body weight. Physical manifestations (Fig. 29–4) include dry skin, pallor, bradycardia, hypotension, intolerance to cold, constipation, and amenorrhea.

Clinical manifestations of bulimia nervosa include episodes of binge eating followed by self-induced vomiting. The eating and vomiting episodes occur most often in the late afternoon and evening and are done in secret. Some clients may abuse laxatives and diuretics as well. Personality characteristics typical of clients with bulimia are related to depression. Physical manifestations may not be as obvious, since the client with bulimia may be of normal weight without any depletion of fat stores. Less obvious clinical manifestations are erosion of tooth enamel, from frequent vomiting, and esophageal and throat irritation.

Outcome Management

■ Medical Management

The medical management of eating disorders must include physical and psychological components. Psychotherapy should focus on the underlying problems causing the disordered eating behavior. The physical rehabilitation of nutritional status targets ways to normalize the client's eating pattern and to help the client begin regaining weight, if needed. Excessive caloric intakes are not necessary in clients with anorexia and can actually be harmful in the severely malnourished client. A registered dietitian

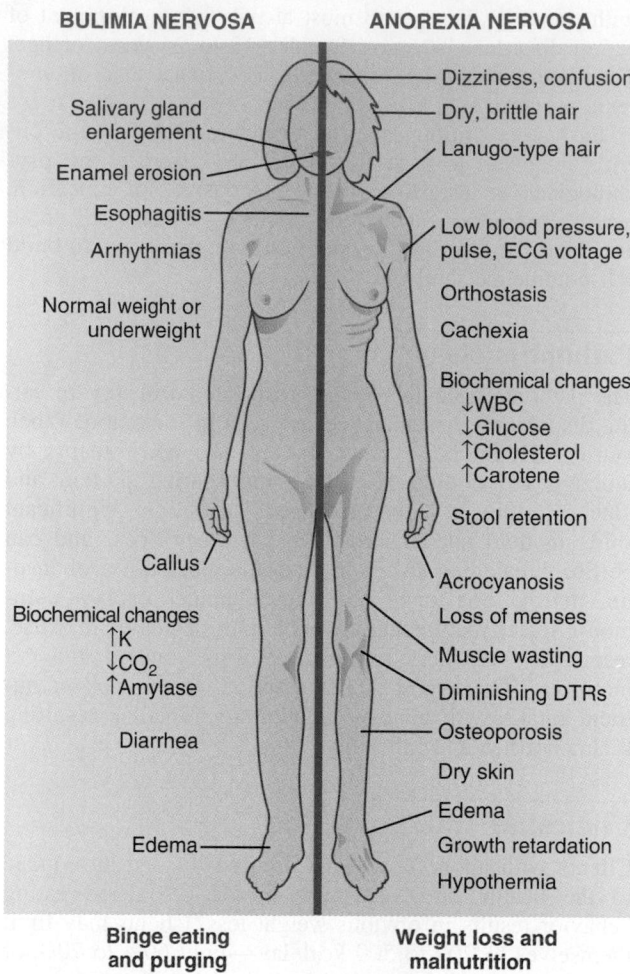

BULIMIA NERVOSA | ANOREXIA NERVOSA

Salivary gland enlargement
Enamel erosion
Esophagitis
Arrhythmias

Normal weight or underweight

Callus

Biochemical changes
↑K
↓CO₂
↑Amylase

Diarrhea

Edema

Dizziness, confusion
Dry, brittle hair
Lanugo-type hair

Low blood pressure, pulse, ECG voltage
Orthostasis
Cachexia

Biochemical changes
↓WBC
↓Glucose
↑Cholesterol
↑Carotene

Stool retention

Acrocyanosis
Loss of menses
Muscle wasting
Diminishing DTRs
Osteoporosis
Dry skin
Edema
Growth retardation
Hypothermia

Binge eating and purging | Weight loss and malnutrition

FIGURE 29–4 Physical manifestations of anorexia nervosa and bulimia nervosa. CO₂, carbon dioxide; DTRs, deep tendon reflexes, ECG, electrocardiographic; K, potassium; WBC, white blood cell. (From Mahan, L. K., & Escott-Stump, S. E. [2000]. *Krause's food, nutrition, & diet therapy* [10th ed., p. 521]. Philadelphia: W. B. Saunders.)

should be part of the treatment team and assist in the determination of caloric goals.

Hospitalization is necessary when malnutrition is severe enough to result in serious fluid and electrolyte disturbances. Enteral or parenteral therapy may be needed in extreme cases when the client has not responded to strategies to encourage and improve oral intake. Nutritional support therapies should be introduced slowly in severely malnourished clients to avoid complications of refeeding syndrome. Refeeding syndrome is characterized by precipitous drops in serum potassium, magnesium, and phosphorus when nutrients are administered to depleted clients.

■ Nursing Management of the Client with Eating Disorders

ASSESSMENT

A comprehensive history will help identify the type of eating disorder (see Chapter 28). Collect details of weight history and eating patterns to successfully identify the problem and help develop an appropriate plan of care.

Have the client describe her typical pattern of eating, and ask about the use of appetite-suppressing medication, laxatives, and self-induced vomiting. Other pertinent data to gather include exercise patterns and menstrual history.

DIAGNOSIS, OUTCOMES, INTERVENTIONS

Altered Nutrition: Less Than Body Requirements. The client with anorexia nervosa often experiences *Altered Nutrition: Less Than Body Requirements related to inadequate food intake (anorexia nervosa).*

Outcomes. The client will be able to resume normal eating behaviors. In clients with severe nutritional depletion, the client will be able to regain weight at a safe rate (1 to 2 pounds/week).

Interventions. When caring for a client with anorexia nervosa, help the client select foods from the Food Guide Pyramid for a nutritionally balanced diet. The client is usually allowed to refuse a specific number of foods (such as two or three) so that some sense of control is felt. Observe the client during mealtimes. Be supportive during mealtimes and, if needed, stay with the client after she eats to prevent her from purging. Education related to nutrition must include the client's family, caregivers, or co-residents. An accurate calorie count and regular monitoring of weight are other important interventions. TPN or TEN may be required if the client is severely malnourished.

Altered Nutrition: More Than Body Requirements. Clients with bulimia nervosa and obesity often experience *Altered Nutrition: More Than Body Requirements related to increased food intake.*

Outcomes. The client will lose 1 to 2 pounds per week until ideal body weight is achieved and maintain ideal body weight thereafter.

Interventions. Teach the client how to use the Food Guide Pyramid to select a healthy diet with portions of appropriate size. Encourage the client to eat slowly and to develop a regular exercise pattern. Encourage the client to approach food, eating, and self-image in a new way. Provide emotional support and supervision for the client to overcome stressful periods and break the binge-and-purge cycle.

Body Image Disturbance. The client with an eating disorder often has a *Body Image Disturbance related to misconception of body size or negative feelings (all disorders).*

Outcomes. The client will develop a more normal image of self, as evidenced by statements concerning self and by the client's ability to overcome the eating disorder.

Interventions. Recognize that clients suffering from eating disorders typically have low self-esteem. These clients see the regulation of food and exercise of self-control in eating patterns and amounts as ways to prove themselves successful. It is important that the client's significant others help the client find other areas of self-regard.

Risk for Injury: Dysrhythmias. Both anorexia and bulimia lead to altered fluid and electrolyte balance. This puts them at *Risk for Injury: Dysrhythmias related to hypokalemia.*

Outcomes. The client will maintain normal cardiac output, as evidenced by the absence of cardiac dysrhythmias and adequate tissue perfusion.

Interventions. Monitor the client's serum potassium level at regular intervals. If the potassium level is low, administer potassium supplements as prescribed. If the level is dangerously low, IV replacement may be required.

EVALUATION

It is expected that the client will overcome the eating disorder with consistent and continued treatment and that weight will return to normal.

CONCLUSIONS

The nutritional care of the adult medical-surgical client is an important part of a comprehensive treatment plan. Preventing and treating malnutrition is just one way to facilitate recovery from acute and chronic illness. As a nurse, you have a vital role in nutritional assessment as well as in the prevention and treatment of malnutrition. Clients with eating disorders, such as obesity, anorexia nervosa, and bulimia nervosa, require both medical-surgical and psychological interventions.

THINKING CRITICALLY

1. **You are caring for a 62-year-old client in a nursing home. She has had a cerebrovascular accident and is paralyzed, sometimes confused, and incontinent. She refuses to eat and drink after many episodes of coughing and choking at mealtimes. A small-bore feeding tube has been inserted. When you check the tube for aspirate to confirm patency, you are unable to obtain any return aspirate. What nursing measures should be instituted to determine the problem? What is the priority nursing intervention?**

Factors to Consider. What conditions contribute to the lack of aspirate return? What is your decision if the tube remains occluded?

2. **You are assigned to care for two clients. One is an older man with a 6-month history of difficulty swallowing and a weight loss of 25 pounds. The other client, a woman in her mid-30s, has Crohn's disease and has been admitted with an exacerbation of the disease. How should nutritional needs be addressed for each client?**

Factors to Consider. How should nutritional needs be met for the client with an upper gastrointestinal tract disorder? With a lower gastrointestinal tract disorder?

3. **D. A. is a 20-year-old white woman who is a sophomore in college and living away from home. She is 5 feet 1 inch tall. She has been steadily losing weight, although she participates in the campus meal plan and takes her meals in the dormitory cafeteria. She plays on the college volleyball and basketball teams. Most of the students are excited about Thanksgiving holiday plans, but the dormitory counselor noticed that D. A. has not voiced any plans. She is found unconscious on the floor in the dormitory communal bathroom. She is taken by ambulance to the community hospital. Her college physical health record states that she weighed 98 pounds in June and had no known medical problems. On admission to the hospital, she weighs 79 pounds. What is her percentage of weight loss? What additional data need to be collected?**

Factors to Consider. What interventions can be used to increase D. A.'s food intake? Is it feasible for a nurse on a busy medical-surgical unit to stay with D. A. during and after her meals? What alternatives might be used?

BIBLIOGRAPHY

1. ASPEN Publications. (1998). *The ASPEN nutrition support practice manual.* Silver Spring, MD: Author.
2. ASPEN Publications. (1998). *Clinical pathways and algorithms for delivery of parenteral and enteral nutrition support in adults.* Silver Spring, MD: Author.
3. Bistrian, B., et al. (1974). Protein status of general surgical patients. *Journal of the American Medical Association, 230,* 858–860.
4. Bistrian, B., et al. (1976). Prevalence of malnutrition in general medical patients. *Journal of the American Medical Association, 235,* 1567–1570.
5. Blackburn, G., Miller, D., & Chan, S. (1997). Pharmaceutical treatment of obesity. *Nursing Clinics of North America 32*(4), 831–848.
6. Bowers, S. (1999). Nutrition support for malnourished acutely ill adults. *MEDSURG Nursing, 8*(3), 145–161.
7. Centers for Disease Control and Prevention. (1996). The Hospital Infection Control Practices Advisory Committee: *Guidelines for the prevention of intravascular device–related infections.* Atlanta: Author.
8. Centers for Disease Control and Prevention. (1997). Prevalence of overweight among children, adolescents, and adults—United States, 1988–1994. *Morbidity and Mortality Weekly Report, 46*(9), 198–202.
9. Edington, J., Kon, P., & Martyn, C. (1996). Prevalence of malnutrition in patients in general practice. *Clinical Nutrition, 15,* 60–63.
10. Guenter, P., et al. (1997). Delivery systems and administration of enteral nutrition. In J. Rombeau & R. H. Rolandelli (Eds.), *Clinical nutrition: Enteral and tube feeding* (3rd ed., pp. 240–267). Philadelphia: W. B. Saunders.
11. Huse, D., & Lucas, A. (1999). Behavioral disorders affecting food intake: Anorexia nervosa, bulimia nervosa and other psychiatric conditions. In M. Shils, et al. (Eds.), *Modern nutrition in health and disease* (9th ed., pp. 1513–1522). Baltimore: Williams & Wilkins.
12. Kannel, W., & Gordon T. (1979). Physiologic and medical concomitants of obesity: The Framingham Study. In G. Bray (Ed.), *Obesity in America.* National Institutes of Health, Pub. No.79. Washington, DC: Department Health, Education, and Welfare.
13. Metheny, N. (1997). *Minimum Data Set, version 2.* Des Moines, IA: Briggs Corporation.
14. Metheny N., et al. (1999). pH and concentration of bilirubin in feeding tube aspirates as predictors of tube placement. *Nursing Research, 48*(4), 189–197.
15. National task force on the prevention and treatment of obesity. (1996). Long term pharmacotherapy in the management of obesity. *Journal of the American Medical Association, 276,* 190–196.
16. Poppit, S., & Prentice, A. (1996). Energy density and its role in the control of food intake: Evidence from metabolic community studies. *Appetite, 26,* 153–156.
17. Rombeau, J. L., & Rolandelli, R. H. (1997). *Clinical nutrition: Enteral and tube feeding* (3rd ed.). Philadelphia: W. B. Saunders.
18. Saltzman, E., & Mason, J. (1997). Enteral nutrition in the elderly. In J. L. Rombeau & R. H. Rolandelli (Eds.), *Clinical nutrition: Enteral and tube feeding* (3rd ed., pp. 385–401). Philadelphia: W. B. Saunders.
19. Stoner, N. E. (1997). Nutrition assessment: A practical approach. *Nursing Clinics of North America, 32*(4), 637–650.
20. Torun, B., & Chew, F. (1999). Protein-energy malnutrition. In M. Shils, et al. (Eds.), *Modern nutrition in health and disease* (9th ed., pp. 963–988). Baltimore: Williams & Wilkins.
21. Veterans Affairs Total Parenteral Nutrition Cooperative Study Group. (1991). Perioperative total parenteral nutrition in surgical patients. *New England Journal of Medicine, 325,* 525–532.

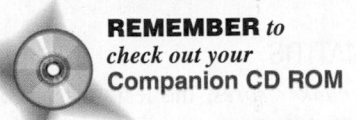

REMEMBER *to*
check out your
Companion CD ROM

CHAPTER
30

Management of Clients with Ingestive Disorders

Elizabeth A. Murphy-Blake

NURSING OUTCOMES CLASSIFICATION (NOC)
for Nursing Diagnoses—Clients with Ingestive Disorders

Altered Nutrition: Less Than Body Requirements	**Swallowing Status: Pharyngeal Phase**	**Nutritional Status: Biochemical Measures**
Nutritional Status	**Impaired Verbal Communication**	Tissue Integrity: Skin and Mucous Membranes
Nutritional Status: Food and Fluid Intake	Communication Ability	Wound Healing: Secondary Intention
Nutritional Status: Nutrient Intake	Communication: Expressive Ability	**Risk for Ineffective Individual Coping**
Altered Oral Mucous Membrane	**Knowledge Deficit**	Coping
Oral Health	Knowledge: Illness Care	Decision Making
Tissue Integrity: Skin and Mucous Membrane	Knowledge: Treatment Procedure	Information Processing
	Knowledge: Treatment Regimen	Role Performance
Impaired Swallowing	**Pain**	Social Support
Swallowing Status	Comfort Level	**Risk for Injury**
Swallowing Status: Esophageal Phase	Pain: Disruptive Effects	Risk Control
Swallowing Status: Oral Phase	**Risk for Impaired Skin Integrity**	Risk Detection
	Nutritional Status	

The client with an ingestive disorder, regardless of the cause, may have a problem in the oral cavity or esophagus that indicates a common nursing diagnosis, such as *Altered Oral Mucous Membrane; Pain; Altered Nutrition: Less than Body Requirements; Impaired Verbal Communication;* or *Impaired Swallowing.* Usually, the client first experiences pain in the mouth or esophagus or difficulty with swallowing. Shortly thereafter, oral communication and nutritional intake may be compromised. These complications may also result in the development of personal and family coping problems as well as a lack of knowledge related to the treatment required for the disorder.

DENTAL DISORDERS

A person must have healthy teeth and gums for good general health. Health care providers strive to preserve healthy gums and natural teeth for as long as possible for these reasons:

- Natural teeth are almost always more functional in masticating food than is a dental prosthesis.
- Effective mastication of food helps promote efficient digestion.

- Efficient digestion of food results in healthy gastrointestinal (GI) function and good general health.

The most frequent causes of tooth loss are dental decay and periodontal disease. Plaque is the major cause of both caries (decay) and periodontal disease. The best treatment for dental caries is prevention. Encourage clients to brush and floss regularly, eat a diet low in simple carbohydrates, use fluoride, and schedule regular visits to the dentist for examination, cleaning, and treatment of dental caries.

Increasing the resistance of the enamel also helps prevent caries. The resistance of enamel increases with the ingestion of fluoridated water during tooth formation and the continued use of fluoride throughout life. The daily use of fluoride rinses produces a more acid-resistant structure, enhances tooth mineralization, and interferes with bacterial growth. In addition, the dentist may apply topical fluoride to the teeth.

Treatment of dental caries may include drilling out cavities and filling them with material to restore the tooth, extraction (removal) of the entire tooth, and preservation of the tooth by *root canal therapy* (pulpectomy) followed by proper restoration. Any number of teeth can be removed because of disease. They are usually replaced with some type of dental prosthesis (crowns, dentures, dental implants). If only one tooth or a few teeth are removed,

---

This chapter incorporates material written for the fifth edition by Jane Hokanson Hawks.

local anesthesia is usually used. Removing several teeth or having a full-mouth extraction may require sedation or general anesthesia. Potential complications include hemorrhage and abscess formation.

During root canal therapy, the entire pulp of the tooth is removed. The canal space within the roots is filled aseptically and sealed to prevent infection. The tooth remains rooted in the gingiva and can still be used. Subsequent restoration of the tooth is essential to retain the tooth in a normal functional relationship with the rest of the teeth.

Periodontal disease, caused by plaque formation and bacterial colonization, results in gingival inflammation if the plaque is not removed by proper brushing and flossing. Eventually, inflammation destroys the underlying tissues and separates the gingiva from the tooth. In periodontitis, the inflammation extends from the gums into the alveolar bone and periodontal ligament, destroying the supporting structures of the teeth. As a result, the teeth loosen and extraction may be required.

Postoperative care of a tooth extraction includes assessing the oral cavity for bleeding and monitoring vital signs (if the client stays in an inpatient facility or recovery area). A gauze pad is usually placed over the extraction site, and the client is instructed to bite down gently on the pad to maintain pressure. Ice may be applied to the jaw over the site to decrease the blood flow and edema. Small amounts of bleeding may be normal, but you should notify the dentist or physician (or instruct the client to do so) if bleeding lasts longer than 1 hour.

The client usually requires analgesics to control pain. Instruct the client to eat soft foods and to avoid hot or cold foods for several days. The client should gently rinse the mouth with normal saline but should avoid brushing any remaining teeth for about 24 hours.

ORAL DISORDERS

STOMATITIS

Stomatitis, an inflammation of the oral cavity, may be of infectious origin or a manifestation of a systemic condition. It may be caused by *mechanical* trauma, such as injury, or *chemical* trauma, such as drugs given for cancer treatment. Jagged teeth, cheek-biting, and mouth-breathing also may result in mechanical trauma. Certain foods and drinks and sensitivity to mouthwashes or toothpaste may produce chemical trauma. The imflammatory sloughing of tissue allows organisms to multiply; thus, stomatitis may lead to infection by viruses, bacteria, yeasts, or fungus.

Stomatitis is classified as primary or secondary, depending on the cause. Primary stomatitis includes aphthous stomatitis (canker sore), herpes simplex, and Vincent's angina. Secondary stomatitis results when a client's lowered resistance allows an opportunistic infection to develop. Secondary stomatitis can be caused by a local or systemic disorder. Systemic disorders that can affect the oral mucous membranes include (1) allergies, (2) bone marrow disorders, (3) nutritional disorders, (4) immunodeficiency disorders, and (5) chemotherapy, radiation therapy, or immunosuppressive therapy.

■ APHTHOUS STOMATITIS

Commonly known as *canker sores,* the lesions caused by aphthous stomatitis are recurrent, small, and ulcerated. They develop in the soft tissues of the mouth, including the lips, tongue, and insides of the cheeks. Canker sores affect people of all age groups, although young adult women are more frequently affected. The cause of canker sores is unknown, but they may be related to emotional stress, trauma, vitamin deficiency, food and drug allergies, endocrine imbalances, and viral infections. Prevention is almost impossible because the exact cause is unknown.

These lesions start as small, reddened areas that undergo central necrosis and ulceration. The lesions are not infectious but are simply inflammatory. They heal within 1 to 3 weeks without treatment. Assessment usually reveals a well-circumscribed erythematous macule that undergoes necrosis, creating a well-defined pseudomembranous ulcer with an erythematous border.

Medical treatment involves topical application of amlexanox (Aphthasol) to the ulcer. Topical or systemic steroids may shorten the healing time. In addition, to suppress recurrence, teach clients prone to allergic reactions to avoid tomatoes, chocolate, eggs, shellfish, milk products, nuts, and citrus fruits.

■ HERPES SIMPLEX

Herpes simplex stomatitis is a form of inflammation and ulceration caused by the herpes simplex virus (HSV). By age 5 years, 90% of the population has been infected with *primary* herpes simplex. When the client is first infected with the primary herpes virus, lesions appear in the oral cavity. These vesicles, which can appear throughout the oral cavity, rupture to form ulcerated areas that resemble canker sores and heal within several weeks. The client's tongue has a characteristic heavy white coating. The client may have manifestations of generalized infection as well.

Secondary herpes is a recurrent infection that appears to lie dormant after the primary herpes infection. Secondary herpes takes the form of herpes labialis (fever blister, cold sore) and is often seen in clients receiving immunosuppressants and in those with human immunodeficiency virus (HIV) infection or acquired immunodeficiency syndrome (AIDS). Any infection, especially upper respiratory infections, fever, stress, or even sunlight, can reactivate the virus.

Assessment reveals clear, vesicular lesions, most often appearing at the mucocutaneous junction of the lips (Fig. 30–1) and face. The lesions are contagious, last about 1 week, and heal without scarring. Later in the course of the infection, the tongue may appear coated and the client may complain of a foul breath odor.

General pain may be treated with analgesics. Local ointments and anesthetics may soothe lesions. Clients who are immunocompromised are started on intravenous (IV) acyclovir (Zovirax). Clients with competent immune systems may be given acyclovir in oral or topical forms or penciclovir (Denavir) topical cream. Unless the ulcer is secondarily infected, antimicrobial treatment does not affect the progress of the ulcer.

■ VINCENT'S ANGINA

Vincent's angina (necrotizing ulcerative gingivitis, trench mouth) is an acute bacterial infection of the gingivae

FIGURE 30–1 Herpes simplex of the lip. (From Hurwitz, S. [1993]. *Clinical pediatric dermatology* [2nd ed., p. 321]. Philadelphia: W. B. Saunders.)

caused by resident flora in the mouth, fusiform bacteria, and spirochetes. Precipitating factors include poor oral hygiene, increased age, nutritional deficiencies, lack of rest and sleep, local tissue damage, and debilitating diseases, such as infectious mononucleosis, nonspecific viral infections, bacterial infections, blood dyscrasias, and diabetes mellitus. Most of these factors are unavoidable and therefore unpreventable. This condition is not contagious.

The disease is of sudden onset, causes erythema and ulceration of the gingivae, and affects the entire oropharynx. Once the tonsils are removed, this disorder rarely recurs. Assessment reveals ulcers covered with a pseudomembrane. A smear from an ulcer exudate identifies the causative organisms. Clients often have an elevated white blood cell (WBC) count. The client may complain of a foul taste, pain, a choking sensation, fever, thick secretions, anorexia, and occasionally, lymphadenopathy.

Management consists of removing the devitalized tissue and correcting the underlying cause with rest, improved oral hygiene, a bland diet, and vitamins. Pain medications and saline, peroxide, or half-saline half-peroxide mouthwashes promote comfort.

CANDIDIASIS

Candidiasis (moniliasis, thrush) is caused by the organism *Candida albicans,* a yeast-like fungus that is part of the normal flora of the oral cavity. Candidiasis of the oral cavity is commonly seen in immunosuppressed clients, such as those receiving chemotherapy or those with HIV infection or AIDS. The incidence is also increased in clients with diabetes mellitus and those who are pregnant, under stress, receiving high-dose or long-term antibiotic therapy, or receiving long-term tube feeding.

Etiology and Risk Factors

When the client is in a state of immunosuppression or has decreased levels of some normal oral flora, an overgrowth of the normal flora *Candida* can occur. Candidiasis commonly occurs in critically ill clients with prolonged intubation. The major risk factors are immunosuppression and prolonged use of antibiotics that disrupts the normal flora. Clients with either risk factor should be monitored

closely. Prophylactic treatment is often started for these high-risk clients.

Pathophysiology

Candidiasis is a secondary infection resulting from either an immunodeficiency or prolonged use of antibiotics. When the normal flora is disrupted, an overgrowth of the *Candida* organism may occur.

Clinical Manifestations

Assessment reveals white patches on the tongue, palate, and buccal mucosa (Fig. 30–2). These lesions adhere firmly to the tissues and are difficult to remove. The lesions are often referred to as "milk curds" because of their appearance. Clients describe the lesions as dry and hot. Clients who have recurrent candidiasis infections should be examined for a possible systemic cause.

Outcome Management

■ Medical Management

Medical management includes topical antifungal agents as well as other topical agents to alleviate the infection and provide pain relief. Analgesics, such as acetaminophen or aspirin, may also be administered to promote pain relief. Mouthwashes of warm saline (or water) or half warm saline (or water) and half hydrogen peroxide are often ordered as part of an oral hygiene regimen. A bland liquid or puréed diet may be necessary. Prophylactic use of antifungal agents is indicated for high-risk clients. Oral pharyngeal cultures should be taken if infection is suspected.

■ Nursing Management of the Medical Client
ASSESSMENT

Clients with the risk factors of immunosuppression or prolonged antibiotic use should be monitored closely. Assess whether the client has pain, tenderness, or bleeding in any part of the oral cavity or has had any febrile episodes. Ask about a history of previous infection elsewhere in the body and the use of any medications, especially antibiotics. Ask the client about a history of treatment with radiation or chemotherapy because both can

FIGURE 30–2 Oral candidiasis. Note the small white patches on the buccal mucosa. (From Moschella, S. L., & Hurley, H. J. [1992]. *Dermatology* [3rd ed., p. 231]. Philadelphia: W. B. Saunders.)

affect the oral mucosa. Prophylactic treatment for these high-risk clients may have been instituted.

To perform the oral assessment, have a tongue blade and good lighting and wear gloves. Inspect the oral cavity, noting any areas of inflammation, vesicular eruptions, ulcers, white patches, or erythema of the gingivae.

DIAGNOSIS, OUTCOMES, INTERVENTIONS

Pain. A common nursing diagnosis for the client with candidiasis is *Pain related to altered oral mucous membrane and ulcerations.*

Outcomes. The client's pain will be relieved or controlled, as evidenced by expressions of pain relief and demonstrating the ability to maintain normal nutrition.

Interventions

Minimize Pain. Assess for oral pain using a pain scale, and administer analgesics, such as aspirin or acetaminophen, as ordered. Topical agents and topical mouth rinses often provide pain relief. Antifungal agents to rinse with and swallow are used to alleviate the infection. A change in diet to liquid or puréed foods often eases the discomfort of eating. The client should avoid spicy foods, citrus juices, and hot liquids.

Provide Oral Care. Clients with painful lesions cannot tolerate commercial mouthwashes because of the high alcohol level in these products. A solution of warm saline (or water), half-strength hydrogen peroxide, or mouthwash formulas specific to many institutions are better tolerated and may promote healing. If painful oral lesions are present, suggest modifications in the client's oral hygiene regimen. Gauze pads may replace toothbrushes, and oral rinses may be needed to clean the area of debris and promote healing.

■ Promote Self-Care

Give the client oral and written instructions regarding a dental hygiene regimen, diet, medications, and manifestations of complications. The client should demonstrate proper techniques of dental hygiene. Minimal home health care preparation is required unless the client requires alternative feeding routes. If the client is receiving tube feedings, referral to a home health agency may be appropriate. If home care is not affordable, teach the client or significant other how to perform the tube feedings (see Chapter 29). The client should be scheduled for follow-up to assess for recurrence.

EVALUATION

The infection should clear up within a few days to a week in most clients. Assess the client for other risk factors if reinfection occurs. Educate the client about the signs of infection and what to report to the health care practitioner.

TUMORS OF THE ORAL CAVITY

■ BENIGN TUMORS OF THE ORAL CAVITY

The most common benign tumors of the mouth are fibromas, lipomas, neurofibromas, and hemangiomas. As with benign tumors in other parts of the body, oral tumors cause problems primarily by occupying space and causing

pressure. Benign tumors are usually excised if they cause functional or cosmetic problems.

■ PREMALIGNANT TUMORS OF THE ORAL CAVITY

LEUKOPLAKIA. Leukoplakia, a potentially precancerous, yellow-white or gray-white lesion, may occur in any region of the mouth. The size and shape of lesions vary, but they are usually elevated and have a roughened or leathery surface and clearly defined borders (Fig. 30–3). Leukoplakia is a common disorder of the oral mucous membranes, usually seen in people in their 30s and 40s. Men are affected twice as often as women; however, the incidence in women is increasing because of the increasing number of women who smoke.

Leukoplakia results from chronic irritation of the mucosa by physical, chemical, or thermal factors. Physical factors include poorly fitting dentures, broken teeth, cheek nibbling, and occlusion problems. Chemical and thermal factors arise from the use of tobacco products, both inhaled and chewing products. Ingestion of excessively hot food and beverages also places the person at risk. This condition may also develop from systemic factors such as poor nutrition or syphilis.

ERYTHROPLAKIA. Erythroplakia is a red, velvety-appearing patch that commonly indicates early squamous cell carcinoma. It occurs most frequently in people ages 50 to 60, with men and women equally affected. Risk factors are the same as those for squamous cell carcinoma.

■ MALIGNANT TUMORS OF THE ORAL CAVITY

Cancers of the oral cavity account for fewer than 3% of total cases of body malignancies. Cancers in this area most frequently are seen in people in their 40s and 50s and in men more frequently than women. Cancers of the oral cavity are most often associated with alcohol consumption and tobacco use. With the increase of tobacco use by younger people, especially the use of smokeless (chewing) tobacco, and by women, the age and sex ratios are changing.

Health promotion actions are to teach clients to avoid excessive use of tobacco, alcohol, and very hot beverages and foods. Encourage clients to maintain meticulous oral hygiene, to eat a well-balanced diet, and to use sunscreen

FIGURE 30–3 Leukoplakia of the lateral edge of the tongue. (From Sleisenger, M. H., & Fordtran, J. S. [1989]. *Gastrointestinal disease: Pathophysiology, diagnosis, and management* [4th ed.]. Philadelphia: W. B. Saunders.)

during exposure to sunlight. Health maintenance activities involve oral screening of smokers and drinkers of alcohol and teaching these high-risk people to observe for early manifestations of oral cancer. Health restoration interventions include the management of chemotherapy and radiation for clients after tumor excision and providing nutritional support as needed.

BASAL CELL CARCINOMA. Basal cell carcinoma of the oral cavity, the second most common oral cancer, occurs primarily on the lips. It starts as a small scab that develops into an ulcer with a characteristic pearly border. Basal cell carcinoma primarily occurs as a result of excessive exposure to sunlight, tending to occur more commonly in fair-skinned people who are exposed to sunlight.

SQUAMOUS CELL CARCINOMA. Squamous cell carcinoma is a malignant growth arising from tiny flat squamous cells that line mucous membranes. Squamous cell carcinoma is the leading type of oral cancer. Most tumors occur in clients older than age 45. Common sites include the lower lip and tongue. About 95% of cancers found on the tongue are squamous cell carcinomas. Malignancies of the tongue represent 1% to 1.5% of all malignancies in the United States.

The primary cause of squamous cell carcinoma is chronic irritation of the mucous lining of the mouth and oral cavity. Overuse of alcohol and tobacco is the primary cause of oral irritation. In combination, tobacco and alcohol are extremely destructive to the oral mucosa.

Squamous cell carcinoma develops from tiny cells that line the oral cavity. It can occur on the lips, buccal mucosa, tongue (Fig. 30–4), floor of the mouth, and tonsils. It is usually well differentiated, and the rate of metastasis is less than 10%. Cells metastasize by direct infiltration of local lymph nodes and can extend into the buccal fat and even to the mandible.

Manifestations may include a sore or lesion in the oral cavity. Red-appearing (erythroplakia) squamous cell carcinomas may not be well delineated and often bleed easily. Because squamous cell carcinomas usually grow slowly, they may be large before manifestations are detected. Other manifestations can include a mild irritation of the

FIGURE 30–4 Oral squamous cell carcinoma. This is an ulcerated lesion with surrounding leukoplakia on the posterior lateral and ventral portions of the tongue. (From Neville, B. W., et al. [1995]. *Oral and maxillofacial pathology.* Philadelphia: W. B. Saunders.)

tongue, sore throat, trouble with wearing dentures, or pain in the tongue or ear.

Only a biopsy of lesions positively confirms a diagnosis of oral cancer. Cytologic examination of mucosa thought to be malignant, while valuable in screening, unfortunately is not used widely enough to reduce the mortality rate. To be a valuable diagnostic aid, cytologic examination must be followed by biopsy when questionable cells are found. Biopsies may be performed with local or general anesthesia. To diagnose carcinoma at the base of the tongue, a laryngoscopic examination must be performed.

Outcome Management

■ Medical Management

INHIBIT TUMOR GROWTH

The survival rate of clients with oral cancer depends on the site and staging of the tumor. The tumor-node-metastasis (TNM) staging system (see Chapter 19) is used to stage oral cancers. Of the oral cancers, cancer of the lip carries one of the highest cure rates. Squamous cell carcinoma of the tongue carries the poorest prognosis because of the tongue's extensive vascular and lymphatic supply. Management of oral cancers includes radiation therapy, chemotherapy, and surgery and, again, depends on the site and staging of the tumor.

RADIATION THERAPY. Oral cancers can be treated with *external beam therapy* or *interstitial radiation therapy (brachytherapy).* The external beam passes through the skin or mucous membrane to the tumor. Interstitial radiation involves implanting radioactive seeds into the tissue for a prescribed period of time. Because interstitial radiation affects local tissue, it is used for small lesions that have not infiltrated the surrounding tissue. The client undergoing interstitial radiation is hospitalized and placed on radiation precautions (see Chapter 19) while the materials are active.

CHEMOTHERAPY. The effectiveness of chemotherapy for the treatment of oral cancers is unknown. Several drugs are used to treat head and neck cancers. They include bleomycin (Blenoxane), cisplatin (Platinol), cyclophosphamide (Cytoxan), doxorubicin (Adriamycin), 5-fluorouracil (5-FU), hydroxyurea (Hydrea), methotrexate (Folex), and vincristine (Oncovin).

■ Nursing Management of the Medical Client

ASSESSMENT

Carefully question the client about manifestations. A common finding is that of a painful ulcer. Assess the client for difficulty in swallowing, white or red patches on the oral mucosa, bleeding in the mouth, lumps in the neck, pain referred to the ear, foul odor, and hoarseness. Ask about the use of alcohol and tobacco, oral hygiene habits, and sun exposure. Assess the client's rehabilitative needs. Surgery can cause disfigurement and may alter speech; the client may experience depression from a change in body image and the diagnosis of cancer.

DIAGNOSIS, OUTCOMES, INTERVENTIONS

Altered Oral Mucous Membrane. A common nursing diagnosis for the client who has oral cancer or who is at risk for oral cancer is *Altered Oral Mucous Membrane related to irritants such as alcohol or tobacco, chemotherapy, radiation therapy, ill-fitting dentures, poor nutrition, and knowledge deficit of prevention and treatment of oral lesions.*

Outcomes. The client will understand and comply with measures to maintain the oral mucosa, as evidenced by statements of understanding of the substances and activities to avoid. The client will also be able to discuss the treatment regimen.

Interventions

Avoid Oral Irritants. Teach the client about the disease and treatment protocols. Advise the client to avoid chemical, physical, and thermal oral trauma; to perform careful, frequent oral hygiene, preferably three times daily; to see a dentist about ill-fitting dentures; and to see a physician about any mouth lesion that does not heal in 2 to 3 weeks.

Promote Comfort. If the client is receiving radiation therapy or chemotherapy, discuss possible side effects of these forms of treatment. Provide the client with comfort measures to minimize side effects, such as frequent oral hygiene and antiemetics to prevent nausea and vomiting.

Altered Nutrition: Less Than Body Requirements.
Clients with oral cancers often have nutritional difficulties, and a usual nursing diagnosis is *Altered Nutrition: Less than Body Requirements related to oral pain and difficulty eating and swallowing.*

Outcomes. The client will maintain weight or show weight gain before surgery, as evidenced by an increase in intake, maintenance of weight, or a weight gain of 1 pound per week preoperatively.

Interventions

Promote Nutrition. The location and size of a tumor, and the pain it causes, commonly interfere with a client's ability to eat. Small, frequent feedings can promote intake. Giving an analgesic 30 to 45 minutes before a meal can decrease the pain associated with eating. Provide oral care before and after meals to remove debris and minimize oral odors. Give the client with poor nutrition guidelines for improving the diet. Supply pamphlets outlining the basic nutrients for good health, and refer the client to a dietitian as needed.

Relieve Mouth Dryness. Unfortunately, treatments such as radiation alter salivation and taste perception. Xerostomia (dryness of the mouth) usually lessens with the use of pilocarpine and artificial saliva. Suggest that the client chew sugarless gum or suck on sugar-free hard candy to increase moisture. The client should perform frequent oral rinses with cool water to reduce dryness.

EVALUATION

The best outcome is for the client to stop high-risk behaviors for oral cancer, undergo successful treatment, and maintain nutritional status.

■ Surgical Management

Surgical management of oral cancers can range from local excision of small tumors to extensive surgery for invasive tumors. Small tumors can be treated in outpatient facilities by local excision, radiation, or laser therapy. Small tumors of the floor of the mouth can be locally excised with or without removing a portion of the mandible. Small tumors in the anterior floor of the mouth can be excised, and the area can be reconstructed with the use of a split-thickness skin graft.

A thin layer of skin, usually from the anterior thigh, can line the surgical site, allowing the client to maintain good mobility and function of the tongue. Xeroform gauze is usually placed over the skin graft and sutured into place. This can restrict the tongue, causing aspiration of secretions. Because of this packing and as a result of postoperative edema, a tracheostomy tube (see Chapter 60) is usually placed until edema subsides and the oral airway is patent. The client receives nothing by mouth (NPO) for 7 to 10 days after surgery to allow for healing. A nasogastric (NG) feeding tube, gastrostomy, or percutaneous endoscopic gastrostomy (PEG) is used to provide nutrition until the client can resume oral feedings (see Chapter 29).

Clients with invasive tumors require extensive surgical excision, usually involving removal of associated lymph nodes. Depending on the location, glossectomy (removal of the tongue), mandibulectomy (removal of the mandible), hemiglossectomy (removal of part of the tongue), or radical neck dissection may be performed. A radical neck dissection is an extensive procedure that involves removal of all tissue under the skin, from the jaw down to the clavicle, and from the anterior border of the trapezius muscle to the midline. To remove the cervical lymph nodes in this procedure, the surgeon must remove the sternocleidomastoid muscle, the spinal accessory nerve, and the jugular vein. A modified radical neck dissection involves removal of the lymph nodes only and is preferred when the disease is confined to mobile lymph nodes (see Chapter 60 for surgical management of cancer of the larynx). The Commando procedure is an extensive oral operation in which part of the mandible is excised along with the oral lesion. This procedure is often combined with a radical neck dissection.

■ Nursing Management of the Surgical Client

ASSESSMENT

Assessment of the surgical client is similar to assessment of the medical client. Complete routine preoperative and postoperative assessments, and ensure that the client understands the implications of the selected surgical approach and the associated postoperative assessments and treatments. Assessment of rehabilitative needs, such as speech therapy and coping with disfigurement, may also be required.

DIAGNOSIS, OUTCOMES, INTERVENTIONS

Risk for Injury. Surgery for oral cancer involves many potential risks. *Risk for Injury related to surgical procedure, including hemorrhage, ineffective airway clearance and possible wound infection* is an appropriate nursing diagnosis.

Outcomes. The client will remain free from injury, as evidenced by absence of excessive bleeding, maintenance of a patent airway, and wound healing without manifestations of infection.

Interventions

Maintain Airway. The most critical postoperative intervention is to maintain a patent airway. If the surgical procedure has been extensive, a tracheostomy is usually in place to help prevent respiratory difficulty from edema of the oral and pharyngeal structures. Clients at risk for ineffective airway clearance should be in a semi-Fowler to a high Fowler position after surgery to promote venous lymphatic drainage. The client may have a dusky appearance about the face from venous congestion. Pulse oximeter readings also should be used to determine whether the client is sufficiently oxygenated.

For the client with a tracheostomy, some blood-tinged mucus is normal in tracheal secretions for the first 48 hours after surgery. Bright red bleeding from the tracheostomy tube or site is a manifestation of hemorrhage. Notify the physician immediately if this occurs.

Provide Wound Care. The amount of nursing care required by the client after surgery depends on the extent of the procedure. After local excisions, teach the client how to perform hygiene gently. If a dressing and packing are in place, monitor the amount of drainage. After the dressing and packing are removed, the client should rinse the oral cavity with a mild half-strength form of hydrogen peroxide and water or saline solution every 4 hours to remove debris and promote healing. If half-strength hydrogen peroxide and water is used, it should be followed with normal saline or water to prevent drying.

With more extensive surgery, the suture lines must be protected from trauma. Oral hygiene and oral suctioning are usually not implemented until healing has begun and the physician decides that this type of cleaning can be performed.

Monitor for Bleeding. Hemorrhage may occur at any time after surgery, especially with extensive resection of the tongue. Hemorrhage can be massive because of the large vessels that supply the mouth and oral area. If bleeding occurs, apply pressure on the site until the bleeding stops spontaneously or stops with medical or surgical intervention. Surgical repair may be required. If an extensive resection is performed requiring skin grafts, monitor the site every 4 to 8 hours for drainage and manifestations of infection.

Altered Nutrition: Less Than Body Requirements.
After surgical intervention for oral cancers, the client often continues to have difficulties with nutrition. *Altered Nutrition: Less Than Body Requirements related to altered oral mucosa and surgical procedure* is an appropriate nursing diagnosis.

Outcomes. The client will maintain or gain weight after surgery, as evidenced by stabilization of weight and, possibly, a weight gain of 1 pound per week.

Interventions
Administer Supplemental Nutrition. Immediately after surgery, monitor IV hydration. Assess bowel sounds every shift. The return of bowel sounds is often an indication to begin tube feedings. When adding each feeding to the feeding bag, assess the client for proper tube placement and retention of stomach contents. Administer nutritional supplements by pump or bolus feedings. In addition, the physician may order total parenteral nutrition (TPN) as the first line of nutritional management (see Chapter 29 and the achalasia discussion in this chapter).

Discuss Eating Modifications. Once the edema has subsided, healing has occurred, and the tracheostomy tube

has been removed, the client may resume oral feedings. Caution the client about a decrease in sensation in the oral cavity after surgery. Assess swallowing carefully before eating begins. Instruct the client to avoid putting food directly on the surgical resection site. After meals, the client should always perform oral hygiene to remove any particles that remain and that may cause problems with the incision.

Impaired Verbal Communication. When the client has a tracheostomy after surgery, a common diagnosis is *Impaired Verbal Communication related to the presence of tracheostomy.*

Outcomes. The client will use alternative forms of communication to communicate with staff and significant others.

Interventions
Promote Alternate Forms of Communication. Assess the client's literacy, and provide paper and pencil, magic slate, chalkboard or a marker board for the client to write on as a substitute for talking. An alternative is to provide the client with a picture board to use for communicating any needs. Ideally, the assessment and instruction are completed preoperatively. The client should be allowed to communicate by gestures or written notes if this approach puts the client at ease. Most important, your manner should communicate acceptance, compassion, and caring. It is common to treat clients who cannot talk as though they cannot hear or understand. Be alert to any tendency to treat these clients as though they were mentally incompetent or deaf. Help the client avoid social isolation by taking the client for walks and meeting others. Friendly social encounters and physical activity can help alleviate depression.

Relieve Anxiety. Help clients who cannot speak to express their needs, concerns, and feelings. Check on the client frequently to reduce anxiety and loneliness. Place the call light within easy reach, and respond to the light promptly. If an intercom is used, it should be appropriately labeled regarding the client's limited ability to speak.

EVALUATION
The most favorable outcome is that the client heals within 6 weeks to 3 months, according to the extent of the radical surgery, and without complications. If complications develop, provide the name of the person to call. Also evaluate the client's ability to maintain intake of nutrients. If the client can self-feed via a tube until healing occurs and then increase oral intake, nutritional status should remain adequate. All clients also need tremendous emotional support with this type of surgical intervention and need to be evaluated for possible complications related to lack of support from family or significant others.

■ Self-Care
On discharge, supply the client and family with complete instructions regarding diet, medications, manifestations of complications, and any treatments, such as care of the wound or tracheostomy. Explain how and when to contact health care practitioners. The client needs to be seen by the physician after discharge to ensure complete healing of any extensive surgical wounds. If the client has a

tracheostomy, it may be permanent or may be closed at a later date. Clients who have undergone extensive surgery may need a referral to a home health agency for possible assistance with respiratory support (home oxygen), suctioning, nutritional support, and wound and tracheostomy care.

DISORDERS OF THE SALIVARY GLANDS

INFLAMMATION

Parotitis ("surgical mumps") is an inflammation of the parotid glands. It is the most common inflammatory condition affecting the salivary glands and probably results from inactivity of the glands caused by certain medications (such as diuretics), prolonged NG intubation, and lack of oral intake, such as that seen in postoperative clients. As secretions of the salivary gland diminish, oral bacteria have an opportunity to invade the gland and multiply. Interventions involve:

- Administering frequent oral hygiene to keep the bacterial count of the mouth low
- Keeping the client well hydrated
- Suggesting that the client use sugarless hard candies or chew sugarless gum to stimulate secretion of saliva

CALCULI

Stones, or calculi, form in the salivary glands when the glands are inactive and a metabolic condition favors the precipitation of salts. A nidus, or focus of origin, is necessary for stimulating salt precipitation. Assessment reveals that irritation from the stones causes local inflammation, swelling, and pain when the gland is stimulated to secrete, as during chewing. Intervention requires local excision by a physician. Stones occur most commonly in the submaxillary glands, probably because of the longer length of the duct and production of viscous alkaline secretions.

TUMORS

Most tumors in the salivary glands are benign. The most frequently seen malignant tumor is adenocarcinoma. Both benign and malignant tumors are characterized by enlargement of the gland. Pain occurs when expansion within the capsule of the gland creates pressure on sensory nerves. The treatment of choice for both benign and malignant tumors is usually surgical excision. If the tumor has recurred or is highly malignant, radiation therapy may also be used.

DISORDERS OF THE ESOPHAGUS

The most common manifestation of esophageal disease is dysphagia (difficulty with swallowing). Other manifestations include regurgitation, pain (which is probably linked with spasm), and heartburn.

DYSPHAGIA

Dysphagia can be caused by any esophageal disorder. Specific causes include neuromotor malfunction, mechani-

cal obstruction, cardiovascular abnormalities, and neurologic diseases.

■ DYSPHAGIA CAUSED BY MECHANICAL OBSTRUCTIONS

Mechanical obstructions causing dysphagia include congenital defects, cancer, and acquired conditions such as hiatal hernia. When an obstruction narrows the esophageal lumen, clients first experience dysphagia only with solid foods. Later, dysphagia becomes associated with semisolid foods and liquids. Finally, clients are unable to swallow their own saliva. Obstructive disorders, particularly esophageal cancer, may be accompanied by weight loss and cachexia.

■ DYSPHAGIA CAUSED BY CARDIOVASCULAR ABNORMALITIES

Dysphagia also may result from cardiovascular abnormalities, particularly in older people. Specific conditions causing vascular dysphagia include an enlarged heart, an aortic aneurysm, and calcification of the descending aorta. Figure 30–5 shows the relationship of the heart and great arteries to the esophagus.

■ DYSPHAGIA CAUSED BY NEUROLOGIC DISEASES

Dysphagia also may be caused by certain neurologic diseases, such as cerebrovascular accident (CVA), multiple

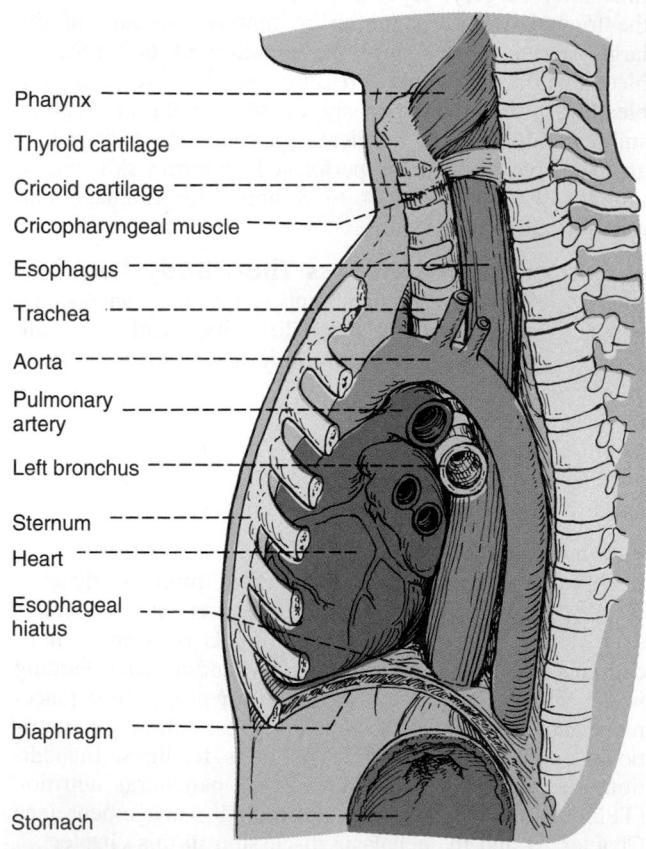

Pharynx
Thyroid cartilage
Cricoid cartilage
Cricopharyngeal muscle
Esophagus
Trachea
Aorta
Pulmonary artery
Left bronchus
Sternum
Heart
Esophageal hiatus
Diaphragm
Stomach

FIGURE 30–5 Relationship of the heart and great arteries to the esophagus.

sclerosis, poliomyelitis, and amyotrophic lateral sclerosis (ALS). CVA is the most frequent cause of dysphagia.

■ DYSPHAGIA FROM OTHER CAUSES

Dysphagia can be experienced after swallowing if food gets caught in the esophagus. Clients may obtain relief by drinking liquids to force the impacted bolus through the narrow segment or by retching to dislodge the food. If vomiting does not succeed, endoscopy may be used to remove food lodged in the esophagus.

REGURGITATION

Regurgitation is the ejection of small amounts of chyme or gastric juice from the mouth without antecedent nausea. It is usually caused by an incompetent lower esophageal sphincter (LES). Regurgitation occurring immediately after swallowing results from structural or motor abnormality in the LES. Contributing factors include abnormal motor activity, increased abdominal pressure, and sphincter abnormality. Regurgitation occurs with achalasia, pylorospasm, lesions proximal to the cardia, hiatal hernia, reflux esophagitis, and esophageal ulcer or cancer. Stooping or lying down facilitates the flow of gastric contents into the esophagus, thus exacerbating regurgitation.

PAIN

Pain, which may be constant or may occur only with swallowing, suggests diffuse esophageal spasm. Pain may result from alterations of the mucosa from reflux disease, radiation, or viral infection. Pain that affects the esophageal mucosa and occurs with swallowing is called *odynophagia*. The client usually describes the pain as sharp, constricting, sticking, crushing, stabbing, or knife-like. Odynophagia is usually severe, quite distressing, and often associated with a deep and long-lasting pain. The pain, located substernally, may radiate to the neck, back, and shoulder. Pain may occur throughout the day and can be confused with angina. Odynophagia can be triggered by a cold or carbonated beverage or by solid food passing through the esophagus. The most common cause is the reflux of gastric contents into the esophagus.

HEARTBURN

Heartburn (pyrosis, indigestion, or dyspepsia) is another common manifestation of esophageal disease. Generally, it is a painful sensation of warmth and burning in the lower retrosternal midline. Because clients may use the word "heartburn" to describe very different sensations, it is essential to find out exactly what this term means to the client using it. Heartburn usually means substernal, midline burning that tends to radiate, generally in waves, upward to the neck, resulting from abnormalities of the LES. Clients often describe this discomfort as cramping or knotting.

Heartburn is commonly experienced with postural changes (such as bending, stooping, and lifting) gulping of food or liquids, or ingestion of alcohol. Manifestations often are relieved by standing or eructing. Heartburn also arises in the presence of refluxed gastric or duodenal contents. Disorders most commonly associated with heartburn are reflux esophagitis, hiatal hernia, achalasia, and gastric stasis. Heartburn is common in people with pyloric or duodenal ulcers and LES disorders.

ACHALASIA

Achalasia is a disorder characterized by progressively increasing dysphagia, with the client eventually having great difficulty swallowing and expressing the feeling that "something is stuck in the throat." Achalasia commonly occurs in people in their 20s and 30s and appears equally often in men and women.

Etiology and Risk Factors

Achalasia is a chronic, progressive disease of unknown cause. Occasionally, the client can relate the onset to an episode of acute dysphagia, but usually the onset is obscure. The disease is noticed only when dysphagia becomes severe. Because achalasia is idiopathic, there are no identified risk factors. There may be a familial component.

Pathophysiology

Achalasia is characterized by impaired motility of the lower two thirds of the esophagus. The LES fails to relax normally with swallowing. Inadequate functioning occurs because nerve impulses cannot pass through the esophagus or sympathetic receptors are absent from the LES. There also may be degeneration of the ganglion cells or impairment of impulses from Auerbach's plexus. Impaired propulsion and a constricted LES result in accumulation of food and fluid within the lower esophagus. When hydrostatic pressure exceeds the force of resistance of the LES, the contents pass into the stomach. Reflux esophagitis with resultant ulceration (Fig. 30–6) is a possible complication (see Gastroesophageal Reflux Disease). Aspiration of regurgitated esophageal contents may result in atelectasis and other pulmonary problems.

Clinical Manifestations

The initial manifestation of achalasia is dysphagia. It is difficult for food and fluid to pass through the LES. In the early stages of achalasia, the client may have subster-

FIGURE 30–6 Endoscopic view of severe esophagitis.

nal pain because of spasms of the esophagus or may be unable to eructate (belch). The client may regurgitate undigested food eaten many hours earlier as well as large amounts of mucus that have been stimulated by esophageal irritation. As achalasia progresses, manifestations increase in frequency and severity. Upper respiratory infections, emotional disturbances, overeating, and pregnancy may exacerbate the problem.

Diagnostic tests used to determine the presence of achalasia include barium swallow, endoscopy, and manometry. The barium swallow is considered positive for achalasia if it reveals nonpropulsive waves and esophageal dilation. Barium may also be retained in the esophagus. Endoscopy helps determine the status of the LES, the amount of dilation, and the presence of food. Manometry (measurement of pressure in the esophagus) confirms the diagnosis with elevated resting pressures in the LES or slow, low-amplitude, or absent peristalsis.

Outcome Management

Medical Management

RELIEVE MANIFESTATIONS
Treatment of achalasia is aimed at relieving clinical manifestations. Management usually begins with medical treatment on an outpatient basis. Often, as the problem progresses, hospitalization is required for surgical procedures or for placement of a gastrostomy, PEG, or percutaneous endoscopic jejunostomy (PEJ) tube for nutritional support.

ADMINISTER MEDICATIONS
Medications that relax the LES or lower esophageal pressures (such as anticholinergic drugs, nitrates, gastrointestinal hormones, and calcium-channel blockers) have been studied, but none of them have proved to be of consistent value or effectiveness. Pain is managed with antacids, H_2 receptor antagonists, and proton pump inhibitors.

MODIFY DIET
Changes in diet may ease the pressure and reflux in the client with achalasia. Small, frequent feedings ease the passage of food, and semisoft, warm foods are better tolerated than cold, hard foods. The client should avoid hot, spicy, and iced foods as well as alcohol and tobacco. Foods should be chewed thoroughly to add saliva to the mixture for lubrication and allowing the bolus to pass more easily from the esophagus to the stomach.

ALTERNATE POSITIONS
The client should experiment with different positions to reduce pressure while eating. Some clients benefit from arching the back while swallowing. After eating, the client should remain upright by standing or sitting. Restrictive clothing, which may increase esophageal pressure and regurgitation, should be avoided.

To prevent nocturnal reflux of food, the client should sleep with the head of the bed elevated. You may place the client in a semi-Fowler position, using a wedge pillow to keep the head higher than the LES, or may elevate the head of the bed on 4- to 6-inch blocks.

Nursing Management of the Medical Client
ASSESSMENT
Obtain a history, noting the manifestations the client is experiencing, onset and duration of aggravating factors,

and any methods the client uses for relief. Assess respiratory manifestations because reflux or regurgitation can affect the respiratory tract. Assess the client's nutritional status, noting any weight changes and the effects of esophageal manifestations on dietary habits.

DIAGNOSIS, OUTCOMES, INTERVENTIONS
Altered Nutrition: Less Than Body Requirements. The client with achalasia experiences a great deal of difficulty swallowing, leading to the diagnosis of *Altered Nutrition: Less Than Body Requirements related to dysphasia.*

Outcomes. The client will maintain an adequate nutritional intake, as evidenced by maintenance of ideal body weight or gaining back any weight lost at a rate of 1 pound per week.

Interventions. Consult with the client concerning dietary habits and daily intake of nutrients. Obtain a baseline weight and daily weights. Teach the client about changes in dietary habits that may relieve manifestations, as discussed under Medical Management. A gastrostomy tube, PEG tube, or PEJ tube may be used to provide adequate nutritional support if dysphagia continues to be a problem. Nursing management of feedings is discussed in Chapter 29 and later in this chapter under Nursing Management of the Surgical Client.

Pain. When the client experiences gastric reflux, the acid in the esophagus causes *Pain related to episodes of gastric reflux,* making this an appropriate nursing diagnosis.

Outcomes. The client will experience a decrease in pain or an absence of pain, as evidenced by verbalizing a reduction in or an absence of pain and an ability to maintain oral intake.

Interventions. Pain can be decreased or relieved through the use of medications (such as antacids, histamine H_2 receptor antagonists, and proton pump inhibitors), dietary changes, and repositioning. Assess the client every shift to determine whether medications, changes in diet, and repositioning are effective in controlling or relieving pain.

EVALUATION
The most appropriate outcome would be that the achalasia is controlled with medical treatment and the client's nutritional status is maintained. If the client's manifestations cannot be controlled with medical treatment, surgical intervention may be necessary.

Surgical Management
Surgical management of achalasia may involve dilating the LES (esophageal dilation) or enlarging the sphincter (esophagomyotomy). Esophageal dilation (bougienage) forcefully dilates the LES (Fig. 30–7). This procedure, which is usually done on an outpatient basis, is used to help correct not only achalasia but also esophageal spasms and strictures. Vigorous dilation is associated with a 75% success rate. Local anesthesia is used under radiologic guidance.

In the more complex procedure, esophagomyotomy (Heller's procedure), the surgeon enlarges the vestibule by incising the circular muscle fibers down to the mucosa

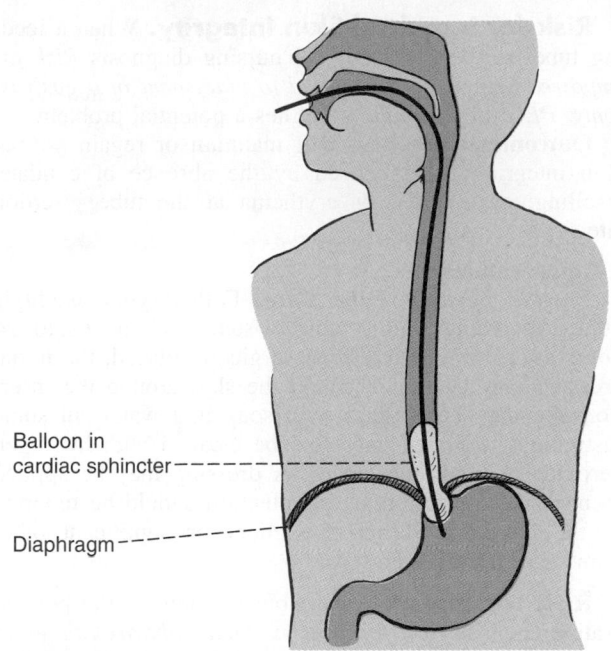

FIGURE 30–7 Bougienage (passage of a bougie) relieves dysphagia by dilating the lower esophageal sphincter.

(Fig. 30–8). Complications may include reflux esophagitis and restenosis.

If a client cannot swallow for long periods, a gastrostomy tube, PEG, or PEJ may be inserted. The tubes may be inserted surgically, laparoscopically or via percutaneous endoscopy.

For the laparoscopic or surgical method, the physician makes an incision in the wall of the abdomen and sutures the tube to the gastric wall.

For a percutaneous endoscopic approach, the physician uses local anesthesia and inserts a cannula into the stomach through a small abdominal incision. A suture is threaded through the cannula. A second physician uses an endoscope to pull the suture through the client's mouth. The PEG tube is attached and advanced down the esophagus, through the abdominal incision, where crossbars (Fig. 30–9) secure it internally and externally. Some tubes contain an internal balloon instead of an internal crossbar, while other tubes contain internal and external crossbars and an internal balloon. Skin care around the percutaneous site is necessary postoperatively. In the PEJ procedure, the tube is inserted into the jejunum instead of the stomach. See Chapter 29 for a comparison of enteral feeding routes.

Nursing Management of the Surgical Client
PREOPERATIVE CARE
ASSESSMENT

Obtain a history, noting the onset and duration of manifestations the client is experiencing, aggravating factors, and any methods the client uses for relief. Assess the client's respiratory status and nutritional status in addition to the routine preoperative assessments.

DIAGNOSIS, OUTCOMES, INTERVENTIONS

Knowledge Deficit. To prepare the client for surgery, consider the nursing diagnosis *Knowledge deficit related to preoperative preparation and postoperative care.*

Outcomes. The client will understand and be prepared for surgery, as evidenced by asking questions and expressing statements of understanding.

Interventions
Teach about Esophageal Dilation. If your client is to undergo esophageal dilation, explain that the client will be awake during the procedure. A local anesthetic solution is sprayed on the throat, and an analgesic or tranquilizer may be given. The client should take long, slow breaths during passage of the bougies. As the bag is inflated, the client may feel brief discomfort. Weighted

FIGURE 30–8 *A* and *B,* Esophagomyotomy (Heller's procedure) is the surgical procedure of choice when a segment of esophagus narrows and causes functional obstruction.

A
Line of incision
into constricted
section of muscle

B
Esophageal mucosa
pouches through
incision in muscle

FIGURE 30–9 Percutaneous endoscopic gastrostomy tube in place for a client with achalasia.

bougies with increasing weight can also be used for dilation. Esophageal dilation is often performed on an outpatient basis.

Explain Esophagomyotomy. Esophagomyotomy is a more complex procedure. The client will require a general anesthetic and remain hospitalized for more than 24 hours. Instruct the client undergoing an esophageal procedure about the usual preoperative procedures, such as an NPO status after midnight, IV fluids, and preoperative medications. Discuss pain control, drains, surgical dressings, and the presence of an NG tube, a gastrostomy tube, a PEG tube, or a PEJ tube. The possibility of a thoracotomy approach being used to reach the esophagus requires instruction concerning chest tubes. Discuss manifestations of respiratory complications related to esophageal reflux and aspiration.

Instruct clients who have undergone an esophagomyotomy to sleep with the head of the bed elevated and to recognize manifestations of respiratory complications. Explain the manifestations of infection and esophageal perforation; urge the client to notify the physician if any of these problems occur.

POSTOPERATIVE CARE
ASSESSMENT

Routine postoperative assessments, such as monitoring vital signs, pain, and drainage tubes placed during surgery, are required. In addition, monitor the client's respiratory and nutritional status and the site of the feeding tube (if placed).

DIAGNOSIS, OUTCOMES, INTERVENTIONS

Altered Nutrition: Less Than Body Requirements. For the client experiencing dysphagia, the nursing diagnosis *Altered Nutrition: Less Than Body Requirements related to dysphagia and placement of a gastrostomy, PEG, or PEJ tube* is appropriate.

Outcomes. The client will maintain an adequate nutritional intake, as evidenced by maintaining ideal body weight or gaining weight at a rate of 1 pound per week to replace previous weight loss.

Interventions. A baseline weight and daily weight should be obtained.

Maintain Feeding Tube. Follow institutional policy regarding care for the client with a gastrostomy, PEG, or PEJ tube. Typically, the client is on NPO status for at least 24 hours before continuous or bolus tube feedings begin. Nursing interventions include checking tube placement via measurement of the tube and checking pH of stomach contents and residual amounts every 4 hours. (Do not assess this via aspiration if the tube is placed in the jejunum, because these tubes are flushed, not aspirated.) If the gastric return is more than 100 ml, hold the feeding for 1 hour and repeat aspiration before continuing the feeding. After checking placement and administering bolus feedings or medications, flush the tube with 50 to 100 ml of normal saline or water. Keep the head of the bed elevated at least 30 degrees at all times for continuous feedings or for 1 hour after completion of intermittent bolus feedings. Change the enteral feeding bag and tubing every 24 hours, and rinse them with water every 4 hours or after each intermittent feeding to decrease the risk of bacterial contamination. (See Chapter 29 for additional information about enteral feedings.)

Risk for Impaired Skin Integrity. When a feeding tube has been placed, the nursing diagnosis *Risk for Impaired Skin Integrity related to placement of a gastrostomy, PEG, or PEJ tube* identifies a potential problem.

Outcomes. The client will maintain or regain normal skin integrity, as evidenced by the absence of exudate, swelling, excoriation, or erythema at the tube insertion site.

Interventions
Provide Feeding Tube Care. Follow your facility's policy regarding routine care. Usually, about 12 to 24 hours after the tube has been surgically placed, the initial dressing may be removed and the skin around the insertion site may be washed with soap and water. In some institutions, the area may also be cleaned with hydrogen peroxide or other substances. A dressing may be applied as needed. Manifestations of infection should be reported to the physician. Teach the client or significant other home care management.

Risk for Injury. A possible problem in the postoperative client is *Risk for Injury: Pneumothorax related to surgical procedure and presence of chest tubes.*

Outcomes. Injury will be prevented, as evidenced by absence of hemorrhage, absence of manifestations of perforation, normal temperature, and absence of problems associated with chest tubes, such as respiratory distress.

Interventions
Monitor for Complications. After esophageal dilation, monitor the client for manifestations of perforation, such as elevated temperature, chest or shoulder pain, and subcutaneous emphysema. If any of these manifestations are noted, notify the physician immediately. The client will require an x-ray study to determine whether air is in the mediastinum, indicating perforation.

Maintain Chest Tubes. After an esophagomyotomy, a thoracotomy incision and chest tubes are in place. Maintain chest tube drainage and the NG or gastric drainage system, and manage the client's pain see Chapter 62 for care of the client with chest tubes.

EVALUATION

An appropriate outcome is that the client will maintain adequate nutrition and that the condition will be reversed with surgery. The esophagus must heal completely before the client can return to eating the usual foods. An acceptable evaluation is that the client or significant others have been able to continue tube feedings for at least 6 weeks after surgery.

▉ Modifications for Elderly Clients

An attempt is made to treat older clients with more local measures (pain medications, positioning, and dietary modification) and possibly esophageal dilation. The older adult is less likely to tolerate the more complicated procedures and, therefore, more likely to experience complications.

▉ Self-Care

The client or significant others will require teaching if the feedings are required after discharge. Initially, home visits by a nurse may be necessary to assist the client with any home care needs related to tube feedings, diet, medications, and wound care and to provide an ongoing evaluation of the client's condition. A referral to a social worker may be needed to assist the client with financial assistance, community resources, counseling, and specialized equipment (see Chapter 29).

GASTROESOPHAGEAL REFLUX DISEASE

Esophageal reflux is a backward flow of gastric contents into the esophagus. Gastroesophageal reflux disease (GERD) refers to a syndrome resulting from esophageal reflux. Reflux exposes the esophageal mucosa to the gastric contents, which gradually breaks down the esophageal mucosa. This condition, sometimes called *reflux esophagitis,* is often associated with a sliding hiatal hernia. However, complications causing reflux can occur without a hiatal hernia, and people with a hiatal hernia may not have manifestations of reflux.

GERD can occur in any age group. About 10% of the population have daily manifestations of GERD, and as much as one third of the population have monthly manifestations. Manifestations are often overlooked and attributed to stress.

Etiology and Risk Factors

The cause of GERD seems to be an inappropriate relaxation of the LES (Fig. 30–10). The exact cause of the relaxation is unknown, but reflux occurs with:

- An alteration in the innervation of the pressure zone in the region of the gastroesophageal sphincter
- Displacement of the angle of the gastroesophageal junction
- An incompetent LES

Risk factors and health promotion and maintenance behaviors are important teaching topics. These factors include obesity and weight gain, pregnancy, chewing tobacco, smoking, high-fat foods, theophylline, caffeine, chocolate, and high levels of estrogen and progesterone. Teaching clients to limit smoking, caffeine, chocolate, and high-fat foods helps to prevent GERD. Eating small meals and increasing dietary protein also helps. Losing weight, elevating the head of the bed for sleeping, and avoiding lifting, straining, bending, and tight or constrictive clothing can further help prevent the problem. Once GERD has developed, a health restoration action is to instruct the client on how to take prescribed medications.

Pathophysiology

Normally, a high-pressure zone exists in the region of the gastroesophageal sphincter. High pressure prevents reflux but permits the passage of food and liquids. When there is an alteration in this region, reflux occurs.

Reflux esophagitis may also occur with gastric or duodenal ulcer, after esophageal or gastric surgery, after prolonged vomiting, or after prolonged gastrointestinal intubation. The reflux most often consists of hydrochloric acid or gastric and duodenal contents containing bile acid and pancreatic juice. Frequent or prolonged reflux results in inflammation of the esophageal mucosa (esophagitis). The degree of reflux esophagitis present depends on (1) frequency of the reflux, (2) contents of the reflux, (3) buffering ability of the saliva and mucous secretion, and (4) rate of gastric emptying.

Clinical Manifestations

GERD may begin suddenly or gradually. The client may complain of heartburn, odynophagia, dysphagia, acid regurgitation, water brash (the release of salty secretions in the mouth), or eructation. Pain in GERD is typically described as a burning sensation that moves up and down. If the condition is severe, the pain may radiate to the back, neck, or jaw. Pain usually occurs after meals and is relieved with antacids or fluids. Discomfort sometimes accompanies activities that increase intra-abdominal pressure, such as lifting or straining. The client may state that discomfort occurs when lying supine or when the stomach is distended. Standing and walking may relieve it. Dysphagia resulting from edema, spasm, or a narrowed lumen is intermittent and worse at the beginning of meals. Responses to pain-relieving measures (such as nitroglycerin) help to differentiate between esophagitis and problems of cardiac origin (such as angina pectoris).

Diagnosis rests on the demonstration of reflux. Barium swallow, esophageal manometry, esophagoscopy, esophageal biopsy, cytologic examination, analysis of gastric secretions, and acid perfusion tests confirm the diagnosis of GERD (see Chapter 28).

Outcome Management

■ Medical Management

DECREASE REFLUX WITH MEDICATIONS

Of the many medications used to treat GERD, only one drug of its class is discussed. A more detailed description of these classifications of drugs is provided in Chapter 31. For people receiving long-term therapy with nonste-

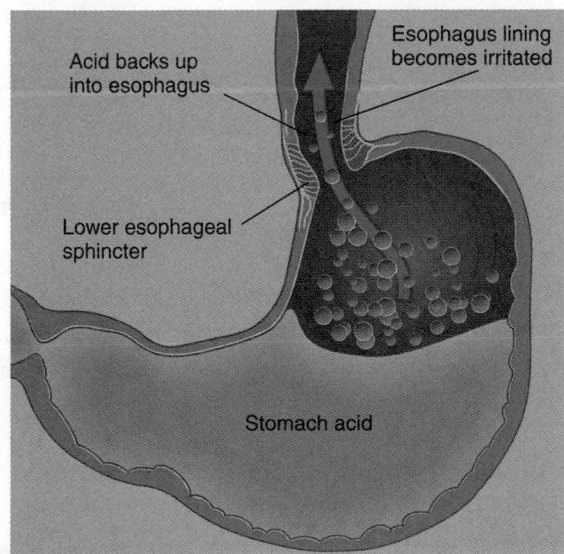

FIGURE 30–10 Anatomy of gastroesophageal reflux disease (GERD): Relaxed lower esophageal sphincter, displaced angle of the gastroesophageal junction, and altered nerve innervation in the region of the gastroesophageal sphincter.

roidal anti-inflammatory drugs (NSAIDs), misoprostol (Cytotec) is useful for preventing gastric ulcer formation and, in some instances, GERD manifestations. Anticholinergic drugs, calcium-channel blockers, and theophylline should be avoided because they appear to decrease LES pressure or delay gastric emptying.

ANTACIDS. Drug therapy for GERD usually starts with an antacid, which commonly provides prompt relief. Typically, the client takes 30 ml of antacid 1 hour before and 2 to 3 hours after each meal to neutralize gastric acid secretions. Clients typically tolerate combination products such as calcium carbonate–magnesium carbonate (Mylanta) or magnesium hydroxide–aluminum hydroxide (Maalox). Aluminum hydroxide–magnesium carbonate (Gaviscon) is another excellent antacid because of its foaming action. A major disadvantage of antacids is that their effects last only about a half-hour.

HISTAMINE RECEPTOR ANTAGONISTS. If manifestations are severe or persist, the client may be prescribed histamine receptor antagonists such as ranitidine (Zantac) or famotidine (Pepcid) to decrease gastric acid secretions.

CHOLINERGICS. Bethanechol (Urecholine) may be added for clients with severe manifestations because it has been found to increase LES pressure and prevent reflux. Because bethanechol is a cholinergic drug, it is usually given with antacids and a histamine receptor antagonist because it can increase the secretion of gastric acid. It should be taken before meals.

GASTROINTESTINAL STIMULANTS. Metoclopramide (Reglan) may be prescribed because it increases LES pressure by stimulating the smooth muscle of the GI tract and increases the rate of gastric emptying. This medication is taken before meals.

Cisapride (Propulsid) was pulled in July 2000 by the FDA because of problems with dysrhythmias, and is used only when no other drug is effective and the client has no contraindications and is closely supervised.

PROTON PUMP INHIBITORS. Lansoprazole (Prevacid), a proton pump inhibitor, suppresses secretion of gastric acid. It has been effective for short-term treatment of GERD.

DECREASE REFLUX WITH LIFESTYLE AND DIET CHANGES

In mild GERD, diet and lifestyle changes may be sufficient to relieve manifestations. Instruct the client to follow this regimen:

- Restrict the diet to small, frequent feedings (four to six per day).
- Drink adequate fluids at meals to assist food passage.
- Eat slowly and chew thoroughly to add saliva to the food.
- Avoid extremely hot or cold foods, spices, fats, alcohol, coffee, chocolate, and citrus juices.
- Avoid eating and drinking for 3 hours before retiring to prevent the common problem of nocturnal reflux.
- Elevate the head of the bed 6 to 8 inches to prevent nocturnal reflux.
- Lose weight, if overweight, to decrease the gastroesophageal pressure gradient.

- Avoid tobacco, salicylates, and phenylbutazone, which may exacerbate esophagitis.

■ Nursing Management of the Medical Client

ASSESS MANIFESTATIONS

Identify specific manifestations the client has been experiencing. Document when manifestations started, their frequency and severity, and the relationship of manifestations to food and various food products. Assist in maintaining the client's general appearance and nutritional status. Help the client identify risk factors for GERD, and instruct the client about lifestyle changes to reduce those risk factors.

PROVIDE TEACHING

Instruct the client in the prescribed diet regimen, and evaluate both the client's understanding of treatment and its effectiveness. Administer medications ordered for the pain, and document their effectiveness. Instruct the client in the prescribed medication regimen, and evaluate the client's understanding of the treatment.

■ Surgical Management

Clients who do not respond to medical management undergo one of three surgical procedures: the Nissen fundoplication, the Hill operation, or the Belsey operation. The surgeon may use an open surgical approach or a laparoscopic approach to complete these procedures. Recovery is usually faster with the laparoscopic approach.

The *Nissen fundoplication* is most common and involves suturing the fundus around the esophagus (Fig. 30–11). An abdominal approach is usually used. An increase in pressure or volume in the stomach closes the cardia and blocks reflux into the esophagus. The surgeon creates a valve-like substitute sphincter with inherent contractility.

The *Hill operation* narrows the esophageal opening and anchors the stomach and distal esophagus to the median arcuate ligament (posterior gastropexy). This procedure reinforces the sphincter and recreates the gastro-

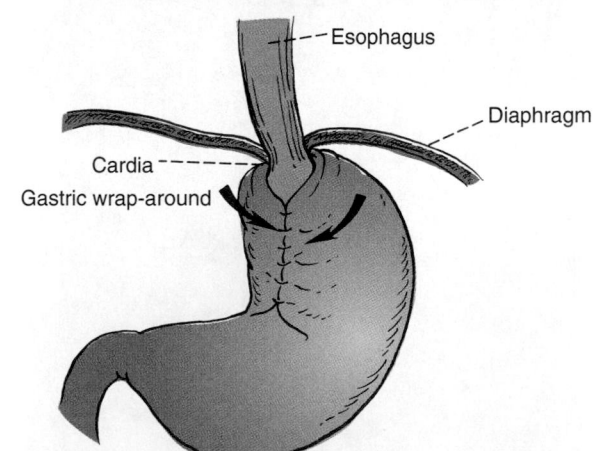

FIGURE 30–11 Nissen fundoplication for hiatal hernia. The gastric fundus is wrapped around the distal esophagus and sutured to itself.

esophageal valve. A partial wraparound (180 degrees) of the stomach around the esophagus is created via an abdominal approach.

The *Belsey (Mark IV) repair* consists of plication of the anterior and lateral aspects of the stomach onto the distal esophagus. The surgeon creates the esophagogastric angle without opening the esophagus or the diaphragm. A 280-degree esophageal wraparound is created via a thoracic approach.

In clients with severe reflux, an Angelchick prosthesis may be inserted. A laparotomy is performed, and a synthetic C-shaped silicone prosthesis is tied around the distal esophagus (Fig. 30–12). The prosthesis anchors the LES in the abdomen and reinforces sphincter pressure. The success of this procedure is variable, depending on the severity of the problem. In clients with severe reflux, this procedure may be unsuccessful.

Clients undergoing a surgical procedure are encouraged to follow the GERD antireflux medical regimen (medications, diet changes, lifestyle changes) because the recurrence rate is significant.

■ Nursing Management of the Surgical Client

COMPLETE POSTOPERATIVE ASSESSMENTS
The surgical client requires the same assessments as those for the medical client as well as routine preoperative and postoperative assessments. If chest tubes are placed postoperatively, monitor the client for respiratory distress. An abdominal incision results in a greater chance of a wound infection. Assess the wound drainage for signs of infection. The client will have an NG tube, and tube patency must be maintained to avoid stomach distention.

PREVENT RESPIRATORY COMPLICATIONS
Teach the client the importance of coughing and deep breathing after surgery to prevent respiratory complications. Because postoperative breathing can be painful, the client must cough and deep-breathe to avoid respiratory complications. The use of an incentive spirometer may be ordered by the surgeon. If a thoracic approach is used, explain the purpose of the chest tubes and the care needed (see Chapter 62).

PREVENT GAS-BLOAT SYNDROME
Fluids are usually resumed after 24 hours, and the diet is progressively advanced as tolerated when peristalsis returns. Small, frequent meals are provided to avoid overloading the stomach. After fundoplication, the client may experience gas-bloat syndrome if the wrap of the fundus is too tight, causing bloating and an inability to eructate. Clients should avoid carbonated beverages and gas-producing foods and should drink with a straw. Ambulating can assist peristalsis in removing air from the GI tract. The condition is usually temporary. Instruct clients to report dysphagia, epigastric fullness, bloating, or excessive borborygmi to their physician or health care practitioner.

HIATAL HERNIA

A hiatal hernia (diaphragmatic hernia) is a condition in which the cardiac sphincter becomes enlarged, allowing a part of the stomach to pass into the thoracic cavity. There are two major types of hernias: *sliding* hernias (type I) and *rolling* or *paraesophageal* hernias (type II). In a sliding hernia, the upper stomach and the gastroesophageal junction are displaced upward into the thorax (Fig. 30–13). Sliding hernias account for about 90% of the total cases of esophageal hiatal hernias. With a rolling hernia, the gastroesophageal junction stays below the diaphragm but all or part of the stomach pushes through into the thorax (see Fig. 30–13).

The incidence of hiatal hernia is estimated as 5 per 1000 in the general population and may be as high as 60% in clients over age 60 years. Women tend to be affected more often than men, and the incidence increases significantly with age.

Etiology and Risk Factors

Hiatal hernias are related to muscle weakness in the esophageal hiatus, which loosens the esophageal supports and allows the lower portion of the stomach to rise into the thorax. As with other hernias, the muscle weakness is caused by a variety of conditions, such as aging, trauma, congenital muscle weakness, surgery, or anything that increases intra-abdominal pressure such as lifting or coughing.

Risk factors are those that weaken the diaphragm and increase intra-abdominal pressure. Pressure may be increased by conditions such as obesity, pregnancy, or ascites.

Health promotion behaviors to prevent or at least delay a hiatal hernia include avoiding any activities that increase intra-abdominal pressure. These activities include heavy lifting and wearing tight constrictive clothing, especially around the waist. Other than these measures, hiatal hernias are not preventable.

Pathophysiology

A hiatal hernia involves protrusion of part of the stomach through a weakness in the diaphragm. The resulting re-

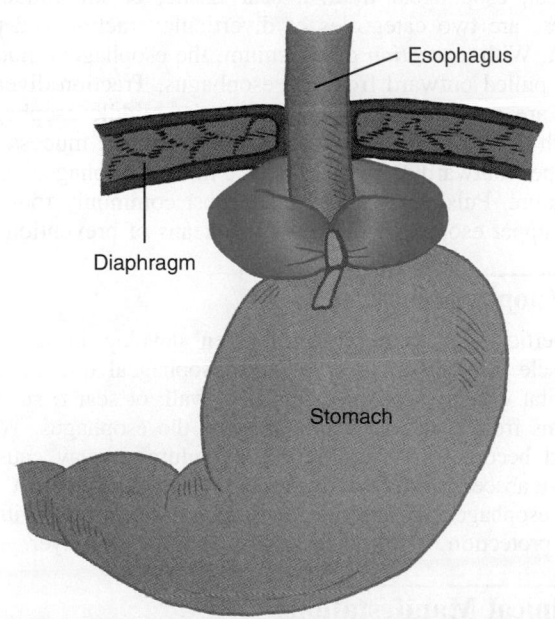

Esophagus

Diaphragm

Stomach

FIGURE 30–12 Angelchick antireflux prosthesis in place.

FIGURE 30-13 *A,* A sliding hiatal hernia. *B,* A rolling hiatal hernia.

gurgitation and motor dysfunction cause the manifestations associated with hiatal hernia. The major problem with a sliding hernia is reflux (GERD), which appears to be caused by the exposure of the LES to the low pressure in the thorax.

With a rolling hernia, the LES remains below the diaphragm and reflux is not a problem. Complications of a rolling hiatal hernia include obstruction, strangulation, and the development of a volvulus.

Clinical Manifestations

Manifestations of hiatal hernia vary in kind and severity. In sliding hiatal hernias, the client may experience heartburn 30 to 60 minutes after meals. Reflux may also result in substernal pain.

The client with a rolling hiatal hernia does not have manifestations of reflux. The client may complain of a feeling of fullness after eating or may have difficulty breathing. Some clients experience chest pain similar to that of angina. Pain is usually worse when the client lies down.

A barium swallow with fluoroscopy can reveal a hiatal hernia by showing the position of the stomach in relation to the diaphragm.

Outcome Management

■ Medical and Surgical Management

The medical and surgical management for the client with a hiatal hernia is the same as that for the client with GERD.

■ Nursing Management of the Medical or Surgical Client

The nursing care of the client with a hiatal hernia is the same as that for a client with GERD.

DIVERTICULA

An esophageal diverticulum is a sac-like outpouching in one or more layers of the esophagus. As food is ingested, it becomes trapped in a diverticulum and can later be regurgitated. The most common type of esophageal diverticulum is esophageal pulsion (Zenker's) diverticulum. Esophageal diverticula are considered rare. Zenker's diverticula occur three times more often in men as in women.

Etiology and Risk Factors

The cause of esophageal weakness may be a congenital defect, esophageal trauma, scar tissue, or inflammation. There are two categories of diverticula: traction and pulsion. With a *traction* diverticulum, the esophageal mucosa has pulled outward from the esophagus. Traction diverticula are most commonly found in the middle esophagus. With a *pulsion* diverticulum, the esophageal mucosa has pushed outward through a defect in the esophageal musculature. Pulsion diverticula are most commonly found in the upper esophagus. There is no means of prevention.

Pathophysiology

Diverticula in the esophagus often develop in areas of muscle weakness that arise from esophageal trauma, congenital weakness of the esophageal wall, or scar tissue that forms from chronic inflammation of the esophagus. When food becomes trapped in a diverticulum, it may cause a local abscess. Infected diverticula place the client at risk for esophageal perforation because the mucosa is without the protection of the normal esophageal muscle layer.

Clinical Manifestations

Initially, the client usually complains of difficulty swallowing. Other manifestations may include eructation, regurgitation of undigested food, halitosis, and a sour taste in the mouth. Coughing also may occur because of irritation of the trachea from regurgitated food.

A barium swallow is performed to locate the diverticulum. Endoscopy is usually contraindicated because the diverticulum may be perforated by the endoscope.

Outcome Management

Medical Management

Medical management of esophageal diverticula includes dietary management and positioning. Small, frequent meals of semi-soft foods often facilitate passage of food. The client should note which foods ease or worsen the manifestations.

To prevent reflux of food, the caregiver should raise the head of the bed for 2 hours after meals. Sleeping with the head of the bed elevated can often prevent nocturnal reflux. The client also should avoid constrictive clothes and vigorous exercise after eating.

Nursing Management of the Medical Client

Obtain a history from the client, noting the onset and duration of manifestations and whether they occur at mealtimes or at night. Assess the client's respiratory status because regurgitation can cause respiratory complications.

Teach the client how changes in diet and positioning can control manifestations. Encourage the client to try various foods and various positions to evaluate which are most effective.

Surgical Management

When manifestations become severe, surgery may be indicated. A cervical approach is used for Zenker's diverticulum, whereas a thoracic approach is used for diverticula located lower in the esophagus. In both procedures, the diverticulum is excised and the esophageal mucosa is reanastomosed.

Nursing Management of the Surgical Client

ASSESSMENT

Obtain a history, noting the onset and duration of manifestations, aggravating factors, and any methods the client uses for relief. In addition, routine preoperative and postoperative assessments are required.

DIAGNOSIS, OUTCOMES, INTERVENTIONS

Risk for Injury. When an esophageal diverticulum is treated surgically, the nursing diagnosis *Risk for Injury related to surgical procedure and presence of chest tubes* is appropriate.

Outcomes. Injury will be prevented, as evidenced by a normal temperature and an absence of hemorrhage, infection, and problems associated with the chest tubes, such as respiratory distress.

Interventions
Provide Teaching. Discuss the normal preoperative routines. Explain that the client will be taking nothing by mouth after surgery and that an NG tube will be present until healing occurs. If a thoracic approach is used, preoperative and postoperative nursing care is similar to that

for clients having thoracic surgery and chest tubes (see Chapter 62).

Maintain the NG Tube. After surgery, the client's NG tube is attached to low intermittent suction to avoid trauma to the stomach lining. Assess the amount and color of drainage during each shift. Check for continued bloody NG drainage as well as for external bleeding. Do not irrigate or reposition the NG tube unless told to do so by the physician. Moving the NG tube can perforate the esophagus or stomach (see Chapter 31 on irrigation of tubes if ordered by the surgeon). Assess the client for manifestations of esophageal perforation, such as chest pain, fever, and subcutaneous emphysema. The client will receive IV fluids until tube feedings begin. Once fluids and supplemental feedings begin, record the client's response.

After surgery, the client may be discharged with an NG or a gastrostomy tube in place to allow for esophageal healing. Give the client written and verbal instructions about tube feedings, diet, and positioning. A visiting nurse should see the client at home to ensure that tube feedings are being tolerated well and should continue visits until the feeding tube is removed.

Promote Comfort. Assess the client's pain, and administer and evaluate prescribed analgesics. After surgery, the head of the bed should be elevated 30 degrees to reduce edema around the neck and upper chest. Frequent oral hygiene increases the client's comfort.

EVALUATION

An appropriate outcome for the client with a diverticulum is that the altered diet will control the problem. If surgery is required, the client's nutritional intake should return to normal after healing occurs.

Modifications for Elderly Clients

Older adults are treated more conservatively, with an emphasis on diet and positioning rather than surgery. Surgery may entail too much risk for older clients.

ESOPHAGEAL CANCER

Cancer of the esophagus takes the form of either squamous cell carcinoma or adenocarcinoma of the esophageal mucosa. An estimated 12,300 new cases of esophageal cancer are diagnosed each year in the United States.[1] The incidence is three times as high in men as in women, and it is higher in African American and Asian men than in white men. Adenocarcinoma of the esophagus occurs less often than squamous cell carcinoma and develops primarily in the distal esophagus.

Etiology and Risk Factors

The cause of esophageal cancer is unknown, but researchers are studying environmental differences between locations with a low and a high incidence. In the Western world, evidence points to heavy smoking, nutritional deficiencies, and habitual ingestion of alcohol, hot foods, and hot drinks as underlying etiologic factors.

In other parts of the world, contaminants in the soil and food, high levels of nitrosamines, smoking opium, and nutritional deficiencies (especially of fruits and vegetables) have been linked to the condition. Chronic irritation from other esophageal problems, such as achalasia, hiatal hernia, and stricture, plays a minor role in the development of esophageal cancer.

These are very preventable causes. Prevention should be targeted particularly toward the African American population because their risk is higher. Risk factors include smoking tobacco or opium, nutritional deficiencies, ingestion of hot foods and beverages, habitual ingestion of alcohol, ingestion of smoked meats or meats cooked over very high heat, irritation from GERD, hiatal hernia, or achalasia. Health promotion and maintenance behaviors involve limiting or stopping smoking and avoiding chronic ingestion of alcohol, hot foods, and hot beverages. Restorative behaviors include advising the client to follow the appropriate medical or surgical regimen for treatment of the specific condition.

Pathophysiology

Cancer of the esophagus begins as slow-growing benign tissue changes. Most of these cancers are squamous epidermoid tumors that are commonly found in the middle or upper third of the esophagus. Because the esophagus has no serosal layer to limit its extension, esophageal tumors expand locally and very rapidly. Early spread to the lymph nodes is common. The rich lymphatic supply to the mucosa provides an excellent means for the cancer to metastasize widely. The cancers are typically intraluminal, ulcerating lesions that encircle the esophageal wall and extend upward and downward.

The disease is progressive and almost always fatal. As it progresses, most clients experience some pulmonary complications because of the formation of tracheoesophageal fistulae that result in aspiration. If the condition is not treated, total esophageal obstruction is the inevitable outcome of the disease. Infiltration into blood vessels may predispose the client to hemorrhage. Metastasis is common because of the large supply of lymph channels in the area.

Clinical Manifestations

Typically, the first manifestations are dysphagia or odynophagia. Unfortunately, they are usually not apparent until the cancer involves the circumference of the esophagus. By the time the client becomes aware of a swallowing problem and seeks medical care, the cancer frequently has invaded the deeper layers of the esophagus and, sometimes, adjacent structures such as the bronchus.

At first, dysphagia is usually mild and intermittent, occurring only after ingestion of solid food (especially meat). Soon, dysphagia becomes constant and manifestations of esophageal obstruction appear. These manifestations include an increase in salivation and mucus in the throat, nocturnal aspiration, regurgitation, and an inability to swallow even liquids.

Barium swallow, endoscopy, cytologic examination, and direct biopsy confirm the diagnosis. Computed tomography (CT) scans provide an excellent definition of the size of the primary lesion and reveal the extent of nodal involvement.

Outcome Management

▄ Medical Management
INHIBIT TUMOR GROWTH
Treatment of esophageal cancer depends on the tumor's location and size, metastases, and the condition of the client. If the cancer is found in an early stage, treatment is directed toward cure; however, it is usually detected in the late stages, when treatment becomes palliative, aimed specifically at allowing the client to continue eating.

RADIATION THERAPY. Radiation therapy can be used alone or before or after surgery. It provides palliation by reducing tumor size and slowing tumor growth. Because high-dose radiation therapy may cause stenosis of the esophagus, treatments are usually administered over 6 to 8 weeks to minimize this effect.

CHEMOTHERAPY. Chemotherapy, combining several drugs, provides symptomatic relief. Neoadjuvant chemotherapy with cisplatin (Platinol) and 5-fluorouracil (5-FU) before surgery can facilitate surgical resection by decreasing tumor size and invasiveness of the disease in about 50% of clients treated. Chemotherapy, combined with radiation and followed by surgery, shows promising early results.[3, 19]

PHOTODYNAMIC THERAPY. Photodynamic therapy is a relatively new therapy for palliative treatment of esophageal cancer in clients who are not surgical candidates. The client receives an injection of a light-sensitive drug (Photofrin), which is followed 2 days later with a special fiberoptic probe with a light-bearing tip placed in the esophagus. The light activates the Photofrin and kills only cancer cells. This outpatient procedure utilizes conscious sedation, takes about 13 minutes to perform, and enables about 1 inch of tumor to be removed. Clients return home the same day and resume their usual activities the next day.[19]

MAINTAIN NUTRITION
Maintaining nutrition is a major goal for the client with esophageal cancer. Early in the disease, the client may be able to tolerate small, frequent feedings of soft or semisoft foods. As the disease progresses, feeding tubes may be needed. If necessary, a feeding gastrostomy or jejunostomy may be created. Short-term TPN may be used to improve the client's nutritional status before surgery. Proper positioning after meals is necessary if the client is experiencing frequent regurgitation or wearing a prosthesis. The head of the bed should always be elevated 30 degrees.

▄ Nursing Management of the Medical Client
ASSESSMENT
Obtain data concerning the client's nutritional status. Most clients complain of dysphagia that is both persistent and progressive. The client initially may have difficulty swallowing solid foods and then may have difficulty swallowing soft foods and liquids.

A careful assessment of dysphagia is important. Other manifestations, such as odynophagia, regurgitation, chronic cough, increased secretions, and hoarseness (from involvement of the larynx), also are important to assess.

DIAGNOSIS, OUTCOMES, INTERVENTIONS

Altered Nutrition: Less Than Body Requirements.

Because of the progressively worsening dysphagia, the client with esophageal cancer exhibits the nursing diagnosis *Altered Nutrition: Less Than Body Requirements related to the client's inability to swallow.*

Outcomes. The client will maintain an adequate nutritional status, as evidenced by maintenance of stable body weight or slowed weight loss.

Interventions. Monitor the client's nutritional status throughout treatment, including daily weights, intake and output, and calories consumed. In the beginning, teach the client about diet changes that can make eating easier.

As the disease progresses, you may have to provide tube feedings. Assess the skin around the feeding tube for impairment of skin integrity caused by leakage of gastric juices. Wash the skin around the opening with a gentle soap and dry thoroughly twice daily or as needed. Apply a protective ointment, such as zinc oxide or karaya gum, to the skin for further protection.

Risk for Impaired Swallowing.

The client with esophageal cancer experiences increasing dysphagia that may lead to the diagnosis *Risk for Impaired Swallowing related to esophageal obstruction from tumor.*

Outcomes. The client will not suffer from impaired swallowing, as evidenced by an absence of choking and maintenance of a patent airway.

Interventions. Many problems arise when the client is unable to swallow. The client can easily choke on saliva and mucous secretions and must spit frequently or drool. Constant wiping of saliva from the lips can cause irritation, cracking of the skin, and open lesions. Because it is impractical to collect this quantity of secretions in tissues, the client should carry a receptacle to receive the saliva. While hospitalized, clients are often taught to do self-suctioning. To prevent oral lesions and infections and to provide comfort, you should administer or assist with frequent oral care.

Risk for Ineffective Individual Coping.

The client with cancer of the esophagus has many problems associated with both the disease and its treatment. This can lead to a nursing diagnosis of *Risk for Ineffective Individual Coping related to changes in body image and potentially terminal prognosis.*

Outcomes. The client will effectively cope with the alterations in body image and potentially terminal prognosis, as evidenced by maintenance of activities and continued social interaction.

Interventions. In addition to meeting the client's physical needs, you must provide emotional support. The gastrostomy tube may cause an alteration in body image and increased dependency. The drooling or need to spit constantly also may cause the client a great deal of emotional distress. The poor prognosis of esophageal cancer necessitates psychological support and interventions aimed at helping the client and significant others prepare for the client's death (see Chapters 19 and 22).

EVALUATION

Successful control of manifestations and prevention of extensive weight loss, as the client is supported to a peaceful death, may be the desired outcomes. Few clients survive for 5 years.

▮ Surgical Management

Esophageal dilation may be necessary throughout the course of the disease to treat strictures and obstruction caused by the tumor. The physician should perform the treatment as often as needed to relieve dysphagia.

In advanced disease, a prosthesis may be inserted to bypass the tumor or to prevent aspiration in clients with fistulae. The prosthesis can maintain esophageal patency but can perforate the esophagus if it becomes dislodged or the tumor increases in size.

Surgery may be performed for prophylaxis, cure, or palliation, depending on the extent of the disease. For high-risk clients with Barrett's esophagus, a premalignant healing process that occurs in association with GERD, the lower third of the esophagus is removed prophylactically.[19] Three surgical procedures can be performed:

1. An *esophagectomy* consists of the removal of all or part of the esophagus. The resected esophagus is replaced with a polyester (Dacron) graft. This procedure is usually performed via a thoracotomy, but it may be performed transhiatally, which eliminates the need for a thoracotomy.
2. An *esophagogastrostomy* involves resection of the lower portion of the esophagus and anastomosis of the remainder to the stomach, brought up into the thorax.
3. In an *esophagoenterostomy* (colon interposition), the esophagus is resected and replaced with a segment of the descending colon.

▮ Nursing Management of the Surgical Client

ASSESSMENT

Obtain data about the client's nutritional status, ability to swallow, respiratory status, and ability to cope with the diagnosis. In addition, routine preoperative and postoperative assessments are required.

DIAGNOSIS, OUTCOMES, INTERVENTIONS

Risk for Injury.

Surgery to treat esophageal cancer is often extensive, necessitating a thoracic approach and leading to the nursing diagnosis *Risk for Injury related to surgical procedure.*

Outcomes. Injury will be prevented, as evidenced by an absence of atelectasis, fever, wound infection, or problems associated with the chest tubes.

Interventions

Improve Nutritional Status before Surgery. Before surgery, clients usually require 2 to 3 weeks of nutritional support. Often, this support includes tube feedings or TPN. The client's weight and fluid and electrolyte status are monitored.

Provide Preoperative Teaching. Provide extensive instruction on postoperative respiratory care, including turning, coughing, deep breathing, and chest physiotherapy. Teach the client about all incisions, wound drainage tubes, feeding tubes, and chest tubes that may be present after surgery. Oral care should be performed four times a day to help prevent infection postoperatively. If an esophagoenterostomy is performed, a complete bowel preparation is performed before surgery.

Maintain Airway. After surgery, respiratory care is a high priority. The client may be placed on a ventilator in a critical care unit (see Chapter 62 for care of a client receiving mechanical ventilation). Otherwise, the client must turn, cough, and deep-breathe every hour. Carefully assess the client's respiratory status, report any manifestations of atelectasis or pneumonia, and administer supplemental oxygen. Administer pain medication frequently, and assist the client in splinting the incision while coughing. Place the client in a semi-Fowler position to prevent reflux. Continually monitor the chest tube drainage for amount, color, and patency.

Maintain Fluid and Electrolyte Balance. Assess the client's fluid and electrolyte status. Monitor drainage from the NG, gastric, and all drainage tubes at least every shift. The client will be NPO for 4 to 5 days until peristalsis returns. During the first 24 hours after surgery, NG or gastric drainage is bloody but should then change to a greenish yellow color. If bloody drainage continues, it may indicate bleeding at the suture line and should be reported.

Leakage at the site of anastomosis may appear about 5 to 7 days after surgery. Assess the client for early manifestations of shock as well as for fever, fluid accumulation at the wound site, and inflammation. Check all dressings for bleeding, drainage, or separation of the suture lines.

Advance Diet as Tolerated. The client should be started on small sips of water. If this intake is tolerated, the quantity is slowly increased. Supervise the client, making sure the client stays in an upright position, and monitor for manifestations of leakage at the anastomosis site. If this is tolerated, the client gradually progresses to puréed and semi-solid foods. Explain the importance of small, frequent feedings, and advise the client to sit upright at meals and for 1 hour after meals to prevent overdistention of the stomach and reflux.

EVALUATION

The poor prognosis associated with the illness means that successful control of manifestations and prevention of extensive weight loss may be the only reasonable outcomes for these clients. Few clients survive for 5 years. They should receive support during the process of dying.

■ Self-Care

Upon discharge, give the client and family written and oral instructions concerning wound healing, nutritional support, respiratory care, and medications. Teach the client about possible wound and respiratory complications, manifestations that should be reported immediately, and how to contact appropriate members of the health care team.

Make appropriate referrals to community agencies. Most clients need a great amount of assistance at home. Provide information about services offered by the American Cancer Society and local hospice (see Chapter 19), if it becomes apparent that hospice care is necessary. End-of-life care is discussed in Chapter 22.

VASCULAR DISORDERS

The principal vascular disorder of the esophagus is varices. Because esophageal varices result from portal hyper-

tension, this condition is discussed with liver disorders in Chapter 47.

TRAUMA

Major traumatic conditions of the esophagus include chemical burns, the presence of foreign bodies, and injuries from external forces, such as endoscopic equipment. Chemical burns result from the ingestion of acids or alkalis and sometimes from highly spiced foods. Thermal burns can occur after drinking extremely hot liquids, accidental ingestion of foreign bodies that lodge in the natural narrow spots of the esophagus, and self-mutilation related to suicide attempts. Trauma can cause esophageal perforation, with resultant contamination of the mediastinum and stricture formation as a complication of the healing process. Treatment of esophageal strictures involves dilation of the esophagus or surgical excision of the diseased portion and reanastomosis or interposition of a piece of gut from the stomach or colon (see Esophageal Cancer).

CONCLUSIONS

Disorders of the mouth and esophagus range from fairly simple problems, such as dental caries, to complex and potentially lethal problems, such as cancer of the esophagus. No matter how minor, disorders throughout the oral-esophageal area can interfere with the client's nutritional intake. Always keep this fact in mind when assessing and caring for clients with these disorders.

THINKING CRITICALLY

1. **The client is a 72-year-old retired schoolteacher who lives with her 70-year-old sister. She is being evaluated for complaints of chest pain, which have become increasingly more frequent. Yesterday, while she was lifting flats of bedding plants to prepare for planting, she became dyspneic and collapsed. Her sister called the ambulance, and the client was admitted to a medical-surgical unit. This morning, she underwent an abdominal ultrasound prior to an upper GI series. An electrocardiogram (ECG) followed the tests. When the nurse last checked, the client was sleeping soundly. Now the client's call light is on. When entering the room, the client is gasping, clutching at her chest, and attempting to get out of bed, saying, "Please help me! I can't catch my breath!" What is your first priority?**

Factors to Consider. Is the client experiencing manifestations of a cardiovascular problem or a gastrointestinal one? How can the nurse tell the difference?

2. **A 61-year-old woman is being treated as an outpatient for gastroesophageal reflux disease. She tells the nurse that the doctor told her to take Maalox but did not tell her how else to treat her condition. What would you teach her?**

Factors to Consider. What lifestyle changes might help the client manage her condition?

3. An 18-year-old man is seen at a dental clinic following the blow of a soccer ball to the head. Several teeth were loosened by the impact. During the oral examination, the nurse notes that the gums are reddened and tender and bleed easily when probed with a tongue blade. The area under the left premolar is swollen, tender, and abscessed. The client pulls away and tells the nurse to stop because it hurts too much to touch that tooth and states, "It's been hurting for the past several weeks." When questioned, the client states that he brushes his teeth once a day or every other day, has never flossed, and usually eats several candy bars a day. What nursing interventions are appropriate?

Factors to Consider. What might be the problem with the client's tooth? What could be the cause of his gingival problems?

BIBLIOGRAPHY

1. American Cancer Society. (2000). *Cancer facts and figures.* Atlanta: Author.
2. Ault, D. L., & Schmidt, D. (1998). Diagnosis and management of gastroesophageal reflux. *Nurse Practitioner, 23*(6), 81–82, 88–89.
3. Cooper, J., et al. (1999). Chemoradiotherapy of locally advanced esophageal cancer. *JAMA, 281*(17), 1623–1627.
4. Copstead, L. (1999). *Perspectives on pathophysiology* (2nd ed.). Philadelphia: W. B. Saunders.
5. Feldman, M., Scharschmidt, B., & Sleisenger, M. (Eds.). (1997). *Gastrointestinal and liver disease: Pathophysiology/diagnosis/management* (6th ed.). Philadelphia: W. B. Saunders.
6. Gavaghan, M. (1999). Anatomy and physiology of the esophagus. *AORN Journal, 69*(2), 372–386.
7. Goldsmith, C. (1998). Gastroesophageal reflux disease. *American Journal of Nursing, 98*(9), 44–45.
8. Graling, P. R. (1998). Managing the patient with perforated intrathoracic esophagus. *AORN Journal, 68*(1), 56–58, 61–61, 67.
9. Hansen, M. (1998). *Pathophysiology: Foundations of disease and clinical intervention.* Philadelphia: W. B. Saunders.
10. Heuman, D., Mills, S., & McGuire, H. (1997). *Gastroenterology.* Philadephia: W. B. Saunders.
11. Lehne, R. (1998). *Pharmacology for nursing care* (3rd ed.). Philadelphia: W. B. Saunders.
12. McCorkle, R., et al. (1996). *Cancer nursing: A comprehensive textbook* (2nd ed.). Philadelphia: W. B. Saunders.
13. McHale, J. M., et al. (1998). Expert nursing knowledge in the care of patients at risk of impaired swallowing. *Image, 30*(2), 137–141.
14. Metheny, N., et al. (1997). pH and concentrations of pepsin and trypsin in feeding tube aspirates as predictors of tube placement. *Journal of Parenteral and Enteral Nutrition, 21,* 279–285.
15. Metheny, N., et al. (1999). pH and concentration of bilirubin feeding tube aspirates as predictors of tube placement. *Nursing Research, 48*(4), 189–197.
16. Mittal, R., & Balaban, D. (1997). The esophagogastric junction. *New England Journal of Medicine, 336*(13), 924–932.
17. Moody, F. (1999). *Atlas of ambulatory surgery.* Philadelphia: W. B. Saunders.
18. Pehl, C., et al. (1999). Effect of low and high fat meals on lower esophageal sphincter motility and gastroesophageal reflux in healthy subjects. *American Journal of Gastroenterology, 94*(5), 1190–1196.
19. Quinn, K. L., & Reedy, A. (1999). Esophageal cancer: Therapeutic approaches and nursing care. *Seminars in Oncology Nursing, 15*(1), 17–25.
20. Rombeau, J., & Rolandelli, R. (1997). *Clinical nutrition: Enteral and tube feeding* (3rd ed.). Philadelphia: W. B. Saunders.
21. Sabiston, D., & Lyerly, H. (Eds.). (1997). *Textbook of surgery: The biological basis of modern surgical practice* (15th ed.). Philadelphia: W. B. Saunders.
22. Schlomer, P. (1998). Using a prosthesis to treat gastroesophageal reflux. *AORN Journal, 68*(1), 93–96.
23. Spiess, A., & Kahrilas, P. (1998). Treating achalasia. *JAMA, 280*(7), 638–643.
24. Steele, G., & Katz, J. (1996). *Primary Care: Gastroenterology, 23*(3), 417–648.
25. Whitney, L. (1995). Vincent's angina, periodontitis, and stomatitis. *Nursing, 25,* 32.

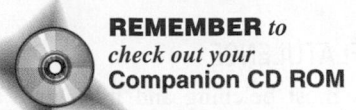

C H A P T E R

31

Management of Clients with Digestive Disorders

Elizabeth A. Murphy-Blake

NURSING OUTCOMES CLASSIFICATION (NOC)
for Nursing Diagnoses—Clients with Digestive Disorders

Altered Nutrition: Less Than Body Requirements
Knowledge: Diet
Nutritional Status
Nutritional Status: Food and Fluid Intake
Nutritional Status: Nutrient Intake
Fear
Fear Control
Anxiety Control
Coping
Ineffective Management of Therapeutic Regimen (Individual)

Compliance Behavior
Knowledge: Treatment Regimen
Participation: Health Care Decisions
Treatment Behavior: Illness or Injury
Risk for Injury: Postoperative Complications
Circulation Status
Risk Control
Risk Detection
Safety Status: Physical Injury

Symptom Control
Tissue Perfusion: Abdominal Organs
Tissue Perfusion: Peripheral
Vital Signs Status
Pain
Comfort Level
Pain Control
Pain: Disruptive Effects
Pain Level

The client with a gastric disorder usually has a problem with nutritional intake. As a result, the most common nursing diagnoses are *Altered Nutrition: Less Than Body Requirements* and *Pain*. Additional nursing diagnoses (e.g., *Ineffective Management of Therapeutic Regimen [Individuals] related to dietary changes and pharmacologic management, Fear,* and *Risk for Injury related to complications)* are also possible.

GENERAL CLINICAL MANIFESTATIONS OF GASTROINTESTINAL DISORDERS

Manifestations of gastrointestinal (GI) tract dysfunction are caused by excessive gastric secretions that erode stomach mucosa, excessive motility, and retention of gastric contents. The most prominent clinical manifestations are pain, acid reflux, anorexia, belching and flatulence, nausea, vomiting, bleeding, indigestion, and diarrhea.

■ PAIN

Pain is the most characteristic clinical manifestation; it usually results from chemical irritation of nerve endings. Nerve irritation occurs when acid comes into contact with the eroded stomach mucosa. It also results from stretching and contracting of the stomach, caused in turn by increased motility and increased smooth muscle tension, as found in an obstruction.

■ ANOREXIA

Anorexia, or loss of appetite, is often experienced by clients with malignancy or various other disorders. Hunger is normally caused by several stimuli, including contraction of the empty stomach. When the stomach empties slowly or when gastric stasis occurs because of a gastric disorder, anorexia can result.

■ NAUSEA AND VOMITING

Nausea is a result of conditions that increase tension on the walls of the stomach, duodenum, or lower end of the esophagus. Unpleasant stimuli, distention, gastritis, and carcinoma of the stomach can produce nausea. Vomiting

This chapter incorporates material written for the fifth edition by Jane Hokanson Hawks.

may follow nausea or occur without it. Vomiting is caused by stimulation of the emetic center:

1. The chemoreceptor trigger zone (CTZ) in the fourth ventricle. The CTZ is stimulated by various drugs and body toxins. Conversely, medications of the phenothiazine derivative groups, such as chlorpromazine (Thorazine) and prochlorperazine (Compazine), depress vomiting caused by chemoreceptor stimulation. Serotonin antagonists, such as ondansetron (Zofran), block serotonin receptors in the vagus nerve and CTZ.
2. Nerve impulses, which can be excited by
   a. Direct mechanical stimuli, as in increased intracranial pressure
   b. Chemical stimuli from blood-borne metabolites or toxic substances
   c. Sympathetic and parasympathetic afferent nerve impulses through the vagus, glossopharyngeal, vestibular, and splanchnic nerves (the most sensitive receptors are located in the proximal duodenum)
3. Unpleasant odors, subjects, and sights that stimulate higher center impulses
4. Distention of stomach or duodenum
5. Decreased gastric motility
6. Pain, because the pain centers are close to the vomiting centers in the medulla
7. Increased intracranial pressure

■ BLEEDING

Bleeding results from local trauma or irritations that cause erosion or ulceration of the GI tract mucosa. The disorders involved include stomach neoplasms, gastric ulcer, gastritis, anastomotic (marginal) ulcers, and duodenal ulcers. Duodenitis can also cause bleeding. Although bleeding may have numerous causes, up to 75% of all cases of upper GI tract bleeding result from esophagogastric varices (venous), hemorrhagic gastritis (capillary), or peptic ulcer. Ulcers account for 80% of all upper GI tract hemorrhage.

■ DIARRHEA

Diarrhea can be caused by increased peristalsis resulting from an increased gastrocolic reflex or from the effort of the stomach and intestines to eliminate a local irritant.

■ BELCHING AND FLATULENCE

Swallowed air causes most belching and flatulence. It is easy to swallow air during eating and drinking, especially when food is ingested rapidly. Frequently, clients attempt to belch to relieve a vague feeling of distress in the stomach caused by swallowed air. Attempting to belch with the mouth closed sometimes adds more air to the stomach than it removes.

■ INDIGESTION

Indigestion or dyspepsia can be caused by such factors as strong emotions, GI tract disease, eating too rapidly, chewing inadequately, gas-forming foods (e.g., beans and cabbage), and food allergy.

GASTROINTESTINAL INTUBATION

Gastric and intestinal tubes are inserted for several purposes: (1) decompression, (2) lavage, (3) gastric analysis, and (4) tube feedings.

Decompression relieves the pressure caused by contents and gases that remain in the stomach or bowel because of some obstruction. Long intestinal tubes are sometimes used to dilate the lumen or to release an obstruction. Postoperative decompression removes secretions that cannot pass through the GI tract because of edema and decreased gastric motility. The placement of a tube (intubation) helps prevent vomiting, distention, and obstruction.

Lavage is the irrigation or washing out of an organ. Gastric lavage washes out the stomach. It is used most frequently as an emergency treatment in poisoning. Lavage is also used for exfoliative cytology to determine the presence of abnormal cells.

Tube feeding or *gavage feeding,* referred to as *enteral nutrition,* is a method of giving clients fluids and nutrients via a tube when oral intake is inadequate or impossible.

■ TYPES OF TUBES

Three types of tubes are used for decompression: (1) *short* nasogastric (NG) tubes are used for the stomach, (2) *medium* tubes extend into the duodenum or jejunum, and (3) *long* tubes are used for the rest of the GI tract (see Table 31–1).

TABLE 31–1	GASTRIC AND INTESTINAL TUBES				
		Length	Size (French)	Lumen	Other Characteristics
SHORT TUBES					
	Levin type (plastic or rubber)	125 cm (50 inches)	12, 16, 18	Single	
	Salem sump	120 cm (48 inches)	12, 14, 16, 18	Double	Sump-type suction
MEDIUM TUBES					
	Dobhoff (nasoduodenal or nasojejunal)	160–175 cm (60–66 inches)	8, 10, 12	Single	Radiopaque, tungsten-weighted
LONG TUBES					
	Cantor	300 cm (10 feet)	16	Single	Mercury weighted
	Harris	180 cm (6 feet)	14, 16	Single	Mercury weighted
	Miller-Abbott	300 cm (10 feet)	12, 14, 16, 18	Double	Mercury weighted

Short Tubes

Short tubes include the Levin and Salem sump tubes. Short tubes are long enough to extend into the stomach but not into the bowel. These tubes are usually attached to suction. Occasionally, they may be used for short-term enteral feedings over a brief period. However, nasoduodenal tubes are preferred for feedings because of the high rate of aspiration pneumonia associated with NG tube feedings.

LEVIN TUBE. The Levin tube is a single-lumen tube used to remove fluid or gas or to obtain a specimen of gastric contents. Because the tube has only one lumen, low intermittent suction is required to minimize the irritation of the gastric mucosa. Levin tubes may be made out of plastic, rubber-like silicone (Silastic), or rubber.

SALEM SUMP TUBE. The Salem sump tube is a double-lumen tube used to empty and decompress the stomach. Low, continuous suction is used because the "pigtail" lumen on the Salem sump tube vents the tube and protects gastric mucosa from being sucked against the tube. The pigtail lumen should not be clamped or irrigated and should be kept higher than the client's stomach to prevent drainage.

Medium Tubes

Medium tubes include a variety of nasoduodenal (e.g., Dobhoff) tubes that extend into the duodenum and are designed for short-term feeding. They are less likely to cause aspiration pneumonia because of their small size and weighted tip. Placement is verified by abdominal x-ray study (radiography).

Long Tubes

The long tubes extend into the small bowel, sometimes for its entire length. They are between 1.8 and 3.0 m (6 and 10 feet) long and are used to prevent gas and fluid accumulation in the intestine, which is usually caused by intestinal obstruction. The more common long tubes are the Miller-Abbott, Cantor, and Harris tubes.

MILLER-ABBOTT TUBE. The Miller-Abbott tube is a double-lumen tube, 3 m (10 feet) long. One lumen is used to introduce mercury or to inflate the balloon at the end of the tube, and the other is used for aspiration. Markings on the tube indicate the distance the tube has been passed. Initial placement of the tube is completed by a physician. The nurse is responsible for advancing the tube as ordered.

CANTOR TUBE. The Cantor tube is used for aspirating intestinal contents and has only one lumen. It is 3 m (10 feet) long and is larger than the other tubes. It has 4 to 5 ml of mercury in a bag at the end, which is wrapped about the tube before insertion. For intestinal intubation, the tube is threaded through the nose into the stomach and then through the pylorus, where peristaltic activity of the bowel carries it to the desired intestinal area.

HARRIS TUBE. The Harris tube is a single-lumen, mercury-weighted tube, 1.8 m (6 feet) long. A metal tip is introduced into the nostril after it is lubricated. The weight of the mercury carries the tube by gravity. This tube is used for suction and irrigation.

Sometimes it is difficult to get intestinal tubes to pass through the pylorus. The client is instructed to lie on the right side in order to facilitate passage. When the tube has passed into the duodenum, it is advanced, as ordered, an additional 4.8 to 9.6 cm (2 to 4 inches) every hour or half-hour. When the tube has reached the desired location, tape it securely to the client's face to prevent further advancement.

Other Tubes

For long-term enteral feedings, gastrostomy tubes (GTs or G tubes) or jejunostomy tubes (JTs or J tubes) are often placed surgically. The GT and JT (see Chapter 29) can be inserted surgically or laparoscopically. The percutaneous gastrostomy (PEG), which is the most common, and the percutaneous jejunostomy (PEJ) have been discussed in Chapter 29.

■ INSERTING GASTROINTESTINAL TUBES

GI tubes are generally inserted through the nose into the stomach or small intestine; they are rarely inserted through the mouth. Explain each step of the intubation procedure at the client's level of understanding. Assist the client to assume a high Fowler's position, which makes intubation easier. Measure the distance on the tube from the tip of the nose to the ear lobe plus the distance from the ear lobe to the tip of the xiphoid process (the NEX measurement). This approximates the distance that the tube must be passed to reach the stomach. Mark this distance on the tubing with adhesive.

After measuring the tube, lubricate and gently insert the tube through the nares and posterior nasal pharynx and into the oropharynx. When the tube is in the oropharynx, instruct the client to swallow; sometimes the client is allowed to drink water at this point to help with tube passage. Having the client swallow is important, because the sphincter at the proximal end of the esophagus remains closed except during swallowing. The larynx rises during swallowing, stretching the cricopharyngeal muscle and causing it to relax, thus reducing resistance to the tube. Swallowing also enables the tube to enter the esophagus rather than the trachea. After the tube passes the sphincter, advance it into the stomach.

To verify placement, perform at least two of these activities:

1. Aspirate gastric contents.
2. Measure the pH of the aspirant; the pH of the stomach is less than that of the lungs.
3. Instill air into the tube with a syringe and listen with a stethoscope for air passing into the stomach.
4. Check with an x-ray study for the radiopaque lines on the tube.

After confirming placement, secure the tube to the nose with hypoallergenic tape. (This procedure is used for short tubes only; medium tubes are checked with an x-ray and long tubes need to be able to advance.)

■ SUCTIONING GASTROINTESTINAL TUBES

When suction is applied to a GI tube to remove accumulated gas and fluid, ensure that the GI mucosa is not traumatized. Excessive negative pressure causes the mucosa to be sucked into the openings on the tube, impairing suction and injuring the mucosa. Intermittent suction is used to avoid this problem unless a double-lumen tube, such as the Salem sump, is used. Mucus tends to plug the openings of these tubes, making it necessary to irrigate with saline as ordered to maintain or to check tube patency (usually every 4 hours).

■ NURSING MANAGEMENT OF CLIENTS WITH GASTROINTESTINAL TUBES

Maintain the client's comfort while the tube is in place. Some helpful nursing interventions include these steps:

1. Clean and lubricate external nares. The nares may become sore because of crusted secretions around the tube. Always use a water-soluble lubricant to avoid the possibility of lipid pneumonia when using an oil-based lubricant.
2. Tape the tube in a manner that prevents irritation of the nares.
3. Administer frequent oral hygiene to remove debris, increase comfort, maintain a healthy oral cavity, and stimulate saliva secretion. The client's mouth is usually dry because the absence of chewing prevents the normal stimulus to salivary secretions and the presence of the tube causes mouth breathing.
4. Permit the client, if possible, to chew gum or suck on sour candies or ice chips to help stimulate salivation. Excessive use stimulates gastric secretions and causes electrolyte loss through the suction.
5. Brush the client's teeth or assist the client in brushing teeth.
6. Request an order for anesthetic mouth rinses or lozenges because the presence of the tube frequently causes sore throat.

Placement of the tube in the throat may result in cricoid chondritis (irritation of the cricoid cartilage of the larynx) and laryngeal injuries. Presenting clinical manifestations include:

- Localized odynophagia
- Pain radiating to the ears
- Sore throat
- Stridor
- Bloody sputum
- Mild hoarseness

Assess for these potential complications and report the findings immediately. An order for anesthetic lozenges or gargles to relieve manifestations may be needed. Frequent assessment of secretions for color, odor, and quantity is essential. Report any changes to the physician. It may be necessary to send samples of these secretions to the laboratory for analysis. Measure the contents of the suction containers to maintain an accurate record of GI losses. Metabolic alkalosis may result from a major loss of water and electrolytes. Monitor potassium levels, since potassium is one of the major electrolytes lost through suctioning.

The irrigating solution instilled into a GI tube is counted as intake if it is not removed when contents are aspirated. Keep accurate records of the amount instilled and the amount aspirated from the tube during irrigations.

Normal saline is the preferred irrigating solution because water, a hypotonic solution, increases electrolyte loss through osmotic action if the tube is irrigated frequently.

GASTRITIS

ACUTE GASTRITIS

Gastritis, an inflammation of the gastric mucosa, is classified as either acute or chronic. The incidence of gastritis is highest in the fifth and sixth decades of life; men are more frequently affected than women. The incidence is greater in clients who are heavy drinkers and smokers.

Etiology and Risk Factors

The acute form of gastritis may be seen with nausea and vomiting, epigastric discomfort, bleeding, malaise, and anorexia. It usually stems from ingestion of a corrosive, erosive, or infectious substance. Aspirin and other nonsteroidal anti-inflammatory drugs (NSAIDs), digitalis, chemotherapeutic drugs, steroids, acute alcoholism, and food poisoning (typically caused by *Staphylococcus* organisms) are common causes. In addition, food substances, including excessive amounts of tea, coffee, mustard, paprika, cloves, and pepper, can precipitate acute gastritis. Foods with a rough texture or those eaten at an extremely high temperature can also damage the stomach mucosa. Ingestion of corrosive agents, such as lye or drain cleaner, also causes acute gastritis.

Disorders linked with acute gastritis include uremia, shock, central nervous system lesions, hepatic cirrhosis, portal hypertension, and prolonged emotional tension. Acute gastritis is usually of short duration unless the gastric mucosa has suffered extensive damage.

Health promotion behaviors include limited use of NSAIDs, alcohol, and caffeine and avoidance of nicotine products. Health maintenance behaviors include use of enteric-coated aspirin, misoprostol (Cytotec) to protect against NSAIDs, histamine-receptor antagonists to decrease gastric acidity, or proton pump inhibitors to block gastric acid production. Clients with medical disorders that may lead to gastritis should follow orders for prescribed medications to minimize stomach irritation.

Pathophysiology

The mucosal lining of the stomach normally protects it from the action of gastric acid. This mucosal barrier is composed of prostaglandins. If this barrier is penetrated, gastritis occurs, with resultant injury to the mucosa. When hydrochloric acid comes into contact with the mucosa, injury to small vessels occurs with edema, hemorrhage, and possible ulcer formation. The damage associated with acute gastritis is usually limited.

Clinical Manifestations

Assessment typically reveals epigastric discomfort, abdominal tenderness, cramping, belching, reflux, severe nausea and vomiting, and sometimes hematemesis. Sometimes GI bleeding is the only manifestation. When contaminated food is the cause of gastritis, the client usually develops diarrhea within 5 hours of ingestion of the offending substance.

Diagnosis is based on a detailed history of food intake, medications taken, and any disorders related to gastritis. The physician may also perform a gastroscopic examination with a biopsy.

Outcome Management

■ Medical Management

Intervention involves removing the cause and treating the manifestations. Vomiting frequently responds to medications of the phenothiazine group; pain responds to antacids or histamine (H_2) receptor antagonists (see Table 31–2). If ingestion of NSAIDs is a problem, a prostaglandin E_1 (PGE_1) analog may be prescribed to protect the stomach mucosa and inhibit gastric acid secretion.

Initially, foods and fluids are withheld until nausea and vomiting subside. Once the client tolerates food, the diet includes decaffeinated tea, gelatin, toast, and simple, bland foods. The client should avoid spicy foods, caffeine, and large, heavy meals. In the continued absence of nausea, vomiting, and bloating, the client can slowly return to a normal diet.

■ Nursing Management of the Medical Client

Nursing management of the medical client with acute gastritis is described in the section on chronic gastritis.

CHRONIC GASTRITIS

This condition appears in three different forms:

- *Superficial gastritis,* which causes a reddened, edematous mucosa with small erosions and hemorrhages
- *Atrophic gastritis,* which occurs in all layers of the stomach, develops frequently in association with gastric ulcer and gastric cancer, and is invariably present in pernicious anemia; it is characterized by a decreased number of parietal and chief cells
- *Hypertrophic gastritis,* which produces a dull and nodular mucosa with irregular, thickened, or nodular rugae; hemorrhages occur frequently

Etiology and Risk Factors

Peptic ulcer disease (PUD), infection with *Helicobacter pylori* bacteria, or gastric surgery may lead to chronic gastritis. Other risk factors are similar to those for acute gastritis. Chronic gastritis is associated with atrophy of the gastrin glands. After gastric resection with a gastrojejunostomy, bile and bile acids may reflux into the remaining stomach, causing gastritis. *H. pylori* infection can lead to chronic atrophic gastritis, which predisposes to the development of gastric cancer. Age is also a risk factor; chronic gastritis is more common in older adults.

Pathophysiology

The initial pathophysiologic changes associated with chronic gastritis are the same as with acute gastritis. The stomach lining first becomes thickened and erythematous and then becomes thin and atrophic. Continued deterioration and atrophy lead to loss of function of the parietal cells. When the acid secretion decreases, the source of intrinsic factor is lost, which results in inability to absorb vitamin B_{12}; this leads to the development of pernicious anemia.

In chronic gastritis the mucosa usually heals without scarring, but ulcer formation and bleeding can occur. The atrophic changes eventually result in a minimal amount of acid being secreted into the stomach (achlorhydria), which is a major risk factor for the development of gastric cancer.

Clinical Manifestations

Manifestations are vague and may be absent (because the problem does not cause an increase in hydrochloric acid). Assessment may reveal anorexia, a feeling of fullness, dyspepsia, belching, vague epigastric pain, nausea, vomiting, and intolerance of spicy or fatty foods.

Complications of Gastritis

The clinical course of clients with chronic gastritis may include such complications as bleeding, pernicious anemia, and gastric cancer. Bleeding can be a complication of gastritis, especially when the stomach mucosa becomes denuded or erosive. Bleeding is common with use of alcohol, aspirin, or NSAIDs. The client should undergo an endoscopic examination to determine the source of the bleeding. Another possible complication of atrophic gastritis is diminished ability of the stomach to secrete intrinsic factor, resulting in malabsorption of vitamin B_{12}, which is confirmed by Schilling's test. Gastric cancer may be suspected in a client whose gastritis does not heal with therapy. (See Gastric Cancer later in this chapter.)

Outcome Management

■ Medical Management

Intervention begins when the health care provider rules out cancer as a causative factor. Discomfort may lessen with a bland diet, small frequent meals, antacids, anticholinergics, and sedatives and with avoidance of foods that cause manifestations.

If *H. pylori* bacteria are present, a combination of clarithromycin (Biaxin), metronidazole (Flagyl), and omeprazole (Prilosec) is administered to eliminate the bacteria. If 1 week of this regimen does not succeed eliminating the bacteria, it may be repeated for an additional week.

Medications used to treat chronic gastritis are the same as those given in Table 31–2 for treatment of PUD. Corticosteroids are sometimes prescribed in the hope of inducing some parietal cell regeneration. Intramuscular injections of vitamin B_{12} may be administered monthly if the client has pernicious anemia.

■ Nursing Management of the Medical Client

When assessing the client with acute or chronic gastritis, carefully focus on risk factors. Consider the client's diet, patterns of eating, use of prescription and over-the-

TABLE 31-2   MEDICATIONS COMMONLY USED TO TREAT PEPTIC ULCERS

Class	Action	Therapeutic Outcomes	Adverse Outcomes	Dosing
ANTIBACTERIAL REGIMEN TO ERADICATE *H. PYLORI*				
Clarithromycin (Biaxin); metronidazole (Flagyl); and omeprazole (Prilosec) or ranitidine (Zantac)	Eradicate *H. pylori* bacteria that cause peptic ulcer disease and gastritis	Reduced gastric pain and bleeding. Elimination of *H. pylori*	Diarrhea, suprainfection with *Clostridium difficile*	Instruct client to take as ordered (usually twice daily for 7 days); monitor for diarrhea and signs of suprainfection; encourage client to take entire prescribed regimen.
HYPOSECRETORY AGENTS				
Histamine (H$_2$) Receptor Antagonists				
Ranitidine hydrochloride (Zantac)	Inhibits gastric acid secretion by blocking H$_2$-receptors on parietal cells	Reduced gastric pain and bleeding. Short-term and maintenance treatment of duodenal and gastric ulcers. Prevention of PUD with NSAIDs and stress ulcers	All side effects rare including nausea, constipation, bradycardia, increased liver enzymes, and headache	Give IM, IV, or PO 1 hr before meals or as maintenance dose at bedtime. Give antacids at least 1 hr before or 2 hr after ranitidine; use cautiously in clients with liver or renal disorders; absorption not affected by food; interacts minimally with diazepam (Valium), glipizide (Glucotrol), theophylline, and warfarin (Coumadin).
Prostaglandin Analogs				
Misoprostol (Cytotec)	Suppresses secretion of gastric acid and stimulates production of cytoprotective mucus	Prevention of aspirin and NSAID-induced gastric ulcers. Relief of pain and bleeding for PUD	Diarrhea, nausea, abdominal discomfort, headache, and dizziness Cannot be used in pregnancy because it stimulates uterine contractions	Give with meals qid (last dose at bedtime). Avoid with Mg$^+$ antacids and pregnancy.
Anticholinergics				
Dicyclomine hydrochloride (Bentyl)	Muscarinic antagonist; inhibits secretion of gastric acid in large doses	Decreases motility and spasms of GI tract	Headache, palpitations, dizziness, constipation, paralytic ileus, urinary hesitancy and retention, and dry mouth	Give 1 hr before meals and at bedtime. Do not give if active bleeding. Do not use in clients with obstructive uropathy, gastrointestinal obstruction, ulcerative colitis, unstable cardiovascular status, or toxic megacolon; use carefully in clients with narrow-angle glaucoma, hyperthyroidism, hiatal hernia, congestive heart failure, hepatic or renal disease.

Drug	Action	Use	Side/Adverse Effects	Nursing Implications
Proton Pump Inhibitors				
Omeprazole (Prilosec)	Suppression of acid secretion by inhibiting H+, K+-ATPase (the enzyme that makes gastric acid)	Short-term (4–8 weeks) treatment of active duodenal ulcer, active benign gastric ulcer, and heartburn associated with gastroesophageal reflux disease	Headache, diarrhea, nausea, vomiting. Gastric cancer is a risk factor with long term use	Give once a day for 4–8 weeks before breakfast or at bedtime.
Antacids				
Aluminum-magnesium combinations (Riopan, Maalox, Mylanta, Gelusil)	Increases gastric pH to reduce pepsin activity; strengthens gastric mucosal barrier and esophageal sphincter tone; direct H+ ion buffering	Short-term treatment of duodenal ulcer. Hasten healing of gastric ulcers. Treatment of reflux disease	Mild constipation or diarrhea	Give 1 hr before meals and at bedtime. Do not use in clients with renal disease; monitor bowel movements and signs of hypermagnesemia; Riopan low in sodium; do not give within 1 to 2 hr of H₂-receptor antagonists, tetracycline; causes decreased absorption of many drugs.
MUCOSAL BARRIER FORTIFIERS				
Sucralfate (Carafate)	In presence of mild acid condition, forms viscid and sticky gel and adheres to ulcer surface, forming a protective barrier	Short-term treatment of active gastric ulcers. Maintenance treatment of PUD	Dizziness, constipation, sleepiness, nausea, and gastric discomfort	Give on empty stomach 1 hr before meals and at bedtime. Do not give within 30 min of antacids. Urge client to take entire prescribed regimen.

ATP, adenosine triphosphate; GI, gastrointestinal; IM, intramuscularly; IV, intravenously; NSAIDs, nonsteroidal anti-inflammatory drugs; PO, orally; qid, four times a day; PUD, peptic ulcer disease.

counter drugs, and lifestyle, including alcohol consumption and cigarette smoking.

REDUCE PAIN

Focus on teaching the client about the causes of gastritis and foods that may worsen the disease. Help the client assess factors that increase manifestations, such as stress or fatigue, taking certain medications on an empty stomach, ingestion of foods and beverages, alcohol consumption, and smoking. Encourage the client to avoid these agents.

Aluminum hydroxide with magnesium trisilicate (Gaviscon), which produces a soothing foam, is the best antacid for gastritis. H_2-receptor antagonists, proton pump inhibitors, antisecretory agents, and drugs that enhance mucosal defenses also provide pain relief (Table 31–2).

If the nausea and vomiting are severe, the client may be given nothing by mouth until these problems decrease in severity. When the pain and nausea associated with gastritis have subsided, the client is instructed to have a well-balanced diet and avoid irritating foods and beverages.

PROMOTE SELF-CARE

Clients with acute and chronic gastritis are managed at home unless complications develop. Instruct the client with chronic gastritis to see the health care provider at regular intervals. This is particularly important if the diagnosis is *H. pylori* infection and atrophic gastritis, because these problems are closely related to gastric cancer. Teach the client to use medications correctly, to maintain adequate nutrition, and to control risk factors that contribute to gastritis.

■ Surgical Management

If conservative measures have not controlled bleeding, surgery may be necessary. Subtotal gastrectomy, pyloroplasty, vagotomy, or total gastrectomy may be indicated with severe erosive gastritis. These procedures are discussed in the section on peptic ulcer disease.

PEPTIC ULCER DISEASE

Peptic ulcer disease (PUD) involves a break in continuity of the esophageal, gastric, or duodenal mucosa. It may occur in any part of the GI tract that comes into contact with gastric juices (hydrochloric acid and pepsin). The ulcer may be found in the esophagus, stomach, duodenum, or the jejunum after gastroenterostomy.

PUD occurs in approximately 10% of the population. Gastric ulcers are more likely to occur during the fifth and sixth decades of life; duodenal ulcers more commonly occur during the fourth and fifth decades for men. For women, the occurrence is about 10 years later in life. Men are more likely to have both gastric and duodenal ulcers.

■ DUODENAL ULCERS

Duodenal ulcers, which have a higher incidence than gastric ulcers, usually occur within 1.5 cm (0.6 inch) of the pylorus. These ulcers are usually characterized by high gastric acid secretion. Some are associated with normal gastric secretion associated with rapid emptying of the

stomach. Hypersecretion of acid is attributed to a greater mass of parietal cells. Stimuli for acid secretion include protein-rich meals, alcohol consumption, calcium, and vagal stimulation.

Clients with a duodenal ulcer experience low pH levels in the duodenum for longer periods. The stomach lining is more sensitive to gastrin and secretes excess gastrin.

Finally, clients with duodenal ulcers have more rapid gastric emptying. The combined effect of hypersecretion of acid and rapid emptying of food from the stomach reduces the buffering effect of food and results in a large acid load in the duodenum. Within the duodenum, inhibitory mechanisms and pancreatic secretion may be insufficient to control the acid load.

■ GASTRIC ULCERS

Gastric ulcers, which tend to heal within a few weeks, form within 1 inch (2.5 cm) of the pylorus of the stomach in an area where gastritis is common. Gastric ulcers are probably caused by a break in the mucosal barrier. The barrier, which differs from the layer of glycoprotein mucus that overlies the gastric epithelium, normally allows hydrochloric acid to be secreted into the stomach without injury to the epithelial cells. An incompetent pylorus may decrease production of mucus, the usual gastric defense. The reflux of bile acids through an incompetent pylorus into the stomach may break the mucosal barrier. Decreased blood flow to the gastric mucosa may also alter the defensive barrier and may make the duodenum more susceptible to gastric acid and pepsin trauma. The recurrence rate of gastric ulcer is lower than that of duodenal ulcer.

Table 31–3 distinguishes gastric from duodenal peptic ulcers.

■ STRESS-INDUCED AND DRUG-INDUCED ULCERS

Besides peptic ulcers, acute gastric erosion, frequently called *stress ulcers* or *stress erosive gastritis*, can occur after an acute medical crisis. Major assaults that give rise to gastroduodenal ulcerations include:

- Severe trauma or major illness
- Severe burns (may cause what is known as Curling's ulcers)
- Head injury or intracranial disease (frequently called Cushing's ulcers)
- Ingestion of a drug (e.g., aspirin, NSAIDs, steroids, and alcohol) that acts on the gastric mucosa (Fig. 31–1)
- Shock
- Sepsis

Etiology and Risk Factors

The causal factor in more than 90% of all peptic ulcers has been attributed to *H. pylori*. Eradication of the organism usually results in resolution of gastritis and subsequent ulcer healing. Multiple studies support this finding, which calls into question earlier theories about the causes of PUD.

The occurrence of PUD depends on the defensive resistance of the mucosa in relation to the aggressive force of secretory activity. The defensive resistance of the mu-

TABLE 31–3	CLASSIFICATION OF PEPTIC ULCERS	
Assessment Data	**Duodenal Ulcers**	**Gastric Ulcers**
Location of ulcer	¼ to 1 inch from pylorus	Junction of fundus and pylorus, some in antrum
Acid secretion	Increased	Normal to decreased
Serum pepsinogen I	Increased	Normal
Serum gastrin		
Fasting	Normal	Elevated
Postprandial	Elevated	
Blood group	Most frequently type O	No difference
Age at onset	25–50 years	Peaks at 45–54 years
Gender predominance	Men to women, 4 : 1	Men to women, 2 : 1
Associated gastritis	None	Common and increased
Pain	Occurs on empty stomach, 2–3 hr after meals or in middle of night; relieved by food and antacids	Variable pain pattern; may be made worse by food; antacids ineffective
Nutritional status	Usually well nourished	Probably malnourished
Malignancy potential	Rare, no increase in incidence	Occurs in approximately 10% of clients
Bleeding pattern	Melena more common than hematemesis	Hematemesis more common than melena
Recurrence	May occur as marginal ulcers after surgery	Recurrence unlikely after surgery

cosa depends on mucosal integrity and regeneration, presence of a protective mucous barrier, adequate blood flow to the mucosa, ability of the duodenal inhibitory mechanism to regulate secretion, and the presence of adequate gastromucosal prostaglandins. The aggressive factors of PUD are related to the presence of *H. pylori* and the volume of hydrochloric and biliary acids. Ulceration occurs when aggressive factors exceed the defensive barrier. The aggressive nature of the gastric juice may be the result of hypersecretion of gastric juices, increased stimulation of the vagus nerve, decreased inhibition of gastric secretions, increased capacity or number of the parietal cells secreting hydrochloric acid, or increased response of the parietal cells to stimulation.

Risk factors that contribute to PUD include smoking (nicotine), steroids, aspirin, NSAIDs, caffeine, alcohol, and stress. Certain medical conditions, including Crohn's disease, Zollinger-Ellison syndrome, and hepatic and biliary disease, may also play a role.

Health promotion and health maintenance actions for clients with PUD are the same as those discussed for acute gastritis. Health restoration for clients involves treating medical disorders that cause secondary PUD. En-

sure that the client complies with the prescribed medication regimen to minimize stomach irritation. Treat aggressively any disorders that result in the development of PUD, for example, long-term use of steroids, severe burns, and chronic renal failure.

Pathophysiology

In addition to *H. pylori* inflammation as the primary pathophysiologic change, two different mechanisms for the development of PUD have been proposed. In the stomach, it is thought that a breakdown of the normally protective epithelial lining causes gastric ulcers. Under normal circumstances, flow of hydrochloric acid from the lumen of the stomach is prevented by the presence of tight, nonpermeable junctions between the epithelial cells and by the slightly alkaline layer of mucus that coats the surface of the gastric epithelium.

In the formation of a gastric peptic ulcer, this diffusion barrier may be interrupted by the chronic presence of such injurious substances as aspirin, NSAIDs, cortisone, adrenocorticotropic hormone (ACTH), caffeine, phenylbutazone (Butazolidin), alcohol, and chemotherapeutic agents. These substances may stimulate acid production, cause local mucosal damage, and suppress mucus secretion. The substances strip away surface mucus and cause degeneration of epithelial cell membranes with massive diffusion of acid back into the gastric epithelial wall.

The pathogenesis of duodenal peptic ulcers has a different proposed mechanism, as excess acid secretion is responsible for ulcer development. Activity of the vagus nerve is increased in people with duodenal ulcers, particularly during a fasting state and at night. The vagus nerve stimulates the pyloric antrum cells to release gastrin, which travels via the bloodstream and acts on the gastric parietal cells to stimulate the release of hydrochloric acid.

Another factor in PUD is emotional stress, which can cause an increase in gastric secretion, blood supply, and gastric motility by thalamic stimulation of the vagal nerves. Hormonal influence takes place via the hypothala-

FIGURE 31–1 Gastric peptic ulceration caused by nonsteroidal anti-inflammatory drugs.

mus through the pituitary adrenal route. In clients with stress reactions, the sympathetic nervous system causes the blood vessels in the duodenum to constrict, which makes the mucosa more vulnerable to trauma from gastric acid and pepsin secretion. On activation of the adrenal cortex, mucus production decreases and gastric secretion increases. Together, these factors result in increased vulnerability to ulceration. Stress reactions thus upset the aggressive-defensive balance. Prolonged stress associated with burns, severe trauma, and other conditions can produce stress ulcers, or stress erosive gastritis, in the GI tract.

Zollinger-Ellison syndrome is characterized by abnormal secretion of gastrin by a rare islet cell tumor in the pancreas. Pathophysiologic changes associated with this syndrome include hypergastrinemia and diarrhea secondary to fat malabsorption resulting from decreased duodenum-inactivating pancreatic lipase or acid-induced injury of the villi. In addition to increased gastric secretion, hyperplasia of the gastric mucosa is induced by the trophic effects of gastrin. Treatment of the Zollinger-Ellison syndrome is aimed at suppression of acid secretion.

Treated ulcers usually heal without difficulty. Untreated ulcers or those that do not respond to treatment can result in perforation, hemorrhage, or obstruction, which may require surgical treatment. Some ulcers recur after healing, particularly if the risk factors associated with their development are not modified.

Critically ill clients are susceptible to *stress ulcers*. For example, gastric mucosal changes caused by stress develop within 72 hours in 78% of clients with greater than 35% burns on their body. Stress ulcers manifest with superficial gastric erosions, often accompanied by painless massive gastric hemorrhage. The client characteristically has multiple lesions, usually small and superficial, that do not extend through the muscularis mucosae. These lesions may appear to ooze blood. The mechanism causing stress ulcerations is unknown, but it probably involves ischemia. In the presence of acid, ischemia can produce erosive gastritis and ulcerations. Increased hydrogen ion back-diffusion and decreased mucosal perfusion may also contribute to stress ulcer formation. Low gastric pH (high acidity) is necessary for development of stress ulcers.

Researchers continue to seek the precise mechanism by which stress ulcers occur. Few manifestations accompany stress ulcer. These ulcerations are typically painless unless perforation occurs, which is rare. Upper GI tract hemorrhage is the major manifestation of stress ulcers. About 10% of clients experience dyspepsia before hemorrhage, but typically there are no warning manifestations. When stress ulcers cause profound hemorrhage, the mortality rate rises to about 50%.

Clinical Manifestations

PAIN. The principal manifestation of ulcers is an aching, burning, cramp-like, gnawing pain. The pain has a definite relationship to eating. With gastric ulcers, food may cause the pain and vomiting may relieve it. Clients with duodenal ulcers have pain with an empty stomach, and discomfort may be relieved by ingestion of food or antacids. Clients usually describe the pain as circumscribed in an area 2 to 10 cm (0.8 to 4 inches) in diameter, between the xiphoid cartilage and the umbilicus. Gastric ulcer pain often occurs in the upper epigastrium, with localization to the left of the midline, whereas duodenal pain is in the right epigastrium. Ulcer pain also varies with the site, size, or penetration of the ulcer or the amount of surrounding fibrotic tissue.

In duodenal ulcers, steady pain near the midline of the back between the sixth and 10th thoracic vertebrae with radiation to the right upper quadrant may indicate perforation of the posterior duodenal wall. Fullness or hunger may also be present. Distention of the duodenal bulb produces epigastric pain, which may radiate to the back and thorax. Hydrochloric acid secretion may produce edema and inflammation, with resultant pain, or may activate motor changes with increased spasm, intragastric pressure, and increased motility, also with resultant pain. In addition, ulcer pain tends to occur in distinct periods (periodicity).

NAUSEA AND VOMITING. Clients with a duodenal ulcer usually have a normal appetite unless pyloric obstruction is present. Carcinoma, gastric ulcers, or gastritis may be associated with anorexia, weight loss, and dysphagia. Vomiting occurs more often with gastric ulcer than with uncomplicated duodenal ulcer. It also occurs more frequently when the ulcer is in the pylorus or antrum of the stomach. Vomiting results from gastric stasis or pyloric obstruction, and the client typically vomits undigested food. Severe retching and vomiting may suggest an esophageal tear.

BLEEDING. Clients with ulcers often bleed when the ulcer erodes through a blood vessel. Bleeding may occur as massive hemorrhage or may be occult, with slow oozing. Approximately 25% of clients with gastric ulcers may experience bleeding.

The diagnosis of ulcers is confirmed on the basis of manifestations, x-ray evidence, and endoscopy. The history and physical examination do not yield much significant information in a client with uncomplicated peptic ulcer. A complete blood count with decreased hematocrit and hemoglobin values may indicate bleeding. Stool testing for occult blood might also be positive if bleeding is present. Testing for the presence of *H. pylori* can be done via urea breath tests or identification of *H. pylori* serum antibodies in addition to esophagogastroduodenoscopy (EGD) with biopsy.

The major diagnostic tests include EGD and an upper GI tract x-ray series. The EGD has several advantages. It allows the physician to take tissue specimens and to treat the ulcer with either multipolar electrocoagulation (MPEC) or heater-probe therapy (see complications under Medical Management).

Outcome Management

■ Medical Management

The primary objective of intervention for peptic ulcer is to provide stomach rest. Approaches include neutralizing or buffering hydrochloric acid, inhibiting acid secretion, decreasing the activity of pepsin and hydrochloric acid, and eradicating *H. pylori* from the GI tract. Specific measures include medications, physical and emotional rest, dietary management, and stress reduction.

Response to the therapeutic program varies with clients' perception of their health status and the degree to which lifestyle influences the ulcer disease. The following list outlines the hallmarks of successful interventions:

- The client experiences a decrease in pain with eventual elimination of all ulcer pain and related manifestations.
- The client eats a nutritionally sound diet and reports increased tolerance of food.
- The client complies with the medication schedule (see Table 31–2).
- The client identifies stressors and develops ways to modify stress and make necessary lifestyle changes.

ELIMINATE *H. PYLORI* BACTERIA

The antibacterial regimen used for treatment of *H. pylori* consists of clarithromycin (Biaxin), 250 mg twice a day, plus metronidazole (Flagyl), 250 mg four times daily, plus omeprazole (Prilosec), 20 mg twice a day or ranitidine (Zantac) twice a day (see Table 31–2). More than 90% of clients are cured by using this protocol for 1 week. Fewer than 10% of clients require a second week of treatment or a variation of pharmacologic agents.

REDUCE GASTRIC SECRETIONS

Hyposecretory agents cause a reduction in acid secretions. These agents include H_2-receptor antagonists, prostaglandin analogs, anticholinergics, proton pump inhibitors, and antacids (the drugs are shown in Table 31–2).

STRENGTHEN MUCOSAL BARRIER

Mucosal barrier fortifiers prevent hydrogen ion back-diffusion into the mucosa and stimulate mucus production, which results in accelerated gastric ulcer healing (see Table 31–2). Prostaglandin analogs, in addition to decreasing acid secretion, stimulate production of cytoprotective mucus.

MODIFY DIET

For uncomplicated ulcer disease, few physicians or advanced practitioners favor strict dietary changes. There is scant evidence that diet treatment promotes or accelerates healing. Foods known to increase gastric acidity or cause discomfort should be avoided, such as coffee, alcohol, protein foods, and milk.

PREVENT AND TREAT COMPLICATIONS

Hemorrhage, perforation, and obstruction are the main complications that develop after PUD.

Hemorrhage

ASSESS BLEEDING. Hemorrhage varies in degree from minimal, manifested by the presence of occult blood in the stool (melena), to massive, manifested by vomitus containing bright red blood (hematemesis). The usual manifestation of GI tract bleeding is either vomiting of coffee ground–like material or passing of tarry stools. Acid digestion of blood in the stomach results in a granular dark emesis, whereas digestion in the duodenum or below may result in a black stool. Hemorrhage tends to occur more often with gastric ulcers (Fig. 31–2), especially in the elderly population. Although the onset of hemorrhage may be associated with fatigue, nervous tension, upper respiratory tract infection, dietary indiscretion, alcoholism, or irritating drugs, there may be no known precipitating factor.

Manifestations depend on the severity of the hemorrhage. With mild bleeding (< 500 ml), the client may

FIGURE 31–2 Bleeding ulcer on gastric mucosa.

experience only slight weakness and diaphoresis. Severe loss of more than 1 L of blood per 24 hours may cause manifestations of shock (see Chapter 81).

PREVENT SHOCK. Intervention for massive bleeding aims to treat hypovolemic shock, prevent dehydration and electrolyte imbalance, and stop the bleeding. The client, who should be fasting, receives intravenous fluids until the bleeding subsides. The nurse or the physician may insert an NG tube in the presence or absence of blood in

---

GUIDE TO CLINICAL PATHWAY

GI Hemorrhage

GI hemorrhage is an acute condition that requires a complete assessment of the client. This care map indicates a 3 day hospital stay in order to diagnose and treat the bleeding. Some of the assessments are completed in the laboratory, where the client may undergo endoscopy to determine the cause and location of the bleeding. Ensure that the client will be ready for the endoscopy by maintaining NPO status.

A second major nursing focus is assessment of the influence of blood loss on activity and oxygenation. Note the client's hemoglobin levels, reports of fatigue at rest and during activity, and oxygenation levels at rest and during activity with and without oxygen (using pulse oximetry). If oxygen saturation cannot be kept above 92%, transfusion may be required. Blood loss may be occult, and the client should be assessed for changes in vital signs, and presence of blood in vomitus or stool.

Discharge to self-care is the goal, but only if the cause and location of the bleeding are determined and only if the client can provide self-care. If the bleeding is a result of suspected or confirmed alcohol abuse, consult the discharge coordinator or social worker early in the hospital stay to determine discharge needs.

The CareMap is reprinted with permission from Baptist Health Center–Montclair. The CareMap shown is an excerpt of one covering emergency department admission through discharge.

Helen Andrews, BSN, RN, *Care Manager, Alegent Health Bergan Mercy Medical Center, Omaha, Nebraska,* and
Linda R. Haddick, MSN, RN, *Clinical Nurse Specialist, Alegent Health Home Care & Hospice, Omaha, Nebraska*

✞ BAPTIST
HEALTH SYSTEM

GI HEMORRHAGE CAREMAP

(Addressograph)

	Phase I - ER Adm 0-24 Hrs.: Date: _____	INITIAL Met	Not Met	Phase II - 24-48 Hrs.: Date: _____	INITIAL Met	Not Met
General Safety:	Bed rails up Fall precautions Bleeding precautions Airway precautions Call light within reach			Bed rails up Fall precautions Bleeding precautions Call light within reach		
Activity	Advance as tolerated.			Advance as tolerated.		
	Goal: Tolerates activity without SOB.	___	___	**Goal:** Tolerates activity progression.	___	___
Dietary: Consult Date/Time Completed _____	NPO except meds. Advance per orders **Goal:** Tolerates 50% of diet as ordered.	___	___	Advance as ordered. **Goal:** Tolerates po intake.	___	___
Respiratory: Consult Date/Time Completed _____	Check SaO2 on RA: if < 92%, start O2 at 2 L/M. Wean O2 per protocol.			Wean O2 per protocol as indicated.		
	Goal: SaO2 ≥ 92%; No SOB.	___	___	**Goal:** SaO2 ≥ 92% on RA.	___	___
Rehab: Consult Date/Time Completed _____	**Goal:**	___	___	**Goal:**	___	___

Discharge Planning:
Consult Date/Time
Completed _____
	1. Identify DCP needs & initiate plan.
	  Notify Social Worker if:
	   • patient has HHC
	   • patient is from a Nursing Home or
	     Assisted Living facility
	   • patient has other discharge/social needs
	2. Initiate Teaching For:
	  • Diet • NSAID use
	  • ETOH use • Smoking cessation
	  • Treatment for PUD
	3. Discharge Instruction sheet (if discharged)
	4. Distribute Patient/Family CareMap.
				Continue DCP plan.
				Reinforce Teaching For:
				  • Diet • NSAID use
				  • ETOH use • Smoking cessation
				  • Treatment for PUD
				Discharge Instruction sheet (if discharged)		

	Goal: DCP needs identified; plan initiated. **Goal:** Teaching plan initiated.	___	___	**Goal:** Discharge/Teaching Plan continued. **Goal:** Prepare for D/C in AM.	___	___
Nursing: Consult Date/Time Completed _____	Vital signs: frequency per MD orders. Assess GI function, bowel sounds, N/V/D. Document color/character of emesis/stool. Document use of NSAIDS, antiplatelets, anticoagulants. Have transfusion consent signed. I & O Q shift. Verify MD consults.			Assess GI function, bowel sounds, N/V/D. VS q shift. Document color/character/amount of aspirate, emesis, stool. I & O Q shift.		
	Goal: No signs/symptoms of GI bleeding. **Goal:** No vomiting or diarrhea **Goal:** VS stable.	___	___	**Goal:** No signs/symptoms of GI bleeding. **Goal:** No vomiting or diarrhea **Goal:** VS stable.	___	___
Tests:	CBC; Basic Metabolic Profile; PT with INR; Colonoscopy; Hemoccult Stool; Type & Screen; Hct now then Q 8 h x 24 hr then QD. Permit for EGD, Colonoscopy, Routine pre- post procedure orders. Transfuse per orders			HCT QD		
	Goal: Initial diagnostic test completed w/i 24 hours. **Goal:** Site identification via diagnostic procedure. **Goal:** No adverse reaction to blood components.	___	___	**Goal:** Hct stable and increasing.	___	___
Other:						
	Goal:	___	___	**Goal:**	___	___

GI HEMORRHAGE CAREMAP

G-99-5149-2 PG REV. 9/22/99 P

the stomach to assess the rate of bleeding, prevent gastric dilation, and administer room temperature saline to remove blood from the stomach. The room temperature saline is cooler than the body temperature, which creates mild vasoconstriction. Gastric cooling may also be promoted by cool saline lavage, which, although controversial, further curtails hemorrhage through its vasoconstric-

tive effect. Iced saline is rarely used because it may lead to more mucosal damage by decreasing perfusion to the gastric mucosa and may cause a vagal response, decreasing systemic perfusion.

REPLACE FLUIDS. Blood volume depletion is a major problem for the client with severe hemorrhage. For those who have suffered a massive upper GI tract hemorrhage, a primary objective of intervention is to replace blood volume. Restlessness and tachycardia are the earliest manifestations of hypovolemia. The client also has a greatly decreased urine output, which should be monitored with a Foley catheter and hourly urine measurement. This is important because fluids must be replaced to prevent damage to the kidneys.

ADMINISTER VASOPRESSIN. Arterial administration of vasopressin (via an infusion pump) can also control acute hemorrhage. Vasopressin produces few complications if given intravenously for less than 36 hours to control bleeding.

INJECT ARTERY WITH EMBOLI. Another approach to control of bleeding is selective arterial embolization with angiography. The emboli may consist of autologous blood clots with or without an absorbable gelatin sponge. A modified clot may be made with a mixture of the client's own blood, aminocaproic acid, and platelets. Fibrin glue has also been used.

MAINTAIN REST. The client must have absolute bed rest for several days after bleeding has subsided. Rest decreases blood pressure and GI tract activity. When bleeding stops, the client is allowed bathroom privileges. If the client requires narcotics, administer with caution. Morphine sulfate can cause nausea and vomiting; however, the drug may calm the client who is extremely restless and apprehensive. A better alternative is to manage anxiety with non-narcotic alternatives.

MAINTAIN HIGH GASTRIC PH. During the first few days of hemorrhaging, gastric pH should be maintained between 5.5 and 7.0. To maintain the pH at this level, administer H_2-receptor antagonists intravenously for 4 days or as prescribed and advance to oral administration. Monitor gastric pH at least each shift. Anticholinergics are not recommended. Administer antacids for 1 week to complement the H_2-receptor antagonists. Give antacids 1 hour before or 2 hours after the H_2-receptor antagonists so that the antacids do not interfere with absorption of drugs. The client may require antacids every 30 minutes after starting intake of food or fluids.

STOP BLEEDING SURGICALLY. If bleeding continues beyond 48 hours, recurs, or is associated with perforation or obstruction, surgery may be indicated. Increased surgical risk is associated with prolonged bleeding, multiple transfusions, debilitation, electrolyte imbalances, and increased age. Surgical procedures include partial gastric resection, excision of the ulcer, and vagotomy and pyloroplasty.

PERFORM MULTIPOLAR ELECTROCOAGULATION OR HEATER-PROBE THERAPY. Two endoscopic procedures have been effective in treating bleeding ulcers: MPEC and heater-probe therapy. In MPEC, a bipolar electric current cauterizes the bleeding lesion; in heater-probe therapy, direct heat cauterizes the lesion.

Perforation

Perforation is usually a surgical emergency. When the ulcer perforates, gastroduodenal contents empty through the anterior wall of the stomach into the peritoneal cavity, resulting in chemical peritonitis, bacterial septicemia, and hypovolemic shock. Peristalsis diminishes, and paralytic ileus develops. Posterior perforation is not as clear and often results in pancreatitis, because the pancreas plugs the perforation.

ASSESS PAIN. Perforation occurs most frequently with duodenal ulcers (Fig. 31–3). It occurs when the ulcer erodes through the tunica muscularis. The client experiences sudden, sharp, severe pain beginning in the midepigastrium. As peritonitis develops, the pain spreads over the entire abdomen, which becomes tender, hard, and rigid. (See discussion of peritonitis in Chapter 33.)

The degree of pain depends on the amount and type of contents that are spilled. The pain often causes the client to bend over or draw the knees up to the abdomen in an effort to decrease the tension on the abdominal muscles. If the perforation occurs on the posterior gastric wall, it may erode through to adjacent organs and become sealed, causing few manifestations. When a perforation erodes into the pancreas, manifestations of pancreatitis (see Chapter 46) develop.

REPLACE FLUIDS. If perforation occurs, the client needs immediate replacement of fluids, electrolytes, and blood as well as administration of antibiotics. Nasogastric suction should be instituted to drain gastric secretions and thus prevent further peritoneal spillage. A small perforation that closes immediately by adhering to adjacent tissues causes only a small loss of gastric contents.

CORRECT PERFORATION SURGICALLY. When surgery is necessary, the surgeon evacuates the escaped gastric contents, cleans the peritoneal cavity by flushing it out with normal saline or an antibiotic or both, and closes the perforation by patching it with omentum. Vagotomy and hemigastrectomy or vagotomy and pyloroplasty provide definitive control of both the ulcer and the complications. The Case Study describes the treatment of a client whose perforated ulcer was surgically managed. After surgery, antibiotics are given to combat peritonitis. The NG tube remains in the stomach until peristalsis returns. Postoperative complications include subphrenic abscess, hemorrhage, duodenal or gastric fistula, atelectasis, and pneumonia.

Obstruction

Long-standing ulcer disease causes scarring because of repeated ulcerations and healing. Scarring at the pylorus frequently causes pyloric obstruction, manifested most often by pain at night, when the stomach cannot be emptied by peristalsis. Pyloric obstruction can also lead to vomiting. Surgery (pyloroplasty) is usually required to correct the problem.

FIGURE 31–3 Perforation of a duodenal ulcer.

■ **Nursing Management of the Medical Client**

ASSESSMENT

Nursing assessment involves gathering both psychosocial and pathophysiologic data concerning the client. To assess psychosocial aspects of ulcer disease, ask the client about a familial incidence of ulcer, ingestion of medications that cause gastric irritation, cigarette smoking, alcohol intake, stressors, and coping patterns. Questions about lifestyle, occupation, work, and leisure activities can yield valuable information.

Physical assessment includes accurately observing and immediately reporting manifestations that help pinpoint the diagnosis or that might indicate the presence of a complication. Manifestations include pain, vomiting, and, occasionally, bleeding and changes in appetite. Always obtain a complete history of previous ulcer attacks, including frequency, duration, manifestations, and response to intervention.

Monitor for the development of complications of ulcers, such as hemorrhage, perforation, or obstruction. Assessment also involves describing the bleeding, including hematemesis and melena. Note such factors as color, amount, consistency, and frequency. Bright red blood usually signifies new bleeding; dark red blood indicates old bleeding. If bleeding is severe, always maintain a current and accurate record of the client's hemoglobin, hematocrit, red blood cell count, and fluid intake and output. Monitor the client closely for the development of manifestations of shock that might occur if bleeding is present.

Because of shock, the client may experience decreased renal blood flow, which causes a decrease in the glomerular filtration rate and in renal excretion. As the body absorbs the by-products of erythrocyte destruction and renal blood flow decreases, watch for an increase in blood urea nitrogen (BUN), creatinine, and ammonia levels. An elevated BUN may follow dehydration from vomiting. In addition, carefully assess the client for metabolic acidosis caused by vomiting.

Monitor the client for the development of perforation. Assess the abdomen for pain, tenderness, or rigidity. Report suspected perforation to the physician immediately, and prepare the client for possible surgery.

Monitor the client for the development of gastric obstruction. If the client vomits, record the frequency and the consistency (digested or undigested food or hematemesis) of the vomitus. If pyloric obstruction is present, nasogastric tube and intravenous fluids and electrolytes are needed until the problem is corrected surgically.

DIAGNOSIS, OUTCOMES, INTERVENTIONS

Pain. One of the most common nursing diagnoses for the client with a peptic ulcer is *Pain related to gastric mucosal injury.*

Outcomes. The client's pain will be relieved, as evidenced by healing of gastric or duodenal mucosal injury and the client's statement of decreased pain on a pain scale of 1 to 10 with the pain being less than 2 or 3.

Interventions

Administer Prescribed Medications. Administer medications as ordered to relieve the client's pain. The following medications may be used:

- Eliminate *H. pylori* (triple therapy)
- Neutralize gastric acids (antacids)
- Reduce secretions (H$_2$-receptor antagonists, prostaglandin analogs, proton pump inhibitors)
- Protect the gastric mucosa (mucosal barrier fortifiers, prostaglandin analogs)

Assess the effectiveness of the medications that the client is taking, and notify the physician if the pain is not relieved by the medications used in the treatment regimen.

Promote Rest and Relaxation. Avoidance of strenuous physical activity decreases gastric secretions and peristalsis. Help the client achieve rest, both physically and mentally. Be alert for factors that interfere with the client's rest. Arrange the environment to encourage relaxation. If certain visitors or telephone calls agitate the client, discourage these visits or calls until the client improves.

Encourage clients who attempt to carry on their normal work routine (despite prescribed rest) to schedule physical and mental relaxation. Explore with the client and significant others or co-workers ways to reduce work responsibilities temporarily.

Modify Diet. The diet must meet basic nutritional needs. Because an empty stomach stimulates gastric acid secretion, advise the client to eat small amounts at frequent, regular intervals. Discourage ingestion of alcohol, cola, tobacco, caffeine, milk, and foods that cause discomfort. The client may drink decaffeinated beverages.

During the acute phase, the client often requires a bland, nonirritating, low-fiber diet. Clients and their significant others need to learn the modifications in the diet. Also, have the dietitian review the home diet with the client or whoever will be cooking for the client.

Ineffective Management of Therapeutic Regimen (Individuals). For the client with an uncomplicated ulcer, most of the care must be done by the client at home. Write the nursing diagnosis as *Risk for ineffective management of therapeutic regimen (individual) related to lack of knowledge of cause of ulcer and measures to treat and prevent recurrence.*

Outcomes. The client will understand and be able to discuss the cause of the ulcer and the treatment and ways to prevent recurrence.

Interventions

Provide Teaching. Treatment of PUD places the responsibility for self-care on the client. To maintain good self-care, the client must understand the process underlying ulcer development and the rationale underlying interventions.

Help the client to:

- Understand the pathogenesis of the ulcer and the significance of the pain
- Realize that healing takes place rapidly when the irritating effect is removed
- Understand what caused the condition to develop and what must be done to lessen the stimulation
- Discover which substances cause pain by stimulating secretion of gastric juices and to eliminate the substances from the diet until the ulcer heals
- Understand the importance of continuing the medical regimen, although the pain is gone, until healing is completed

- Recognize that once maintenance therapy stops, the ulcer may recur

Instruct the client to use acetaminophen instead of aspirin preparations when these medications are needed. Teach the client to examine the labels of all nonprescription medications, particularly cold remedies, for aspirin (acetylsalicylic acid), other salicylates, NSAIDs (ibuprofen, phenylbutazone), adrenocorticosteroids, and ACTH. These medications are ulcerogenic (ulcer causing), particularly when combined. If any of these medications must be taken, advise the client to check with the physician first, to eat between meals, and to use H_2-receptor antagonists or antacids to protect the stomach lining.

Provide Support. Helping clients with PUD cope with psychosocial problems is a vital part of intervention. Encourage the client to learn about the stressors that may be causing the development of ulcers. Discussing coping and relaxation techniques may enable clients to better deal with problems.

EVALUATION

Medical management usually controls PUD, often within a few weeks. Many clients must continue treatment to remain ulcer-free. The client must follow the therapeutic regimen and practice good health maintenance and restoration behaviors in order to avoid complications and prevent future recurrence of PUD.

■ Surgical Management

GASTRIC SURGICAL PROCEDURES

INDICATIONS. Various types of gastric surgery are performed to reduce the stomach's acid-secreting ability, to remove a malignant or potentially malignant lesion, to treat a surgical emergency that develops as a complication of PUD, or to treat clients who do not respond to medical intervention. Most chronic, recurring ulcers are eventually managed surgically.

Surgery for prevention of ulcer recurrence is performed to:

- Facilitate enterogastric regurgitation of mucous secretions, bile, and pancreatic juice
- Decrease the secretory capacity of the stomach by removing parietal cells
- Remove stimuli for hydrochloric acid secretion by cutting the vagus nerve;
- Eliminate the gastrin hormone mechanisms by antrectomy

CONTRAINDICATIONS. Most contraindications to gastric surgery involve the client's age and physical condition. Any life-threatening disease process, such as chronic obstructive pulmonary disease (COPD) or heart failure, may be a contraindication to surgery.

COMPLICATIONS. Complications are discussed after the types of surgeries.

OUTCOMES. The outcomes desired from the various surgeries are that the client will survive and recover from the surgery without further injury related to surgery. After most procedures, the client will return home in 7 days or less and resume the previous lifestyle within 6 to 12 weeks. It may take 3 months to a year before the client can eat normally.

TYPES OF OPERATIONS

VAGOTOMY. Vagotomy is performed to eliminate the acid-secreting stimulus to gastric cells. There are three types of vagotomy (Fig. 31–4A):

1. *Truncal vagotomy.* Each vagus nerve is completely cut.
2. *Selective vagotomy.* The surgeon partially severs the nerves to preserve the hepatic and celiac branches.
3. *Proximal* vagotomy. Partial cutting is performed, but only the parietal cell mass is denervated; innervation of both the antrum and the pyloric sphincter is preserved. Cutting the vagal nerve fibers selectively avoids the problems of impaired emptying and diarrhea that follow the truncal vagotomy. It

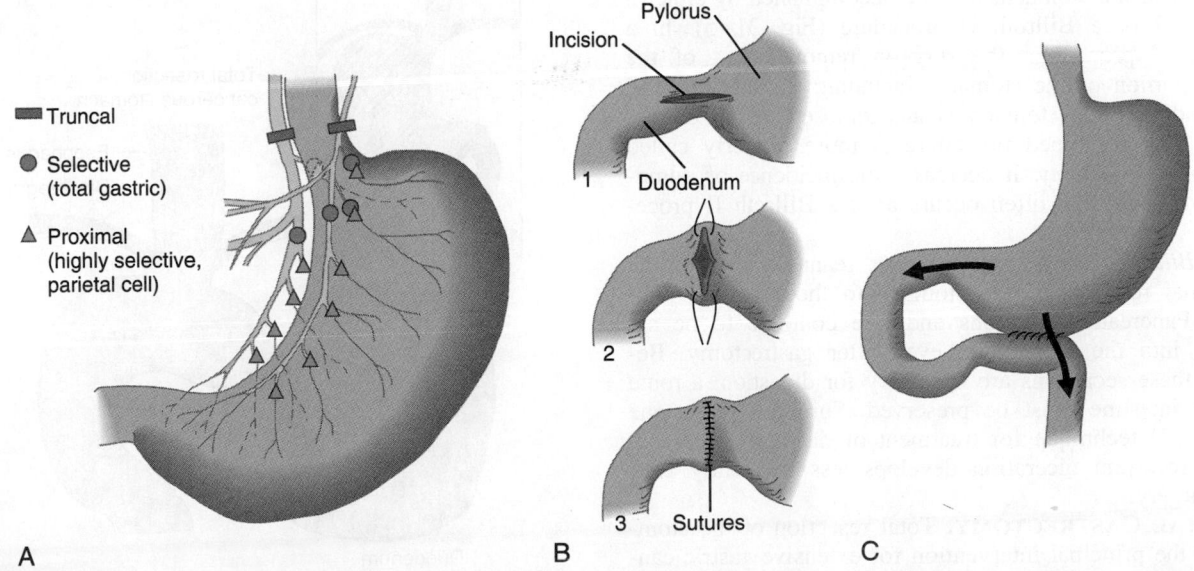

FIGURE 31–4 Vagotomy and drainage. *A,* Sites at which the three types of vagotomy are performed. *B,* Pyloroplasty provides a larger opening from stomach to duodenum to enhance emptying after vagotomy. *C,* Gastroenterostomy, another associated surgical procedure, creates a passage between the body of the stomach and the jejunum.

also eliminates the necessity for a drainage anastomosis to offset gastric stasis. Proximal vagotomy also reduces acid secretion and preserves the function of the antrum.

VAGOTOMY WITH PYLOROPLASTY. Vagotomy with pyloroplasty involves cutting the right and left vagus nerves and widening the existing exit of the stomach at the pylorus. This procedure prevents stasis and enhances emptying, thereby preventing belching, weight loss, and feelings of fullness (see Fig. 31–4*B*).

GASTROENTEROSTOMY. A simple gastroenterostomy (Fig. 31–4*C*) permits regurgitation of alkaline duodenal contents, thereby neutralizing gastric acid. A drain is made in the bottom of the stomach and sewn to an opening made in the jejunum. Because this neutralization interferes with the inhibition of gastrin release, a net increase in acid secretion may result. If the gastroenterostomy drains the stomach, it reduces motor activity in the pyloroduodenal area. Drainage also diverts acid away from the ulcerative area, which facilitates healing. A gastroenterostomy does not reduce the secretory capacity of the parietal cell mass, and the gastrin mechanism continues to function. Gastroenterostomy should be combined with vagotomy to reduce vagal influences.

ANTRECTOMY. Antrectomy is performed to reduce the acid-secreting portions of the stomach. The procedure removes the entire antrum of the stomach; thus, the cells that secrete gastrin are excised. This delays or eliminates the gastric phase of digestion by withdrawing the source of stimulation for acid release and slows the direct response to protein. The surgeon then anastomoses the remaining portion of the stomach to the duodenum.

Antrectomy is often accompanied by vagotomy; thus, the cephalic and gastric phases of gastric secretion are eliminated and GI tract motor activity is decreased. This surgical procedure usually prevents recurrence and is probably superior to more extensive operations.

SUBTOTAL GASTRECTOMY. Subtotal gastrectomy, a generic term referring to any surgery that involves partial removal of the stomach, may be accomplished by either a Billroth I or a Billroth II procedure (Fig. 31–5). In a *Billroth I* procedure, the surgeon removes part of the distal portion of the stomach, including the antrum. The remainder of the stomach is anastomosed to the duodenum. This combined procedure is more properly called *gastroduodenostomy*. It decreases the incidence of dumping syndrome that often occurs after a Billroth II procedure.

A *Billroth II* resection involves reanastomosis of the proximal remnant of the stomach to the proximal jejunum. Pancreatic secretions and bile continue to be secreted into the duodenum, even after gastrectomy. Because these secretions are necessary for digestion, a route to the intestine must be preserved. Surgeons prefer the Billroth II technique for treatment of duodenal ulcer because recurrent ulceration develops less frequently after this surgery.

TOTAL GASTRECTOMY. Total resection of the stomach is the principal intervention for extensive gastric cancer. This surgery involves removal of the stomach, with anastomosis of the esophagus to the jejunum, an esophagojejunostomy (Fig. 31–6). To perform total gastrectomy,

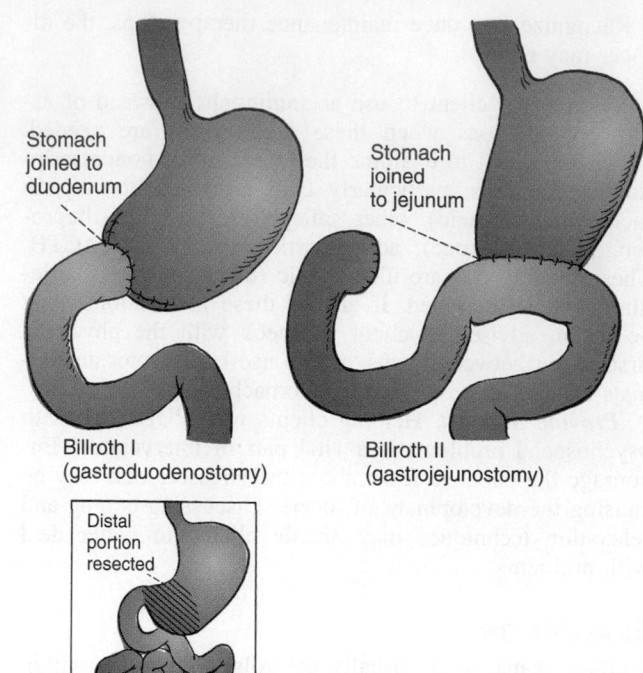

Stomach joined to duodenum

Stomach joined to jejunum

Billroth I (gastroduodenostomy)

Billroth II (gastrojejunostomy)

Distal portion resected

FIGURE 31–5 Subtotal gastrectomy removes acid-secreting portions of the stomach. After removing the distal stomach (*inset*), a surgeon sutures the remaining portion of the stomach to the duodenum (Billroth I procedure) or to the proximal jejunum (Billroth II procedure).

the surgeon enters the chest; thus, the client returns to the recovery room with chest tubes.

COMPLICATIONS OF GASTRIC SURGERIES

MARGINAL ULCERS. A marginal ulcer can develop where gastric acids come in contact with the operative site, either at the site of the anastomosis or in the jeju-

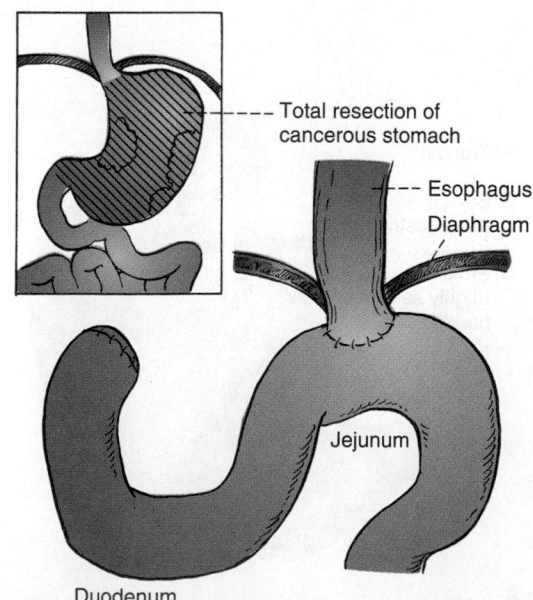

Total resection of cancerous stomach

Esophagus

Diaphragm

Jejunum

Duodenum

FIGURE 31–6 Total gastrectomy (*inset*) with anastomosis of esophagus to jejunum (esophagojejunostomy), which is the principal intervention for extensive gastric cancer.

num. Ulceration may cause scarring and obstruction. Hemorrhage and perforation can also occur at the surgical site.

HEMORRHAGE. The reported incidence of hemorrhage after gastric surgery is 1% to 3%. Bleeding is usually caused by a splenic injury or slippage of a ligature. Assess the client postoperatively for manifestations of bleeding and intraperitoneal hemorrhage.

ALKALINE REFLUX GASTRITIS. Alkaline reflux gastritis caused by duodenal contents occurs after gastric surgery in which the pylorus has been bypassed or removed. It also occurs after pyloroplasty and gastrojejunostomy. Usually, an associated vagotomy has been performed, which decreases gastric motility, allowing reflux of duodenal contents into the stomach.

ACUTE GASTRIC DILATION. In the immediate postoperative period, distention of the stomach produces epigastric pain, tachycardia, and hypotension. The client complains of a feeling of fullness, hiccups, or gagging. Gastric dilation rapidly improves after insertion of a nasogastric tube or clearing of a plugged nasogastric tube.

NUTRITIONAL PROBLEMS. Nutritional problems common after stomach removal include vitamin B_{12} and folic acid deficiency, calcium metabolism disorders, and reduced absorption of calcium and vitamin D. Such problems result from a shortage of intrinsic factor and inadequate absorption because of rapid entry of food into the bowel. With the Billroth II gastric resection, pancreatic juice and bile secretion are reduced because the usual stimulus of food passing through the duodenum is missing.

DUMPING SYNDROME. This postprandial problem occurs after gastrojejunostomy because ingested food rapidly enters the jejunum without proper mixing and without the normal duodenal digestive processing. It usually subsides in 6 to 12 months. Early manifestations, which occur 5 to 30 minutes after eating, involve the vasomotor disturbances of vertigo, tachycardia, syncope, sweating, pallor, palpitation, diarrhea, and nausea with a desire to lie down. The client's blood pressure and pulse may either rise or fall.

Dumping syndrome is most common after the Billroth II procedure. Intestinal manifestations include epigastric fullness, distention, abdominal discomfort, abdominal cramping, nausea (with only occasional vomiting), and borborygmi (rumbling sounds in the bowel). The client may experience tenesmus (ineffectual and painful straining to defecate). Pain is not present.

Early manifestations are probably caused by rapid movement of extracellular fluids into the bowel to convert the rapidly entering hypertonic bolus into an isotonic mixture. This rapid fluid shift decreases the circulating blood volume. A jejunum distended with food and fluid increases intestinal peristalsis and motility. Late manifestations, which occur 2 to 3 hours after eating, are a result of rapid entry of high-carbohydrate food into the jejunum, a rise in blood glucose level, and excessive insulin levels.

Management involves decreasing the amount of food taken at one time and maintaining a high-protein, high-fat, low-carbohydrate, dry diet. Gastric emptying can be delayed by eating in a recumbent or semi-recumbent posi-

tion, lying down after meals, increasing the fat content in the diet, and avoiding fluids 1 hour before, with, or 2 hours after meals. The Client Education Guide provides a diet for clients with dumping syndrome.

The client may also be given sedatives and antispasmodic agents to delay gastric emptying. When manifestations persist, surgical intervention may include reducing the size of the gastroenterostomy or converting a Billroth II resection to a Billroth I by inserting a short segment of jejunum between the duodenal stump and the stomach.

GASTROJEJUNOCOLIC FISTULA. This postoperative complication follows recurrent PUD. The fistulae arise from perforation of a recurrent ulceration at the gastrojejunal anastomosis site. The perforation forms a fistula between the ulcer and adjacent bowel. Manifestations are variable but include fecal vomiting, diarrhea, weight loss, and anorexia. Belching of gas that has a fecal odor may also occur. The manifestations are caused by bacterial overgrowth in the small intestine.

PYLORIC OBSTRUCTION. Pyloric obstruction, manifested by vomiting, occurs at the pylorus and is caused by scarring, edema, inflammation, or a combination of these conditions. When vomiting persists, alkalosis tends to develop because large quantities of acid gastric juice are vomited. A client who vomits persistently is usually hospitalized to receive intravenous fluids with electrolytes added.

Pyloroduodenal obstruction can cause gastric dilation, gastritis, and gastric stasis. These mechanisms create

---

CLIENT EDUCATION GUIDE

Diet for Dumping Syndrome
Client Instructions

Eat five to six small meals every day.

Eat high-fat, high-protein, low-carbohydrate foods.

Do not eat much roughage.

Avoid milk, sweets, and sugars.

Drink liquids between meals only (avoid liquids 1 hour before and 2 hours after meals).

Eat meat (beef, fish, pork, and poultry) and meat substitutes (cheese, peanut butter, and eggs); potatoes, rice, pasta, and starchy vegetables; white bread, rolls, muffins, cracker, and cereals; cooked vegetables; unsweetened cooked or canned fruits; dietetic drinks, jellies, and syrups; margarine, oils, butter, and salad dressings.

Eat the following foods with caution: Drink fluids 1 hour before and/or 2 hours after meals. Whole-grain breads, rolls, cereals, and pasta; foods made with milk; gas-producing vegetables (cabbage, onions, and broccoli); raw vegetables; fresh fruit; caffeinated beverages; mayonnaise; and salt.

Avoid spicy meats, soups, and potatoes; breads with frosting or jelly; sweetened fruit or fruit juice, cakes, pies, cookies; malts, milk shakes and milk products; carbonated beverages; alcoholic beverages; and spices, sugar, jelly, syrup, molasses, and honey.

manifestations that gradually make it more difficult for the stomach to empty. Assess the client for feelings of fullness, distention, or nausea after eating, with loss of appetite and weight loss.

Management of obstruction focuses on restoring fluid and electrolytes and decompressing the dilated stomach; if necessary, surgical intervention is instituted.

▓ Nursing Management of the Surgical Client

PROVIDE SUPPORT

Surgical intervention for gastric and duodenal conditions may be either a planned procedure or an emergency. When emergency surgery is required (e.g., for acute obstruction, perforation, or hemorrhage), the client is very ill and is usually frightened. Provide calm, efficient, knowledgeable care, and explain what is being done. Note and respond to the client's nonverbal behavior. Help significant others provide the client with empathy and emotional support.

When cancer is suspected, the client may want to talk about fears and concerns. Listen to the client carefully, respond to cues, and offer support and understanding. The client may wish to attend to personal matters before surgery (e.g., review a will, see a clergyperson).

When elective surgery is done, the client will have an extensive series of preoperative tests, such as a GI tract x-ray series, endoscopy, and perhaps acid secretion studies (see Chapter 28).

PROVIDE TEACHING

Preoperative teaching should include an explanation of the surgery. Explain that the client will have either an NG tube or a gastrostomy tube with suction. An intravenous infusion line is placed in the client's hand or arm for fluids until the surgical site heals. Thoroughly demonstrate and discuss the importance of deep-breathing exercises or use of an incentive spirometer or both. Warn clients that the high abdominal incision makes deep breathing uncomfortable and that the high incision increases the risk of respiratory complications.

ASSESSMENT

Assess the client with surgical management of PUD in the same way as for the client being managed medically. In addition, perform routine preoperative and postoperative assessments (see Chapter 15).

DIAGNOSIS, OUTCOMES, INTERVENTIONS

Risk for Injury. After surgery, the client is susceptible to postoperative complications. The diagnosis is *Risk for Injury: Postoperative complications (immediate and delayed) related to bleeding, distention and atelectasis.*

Outcomes. The client will not suffer injury related to postoperative complications (immediate and delayed) as evidenced by decreasing bloody drainage from the NG tube, absence of abdominal distention, and normal breath sounds.

Interventions. Nursing care after gastric surgery is the same as postoperative care for any client recovering from major abdominal surgery.

Maintain Nasogastric Tube. In addition to general postoperative care, perform the following functions:

- Check drainage from the NG tube
- Maintain NG tube patency with saline irrigations, as ordered
- Ensure that the NG tube is attached to suction, as ordered
- Assess the operative site for excessive drainage; too much fluid in the remaining gastric stump may cause increased pressure and injury
- Note the color and consistency of drainage from the operative site, and report bleeding or hemorrhaging

The client will return from surgery with an NG or gastrostomy tube to prevent retention of gastric secretions. Carefully assess for abdominal distention. Do not reposition the NG or gastrostomy tube after gastric surgery because it is placed directly over the suture line. Gently irrigate with saline *only* if specifically ordered to do so by the physician.

The color of the drainage in the NG tube may be bright red during the early hours after surgery but should become dark red by the end of 24 hours. The drainage has the appearance of coffee grounds for several days after surgery.

Monitor for Complications. Immediate complications after gastric surgery include hemorrhage, gastric distention, obstruction, and disruption of the suture line. Also, observe for general surgical complications, such as shock, hemorrhage, pulmonary problems, thrombosis, infection (peritonitis), evisceration, and paralytic ileus. Nausea and vomiting should not occur if the nasogastric tube is patent. Carefully measure and document intake (oral and intravenous) and output (urine, suction and wound drainage).

Promote Comfort. Keep the client comfortable with liberal administration of pain medications; this helps the client to cooperate more fully during deep-breathing and coughing exercises. Give fluids by intravenous infusion, as ordered, until edema and swelling have diminished enough to allow fluids to pass the operative area (seen as a decrease in the gastric tube output and return of bowel sounds).

Altered Nutrition: Less Than Body Requirements. After surgery the client is at risk for *Altered Nutrition: Less Than Body Requirements related to decreased nutrient absorption secondary to dumping syndrome.*

Outcomes. The client will maintain adequate nutrition, as exhibited by maintaining weight and with no evidence of dumping syndrome.

Interventions. When healing has occurred, clamp the NG or gastrostomy tube and begin oral intake by giving the client clear water, usually 30 ml at a time. Aspirate the tube an hour or so later to see whether the fluid has been retained. When GI function has returned (e.g., active bowel sounds, passage of flatus) and the client tolerates clear water, the NG tube is usually removed and the diet progresses to soft foods; eventually, a regular diet of five or six small meals a day is given. The diet should not begin too early or progress too rapidly. At first, the client may experience discomfort if too much food is taken at one time.

EVALUATION

Postoperatively, some clients need help to reduce the number of stressors in their lives. Strategies for altering

Perforated Ulcer Managed Surgically

Mr. Fong is a 50-year-old, divorced, second-generation Asian American who is the chief executive officer of a local telecommunications firm. He has a history of peptic ulcer disease. Mr. Fong has been taking clarithromycin (Biaxin), 250 mg bid; metronidazole (Flagyl), 250 mg bid; and omeprazole (Prilosec), 20 mg bid, for 1 week. He reports that he has not been able to eat breakfast or lunch on a regular basis and has subsequently not taken sucralfate (Carafate) as ordered. He was taken to the emergency department today via rescue squad with complaints of sudden onset of severe abdominal pain accompanied by emesis of bright red blood at his office. He is admitted to the hospital unit for preoperative diagnostic evaluation and preoperative preparation.

- Endoscopic view of a perforated peptic ulcer.

Nursing Admission

Assessment

Mr. Fong arrives at the unit accompanied by his girlfriend. He vomits bright red blood on admission and is unable to answer questions. He assumes the fetal position and clutches his abdomen.

Mr. Fong's girlfriend tells the nurse that she is not aware of any allergies. She states that he did take his medicine and ate breakfast this morning, but she is uncertain whether he ate lunch. Other pertinent preoperative assessment data include that Mr. Fong smokes two packs of cigarettes a day and drinks one or two alcoholic beverages every evening before dinner. He practices Buddhism.

In addition to his anti-ulcer medications, he has been taking ibuprofen-pseudoephedrine (Advil Cold & Sinus) three or four times a day for 5 days. Mr. Fong removed his partial bridge when he vomited the first time at the office. His contact lenses are still in place. Mr. Fong's

girlfriend is concerned that his two teenage children will not arrive before their father goes to surgery.

Emergency Department Diagnostic Test Results

- Red blood cells (RBCs): 4.8 million/mm^3 L
- Hemoglobin (Hg): 13.5 g/dl
- Hematocrit (Hct): 40%
- White blood cells (WBCs): 8000/mm^3
- Sodium: 140 mEq/L
- Potassium: 4 mEq/L
- Chloride: 101 mEq/L
- Glucose: 90 mg/dl
- Prothrombin time (PT): 15 seconds
- Partial thromboplastin time (PTT): 40 seconds
- Electrocardiogram (ECG): Normal sinus rhythm (NSR)
- Chest x-ray: Within normal limits

Nursing Physical Examination

Assessment

- Height: 5 feet, 9 inches
- Weight: 150 lb (68.2 kg)
- Vital signs: Blood pressure, 90/50; temperature, pulse, and respirations, 99, 120, 22
- Level of consciousness (LOC): Awake, restless, complaining of severe abdominal pain
- Eyes, ears, nose, throat (EENT): Within normal limits
- Cardiac: Tachycardia, regular rate and rhythm without gallop or murmur
- Pulmonary: Lung sounds coarse and diminished bilaterally
- Abdominal: Rigid, board-like abdomen without bowel tones
- Genitourinary: No urine output since admission; client denies urge to void
- Peripheral pulses: 2/2 without edema

Initial Treatment Plan

- Medications: Preoperative medications per anesthesia
- Intravenous: D$_5$LR (lactated Ringer's) at 100 ml/hr
- Diet: nothing by mouth (NPO)
- Activity: bed rest
- Other: surgical permit for upper gastrointestinal endoscopy with possible gastric or duodenal resection

Mr. Fong's endoscopy revealed a perforated peptic ulcer and he was taken to the operating room for resection of the ulcer. He returns to the surgical unit after 2 hours in the postanesthesia care unit. Consider the postoperative orders and related assessments and interventions expected in the care of Mr. Fong.

Case Study continued on following page

Nursing Assessments and Interventions Expected in the Postoperative Care of Mr. Fong

Mr. Fong is reluctant to take his pain medication because he is afraid of addiction. Two days postoperatively, he has a temperature spike of 101.6° F. On occasion, his cough is productive of thick, white sputum. His lungs remain coarse and diminished with scattered rhonchi and occasional wheezes bilaterally. A chest x-ray film reveals bilateral atelectasis. Discuss how the nurse might have intervened to prevent this situation.

Mr. Fong's incision is clean, dry, and intact. His abdomen is tender but soft. Bowel sounds remain absent and Mr. Fong denies flatus. Nasogastric intubation returns moderate amounts of green drainage. Consider the pathophysiology related to the continued absence of bowel tones.

Three days after the surgery, Mr. Fong continues to receive an IV infusion and IV antibiotics. His hemoglobin is 7.6 g/dl, and hematocrit is 24%. He complains of being very thirsty and asks when he will be able to eat and drink. Discuss appropriate medical and nursing interventions.

Eight days after the surgery, Mr. Fong is taking a soft diet and ambulating in the halls with good tolerance. He is scheduled for discharge in the morning.

Discharge Criteria

- Average length of stay: 6.7 days without complications; 12.1 days with complications
- Complete discharge teaching (includes diet, medications, activity, stress management, and follow-up appointments)
- Community referral: smoking cessation program

Questions to Be Considered

1. Categorize Mr. Fong's surgeries according to the Categories of Surgical Procedures (Table 15–4). Define Mr. Fong's surgical procedures. Review the roles of the nurses on the perioperative team.
2. Compare and contrast local versus general anesthesia. Identify which type would be used for each of Mr. Fong's surgeries. Why?
3. Discuss the principles of surgical positioning. How would Mr. Fong be positioned for each of his surgical procedures? Include the rationale for your answer.
4. How is the routine preoperative abdominal surgery client prepared for surgery? Discuss how Mr. Fong's preparation was different and the implications this would have for his recovery.
5. Explain informed consent. Describe the nurse's role in obtaining and completing informed consent forms.
6. Discuss the nurse's role in the promotion of wound healing. Include dietary management, wound care, positioning, rest, pain management, and pulmonary hygiene.
7. Discuss the psychosocial, spiritual, and cultural factors that may influence clients' attitudes about surgery and recovery. Apply these factors to Mr. Fong.
8. Compare and contrast the etiology, clinical manifestations, and management of peptic ulcer disease (gastric versus duodenal).

lifestyle may be an important part of the rehabilitation and recovery plan. Clients need to know that convalescence after gastric surgery tends to be slow. It may be 3 months before they regain strength and even partial ability to eat in a more normal manner. It may take a year or so before clients can eat three normal meals a day, and they may need to eat five times per day to accommodate changes in the anatomic structures. When complications such as dumping syndrome occur, clients may feel disappointed. Many clients expect a rapid recovery and may be unprepared when complications develop. Most clients can learn to control manifestations and lead a fairly normal life.

GASTRIC CANCER

Gastric cancer refers to the malignant neoplasms found in the stomach, usually adenocarcinoma, although there may be malignant lymphomas. For unknown reasons, the incidence of stomach cancer in the United States has diminished steadily since 1960.

The American Cancer Society estimated that 21,500 new cases of gastric cancer would be diagnosed in 2000, with 13,000 deaths attributed to gastric cancer. Stomach cancer is twice as common in men as in women, more common in whites in the United States, and more frequent in clients who have pernicious anemia.

Etiology and Risk Factors

Although no specific cause of gastric cancer has been identified, several factors are associated with the development of the disease. The latest research indicates that the presence of *H. pylori* in the stomach increases the incidence of gastric cancer. Gastric cancer often develops in conjunction with chronic atrophic gastritis and affects individuals who live in urban areas, have a low socioeconomic status, eat smoked fish or meats, and have a history of exposure to background radiation or trace metals in soil. The changes in the mucosa may lead to an increase in absorption of carcinogens from the diet, such as pickled foods, salted fish, and nitrates. Other etiologic factors include achlorhydria, pernicious anemia, and smoking. There may also be a genetic factor because the disease seems to run in families. Metalcrafts workers, coal miners, bakers, and those working in dusty, smoky, and sulfur dioxide–containing environments are at increased risk. Wood or tobacco smoke, nitrite food preservatives, and overheated fat products may predispose clients to gastric cancer.

Avoidance of the carcinogenic agents is important, especially in clients with other risk factors, such as chronic gastritis, *H. pylori* infection, and pernicious anemia. Cessation of smoking is an excellent health promotion behavior. The American Cancer Society recommends screening for cag A strain of *H. pylori* bacteria in people with a family history of gastric cancer.

Pathophysiology

Gastric cancer most often arises from the mucous lining of the stomach. Most of these cancers occur in the lesser curvature of the stomach in the pyloric and antral regions. Prognosis is best for stomach cancer involving polypoid lesions; it is poor for ulcerating cancers and poorest for infiltrating forms. Stomach cancer spreads by direct extension into the pancreas via the lymphatics and by hematogenous infiltration of the liver, lungs, and bones. The particular route depends on the location and the type of tumor. Some tumors penetrate, some ulcerate, and some spread along the tissue planes.

Gastric cancer is staged using the tumor, nodes, and metastasis (TNM) classification with stages I to IV (see Chapter 19). The cancer is resectable in early stages before it has invaded the wall of the stomach. The 5-year survival rate is about 90% for local disease and drops below 10% for stage III disease. In advanced gastric cancer, the survival rate is almost zero.

Clinical Manifestations

Because clinical manifestations occur late in the course of the disease, stomach cancer is seldom detected in an early stage. Unless hemorrhage or perforation occurs, manifestations are vague and indefinite. The presence of a palpable mass, ascites, or bone pain caused by metastasis may be the first manifestation. Manifestations vary, depending on the location of the tumor in the stomach. If the cancer grows near the cardia, the client may experience dysphagia because of early involvement of the esophagus. If the cancer is near the pylorus, manifestations may result from obstruction.

Assessment reveals weight loss, vague indigestion, anorexia, or a feeling of fullness or mild discomfort so insidious that the client does not recognize it as abnormal or seek medical assistance. Discomfort may be brought on or relieved by eating. Anemia from blood loss commonly occurs, and occult blood may be present in the stool. The presence of lactic acid and a high lactate dehydrogenase (LDH) level in the gastric juice suggests carcinoma.

The diagnosis of gastric cancer is confirmed by upper GI tract x-ray examination and gastroscopy. Gastroscopy allows direct visualization and permits cytologic brushing or biopsies to facilitate retrieval of cells for cytologic examination.

Outcome Management

■ Medical Management

Little effective medical treatment is available for gastric cancer. Clients may receive chemotherapy and radiation therapy, but the primary treatment is surgical resection. At present, best results are achieved with multiple drug combinations. Drugs giving the best results are 5-fluorouracil, mitomycin C, cisplatin, etoposide, leucovorin, and doxorubicin (Adriamycin). A combination of radiation and chemotherapy after surgery may be used. Total parenteral nutrition (TPN) (see Chapter 29) is a method for providing nutrition to the client intravenously, bypassing the GI tract.

■ Surgical Management

Surgery is the only intervention that effectively treats stomach cancer. Unfortunately, because the diagnosis is usually late, surgery is more often palliative than curative. Gastrectomy, either partial (with Billroth I or II reconstruction) or complete depending on tumor location, is the usual procedure. Ideally, the surgeon removes all local growth and associated lymph nodes. When an extensive tumor makes resection impractical or impossible and the pylorus is obstructed, the surgeon may perform a palliative gastroenterostomy (surgical creation of a passage between the stomach and small intestine).

■ Nursing Management of the Surgical Client
ASSESSMENT

Clients may present with manifestations similar to those of PUD, but frequently manifestations are not present until the tumor is advanced. While assessing the client, note any history of risk or factors predisposing to the development of gastric cancer. These include a history of chronic gastritis, pernicious anemia, previous gastric surgery, presence of *H. pylori* infection, or smoking. Ask the client if there is a history of ingestion of large amounts of nitrates, smoked fish, salty foods, or pickled foods.

DIAGNOSIS, OUTCOMES, INTERVENTIONS

Pain. Both before and after surgery, a primary nursing diagnosis for the client is *Pain related to gastric erosion and postoperative pain related to high surgical incision.*

Outcomes. The client will have pain controlled or experience a reduction in pain, as evidenced by the client's use of a pain scale of 1 to 10 and stating a pain score of less than a 2 or 3.

Interventions. It is important that the client receive pain relief. Pain that is not controlled can interfere with sleep and eating and contributes to overall physical and mental deterioration. (Chapter 23 describes pain control in detail.) The client should have verbal and written instructions regarding medications, treatments, and follow-up care.

Altered Nutrition: Less Than Body Requirements. An important nursing diagnosis for the client with gastric cancer is *Altered Nutrition: Less Than Body Requirements related to decreased appetite, pain, possible gastric obstruction and nausea and vomiting.*

Outcomes. The client will maintain nutritional intake to meet metabolic requirements, as evidenced by maintenance of normal body weight.

Interventions. Nutritional therapy is an important aspect of management of the client with gastric cancer. TPN or jejunostomy tube feedings may be used postoperatively (or for clients with inoperable disease) to maintain the nutritional status (see Chapter 29).

Fear. Because of the uncertainty of the disease, an appropriate nursing diagnosis for the client with gastric cancer is *Fear related to knowledge deficit, body image changes, treatment and life-threatening illness.*

Outcomes. The client will have reduced or controlled fear, as evidenced by the client's ability to understand and discuss disease and treatment options.

Interventions. The client needs an explanation of the disease and all treatment options. Reinforce information to the client as needed. The client also needs information concerning operative procedures and postoperative interventions (nothing by mouth [NPO] status, NG tubes, other drains, intravenous infusions). This information will help decrease the client's fear.

Postoperative complications include hemorrhage, obstruction, anemia, nutritional deficiency, dumping syndrome, duodenal stump leakage, gastric dilation, and delayed gastric emptying. A home health care referral can assist the client with emotional support and treatments and provide an ongoing assessment of the client's condition. Referring the client to a dietitian, member of the clergy, and hospice team may also be necessary. Various community support groups are also available (e.g., I Can Cope). For terminal cancer care, see Chapters 19 and 22.

EVALUATION

The prognosis for clients with gastric surgery is poor. Generally, surgery is performed to provide a palliative means of assisting the client to be more comfortable rather than a cure of the stomach cancer. Therefore, the only appropriate outcome may be as good a quality of life as possible and adequate control of manifestations.

CONCLUSIONS

Gastric disorders are common; unless treated promptly and completely, they can continue to cause problems throughout the client's life. Assist clients to learn a new way of eating to achieve and maintain health and to make necessary lifestyle changes. This is a difficult task; however, unless the client modifies behavior, especially eating behaviors, many of the gastric disorders recur. The foci of nursing interventions are education and modifications of the client's behavior to promote a healthier lifestyle pattern.

THINKING CRITICALLY

1. **A young female executive comes to the health clinic with complaints of epigastric pain and malaise. She works under stress and smokes heavily. She is in a hurry and wants quick action. The physician or advanced health practitioner recommends ranitidine (Zantac) for pain relief and an upper gastrointestinal x-ray film to rule out a duodenal ulcer. What further nursing assessment is required? What nursing interventions should be planned?**

Factors to Consider. What places the client at risk for a duodenal ulcer? What teaching is required for medication and dietary management? How should changes in lifestyle be addressed?

2. **A 43-year-old male client is being evaluated for intractable peptic ulcer disease. He has a history of recurrent duodenal ulcers. Last night he awakened at 2:00 AM and requested an antacid. This morning after breakfast, he passed a large, dark, liquid stool that tested positive for occult blood. Just before his 11:00 AM H_2-receptor antagonist, he turns on his call light. When the nurse enters the room, he is lying on his side with his knees drawn up, moaning and holding his pillow against his abdomen. He is diaphoretic, pale, and breathing rapidly and shallowly. The client states, "It's never hurt like this before. I feel as though I've been stabbed." What should the nurse's first actions be? What has probably happened to this client? Will he need surgery?**

Factors to Consider. What type of surgery will be performed? What are the expected nursing assessments postoperatively? What complications is he at risk for? What discharge teaching will be needed to enhance his health maintenance and prevent recurrence of PUD?

3. **A 52-year-old man who had a subtotal gastrectomy for stage III gastric cancer 10 weeks ago is having difficulty maintaining his body weight. His usual body weight is 190 pounds; he currently weighs 165 pounds. His wife reports that her husband is depressed, will not eat, and sleeps all day in his chair. She states, "I don't know what to do anymore! I think he just wants to die." She then starts crying. What should the nurse say to the client's wife? Whom should the nurse contact to assist the family?**

Factors to Consider. Why is the client at nutritional risk? What is his percentage of weight loss? What measures might be initiated to facilitate nutrition?

BIBLIOGRAPHY

1. American Cancer Society. (2000). *Cancer facts and figures.* Atlanta: Author.
2. Aronson, B. (1998). Update on peptic ulcer drugs. *American Journal of Nursing, 98*(1), 41–47.
3. Bode, C., & Bode, J. C. (1997). Alcohol's role in gastrointestinal tract disorders. *Alcohol Health and Research World, 21*(1), 93–96.
4. Branicki, F., et al. (1998). Quality of life in patients with cancer of the esophagus and gastric cardia: A case for palliative resection. *Archives of Surgery, 133,* 316–322.
5. Brooks, M., Maxson, C., & Rubin, W. (1996). The infectious etiology of peptic ulcer disease: Diagnosis and implications for therapy. *Primary Care, 23*(3), 443–454.
6. Copstead, L. (1999). *Perspectives on pathophysiology* (2nd ed). Philadelphia: W. B. Saunders.
7. Djonret, L. L. (1998). Perspectives: An unexpected outcome after gastroesophagogastroduodenoscopy. *Gastroenterology Nursing, 21*(3), 29–30.
8. Erstad, B., et al. (1997). Impacting cost and appropriateness of stress ulcer prophylaxis at a university medical center. *American Journal of Industrial Medicine, 25,* 1678–1684.
9. Feldman, M., et al. (1998). Role of seroconversion in confirming cure of *Helicobacter pylori* infection. *Journal of the American Medical Association, 280*(4), 363–365.
10. Gillen, D., et al. (1999). Rebound hypersecretion after omeprazole and its relation to on-treatment acid suppression and *Helicobacter pylori* status. *Gastroenterology, 116*(2), 239–247.

11. Hansen, M. (1998). *Pathophysiology: Foundations of disease and clinical intervention.* Philadelphia: W. B. Saunders.

12. Hay, J., et al. (1997). Prospective evaluation of a clinical guideline recommending hospital length of stay in upper gastrointestinal tract hemorrhage. *Journal of the American Medical Association, 278*(24), 2151–2156.

13. Heslin, J. (1997). Peptic ulcer disease. *Nursing, 27*(1), 34–37.

14. Laine, L., et al. (1998). Has the impact of *Helicobacter pylori* therapy on ulcer recurrence in the United States been overstated? A meta-analysis of rigorously designed trials. *American Journal of Gastroenterology, 93,* 1409–1415.

15. Lehne, R. (1999). *Pharmacology for nursing care* (3rd ed.). Philadelphia: W. B. Saunders.

16. Levenstein, S., et al. (1999). Stress and peptic ulcer disease. *Journal of the American Medical Association, 281,* 10–11.

17. Lind, T., et al. (1999). The MACH2 study: Role of omeprazole in eradication of *Helicobacter pylori* with 1-week triple therapies. *Gastroenterology, 116*(2), 249–253.

18. McConnell, E. (1997). How to determine gastric pH. *Nursing, 27*(8), 26.

19. McCorkle, R., et al. (1996). *Cancer nursing: A comprehensive textbook* (2nd ed.) Philadelphia: W. B. Saunders.

20. Metheny, N., et al. (1994). Visual characteristics of aspirates from feeding tubes as a method for predicting tube location. *Nursing Research, 43*(5), 282–287.

21. Metheny, N., et al. (1993). Effectiveness of pH measurements in predicting feeding tube placement: An update. *Nursing Research, 42*(6), 314–331.

22. Metheny, N., et al. (1993). How to aspirate fluid from small-bore feeding tubes. *American Journal of Nursing, 93*(5), 86–88.

23. Miller, D., & Miller, H. (1995). Giving meds through the tube. *RN, 58*(1), 44–48.

24. Nardone, G., et al. (1999). Effect of *Helicobacter pylori* infection and its eradication on cell proliferation, DNA status, oncogene expression in patients with chronic gastritis. *Gut, 44*(6), 789–799.

25. O'Connor, K. (1999). Gastric cancer. *Seminars in Oncology Nursing, 15*(1), 26–35.

26. Ohkusa, T., et al. (1998). Disappearance of hyperplastic polyps in the stomach after eradication of *Helicobacter pylori:* A randomized, controlled trial. *Annals of Internal Medicine, 129,* 712–715.

27. Onishi, K., & Miaskowski, C. (1998). Mechanisms and management of gastric cancer. A comparison between the Japanese and U.S. experiences. *Cancer Nursing, 19*(3), 187–196.

28. Pehl, C., et al. (1999). Effect of low and high fat meals on lower esophageal sphincter motility and gastroesophageal reflux in healthy subjects. *American Journal of Gastroenterology, 94*(5), 1192–1196.

29. Peterson, W., & Cook, D. (1998). Antisecretory therapy for bleeding peptic ulcer. *Journal of the American Medical Association, 280*(10), 877–878.

30. Rutgeerts, P., et al. (1997). Randomized trial of single and repeated fibrin glue compared with injection of polidocanol in treatment of bleeding peptic ulcer. *Lancet, 350,* 692–696.

31. Sabiston, D. (1997). *Textbook of surgery: The biological basis of modern surgical practice* (15th ed.). Philadelphia: W. B. Saunders.

32. Smith, A. D., et al. (1999). Dyspepsia on withdrawal of ranitidine in previously asymptomatic volunteers. *American Journal of Gastroenterology, 94*(5), 1202–1213.

33. Soll, A., et al. (1996). Gastrointestinal Diseases. In J. Bennett & F. Plum (Eds.), *Cecil textbook of medicine* (20th ed.). Philadelphia: W. B. Saunders.

34. Vakil, N., & Cutler, A. (1999). Ten-day triple therapy with ranitidine, bismuth, amoxicillin, and clarithromycin in eradicating *Helicobacter pylori. Gastroenterology, 116*(3), 1197–1199.

35. Veldhuyzen van Zanten, S., et al. (1998). Adding once-daily omeprazole 20 mg to metronidazole/amoxicillin treatment for *Helicobacter pylori* gastritis: A randomized, double-blind trial showing the importance of metronidazole resistance. *American Journal of Gastroenterology, 93,* 5–10.

36. Wagner, S., et al. (1997). Regulation of gastric epithelial cell growth by *Helicobacter pylori:* Evidence for a major role of apoptosis. *Gastroenterology, 113,* 1836–1947.

Feeding Tube Placement Errors

QUESTIONS

What is the prevalence of feeding tube placement errors?
What are the risk factors associated with misplacement at the time of insertion and subsequent displacement from the intended site?
How accurate and reliable is gastric pH measurement as a method for verifying placement?

CITATIONS

Ellet, M. L. C. (1997). What is the prevalence of feeding tube placement errors and what are the associated risk factors? *Online Journal of Knowledge Synthesis for Nursing, 4*(5).
Chen, C. A., Paxton, P., & Williams-Burgess, C. (1996). Feeding tube placement verification using gastric pH measurement. *Online Journal of Knowledge Synthesis for Nursing, 3*(10).

STUDIES*

For the Ellet review, study reports were located by searching *MEDLINE* (1966–1996) and *CINAHL* (1982–1996) using the terms feeding tube, tube placement determination, risk factors, and enteral nutrition. Five studies addressed placement insertion errors, and two addressed tube displacement in adults. Six studies addressed risk factors associated with feeding tube placement errors.

For the Chen review, study reports were located by searching *MEDLINE* and *CINAHL* (1988–1995) using the terms feeding tube, feeding tube placement, gastric pH, nasogastric tube, pH measurement, pH sensor, and pH paper. Nursing, medical, and interdisciplinary studies were included.

Summary of Findings from the Ellett Review

Prevalence of Misplacement and Displacement

In two studies of small-bore feeding tubes in critically ill adults, the rates of misplacement at time of insertion were 4.4%[6] and 1.3%.[12] By radiologic detection, tubes were found to be inadvertently placed into the esophagus, lungs, pleural space, and brain.[7, 16] The latter errors occurred in clients with severe traumatic craniofacial injuries.[5, 10] The rate of displacement of gastric feeding tubes, after confirmation of correct original placement, was 15% in one study[14] and 18% in another[3]; most displacements involved upward migrations of the tube. The small-bore feeding tubes in use today are more prone to misplacement and displacement than the larger tubes formerly used.[8]

Feeding tubes intended to terminate in the small intestine are even more subject to placement errors.[9, 11, 14] The most common problems are that (1) the tubes never pass through the distal part of the stomach (i.e., the pylorus) into the small intestines, or (2) once in place they migrate upward (i.e., backward) into the stomach or esophagus.

In a comparison of weighted and unweighted duodenal tubes,[11] only 57% of the weighted tubes and 67% of the un-

weighted tubes were in the desired location. In another study of intestinal tubes,[14] 27% of the weighted tubes and 50% of the unweighted tubes were not in the correct position.

Risk Factors Associated with Placement Errors

Several factors are related to incorrect tube position and subsequent aspiration. One risk factor associated with misplacement into the tracheobronchial tree is the presence of a high-compliance, low-pressure cuffed endotracheal tube.[7, 15] During insertion, the feeding tube follows the endotracheal tube past the cuff and into the trachea.

Other risk factors include decreased levels of consciousness, impaired gag and cough reflexes, coughing, tracheal suctioning, retching, vomiting, failure to maintain elevation of the head of the bed, restlessness, and recent extubation.[1, 2, 4, 7, 14] In one study, 41% of clients with feeding tubes pulled out at least one tube[4]; restlessness and disorientation were significant associated factors.

Summary of Findings from the Chen, Paxton, & Williams-Burgess Review

Accuracy and Reliability of Placement Verification Methods

Various nonradiologic methods have been used to test feeding tube placement, including aspiration of recognizable gastric contents, auscultation of air introduced via syringe into the tube, and measurement of pH of fluid aspirated via syringe.

Inadvertent respiratory placement can also be ruled out by observing for coughing, choking, or cyanosis; asking the client to speak; and observing for bubbles caused by exhaled air when the end of the tube is held under water.

The research findings indicate a low level of accuracy in predicting feeding tube location[21–23]; however, several of these studies used simulations rather than actual clinical situations. In 1988, Metheny and coworkers[14] pointed out that many of the verification methods were developed for use with large-bore feeding tubes and thus might be inaccurate for use with the small-bore feeding tubes in use today.

---

*The findings of the two reviews are presented separately; the research-based care actions are combined.

Feeding Tube Placement Errors *Continued*

Use of Gastric pH Measurement

A study of gastric and intestinal readings demonstrated that the two placements could be differentiated based on pH values.[24] pH values below 4.0 indicated gastric placement, whereas pH values above 4.0 indicated intestinal placement; these parameters were adjusted if the patient was receiving medications to prevent gastric stress ulcers. In a follow-up study of 405 aspirates from nasogastric tubes and 389 aspirates from nasointestinal tubes, gastric placement was successfully distinguished from intestinal placement using pH meter readings in both the presence and absence of acid inhibitors.[25] Although it was hypothesized that gastric and respiratory aspirates could be differentiated based on pH levels, this hypothesis was not tested because of a very low number of readings from tubes in the respiratory tract; however, the average pH of tracheobronchial fluid aspirates was 7.81 (alkaline)—much higher than that of gastric contents.

The pH of aspirated gastric contents can be measured using pH paper or a tube having a built-in probe and pH meter. The accuracy of pH paper is not clear. In one study, paper determinations were accurate in obtaining both true low pH results and true high pH results.[20] In another study, however, in which the goal was to maintain a gastric pH of greater than 3.5 to prevent upper GI bleeding in critically ill clients,[19] the pH paper accurately determined the pH of gastric contents with values of less than 4 only 67% of the time; with pH values of 4 or more, the paper was accurate 95% of the time. It was concluded that using pH paper lacks accuracy and reliability in the clinical setting and may result in significant undertreatment.

Three studies have compared the values of pH determination by color-coded pH paper with the values produced by the pH probe and meter.[17, 18, 20] One study revealed that the pH probe and meter were more accurate, especially in clients with decreased amounts of gastric acid.[18] The other study[20] found a high correlation between the two measurements. One research group noted that differences between the two ways of measuring gastric pH may be related to the fact that the probe samples gastric contents right next to the mucosa, whereas the paper measures pooled gastric contents.[26] Use of the gastric pH probe and pH meter required less staff contact with gastric aspirates and required less time to perform than pH paper measurements.[26]

Limitations/Reservations: It was not clear whether all the studies examined small-bore tubes; it is possible that some of the older studies involved large-bore enteral tubes. Several studies demonstrated that what worked under controlled laboratory conditions did not necessarily work well in clinical situations; thus, research regarding accuracy of determinations at the bedside is needed. Studies differentiating respiratory from intestinal placement are also lacking; this is important because the pH levels of their aspirates overlap.

Research-Based Practice (From Both Reviews Combined)

It is evident that some feeding tubes either never reach their intended destination or become displaced after insertion. The tube can be placed or can migrate into the respiratory tract, the esophagus, or traumatized craniofacial spaces. After being placed, a tube can move back from the intestines into the stomach, or it can migrate from the stomach into the distal esopha-gus. Tubes passed with the aid of a guide wire tend to perforate the wall of the bronchus or the lung, causing a pneumothorax. The actual rate of insertion and displacement errors is not known.

Clients who are at risk for incorrect tube position include those who (1) have low-pressure cuffed endotracheal tubes, (2) cough a lot or have a depressed cough reflex, and (3) have a decreased level of consciousness. Elevating the head of the bed may help prevent tube displacement. Even though feeding tubes are often taped where they exit from the nose, this is not a guarantee that the end point of the tube is in the correct location. Check the location frequently to prevent aspiration or other problems associated with incorrect location.

Clearly, radiographic studies can accurately demonstrate the location of feeding tubes; however, clients should not be required to undergo repeated x-ray examinations for this purpose. An easy-to-use, accurate, and dependable bedside method is needed to monitor tube placement on an ongoing basis. Many of the commonly used monitoring signs and methods (e.g., coughing, auscultation of inserted air, and visual identification of gastric contents) are probably not dependable with small-bore tubes. At this point, small-bore tubes with a probe and pH meter provide the easiest and most accurate method of pinpointing the location of a tube. Advantages include the ability to continuously monitor tube location and to measure gastric pH right next to the mucosa rather than pooled gastric secretions, as with the aspirate method. The latter feature is a benefit when the client is receiving anti-ulcer therapy. Although using pH paper to determine gastric acidity may not be as accurate as using a pH probe and sensor, pH paper has been found to be more accurate than most of the other methods.

More recently, determining the pH of the aspirate combined with a laboratory measurement of pepsin and trypsin levels has been found to be very accurate in confirming the location of a tube. The pattern of presence or absence of the two enzymes and the pH level of the aspirate enable 100% accuracy in determining respiratory locations and a high level of accuracy in distinguishing between gastric and intestinal locations.[27] The ability to determine pepsin and trypsin levels as well as pH levels at the bedside would provide even better ongoing monitoring of feeding tube locations.

Cited References from the Ellet Review

1. Arms, R. A., Dines, D. E., & Tinstman, T. C. (1974). Aspiration pneumonia. *Chest, 65,* 136–139.
2. Bartlett, J. G., & Gorbach, S. L. (1975). The triple threat of aspiration pneumonia. *Chest, 68,* 560–566.
3. Crocker, K. S., Krey, S. H., & Steefee, W. P. (1981). Performance evaluation of a new nasogastric feeding tube. *Journal of Parenteral and Enteral Nutrition, 5,* 80–82.
4. Eisenberg, P., Spies, M., and Metheny, N. A. (1987). Characteristics of patients who remove their nasal feeding tube. *Clinical Nurse Specialist, 1,* 94–98.
5. Fletcher, S. A., et al. (1989). The successful surgical removal of intracranial nasogastric tubes. *Journal of Trauma, 27,* 948–952.
6. Ghahremani, G. G., & Gould, R. J. (1986). Nasoenteric feeding tubes: Radiographic detection of complications. *Digestive Diseases and Sciences, 31,* 574–585.
7. Harris, M. R., & Huseby, J. S. (1989). Pulmonary complications from nasoenteral feeding tube insertion in an intensive care unit: Incidence and prevention. *Critical Care Medicine, 17,* 917–919.

Bridge continued on following page

Feeding Tube Placement Errors *Continued*

8. Keohane, P. P., et al. (1983). Limitations and drawbacks of "fine bore" nasogastric feeding tubes. *Clinical Nutrition, 2,* 85–86.
9. Kiver, K. F., et al. (1984). Pre- and postpyloric enteral feeding: Analysis of safety and complications (Abstract). *Journal of Parenteral and Enteral Nutrition, 8,* 95.
10. Koch, K. J., et al. (1989). Intracranial placement of a nasogastric tube. *American Journal of Neuroradiology, 10,* 443–444.
11. Levenson, R., et al. (1988). Do weighted nasoenteric feeding tubes facilitate duodenal intubations? *Journal of Parenteral and Enteral Nutrition, 12,* 135–137.
12. McWey, R. E., et al. (1988). Complications of nasoenteric feeding tubes. *American Journal of Surgery, 155,* 253–257.
13. Metheny, N. A. (1993). Minimizing respiratory complications of nasoenteric tube feedings: State of the science. *Heart and Lung, 22,* 213–223.
14. Metheny, N. A., Spies, M., & Eisenberg, P. (1986). Frequency of nasoenteral tube displacement and associated risk factors. *Research in Nursing and Health, 9,* 241–247.
15. Scholten, D. J., Wood, T. L., & Thompson, D. R. (1986). Pneumothorax from nasoenteric feeding tube insertion: A report of five cases. *American Surgeon, 52,* 381–385.
16. Woodall, B. H., Winfield, D. F., & Bissett, G. S. III. (1987). Inadvertent tracheobronchial placement of feeding tubes. *Radiology, 165,* 727–729.

Cited References from the Chen, Paxton, & Williams-Burgess Review

17. Botoman, V. A., Kirtland, S. H., & Moss, R. L. (1994). A randomized study of a pH sensor feeding tube vs. a standard feeding tube in patients requiring enteral nutrition. *Journal of Parenteral and Enteral Nutrition, 18,* 154–158.

18. Caballero, G. A., et al. (1990). Gastric secretion pH measurement: What you see is not what you get. *Critical Care Medicine, 18,* 396–399.
19. Dobkin, E. D., et al. (1990). Does pH paper accurately eflect gastric pH? *Critical Care Medicine, 18,* 985–988.
20. Levine, R. L., et al. (1994). Equivalence of litmus paper and intragastric pH probes for intragastric pH monitoring in the intensive care unit. *Critical Care Medicine, 22,* 945–948.
21. Metheny, N., et al. (1990). Detection of inadvertent respiratory placement of small-bore feeding tubes: A report of 10 cases. *Nursing Research, 37,* 324–329.
22. Metheny, N., et al. (1990). Effectiveness of the auscultatory method in predicting feeding tube location. *Nursing Research, 39,* 262–267.
23. Metheny, N., et al. (1994). Visual characteristics of aspirates from feeding tubes as a method for predicting tube location. *Nursing Research, 43,* 282–287.
24. Metheny, N., et al. (1989). Effectiveness of pH measurement in predicting feeding tube placement. *Nursing Research, 38,* 280–285.
25. Metheny, N., et al. (1993). Effectiveness of pH measurements in predicting feeding tube placement: An update. *Nursing Research, 42,* 324–331.
26. Neill, K. M., Rice, K. T., & Ahern, H. L. (1993). Comparison of two methods of measuring gastric pH. *Heart and Lung, 22,* 349–355.

Added Reference

27. Metheny, N. A., et al. (1997). pH and concentrations of pepsin and trypsin in feeding tube aspirates as predictors of tube placement. *Journal of Parenteral and Enteral Nutrition, 21,* 279–285.

Sarah Jo Brown, PhD, RN, *Principal and Consultant, Practice-Research Integrations, Norwich, Vermont*

Elimination Disorders

Anatomy and Physiology Review: The Elimination Systems

32 Assessment of Elimination

33 Management of Clients with Intestinal Disorders

34 Management of Clients with Urinary Disorders

35 Management of Clients with Renal Disorders

36 Management of Clients with Renal Failure

Anatomy and Physiology Review:
The Elimination Systems
Robert G. Carroll

The urinary tract is composed of four structures:

- Kidneys
- Ureters
- Bladder
- Urethra

The *kidneys* balance the urinary excretion of substances against the accumulation within the body through ingestion or production. Consequently, they are a major controller of fluid and electrolyte homeostasis. The kidneys also have several nonexcretory metabolic and endocrine functions, including blood pressure regulation, erythropoietin production, insulin degradation, prostaglandin synthesis, calcium and phosphorus regulation, and vitamin D metabolism.

Filtration at the renal glomerulus is the first step in urine formation. Normally, a volume equal to plasma volume is filtered every 24 minutes and a volume equal to total body water is filtered every 6 hours. This glomerular filtrate is similar to plasma, but it lacks cells and large-molecular-weight proteins. The glomerular filtrate is modified by active transport, diffusion, and osmosis as it passes through the renal tubules. *Reabsorption* of filtrate components enhances conservation of glucose, amino acids, and electrolytes. *Secretion* of plasma components enhances elimination of organic acids and bases (and some drugs). The remnants of the glomerular filtrate exit the kidney through the ureters.

The *ureters* conduct urine from the kidneys to the bladder by peristaltic contraction. The *bladder* is a distensible chamber that stores urine until it is *excreted*. The *urethra* is the exit passageway from the bladder that carries urine for elimination from the body.

STRUCTURE OF THE ELIMINATION SYSTEM

KIDNEYS

The kidneys are located retroperitoneally, in the posterior aspect of the abdomen, on either side of the vertebral column (Fig. U7–1). They lie between the 12th thoracic and the third lumbar vertebrae. The left kidney is usually positioned slightly higher than the right. Adult kidneys average approximately 11 cm in length, 5 to 7.5 cm in width, and 2.5 cm in thickness. Affixing the kidneys in position behind the parietal peritoneum is a mass of perirenal fat (adipose capsule) and connective tissue called *Gerota's (subserosa) fascia*. A fi-

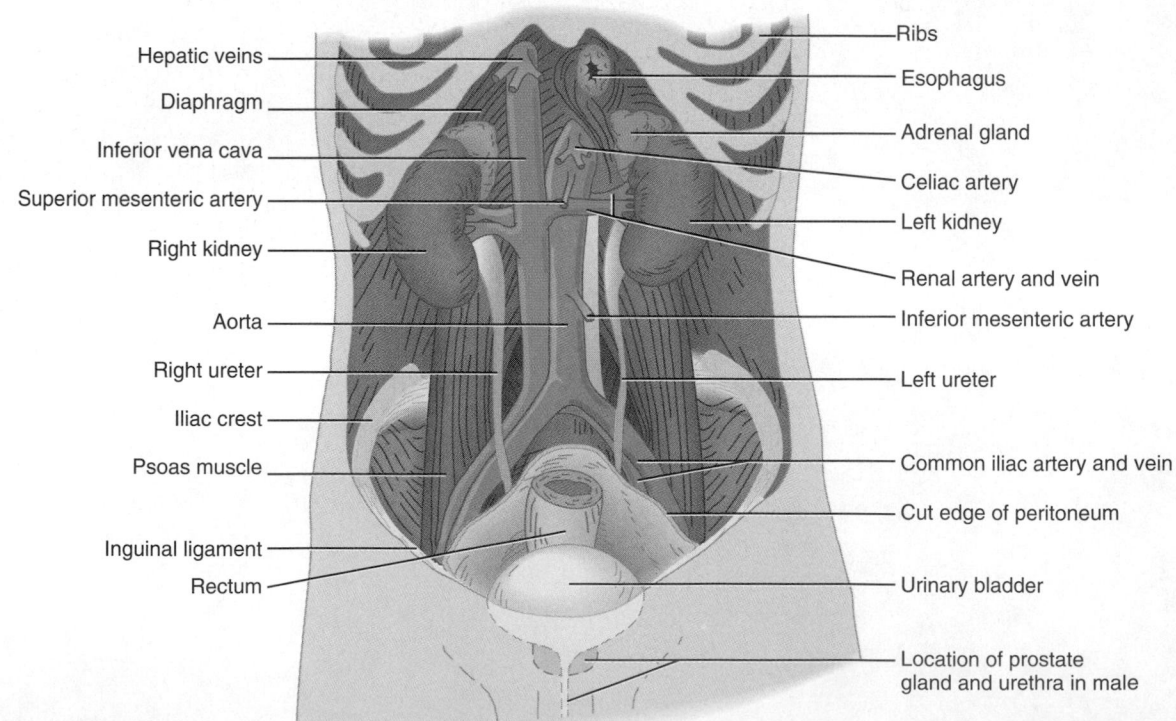

Hepatic veins
Diaphragm
Inferior vena cava
Superior mesenteric artery
Right kidney
Aorta
Right ureter
Iliac crest
Psoas muscle
Inguinal ligament
Rectum

Ribs
Esophagus
Adrenal gland
Celiac artery
Left kidney
Renal artery and vein
Inferior mesenteric artery
Left ureter
Common iliac artery and vein
Cut edge of peritoneum
Urinary bladder
Location of prostate gland and urethra in male

FIGURE U7–1 Anatomic relationship of the kidneys and related structures.

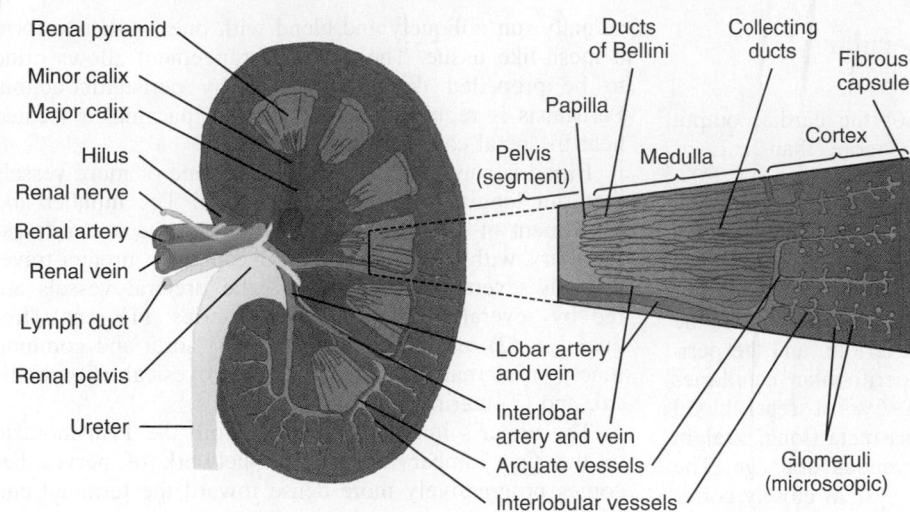

Renal pyramid
Minor calix
Major calix
Hilus
Renal nerve
Renal artery
Renal vein
Lymph duct
Renal pelvis
Ureter

Ducts of Bellini
Papilla
Pelvis (segment)
Collecting ducts
Fibrous capsule
Medulla
Cortex

Lobar artery and vein
Interlobar artery and vein
Arcuate vessels
Interlobular vessels
Glomeruli (microscopic)

FIGURE U7–2 Anatomy of the kidney. *Inset,* Enlargement of a segment of the kidney.

brous capsule (renal capsule) forms the external covering of the kidney, except for the hilum. The kidney is further protected by layers of muscle of the back, flank, and abdomen as well as by layers of fat, subcutaneous tissue, and skin.

The kidney has a characteristic curved shape, with a convex distal edge and a concave medial boundary. In the innermost part of the concave section is the *hilus,* through which pass the renal artery, renal vein, lymphatics, nerves, and the renal pelvis (the natural upper extension of the ureter). A fibrous capsule surrounds each kidney and adheres to the renal parenchyma. Each kidney is divided into three major areas: (1) cortex, (2) medulla, and (3) pelvis (Fig. U7–2).

The *cortex* of the kidney lies just under the fibrous capsule, and portions of it extend down into the medullary layer to form the renal columns (columns of Bertin) or cortical tissue that separates the pyramids. The *medulla* is divided into eight to 18 cone-shaped masses of collecting ducts called the *renal pyramids.* The bases of the pyramids are positioned on the corticomedullary boundary. Their apices extend toward the renal pelvis, forming papillae. The papillae have 10 to 25 openings each on the surface, through which the urine empties into the renal pelvis (see *inset,* Fig. U7–2). Eight or more groups of papillae are present in each pyramid; each empties into a *minor calix,* and several minor calices join to form a *major calix.* The two to three major calices are outpouchings of the *renal pelvis* (the inner area of the kidney). They channel the urine from the pyramids to the renal pelvis. The *renal pelvis* is a cavity lined with transitional epithelium. The combined volume of the pelvis and calices is approximately 8 ml. Volumes in excess of this amount damage the renal parenchymal tissue. The renal pelvis narrows as it reaches the *hilus* and becomes the proximal end of the ureter.

Within the cortex lies the *nephron,* the functional unit of the kidney, consisting of both vascular and tubular elements (Fig. U7–3). Filtration begins at the renal *glomerulus.* The glomerular tuft (glomerulus) contains capillaries and the beginning of the tubule system, Bowman's capsule. Filtrate from the glomerulus enters Bowman's capsule and then passes through a series of tubule seg-

ments that modify the filtrate as it passes through the renal cortex and medulla and, finally, flows into the renal calices. A second capillary bed, the peritubular capillaries, carries the reabsorbed water and solutes back toward the vena cava.

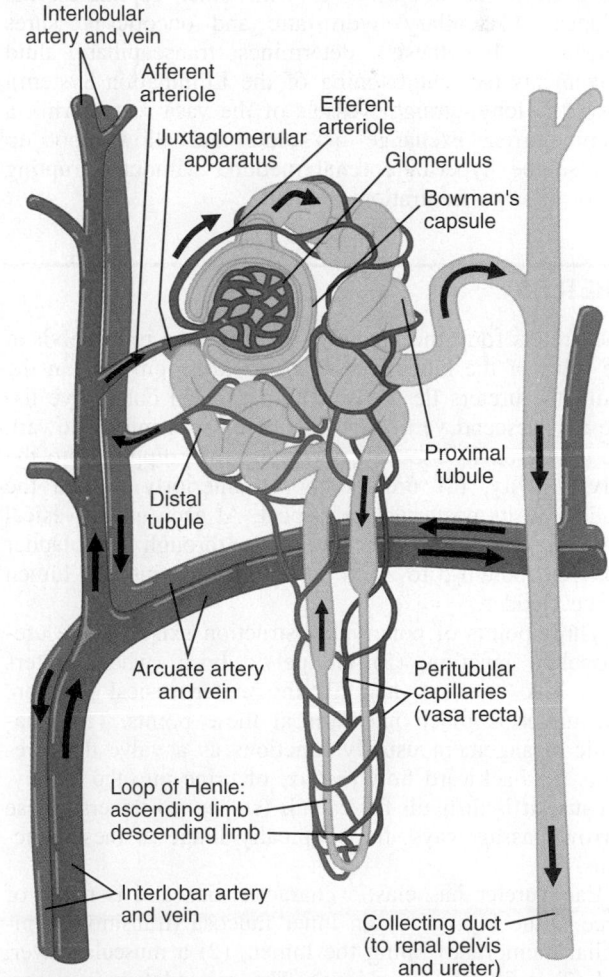

Interlobular artery and vein
Afferent arteriole
Juxtaglomerular apparatus
Efferent arteriole
Glomerulus
Bowman's capsule
Proximal tubule
Distal tubule
Arcuate artery and vein
Peritubular capillaries (vasa recta)
Loop of Henle: ascending limb descending limb
Interlobar artery and vein
Collecting duct (to renal pelvis and ureter)

FIGURE U7–3 Diagram of a nephron and associated vascular structures.

Renal Blood Flow and Glomerular Filtration

The kidneys receive 20% to 25% of the cardiac output under resting conditions, averaging more than 1 L of arterial blood per minute. The renal arteries (see Fig. U7–2) branch from the abdominal aorta at the level of the second lumbar vertebra, enter the kidney, and progressively branch into lobar arteries, interlobar arteries, arcuate arteries, and interlobular arteries. Blood flows from the interlobular arteries through the afferent arteriole, the glomerular capillaries, the efferent arteriole, and the peritubular capillaries. Some of the peritubular capillaries carry a small amount of blood (~5% of renal blood flow) to the renal medulla in the vasa recta (long, straight blood vessels) before entering the venous drainage. The blood leaves the kidney in a venous system closely corresponding to the arterial system: interlobular veins, arcuate veins, interlobar veins, and the renal vein. The renal circulation then empties into the inferior vena cava.

The arrangement of the two capillary beds in series in the nephron allows most of the large volume of filtrate at the glomerular capillaries to be reabsorbed by the peritubular capillaries. The normal glomerular filtration rate (GFR) is 125 ml/min, but because of filtrate reabsorption at the peritubular capillaries only about 1 ml/min of urine flows from the kidneys. As with other capillaries, the balance of capillary hydrostatic and oncotic pressures (Starling's hypothesis) determines transcapillary fluid movements (see Functioning of the Elimination System). Also, the long, straight vessels of the vasa recta permit a countercurrent exchange of solute and allow blood to perfuse the hypertonic renal medulla without disrupting the osmotic concentration gradient.

URETERS

The ureters form the medial tapering of the renal pelvis at the hilus of the kidney. Usually 25 to 35 cm long in the adult, the ureters lie in the extraperitoneal connective tissue and descend vertically along the psoas muscle toward the pelvic cavity (see Fig. U7–1). After dipping into the pelvic cavity, the ureters course anteriorly to join the bladder in its posterolateral aspect. At each ureterovesical junction, the ureter runs obliquely through the bladder wall for about 1.5 to 2 cm before opening into the lumen of the bladder.

Three points of potential obstruction exist: (1) the ureteropelvic junction, (2) the pelvic brim (where ureters cross iliac arteries), and (3) the ureterovesical junction. The ureter is much narrower at these points. This anatomic arrangement usually functions as a valve that prevents the backward flow *(reflux)* of urine into the kidney. Because it is difficult for calculi (stones) to traverse these narrow passageways, they typically lodge at these junctions.

Each ureter has elastic characteristics and is made of three tissue layers: (1) an inner mucosa (transitional epithelial membrane) lining the lumen, (2) a muscular layer, and (3) a fibrous outer layer. The musculature is generally designated as *inner longitudinal* and *outer circular.* Along most of the ureter, however, the muscle fibers actually run obliquely and blend with one another to form a mesh-like tissue. The muscle arrangement allows urine to be propelled down the ureter by peristaltic action. Peristalsis is regulated by a myogenic pacemaker located near the renal calices.

Blood is supplied to the ureters by one or more vessels that run longitudinally along the tube. The number and assortment of arteries anastomosing with the ureteric vessels vary with each individual. Because the ureters travel through several anatomic areas, the ureteral vessels are fed by several of the following arteries: (1) renal (frequently), (2) testicular or ovarian, (3) aorta and common iliac, (4) internal iliac (frequently), (5) vesical, (6) umbilical, and (7) uterine.

The ureter's innervation comes from the 11th thoracic to the first lumbar nerves. The network of nerves becomes progressively more dense toward the terminal end of the ureters.

BLADDER

The *urinary bladder* is a hollow organ located in the anterior half of the pelvis behind the symphysis pubis (see Unit 8 review, Figs. U8–1B and U8–4, for a discussion of anatomic structures). The space between the bladder and the symphysis pubis is filled with a loose connective tissue that allows the bladder to stretch cranially as it fills. The peritoneum covers the top border of the bladder, and the base is held loosely in place by the true ligaments. The bladder is also enveloped by a loose fascia.

The bladder wall has several tissue layers. The internal lining of the vesical wall is transitional epithelium with some mucus-secreting glands. There are three ill-defined muscle layers: the inner and outer layers (longitudinal) and middle layer (circular). The fibers from these layers interweave to form a mesh-like muscle layer called the *detrusor muscle.* This arrangement allows the bladder wall to be elastic while maintaining strength. Bundles of these smooth muscle layers come together at the base of the bladder to form the internal sphincter, or opening into the urethra. The *trigone* is the triangular area formed by the ureterovesical junctions and the internal sphincter.

The superior and lateral aspects of the bladder are served by the superior vesical artery, which branches from the umbilical artery and internal iliac artery. The inferior vesical artery, which supplies the underside of the bladder, may arise independently or in common with the middle rectal artery. The veins draining the bladder pass to the internal iliac trunk.

Innervation for the bladder comes from the hypogastric sympathetic, pelvic parasympathetic, and pudendal somatic nerves. Ganglia are most commonly found in the bladder base and around the urethral orifice. These areas tend to act in continuity with each other, and their functions seem to be coordinated by both the sympathetic and parasympathetic nervous systems.

URETHRA

The urethra is a tube that extends from the base of the bladder to the surface of the body. The urethra differs greatly in females and males.

FEMALE URETHRA

The female urethra is approximately 4 cm long and curves slightly forward as it reaches the external opening, or *meatus,* located between the clitoris and the vaginal orifice. The urethra is lined with epithelium, which contains some mucus-secreting glands. The longitudinal muscle layer is a continuation of longitudinal layer of bladder muscle. The circular muscle fibers encompass the urethra and meet with the circular bladder muscle. This muscle thins out near the meatus. As the urethra passes through the urogenital diaphragm, the circular muscle fibers form the external sphincter.

MALE URETHRA

In males, the urethra is a common outlet for the reproductive system and urinary elimination. The *prostate gland,* although not a direct part of the urinary system, is a major cause of urinary dysfunction in men. Located below the bladder neck, the prostate completely surrounds the urethra. Normally, this relationship causes no problem, but if the prostate enlarges, it constricts the urethra and obstructs the outflow of urine (see Chapter 38).

The male urethra is about 20 cm long and is divided into three main sections. The *prostatic urethra* extends about 3 cm below the bladder neck, through the prostate gland, to the pelvic floor. The ejaculatory ducts of the reproductive system empty into its posterior wall. The *membranous urethra* is about 1 to 2 cm in length and ends where the muscle layer forms the external sphincter. The distal portion is the *cavernous (penile) urethra.* Approximately 15 cm long, it travels through the penis to the urethral orifice at the tip of the penis; it is also lined with epithelial cells.

FUNCTION OF THE ELIMINATION SYSTEM

TRANSCAPILLARY FLUID EXCHANGE

Fluid movement at each capillary bed depends on the balance of fluid pressures and osmotic pressures. Glomerular capillary blood pressure reflects resistance to flow at afferent and efferent arterioles. *Preglomerular contraction* (primarily afferent arteriole), such as caused by renal sympathetic nerves, decreases flow of blood into the glomerular capillaries and decreases glomerular capillary blood pressure and GFR. *Postglomerular contraction* (primarily efferent arteriole), such as caused by angiotensin II, traps blood in the glomerulus and increases glomerular capillary pressure and GFR. Peritubular capillary blood pressure, because the peritubular capillaries are located downstream of the glomerulus, decreases following either afferent or efferent arteriolar contraction. A decrease in peritubular capillary pressure facilitates reabsorption of glomerular filtrate.

Plasma oncotic pressure, due primarily to albumin, attenuates filtration at the glomerular capillaries. If the glomerular barrier is damaged, the permeability of the glomerular capillary to protein decreases the normal oncotic reabsorptive forces and GFR is increased. The primary barrier to protein filtration is the negatively charged endothelium and basement membrane of the glomerular capillaries. A loss of this negative charge, such as occurs in diabetes, allows some proteins to pass into the urine (proteinuria).

TUBULAR MECHANISMS FOR SECRETION AND REABSORPTION

The renal tubules are lined with epithelial cells that selectively secrete or reabsorb compounds (Table U7–1). This blind-ended tubular segment originates at the glomerulus. Transport proteins and tightness of tight junctions help define segments of the tubules. Because the renal tubules and urinary tract are lined with epithelial cells, tubular fluid is functionally outside of the body (as with the gastrointestinal tract).

Modification of ultrafiltrate occurs by *diffusion* and *selective transport* in tubules. Diffusion is quantitatively the most important process. Some compounds are absorbed by carrier-mediated transport, such as sodium (Na^+)-coupled glucose transport.

Glomerular filtrate travels progressively through Bowman's capsule, the proximal tubules, the loop of Henle, the distal tubules, the connecting segment, and the collecting duct; it then enters renal medullary space, passes into ureter, and is stored in the bladder before exiting body as urine. The tubule segments are anatomically adjacent to the vascular supply for that nephron. The juxtaglomerular apparatus consists of the glomerulus and the distal tubule that originated from that glomerulus. This arrangement allows negative feedback control of glomerular filtrate formation at the individual nephron level.

Water reabsorption is driven by osmotic gradients. The osmolality of the renal cortex is 300 mOsm, similar to that in most areas of the body. Osmolality of the renal medulla, however, can reach 1500 mOsm, as a result of the high concentrations of urea, Na^+ and chloride (Cl^-) in the intersitial spaces. Two tubular segments, the loop of Henle and the collecting ducts, pass through the renal medulla and, consequently, play a major role in determining urine volume and osmolality.

Renal Tubular Segments

The proximal tubules reabsorb 65% of filtered water, Na^+, Cl^-, and potassium (K^+). This segment also reabsorbs 100% of filtered hexoses (glucose), amino acids, and small peptides by Na^+-coupled co-transport. Because this mechanism exhibits saturation kinetics, glucose can pass into the urine if the filtered load (plasma concentration $\times$ GFR) exceeds the renal reabsorptive capacity (T_{max}). This situation occurs in diabetes mellitus, generally when the plasma glucose concentration exceeds 300 mg/dl.

The thin limb of the loop of Henle is water-permeable, allowing water to exit the tubule as the filtrate passes into the osmotically concentrated renal medulla. Sodium chloride (NaCl) and urea, the osmotic particles of the medulla, can also enter the tubule in this segment. The thick ascending limb of the loop of Henle is water-impermeable, as—in the absence of antidiuretic hormone (ADH)—are the remaining segments of the urinary system. The $Na^+/K^+/2Cl^-$ transporter reabsorbs electrolytes. This solute transport without water movement results in hypotonic filtrate (100 mOsm); thus, this tubule segment is sometimes called the *diluting segment.*

Transport in the distal tubule and collecting duct represents the final chance to modify the tubular fluid before it is lost from the body as urine. Aldosterone promotes K^+

TABLE U7–1	KIDNEY REABSORPTION AND SECRETION	
Compound	Mechanism	Blocker
PROXIMAL TUBULE REABSORPTION		
Na^+	Facilitated diffusion	Amiloride
HCO_3^-	Na/H antiport	Carbonic anhydrase inhibitors
Cl^-	Diffusion	
K^+	Diffusion	
Water	Osmosis	
Glucose	Na-coupled transport	Phloritine
Amino acids	Na-coupled transport	
Urea	Diffusion	
Urate	Diffusion	
PROXIMAL TUBULE SECRETION		
Penicillin	Active transport	Probenecid
Para-amino hippuric acid (PAH)	Active transport	
Quinine, choline, thiamine, others	Active transport	
Creatinine	Active transport	
H^+	Na^+/H^+ antiport	Carbonic anhydrase inhibitors
THICK ASCENDING LIMB OF THE LOOP OF HENLE REABSORPTION		
Na^+	Na/K/2Cl transporter	Furosemide and bumetanide
K^+	Na/K/2Cl transporter	Furosemide and bumetanide
Cl^-	Na/K/2Cl transporter	Furosemide and bumetanide
Mg^{2+}	Electrochemical gradient	
NH_4	Na/K/2Cl transporter	Furosemide and bumetanide
THICK ASCENDING LIMB OF THE LOOP OF HENLE SECRETION		
H^+	H^+ ATPase	
DISTAL TUBULE REABSORPTION		
Na^+/Cl^-	NaCl symport	Thiazides
Na^+	Diffusion (aldosterone)	Amiloride, spironolactone
H^+ or HCO_3^-	Intercalated cells	Carbonic anhydrase inhibitors
DISTAL TUBULE SECRETION		
K^+	Aldosterone Na^+ reabsorption	Amiloride, spironolactone
H^+	H^+ ATPase	
COLLECTING DUCT REABSORPTION		
Urea	Transporters (ADH control)	
Water	Aquaporins, osmosis (ADH control)	
NaCl	NaCl symport	Thiazides

secretion in the distal tubule, and ADH increases water reabsorption. The filtrate that flows from the collecting duct into the ureter is the final excretory product or *urine*. The bladder stores urine for elimination but does not further modify urine composition.

Renal Mechanisms in Acid-Base Balance

Renal acid-base excretion complements pulmonary carbon dioxide (CO_2) elimination to regulate body acid-base status. Renal acids are hydrogen (H^+), ammonium, phosphate, and sulfate buffers. The renal base is predominantly bicarbonate (HCO_3^-). Because of the high HCO_3^- filtered load, reabsorption of HCO_3^- is the primary task of the tubule segments. This is accomplished in the proximal and distal tubules by H^+ secretion, and carbonic anhydrase–mediated CO_2 formation. Ultimately, urinary acid secretion is determined by plasma CO_2 levels.

Ammonium (NH_4^+) formation in the proximal tubule augments acid secretion, particularly in chronic acidosis. The proximal tubule cells metabolize glutamine to form ammonia (NH_3). NH_3 is uncharged and diffuses into tubular lumen, where it combines with secreted H^+ to form NH_4^+. Ionic NH_4^+ does not freely diffuse, and it remains in the lumen in a process termed *ammonia trapping*.

Distal nephron pH is regulated by intercalated cells. There are two populations of intercalated cells: one is oriented for HCO_3^- secretion, the other for H^+ secretion. Increased plasma CO_2 causes net sodium bicarbonate ($NaHCO_3$) reabsorption, correcting the acidosis. Decreased plasma CO_2 promotes net hydrochloric acid (HCl) reabsorption, correcting the alkalosis.

Clearance

The clearance principle assumes that the substance being cleared has been completely removed from a hypothetical amount of plasma. Clearance is the minimum flow of plasma required to deliver that substance to the kidney and is calculated as

$$C_x = \frac{U_x \dot{V}}{P_x}$$

$$clearance = \frac{urine\ concentration \times urine\ flow\ rate}{plasma\ concentration}$$

where U_x is urine concentration and $\dot{V}$ is urine minute volume.

Clearance of inulin or creatinine provides a noninvasive measurement of GFR, and clearance of para-aminohippurate (PAH) or Diodrast provides an estimate of renal plasma flow.

Free water clearance is the rate of solute-free plasma (water) added to or subtracted from urine flow necessary to make the urine isosmotic to plasma. It provides a measure of water balance. A client may be in *positive* free water clearance if urine osmolarity is less than plasma osmolarity or in *negative* free water clearance if urine osmolarity is greater than plasma osmolarity.

Urinary Concentration and Dilution

Urine osmolarity reflects the balance of water and solute reabsorption rates. It is determined by the medullary osmolarity and the amount of ADH acting on the collecting ducts. Glomerular filtrate is isosmotic with plasma (300 mOsm), and the filtrate osmolarity remains unchanged in the proximal tubule. Osmolarity increases in the descending loop of Henle. The ascending loop of Henle, where the Na/K/2Cl transporter removes ions but not water, causes the filtrate osmolarity to drop to 100 mOsm. This value is close to the lower limit of urine osmolarity, but some additional NaCl can be reabsorbed in the distal tubule and collecting duct. ADH acts on the distal tubule and collecting duct to increase water and urea permeability, allowing the filtrate to become isosmotic with the cortex (300 mOsm); if a large amount of ADH is present, filtrate becomes isosmotic with the inner medulla (1500 mOsm). The inner medulla osmolarity represents the upper limit on urine osmolarity.

REGULATION OF URINE FORMATION

Renal perfusion pressure is the dominant long-term regulator of glomerular filtrate formation and urine production (pressure diuresis and pressure natriuresis). However, other mechanisms also alter the rate of filtrate formation and the efficiency of filtrate reabsorption.

Tubuloglomerular feedback at the juxtaglomerular apparatus provides negative feedback control of filtrate formation. The juxtaglomerular apparatus is formed by the junction of the glomerular afferent arteriole and the macula densa of the distal convoluted tubule. A decrease in distal tubule NaCl delivery causes a reflex increase in GFR, both by afferent arteriolar dilation and an angiotensin II–mediated efferent arteriolar constriction. Blockade of angiotensin II formation reduces the effectiveness of this system and may cause a drop in GFR.

Neural regulation by the sympathetic nervous system also regulates urine formation. Sympathetic contraction of afferent arterioles reduces filtrate formation and enhances salt and water conservation. Renal sympathetics are activated in response to hypotension sensed by arterial baroreceptors and in response to hypovolemia sensed by cardiopulmonary volume receptors.

RENAL ENDOCRINE AND METABOLIC ACTIONS

Most endocrine actions of the kidney are tied to the cardiovascular system. The kidneys synthesize and secrete *erythropoietin,* the hormone that increases blood cell synthesis in the bone marrow. *Renin* release from the afferent arteriole ultimately leads to formation of vasoconstrictor angiotensin II and release of aldosterone. *Intrarenal prostaglandin* production assists the regional distribution of renal blood flow. One exception to the renal-cardiovascular connection is vitamin D. Vitamin D_3 is activated to 1,25-dihydroxycholecalciferol by renal proximal tubules to enhance calcium (Ca^{2+}) absorption.

Second only to the liver, the kidney has a powerful capacity for *gluconeogenesis.* Urine represents a possible loss pathway for nutrients, especially in disease. Proteinuria may cause a greater loss of protein than may be offset by ingestion. The glucosuria of diabetes may also represent a significant loss of potential calories.

MICTURITION

Urine production by the kidneys is relatively constant (~ 1 ml/min) but can vary from 0.5 to 20 ml/min. Flow through ureters is intermittent and is controlled by the rate of peristaltic wave generation. The peristalsis that forces the urine into the bladder for storage occurs every 10 to 150 seconds. Parasympathetic activation increases frequency of peristalsis, and sympathetic stimulation decreases frequency. Afferent (pain) nerves initiate the *ureterorenal reflex.* This reflex, activated by obstruction, causes ureter constriction and also causes afferent arteriolar constriction to decrease urine production. Lodging of kidney stones in the ureter is a major cause of this response.

Both sensory and motor components of the pelvic nerves supply the bladder. Activation of the parasympathetic nerves causes a contraction of the detrusor muscle (bladder). The internal sphincter at neck of bladder is normally contracted, but it is relaxed when the bladder muscle contracts. The external sphincter is skeletal muscle under voluntary control, innervated by pudendal nerves. These nerves are tonically active, but activity can be decreased when controlled from higher central nervous system (CNS) centers.

The *micturition reflex* is initiated when bladder filling increases wall tension above a threshold point. Sensory nerves transmit tension information to the spinal cord, where an increase in parasympathetic activity causes contraction of the detrusor muscle. This contraction further increases wall tension, increasing reflex parasympathetic activity and enhancing the contraction. The process repeats until tension plateaus (for a minute or so), the reflex fatigues, or the external sphincter is relaxed and the bladder empties. If emptying does not occur, the process begins again after a few minutes.

Urination is facilitated by abdominal contraction, which compresses the bladder and increases wall tension, initiating the reflex. The micturition reflex is modulated by descending inputs from higher CNS structures. The pons has both strong facilitatory and inhibitory centers. The cerebral cortex also can modulate the reflex, allowing voluntary control of the timing of urination.

EFFECTS OF AGING AND NUTRITION

Aging causes atrophy of the kidneys and a progressive loss of renal function. This change is usually not critical, because the kidneys have an excess function capacity. Damage or loss of one kidney, however, may allow the age-related changes to impair renal function in the remaining kidney. The increased capillary hydrostatic pressure caused by hypertension or protein ingestion causes progressive damage to glomeruli and accelerates the age-related decrease in renal function. Low-protein diets attenuate the age-related decrease in renal function and are recommended for clients with damaged kidneys.

The aging process also affects micturition. The bladder becomes funnel-shaped as a result of alterations in the connective tissue and weakening of the pelvic floor muscles. Irritability of the bladder wall often increases, adding more urgency to the normal desire to void. Finally, impairment of the detrusor muscle's ability to elongate results in decreased bladder capacity. Because of these changes, older people may have problems with incontinence, frequency, urine retention, or dysuria.

Dietary components can alter renal function at the glomerular and tubular levels. Ingestion of a protein-rich meal dilates the afferent arteriole and increases renal blood flow. The increase in glomerular capillary pressure increases the GFR. These responses are termed *postprandial renal hyperemia*.

CONCLUSIONS

The four organs of the urinary elimination system—kidneys, ureters, bladder, and urethra—work together to filter liquids and to remove waste from the body in the form of urine. The kidneys control fluid and electrolyte homeostasis and play a role in blood pressure regulation, red blood cell production, insulin degradation, prostaglandin synthesis, calcium and phosphorus regulation, and vitamin D metabolism. The body can survive minimal kidney dysfunction because of its excess-function capacity. However, serious renal dysfunction is life-threatening, requiring dialysis or transplantation.

BIBLIOGRAPHY

1. Fauci, A. S. (1998). *Harrison's principles of internal medicine.* New York: McGraw-Hill.
2. Guyton, A. C., & Hall, J. (1996). *Textbook of medical physiology* (9th ed.). Philadelphia: W.B. Saunders.
3. Silverthorn, D. (1998). *Human physiology.* Upper Saddle River, NJ: Prentice Hall.
4. Valtin, H., & Schaffer, J. A. (1995). *Renal function* (3rd ed.). Boston: Little, Brown.

CHAPTER 32

Assessment of Elimination

Roberta Jorgensen
Karen A. Hanson

In spite of advanced technology for diagnosing problems of elimination, every diagnostic evaluation is guided by an accurate, thorough, and documented assessment. Assessment of elimination is fundamental to the evaluation of the client.

Taking a health history requires exceptional skills in speaking, listening, observing, and interpreting the client's communication because anxiety and embarrassment often accompany discussion of bowel, urinary, or genital problems. Language and semantic barriers can interfere with communication, especially with the variety of terms used to describe bowel and urinary elimination. Differences in educational background can result in fear and poor communication when the client has difficulty understanding medical terminology. A calm, caring, and accepting atmosphere during the interview promotes communication. The client may wish to have a family member present to assist with describing the details of the problem or health history.

BOWEL ELIMINATION

HISTORY

Assessment of the lower gastrointestinal (GI) system begins with the health history, followed by physical examination of the abdomen, anus, and rectum and diagnostic studies. Review previous hospitalizations, surgery, recent exposure to infection, recent travel, current medications, habits, and family history. Explore family risk factors for lower GI disorders, such as a history of colon cancer. Determine whether the client has regular screening for colon cancer.

■ BIOGRAPHICAL AND DEMOGRAPHIC DATA

A thorough review of biographical and demographic characteristics helps to elicit data related to disorders that are more likely to occur. Many lower GI disorders are associated with age and sex. For example, colorectal cancer is predominantly a disease of older adults, peaking in the seventh decade.[19] Ulcerative colitis occurs more frequently in whites and in those of Jewish descent. Diver-

ticular disease is most common in individuals living in developed countries whose diets consist primarily of refined foods. Diverticular disease is also more common in older people. In the United States, diverticulitis develops in approximately one third of the population by age 50 and in almost two thirds by age 80.[13]

■ CURRENT HEALTH

A simple, open-ended question, such as "How are you feeling?" may elicit concerns about conditions that contribute to the current health problem. Explore potentially relevant areas such as the client's social situations, life events, and difficulties surrounding the health problem. Many lower GI manifestations are vague and have various causes.

Chief Complaint

Allow clients to describe the chief complaint in their own words. Elicit information about and learn to recognize a wide variety of manifestations that are potentially associated with a specific GI disorder. Manifestations include abdominal cramping, gaseousness, or rectal pain and may be influenced by socioeconomic status and culture. Objective findings, such as ascites and rebound tenderness, may be observed upon physical examination. For any lower GI disorder, some manifestations may occur together. With experience, you will learn to recognize these as they relate to a specific GI disorder.

Symptom Analysis

Obtain more specific information about the problem by means of a symptom analysis (see Chapter 9). Include the following.

TIMING. When was the problem first noticed? How long did it last? Was the onset abrupt or insidious? Where was the client when it occurred? Has the problem been present since that time? Abrupt onset of abdominal pain could indicate emergent conditions such as appendicitis, volvulus, or bowel obstruction. Pain of gradual onset may be related to acute inflammation of the colon or diverticula, severe gastroenteritis, or constipation and gas.

Is the problem related to food intake? If diarrhea is present, ask about awakening during the night because of diarrhea. If this is the case, it may indicate *inflammatory bowel disease* rather than *irritable bowel syndrome* (IBS).[22]

QUALITY AND QUANTITY. Ask the client to describe the problem in detail. If the complaint is lower abdominal pain, determine whether it is sharp, dull, aching, burning, intermittent, or spasmodic. If the pain is deep, dull, and diffuse, it is probably visceral in origin, that is, the result of localized inflammation or ischemia. Pain that is sharp and more localized may be parietal or peritoneal pain that might be the result of generalized inflammation. If the client has noticed bloody stools, ask whether bleeding occurs with every bowel movement or only on occasion. Ask whether the blood is mixed in with the stool or present only on the surface.

LOCATION. Assist the client in defining and locating abdominal pain. Does the pain radiate? The location of pain provides clues to common causes. Right upper quadrant pain may be hepatic in origin, resulting from disorders such as hepatitis, liver abscess, or perihepatitis. Right lower quadrant pain may indicate appendicitis. Left upper quadrant pain may result from splenic rupture, infarct, or abscess. Left lower quadrant pain suggests a left colon origin and may indicate diverticulitis or ischemic colitis.[22] Generalized abdominal pain suggests a number of possible causes such as appendicitis, intestinal obstruction, inflammatory bowel disease, or generalized peritonitis.

PRECIPITATING FACTORS. Are there events that occur in relation to or before the problem onset, such as stress, specific foods, medications, or activity? Does the problem occur at a certain time of the day? In cases of suspected gastroenteritis, has the client's source of drinking water changed recently, or has the client eaten unusual foods such as wild mushrooms or improperly handled food?

AGGRAVATING AND RELIEVING FACTORS. Are there situations that worsen the problem? Are there particular medications or actions that have provided relief? What has the client done to make the situation better?

ASSOCIATED MANIFESTATIONS. Has the client noticed other manifestations that have become apparent recently? Disturbances in lower GI elimination may affect appetite, energy level, and weight. In addition to or in association with the problem, are there other GI manifestations such as nausea, vomiting, early satiety, anorexia, eructation (belching), flatulence, diarrhea, constipation, abdominal distention, heartburn, or indigestion? Does the client have food intolerances, abdominal cramping, weight gain or loss, hematemesis (vomiting of blood), melena (black, tarry stools), rectal pain, or anal pruritus? Other lower GI manifestations related to hepatic, biliary, or pancreatic disorders include jaundice, ascites, fatty stools, and colicky, abdominal pain. (Metabolic system assessment is discussed in Chapter 42.)

Abdominal pain that accompanies diarrhea is frequently associated with infectious gastroenteritis, inflammatory bowel disease, diverticulitis, and early intestinal obstruction. Constipation preceding abdominal pain by several days may be associated with diseases of the colon or rectum.

Explore all manifestations because a health problem related to the GI system rarely occurs in the absence of other manifestations or etiologic events. Clients may be aware of other relevant symptoms. Review the client's health status, discussing general health, diet, lifestyle, and health risk factors. It is an opportune time to assess the client's health awareness and implement health promotion teaching. (See Chapters 9 and 28 for discussions of diet history and nutritional assessment and this chapter for assessment of elimination patterns.)

■ PAST HEALTH HISTORY

The past health history includes information about the client's general state of health, past illnesses, immunizations, injuries, hospitalizations, surgeries, current medications, and allergies.

Childhood and Infectious Diseases

Inquire about both childhood and adult problems. In addition to asking about common childhood infectious diseases, specifically question the client about hepatitis, intestinal infections, encephalitis, sexually transmitted diseases, and human immunodeficiency virus (HIV) infection.

Immunizations

Record the immunization history. Inquire whether the client has received routine childhood immunizations including *Haemophilus influenzae* type b (Hib) conjugate. Everyone should be immunized against hepatitis B, particularly people whose lifestyles put them at risk. In addition, inquire about hepatitis A vaccination, which is indicated for international travelers or those employed in day care settings. Ask whether immunizations are current, and note dates of the last tetanus booster and influenza vaccination.

Major Illnesses and Hospitalizations

Note all hospitalizations and major illnesses. Has the client been hospitalized or treated for abdominal pain, anemia, GI bleeding, change in bowel habits, colitis, unexplained weight loss, or colon cancer? What was the plan of care, and what was found? Ask for a summary of the hospitalization experience, including laboratory tests, diagnostic procedures, and the results obtained. Ask about previous operations, particularly those involving the GI tract or accessory organs.

Try to determine what was found as a result of hospitalization. A discharge summary may be beneficial in treating the current health problem. How has the client been since having an operation performed? If the colon was resected, as for cases of severe chronic ulcerative colitis, the client may be functioning and feeling much improvement.

Medications

Note all current medications and how they are taken. Ask about over-the-counter medications, such as vitamins, antacids, laxatives, enemas, pain relievers, herbal remedies, and nutraceuticals (health food supplements). Often, clients consider these medications and natural remedies not worth mentioning. Be aware of potential relationships between what is taken and the client's current GI manifestations. For example, nonsteroidal anti-inflammatory drugs (NSAIDs) can contribute to epigastric pain, gastric ulcers, and bleeding. Calcium preparations can cause constipation, as can iron preparations. Magnesium preparations can contribute to diarrhea. Soluble fiber products such as oat bran, dried beans, and psyllium reduce fat absorption and have a laxative effect. Herbs that can cause GI upset include milk thistle (*Silybum marianum*), goldenseal (*Hydrastis canadensis*), ginger (*Zingiber officinale*), kelp (*Fucus vesiculosus*), comfrey (*Symphytum officinale*), chaparral (*Larrea divaricata*), cayenne (*Capsicum*), and alfalfa (*Medicago sativa*).

Allergies

Ask about allergies that are related to the environment, food, or drugs. Seek specific details to determine the client's allergic response. Be careful to distinguish between foods that are merely difficult to tolerate and those that induce an actual allergic reaction. Ask what types of lower GI problems occur when the client ingests a particular food. Note allergic manifestations such as abdominal cramping, belching, or diarrhea.

■ FAMILY HEALTH HISTORY

A number of GI disorders have a familial association. Inquire whether any family members have been diagnosed with Crohn's disease, chronic ulcerative colitis (CUC), intestinal polyps, or colon cancer. Information about the family incidence of other GI-related disorders such as jaundice, hepatitis or other liver disease, bleeding ulcers, or irritable bowel syndrome is also relevant.

■ PSYCHOSOCIAL HISTORY

The psychosocial history includes information on occupation, current environment, life experiences, personal relationships, and lifestyle habits. Determine the client's knowledge about the manifestations and illness. Has the illness caused the client to lose time from work? Does the client have insight into the symptoms? Are there environmental or psychosocial factors that have changed recently in the client's situation?

Occupation and Environment

Explore the client's occupational and environmental history to determine whether exposure to disease-provoking substances or environments has occurred. Ask about occupational exposure to substances that may be toxic if ingested or absorbed. If travel is a regular part of the client's job, has there potentially been exposure to unusual or improperly handled foods or contaminated water? Does the client have any hobbies that involve possibly hazardous materials? Has there been increased stress in the workplace?

Geographical Location

Has the client recently traveled abroad and been exposed to contaminated food or drink? The enteropathogens most commonly responsible for traveler's diarrhea are transmitted via contaminated food or drink. The most frequent causes are bacterial pathogens, of which *Escherichia coli* is the most common. The most common protozoal infectious agent in travelers is *Giardia intestinalis (Giardia lamblia)*. Protozoa and helminths account for a greater proportion of cases of prolonged diarrhea after travel abroad.[19]

Exercise

Ask whether the client has a regular exercise program or whether physical activity is part of the daily routine. A sedentary lifestyle can be a causative factor in certain types of lower GI disorders, particularly constipation.[23]

Nutrition

Thorough assessment of dietary habits is essential when evaluating GI elimination disorders. The diet may be a causative factor, or it may have been altered in an attempt to ameliorate the manifestations. GI disorders may cause significant impairment of normal digestive function. In addition, nutritive factors may be responsible for GI disease, as exemplified by the relationship between a high-fat diet and the development of colorectal cancer and that between lack of dietary fiber and the development of diverticulosis.[15]

When assessing the diet, ask the client to describe what was eaten the previous day, as this is usually easiest to recall. Ask about consumption of high-fiber foods such as fruits and vegetables, whole grains, breads and cereals, red meats, and saturated fats. Are most of the meals eaten at home or at a restaurant, where there is a greater likelihood of high fat and sodium content? Assess the client's knowledge of what constitutes a healthy diet. Are there dietary modifications that might be made to improve the client's nutritional intake?

What fluids are consumed in a day and in what amounts? Ask about water, coffee, cola, and alcohol intake in a 24-hour period. Many GI symptoms attributed to irritable bowel syndrome may be related to excess alcohol and caffeine intake.[19]

Assess the relationships between dietary intake and resultant GI manifestations. Excessive ingestion of synthetic, nonabsorbable sugars such as sorbitol may cause diarrhea. Lactose intolerance occurs when the intestine does not produce enough lactase to digest lactose (milk sugar), resulting in abdominal bloating and cramping. It is the most common cause of osmotic diarrhea.[13] Chapter 28 discusses nutritional assessment.

Habits

Certain lifestyle habits may contribute to GI manifestations. Lack of a regular bowel elimination routine in the daily schedule can lead to chronic constipation. Excessive alcohol consumption, if not curtailed, may lead to gastritis and eventual hepatic damage.

Inquire whether the client is experiencing increased stress either at home or at work. Altered stress levels can bring about GI-related manifestations such as epigastric pain, ulcers, and diarrhea.

■ REVIEW OF SYSTEMS

Review possible GI manifestations, and check each system to uncover additional symptoms of "unrelated" illness. Are there problems in chewing or swallowing food? Ask about the condition of the teeth or whether dentures (if worn) fit properly. Are there sores in the mouth or on the tongue, or has there been difficulty with mouth dryness and odor?

Determine whether there has been a change in appetite, either excessive hunger or anorexia, or problems with indigestion such as excessive belching or heartburn. Has the client experienced abdominal pain, nausea, or vomiting? If there was vomiting, what was the character of the vomitus? Has there been a change in bowel movements such as change in color, consistency, or caliber? Has there been rectal bleeding or black, tarry stools? Does the client experience rectal pain or pruritus? In addition, determine whether there have been any manifestations related to the accessory organs of digestion, such as the development of jaundice, ascites, peripheral edema, generalized intractable pruritus, clay-colored stools, or dark urine.

PHYSICAL EXAMINATION

Physical examination of the lower GI tract includes the abdomen, anus, and rectum. Discussions of upper GI tract, liver, and spleen assessment appear in Chapters 28 and 42. An example of an abdominal assessment recording is given in Chapter 28.

■ ABDOMEN

Lower GI tract assessment begins with the abdomen. The abdomen is divided into either four quadrants or nine regions for descriptive purposes. Be familiar with the abdominal structures located in each of these areas. Figure 28–5 shows the quadrants and anatomic regions of the abdomen and their underlying organs.

The equipment for the examination of the abdomen and rectum includes a stethoscope, gloves, lubricant, tissues, materials for occult blood testing, and reagent. The client should be supine, with the abdomen fully exposed from the sternum to the knees (see Fig. 10–6). A sheet or towel may be placed over the genitalia. The arms should be at the sides and the legs extended. A pillow under the knees aids in relaxing the abdominal muscles. Stand at the client's right side. If the current problem is one of abdominal pain, examine the area of pain last to avoid stimulating tightening of the abdominal muscles (guarding). Proceed as follows: inspection, auscultation, percussion, palpation, and rectal examination.

Inspection

Inspect the abdominal contour for evidence of distention, masses, asymmetry, or visible peristaltic waves, which are abnormal and should be reported. In addition, note scars, striae, petechiae, and the presence of dilated veins. Note the shape, position, and color of the umbilicus. A protruding umbilicus may indicate ascites, mass, or an umbilical hernia.

Assess for inguinal, umbilical, and femoral hernias by asking the client to cough. A sudden bulge may indicate a hernia. In addition, coughing may elicit localized pain. Lastly, ask the client to perform the Valsalva maneuver (if not contraindicated) or attempt a stomach curl. Look for a separation of the rectus muscles at the midline (*diastasis recti*), which may be accompanied by a bulge. This condition results from obesity, pregnancy, or problems in which sustained elevated intra-abdominal pressure weakens the muscles.

Auscultation

Auscultation of bowel sounds provides information about the motion of liquid and air through the intestinal tract. Perform auscultation before percussion and palpation. Palpation and percussion may affect intestinal motility and therefore alter bowel sounds.

While the client is supine, place the diaphragm of the stethoscope over the midabdomen. Normal bowel sounds are high pitched and heard every 5 to 10 seconds. If no sounds are heard after listening for at least 2 minutes, bowel sounds are considered absent. The absence of bowel sounds suggests a paralytic ileus that may be related to diffuse peritoneal irritation.[20] Rushes of rapid high-pitched bowel sounds or *borborygmi* are associated with hyperperistalsis and may be present in gastroenteritis or early intestinal obstruction.

Auscultation helps to determine whether an abdominal *bruit* is present. Place the diaphragm of the stethoscope in the midline of the abdomen 2 inches above the umbilicus, and listen carefully for an aortic bruit. Next, listen at a point 2 inches above the umbilicus and 1 to 2 inches laterally on both sides of midline for a renal bruit. A renal bruit may indicate renal artery stenosis. Bruit is discussed further in Chapter 51.

A *peritoneal friction rub*, like a pleural or pericardial rub, indicates inflammation. During respiration, a friction rub may be heard in the right or left upper quadrant, suggesting hepatic or splenic pathology.[20] A rub is described further in Chapter 10.

Percussion

Percussion is used to detect the presence of fluid, gaseous distention, or solid masses and to determine the location and size of abdominal organs, primarily the liver and spleen. At times, it may be preferable to palpate before percussion, especially if the client is complaining of abdominal pain.

The client should be supine. Evaluate all four quadrants. The most common percussion note heard in the abdomen is *tympany* (high pitched, loud, or musical), which is due to the presence of gas in the stomach, small bowel, and colon. If the bladder is full, the suprapubic area may sound *dull* (thud-like sounds over fluid or solid organs) when percussed (see the discussion of bladder percussion later). Percussion of the liver and spleen is discussed in Chapter 42.

If ascites is suspected, a special percussion test for *shifting dullness* may be performed by nurses who have advanced assessment skills. Ascitic fluid sinks to the lower abdomen as a result of gravity (when standing), shifts to the side of the abdomen (when lying on one's side), and bulges in the flanks (when supine). While the client is supine, the borders between the areas of tympany and dullness are percussed. The area of tympany is due to gas in the bowel present above the ascites and is located above the area of dullness. The client is then asked to turn on the side, and the nurse again percusses the abdomen. If ascites is present, the area around the umbilicus that was initially tympanic becomes dull because the ascites has shifted to the more dependent position.[20] Ascites may also be detected by determining the presence of a *fluid wave*. This advanced assessment technique is discussed in Chapter 42.

Palpation

Abdominal palpation usually proceeds from light to deep and then to the liver, spleen, and kidneys. The client is supine, and the examination begins with the area of the abdomen that is farthest from the area of pain, if present.

Light palpation is used to detect masses, areas of muscular spasm or rigidity, and areas of direct tenderness. Deep palpation is used to determine the size and shape of abdominal organs and masses. Deep palpation is used primarily by nurses in advanced practice areas. Palpation techniques are discussed in detail in Chapter 10.

If the abdominal rectus muscles do not relax and soften during expiration, abdominal *rigidity* is present. Rigidity may indicate peritoneal irritation if diffuse or an inflamed gallbladder if localized. In clients who complain of abdominal pain, palpation is performed gently.

Perform a test for *rebound tenderness* if the client has abdominal pain. Palpate slowly and deeply away from the area of suspected inflammation; then quickly withdraw the palpating hand. The feeling of pain on the side of the inflammation that occurs when the palpating hand is withdrawn is called rebound tenderness. Because this maneuver may induce generalized pain, perform this test at the end of the abdominal examination.

Palpation of the liver and spleen is discussed in Chapter 42, and palpation of the kidneys is discussed later in this chapter.

■ ANUS AND RECTUM

The abdominal examination concludes with examination of the anus and rectum. Maintain a calm, matter-of-fact approach because it is often embarrassing for the client.

Most nurses perform only a visual inspection of the perianal area, but advanced practice nurses can perform a complete digital examination of the rectum. Be familiar with rectal anatomy and expected physical findings. This information is necessary when digitally assessing for rectal impaction or administering rectal medications (Fig. 32–1).

Inspection

Perform the rectal examination with female clients in the lithotomy position immediately after the pelvic examination, in Sims' position, or in a dorsal recumbent position.

Male clients may be examined either in Sims' position or standing and leaning across the examination table, which makes examination of the prostate gland easier. Spread the buttocks apart with the gloved nondominant hand, and examine the anus and surrounding tissue.

Inspect perianal skin for signs of inflammation, rashes, nodules, ulceration, fissures (cracks), fistulous openings, and hemorrhoids (dilated veins seen as reddened skin protrusions). Normally, the anus looks moist and hairless with coarse folded skin that is more darkly pigmented than the perianal skin. The anal opening should be tightly closed. No lesions should be present. Inspect the sacrococcygeal area, which is normally smooth and even. Ask the client to strain while you look for evidence of rectal prolapse (protrusion of rectal mucosa through the anal opening), internal hemorrhoids, polyps, or fissures. There should be no break in the skin integrity or protrusion through the anal opening.

Palpation

Inform the client that a rectal examination will be performed. Tell the client that there will be the sensation of a cool lubricant and a feeling as if having a bowel movement.

Use the gloved nondominant hand to spread the buttocks apart, and place the lubricated index finger of the other hand on the anus. Apply gentle pressure over the anus, thereby relaxing the sphincter. Instruct the client to take a deep breath as the index finger is inserted into the anal canal. The anal sphincter should close completely around the examining finger, at which time sphincter tone may be assessed. Advance the examining finger approximately 6 to 10 cm (2 to 4 inches) into the rectum in the direction of the umbilicus. The rectal mucosa should feel smooth and be nontender. Note irregularities such as polyps, masses, or undue tenderness, and describe their location and characteristics. Once the index finger is fully inserted, instruct the client to bear down again and feel for a mass descending from above against the palpating finger. A mass should be absent.

In a female client, the cervix of the uterus may be felt through the rectovaginal wall along the anterior rectum (see Chapter 37). The rectovaginal wall is firm, smooth, and resilient. In a male client, the prostate gland may be palpated through the anterior rectal wall. This part of the examination is discussed in Chapter 37.

Note the color of the fecal material present on the glove when you withdraw your finger. Mucus; blood; or tan, gray, or black tarry stool is abnormal. Test the fecal material for occult blood (described later in this chapter). If a sexually transmitted disease is suspected, obtain a rectal culture (see the discussion later in this chapter). Wipe the perianal area clean, and inform the client that the examination is completed.

DIAGNOSTIC TESTS

Diagnostic tests are performed to determine the nature of the lower GI disorder. The general methods of diagnosis include laboratory tests (Table 32–1), radiographic stud-

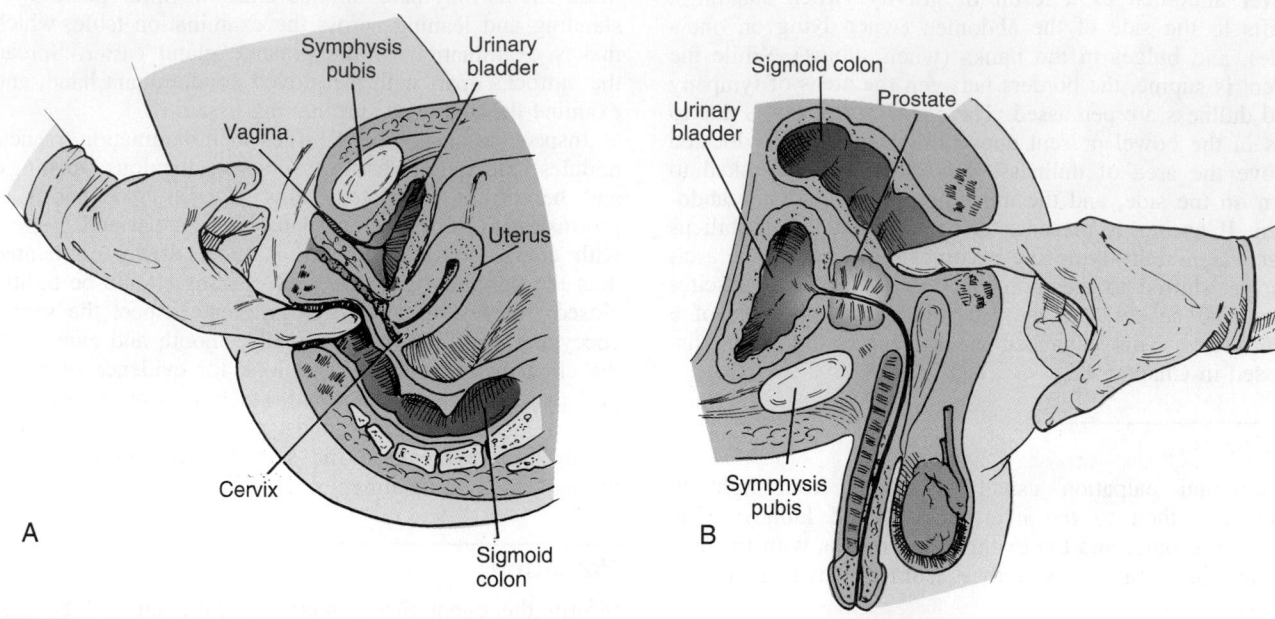

FIGURE 32–1 Palpation of the rectum in female *(A)* and in male *(B)* clients.

TABLE 32–1	LABORATORY TESTS USED TO ASSESS LOWER GASTROINTESTINAL (GI) FUNCTION	
Test	**Normal Findings**	**Abnormal Findings**
COMPLETE BLOOD COUNT		
Red blood cells	4.2–5.4 million/mm³ (women) 4.5–6.2 million/mm³ (men)	Decreased values may indicate anemia or hemorrhage
Hemoglobin	12–16 g/dl (women) 14–18 g/dl (men)	Increased values indicate possible hemoconcentration, caused by dehydration
Hematocrit	38%–46% (women) 42%–54% (men)	
ELECTROLYTES		
Potassium	3.5–5.0 mEq/L	Decreased values indicate possible GI suction, diarrhea, vomiting, intestinal fistulas
Calcium	8.0–10.5 mg/dl	Decreased values indicate possible malabsorption
Sodium	135–145 mEq/L	Decreased values indicate possible malabsorption and diarrhea
CEA		
	<5 ng/ml (nonsmokers)	Increased values indicate possible colorectal cancer and inflammatory bowel disease
FECAL ANALYSIS		
Stool for occult blood	Negative	Presence indicates possible peptic ulcer, cancer of the colon, ulcerative colitis
Stool for ova and parasites	Negative	Presence of *Entamoeba histolytica* (amebiases) or *Giardia lamblia*
Stool cultures	No unusual growth	Presence of *Salmonella typhi* (typhoid fever), *Shigella* (dysentery) *Escherichia coli* (gastroenteritis), *Staphylococcus aureus* (food poisoning), *Clostridium botulinum* (food poisoning), or *Aeromonas*
Stool for lipids	2–6 g/24 hr (normal diet)	Steatorrhea (increased values) can result from intestinal malabsorption or pancreatic insufficiency

ies, ultrasonography, and endoscopy. Hematologic studies and electrolyte determinations offer additional information; however, these reflect primarily general health status.

■ LABORATORY TESTS

Carcinoembryonic Antigen

Carcinoembryonic antigen (CEA) is a glycoprotein secreted on the glycocalyx surface of cells lining the GI tract and is normally produced during the first or second trimester of fetal life. High CEA levels are characteristic of various malignant conditions such as cancer of the colon, lung, or breast and of certain nonmalignant conditions such as liver disease, cirrhosis, alcoholic pancreatitis, heavy smoking, and inflammatory bowel disease.

CEA levels cannot be used as a general indicator of cancer, but they are useful for preoperative staging of colorectal cancer and assessing the adequacy of surgical resection. Often called a tumor marker, CEA is used to monitor the effectiveness of colorectal cancer therapy. Serum levels usually return to normal within 6 weeks if cancer treatment is successful.

Perform venipuncture and collect the sample in a 7-ml red-top tube. Handle the sample gently to prevent hemolysis, which may alter test results. There is no postprocedure care.

■ FECAL ANALYSIS

Fecal analysis aids evaluation of digestive efficiency and the integrity of the stomach and intestines. Analysis begins with gross examination of stool color, consistency, odor, and other characteristics and concludes with microscopic, chemical, or bacterial analysis.[22]

If the colon is partially obstructed or loses its elasticity, stool in transit may cause bleeding. Blood in the stool also may result from hemorrhoids. A black, tarry stool can result from upper GI bleeding. A large, bulky, foul-smelling stool that floats in the toilet may indicate fat malabsorption. Diarrhea is a result of too rapid transit of food in the GI tract, often caused by a viral infection. Mucus or pus in the stool may be a result of rectal abscesses or ulcerative colitis. A stool specimen is often required for diagnosis of infectious diseases, GI bleeding, and other GI tract disorders. Because stool specimens cannot be obtained on demand, close cooperation is necessary to secure a suitable specimen.

Fecal Occult Blood Tests

Fecal occult blood tests are most useful in screening asymptomatic clients at risk for developing colorectal cancer or in detecting GI bleeding. The Hemoccult test is widely used to detect occult blood in the feces. It is based on the change in color of a guaiac-based colorless dye to blue caused by the peroxidase activity of hemoglobin.

The Hemoccult test has been used in screening programs for colon cancer. Annual fecal occult blood testing, in conjunction with flexible sigmoidoscopy every 3 to 5 years, has been recommended by the American Cancer Society for screening people between 40 and 50 years of age.[12]

The fecal occult blood test can be performed immediately after the rectal examination or on stool specimens collected over 3 days. Two samples from each of the consecutive stools are tested to avoid false-positives. A wooden applicator is used to apply stool to one side of guaiac-treated paper. Developing solution is applied, and the result is immediately noted. Blue indicates a positive reaction and should be reported.

The client should abstain from rare meat and peroxidase-rich foods such as raw fruits and vegetables for 3 days before the test. Aspirin and NSAIDs, which may increase GI bleeding, should be withheld, although clients with painful arthritis may find this difficult. There is no postprocedure care.

Stool Examination for Ova and Parasites

Examination of a stool specimen can detect intestinal infection caused by several types of parasites and their ova (eggs). Wear gloves, and collect the stool specimen directly in the container. Note the date and time of the collection, the consistency of the specimen, pertinent dietary history, and recent or current antimicrobial therapy. The specimen should be sent to the laboratory within 30 minutes of passage or refrigerated if it is not examined immediately.

Instruct the client to avoid treatments with castor oil or mineral oil, bismuth, magnesium or antidiarrheal compounds, barium enemas, and antibiotics for 7 to 10 days before the test. Three specimens should be tested by collection of a stool every other day or every third day. There is no postprocedure care.

Stool Cultures

Bacteriologic examination of the stool identifies pathogens that may be causing overt GI disease. Identifying these organisms is necessary to treat the client and thereby prevent potentially serious complications. A sensitivity test may follow isolation of the pathogen. Some viruses may also cause GI symptoms, but these viruses can be detected only by immunoassay or electron microscopy.

A stool specimen is collected on 3 consecutive days. Wear gloves to obtain the specimen, which is collected directly in the container. Stool may also be collected by means of a rectal swab inserted past the anal sphincter, rotated gently, and withdrawn. Place the swab in the appropriate container, and send immediately to the laboratory. Note the dietary history, recent antimicrobial therapy, and any recent travel that might indicate endemic infection or infestation. There is no postprocedure care.

Fecal Lipids

Dietary lipids, emulsified by bile, are almost completely absorbed in the small intestine provided that there are adequate biliary and pancreatic secretions. However, both digestive and absorptive disorders may cause *steatorrhea* (excessive secretions of fecal lipids). A quantitative test performed on stool collected over a 72-hour period confirms the presence of steatorrhea. Collect the stool in a non-wax container and keep refrigerated.

Instruct the client to abstain from alcohol and to consume a high-fat diet (100 g/day) for 3 days before the test and during the collection period. Drugs that may affect test results, such as mineral oil, potassium chloride, and neomycin, should be withheld. There is no postprocedure care.

■ RADIOGRAPHY

Flat Plate of the Abdomen

A flat plate of the abdomen is an x-ray film of the abdominal organs. It is used to help identify tumors, obstructions, abnormal gas collections, and strictures.

Lower Gastrointestinal Series (Barium Enema)

PROCEDURE

A barium enema is administered for the radiographic examination (with or without fluoroscopy) of the large intestine. Barium sulfate (single-contrast technique) or barium sulfate and air (double-contrast technique) are instilled rectally. The test is indicated for clients with a history of altered bowel habits, lower abdominal pain, or passage of blood, mucus, or pus in the stools. The test helps detect tumors, diverticula, stenoses, obstructions, inflammation, ulcerative colitis, and polyps.

PREPROCEDURE CARE

Adequate preparation is essential and varies among agencies. Typical preparation includes a low-residue or clear liquid diet for 2 days before the test to reduce feces volume. The client usually receives a potent laxative and an oral liquid preparation for cleaning the bowel the day before the test and has nothing by mouth (*nil per os*, NPO) after midnight. The morning of the examination, a suppository or cleansing enema may be administered. If the client has active bleeding or an ileostomy, different bowel preparations may be needed. *If ultrasonography, an abdominal scan, or colonoscopy is also indicated, it should be performed first because barium interferes with these tests.* The procedure is uncomfortable and takes 60 to 90 minutes.

POSTPROCEDURE CARE

Barium impaction is a serious complication after a lower GI series if the barium is not evacuated. A laxative or cleansing enema is often given after the test to empty the large bowel. Stools are white for 24 to 72 hours after the examination. Encourage the client to increase liquid intake to prevent fecal impaction. Instruct the client to report any pain, bloating, absence of stool, or bleeding.

Computed Tomography

Computed tomography (CT) is a complementary test in assessing acute diverticulitis and abscess formation, diagnosing colorectal cancer, and staging rectal tumors. CT is a useful alternative to barium enema for clients who are unable to retain barium. CT is used primarily to identify masses such as neoplasms, cysts, focal inflammatory lesions, and abscesses of the liver, pancreas, and pelvic areas (see Chapter 11).

Ultrasonography

Ultrasonography is used to identify pathophysiologic processes in the pancreas, liver, gallbladder, spleen, and retroperitoneal tissues. Gas in the abdomen may interfere with the ultrasound waves (see Chapter 11).

■ ENDOSCOPY

Endoscopy is the direct visualization of the GI system by means of a lighted, flexible tube. The physician can directly observe sources of bleeding and surface lesions and determine the status of healing tissues.

Proctosigmoidoscopy

PROCEDURE

Proctosigmoidoscopy is the endoscopic examination of the lining of the distal sigmoid colon, the rectum, and the anal canal using two instruments: a proctoscope and a sigmoidoscope. Indications include a recent change in bowel habits, lower abdominal and perineal pain, prolapse on defecation, anal pruritus, and passage of mucus, blood, or pus in the stool. This procedure involves three steps: a digital examination, sigmoidoscopy, and proctoscopy.

During digital examination, the anal sphincters are dilated to detect any obstruction that might hinder the passage of the endoscope. During sigmoidoscopy, a 25- to 30-cm (10- to 12-inch) rigid sigmoidoscope is inserted into the anus to allow visualization of the distal sigmoid colon and rectum. The flexible sigmoidoscope also permits visualization of the descending colon. During proctoscopy, a 7-cm (2-inch) rigid proctoscope is inserted into the anus to aid examination of the lower rectum and anal canal. Specimens may be obtained by biopsy, lavage, cytology brush, or culture swab at any point during the procedure from the mucosal areas under suspicion.

PREPROCEDURE CARE

Explain to the client that proctosigmoidoscopy allows visual examination of the lining of the distal sigmoid colon, the rectum, and the anal canal. Describe the preparation for the procedure and the position assumed (knee-chest or left lateral). In addition, explain that some colicky, abdominal pain may result from passage of the instrument and introduction of air into the intestines. Reassure the client that there will be adequate draping to avoid embarrassment during the procedure. Obtain consent.

Agencies may specify various dietary and bowel preparations for this procedure. Clients are usually required to maintain a clear liquid diet for 24 to 48 hours before the test and to fast on the morning of the procedure. If a special bowel preparation is ordered, explain that this clears the intestine to provide a better view. A warm tap water or Fleet enema may be administered as ordered on the morning before the procedure.

POSTPROCEDURE CARE

Observe closely for signs of bowel perforation (malaise, rectal bleeding, abdominal distention and pain, mucopurulent drainage, and fever) and for vasovagal attack related to emotional stress (depressed blood pressure, pallor, diaphoresis, and bradycardia). If the knee-chest position was used, instruct the client to rest supine for several minutes before standing to avoid postural hypotension. As ordered, the client is given nothing by mouth and vital signs are monitored every 30 minutes until the client is alert.

Colonoscopy

PROCEDURE

Colonoscopy is the visual examination of the lining of the large intestine with a flexible fiberoptic endoscope. This procedure is indicated for clients with a history of constipation and diarrhea, persistent rectal bleeding, or lower abdominal pain when results of proctosigmoidoscopy and a barium enema are negative or inconclusive. Colonoscopy is also used to screen clients at high risk for colon cancer.

PREPROCEDURE CARE

The client is sedated and placed on the left side. After the colonoscope is inserted through the anus, a small amount of air is insufflated to locate the bowel lumen. The scope is advanced through the rectum into the sigmoid colon under direct visualization. When the instrument reaches the descending sigmoid junction, the client may be assisted to the supine position to aid the scope's advance past the splenic flexure. After the scope has passed the splenic flexure, it is advanced through the transverse colon and past the hepatic flexure into the ascending colon and cecum. Abdominal palpation or fluoroscopy may help guide the colonoscope through the large intestine.

POSTPROCEDURE CARE

Observe the client closely for signs of bowel perforation (malaise, rectal bleeding, abdominal pain and distention, fever, and mucopurulent drainage). Monitor vital signs as ordered until they are stable.

URINARY ELIMINATION

HISTORY

Urologic assessment includes assessment of elimination as well as sexual and reproductive function. This chapter describes urologic assessment, and Chapter 37 describes reproductive assessment.

■ BIOGRAPHICAL AND DEMOGRAPHIC DATA

Biographical and demographic data, such as age, gender, marital status, race, occupation, and geographical location, provide the framework for the health history. Gather specific information regarding sexual preference or practices to assess the client's risk of venereal disease or HIV infection. Certain diseases and health states are more common in specific groups of people. For example, urinary incontinence affects approximately 13 million Americans, with the highest prevalence in the elderly population. It is more common in women than in men (10% to 30% versus 1.5% to 5%) and often affects older multiparous women (who have had multiple pregnancies) in the form of stress incontinence.[3]

Benign prostatic hyperplasia (BPH), a benign growth of the prostate, occurs in men older than 50 years and often coincides with prostate cancer, possibly because of a common hormonal cause.[18] BPH is usually the cause of irritative and obstructive voiding manifestations in older adult men. Prostatitis can mimic some of the manifestations of BPH but is more likely to be the diagnosis if the client is younger than 40 years of age.

Black males and men older than age 40 are at risk for adenocarcinoma of the prostate. The incidence of prostate cancer doubles with each decade of life after age 40.[18] Testicular cancers most often occur in young men between ages 25 and 35. Bladder cancer occurs more often in men than in women and in white than in black males. Bladder cancer has been linked to a variety of environmental factors, such as aromatic amines in certain dyes and organic chemicals such as pesticides.[18]

■ CURRENT HEALTH

Clients with urologic complaints may find it embarrassing to discuss their problems. Establish a private, confidential, unhurried atmosphere when obtaining the history. Continually assess verbal and nonverbal feedback, evaluate nonjudgmentally and objectively, and provide information using language and diagrams that the client understands.

Chief Complaint

Upon identifying the chief complaint, ask specific questions about common urologic manifestations. Clients who have a urologic chief complaint describe manifestations in the categories of disturbances of voiding, alterations in urine characteristics, pain or referred pain, and systemic or GI manifestations.[24] More than one manifestation may be present. Explore each one.

Symptom Analysis

DISTURBANCES IN URINATION

Disturbances in urination include changes in urinary volume, irritative or obstructive manifestations, and urinary incontinence. Normal adult bladder capacity is about 300 to 500 ml. Adults normally void five or six times per 24 hours, more during the day than at night. Total daily urine output ranges between 800 and 1800 ml.[2] This amount varies with changes in the amount and type of fluid intake, amount of perspiration, environmental or ambient temperature, and the presence of vomiting or diarrhea. It may also be affected by pathologic changes in the urinary system.

CHANGES IN URINARY VOLUME. *Anuria* refers to a total urine output of less than 100 ml per 24 hours, and *oliguria* refers to a total urine output of 100 to 600 ml per 24 hours. Anuria and oliguria are associated with acute or chronic renal failure secondary to systemic events (shock, dehydration, reduced cardiac output), renal injury (glomerulonephritis, acute interstitial nephritis, renal artery aneurysms or emboli), or postrenal obstruction (ureteral, bladder outlet, or urethral).[10] *Polyuria* (voiding in unusually large daily amounts) may be associated with systemic disease (diabetes mellitus or diabetes insipidus, adrenal insufficiency), diuretic medication, or chronic renal disease resulting in electrolyte imbalance.

Review the client's health history to determine any known precipitating medical causes of urine volume changes. Inquire about the onset and duration of the urinary volume change to establish whether it is acute or chronic in nature or reflects an acute exacerbation of a chronic disease. Assess fluid intake, noting the amount and timing of consumption, especially of caffeinated and alcoholic beverages.

IRRITATIVE AND OBSTRUCTIVE MANIFESTATIONS. Irritative voiding symptoms of urgency, frequency, nocturia, and dysuria can occur with infection, inflammation, calculus, cancer, obstruction, or neurogenic dysfunction of the lower urinary tract (bladder, prostate, and urethra). Urgency and frequency are often present regardless of etiology and often appear in combination.

Urinary frequency, voiding more often than every 2 hours, is a common manifestation. It can occur because of changes in urine volume, decreased bladder capacity (such as with prostatic enlargement or detrusor instability), increased postvoid residual urine, inflammatory irritability of the bladder mucosa, and psychological disorders.

Urgency is a sudden strong desire to void that can usually be controlled. Urgency is caused by irritation of the lower urinary tract secondary to inflammation, calculus, bladder cancer, or neurogenic dysfunction.

Nocturia is excessive urination during the night (awakening with the need to urinate more than twice nightly). Nocturia may be related to the same urinary conditions listed for urinary frequency. It may also occur in clients who have circulatory problems that result in dependent edema during the day. The recumbent position helps to mobilize the sequestered fluids, resulting in increased venous return to the circulatory system and subsequent increased renal perfusion.

Dysuria, described as a burning sensation on initiation of, during, or at the end of urination, is usually associated with infection, inflammation, or, rarely, cancer of the bladder or urethra. It is usually accompanied by urgency and frequency.

Irritative manifestations may be accompanied by obstructive manifestations, such as hesitancy, straining to begin urination, intermittency, decreased force and caliber of the urinary stream, high postvoid residual, and urine retention. The cause is usually bladder outlet obstruction secondary to prostatic enlargement (in men), congenital urethral valves, urethral meatal stenosis, or urethral stricture. Symptom severity can be established for BPH by reference to the American Urologic Association (AUA) symptom index (Fig. 32–2). Neurologic diseases may mimic obstructive symptoms by affecting the innervation of the striated or smooth muscle components of the bladder and external sphincter, thereby impairing bladder contractility.

Hesitancy refers to delay in initiation of urination of at least 10 seconds. It is not associated with "bashful bladder," which can occur when urinating in a public restroom. It often leads to straining or pushing, which voluntarily increases intra-abdominal pressure to start the *urinary stream*. With prostatic obstruction or urethral stricture, straining is rarely helpful in initiating the stream.

When the client presents with obstructive manifestations, ask for a description of the urinary stream. Note whether (1) there is decreased force and caliber, (2) the stream is intermittent or interrupted (bladder stones or impaired bladder contractility), and (3) the stream is bifurcated or spraying (commonly seen with urethral stricture or meatal stenosis).

FIGURE 32–2 American Urologic Association (AUA) Symptom Index. (Modified from Barry, M. J., et al. [1992]. The American Urologic Association symptom index for benign prostate hyperplasia. *Journal of Urology, 148,* 1549–1557.)

Clients who have significant amounts of *postvoid residual* urine or *urinary retention*, usually greater than 100 ml, may describe a sense of incomplete bladder emptying. This is noted either as bladder fullness after urinating or more commonly as "double voiding," a second urination necessary within 5 to 15 minutes after the initial void. When clients experience long-standing high residual urine volumes, sometimes more than 1000 ml, they are considered to have *chronic urinary retention*. These clients experience little or no pain but may demonstrate other obstructive manifestations. Continual overflow incontinence is common because the bladder remains full to capacity at all times.

Acute retention is a sudden inability to void, accompanied by severe suprapubic pain (which distinguishes it from anuria) and urgency. It may occur postoperatively or post partum (after delivery), with use of certain medications, or with worsening of bladder outlet obstruction. It is a medical emergency requiring immediate intervention (e.g., urethral or suprapubic catheterization).

URINARY INCONTINENCE. *Urinary incontinence* refers to involuntary loss of urine. According to the Agency of Health Care Evaluation Clinical Practice Guidelines, urinary incontinence plagues 10% to 35% of adults and is widely underreported and underdiagnosed.[3] The social stigma and embarrassment of urinary incontinence result in loss of self-esteem and decreased ability to maintain an independent lifestyle. Decreased social interactions and decreased sexual activity are commonly reported. Considering the impact on one's quality of life, thoroughly investigate any mention of urinary incontinence by the client.

Urinary incontinence can be divided into several types: urge, reflex, stress, mixed, overflow, and functional.

Urge incontinence is the involuntary loss of urine associated with a strong desire to void. It is present with *detrusor instability* (DI) and normal bladder sensation.

Urge incontinence resulting from DI that is present without normal bladder sensation is considered *reflex incontinence*. Diseases of the spinal cord above the sacral micturition center (S2-4) produce reflex incontinence. DI with a neurologic cause is commonly referred to as *detrusor hyperreflexia*. It may also be accompanied by poor detrusor contractility and thus may contribute to difficulty emptying the bladder completely. Ask, "Are you able to feel when your bladder is full?" "Are you aware of urinary leakage when it happens?" "Do you still feel fullness in the bladder after you urinate?"

Stress incontinence is the leakage of urine with physical exertion or with an increase in intra-abdominal pressure but without actual detrusor contraction. Stress incontinence in women is most often due to urethral hypermobility associated with the pelvic descent that occurs after childbearing. In both sexes, it may be due to

intrinsic urethral sphincter deficiency (ISD), congenital or acquired, in which the sphincter cannot create enough resistance to retain urine. Ask when the urine loss occurs. Is it with coughing, sneezing, laughing, or other physical activity?

A combination of stress and urge incontinence, or *mixed incontinence*, typically occurs in older women. Urge incontinence is more distressing for the client, probably because there is less control in social situations.

Overflow incontinence is associated with chronic overdistention of the bladder secondary to impaired bladder contractility or bladder outlet obstruction. Clients present with frequent or constant dribbling or may have stress or urge incontinence.

Functional incontinence is associated with cognitive or physical impairments outside the lower urinary tract and is often seen in nursing home clients. It can often be remedied, even when it coexists with other types of incontinence, by changes in medications, improvements in hydration status, and removal of environmental barriers to toileting.

A careful interview and health history are instrumental in differentiating between the types of incontinence so that the appropriate diagnostic evaluation can be performed.

ALTERATIONS IN URINE CHARACTERISTICS

When evaluating urine characteristics, ask the client to describe (1) the color, (2) the clarity, and (3) the odor of the urine.

Urine *color* is affected by blood, changes in hydration status, certain diseases, and ingestion of certain foods or medications (Table 32–2). Color can be clinically significant, especially if the client reports even a single episode

TABLE 32–2	CAUSES OF URINE DISCOLORATION	
Color	**Disease Etiology**	**Medication, Dyes, Dietary**
Colorless	Chronic glomerulonephritis	Excessive fluid intake, alcohol, diuretics
	Diabetes mellitus	
	Diabetes insipidus	
Cloudy white	Phosphate in alkaline urine	
	Epithelial cells	
	Bacteria, pus, chyle	
Yellow	Concentrated urine	Tetracycline, rifampin
Dark yellow	Urobilinogen	Santonin, phenindione, rhubarb (in acid urine), nitrofurantoin, sulfasalazine, docusate calcium, thiamine (multivitamins)
Pink or red	Red blood cells	Beet ingestion, vegetable dyes, phenolphthalein laxatives (in alkaline urine), cascara (in alkaline urine), senna (X-Prep, Senokot), rhubarb (in alkaline urine)
	Hemoglobin	
	Urate excretion	
	Myoglobin	
	Serratia marcescens	
	Menstrual contamination	
Brown	Highly concentrated urine	Metronidazole (left standing), porphyrin
	Red blood cells	
Dark brown or black	Highly concentrated urine	Porphyrin (after standing), tyrosine, phenacetin, quinine, senna, methyldopa
	Bilirubin	
	Melanin	
	Red blood cells (old)	
Blue-green	Bilirubin	Methylene blue, indigo carmine, thymol, phenol, amitriptyline
	Pseudomonas	

of "bloody urine" (*hematuria*), which can be pink, red, tea colored, dark brown, or maroon and may or may not be accompanied by blood clots. Gross hematuria is often the only presenting manifestation of bladder cancer. If clots are present, question the client regarding their appearance. Clots from the ureter or kidney are often long and stringy, whereas those from the bladder or prostate are large and amorphous. Further define the hematuria by asking at which point during voiding it occurs. *Initial* hematuria indicates a urethral, prostatic, or seminal vesicle origin. *Terminal* hematuria indicates bleeding from the bladder neck, trigone, or posterior urethra. Hematuria throughout the stream may indicate glomerulonephritis. *Total* hematuria indicates profuse bladder, ureteral, or kidney hemorrhage. Rule out menstrual contamination in female clients. Urinary tract infection is a common cause of hematuria in women.

Urine *clarity* is affected by infection or inflammation of the urinary tract that results in bacteriuria and *pyuria* (white blood cells in the urine). Most typically, cloudy urine is due to amorphous phosphates in alkaline urine. Other causes of hazy or cloudy urine are epithelial cells from the lower urinary tract (contamination only), yeast, crystals, mucus, or fecal material. Milky urine results from prostatic fluid or semen, lipids, lymphatic fluid (chyle), or blood. Microscopic urinalysis determines the cause of the cloudiness. Figure 32–3 depicts examples of urine casts and crystals.

Urine *odor* is rarely of clinical significance, but strong-smelling or foul-smelling urine may indicate infection, and a sweet or fruit-like odor can be due to ketonuria. A strong ammonia odor may occur if the urine is left standing too long. Medications and dehydration can also affect urine odor.

Pneumaturia is the presence of gas in the urine during voiding. Pneumaturia suggests fistula formation between the bladder and bowel.

CRYSTALS

Cystine   Calcium   Uric acid   Triple-phosphate
           oxalate   (struvite)

A

CASTS

Hyaline cast   RBC cast   WBC cast

B

FIGURE 32–3 Urine clarity can be affected by crystals (A) and casts (B). RBC, red blood cell; WBC, white blood cell. (400× magnification.) (Modified from Walsh, P. C., et al. [Eds.]. [1998]. *Campbell's urology* [7th ed.]. Philadelphia: W. B. Saunders.)

PAIN OR REFERRED PAIN

Urinary tract disease does not always cause pain. When pain is present, ask the client to describe the location, intensity, onset, and duration to define the etiologic mechanism further. What seems to alleviate or worsen the pain? Is the pain affected by bladder fullness or urination? Is it better or worse with position change, ejaculation, or bowel movement?

Pain in the upper urinary tract (kidney and ureter) is frequently felt locally as a dull, constant ache in the costovertebral angle just lateral to the sacrospinal muscle and beneath the 12th rib posteriorly. Sudden distention of the renal capsule secondary to acute pyelonephritis or ureteral obstruction is typically the cause of renal pain. Renal distention may refer pain to the epigastric area as well as to the subcostal area toward the umbilicus and lower abdominal quadrant. Ask when the pain occurs. Costovertebral pain caused by mechanical back pain and radiculitis differs from renal pain in that it becomes worse with heavy physical work and position changes of the spine.

If the pain is colicky in nature, the ureter is probably involved. Ureteral colic may radiate to the bladder, scrotum, and testicle in a male and to the vulva in a female. Colicky pain can be continuous, spasmodic, severe, and unbearable. If ureteral stones are suspected, ask the client to identify the site of referred pain to help identify the location of the stone. Upper ureteral stones result in pain referred to the testicles, midureteral stones cause pain referred to the intestine, and stones near the ureteral orifices in the bladder cause irritative bladder symptoms. Manifestations tend to be localized in adults but are more generalized in children, who often present with only GI symptoms of abdominal pain, nausea, and vomiting.

Bladder pain is usually associated with acute overdistention, infection, or irritation of the bladder wall. Acute urinary retention causes agonizing suprapubic pain and sometimes bladder spasms, which are experienced as intermittent, cramping, severe pain in the bladder. Bladder spasms also result from irritation of the bladder wall by a foreign body, such as an indwelling urinary catheter, infection, or bladder tumors. With bladder infections there may be only pain referred to the distal urethra, causing dysuria while voiding.

In the absence of a bacterial infection, symptoms of urgency and frequency can be caused by *interstitial cystitis,* a type of local autoimmune disorder that occurs most often in middle-aged women. Interstitial cystitis is often debilitating and poorly understood.[10] Pain in the spine or bony structure of the pelvis or pain that radiates down one or both legs may be due to metastasis of prostate, kidney, or bladder cancer.

Prostate pain is not common. Men with acute prostatitis may feel fullness in the rectum or perineum, have irritative voiding manifestations, and have postejaculatory pain. Testicular pain secondary to orchitis, trauma, or torsion of the spermatic cord is usually localized and severe and may radiate along the spermatic cord to the lower abdomen. Pain may be referred to the testicle from an inguinal hernia or upper ureteral stone.

Epididymal pain results from acute infection and initially occurs as local pain and swelling in the scrotum.

The pain can progress to an exquisitely painful mass involving the entire hemiscrotum, possibly radiating to the groin and lower abdomen. Epididymal pain is relieved by elevating the scrotum (Prehn's sign).

Pain in the urethra is localized and results from inflammation and irritation of the urethral mucosa. It occurs with urethral stricture, urethritis, or urethral cancer. Urethral pain may be more apparent before and after voiding.

SYSTEMIC MANIFESTATIONS

Fever and chills are usually associated with acute, not chronic, infectious processes in the urinary tract such as cystitis, pyelonephritis, prostatitis, and epididymitis. GI manifestations such as nausea, vomiting and diarrhea, abdominal distention, and pain commonly occur with many urinary tract disorders. With "silent" urologic disease, GI manifestations may be the only presenting complaint.

Renal pathology causes GI symptoms for several reasons. The renointestinal reflexes, which arise from common autonomic and sensory innervations of the urinary and GI tract, can trigger pylorospasm or changes in the smooth muscle of the GI tract when there is distention of the renal capsule. The kidneys are anatomically related to the colon, duodenum, liver, spleen, pancreas, diaphragm, and psoas muscle; inflammation of the kidney may create manifestations in any of these intraperitoneal or retroperitoneal organs. Anteriorly, the kidneys are covered by the peritoneum; thus, renal inflammation may provoke muscle rigidity and rebound tenderness.

Evaluate the client carefully for signs of infection if renal failure is suspected or confirmed. Sepsis is the most common cause of death in clients with renal failure.[11] Observe for manifestations of end-stage renal disease, such as edema, confusion, lethargy, weakness, and muscle twitching or cramps. Weight loss and lethargy can occur with advanced stages of urinary cancer.

■ PAST HEALTH HISTORY

In obtaining the past health history, inquire about coexisting systemic disease. Many disorders affect urinary function. Because urinary tract infection, retention, urinary calculi, or incontinence can be chronic or recurrent, explore any history of these disorders, including treatments implemented and their outcomes.

Childhood and Infectious Diseases

Congenital anomalies of the urinary tract are common but range in severity from being incidental radiologic findings to being incompatible with life. The kidney may be absent (renal agenesis), dysplastic or atrophic, ectopic (located outside the flank position), or fused (joined, as in "horseshoe" kidney). Note when a client has a solitary kidney because treatment must be tailored to preserve optimal renal function. Children with ectopic or fused kidneys are likely to have other genitourinary, skeletal, GI, or cardiovascular anomalies. When ectopia or fusion occurs alone, it is often asymptomatic. Ureters can be ectopic, incomplete, or absent (agenesis); duplicated; or markedly dilated (megaureter). Bladder extrophy, persistent urachus, and epispadias are congenital anomalies that require reconstructive surgery and potentially lead to long-term problems with urinary incontinence.

Malformations of the spinal cord, such as meningomyelocele and spina bifida, can cause neuropathic voiding disorders. Childhood streptococcal infections, mononucleosis, mumps, measles, and cytomegalovirus infections can result in acute glomerulonephritis.

Trauma

Is there a history of a motor vehicle accident, falls, straddle injury, penetrating abdominal injury, or contact sports injury? Assess the injury, how long ago it occurred, and the medical or surgical management that followed. The most frequent renal injury is blunt trauma, which is often managed conservatively, whereas penetrating trauma is usually explored surgically. Assessment of blunt or penetrating renal injury involves observing for a flank mass, tenderness, or bruising, especially when there is visible evidence of abdominal trauma. Long-term complications are rare with early intervention and careful follow-up.

Injury to the ureters is rare and most often occurs after penetrating wounds or complicated pelvic surgery. If ureteral injury is promptly corrected surgically, long-term complications are rare. When treatment is delayed, the client may experience flank or abdominal pain, peritonitis, paralytic ileus, fever, and possibly fistulae. Delayed diagnosis increases the risk of renal damage secondary to infection, hydronephrosis, abscess formation, and ureteral stricture.

Bladder trauma is related to the amount of urine in the bladder at the time of the injury; the bony pelvis protects the empty bladder. Suspect trauma anytime a pelvic fracture has occurred. If the bladder wall is ruptured by a penetrating or blunt injury to the lower abdomen, urine may extravasate into the peritoneal cavity and cause an acute abdomen or peritonitis if the urine is contaminated. Typically, the client has suprapubic pain or is unable to void. Gross hematuria is usually present. Complications of bladder injury are rare if it is treated promptly but can include temporary incontinence.

Urethral injuries are more common in males than females and can occur with instrumentation such as endoscopy or catheterization, straddle injury of the anterior urethra (distal to the urogenital diaphragm), or pelvic fracture in the posterior urethra (proximal to the urogenital diaphragm). In females, urethral injury is sometimes seen after traumatic intercourse, childbirth, or vaginal surgery. Assess for blood at the meatus, urinary retention, and bladder distention. Partial or complete disruption of the urethra may lead to urethral stricture, which can restrict urinary flow and predispose to urinary tract infections.

Major Illnesses and Hospitalizations

Ask about recent illnesses, including diarrhea, vomiting, trauma (abdominal, pelvic, or vascular), and any associated manifestations such as visual disturbances or excessive thirst. Include chronic diseases that may affect urinary function. Hypertension, diabetes, electrolyte imbalance, coronary artery disease, heart failure, and anemia worsen renal disease. Diabetes mellitus and multiple sclerosis can impair urinary and erectile function by interfering with autonomic function of the bladder.

A history of tuberculosis is significant when a client reports manifestations of renal insufficiency or failure, ureteral obstruction, or chronic urinary tract infections. *Mycobacterium tuberculosis* may travel from the lungs to the genitourinary organs and cause a chronic granulomatous infection. A history of tuberculosis helps to differentiate between tuberculosis of the bladder and interstitial cystitis.

Clients with a history of sickle cell anemia are at risk for papillary necrosis of the kidney and erectile dysfunction secondary to recurrent priapism. If renal neoplasm is suspected, inquire whether the client has von Hippel–Lindau syndrome, an autosomal dominant disorder that causes angiomatous cerebellar cysts, angiomatosis of the retina, and tumors of the pancreas; it is associated with cysts or adenocarcinoma of the kidneys. Disorders of the central nervous system can also affect innervation of the bladder. Disorders leading to hypercalcemia, such as hyperparathyroidism, limited mobility, and excessive vitamin D intake, can predispose to renal stones, obstruction, and subsequent renal failure. External beam radiation therapy for bladder or prostate cancer can cause radiation cystitis.

Scleroderma, an autoimmune disorder characterized by massive deposits of collagen, may involve the kidneys. Erythema multiforme, an inflammatory disorder of the skin associated with allergic or toxic reactions to drugs or microorganisms such as *Mycoplasma pneumoniae* and herpes simplex virus, can involve the kidneys of young adults and children in its most severe form (Stevens-Johnson syndrome). Systemic lupus erythematosus may lead to glomerulonephritis with hypertension and nephrotic syndrome.

Operations

Previous abdominopelvic or genitourinary procedures can affect urinary function through accidental trauma to the ureters and bladder. Document all invasive procedures, especially if the client may need surgery again. Ask about previous surgery for urinary calculus, obstruction, or incontinence. Surgical management of urologic cancers includes radical nephrectomy, transurethral resection and fulguration of bladder tumors, radical cystectomy with urinary diversion, and radical prostatectomy with pelvic lymphadenectomy. Has the client had a hysterectomy? Other operations that may interfere with the innervation of the urinary tract include neurosurgical and orthopedic procedures of the spine. Colon and rectal surgery can lead to a neurogenic bladder or erectile dysfunction.

Medications

Many medications can affect urinary function. Obtain a complete history of prescription and nonprescription medications, including herbs and nutraceuticals. Medications that can worsen some urinary conditions may be helpful in others. For example, anticholinergics and alpha-sympathomimetics can relieve urinary incontinence in some clients but may lead to urinary retention in others. If the client presents with urinary calculi, inquire about antihypertensives, diuretics, or silica antacids. Prolonged consumption of analgesics containing acetaminophen, aspirin, caffeine, and phenacetin may be associated with an increased risk of upper tract urothelial cancers. Determine the medication, dose, dosage changes, length of time taken, type, and frequency to ascertain a possible relationship to the onset of the chief complaint. Medications that are known to alter urinary function are listed in Table 32–3.

Allergies

Document allergies to antibiotics. Penicillin, cephalosporins, sulfonamides, and quinolones are often used in treatment of urinary tract infections. Aminoglycosides are used when less toxic antibiotics are ineffective or contraindicated; however, they pose a greater risk of allergic reaction. Inquire about allergies to radiographic contrast dyes as well as to iodine, as iodine dyes are used in some of the radiologic diagnostic tests routinely performed in a urologic evaluation.

■ FAMILY HEALTH HISTORY

Ask about a family history of urinary calculi and renal or sickle cell disease when clients present with pain or hematuria or both. The client who has stones is twice as

TABLE 32–3	MEDICATIONS THAT AFFECT URINARY ELIMINATION
Medication Type	**Effect on Urination**
Anticholinergics	Decreased detrusor contractility (oxybutynin, methantheline), urinary retention, hesitancy
Antispasmodics	Decreased detrusor contractility (dicyclomine, belladonna), urinary retention, urinary hesitancy
Tricyclic antidepressants	Decreased detrusor contractility (imipramine), urinary retention, less incontinence
Cholinergics	Increased detrusor contractility (bethanechol chloride), incontinence, urgency
Alpha-sympathomimetics	Increased sphincter resistance (pseudoephedrine), urinary retention, dysuria
Alpha-blockers	Reduced sphincter resistance (prazosin, terazosin), frequency, incontinence
Estrogens (women)	Increased urethral muscle tone (progestin, estriol), reduced incontinence
Antiandrogens (men)	Improved urinary flow (flutamide, bicalutamide)
Sedatives-hypnotics	Urinary incontinence
Nonsteroidal anti-inflammatories	Renal papillary necrosis (long term)
Diuretics	Polyuria, urinary incontinence (hydrochlorothiazide)
Aminoglycoside antibiotics	Nephrotoxicity (gentamicin, amikacin)
Calcium channel blockers	Urinary retention (diltiazem, verapamil)
Alcohol	Polyuria, frequency, urgency

likely as one who does not to have a first-degree relative with renal stones.[24] Certain other diseases, such as prostate or testicular cancer and BPH, tend to be familial.[18] Hypertension and diabetes are often inherited and can have a significant effect on renal function. Well-known genetic urinary disorders include adult polycystic kidney disease, tuberous sclerosis, von Hippel–Lindau disease, renal tubular acidosis, and cystinuria.

■ PSYCHOSOCIAL HISTORY

Psychosocial assessment is ongoing throughout the interview. Observe and assess for impairments in vision, hearing, or speech. Assess the level of mobility and social factors of living and work environment, caregivers, social contacts, and family. For clients who report (or you suspect have) involuntary incontinence, evidenced as wetness of clothing or odor, assess access to toilets and overall hygiene. Ask about positive or negative childhood experiences with toilet training that may have had a long-term effect on urination patterns.

Assess the client's knowledge of variables in daily life at home and at work that may contribute to the urinary problem. Is the client anxious about urinating in a public place? Anxiety and stress can stimulate or inhibit urination and provoke urgency and frequency. Establish how the client recognizes and manages stress, particularly when the presenting manifestation is worsened by anxiety and stress. Clients may be unaware of lifestyle changes that they might make to improve their urinary problem.

Ascertain the client's knowledge and anxiety about a potential cancer diagnosis. Provide information and feedback according to the client's educational and emotional needs. Some clients have misconceptions or fears regarding their problem and treatments available. Address fear of surgery and changes in body functions, which can seriously alter body image, so that support can be provided throughout the treatment process.

Occupation

Occupation can play a role in urinary function. Exposure at work to toxic chemicals (e.g., aniline dyes in the automobile industry, polycyclic aromatic hydrocarbons in motor exhaust, and benzidine in paint) can lead to bladder cancer. The prevalence of bladder cancer is significant enough in some occupational groups to warrant closer surveillance and possible screening of such populations.[18] Assess the accessibility of toilets in the workplace, especially for clients who have urgency and urge incontinence. Prolonged exposure to heat or cold can affect urination. An increased risk of renal adenocarcinoma has been reported among shoe workers, leather tanners, and those exposed to cadmium, petroleum products, and asbestos.[18]

Geographical Location

Hot climates can lead to chronic dehydration if fluid intake is inadequate. This, along with increased exposure to sunlight, can increase the risk of urinary calculi. People who live in warm climates are at increased risk for infection in larva-infested water used for swimming, bathing, and farming. Larvae may cause the disease schistosomiasis, which predisposes to urinary obstruction and bladder cancer.

Exercise

The positive effects of regular exercise on physical and psychological well-being cannot be overstated. What type of exercise does the client participate in regularly? How strenuous is the exercise? Does exercise affect the urinary problem in any way, or does the urinary problem prohibit participation? Does the client become rehydrated as needed after heavy physical exertion? Long-distance runners sometimes have hematuria, which may originate from the kidney or bladder or may be a sign of underlying glomerular disease.

Nutrition

Nutritional status can have a significant impact on urinary elimination. Diets rich in saturated and unsaturated fats, animal protein, and sugar and deficient in vegetable protein and unrefined carbohydrates (as seen in more affluent countries) can increase the risk of renal stone formation. Ask about dietary habits that may increase the risk for urinary stones, such as dairy products; purine in meats, fish, and poultry; and oxalate in tea, chocolate, and nuts. Excessive dietary intake in obesity may predispose the client to urinary tract carcinogenesis by promoting hormonal changes and arteriosclerosis of the renal arteries.[18]

Ingestion of spicy foods and caffeine can lead to bladder irritation and may exacerbate conditions such as interstitial cystitis (Table 32–4). For the client who complains of nocturia, assess when and what type of fluids are consumed during the evening. Coffee, tea, and caffeinated sodas can have a diuretic effect on the urinary tract. Some studies have linked coffee consumption, diuretic use, and obesity to renal cell adenocarcinoma. High-fat diets have been implicated in increased risk of prostate cancer in the United States.[18]

Habits

Obtain a history of tobacco, alcohol, and recreational drug use. Cigarette smoking has been consistently shown

TABLE 32–4	DIETARY IRRITANTS OF THE URINARY TRACT
Irritant*	**Possible Substitutes**
Alcohol	Late harvest dessert wines
Apples, apple juice	Apricot or pear nectar, papaya juice
Coffee, tea	Kava, cold brewed coffee, herbal tea
Chocolate	Carob
Carbonated beverages	
Chilies, spicy foods	
Aspartame (NutraSweet)	Fructose
Strawberries, cranberries	
Grapes, guava, cantaloupe	
Peaches, pineapples, plums	
Tomatoes, onions	
Vinegar	

*Not all irritants have a corresponding substitute.

to be a risk factor for urothelial cancers, increasing the risk two or three times over a nonsmoker's risk.[18] Smoking can also lead to peripheral vascular disease and to subsequent erectile dysfunction. The risk associated with cigarette smoking declines significantly with years of smoking cessation.

Alcohol can irritate the bladder and increase urinary output. Chronic alcoholism may lead to autonomic and peripheral neuropathy that impairs urinary and sexual function and to decreased serum testosterone, testicular atrophy, and decreased libido. If the client is scheduled for surgery, heavy tobacco and alcohol use can increase the risk of perioperative complications significantly. (See Chapter 15 for a discussion of the effects of tobacco and alcohol on perioperative outcomes.)

■ REVIEW OF SYSTEMS

Ask about symptoms such as GI complaints, blood pressure changes, weight loss or gain, edema, fatigue, lethargy, headaches, blurred vision, changes in mentation, numbness or tingling of the extremities, pruritus, bleeding tendencies, exposure to infectious disease, and allergies that may be associated with urologic disorders. See Table 9–2 for additional questions to include in the review of systems.

PHYSICAL EXAMINATION

The urologic physical examination typically includes:

- Temperature, pulse, blood pressure, height, and weight
- General inspection of the skin for integrity, color, and peripheral edema
- Examination of the abdomen, pelvis, genitalia, and rectum

The examination may be tailored to the client's specific complaint or condition. Instruct the client to empty the bladder before the examination. When the physical examination is completed, document findings using the Physical Assessment Findings in the Healthy Adult feature as a guide.

PHYSICAL ASSESSMENT FINDINGS IN THE HEALTHY ADULT

Urinary System

Inspection

Lower abdomen flat, nondistended. External urethral orifice pink without discharge.

Auscultation

No renal bruit noted anteriorly or posteriorly over the right or left costovertebral angle.

Percussion

Flat note over symphysis pubis and tympany over lower abdomen. No tenderness posteriorly over the right or left costovertebral angle.

Palpation

Lower pole of right kidney palpable, smooth, nontender. Left kidney nonpalpable.

■ ABDOMEN

Inspection

Have the client lie in a supine position with arms at the sides and knees slightly flexed to relax the abdominal muscles. If the client has complained of abdominal, back, or flank pain, note whether there is guarding or restlessness in this position. Inspect the abdomen for symmetry and contour. Asymmetry or a mass in the upper quadrants may indicate a renal tumor or hydronephrosis, although only a very large renal or adrenal mass in a very thin client would potentially be visible. Fullness in the suprapubic area may indicate a distended bladder.

Note any surgical or traumatic scarring that may have affected the urinary or GI tract or caused adhesions, especially if the client presents with abdominal complaints. Also note any herniation, either at the site of surgical scarring, around a stoma, or in the ventral area (epigastric or umbilical region), particularly with straining (see discussion under lower GI elimination physical examination).

For clients who have had previous urologic surgery, note the presence of a stoma, the type, whether it is a continent urinary diversion, and the appearance of the stoma and surrounding skin. Observe the size and contour of the stoma, and note the color of the mucosa. Observe for abnormal findings such as retracted or prolapsed stomal mucosa, lesions, inflammation, or macerated skin. Document the type of ostomy appliance or stomal covering, if used. Also note the presence of an indwelling urethral or suprapubic catheter, its patency, and the color and odor of the urine. Document the presence of sediment in the drainage collection system. Evaluate the drainage system for cleanliness and closed system integrity.

Auscultation

Auscultation is performed before palpation to avoid disruption of vascular murmurs and bowel sounds. Renal artery bruits are most commonly heard just above and slightly left of the umbilicus and can indicate renal artery stenosis or aneurysm or arteriovenous malformation. If a bruit is heard, avoid deep palpation. Evaluate bowel sounds in all four quadrants for frequency, intensity, and pitch, especially in the presence of GI manifestations (see lower GI tract physical examination earlier).

Percussion

Percussion is valuable in identifying a bladder containing at least 150 ml of urine. The percussion sound changes from tympanic to dull over a full bladder. Blunt percussion can also be valuable if performed anteriorly and posteriorly to identify renal masses or tenderness when renal trauma and hemorrhage prevent deep palpation. With the client sitting, place one hand over the costovertebral angle on the left side and strike the hand lightly with the opposite fisted hand. The effect is perceived as a dull thud in a normal kidney but as sharp pain or tenderness in a distended kidney. Repeat for the right kidney. Figure 32–4 illustrates this maneuver, and Chapter 10 describes the blunt percussion technique.

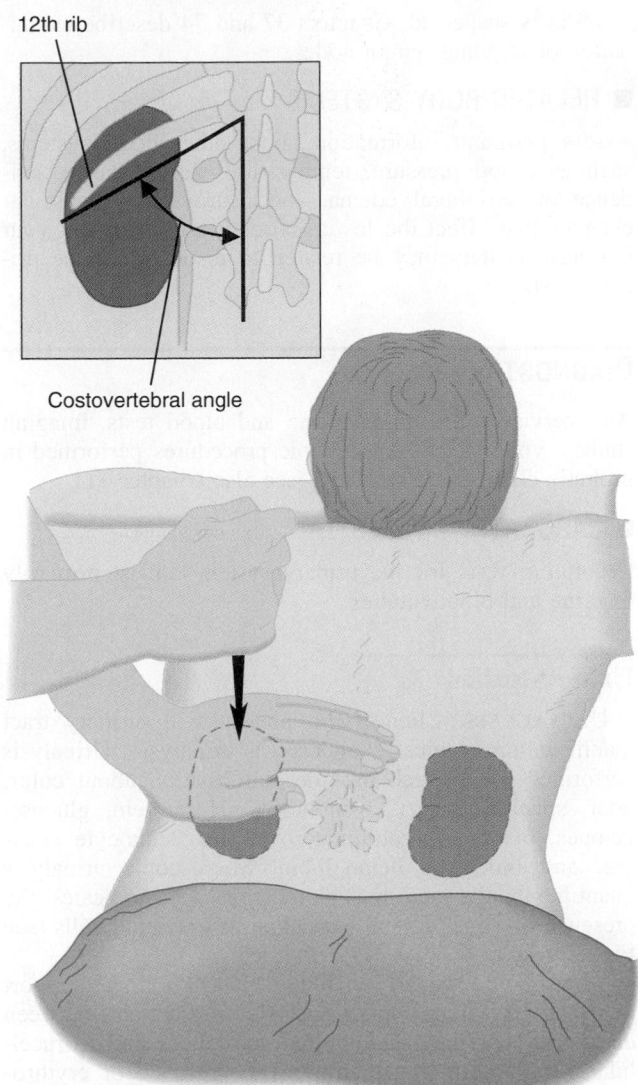

FIGURE 32–4 Percussion over the costovertebral angle.

Palpation

Begin palpation with a *light* touch, depressing the skin no deeper than 1 to 2 cm, to assess tenderness and muscle resistance or guarding, which might be a sign of peritoneal irritation. Light palpation allows examination of tender abdominal areas with minimal production of pain. Such pain may cause voluntary muscle rigidity and reduce the effectiveness of deep palpation.

Examine each of the four quadrants noting areas of muscle resistance, which may indicate a superficial or large pelvic mass, either infectious or neoplastic, or bladder distention if it is in the suprapubic area. Involuntary muscle rigidity is usually unilateral, whereas voluntary rigidity is symmetrical. To differentiate between a rigid muscle and a mass, note whether the area of resistance follows an abdominal muscle or is lobular in shape.

Last, palpate any region under suspicion on the basis of the health history and previous inspection.

Deep palpation follows light palpation and is used primarily to detect renal enlargement or masses. The technique is similar to that of light palpation, but the depth is 4 to 5 cm. Reinforced (bimanual) palpation is used in cases of more resistant muscle tone. (See Chapter 10 and Figure 10–3 for a discussion of bimanual palpation.)

Describe identified masses in terms of location, size, consistency, surface characteristics, tenderness, mobility, and pulsation. Assess rebound tenderness to determine the presence of peritoneal inflammation. Deep palpation should never be used in cases of known renal trauma, polycystic kidneys, abdominal aortic aneurysm, kidney transplantation, or appendicitis.

The kidneys are normally well protected by the diaphragm and lower ribs and cannot be palpated easily. The right kidney is slightly lower than the left because of the presence of the liver. In a thin client, the lower pole of the right kidney can sometimes be detected with deep palpation. Palpate the kidney bimanually, with one hand on the costovertebral angle posteriorly and the other hand pushing firmly and deeply under the costal margin anteriorly, while instructing the client to inhale deeply. As the client inhales, the right kidney descends and may be felt by the anterior hand as it slides between the hands. A normal kidney feels smooth, firm, and rounded (Fig. 32–5). The left kidney is usually not palpable because it lies higher up under the rib cage. In older adults, the kidneys may be palpated more readily because of loss of abdominal muscle firmness.

An empty bladder cannot be palpated. In acute or chronic urinary retention, the bladder rises up out of the pelvis at the midline toward the umbilicus. It may be seen and usually felt. When there is chronic urinary retention, the bladder is atonic and difficult to palpate.

■ GENITALIA

Use inspection and palpation to examine the genitalia. Clients tend to be more anxious about examination of the genitalia. Therefore, remain straightforward and professional and perform this part of the examination after establishing rapport.

MALE CLIENTS

While the male client lies supine, inspect the perineum and groin area for signs of skin irritation or excoriation, especially if he has reported urinary incontinence. Examine the glans meatus. Circumcised males have a dry glans, whereas uncircumcised males have a relatively moist and pink glans. Examine the urethral meatus after carefully retracting the foreskin (in uncircumcised males).

FIGURE 32–5 Palpating the kidneys.

The foreskin should retract easily. Normally, the meatus is located centrally on the glans and the mucosa is pink and moist, readily separating when the glans is pressed between the thumb and forefinger.

A meatus opening dorsally on the glans, penile shaft, or penoscrotal junction indicates *epispadias. Hypospadias* is an anomaly in which the urethra opens on the ventral aspect of the glans, penile shaft, or penoscrotal junction. Malposition of the urethral meatus can interfere with normal voiding and can be associated with curvature of the penis that is called *chordee.* Note the presence of any urethral discharge or reddened edematous meatal edges that indicate urethritis. Difficulty exposing the distal meatal mucosa (fossa navicularis) may indicate stenosis. Next, palpate the penile shaft ventrally along the urethra for tenderness, swelling, or mass. (Chapter 37 covers the examination of the genitalia.)

FEMALE CLIENTS

Urologic examination of the female genitalia includes examination of the external genitalia and in some cases a complete pelvic examination (see also Chapter 37). For an examination of the external genitalia, position the client in a supine recumbent position with knees and feet apart and knees flexed. Examine the urethral meatus for eversion or redness, which may indicate urethritis.

Palpate the urethra by inserting a gloved index finger into the vagina and palpating the anterior vaginal wall for induration or mass from the bladder to the meatus. Inspect for the presence of urethral discharge indicative of infection.

Ask the client to cough or strain, and note any bulging of the vaginal walls. Bulging of the anterior vaginal wall can indicate a *cystocele* and that of the posterior wall a *rectocele.* Cystocele is seen with relaxation of the pelvic floor musculature and may be the source of irritative voiding symptoms and stress incontinence.

■ RECTUM

MALE CLIENTS

The urologic digital rectal examination of the male client is done to evaluate the prostate gland. Although the prostate is primarily a reproductive organ, disorders of the gland can affect urination. Disorders include BPH, prostatitis, prostatodynia, and prostate adenocarcinoma. Examination of the prostate is discussed in Chapter 37.

Depending on the skill of the examiner, the bulbocavernosal reflex can be assessed for neurologic abnormalities. Evaluate the reflex by gently compressing the glans penis with the thumb and forefinger of the opposite hand while the index finger remains in the rectum. When the reflex arc is intact, the sphincter contracts.

FEMALE CLIENTS

In the female client, the examiner can duplicate the evaluation performed for the male client by gently flicking the clitoris during the rectal examination. A rectal examination of the female urologic client is done primarily to assess sphincter tone and the bulbocavernosal reflex (see the earlier discussion of the rectal examination).

■ LYMPH NODES

Inspect and palpate the supraclavicular and inguinal groups of lymph nodes if metastatic cancer of the prostate or testis is suspected. Chapters 37 and 74 describe examination of inguinal lymph nodes.

■ RELATED BODY SYSTEMS

Assess pertinent information about other body systems, such as blood pressure, temperature, fluid balance, evidence of peripheral edema, and neurologic or vascular changes that affect the lower extremities. Document your findings, as they may be related to disorders of the urinary tract.

DIAGNOSTIC TESTS

An overview of common urine and blood tests, imaging studies, voiding, and endoscopic procedures performed in urologic clients, is given next (see also Chapter 11).

■ LABORATORY TESTS

Laboratory tests for the urinary system consist primarily of urine and blood studies.

Urine Studies

URINALYSIS. Clients who present with urinary tract manifestations typically undergo a urinalysis. Urinalysis performed by dipstick provides information about color, odor, specific gravity, osmolality, pH, protein, glucose, ketones, bilirubin, urobilinogen, nitrites, leukocyte esterase, and blood or hemoglobin. Microscopic urinalysis quantifies white and red blood cells and indicates the presence of casts, crystals, bacteria, or epithelial cells (see Fig. 32–3).

Microscopic urinalysis should always follow a report of red urine. Microscopic urinalysis differentiates between discoloration related to ingested substances and extracellular hemoglobin in the urine. The presence of erythrocyte casts indicates a renal origin of the blood. Gross hematuria and microscopic hematuria, defined as more than three red blood cells per high-power field (HPF), can indicate trauma, infectious processes, toxicity, calculus, and benign and malignant neoplasms (Table 32–5).

Specific gravity indicates the concentration of urine and reflects the client's hydration status as well as renal function. For example, clients who have diabetes insipidus consistently have specific gravity values less than 1.010. Clients with extensive tubular damage or endocrine disease involving antidiuretic hormone (ADH) insufficiency have specific gravity fixed at 1.010, the level of the plasma.

Osmolality is a measure of the concentrating ability of the kidney. Osmolality increases in hypernatremia, acidosis, and shock. It decreases in diabetes insipidus, hypercalcemia, excessive hydration, and renal tubular acidosis.

Urine pH can fluctuate with fluid intake but is important in a few specific clinical situations. Clients with uric acid stones usually have more acidic urine with a pH less than 6.5. In clients who have renal tubular acidosis, the pH of the urine cannot be less than 6.0. Urinary tract infections caused by urea-splitting organisms (e.g., *Proteus*) cause the urinary pH to rise above 7.0. Urine left standing more than 2 hours or collected after a large meal may be more alkaline.

TABLE 32-5	UNDERSTANDING URINALYSIS	
Variable	Normal Values	Causes of Abnormal Values
Specific gravity	1.001–1.035	Decreased: increased fluid intake, diuretics, decreased renal concentration, diabetes insipidus
		Increased: dehydration, diabetes mellitus, increased ADH secretion, iodine contrast
Osmolality	50–1200 mOsm/L	Varies with hydration
pH	5.5–6.5	<5.5: metabolic or respiratory acidosis, renal tubular acidosis type II
		>7.5: presence of urea-splitting organism (Proteus), renal tubular acidosis type I
Blood	None	Carcinoma, renal lithiasis
Protein	<20 mg/dl	Glomerular disease, nephropathy, interstitial disease, strenuous exercise, multiple myeloma
Glucose	Negative	Diabetes mellitus
Ketones	Negative	Diabetic ketoacidosis
Bilirubin	Negative	Intrinsic hepatic disease, bile duct obstruction
Urobilinogen	Trace	Hemolysis, hepatocellular disease
Nitrites	Negative	Bacteriuria
Leukocyte esterase	Negative	Bacteriuria
Red blood cells	<3 RBCs/HPF	Urinary tract cancer, IgA nephropathy, lithiasis, prostate enlargement, menstrual contamination, infection, papillary necrosis, renal artery embolism or thrombosis
White blood cells	0–5 WBCs/HPF	Infection
Bacteria	None	Urinary tract infection
Casts	0–4 hyaline/HPF	Red blood cell casts: glomerular bleeding
		White blood cell casts: glomerulonephritis
		Fatty casts: nephrotic syndrome
Crystals	Varies	Significant in renal lithiasis

ADH, antidiuretic hormone; HPF, high-power field; IgA, immunoglobulin A; LPF, low-power field; RBC, red blood cell; WBC, white blood cell.

Proteinuria or persistent elevation of protein in the urine may be glomerular, tubular, or overflow in origin. Glomerular proteinuria occurs with immunoglobulin A (IgA) nephropathy or diabetes mellitus. Tubular proteinuria results from failure to resorb immunoglobulins because of defective tubular function. Overflow proteinuria is due to an increase in abnormal immunoglobulins and is often seen with multiple myeloma. Prolonged fever and excessive physical exertion can cause a transient elevation of urinary protein levels. Orthostatic proteinuria occurs occasionally when the client has been standing for several hours. A false-positive result for urine protein may be obtained when the urine is concentrated or contains white blood cells or vaginal secretions.

Glucosuria (glucose in the urine) most often occurs in clients with diabetes mellitus, which may result in renal papillary necrosis and recurrent urinary tract infections. Glucosuria occurs when the serum glucose level exceeds the resorptive capacity of the kidneys, a level of 180 mg/dl. *Ketonuria* (ketones in the urine) occurs when body fat is metabolized for energy, as in cases of diabetic ketoacidosis, fasting, pregnancy, vomiting, and diarrhea.

Direct bilirubin is made in the hepatocyte and appears in the urine only when extrahepatic biliary tract obstruction or intrinsic hepatic disease is present. *Urobilinogen* is the end product of conjugated bilirubin metabolism, and a small amount, 1 to 4 mg/day, is excreted in the urine.

Leukocyte esterase indicates white blood cells in the urine. *Nitrites* in the urine strongly suggest bacteriuria. Epithelial cells are often present in urinary sediment. Renal tubular cells are least often seen but are indicative of renal disease.

Casts are formed in the distal tubules and collecting ducts of the kidneys and signify renal disease when found in the urine. Red blood cell casts indicate glomerulitis or vasculitis. White blood cell casts indicate bacterial infection but are often difficult to distinguish from epithelial casts. Granular casts often represent disintegrated epithelial cells, leukocytes, or protein associated with renal tubular disease. Hyaline casts represent a mixture of mucus and globulin from the tubules and are not significant in small numbers.

Depending on the test ordered, urinalysis may be performed on a clean catch specimen, midstream specimen, fresh urine specimen, first morning specimen, 12- or 24-hour collection, multiple bottle voidings (serial urine collections), or a specimen obtained with a catheter. First voided morning specimens are helpful in evaluation of renal function. Ideally, the urine should be obtained several hours after eating because postprandial specimens may contain lysed blood cells and disintegrated casts. Clean catch continues to be the standard method for obtaining urine specimens. Several studies have shown that there is little difference in contamination levels between a clean catch and a midstream urine specimen collected without previous cleansing with an antiseptic towelette.[17]

Instruct female clients to separate the labia and uncircumcised males to retract the foreskin. For a catheterized client, collect urine from the port on the tubing, not the urinary drainage bag, because this urine may be contaminated. Use a drip method to collect urine from a urostoma. Approximately 10 ml is required. In some situations, catheterization for a urine sample may be required. In these cases, follow universal precautions and maintain sterile technique (see Chapter 11 for additional discussion of urinalysis). Refer to a nursing fundamentals textbook for specific information about the techniques for collecting urine specimens (random, clean catch, catheterized, timed, and from a urostomy). Always follow protocol for specimen collection and handling.

URINE CULTURE. When urinary tract infection is suspected from the client's history or the presence of bacteria or significant white blood cells on urinalysis, a urine culture is necessary. This test identifies the offending organism and quantifies the amount of colonization. Generally, the presence of organisms in a concentration greater than 100,000/ml indicates infection, although the value may vary, depending on the method of collection and symptoms of infection.

Collection technique is as for midstream clean catch or catheter specimens for urinalysis. Determining the sensitivity of the organism to specific antibiotics is not usually necessary because *E. coli,* known to cause 85% of routine infections, is sensitive to most oral antibiotics. Identifying the drugs to which the bacteria are sensitive is done in cases with recurrent or persistent symptoms of urinary tract infection.

URINE CYTOLOGY. When urinary tract carcinoma is known or suspected, urine cytologic evaluation is performed. The specimen may be voided or a bladder washing obtained either by catheterization or cystoscopically. Transitional cell carcinoma of the bladder typically sheds cells into the urine more than upper tract carcinomas, but the amount of cells retrieved for study depends on the adequacy of the specimen and the grade and volume of the tumor.

CLEARANCE STUDIES. Urine clearance studies determine the glomerular filtration rate and tubular excretion ability of the kidney. Creatinine clearance is the most accurate measure of glomerular filtration rate, although urea, insulin, para-aminohippuric acid, and phenolsulfonphthalein can also be measured. Radioisotopes may also be used to determine clearance rates. Renal excretory function is measured as the difference between the filtration rate of a substance and the rate of excretion in the urine.

For a creatinine clearance test, collect the urine specimen for 12 or 24 hours as ordered (see Chapter 11). A blood sample is drawn at any point during the collection period in a 7-ml red-top tube. There is no postprocedure care.

CONCENTRATION AND DILUTION STUDIES. Loss of ability to concentrate and dilute urine indicates significant renal tubular damage. Several tests can be performed to evaluate the ability of the kidneys to concentrate and dilute the urine. Many of these tests can be risky for clients who have compromised renal or cardiac function because of the severe fluid loading or fluid deprivation that is part of the procedure. Carefully assess and monitor the client's fluid balance and cardiovascular status (pulse, blood pressure, lung sounds) during urine concentration and dilution testing.

Blood Studies

BLOOD UREA NITROGEN. Blood urea nitrogen (BUN) is a measure of renal function because urea is the primary end product of protein metabolism and is excreted by the kidneys. An elevated BUN level may indicate impaired renal function, although it is not specific for the kidneys. BUN may be elevated because of systemic factors such as sepsis, excess protein consumption, starvation, dehydration, and cardiac failure.

SERUM CREATININE. Serum creatinine is more specific for renal function because it is not affected by dietary intake or hydration status. It can be elevated in cases of glomerulonephritis, pyelonephritis, acute tubular necrosis, nephrotoxicity, renal insufficiency, and renal failure. Elevations are also seen in clients who have renal failure secondary to outlet obstruction. Some studies suggest that the elevated serum creatinine levels seen with urinary obstruction are related to coexisting hypertension or diabetes rather than the obstruction.[17] The normal ratio of BUN to creatinine is 10:1.

■ RADIOGRAPHY

Kidney-Ureter-Bladder X-ray Study

The kidney-ureter-bladder (KUB) x-ray study provides an anteroposterior film of the kidneys, ureters, and pelvis taken without contrast medium. It is used to evaluate suspected radiopaque urinary calculi or masses and as a preliminary study for other radiologic tests of the abdomen.

Client preparation includes bowel preparation if the KUB study is done as a preliminary evaluation test. Advise the client that the x-ray procedure is painless.

Intravenous Pyelography or Excretory Urography

Intravenous pyelography (IVP) or excretory urography (EXU) is a study in which a series of radiologic films are obtained after intravenous injection of contrast medium. IVP or EXU provides information about the entire urinary tract because films are taken at regular intervals as the contrast medium moves through the tract. The final film is taken after the client voids to evaluate the ability of the bladder to empty. Pressure applied across the client's lower abdomen to compress the ureters allows enhancement of the renal pelvis and proximal ureters. This test is used to evaluate renal stones, masses, hematuria, obstructive uropathy, congenital anomalies, infection, and renal function.

PREPROCEDURE CARE

Client preparation includes careful screening for potential allergies or sensitivity to contrast medium and iodine. A steroid may be given before injection of contrast medium in cases of sensitivities. Instruct clients about the necessary bowel preparation. This includes a liquid meal before 6 PM the preceding evening, followed by a laxative such as senna extract (X-Prep). Fluids are withheld after 10 PM the evening before the procedure to promote greater concentration of the contrast medium in the kidneys.

Explain that there may be a sensation of flushing and warmth, an unpleasant or salty taste in the mouth, or nausea when the contrast dye is administered. Allergic reactions (e.g., urticaria, itching, and respiratory distress or failure) occur in about 5% of clients. Because reactions happen immediately after injection of the contrast medium, antihistamines, steroids, and an emergency cart must be readily available. IVP or EXU is not recommended for clients who have renal insufficiency or failure.

POSTPROCEDURE CARE
Monitor the hydration status of the client after IVP or EXU to reduce the risk of renal failure in susceptible clients. Unless there is a contraindication, force fluids to promote renal clearance of the contrast medium. Monitor output.

Retrograde Urography

For clients who are allergic to iodine-based contrast media, a *retrograde pyelogram* can be obtained. Contrast medium is administered directly into the urinary tract (rather than intravenously) during endoscopic visualization via cystoscopy. (Cystoscopy is discussed later in this chapter.) A retrograde pyelogram details the ureter, ureteropelvic junction, renal pelvis, and calices.

A *cystogram* is obtained after instillation of contrast medium directly into the bladder via a catheter. Cystographic studies are used to evaluate recurrent urinary tract infections, vesicoureteral reflux, hematuria, trauma, postsurgical healing, and stress urinary incontinence.

A *voiding cystourethrogram* is similar to a cystogram, except that films are taken while the client is voiding. A *retrograde urethrogram* is indicated when there is suspicion of urethral stricture, fistula, trauma, diverticulum, or tumor. Oblique x-ray films are taken after instillation of 15 to 30 ml of contrast medium into the urethra via a catheter in the fossa navicularis or a catheter-tip syringe.

Urinary tract infection should be ruled out before any of these procedures. Instruct clients to watch for and report symptoms of infection, which may occur for up to 24 to 48 hours after the procedure (flank pain, dysuria, chills, fever). Encourage consumption of fluids. Transient flank pain, bladder, or urethral discomfort may occur but should resolve in 24 to 48 hours.

Computed Tomography

CT is used in urology to evaluate the kidneys, major renal vessels, ureters, and bladder as well as the abdominal and pelvic contents for malignant masses, metastases, or lymphadenopathy. It is used primarily for tumor staging and identifying abscesses. Other uses for CT are to evaluate a nonfunctioning kidney, urinary tract trauma, a transplanted kidney, renal calculi, and infections. Clients should fast for 4 hours before the procedure. (See Chapter 11 for general care of the client having a CT scan.)

Magnetic Resonance Imaging

Magnetic resonance imaging (MRI) is used to visualize the kidneys, retroperitoneum, bladder, prostate, testes, and penis. It is used in urology to stage cancers of the kidney, bladder, and prostate. MRI has become increasingly useful when gadolinium, an extracellular contrast agent, is used.[24] (See Chapter 11 for general care of the client undergoing MRI.)

Renal Angiography

Angiography is the visualization of blood vessels by the use of radiopaque contrast media. This modality is used to visualize renal and penile structures but has little use in evaluation of the ureter, bladder, and prostate. Renal arteriography is used to evaluate renal tumors, to obtain vascular maps preoperatively, or to evaluate potential kidney donors. Angiography is rarely used in urology for strictly diagnostic purposes because it is expensive and invasive compared with other imaging procedures. A safer technique, *digital angiography*, uses computerized radiographic subtraction to obtain images of renal arteries with an intravenous injection of contrast medium instead of femoral artery puncture and catheterization. (Chapter 11 describes general care of the client undergoing angiography.)

■ ULTRASONOGRAPHY

Ultrasonography is used in urology to evaluate the kidneys, ureters, bladder, prostate, testes, and penis. In a renal scan, the client's abdomen and back are scanned in the longitudinal and transverse planes. The kidneys can be evaluated for size, hydronephrosis, calculi, solid tumors, and cysts. Renal ultrasonography is used to differentiate simple cysts from other types of mass lesions in the kidney. Other uses include localizing and mapping the kidneys before biopsy and evaluating transplanted kidneys.

The bladder may be scanned for residual urine volume, bladder wall thickness, bladder calculi, tumors, and diverticula with an ultrasound probe over the suprapubic area. A portable ultrasound instrument exists that computes bladder volume from 12 cross-sectional readings. It is used to determine postvoid residual accurately and has been shown to reduce the risk of nosocomial (hospital-acquired) urinary tract infection associated with catheterization for postvoid residual.[16]

Prostate ultrasonography is performed transrectally with a transducer probe inserted 4 to 5 inches into the rectum. Images are obtained in the anterior-posterior (AP), coronal, and sagittal planes to approximate size with an ellipsoid volume equation:

$$volume = AP \times coronal \times sagittal \times 0.5236$$

Prostate ultrasonography is also used to evaluate the peripheral zone for hypoechoic areas that may be associated with prostate cancer. (Chapter 37 describes ultrasonography of the testes and penis.)

Reassure clients that ultrasonography is painless and not invasive. An exception is transrectal ultrasonography, which can cause discomfort and pressure when the anus is dilated. For prostate ultrasonography, instruct the client to evacuate the rectum by administering a Fleet enema about 45 minutes before the procedure. No colon or proctologic examinations should be performed on the same day.

■ RADIONUCLIDE STUDIES

Nuclear medicine studies are performed in urology to evaluate renal failure, masses, hydronephrosis, and renal blood flow and to rule out metastatic bone disease in genitourinary cancers. Clients receive an injection of a technetium-based isotope. This is followed by a nuclear scan 3 hours later when the radioactive tracer has concentrated in the target organ. Encourage clients to force fluids before the scan. (See Chapter 11 for a general discussion of radionuclide studies.)

■ ENDOSCOPY

Cystourethroscopy and Urethroscopy

Endoscopy (see Chapter 11) is utilized in urology most commonly in *cystourethroscopy*. This endoscopic study is used to evaluate the anterior and prostatic urethra, bladder urothelium and trigone, and the ureteral orifices in the bladder. The procedure is performed transurethrally, by either a rigid or flexible cystoscope (Fig. 32–6). Cystoscopy allows diagnostic inspection of the urinary tract for evidence of urinary calculi, infection, vesicoureteral reflux, prostatic obstruction, bladder tumor, and urethral stricture. A variation of cystourethroscopy is *urethroscopy*, in which only the urethra is visualized.

PREPROCEDURE CARE

Before the procedure, a urine culture or Gram stain must be negative because an active urinary tract infection is a contraindication to the test. The procedure is usually performed with the client in the lithotomy position, and the urethra is prepared with a water-soluble lubricant containing 2% lidocaine. A spinal or general anesthetic is administered if the cystoscopy is done before a surgical procedure such as transurethral resection of the prostate (TURP) or bladder tumor. Instruct the client in the preoperative protocol for spinal or general anesthesia and obtain consent (see Chapter 15). Clients who have artificial joints, cardiac valvular disease, or valve replacement require prophylactic antibiotic therapy before the procedure to prevent the development of subacute bacterial endocarditis.

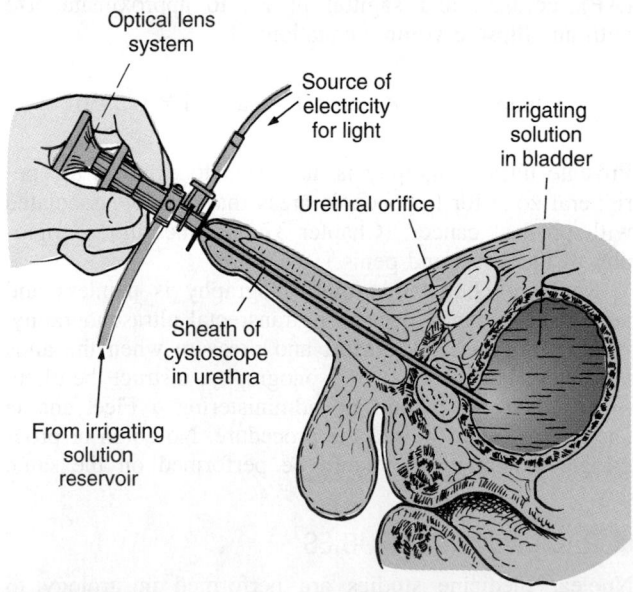

Optical lens system

Source of electricity for light

Irrigating solution in bladder

Urethral orifice

Sheath of cystoscope in urethra

From irrigating solution reservoir

FIGURE 32–6 Cystoscope in the male bladder.

POSTPROCEDURE CARE

Hematuria (pink-tinged urine) is expected after cystoscopy. Instruct the client to force fluids and to report any frank bleeding or clots in the urine or symptoms of urinary tract or systemic infection (e.g., dysuria, fever, or chills). Warm baths and NSAIDs may relieve dysuria. If acute urinary retention occurs after cytoscopy, intermittent bladder catheterization is required. Belladonna and opium suppositories or antispasmodics, such as propantheline bromide, may relieve bladder spasms.

Ureteroscopy, Nephroscopy, and Ureterorenoscopy

Endoscopic procedures for the upper urinary tracts (see Chapter 34) include the following:

- *Ureteroscopy,* performed for diagnostic as well as therapeutic purposes, is used to evaluate radiologic filling defects, gross hematuria, and malignant cytology. Additional information regarding the grade and extent of malignant tumors can be obtained with ureteroscopic biopsy.
- *Nephroscopy* is used to evaluate the renal pelvis for abnormalities.
- *Flexible deflectable ureterorenoscopy* is used for biopsy of interstitial lesions in the outflow tract as well as to retrieve stones up to the level of the calices.

These procedures are performed transurethrally with a flexible or rigid ureteroscope and allow direct visualization of the ureter and renal pelvis. The client is placed in a Trendelenburg position, and general or regional anesthesia or intravenous sedation is administered. Manipulation of the lower urinary tract, especially dilation of the ureteral orifice, can cause discomfort.

PREPROCEDURE CARE

Client preparation includes ensuring sterile urine, administering a perioperative broad-spectrum antibiotic, giving the client nothing by mouth, and obtaining consent. A history of previous radical surgery or ureteral manipulation should be known before ureteroscopic examination because it may make the procedure more difficult or impossible to complete successfully.

POSTPROCEDURE CARE

Because of the ureter's smaller anatomic size, observe for possible complications including perforation and urinary extravasation into the abdomen, which occur in about 4% of clients, as well as infection, renal colic, and bleeding. Typically, a ureteral stent or temporary diversion catheter is left in place for at least 48 hours. The time may be extended if minor perforations have occurred with urinary extravasation. Encourage the client to force fluids, and continue prophylactic antibiotics as ordered after the procedure.

■ BIOPSY

Biopsies for malignancy in the urinary tract can be done transurethrally (kidney, ureter, bladder, and urethra) and percutaneously (prostate). Biopsy of the kidney can be performed by either a percutaneous or an open surgical approach.

Transurethral Biopsy

Biopsy of a suspicious lesion in the bladder that is discovered during cystourethroscopy is done with the client under regional or general anesthesia. Biopsy specimens of surrounding bladder tissue are also taken randomly to evaluate the rest of the bladder. Care of the client is the same as for the client undergoing endoscopy but also involves preparation for anesthesia (see Chapter 15).

Intervention includes assisting the client in anesthesia recovery as well as using comfort measures for urethral pain, bladder spasms, flank pain, and dysuria, which are commonly experienced after biopsy. Instruct the client to watch for signs of urinary tract infection or infection of the puncture site and to report these promptly after the procedure.

Transrectal Prostate Biopsy

Biopsy of the prostate gland is performed via a rectal approach. The biopsy specimen is usually obtained with a multiple-core biopsy needle guided by ultrasonography. The procedure is done in an outpatient setting when preliminary tests indicate the presence of prostate cancer. Before the procedure, instruct the client to avoid aspirin for 10 days and NSAIDs for 24 hours. A urine specimen is obtained for culture to ensure sterile urine. Prophylactic antibiotics are given.

Instruct clients that they may experience dysuria, hematuria, hematospermia, rectal bleeding, or urinary retention for 24 to 48 hours after the procedure. (See Chapter 37 for additional discussion of prostate biopsy.)

Percutaneous Renal Biopsy

Percutaneous biopsy of the renal pelvis is used to diagnose benign and malignant masses, establish a prognosis, and follow progression and response to treatment. Renal biopsy is contraindicated for clients who have a solitary kidney, malignant tumors, hydronephrosis, infection or abscess, serious hypertension, or coagulation disorders. Small-gauge (21- to 25-gauge) needles are used for cytologic examination, and larger-gauge (14- to 20-gauge) needles are used to obtain tissue cores for histopathologic examination (Fig. 32–7). Guided imaging such as fluoroscopy, ultrasonography, CT scanning, or MRI is used to help avoid large blood vessels. The physician inserts the biopsy needle as the client inspires deeply, and the client must be able to cooperate. Complications after biopsy include pneumothorax, hemorrhage, infection, and laceration or perforation of the kidney.

Brush biopsies of lesions of the upper tract urothelium are performed with a steel or nylon brush inserted via a ureteral catheter with endoscopic guidance. Biopsies of the renal pelvis, calices, and ureter can be obtained with this approach (see earlier discussion of ureteroscopy).

PREPROCEDURE CARE

Prepare the client for local anesthesia (see Chapter 15), obtain consent, and give nothing by mouth. Determine that results of coagulation studies are in the client's record. Obtain and record baseline vital signs. Clients are often managed in an outpatient setting with conscious sedation.

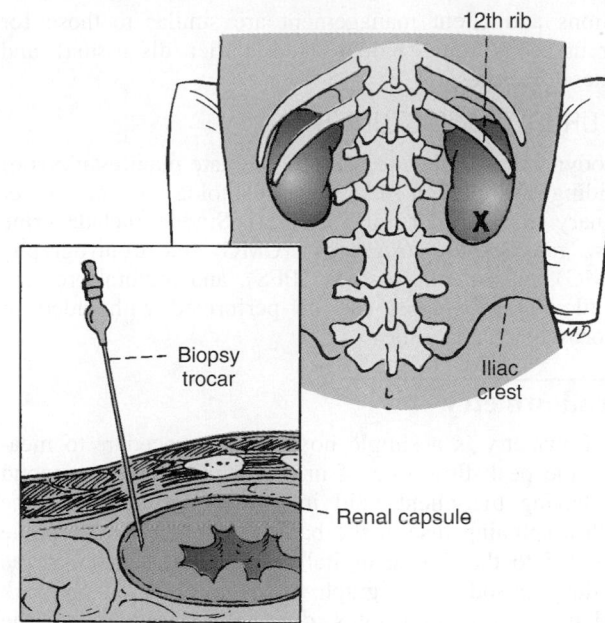

FIGURE 32–7 Percutaneous renal biopsy showing location of the trocar.

POSTPROCEDURE CARE

Immediately after the biopsy, apply pressure to the puncture site for 20 minutes. Apply a sterile dressing. Pressure may be maintained by having the client lie on a sandbag placed against the biopsy site. Check the puncture site for bleeding and monitor vital signs according to agency protocol. Force fluids to promote urination and to prevent clot formation, which can lead to urine obstruction.

Observe each voiding for hematuria; protocol may require checking each specimen with a dipstick for microscopic blood. Postbiopsy hematocrit levels are usually monitored.

The time for bed rest varies; clients may be discharged between 4 and 24 hours after biopsy. Encourage limited activity for the first 24 hours to prevent bleeding.

Complications after renal biopsy include gross hematuria, pain, infection, decreased hematocrit, and hypotension indicative of hemorrhage. Instruct the client to report immediately fever, increasing pain levels (back, flank, or shoulder), bleeding from the puncture site, weakness, dizziness, grossly bloody urine, or dysuria. Activity should be restricted if blood is seen in the urine. Advise the client to avoid strenuous lifting, physical exertion, or trauma to the biopsy site for up to 2 weeks after discharge.

Open Renal Biopsy

An open biopsy approach is indicated for diagnosis of renal diseases when tissue sampling by other methods is inadequate. The client requires preparation for general anesthesia (see Chapter 15) as well as renal function and coagulation studies. The procedure requires a nephrotomy via a flank incision to permit direct visualization of the kidney.

After surgery, monitor vital signs, fluid balance, wound hemostasis, urine color, and pain levels. Complications and client management are similar to those for percutaneous renal biopsy (see earlier discussion) and general anesthesia.

■ URODYNAMIC STUDIES

Urodynamic studies are used to evaluate manifestations of voiding dysfunction related to pathology of the lower urinary tract (bladder and urethra). Studies include urine flow rate, cystometrography (CMG), electromyography (EMG), pressure flow study (PFS), and urethral pressure profile. These studies can be performed with video or fluoroscopic capabilities.

Uroflowmetry

Uroflowmetry is a simple noninvasive procedure to measure the peak flow rate of urine in milliliters per second by having the client void into a special funnel device with a spinning disc at the base. A computerized module attached to the device digitally calculates a graph of the voiding episode. The graph yields information on peak and mean urine flow rates, duration of voiding, and the volume voided (Fig. 32–8). Peak flow may be diminished in clients with bladder outlet obstruction or poor detrusor contractility.

Instruct the client to prepare for the test by having a full bladder. Accuracy of the measurement depends on a voided volume of at least 125 ml, although clients should avoid overfilling the bladder. Complications or risks associated with this test are minimal. The bladder may be further evaluated for postvoid residual volume with ultrasonography (see earlier discussion of ultrasonography of the bladder).

Cystometrography

CMG involves the use of at least one urethral catheter to measure bladder pressure and a second catheter in the rectum or vagina to measure intra-abdominal pressure. The abdominal pressure measurement is then subtracted from the bladder pressure measurement to obtain an accurate representation of the detrusor pressure and the reaction of the smooth muscle of the bladder wall during filling and voiding. CMG is performed in both the filling and voiding phases to evaluate bladder compliance, ca-

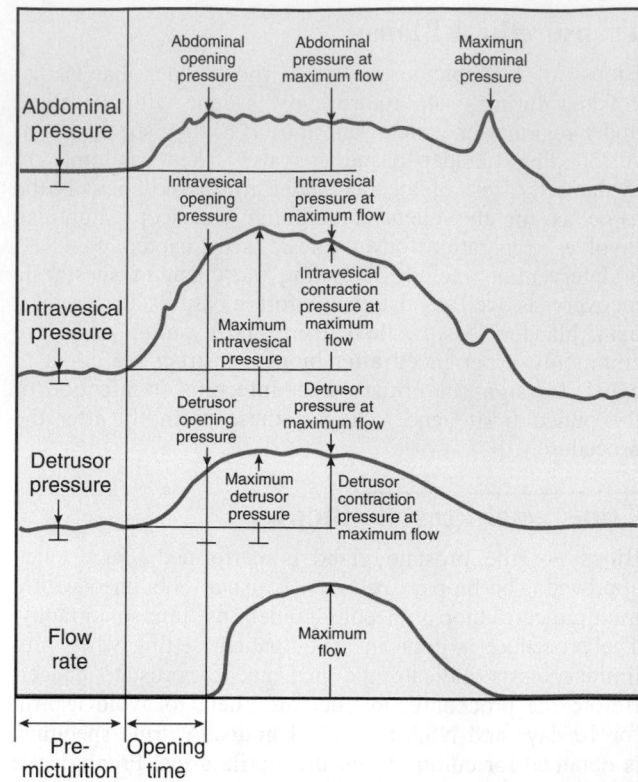

FIGURE 32–9 Diagram of a pressure flow study graph. (Modified from Walsh, P. C., et al. [Eds.]. [1998]. *Campbell's urology* [7th ed.]. Philadelphia: W. B. Saunders.)

FIGURE 32–8 Diagram of terminology used in urodynamic studies. *Shaded area* shows voided volume. *Dotted lines* show how voided volume is divided into time and flow rate.

pacity, stability, and sensation. CMG is indicated for evaluating bladder outlet obstruction and urinary incontinence.

Sphincter Electromyography

EMG is performed at the same time as CMG. EMG evaluates for detrusor or sphincter dyssynergia, which occurs when the sphincter cannot relax or becomes overactive during detrusor contraction with voiding. This disorder can cause elevated postvoid residual volumes, urinary tract infection, or urinary retention and occurs in neurologic disorders.

Patch, wire, or needle electrodes are positioned on the perineum to monitor the response of the pelvic floor muscles to bladder filling and voiding. The patch and wire electrodes are painless but are prone to recording artifact. The needle electrodes provide detailed information but can cause discomfort and limit mobility. The integrity of the sacral reflex arc may be tested by eliciting the bulbocavernosal reflex during EMG (see earlier discussion of assessment of this reflex).

Pressure Flow Study

The pressure flow study is performed with the voiding cystometrogram and simultaneously illustrates graphically a comparison of the detrusor pressure, abdominal pressure, urine flow rate, and electromyogram. It can help to distinguish between poor detrusor contractility and bladder outlet obstruction (Fig. 32–9).

Video-Fluoroscopic Urodynamics

The lower urinary tract can be directly visualized during CMG and EMG by filling the bladder with a radiologic contrast medium instead of sterile water, saline, or carbon dioxide. This technique provides more information about voiding disorders. Results can be recorded on videotape for later evaluation.

Urethral Pressure Profile

The urethral pressure profile measures sphincter closure pressure and evaluates urethral incompetence. The urethral length and continuous urethral response to filling, voiding, and provocative measures, such as coughing, may be assessed. A specialized catheter, either a membrane catheter or a catheter mounted with microtransducers, is withdrawn slowly through the urethra while recording pressure readings at every level. This test can be done in cases of sphincter dysfunction, urinary incontinence, or detrusor or sphincter dyssynergia.

PREPROCEDURE CARE

All urodynamic testing except uroflowmetry requires a negative Gram stain or urine culture. Advise clients to force fluids and to abstain from voiding approximately 1 to 2 hours before the procedure if possible. Clients may be advised to discontinue any medications that may affect urinary function before the study. The study should not be performed after recent cystoscopy or prostate biopsy. Clients who have artificial joints or cardiac valvular disease or replacements should have appropriate prophylactic antibiotics.

Explain how the procedure is performed, the catheters and equipment used, the client's role in the study, and what the client can expect to feel during and after the study. If videourodynamics are measured, explain the need to have two or three people in the room (the nurse or technician performing the study, a radiologic technician, and possibly a urologist). Reassure the client that every effort will be made to preserve privacy.

POSTPROCEDURE CARE

Teach the client to watch for and report manifestations and symptoms of urinary tract infection, urgency, and frequency persisting after 24 hours. Encourage the client to drink at least two 8-ounce glasses of water each hour for 4 hours after the procedure. A warm bath or washcloth applied to the perineum may help alleviate the urethral irritation that is common after the procedure.

CONCLUSIONS

A thorough knowledge of the potential causes of elimination disorders is essential in order to obtain a pertinent health history and to perform an accurate physical assessment. Careful assessment facilitates formulation of accurate nursing and medical diagnoses and planning for the optimal treatment of the client. Knowledge of diagnostic testing is necessary to prepare the client for the tests and to facilitate the diagnostic process.

BIBLIOGRAPHY

1. Chiverton, P. A., et al. (1996). Psychological factors associated with urinary incontinence. *Clinical Nurse Specialist, 10*(5), 229–233.
2. DeGowin, E. L., & DeGowin, R. L. (1971). *Bedside diagnostic examination.* New York: Macmillan.
3. Fantl, J. A., et al. (1996). *Urinary incontinence in adults: Acute and chronic management* (Clinical Practice Guideline No. 2, AHCPR Publication No. 96-0682). Rockville, MD: Agency for Health Care Policy and Research, Public Health Service, U.S. Department of Health and Human Services.
4. Gallo, M. L., Fallon, P. J., & Staskin, D. R. (1997). Urinary incontinence: Steps to evaluation, diagnosis, and treatment. *The Nurse Practitioner, 22*(2), 21–42.
5. Goroll, A. H., May, L. A., & Mulley, A. G. (Eds.). (1995). *Primary care medicine: Office evaluation and management of the adult client* (3rd ed.). Philadelphia: J. B. Lippincott.
6. Gray, M. (1992). *Genitourinary disorders.* St. Louis: Mosby–Year Book.
7. Hanson, K. A., & Blute, M. L. (1994). Endourologic diagnosis and conservative management of upper tract urothelial cancer. *Urologic Nursing, 14*(4), 159–163.
8. Heitkemper, M., et al. (1995). Interventions for irritable bowel syndrome: A nursing model. *Gastroenterology Nursing, 18*(6), 224–230.
9. Holmes, H., et al. (1998). *Illustrated guide to diagnostic tests* (2nd ed.). Springhouse, PA: Springhouse Publishing.
10. Karlowitz, K. A. (1995). *Urologic nursing: Prevention and practice.* Philadelphia: W. B. Saunders.
11. Kelly, M. (1996). Chronic renal failure. *American Journal of Nursing, 96*(1), 36–37.
12. Khullar, S., & DiSario, J. (1997). Colon cancer screening: Sigmoidoscopy or colonoscopy. *Gastrointestinal Endoscopy Clinics of North America, 7*(3), 365–386.
13. McCance, K., & Huether, S. (1994). *Pathophysiology: The biologic basis for diseases in adults & children* (2nd ed.). St. Louis: Mosby–Year Book.
14. McConnell, J. D., et al. (1994). *Benign prostatic hyperplasia: Diagnosis and treatment* (Clinical Practice Guideline No. 8, AHCPR Publication No. 94-0582). Rockville, MD: Agency for Health Care Policy and Research, Public Health Service, U.S. Department of Health and Human Services.
15. McQuaid, K., & Friedman, S. (1996). *Current diagnosis and treatment in gastroenterology.* Norwalk, CT: Appleton & Lange.
16. Moore, D. A., & Edwards, K. (1997). Using a portable bladder scan to reduce the incidence of nosocomial urinary tract infections. *MEDSURG Nursing, 6*(1), 39–43.
17. Prandoni, D., et al. (1996). Assessment of urine collection technique for microbial culture. *American Journal of Infection Control, 24*(3), 219–221.
18. Schottefeld, D., & Fraumeni, J. F. (1996). *Cancer epidemiology and prevention.* New York: Oxford University Press.
19. Shearman, D., et al. (1997). *Diseases of the gastrointestinal tract and liver* (3rd ed.). New York: Churchill Livingstone.
20. Swartz, M. (1994). *Textbook of physical diagnosis, history and examination* (2nd ed.). Philadelphia: W. B. Saunders.
21. Tanagho, E. A., & McAninch, J. W. (1995). *Smith's general urology.* Norwalk, CT: Appleton & Lange.
22. Uphold, C., & Graham, M. (1994). *Clinical guidelines in family practice* (2nd ed.). Gainesville, FL: Barmarrac Books.
23. Vickery, G. (1997). Basics of constipation. *Gastroenterology Nursing, 20*(4), 126–128.
24. Walsh, P. C., et al. (1998). *Campbell's urology* (7th ed.). Philadelphia: W. B. Saunders.
25. Wozniak-Petrofsky, J. (1997). Urodynamic tests: Client preparation, assessment, and follow-up. *The Nurse Practitioner, 22*(3), 70–91.

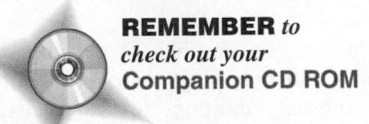

CHAPTER

33

Management of Clients with Intestinal Disorders

Helen Murdock Rogers

NURSING OUTCOMES CLASSIFICATION (NOC) for Nursing Diagnoses—Clients with Intestinal Disorders

Altered Nutrition: Less Than Body Requirements
Nutritional Status
Bowel Incontinence
Bowel Elimination
Bowel Continence
Tissue Integrity
Constipation
Bowel Elimination
Hydration
Diarrhea
Fluid Balance
Hydration
Symptom Severity
Fluid Volume Deficit
Bowel Elimination

Fluid Balance
Hydration
Knowledge Deficit
Knowledge: Treatment Procedures
Pain
Comfort Level
Pain: Disruptive Effects
Risk for Body Image Disturbance
Grief Resolution
Psychosocial Adjustment: Life Change
Self-Esteem
Risk for Ineffective Individual Coping
Coping
Decision-Making
Role Performance
Social Support

Risk for Ineffective Management of Therapeutic Regimen (Individuals)
Health Beliefs: Perceived Ability to Perform
Knowledge: Treatment Regimen
Participation: Health Care Decisions
Risk for Infection
Risk Detection
Risk for Injury
Risk Control
Safety Status: Physical Injury
Risk for Sexual Dysfunction
Sexual Functioning
Body Image
Self-Esteem

The client with an intestinal disorder usually has a problem with bowel elimination. Hence, the most common nursing diagnoses are *Constipation, Bowel Incontinence,* and *Diarrhea.* Additional nursing diagnoses are *Pain, Altered Nutrition: Less Than Body Requirements, Fluid Volume Deficit,* and *Body Image Disturbance.*

GENERAL CLINICAL MANIFESTATIONS

Disorders of the intestine disrupt one or more of its functions. They can slow, obstruct, or accelerate the movement of intestinal contents (*chyme*) through the intestine, or they can disrupt secretion, motility, and absorption of intestinal contents. Disorders occur in response to inflammation, tumors, infections, obstructions, and changes in the structure of the intestine. Manifestations of intestinal disorders vary according to which function (motility, digestion, or absorption) is disturbed. The major manifestations of dysfunction are hemorrhage, pain, nausea and vomiting, distention, constipation, diarrhea, and abnormal fecal contents.

HEMORRHAGE. Bleeding may be caused by trauma, ulceration, inflammation, or a growth that erodes through

a blood vessel. The usual manifestation is blood in the stool (*hematochezia*) rather than in vomitus (*hematemesis*). The amount of bleeding varies from a minute quantity that is invisible except by testing (*occult blood*) to large quantities that cause stools to be bright red to tarry-black (*melena*). The stool color is affected by (1) the digestive processes acting on the blood and (2) the rapidity with which chyme passes through the bowel. For instance, slow bleeding from the duodenum may not increase peristalsis and may produce a tarry stool. If the rate of bleeding or of peristalsis increases, subsequent stools may become brighter red.

PAIN. Mechanical, inflammatory, or ischemic changes cause pain by stimulating the nerve endings in the muscular or submucosal layers of bowel wall. Mechanical factors cause pain by stretching and distending the bowel; these actions then activate nerve endings. For example, edema and vascular congestion cause painful stretching. Biochemical mediators that are released during the inflammatory process cause pain by stimulating nerve endings.

Obstruction of blood supply to the intestine (*ischemia*) also can cause pain. Acute or partial occlusion of the mesenteric artery causes intermittent pain during digestion because of the greater need for blood at that time. Occlusion can occur in the major artery or one of the smaller branches.

Discomfort occurs in various places and is characterized as three types:

- *Visceral pain* arises from a stimulus acting on the involved portion of the bowel. It results in a diffuse, poorly localized pain that clients describe as gnawing, burning or cramping.
- *Somatic pain* arises from the parietal peritoneum and is more localized and intense than visceral pain.
- *Referred pain* is visceral pain felt at a distance from an affected organ.

NAUSEA AND VOMITING. In intestinal disorders, nausea results from distention of the duodenum. Vomiting may occur from changes in the integrity of the intestinal wall (as in gastroenteritis) or from changes in the motility of the bowel (such as caused by an obstruction). Vomitus that contains fecal matter usually indicates a distal obstruction in the small intestine.

DISTENTION. Distention is caused by excessive gas in the intestines. It may be due to the inability to adequately digest a specific nutrient, such as lactose, or may result from a defect in intestinal motility. *Flatus* (passing of bowel gas) may be another clinical manifestation.

DIARRHEA. *Diarrhea* is defined as an increase in the frequency, volume, and fluid content of stool. Rapid propulsion of intestinal contents through the small bowel results in diarrhea and may lead to a serious fluid volume deficit. Common causes are infections, malabsorption syndromes, medications, allergies, and systemic diseases.

CONSTIPATION. *Constipation* is the infrequent or difficult passage of stools. It is a very common manifestation that can be caused by inadequate fluid or bulk, mechanical blockage of the passage of intestinal contents (by a tumor), or slow peristalsis.

ABNORMALITIES IN FECAL CONTENT. The presence of fats or other abnormal constituents, normally absorbed from the stool, indicates malabsorption. Other fecal abnormalities that may aid in diagnosis are bacteria, parasites, pus, blood, and abnormal quantities of mucus from the colon.

DISORDERS OF THE LARGE AND SMALL BOWEL

INFLAMMATORY DISORDERS

Inflammation can occur in any portion of the bowel and can be caused by organisms, toxins produced by organisms, infiltration of the bowel wall by granulomatous processes, injury from radiation, trauma, and medications.

INFECTIONS AND INFESTATIONS

■ VIRAL AND BACTERIAL INFECTIONS: GASTROENTERITIS

Gastroenteritis is an inflammation of the stomach and intestinal tract that primarily affects the small bowel. The major clinical manifestations are diarrhea of varying degrees and abdominal pain and cramping. Associated clinical manifestations are nausea, vomiting, fever, anorexia, distention, *tenesmus* (straining on defecation), and *borborygmi* (hyperactive bowel sounds).

Gastroenteritis occurs throughout the world, often in epidemic outbreaks. Contaminated food and water are major sources of these diseases and cause thousands of deaths yearly. The incidence of infections caused by food-borne diseases is rising; only respiratory infections are more common. Eighty million cases of food-borne disease occur annually in the United States, costing society billions of dollars each year. *Campylobacter* causes an estimated 2 million illnesses each year. Another bacteria, *Escherichia coli 0157:H7*, causes an estimated 30,000 infections and 250 deaths annually.

Infection with *Clostridium difficile,* also known as pseudomembranous colitis, is a bacterial dysentery commonly seen in clients who have been receiving large doses of antibiotics or who have taken antibiotics for a long time. The condition is becoming more common in hospitalized clients.

Etiology and Risk Factors

Pathogens that cause gastrointestinal (GI) disease are transmitted by the fecal-oral route, from person to person, and through ingestion of fecally contaminated food and water. GI infections are often referred to as "food poisoning" because food is frequently the vehicle for transmission of actively growing microbes or their toxins. Common bacterial sources of contaminated foods are eggs (*Salmonella*), raw or undercooked meat (*E. coli*), and chicken (*Campylobacter*). Outbreaks of food-borne viral infections are almost entirely caused by fecally contaminated shellfish. Unpasteurized milk, apple juice, and ice cream are also sources of food-borne infection. Other causative organisms are *Vibrio cholerae* (cholera), *Shigella* bacilli (dysentery) and *Staphylococcus aureus* (staphylococcal food poisoning). The incubation period for all viral and bacterial infections ranges from 6 hours to 3 or 4 days.

Health promotion actions for avoiding such GI infections involve instructing clients about (1) good handwashing technique after defecation and before handling food and (2) obtaining available vaccinations against bacterial and viral gastroenteritis. Encourage cleanliness and sanitation as well as proper food handling, preparation. and storage techniques, such as cooking meats to 150° F, cooking chicken to 170° F, and not allowing food to sit at room temperature for long periods. Advise clients to avoid the use of antibiotics over a long time. Teach travelers going to developing countries about safe food practices, such as avoiding tap water, milk products, raw seafood, and foods that cannot be cooked or peeled.

Health maintenance activities include the assessment of clients who are receiving high or continued doses of antibiotics for manifestations of *C. difficile* infection and other manifestations of GI infection secondary to antibiotic use. Health restoration interventions involve client self-management of manifestations. Instruct clients to follow their medication regimen and to call their health care provider if (1) manifestations continue for several days, (2) they might be dehydrated, or (3) body temperature is higher than 100° F. Promote bowel rest and replacement of fluids and electrolytes as needed.

Pathophysiology

Normally, human intestinal flora protect the bowel from colonization of pathogens. However, the intestinal flora can be (1) disrupted by harmful bacteria and viruses that cause tissue damage and inflammation or (2) depressed by antibiotic therapy. Antibiotics most often implicated in the depression of normal flora are clindamycin, penicillins, cephalosporins, and aminoglycosides.

Pathogens cause tissue damage and inflammation by releasing endotoxins that stimulate the mucosal lining of the intestine, resulting in greater secretion of water and electrolytes into the intestinal lumen. The active secretion of chloride and bicarbonate ions in the small bowel leads to inhibition of sodium reabsorption. In order to balance the excess sodium, large amounts of protein-rich fluids are secreted in the bowel, overwhelming the large bowel's ability to reabsorb the fluid and leading to diarrhea. Pathogens also cause damage and inflammation by invading and destroying the mucosal lining of the bowel, resulting in bleeding and ulceration. When the integrity of the GI tract is impaired, its ability to carry out digestive and absorptive functions may be affected.

Clinical Manifestations

The universal manifestation of gastroenteritis is diarrhea, which occurs in varying intensity depending on the organism involved and the health status of the individual. The diarrhea may be mild (two to three stools per day) or intense (>10 watery stools per day). Nausea, vomiting, and anorexia may occur from abdominal distention caused by increased fluid content and undigested food. Abdominal pain, cramping, and borborygmi may occur from gas released from undigested food, irritation of bowel mucosa, and distention of the intestines. The client may have a fever, depending on the causative organism. The stool may test positive for leukocytes and may contain the causative organism as well as mucus and varying amounts of blood.

Prognosis

Most cases of gastroenteritis are temporarily disabling and self-limiting, with resolution in 1 to 5 days. However, gastroenteritis can be fatal in debilitated, older, or very young people. Early detection and treatment with fluids and electrolytes are critical to prevent death or disability in such cases. Up to 10% of clients infected with *E. coli 0157:H7* develop hemolytic uremic syndrome (HUS), which causes death in 3% to 5% of the people it affects and chronic renal failure in 10% to 30% of those who survive it.

■ PARASITIC INFECTIONS
Protozoa

Protozoa are parasites that replicate in the intestines of infected hosts and are excreted in the feces. They are transmitted in the same way as bacterial and viral pathogens; however, fewer numbers or organisms are needed to produce clinical manifestations. Enteric protozoa are the leading cause of water-borne disease and are becoming more frequently implicated as causes of food-borne infections. Several new protozoa have been identified; for example, *Cyclospora*, which has been linked to contaminated raspberries. Some protozoa are becoming resistant to methods used to eliminate them, such as chlorination.

Giardiasis, the most common protozoal diarrheal illness in the United States, is caused by the protozoan *Giardia lamblia.* It generally spreads through the water system or spoiled food. Most infected people are asymptomatic. However, those with manifestations may present several weeks after exposure with nausea, vomiting, excessive foul flatulence, and malabsorption, which results in weight loss and copious, foul-smelling, greasy stools. Organisms infect the small intestine mucosa and submucosa and are found in the stool. The medications used for treatment include metronidazole (Flagyl), quinacrine (Atabrine) and furazolidone (Furoxone). A new vaccine may be available in the near future; however, at present, no agent is effective in preventing giardiasis.

Cryptosporidium is associated with water-borne and food-borne outbreaks in nursing homes and day care centers. It is spread by drinking contaminated water or swimming in infected lakes or swimming pools. The organism attaches itself to the intestinal epithelium, causing surface damage, inflammation, and watery diarrhea.

Amebiasis produces diarrhea when a protozoan *(Entamoeba histolytica)* invades the lining of the colon. Manifestations include rectal inflammation as well as blood, pus, and amebae in the stool. Metronidazole (Flagyl) is the drug of choice for treatment.

Helminths

The intestinal tract may be infested with any of several species of helminths or parasitic worms, including *Ascaris* (roundworms), *Enterobius* (pinworms), *Trichinella spiralis* (which causes trichinosis), and various species of *Cestoda* (tapeworms). These parasites are found worldwide. Worm infestations, contracted through the skin or from ingesting contaminated food or water, can cause serious and even fatal disease if the parasites are not eradicated from the intestinal tract. Worms also may cause urinary tract infections or pruritus ani. Fortunately, most of these parasites are susceptible to medications such as mebendazole and pyrantel pamoate. Piperazine and quinacrine hydrochloride also may be used, but they have more side effects. Treatment of all household members may reduce reinfection.

Schistosomiasis is caused by a blood fluke (a parasitic flatworm). The infection is prevalent worldwide, occurring in about 1 in 30 people. The cercariae (larvae) of the parasite penetrate the skin, migrate to the liver via the lungs, and remain in intrahepatic portal venules until the worm matures. The mature worm, which does not multiply within humans, then moves into its final habitat. Depending on the species involved, the worm may settle in the veins of the large bowel, small bowel, or bladder, where it lays eggs. These eggs, which form pseudotubercles (small, nobby prominences), have been found in every system of the body. Schistosomiasis may have mild or severe manifestations, depending on the species of worms involved and the number present. Laboratory studies to identify the species are completed before pharmacologic treatment with oxamniquine, metrifonate, praziquantel, or niridazole is started.

Outcome Management for Viral, Bacterial, and Parasitic Infections

■ Medical Management

REST THE BOWEL

Rest, with nothing by mouth (NPO [from the Latin *nil per os*]) until the vomiting has stopped, is the best intervention.

DECREASE DIARRHEA

When diarrhea is severe and does not resolve within 2 to 3 days, the infecting organism needs to be identified from stool specimens and blood samples. Medications to decrease intestinal motility are usually not administered because the infecting agents need to be eliminated; this is particularly true with *C. difficile* infection because the bacteria multiply if GI motility is slowed and the bacteria are retained. Anti-infective agents are chosen on the basis of the organism identified.

RESTORE FLUIDS AND ELECTROLYTES

The client is started on small amounts of clear liquids as tolerated. An electrolyte replacement beverage may be given. The diet is advanced after 24 hours as tolerated. If the client has a severe fluid depletion, an intravenous (IV) agent such as 0.45% sodium chloride may be required. A potassium supplement may be ordered if the client's serum potassium level is low.

■ Nursing Management of the Medical Client

Most clients present with an acute onset of diarrhea. Carefully note a description of the diarrhea, including (1) onset, (2) number, color, and consistency of stools, and (3) accompanying manifestations, such as nausea and vomiting. Ask the client about recent foreign travel, eating habits, and antibiotic use.

Assess the client's abdomen. Examination may reveal hyperactive bowel sounds, distention, and tenderness. Dehydration and electrolyte imbalance may be present, depending on the amount of fluids and electrolytes lost. Assess muscle weakness and fatigue due to hypokalemia. Metabolic alkalosis from bicarbonate loss is also a potential problem. Carefully examine all stool for blood and mucus, and record intake and output. Examine the client's anal area for irritation. After cleaning the area, apply a protective moisture barrier product for clients with irritation.

Administer anti-infective medications, such as antibiotic and antiparasitic agents, to treat the specific cause of the diarrhea. Antidiarrheals may be ordered if the diarrhea is uncontrollable. If there are manifestations of fluid and electrolyte imbalance, start IV fluids until oral fluids are tolerated. Begin clear liquids with electrolytes in small amounts until the client can tolerate toast and crackers. Advance the diet as tolerated.

Provide written and oral instructions regarding medications, diet, and rest as well as about when and how to report any continued problems. If other family members are sharing the bathroom, the client must be reminded to wash the hands well and to maintain absolute cleanliness.

APPENDICITIS

Appendicitis is an inflammation of the vermiform appendix that develops most commonly in adolescents and young adults. It can occur at any age but is rare in clients younger than 2 years and reaches a peak incidence in clients between 20 and 30 years. It is not common in older adults; however, when it does occur in such clients, rupture of the appendix is more common. Appendicitis affects 7% to 12% of the population.

Etiology and Risk Factors

Appendicitis can be caused by:

- A fecalith (a fecal calculus, or stone) that occludes the lumen of the appendix
- Kinking of the appendix
- Swelling of the bowel wall
- Fibrous conditions in the bowel wall
- External occlusion of the bowel by adhesions

There are no particular risk factors for appendicitis. Because it is not preventable, early detection of the condition is important.

Pathophysiology

When the appendix becomes obstructed, the intraluminal pressure increases, leading to decreased venous drainage, thrombosis, edema, and bacterial invasion of the bowel wall. After the initial obstruction, the appendix becomes increasingly hyperemic, warm, and covered with exudate, progressing to gangrene and perforation.

Clinical Manifestations

The classic manifestations of appendicitis begin with acute abdominal pain that comes in waves. At first, the pain may be perceived merely as discomfort that makes the client feel that passing flatus or having a bowel movement will bring relief. Unfortunately, many clients take a laxative during this period, which may lead to rupture of the appendix and peritonitis.

The pain typically starts in the epigastrium or periumbilical region. It then shifts to the right lower quadrant as the inflammatory process spreads to involve the serosal layers of the bowel, thereby bringing the inflammatory process into contact with the peritoneum. The pain becomes steady rather than intermittent, and the client often *guards* or protects the area by lying still and drawing the legs up to relieve tension on the abdominal muscles.

Assessment also may reveal vomiting that begins after the pain starts, loss of appetite, low-grade fever, coated tongue, and bad breath. Mild leukocytosis is usually present, with the white blood cell (WBC) count between 10,000 and 15,000/mm³. Pain at McBurney's point, which lies midway between the right anterior superior iliac crest and the umbilicus, confirms the diagnosis.

Outcome Management

■ Surgical Management

APPENDECTOMY

There is no medical treatment for appendicitis. Preoperatively, IV fluids and antibiotics are administered. Pain medication is withheld until the diagnosis is confirmed.

INDICATIONS. Surgical intervention involves removal of the appendix (*appendectomy*) within 24 to 48 hours of onset of the manifestations. The surgery can be performed through a small open incision or a laparoscope (a lighted scope used to visualize and remove the appendix). When the operation is performed in time, the mortality rate is less than 0.5%. Delay usually causes rupture of the organ and resultant peritonitis (see "Peritonitis").

COMPLICATIONS. Perforation of the bowel is the most common complication. Antibiotics and surgical drainage are required if perforation occurs. Peritonitis may develop after perforation.

OUTCOMES. Following a laparoscopic procedure, the client is usually dischargeded in 24 to 48 hours. Another day of hospitalization may be indicated after an open surgical procedure. Lifting is restricted for 2 to 4 weeks. The client can resume all activities 4 to 6 weeks after surgery.

■ Nursing Management of the Surgical Client

ASSESSMENT

The client is usually admitted with severe abdominal pain. Carefully assess the pain, especially to determine its location. Also assess the client for rebound tenderness (sharp pain when pressure is released on abdomen after deep palpation) and the presence of peritonitis (see "Peritonitis"). Carefully assess the client's vital signs, fluid and electrolyte status, and laboratory data. The client with appendicitis should fast preoperatively.

DIAGNOSIS, OUTCOMES, INTERVENTIONS

Pain. One of the most appropriate nursing diagnoses for the client with acute appendicitis is *Pain related to inflammation*.

Outcomes. The client describes decreased postoperative pain.

Interventions. An abrupt change in the character of the pain preoperatively may indicate perforation. Postoperatively, pain control, as described in Chapters 15 and 23, should be practiced. Sometimes, pain medication is not given until the client is actually ready for surgery. Never give an enema or a laxative or apply heat to the abdomen of the client with appendicitis, because any one of these actions may lead to bowel perforation.

Risk for Fluid Volume Deficit. Another appropriate nursing diagnosis for the client with acute appendicitis is *Risk for Fluid Volume Deficit related to vomiting*.

Outcomes. The client maintains fluid and electrolyte balance, as evidenced by balanced intake and output and electrolyte levels within normal limits.

Interventions. As soon as the client is admitted, IV fluids are started to maintain fluid balance, with electrolytes added as needed. If the client is vomiting, a nasogastric (NG) tube may be inserted. Carefully measure intake and output.

Risk for Infection. The diagnosis *Risk for Infection related to rupture of appendix* is common.

Outcomes. An infection will not develop, or rupture will be diagnosed early, as evidenced by (1) removal of the appendix before rupture or (2) prompt treatment of the rupture.

Interventions. Check the client's vital signs regularly, monitoring closely for an increase in temperature and a change in pulse and blood pressure, which may signify a ruptured appendix. Preoperative antibiotics are usually administered to reduce the infection. Monitor pain closely. If the pain becomes generalized throughout the abdomen and the abdomen becomes rigid and board-like, the appendix may have ruptured.

After surgery, monitor vital signs, urine output, level of consciousness, and IV therapy and assess the client's respiratory status and the surgical wound. The client may have a drain, and if the appendix ruptured, packing may be present. Assess the dressings, provide wound care, reposition the client approximately every 2 hours, and adequately manage the client's pain.

The client who has had a ruptured appendix with an infected wound needs to be taught the proper way to care for the wound. Wound care usually involves irrigation of the wound with sterile saline and application of a sterile dressing at least several times a day. Assess the client's ability to function at home and to care for the wound. A home health care referral may be needed to assist the client with physical needs and to ensure that the wound is healing properly.

EVALUATION

The usual outcome after an uncomplicated appendectomy is healing within a few weeks. If the appendix has ruptured, however, healing takes longer. With a ruptured appendix, healing cannot occur until the infection has cleared and the wound is clean. A secondary closure may be required after the wound is clean. Some incisions are left open to heal through granulation (regeneration) of tissue.

PERITONITIS

Peritonitis is inflammation of the peritoneal membrane. The *peritoneum* is a semipermeable two-layered sac filled with approximately 1500 ml of fluid. This sac covers all the organs in the abdominal cavity. Because it is well supplied with somatic nerves, stimulation of the parietal peritoneum that lines the abdominal and pelvic cavities causes sharp, well-localized pain. The visceral peritoneum is relatively insensitive.

Etiology and Risk Factors

Peritonitis can be primary or secondary. Major sources of inflammation are from the gastrointestinal tract, from the external environment, and through the bloodstream. Normal flora of the intestine become a source of infection when they enter the sterile peritoneal cavity. The most common organism is *E. coli*, although streptococci, staphylococci, and pneumococci also may be involved. The peritoneum may produce an inflammatory reaction and wall off (prevent the spread of) a localized process to combat an infection if the stimulus is not too massive and if the source of infection does not continue.

There are no risk factors for peritonitis because the condition is a result of another problem. Causes include ruptured or gangrenous gallbladder, perforated peptic ulcer, perforated stomach or intestine secondary to cancer or inflammatory bowel disorders, bowel obstruction, penetrating wounds, and other conditions (such as acute pancreatitis and mesenteric thrombosis). The major preventive measures are early diagnosis of clients at risk for peritonitis and initiation of early treatment help to prevent spread of the infection.

Pathophysiology

Peritonitis produces severe systemic effects. Circulatory alterations, fluid shifts, and respiratory problems can cause critical fluid and electrolyte imbalances. The inflammatory response shunts (diverts) extra blood to the inflamed area of the bowel to combat the infection. Peristaltic activity of the bowel ceases. Fluids and air are retained within its lumen, raising pressure and increasing fluid secretion into the bowel. Thus, circulating blood volume diminishes. The inflammatory process increases oxygen requirements at a time when the client has difficulty ventilating (breathing) because of abdominal pain and increased abdominal pressure, which elevates the diaphragm.

Clinical Manifestations

Manifestations of peritonitis vary according to the cause. Pain may be localized or generalized. Well-localized pain that causes rigidity of abdominal muscles and pain that increases with any pressure or motion of the abdomen are characteristic of peritonitis. Also, the client usually experiences nausea, vomiting, and, possibly, a low-grade fever. Assessment reveals absence of bowel sounds and shallow respirations because the client is trying to avoid the pain caused by body movement.

The client with peritonitis commonly has an elevated WBC count (20,000/mm^3) with a high neutrophil count. Abdominal x-ray studies are performed, which may show dilation and edema of the intestines or free air or fluid in the abdominal cavity. If the client is vomiting, manifestations of altered fluid and electrolyte balance also may be present.

Outcome Management

■ Medical Management

MAINTAIN FLUID AND ELECTROLYTE BALANCE
If peritonitis is advanced and if surgery is contraindicated by shock and circulatory failure, oral fluids are prohibited. IV fluids are necessary for replacement of electrolyte and protein losses. An NG tube or a long intestinal tube may be inserted to reduce pressure within the bowel. See Chapter 31 for nursing care of a client with an NG or intestinal tube.

CONTROL INFECTION
Once the infection has been walled off and the client's condition improves, surgical drainage and repair can be

attempted. The other major treatment of peritonitis is IV antibiotic therapy with potent broad-spectrum agents.

■ Surgical Management

Surgery may be performed to prevent peritonitis, such as an appendectomy for an inflamed appendix or a colon resection (surgical removal) for inflamed diverticulum. If the perforation is not prevented, the major surgical intervention is incision and drainage of the abscess once it is walled off.

■ Nursing Management of the Surgical Client

Preoperatively, obtain a thorough history, including specific information about the client's pain. Assess the abdomen, noting the presence or absence of bowel sounds. Palpate the abdomen, noting whether the abdomen is firm, distended, or rigid. Note areas of rebound tenderness.

Clients with peritonitis are acutely ill and are given broad-spectrum antibiotics immediately. The perforated organs are usually repaired as soon as the client is stable enough to withstand the stress of surgery. During surgery, any leakage can be sampled for culture so that specific antibiotic therapy can be implemented. The peritoneal cavity is irrigated with an antibiotic solution to reduce the bacterial count. Often, the wound is packed open or drains are placed so that infection can be treated.

Postoperatively, carefully monitor clients for the development of postoperative complications, such as adult respiratory stress syndrome (ARDS), sepsis, and shock. Closely monitor the client's fluid balance by assessing vital signs, bowel sounds, urine output, skin turgor, mucous membranes, and weight. Immediately report any manifestations of sepsis, such as a drop or rise in temperature or a drop in blood pressure. IV fluids are administered along with antibiotic therapy. Upon discharge, provide the client with oral or written instructions regarding wound care, medications, activity restrictions, and follow-up visits.

INFLAMMATORY BOWEL DISEASE

Inflammatory bowel disease (IBD) affects approximately 2 million Americans, or 1 of every 125 people. Each year, 30,000 people learn that they have this chronic disease. It is estimated that IBD costs between $1.8 and 2.6 billion annually in lost wages and disability and health care payments. Relatives of clients with IBD are 10 times more likely to experience IBD than the general population.

IBD consists of two chronic inflammatory disorders: Crohn's disease (regional enteritis) and ulcerative colitis. These chronic, recurrent diseases predominantly affect younger people. Treatment is symptomatic, and responses are often unpredictable. Frequently, clients with IBD require surgery, which may be followed by recurrence. Because of the similarities between Crohn's disease and ulcerative colitis, the two conditions are compared throughout the following discussion and in Table 33–1.

CROHN'S DISEASE
Crohn's disease is a chronic relapsing disease that may develop discontinuously (without sequence and skipping

TABLE 33-1	DIFFERENTIATION BETWEEN CROHN'S DISEASE AND ULCERATIVE COLITIS	
Characteristic	**Regional Enteritis (Crohn's Disease)**	**Ulcerative Colitis**
GENERAL DESCRIPTION		
Age at onset	Young	Young to middle age
PATHOLOGY AND ANATOMY		
Depth of involvement	Transmural (all layers of submucosa)	Mucosa and submucosa
Rectal involvement	50%	95%
Right colon involvement	Frequent	Occasional
Small bowel involvement	Involved, ileum narrow	Usually normal
Distribution of disease	Segmental	Continuous
Inflammatory mass	Chronic and extensive	Rare (crypt abscess)
Cobblestone-like mucosa and granuloma	Common	Absent
Mesentery lymph involvement	Edema and hyperplasia	Not involved
Toxic megacolon	Occasional	Occasional
Steatorrhea	Frequent	Absent
Malignancy results	Rare	After 10 years
Fibrous stricture	Common	Absent
CLINICAL CHARACTERISTICS		
Course of disease	Slowly progressive	Remissions and relapses
Rectal bleeding	Occasional	Common (90%–100%)
Abdominal pain	Colicky (45%)	Predefecation (60%–70%)
Hematochezia	Unusual or absent	Almost always present
Diarrhea	Present (65%–85%)	Early and frequent (80%–95%)
Vomiting	Present (35%)	Present (15%)
Nutritional deficit	Common	Common
Weight loss	Present (60%–70%)	Present (10%)
Fever	Present (35%)	Present (10%)
Anal abscess	Common (75%)	Occasional (10%)
Fistula and anorectal fissure fistula	Common (80%)	Rare (10%–20%)
SYSTEMIC MANIFESTATIONS		
Arthritis	20%	Uncommon (10%)
Peripheral sacroiliitis	18%	18%–20%
Hepatobiliary involvement	Uncommon	15% cholestatic dysfunction
		19%–38% fatty liver
		30%–50% pericholangitis
Skin: erythema nodosum, pyoderma gangrenosum	Common	Present (5%–10%)
Nephrolithiasis	Occasional	Rare

sections) in any segment of the alimentary tract. The most common location is the terminal ileum. Crohn's disease more characteristically involves the entire thickness of the bowel wall (*transmural*), particularly the submucosa. The mortality rate is not high, but recurrences and complications can result in disability. Crohn's disease is more common in whites and among Ashkenazi Jews. There is a higher incidence within families. The disorder occurs at all ages but more often in people between 20 and 30 years old. The two sexes are affected equally.

ULCERATIVE COLITIS
Ulcerative colitis is a disease that spans the entire length of the colon and involves only the mucosa and submucosa. The disease usually starts in the rectum and distal colon, spreading upward beyond the rectosigmoid valve to involve most of the sigmoid and descending colon. Ulcerative colitis causes inflammation, thickening, congestion, edema, and minute lacerations that ooze blood and eventually develop into abscesses. The edema may lead to extreme friability of the mucosa, and bleeding can thus occur from any minor trauma. Ulcerative colitis is

more common than Crohn's disease. It occurs at all ages, but the incidence is higher among young adults, women, and Jews. The disorder has demonstrated a familial tendency.

Etiology and Risk Factors
CROHN'S DISEASE
The cause of Crohn's disease is unclear, although there may be a genetic or hereditary basis. It is also considered an autoimmune disease. The only risk factors identified for Crohn's disease are genetic. There are no preventive measures.

ULCERATIVE COLITIS
Several theories have been advanced to explain the cause of ulcerative colitis. One theory is that the disease is of bacterial origin, because many clients have a history of bacterial infection before the onset of the condition. Researchers have also suspected an allergic reaction as a basis of the disease. Others believe that ulcerative colitis may be due to an altered immune status because antibodies

have been found in the colon. Still others suggest that destructive enzymes and a lack of protective substances in the bowel wall cause the inflammatory process. An emotional disturbance can precipitate an exacerbation or prolong an attack of the disorder, but it is not the primary cause.

No preventable risk factors are associated with ulcerative colitis. Once the client has the disease, controlling stress can help keep the disease in remission.

Pathophysiology

CROHN'S DISEASE

Lesions typically develop in several separated segments of bowel. They are visible on gross examination (without aid of a microscope), and their color is dramatically different from that of normal tissue. Examination of the bowel tissue by endoscopy reveals edematous, heavy, reddish purple areas. Granular spots also may be present. Enlarged lymph nodes appear in the submucosa, and Peyer's patches are seen in the intestinal mucous membrane. These areas undergo small superficial ulcerations with granulomas and fissures. Fissures may completely penetrate the bowel wall, leading to fistulas and abscesses. Collections of lymphocytes throughout the mucosa, submucosa, and serosa are the only microscopic features of Crohn's disease. The small bowel wall becomes congested and thickened, narrowing the lumen.

Small bowel–related complications include malabsorption, kidney stones, gallstones, and hydronephrosis. Anorectal problems include internal fistulae and abscesses. Anal fissure (see later) is common and is directly related to the severity of the diarrhea, which produces ulceration of the perianal skin. Pain is aggravated by walking, sitting, and defecation.

ULCERATIVE COLITIS

The appearance of the colon depends on the stage, activity, and severity of the disease. The most characteristic lesion of ulcerative colitis is an inflammatory infiltrate called a *crypt abscess*. This abscess consists of polymorphonuclear leukocytes, lymphocytes, red blood cells, and cellular debris appearing at the base of the crypts of Lieberkühn. Secretions from crypt abscesses result in purulent discharge from the bowel mucosa. Abscesses may become necrotic and may ulcerate.

Infections secondary to ulcerative colitis produce further inflammatory reactions in the mucosa and submucosa. When the inflammatory lesions heal, scarring and fibrosis, with narrowing, thickening, and shortening of the colon and loss of haustral folds, may follow.

Cancer of the colon is more common among clients with ulcerative colitis than in the general population. The incidence is greatly increased when ulcerative colitis develops before the client is 16 years of age and in clients who have had the condition for more than 20 years.

Toxic megacolon is an extreme dilation of a segment of the diseased colon (often the transverse segment) that results in complete obstruction. Toxic megacolon usually occurs during an acute exacerbation of ulcerative colitis, and it may follow hypokalemia, a barium enema, or the use of anticholinergics, narcotics, corticosteroids, or antibiotics. Bacterial overgrowth contributes to this complication. Perforation and peritonitis may complicate the condition.

Clinical Manifestations

Crohn's disease and ulcerative colitis produce similar manifestations. Clients suffer from abdominal pain, diarrhea, fluid imbalances, and weight loss. Severe diarrhea or vomiting may cause metabolic acidosis. Remissions are followed by exacerbations of acute disease. When the disease is acute, the client has a fever. The general appearance of clients with IBD varies from reasonably healthy to wasted, drawn, and malnourished, with varying degrees of pallor. They usually report a steady and progressive weight loss. Inspection reveals a flat or concave shape to the abdomen, with visible peristaltic activity. Palpation of the abdomen reveals tenderness over the area of inflamed bowel. Increased bowel sounds are heard on auscultation. Hemorrhoids and, in Crohn's disease, perianal abscess, fistula, and ulcers may be apparent.

Hematocrit and hemoglobin values are usually decreased. A barium enema study with air contrast is often performed to differentiate ulcerative colitis from Crohn's disease. The client with suspected IBD routinely undergoes colonoscopy. Biopsy and cytologic studies also help distinguish among carcinoma, ulcerative colitis, and Crohn's disease. The clinical manifestations of Crohn's disease and ulcerative colitis are compared in Table 33–1.

CROHN'S DISEASE

Diarrhea in Crohn's disease is usually less severe than that in ulcerative colitis. Stool consistency is typically soft or semiliquid. Urgency to expel stools may awaken the person at night. The client rarely passes gross blood unless ulceration is present. Malabsorption, associated with steatorrhea, may develop. If so, stools may be foul-smelling and fatty.

The client with severe steatorrhea, diarrhea, or long-standing enteritis may have associated nutritional deficits, weight loss, anorexia, pain, anemia, debility, fatigue, and metabolic disturbances. Nutritional deficits arise from (1) a reduction in the intestinal absorptive surface, (2) malabsorption of protein and carbohydrates, and (3) impaired absorption of fat, folic acid, iron, calcium, and vitamins A, B_{12}, C, D, E, and K. Alterations in bile salt and vitamin metabolism may result from surgery or mucosal defects. Metabolic requirements increase because of the inflammatory process and infection, the decrease in food intake, and the loss of nutrients in the feces due to rapid gastrointestinal transit time. Electrolytes lost from diarrhea include sodium, potassium, chloride, the trace elements (magnesium, zinc, copper), and minerals. Nitrogen excretion remains normal if there is no loss of protein from the inflammatory exudate. The consequences of malnutrition include:

- Loss of immunocompetence
- Decreased resistance to infection
- Diminished wound healing
- Reduced pancreatic enzyme output
- Impaired healing (fistula and surgical wounds)
- Decreased iron-binding capacity resulting from chronic infection or blood loss

ULCERATIVE COLITIS

The predominant manifestation of ulcerative colitis is rectal bleeding. Clients often experience diarrhea, possibly

20 or more stools per day. The severity and frequency of diarrhea depend on the extent of involved colon. Severe diarrhea can cause a loss of 500 to 17,000 ml of water in 24 hours. Liquid stools occur with tenesmus and may contain blood, mucus, and pus. A sense of urgency and cramping abdominal pain may occur with the diarrhea. The client typically experiences colicky pain in the lower left quadrant.

Nausea, vomiting, anorexia, weight loss, and decreased serum potassium concentration may occur with severe disease. In addition, the client loses plasma proteins, prothrombin, and fluids. Anemia may develop with severe blood loss and decreased dietary iron intake.

Physical findings include tenderness in the lower left quadrant, guarding, and (in severe ulcerative colitis) abdominal distention. Following remissions, ulcerative colitis may recur after bouts of emotional stress, dietary indiscretion, or the ingestion of irritants such as laxatives and antibiotics. Physical exertion, respiratory infections, and overfatigue also may cause an attack.

Prognosis

Remissions and exacerbations characterize both types of IBD. The only known cure for ulcerative colitis is surgical removal of the colon. Surgical procedures and medication therapy can control the manifestations in Crohn's disease, but currently there is no known cure.

Outcome Management

▆ Medical Management

DECREASE DIARRHEA

Medical treatments, which primarily aim to control the manifestations, are similar for ulcerative colitis and Crohn's disease. Because the inflammatory process in Crohn's disease involves deeper layers of the bowel wall and is more chronic, healing may occur more slowly than in ulcerative colitis. Thus, anti-inflammatory therapy, including steroids, is required for longer periods in Crohn's disease than in ulcerative colitis.

Fluids, electrolytes, and blood are replaced as needed to maintain the client's homeostasis. Physical activity should be kept to a minimum during an acute attack to decrease intestinal motility. The client with a mild attack may work but needs extra rest. The client with fever, toxemia, frequent bowel movements, bleeding, or pain requires bed rest. Failure of the inflamed colonic mucosa to reabsorb water and electrolytes, bile salts, and lactose interferes with control of diarrhea. The extent of large bowel involved by the disease influences the severity of diarrhea. The client should keep a record of the number of stools, their consistency and color, and the presence or absence of blood.

Bowel rest and parenteral hyperalimentation may result in restored immunocompetence, greater resistance to infection, correction of nutritional deficiencies, and relief of edema and bowel inflammation.

Pharmacologic Agents

ANTIDIARRHEAL MEDICATIONS. Antidiarrheal preparations may provide symptomatic benefit. Loperamide (Imodium) is superior to atropine-diphenoxylate (Lomotil)

in controlling the diarrhea of Crohn's disease, with fewer side effects. Use of opiates for diarrhea control may cause distention and megacolon. Hydrophilic mucilloids, such as psyllium (Metamucil), may improve consistency of stools and control incontinence. Antispasmodic medications, such as propantheline bromide, glycopyrrolate, and dicyclomine hydrochloride, may reduce postprandial (after-meal) pain and diarrhea.

AMINOSALICYLATES. Diarrhea associated with IBD may be treated successfully with agents that inhibit prostaglandin synthesis and reduce inflammation. Examples are sulfasalazine (Azulfidine), mesalamine (5-ASA), and olsalazine (Dipentum). Mesalamine is available orally as Asacol and Pentasa and rectally as Rowasa. The oral tablets should not be crushed because they are coated for release of the drug in the colon. Rowasa suppositories and rectal suspension are used when disease is contained in the rectum or distal colon. The suppository should be retained in the rectum for 1 to 3 hours, and the suspension should be retained for 8 hours.

CORTICOSTEROIDS. Clients whose IBD fails to respond to the previously discussed measures may require corticosteroid medications. Adrenal steroids and corticotropin may be used with other therapy to reduce the body's response to inflammation. Steroids may be given orally, intravenously, intramuscularly, or rectally. Oral forms include hydrocortisone, prednisolone, and prednisone. Hydrocortisone also can be administered rectally as an enema or suppository. Steroids do not cure IBD, but they modify its course. Long-term complications associated with steroid use must be weighed against the relief of manifestations of IBD. Antacids or histamine receptor antagonists should be given during steroid therapy to prevent gastric ulceration. Steroids reduce adrenal function and may impair resistance, causing defective healing of abscesses and fistulas.

IMMUNOSUPPRESSIVE AGENTS. 6-Mercaptopurine (Purinethol) is used when other treatment modalities fail and can be effective against chronic, unrelenting Crohn's disease. Methotrexate (Folex) and azathioprine (Imuran) are now widely accepted as therapies for IBD. Cyclosporine (Sandimmune) is an effective agent but is associated with much toxicity. Infliximab (Remicade) is a new drug for Crohn's disease that blocks the action of tumor necrosis factor—a natural protein that causes intestinal inflammation. This agent is given by a single IV infusion that may be repeated every 2 to 3 months. Several new drugs, currently in clinical trials, are the selective cytokine-inhibiting drug CDC 801 (SelCID) and two successor compounds to SelCID called inflammation modulator imidazoles (IMIDs).

ANTICHOLINERGIC MEDICATIONS. During acute exacerbations, the client is given anticholinergic medications to relieve abdominal cramps and help control diarrhea. Anticholinergic, antidiarrheal, and antispasmodic agents allow the colon to rest. Withhold these medications if there are manifestations of obstruction.

ANTI-INFECTIVE MEDICATIONS. Medications commonly used to prevent or control infections include sulfonamides and antibiotics such as metronidazole (Flagyl) and ciprofloxacin (Cipro). Antibiotics may be given to control secondary bowel inflammation and infection.

INCREASE NUTRITIONAL INTAKE

Nutritional deficiencies are the most common complications of IBD. These deficits derive from decreased intake, increased losses, greater nutritional requirements, and side effects of certain medications. Diarrhea leads to fluid and electrolyte losses with resultant muscle wasting and edema. Malabsorption due to bacterial overgrowth or mucosal involvement of the bowel may cause further problems. Deficiencies of fat-soluble vitamins (A, D, E, and K) and folate may develop. Vitamin K deficiency causes bleeding tendencies.

DIET AND SUPPLEMENTS. A diet high in protein and calories is given in an attempt to restore normal nutritional levels but is not always well tolerated. Liquid supplements are residue free, low in fat, and digested mainly in the upper jejunum.

Anemia and vitamin deficiencies should be corrected nutritionally or with supplements. Folate deficiency, which may be due to the therapeutic use of sulfasalazine, may be prevented by (1) increasing dietary intake of folate, (2) having the client take sulfasalazine between meals, or (3) supplementing the intervention regimen with folic acid.

TOTAL PARENTERAL NUTRITION. Total parenteral nutrition (TPN) is indicated when a client has not responded to medical intervention, is being prepared for surgery, or has undergone intestinal resection. TPN provides bowel rest by removing all stimulation of secretion and by decreasing fecal bulk. Weight gain, positive nitrogen balance, and a temporary remission of manifestations can occur. TPN appears to be more useful in Crohn's disease than in ulcerative colitis.

When oral food and fluids are resumed, they should be chemically and mechanically nonirritating and high in calories, protein, and minerals. The client should avoid cocoa, chocolate, citrus juices, cold or carbonated drinks, nuts, seeds, popcorn, and alcohol.

◼ Nursing Management of the Medical Client

ASSESSMENT

Assess the client's bowel elimination pattern, noting the number of stools, their color and consistency, and the presence or absence of blood or steatorrhea. Also assess the client's abdomen. Note bowel sounds and the location of pain. Complete a nutritional assessment, as directed in Chapter 29.

DIAGNOSIS, OUTCOMES, INTERVENTIONS

Diarrhea. Diarrhea is the most common manifestation of IBD, so the primary nursing diagnosis is *Diarrhea related to inflamed intestinal mucosa.*

Outcomes. The client will experience a decrease in diarrhea, as evidenced by a decrease in number and a more solid consistency of stools.

Interventions. Antidiarrheal medications may be administered to control the client's diarrhea. Perianal excoriation often occurs with diarrhea. After every bowel movement, gently clean the skin with warm water and apply a protective moisture barrier product.

See the Management and Delegation feature (p. 799).

Altered Nutrition: Less Than Body Requirements. The client with inflammatory bowel disease has many difficulties with nutrition, making *Altered Nutrition: Less Than Body Requirements related to diarrhea and malabsorption* a common nursing diagnosis.

Outcomes. The client will increase nutritional intake to meet metabolic requirements, as evidenced by weight stabilization and, possibly, weight gain.

Interventions. Monitor the client's nutritional intake. The type of diet ordered depends on the client's condition. If the client can tolerate a diet, encourage intake of fluids and food. Because eating stimulates the gastrocolic reflex and the urge to defecate, many people are afraid to eat; small servings may enable the client to avoid this problem. Foods should be easily digested to promote absorption during the short time the food remains in the bowel.

Clients with Crohn's disease are often receiving home TPN because they cannot tolerate foods for long periods as a result of disease exacerbation (see Chapter 29). These clients also may have undergone multiple bowel resections, resulting in short-bowel syndrome and problems of malabsorption.

Pain. Another common nursing diagnosis for the client with inflammatory bowel disease is *Pain related to inflamed mucosa.*

Outcomes. The client will experience a relief in abdominal pain, as evidenced by the client's statement of pain relief.

Interventions. Assess the client's pain, and give pain medications as ordered. Note any changes in the client's complaints of pain because they may indicate the development of complications. Narcotics are generally used sparingly so that they do not mask manifestations.

Risk for Ineffective Individual Coping. Stress is associated with inflammatory bowel disease. Write the nursing diagnosis as *Risk for Ineffective Individual Coping related to stress of disease and exacerbations related to stress.*

Outcomes. The client will cope effectively with the disease, as evidenced by fewer exacerbations and an improved coping style.

Interventions. Although emotional factors may not contribute to the cause of the disease, they do influence its course. Prolonged stress often precedes the onset of IBD and exacerbations. Recommend that the client schedule a follow-up physical examination and colonoscopy every 1 to 2 years. Refer clients with IBD to the Crohn's and Colitis Foundation of America (386 Park Ave. S., New York, NY 10016-8804) to learn about the condition and about meetings of local support groups. Instruct the client to call the physician at the first manifestation of IBD recurrence.

EVALUATION

It is hoped that the client's disease will respond to medical management and that the client will achieve remission, improved coping, and adequate nutritional intake. If the client's IBD does not respond to medical management, surgical intervention may be required.

◼ Surgical Management

Surgery, the only cure for ulcerative colitis, is usually indicated when medical management fails and the condition is intractable. Twenty-five per cent to 40% of clients with ulcerative colitis must undergo surgical removal of the colon with a permanent ileostomy or a restorative procedure, such as an ileal pouch–anal anastomosis (suturing two loops of bowel together) or a Kock pouch, or continent ileostomy. Surgery is not indicated in Crohn's disease except to treat complications. An operation may be indicated in either or both conditions, however, for complications, such as perforation, hemorrhage, obstruction, toxic megacolon, abscess, fistula, and disease intractability.

TOTAL PROCTOCOLECTOMY

In a total proctocolectomy, the colon and rectum are removed and the anus is closed. The terminal ileum is brought out through the abdominal wall, and a permanent ileostomy is formed.

ILEORECTAL ANATOMOSIS

Ileorectal anastomosis is another form of surgical management. The colon is resected, leaving a rectal stump. The terminal ileum is then anastomosed to this stump. The client has diarrhea postoperatively; in time, however, the stool usually becomes more solid.

Ileorectal anastomosis, an early alternative to total proctocolectomy, is associated with several problems, however. The remaining rectum is often still affected by the disease, and further treatment, even eventual resection, is often required. There is also a significant incidence of rectal cancer among clients who have undergone this procedure. The need for ileorectal anastomosis has essentially been eliminated because safer, more effective procedures are now available.

CONTINENT ILEOSTOMY

INDICATIONS. A continent ileostomy, or Kock pouch, is a procedure in which a reservoir or pouch is constructed from a loop of ileum. This allows stool to be stored intra-abdominally until it is drained through a nipple valve made from an intussuscepted portion of ileum (prolapse of one part of intestine into an adjacent section) (Fig. 33–1). The client has a flat stoma on the right side of the abdomen. Advantages of the continent ileostomy are (1) no need to wear an external pouch, (2) minimal skin problems, and (3) usually, no flatus or leakage of

stool. The client drains the pouch several times a day using a catheter, usually in response to a feeling of fullness.

CONTRAINDICATIONS. A continent ileostomy should not be performed for Crohn's disease. If the client has malnutrition, TPN may be required to improve the outcome of surgery and promote wound healing.

COMPLICATIONS. After the formation of the Kock pouch, suture line leakage with local or generalized peritonitis may occur in the early postoperative period. Other complications, including fistula formation, sliding of the valve, and obstruction by food residue, may occur late in the recovery period.

OUTCOMES. The client resumes usual activities within 4 to 6 weeks. Nutritional status also improves. The client experiences improved quality of life without the necessity of frequent trips to the bathroom.

ILEAL POUCH–ANAL ANASTOMOSIS

INDICATIONS. Ileal pouch–anal anastomosis is the preferred surgical procedure for clients with ulcerative colitis. The procedure (the J pouch) avoids an ostomy and preserves the rectal sphincter muscle.

The rectal mucosa is excised, and the colon removed. An ileoanal reservoir is then created in the anal canal, and a temporary loop ileostomy is formed. After healing has taken place, usually in 2 to 3 months, the ileostomy is reversed, so that stool drains into the reservoir, which is created by suturing two loops of bowel together (Fig. 33–2). Some surgeons are completing this procedure in one operation so that a temporary ileostomy is not required.

CONTRAINDICATIONS. This anastomosis should not be performed for Crohn's disease. If malnutrition is a problem, TPN may be needed to improve the outcome of surgery and promote wound healing.

COMPLICATIONS. Complications include anastomotic leakage, pouchitis (inflammation of the pouch), and bowel obstruction.

OUTCOMES. The client resumes regular activities in 4 to 6 weeks after the second procedure or after the first procedure if a temporary ileostomy has not been performed. Nutritional status improves, and the client experi-

FIGURE 33–1 Continent ileostomy (Kock pouch). *1,* Loop of terminal ileum is sutured together and cut open. Using forceps, the surgeon intussuscepts the distal ileum to form a nipple valve. *2,* Free edges are sutured together to form the reservoir, the stoma is sutured flush with the skin, and the pouch is sutured to the abdominal wall.

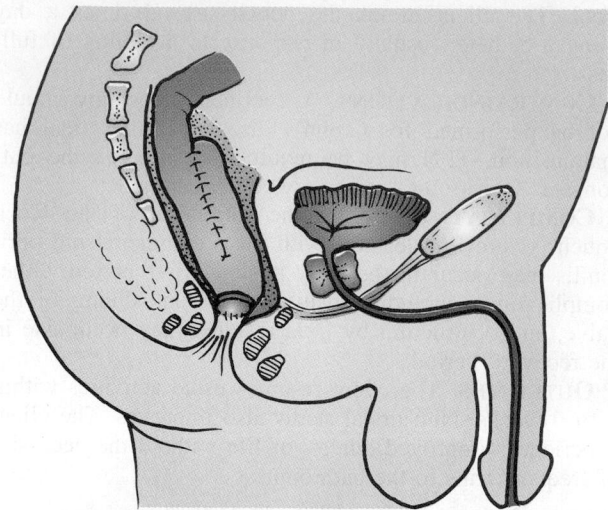

FIGURE 33–2 Ileal J pouch–anal anastomosis. The two-loop ileal pouch is simple to construct, provides adequate storage capacity, and is evacuated spontaneously and fully.

ences improved quality of life with nearly normal bowel movements and fewer trips to the bathroom.

SURGICAL RESECTION OF SMALL BOWEL

INDICATIONS. In Crohn's disease, surgery is used only to treat the complications, because even when the diseased portion is removed, the incidence of recurrence is 50%. The physician may prescribe antibiotics to control infection. During surgical resection for Crohn's disease, attempts are made to preserve as much of the small intestine as possible. Two thirds of the small intestine may be removed with no ill effects if the remaining portion is normal.

CONTRAINDICATIONS. Clients may be too malnourished to undergo surgery. TPN is needed to prepare the client for surgery and to improve wound healing.

COMPLICATIONS. With resection of the distal ileum, the client cannot absorb vitamin B_{12} and removal of more than 6 to 8 feet results in impaired absorption of glucose, fat, and protein. If the colon is diseased, an ileotransverse colectomy (right colon and ileum), segmental colectomy, or total colectomy may be performed. A total colectomy with ileorectal anastomosis may be the surgery of choice.

For 1 to 3 weeks after extensive small bowel resection, the client may be unable to tolerate oral intake and may experience further losses in body protein or lean body mass. TPN is given until oral intake can be resumed. Diarrhea usually occurs during the first 6 weeks after surgery. Anemia (from iron deficiency, steatorrhea, or decreased protein absorption) also may ensue. Paralytic ileus (see later) is another possible complication.

Clients with either irreversible intestinal failure or short-bowel syndrome resulting from multiple bowel resection, may be candidates for small bowel transplantation (SBT). This procedure is an alternative therapy for clients who might otherwise face the prospect of lifelong TPN. In the past, cadaver donors were used, but more recently a living-related intestinal transplantation has been accomplished. Clients undergoing SBT have a difficult postoperative course and long-term complications of im-

munosuppression, and they are at risk for graft rejection (see Chapter 80).

OUTCOMES. It is hoped that the client can return to regular activities with complete wound healing and adequate nutrition 4 to 6 weeks after surgery.

■ Nursing Management of the Surgical Client

ASSESSMENT

Assessment of the surgical client is similar to assessment of the medical client. However, routine preoperative and postoperative assessments as discussed in Chapter 15 are also necessary. If the client is malnourished, TPN may be required preoperatively to improve nutritional status.

DIAGNOSIS, OUTCOMES, INTERVENTIONS

PREOPERATIVE CARE

Knowledge Deficit. The client who is to undergo surgical resection for inflammatory bowel disease has many learning needs. The nursing diagnosis is *Knowledge Deficit related to surgical procedure and possible ileostomy or other bowel resection.*

Outcomes. The client will understand the surgical procedure and implications of bowel resection, as evidenced by the ability to describe the procedure and perform a demonstration of ileostomy care.

Interventions. Describe the anticipated postoperative course, including types of tubes that will be in place. Ostomy care must be fully explained to the client scheduled for ileostomy surgery. A preoperative visit from a member of any ostomy association may be helpful. An enterostomal therapy nurse should assist with the preoperative preparation. Before surgery, the site of the ileostomy is selected, with consideration being given to the location of the disease, body contours, convenience, and type of clothing the client wears. The client may wear the pouch for 1 to 2 days before surgery to ensure comfort with the site selected. In order to provide assistance and support, assess the client's body image as well as feelings about loss of a major body part and wearing a pouch for a lifetime.

If the client is having a continence-sparing surgery, extensive teaching is still required. The client needs to understand the type of bowel resection to be performed and the implications of the surgery. With some procedures, a temporary ileostomy (ileal pouch–anal anastomosis) may be necessary; with other procedures (e.g., the Kock pouch), the client's method of waste elimination is altered permanently.

POSTOPERATIVE CARE

Risk for Injury: Postoperative Complications (Stomal Necrosis, Retraction, Prolapse, Stenosis, Obstruction). The client undergoing stoma formation is prone to complications. The nursing diagnosis is *Risk for Injury related to postoperative complications of stomal necrosis, retraction, prolapse, stenosis, or obstruction.*

Outcomes. The client will not suffer injury, as evidenced by minimal distention, rapid return of normal peristalsis, and absence of fluid and electrolyte imbalance.

Interventions

Monitor Stoma. Monitor the stoma after surgery. Ensure that there is no pressure on the stoma that could interfere with circulation. Assess the color of the stoma frequently (see Fig, 33–7 for appearance of a normal stoma). If the stoma becomes pale, dusky, or cyanotic, notify the physician immediately. When blood supply to the stoma is compromised, surgical revision is required.

Advance Diet. An NG tube is in place for several days after surgery to remove gases and fluids that would increase intestinal distention and put pressure on the suture line. The drainage must be accurately noted. The passage of flatus indicates return of peristalsis. As bowel sounds return, clamp the tube as prescribed, and give the client ice chips and water. When the client has tolerated ice chips and water for a minimum of 24 hours, the tube is usually removed, and clear liquids are given.

Monitor for Complications. Although the postoperative course for most clients with ileostomies is uneventful, several complications can occur. The most common is an intestinal obstruction, which may be caused by obstruction of the lumen, adhesions, food, or stomal edema. Early manifestations of obstruction are (1) anorexia, (2) abdominal cramps, (3) absence of ileostomy drainage or a foul, brown, watery discharge in the pouch, and (4) visible peristalsis. Other early postoperative complications are hemorrhage, hypoxia, and fluid and electrolyte imbalance. If there are severe or prolonged problems with absorption, parenteral nutrition may be necessary.

Risk for Body Image Disturbance.
The client with an ostomy has to face alterations in self-concept and body image. Write the nursing diagnosis as *Risk for Body Image Disturbance related to alteration of lifestyle secondary to ostomy.*

Outcomes. The client experiences a positive body image and self-concept, as evidenced by the client's statements and the ability to care for the ostomy without embarrassment.

Interventions. A few days after surgery, the client needs to begin to (1) confront the stoma and (2) integrate its function and appearance into his or her body image. Help the client look at and touch the stoma as soon as possible. Always use proper terms for the stoma and equipment.

Because clothing can be a concern for the client with an ostomy, clothing options should be discussed. Discourage the client from wearing a tight waistband, which might rub on the stoma. Encourage the client to try on various outfits to ensure that the stoma and pouch are not visible. A visit from another person with an ostomy, usually available through the local chapter of the American Cancer Society, often helps the client realize that the ostomy is easily hidden beneath clothing.

Encourage the client to verbalize feelings about the stoma and its appearance. The client may be very accepting of the stoma because the illness (ulcerative colitis) is now gone and his or her life may be more normal and productive than it had been with the disease. Young men and unmarried women may express the greatest concern about body image. Find out how family or significant others now view the client. Their response might be positive because the client may have been chronically ill prior to surgery and now appears much healthier.

Risk for Ineffective Management of Therapeutic Regimen (Individuals).
The client with a new stoma has much to learn about self-care. The nursing diagnosis is *Risk for Ineffective Management of Therapeutic Regimen (Individuals) related to ileostomy care, care following ileorectal anastomosis, care of an ileal pouch–anal anastomosis, or care of a continent ileostomy.*

Outcomes. The client will understand proper care of the chosen surgical procedure, as evidenced by (1) the ability to apply the appliance correctly, without leakage, and to empty the pouch appropriately, and (2) absence of perianal breakdown.

Interventions

Ileostomy

Teach ostomy care. The client must master the skills needed to provide self-care. Stoma care is the area of greatest concern to the client with an ileostomy. Consultation with an enterostomal therapy nurse, if available, may enhance teaching and care (see Management and Delegation: Stoma Care). Initially, the client can simply observe care of the stoma. Begin by telling the client what the stoma looks like; that it extends ½ to ¾ inch beyond the abdominal wall, is 1 to 1½ inches in diameter, and is very red and swollen at first. Assure the client that permanent changes in stoma size occur within the first 3 months after surgery as the swelling subsides.

The frequency with which the ileal pouch needs to be emptied varies with each client. It should be emptied whenever it is approximately one-third to one-half full. Instruct the client to empty the pouch during times of low output, usually before meals, at bedtime, and upon arising in the morning. It is best to change the pouch when the ileostomy is the least active, usually first thing in the morning.

When changing the pouch, have all equipment ready before removing the old pouch. Remove the old pouch carefully using a moist cloth. A piece of gauze may be held over the stoma until the new pouch is attached. Encourage the client to inspect and touch the stoma at this time. Remind the client with a new ileostomy to take ostomy supplies along when traveling. The client may want to keep supplies handy in a shaving or cosmetic case instead of a suitcase. Many different types of pouches are available (Fig. 33–3). Clients should try to find the best pouch for their needs.

Teach stoma assessment. When changing the pouch, the client should learn to check the size and color of the stoma, assess the odor of the drainage, and observe for manifestations of irritation. When the ileostomy begins to function, the output is minimal. As the client takes in more food, the drainage becomes thicker and has a weak odor. Because an ileostomy may drain continuously (drainage is related to eating patterns), a pouch must be worn continuously, and the stoma must be covered with gauze when the pouch is being changed.

Prevent skin irritation. The pouch should be cut to fit the stoma, allowing only 1/16 inch of room around the stoma. If the pouch does not fit well, severe skin irritation can occur because of the alkalinity of the effluent. Skin irritation can vary from redness to weeping dermatitis or ulceration. Irritation also can result from adhesives or frequent removal of the appliance. The skin should be washed and rinsed thoroughly between removing one pouch and applying another. With a two-piece setup, a pouch is snapped onto the faceplate, which is applied to

MANAGEMENT AND DELEGATION

Stoma Care and Application of Ostomy Appliances

The care of a mature stoma and the application of an ostomy appliance may be delegated to unlicensed assistive personnel. The assessment and care of a newly created ostomy, however, should be performed only by a Registered Nurse. Before delegating stoma care and applying an ostomy appliance, consider the following:

- The age of the ostomy. Is this a postsurgical client with a new ostomy, or a client with an ostomy that is several weeks, months, or years old? For the client with a new ostomy, you or a trained ostomy nurse should provide care. For the client with a long-standing ostomy, assess the ostomy to ensure that the client is caring for it properly and that the stoma and surrounding skin are intact before you delegate ostomy care to assistive personnel.
- The client's need to learn self-care of the stoma and ostomy. You or a trained ostomy nurse should provide this instruction for a client needing to learn self-care.
- The client's acceptance of the ostomy, altered appearance, and bowel function. Clients having difficulty accepting their altered body image would benefit from having you or an ostomy nurse help them increase the acceptance and their ability to cope with the new ostomy.
- The competency level of the unlicensed assistive personnel who will potentially perform this task.

The assistive personnel providing stoma care and applying ostomy appliances should be instructed to:

1. Provide privacy for the client.
2. Place a waterproof pad around the ostomy or under the client, to protect the skin and bed linens.
3. Empty the contents of the ostomy bag prior to removing the bag, noting the consistency, color, volume, and odor of the feces.
4. Loosen the skin barrier with alcohol or another adhesive.
5. Gently remove the barrier and bag while supporting the client's skin.
6. Place a gauze pad or tissues over the exposed stoma to avoid soiling from leakage.
7. Wash the skin around the stoma with warm water and a mild soap, and wash the stoma with clear water.
8. Rinse the area with water and pat it dry.
9. Note the color, moisture, and protrusion of the stoma and the condition of the surrounding skin.
10. Create a circle 14 to 18 inches larger than the size of the stoma on the back of the appliance. A stoma-measuring guide may be helpful for this procedure.
11. Prepare the barrier and appliance as a unit.
12. Smooth the barrier to remove all air bubbles.
13. Fill in irregular stoma borders with skin paste.
14. Apply the unit, skin barrier, appliance, and bag around the stoma. Position the bag to hang in a dependent position. If the client is ambulatory, remember to position the bag for optimal drainage while the client is upright.
15. Dispose of the soiled bag and appliance properly. Do this outside the client's room to prevent embarrassment about any odors.

Assistive personnel should also be taught to report immediately to you if they find black, tarry stools or overt signs of blood in the bag or bleeding from the stoma. Reddened, inflamed skin surrounding the stoma should also be brought to your attention. Information pertaining to the care and condition of the stoma should be recorded.

Donna W. Markey, MSN, RN, ACNP-CS, *Clinician IV, Surgical Services, University of Virginia Health System, Charlottesville, Virginia*

---

the skin. This arrangement allows for easy emptying of the pouch. The faceplate usually remains adherent to the skin for 5 to 7 days. It may need to be changed sooner if it becomes loose or if leakage occurs.

FIGURE 33–3 Natura brand ostomy products. (Courtesy of ConvaTec, Bristol-Myers Squibb, Skillman, NJ.)

Treat skin problems. If skin irritation does occur, first check the fit of the pouch. The best initial treatment for this problem would be to reapply the ostomy appliance, ensuring a proper fit and seal. The skin barrier of the appliance is usually sufficient to protect and heal the skin. If this method does not work, other barriers must be used. A wide variety of skin care products are available. If the problems continue, consult an enterostomal therapy nurse for further assistance.

Skin infection also can occur. *Candida* is the most common cause. The peristomal skin takes on a rash-like appearance. An antifungal powder should be rubbed onto the affected skin area. The barrier can then be applied over the powder.

Reduce odor. Foods such as eggs, fish, onions, cabbage, and some greens cause stool odor; therefore, deodorizing solutions and tablets may be placed in the pouch. Spinach, parsley, yogurt, and buttermilk reduce drainage odor.

Discuss medications. The client also needs special instructions regarding prescription and over-the-counter medications. Enteric-coated tablets, such as iron preparations, vitamins, and hormones, multilayer tablets, timed-release capsules, and gelatin capsules may not be absorbed in the small intestine. The client should note whether any medications are obvious in pouch drainage;

if so, the physician must prescribe different medications or different forms of medication.

Emphasize fluid intake. The client who has had an ileostomy needs to pay close attention to fluid intake. It is very easy for such a client to become dehydrated. The approximate output from an ileostomy is 1200 to 1500 ml/day. The client must monitor this output for any increase that could lead to severe fluid and electrolyte imbalance.

Explain dietary recommendations. A low-residue diet that is high in protein, carbohydrates, and calories is recommended after ileostomy surgery. Supplemental vitamins A, D, E, K, and B$_{12}$ may be needed. Berries, whole-grain cereals, and raw fruits and vegetables can cause problems for the client with an ileostomy. Any foods that cause discomfort or diarrhea should be omitted. Ingested foods pass through the ileostomy within 4 to 6 hours. It is not advisable to eat a large meal close to bedtime.

The client with an ileostomy must learn to chew food well because the shortened bowel transit time would caused poorly chewed food to be passed undigested. High-fiber and high-cellulose foods may absorb excessive moisture, leading to swelling and possibly constipation or even obstruction. Foods that should be avoided or limited, at least initially, include popcorn, peanuts, tough fibrous meats, vegetables with skins, rice, bran, and coconuts.

Clients may find that the postoperative diet is less restrictive than the diet they followed before the operation. The diet required by the presence of the disease was often very restricted because so many foods increased the diarrhea and other manifestations. Clients with ileostomies often gain weight after surgery, sometimes to the point of having to restrict caloric intake.

Prevent urolithiasis. Some clients with ileostomies tend to have calcium oxalate, uric acid, or urinary calculi because greater amounts of fluid are lost through the ileostomy, leading to decreased urine output. Uric acid stones tend to form when urine volume is low and the urine is persistently acidic. Ingestion of sodium bicarbonate or potassium citrate alkalinizes the urine. Allopurinol may be used if uric acid levels remain elevated. Fluid intake should be at least 2000 ml/day.

Ileorectal Anastomosis. The client with an ileorectal anastomosis does not have to learn about stoma or pouch care unless a temporary ileostomy is present. The major goal of teaching centers on the importance of defecating before the rectum becomes overly distended. Most clients find that they have four to five stools per day once their bodies have adjusted to the surgical alteration. The feces of these clients are often described as pasty in consistency, and they appear to contain fewer electrolytes than the drainage from a traditional ileostomy. It may take up to 1 year for the client's altered bowel to adapt.

Encourage follow-up. Clients with ileorectal anastomoses must understand the importance of follow-up meetings with the physician. They must understand that the remaining mucosa can become diseased with ulcerative colitis or Crohn's disease, requiring further resection and, possibly, formation of an ileostomy. They also need to know that they are at increased risk for development of rectal cancer. Such clients must undergo regular proctoscopic examinations following surgery.

Avoid irritating foods. The client should learn to avoid foods that may cause diarrhea. It is best to try new foods one at a time so the effect can be determined. The diet is usually not limited; however, it should include adequate fluids to avoid dehydration.

Ileal Pouch–Anal Anastomosis. The client with an ileal pouch–anal anastomosis also has no need to learn about stoma or pouch care unless a temporary ileostomy was created. The client will learn to respond to the sensation to defecate so that spillage does not occur. After the bowel adapts to the surgical alteration, the stool becomes more formed, and many clients have only five or six stools per day. The client should maintain an adequate fluid intake.

Continent Ileostomy (Kock Pouch)

Maintain ileal drainage. During surgical formation of the Kock pouch, an evacuation catheter is inserted. A skin barrier and special gauze dressing are then applied. These hold the catheter in an upright position to avoid stress on a healing nipple valve. It is imperative to avoid distention of the ileostomy reservoir in the early postoperative period because of the pressure it would put on the suture line. Thus, the reservoir is attached to straight drainage for several days after surgery. Then it is emptied every 2 hours for about 2 weeks.

Carefully observe for the start of ileal drainage, which usually begins 3 or 4 days postoperatively. About 2 weeks after surgery, the catheter is removed from the pouch. The catheter may then be used to drain the pouch. The intervals between drainings are gradually increased each week until the ileostomy is emptied four to six times per day and once or not at all at night.

Teach Reservoir Catheterization. Explain the following procedure for emptying the reservoir, which should be performed with the client sitting on the toilet:

1. Lubricate the catheter with a water-soluble lubricant, and insert it into the stoma through the valve.
2. Allow the contents to drain by gravity through the catheter into the bathroom toilet; drainage should be complete in 3 to 5 minutes.
3. Apply a small gauze dressing over the stoma.
4. Clean the equipment with mild soap, and rinse it; the equipment can be carried in a plastic case.

The reservoir volume continues to increase to a maximum of around 600 ml in 6 months.

Explain dietary recommendations. The client needs an oral intake of at least eight 8-oz glasses of fluid per day. Foods that could cause a blockage of the valve and the stoma, including mushrooms and nuts, may need to be avoided. All foods need to be chewed thoroughly because partly digested food may occlude the stoma.

Risk for Sexual Dysfunction. In the client with an ileostomy, there are no physiologic reasons for sexual dysfunction; however, psychological changes may lead to sexual dysfunction. In this case, the nursing diagnosis is *Risk for Sexual Dysfunction related to concern about ileostomy and altered body image and self-concept.*

Outcomes. The client will not have a sexual dysfunction, as evidenced by the ability to resume pre-ileostomy sexual functioning and role.

Interventions. The client with an ileostomy may be concerned about sexual activity and pregnancy. Encourage the client to express any such concerns and to discuss them with the sexual partner. Clients can be taught activities to lessen the intrusiveness of the pouch during intercourse, such as emptying the pouch before intercourse, wearing a soft flannel pouch cover, and being open to using different positions for intercourse. If there are problems, a sexual therapist should be consulted for further information and assistance. Impotence is uncommon; psychological reasons should be explored if it does occur.

Pregnancy and normal vaginal delivery are possible for a client with an ileostomy. The United Ostomy Association has a wide variety of booklets available for clients with an ostomy. Titles include *Sex, Pregnancy and the Female Ostomate; Sex, Courtship and the Single Ostomate; Sex and the Male Ostomate;* and *Insight into the Emotional Aspects of Ileostomies and Colostomies.* Similar resources are available from the American Cancer Society.

EVALUATION

If teaching was adequate, the client should be able to care for the ostomy and to handle the altered elimination. Preoperative activities may be resumed within 6 weeks.

Self-Care

Postoperative care and care of the stoma or diversion should be reinforced before the client is discharged. The client with an ileostomy should be encouraged to join the United Ostomy Association. This organization often helps clients regain self-esteem and improve self-concept and body image. The successful rehabilitation of others helps clients believe that they, too, can return to a normal lifestyle.

The Client Education Guide: Ostomy Supplies mentions the equipment needed to care for an ileostomy. The client should be aware of the nearest ostomy supply center so that equipment will be easy to obtain. If the client experiences difficulty with self-care, a visiting nursing or enterostomal therapy nurse should visit the client at home to follow up on learning needs.

No long-term restrictions are placed on physical activities. Tell the client to wear a medical alert identification bracelet and to carry a brief description of the pouch and drainage procedure in case of emergency.

NEOPLASTIC DISORDERS

BENIGN TUMORS OF THE BOWEL

Various kinds of benign tumors are found in the bowel. Polyps are the most commonly found benign tumor of the large bowel. A *polyp* is a lesion that projects into the lumen of the bowel. Some polyps have stems (*pedunculated*), whereas others do not (*sessile*). Polyps are usually benign lesions, but some types are precursors of cancer (i.e., premalignant tumors). Polyps are dangerous because (1) they can mask the presence of a malignant tumor and (2) they may serve as the focus for bowel obstruction or intussusception. Benign bowel tumors have clinical manifestations similar to those of malignant tumors. Some benign tumors bleed profusely and cause abdominal discomfort. Bleeding benign tumors are usually removed surgically.

CANCER OF THE BOWEL

■ CANCER OF THE SMALL BOWEL

Fewer than 5% of all gastrointestinal cancers involve tumors of the small bowel. It was estimated that, in 2000, 4700 people would have cancer of the small bowel and 1200 will have died of it.[1] The average age of onset is 53 to 58 years. Most tumors are in the ileum, with the remainder almost equally divided between the duodenum and jejunum. Manifestations are vague and nonspecific; they include weight loss, pain, anemia, nausea, vomiting, obstruction, a palpable mass, and hemorrhage.

Surgery is the only intervention that offers hope of cure. Unfortunately, even with early diagnosis and bowel resection, only about 20% of clients small bowel cancer survive 5 years. With late diagnosis, the 5-year survival rate decreases to about 5%.

■ COLORECTAL CANCER

More than 95% of cancers of the colon are adenocarcinomas. In both sexes, colon and rectal (colorectal) cancer is the third most common cause of death from cancer in the United States.[1] Men are more likely to have colorectal cancer than women. In 2000, it was estimated that about 130,200 new cases of colorectal cancer, including 93,800 of colon cancer and 36,400 of rectal cancer, will have been diagnosed. About 56,300 people will have died from colorectal cancer, accounting for about 11% of all cancer deaths. The incidence rates have been declining in the last 20 years, a trend most likely attributable to increases in screening and polyp removal. Likewise, mortality rates have also been declining, most likely a reflection of falling incidence rates and rising survival rates from early diagnosis and treatment.

Most tumors are found in the distal portion of the large bowel, from the sigmoid colon to the anus. In the 1990s, the incidence of carcinoma of the right colon increased, whereas that of the rectosigmoid area decreased.

Survival following diagnosis correlates with the stage of tumor invasion (Fig. 33–4). The 5-year survival rate for colorectal cancer is 90% when disease is diagnosed and treated in the early stage. Once the cancer has spread to other organs, the 5-year survival rate decreases to 65%. For clients with metastasis to distant organs, the 5-year survival rate is 8%.

Etiology and Risk Factors

The cause of colorectal cancer is not definitely known. It may be related to low-residue, high-fat diets and highly refined foods with an inadequate intake of fruits and vegetables. There is a higher incidence in cities and industrialized countries. Genetic mutations are involved in hereditary forms of colorectal cancer; there also is a familial tendency. Gene mutations found in people with hereditary nonpolyposis colorectal cancer (HNPCC) suggest a lifetime risk of colon cancer of 80% to 85%. The risk of cancer increases with age and in those who have ulcerative colitis or familial polyposis.

Epidemiologic studies indicate that diet may be a major factor in the development of cancer of the large bowel. Studies on bulk in stool and the rate of transit of fecal matter have so far given mixed results. Some re-

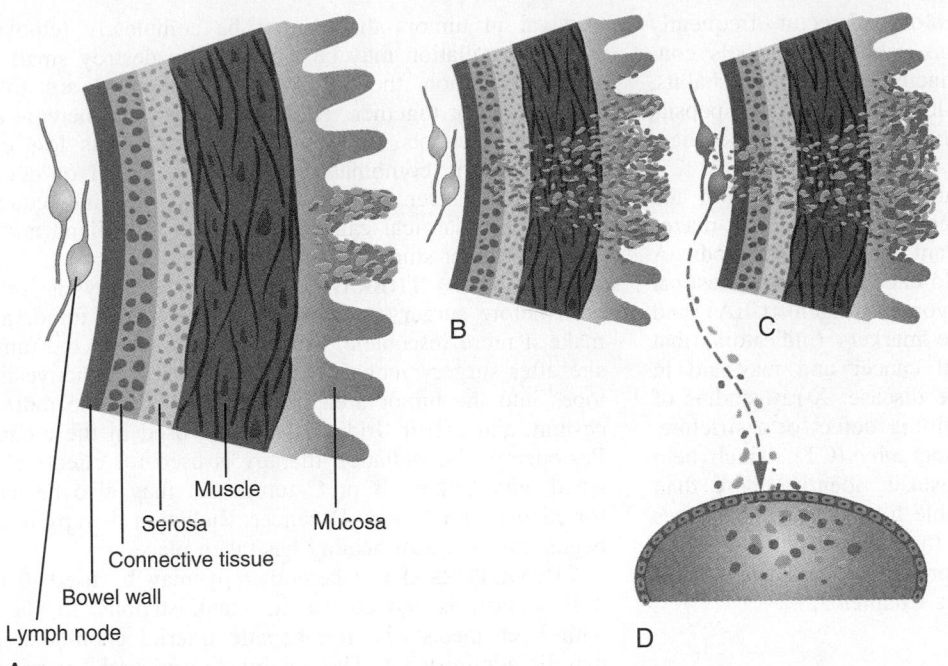

FIGURE 33-4 Stages of colon cancer, tumor (T), node (N), metastasis (M) system. *A*, Dukes' A or TNM I. Cancer is confined to bowel mucosa. *B*, Dukes' B or TNM II. Cancer extends into muscle, serosa, and connective tissue or adheres to or invades adjacent organs. *C*, Dukes' C or TNM III. Cancer penetrates the bowel wall and adheres to or invades adjacent organs; lymph nodes are positive. *D*, Cancer metastasizes to distant organs.

searchers propose that metabolic and bacterial end products are carcinogenic and that constipation allows a longer contact with the bowel wall, thus raising the probability that cancer will develop. Increasing fiber in the diet may reduce exposure to carcinogens by speeding stool transit through the intestines. Folate and selenium have been found to possibly prevent colon cancer.

Some studies have indicated that hormone replacement therapy and regular use of nonsteroidal anti-inflammatory drugs (NSAIDs) may reduce the risk of colon cancer. Uses of these agents are health promotion actions, as are regular physical activity and the identified diet changes.

Health maintenance activities include yearly screening with fecal occult blood test (FOBT) and digital rectal examination (DRE) for people at average risk for colorectal cancer who are older than 50 years of age. A flexible sigmoidoscopy, colonoscopy, or double-contrast barium enema study should be performed every 5 to 10 years in clients with normal screening results and more frequently in clients from whom polyps have been removed. Clients should begin colorectal cancer screening at a younger age, should undergo screening more frequently, or both if they have a family or personal history of colorectal cancer, polyps, or IBD, or genetic indicators for colorectal cancer. It is vital to explain to all clients the necessity for early detection and the importance of reporting manifestations such as rectal bleeding and a change in bowel habits to a health care provider.

Pathophysiology

Most malignant tumors (at least 50%) occur in the rectal area; another 20% to 30% are found in the sigmoid colon and descending colon. The remainder are found in the transverse colon and ascending colon, with twice as many found in the ascending colon as in the transverse colon.

Cancers of the colon almost always develop from ade-

nomatous polyps. As a polyp becomes malignant, it increases in size within the lumen and begins to invade the bowel wall. Tumors in the right intestine tend to be bulky and to cause necrosis and ulceration. Tumors in the left intestine start as small, button-like masses that cause ulceration of the blood supply.

Colon cancer is staged using the TNM (tumor-node-metastasis) or Dukes' classification system. The TNM system is described in Chapter 19. Figure 33-4 compares the TNM system with the Dukes system, the system most commonly used for colon cancer. Dukes' classifications (A, B, C, D) correlate with the TNM stage groupings (I, II, III, IV).

Malignant bowel tumors spread by (1) direct extension to a nearby organ, such as to the stomach from the transverse colon, (2) lymphatic and hematogenous channels, usually to the liver, and (3) seeding of, or implanting of cells into, the peritoneal cavity. The urinary bladder, ureters, and reproductive organs are frequently involved by direct extension. Blood-borne metastasis extends most commonly to the liver but also may involve the lungs, kidneys, and bones.

Clinical Manifestations

Manifestations of colon cancer include rectal bleeding, changed bowel habits, abdominal pain, weight loss, anemia, and anorexia. In general, tumors in the small bowel and right colon are more likely to cause abdominal pain and cramping, nausea, and vomiting. Because the large intestine distends, cancer located there has fewer early manifestations. At this location, lesions often ulcerate, resulting in anemia and dark, reddish brown stools. Anorexia, weight loss, weakness, debility, and a palpable mass in the right lower quadrant may be present at the time of diagnosis. Lesions of the ascending colon and transverse colon often manifest as progressive obstruction.

Tumors in the descending colon and rectum frequently cause obstructive manifestations, ribbon-like stools containing bright red blood and mucus, altered bowel habits, and tenesmus, but not weight loss, anemia, or dyspepsia. Bleeding is the manifestation that often prompts the client to seek health care.

One third of malignant tumors of the distal colon and rectum can be felt with an examining finger. This makes DRE one of the more important diagnostic methods. A stool guaiac test is performed to check for gastrointestinal bleeding. Serum carcinoembryonic antigen (CEA) and cancer antigen (CA) 19–9 are markers (indicators) that may be elevated in colorectal cancer and may aid in determining the progress of the disease. X-ray studies of the colon may show either a filling defect or a stricture. Ultrasound and computed tomography (CT), which help establish tumor size and metastasis, identify more than half of colorectal tumors. Flexible fiberoptic colonoscopes permit better visualization into the right colon, extend the diagnostic capabilities of the procedure, and enable collection of biopsy specimens (see Chapter 32).

Prognosis

The prognosis in colorectal cancer depends on (1) the health of the client, (2) how early the disease is diagnosed, and (3) how effective the treatment is. The 5-year survival rates, listed according to Dukes' classification, are as follows: Dukes' A, 80% to 90%; Dukes' B, about 60%; Dukes' C, 25% to 40%; Dukes' D, less than 5%. Overall, 51% of clients with a diagnosis of colorectal cancer survive for 10 years. Early diagnosis and treatment are essential for a good outcome. However, only 37% of colorectal cancers are identified in the early stages.

Outcome Management

■ Medical Management

DECREASE TUMOR GROWTH
The primary treatment for colon cancer is surgery; however, medical treatment is used as an adjunct to improve survival in tumors that cannot be completely removed. Electrocoagulation may be employed to destroy small tumors. Radiation therapy and chemotherapy are often given alone or together. The combination can increase the survival of clients with rectal cancer; there is less evidence that the combination increases survival of clients with colon cancer. A new custom-made vaccine reduced stage B postsurgical cancer recurrence in Holland and is currently under study in the United States.

RADIATION THERAPY. Radiation therapy is often used before surgery to reduce the size of the tumor and make it more resectable. Local interventions at the tumor site after surgery include implantation of radioactive isotopes into the tumor area. Isotopes used include radium, cesium, and cobalt. Iridium has been used in the rectum. Postoperatively, radiation therapy is used for clients classified with Dukes' B or C tumors. It may also be used for clients with Dukes' D cancer. Radiation therapy is not begun until surgical healing has taken place.

CHEMOTHERAPY. Chemotherapy may be used to reduce metastasis and control its manifestations. In clients with liver metastasis, intrahepatic arterial chemotherapy may be administered. The combination of oral levamisole (Ergamisol) and IV 5-fluorouracil (5-FU) has improved survival in Dukes' C tumors. Leucovorin (folinic acid) also may be given with 5-FU, with or without levamisole, to increase its effects. Irinotecan (Camptosar) has been effective when colorectal cancer recurs after treatment with 5-FU.

■ Nursing Management of the Medical Client

Care of the client undergoing medical treatment for colon cancer revolves around care of a client undergoing chemotherapy and, occasionally, radiation therapy. See Chapter 19 for further information on the care of these clients.

■ Surgical Management

Intervention depends on the type of tumor, its location and stage, and the client's general condition. A variety of surgical procedures are performed to treat colorectal cancer (Figs. 33–5 and 33–6). Early colorectal cancers can

  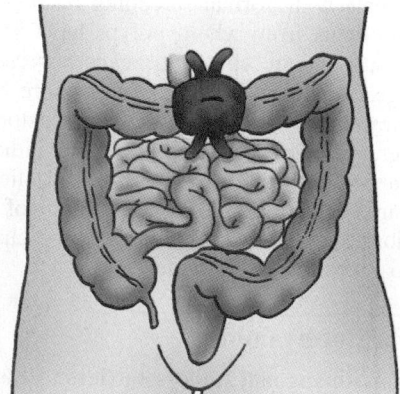

Single-barrel · Double-barrel · Loop

FIGURE 33–5 Types of colostomies. Single-barreled colostomies are usually permanent. Double-barrel colostomies are usually temporary, and stomas may be adjacent or several inches apart. Loop colostomies are temporary and are formed by bringing a loop of colon through the abdominal wall and supporting it with a plastic brace.

FIGURE 33–6 Resecting malignant tumors in the rectosigmoid segment of the bowel. *A,* Anterior resection with primary anastomosis is used for cancer at any point in the bowel except the terminal rectum. Associated lymph nodes are resected, *B,* Abdominoperineal (anteroposterior) resection with formation of permanent colostomy (Miles' operation) for cancer involving the anus and terminal portion of the rectum. *C,* Proctosigmoidectomy with pull-through and preservation of external sphincter muscles is appropriate when the tumor is in the proximal rectum and unlikely to metastasize further.

be excised and removed through a colonoscope; however, most procedures entail colon resection. The tumor is removed with several inches of colon on either side of the tumor. An end-to-end anastomosis is performed, if possible. A sleeve resection may be performed for clients with advanced disease; it is a less involved procedure in which segments of the intestine are resected to relieve obstruction and bleeding.

Several different procedures are used for rectal cancer, depending on tumor location. It may be possible to preserve sphincter function by resecting tumors located in the proximal area. However, sphincter function may not be preserved if tumors are less than 2 to 2.5 cm from the anal opening.

COLOSTOMY

INDICATIONS. A colostomy may have to be performed for colorectal cancers. This procedure involves creating an opening between the colon and abdominal wall, from which fecal contents will pass. Because the main function of the large bowel is to absorb water, the colostomy is easier to manage nearer the sigmoid colon, because the stool is more formed here than in the transverse or right colon. A colostomy can be located in the ascending, transverse, descending, or sigmoid colon and can be permanent or temporary.

A temporary colostomy allows the bowel to rest and may later be reanastomosed. The temporary colostomy also can be used to treat inoperable bowel cancer, with the ostomy placed proximal to the cancer. A temporary colostomy is made most commonly at the midpoint of the left colon or transverse colon, whereas a permanent colostomy is usually placed in the sigmoid colon. When creating a temporary loop colostomy, the surgeon brings a loop of bowel out through a wound that is separate from the surgical incision. To keep the loop from slipping back into the abdominal cavity, the surgeon places a rod or bridge beneath it. Although the bowel is usually opened with a cautery in surgery, the surgeon may wait 2 or 3 days postoperatively to open the bowel. Because there are

no sensory nerve endings in the bowel wall, this procedure is essentially painless, except for some cramping. The surgeon usually indicates which is the proximal loop and which is the distal loop.

A colostomy may also be single-barreled or double-barreled. When only one loop end of bowel is opened onto the abdominal surface, the result is called an *end* or *single-barreled colostomy*; the client has only one stoma. An end colostomy is permanent if the bowel distal to it has been resected. A *double-barreled colostomy* is one in which both loops, distal and proximal, are open onto the abdominal wall. It may be closed later, depending on the disease present. A double-barreled colostomy can be two separate stomas, a loop with one stoma and two openings, or one stoma and a mucus fistula. The fistula expels mucus and is covered with a gauze dressing or pouch.

CONTRAINDICATIONS. Any health condition that makes the client a poor surgical risk is a contraindication to a colostomy procedure.

COMPLICATIONS. Suture line leakage with local or generalized peritonitis may occur in the early postoperative period. Other complications are hemorrhage and stomal necrosis, retraction, prolapse, and stenosis. Stomal complications may require additional surgery to revise the stoma.

OUTCOMES. The client resumes usual activities within 4 to 6 weeks and is able to perform self-care of the stoma. If needed, radiation therapy and chemotherapy are initiated.

ABDOMINAL-PERINEAL RESECTION

Rectal tumors may require an abdominal-perineal resection, with the formation of a permanent or end colostomy. The affected colon and entire rectum are excised, and the anus is closed. The colon is removed through an abdominal incision, and the rectum through a perineal incision. Newer surgical techniques allow removal of low sigmoid tumors while leaving the rectal sphincter intact; normal bowel elimination is maintained.

■ Nursing Management of the Surgical Client
PREOPERATIVE CARE

The client often presents with weight loss and a change in bowel habits. Obtain accurate descriptions of manifestations as well as an assessment of major risk factors, such as a family history of colon cancer, ulcerative colitis, or familial polyposis. Assess the abdomen, noting any abnormalities, such as pain, distention, and masses.

Preoperatively, a diet high in calories, protein, and carbohydrates but low in residue may be given to provide nutrition and reduce peristalsis. TPN may be necessary to provide nutrients and vitamins the client requires.

The bacteria level in the bowel must be lowered preoperatively to decrease the risk of infection. Clients needing a bowel resection must undergo a bowel preparation to minimize bacterial growth in the bowel and postoperative wound infection. This preparation usually involves:

- A low-residue or liquid diet to reduce the fecal contents of the bowel
- Oral administration of cathartics, such as polyethylene glycol–electrolyte solution (GoLYTELY) or a pre-procedure bowel evacuator (Fleet Prep Kit No. 2), which is started at least 12 to 24 hours preoperatively
- Administration of antibiotics, such as sulfonamides and possibly neomycin and cephalexin, usually by mouth, for 12 to 48 hours preoperatively
- Administration of enemas to clean the bowel (the inside of the bowel lumen should be as clean and as bacteria-free as possible)
- Blood transfusions to correct severe anemia

Identify the client's level of anxiety and provide supportive efforts. Explain all treatments and procedures fully. Clarify and reinforce the information provided by the physician. Encourage clients to ventilate their feelings and meet with health team members to discuss treatments and prognosis. The client also needs to know how treatment decisions will be made when the results of pathologic study are available and what to expect after the operation, such as placement of tubes and measures to prevent postoperative complications.

If a colostomy is necessary, an enterostomal therapy nurse should be asked to educate the client about the ostomy, answer questions, and advise on optimal placement of the stoma. If an enterostomal therapy nurse is not available, assume the responsibility for teaching the client about the stoma. The risk of sexual dysfunction should be explained to the client in a supportive atmosphere.

POSTOPERATIVE CARE
ASSESSMENT

Immediate postoperative assessments are as discussed in Chapter 15. Assess for the return of peristalsis; indications are passage of flatus and return of bowel sounds, heard during auscultation of the abdomen. Gastric suction may be continued until peristalsis returns. Make sure the NG tube is patent.

Additionally, if a colostomy was created, monitor the colostomy output, and use special care to keep fecal contents from the colostomy (which contain bacteria) away from the surgical incision. Assess the client's stoma closely for the presence of stomal ischemia. The stoma should be red and moist. If it becomes dark or dusky, report this change to the surgeon immediately.

If an abdominal-perineal resection with creation of an end colostomy was performed, assess both the abdominal and perineal wounds. The incision may be sutured completely closed. However, sometimes drains are left in the incision and may be attached to a suction device such as a Hemovac. When suction is not used, a Penrose drain may be placed in the wound; change the dressing frequently or as ordered. A large amount of serous drainage can be expected from the perineal wound. It often takes several weeks to months for the wound to heal completely because of its size.

DIAGNOSIS, OUTCOMES, INTERVENTIONS

Risk for Injury. The postoperative client is at risk for the development of postoperative complications. The nursing diagnosis is *Risk for Injury related to postoperative complications, including infection, hemorrhage, wound disruption, thrombophlebitis, and abnormal stomal function.*

Outcomes. The client does not experience an injury, as evidenced by absence of manifestations of infection, bleeding, and evidence of wound disruption, thrombophlebitis, stomal ischemia, and bowel spillage.

Interventions

Monitor Vital Signs. Immediate postoperative interventions are the same as those used for any major abdominal procedure; they involve monitoring vital signs for manifestations of infection and shock.

Advance Diet as Tolerated. An NG tube is usually in place until peristalsis returns. It is usually several days before the NG tube is discontinued and the client begins to consume fluids and food. As the client tolerates food, he or she is slowly advanced to a regular diet.

Decrease Cramping. Abdominal cramps commonly occur after surgery, as does distention of the bowel. Distention is uncomfortable and may put pressure on suture lines. The insertion of a rectal tube for 20 to 30 minutes per physician order will help if the rectum contains gas. Early ambulation helps relieve distention and promotes peristalsis.

Apply Rectal Dressing. Prepare the client to wear a rectal dressing throughout the healing period. The character, volume, and odor of the drainage should be assessed. If the drainage in any way suggests a developing infection, arrange for a culture of the wound to identify the organism.

Occasionally, in the immediate postoperative period, sump drainage is placed in the perineal wound. This is also indicated if the wound becomes infected. The sump tube is attached to suction, allowing the wound to heal from its deepest portion without forming an abscess.

Reduce Pain. The perineal wound can be very painful, and the client should receive sufficient medication to control the pain. Once the packing is removed, the wound is irrigated, and the client should take a sitz bath three or four times a day. The client will find a side-lying position in bed most comfortable.

Monitor Stoma Drainage. There may be a colostomy pouch over the stoma. Make sure that this pouch is not applying pressure to the stoma, which would interfere with its blood supply. When changing or emptying the pouch, prevent contamination of the surgical wound by fecal discharges. Monitor the return of bowel function by observing the type and quantity of discharges from the stoma.

Prevent Thrombophlebitis. The high lithotomy position associated with the abdominal-perineal resection is associated with an increased risk of development of postoperative phlebitis. To prevent this problem, subcutaneous injections of heparin, usually 5000 units every 12 hours after surgery, are often prescribed. Sequential pressure stockings or thigh-high antiembolic hose also must be worn. The client must perform leg exercises before and after surgery. Monitor the client for manifestations of thrombophlebitis.

Risk for Body Image Disturbance.
The client with an ostomy must face alterations in self-concept and body image. Write the nursing diagnosis as *Risk for Body Image Disturbance related to colostomy and lifestyle changes.*

Outcomes. The client adjusts to changes in body image, as evidenced by the ability to identify and use effective coping methods in dealing with the disease and losses experienced.

Interventions. Give emotional support while the client begins the process of adjusting to the colostomy. It is also important to provide extensive teaching about how to care for the colostomy. The client's significant others also must adjust to the colostomy; help them by listening to their reactions and explaining the client's problems to them.

A client's reactions to a new colostomy may range from apparently easy acceptance to total withdrawal from social contacts. How well clients adjust depends partly on their attitudes toward excretory functions, previous knowledge about colostomies, and general ability to adjust to stressful situations.

Some clients refuse to look at the stoma and find it very difficult to accept its presence, whereas others begin to participate in stoma care almost immediately. Your reactions to and manner toward the client and the care required can affect the client's adjustment. For some clients, the colostomy represents a "cure"; for others, it is palliation when the cancer has spread.

Continuing sexual relationships is a major concern for the client with a colostomy and the significant other. There is no physical reason that a client cannot enjoy normal sexual relations, although a small number of men become impotent after a radical perineal dissection. If this complication occurs, the physician may recommend a urology consultation to discuss treatment options for impotence (see Chapter 38). Psychological barriers may cause problems. With love, patience, understanding, and good hygienic practices, there should be no problem. However, it may be several months after surgery before a couple manages to reestablish a satisfactory sexual relationship. Referral to a social worker, counselor, psychiatric liaison, sex therapist, or registered nurse with a counseling background may be beneficial.

Risk for Ineffective Management of Therapeutic Regimen (Individuals).
The client with a colostomy needs to learn about self-care. The nursing diagnosis is *Risk for Ineffective Management of Therapeutic Regimen (Individuals) related to colostomy care, irrigation, and possible complications associated with colostomies.*

Outcomes. The client understands care of the colostomy, as evidenced by the ability to (1) apply the pouch, (2) care for peristomal skin, (3) irrigate the colostomy, if applicable, and (4) prevent or treat any associated problems.

Interventions. Carefully assess the client's physical condition and emotional and mental attitude toward the colostomy before attempting to teach ostomy self-care. Pace the teaching to the client's level of acceptance of the colostomy and ability to manage it.

Teach Ostomy Care. Teach the client how to correctly apply the pouch to the stoma. The client first should be taught how to examine the stoma. A healthy stoma is red and slightly raised. (Figure 33–7 shows a colostomy during application of an appliance.) The skin around the stoma (*peristomal skin*) should be clear, without evidence of irritation. The peristomal area should be cleaned well with a mild soap and water and dried well before the new pouch is applied. The skin should be treated with a skin barrier and the new pouch applied, cut about 1/16 to 1/8 inch larger than the stoma. The pouch should be changed every 4 to 5 days or when leakage occurs. If a two-piece system is used, the faceplate may stay in place for 7 days. Types of pouches are shown in Figure 33–3.

Teach the client to empty the pouch when it is about half full and how to clean out the pouch when emptying it. The client should demonstrate the ability to empty and change the pouch independently before being discharged. See the discussion of ileostomy care for further information.

Teach Stoma Irrigation. Clients with end sigmoid colostomies can be taught to regulate the colostomy through regular irrigation. Clients who are physically, mentally, and emotionally capable should be encouraged to attempt irrigation and regulation. Some clients, in spite of irrigation, may never achieve regularity of elimination. If they have not achieved regularity within 6 months, they probably never will.

The Client Education Guide: Colostomy Irrigation lists the steps involved in irrigation. The best time for irriga-

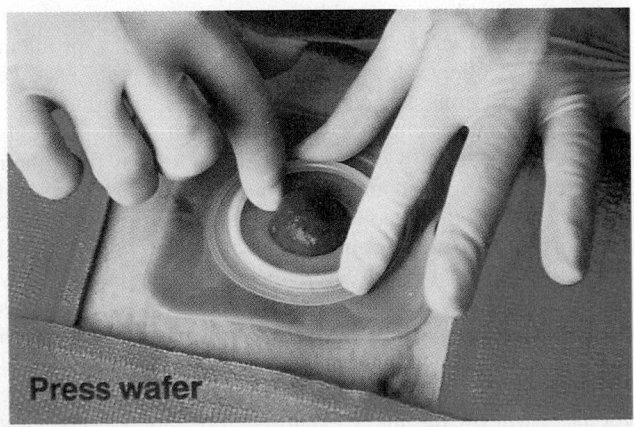

Press wafer

FIGURE 33–7 Healthy stoma during application of wafer. (Courtesy of ConvaTec, Bristol-Myers Squibb, Skillman, NJ.)

CLIENT EDUCATION GUIDE

Colostomy Irrigation

1. Assemble all the irrigation equipment and skin care products, and new colostomy pouch.
2. Remove and discard the old pouch.
3. Clean the peristomal skin.
4. Apply the irrigating sleeve, and close off the distal end or place it in the toilet.
5. Using 500 to 1000 ml of warm tap water, suspend the solution container about 18 inches above the stoma. Clear the air from the irrigation tubing. Insert the lubricated cone (water-soluble lubricant) 2 to 4 inches into the stoma (*never force the cone*), and allow the solution to flow gently into the colon.
6. Once all solution has been instilled for 6 to 8 minutes, either allow most of the stool to pass into the toilet and then close off the pouch for another 30 to 45 minutes, or simply close off the end of the pouch until the bowel has evacuated.
7. Once the bowel has emptied, simply remove the sleeve, clean the stoma, and cover it with a small pouch or gauze pad.

tion is when the client formerly had a daily bowel movement, because the bowel is already "trained" to evacuate at this time. If there is difficulty inserting the catheter, let a little solution flow in, and rotate the catheter. If the catheter will not go in, teach the client to apply gloves or a finger cot, lubricate the finger, and gently pass it into the stoma. This method often dislodges any feces that may be near the stoma. If the client cannot pass a catheter and no obstruction is felt digitally, the client should notify the health care provider.

If cramping occurs, the client should stop the solution temporarily, take a few deep breaths, and restart the solution slowly. The client should *never* (1) use more than 1000 ml, (2) irrigate the colostomy more than once a day, or (3) irrigate the colostomy if diarrhea is present.

If there is no return after irrigation, the client should ambulate, gently massage the abdomen, and try drinking some warm water. If there is still no return, the client should apply a pouch and try the irrigation again the next day. If there is no return the second day, the client should notify the health care provider.

Minimize Flatus. Flatus is an embarrassing problem because the client may have no control over its passage and no sensations to indicate when it is about to pass. Flatus can make clients avoid social situations. Clients can be taught how to muffle the passage of gas from their colostomies. Women may hold their purses or arms, and men their folded jackets or hats, over the stoma to muffle the noise. Odor-proof pouches and pouches with charcoal filter discs are available, but the most satisfactory way to control flatus is through diet. Because everyone is different, clients must learn by trial and error which foods cause gas. In general, nuts, corn, cabbage, sauerkraut, broccoli, cauliflower, and legumes are gas-forming foods. Swallowing air by eating too rapidly, chewing gum, and drinking carbonated beverages also cause intestinal gas.

EVALUATION

The client should recover from surgery without complications and should resume usual activities within 6 weeks. When a colostomy has been performed, the client should be able to manage it within 2 months. If the client is unable to accomplish self-care, the need for further teaching should be explored.

■ Self-Care

In preparation for discharge, clients need support and knowledgeable advice as they learn to live with their colostomies. The client needs to know the nearest location for purchase of ostomy supplies (see Client Education Guide: Ostomy Supplies). Immediately after dismissal, home delivery of supplies may be necessary. The enterostomal therapy nurse can help the client learn to manage and accept the ostomy and to achieve a smooth transition from the health care facility to the home. Some cities have established ostomy rehabilitation clinics to help clients, and most large communities have an ostomy association that maintains contact with the American Cancer Society. These support groups are helpful because clients can share their ostomy concerns with others who have similar problems. A home health care referral can add to the client's peace of mind, identify problems that might not otherwise be known, and ensure necessary follow-up care. See to Bridge to Home Health Care.

Before discharge, advise clients that it may take several weeks for them to regain their strength after major bowel surgery; further, when segments have been removed from the bowel, bowel habits may alter until the body adjusts to the situation. You may need to teach the client and significant others how to change dressings at home, because wounds may not be healed totally by the time the client is discharged. In general, teaching should cover (1) dressing changes, (2) dietary or activity restrictions, (3) colostomy care if applicable, and (4) manifestations of intestinal obstruction and perforation.

CLIENT EDUCATION GUIDE

Ostomy Supplies

Before you leave the hospital, find out where to purchase supplies for your ostomy. Obtain written instructions, including the brand name, order number, size of pouch, skin barrier, and pouch deodorants, as well as the name, address, and telephone number of a local medical supply facility. Ostomy supplies are very expensive; the following resources may help you obtain them more economically:

- *Ostomy Quarterly*, which lists mail order houses selling equipment at a discount (telephone: 1-800-826-0826)
- Talking with other ostomates at a local meeting of the United Ostomy Association (telephone: 1-800-826-0826)
- *The Ostomy Book,* by Barbara Dorr Mullen and Kerry Anne McGinn, an excellent publication written especially for clients and their families (Palo Alto, CA, Bull Publishing Co., 1992).

BRIDGE TO HOME HEALTH CARE

Adjusting to Life with a Colostomy

When you visit a client who has a new colostomy, assess the stoma and peristomal skin thoroughly before selecting a pouch. The stoma should be beefy red; a pale red or pale pink stoma indicates a limited blood supply. A healthy stoma is moist; dryness suggests dehydration. Note whether the outer edges are intact and attached to the peristomal skin. The stoma should be round and raised; it will shrink during the next 4 to 6 weeks. Assess the stoma when the pouch is off and the client is lying down; repeat when the client sits. Watch for (1) changes in stoma shape, (2) skin folds, (3) creases, and (4) dimpling of the peristomal skin.

Clients and caregivers are more likely to manage a colostomy independently if they understand and follow your instructions and participate in care. Demonstrate how to clean the stoma; request return demonstrations. Some bleeding is normal; applying pressure should stop the bleeding. Excessive bleeding is abnormal; if this happens, they should call the physician immediately. Tell client and caregiver to expect output (effluent) daily. The effluent will by runny initially but will thicken within 2 to 4 weeks. Expect excessive flatulus (bowel gas) for 4 to 8 weeks. Teach clients and caregivers to watch for manifestations of intestinal obstruction that require immediate medical care, such as nausea or vomiting, body temperature exceeding 101° F, severe abdominal pain, distention, limited or no output, and decreased bowel sounds.

Leakage is a common problem. To minimize leakage, provide detailed instructions about pouch fit and care; the pouch should be changed twice a week. *Do not* assume that the appliance the client took home from the hospital will fit when the stoma shrinks. If the peristomal skin

retracts, the client needs a pouch with a convex wafer, not a flat wafer. If the stoma is round, you may use a precut pouch; if it is not round, use a cut-to-fit pouch. Make and date a pattern of the stoma by tracing the outline of the stoma on a clear piece of rigid plastic with an indelible marker. Cut out the pattern and check it for proper fit against the stoma; it may not fit when the stoma shrinks. Use an ostomy belt that is snug but not tight to improve the bond between the pouch and peristomal skin. If the client is using a two-piece pouch system, make sure that there is a good seal between the pouch and the wafer.

To reinforce instructions between your visits, leave simple, step-by-step directions for pouch changing for clients and caregivers. Also leave written details about purchasing ostomy supplies locally or by mail order. Provide verbal and written diet and hydration information. Suggest that the client avoid foods high in fiber initially, such as corn, popcorn, mushrooms, peanuts, and Chinese foods; these foods can cause the bowel to swell and become obstructed. When the swelling decreases in 4 to 8 weeks, clients should be able to gradually resume eating a regular diet and to increase fluid consumption to prevent constipation at resumption of regular diet.

Refer clients with a colostomy and their family members to organizations that can help them cope with the colostomy diagnosis and changed body image, such as the United Ostomy Association (1-800-826-0826), the American Cancer Society (1-800-227-2345), and the National Wound, Ostomy, and Continence Nurses Association (1-888-224-9626). Nurse members of the last group can provide valuable information about resuming a normal lifestyle and can help manage complicated ostomies.

James McLean, RN, BSN, WOCN, *Enterostomal Therapist, Fort Worth, Texas*

The client who is having a problem with the colostomy should see an enterostomal therapy nurse. The client with an abdominal-perineal resection needs follow-up from the surgeon to ensure that the perineal wound is healing properly.

OTHER DISORDERS OF THE LARGE AND SMALL BOWEL

HERNIATIONS

A *hernia* is the abnormal protrusion of an organ, tissue, or part of an organ through the structure that normally contains it. Hernias most commonly occur in the abdominal cavity when a section of the bowel protrudes through as a result of a congenital or acquired weakness of abdominal musculature. Hernias can occur at any age and in either sex. Approximately 700,000 inguinal herniorrhaphies are performed in the United States each year. Indirect inguinal hernias, the most common type, typically occur in men. Direct inguinal hernias are found more commonly in older people. Incisional or ventral hernias occur most often in clients who had poor wound healing

after surgery. Obese or pregnant clients are more likely to develop umbilical hernias.

Etiology and Risk Factors

Hernias develop when there is a defect in the integrity of the muscular wall accompanied by increased intra-abdominal pressure. Congenital muscle weakness is one risk factor as are any factors that increase intra-abdominal pressure. The muscle weakness cannot be prevented, but exercises can be performed to strengthen weak muscles. Because obesity is one cause of increased intra-abdominal pressure, such an increase can be prevented by weight control. Avoiding heavy lifting and straining also reduces intra-abdominal pressure. Early diagnosis is important to prevent incarceration and strangulation of the herniated tissue.

Pathophysiology

Defects in the muscular wall may be congenital and due to weakened tissue or a wide space at the inguinal ligament or may be caused by trauma. Intra-abdominal pressure increases with pregnancy, obesity, heavy lifting, coughing, and traumatic injuries from blunt pressure. When two of these factors coexist with some tissue weakness, a hernia may occur. Increased pressure without a weakness is not likely to cause a hernia. Weakness, in addition to being present from birth, is acquired as part of the aging process. As clients age, muscular tissues become infiltrated and are replaced by adipose and connective tissues.

When the contents of the hernial sac can be replaced into the abdominal cavity by manipulation, the hernia is said to be *reducible*. *Irreducible* and *incarcerated* are terms that refer to a hernia in which the contents of the sac cannot be reduced or replaced by manipulation. When pressure from the hernial ring (the ring of muscular tissue through which the bowel protrudes) cuts off the blood supply to the herniated segment of bowel, the bowel becomes *strangulated*. Incarcerated hernias usually become strangulated. This situation is a surgical emergency because unless the bowel is released, it soon becomes gangrenous because of the lack of blood supply.

Hernias may penetrate through any defect in the abdominal wall, through the diaphragm, or through some internal structure within the abdominal cavity (Fig. 33–8). This discussion covers only the more common types of hernias: inguinal (both indirect and direct), femoral, umbilical, and incisional. (Hiatal hernia is discussed in Chapter 30.)

INDIRECT INGUINAL HERNIA. An indirect inguinal herniation occurs through the inguinal ring and follows the spermatic cord through the inguinal canal. It is more common in males than females because of the space allowed for the testicles to descend. There is a high incidence of indirect inguinal hernia in young people. The incidence is also high among clients 50 to 60 years of age and then gradually decreases in older age groups. These hernias can become extremely large and often descend into the scrotum.

DIRECT INGUINAL HERNIA. In a direct inguinal hernia, bowel passes through the abdominal wall in an area of muscular weakness, not through a canal as do indirect inguinal and femoral hernias. This type of hernia is more common in the elderly. Direct inguinal hernia gradually develops in an area that is weak owing to a congenital deficiency in the number of fibers it contains.

FEMORAL HERNIA. A femoral hernia occurs through the femoral ring and is more common in females than in males. It begins as a plug of fat in the femoral canal that enlarges and gradually pulls the peritoneum, and almost inevitably the urinary bladder, into the sac. There is a high incidence of incarceration and strangulation with this type of hernia.

UMBILICAL HERNIA. Umbilical herniation in the adult is more common in women and is due to increased abdominal pressure. It usually occurs in obese clients and in multiparous women.

INCISIONAL OR VENTRAL HERNIA. The incisional or ventral hernia occurs at the site of a previous surgical incision that has healed inadequately because of a postoperative problem, such as infection, inadequate nutrition, extreme distention, or obesity.

Outcome Management

■ Medical Management

Hernias that are not strangulated or incarcerated can be mechanically reduced. A truss, a firm pad held in place by a belt, also can be used to keep the hernia reduced. The pad is placed over the hernia after it has been reduced and is left in place to prevent the hernia from recurring. The client is taught to apply the truss daily before arising. The client should carefully inspect the skin under the truss for any manifestation of breakdown.

■ Surgical Management

A hernia repair is performed using a small incision directly over the weakened area. The intestine is then returned to the perineal cavity, the hernia sac is excised, and the muscle is closed tightly over the area. Hernias in the inguinal region are usually repaired with the use of

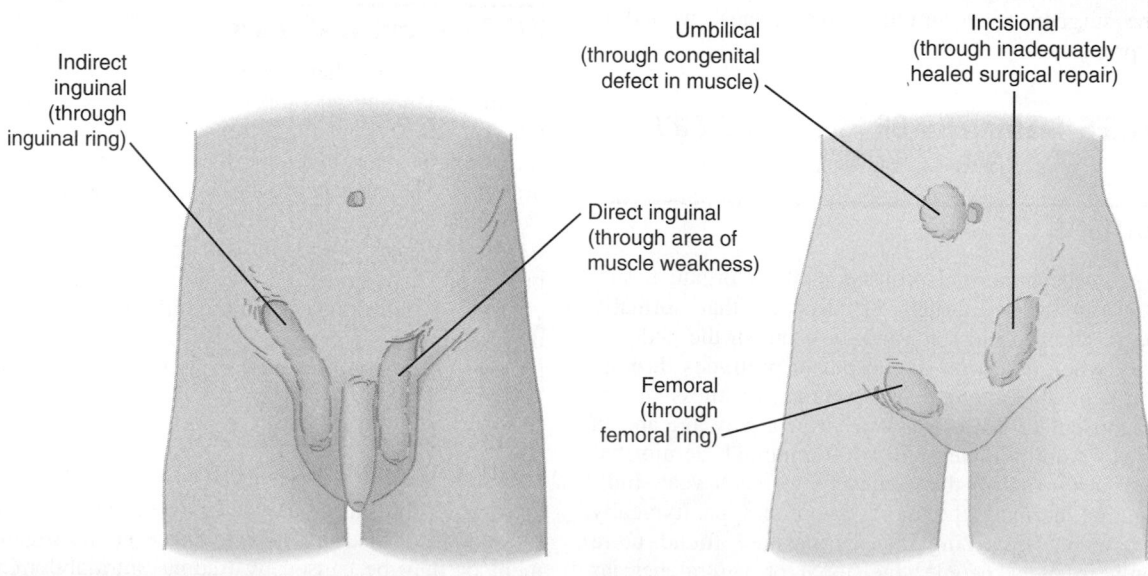

Indirect inguinal (through inguinal ring)

Umbilical (through congenital defect in muscle)

Incisional (through inadequately healed surgical repair)

Direct inguinal (through area of muscle weakness)

Femoral (through femoral ring)

FIGURE 33–8 Common types of herniation.

spinal or local anesthesia. Most hernia repairs are now performed as outpatient procedures. Laparoscopic extra-peritoneal (LEP) herniorrhaphy is a newer technique that results in higher success rates with less recurrence, less pain, and shorter postoperative recovery periods.

Some repairs are difficult because there is insufficient muscle mass to keep the intestines in place. In this case, mesh grafts are used to reinforce the area of herniation. Clients with difficult repairs are usually hospitalized for 1 to 2 days to receive prophylactic antibiotics.

▇ Nursing Management of the Surgical Client

Make certain the client voids after hernia surgery, because urinary retention is a common problem, especially in males. Return the client to a general diet as soon as he or she tolerates food. When general anesthesia is used, postoperative progress is slower. Assure the client that during the immediate postoperative period, the hernia will not recur. Some clients hesitate to become active because of this fear. The client should be told not to engage in any lifting for 4 to 6 weeks after surgery. Obese clients progress more slowly, heal more slowly, and may need more encouragement to participate in postoperative activities.

Following an inguinal hernia repair, an ice pack is usually applied to the incisional area to control pain and reduce swelling. In males, the scrotal area should be carefully assessed for swelling. An ice pack also can be applied to the scrotal area. To reduce scrotal swelling, position the client so as to elevate the scrotum and have the client wear a scrotal support when out of bed.

DIVERTICULAR DISEASE

Diverticular disease refers to two disorders, diverticulosis and diverticulitis. A *diverticulum* is a blind outpouching or herniation of intestinal mucosa through the muscular coat of the large intestine, usually the sigmoid colon. *Diverticulosis* is the presence of non-inflamed diverticula. *Diverticulitis* is inflammation of a diverticulum. Diverticular disease is common in men and women older than 45 years and in the obese. It is present in approximately one third of the population older than 60 years.

Etiology and Risk Factors

Low-fiber diets have been implicated in the development of diverticula, because such diets decrease bulk in the stool and predispose to constipation. In the presence of muscle weakness in the bowel, this increase in intraluminal pressure can lead to the formation of diverticula.

Diverticulitis occurs when undigested food blocks the diverticulum, leading to a decrease in blood supply to the area and predisposing the bowel to invasion of bacteria into the diverticulum.

Pathophysiology

Diverticula have a narrow neck like that of a flask that communicates with the bowel lumen. Weak points in the bowel musculature exist where branches of the blood vessels penetrate the colonic wall. These weak points create areas for bowel protrusion when there is increased intraluminal pressure. Diverticula frequently develop in the sigmoid colon because of the high pressures required in this area to move the stool into the rectum.

Diverticulitis may be acute or chronic. If the diverticulum is not infected, it causes few problems. However, when fecaliths do not liquify and drain from the diverticulum, they may become trapped, causing irritation and inflammation (diverticulitis). The inflamed area becomes congested with blood and may bleed or perforate. Chronic diverticulitis results in increased scarring and eventual narrowing of the bowel lumen, potentially causing obstruction.

Clinical Manifestations

The manifestations of diverticulitis depend on the extent of the inflammation and the site of occurrence. Discomfort consists of dull, episodic or steady, left quadrant or midabdominal pain. Assessment also reveals alteration in bowel habits (constipation, diarrhea, or both), increased flatus, anorexia, and low-grade fever. The inflammatory process usually subsides within several weeks. If the infection penetrates the pelvic floor or retroperitoneal tissues, abscesses may result. Extension of the inflammation to adjacent organs can lead to fistulas of the bladder or vagina and peritonitis. Repeated inflammation can result in narrowing and obstruction of the bowel.

Rectal bleeding occurs in about 15% of clients. Stools also may contain mucus. Urinary frequency can occur if the inflammation is in the proximity of the bladder. Straining, coughing, or lifting causes an increase in intra-abdominal pressure and manifestations such as diarrhea, constipation, pain, mucus and flatus. The clinician may palpate a tender mass on digital rectal examinations.

Outcome Management

▇ Medical Management

Asymptomatic diverticular disease requires no specific therapy other than diet modification. Mild disease can be treated by adherence to a high-fiber diet and prevention of constipation with bran and bulk laxatives (hydrophilic colloids). Advise clients to notify the physician of any change in bowel movement pattern (constipation or diarrhea) or character (presence of mucus or blood), or if fever, abdominal pain, or urinary manifestations develop.

Diverticulitis may be treated conservatively with medical intervention by allowing the colon to rest. Clients with acute diverticulitis are assigned to NPO status, may have an NG tube, and receive parenteral fluids and antibiotics until pain, inflammation, and temperature decrease. When the acute episode subsides, oral liquids and, later, a progressively more inclusive diet can be added. Nursing care involves the preceding interventions and client teaching about diet changes.

▇ Surgical Management

Surgery is indicated for diverticular disease with complications, such as hemorrhage, obstruction, abscesses, and perforation. Surgical procedures usually involve ligation and removal of the sac or resection of involved bowel if there are complications. With abscess or obstruction, the surgeon performs a colon resection with a temporary co-lostomy, which is left in place until the client's condition improves. For some clients, the temporary colostomy alone allows the bowel to rest and heal. For nursing care, see the earlier discussion of bowel resection.

MECKEL'S DIVERTICULUM

Meckel's diverticulum, an outpouching of the bowel, is a vestige of embryonic development found on the ileum within 10 cm of the cecum. The pouch may be lined with gastric mucosa or may contain pancreatic tissue. The gas-tric mucosal lining sometimes ulcerates and bleeds or perforates. In addition, the diverticulum may become in-flamed and may mimic appendicitis. Meckel's diverticu-lum is sometimes attached to the umbilicus by a fibrous band and may be the focus around which the bowel twists, causing obstruction. Treatment involves surgical excision of the diverticulum.

OBSTRUCTION

Partial or complete impairment of the forward flow of intestinal contents is known as an intestinal obstruction. Approximately 90% of bowel obstructions occur in the small bowel, especially in the ileum, which is the narrow-est segment. Obstructions of the small intestine are a common surgical emergency. Obstruction produces nau-sea, vomiting, dehydration, and severe pain. Intestinal ob-struction has a high mortality rate if it is not diagnosed and treated within 24 hours.

Etiology and Risk Factors

Obstruction of the small intestine may be caused by nar-rowing of the intestinal lumen due to inflammation, neo-plasms, adhesions, hernia, volvulus, intussusception, food blockage, or compression from outside the intestine. Para-lytic ileus (see later discussion), vascular problems such as mesenteric embolus and thrombus, and hypokalemia from diuretics or antihypertensive agents also may result in small bowel obstructions. Lobar pneumonia, peritonitis, and pancreatitis frequently produce an ileus (see later discussion) of infectious origin.

Cancer accounts for approximately 80% of obstruc-tions of the large intestine, most occurring in the sigmoid colon. Other causes are diverticulitis, ulcerative colitis, and previous abdominal surgery. Factors causing intesti-nal obstructions may be mechanical, neurogenic, or vas-cular.

Mechanical Factors

ADHESIONS. Adhesions are probably the most com-mon cause of obstruction in both the small and large intestines. Adhesions form after abdominal surgery, and for unknown reasons, some clients have massive adhe-sions. Irritants that remain in the abdomen following sur-gical procedures enhance the formation of adhesions. These fibrous bands of scar tissue can become looped over a portion of the bowel. The loops can then become either the focus around which the bowel can twist (*volvu-lus*) (Fig. 33–9) or the band that mechanically obstructs

FIGURE 33–9 Volvulus. Intestine twists at least 180 degrees, causing obstruction and ischemia.

the bowel by external pressure. The presence of multiple adhesions increases the risk of obstruction.

HERNIA. An incarcerated hernia may or may not cause obstruction, depending on the size of the hernial ring. However, the potential for obstruction is always present in any hernia. A strangulated hernia is always obstructed, because the bowel cannot function when its blood supply is cut off.

VOLVULUS. Volvulus is a twisting of the bowel that commonly occurs about a stationary focus (e.g., tumor or Meckel's diverticulum) in the abdominal cavity (see Fig. 33–9). It can cause infarction of the bowel and can occur in either the large or small bowel. Volvulus can some-times be corrected without surgical intervention. Success-ful decompression of the bowel with a long tube (Cantor or Miller-Abbott tube) releases pressure against the proxi-mal end of the loop, thus allowing a small bowel volvu-lus to relax.

INTUSSUSCEPTION. *Intussusception,* which sometimes complicates IBD, is a telescoping of the bowel (slipping of a section of bowel into an adjacent section) (Fig. 33–10). The condition is often associated with tumor of the large bowel. Peristaltic action telescopes the proximal bowel into the bowel distal to it. Intramural lesions often cause intussusception.

CANCERS. In the large bowel, cancer is the chief cause of obstruction. Carcinogenesis is slow and, because of the large lumen of the bowel, may become advanced before a fecal mass lodges at the constricted site and

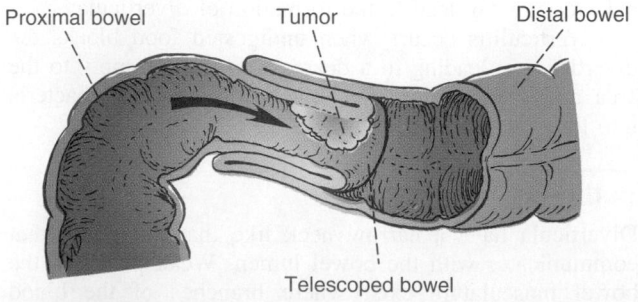

Proximal bowel   Tumor   Distal bowel

Telescoped bowel

FIGURE 33–10 Intussusception. A portion of bowel telescopes into adjacent (usually distal) bowel.

precipitates an acute obstructive process. In the small bowel, obstructive manifestations are frequently the first indication of a tumor. Even though the lumen of the small bowel is smaller, manifestations do not appear early in the process because the intestinal contents are liquid.

Neurogenic Factors

An *adynamic* (or functional) obstruction, sometimes called a *paralytic ileus*, is caused by lack of peristaltic activity. Paralytic ileus commonly occurs after abdominal surgery. The bowel ceases to function for a few hours to several days. Extensive surgical procedures in the bowel and in the retroperitoneal area may cause a postoperative neurogenic problem. Treatment involves aspiration of secretions by NG suction until the bowel begins to function.

Vascular Factors

When the blood supply to any part of the body is interrupted, the part ceases to function, and pain occurs. Blood is supplied to the bowel by way of the celiac and superior and inferior mesenteric arteries. These vessels have anastomotic intercommunications at the head of the pancreas and along the transverse bowel. Obstruction of blood flow can arise as a result of complete occlusion (mesenteric infarction) or partial occlusion (abdominal angina).

COMPLETE OCCLUSION (MESENTERIC INFARCTION). Any occlusion of arterial blood supply to the bowel, as in mesenteric thrombosis, effectively stops bowel function. The usual cause is an embolus. An acute occlusion, at its onset, causes intense abdominal pain. Usually, there are no manifestations of advanced intestinal obstruction because the pain results from ischemic tissue rather than from obstruction. As the process advances, fever, leukocytosis, shock, and other manifestations of bowel gangrene appear. Acute mesenteric obstruction constitutes a surgical emergency and carries a high mortality rate (approximately 75%). Surgical intervention must be initiated early. Sometimes, an embolectomy can restore circulation. The surgeon also must resect necrotic (dead) segments of the bowel.

PARTIAL OCCLUSION (ABDOMINAL ANGINA). Abdominal angina usually results from atherosclerosis of the mesenteric arteries. It is a common, although often asymptomatic, problem, being found in 33% of routine autopsies. Because there is a greater need for oxygenation during the digestive process, pain may develop 15 to 30 minutes after eating in a client with abdominal angina. Initially, pain may occur only after ingestion of a large meal. However, as the arterial process extends, it may occur even after a small meal, and eventually, the pain becomes almost continuous.

Manifestations arise only when interruption of blood supply is sufficient to compromise bowel function. At this time, in addition to pain after eating, assessment reveals a change in bowel habits, nausea and vomiting, and weight loss due to the client's restriction of intake to avoid the discomfort of eating. Vascular or bypass grafts can sometimes improve the blood supply to the affected portion of the bowel.

Pathophysiology

Normally, 7 to 8 L of electrolyte-rich fluid is secreted by the bowel, and most of the fluid is reabsorbed. When the bowel is obstructed, this fluid is partially retained within the bowel and partially eliminated by vomiting, causing severe reduction in circulating blood volume, which results in hypotension, hypovolemic shock, and diminished renal and cerebral blood flow. Because fluid is lost but blood cells are not, hematocrit and hemoglobin values rise, thus increasing the potential for vascular occlusive disorders, such as coronary, cerebral, and mesenteric thromboses.

For instance, with the onset of an obstruction, fluids and air collect proximal to the site of the problem, causing distention. Manifestations occur sooner and are more intense in a small bowel blockage because the small bowel is narrower and normally more active. The large volume of secretions from the small bowel adds to the distention. The only significant secretion from the large bowel is mucus.

Distention causes a temporary increase in peristalsis as the bowel attempts to force the material through the obstructed area. Within a few hours, the increased peristalsis ends and the bowel becomes flaccid, thus reducing pressure within the lumen and slowing the process caused by the obstruction. Greater pressure within the bowel reduces its absorptive ability, which increases the fluid retention still further. Soon the intraluminal pressure reduces venous return, increasing venous pressure, congestion, and vessel fragility. This process, in turn, raises capillary permeability and allows plasma to extravasate (escape) into the bowel lumen and the peritoneal cavity. The bowel wall becomes permeable to bacteria, and bowel organisms enter the peritoneal cavity. Rising pressure in the bowel wall soon slows arterial blood flow, causing necrosis and, in some cases, toxemia and peritonitis.

Strangulation of the bowel results in decreased arterial blood supply. Necrosis and perforation may force the intestinal contents into the peritoneal cavity, causing peritonitis. Bacteria proliferate in the strangulated bowel and may form endotoxins. When the endotoxins are released into the peritoneal cavity or systemic circulation, there is rapid circulatory collapse with endotoxic shock, accounting for the high mortality rate associated with this condition. These complications are especially likely to occur in older adults, who tend to have atherosclerotic narrowing of these vessels, making thrombosis more likely.

Clinical Manifestations

Manifestations of intestinal obstruction depend on the level and length of bowel involved, the extent to which the obstruction interferes with blood supply, the completeness of the obstruction, and the type of lesion producing the obstruction. Local changes in the bowel wall include congestion, fragility, reduced circulation, and increased pressure. Increased pressure leads to reverse peristalsis, producing vomiting that helps prevent overdistention of the bowel. These local effects result from (1) loss of fluids, electrolytes, and plasma, (2) bacterial proliferation, and (3) perforation. Systemic effects include a reduction in extracellular fluid and circulating blood volume, toxemia, and peritonitis.

The client with small bowel obstruction typically experiences abdominal pain in rhythmically recurring waves. The pain results from distention and the small intestine's peristaltic efforts to push its contents past the obstruction. Small intestinal pain is felt in the upper and midabdomen, whereas colonic pain is experienced in the lower abdomen. Soon after the small intestine becomes distended, the peristaltic waves are visible, accompanied by high-pitched tinkling sounds. The client usually becomes nauseated and vomits, bringing some relief from the pain if the obstruction is high or proximal to the ileum.

If the obstruction is distal to the ileum, vomiting fails to empty the bowel completely, allowing the accumulation of fluids, residue, and gases. As the muscles become atonic, loops of small bowel dilate, compounding the problem of distention. Eventually, severe distention may raise the diaphragm, thereby inhibiting respirations. Hypoxia (due to inadequate respirations, decreased circulating blood volume, and hypotension) often develops. Vomiting is more severe if the obstruction is located high in the small bowel. At first, vomitus is composed of semidigested food and chyme; later, it becomes watery and contains bile. Finally, the client vomits dark fecal material, the result of bacterial growth in the fluid that has stagnated in the obstructed bowel.

When the colon is obstructed, the competent ileocecal valve prevents regurgitation (and vomiting), and pressure within the lumen increases, resulting in distention. The cecum may perforate. Obstruction of the colon results in altered bowel habits, lower abdominal pain, a desire to defecate, distention, and borborygmi. In the presence of an incompetent ileocecal valve, distention progresses to the small intestine. Vomiting that accompanies large intestine obstruction is a very late manifestation, and occurs only from a distended small intestine.

Clients with vomiting may experience severe fluid and electrolyte imbalances. They lose not only water but also sodium, chloride, potassium, and bicarbonate. The result is an acute extracellular volume deficit (dehydration), which in turn lowers the circulating blood volume. Hydrogen ion imbalances frequently occur in intestinal obstructions, with metabolic acidosis being the most common problem.

Specific diagnostic tests for possible bowel obstruction consist of a plain x-ray film, which shows gas shadows, barium or radiopaque x-ray studies, and complete blood studies. Increased hemoglobin and hematocrit values may indicate dehydration. Leukocytosis may point to a strangulated bowel. A decrease in sodium, potassium, and chloride levels and a rise in nonprotein nitrogen and blood urea nitrogen (BUN) levels may indicate small bowel obstruction.

Outcome Management

■ Medical Management

DECOMPRESS THE BOWEL
The major treatment for an intestinal obstruction is the insertion of an intestinal tube (see Chapter 31). Often, an intestinal tube both decompresses the bowel and breaks up the obstruction.

In adynamic ileus, the best intervention is bowel rest and prevention of distention by gastric suction. Medications are not effective in stimulating bowel activity. The bowel will respond when it recovers completely from the effects of obstruction.

■ Nursing Management of the Medical Client

ASSESSMENT
Obtain a complete history of the onset of manifestations, eating patterns, food tolerance, vomiting episodes, stools (number per day and appearance), distention, and factors that increase or decrease pain.

During physical assessment, note abdominal distention, quality of bowel sounds, presence and extent of dehydration, and manifestations of abdominal pain, such as muscle guarding. A lack of bowel sounds indicates peritoneal irritation or adynamic ileus. Usually, in the case of bowel obstruction, auscultation reveals high-pitched peristaltic rushes with high, metallic tinkling sounds.

DIAGNOSIS, OUTCOMES, INTERVENTIONS
Fluid Volume Deficit. A priority nursing diagnosis for the client with an intestinal obstruction is *Fluid Volume Deficit related to vomiting, decreased intestinal reabsorption of fluid, and decreased intestinal secretions.*

Outcomes. The client maintains fluid balance, as evidenced by balanced intake and output, no manifestations of dehydration, and blood pressure within the client's normal range.

Interventions
Maintain Fluid Balance. Maintain good fluid balance in the client with an obstruction by carefully replacing fluids and electrolytes. Administer parenteral fluids with sodium chloride, bicarbonate, and potassium added as ordered.

Decompress the Bowel. An intestinal tube is inserted and attached to suction to relieve the vomiting and distention. If the obstruction is not mechanical, an intestinal tube can achieve decompression. If the obstruction is due to adhesions, hernia, or tumors, the tube stops at the point of obstruction and keeps the bowel decompressed above the obstruction.

Note the progress of an intestinal tube, the amount and type of drainage, and whether or not relief of distention and nausea occurs. Assess and measure drainage from the intestinal tube; document color, odor, consistency, and volume. Inform the physician of blood levels of sodium, potassium, and bicarbonate, and the pH of the blood, all of which reflect fluid and electrolyte balance.

Provide Discharge Teaching. For dismissal following medical resolution of the obstruction, the client needs to learn ways to prevent recurrence and to maintain bowel elimination. The client must be seen by a primary health care provider at intervals after the obstruction is relieved to confirm that it has not recurred. The client's nutritional status also should be monitored to ensure that adequate nutrition is maintained.

EVALUATION
Once the obstruction is relieved medically, bowel function should return to normal within a matter of days. If the obstruction cannot be relieved medically, surgery is required.

■ Surgical Management

If intestinal intubation does not relieve the obstruction, surgery is the only remaining option. The major objective in treating bowel obstruction is to relieve the cause and thus eliminate the problem. However, the cause is not always immediately obvious. Diagnosis of the cause of the acute abdominal condition may be difficult and commonly can be made only during surgery. Document specific observations to aid in the diagnosis.

In most vascular and mechanical obstructions, surgical excision of the cause is the only intervention. Surgery relieves the obstruction and removes any ischemic bowel. Relieving the obstruction should reestablish bowel patency. The type of surgery depends on the location and type of obstruction. The surgeon may perform bowel resection, colostomy, or a bypass procedure.

■ Nursing Management of the Surgical Client

Assessment of the surgical client is the same as assessment of the medical client. In addition, routine preoperative and postoperative assessments are required. Additional nursing interventions are the same as those discussed for other GI procedures.

IRRITABLE BOWEL SYNDROME

Irritable bowel syndrome (IBS) is a functional disorder of motility in the intestines. There is no organic disease or anatomic abnormality. Other descriptive names for this condition are: spastic colon, irritable colon, nervous indigestion, spastic colitis, intestinal neurosis, and laxative or cathartic "colitis." IBS is the most common gastrointestinal disorder in Western society, accounting for 50% of subspecialty referrals. It is more common in women than men and occurs during middle age. It is estimated to affect 17% to 20% of the American population.

Etiology and Risk Factors

Clients at risk for IBS are those who consume diets high in fat, fresh fruits, gas-producing foods, carbonated beverages, and alcohol. Also at risk are clients who smoke, are lactose intolerant, have high stress in their lives, or complain of alterations in sleep and rest.

Health promotion strategies are to instruct clients to consume a high fiber, low-fat, well-balanced diet that avoids problematic foods and carbonated beverages. Also encourage clients to reduce stress, limit smoking and alcohol consumption, engage in regular exercise, and get 8 hours of sleep each night. To promote health maintenance, advise clients to stop smoking and to follow diet and fluid recommendations previously described. Encourage clients to practice stress relaxation techniques. Health restoration actions are to administer sedative and antispasmodic medications. Encourage clients to follow diet, exercise, and relaxation regimens and to increase fiber in their diets.

Pathophysiology

IBS appears to be a disorder of gastrointestinal motility. Motility may be altered by any number of factors, including diet and emotions. The alteration in motility can cause diarrhea, constipation, or alternating diarrhea and constipation. The structure of the bowel mucosa is not changed, although the disease continues whenever the client is exposed to the causative agents. Causative agents vary among clients; however, most clients can clearly identify them.

Clinical Manifestations

The client with IBS is usually found to have some combination of the following manifestations: abdominal pain, altered bowel function, constipation or diarrhea, hypersecretion of colonic mucus, dyspeptic manifestations (flatulence, nausea, anorexia), and some level of anxiety or depression. Manifestations vary in intensity. Fiber, fruits, alcohol, and fatigue may aggravate or precipitate manifestations.

Emotional disturbances affect the autonomic nervous system (ANS) and its innervation of the bowel. Disturbances of ANS function probably alter motor activity and bowel transit time. Manifestations may mimic various organic and systemic diseases. Pain may be steady or intermittent, and there may be a dull deep discomfort with sharp cramps in the morning or after eating. The typical pattern consists of lower left quadrant abdominal pain and constipation or diarrhea. There may be tenderness over the sigmoid area.

Diarrhea tends to be the major problem but does not usually occur at night; nocturnal diarrhea tends to be associated with organic disease of the bowel. Examination of the stool reveals mucus but not blood. Eating may aggravate pain and defecation, and passing flatus or stool may provide temporary relief. Spastic contractions sometimes occur with stools that are small, dry, hard, and pellet-like. Other manifestations are abdominal disturbances such as nausea, distention, dyspepsia, eructation (belching), and borborygmi due to aerophagia (swallowing of air) and decreased gas motility. Anorexia, foul breath, sour stomach, flatulence, and cramps also may be present. Associated behavioral disturbances are anxiety, tension, nervousness, depression, sleep disturbances, weakness, and difficulty concentrating.

Because there are no confirmatory diagnostic tests for or histologic features of IBS, diagnosis generally is made by excluding other diseases. Diagnostic techniques, therefore, must eliminate the possibility that the client has organic GI disease.

Clients older than 50 years in whom IBS is suspected must be carefully evaluated to rule out malignancy and diverticular disease. When functional bowel disease develops, the client usually gives a history of nervousness and emotional disturbance. The client also may be bowel-conscious and a frequent user of cathartics and enemas. Palpation may demonstrate abdominal tenderness, particularly along the course of the colon.

Sigmoidoscopy or colonoscopy may reveal spasm and mucus in the colonic lumen. A barium enema study is usually performed. A complete blood count and stool examination are needed to rule out occult blood, ova, parasites, and pathogenic bacteria.

Outcome Management

■ Medical Management

ENCOURAGE LIFESTYLE CHANGES
Treatment is supportive. Advise the client to limit responsibilities, seek rest, and adopt measures to reduce stress, such as progressive relaxation, biofeedback, and a regular exercise routine. The client can control manifestations through diet, medication, and regular physical activity. The client must continue with routine follow-up assessment and care.

ADMINISTER MEDICATIONS

Sedative and antispasmodic medications may help the client feel more relaxed. Vegetable mucilages, such as psyllium hydrophilic mucilloid (Metamucil), can increase stool bulk.

MODIFY DIET

A high-fiber diet helps control IBS through the production of bulkier stools and reduction of tension in the walls of the sigmoid colon. Fiber helps manage both constipation and diarrhea. In constipation, the softer, bulkier, and heavier stools produced by dietary fiber tend to decrease transit time. In diarrhea, the fiber diet helps absorb water, giving form to the stool and increasing transit time.

Sources of fiber include unprocessed miller's bran, bran cereals, whole wheat, other whole grains such as brown rice, and fresh vegetables. Clients should drink six to eight 8-oz glasses of water daily, because water helps regulate stool consistency and frequency. If diarrhea is a problem, the client needs to avoid foods that may cause it, such as carbonated beverages, and to drink liquids between meals rather than at mealtime.

◼ Nursing Management of the Medical Client

Reinforce the physician's explanation of the nature of the disorder, the intervention plan, and the prognosis. Make it clear to the client that the bowel responds to stress, foods, and medications. Emphasize the importance of regular hours, nourishing meals, and adequate sleep, exercise, and recreation. Help the client establish a regular bowel routine. Advise the client with diarrhea to limit foods that are gas-producing or irritating and to avoid (1) caffeinated and carbonated beverages, (2) alcohol, (3) foods containing nondigestible carbohydrates, such as beans, and (4) milk and milk products. Provide empathy and support.

For alternative therapeutic interventions, see the Alter-

ALTERNATIVE THERAPY

Alternative Treatments for Irritable Bowel Syndrome

The pathophysiology, incidence, and medical and nursing treatments of irritable bowel syndrome (IBS) have been discussed in this chapter. A number of alternative treatments may be helpful for this condition. *Traditional Chinese medicine* has long been used to treat a variety of gastrointestinal complaints.[2] Herbal formulas are generally administered, being chosen according to the specifics of the diagnostic patterns of traditional Chinese medicine. Most of the literature about such usage appears either in Chinese or Japanese journals or in textbooks of Chinese medicine, some of which are now available in English translations. As the number of English language journals of traditional Chinese medicine increases, articles on disorders such as IBS are appearing.[1]

Results of a randomized, double-blind, placebo-controlled trial appeared in *JAMA* in late 1998. This trial, conducted in Australia, showed that Chinese herbal formulations were able to offer improvement in manifestation management for clients with IBS.[3] Participants, other than those receiving placebos, received herbs for 16 weeks. Interestingly, some experienced relief of symptoms for up to 14 weeks after completing the herb therapy. Also of note is that two groups in the study received herbs: one received a standardized formula for that group, and the second received herbs chosen on the basis of individual traditional Chinese medicine diagnoses. The researchers noted that although there was no significant difference in outcome between the two groups at the end of the treatment period, the group receiving individually prescribed herbs maintained the greatest improvement at the 14-week follow-up.

Peppermint oil, an herbal extract, has also been studied for its use in IBS. A meta-analysis of prior trials showed that there was a significant improvement in IBS manifestations with peppermint oil preparations,[7] but the researchers cautioned that study design flaws make a fully positive conclusion difficult. They judged that further well-designed trials were necessary to determine the true effectiveness of peppermint oil for IBS. A later randomized, double-blind, placebo-controlled trial not included in their analysis concluded that peppermint oil capsules were both effective in treating IBS manifestations and well tolerated.[6]

Another area of research that has shown good results in the treatment of IBS is biofeedback. Also called "psychophysiologic self-regulation," biofeedback is a relaxation training method that gives individuals a greater degree of awareness and control of physiologic function. Usually, computer-based biofeedback equipment is used, which gives immediate feedback to the client as to progress in influencing certain parameters, such as muscle electrical activity and skin temperature. Numerous studies have shown that biofeedback training leads to reduction in IBS manifestation scores, even in cases refractory to medical therapy.[5, 8]

Other similar interventions have utilized variously psychotherapy, stress management, and relaxation exercises, often in combination. As many as two thirds of participants in some studies achieved some relief of their IBS manifestations.[4, 9]

References

1. Bean, J. (1999). Irritable bowel syndrome. *California Journal of Oriental Medicine, 10*(2), 30–34.
2. Bensky, D., & Barolet, R. (1990). *Chinese herbal medicine— formulas and strategies.* Seattle: Eastland Press.
3. Bensoussan, A., et al. (1998). Treatment of irritable bowel syndrome with Chinese herbal medicine—a randomized controlled trial. *Journal of the American Medical Association, 280,* 1585–1589.
4. Guthrie, E., et al. (1991). A controlled trial of psychological treatment for the irritable bowel syndrome. *Gastroenterology, 100,* 739–740.
5. Leahy, A., et al. (1998). Computerised biofeedback games: A new method for teaching stress management and its use in irritable bowel syndrome. *Journal of the Royal College of Physicians of London, 32,* 552–556.
6. Lilu, J. H., et al. (1997). Enteric-coated peppermint-oil capsules in the treatment of irritable bowel syndrome: A prospective, randomized trial. *Journal of Gastroenterology, 32,* 765–768.
7. Pittler, M. H., & Ernst, E. (1998). Peppermint oil for irritable bowel syndrome: A critical review and meta-analysis. *The American Journal of Gastroenterology, 93,* 1131–1135.
8. Schwarz, S. P., et al. (1990). Behaviorally treated irritable bowel syndrome. A four-year follow-up. *Behavioral Research and Therapy, 28,* 331–335.
9. Shaw, G., et al. (1991). Stress management for irritable bowel syndrome: A controlled trial. *Digestion, 50,* 36–42.

James Higgy Lerner, RN, LAc, *Private practice of acupuncture, traditional Oriental medicine, and biofeedback* native Therapy feature, Alternative Treatments for Irritable Bowel syndrome.

DISORDERS OF THE ANORECTAL AREA

The major function of the rectum is to store feces until evacuation. When feces enter the rectum, peristalsis occurs. Many disorders in the rectal area result from constipation or failure to empty the rectum when peristalsis occurs.

At the mucocutaneous border of the anal canal, the mucous membrane changes to skin that has cutaneous somatic nerve endings. Because of this anatomic structure, lesions of the external anal canal are very painful. The two most common manifestations are bleeding and pain. Drainage of mucus and fecal matter and irritation of the skin by organisms can cause intense itching.

Hemorrhoids and skin tags may protrude from the anal opening, and there may be drainage of pus from abscesses. Bright-red blood per rectum usually indicates a lesion of the left colon or anorectal region. Blood on the toilet paper alone usually indicates perianal disease, whereas blood on the surface of a formed stool may suggest a polyp or carcinoma of the left colon or rectum. Blood mixed with the stool suggests inflammatory bowel disease or carcinoma of the proximal colon. Blood in the toilet bowl after the passage of formed stool suggests hemorrhoidal bleeding, the most common source of bright-red blood in the stool. All rectal bleeding must be evaluated by a physician.

HEMORRHOIDS

Hemorrhoids are perianal varicose veins. Hemorrhoids may be internal or external (Fig. 33–11). Internal hemorrhoids are varicosities of the superior hemorrhoidal plexus occurring above the mucocutaneous border (pectinate line); they are covered by mucous membrane and are innervated by the autonomic nervous system. Hemorrhoids are a common disorder, affecting both men and women of any age, but the incidence is higher in people between 20 and 50 years old.

Etiology and Risk Factors

Enlargement of hemorrhoids is caused by increased intra-abdominal pressure. Pregnancy, constipation with prolonged straining, obesity, congestive heart failure, prolonged sitting or standing, and cirrhosis with portal hypertension also raise the incidence of hemorrhoids. Any condition that increases constipation, intra-abdominal pressure, or hemorrhoidal venous pressure raises the risk of development of hemorrhoids. Prevention of constipation through more fiber in the diet is an excellent measure to reduce the risk of hemorrhoids.

Pathophysiology

Tenesmus increases intra-abdominal and hemorrhoidal venous pressures, leading to distention of the hemorrhoidal veins. When the rectal ampulla (pouch) is filled with formed stool, venous obstruction is believed to occur. As a result of the repeated and prolonged increase in this pressure and the obstruction, hemorrhoidal veins become permanently dilated. As a result of the distention, thrombosis and bleeding also may occur.

Clinical Manifestations

The major manifestation of external hemorrhoids is an enlarged mass at the anus. Internal hemorrhoids are characterized by bleeding and prolapse (protrusion outside the

FIGURE 33–11 Structure of the anus and common disorders: internal hemorrhoids, external hemorrhoids, and anal fissures.

anus). Other manifestations are rectal itching and constipation. Pain may be present if there is associated thrombosis. The blood is bright red and may be seen in the stool or on toilet tissue. A prolapse may occur in severe cases after exercise or after prolonged standing. Hemorrhoids may prolapse during defecation and spontaneously return, or the client may need to replace them manually. In some clients, hemorrhoids are prolapsed at all times.

External hemorrhoids are diagnosed by visual examination; internal hemorrhoids are diagnosed through history, digital palpation, and proctoscopy. Asking the client to strain during assessment causes the veins to enlarge, thus aiding diagnosis.

Complications of hemorrhoids are bleeding, thrombosis, and hemorrhoidal strangulation. Severe bleeding from prolonged trauma to the vein during defecation can cause iron deficiency anemia. Blood oozes or may even spurt out following a bowel movement. Thrombosis within the hemorrhoids can occur at any time and manifests as intense pain. Strangulated hemorrhoids, prolapsed hemorrhoids in which the blood supply is cut off by the anal sphincter, can result in thrombosis when blood within the hemorrhoid clots. Assessment reveals severe pain, extreme edema, and inflammation.

Outcome Management

■ Medical Management

Medical therapy is used for small, uncomplicated hemorrhoids with mild manifestations.

PREVENT CONSTIPATION

Dietary changes used to treat constipation include increasing fluids and fiber in the diet. Constipation unrelieved by diet may require use of a stool softener (docusate sodium) or a hydrophilic psyllium preparation (e.g., Metamucil).

RELIEVE PAIN

For pain, an initial application of cold packs, followed by warm sitz baths three or four times a day, should help. A topical anesthetic or steroid preparation, such as lidocaine (Xylocaine) or steroid cream, also reduces pain and itching.

■ Nursing Management of the Medical Client

PREVENT CONSTIPATION

The client with hemorrhoids should take measures to avoid constipation. The anal area is very painful, and the client may avoid defecating, resulting in hard stool or fecal impaction. Encourage the client to take bulk laxatives, stool softeners, or mineral oil as prescribed to promote stool passage. Monitor the stool for consistency and blood.

Counsel the client to (1) eat fiber-containing foods and drink ample fluids to prevent straining and (2) avoid laxatives as much as possible. Remind the client not to sit on the toilet longer than necessary; this position impairs blood flow and puts added pressure on anal vessels.

RELIEVE PAIN

Encourage warm sitz baths three or four times per day for 15 minutes. The use of witch hazel compresses are soothing to the mucosa. Other over-the-counter preparations may temporarily relieve pain.

■ Surgical Management

Several surgical procedures are used to treat hemorrhoids. Most are performed as outpatient or clinic procedures.

SCLEROTHERAPY

Sclerotherapy is performed by the injection of a sclerosing agent (substance that causes formation of scar tissue) between and around the veins. This produces an inflammatory reaction that leads to thrombosis and fibrosis. This procedure can be performed on an outpatient basis but requires one to four injections 5 to 7 days apart. The sclerosing agent can scar the anal canal.

LIGATION

Ligation, a common procedure for internal hemorrhoids, is performed in the office setting. The client can usually resume normal activities immediately after the treatment. Unfortunately, the procedure cannot be used for external hemorrhoids and may be only temporarily effective. The surgeon inserts a ligator, a small, double-lumen cylinder with a small rubber band on the inner layer, through an anoscope. The hemorrhoid is then grasped with forceps and pulled through the ligator. The rubber band is placed around the neck of the hemorrhoid. Although bleeding can occur, the most common problem is some pain during ligation. The client takes a bulk laxative after the procedure to avoid local trauma from a hard fecal mass. In 8 to 10 days, the rubber band cuts through the neck of tissue, and the tissue sloughs.

CRYOSURGERY

Cryosurgery (freezing) of hemorrhoids is performed less commonly today. It is also an outpatient procedure. The freezing of the tissue leads to necrosis and sloughing of the hemorrhoids. The problems associated with this procedure are the prolonged periods of drainage, the amount of foul drainage, the presence of large residual skin tags, and possibly, incomplete destruction of the hemorrhoids.

LASER

Laser removal of hemorrhoids is also is performed on an outpatient basis. The hemorrhoid is burned off with the laser. There is minimal bleeding, although the procedure causes some pain.

HEMORRHOIDECTOMY

With a hemorrhoidectomy, the vein is excised, and the area either is left open to heal by granulation or is closed with sutures. The open method is very painful but has a high rate of success. The suture method, although far less painful, is more likely to cause infection and result in poor healing. Complications include infection, stricture formation as the lesion heals, and hemorrhage. Hemorrhage may occur immediately after surgery or about 10 days later as a result of sloughing of tissue. Also, bleeding may not be evident because it can occur into the rectum without being passed immediately.

■ Nursing Management of the Surgical Client

PROMOTE HEALING

After the client has undergone a procedure to remove hemorrhoids, stress the importance of keeping the area clean and the stool soft but formed, to help prevent strictures. Encourage the client to wash the area after defecation and to pat it dry. Local moist heat, applied with a washcloth or piece of cotton to the anal opening for a few minutes, cleans, soothes, and promotes healing. Never apply heat in the immediate postoperative period because of the increased risk of hemorrhage. Beginning 12 hours after surgery, sitz baths three or four times a day, as the client desires, and after each bowel movement are encouraged. A sanitary napkin is the most convenient perianal dressing if one is required.

PREVENT COMPLICATIONS

Postoperative complications requiring nursing assessment include hemorrhage and urinary retention. The proximity of the bladder and tenderness in the area sometimes make urination difficult. Reestablishment of bowel habits is another potential postoperative problem. The client may need instruction on the relationship of proper diet and adequate fluid intake to bowel regularity, the physiology of defecation, and the importance of establishing a regular bowel routine.

RELIEVE PAIN

Postoperative pain can be controlled with parenteral and then oral analgesics. Warn the client to avoid vigorous perianal wiping during the immediate postoperative period. The client is usually given a stool softener and mineral oil to soften and lubricate the first stool. Warn clients that fainting can occur, from pain and vagal stimulation, during the first postprocedure bowel movement.

PILONIDAL CYST

A *pilonidal cyst* occurs at the base of the sacrum, usually contains hair, and becomes infected, forming an abscess and then a sinus tract. It is most common in young adults, especially men. It may result from hairs that penetrate the skin and cause sinus tracts to form. Constant irritation (e.g., from clothing and perspiration from activity) can cause hairs to become embedded and then infected. Acute pain and swelling result, followed by a discharge. Treatment involves surgical excision of the abscess. Healing is slow, and if the infectious process is not completely removed, the condition may recur. The client also may receive antibiotics.

ANAL FISSURE

An *anal fissure* is an ulceration or tear of the lining of the anal canal, usually the posterior wall, that occurs as a result of excessive tissue stretching and possibly from passage of a hard or large stool. The skin tear is tender and tends to reopen at subsequent defecation.

Chronic fissures are usually secondary to infectious material retained in the anal crypts. Sharp pain accompanies defecation, followed by burning. Severe muscle spasm of the sphincter usually accompanies chronic conditions. The client may try to avoid defecation, aggravating the conditions.

If the acute lesion does not heal with local dilations, cleaning, and control of constipation, the tract can be excised surgically. A chronic fissure usually does not heal spontaneously and requires surgery.

Advise the client to (1) keep the stool soft with psyllium hydrophilic mucilloid (Metamucil), mineral oil, or

docusate sodium, as prescribed, (2) have a bowel movement daily, and (3) clean the area after defecation, preferably with warm water. Sitz baths aid healing and may relieve pain. Suppositories with a local anesthetic may relieve constipation.

ANAL FISTULA

A *fistula* is a sinus tract that develops between two body cavities or between a body cavity and the surface of the body. A rectal fistula is a tract that leads from the anal canal to the skin outside the anus, or from an abscess to either the anal canal or the perianal area. It usually is preceded by an abscess. A fistula may heal over temporarily and then open and drain periodically.

Anal fistula is a chronic condition for which surgery is the only cure. The surgeon excises the tract and cleans the area, leaving it open to heal by granulation. It may heal very slowly and be very painful. Advise the client to keep the area clean, especially after a bowel movement.

ANORECTAL ABSCESS

Anorectal abscesses form in several locations. Most abscesses begin as cryptitis, with the formation of cysts that extend through the tubular ducts into the submucosal spaces. They also may originate from abrasions of the local tissues, with entry of a virulent organism. Anal intercourse may also cause a rectal abscess. Treatment involves drainage of the abscess and surgical excision of any associated fistulas. Two stages of surgery may be required to accomplish the needed resection.

CANCER

Carcinoma and melanoma can occur at the anus but are rare, constituting less than 5% of anorectal cancers. They spread by local extension into the perirectal spaces and then to the inguinal nodes. Cancer of the anal canal or lower rectum can coexist with other rectal conditions, and the client may falsely attribute bleeding to a hemorrhoid instead of carcinoma. Anal cancers are more common in blacks and usually occur in clients with preexisting anal and perianal problems, such as fistula.

Bleeding, pain, and tenesmus are characteristic manifestations. The client is usually aware of a lump near the anus that has bled and gradually becomes more and more painful, particularly during or just after a bowel movement. Many cancers are not diagnosed until they are large, and by then the prognosis is poor. Some tumors are treated with radiation and chemotherapy, whereas others may require surgical excision. Surgical intervention involves excision of the anus with an abdominoperineal resection.

BOWEL INCONTINENCE

Bowel incontinence may develop in clients as a result of aging, trauma, diabetes, rectal prolapse, or childbirth injuries or a neurogenic cause, such as spina bifida. Clients with cancer in the lower pelvic and rectal areas or with a history of radiation therapy to the rectal region are also at risk for bowel incontinence.

As an aid to promote continence, a new device called an artificial rectal sphincter (ARS) has been used successfully to promote bowel continence in almost all clients except those who have a history of cancer or radiation and who would be unable to activate the pump. The device mimics the natural process of bowel control and elimination.

The ARS consists of three parts: (1) a cuff, placed under the skin to fit around the anal canal for an artificial rectal sphincter, (2) a pressure-regulating balloon, placed in the abdominal wall and filled with liquid such as a contrast agent that can be seen on x-ray, and (3) a control pump, placed in the scrotum or labia to inflate the cuff. The cuff inflates like a balloon to prevent passage of stool and to promote continence. To evacuate the rectum, the client deflates the plastic ring and stool is able to pass through. After a bowel movement, the cuff automatically inflates in 10 minutes.

General or spinal anesthesia is used for surgical implantation of the ARS, and the procedure takes about 1 hour. The bowel is cleaned with antibiotics, laxatives, and enemas (see preparation for bowel surgery).

Postoperatively, the client is given IV antibiotics for several days to prevent infection. The nurse teaches the client how to deflate the cuff for bowel evacuation and monitors the client's bowel patterns as well as for complications such as mechanical failure, infection, and ulceration. If mechanical failure is suspected, manometry is used to measure the closing pressure of the ARS. Client satisfaction has been reported.

(See also the Management and Delegation feature on rectal pouches for clients with diarrhea.)

BLUNT OR PENETRATING TRAUMA

Blunt or penetrating trauma to the abdomen refers to accidental or intentional trauma causing internal injuries. Most blunt abdominal trauma is caused by automobile steering wheel or pedestrian accidents, whereas most penetrating trauma is caused by gunshot wounds or stabbings.

Etiology and Risk Factors

Almost any kind of injury can cause blunt trauma to the abdomen. In automobile accidents, rapid, uncontrolled deceleration is the force that produces the trauma, when the client's body hits the steering wheel or some other object. Penetrating trauma commonly results from gunshot wounds, which cause a great deal of internal damage. Stabbings are the next most common cause of penetrating abdominal wounds, although the wounds are less traumatic.

Trauma is the leading cause of death in adults younger than 40 years and the fifth leading cause of death in all adults. Although not all cases of trauma involve abdominal trauma, abdominal injuries are common with motor vehicle accidents. One method of prevention is wearing seat belts, which could decrease abdominal trauma during accidents.

Pathophysiology

Blunt trauma to the abdomen can cause shearing, crushing, or compressing forces that rupture the bowel and

other abdominal structures. Gunshot wounds can damage every structure in the abdomen. The bullets may perforate the stomach or bowel, causing peritonitis and sepsis.

Stab wounds produce less trauma to internal abdominal structures because the abdominal organs have more time to shift out of the way of the penetrating instrument.

Clinical Manifestations

Assessment of the client first involves obtaining a thorough history of the accident so that the extent of blunt trauma can be estimated. For penetrating trauma, careful assessment of the position of entry and possibly exit wounds is vital.

The client may show manifestations of an acute abdomen with either type of trauma. With both injuries, either internal or external hemorrhage may occur. If the bowel is ruptured, manifestations of peritonitis are present. All abdominal drainage is closely assessed for the presence of bowel contents.

Abdominal lavage is commonly used to assess the presence of bleeding in all abdominal wounds. This procedure involves instillation of a crystalloid solution into the peritoneal cavity followed by paracentesis (drainage of contents). Note and record the color and amount of the drainage.

A CT scan of the abdomen is now considered the base assessment of intra-abdominal injury. Angiography, intravenous pyelography (IVP), and other studies may be performed to assess different organs and the degree of trauma suffered.

Outcome Management

Medical Management

If minimal blunt trauma was sustained without severe injury to any abdominal organs, the client may simply be observed for problems once the diagnostic tests have been performed. Penetrating trauma always requires surgical intervention. The major complications of trauma are hemorrhage, shock, peritonitis, and sepsis.

The client's pain is treated conservatively until the severity of trauma has been determined. If the bowel has been ruptured, large doses of IV antibiotics are given to control infection. If hemorrhage and shock are present, IV fluids, colloids, and vasopressors may be used. The client is assigned to NPO status until the abdomen has been assessed and found to be intact.

Surgical Management

The treatment of choice for abdominal trauma with injury is an exploratory laparotomy. Depending on the injury, the surgery may be as simple as a closure of tears or as complex as a bowel resection and even a temporary colostomy.

Nursing Management of the Medical-Surgical Client

Careful assessment of the client's injury is vital. The client often must be prepared for immediate emergency surgery. Prepare the client as quickly as possible, knowing that postoperatively, much more teaching and support will be required.

MANAGEMENT AND DELEGATION

Application and Care of Rectal Pouches and Rectal Tubes

Diarrhea is the rapid movement of fecal matter through the gastrointestinal (GI) tract, resulting in poor absorption of nutrients, water and electrolytes. Because of this rapid transit, the client experiences frequent evacuation of watery, liquid, or unformed stools. The stool in diarrhea is usually alkaline because it contains digestive enzymes. Skin breakdown results if there is prolonged or frequent cutaneous contact. A rectal pouch may be applied to collect feces, to protect the skin from prolonged contact with fecal material, and to prevent subsequent skin breakdown.

You may delegate the application and care of rectal pouches to unlicensed assistive personnel.

Application of Rectal Pouches

Instruct assistive personnel to:

- Wash hands and don gloves.
- Provide privacy for the client.
- Wash and dry the rectal area thoroughly with soap and water.
- Assist the client to a side-lying position, with upper knee drawn to the chest to expose the perineal area.
- Remove the rectal pouch from packaging, and enlarge the opening in the skin barrier with scissors if necessary.
- Remove paper backing from the skin barrier.
- Spread the patient's buttocks, then apply the adhesive backing to the perineal area; apply firm, gentle pressure to ensure adherence.
- Release the buttocks, allowing them to assume a relaxed position.
- Assist the client to a comfortable position, returning the bed to its lowest position.
- Remove gloves and wash hands.

Emptying the Collection Bag

- Wash hands and don gloves.
- Empty the collection bag by opening the cap on the drain and by directing stool into a collection container or bedpan.
- Remove gloves and wash hands.
- Record stool volume per physician's order.

Removing the Rectal Pouch

- Wash hands and don gloves.
- Empty and reseal the collector bag.

- Gently ease the skin barrier away from the client's skin.
- Discard the pouch into an appropriate receptacle.
- Wash and dry the perineal area thoroughly with soap and water.
- Assist the client to a comfortable position, returning the bed to its lowest position.
- Remove gloves and wash hands.

Rectal Tubes

Flatulence (presence of abnormal amounts of gas in the GI tract) may occur any time peristalsis is decreased or absent. Excess gas may lead to a bloated feeling, abdominal distention, and cramping pain. A rectal tube may be inserted and left in place for 20 to 30 minutes to facilitate the client's passage of excessive flatus. You may delegate the skin care and positioning of a client with a rectal tube to unlicensed assistive personnel.

Skin Care and Positioning of a Client with a Rectal Tube

- Wash hands and don gloves.
- Provide privacy for the client.
- Wash the patient's rectal area with soap and water.
- Place a water proof pad under the client's hips and buttocks.
- Assist the patient to a left Sims position.
- Assist the Registered Nurse with insertion of the rectal tube as needed.
- Instruct the client to remain in a side-lying position to prevent dislodgment of the tube.
- Wash hands and don gloves before assisting with removal of the rectal tube after 20 to 30 minutes.
- Wash and dry the perineal area thoroughly with soap and water if needed.
- Assist the client to a comfortable position, returning the bed to its lowest position.
- Remove gloves and wash hands.

Describe findings that are immediately reportable to you for assistive personnel, including any difficulty with application of the rectal pouch, continued complaints of abdominal pain or discomfort by the client, and any areas of skin breakdown.

Verify competence of assistive personnel in performing these tasks during orientation and annually thereafter.

Hilary S. Blackwood, MSN, RN, Clinician IV, Surgical Nutrition Support, Services, University of Virginia Health System, Charlottesville, Virginia

Usually, once the injuries and repair have had sufficient time to heal and the infection has been adequately treated, the client returns to the hospital so that the temporary ostomy may be closed and the bowel returned to normal.

DISCHARGE TEACHING
Prior to discharge, the client may need education regarding home health care, which may include ostomy care and extensive wound care. The client or significant others may have to learn to change dressings and to care for an open, draining wound. Follow-up care from a visiting

nurse may also be required for the administration of antibiotics at home, further ostomy teaching, or wound care for an open draining wound.

CONCLUSIONS

Intestinal disorders are common and may cause problems for the client throughout life if they are not treated promptly and completely. Even with early treatment, many clients require ostomies for treatment of large and small bowel disorders. The resultant body image changes are the focus of nursing interventions to educate the client and facilitate modifications in behavior to promote health and adaptation to the changes.

THINKING CRITICALLY

1. **A young man is admitted with an exacerbation of inflammatory bowel disease. He reports frequent watery stools, general weakness, lack of appetite with a loss of 5 lb in a week, and cramping abdominal pain. What nursing history and physical assessment are required? How will his exacerbation be treated?**

Factors to Consider. What are the clinical manifestations of inflammatory bowel disease? What are priority nursing interventions?

2. **An elderly client has undergone a bowel resection with placement of a temporary transverse colostomy for treatment of colon cancer. He lives with his wife of 25 years. She is very interested in learning how to help her spouse manage care for the stoma and how to change the colostomy bags. What is your priority assessment? What teaching methods should you use to teach the client and his wife?**

Factors to Consider. What is the appearance of a healthy stoma and healthy skin around the stoma? What dietary management is important?

3. **A young man arrives in the emergency department in a highly anxious state. He has a history of numerous abdominal operations and now eliminates fecal material through a colostomy. He is handsome, appears very thin, and cannot sit still. He has a paper bag which he says contains a gun. He wants to shoot the doctor who did this to him. He wants to be admitted for a revision and asks that his bowel be "reconnected." What is your priority intervention? What psychosocial assessment should you pursue?**

Factors to Consider. How is the client coping with his changed body function? What are relationships with others his age, especially women?

BIBLIOGRAPHY

1. American Cancer Society. (2000). *Cancer facts and figures.* Atlanta: Author.
2. Botoman, V., Bonner, G., & Botoman, D. (1998). Management of inflammatory bowel disease. *American Family Physician, 57*(1), 57–68, 71–72.
3. Bradley, M., & Pupiales, M. (1997). Essential elements of ostomy care. *American Journal of Nursing, 97*(7), 38–46.
4. Carlson, E. (1998). Irritable bowel syndrome. *Nurse Practitioner, 23*(1), 82–91.
5. Cavalieri, J., & Franklin, B. (1998). Hereditary nonpolyposis colon cancer. *American Journal of Nursing, 98*(10), 42–43.
6. Climo, M., et al. (1998). Hospital-wide restriction of clindamycin: Effect on the incidence of *Clostridium difficile*-associated diarrhea and cost. *Annals of Internal Medicine, 128,* 989–995.
7. Crohn's & Colitis Foundation. (1998). *Crohn's disease and ulcerative colitis.* New York: Author.
8. Dunn, D. (1997). Common questions about ileoanal reservoirs. *American Journal of Nursing, 97*(11), 67–75.
9. Fathi, J., Isler, J., & Billingham, R. (Eds.). (1999). *Primary care: Office management of common anorectal problems, 26*(1), 1–187.
10. Ferzoco, L., Raptopoulos, V., & Silen, W. (1998). Acute diverticulitis. *New England Journal of Medicine, 338*(21), 1521–1526.
11. Gastrointestinal illness appears to be increasing. (1999). *Infectious Disease News* (On-line). Available: *http://www.slackinc.com.*
12. Gefland, D. (1997). Colorectal cancer: Screening strategies. *Radiology Clinics of North America, 35*(2), 431–438.
13. Giovannucci, E., et al. (1998). Folate: Is there a colon cancer connection? *Annals of Internal Medicine, 129,* 517–524.
14. Glaser, E., & Grogan, L. (1999). Molecular genetics of gastrointestinal malignancies. *Seminars in Oncology Nursing, 15*(1), 3–9.
15. Gruessner, R., & Sharp, H. (1997). Living-related intestinal transplantation: First report of a standardized surgical technique. *Transplantation, 64* 11), 1605–1607.
16. Guyton, A. C., & Hall, J. E. (1996). *Textbook of medical physiology* (9th ed.). Philadelphia: W. B. Saunders.
17. Hansen, M. (1998). *Pathophysiology: Foundations of disease and clinical intervention.* Philadelphia: W. B. Saunders.
18. Held, J. (1997). Caring for a patient with colon cancer. *Nursing, 27*(4), 34–39.
19. Howe, J., & Guillem, J. (1997). The genetics of colorectal cancer. *Surgical Clinics of North America, 77*(1), 175–195.
20. Klonowski, E., & Masoodi, J. (1999). The patient with Crohn's disease. *RN, 62*(3), 32–37.
21. Lehne, R. (1998). *Pharmacology for nursing care* (3rd ed.). Philadelphia: W. B. Saunders.
22. Lerman, C., et al. (1999). Genetic testing in families with hereditary nonpolyposis colon cancer. *Journal of the American Medical Association, 281*(17), 1618–1622.
23. Levin, T., et al. (1999). Predicting advanced proximal colonic neoplasia with screening sigmoidoscopy. *Journal of the American Medical Association, 281*(17), 1611–1617.
24. Mamounas, E., et al. (1997). Future directions in the adjuvant treatment of colon cancer. *Oncology, 11*(9 Suppl 10), 44–47.
25. McCorkle, R., et al. (1996). *Cancer nursing* (2nd ed.). Philadelphia: W. B. Saunders.
26. Moody, F. (1999). *Atlas of ambulatory surgery.* Philadelphia: W. B. Saunders.
27. Newland, J. (1997). Traveler's diarrhea. *American Journal of Nursing, 97*(4), 161–162.
28. Outbreak of *Campylobacter* reported in Oklahoma. (1998). *Infectious Disease News* (On-line). Available: *http://www.slackinc.com.*
29. Pastore, R., Wolff, B., & Hodge, D. (1997). Total abdominal colectomy and ileorectal anastomosis for inflammatory bowel disease. *Diseases of the Colon and Rectum, 40*(12), 1455–2464.
30. Sabiston, D. C., Jr. (1997). *Textbook of surgery* (15th ed.). Philadelphia: W. B. Saunders.
31. Saddler, D., & Ellis, C. (1999). Colorectal cancer. *Seminars in Oncology Nursing, 15*(1), 58–69.
32. Schoemaker, D., et al. (1998). Yearly colonoscopy, liver CT, and chest radiography do not influence 5-year survival of colorectal cancer patients. *Gastroenterology, 114,* 7–14.
33. Warmkessel, J. (1997). Caring for a patient with colon cancer. *Nursing, 27*(4), 34–39.
34. Wellwood, J., et al. (1998). Randomized controlled trial of laparoscopic versus open mesh repair for inguinal hernia: Outcome and cost. *British Medical Journal, 317,* 103–110.
35. Wyngaarden, J. B., et al. (Eds.). (1996). *Cecil textbook of medicine* (20th ed.). Philadelphia: W. B. Saunders.

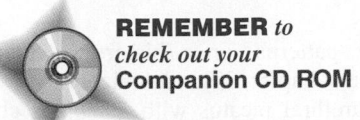

Management of Clients with Urinary Disorders

Francie Bernier

NURSING OUTCOMES CLASSIFICATION (NOC)
for Nursing Diagnoses—Clients with Urinary Disorders

Altered Urinary Elimination
Urinary Continence
Urinary Elimination
Effective Management of Therapeutic Regimen
Adherence Behavior
Compliance Behavior
Family Participation in Professional Care
Knowledge: Treatment Regimen
Participation: Health Care Decisions
Risk Control
Symptom Control
Functional Urinary Incontinence
Urinary Continence
Urinary Elimination
Knowledge Deficit
Knowledge: Disease Process
Knowledge: Health Behaviors
Knowledge: Health Resources
Knowledge: Illness Care
Knowledge: Medication
Knowledge: Prescribed Activity
Knowledge: Treatment Procedure
Knowledge: Treatment Regimen
Pain
Comfort Level
Pain Control

Pain: Disruptive Effects
Pain Level
Powerlessness
Depression Control
Depression Level
Family Participation in Professional Care
Health Beliefs
Health Beliefs: Perceived Ability to Perform
Health Beliefs: Perceived Control
Health Beliefs: Perceived Resources
Participation: Health Care Decisions
Reflex Urinary Incontinence
Neurologic Status: Autonomic
Urinary Continence
Urinary Elimination
Risk for Body Image Disturbance
Body Image
Grief Resolution
Psychosocial Adjustment: Life Change
Self-Esteem
Risk for Injury
Risk Control
Risk Detection
Symptom Control
Risk for Impaired Skin Integrity
Nutritional Status

Risk Detection
Tissue Integrity: Skin and Mucous Membranes
Tissue Perfusion: Peripheral
Wound Healing: Primary Intention
Wound Healing: Secondary Intention
Risk for Sexual Dysfunction
Body Image
Role Performance
Self-Esteem
Stress Incontinence
Urinary Continence
Urinary Elimination
Total Incontinence
Tissue Integrity: Skin and Mucous Membranes
Urinary Continence
Urinary Elimination
Urge Incontinence
Tissue Integrity: Skin and Mucous Membranes
Urinary Continence
Urinary Elimination
Urinary Retention
Urinary Continence
Urinary Elimination

Nurses commonly provide the initial assessment, diagnosis, and outcome management of altered urinary elimination and related nursing diagnoses. *Altered urinary elimination* is a nursing diagnosis used for dysfunction involving the urethra, bladder, or ureters. More specific nursing diagnoses include *Stress Incontinence, Reflex Urinary Incontinence, Urge Incontinence, Functional Urinary Incontinence, Total Incontinence,* and *Urinary Retention.* Several additional nursing diagnoses are discussed throughout the chapter.

Because of the personal nature of the urinary system, its proximity to the reproductive system in females, and the shared urinary and reproductive system of males, urinary disorders commonly lead to feelings of shame, isolation, and embarrassment. It is vital that you be sensitive to the psychosocial needs of any client with a urinary disorder.

It is also important to recognize that urinary diagnoses may signal other medical conditions as well. Long-term sequelae or conditions occurring as a consequence of altered urinary elimination may include such problems as impaired kidney function, changes in fluid volume and electrolytes, skin breakdown, changes in quality of life, and other associated conditions.

INFECTIOUS AND INFLAMMATORY DISORDERS

CYSTITIS

The diagnosis of a *urinary tract infection* (UTI) is typically confirmed on the basis of a certain number of microorganisms in the urinary system (usually 10^5 organisms), although manifestations may begin with many fewer organisms than that. The infectious process usually affects the bladder, but the urethra, ureters, and kidneys may be involved. *Cystitis,* the most common type of UTI, is an inflammation of the bladder wall, usually caused by ascending bacteria or obstructive voiding patterns that lead to decreased flow or stasis of urine. *Urethritis,* inflammation of the urethra, may cause the same manifestations as cystitis.

UTI is one of the most common infections treated by primary care providers. Untreated, it has the potential for serious consequences, such as pyelonephritis (inflammation of the kidney) (see Chapter 35) and bacteremia (bacteria in the blood). On rare occasions, complications of a UTI can lead to death.

The prevalence of UTIs is about eight times higher in women than in men, probably because the female urethra is shorter and lies closer to the anal and vaginal openings. This position increases the risk of bacterial contamination of the lower urinary tract. About 6 to 7 million young women see physicians for UTIs each year, second in frequency only to upper respiratory infections.[22] In 5% to 10% of cases, the UTI recurs after initial treatment.

UTIs rarely develop in men before age 50 years because of the length of the male urethra and the antibacterial properties of prostatic fluid. The incidence of UTIs in men rises with age, as does the incidence of prostate disease. This medical problem leads to dysfunctional voiding patterns with incomplete emptying of the bladder. Stasis of urine in the bladder raises the risk of cystitis.

The incidence of UTIs increases during hospitalization, usually from catheterization procedures and possibly from inadequate catheter care. Nosocomial (hospital-acquired) UTIs occur in about 2% of inpatients. About 1% of nosocomial UTIs (5000 each year) become life-threatening.[29]

Etiology and Risk Factors

The most common UTI-causing bacteria are gram-negative organisms found in the intestine. *Escherichia coli* probably causes about 80% of UTIs, and *Klebsiella* causes about 5% of reported UTIs. *Enterobacter* and *Proteus* are found in about 2% of reported cases.[22]

Women with vaginal *candidiasis* commonly complain of UTI manifestations. Other causative organisms, such as *Chlamydia trachomatis, Trichomonas vaginalis, Neisseria gonorrhoeae,* and herpes simplex, may be responsible for UTI manifestations as well. Therefore, ask female clients about any gynecologic manifestations when clients present with potential UTIs.

Besides the shorter urethra and its proximity to the vagina and anus, other risk factors for women may be related to sexual intercourse, pregnancy, poor hygiene, dysfunctional voiding patterns, or a history of female genital mutilation (see Chapter 39). Colonization of the vaginal opening and urethral meatus with *E. coli* is characteristic of women who have recurrent UTIs. Hormonal changes in pregnant and postmenopausal women alter the vaginal pH, change the vaginal flora, and may allow abnormal levels of normal bacteria to grow.

In addition, shrinkage of the mucosal layer of the lower urogenital system of postmenopausal women increases the risk of urethral irritation during intercourse. In fact, sexual intercourse may increase the risk of UTI in all women. The thrusting motion during coitus can push organisms up the urethra and into the bladder, which can lead to cystitis if the woman does not void after intercourse. The term "honeymoon cystitis" is frequently used to describe this phenomenon.

A poorly fitting contraceptive diaphragm or pessary may lead to recurrent UTI as well. Pressure against the urethra may obstruct the flow of urine, leading to irritation and incomplete emptying of the bladder. Spermicides are also associated with increased UTIs. They seem to increase the vaginal pH, alter the normal vaginal flora, and increase colonization of *E. coli.*

In women, synthetic underwear and pantyhose, tight jeans, and wet bathing suits can also foster the development of cystitis. Allergens or irritants—such as feminine hygiene sprays, bubble baths, perfumed toilet paper, sanitary napkins, and soaps—contribute to the development of cystitis in some women.

Indwelling urethral catheters dramatically increase the occurrence of UTIs. Indeed, UTIs are the most common nosocomial infection. Among catheterized clients, the rates for UTIs in most hospitals are well above 50%, with some rates reported as high as 100%. Indwelling catheters can introduce bacteria into the urinary tract, possibly from poor insertion technique, irritation and consequent inflammation of the urethra, and ascension of bacteria along the length of the catheter. The rate of infection rises significantly if the drainage system does not remain closed.

Diabetic clients are at increased risk for UTIs because increasing neuropathy can keep the bladder from emptying completely. Anything that interrupts the integrity of the bladder lining opens the way to possible infection. Loss of integrity of the mucosal lining may be caused by an indwelling catheter, calculus, tumor, or diminished estrogen levels. In addition, anything that contributes to urinary stasis significantly increases the risk of UTI.

In older men, obstructive uropathy, loss of the bactericidal properties of prostatic secretions, poor bladder emptying, and other medical disorders contribute to the development of UTIs. The incidence of UTI in older men is about 15%.

Health promotion and health maintenance strategies are discussed under Nursing Management of the Medical Client.

Pathophysiology

The most common mechanism by which a UTI develops is via ascending and invading bacteria. The organism triggers an inflammatory response in the lining of the urinary tract. This irritation leads to pain, frequent voiding, and other clinical manifestations.

Clinical Manifestations

Any change in a client's voiding habits should alert you to a possible UTI. The most common clinical manifestations of cystitis are burning pain on urination (dysuria), frequency, urgency, voiding in small amounts, an inability to void, incomplete emptying of the bladder, cloudy urine, and hematuria (blood in the urine). Lower back or suprapubic pain may be present as well. Other manifestations may include malaise and abdominal and flank pain related to upper tract infection. Manifestations of ureteral involvement may include abdominal distention, nausea, and diarrhea.

Asymptomatic bacteriuria (bacteria in urine) is seen in about 10% of cases, most often in older adults. The only reported manifestation of asymptomatic bacteriuria in an older client may be a change in the mental status with or without fever.

A urine culture is the most accurate diagnostic tool. Initially, a dipstick test for leukocyte esterase and nitrite activity may detect bacteriuria, allowing for immediate broad-spectrum antibiotic therapy to begin. However, the dipstick test should not be used as the exclusive diagnostic tool for a UTI. Some bacteria, such as enterococci, do not convert from nitrates to positive nitrites. Therefore, a urine culture is essential for all clients with evidence of cystitis or a positive dipstick test. Sensitivity testing can determine which antibiotics the bacteria will respond to. A urine specimen drawn by catheter yields a more accurate test than a voided specimen does.

An area of controversy arises in asymptomatic clients with indwelling urinary catheters and a high bacterial count. Some believe that the UTI should not be treated until the catheter is removed or manifestations develop. Others say that the infection should be treated when a culture is found to grow bacteria. However, most clinicians believe that specimens must be obtained for culture before antibiotics are started.

Traditionally, a bacterial count above 100,000/ml for voided specimens has been considered appropriate for antibiotic intervention. However, symptomatic clients may need treatment even with bacterial counts as low as 1000 to 10,000/ml.

Diagnostic testing, such as an intravenous pyelogram (IVP), voiding cystourethrogram (VCUG), retrograde pyelogram, or cystoscopy, may be used to evaluate clients with recurrent UTIs or clients at risk for strictures from previous interventions that have been used to identify structural abnormalities, stones, tumors, or foreign bodies in the lower urologic tract. The VCUG detects obstructive voiding patterns, as from an enlarged prostate, that increase the client's risk for recurrent cystitis.

Outcome Management

■ Medical Management

INHIBIT BACTERIAL GROWTH

To promote comfort and decrease complications, broad-spectrum antibiotics typically begin before the culture and sensitivity results are known. Later, on the basis of the sensitivity report, a more specific antibiotic may be prescribed. Fosfomycin (Monurol), a single-dose medication,

is commonly used for an initial uncomplicated infection of the lower urinary tract. Single-dose therapy does not suppress the client's normal flora, including altered vaginal flora leading to yeast infections, to the same degree as long-term therapy, and it reduces the development of resistant organisms.[22] Other commonly used pharmacologic agents include urinary antiseptics, sulfonamides, fluoroquinolones, and other antibiotics, such as aztreonam (Azactam), ampicillin (Omnipen), and cephalexin (Keflex). Medications containing azo dyes, such as phenazopyridine (Pyridium), have an anesthetic effect on the urinary tract mucosa and are used to treat the burning sensation often felt with cystitis (Table 34–1).

Simple, acute bacterial cystitis may also be treated with a 3-day course of antibiotic therapy. Treatment failures and recurrences are treated with a 7- to 10-day antibiotic regimen. Some clients may be treated for 14 days if they are medically compromised, such as a hospitalized client with an indwelling catheter or a client with a history of diabetes or immunosuppression.

A client who reports continued manifestations after completing an antibiotic course or who complains of recurrent UTIs should return for a follow-up culture after antibiotic therapy. If the urine is not yet sterile, antibiotic therapy may be continued with the same or another antibiotic, based on the sensitivity report of the repeated culture.

Chronic or recurrent infections are a frustrating problem. Each infection must be treated with antibiotics. Persistent infections may call for suppression to keep the urine sterile. This measure consists of a small dose of antibiotic taken once daily or several times a week. Clients should be educated to avoid self-diagnosis and self-treatment with over-the-counter products, such as phenazopyridine. Each infection necessitates culture and sensitivity testing with specific treatment. The primary caregiver either may prescribe continuous suppression therapy or may continue episodic administration of antibiotics when a UTI recurs.

There is a growing trend to provide self-care for medication administration in clients with chronic infections. For example, women who experience UTIs in relation to sexual activity may receive a prescription for an antibiotic and instructions to take the medication after coitus. Other clients with frequent recurrences are:

- Given a prescription for medication
- Taught to recognize early manifestations of a UTI
- Instructed to begin antibiotic therapy at the first hint of infection
- Reminded to complete the full course of antibiotics even if the manifestations disappear

Treating the client with asymptomatic bacteriuria is yet another problem. Some clinicians suggest that an asymptomatic infection be treated only if intervention is certain to prevent further morbidity or if the client is medically compromised. Others suggest immediate antibiotic treatment to reduce the risk of damage to the upper urinary tract.

MODIFY DIET

Certain foods are known to irritate the bladder, such as caffeine, alcohol, tomatoes, spicy food, chocolate, and

TABLE 34–1	**MEDICATIONS USED TO TREAT CYSTITIS**			
Class	**Action**	**Therapeutic Outcome**	**Adverse Outcome**	**Dosing**
URINARY ANTISEPTICS				
Cinoxacin (Cinobac)	Antibacterial action in urine with little or no systemic action. Effective against *Escherichia coli, Klebsiella, Enterobacter, Pseudomonas mirabilis,* and other gram-negative organisms.	Reduce or eliminate bacteria for treatment of initial, uncomplicated acute UTI. Sometimes used to prevent reinfection with persistent bacteriuria.	Monitor for photosensitivity, GI upset, and rash.	Administer 2–4 times daily P.O. for 7–14 days with meals. Maintain urine output of at least 2500 ml/day. Avoid sunlight. Most antiseptics require acidic urine for best effectiveness. Some antiseptic drugs discolor urine, such as nitrofurantoin (Macrobid).
SULFONAMIDES				
Trimethoprim-sulfamethoxazole (Bactrim, Septra)	Antibacterial action. Effective against *E. coli, Morganella morganii, Pseudomonas mirabilis, Pseudomonas vulgaris, Enterobacter,* and other organisms.	Reduce or eliminate bacteria for treatment of initial, uncomplicated acute UTI. Sometimes the drug is used to treat reinfection or as prophylactic treatment of bacteriuria.	Monitor for photosensitivity, GI upset, and rash.	*Acute UTI:* Administer 2 double-strength (DS) tablets P.O. × 1 or 1 DS tablet P.O. every 12 hours for 3 days. *Persistent UTI or reinfection:* 1 DS tablet P.O. every 12 hours for 7 days. *Prophylaxis:* ½ single strength tablet at bedtime or after intercourse. Give with large amounts of water to maintain urine output >2500 ml. Monitor serum glucose. Avoid sunlight. Most sulfonamides require alkaline urine for best effectiveness. Some may discolor urine, such as sulfisoxazole (Gantrisin).

berries. Cranberry juice and ascorbic acid (vitamin C) have been used to acidify the urine. However, research findings disagree as to whether these remedies adequately reduce the urinary pH and suppress infection. Although cranberry juice can acidify the urine, some commercial products do not contain a high enough concentration of pure juice to reduce the pH. In addition, the effectiveness of some antibiotics, such as nitrofurantoin (Macrodantin), is diminished by acidic urine.

INCREASE FLUID INTAKE
To treat and prevent UTI, encourage increased fluid intake, especially water, if the client is not required to restrict fluids. The desired amount is 3 to 4 liters per day (L/day). Research suggests that calculating ½ ounce of fluid per pound of body weight (or dividing body weight in half to find the ounces of fluid needed) is an easy way to individualize fluid intake. Increased fluids flush the urinary system and are important in preventing *urolithiasis* (urinary calculi, or stones) in clients treated with sulfa drugs. Fluids containing alcohol and caffeine should be avoided because they increase mucosal irritation.

PREVENT COMPLICATIONS
Broad-spectrum antibiotic therapy may destroy normal flora in the body and allow an overgrowth of opportunistic organisms. On occasion, diarrhea, associated bowel problems, and vaginal candidiasis may develop. Some antibiotics may reduce the effectiveness of oral contraceptives and estrogen, whereas sulfa drugs increase sensitivity to the effects of the sun.

Complications can also occur if the infection is not completely eradicated. An ascending infection can migrate from the bladder to the kidneys, resulting in pyelonephritis. Recurrent pyelonephritis can predispose the client to renal scarring and chronic renal failure if damage to the

TABLE 34–1	MEDICATIONS USED TO TREAT CYSTITIS *Continued*			
Class	**Action**	**Therapeutic Outcome**	**Adverse Outcome**	**Dosing**
FLUOROQUINOLONES				
Ciprofloxacin (Cipro)	Antibacterial action. Effective against Enterobacteriaceae staphylococci, some enterococci, *Pseudomonas aeruginosa.*	Reduce or eliminate bacteria for treatment of complicated UTI or when parenteral treatment is needed. (To prevent organism resistance, use the drug rarely for uncomplicated UTI.)	Monitor for GI upset, dry mouth, and oral and vaginal fungal infections.	Give P.O. every 12 hours for 3 days for uncomplicated UTI and every 12 hours P.O. or IV for 7–10 days for complicated UTI. Avoid aluminum antacids, which may hinder fluoroquinolone absorption. Avoid in pregnancy. Give with large amounts of water to maintain urine output >2500 ml/day.
ANTIBIOTICS				
Aztreonam (Azactam)	Antibacterial action. Effective against *E. coli, Klebsiella, Serratia, Enterobacter, Shigella, Providencia.*	Reduce or eliminate bacteria for treatment of complicated, drug resistant UTI.	Monitor for GI upset and rash.	Give IM or IV every 8–12 hours for 7–14 days. Contraindicated in clients allergic to penicillins and cephalosporins or if creatinine clearance <30 ml/min. Probenecid and furosemide increase effects of aztreonam.
URINARY ANALGESICS				
Phenazopyridine (Pyridium)	Topical analgesic and anesthetic	Relieves pain, itching, burning, urgency, and frequency associated with UTI.	Monitor for GI upset, rash, and blue to purple skin discoloration.	Give P.O. 3 times daily for 2 days. Teach to not self-medicate when manifestations appear. Causes bright red-orange urine that stains clothing. Interferes with urine tests based on color reactions. Avoid in renal insufficiency.

UTI, urinary tract infection; GI, gastrointestinal.

kidneys is severe enough. In clients with a history of recurrent or chronic infections, diagnostic testing is necessary to prevent complications associated with recurrent UTIs.

■ Nursing Management of the Medical Client

ASSESSMENT

Direct the initial nursing assessment at the history and clinical manifestations, as described earlier, to determine whether the problem is acute or chronic in nature. Also take a gynecologic, sexually transmitted disease (STD), and contraceptive history from female clients. Question male clients about presenting manifestations, and take an STD history.

A key nursing responsibility is to instruct the client about clean-catch urine collection to minimize contamination from surface organisms. Appropriate collection of a

clean catch urine specimen for a dipstick test and culture and sensitivity should be included in the assessment. The urine specimen should initially be checked for leukocytes, blood, and nitrites. Color, odor, and clarity should also be evaluated. The urine specimen should then be sent for culture and sensitivity testing. If a client presents with chronic manifestations, additional radiologic diagnostic testing may be ordered to locate the origin of the disease process.

DIAGNOSIS, OUTCOMES, INTERVENTIONS

Altered Urinary Elimination. The primary nursing diagnosis when a client is experiencing problems related to cystitis is *Altered Urinary Elimination related to irritation and inflammation of the bladder mucosa.*

Outcomes. The client will have return of normal voiding habits within 3 days of starting antibiotic treatment, as evidenced by an absence of fever, pain, burning, frequency, and urgency.

Interventions

Inhibit Bacterial Growth. Give adequate instructions to the client regarding antibiotic therapy and dietary and activity restrictions needed during antibiotic therapy. Make sure the client understands the drug, its side effects, and the importance of taking the full course of the drug even after manifestations disappear. Have the client restate the antibiotic instructions by asking questions to ensure that the instructions have been understood.

Modify Diet. Provide information about dietary changes needed to keep the urine acidic and to reduce bladder irritation, such as avoiding alcohol and caffeinated beverages. Caffeine is found in coffee, tea, chocolate, some carbonated beverages, and some over-the-counter medications. Spicy foods and tomatoes are also associated with increased irritation.

Increase Fluid Intake. In an effort to control the urgency and frequency caused by a UTI, clients may limit rather than increase fluid intake. Instruct your client to eliminate fluids that increase urgency and frequency, such as caffeinated beverages, and to increase the intake of other fluids to 3 to 4 L/day to flush the urinary system. To treat infection and prevent recurrence, teach the client how to calculate an appropriate fluid intake: ½ ounce of fluid per pound of body weight per day unless this amount is contraindicated.

Prevent Complications. Tell the client about the increased manifestations that might result from infection of the upper urinary tract and what to do if those manifestations occur. You should maintain a closed urinary drainage system and provide meticulous perineal care with mild soap and water for clients with an indwelling catheter. Keep the catheter bag below the level of the bladder at all times.

Teach Health Promotion Strategies. Encourage the client to engage in health promotion activities to prevent UTIs. For example, encourage a fluid intake of at least 3 L/day, especially of water and acid-ash items to acidify the urine (such as cranberry juice and vitamin C). Advise clients to avoid caffeinated and alcoholic beverages that may irritate the bladder lining.

An important health promotion activity centers on client teaching to prevent recurrence of UTI. Female clients should learn the risks associated with chemical irritants, intercourse, poorly fitted vaginal devices, and the additional risk of lowered estrogen levels associated with menopause. A review of correct hygienic practices should also be included. Alert both male and female clients that STDs can cause manifestations similar to those of a UTI. Inform male clients about obstructive voiding problems, caused by benign prostatic hypertrophy (BPH), that lead to urinary stasis.

Emphasize the importance of increased fluids and avoidance of foods and fluids that increase irritation. Also remind the client to void every 2 to 4 hours during the day (unless the bladder program is planned otherwise) to keep the urinary system flushed. Pregnant women should void every 2 hours.

Encourage women to void before and after coitus. Suggest that sexually active women use positions that minimize pressure on the anterior vaginal wall during intercourse. Also emphasize the need to maintain good perineal hygiene. For example, instruct women to wipe the urinary meatus from front to back. Encourage women who experience frequent UTIs to shower rather than take tub baths, and urge them to avoid bubble baths, salts, and scented feminine hygiene products. Wearing cotton underpants, which are more absorbent and breathable or porous than synthetic undergarments, and avoiding pantyhose with slacks, a practice that can trap moisture in the perineal region, are additional ways to lower the risk of UTI in women.

The application of vaginal estrogen increases circulation to the lower urogenital system and increases the mucosal layer of atrophic tissues commonly seen in postmenopausal women. Since the lower urogenital system is heavily enriched with estrogen receptors before menopause, women should be informed about the need for topical estrogen and systemic estrogen in the postmenopausal period. Using a vaginal lubricant during intercourse is helpful as well.

Health maintenance activities include (1) monitoring pregnant women and older male clients (especially those with BPH) for the presence of UTI, (2) teaching high-risk clients the clinical manifestations of infection, and (3) monitoring clients with an indwelling catheter for the presence of infection. Many postoperative clients receive prophylactic antibiotics while an indwelling catheter is in place.

Finally, clients with a UTI are managed with antibiotics and increased fluid intake. To restore health, clients should be taught ways to prevent recurrence and the importance of taking all antibiotics, followed with repeated cultures and sensitivity testing as ordered.

Pain. Another common nursing diagnosis for clients with cystitis is *Pain related to irritation and inflammation of bladder and urethral mucosa.*

Outcomes. The client will be able to urinate without discomfort within 24 hours after treatment begins and will return to normal voiding habits within 3 days, as evidenced by an absence of pain and burning on urination.

Interventions. Medications prescribed specifically to treat pain, such as phenazopyridine (Pyridium), should be administered. Other comfort measures include forcing fluids to dilute urine and taking a warm sitz bath to decrease urethral smooth muscle spasms. Some clients find a heating pad applied to the suprapubic area helpful in reducing bladder spasms and suprapubic pain.

EVALUATION

After the first 24 hours of treatment, the client should be able to report a reduction in pain, burning, urgency, and frequency. Antibiotic therapy usually brings about complete resolution of irritation and pain within 3 days. If indicated, urine culture specimens should be negative after 1 week of treatment or after the course of antibiotics is completed.

■ Surgical Management

The need for surgery is rare, and operations are performed only to address structural anomalies that cause repeated infections. Strictures of the bladder neck or urethra are the most common problems requiring surgical intervention. BPH may also be treated surgically (see Chapter 38). Correction of structural abnormalities or obstruction should resolve recurrent UTIs. Nursing care of clients after surgery is discussed under the specific disorder. Chapter 38 describes nursing care of men after surgery for BPH.

Self-Care

Promotion of self-care for a client with a UTI includes recognition of lifestyle changes needed to decrease risk factors, the ability to restate the medication protocol, and return for follow-up urine cultures, if indicated. Explain risk factors for UTIs and health promotion strategies to prevent recurrence. These strategies include increased fluid intake, fluid and diet modifications, voiding every 2 hours, and lifestyle modifications, as previously discussed. Advise the client to seek care if manifestations recur.

Modifications for Elderly Clients

In older people, cystitis may occur more often than in younger people but for different reasons. Such a cause might be immobility, constipation, fecal and urinary incontinence, urinary retention (incomplete voiding), altered mental status, or systemic disease.

In older women, atrophic changes resulting from decreased estrogen affect the vagina and urethra. This alteration causes bladder dysfunction, which may predispose this population to infection.

In older men, BPH is one of the main risk factors for UTIs. BPH becomes more common with increased age. Management of recurrent UTIs in men involves treatment of BPH. Once BPH is treated, the infections should diminish.

When administering medications to older or compromised clients, you must consider their renal and hepatic status. Many drugs used to treat UTIs necessitate that the client have adequate renal and hepatic function, particularly with long-term administration. Also, consider any changes in cardiovascular status that might prevent an increase in fluid intake.

INTERSTITIAL CYSTITIS

Cystitis may be noninfectious or abacterial. One type, interstitial cystitis (IC), is also called painful bladder disease (PBD), Hunner's ulcer, urethral syndrome, pseudomembranous trigonitis, and other names. This greatly underdiagnosed condition involves urgency, frequency, and a painful bladder despite a lack of bacteria in the urine culture. The most severe forms of this disease involve ulcerations and hemorrhages in the bladder wall. The cause of these ulcers is unknown, but the ulcers may stem from a defect in the epithelial molecular layer of the bladder wall.

Etiology and Risk Factors

IC occurs mainly in young women (90% to 95% of all cases), usually white but occasionally African American. The disease is increasing significantly among Jewish women, which may be somehow related to the increase in inflammatory bowel disease associated with autoimmune disorders in this population.[25]

Pathophysiology

IC is a poorly understood disorder with an unclear pathophysiology. It may be a local autoimmune phenomenon. Despite clinical manifestations, the urine is usually sterile. The most current theory seems to be associated with a breakdown in the permeability of the glycosaminoglycan layer of the bladder mucosa, which is usually impermeable to urea and bacteria. This theory has been questioned in some studies, which suggest that the permeability of the bladder in clients with IC is no greater than that in normal people.[25]

Characteristic pathologic changes are found in more severe forms of IC, including nonspecific chronic inflammatory infiltrate, edema, vasodilation, and eventually fibrosis of the submucosa and detrusor layers of the bladder wall. The fibrosis of the submucosa seems to decrease the elasticity of the detrusor muscle, which decreases bladder capacity.

Mast cell infiltrates have been identified in the bladders of clients with IC, particularly in the detrusor layer. Because mast cells are associated with allergic reactions, it is worth noting that about half of clients with IC are reported to have allergies and 30% have inflammatory bowel disease.[25] Finally, another hypothesis is that bacteria are found only in the wall of the bladder and not in the urine.[25]

Clinical Manifestations

The clinical manifestations of IC are tenderness in the area of the bladder trigone during anterior palpation during a vaginal examination, complaints of lower abdominal or pelvic pain, urinary urgency, and frequency (up to 60 times a day), *nocturia* (excessive urination at night), and, in some women, dyspareunia (painful intercourse). Presenting manifestations and their severity vary from client to client. Some women find the disorder debilitating. Manifestations may be present for years and treated as bacterial cystitis before an appropriate diagnosis is made.

The National Institute of Arthritis, Diabetes, Digestive, and Kidney Diseases recommends specific diagnostic criteria for identifying clients with clinical manifestations. These criteria include:

- A detailed client history
- A completed bladder diary
- Urine cytology
- Urodynamic evaluation to determine bladder capacity and evaluate bladder function
- Cystoscopy with the client under anesthesia and with hydrodistention of the bladder
- Bladder biopsy

During cystoscopy and hydrodilation of the bladder, the presence of outpouches in the bladder wall, Hunner's ulcers, and a severely decreased bladder capacity is considered by many physicians to be the clinical diagnostic feature of IC. Others believe that IC may be present even without these findings.

Outcome Management

■ Medical Management

REDUCE PAIN

The treatment of IC is controversial, with no single accepted treatment. Anti-inflammatory, antispasmodic, antidepressant, and antihistamine medications and, occasionally, tranquilizers or narcotics may be used.

Pentosan polysulfate sodium (Elmiron) is the newest oral medication of choice. This drug increases the bladder defense mechanism or detoxifies irritants in urine that might break down the bladder lining. The mechanism of action is like heparin, with anticoagulant and antifibrin effects. Relief of manifestations may take up to 3 months.

Other treatments include instillation of a variety of agents into the bladder to promote healing and pain relief, such as sodium oxychlorosene (Clorpactin), silver nitrate, and dimethyl sulfoxide (DMSO). Heparin itself has been instilled in the bladder, initially daily for 3 to 4 months. Therapy is continued three times a week for 3 to 6 months. Some clients may not notice any improvement in manifestations until after the first 2 to 4 months of treatment.[25] All of these treatments are designed to decrease the permeability of the bladder mucosa so that the causative agent has more difficulty penetrating the lining.

Although the mechanism of action is unclear, bacille Calmette-Guérin (BCG) has been effective as an intravesical agent administered weekly. BCG instillations for 6 weeks have led to a decreased need for pain medications, a doubling of cystometric capacity, and sometimes a decrease in client discomfort.[25]

Referrals to centers providing conservative management programs with behavioral intervention, electrical stimulation, and biofeedback to the pelvic floor musculature may also alleviate manifestations of IC. Because of the chronic nature of the disorder, physicians are reluctant to offer narcotics for pain relief. During severe exacerbations, however, narcotics may be appropriate.

IMPROVE COPING

Many clients with IC complain of exhaustion and depression. The exhaustion usually stems from poor sleep patterns caused by nocturnal urgency, frequency, and pain. Depression can result from frustration, exhaustion, chronic pain, and difficulty in obtaining effective medical care.

During the acute phase, these clients may require medications to improve sleep as well as antidepressant therapy to increase coping ability. Referrals to social workers or other health care professionals to improve coping strategies and mental status may be needed. You also may need to refer the client to a center that specializes in treating IC.

■ Nursing Management of the Medical Client

REDUCE PAIN

Nurses provide a great deal of education about drug therapy. Many of the medications have a cumulative effect, making long-term therapy necessary for maximal results. You may need to continuously reinforce this point if the client grows frustrated with pharmacologic intervention. You also should counsel the client before narcotic intervention. Because IC is a chronic problem, inform the client about risk factors associated with narcotic drugs.

IMPROVE COPING

Your major responsibility is to support the client through diagnosis and treatment. Because the cause of IC is unclear, few nursing interventions are aimed at prevention. IC is a chronic disorder requiring long-term client support. Clients may need additional psychological counseling to help with stress-related coping strategies. Become familiar with national and local resources for clients with IC or painful bladder disease (Interstitial Cystitis Association), and refer clients as appropriate.

Bladder retraining with conservative management programs can help to reduce clinical manifestations. Teaching clients to void by the clock rather than by urge will gently and slowly increase bladder capacity. Biofeedback-directed pelvic floor exercises teach the client the urge suppression technique. This process decreases episodes of urgency and frequency and promotes control of manifestations. The additional use of transvaginal or transanal electrical stimulation may help to override bladder spasms and can increase the quality of pelvic floor contractions.

■ Surgical Management

Surgery is rarely used to manage the client with IC. The traditional therapy is hydraulic distention of the bladder, with or without instillation of DMSO to increase the bladder's functional capacity. Clients with severely reduced bladder capacity and incapacitating manifestations may be candidates for a transurethral resection (TUR), laser surgical resection of the lesions, a partial or complete *cystectomy* (resection of the bladder), and *urinary diversion* (surgical rerouting of the normal urinary flow) (see bladder cancer later).[55]

UROSEPSIS

Urosepsis is a gram-negative bacteremia originating in the genitourinary tract. The most common predisposing factor is an indwelling catheter or an untreated UTI in a medically compromised client. Other primary risk factors include immunosuppression therapy and chemotherapy. The most common organism responsible for gram-negative bacteremia is *E. coli,* which has the ability to develop resistant strains.

The pathophysiologic mechanisms of urosepsis are complex and not fully understood. The disorder can lead to septic shock if it is not treated immediately and aggressively (see Chapter 81). The cell wall of the gram-negative bacillus is composed of a lipid-carbohydrate complex. Bacteria release endotoxins, which damage cells. The cells release lysosomes, which further damage tissues and set off the kinins and complement cascade. Cellular metabolism becomes anaerobic, and lactic acidosis develops. Fever is the most common early manifestation; in older adults, however, fever and altered mental status are the first clinical signs.

To prevent sepsis and shock, treatment of gram-negative urosepsis must be instituted right after specimen collection for culture and sensitivity testing. Initial treatment consists of intravenous (IV) aminoglycosides, beta-lactam antibiotics (such as aztreonam), or third-generation cephalosporins until culture results are available. As soon as culture and sensitivity results are available, the antibiotic may be changed if necessary. IV treatment is directed by the status of the client and continued for 3 to 5 days once the client becomes afebrile. Oral antibiotics are continued for the duration of therapy.

URETHRITIS

Urethritis, or inflammation of the urethra, is commonly associated with STDs or sexually transmitted infections (see Chapter 41) and is an associated manifestation of cystitis. The most common causes of urethritis are gonorrhea, chlamydial infection, and other bacterial infections. Among women, common causes also include feminine hygiene sprays, scented toilet paper, sanitary napkins, spermicidal jellies, UTIs, and changes in the vaginal mucosal lining. In short, any irritant that comes into contact with the urethra can cause urethritis.

Exposure to irritants causes the mucosal lining of the urethra to become inflamed. The mucosal lining becomes swollen, painful, red, and irritated. Pus may be produced. *Pyuria*, the presence of pus in the urine, is a common indication of urethritis. Manifestations are similar to those described for cystitis. Frequently, women reveal a history of chemical irritant exposure. Male clients frequently exhibit a urethral discharge.

The diagnosis is often confirmed on the basis of the client's history and clinical manifestations. Culture and sensitivity testing of the urine should be performed, and culture specimens should be obtained to exclude STDs if indicated.

Management of urethritis includes removing the etiologic mechanism. If a microorganism is the cause, administration of systemic and topical antibiotics is essential. Sitz baths and an increased fluid intake are also encouraged. Advise the client to avoid coitus until the manifestations subside or treatment of the STD is completed. The use of lubricants with intercourse decreases irritation in women who have had frequent episodes. Common medications are the same as those used to treat cystitis. The physician may also prescribe topical estrogens for a menopausal woman.

Prevention of urethritis by decreasing exposure to STDs is essential. Inform women about the increased risk of urethritis from spermicides and about the need to avoid feminine hygiene sprays, perfumed toilet paper, and scented sanitary napkins.

URETERITIS

Ureteritis, or inflammation of the ureter, is commonly associated with pyelonephritis (see Chapter 35). Once the kidney infection is treated, ureteral inflammation usually subsides. Chronic pyelonephritis can cause the ureter to become fibrotic and narrowed by strictures, which in turn can continue to foster this condition.

OBSTRUCTIVE DISORDERS

BLADDER CANCER

Most bladder cancers are transitional or papillary tumors in the bladder urothelium. These tumors may infiltrate the bladder wall. Bladder cancer is the most frequent neoplasm of the urinary tract, accounting for about 6% of all cancer cases in men and 2.5% in women. It is rarely seen in adults younger than 40 years of age and occurs most frequently in 50- to 60-year-old adults. Now the fourth most common cancer in men and the eighth most common cancer in women,[1] it affects whites twice as often as blacks. Bladder cancer is more common in people living in urban, industrialized northern states than those living in southern states.[32] In addition, the incidence is higher in people of Jewish descent than in non-Jewish persons. Heredity has not been linked to the development of bladder cancer.

Etiology and Risk Factors

The disease process has several possible causes. There is a strong correlation between cigarette smoking and bladder cancer. Hence, a health promotion and health maintenance strategy is to encourage smokers to stop smoking and to be screened regularly after age 50 years for hematuria and other manifestations of bladder cancer.

Industrial exposure to certain substances, such as aniline dyes, asbestos, and aromatic amines (e.g., benzidine and 2-naphthylamine) may also result in bladder cancer. The latency period of industrial exposure can be as long as 18 to 45 years. Workers in this high-risk group should also be screened regularly after age 50 for hematuria and other manifestations of bladder cancer.

Artificial sweeteners have been weakly linked to the development of bladder cancer. Attempts to connect coffee consumption and bladder cancer have produced contradictory findings because of the increased use of artificial sweeteners and cigarettes associated with coffee consumption. Use of the drug phenacetin has also been debated. Other risk factors may be chronic cystitis, pelvic radiation, and the chemotherapeutic drug cyclophosphamide (Cytoxan).

Clients who have undergone transurethral resection or removal of superficial bladder cancer should return for regular cystoscopic follow-up as a health maintenance and restoration activity. Teaching clients to care for a urinary diversion is a health restoration activity provided by nurses.

Pathophysiology

Bladder cancer appears to result from exposure of the bladder wall to a *carcinogen* (a cancer-causing agent). Cigarette smoking or second-hand smoke may result in carcinogenic metabolites produced by abnormal tryptophan metabolism, with the metabolite excreted in the urine. Cigarette smoke also contains nitrosamines as well as 2-naphthylamine (both carcinogens), which are also excreted in the urine.

Premalignant proliferative changes are often found in the transitional cell layer. These changes are called *dysplasia* and refer to abnormal cell configuration found in several degrees of severity. The extent of dysplasia may be described as mild, moderate, or severe, leading to carcinoma in situ (localized).[44] Most bladder cancers start as papillary or transitional cell tumors and account for 70% of bladder tumors. These tumors are most commonly found in the trigone of the bladder and lateral wall of the bladder.

Staging of a tumor indicates the depth of penetration into the bladder wall and degree of *metastasis*. Staging must be done to determine the treatment modality. Clinical staging includes the results and review of an excretory urogram, cystoscopy, biopsy, and bimanual examination with the client under anesthesia. For evaluation of specific areas of metastasis as well as for staging, chest radiography, lymphangiography, isotope bone scans, computed tomography (CT), and liver function analysis are needed. The most frequently used staging systems are the Jewett-Marshall-Strong System and the tumor-node-metastasis (TNM) classification.[17] The stages refer to the depth of invading tumor found during biopsy (Fig. 34–1).[17]

Metastasis to other organs begins once the invading cancer penetrates the submucosal and muscular layer of the bladder. The invasion progresses through pelvic lymph nodes and spreads to liver, bones, and lungs. As metastasis progresses, it can extend into the rectum, vagina, other pelvic soft tissues, and retroperitoneal structures. The prognostic "dividing line" lies between stages B1 and B2; stage C and D tumors portend a much poorer prognosis. Clients with superficial bladder tumors have a survival rate of 70% after 5 years. Other clients with muscle invasive disease experience tumor recurrence within 18 to 24 months of the diagnosis.[17, 44]

Superficial tumors have a good chance of being eradicated or stabilized; however, recurrence is frequent. Therefore, it is crucial to do follow-up cystoscopic examinations every 3 months for 2 years, with additional cystoscopic examinations every 6 months for 2 years, then yearly.[17, 44] In a study of 114 clients, the interval between the original intervention and recurrence ranged from 3 months to 27 years. Nineteen per cent involved a new tumor of a higher grade, and 22% of the tumors were of a more advanced stage. Most recurrences of superficial tumors represent lesions that can be controlled by transurethral resection.[17, 44]

Clinical Manifestations

Gross painless hematuria is most frequently the first manifestation of bladder cancer, occurring in 85% of all cases. Unfortunately, the bleeding is usually intermittent initially, which may often lead a client to delay seeking health care. As the disease becomes more invasive, the client may experience frequent bladder irritability with dysuria, frequency, and urgency. Frequently, gross hematuria or obstruction in voiding forces the client to seek help. The amount of hematuria does not correlate with stage of disease.

When gross or microscopic hematuria is identified without any known etiologic agent, an extensive evaluation is necessary. Cystoscopy is indicated to identify and visualize the tumor directly and to obtain a biopsy specimen of the lesion for cytologic study. Flow cytometry can be done to examine the deoxyribonucleic acid (DNA) content of the cells in the urine. Bladder washings during cystoscopy produce more accurate specimens compared with a voided specimen. The mechanical action resulting from saline washings enhances tumor shedding, with better-quality specimens sent for cytologic study.

Another examination, IVP, is a dye-enhanced x-ray examination that allows one to evaluate not only the bladder but also the ureters and kidneys. CT, magnetic resonance imaging (MRI), and ultrasonography also may be done to assess the bladder and surrounding structures, such as the rectum or uterus, possible sites of spread. A tumor marker, serum carcinoembryonic antigen (CEA), which is present with adenocarcinomas of the bladder, can also be evaluated.

Outcome Management

Medical Management

The outcome desired with medical management is to eradicate the bladder of transitional or papillary cell carcinoma in situ in the early stages. This is best achieved with alkylating intravesical chemotherapy or BCG instillations, which are the first-line and most common therapies. Advanced cancer that has invaded muscle is usually treated surgically with a radical cystectomy. Radiation therapy is rarely used except for advanced disease or as palliative treatment.

CHEMOTHERAPY ADMINISTRATION

Intravesical therapies can be administered for superficial tumors, such as transitional cell, papillary cell, or Stage

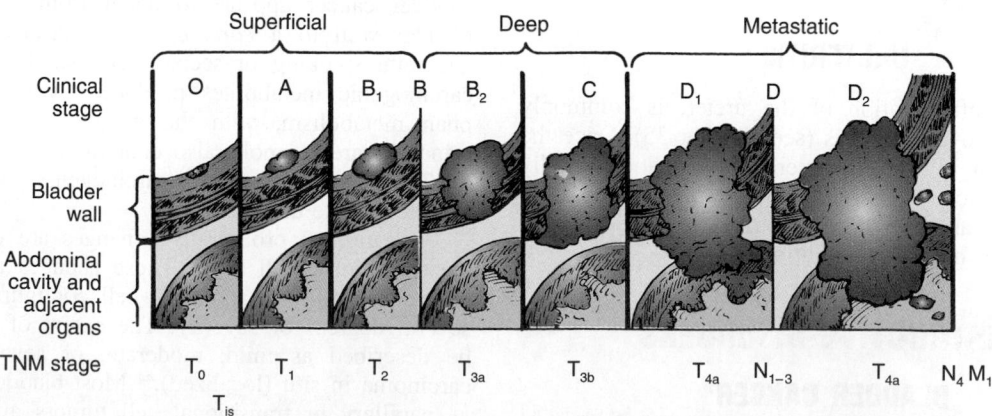

FIGURE 34–1 The Jewett-Marshall-Strong clinical staging of bladder cancer. The diagram shows the degree of tumor infiltration at each stage and compares it with the tumor, node, metastasis (TNM) system. (Adapted from K. Karlowicz (Ed.) [1995]. *Urologic nursing: Principles and practice.* Philadelphia: W. B. Saunders.)

0-A tumors. Intravesical BCG therapy appears to be quite successful in treating carcinoma in situ. The best results have been obtained with BCG as an intravesical agent for transitional cell tumors, although it has also been used for papillary tumors, adenocarcinoma, and squamous cell carcinoma.

Usually, BCG is instilled into the bladder through a urethral catheter. The catheter is clamped or removed. The client is directed to retain the fluid for 2 hours, with side-to-side position changes or supine-to-prone changes required every 15 to 30 minutes. Once the 2 hours have passed, the client voids in a sitting position or the catheter is unclamped to allow drainage. Finally, the client is instructed to drink two glasses of water to help flush the bladder. Steroids and ciprofloxacin (Cipro) have sometimes been given after intravesical BCG treatment to prevent recurrence. If two treatments of intravesical BCG have been ineffective, most urologists recommend a cystectomy.

Intravesical instillation of an alkylating chemotherapeutic agent, another common practice, provides concentrated topical treatment with relatively little systemic absorption. Thiotepa, mitomycin, doxorubicin (Adriamycin), and cyclophosphamide (Cytoxan) are all used for low-grade, superficial, papillary tumors. Systemic chemotherapy drugs are used for more advanced disease, to treat the metastasis of the bladder tumor, and to prolong life. However, surgical removal of the bladder is the most common approach in advanced disease when tumor has invaded muscle.

The major side effects or complications of intravesical chemotherapy or BCG instillation include bladder irritation, frequency, urgency, and dysuria. These manifestations usually resolve within 1 or 2 days. Occasionally, hematuria, fever, malaise, nausea, chills, arthralgia (joint pain), and pruritus (itching) are reported. These manifestations are more representative of systemic reaction and should be reported to the physician.

RADIATION THERAPY

Radiation therapy alone is not as effective a treatment for bladder cancer as surgery and chemotherapy; the 5-year survival after radiation alone is less than 40%. Radiation therapy is rarely used except as palliation for advanced disease that cannot be eradicated by intravesical chemotherapy or radical surgery. Most bladder cancers are poorly radiosensitive, and high doses of radiation are necessary.

External supervoltage radiation, somewhat unsuccessful by itself, is effective when used in combination with surgery or chemotherapy. Hyperbaric radiation therapy increases the oxygen tension of the tumor cells and their radiosensitivity. Palliative radiation may be used to relieve pain, to prevent and relieve bowel obstruction, to control potential hemorrhage, and to alleviate leg edema secondary to venous or lymphatic obstruction.

The major side effects of radiation are hemorrhagic cystitis and bladder irritation. Local instillation of formalin may control bladder hemorrhaging resulting from the cancer or the treatments. Hemorrhagic cystitis may occur even as late as 10 years after pelvic radiation. Other complications include manifestations of cystitis and proctitis, such as dysuria, frequency, urgency, nocturia, and

diarrhea. Delayed adverse effects, such as ileitis, colitis, persistent cystitis, bladder ulceration, and fistula formation, may occur as late as 6 to 12 months after radiation.

A *fistula* is an abnormal passage between two organs or between an organ and the skin. It allows for intercommunication of secretions and other substances. After radiation to the bladder, a vesicovaginal fistula may be found in women or a colovesical fistula may develop. A fistula is suspected when urine leaves the body from an unnatural site, such as the vagina, when fecal material or air appears in the urine, or when the client has recurrent UTIs. Diagnosis is confirmed by IVP, cystography, cystoscopy, or sigmoidoscopy. To further delineate the path of a fistula, a dye, such as Congo red or indigo carmine, is instilled into the bladder and all outlets are identified.

Before surgical repair of a fistula, the client must maintain a continuous flow of urine from the kidney through temporary urinary diversion, either externally or with a catheter. Surgical repair often requires a long and slow surgical procedure and may require several procedures. The primary goals are to excise the fistula and to reestablish tissue integrity.

◼ Nursing Management of the Medical Client

ASSESSMENT

Begin your assessment of a client being evaluated for bladder cancer with a careful health, medical, and surgical history. Because this client will be undergoing extensive diagnostic evaluation, be sure to collect additional information about drug, chemical, and food allergies. Explain risk factors from exposure to known carcinogens. Ask the client about changes in urine or urination patterns, noting changes in color, frequency, and amount.

DIAGNOSIS, OUTCOMES, INTERVENTIONS

Powerlessness. The client with bladder cancer will experience *Powerlessness related to lack of knowledge of disease process, options, treatment, and side effects of therapy; fear of the disease process and treatment; and loss of control following the diagnosis and decisions regarding treatment offered.*

Outcomes. The client will learn about the medical management of the disease process, with a full understanding of client responsibilities during the treatment. The client and family will be involved with decisions about therapies and care. The client will also be encouraged to help direct care with involved health care professionals.

Interventions
Provide Education. To increase knowledge, educate the client and family about the use, rationale, risks, side effects, and expected outcomes of intravesical chemotherapy, BCG instillation, radiation, and surgery. You play an important role in client education of treatment modalities and complications that may accompany them.
Encourage Decision-Making. Encourage the client to discuss and make decisions about care. Provide opportunities for the client to express desires for care as well as time to discuss what the diagnosis and treatment mean personally.

Altered Urinary Elimination. *Altered Urinary Elimination related to urgency, frequency, dysuria, and* *hematuria resulting from chemotherapy, radiation, or BCG instillation for treatment of bladder cancer.*

Outcomes. Normal voiding will resume by day 3 after removal of the catheter, and the client will not experience sequelae to BCG instillation, chemotherapy, or radiation therapy.

Interventions. Nursing management of intravesical chemotherapy includes client education, administration of the chemotherapy agent, care of the client throughout the procedure, and monitoring for complications after administration.

Provide Education. Preparation before BCG or chemotherapy bladder instillation requires fluid restriction for 4 hours before the procedure to decrease the need to void for 2 hours afterward. Tell the client that a catheter will be inserted before the instillation and that it will be necessary to rotate and change positions every 15 to 30 minutes during treatment. After the 2-hour instillation, fluids are encouraged to flush the urinary system. Explain that treatments are typically repeated weekly for 4 to 8 weeks and then monthly for varying periods. Follow-up cystoscopy is required to monitor tumor growth.

Promote Safety. Because of the toxicity of the intravesical chemotherapy or BCG instillation, it is important to provide a safe environment for health care workers who may come in contact with the chemotherapeutic agent. For 6 hours after treatment, urine and the toilet bowl must be disinfected with bleach.

Promote Comfort. Dysuria or irritation while voiding may result from the side effects of chemotherapy, placement of an indwelling catheter, and the presence of the tumor, and it must be managed. Tumor pain is managed with analgesics. Irritative problems of dysuria, frequency, and urgency from the catheter will diminish when the catheter is removed. Irritation from the chemotherapy will decrease after about 2 days.

Reassure the client that dysuria, frequency, and urgency from catheter placement and intravesical treatment will diminish over 2 days. Discuss prescribed analgesics, antispasmodics, or anticholinergics, and explain how they should be taken.

Risk for Injury. The client who undergoes chemotherapy, BCG instillation, or radiation therapy is at *Risk for Injury from side effects of these treatments.*

Outcomes. Complications resulting from these treatments will be minimized. The client will verbalize an understanding of risk and side effects following the selected treatment option.

Interventions. Explain expected and unexpected outcomes of BCG instillation, chemotherapy, or radiation therapy. Inform the client and family how and when to alert medical staff to potential complications. Interventions for side effects include administration of antispasmodics, increasing fluid intake, and administering urinary tract antiseptics or analgesics.

If a high fever develops after BCG instillation, treatment with isoniazid or other medications used to treat tuberculosis may be indicated.

For radiation proctitis, the client will require a low-residue diet and drugs to decrease intestinal motility. For complete information on nursing care for clients receiving radiation therapy, see Chapter 19.

Urine from a client undergoing this intervention should be sent to the radioisotopes laboratory for monitoring. A client with radioactive implants is typically placed in a private room with limited visitation, but hospital policies may vary.

EVALUATION

Complications that arise from medical treatment may be difficult to manage, but they typically resolve after the treatment has ended. Evaluation of the nursing management of radiation therapy and intravesical BCG and chemotherapy will be based on the client's ability to restate personal responsibilities, to verbalize an understanding of the disease process, and to participate in care.

Because clients with bladder cancer require long-term follow-up care and continuous evaluation, they must understand the disease process and long-term follow-up responsibilities needed to maintain optimal health. If medical therapies are unsuccessful, surgical removal of the bladder may be required.

■ Surgical Management

Several surgical options may be used to treat bladder cancer that has not responded to medical therapies or that has invaded the bladder muscle. Surgical intervention ranges from local resection and fulguration of the tumor (destruction of tissue by electrical current through electrodes placed in direct contact with the growth) to total cystectomy, which requires diversion of normal urinary flow.

TRANSURETHRAL RESECTION

The simplest procedure is transurethral resection of the bladder tumor and fulguration done for low-grade, superficial, isolated papillary tumors or, sometimes, for inoperable tumors for palliation. The bladder is accessed through a cystoscope, which has been inserted through the urethra (see Chapter 38). This procedure is commonly followed by intravesical BCG or chemotherapy to prevent recurrence from reattachment of loose bladder cancer cells.

PARTIAL CYSTECTOMY

A segmental or partial cystectomy may be done if the client cannot tolerate a radical cystectomy and for isolated tumor which cannot be treated by transurethral resection. Up to half the bladder can be removed. This procedure is appropriate for 10% to 15% of clients. The recurrence rate can be high.

During the initial postoperative period, bladder capacity is markedly reduced. The postoperative bladder may be able to hold no more than 60 ml. Over several months, bladder tissue expands, increasing its capacity from 200 to 400 ml.

RADICAL CYSTECTOMY AND URINARY DIVERSION

A radical cystectomy with urinary diversion is the procedure of choice when potentially curable stage B disease is too advanced for transurethral resection or intravesical chemotherapy. The procedure may also be performed for treatment of:

● Neurogenic bladder (see Neurogenic Bladder Dysfunction later on)

- IC or radiation-induced cystitis with severely reduced bladder capacity
- Congenital anomalies of the lower urinary tract, such as bladder exstrophy

Radical cystectomy entails removal of the bladder, urethra, uterus, fallopian tubes, ovaries, and anterior segment of the vagina in women. In men, the bladder, urethra, and usually the prostate and seminal vesicles are removed. Cystectomy also involves removal of perivesical fat and dissection of the pelvic lymph nodes. This procedure is necessary when the tumor has invaded the bladder wall, involves the trigone, or cannot be treated adequately by less radical methods. When the bladder and urethra are removed, permanent urinary diversion is required. The entire surgical procedure is done in one step, with urinary diversion and cystectomy performed at the same time.

Ileal Conduit

An ileal conduit (also called ureteroileostomy, ileal bladder, or Bricker's procedure) is one type of urinary diversion. Using a segment of the intestine as a conduit, the surgeon constructs a system in which urine empties through an artificial opening in the skin called a *stoma* (Fig. 34–2). Usually, a portion of the terminal ileum, which has the least reabsorptive power, is used for the conduit. After the continuity of the remaining intestine is reestablished with end-to-end anastomosis, the proximal end of the segment is closed. The distal end is brought out through a hole created in the abdominal wall, folded back, and sutured to the skin to form a stoma. The ureters are then implanted into the ileal segment. Urine flows into the conduit and is continually propelled out through the stoma by peristalsis. Mucous shreds will always be present in the urine because of the mucus produced by the lining of the bowel.

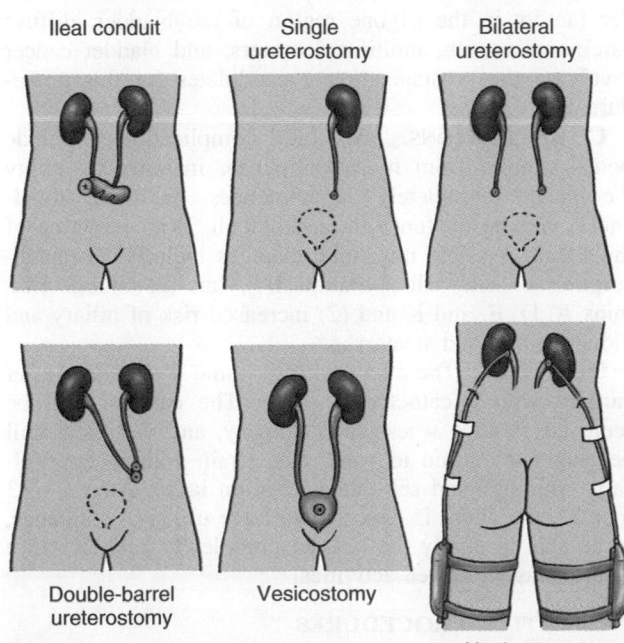

Ileal conduit   Single ureterostomy   Bilateral ureterostomy

Double-barrel ureterostomy   Vesicostomy   Nephrostomy

FIGURE 34–2 Some older surgical alternatives for urinary diversion.

INDICATIONS. The client who has undergone an ileal conduit must wear an appliance over the stoma to collect the urine. This treatment is rarely selected for clients with a life expectancy of more than 1 to 2 years. The procedure involves less time, and the conduit is easier to construct compared with other diversion procedures, which makes it an excellent choice for older clients who are unable to tolerate a lengthy surgery because of other medical conditions. Because the ileal segment is not a reservoir, absorption of electrolytes and the frequency of other complications are minimal.

CONTRAINDICATIONS. Clients who cannot maintain follow-up care or treatment because of physical limitations or mental impairment are not candidates for an ileal conduit; clients with chronic bowel disease or colon cancer may not be candidates either. Any medical condition that prevents a major surgical procedure would also be a contraindication.

COMPLICATIONS. Several complications related to stoma management (e.g., skin irritation, stomal defects, and stomal pouching problems) may arise. Leakage at the anastomosis site, stenosis, peristomal hernia, ulceration, and obstruction at the ureteroileal anastomosis may develop. Finally, clients who have undergone an ileal conduit procedure are at increased risk for pyelonephritis, hydronephrosis (distention of renal pelvis and calices with urine), and formation of calculi.

OUTCOMES. Eight weeks after surgery, it is expected that the client will adjust to the stoma and appliance, maintain stoma and appliance care, have a urine output of ½ ml/kg/hr, and return to most previously enjoyed activities.

Indiana Pouch

Other diversionary procedures are the Indiana pouch, Florida pouch, Kock pouch, and continent internal ileal reservoir. A reservoir is created from the ascending colon and terminal ileum. The Indiana pouch is an improved and larger version of the original Kock pouch (Fig. 34–3). Other continent reservoir operations vary slightly regarding surgical technique and the portion of the colon and ileum used.

Once the reservoir has been created, the ureters are implanted into the side of the diversion. A special nipple valve is then constructed and used to attach the reservoir to the skin. Several weeks after surgery, the client is taught to use a catheter to drain the reservoir at 3- to 4-hour intervals. Internal storage of up to 800 ml of urine is possible, with a daytime continence rate of up to 93% and a nighttime continence rate of up to 76%.

INDICATIONS. Because this procedure involves no appliance for collecting urine, it is preferred for clients with a life expectancy of more than 2 years. Creation of the reservoir and nipple valve requires 1 to 3 more hours more surgical time compared with the time needed to construct an ileal conduit. The client's serum creatinine level should be 2.5 mg/dl or less. The client will need gross and fine motor coordination to catheterize the nipple valve and must be willing and able to participate in self-care. Electrolyte reabsorption is minimal with this diversion technique as long as the urine is drained regularly.

CONTRAINDICATIONS. Clients with a history of significant bowel resection and malabsorption related to diar-

FIGURE 34–3 Indiana pouch procedure.

rhea, irritable bowel syndrome, ulcerative colitis, diverticular disease, bowel cancer, Crohn's disease, progressive neurologic disorders, morbid obesity, kidney disease (creatinine > 2.5 mg/dl) and pelvic radiation are not candidates for an Indiana pouch.

COMPLICATIONS. Possible complications include incontinence, difficult catheterization, urinary reflux, anastomotic leaks, pyelonephritis, obstruction, bacteriuria, calculi, erectile dysfunction, electrolyte imbalances, and rupture of the reservoir.

OUTCOMES. About 8 to 10 weeks after surgery, the client will have urinary continence, will remain free of urinary tract infection, and will return to activities pursued before surgery. Self-catheterization should begin 3 weeks postoperatively.

Neobladder
Sometimes the urethra can be spared, allowing the creation of a *neobladder,* also known as an ileal W-bladder. This operation is the treatment of choice for a client with bladder cancer that has invaded the bladder muscle. Although this procedure differs from one in which the reservoir empties through an abdominal stoma, a neobladder empties via a pelvic outlet to the urethra. Maintaining continence can be a problem unless the lower portion of the bladder can be spared.

Some surgeons believe that the urethra should be removed because of the risk of tumor recurrence. If the urethra is resected, a reconstructed neourethra together with an artificial sphincter is created. This procedure is more successful in males because of the longer urethra.

Several weeks after surgery, the catheter is removed and the client empties the neobladder by relaxing the external sphincter and creating abdominal pressure. The client will have to learn intermittent self-catheterization to cope with any voiding difficulties. Even with the potential postoperative problems that may be encountered, accep-

tance of this procedure is very high because it allows a more normal anatomy to be maintained for the client. Total continence is achieved in 84% to 96% of clients at 5 years.

INDICATIONS. Because an appliance is not required and normal anatomy is maintained, the neobladder technique is the preferred urinary diversion for clients with a life expectancy of more than 2 years and with no contraindications. Other indications are as described for an Indiana pouch.

CONTRAINDICATIONS. In addition to the contraindications listed for an Indiana pouch, the client with bladder tumors in the trigone region of the bladder, diffuse carcinoma in situ, multifocal tumors, and bladder cancer involving the prostate are not candidates for this procedure.

COMPLICATIONS. Possible complications include pouch rupture from hypercontinence, inability to empty the bladder completely, incontinence, electrolyte imbalances, erectile dysfunction, and calculi. With resection of the ileum, possible metabolic changes include (1) malabsorption of bile salts; vitamin B_{12}; fat; fat-soluble vitamins A, D, E, and K and (2) increased risk of biliary and kidney stones and steatorrhea.

OUTCOMES. The client will go home 4 to 8 days after surgery with a catheter in place. The catheter will be removed about 4 weeks after surgery, and the client will be taught to "strain to void" (see strain voiding or "Valsalva voiding" and self-catheterization later). After 2 to 3 months, the client is expected to have urinary continence, to be able to empty the bladder completely, and to return to previously pursued activities.

PALLIATIVE PROCEDURES
Percutaneous Nephrostomy or Pyelostomy
For the client with inoperable bladder cancer, a percutaneous nephrostomy (see Fig. 34–2) or pyelostomy may

be performed to prevent obstruction. A catheter is inserted into the renal pelvis by surgical incision or, more likely, a percutaneous puncture procedure. In the surgical approach, a balloon-tipped or mushroom-tipped catheter is connected to an external drainage system.

In the percutaneous nephrostomy procedure, a trocar is inserted under fluoroscopy by direct puncture into the renal pelvis or calix. A flexible small-gauge needle is then used to instill contrast material to verify proper location. Using angiographic wire as a guide, the surgeon places the nephrostomy tube and connects it to a closed drainage system. The entire procedure is done with the client under local anesthesia. It is important to stabilize the tube to prevent dislodgment.

Ureterostomy

A ureterostomy may be performed as a palliative procedure if the ureters are obstructed by tumor. During a cutaneous ureterostomy, the surgeon attaches the ureter to the surface of the abdomen where urine flows directly into a drainage appliance without an intermediary conduit. For clients with ureterostomies, infection, obstruction to urine flow secondary to strictures at the opening, and skin irritation are potential problems. This procedure includes several variations (see Fig. 34–2).

■ Nursing Management of the Preoperative Client

ASSESSMENT

Preoperative nursing management of the client with bladder cancer is directed at educating the client and family. Assess the client and family's understanding of pending diagnostic testing, bladder cancer, and proposed surgical procedure. Evaluate the client's anxiety level by providing opportunities to talk about feelings and to ask questions about the upcoming surgery, potential for distorted body image, and support systems outside the hospital.

In addition to educating and counseling the client, obtain physical assessment findings. Check for (1) costovertebral tenderness and masses in the upper abdomen and flank, (2) distention before and after urination, (3) vaginal or rectal masses, and (4) signs of discharge in urethral meatus and perianal areas. Assessment of other body systems includes (1) monitoring vital signs; (2) measuring intake and output; (3) examining skin for color, bruises, petechiae, and hydration; and (4) auscultating heart and lung sounds.

Complete a self-care or functional assessment to determine whether the client can manage drains and indwelling catheters and is able to catheterize a continent stoma or urethra. Finally, determine whether a family member can provide care or whether home health care is available to the client.

DIAGNOSIS, OUTCOMES, INTERVENTIONS

Knowledge Deficit. The most common nursing diagnosis preoperatively is *Knowledge Deficit related to bladder cancer and diagnostic testing, possible bowel preparation prior to surgical intervention, and surgical intervention with associated expected course of treatment.*

Outcomes. Preoperative education will bring about an increased awareness of the procedure and lowered anxiety preoperatively and postoperatively. The client will under-

stand diagnostic tests, bowel preparation, surgical intervention, and the anticipated postoperative course, as evidenced by statements and demonstrations of self-care.

Interventions

Provide Preoperative Teaching. Assess the client's educational deficits surrounding bladder cancer, proposed treatment, and expected outcomes by encouraging discussion. Include the family in the discussion to review diagnostic evaluation, preoperative treatment, and postoperative expectations. Explain the purpose of various tubes, such as IV lines, the nasogastric (NG) tube, stents, drains, and catheters that will be present after surgery and when they will be discontinued. As needed, discuss support services available after discharge.

Discuss Bowel Preparation. If a diversion or pouch procedure has been chosen as the appropriate surgical intervention, discuss the preoperative bowel preparation ("bowel prep"). Because a segment of bowel will be used to create the conduit or reservoir, this measure relates to the segment of intestine to be used in the procedure.

Bowel preparation calls for a clear liquid diet for 1 to 3 days, laxatives and enemas to clear the bowel, and antibiotics to lower the bacterial count in the bowel. Because this step takes several days and includes enemas, dietary restrictions, and medications, it is extremely important to teach the client and family to strictly adhere to the directions.

Provide Enterostomal Nurse Visitation. If the client will have a pouch or diversion procedure, a visit from an enterostomal nurse may be reassuring for the client and family. This visit allows the client and family to interact and learn the expected postoperative course with a nurse with expertise in this field.

Before surgery, the enterostomal nurse selects and marks the best site for ostomy placement if the surgeon plans to construct a stoma. The main criterion for stomal placement is finding a site that allows the faceplate of the drainage appliance to bind securely to the surface of the abdomen.

The stoma must be clearly visible to the client. This means that the surgeon should avoid the umbilicus, rib margins, pubis, iliac crests, and pre-existing scars, wrinkles, or crevices. Placing the stoma directly on the client's waistline can cause excessive pressure from clothing.

The client is observed in the supine, standing, and sitting positions during the selection process. Stoma placement is usually on the right lower quadrant of the abdomen, in the abdominal rectus muscle, about 2 inches below the waist and 2 inches from the midline. Explain the proper way to care for the urinary diversion.

Risk for Body Image Disturbance. The client is at *Risk for Body Image Disturbance related to surgery, possible stoma formation, possible sexual dysfunction, and potential change in urinary elimination.*

Outcomes. The client will not experience body image disturbance postoperatively, as evidenced by the ability to discuss concerns regarding altered body image, stoma placement, change in urination pattern, risk of sexual dysfunction, and verbalization of fears.

Interventions. Identify factors that reveal the client's difficulty in coping with anticipated changes in body image. Should a diversion procedure be necessary, in addition to a preoperative visit from an enterostomal nurse, you may want to suggest a visit from a client with a similar diagnosis and procedure. These visits provide the client with a comfortable opportunity to ask questions, to experience a sense of comfort and support, and to receive information.

Preoperative teaching should include explanations of the expected anatomic and physiologic alterations and possible effects for the client. Because of the lifestyle changes that are required by diversion or pouch surgery, be sure to offer support and refer the client for additional counseling if indicated. Community associations, such as the United Ostomy Association and the American Cancer Society, provide tremendous help for clients undergoing urinary diversion.

Radical bladder surgery may cause a disturbance in sexual function. Because of the private and personal nature of this surgery, you should use this opportunity to discuss potential sexual dysfunction following radical surgery for bladder cancer. Although nerve sparing procedures and vaginal reconstruction procedures can reduce sexual dysfunction, clients should be prepared to take advantage of available resources in case impotence or difficulty with intercourse develops after surgery.

EVALUATION

It is expected that the client will be prepared for and will undergo the selected surgery successfully. The client will restate information about bladder cancer, diagnostic testing, the bowel preparation, and surgical intervention. In addition, the client will be able to voice concerns about body image disturbance and sexual dysfunction after surgery. The client will be aware of outside resources available following discharge.

■ Nursing Management of the Postoperative Client

ASSESSMENT

Routine postoperative evaluation and care involve the usual assessments for a client after major abdominal surgery. The stoma, if present, should be inspected hourly for 24 hours after surgery, then every 4 hours for 24 hours, then every 8 hours. The stoma should be red and moist at all times and will be edematous just after surgery. The edema will diminish by 200% to 500% within a few weeks. Peristomal sutures may be seen adhering to the skin and mucosal bowel edge. Any sign that the stoma is becoming pale, dark, dusky, gray, or cyanotic may mean loss of vascular supply; this event must be corrected immediately to avoid necrosis.

Peristalsis in the intestinal tract will be absent for several days because of the manipulation and resection of the bowel. The client will continue to receive nothing by mouth (i.e., will remain on NPO status) with IV lines and a nasogastric tube in place until peristalsis returns. Assessment of bowel sounds and nasogastric contents is required.

Urine flow never stops after surgery. Ureteral stents originating in the renal pelvis extend through the ureters and through the reservoir, conduit, or neobladder. The stents that exit through a stoma are contained in the

pouch. With continent reservoirs, a catheter is placed through the nipple valve to drain the internal reservoir for 2 to 3 weeks until healing occurs. For a neobladder, a suprapubic catheter may be placed through the abdominal wall into the reservoir to keep it drained while another catheter is placed through the urethra and used as a stent. This protects the anastomosis of the urethra and neobladder.

In some instances, ureteral stents or catheters may drain urine after neobladder or continent reservoir surgery. The stents and catheter are removed once adequate healing has occurred; this is usually in 3 to 4 weeks. The catheter is usually the last tube to be discontinued. Constantly monitor the tubes for patency and continuous drainage, usually in separate closed gravity systems. For the first 24 to 48 hours, hourly intake and output records may be required. Clients should be kept from manipulating tubes immediately after surgery.

HEMATURIA. Assess for hematuria, stenosis, and other complications after surgery. Hematuria, a common problem after transurethral resection, is controlled with a three-way indwelling catheter and, if necessary, bladder irrigation. The greatest potential problems after any diversion or pouch procedure are infection, wound dehiscence, skin irritation, ulceration, and stomal defects. Later complications are renal deterioration caused by reflux, stenosis of the stoma, strictures at the site of the anastomosis, hydronephrosis, calculi, and peristomal hernia.

STENOSIS. Stenosis of the stoma may occur from scarring during stomal maturation. If the opening on the faceplate is too large, epithelial hyperplasia or thickening of the peristomal skin may contract the stoma. Clients with urinary diversion are also susceptible to uric acid and calcium stone disease. The onset of urinary stone development usually occurs at least 2 years postoperatively and sometimes as long as 5 to 10 years later. UTI is a perpetual threat because of the exposure of the urinary tract. Obstruction anywhere in the urinary tract may interfere with normal urine flow.

OTHER COMPLICATIONS. The potential complications of continent reservoirs or pouch procedures include incontinence, difficult catheterization, urinary reflux, and possible pyelonephritis, obstruction, bacteriuria, electrolyte imbalances, urolithiasis, or absorptive problems. The reservoir may rupture if the client does not comply with the self-catheterization protocol.

Monitor the client for other complications as well following a radical cystectomy. Cystectomy is a very invasive surgery that puts the client at risk for most of the usual postoperative complications, including shock and hemorrhage. The extensive pelvic dissection associated with this surgery can increase the risk of thrombophlebitis. Additionally, pelvic lymph node dissection can predispose the client to lymphedema in the lower limbs. You may need to assess calf circumference during each shift.

DIAGNOSIS, OUTCOMES, INTERVENTIONS

Risk for Injury: Occlusion of Urinary Drainage. A potential problem for the postoperative client is *Risk for Injury: Occlusion of urinary drainage device related to hematuria, clot formation, and swelling following the surgical procedure.*

Outcomes. Catheters and other drainage tubes will not become obstructed, and urine will flow freely.

Interventions. After transurethral resection of the bladder, the client will usually have hematuria. A three-lumen, indwelling urethral catheter will be attached to a continuous or intermittent closed bladder irrigation system to facilitate urine flow, minimize blood clots, and monitor for postoperative bleeding. Nursing care is similar to that after transurethral resection of the prostate (see Chapter 38). Bright red or pink urine will fade to clear in about 3 days.

Nursing care after segmental bladder resection centers on maintaining constant urinary drainage to ensure that the remaining bladder does not become distended, putting strain on the suture line. The client usually has both urethral and suprapubic catheters. The client is discharged with the catheter in place, and it remains in place for about 2 weeks or until complete healing has occurred.

As with any major abdominal surgery, clients who undergo a radical cystectomy and urinary diversion are at an increased risk for hemorrhage. Monitor the client's vital signs, the incision, and the drainage tubes closely for early signs of excessive bleeding. If an ileal conduit is formed, the client will have a pouch in place to collect urine from the ileal conduit or ureteral catheters or stents.

After a continent diversion, make sure that the catheter is draining urine freely. If any obstruction occurs, the newly created reservoir can become damaged and internal leakage along the suture line can occur. Monitor the catheter output closely, and perform irrigations at regular intervals as directed. Perform catheter irrigation gently in the immediate postoperative period, using about 60 ml of normal saline solution. Irrigation is necessary to help prevent obstruction from clots or mucus.

After neobladder surgery, one or two catheters will be in place to prevent overdistention of the newly created bladder. These catheters are treated as closed drainage systems. Carefully monitor the neobladder for possible obstruction. Regular irrigation is needed to rid the neobladder of mucus.

When ureteral stents or catheters are placed, patency is very important to prevent hydronephrosis and pyelonephritis. Because there is no mucus in urine from the kidney, irrigation is usually not required and is kept to a minimum to prevent pyelonephritis and hydronephrosis. In fact, do not irrigate ureteral catheters unless you have a specific order to do so, and then only with 5 to 10 ml of sterile saline solution. Urine output from each ureteral catheter should be ¼ ml/kg/hour or roughly half of the ½ ml/kg/hr normally expected from a urethral catheter. Ureteral catheters may drain into a pouch when a stoma is present (see Critical Monitoring feature).

If the client has a stoma, a temporary, clear urostomy pouch over the stoma will be connected to a gravity drainage system. Sometimes ureteral catheters are used to splint the ureters while they heal. These catheters, usually removed before the client is discharged, may extend through the stoma.

Label all catheters, stents, and drainage tubes to prevent errors in irrigation and output calculations. Secure all tubes. Use a separate closed gravity drainage system for each tube unless, as with an ileal conduit, ureteral catheters exit into the pouching system until they are discon-

---

CRITICAL MONITORING

Postoperative Monitoring After Urinary Diversion Procedures

- Measure urine output every hour for the first 24 hours, and at least every 8 hours thereafter; report any amount less than ½ ml/kg/hour (~30 ml/hr) or no output for more than 15 minutes.
- Check the ostomy pouch for leaks and the skin under it for irritation every 4 hours initially, then every 8 hours.
- Inspect the stoma every hour for the first 24 hours after surgery. (This will give you a baseline from which you can quickly detect deviations. The stoma should be red and moist.) If you find no problems, extend intervals to every 4 hours, then to every 8 hours.
- Note the stoma's size, shape, and color. Expect it to be edematous in the immediate postoperative period. However, other changes may indicate complications, warranting action from the physician. A dusky or cyanotic stoma color may denote an insufficient blood supply and the onset of necrosis. This is an emergency. The reduced blood supply may result from surgical technique, from an appliance faceplate that is too small or improperly centered, or from peristomal protective materials that have been poorly applied. Other complications with the stoma include prolapse (protrusion from the skin) or retraction into the abdomen beneath the skin.
- Watch for manifestations of peritonitis, such as fever and abdominal pain and rigidity. Leakage at the site of the anastomosis or ureteral separation from the conduit may allow urine to seep into the peritoneal cavity, leading to peritonitis.
- Observe for bleeding. Although bleeding from the stoma may indicate a surgical defect, it is also common for the intestinal mucosa, which is very fragile, to bleed during a change of appliance or because of a poorly fitted collection pouch.

---

tinued. A separate system for each tube minimizes the risk and extent of bacterial infection.

Effective Management of Therapeutic Regimen. Clients undergoing any type of urinary diversion need to learn new self-care strategies. The nursing diagnosis of *Effective Management of Therapeutic Regimen related to complexity of therapeutic regimen* is applicable for this client.

Outcomes. The client will effectively manage the urinary diversion or neobladder, as evidenced by the ability to describe the regimen and to perform the required care successfully.

Interventions

Ileal Conduit. For a client with an ileal conduit, teach stoma care and skin care, promote self-care of the collection device, prevent odor, promote independence, and encourage follow-up.

Teach stoma care. The client will need to learn to care for the stoma and skin with proper application of a urinary pouch (see Bridge to Home Health Care). An opening must be cut in the skin barrier just large enough to fit over the stoma. The barrier is then applied to the

BRIDGE TO HOME HEALTH CARE

Managing an Ileal Conduit

When clients first come home from the hospital, they need your help to get organized and feel in control. Use a small plastic basket, such as one purchased at a discount store, to store small supplies, such as adhesive tape, stoma adhesive, a pen, and a small scissors. A wash basin, a small box, or a small organizer on wheels works well for the larger items, such as faceplate or wafers, skin barriers, pouches, and paper towels.

Typically, clients are taught about stoma care before discharge, but they may have been so overwhelmed that they did not hear or remember instructions. Once home, they may have many questions. While you change the appliance, have your clients lie down with a mirror positioned so they can become accustomed to seeing the stoma and can learn to care for the stoma without experiencing side effects such as faintness or dizziness. Eventually, the client should face the toilet while sitting comfortably on a stool or chair.

Before removing the original wafer, cut the new faceplate or wafer to size, snap it on the pouch, and make certain that everything is ready. Some clients may need a circular insert in the wafer to form a convex angle that makes a tighter seal around the small stoma. Once you take off the old appliance, cover the stoma; peristalsis causes urine to squirt out spontaneously.

Do not make your client laugh; pressure will cause urine to leak out. It is frustrating to repeatedly reclean the area. Use thick, absorbent paper towels to cover the stoma; they are also inexpensive and readily available.

Before cleaning the skin surface, make sure that the stoma is open and not becoming filled with mucus from the bowel. Use a small amount of lubricating jelly (e.g.,

K-Y) on your little finger, and gently enter the stoma. Quickly cover the stoma with a paper towel to absorb urine. To keep the skin healthy, wash around the stoma with soap and water, and prepare the skin with a skin barrier. Cover the stoma, and allow the skin barrier to dry. Once you are ready to secure the appliance, remove the paper towel quickly and apply the wafer.

Place your warm hands on the faceplate or wafer for a few minutes to help it adhere to the skin. You may need to apply an extra piece of adhesive tape in the corner or side to prevent leaking. Assess skinfolds before applying the wafer; consider shifting the wafer to a diamond position to decrease the bend at the fold and the potential for leaking.

Leakage is one of the most distressing aspects of the ileal conduit. Instruct clients to attach an overnight Foley bag to the pouch at bedtime and to be sure that there are no kinks in the tubing. Back-pressure and overflow into the pouch will cause the faceplate or wafer to pop off or leak. Until they feel confident, clients may decide to awaken about 2:00 AM to check the pouch. During the day, they need to empty the pouch often because the tension of a full pouch will cause a leak. Clients should change the pouch every 3 to 4 days, the faceplate or wafer once a week to 10 days to avoid odor problems and to decrease the risk of a UTI. The pouch is made with a hard plastic ring that snaps onto the faceplate or wafer because frequent changes are necessary.

Clients may call on enterostomal nurses at local hospitals, the United Ostomy Association, and the American Cancer Society for help in adjusting to an ileal conduit.

Mary M. Stasiak, RN, BSN, PHN, MA, *Case Manager, Allied Health Alternatives, Inc., Rochester, Minnesota*

skin before attaching the pouch or faceplate. A skin cement or adhesive disc may help the faceplate stick more securely to the skin. A non–water-soluble adhesive spray allows the client to go swimming. Most pouches come as two pieces, a faceplate or wafer and a removable pouch. Not having to remove the faceplate or wafer as frequently makes care much easier for many clients.

Teach skin care. Skin irritation or breakdown is a constant threat to a client with a urinary diversion. Advise the client to prevent urine from contacting the skin. This can be achieved in part when a well-fitted and properly attached appliance is used (Fig. 34–4). The opening in the adhesive backing of the faceplate or wafer should be cut no more than 3 mm larger than the stoma. This opening needs to be remeasured after the edema in the stoma recedes.

Each time the faceplate or wafer is changed, the skin around the stoma should be cleaned with a mild, nonresidue soap and water, and thoroughly dried. A gauze pad, absorbent paper towel, or tampon should be held over the stoma during cleaning to prevent urine from flowing out over the skin. Remove this pad or tampon just as the appliance is reapplied. The appliance should be changed early in the morning because urine production is slowest at this time.

Promote self-care of the collection device. Urine pouches have a valve in the bottom for intermittent urine drainage. Alternatively, the pouch may be drained by gravity into a leg or bedside bag, especially at night. The self-contained pouch drainage system allows the client to resume most, if not all, former activities with little or no change in style of dress.

However, instruct clients to empty the pouch when it is one-third to one-half full. The weight of accumulating urine may pull the faceplate away from the skin and cause leakage. Advise clients to check the seal often if they are perspiring heavily.

Prevent odor. Urine odor is a common problem with urinary stomas. Noxious odors result mostly from poor hygiene, alkaline urine, normal breakdown of urine (ammonia), concentrated urine from insufficient fluid intake, and the ingestion of certain foods, such as asparagus.

Because diluted urine has less odor, adequate fluid intake is very helpful. Reusable appliances can be washed with soap and lukewarm water. The pouch can also be soaked in diluted white vinegar or in a commercial deodorant product for 20 to 30 minutes. Rinse the pouch, and allow it to dry. Deodorant tablets are available for placement in the pouch while it is being worn.

FIGURE 34–4 Applying a disposable ostomy pouch. *A,* Gather supplies: ostomy pouch, ostomy belt, skin barrier, stoma template, gauze pads, pouch clip or rubber band, safety pin, and clean gloves. Clamp or wrap rubber band around the end of the pouch to prevent leakage during the procedure. Make sure that lighting is adequate and that the client is comfortable and understands the procedure. Wash your hands, and don clean examining gloves. *B,* Gently remove the old pouch, using warm water or an adhesive solvent around the seal if necessary. Place the gauze pad over the stoma to prevent leakage as you gently clean peristomal area with moist gauze. *C,* Measure the stoma with the stoma template. Trace the shape onto the skin barrier and adhesive, using the template. Cut openings no more than 3 mm larger than the stoma. *D,* Remove backing from the adhesive surface of the disposable ostomy pouch. *E,* Center a pouch opening over the stoma with the pouch drain pointing to floor. (If the client ambulates frequently, the pouch drain should point to the client's feet.) Make sure that the seal is complete. *F,* Connect drainage tubing to the ostomy pouch if appropriate. Secure tubing; with a rubber band around the tubing, pin a rubber band to the sheets if the client is immobile.

Promote independence. Long-term nursing intervention aims to maintain a functional urinary system and prevent complications. It takes time for clients and significant others to adjust to a urinary diversion. Even though counseling may have been excellent during the preoperative period, the reality of the diversion commonly produces anxiety, depression, and anger. The client may need help at first to look at or even talk about the stoma. As soon as possible after surgery, the client must begin to help care for the stoma, peristomal skin, and drainage system, gradually assuming more responsibility until achieving independence (see Client Education Guide).

Encourage follow-up. A client with bladder cancer must receive follow-up at regular intervals to assess for a recurrence of the cancer. The client should also continue

to be seen by an enterostomal therapy nurse to check for problems with the ostomy.

Continent Diversion. Postoperative care for the client with an Indiana pouch is similar to that for any client with a urinary diversion, except there is no external pouch. The client will have a 24 French (F) to 26F or Medina catheter in place to drain urine continuously until the pouch has healed. The reservoir is irrigated through the catheter with about 50 to 60 ml of normal saline every 4 hours to wash out clots or mucus, which may cause obstruction.

Teach reservoir catheterization. After a radiographic study, remove the catheter at 3 to 4 weeks after surgery to make sure that the continent reservoir is functioning properly. The client must learn to empty and irrigate the reservoir at regular intervals before discharge from the hospital. The principles of catheterization of a urinary reservoir are the same as for clean, intermittent urinary self-catheterization.

Using a 16 to 20F catheter with a generous amount of water-soluble lubricant, show the client how to insert the catheter into the nipple valve. Warn against forcing the catheter into the reservoir. If resistance occurs, tell the client to pause and apply only gentle pressure while slightly rotating the catheter. If this does not work, the client should call the physician. Advise the client to insert the catheter every 2 to 3 hours to drain the reservoir. Each week thereafter, the interval is increased by 1 hour, until finally catheterization is completed every 4 to 6 hours during the day.

Teach reservoir irrigation. Once the urine has stopped flowing, the client should take several deep breaths and move the catheter in and out 2 to 3 inches to be sure that the pouch is fully emptied. The catheter should be withdrawn slowly so additional urine can drain.

After urine has been drained from the reservoir, tell the client to leave the catheter in place and to use 50 to 60 ml of normal saline solution to irrigate the reservoir and to prevent excess mucus buildup, which may cause obstruction. The fluid can either be gently aspirated or allowed to drain from the catheter. Once the irrigant is drained, the catheter is removed and the end of the catheter is pinched before removal to prevent dripping. The irrigations may be repeated until the drainage returns free of mucus. If the mucus is very viscous (thick), increasing fluid intake and drinking cranberry juice can decrease the viscosity. Usually, mucus production lessens over time.

Because the catheterization procedure can be unpredictable, advise clients to carry catheterization supplies with them. Most clients develop a sensation of abdominal pressure when catheterization is needed. Regular fluid intake and adherence to the catheterization schedule are important. A full reservoir puts pressure on the nipple valve, making catheterization much more difficult. Clients should be taught to practice these skills before discharge. They may need to be followed up by a visiting nurse for additional help.

Teach strain voiding and intermittent self-catheterization. With a neobladder, the client will have to learn how to *strain void*, relaxing the external sphincter and increasing abdominal pressure to start the urine stream. Show the client how to perform clean self-catheterization in case the bladder cannot be emptied by regular voiding.

Encourage follow-up. Following urinary diversion, the client should be monitored at 3, 6, 9, and 12 months. The assessment includes electrolyte values, serum creatinine and blood urea nitrogen (BUN) values, renal function studies, vitamin B_{12} levels, and urine cultures. Renal damage may occur in noncompliant clients who neglect to empty the pouch and who then develop infection. These clients often experience severe kidney infections and damage, and an ileal conduit must be created to replace the neobladder or Indiana pouch so that urine will drain freely.

Risk for Impaired Skin Integrity. If the client has an ileal conduit, the nursing diagnosis of *Risk for Impaired Skin Integrity related to irritation of peristomal skin* is a potential problem.

Outcomes. The client will not demonstrate altered skin integrity or irritation of peristomal skin, as evidenced by intact, clear skin.

Interventions. Begin interventions for any skin irritation promptly. Check the pH of a urine specimen because strongly alkaline urine irritates the skin and facilitates crystal formation. Encourage the client to drink cranberry juice to help acidify the urine. Any positive urine culture result requires treatment. Check appliances carefully to identify leakage and to detect skin sensitivity.

Skin irritation may result from changing the pouch too frequently. A general recommendation is to leave the pouch in place as long as it is not leaking. During appliance changes, leave the skin open to the air as much as possible. Apply a pouch with a non-karaya (sterculia gum) skin barrier. Karaya cannot be used with urinary pouches because urine erodes karaya.

Skin irritation around the stoma commonly results from a yeast infection. Nystatin creams or powders are effective against topical yeast. Nystatin powder is applied directly over the irritated skin area and sealed to the skin with a liquid skin barrier.

Risk for Sexual Dysfunction. Extensive surgical dissection may alter the reproductive anatomy and may result in *Risk for Sexual Dysfunction related to potential postoperative impotence in men or painful intercourse in women following a radical cystectomy and changes in body image affecting sexuality.*

Outcomes. The client will accept and adopt alternative methods of sexual expression and will obtain additional information about sexuality through questions and statements.

Interventions. Male clients have a risk of impotence after a radical cystectomy related to the resection. Offer counseling both before and after the surgery to help the client adjust to any alterations (see Chapter 38 for information about alterations in male sexuality). Sildenafil (Viagra), 50 to 100 mg three times weekly, is being offered to most male clients immediately after the catheter is removed to maintain blood flow to the corpora cavernosa, so that when sexual intercourse can be resumed the client will have fewer problems with impotence.

For women who have had a total abdominal hysterectomy, bilateral salpingo-oophorectomy, and anterior vaginal resection, the result can be shortening and tightening of the vagina, leading to painful intercourse. Alternative positions, lubricants, topical estrogen, and vaginal dilators may decrease the discomfort. Booklets discussing both female and male sexual dysfunction are available from the American Cancer Society.

For partners of any client, encourage holding, touching, kissing, and other activities to promote intimacy. Partners are often afraid to touch the client for fear of inflicting hurt; embarrassment may also be an issue. Encourage open discussions.

EVALUATION

Carcinoma in situ is considered curable with a simple transurethral resection. Intravesical chemotherapy or BCG may be combined to decrease the risk of recurrence. If the postoperative care of the client has been successful, the client will be able to make the transition to self-care with minimal difficulty. Even with a radical cystectomy, however, the 5-year survival rate for clients with muscle invasive tumor (stage C or greater) is only 40% to 50%.

Self-Care

Motivation to promote preoperative self-care may influence the postoperative course. Direct the client toward self-care by improving knowledge, encouraging independence, and fostering participation in care and treatment. When the client increases self-care, there will be a decreasing need for nursing care and an increase in health promotion activities.

The client will need referrals to durable medical equipment companies for ostomy supplies or catheters for reservoir irrigation or intermittent self-catheterization if needed. These items can be delivered to the client's home. If the client lives alone, it may be necessary to arrange home delivery of groceries and medications.

Housekeeping and lifting are limited for the first 6 to 8 weeks after surgery. Evaluate the client's ability to engage in self-care, and identify the need for additional care from home health nurses. If the client cannot provide care and if a family member is involved with care, respite services may be required. Also consider directing the client and family to local support groups.

Modifications for Elderly Clients

The major modification for older clients with urinary diversion stems from difficulties with self-care. Changing an appliance is one area of difficulty because some dexterity is required. Older clients commonly have arthritis and other disabilities, including decreased visual acuity, that may limit their ability to manipulate catheters and pouches. These concerns must be closely assessed and appropriate assistance offered.

URETERAL TUMORS

Primary tumors of the ureter are rare. In men, ureteral cancer occurs mainly during one's 50s and 60s. This form of cancer rarely affects women. Ureteral neoplasms usually extend from renal or bladder neoplasms or from tumors originating in the bowel, uterus, or ovary. Those primary neoplasms usually occur first as a papillary, transitional cell, or squamous cell carcinoma. These tumors are most frequently found in the lower third of the ureter. In later stages of ureteral cancer, the tumor extends outside the ureter to adjacent structures and regional lymph nodes or to distant sites. Common sites for metastasis include the lungs and liver.

Usually, the first manifestation of ureteral malignancy is gross hematuria. The tumor normally develops painlessly until obstruction occurs. At this point, the client may experience flank pain. Diagnosis is made through urine cytology, IVP, cystoscopy, ultrasonography, and CT scanning.

Treatment of ureteral cancer almost exclusively involves surgical excision and resection. Radiation may also be used in advanced cases with local extension. When the lesion is located in the middle or proximal third of the ureter, the surgical procedure usually involves nephroureterectomy, removal of the kidney, ureter, and attached segment of the bladder on the affected side. If the tumor is in the distal third of the ureter and noninvasive, a more conservative procedure may be used; in this case, just the distal portion of the ureter is resected with ureteral reimplantation.

Silicone rubber (Silastic), polytetrafluoroethylene (Teflon), polytetrafluorourethane, and bovine carotid heterograft are used to replace the resected ureter, facilitating reimplantation in the bladder. A ureter-ureter anastomosis also may be performed. Preoperative and postoperative intervention is similar to that for clients undergoing nephrectomy, ureteral reimplantation, or segmental resection of the bladder.

If the decision is made not to perform any of these procedures, some palliative measure may be needed to prevent or alleviate ureteral obstruction. Urinary diversion may be performed, as described previously, or a ureteral stent catheter may be placed into the ureter during cystoscopy to maintain its patency. The older catheter, a flanged, winged stent (Gibbon's stent), or the newer double J stent is made to prevent migration up the ureter or dislodgment by ureteral peristaltic waves or gravity.

URINARY CALCULI

Urinary calculi (*urolithiasis*) are calcifications in the urinary system. Commonly called stones, calculi form primarily in the kidney (*nephrolithiasis*), but they can form in or migrate to the lower urinary system. They are typically asymptomatic until they pass into the lower urinary tract. Stones are usually managed by a urologist. Primary bladder calculi are rare and usually develop from a history of urinary stasis from obstruction or chronic infection.

Up to 4% of the population in the United States have urolithiasis. About 12% of the male population have a renal stone by age 70. More than 200,000 Americans require hospitalization for treatment of stones each year. Many more people pass stones spontaneously with only minor manifestations that require no treatment, whereas others are treated in an ambulatory setting. The recurrence rate for calcium oxalate stones is about 50% within 5 years.[43]

Etiology and Risk Factors

The two primary causative factors are (1) urinary stasis and (2) supersaturation of urine with poorly soluble crystalloids. Increased solute concentration occurs because of fluid depletion or an increased solute load. This increased concentration leads to the precipitation of crystals, such as calcium, uric acid, and phosphate. Urinary pH influences the solubility of certain crystals, with some crystal types precipitating readily in acid urine and some in alkaline urine. Abnormal pH levels occur in renal tubular acidosis with the administration of carbonic anhydrase inhibitors, in the presence of urea-splitting bacteria, and in severe, chronic diarrhea. Stasis of urine from bladder neck obstruction, continent urinary diversion, and immobilization increases the risk for development of stones because the crystals in unmoving urine precipitate more readily.

Infection, foreign bodies, failure to empty the bladder completely, metabolic disorders, and obstruction in the urinary tract contribute to the formation of calculi as well. The presence of precipitators has been noted in the urine (such as protein matrix and bacteria or inflammatory elements).

Inhibitor substances, such as citrate and magnesium, appear to keep particles from aggregating and forming crystals; a lack of inhibitors increases risk of stone development. Not only does the deficiency of inhibitors predispose the client to calculi, but there may be "anti-inhibitors" in the urine, such as aluminum, iron, and silicone. Certain medications may induce calculus formation, such as acetazolamide, absorbable alkalis (e.g., calcium carbonate and sodium bicarbonate), and aluminum hydroxide. Massive doses of vitamin C increase urinary oxalate levels.

There is an increased risk of calculus formation in the southeast part of the United States—an area known as "the stone belt." Men between ages 30 and 50 years have three times the risk of calculi.[26] Stones are also more common among people of European or Asian descent. Once a client has had calculi, there is an increased risk of additional ones.

Urolithiasis results not from any single factor but from multiple phenomena. One unanswered question is why some clients form calculi whereas others do not. This problem is particularly important with recurrent "stone formers."

Risk factors for stone formation include anything that either causes stasis or supersaturation of the urine, including:

- Immobility and a sedentary lifestyle, which increase stasis
- Dehydration, which leads to supersaturation
- Metabolic disturbances that result in an increase in calcium or other ions in the urine
- Previous history of urinary calculi
- Living in stone-belt areas
- High mineral content in drinking water
- A diet high in purines, oxalates, calcium, animal proteins
- UTIs
- Prolonged indwelling catheterization
- Neurogenic bladder
- A history of female genital mutilation

Health promotion and health maintenance activities are discussed under Nursing Management of the Medical Client.

Pathophysiology

The exact mechanism of stone formation has not been clearly defined. In fact, some researchers believe that a low calcium intake contributes whereas others contend that a high calcium intake contributes. Both groups agree on the role of supersaturation, however. Crystallization appears to be the primary factor in calculus development from[19, 30]:

- Supersaturation of urine with increased solutes
- Matrix formation caused when mucoproteins bind to the mass of the stone
- Lack of inhibitors caused by increased or absent protectors against stone formation
- A combination of these conditions

Generally, crystal growth involves *nucleation*, in which crystals are formed from supersaturated urine. Growth continues by aggregation to form larger particles. One of these particles may travel down the urinary tract until it is trapped at some narrow point where it becomes the nidus for stone formation.

Inhibitor substances (e.g., citrate, pyrophosphate, and magnesium) have been identified as *chelating agents*. When present in adequate amounts, they act to keep crystals from aggregating and forming stones. When inhibitors are absent, stone formation following crystal aggregation is more likely. Also, a fibrous matrix of urinary organic material (mostly mucoproteins) may form in the kidney or bladder, producing a substance into which crystallites are deposited and trapped. This, then, becomes the nidus of the stone. The excessive production of this mucoprotein may, in part, account for a family history of urolithiasis in clients with calculi.

TYPES OF CALCULI

Stones may be of one crystal type or a combination of types.

Calcium

Calcium is the most common substance and is found in up to 90% of stones.[26] Calcium stones are usually composed of calcium phosphate or calcium oxalate. They may range from very small particles, often called "sand" or "gravel," to giant staghorn calculi, which may fill the entire renal pelvis and extend up into the calyces (Fig.

34–5). The peak onset is during a person's 20s, and these stones affect primarily males.

Hypercalciuria (an increased solute load of calcium in the urine), is caused by four main components:

• A high rate of bone reabsorption, which liberates calcium, as in Paget's disease, hyperparathyroidism, Cushing's disease, immobility, and osteolysis caused by malignant tumors of the breast, lung, and prostate
• Gut absorption of abnormally large amounts of calcium, as in milk-alkali syndrome, sarcoidosis, and excessive intake of vitamin D
• Impaired renal tubular absorption of filtered calcium, as in renal tubular acidosis
• Structural abnormalities, such as "sponge kidney"

About 35% of all clients with calcium stones do not have high serum levels of calcium and demonstrate no apparent cause of hypercalciuria.

There are two variants of hypercalciuria:

1. The primary abnormality is increased intestinal absorption of calcium or increased bone reabsorption.

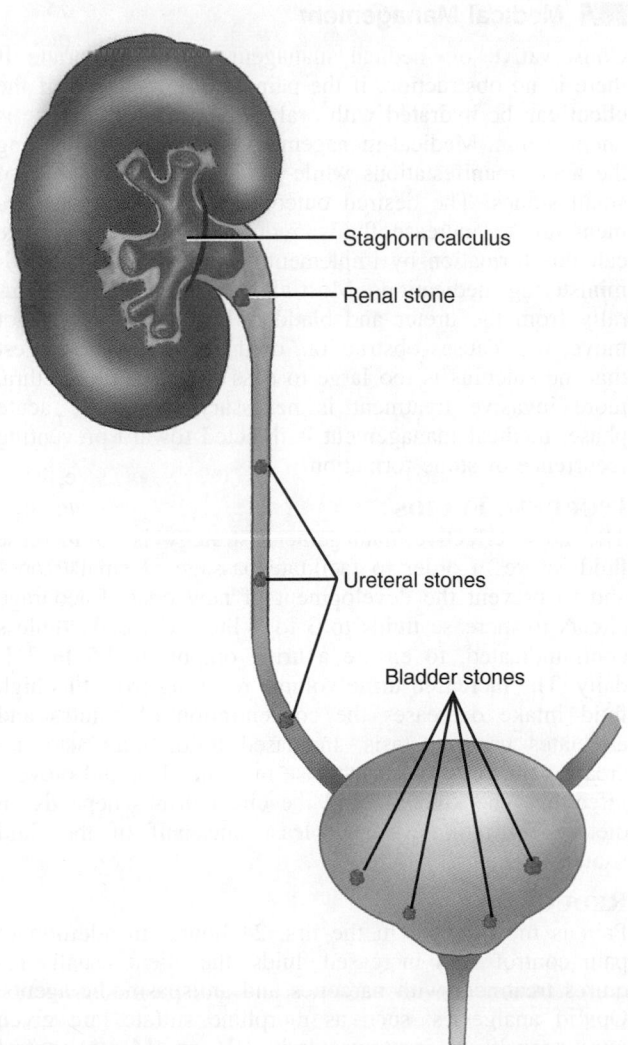

FIGURE 34–5 Staghorn calculus (stone) and other locations of calculi in the urinary tract.

The resulting higher serum calcium level triggers increased renal filtration of calcium and parathyroid hormone (PTH) suppression. This in turn decreases tubular reabsorption, thereby increasing the concentration of calcium in the urine.

2. "Renal leak" of calcium, the other abnormality, is caused by a tubular defect. The resulting hypocalcemia stimulates PTH production, which increases intestinal absorption of calcium. This cycle fits into the previous one, causing an increased solute load of calcium. Clients with this problem are often called "calcium wasters."

Oxalate

The second most frequent stone is oxalate, which is relatively insoluble in urine. Its solubility is affected only slightly by changes in urinary pH. The mechanism of oxalate availability is unclear but may be closely related to diet. The disease is most common in areas where cereals are a major dietary component and least common in dairy-farming regions.

An increased incidence of oxalate stones may be related to:

• Hyperabsorption of oxalate, seen with inflammatory bowel disease
• Postileal resection or small-bowel bypass surgery
• Overdose of ascorbic acid (vitamin C), which metabolizes to oxalate
• Familial oxaluria (oxalate in the urine)
• Concurrent fat malabsorption, which may cause calcium binding, thus freeing oxalate for absorption

Struvite

Struvite stones, also called triple phosphate, are composed of carbonate apatite and magnesium ammonium phosphate. Their cause is certain bacteria, usually *Proteus*, which contain the enzyme urease. This enzyme splits urea into two ammonia molecules, which raises the urine pH. Phosphate precipitates in alkaline urine. This action is responsible for the label "urea-splitter" characterizing these organisms.

Stones formed in this manner are staghorn calculi (see Fig. 34–5). Abscess formation is common. Struvite stones are difficult to eliminate because the hard stone forms around a nucleus of bacteria, protecting them from antibiotic therapy. Any small fragment left after surgical removal of the stone begins the cycle again.

Uric Acid

Uric acid stones are caused by increased urate excretion, fluid depletion, and a low urinary pH. *Hyperuricuria* is the result of either increased uric acid production or the administration of uricosuric agents. Approximately 25% of people with primary gout and about 50% of persons with secondary gout develop uric acid stones. A high dietary intake of food rich in *purine* (a protein) may predispose clients to uric acid stone formation. Also, treating neoplastic disease with agents that cause rapid cell destruction may increase the urinary uric acid concentration. Moreover, a link between hyperuricuria and calcium stone formation may exist. It is hypothesized that uric acid crystals absorb some of the crystal inhibitors normally found in urine.

Cystine

Cystinuria is the result of a congenital metabolic error inherited as an autosomal recessive disorder. Cystine stones typically appear during childhood and adolescence; development in adults is very rare.

Xanthine

Xanthine stones occur as a result of a rare hereditary condition in which there is a xanthine oxidase deficiency. This crystal precipitates readily in acid urine.

SUMMARY

Despite the type of stone that forms, the potential damage is essentially the same: (1) pain, spasm, or colic from peristalsis movements of the ureter contracting on the stone; (2) obstruction with possible hydronephrosis or hydroureter; (3) tissue trauma with secondary hemorrhage; and (4) infection.

Clinical Manifestations

The most characteristic manifestation of renal or ureteral calculi is a sharp, severe pain of sudden onset caused by movement of the calculus and consequent irritation. Depending on the site of the stone, this pain may be either *renal colic* or *ureteral colic*. Renal colic originates deep in the lumbar region and radiates around the side and down toward the testicle in the male and the bladder in the female. Ureteral colic radiates toward the genitalia and thigh.

When the pain is severe, the client usually has nausea, vomiting, pallor, grunting respirations, elevated blood pressure and pulse, diaphoresis, and anxiety. Visceral pain such as renal colic is mediated by the autonomic nervous system via celiac ganglia, which causes nausea, vomiting, decreased intestinal motility, and possibly paralytic ileus. Some people, especially those with bladder stones, experience manifestations of urgency, frequency, hematuria, and chronic cystitis. Pressure against the bladder neck during micturition (voiding) may cause a heavy feeling in the suprapubic region, obstruction in voiding, a decreased bladder capacity, and an intermittent urinary stream. If the stone enters the urethra, urine flow will be obstructed. The pain lasts for minutes to days and can be somewhat resistant to narcotic intervention.

Pain may be intermittent, which usually means that the stone has moved. Physicians hypothesize that the ureter dilates just proximal to the calculus, which allows urine to pass, relieving the ureteral distention. Then, as the stone moves into a new obstruction site, the pain returns. The pain subsides when the stone reaches the bladder.

Pain caused by renal stones is not always severe and colicky. It may be dull or aching or may be experienced as a heavy feeling. This is particularly true during the early stages of hydronephrosis. Sometimes, there may be no sensation, and the first clue the client has is seeing blood in the urine or hearing a "clink" against the toilet when the stone passes.

Other manifestations of calculi include infection with an elevated temperature and white blood cell (WBC) count and urine obstruction that causes hydroureter, hydronephrosis, or both. A flat plate of the abdomen and an x-ray study of the kidney, ureter and bladder (commonly called a KUB) are the standard diagnostic tools. These studies should reveal radiopaque stones and aid in the evaluation of stone size.

Determining the size of the calculus is essential in selecting the treatment. Stones smaller than 4 or 5 mm can pass without intervention. Because some stones, such as uric acid stones, are not radiopaque and not visible on x-ray, it is crucial to note when a client presents with manifestations of calculi. Elevated serum uric acid levels may confirm a suspicion of urinary calculi. In addition, an IVP may show a filling defect at the site of the stone or ultrasonography may reveal the stone. Diagnosis of a bladder stone is confirmed by direct visualization through cystoscopy. Once the stone is retrieved, its components must be analyzed.

Additional studies of blood and urine may be required to determine whether metabolic problems predispose the client to stone formation. Other possible disease processes, such as metastatic bone cancer, must be ruled out as possible causes of calculi.

Outcome Management

Medical Management

Conservative or medical management is appropriate if there is no obstruction, if the pain can be managed, if the client can be hydrated with oral fluids, and if the stone is under 5 mm. Medical management is directed at relieving the acute manifestations while facilitating the passage of small stones. The desired outcomes of medical management are to increase fluids, reduce pain, and minimize calculus formation by implementing diet changes and administering medications. Most clients pass the stone naturally from the ureter and bladder. If the stone does not move, if it causes obstruction, or if x-ray studies suggest that the calculus is too large to pass safely to the urethra, more invasive treatment is necessary. After the acute phase, medical management is directed toward preventing recurrence of stone formation.

INCREASE FLUIDS

The most effective management strategy is to increase fluid intake in order to facilitate passage of small stones and to prevent the development of new ones. Encourage clients to increase fluids to 3 to 4 liters (L) daily, unless contraindicated, to ensure a urine output of 2.5 to 3 L daily. The increased urine volume resulting from this high fluid intake decreases the concentration of solutes and alleviates urinary stasis. Increased fluids may also decrease pain, prevent an increase in stone size, and prevent infection. The kind of fluid the client drinks depends on dietary restrictions, but at least one half of the fluid should be water.

REDUCE PAIN

Pain is most severe in the first 24 hours. In addition to pain control with increased fluids, the client usually requires treatment with narcotics and antispasmodic agents. Opioid analgesics, such as morphine sulfate, are given intravenously or intramuscularly (IV or IM) to control moderate to severe pain. Nonsteroidal anti-inflammatory drugs (NSAIDs) may also be effective.

Antispasmodic agents, such as oxybutynin chloride (Ditropan), are very effective for relieving and controlling colic pain associated with spasms of the ureter. Clients with repeated stone formation may have a family member drive them to a clinic, ambulatory care center, or emergency department for administration of opioid analgesics and antispasmodic agents so that they can relax, go home, and pass the stone naturally. Other clients may require admission to an acute care setting for administration of these medications. For nausea and vomiting associated with colic, antiemetics may also be necessary.

PREVENT STONE RECURRENCE
Diet modifications and medications may be required to prevent further calculus formation in clients who return with repeated stones. Increased fluid intake is still the primary prevention measure. Results of a stone analysis are essential before these recommendations are implemented.

IMPLEMENT DIETARY CHANGES. Some controversy exists over dietary restrictions because of their uncertain effectiveness and the problems clients experience in following the regimen. Calcium stones and hypercalciuria may be controlled by limiting excessive calcium intake, although it should be maintained at about 800 mg daily.

Clients with oxalate stones should avoid high-oxalate foods, such as tea, tomatoes, instant coffee, cola drinks, beer, rhubarb, green beans, asparagus, spinach, cabbage, celery, chocolate, citrus fruits, apples, grapes, cranberries, peanuts, and peanut butter. Megadoses of vitamin C increase oxalate excretion in the urine and should be avoided. If the stone is composed of uric acid, the client should follow a low-purine diet, which involves limiting such foods as aged cheeses, wine, bony fish, and organ meats.

ADMINISTER MEDICATIONS. Following recurrent stone formation, analysis of the stone, or abnormal metabolic findings, medications may be required. For hypercalciuric clients, a thiazide diuretic such as hydrochlorothiazide (HydroDIURIL) will promote calcium resorption from the renal tubules, thereby preventing excess calcium loads in the urine. Potassium citrate is commonly added to the thiazide diuretic to replace potassium as needed.

For low urine citrate levels, potassium or sodium citrate may be ordered. Since these medications can be expensive, many urologists encourage the client to drink a quart of lemonade for both the increased fluid and citrate benefits.

Calcium oxalate stones may be treated with vitamin B_6 (pyridoxine), magnesium oxide, or cholestyramine. For clients with hyperuricosuria and calcium oxalate stones, allopurinol (Zyloprim) is prescribed only if a reduced purine diet fails and stones persist.

Uric acid stones are treated with drugs to lower uric acid, such as allopurinol. In addition, sodium bicarbonate or citrate may be indicated to raise urinary pH because uric acid stones form in acidic urine. This treatment is also effective for xanthine stones, which are inhibited in alkaline urine. Cystine stones are treated with tiopronin (Thiola) and d-penicillamine, which make cystine more soluble for excretion. Long-term antibiotics are used to control the infection that leads to struvite stone formation.

Nursing Management of the Medical Client
ASSESSMENT
Ask the client about any family history of calculi, previous UTIs, immobility, and recent dietary habits. For instance, a large intake of purines may be significant, as would drinking a large amount of fruit juice or tea, which could cause oxalate precipitation. Also assess the amount, pattern, and types of fluids consumed.

Assess the client for the clinical manifestations described earlier. Use rating scales to measure the severity of pain. Many clients describe renal or ureteral colic as "the worst pain I've ever had." Vital signs should be monitored. A decreasing blood pressure may indicate severe pain and impending shock; increased pulse and temperature may result from infection. A sudden onset of little or no urine output suggests obstruction, which is an emergency that must be treated immediately to preserve kidney function. Frequency and dysuria commonly occur when a stone reaches the bladder.

All urine voided should be strained through several layers of gauze or through a commercial urine strainer. Carefully examine all debris caught by straining. Save any stone material so that the stone's composition can be analyzed as a basis for treatment and to show how much has passed through the urinary tract. A routine urinalysis, urine for culture and sensitivity testing, and a 24-hour urine specimen may be needed.

DIAGNOSIS, OUTCOMES, INTERVENTIONS
Pain. The priority nursing diagnosis is *Pain related to irritation and spasm from stone movement in the urinary tract.*

Outcomes. The client will report pain relief or control.

Interventions. During the acute phase of treatment, offer pain medications, antispasmodics, and antiemetics, if necessary. For severe pain, give the medications on a regular schedule. Use a rating scale to help evaluate the client's pain.

Once pain is controlled, the client will be able to force fluids and ambulate, which will facilitate passage of the stone. Relaxation techniques, such as guided imagery or therapeutic or healing touch, can help to relieve pain. Help the client find a comfortable position to alternate with ambulation.

Effective Management of Therapeutic Regimen. More than half of clients with a urinary calculus experience another within 5 years. As a result, an important nursing diagnosis is *Effective Management of Therapeutic Regimen related to prevention of recurrent calculi.*

Outcomes. The number of recurrences will be reduced, and the interval between stones will increase.

Interventions
Increase Fluids. Teach the client to drink 3 to 4 L of fluid daily to flush the urinary system. At least half the fluid consumed should be water. Intake should be as consistent as possible throughout the 24-hour period.

As a rule, encourage the client to drink a full glass of water every hour during the day and two large glasses just before going to bed. This schedule will probably create the need to void during the night, at which time the client should drink another glass of water.

Teach Stone Prevention Measures. Besides increased fluid intake, teach the client other measures to prevent stone recurrence, such as diet modifications, medications if required, and avoidance of urinary stasis (see Client Education Guide). Prompt treatment of urinary tract infections and early recognition of manifestations of stone recurrence are also important.

Health promotion activities include frequent turning and range of motion for immobilized clients, increased fluid intake, and decreased intake of stone-forming solutes in the diet, such as oxalates, purines, and animal proteins. Health maintenance interventions include monitoring high-risk clients with indwelling catheters or obstructions for calculi.

EVALUATION

If medical management is successful, the client's pain will be controlled, the stone will pass unaided, and the client will have no complications of obstruction or infection. The client will be able to describe factors that increase the risk of developing stones and will be able to identify self-care strategies to prevent stone recurrence.

■ Surgical Management

About 20% of stones require additional treatment with shock wave lithotripsy or endourologic or surgical proce-

---

CLIENT EDUCATION GUIDE

Preventing Recurrence of Urinary Stones

Increase your fluid intake to at least 3 L (3 qt) every day.
Be sure to urinate at least every 2 hours.
Remember the early manifestations of urinary stones. If the symptoms occur again, see your physician promptly.
Monitor the pH of your urine with pH paper. If you had calcium stones, keep your urine acidic. If you had uric acid stones, keep your urine basic. Keep urine acidic with high-protein diet. Keep urine basic with a low-protein diet, plenty of vegetables, and citrus fruits.
Be sure to follow your physician's instructions for follow-up urinalysis and blood tests to detect factors that can cause urinary stones.
If manifestations of urinary tract infection develop, see your physician promptly for diagnosis and treatment. Manifestations include pain and burning when you urinate, a sense of urgency to urinate, having to urinate frequently, and a fever.

Stones Other than Uric Acid Stones

Follow your physician's instructions for keeping your urine acidic.

Calcium Stones

Follow an 800-mg calcium diet.

Uric Acid Stones

Follow a low-purine diet.
Take the medications, such as allopurinol (Zyloprim), prescribed to improve your excretion of uric acid.

---

dures. Open surgery is used only for the small percentage of clients who cannot be successfully treated with lithotripsy or endourologic procedures.

ENDOUROLOGIC PROCEDURES

Depending on the position of the calculus, cystoscopy may be done. Small stones may be removed transurethrally with a cystoscope, ureteroscope, or ureterorenoscope. Additionally, one or two ureteral catheters or stents may be inserted past the stone. From this point, several different interventions are appropriate. The catheters may be left in place for 24 hours or longer to drain urine trapped proximal to the stone and to dilate the ureter, which may prompt spontaneous movement of the calculus. Otherwise, the catheter may mechanically guide the stone downward as it is removed.

At times, a continuous chemical irrigation may be used to dissolve uric acid, struvite, and cystine stones. Finally, an attempt may be made to manipulate or dislodge the stone with a variety of special catheters with loops and expanding baskets used to snare the stone. Care of these clients is the same as that following cystoscopy.

Larger stones may be crushed with an instrument called a *lithotrite* (stone crusher) to facilitate removal. *Cystolitholapaxy* is performed when a bladder stone is soft enough to be crushed. In cystoscopic lithotripsy, an ultrasonic lithotrite is placed to pulverize the stone, followed by extensive flushing of the bladder. Possible complications associated with this procedure include hemorrhage, urinary retention, infection, bladder perforation, and possibly retained stone fragments.

A flexible ureteroscope, passed through a cystoscope, is used to collect stones in the ureter. This procedure, called *ureteroscopy*, is used to retrieve 4- to 5-mm stones or, combined with ultrasonic lithotripsy, to remove fragments after treatment. Minimal sedation or anesthesia is necessary, and postoperative complications are usually few.

A flexible ureterorenoscope can be passed for access to the entire upper urinary tract, including the distal ureter and intrarenal collecting system so that stones or lesions in the lower pole or lateral calices can be reached.

A nephroscope may be inserted to retrieve free-lying renal stones. Figure 34–6A shows a nephroscope in place. The stone may be removed with alligator forceps or a stone basket followed by irrigation. Electrohydraulic, laser, or ultrasound lithotripsy may be completed through the nephroscope. After this procedure, a nephrostomy tube remains in place for 1 to 5 days. The client can go home with it in place. Increased fluids are essential to achieve a urine output greater than 3000 ml (3 L). The tube is removed after diagnostic studies determine that all stone fragments have been removed.

LITHOTRIPSY

LASER LITHOTRIPSY. A newer treatment for calculi is laser lithotripsy. Lasers are used together with a ureteroscope to remove or loosen impacted stones. Constant water irrigation of the ureter is required to dissipate the heat. Complications resulting from this procedure are the same as those of any endourologic procedure.

EXTRACORPOREAL SHOCK WAVE LITHOTRIPSY. *Extracorporeal shock wave lithotripsy* (ESWL) is the use of sound waves applied externally to break up stones in

NEPHROSCOPIC REMOVAL

Alligator forceps

Kidney stone fragments

A

B **PYELOLITHOTOMY**

Stone in renal pelvis

C **NEPHROLITHOTOMY**

Stone in renal calyx

FIGURE 34–6 *A–C,* Surgical techniques for removal of kidney stones.

the kidney or ureter (Fig. 34–7). High-energy shock waves, aimed by fluoroscopy, are transmitted to the stone. The shock waves break the stones into small fragments, which are passed or retrieved endoscopically. The client may be strapped to a frame in a water bath or secured on a table, depending on the type of lithotripsy equipment selected or available. The client is usually sedated with regional or general anesthesia.

The procedure lasts 30 to 50 minutes with administration of 500 to 1500 shock waves. Cardiac monitoring is required to synchronize shock waves with the R wave to prevent cardiac dysrhythmias. Complications of ESWL include ecchymosis on the affected flank, retained fragments, urosepsis, perinephric hematoma, and hemorrhage.

Stone fragments may bunch up in the distal ureter, obstructing the kidney. To prevent this accumulation and obstruction, a double J stent is commonly placed via cystoscopy before ESWL for stones larger than 6 mm. The stent is removed during a follow-up visit.

After ESWL, the client may experience renal or ureteral colic that needs to be treated with antispasmodics. Early ambulation and increased fluid intake are important for flushing out stone fragments. The fragments may be passed for up to 3 months after the procedure.

Fractured kidney stone

Electrode

Reflector

FIGURE 34–7 Water bath extracorporeal shock wave lithotripsy. Electrically generated shock waves fracture kidney stones.

PERCUTANEOUS LITHOTRIPSY. Percutaneous lithotripsy involves the insertion of a guide percutaneously (through the skin) under fluoroscopy near the area of the stone. An ultrasonic wave is aimed at the stone to break it into fragments.

OPEN SURGICAL PROCEDURES

If the stone is too large or if endourologic and lithotripsy procedures fail to remove it, an open surgical procedure is performed. Surgery is rarely needed because of the success of modern, less invasive options.

A *ureterolithotomy* is the surgical removal of a stone from the ureter through a flank incision for higher stones or an abdominal incision for lower ones. A Penrose drain and ureteral catheter are usually placed postoperatively for healing and drainage of urine.

Cystolithotomy, removal of bladder calculi through a suprapubic incision, is used only when stones cannot be crushed and removed transurethrally. Stricture (abnormal narrowing) is the most common postoperative complication. A stone is removed from the renal pelvis by *pyelolithotomy* and from the renal calyx by a *nephrolithotomy*. Figure 34–6B and C illustrates these procedures.

Rarely, a partial or total *nephrectomy* (see Chapter 35) is necessary because of extensive kidney damage, overwhelming renal infection, or abnormal renal parenchyma, which can be responsible for stone formation.

◼ Nursing Management of the Surgical Client

ASSESSMENT

Preoperative assessment includes the general condition of the client, including the presence of conditions that may present problems postoperatively. It is a priority to assess the client's understanding of the condition and the procedure to be performed. Other assessments are similar to those described under Nursing Management of the Medical Client.

DIAGNOSIS, OUTCOMES, INTERVENTIONS

Risk for Injury. With any endourologic procedure, lithotripsy, or surgery, the client has a *Risk for Injury related to postoperative complications.*

Outcomes. The client will remain free from injury, as evidenced by absence of hemorrhage, by vital signs within preoperative limits, by normal WBC count and temperature, and by a total urine output of at least ½ ml/kg/hr from all sources.

Interventions

Increase Fluids. Increase the client's IV or oral fluids to 3 to 4 L daily as described earlier, unless contraindicated.

Monitor Urine Output. Maintain the client's urine output at ½ ml/kg/hr or more. Assess any indications of hemorrhage, stone retention, urinary retention, or infection. As needed, irrigate the client's bladder to wash out possible stone fragments. See Chapter 38 for discussion of continuous bladder irrigation (CBI). Continue to strain all urine.

Nursing care after a ureterolithotomy may involve care of a ureteral catheter. Output of at least ¼ ml/kg/hr from the ureteral catheter should be expected and closely monitored. Because the renal pelvis holds only 5 ml, ureteral catheters must be kept patent (open) and are never clamped. Institute prompt intervention with any unexpected reduction in urine flow. Several conditions—such as mucus shreds, blood clots, and chemical sediment—can interfere with the flow of urine through these catheters. Plus, ureteral peristalsis occasionally pushes the catheters out of the ureter into the bladder.

Closely monitor the catheter output. Each ureteral, suprapubic, and urethral catheter should drain into its own collection bag so that the source of the reduced urine flow is noticed immediately. Each tube or bag should be labeled. Measure and record the output of each catheter every hour for the first 24 hours. Output from each catheter should be monitored every 4 to 8 hours until removal. Most of the urine will drain from the ureteral catheters for the first 48 to 72 hours postoperatively. As the inflammation decreases, urine flows around ureteral catheters and is drained by the urethral or suprapubic catheters. Report a total urine output of less than ½ ml/kg/hr or a lack of output from ureteral catheters for more than 15 minutes to the physician immediately.

If the physician orders ureteral catheter irrigation, use strict sterile technique. A maximum of 3 to 5 ml of irrigating solution, usually sterile saline solution, should be allowed to flow in by gravity. Very gentle force should be used. If you cannot confirm patency, notify the physician immediately. Use extreme care to ensure that the catheter is not dislodged. If it is not sutured in place, secure it carefully to the client's skin with tape.

Drainage from a nephrostomy tube should also be carefully monitored and cared for with interventions similar to those used for ureteral catheters. Irrigation amounts, if ordered, are no more than 3 to 5 ml. Because the tube goes directly into the kidney, maintain sterile technique to prevent infection.

Clients with any type of catheter must be taught how to care for them before returning home. They should learn how to clean around them, empty them, prevent kinking, and irrigate them if necessary. A home health nurse may be required to assist with these activities.

Prevent Complications. If a the client has a flank incision, care is similar to that needed after nephrectomy (see Chapter 35). To prevent pneumonia, the client will need to cough and deep breathe 10 to 20 times each hour. To facilitate this, administer opioid narcotics regularly to control incisional pain. Other postoperative interventions are similar to those for a client with any major abdominal incision, such as monitoring bowel sounds, vital signs, and output from drains and nasogastric tube. Antibiotics may be given prophylactically or at the first sign of infection.

EVALUATION

It is expected that surgical intervention for stone removal is completed with the least invasive procedure possible and before renal damage occurs. In most instances the client can go home the day of the procedure and does not need to be hospitalized. Clients may go home with catheters in place for about a week and will need to learn catheter care or have home health follow-up. For major surgical intervention, the client is dismissed 3 to 4 days after the procedure.

Self-Care

A client with urolithiasis is at risk for recurrence. You have a major role in helping the client develop and maintain an effective, individual regimen to prevent stone recurrence. The main components of prevention are (1) increased fluids, (2) dietary modifications, (3) medications as ordered, and (4) prompt treatment of UTIs. The client must understand that these are lifelong changes in lifestyle. If catheters are in place after surgical intervention, client management of the tubes is necessary before discharge from the hospital.

URINARY REFLUX

Urinary reflux is the backward flow of urine in the urinary tract. It usually begins at the vesicoureteral junction. Urine flows back into the ureter and upward into the renal pelvis. The severity of vesicoureteral reflux is stated as grade I, which is least severe, through grade V, which is most severe. There is an increase in the development of reflux in men over 50 years of age because of chronic bladder neck obstruction from BPH. Reflux typically occurs in younger children or in young adults from congenital abnormalities of the vesicoureteral junction.

Etiology and Risk Factors

Reflux can be caused by a congenital abnormality, such as ectopic ureter, chronic bladder infections secondary to dysfunctional bladder, or outlet obstruction in the bladder neck. Urinary reflux is more frequently seen as a result of another condition. Reflux contributes to the increase of intravesical pressure (within the bladder) until it finally overwhelms the resistance of the intramural ureteral sphincters, allowing reflux to occur. Clients with obstructions must be evaluated to have the cause identified and treated to prevent and relieve intravesical pressure.

Pathophysiology

In bladder outlet obstruction, the main result is the continuous presence of residual urine, which leads to chronic UTIs. Continual overdistention of the bladder can also decrease detrusor tone, increasing the bladder's capacity and raising the threshold needed to start the micturition reflex.

Renal damage and pyelonephritis are the two primary problems resulting from vesicoureteral reflux. Because the capacity of the renal pelvis is only 5 ml, larger amounts of urine can cause renal parenchymal changes, hydronephrosis, or hydronephroureterosis if they result from ureteral obstruction or reflux. The increased hydrostatic pressure leads to renal cortical atrophy from ischemia and hypoxia and then to calicectasis (dilation of the renal calices). The destruction of kidney tissue, often asymptomatic and undetected, can progress to end-stage renal disease. The kidneys are usually protected from ascending infections by the intramural portion of the distal ureter. With reflux, however, any pathogens in the bladder are carried through the ureters to the kidney. This problem leads to recurrent pyelonephritis. Chronic pyelonephritis leads to renal failure.

Clinical Manifestations

The major manifestation of reflux in the bladder neck is pyelonephritis. When the obstruction is in the vesicoureteral junction or higher, renal failure may be clinically evident. The major diagnostic studies are (1) the VCUG to visualize the lower urinary system during voiding, (2) cystoscopy to evaluate manifestations of obstruction, (3) ureteroscopy to assess the vesicoureteral junction, (4) ultrasound to assess for hydronephrosis, and (5) IVP to evaluate the entire collecting system. Blood studies of BUN and creatinine levels are also done to assess renal function.

Outcome Management

Surgical Management

Because there are no medical regimens to prevent or treat reflux caused by ectopic ureter, the primary therapy is surgical. Renal damage from the reflux usually calls for surgical intervention. Surgery is also indicated for obstruction at the ureteropelvic junction, for intractable infection, and for a problem not resolved by maturation. Because the most common causes of reflux are ureteral defects, surgical procedures focus on reimplantation or other treatments for the ureter.

Postoperatively, a urethral or suprapubic catheter keeps the bladder empty to reduce tension on the suture line. A ureteral catheter is also inserted into the ureter involved in the surgical procedure. The tip of this tiny, semi-rigid catheter usually rests in the renal pelvis. The distal end extends through the bladder and out through the urethra or through an abdominal incision.

A ureteral catheter provides three benefits: it splints the ureter to facilitate healing, it prevents obstruction from edema after surgery or other trauma in the area, and it drains urine.

Nursing Management of the Surgical Client

Carefully assess any client with a high risk of obstruction for any manifestation of urinary reflux. The client being evaluated for urinary reflux requires support during this diagnostic process. Preoperative preparation for ureteral surgery is similar to that required by any client who needs surgery (see Chapter 15).

Postoperative care is similar to that discussed earlier for urinary calculi. Assess the color of the client's urine frequently. Expect it to progress from bright red to clear yellow over a matter of days. Discharge teaching depends on a variety of factors, including the cause of the reflux, the treatment or procedure done, and the amount of renal damage present. For the client with kidney damage, renal function must be monitored at regular intervals to evaluate any changes in status.

VOIDING DISORDERS

URINARY RETENTION

Urinary retention is the inability of the bladder to empty partially or completely during voiding. Treatment is directed at relieving the cause of the problem.

Etiology and Risk Factors

Detrusor failure is the most common cause of urinary retention in women. Failure of the bladder to contract, demonstrated on urodynamic evaluation, is often associated with neurologic conditions. In men, obstructive voiding due to an enlarged prostate is the frequent cause of retention. Other disorders, urethral strictures, medications, detrusor-sphincter dyssynergia, calculi, blood clots, tumors, bladder neck contractures and history of female genital mutilation may also cause retention. Neuropathies affecting bladder function include diabetes, strokes, and spinal cord injuries. These long-term problems affect the neurologic status of the bladder and interfere with the micturition reflex. Remember, urinary retention is a manifestation of another pathologic condition.

Retention may be caused by decreased sensory input to and from the bladder, muscle tension, anxiety, or other neurologic conditions affecting the bladder. Surgery has traditionally been a factor; spinal anesthesia causes retention more often than general anesthesia does. After surgery, 10% to 15% of clients who received general anesthesia require catheterization because of an inability to void, and 20% to 25% of those who received spinal anesthesia require a catheter.

In women, prolapse of the back wall of the vagina (rectocele or enterocele) increases the risk of retention by exerting pressure against the urethra. Also, a large cystocele may cause kinking of the bladder neck, decreasing the bladder's ability to empty.

More than half of men older than age 50 experience BPH, a common cause of retention. This is not a preventable problem, although the client with an enlarged prostate should be monitored closely for obstruction secondary to the enlargement. Neurologic injury or disease, such as diabetes mellitus, spinal cord injuries, or multiple sclerosis, may lead to urinary retention as well. Other risk factors are a history of structural abnormalities and use of certain medications, such as tricyclic antidepressants. In some clients, a psychogenic origin may be found.

Pathophysiology

Retention of urine is hazardous because the resulting urinary stasis contributes to UTIs, stone formation, and eventual complications of long-term structural damage to the bladder, ureters, or kidneys. Additionally, continued bladder distention leads to loss of bladder tone.

The pathologic process of retention produces a snowball effect. Retained urine increases hydrostatic pressure against the bladder wall, which results in hypertrophy of the detrusor muscle, formation of trabeculae (connective tissue in the bladder wall), or development of diverticula. At the same time, peristalsis in the ureteral musculature increases against the pressure of the accumulating urine. The ureter may gradually become elongated, tortuous, and fibrotic. Increasing pressure is also transmitted through the renal pelvis and calices into the renal parenchyma. The resulting hydronephrosis exerts pressure on the blood vessels, causing ischemia and increasing the renal damage. If the process is not interrupted, it can proceed to renal failure and death. Figure 34-8 demonstrates the sequence. Even after the retention is relieved, when the

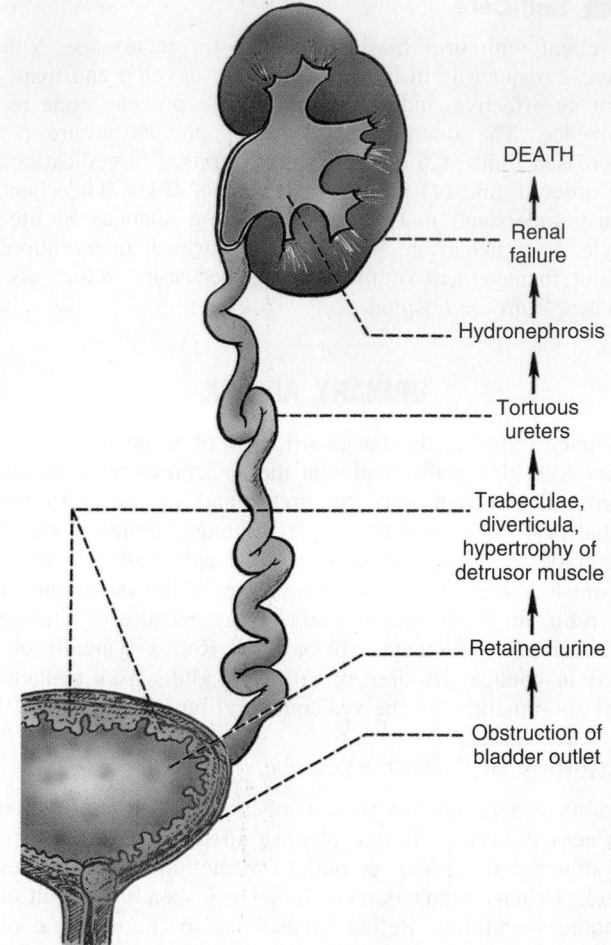

FIGURE 34–8 Potential effects of urinary tract obstruction.

alterations caused by increased pressure reach the renal parenchyma, the damage may be permanent and irreversible.

Medications, such as opiates, tricyclic antidepressants, sedatives, antispasmodics, anti-Parkinson drugs, beta-adrenergic blockers, and psychotropic agents, can interfere with normal neurologic function and the micturition reflex. Diseases with neurologic effects, such as stroke, multiple sclerosis, diabetes mellitus, tabes dorsalis, and spinal cord lesions, also disrupt the micturition reflex.

Urinary retention may result in chronic UTI or a series of UTIs and dysfunctional voiding. Conversely, chronic UTIs and dysfunctional voiding may result in urinary retention. The detrusor muscle may become irritated and fail to function correctly, leading to incomplete bladder emptying. Irritation and scarring of the bladder neck or urethra may develop, thus placing these clients at greater risk for urinary retention.

A disorder of psychogenic origin, such as anxiety or fear of voiding in a public restroom, may lead to distention of the bladder and urinary retention. Inability to relax the urethra because of anxiety or neurologic deficit may lead to urinary retention as well.

Anorectal problems, such as hemorrhoids, abscess, fecal impaction, and vaginal prolapse, can be contributing factors, either from obstruction or from secondary spasms of the perineal musculature that interfere with the urethra during voiding.

Decreased oral or IV fluid intake reduces the glomerular filtration rate (GFR). This causes very slow urine production and overfilling of the bladder. The slow increase allows the detrusor muscle to accommodate the increased volume until the muscle's fibers are stretched beyond their ability to contract, hampering micturition.

Urinary retention with overflow incontinence results from the following events. As the bladder continues filling, the intravesical pressure rises. Eventually, this pressure overcomes the resistance of the sphincter. Urine flows out of the bladder until it reduces the intravesical pressure, but only to the level at which the external sphincter can again control the flow of urine. Most clients report that the bladder does not feel empty. It overfills again, and the cycle is repeated.

Prolonged obstruction leads to increased pressures in the urinary tract and may predispose the client to bladder diverticula. A *diverticulum* is a pouch or sac resulting from the herniation of the mucous membrane lining caused by weakness in the muscular wall of an organ. Bladder diverticula are most common in men. Many diverticula are asymptomatic and are usually discovered by chance during assessment of other conditions.

Bladder diverticula can cause two major problems: (1) UTIs, resulting from stasis of urine, and (2) malignancies, probably a result of chronic irritation by persistent infection. Intervention involves removing the obstruction and relieving the retention, followed by surgical excision of the pouch and reestablishment of normal patency of the urinary tract. Postoperatively, catheter drainage of urine is required to allow complete tissue healing. Clients who have had chronic or recurring infections usually require long-term antibiotic therapy after surgery.

Clinical Manifestations

The primary manifestation of urinary retention is a distended bladder or an inability to empty the bladder completely. Voided amounts of 25 to 50 ml one or more times an hour may indicate retention with overflow. The major diagnostic test is catheterization. A post-void residual amount greater than 100 ml after an attempt to void signals retention. Other diagnostic measures, such as cystoscopy and urodynamic testing to include pressure voiding studies, help to identify the cause of the retention.

Outcome Management

■ Medical Management

Identifying the cause of urinary retention is the first step in determining treatment. Finding the underlying neurologic problem or obstructive disorder is crucial in selecting a treatment plan.

ADMINISTER MEDICATIONS

In some cases, cholinergic medications have been known to help stimulate bladder contractions. If a mechanical obstruction is present, however, cholinergic drug therapy should not be used. In this instance, intravesical pressure increases against an obstructed outlet, causing ureterovesical reflux or a ruptured bladder.

Although their effects are somewhat controversial, bethanechol (Urecholine) and neostigmine (Prostigmin) are commonly given. Bethanechol improves detrusor tone but also increases bladder outlet and urethral resistance. To counteract this, bethanechol is sometimes combined with phenoxybenzamine (Dibenzyline), prazosin (Minipress), and terazosin (Hytrin), which are potent alpha-adrenergic blockers.

URETHRAL DILATIONS

In some instances, urinary retention is relieved by dilation of the urethra by means of the placement of progressively larger urethral sounds. Local or sometimes general anesthesia is used.

■ Nursing Management of the Medical Client

Interventions described next are appropriate for the nursing diagnosis *Urinary Retention.*

ASSESS URINE OUTPUT PATTERNS

It is important to distinguish retention from *oliguria* (diminished urinary secretion) and *anuria* (complete suppression of urinary secretion). In urinary retention, the kidneys are producing a normal amount of urine but the bladder does not function properly. It fills with urine and rises above the level of the pubic symphysis, sometimes being displaced to either side of midline. Percussion over the bladder produces a dull sound. The client may experience increasing discomfort and the need to urinate. The client also may complain of restlessness, sweating, anxiety, bladder pain, and feelings of bladder fullness.

IMPLEMENT MEASURES TO STIMULATE INDEPENDENT VOIDING

Nursing interventions may be used initially to treat retention. Provide privacy, and place the client in a normal sitting or standing position, using gravity and increased intra-abdominal pressure to help relieve an acute problem. Running the water or flushing the toilet within earshot of the client may encourage voiding. Tape-recorded aquatic sounds may be effective. A warm bath or pouring warm water over the perineum often promotes muscle relaxation. Immersing the client's hands in water sometimes works. Applying ice or gently stroking the inner thigh sometimes works as well. These measures may stimulate trigger points of the micturition reflex. If the client is tense and anxious, any measure that induces relaxation may aid in relieving the situation, even a back rub or soothing music.

CATHETERIZE THE CLIENT

For clients with persistent urinary retention, a straight or retention catheter may be inserted through the external meatus, into the urethra beyond the internal sphincter, and into the bladder. A straight catheter is removed after the bladder drains. An indwelling (Foley) catheter is kept in place for continuous or intermittent drainage by inflating a balloon near the catheter's tip. Strict sterile techniques are used for insertion except for clients on an intermittent self-catheterization program; these clients may use clean technique.

The indwelling catheter is attached to either a bedside drainage bag or a leg bag. A leg bag is commonly used for long-term catheterization, especially for a client going home with the catheter in place. This device allows the client more mobility and eliminates the embarrassment of carrying a drainage bag in public view (Fig. 34–9).

Because of the bag's small capacity, it must be emptied frequently. A conventional drainage system is used at night to avoid the need to empty the bag at night. Instruct the client to avoid attaching the rubber straps too tightly, because doing so may cause skin irritation, thrombophlebitis, and ulcer formation. Loose straps tend to tighten as the bag fills. Recent improvements have lead to the use of nylon self-fastening tape (Velcro) leg straps for clients with circulatory problems, latex allergy, and at high risk for skin breakdown. Meticulous skin care and periodic removal of the bag help prevent these problems. Cleanliness and odor control are managed by washing the apparatus with soap and water and soaking the bag in a 1% acetic acid (white vinegar) solution overnight.

PREVENT INFECTION

Prolonged use of an indwelling catheter increases the risk of UTI and tissue trauma. More than 80% of people who develop nosocomial (hospital-acquired) UTIs have undergone urologic instrumentation. Bacteriuria increases in direct relationship to duration of catheter placement; estimates of infection rates range from 4% (within 24 hours) to 95% (within 4 weeks). Organisms enter the catheter through any contamination or break in the system or intrude via the thin layer of fluid and exudate that forms around the outside of the catheter.

Catheter insertion should be avoided unless necessary to monitor urine output. Wash your hands thoroughly before and after handling a catheter or drainage system. In addition:

1. Maintain a closed drainage system.
2. Avoid backflow of urine.
3. Avoid unnecessary manipulation of the catheter during perineal cleaning.

FIGURE 34–9 Condom drainage and leg bag. The bag may be attached to the calf of the leg, as shown, or to the thigh.

4. Prevent microbial invasion and colonization in the urine collection bag.
5. Maintain patency of the catheter.
6. Encourage a high fluid intake.

On occasion, prophylactic antibiotics are given to clients with catheters in place. The practice is not routine, however, because of the threat of resistant organisms and possible adverse reactions.

PREVENT TISSUE INJURY

Tissue trauma may occur during catheterization. Tissue irritation or necrosis may result from:

- Using an oversized catheter
- Continuous pressure and pulling of the catheter between the meatus and the site of taping on the leg or abdomen
- Friction caused by the continuous movement of the catheter, causing tissue breakdown and enhancing encrustation on the outside of the catheter
- Local or systemic allergic reactions to rubber in clients with a history of latex allergy; silicone catheters are available for these clients

The subject of bladder decompression drainage is still misunderstood. In the past, it was incorrectly assumed that rapid emptying of a distended bladder through a catheter could result in bladder hemorrhage and hypotension. Consequently, the catheter was clamped after 1000 ml of urine had been drained, reopened after an hour to drain another 1000 ml, and clamped and reopened again until the bladder was decompressed. Cystometric studies have shown that this problem does not occur with retention. It is now thought that any amount of urine can be drained.[49] Drainage does not occur rapidly, because the usual size of a catheter does not allow rapid drainage.

■ Surgical Management

Surgical intervention is usually employed if a structural defect is found. Intervention may include (1) removal of an enlarged prostate gland or urethral stricture or (2) correction of a structural abnormality.

BLADDER NECK REPAIR

Surgical intervention is sometimes needed for obstructions below the bladder. If the bladder neck becomes rigid as a result of inflammation, cystoplasty may be done by insertion of an elastic wedge into the area. A transurethral incision of the bladder neck might also be done. Excision of urethral strictures, sometimes with a *urethroplasty* (plastic repair of the urethra), helps return proper functioning. Alternatively, a meatotomy may be performed to open the urethral meatus.

SUPRAPUBIC CYSTOTOMY

INDICATIONS. Suprapubic catheterization is sometimes used to relieve urinary retention. Placement of the catheter allows postoperative clients to begin a bladder training program. The catheter is placed when urethral catheterization is difficult, as in clients with a severely enlarged prostate, urethral strictures, or quadriplegia. Local anesthesia is used, although general anesthesia may be used if another surgical procedure is also performed. To facilitate proper placement of the catheter, the bladder must be distended with urine or water before insertion. If the bladder is insufficiently distended with urine, additional fluid is instilled through a catheter or cystoscope.

The suprapubic skin is prepared. Under sterile technique, the suprapubic catheter is inserted through a small surgical incision or by passing a trocar through the skin into the bladder. Once the trocar is in place, the pointed core of the cannula is removed. The catheter is threaded through the cannula and attached to a closed drainage system. The catheter is commonly sutured in place or secured with a commercially made retention seal. When the catheter is removed, the muscle layers of the bladder immediately contract over the puncture site and shrink the surface wound.

CONTRAINDICATIONS. Short-term catheter placement may be a possible contraindication.

COMPLICATIONS. Potential complications of a suprapubic catheter include dislodgment of the catheter, hematuria (especially after the use of a large-bore catheter), bowel perforation during trocar insertion, and failure of the wound to close, which results in a urinary fistula.

OUTCOMES. When a suprapubic catheter is used instead of a urethral catheter, a lower rate of UTIs, increased comfort, and easier implementation of a bladder training protocol are expected.

Nursing Management of the Surgical Client

The client with a suprapubic catheter requires care similar to that needed for clients with a urethral catheter. The most frequent problem is catheter obstruction caused by (1) twisting or kinking or (2) sediment or clots. Disconnecting the catheter from the drainage tubing can disrupt the siphon drainage. When the catheter is removed, dressing changes may be needed to protect the skin from urinary leakage from the site. The suprapubic catheter site usually closes completely immediately or within 24 hours of removal.

Self-Care

The client who is discharged with an indwelling suprapubic or urethral catheter needs to know how to care for the catheter at home. The family and significant others should learn how to empty the drainage bag and how to prevent infection. They should also be taught the clinical manifestations of UTI and instructed to call the physician if they occur. When the client is discharged with a catheter in place, follow-up care is required. Removal of the catheter will depend on the cause of the retention.

Modifications for Elderly Clients

Older clients are more susceptible to urinary retention because of a chronic decrease in bladder tone. Retention leading to infection may also be worse in older clients. Treatment, however, remains the same.

URINARY INCONTINENCE

Urinary incontinence has been defined by the International Continence Society (ICS) as "a condition in which involuntary loss of urine is a social or hygienic problem and is objectively demonstrable."[64] The Agency for Health Care Policy and Research (AHCPR) published a collection of booklets on urinary incontinence in 1996.

Some 10% to 35% of noninstitutionalized adults over age 60 years and at least half of nursing home residents have problems related to incontinence.[60] The annual cost

---

ALTERNATIVE THERAPY

Urinary Disorders

Two common urinary problems that affect women, especially older women, may be helped by relatively simple interventions.

Urinary Tract Infection

Cranberry juice has been used as a folk remedy for prevention and treatment of urinary tract infection (UTI). Initially thought to be of benefit for its acidifying effect on the urine, cranberry seems to prevent microbial adherence to the epithelial cells lining the urinary tract.[3, 5] A randomized, double-blind, placebo-controlled trial using a commercially available cranberry beverage at a dosage of 300 ml/day in a group of older women showed a reduction in bacteria in the urine.[1] Tyler[5] recommends 90 ml/day as a preventive dose, with one third of that being pure cranberry juice, with an increase to 360 to 960 ml/day for UTI treatment. In light of the problem of microbial resistance, cranberry, which has no direct antimicrobial effect, may be a good choice for prevention and initial treatment of UTI.

Urge Incontinence

Urge urinary incontinence is characterized by urgency, frequency of urination, and dysuria. Acupuncture performed at a point approximately 3 inches above the inter-

nal malleolus can be effective in reducing manifestations. In a report of urodynamic studies, 22 of 26 women receiving acupuncture at the point known as Spleen 6, traditionally used for genitourinary complaints, showed improvement, with 17 women showing increased bladder capacity and marked reduction of manifestations after a single treatment.[2] While this report used standard acupuncture, a later one utilized electrical stimulation through needles at the same location, stating that this area is where "nerves that affect bladder control could be stimulated."[4] The authors claim good results in treating urge incontinence in many patients, from children to older adults.

References

1. Avorn, J., et al. (1994). Reduction of bacteriuria and pyuria after ingestion of cranberry juice. *Journal of the American Medical Association, 271*:751–754.
2. Chang, P. L. (1988). Urodynamic studies in acupuncture for women with frequency, urgency and dysuria. *Journal of Urology, 140*:563–566.
3. Kerr, K. G. (1999). Cranberry juice and prevention of recurrent urinary tract infection. *The Lancet, 399*:673.
4. Stoller, M. L., & Harris, M. G. (1998). Needle stimulation (through the skin) for the treatment of incontinence. *Quality Care, 16*(1):1–2.
5. Tyler, V. E. (1994). *Herbs of choice.* Binghamton, NY: Pharmaceutical Products Press.

James Higgy Lerner, RN, LAc, *Private practice of acupuncture, traditional Oriental medicine, and biofeedback* of incontinence exceeds $15 million.[60] Yet most people avoid seeking treatment because they feel shame and embarrassment, which means that the problem is severely underreported and underdiagnosed. Many health care providers do not understand the effects of urinary incontinence on quality of life. Affected people may forfeit their active lifestyles and turn to a reclusive existence because they fear embarrassment.

There are three major types of incontinence: (1) *stress incontinence*, (2) *urge incontinence*, and (3) *overflow incontinence*. Under each of these types are many subtypes that may present in clients as an individual diagnosis or a combination of diagnoses.

Etiology and Risk Factors

Urinary incontinence commonly results from many factors, including anatomic defects and physical, physiologic, psychosocial, and pharmacologic factors. Anatomic and physiologic incontinence results from sphincter weakness or damage, urethral deformity, altered muscle tone at the urethrovesical junction, and detrusor instability.

Stress incontinence is an involuntary loss of urine that occurs without detrusor (bladder) contraction when intravesical pressure exceeds urethral pressure.[9] It commonly results from obstetric or surgical trauma, repeated straining, urogenital prolapse, and congenital weakness. After a suprapubic prostatectomy and transurethral prostatectomy, men may experience some exertional urine loss after the postoperative catheter is removed. Surgical interventions may cause bladder neck damage, with possibly permanent incontinence. A radical perineal or retropubic prostatectomy may cause permanent incontinence if the bladder neck is partially damaged during surgery.

Dysfunction of the urethrovesical junction (the area where the bladder meets the urethra) occurs mainly in women. Common causes include pregnancy, vaginal delivery, menopause, and surgical procedures that damage nerves leading to muscles of the pelvic floor. These injuries may lead to stress incontinence of varying degrees. A change in the angle of greater than 30 degrees from a horizontal plane during straining indicates hypermobility due to relaxation of the urethrovesical junction.

A simple diagnostic test for a hypermobile urethrovesical junction is a *Q-tip test*. A sterile, well-lubricated cotton applicator is placed in the urethra. The client is asked to strain as if to have a bowel movement. More than a 30-degree difference in a horizontal plane indicates a positive result or urethral hypermobility of the urethrovesical junction (Fig. 34–10).

Detrusor instability has many possible causes, although in many cases the cause remains unknown. On occasion, the cause can be identified as a bladder lesion, lower or upper spinal cord lesion, complication of pelvic surgery, or neurologic deficit. The International Continence Society offers two descriptions to characterize detrusor instability. In the first, the bladder contracts either spontaneously or with provocation while the client attempts to inhibit micturition. These contractions are seen during the filling phase of a cystometrogram in a neurologically intact client. In the second, detrusor overactivity results from disturbances of the nervous control mechanism. These clients have objective evidence of bladder dysfunc-

FIGURE 34–10 Diagnostic "Q-tip test" determines the descent of the normal urethrovesical junction contributing to stress incontinence in women. More than a 30-degree increase during exertional activities indicates a hypermobile urethrovesical junction.

tion from a neurologic disorder. This type of detrusor instability, known as *detrusor hyperreflexia*, is commonly seen in the client with a history of a stroke or neurologic impairment.

Urge incontinence occurs randomly when involuntary urination is preceded by the warning of a few seconds to a few minutes. It is caused by uncontrolled contraction or overactivity of the detrusor muscle seen with central nervous system disorders (Alzheimer's disease, brain tumor, Parkinson's disease, multiple sclerosis), bladder disorders (interstitial cystitis, radiation effects, carcinoma in situ), and spinal cord interference with spinal inhibitory pathways (spondylosis, cancer growth in spinal cord).

Overflow incontinence, as defined by International Continence Society, is an involuntary urine loss associated with overdistention of the bladder.[9] The bladder is able to store urine but does not empty completely, causing urine loss as a result of diminishing resistant pressures.

Physical causes of incontinence independent of disorders of the urinary tract are often related to physical immobility, especially with older adults. These clients are often physically unable to get to the toilet independently because of stroke, fractures, or weakness. Failing vision and distances from the bathroom can also contribute to incontinence if the client cannot see the commode or bedpan.

Psychosocial causes of incontinence range from true psychological problems, such as dementia, to simple confusion. Clients may be unaware of the need to void or may be unable to respond appropriately when they feel the urge to empty the bladder. Other possible causes include regression, dependence, insecurity, sensory deprivation, and the disturbance of conditioned reflexes.

Drugs can also contribute to incontinence, especially overflow incontinence. Examples include:

• Narcotics, tranquilizers, sedatives, and hypnotic agents, all of which may affect sensory perception

- Alcohol
- Rapid-acting diuretics
- Antihistamines
- Atropine and atropine-like substances
- Hypotensive agents
- Alpha-adrenergic blockers
- Beta-adrenergic agents
- Ganglionic blockers

Other causative factors include fecal impaction, bladder scarring, urethral adhesions, diabetes mellitus, and obesity. Frequent voiding by clients who fear "accidents" leads to decreased bladder capacity, increased detrusor tone, and thickening of the bladder wall, which only fosters the dysfunction.

Incontinence health promotion activities involve prevention of impaired mobility and UTIs, exercise to minimize muscle weakness, and assisting clients to the bathroom by the clock to prevent accidents. Health maintenance measures are to thoroughly assess clients who report incontinence and monitor high-risk clients for development of incontinence. Teaching clients to perform pelvic muscle exercises (Kegel exercises) to improve muscle tone, follow bladder training protocols, and decrease incontinence by regulating fluid intake (e.g., not drinking large amounts of fluid at bedtime) are examples of health restoration interventions.

Pathophysiology

Pathophysiologic changes associated with incontinence vary with the specific cause of the disorder. In *stress incontinence*, increased vesical pressure commonly stems from such activities as sneezing, coughing, laughing, and exertion. There may be some dysfunction of the urethral sphincter or, in women, changes in the urethrovesical junction caused by weakness of periurethral muscles. Muscle weakness from childbirth, menopause, or other problems loosens the pelvic floor. In addition to the loss of muscle tone supporting the urethrovesical junction, there is increased descent, with a funneling effect of the bladder neck during exertion. In men, the pathophysiologic change usually results from BPH, which causes retention, overflow, and stress incontinence.

Urge incontinence is associated with several pathophysiologic changes. One problem is uninhibited detrusor contraction associated with motor disorders. Another cause is decreased mobility from an upper motor neuron spinal lesion combined with an inability to stop voiding once the impulse is felt.

Overflow incontinence stems from overdistention of the bladder and eventual overflow of the excessive amount of urine. Usually, this problem results from obstruction at the bladder outlet, as with BPH.

If incontinence is not controlled, it can lead to both psychological and physical problems. The psychological consequences of incontinence are serious. Clients may isolate themselves, and the fear of embarrassment may lead to depression. Incontinence is also a leading cause of nursing home admissions. The physical complications of incontinence include infection, skin breakdown, and permanent voiding dysfunctions.

Clinical Manifestations

The major manifestation of urinary incontinence is involuntary urine loss. Manifestations vary from client to client. An excellent diagnostic tool, the *bladder diary*, reveals voiding frequency, fluid intake, patterns of urinary urgency, and number and severity of incontinent episodes. A 7-day diary reveals patterns of incontinence and may be helpful before a diagnostic evaluation.

Urodynamic evaluation provides the best diagnostic information in determining the precise cause of the client's incontinence. The purpose of urodynamics is to reproduce the manifestations. The information collected is used to determine and guide treatment. Additionally, an evaluation of pelvic floor prolapse in women can reveal other contributing factors of urogenital dysfunction.

The variety of urodynamic examinations, including cystometrography and electromyographic (EMG) monitoring, are described in Chapter 32. Urine flow rate studies help identify hypotonic detrusor or an obstructional or dysfunctional voiding mechanism. A urethral pressure profile helps to determine pressure in the urethra, which may contribute to a severe type of stress incontinence (*intrinsic sphincter deficiency*) (see Bladder Neck Suspensions later on). Ultrasonography or catheterization of the bladder can detect elevated residual urine levels. Additionally, cystoscopy can be used to diagnose tumors, foreign bodies (such as stones or sutures), trabeculations, or structural abnormalities in the bladder and urethra.

Outcome Management

Successful management of urinary incontinence requires appropriate diagnostic testing. Treatments include pelvic floor behavioral interventions, drug therapy, and surgery. Naturally, the least invasive treatment should be tried first.[63] Many therapies aimed at improving incontinence can be implemented without risk to the client. Success is based on motivation, competency, and willingness to add these changes to one's lifestyle. Surgery should be performed only when a structural or anatomic defect is found.

The goals of treatment for a client with urinary incontinence include the following:

- Careful evaluation
- Treatment decisions based on the specific abnormalities identified for each client
- Treatment modalities that coordinate with the client's personality, expectations, environment, and clinical status
- A treatment plan that includes ways to circumvent environmental constraints
- Ability of the client to make an informed choice among treatment options

■ Medical Management

Many noninvasive, behavior-based therapies may be effective in controlling some types of incontinence. The AHCPR guidelines provide numerous algorithms that detail the diagnosis and treatment of various forms of incontinence.[63]

PELVIC MUSCLE EXERCISES

Originally designed for postpartum women, these exercises—commonly known as Kegel exercises—have long been the technique of choice for reducing urinary incontinence. Reports of success range from 30% to 90%. New devices have improved the success rate by fostering the correct use of these exercises.

The vaginal cone has been successful in enhancing awareness and in improving the effectiveness of pelvic muscle exercise. The client inserts the cone into the vagina and is instructed to hold the cone in place for 15 minutes twice a day. Correct muscle contraction is required to keep the cone in position. The client advances to a heavier cone once she can retain the lighter cone for the 15 minutes twice a day.

PELVIC FLOOR REEDUCATION

Biofeedback has been used for clients with incontinence to help them learn to reuse the pelvic floor musculature. Clients are educated to control incontinence by isolating and contracting the pelvic floor muscles. The use of biofeedback has been successful in eliminating incontinence in about 54% to 77% of clients who try it.

Biofeedback provides a "relay-like" system by which the client can visualize the isolation and contraction of the pelvic floor musculature. The muscle activity is recorded by either pressure manometry or EMG monitoring.

Clients are taught to use the pelvic floor muscles to override the sense of urgency in an effort to retrain the bladder. They can also be taught to contract the correct muscle group to inhibit urine loss caused by exertion. Biofeedback can also be used to teach clients to relax the pelvic floor if they have problems with urinary retention.

ELECTRICAL STIMULATION

Electrical stimulation of the pelvic floor can be used to inhibit the micturition reflex and to contract the pelvic floor muscles. Delivery of a weak electrical current helps to close the urethra more tightly by direct and reflexogenic contraction of the striated periurethral muscles. Electrical stimulation also helps to increase bladder volume through bladder inhibition and stabilized detrusor activity.

The most common method of delivery is by insertion of a vaginal or anal probe. The procedure can be done in a physician's office or at home. The client inserts the internal device, and the stimulation level is directed at maintaining a synchronous pelvic floor contraction during an on-and-off cycle. Figure 34–11 shows the computerized systems used for biofeedback and electrical stimulation.

BLADDER TRAINING AND BEHAVIORAL TRAINING

The client who uses bladder and behavioral training to address incontinence first voids at short intervals throughout the day—once an hour or less, if necessary. The client then tries to gradually lengthen the time between voiding up to 3 hours. This method seems to benefit 10% to 15% of clients with urge and stress incontinence, and most clients find at least some improvement.

Institutionalized clients can also use a form of bladder training. With these clients, health care workers encour-

FIGURE 34–11 An electrical stimulation and biofeedback system can be used to treat men and women with incontinence. This system is called the InCare PRS 9500 (Hollister Incorporated, Libertyville, IL.)

age voiding at hourly intervals and give positive feedback. The time between voiding can then be gradually increased to 2 hours.

ADMINISTER MEDICATIONS

Drug therapy for incontinence is guided primarily by the following events. During the bladder filling phase, the detrusor relaxes because of beta-adrenergic activity. At the same time, the bladder outlet contracts in response to alpha-adrenergic stimulation. If these actions are insufficient to keep urine in the bladder, drugs can be prescribed to supplement or replacement them (Table 34–2).

Medications are used mainly for urge (overactive bladder) to relax the bladder and, possibly, to increase bladder capacity. The most commonly used medications are anticholinergics and antispasmodics. These medications are contraindicated in clients with bladder outlet obstructions or a weak detrusor muscle. A new antispasmodic medication, tolterodine (Detrol), is reported to produce significantly fewer side effects and to be extremely effective for overactive bladder.

Alpha-adrenergic drugs may alleviate stress incontinence because they tend to increase the uptake of the alpha receptors in the urethra, thus increasing urethral resistance and urinary control.

By increasing circulation to the urogenital system, topical and systemic estrogens can improve function and help relieve manifestations of estrogen deficiency in postmenopausal women.

FLUID INTAKE AND DIETARY CHANGES

The major nutritional aspect of management involves controlling fluid intake. Decreasing fluid intake, especially after dinner, may help decrease nocturia. For obese clients, weight reduction may help decrease stress inconti-

TABLE 34–2	MEDICATIONS USED TO TREAT VOIDING DISORDERS			
Class	**Action**	**Therapeutic Outcome**	**Adverse Outcome**	**Dosing**
ANTISPASMODICS				
Oxybutynin (Ditropan, Ditropan XL) tolterodine (Detrol)	Inhibits muscarinic action of acetylcholine on bladder smooth muscle.	Decreases bladder contractility and promotes urine storage by delaying urge to void and increasing bladder capacity for treatment of urge incontinence (overactive bladder).	Monitor for dry mouth, dry eyes, constipation, headache, drowsiness, tachycardia, blurred vision, and urinary retention.	Give 1 hour before meals. Avoid alcohol and other sedatives that potentiate antispasmodic actions. Avoid with obstructive uropathy. Give hard candy or gum for dry mouth.
ANTICHOLINERGICS				
Propantheline bromide (Pro-Banthine)	Blocks effects of acetylcholine at muscarinic receptors	Decreases bladder contractility and promotes urine storage by delaying urge to void and increasing bladder capacity for treatment of urge incontinence (overactive bladder)	Monitor for dry mouth, dry eyes, constipation, urinary retention, and glaucoma.	Give 1 hour before meals, avoid in clients with glaucoma, ulcerative colitis, heart disease, hypertension, and obstructive uropathy. Give hard candy or gum for dry mouth.
ALPHA-ADRENERGICS				
Pseudoephedrine hydrochloride (Sudafed)	Exaggerates alpha response in bladder neck and urethra to increase bladder outlet resistance.	Increases bladder outlet resistance for relief of stress incontinence and postprostatectomy incontinence.	Monitor for hypertension, tachycardia, urinary retention, insomnia, and restlessness.	Give PO every 4 hours or every 12 hours if extended release form used.
CHOLINERGICS				
Bethanechol (Urecholine)	Stimulates muscarinic cholinergic receptors in bladder to increase bladder tone and sensations to bladder filling.	Stimulates detrusor contractility and promotes bladder emptying for acute postoperative or other urinary retention and neurogenic atony of bladder with retention.	Monitor for increased GI motility, decreased pulse, hypotension, and vasodilation (atropine is antidote).	Give PO 1 hour before meals or SC if client is in NPO status. Contraindicated with bladder obstruction and IM or IV routes.
HORMONES				
Estrogen	Strengthens periurethral blood flow and tissues.	Increases bladder outlet resistance for treatment of incontinence in postmenopausal women.	Monitor for breast tenderness, hypertension, weight changes, and vaginal bleeding.	*Oral:* Once a day cyclically. *Intravaginal:* Daily at bedtime for 12 weeks, then 1–3 times per week. *Topical:* Replace patch weekly.

GI, gastrointestinal; IM, intramuscular; IV, intravenous; NPO, nothing by mouth; PO, by mouth; SC; subcutaneous.

nence by decreasing pressure against the bladder neck during exertion. The client should also avoid bladder irritants, such as alcohol, chocolate, and caffeinated drinks.

BLADDER NECK SUPPORT PROSTHESIS
A bladder neck support prosthesis, a Silastic vaginal device, offers an easy and inexpensive alternative to surgery for certain women with stress incontinence (Fig. 34–12). This ring-shaped device is fitted into the vagina, and the ridges elevate the urethrovesical junction in a manner similar to that of a Burch colposuspension (see Bladder Neck Suspensions later on). The prosthesis reduces incontinence by elevating and supporting the urethrovesical junction during exercise. Every woman requires proper sizing, fitting, and instruction.

Nursing Management of the Medical Client
Multiple nursing diagnoses can be used, depending on the specific type of incontinence: *Stress Incontinence, Reflex Urinary Incontinence, Urge Incontinence,* and *Functional*

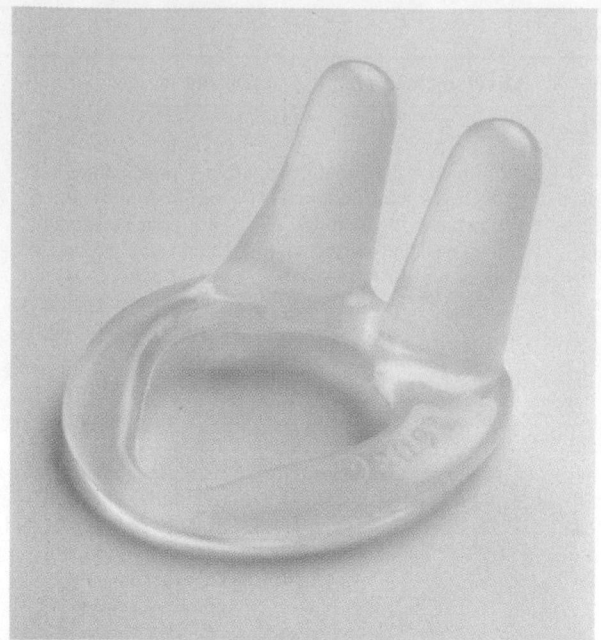

FIGURE 34–12 The bladder neck support prosthesis (Introl). A rubber-like silicone (Silastic) vaginal device supports the urethrovesical junction in women with stress incontinence. The two ridges support the urethrovesical junction during exertional activities.

Urinary Incontinence. All of the following interventions may be implemented as appropriate. Nurses often offer the first intervention for the client with urinary incontinence. The primary intervention is asking about bladder health with sensitivity. Remember, many clients feel shame and embarrassment about incontinence, and they may be reluctant to acknowledge the existence of a bladder control problem.

IMPLEMENT A BLADDER TRAINING PROGRAM

A successful bladder training program requires much patience on everyone's part. The client must accept the program and be a willing and active participant. The first step is to discuss all procedures, expectations, and anticipated outcomes with the client. Do your best to inspire a sense of hope and a positive attitude when discussing the client's prognosis.

A bladder training program involves (1) adequate fluid intake, (2) accessibility to a toilet, (3) muscle-strengthening exercises, and (4) carefully scheduled voiding times. Implementing the program also requires well-organized teaching guidelines. The client also may need behavioral modification or intermittent catheterization.

MONITOR FLUID INTAKE

Many clients with incontinence reduce their fluid intake in an effort to decrease urine production and increase control. Actually, adequate fluid intake and adequate urine production are necessary to stimulate the micturition reflex. Unless the client's physical status is a contraindication, encourage a daily fluid intake of ½ ounce of fluid for every pound of body weight. Carefully space these fluids throughout the day, limiting fluids in the evening to allow longer sleep periods at night. Fluids should be free

of caffeine and alcohol, both of which may irritate the bladder.

TEACH KEGEL EXERCISES

Performed diligently, Kegel exercises strengthen the pubococcygeal muscle, help resolve stress incontinence, and decrease urgency and frequency. Instruct the client to contract the pelvic floor muscles as if to hold back intestinal gas. Do not ask the client to start and stop the urine stream as a way to isolate the correct muscle group. Stopping and starting the urine stream may cause dysfunction of the micturition reflex and may encourage urinary retention.

Once the client can isolate the correct muscle group, he or she should contract these muscles 10 times in sitting, standing, and lying positions, three times a day, working up to 10-second contractions. Then encourage the client to contract the pelvic floor muscles to learn the urge suppression technique or before any exertion that might cause incontinence. As with any exercise program, the program takes a conscious effort and may take months for the muscles to become adequately toned.

DEVELOP A VOIDING SCHEDULE

At the same time that the client is strengthening pelvic floor muscles, the nurse should develop a voiding schedule with the client. Determine how often the client urinates during the day by asking her to maintain a voiding record. Depending on the voiding pattern, help the client to the toilet or commode every 30 minutes, increasing the time to 2 hours. As the program progresses, encourage the client to hold the urine longer. This increases voiding intervals, which increases bladder capacity.

IMPLEMENT BIOFEEDBACK TECHNIQUES

Biofeedback and behavior modification may improve the outcome of the bladder training program. Use biofeedback techniques to help the client regain control over the external urethral sphincter and pelvic floor musculature. An internal probe is placed to measure the pelvic floor muscle activity. As the client contracts the pelvic floor, a Visual Analogue Scale or video graphs indicate the activity, strength, and duration of the muscle contraction. The system gives immediate feedback of progress. The therapy can be offered in the practitioner's office or with the use of a home unit.

USE BEHAVIOR MODIFICATION

Behavior modification is a variation of the voiding schedule. This program conditions the bladder to empty when the client attempts to void. The client is encouraged to void by the clock rather than by urge. The initial time between voiding is based on a completed bladder diary before therapy is begun. The time between voiding may be as little as every 30 minutes, with weekly increases of 15 to 30 minutes between. The gradual increase in time between voiding helps to decrease urge incontinence and to increase bladder capacity.

EXPLORE OBSTRUCTIVE DEVICES

Obstructive devices are sometimes used to interfere with the outflow of urine. For example, certain types of vaginal pessaries can reduce incontinence by obstructing the urethra. Removing the device allows complete emptying of the bladder. Women using such devices must have the dexterity to remove the device for voiding.

A penile clamp can compress the urethra in a male client, but its use is controversial (Fig. 34–13). The clamp should be used only rarely and for short intervals. It must be removed and repositioned frequently to prevent pressure sores and ischemia of the penis.

RECOMMEND COUNSELING

A mental health consultation may help clients with depression that stems from incontinence. Talking to a counselor can help clients manage the fear of embarrassment, sense of increased dependence, and self-image problems accompanying incontinence. Avoid medications such as antidepressants because of the potential for more bladder dysfunction.

USE OTHER INCONTINENCE PRODUCTS

Disposable Pads

Sometimes none of the measures described are effective. Nursing interventions must then be aimed at protecting the client's skin, clothing, and bed linen. Adult-sized disposable pads or briefs help protect and increase the social mobility of clients with chronic incontinence. These commercially available undergarments have elastic legs and cellulose padding that draws fluid away from the skin by capillary action. Some brands include an odor-reducing agent.

Skin Care

If the skin becomes wet, it must be meticulously cleaned with a pH-balanced cleaner and dried to prevent serious rashes and skin breakdown from maceration and ammonia. The skin should then be carefully moisturized. Indwelling catheters to drain urine should be used only in an effort to avoid skin breakdown.

Condom Systems

External condom catheter drainage involves placing a thin rubber or plastic sheath over the penis and connecting it to either a leg bag or a bedside drainage bag (see Fig. 34–9). When the bladder releases urine, it runs down the tube into the collecting device. Problems include leakage (with or without detachment of the condom), twisting of the condom, and stasis of urine, which can macerate the penis.

Select the correct size of sheath, attaching it to stay in place without compromising circulation to the distal penis. Make sure that the sheath is not too tight, particularly at the ring. You may need to remove some of the client's pubic hair before preparing the skin. Wash the penis with soap and water and allow it to dry thoroughly to remove skin oils. If appropriate, apply an adhesive paste or commercial skin barrier.

FIGURE 34–13 A penile clamp compresses the urethra to prevent incontinence.

Many commercially prepared condom systems contain a double-sided adhesive liner that is applied to the penis before the condom. Many newer devices are self-adhesive.

When rolling the condom sheath over the penis, allow at least 1.5 cm between the distal end of the penis and the internal end of the sheath. This reduces skin irritation. Make sure that the foreskin is over the glans.

Use only elastic tape to allow for expansion or erection. Apply this tape in a spiral only. To avoid impaired circulation, never encircle the penis completely with tape. Frequently monitor the patency of the system, and remove the condom daily to clean and dry the skin.

ENCOURAGE FOLLOW-UP

The client should be seen at regular intervals to make sure that interventions are adequate and continence is improved. Referral to a continence clinic may sometimes be appropriate to ensure close follow-up of continuing problems. The National Association for Continence and the Simon Foundation for Continence both publish newsletters containing important information for the incontinent client and family (see Management and Delegation).

■ Surgical Management

Surgical procedures are performed only to correct or compensate for anatomic defects leading to incontinence. After an injury to the bladder neck, the surgeon can resuspend the bladder neck and attempt to recreate normal anatomy. Implantation of an artificial sphincter can bring about opening and closing of the urethra to allow voiding. Other procedures, such as collagen or fat injections, are used to attempt to fill or occlude a urethra that cannot close completely.

BLADDER NECK SUSPENSIONS

Bladder neck suspensions are surgical procedures intended to restore the normal urethrovesical junction or to lengthen and support the urethra. Resuspending the bladder neck allows the urethrovesical junction to function correctly.

The *Burch colposuspension* is a popular surgical procedure for women with stress incontinence. This surgical intervention is a modification of an older procedure known as the MMK (Marshall, Marchetti, Krantz). In the Burch procedure, a surgeon fixes the periurethral tissue to Cooper's ligament, whereas in the MMK procedure, the surgeon sutures the periurethral tissue to the symphysis pubis. After surgery, a suprapubic catheter must usually be in place for up to 14 days. The drainage system must remain patent because the pressure of a filling bladder can inhibit the healing process.

A *sling procedure* is used for intrinsic sphincter deficiency, a severe type of stress incontinence. Material is placed beneath the urethra to elevate it and to increase urethral compression. The sling material may be synthetic or autologous (from one's self), such as fascia from another part of the client's abdomen. There are many variations of the procedure; some present a significant risk of voiding dysfunction.

Other surgical procedures aim to provide an intact, patent route for the transport of urine. Scar tissue that interferes with normal bladder neck function must be removed.

MANAGEMENT AND DELEGATION

Helping Clients with Urinary Incontinence

Various underlying conditions can result in urinary incontinence. Although women are at greater risk than men, incontinence also affects men. You and the physician assess and evaluate the client to determine the appropriate interventions to manage incontinence and may use a bladder record or voiding diary to document patterns and trends. Pelvic muscle rehabilitation, behavior therapy, pharmacologic interventions, and surgical procedures are the recommended treatments. For many, incontinence is an acute problem; for others, it is a chronic one.

Bladder training, assistance with toileting, and providing good skin care are duties that may be delegated to unlicensed assistive personnel. These measures are necessary for improving continence and for keeping clients dry and clean to prevent complications associated with skin irritation and ulceration.

Helping the incontinent client who cannot get out of bed is crucial in preventing skin breakdown and pressure ulcers. Utilizing a bedpan, a bedside commode, or a raised toilet seat may be helpful at times. If the client uses a walking aid to ambulate, ensure that the wheelchair, walker, or cane is near the bed and that the pathway to the bathroom is well lit and clear. Indicate which modality is appropriate for each patient.

Instruct unlicensed assistive personnel to:

- Respond promptly to all call lights in their assigned area.
- Closely measure and record urine output. Cloudy, foul-smelling, or dark urine should be reported immediately to you.
- Give each client plenty of time to void. Create privacy by closing the door or pulling the bedside curtain.
- Never scold a client who is wet. The client may be upset or feel ashamed about incontinence.

With bladder training instruction, direct unlicensed assistive personnel to:

- Assist or prompt the client to the bathroom on a scheduled interval, usually every 1 to 2 hours at the beginning of the training period.
- Increase the interval of time to assist or prompt the client to the bathroom as the client begins to achieve dryness.

Ask unlicensed assistive personnel to:

- Explain when the next bathroom time will be before they leave the room.
- Offer positive reinforcement to the client who can successfully void or asks for assistance to the bathroom to urinate, or has a dry absorbent pad.

- Assist clients with exercises to strengthen pelvic muscles to help minimize incontinence, reinforcing your previous instruction.

Direct unlicensed assistive personnel about which toileting methods to use:

- *Scheduled toileting:* Assist the client to the bathroom every 2 to 4 hours whether or not the client is wet or dry.
- *Prompted voiding:* Check whether the client is wet or dry; ask the client whether he or she needs to void, and help the client to the bathroom if the client answers "yes."
- *Habit training:* Once the client's voiding times each day are determined, help the client to the bathroom at the same times each day.

Maintaining clean, dry, and intact skin is necessary to prevent skin breakdown and unnecessary complications associated with wet skin. Instruct unlicensed assistive personnel to provide proper skin care and to identify any changes such as red, excoriated, or tender skin to you. The regimen may include:

- Cutting back on evening or night fluid intake to decrease voiding accidents during the night.
- Changing disposable wet pads or diapers every time the client is wet.
- Utilizing ointments or creams to protect the skin and to serve as a barrier after cleaning the client.
- Applying absorbent pads or diapers that are not chafing to the skin.

Have unlicensed assistive personnel communicate and report (1) any changes in skin or urine, (2) the client's inability to follow the toileting plan, and (3) any other questions that arise. Remember, you are responsible for assessing, implementing, evaluating, and making all changes to the client's plan of care.

References

1. Agency for Health Care Policy and Research (1996). *Clinical practice guideline: Urinary incontinence in adults: Acute and Chronic Management* (AHCPR Pub. No. 96-0682). Rockville, MD: U.S. Department of Health and Human Services.
2. Agency for Health Care Policy and Research (1996). *Clinical practice guideline: Caregiver guide: Helping people with incontinence* (AHCPR Pub. No. 96-0683). Rockville, MD: U.S. Department of Health and Human Services.

Elizabeth W. Good, MSN, RN, C, *Clinician IV, Urology Care Coordinator, Surgical Services, University of Virginia Health System, Charlottesville, Virginia*

IMPLANTATION OF AN ARTIFICIAL URINARY SPHINCTER

Implantation of an artificial urinary sphincter may help some clients achieve continence. This procedure usually is avoided until all other treatments have failed. Figure 34–14 shows a sphincter device, which consists of an inflatable cuff, a reservoir, and a control pump. The surgeon implants the cuff around the bladder neck or urethra, the deflation (or control) pump in the scrotum or labia, and the fluid reservoir in the abdomen.

The cuff keeps the urethra closed until the client manually squeezes the pump. This moves the fluid from the cuff to the reservoir. The bladder will then drain. The cuff automatically refills after 3 to 5 minutes, again occluding the urethra.

Candidates for this treatment must not have an obstructed lower urinary tract, detrusor hyperreflexia, or progressive neurologic disease affecting bladder function. Clients must have adequate manual dexterity and motivation to manage the system. Failure of the device poses a long-term risk that the client will need more surgery. Clients must be absolutely compliant, or the upper tracts of the urinary system can be damaged by obstruction.

■ Nursing Management of the Surgical Client

Nursing care of clients undergoing surgery focuses on maintaining adequate urinary drainage. With bladder suspension, preventing distention is a priority to help avoid excessive pressure on the healing surgical site. During the immediate postoperative period, a bladder training program is initiated to help the client regain detrusor muscle tone. Clamp the catheter for lengthening intervals while urine collects in the bladder, unclamping it periodically to empty the bladder. If the client reports severe pressure, the catheter should be unclamped immediately.

FIGURE 34–14 Artificial urinary sphincter. This surgically implanted urethral sphincter restores continence. To urinate, the client deflates the cuff around the bladder neck by squeezing the control pump within the scrotum. The cuff reinflates automatically.

*Labels in figure:*
Pressure-regulating reservoir
Urinary bladder
Inflatable cuff
Prostate
Urethra
Control pump
Scrotum

If a suprapubic catheter is used, the client should try to void every 2 to 3 hours. After voiding is attempted, the catheter is drained to measure the residual urine and determine the effectiveness of bladder emptying.

■ Self-Care

The expected outcome is that the client will resume control over bladder function. Many strategies to achieve continence may be tried, and the client will select what is most comfortable and best able to support preferred activities. Management options can be expensive, such as multiple biofeedback sessions. If continence is achieved with any of the described therapies, however, treatment to achieve continence is cheaper than the purchase of adult briefs for daily use; in addition, the client would be free to engage in desired activities. Teach the client about continence options, and help the client make decisions about treatment options.

■ Modifications for Elderly Clients

Incontinence is not a normal part of the aging process, but it is a common problem among older adults. The elderly can be treated with any of the previously mentioned treatments. Because older people are more sensitive to many medications, care should be used when drugs are administered.

NEUROGENIC BLADDER

The term "neurogenic bladder" refers to several bladder dysfunctions caused by lesions of the central or peripheral nervous systems (Fig. 34–15). Their manifestations depend on the site of the lesion. A neurogenic bladder may involve a combination of one or more nervous system dysfunctions. There are five major types of neurogenic bladder dysfunction:

- Uninhibited
- Sensory paralytic (detrusor muscle hyperreflexia)
- Motor paralytic (detrusor muscle areflexia)
- Autonomous
- Reflex

Neurogenic bladder dysfunctions may also be classified according to the level of the lesion in the central nervous system.

Upper motor neuron lesions occur above the sacral segments of the spinal cord. They produce bladders that are spastic or characterized by exaggerated reflexes (hyperreflexia).

Lower motor neuron lesions occur at or below the sacral vertebrae. They produce bladders that are lacking reflexes (areflexic) or tone (atonic).

The incidence of neurogenic bladder dysfunction reflects the incidence and etiology of neurologic injuries or disorders. With certain disorders, a neurogenic bladder may develop in 100% of clients, as with transection of the spinal cord. Clients with conditions such as multiple sclerosis are affected with varying degrees of manifestations.

FIGURE 34–15 Types of neurogenic bladder dysfunction.

Etiology and Risk Factors

Risk factors for neurogenic bladder disorders include tumors, neurologic disorders, and trauma to the nervous system. Accidents are the only preventable cause of this problem.

UNINHIBITED

The uninhibited neurogenic bladder produces "infantile" or uninhibited voiding. The urge to void causes urine to flow. The primary cause is a lesion in the corticoregulatory tracts, as from a cerebrovascular accident or multiple sclerosis.

SENSORY

A sensory paralytic bladder results from an interruption in the lateral spinal tracts, as occurs in tabes dorsalis, diabetic neuropathy, and pernicious anemia. Because of the sensory loss, the client cannot sense the bladder filling. This lack of perception leads to atonic bladder, retention with possible overflow incontinence, and upper tract involvement.

MOTOR

A motor paralytic bladder is the most uncommon type and is caused by lesions in the motor outflow from vertebrae S2 to S4. Disease processes causing this dysfunction include poliomyelitis, tumor, trauma, spina bifida, and infection. This dysfunction may be temporary if a bacterial or viral infection is the cause. Although there is full sensation of bladder filling, even to the point of pain, the client cannot initiate micturition.

AUTONOMOUS

Clients with an autonomous neurogenic bladder cannot perceive bladder fullness, or they cannot start and maintain urination without some type of exertional pressure. Retention and incontinence are common problems. The autonomous type of dysfunction occurs after destruction of all nerve connections between the bladder and the central nervous system at vertebrae S2, S3, or S4 following trauma, inflammatory processes, spinal anesthesia, or malignancy.

REFLEX

Transection of the spinal cord above the sacral segments causes a reflex neurogenic bladder. There is no sensation, and the bladder contracts reflexively but does not empty completely.

Pathophysiology

Lesions at the lower motor neuron level of the spinal cord often directly interfere with the reflex arc leading to inappropriate interpretation of efferent and afferent impulses. When the bladder fills, the message is transmitted through afferent fibers to the brain cortex. The injury keeps these impulses from being correctly interpreted, leading to loss of the micturition reflex. A flaccid bladder with urinary retention is the result.

With upper motor neuron lesions, impulses are not transmitted to or from the lower spinal areas to the cortex. When the bladder distends, no sensation is transmitted. Because the lower cord is intact, activity of the reflex arc can occur. The client would have reflex incontinence as a result.

When the damage is to the cortical area itself, as with a stroke or trauma, the client cannot correctly interpret the impulses that are being transmitted. Unless the client is evaluated and treated appropriately, serious UTIs, skin breakdown associated with incontinence, and even renal failure due to chronic overdistention of the bladder are more likely to develop.

Clinical Manifestations

The major clinical manifestation of neurogenic bladder dysfunction is retention with or without incontinence. The client may or may not feel a need to void or feel a sense of bladder distention. The diagnosis is made from the location of neurologic dysfunction. Urodynamic studies, including EMG monitoring, should be done to determine the extent of neurologic involvement to guide an appropriate treatment plan.

Outcome Management

■ Medical Management

BLADDER TRAINING

If possible, some form of bladder training should be attempted for a client with neurogenic bladder dysfunction. This measure includes a bladder training program, medication, possible intermittent catheterization, and sometimes surgical intervention.

ADMINISTER MEDICATIONS

A number of medications are used to treat neurogenic bladder dysfunction (see Tables 34–1 and 34–2). Antispasmodics and anticholinergics (such as dicyclomine, propantheline, and flavoxate) are given to relieve uninhibited or reflex bladder contractions. Phenoxybenzamine and other alpha-adrenergic blockers may be used. Bethanechol may help stimulate an atonic bladder. Other medications described in the discussion of incontinence may be useful as well.

PREVENT COMPLICATIONS

Autonomic dysreflexia is a serious, potentially life-threatening complication affecting clients who have spinal cord injuries. It may occur during bladder training programs if the urinary system or bowel becomes obstructed. The most frequent cause is bladder distention or feces in the rectum, although autonomic dysreflexia can be triggered by visceral distention or stimulation of pain receptors in the skin. This condition results from an excessive autonomic response to normal stimuli and affects primarily clients with upper motor neuron lesions.

The most common manifestations are severe hypertension, bradycardia, a throbbing headache, flushing, diaphoresis above the level of the lesion, blurred vision, nasal congestion, nausea, and pilomotor spasm ("goose bumps") above the lesion. If left untreated, this problem can lead to retinal hemorrhage, seizures, or stroke. It is important for the client to recognize the earliest manifestations and summon help immediately. Preventing bladder distention is one way to prevent this emergency. If stool is accumulating in the rectum, careful evacuation should be done to avoid either overdistention or overstimulation.

Medications such as diazoxide (Hyperstat), phenoxybenzamine (Dibenzyline), guanethidine monosulfate (Ismelin), propantheline bromide (Pro-Banthine), phentolamine mesylate (Regitine), and mecamylamine (Inversine) relieve both acute manifestations and the chronic recurrence of episodes.

■ Nursing Management of the Medical Client

PREVENT AUTONOMIC DYSREFLEXIA

Always be prepared for the development of autonomic dysreflexia. If severe hypertension (sometimes 300/180 mm Hg), flushing, and a pounding headache suddenly develop, you must address the manifestations immediately.

Nursing interventions involve removal of the triggering stimuli by reestablishing urine flow or removing the fecal impaction. Remove any fecal impaction only after a topical anesthetic agent has been inserted into the rectum to avoid further stimulation. In addition, a catheter may be necessary; if one is already in place, restore its patency by irrigation or by removing kinks and obstructions. Monitor the client's vital signs every 5 minutes, and raise the head of the bed to the semi-Fowler's position. Administer medications as ordered.

TEACH METHODS TO STIMULATE MICTURITION

Neurogenic bladders are difficult to control, but you can teach many clients how to stimulate the micturition reflex and maintain urination. Assist the client by providing external pressure on the abdomen. The client can lean forward or press on the abdomen. Have the client breathe deeply to push the diaphragm downward. Wearing a corset or girdle can provide an extra source of external pressure. The Valsalva maneuver is another method of increasing intra-abdominal pressure on the urinary bladder.

Another method that helps the client learn to empty the bladder is the Credé maneuver. The client places the fingers over the bladder and presses downward slowly toward the symphysis pubis, as though "milking" the urine out of the urinary system. This should be done with great caution. If the client has sphincter dyssynergia (failure of muscle coordination) or if the sphincter does not readily relax, the Credé maneuver can lead to sphincter damage and may cause ureteral reflux if there is any obstruction of outflow. The Credé maneuver is often combined with intermittent self-catheterization.

The client can use several other methods to initiate and maintain micturition. Locate trigger points on the body (lower abdomen, inner thighs, and pubic area), and explain how to stimulate them by stroking, pinching, or applying ice. Stretching the anal sphincter also relaxes the reflexes of the external urethral sphincter because they are both innervated by the pudendal nerve. The client leans forward while sitting on the toilet and inserts two gloved fingers into the anus. The fingers are then either widened apart or pulled posteriorly. Men must be careful to avoid touching the glans penis, which stimulates the bulbocavernosus reflex, contracting the external sphincter.

PERFORM INTERMITTENT CATHETERIZATION

For the treatment of long-term or short-term bladder atony (lack of tone), an intermittent catheterization program is an alternative to indwelling catheterization. A straight urethral catheter is inserted into the bladder at specified intervals, the urine is drained, and the catheter is removed. This may be done in a health care facility or in the client's home (see Bridge to Home Health Care).

TEACH INTERMITTENT SELF-CATHETERIZATION

Clients with bladder atony should be encouraged to learn self-catheterization because it increases independence and mobility. The client or any other person who has been properly educated about the technique may insert the catheter.

Sterile technique is necessary in health care facilities because of the high risk of nosocomial infections. At home, *clean technique* can be used for catheterization

without increasing the rate of UTIs. Clean technique is also easier and less expensive for the client. To reduce the risk of bacteriuria, urinary antiseptics and acidification or bladder irrigation with antibiotics and antiseptics are used with each catheterization.

There are several procedural differences between clean and sterile techniques. For clean technique:

1. Gloves are not worn. The client must perform thorough hand-washing before starting.
2. A clean (rather than a sterile) catheter is used.
3. The catheter can be washed and reused indefinitely.
4. Lubricant should be used because the urethra is susceptible to traumatic urethritis.

The catheter should be washed thoroughly after use with soap and water and stored in a clean sandwich-size plastic bag or other clean container.

During self-catheterization, the client may sit or stand. When a female client stands, she should separate her legs or place one leg on a toilet seat. After separating the labia, she can use a mirror to find the meatus.

Timing is important for successful catheterization programs. Catheterization should be carried out at specified intervals throughout the day until bedtime. The interval between catheterization is set according to the degree of continence. The average interval for adults is every 3 to 4 hours, but the client usually has to start at intervals of 2 to 3 hours. Clients should use the catheter to remove 350 to 400 ml each time. A client who cannot follow a schedule is not an appropriate candidate for the program.

The amount of fluid intake allowed is under debate. Some programs allow fluid as desired; others restrict fluid intake to varying degrees. This aspect of the program requires systematic investigation. Clinicians generally recommend that the client drink about 250 ml of fluid at about 2-hour intervals. Ingestion of large amounts of fluid within a short period can cause bladder distention and reflux. Most clients are urged to drink up to 2 L of fluid daily at regular intervals.

A catheter-free bladder and absence of bacteriuria indicate a successful intermittent catheterization program. Controversy exists about the treatment of asymptomatic bacteriuria. A successful catheterization program may be due to several factors, including intermittent bladder distention, which causes stimulation of the normal micturition reflex and reactivation of the bladder's normal antibacterial properties. Other advantages include continence, independence, good hygiene, prevention of complications arising from urinary stasis or a retention catheter, decreased cost, and comfortable sexual relations.

Intermittent catheterization is not a panacea. The program requires the client to assume a great deal of personal responsibility. Some clients are not sufficiently motivated to fulfill the responsibilities involved in self-catheterization. Also, some problems can occur when the client is away from home.

Clients with high resting pressures in the bladder that are incontinent between catheterizations are likely to have difficulty with intermittent self-catheterization. All clients should be evaluated before starting the program. If urodynamic evaluation reveals high resting pressures, anticholinergic medications are administered.

BRIDGE TO HOME HEALTH CARE

Inserting Urinary Catheters

Indwelling catheters may be inserted to treat urinary incontinence. Indications include pressure ulcers or surgical wounds that do not heal, overflow incontinence associated with obstructions that cannot be removed, and decisions of the client or family that dryness and comfort outweigh the risks, especially in cases of serious or terminal illness.

Catheters affect the client's quality of life and self-esteem and are frequently accompanied by recurrent urinary tract infections (UTIs) that can lead to more serious complications and hospitalization. Therefore, you must evaluate whether a catheter is in the clients' best interest and will adequately meet their needs. Catheters should be the last treatment option; consider a referral to a continence care nurse or continence clinic first. You are responsible for providing instructions about daily cleansing, adequate fluid intake, manifestations of UTI, and indications to call the nurse or physician.

Use the smallest French (F) size catheter to meet the client's needs. A 14F to 16F catheter may be the best size for a woman; a 16F to 18F catheter may be best for a man. The balloon should hold 5 to 10 ml of fluid. A catheter that is too large or is overinflated will cause bladder spasms and urine to leak around the catheter. Men who have an enlarged prostate may need a coudé tip catheter.

Adequate lighting is often a challenge in the home. Consider using a flashlight or small lamp. It may be necessary to ask a family member or informal caregiver to help position the client and to hold the light.

When inserting a urinary catheter, place a female client in the supine position with her knees flexed and separated. Arrange pillows laterally under her knees to provide comfort and increase relaxation. Consider using the posterior approach if the client is obese or has severe

lower extremity contractures; turn her on her side facing the other way.

Using sterile technique, check the catheter balloon for appropriate filling, deflate, and set aside on the sterile field. Cleanse the labia and meatal opening one side at a time, using downward stokes; discard the swabs after each stroke. The last swab may be left slightly inside the vagina as a marker.

Ask the client to breathe deeply, and insert the well-lubricated catheter into the meatal opening. When urine returns, insert the catheter another inch and inflate the balloon with the preattached saline syringe; gently pull back to seal the catheter. If no urine returns, gently insert the gloved little finger into the vagina to assess for slippage of the catheter into the vagina.

If a catheter is accidentally inserted into the vagina, leave it in place as a marker. Never reuse a catheter. Obtain a new catheter, and insert with sterile technique as before.

Place male patients in a supine position. Using sterile technique, check the balloon for appropriate filling, then deflate and set aside on the sterile field. Retract the foreskin, and hold the penis at a 60- to 90-degree angle. Clean the glans penis in circular motion, starting at the meatus and working outward. Using a rotating motion, insert the well-lubricated catheter into the meatus. Do not force the catheter if resistance is met, but maneuver it gently as the client breathes deeply, coughs, or bears down.

When urine returns, inflate the catheter balloon with the saline-filled syringe. If placement cannot be verified, notify the physician. Always hang the drainage bag below the bladder level. Many clients prefer to hang the drainage bag on a clean wastepaper can to prevent urine from leaking on the floor.

Kimberly Stallo, RN, BSN, CETN, *Wound, Ostomy, and Continence Nurse, Fort Worth, Texas*

■ Surgical Management

Surgery is not the primary treatment option for the client with neurogenic bladder. However, if conservative measures are ineffective in treating the neurogenic bladder, surgical intervention may be necessary. External sphincterotomy or incision of the bladder neck may restore normal bladder emptying. Interrupting innervation to the bladder reflex can aid an uninhibited bladder. Injection of alcohol into the subarachnoid space or rhizotomy (cutting) of the sacral nerves increases bladder capacity by inhibiting reflex bladder contractions, without interfering with normal sphincter function. Sometimes a temporary sacral nerve block is performed before surgery to evaluate the potential candidate. Electrodes may be implanted at thoracic or cervical levels of the spinal epidural space and attached to a percutaneous stimulator. As soon as the client learns to regulate the electrical stimulation properly, the device can be used to inhibit or interrupt reflex bladder contractions.

Continuous intrathecal baclofen administered through an implanted infusion pump is another method of treating a neurogenic bladder. Baclofen helps decrease spasms and detrusor sphincter dyssynergia. Clients report improve-

ment in bladder compliance and capacity. Finally, if all else fails, urinary diversion may be performed to provide the client with a more manageable urinary system.

■ Nursing Management of the Surgical Client

Nursing care of the client undergoing surgery for a neurogenic bladder with either an external sphincterotomy or a revision of the bladder outlet is the same as for any client undergoing bladder surgery. Urinary output maintenance is the priority of these clients. A suprapubic or urinary catheter may be needed until healing occurs.

As with the other surgical procedures, focus care on teaching the client self-care. The client needs to learn to regulate electrical stimulation appropriately to inhibit or interrupt the reflex bladder contractions.

Proper care of the implantable infusion pump is another important area of client education. Care of clients undergoing urinary diversion has been discussed under Bladder Cancer.

■ Self-Care

The focus of discharge teaching for the neurogenic bladder client is intermittent self-catheterization. Teach the client and significant others a bladder training program and, possibly, a catheterization program. Assess the client's ability to understand and perform self-care procedures, and ensure that the client understands the self-catheterization program. Written materials, teaching videos, and diagrams can be used to reinforce the teaching.

Clients need to be assessed in the home setting to make sure they can function as well as in the hospital. A visiting nurse may be included to help in the discharge planning of the self-catheterization or bladder training program. The client's urinary function should be monitored at regular intervals, including renal function tests and yearly renal ultrasound studies. Teach the client to call the health care provider if manifestations of a UTI develop.

Modifications for Elderly Clients

Older clients are more likely to have other medical problems, such as arthritis and visual changes, that can interfere with their ability to use the self-catheterization program. However, they may still be able to use this method if they have adequate help.

TRAUMATIC DISORDERS

BLADDER TRAUMA

Bladder trauma is defined as a blunt or penetrating injury to the bladder that may cause bladder rupture. Bladder trauma often results from automobile accidents, when the seat belt compresses the bladder. A bladder distended by urine can rupture with a direct blow to the lower abdomen. The bladder may also be punctured by a bullet, knife, bony splinter from a fractured pelvis, or internal medical instrumentation. When the bladder ruptures, urine spills into the peritoneal cavity. Complications of peritoneal urine accumulation from a ruptured bladder are peritonitis and pelvic cellulitis.

Clinical Manifestations

Bladder injuries usually produce hematuria and pain low in the abdomen or pain referred to a shoulder. The client also may have trouble voiding. Manifestations of peritonitis may develop as well. Fever is usually present as the peritonitis and pelvic cellulitis continue to develop. If the client has had an injury or blow to the abdomen, suspect bladder injury as the cause of the manifestations.

Diagnostic tests include an IVP with lateral views or a CT scan with the bladder full and empty, a cystogram, and a voiding cystourethrogram. If blood is flowing from the meatus, urethral disruption may be present. In this case, catheterization should be avoided until the urethra is evaluated. This allows assessment of both bladder integrity and the bladder's ability to empty.

Outcome Management

Medical Management

The first treatment for suspected bladder injury is insertion of an indwelling or suprapubic catheter to monitor

for hematuria or urine production and to keep the bladder decompressed during healing. Any injury other than a simple contusion or very small perforation will require surgical repair.

Nursing Management of the Medical Client

Immediately assess for a suspected bladder injury if the client has had blunt trauma to the lower pelvis or abdomen. Closely monitor the client's urine output for both amount and the presence of hematuria. Report any decrease in urine output in relation to fluid intake to the physician immediately. Careful catheter insertion is necessary for the client with suspected bladder trauma.

Surgical Management

Clients with bladder injuries usually require surgical intervention. After a urethral or suprapubic catheter has been inserted, surgical repair of the damaged bladder wall is performed. The extravasated urine in the perivesical area is drained. It is important to maintain urinary drainage through a patent catheter to promote healing and to avoid the potential development of fistulas or leakage.

Nursing Management of the Surgical Client

Postoperatively, maintain urinary drainage to prevent tension on the sutures in the bladder. A Penrose drain is left in place to allow drainage of any urine remaining in the pelvis. This may necessitate dressing changes.

Because the client may be discharged with an indwelling or suprapubic catheter, teach catheter care to the client and significant others. Assess the client's self-care abilities to determine a possible need for assistance at home. If the client or significant others cannot care for the catheter, arrange for a home health visit.

Follow-up care is essential after discharge to assess healing. A cystogram may be done before the catheter is removed. If a suprapubic catheter has been placed, the client can begin bladder training before the catheter is removed. If the client has a urethral catheter, the catheter is removed before the client can attempt to void. If clients do not void within 4 to 6 hours after removal, the catheter will need to be reinserted.

URETHRAL TRAUMA

The urethra as well as the bladder may be injured in a pelvic fracture. Falling astride an object, such as the bar on a boy's bike, with sudden force to the groin may cause urethral contusion and laceration. Injury may also occur during medical or surgical interventions, may be self-inflicted, or may occur after female genital mutilation (see Chapter 39). Penetrating wounds also cause urethral damage.

Evaluation of urethral damage is indicated if the client cannot void, has an altered urine stream, or has visible blood at the meatus. Even if the client can pass some urine through the urethra, voiding will cause urinary extravasation, resulting in swelling of the scrotum or inguinal areas, which can lead to sepsis and necrosis. Blood may appear at the external meatus and may also extravasate into the surrounding tissues, giving the area an ecchymotic appearance.

The two most common complications of urethral trauma are (1) development of urethral strictures and (2) risk of impotence in men. Impotence occurs because the corpora cavernosa of the penis, blood vessels, or nerves supplying this area are damaged.

Proper management of urethral injuries is controversial. Clinicians generally agree that urinary drainage must first be established with either a urethral or suprapubic catheter. Some physicians suggest an immediate primary surgical repair of the urethra. Others prefer to wait 2 to 3 weeks to see whether the urethra will heal around the urethral catheter without surgery. During any waiting period, the client must be monitored for developing infection and continuing extravasation of urine.

URETERAL TRAUMA

The ureters are located deep within the abdomen and are protected by the spine and surrounding musculature. Thus, most ureteral trauma takes place accidentally during surgery. Perforation or tearing may occur during manipulation of intraureteral catheters or other instruments. The ureters may be occluded by ligating sutures or a misplaced clamp, or they may be transected during pelvic surgery. Many surgeons insert ureteral stents before pelvic procedures to easily identify the ureters and prevent trauma. Gunshot and stab wounds may also traumatize the ureters. On occasion, blunt trauma from a car accident can tear these structures.

Trauma is often not discovered until a clinical manifestation develops, such as hematuria, flank pain, or the presence of extravasated urine. As the urine seeps out into the tissues, pain may occur in the lower abdomen and flank. As extravasation continues, there may be sepsis, paralytic ileus, a palpable intraperitoneal mass, and the appearance of urine in an external wound. An IVP and ultrasonography are the most definitive means of diagnosis.

Surgical intervention is used to repair the defect, preferably with end-to-end anastomosis. More radical procedures may be needed, such as cutaneous ureterostomy, transureteroureterostomy, and reimplantation. The surgeon may use prosthetic ureteral implants. A nephrectomy is performed if obstruction or sepsis causes severe renal damage. It is essential to treat sepsis aggressively. Significant extravasation of urine may require the surgeon to open the abdomen and drain the urine.

CONGENITAL ANOMALIES

A congenital anomaly of the bladder is exstrophy of the bladder that develops when the symphysis pubis fails to close in utero. The lower anterior abdominal wall and anterior bladder wall are absent, allowing the bladder to protrude through the defective abdominal wall. These conditions are often treated with urinary diversion in childhood, but additional revisions may be needed as the child grows. Children who have had a diversion may be candidates for continent reservoir revisions.

Although congenital anomalies of the ureter are uncommon, several types are described.

1. *Ectopic ureter* occurs when a ureter follows an abnormal course or has an abnormal distal opening. It is the most common congenital ureteral anomaly. An ectopic ureter occurs as a result of the abnormal embryologic development of the ureter. During micturition, this anomaly often results in a back-flow of urine. Misplacement of the meatus (hypospadias and epispadias) is discussed in Chapter 38.
2. *Duplicate ureters,* arising from the same renal pelvis, may develop when the ureters on one side unite at some point, both may open in the normal portion of the trigone or when both may open into the urethra or vagina. This anomaly is not usually recognized unless a radiographic study is done for another reason. Pyelonephritis develops, and an evaluation reveals the anomaly. Surgical intervention is usually not necessary unless complications occur.
3. *Abnormal dilation of the ureter (megaureter)* is characterized by dilation and pouching of the ureteral wall just adjacent to the vesicoureteral junction. Resulting manifestations are seen as reflux or obstructive effects, which predispose the client to recurrent UTIs.
4. *Congenital ureteropelvic obstruction* occurs at the junction of the renal pelvis and the ureter. This anomaly is usually bilateral. A mild obstruction may never cause manifestations of a urinary tract disorder. As long as the kidney produces urine at a rate below 6 ml/minute, the ureter can generally handle the flow; however, urine production above this rate causes urinary stasis in the kidney, which results in hydronephrosis. If the condition is symptomatic, treatment consists of surgical repair of the narrowed section at the ureteropelvic junction.

CONCLUSIONS

Urinary system disorders can be extremely problematic for clients. Nurses play a major role in the diagnosis, prevention, and treatment of these disorders. Many of the disorders of the urinary system are chronic or become chronic problems, leading to renal disease or incontinence. Some of the manifestations of these disorders can drastically alter the client's self-concept and lifestyle. Problems of the lower urinary tract may become life-threatening, and the nurse must ensure that the client receives prompt and adequate treatment of disorders within the lower urinary system.

THINKING CRITICALLY

1. **A 28-year-old newlywed woman has been experiencing pain and burning with urination for the past 24 hours. This is the third episode of urinary manifestations she has had in the past 3 months. What is the probable cause of the urinary manifestations? What further information do you need to assess her problem? What can you do to help her treat this problem and prevent further difficulties?**

Factors to Consider. For what urinary tract problems does the client's status as a newlywed place her at risk?

Which tests would help differentiate an infectious problem from a noninfectious one?

2. The client had a radical cystectomy with formation of an Indiana pouch 12 hours ago. He has a catheter in place, which has drained 10 ml in the last hour. The stoma is a very pale pink. His vital signs are elevated from their preoperative levels. His pulse rate is 100 beats per minute, and his temperature is slightly increased. What actions would be appropriate at this point in the client's care?

Factors to Consider. Is the client's urinary output within expected limits? What color should a fresh stoma normally be?

3. A 69-year-old man with diabetes is admitted with severe left flank pain, nausea, vomiting, and diarrhea. His abdomen is soft and only slightly tender. His urinalysis reveals increased red blood cells, and his KUB shows a large staghorn calculus in the left kidney with hydronephrosis of the left kidney. What would be a priority assessment for this client?

Factors to Consider. What other diagnostic tests should be done? What are the treatment options for large renal stones?

BIBLIOGRAPHY

1. American Cancer Society. (1999). *Cancer facts and figures—1999.* Atlanta: Author.
2. Andriole, V. (1997). Urinary tract infections. *Infectious Disease Clinics of North America, 11*(3).
3. Appell, R. (1998). Periurethral injection therapy. In P. Walsh, et al. (Eds.), *Campbell's urology* (7th ed., pp. 1109–1120). Philadelphia: W. B. Saunders.
4. Atala, A., & Keating, M. (1998). Vesicoureteral reflux and megaureter. In P. Walsh, et al. (Eds.), *Campbell's urology* (7th ed., pp. 1859–1916). Philadelphia: W. B. Saunders.
5. Barrett, D., & Licht, M. (1998). Implantation of the artificial genitourinary sphincter in men and women. In P. Walsh, et al. (Eds.), *Campbell's urology* (7th ed., pp. 1121–1134). Philadelphia: W. B. Saunders.
6. Benson, M., & Olsson, C. (1998). Continent urinary diversion. In P. Walsh, et al. (Eds.), *Campbell's urology* (7th ed., pp. 3190–3246). Philadelphia: W. B. Saunders.
7. Bernier, F., & Harris, L. (1995). Treating stress incontinence with the bladder neck support prosthesis. *Urologic Nursing, 15*(1), 5–9.
8. Bernier, F., & Jenkins, P. (1997). The role of vaginal estrogen in the treatment of urogenital dysfunction in postmenopausal women. *Urologic Nursing, 17*(3), 92–95.
9. Blaivas, J., Ramanzi, L., & Heritz, D. (1998). Urinary incontinence: Pathophysiology, evaluation, treatment overview, and nonsurgical management. In P. Walsh, et al. (Eds.), *Campbell's urology* (7th ed., pp. 1007–1043). Philadelphia: W. B. Saunders.
10. Bowers, V., Hannigan, K. F., & Kushner, K. L. (1995). Bladder exstrophy and epispadias. In K. Karlowicz (Ed.), *Urologic nursing: Practice and principles* (pp. 565–592). Philadelphia: W. B. Saunders.
11. Burgio, K., et al. (1998). Behavioral vs drug treatment for urge urinary incontinence in older women. *Journal of the American Medical Association, 280*(23), 1995–2000.
12. Burton, D. S., et al. (1995). Urinary calculi. In K. Karlowicz (Ed.), *Urologic nursing: Practice and principles* (pp. 177–198). Philadelphia: W. B. Saunders.
13. Button, D., et al. (1998). Consensus guidelines for the promotion and management of continence by primary health care teams: Development, implementation and evaluation. *Journal of Advanced Nursing, 27*, 91–99.
14. Clayman, R., McDougall, E., & Nakada, S. (1998). Endourology of the upper urinary tract: Percutaneous renal and ureteral procedures. In P. Walsh, et al. (Eds.), *Campbell's urology* (7th ed., pp. 2789–2874). Philadelphia: W. B. Saunders.
15. Curhan, G., et al. (1998). Beverage use and risk for kidney stones in women. *Annals of Internal Medicine, 128*, 534–540.
16. Davila, G., & Bernier, F. (1995). Multimodality pelvic physiotherapy for urinary incontinence in women. *International Urogynecology Journal, 6*(4),185–194.
17. Droller, M. (1998). Bladder cancer: State-of-the-art care. *CA: A Cancer Journal for Clinicians, 48*(5), 269–284.
18. Engberg, S., et al. (1998). Treatment of urinary incontinence among caregiver-dependent adults. *Urologic Nursing, 18*(2), 131–136, 155.
19. Fabrizio, M., Behari, A., & Bagley, D. (1998). Ureteroscopic management of intrarenal calculi. *The Journal of Urology, 159*, 1139–1143.
20. Fantl, J. A., et al. (1996). *Urinary incontinence in adults: Acute and chronic management.* AHCPR Publication No. 96-0682. Clinical Practice Guideline, No. 2 (update). Rockville, MD: Agency for Health Care Policy and Research, Public Health Service, U.S. Department of Health and Human Services.
21. Getliffe, K., & Dolman, M. (1997). *Promoting continence: A clinical and research resource.* London: Bailliere Tindall.
22. Giroux, J. A. (1995). Urinary tract infections in adults. In K. Karlowicz (Ed.), *Urologic nursing: Principles and practice* (pp. 141–175). Philadelphia: W. B. Saunders.
23. Ghoniem, G., Elsergany, R., & Lewis, V. (1998). The evolving role of submucosal injectables for treating internal sphincteric deficiency. *Urologic Nursing, 18*(2), 125–130.
24. Gow, J. (1998). Genitourinary tuberculosis. In P. Walsh, et al. (Eds.), *Campbell's urology.* (7th ed., pp. 807–836). Philadelphia: W. B. Saunders.
25. Hanno, P. (1998). Interstitial cystitis and related diseases. In P. Walsh, et al. (Eds.), *Campbell's urology* (7th ed., pp. 631–662). Philadelphia: W. B. Saunders.
26. Hanson, M. (1998). *Pathophysiology: Foundations of disease and clinical intervention.* Philadelphia: W. B. Saunders.
27. Hinman, F. (1998). *Atlas of urologic surgery* (2nd ed.). Philadelphia: W. B. Saunders.
28. Huffman, J. (1998). Ureteroscopy. In P. Walsh, et al. (Eds.), *Campbell's urology* (7th ed., pp. 2755–2785). Philadelphia: W. B. Saunders.
29. Karram, M. M. (1996). Lower urinary tract infection. In D. Ostergard & A. Bent (Eds.), *Urogynecology and urodynamics: Theory and practice* (4th ed., pp. 387–408). Baltimore: Williams & Wilkins.
30. Karlowicz, K., & Meredith, C. (1995). Adult voiding disorders. In K. Karlowicz (Ed.), *Urologic nursing: Principles and practice* (pp. 377–408). Philadelphia: W. B. Saunders.
31. Kuo, R., et al. (1998). Impact of holmium laser settings and fiber diameter on stone fragmentation and endoscope deflection. *Journal of Endourology, 12*, 523–527.
32. Leek, C., et al. (1996). In R. McCorkle, et al. (Eds.), *Cancer nursing: A comprehensive textbook* (2nd ed., pp. 677–697). Philadelphia: W. B. Saunders.
33. Leonetti, F., et al. (1998). Dietary and urinary risk factors for stones in idiopathic calcium stone formers compared with healthy subjects. *Nephrology, Dialysis, and Transplantation, 13*(3), 617–622.
34. Lingeman, J., et al. (1999). Divergence between stone composition and urine supersaturation: Clinical and laboratory implications. *Journal of Urology, 161*, 1077–1081.
35. Lingeman, J., et al. (1998). Medical reduction of stone risk in a network of treatment centers compared to a research clinic. *Journal of Urology, 160*, 1629–1634.
36. Loughrey, L. (1999). Taking a sensitive approach to urinary incontinence. *Nursing, 29*(5), 60–61.
37. Marchiondo, K. (1998). A new look at urinary tract infection. *American Journal of Nursing, 98*(3), 34–39.
38. Marshall, F. (1998). Surgery of the bladder. In P. Walsh, et al. (Eds.), *Campbell's urology* (7th ed., pp. 3274–3298). Philadelphia: W. B. Saunders.
39. Martin, T., & Sosa, R. (1998). Shock-wave lithotripsy. In P. Walsh, et al. (Eds.), *Campbell's urology* (7th ed., pp. 2735–2752). Philadelphia: W. B. Saunders.
40. Massey, L., & Kynast-Gales, S. (1998). Substituting milk for apple juice does not increase kidney stone risk in most normocalciuric

adults who form calcium oxalate stones. *Journal of the American Dietetic Association, 98*(3), 303–308.

41. McDougall, W. (1998). Use of intestinal segments and urinary diversion. In P. Walsh, et al. (Eds.), *Campbell's urology* (7th ed., pp. 3121–3161). Philadelphia: W. B. Saunders.

42. McGuire, E., & O'Connell, H. (1998). Pubovaginal slings. In P. Walsh, et al. (Eds.), *Campbell's urology* (7th ed., pp. 1103–1108). Philadelphia: W. B. Saunders.

43. Menon, M., Parulkar, B., & Drach, G. (1998). Urinary lithiasis: Etiology, diagnosis, and medical management. In P. Walsh, et al. (Eds.), *Campbell's urology* (7th ed., pp. 2661–2734). Philadelphia: W. B. Saunders.

44. Messing, E., & Catalona, W. (1998). Urothelial tumors of the urinary tract. In P. Walsh, et al. (Eds.), *Campbell's urology* (7th ed., pp. 2327–2382). Philadelphia: W. B. Saunders.

45. Montagnino, B., Welch, V., Hoyler-Grant, C. (1995). Congenital anomalies that affect the kidney, ureter, and bladder. In K. Karlowicz (Ed.), *Urologic nursing: Principles and practice* (pp. 526–564). Philadelphia: W. B. Saunders.

46. Moody, F. (Ed.). (1999). *Atlas of ambulatory surgery.* Philadelphia: W. B. Saunders.

47. Morris, R. (1999). Female genital mutilation: Perspectives, risks, and complications. *Urologic Nursing, 19*(1), 13–19.

48. Nicolle, L. E. (1996). Uncomplicated urinary tract infection in women. In W. R. Cattel (Ed.), *Infections of the kidney and urinary tract.* New York: Oxford University Press.

49. Nyman, M., Schwenk, N., & Silverstein, M. (1997). Management of urinary retention: Rapid versus gradual decompression and risk of complications. *Mayo Clinic Proceedings, 72,* 951–956.

50. Parsons, C. L. (1996). Interstitial cystitis. In D. Ostergard & A. Bent (Eds.), *Urogynecology and urodynamics: Theory and practice* (4th ed., pp. 409–425). Baltimore: Williams & Wilkins.

51. Raz, S. (1996). *Female urology* (2nd ed.). Philadelphia: W. B. Saunders.

52. Raz, S., Stothers, L., & Chopra, A. (1998). Vaginal reconstructive surgery for incontinence and prolapse. In P. Walsh, et al. (Eds.), *Campbell's urology* (7th ed., pp. 1059–1094). Philadelphia: W. B. Saunders.

53. Reilly, N. J. (1995). Cancer of the bladder. In K. Karlowicz (Ed.), *Urologic nursing: Principles and practice* (pp. 243–270). Philadelphia: W. B. Saunders.

54. Reilly, N. J. (1995). Genitourinary trauma. In K. Karlowicz (Ed.), *Urologic nursing: Principles and practice* (pp. 411–435). Philadelphia: W. B. Saunders.

55. Rondorf-Klym, L., Colling, J., & Simonson, W. (1998). Medication use by community-dwelling elderly with urinary incontinence. *Urologic Nursing, 18*(3), 201–206.

56. Schaeffer, A. (1998). Infections and inflammations of the genitourinary tract. In P. Walsh, et al. (Eds.), *Campbell's urology* (7th ed., pp. 531–614). Philadelphia: W. B. Saunders.

57. Society of Urologic Nurses and Associates. (1997). *Scope and standards of urologic nursing practice.* Pitman, NJ: Author.

58. Steers, W. (1998). Physiology and pharmacology of the bladder and ureter. In P. Walsh, et al. (Eds.), *Campbell's urology* (7th ed., pp. 870–916.). Philadelphia: W. B. Saunders.

59. Stockert, P. (1999). Getting UTI clients back on track. *RN, 62*(3), 49–52.

60. Stone, J., Wyman, J., & Salisbury, S. (1999). *Clinical gerontological nursing: A guide to advanced practice* (2nd ed.). Philadelphia: W. B. Saunders.

61. Swibold, L. (1999). Maintenance therapy with bacillus Calmette-Guérin in clients with superficial bladder cancer. *Urologic Nursing, 19*(1), 38–41.

62. Urinary Incontinence Guideline Panel. (1992). *Urinary incontinence in adults: A client's guide.* AHCPR Publication No. 92-0040. Rockville, MD: Agency for Health Care Policy and Research, Public Health Service, U.S. Department of Health and Human Services.

63. Urinary Incontinence Guideline Panel. (1992). *Urinary incontinence in adults: Clinical practice guideline.* AHCPR Publication No. 92-0038. Rockville, MD: Agency for Health Care Policy and Research, Public Health Service, U.S. Department of Health and Human Services.

64. Urinary Incontinence Guideline Panel. (1992). *Urinary incontinence in adults: Quick reference guide for clinicians.* AHCPR Publication No. 92-0041. Rockville, MD: Agency for Health Care Policy and Research, Public Health Service, U.S. Department of Health and Human Services.

65. Walsh, P., et al. (Eds.). (1998). *Campbell's urology* (7th ed.). Philadelphia: W. B. Saunders.

66. Webster, G., & Khoury, J. (1998). Retropubic suspension surgery for female sphincteric incontinence. In P. Walsh, et al. (Eds.), *Campbell's urology* (7th ed., pp. 1095–1102). Philadelphia: W. B. Saunders.

67. Wein, A. (1998). Neuromuscular dysfunction of the lower urinary tract and its treatment. In P. Walsh, et al. (Eds.), *Campbell's urology* (7th ed., pp. 953–1006). Philadelphia: W. B. Saunders.

68. Wein, A. (1998). Pathophysiology and categorization of voiding dysfunction. In P. Walsh, et al. (Eds.), *Campbell's urology* (7th ed., pp. 917–926). Philadelphia: W. B. Saunders.

69. Wein, A. (1998). Physiology and pharmacology of the renal pelvis and ureter. In P. Walsh, et al. (Eds.), *Campbell's urology* (7th ed., pp. 839–869). Philadelphia: W. B. Saunders.

70. Wolfish, N. (1997). Caring for the renal client. In D. Levine (Ed.), *Pediatric nephrology* (3rd ed., pp. 108–130). Philadelphia: W. B. Saunders.

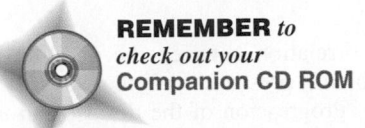

CHAPTER 35

Management of Clients with Renal Disorders

Anita E. Molzahn

NURSING OUTCOMES CLASSIFICATION (NOC)
for Nursing Diagnoses—Clients with Renal Disorders

Altered Health Maintenance
Health-Promoting Behavior
Health-Seeking Behavior
Knowledge: Health Behaviors
Knowledge: Health Promotion
Self-Direction of Care
Altered Nutrition: Less Than Body Requirements
Nutritional Status: Food and Fluid Intake
Anxiety
Anxiety Control
Coping
Fatigue
Activity Tolerance
Endurance

Energy Conservation
Nutritional Status: Energy
Fluid Volume Excess
Fluid Balance
Hydration
Pain
Comfort Level
Pain Control
Pain: Disruptive Effects
Pain Level
Risk for Fluid Volume Deficit
Bowel Elimination
Fluid Balance
Hydration
Knowledge: Medication

Knowledge: Treatment Regimen
Urinary Elimination
Risk for Impaired Skin Integrity
Nutritional Status
Tissue Integrity: Skin and Mucous
   Membranes
Tissue Perfusion: Peripheral
Risk for Infection
Immune Status
Risk Control
Risk Detection
Risk for Injury
Risk Control
Risk Detection
Symptom Control

The kidneys regulate the body's fluid, electrolyte, and acid-base balances while removing toxic substances from the blood and excreting them in urine. The kidneys also play a significant role in erythropoietin and prostaglandin synthesis, in insulin degradation, and in the renin-angiotensin-aldosterone system.

This chapter identifies the common disease processes and injuries that can interfere with normal renal function. Although the effects of extrarenal influences on the kidneys are briefly described, the primary purpose of this chapter is to discuss specific renal pathologic processes. Some of these disorders can result in renal failure (see Chapter 36). Because of the potential seriousness of any renal problem, the client and significant others have physical as well as psychological needs. You need to know about both aspects and should maintain a consistent awareness of the need for appropriate intervention.

EXTRARENAL CONDITIONS

Many conditions primarily located in other parts of the body affect the kidneys, such as diabetes mellitus, hypertension, and sepsis. This chapter provides a brief description of the renal implications of these extrarenal

conditions. For further discussion, see Chapters 45, 52, and 81.

DIABETES MELLITUS

One of the most common extrarenal diseases affecting the kidney is diabetes mellitus. *Diabetic nephropathy*, a progressive process, commonly leads to renal failure. About 30% of clients with end-stage renal disease (ESRD) have diabetes mellitus. Researchers estimate that 25% to 50% of clients with insulin-dependent diabetes mellitus (IDDM, or type 1 diabetes) have end-stage renal disease within 10 to 20 years of beginning insulin therapy. Renal disease can also occur in the non–insulin-dependent diabetic client. The incidence of proteinuria is about 25% after 20 years of diabetes.

Several pathologic changes lead to renal failure in clients who have diabetes mellitus. The most common is a characteristic intercapillary *glomerulosclerosis*, or scarring of the capillary loops. Progressive microangiopathy, called *nephrosclerosis*, affects the afferent and efferent arterioles and eventually scars the glomerulus, tubules, and interstitium. *Pyelonephritis* (kidney infection) can scar the renal parenchyma and lead to ischemia. It may also lead to renal papillary necrosis and sloughing of the papillae. *Neurogenic bladder* dysfunction may contribute to renal failure. The high incidence of urinary tract infection or the increased pressure in the kidney caused by the back-up of urine may also contribute to renal dysfunction.

Initially, the sclerotic, or hardening, process of glomerulosclerosis increases renal vascular resistance, contributing to systemic hypertension. This does not cause renal insufficiency. Indeed, the glomerular filtration rate (GFR) may increase as much as 20% to 50% above the normal GFR during this early "silent" phase. It is now recognized that microalbuminemia (measurable by assay) occurs quite some time before clinical proteinuria. If it is diagnosed, it may be a much earlier indicator of eventual renal failure. As more nephrons are destroyed, available functioning renal tissue decreases and the client begins to show clinical proteinuria (a key manifestation), hypertension, edema, and evidence of renal failure.

The kidney metabolizes 30% to 40% of insulin, and as renal function declines, the degradation of insulin also decreases, resulting in a lower insulin requirement. Renal failure may be initially identified when the client is evaluated for recurrent insulin reactions. Researchers hope the sclerotic process can be slowed by:

- Carefully controlling hypertension
- Adjusting insulin therapy and carefully monitoring blood glucose to maintain euglycemia
- Restricting dietary protein

Regardless of diabetic control, however, renal failure inevitably develops within 5 to 10 years after the appearance of significant proteinuria.

HYPERTENSION

Because the kidneys receive quite a large share of cardiac output, renal function can affect or be affected by cardiovascular changes. Renal blood flow determines the GFR, which directly affects renal function. Hypertension is one condition that can either cause or be affected by renal disease. For example, renovascular hypertension results from renal artery stenosis or renal infarction. The reduction in renal blood flow activates the renin-angiotensin-aldosterone system and increases systemic blood pressure.

Renal hypertension associated with parenchymal renal disease (e.g., glomerulonephritis, polycystic disease, pyelonephritis) usually results from the kidney's decreasing ability to excrete salt and water. Other causes include increased renin release from increased glomerular perfusion and inadequacy of renal vasodilating substances, as occurs with analgesic nephropathy. Among clients with renal failure, 80% to 85% of hypertension results from excess salt and water retention; renovascular hypertension accounts for up to 15% of all systemic hypertension.

On the other hand, sustained systemic high blood pressure adversely affects the kidneys. Researchers report that nephrosclerosis can be seen microscopically in clients who have had uncontrolled hypertension for more than 5 years, although all other renal diagnostic tests may be normal. Kidney damage is the direct result of degenerative changes in the arterioles and interlobular arteries caused by increased blood pressure.

There is a direct correlation between the duration and degree of elevated blood pressure and the severity of renal vascular disease. Progression of the disease can usually be halted or slowed by controlling blood pressure. Client teaching is vital to managing the hypertension and preventing renal failure.

HYPOTENSION

Cardiovascular shock, or hypotension, also affects renal function. Renal vasoconstriction reduces renal blood flow. However, because of the autoregulation capabilities of the kidneys (see Chapters 12, 32, and 81), GFR remains at a functional level until the advanced stages of systemic shock, at which time acute renal failure develops. Restoring systemic blood pressure usually reverses the renal vasoconstriction, and kidney function returns, typically within 2 to 8 weeks as long as prolonged ischemia has not occurred. A period of polyuria (excessive urination) may follow the correction of hypovolemia, although the mechanisms for this are unclear.

Before renal function returns to normal, another oliguric period may occur, followed by a "mobilization phase" in which sequestered fluid is shifted into the intravascular space. The shift may cause some hypertension until the kidneys can remove the extra fluid. Careful assessment of the client's fluid status and meticulous fluid management are crucial during these recovery phases.

RHABDOMYOLYSIS

Rhabdomyolysis is a disorder usually associated with traumatic injury of skeletal muscle tissue, which releases myoglobin and intracellular substances into the blood. It can also occur after serious crush injuries, strenuous exercise, seizures, heat stroke, prolonged coma, and drug overdose. The resulting acute renal failure is usually reversible with treatment.

Clinical evidence of rhabdomyolysis includes fever, malaise, nausea, vomiting, muscular weakness, pain, and swelling. The release of substances from damaged muscles results in myoglobinemia, myoglobinuria (which can be seen as brown urine and confirmed through urinalysis), hyperkalemia, hyperphosphatemia, hyperuricemia, and elevated creatine kinase. Hypocalcemia occurs initially because of the precipitation of calcium with phosphate. Later, in the diuretic phase of acute renal failure, hypercalcemia can occur as calcium is mobilized.

Treatment is typically symptomatic, including bed rest to reduce muscle metabolism and steps to correct acidosis and maintain normal fluid volume.

CARDIOVASCULAR DISEASE

Cardiac disease influences kidney function primarily through its effect on cardiac output and circulating blood volume. The hemodynamic and hormonal changes of cardiac disease may decrease the kidneys' ability to excrete sodium and water. This, in turn, increases intravascular congestion and edema and establishes a pathologic cycle.

Hemodynamic changes also occur with normal aging. Blood flow to the kidneys decreases by up to half by age

70 years, and GFR can decrease by 40% to 50% as well. Renal function deteriorates as glomeruli become sclerotic and atrophy.

PERIPHERAL VASCULAR DISEASE

Thromboembolic disease can affect the renal circulation and cause infarction of the tissue supplied by the affected blood vessel. In clients with sickle cell disease, the interstitial hypertonicity and low oxygen pressure found in the renal medulla seem to favor sickling of red blood cells in the kidney's juxtamedullary region. These cell masses cause gross hematuria as venules rupture, papillary necrosis, renal infarction, concentrating disturbances resulting from interference with the countercurrent mechanism, nephrotic syndrome, pyelonephritis, and, finally, renal failure.

In disseminated intravascular coagulation, in which diffuse clotting consumes clotting factors and causes hemorrhage in affected areas throughout the body, the kidney is the organ most affected.

SEPSIS

Extrarenal sepsis may affect kidney function either through its effect on systemic circulation or by stimulating the immune system. Renal reactions to septic shock are similar to those in hypotension. Immunologic injury can lead to glomerulonephritis (see later). Occasionally, pathogens may break away from extrarenal foci of infection and travel to the kidney to establish additional sites.

PREGNANCY

Pregnancy has a definite influence on kidney function. During the first trimester, the collecting system dilates and the kidneys enlarge, a condition that may persist 9 to 12 weeks after delivery. Renal blood flow and GFR increase by 30% to 50% during pregnancy, contributing to increased creatinine clearance and decreased uric acid excretion. These normal changes (such as lower serum creatinine) must be taken into account in interpreting laboratory findings for pregnant women. Pregnancy also increases the likelihood of proteinuria (usually transient), polyuria, and nocturia (excessive urination at night). These disorders may be caused by external bladder compression and alterations in antidiuretic hormone metabolism.

OTHER CAUSES

Kidney function is influenced by many other extrarenal disease processes, such as cancer, connective tissue disorders, and metabolic disturbances. Many systemic diseases produce clinical manifestations like those of glomerulonephritis, although they typically have other systemic features characteristic of the disease (see glomerulonephritis later). These diseases include systemic lupus erythematosus, systemic scleroderma, polyarteritis nodosa, thrombocytopenic purpura, Wegener's granulomatosis, hemolytic-uremic syndrome, gout, amyloidosis, and Henoch-Schönlein syndrome. Diagnosis can be confirmed by renal biopsy.

Renal disease has become an increasingly common complication for people infected with the human immunodeficiency virus (HIV). Among the several renal disorders associated with HIV and acquired immunodeficiency syndrome (AIDS) are renal tuberculosis and cytomegalovirus, such malignancies as lymphoma and Kaposi's sarcoma, and HIV-associated nephropathy, a focal glomerulosclerosis that is manifested by nephrotic syndrome (see later).

NEPHROTOXINS

Nephrotoxins have specific, destructive effects on renal cells. They can cause the following types of renal injury:

- Acute tubular necrosis
- Defects in the tubular transport system
- Interstitial nephritis
- Vasculitis
- Nephrotic syndrome

Nephrotoxic substances in the environment include heavy metals, such as mercurial compounds, lead, cadmium, bismuth, arsenic, copper, and phosphorus; carbon tetrachloride; ethylene glycol; trichloroethylene; carbon monoxide; and chlorinated hydrocarbons. Exposure to many of these substances occurs in industrial locations. Other environmental nephrotoxins include snake venom and certain mushrooms. Acute tubular necrosis is the most frequent injury resulting from exposure to nephrotoxins. Some nephrotoxins also cause tubular transport defects and nephrotic syndrome. Box 35–1 presents some common nephrotoxic substances.

All five types of kidney damage may result from nephrotoxic reactions to medications. Two types of medications well known to cause renal damage are antibiotics and certain analgesics. Because the kidneys are the major

---

BOX 35–1 Nephrotoxins

Antibiotics	Anesthetics
Aminoglycosides	**Contrast Dyes**
Tetracyclines	
Amphotericin B	**Organic Solvents**
Cephalosporins	Glycols
Sulfonamides	Gasoline
(co-trimoxazole)	Kerosene
Bacitracin	Turpentine
Polymyxin	Tetrachloroethylene
Colistin	
Heavy Metals	**Other Drugs**
Lead	Acetaminophen
Mercury	Nonsteroidal anti-inflammatory
Arsenic	medications
Copper	Salicylates
Gold	Heroin
Lithium	Dextran
	Mannitol
Poisons	Interleukin-2
	Cisplatin
Mushrooms	Amphetamines
Insecticides	
Herbicides	
Snake bites	

route of excretion for many antibiotics, renal tissue is directly exposed to these compounds. The longer the exposure, the higher the risk of renal toxic effects. Pre-existing renal disease, decreased renal blood flow, electrolyte imbalances, and concurrent use of other nephrotoxic medications enhance a medication's nephrotoxic effect.

High-risk antibiotics include cephalosporins, sulfonamides, polymyxins, aminoglycosides, and amphotericin B. Carefully monitor renal function tests to identify early nephrotoxic reactions so that causative medications can be discontinued or the dose decreased. Closely monitor drug levels to make sure that dosages stay in the therapeutic range. Besides using these medications as briefly as possible and at as low a dose as possible, maintaining a high fluid intake may help prevent nephrotoxic effects. A high urine output keeps the medication diluted in the kidney and helps prevent crystallization.

The risk of renal damage caused by excessive use of certain analgesics has been receiving more attention. Salicylates, acetaminophen, phenacetin, and nonsteroidal anti-inflammatory drugs (NSAIDs) are the most common nephrotoxic agents. Short-term overdose or long-term consistent use of these medications may cause acute tubular necrosis or chronic renal failure. Researchers estimate that 5% to 10% of clients with end-stage renal disease have analgesic nephropathy.

Anesthesia reduces the kidney's vasoconstrictive ability, which helps protect it against systemic blood pressure drops; thus, the kidney is made more vulnerable to the effects of shock. In addition, certain anesthetics, particularly methoxyflurane, have a direct nephrotoxic effect. Administration of this general anesthetic agent can cause acute tubular necrosis and has been associated with fatal acute renal failure. Halothane may also adversely affect renal function.

Diuretics may have nephrotoxic effects as well and, when used aggressively, can cause hypovolemia. Other common medications that may have nephrotoxic effects include probenecid, phenytoin, low-molecular-weight dextran, rifampin, phenindione, lithium, and gold. You must know about the possible adverse effects of any medication a client takes so that you can assess and intervene appropriately.

Radioiodinated contrast agents used in radiographic and computed tomographic (CT) studies have been associated with acute tubular necrosis. Risk factors include:

- Age older than 60 years
- Pre-existing renal insufficiency, especially diabetic nephropathy
- Dehydration
- Low cardiac output with pre-existing renal disease
- Proteinuria
- Hypoalbuminemia
- Multiple myeloma
- Multiple contrast studies within a 24-hour period

Using non-dye studies whenever possible and keeping the client well hydrated throughout the test reduce the risk of acute renal failure. Baseline renal function tests before the contrast study should be available to compare with post-test findings. Monitor the client's urine output carefully for several hours after the study is completed.

ACQUIRED DISORDERS

NEPHROLITHIASIS

Although calculi (stones) can form anywhere in the urinary tract, the most frequent site is the kidney. These stones may travel down the urinary tract, lodge anywhere along the tract, and cause obstruction and tissue damage. Or they may stay in the kidney. Urolithiasis is described in detail in Chapter 34.

Treatment and nursing care of clients with renal calculi are similar to those of people with calculi lower in the urinary tract. However, damage to the kidney caused by calculi can be permanent and may require nephrectomy (described later).

PYELONEPHRITIS

Pyelonephritis is an inflammation of the renal pelvis and parenchyma caused by a bacterial infection. The cause may be an active infection in the kidney or the remnants of a previous infection. There are two main types of pyelonephritis: acute and chronic. They differ primarily in their clinical picture and long-term effects.

Etiology and Risk Factors

Sometimes an infection may be a primary disease, as happens with reduced host resistance (e.g., calculi, malignancy, hydronephrosis, or trauma). Most kidney infections, however, are extensions of infectious processes located elsewhere, especially the bladder. Chapter 34 discusses the etiologic mechanism and pathogenesis of infections in the lower urinary tract.

The bacteria spread to the kidney primarily by ascending the ureter to the kidney. Blood and lymphatic circulation also provide channels for the organisms. Ureteral reflux, which allows infected urine back into the ureter, and obstruction, which causes urine to back into the ureter and allows organisms to multiply, are the most common causes of ascending urinary tract infections. *Escherichia coli* is the most common bacterial organism causing pyelonephritis.

Health promotion is key to preventing recurrence of infection and further renal damage. The nurse provides information to clients about health and lifestyle measures to prevent urinary tract infections, including (1) perineal hygiene measures such as wiping from front to back, (2) acidification of the urine (by drinking cranberry juice or taking ascorbic acid), and (3) ensuring adequate fluid intake. Early detection and adequate treatment of lower urinary tract infections greatly reduce the incidence of pyelonephritis.

After infection, health maintenance includes education about the importance of completing the course of antibiotics. Follow-up cultures are important with recurrent pyelonephritis to ensure that the infection has been eradicated. Health restoration measures depend on the extent of renal damage and the cause of the disease. If obstruction precipitated the infection, the cause of the obstruction must be treated.

ACUTE PYELONEPHRITIS. Acute pyelonephritis often occurs after bacterial contamination of the urethra or after introduction of an instrument, such as a catheter or a cystoscope.

CHRONIC PYELONEPHRITIS. Chronic pyelonephritis is more likely to occur after chronic obstruction with reflux or chronic disorders. It is slowly progressive and usually associated with recurrent acute attacks, although there may be no history of acute pyelonephritis.

Pathophysiology

Pyelonephritis occurs when bacteria enter the renal pelvis, causing an inflammatory response and an increase in white blood cells (WBCs). The inflammation leads to edema and swelling of the involved tissue, beginning at the papillae and sometimes spreading to the cortex. The infection can be either ascending, as occurs after cystitis or prostatitis, or descending, as from a streptococcal infection in the bloodstream.

As the infection is treated and the inflammation recedes, fibrosis and scar tissue may develop. The calices become blunted with scarring in the interstitial tissues. If the infection recurs, more and more scar tissue develops; fibrosis and altered tubular reabsorption and secretion lead to decreased renal function.

ACUTE PYELONEPHRITIS. Acute pyelonephritis is associated with the development of renal abscesses, perinephric abscesses, emphysematous pyelonephritis, and chronic pyelonephritis that can lead to renal failure.

Acute pyelonephritis is usually brief. It often recurs, however, either as a relapse of a previous infection not eradicated or as a new infection; 20% of these recurrences take place within 2 weeks after completion of therapy. A client must be treated adequately to prevent the development of chronic pyelonephritis. The infection may also progress to bacteremia.

CHRONIC PYELONEPHRITIS. This disease is characterized by a combination of caliceal abnormalities and overlying cortical scarring. The kidney becomes contracted, and the number of functioning nephrons decreases as they are replaced by scar tissue. Renal failure may ensue, although uremia is less common than once thought.

Clinical Manifestations

ACUTE PYELONEPHRITIS. Acute pyelonephritis is characterized by enlarged kidneys, focal parenchymal abscesses, and accumulation of polymorphonuclear lymphocytes around and in the renal tubules. Typically, the client seems to be in acute distress, although the disorder may cause minimal or no manifestations.

Assessment usually reveals high fever, chills, nausea, flank pain on the affected side (costovertebral angle [CVA] tenderness), headache, muscle pain, and general prostration. The pain commonly radiates down the ureter or toward the epigastrium and may be colicky if the infection is complicated by calculi or sloughed renal papillae. Percussion or deep palpation over the CVA elicits marked tenderness. Commonly, the client has experienced dysuria, frequency, urgency, and other evidence of cystitis for several days. The urine may be cloudy or bloody, is foul smelling, and shows a marked increase in WBCs and casts. Chapter 32 describes assessment of the renal system.

Urine culture and sensitivity studies, along with a physical examination, are the primary diagnostic tests. Studies may be done to detect calculi, especially with recurrent infections, because calculi may seed and cause reinfection, particularly with *Proteus*. X-ray studies, as of the kidney, ureter, and bladder (a KUB study), and intravenous pyelography (IVP) are commonly done. A cystourethrogram may be obtained, especially after an initial episode of pyelonephritis, to look for underlying defects, particularly any cause of reflux. Magnetic resonance imaging (MRI) or a CT scan may also be used to evaluate the kidney size or the presence of other problems.

CHRONIC PYELONEPHRITIS. This disease has no specific manifestations of its own. Thus, it is usually discovered incidentally when the client is being evaluated for hypertension or its complications. Hypertension itself is the most frequent manifestation of the disease.

Abnormal laboratory studies may show azotemia, pyuria, anemia, acidosis, and proteinuria. They may also demonstrate poor urine-concentrating ability.

Outcome Management

▮ Medical Management

ACUTE PYELONEPHRITIS

Ideal outcomes of medical management include:

- Elimination of the pathogenic organisms with appropriate antibiotics, as identified by urine culture and sensitivity studies
- Removal of any factor or disease contributing to decreased host resistance

If calculi or other obstructions are found to be the cause of recurrent infection, appropriate treatment is instituted.

INHIBIT BACTERIAL GROWTH. Antibiotic therapy is based on the results of urine culture and sensitivity tests. Typically, a broad-spectrum antibiotic is prescribed; it may be changed after the results of the culture are available. Sulfonamides or the combination of sulfamethoxazole and trimethoprim is commonly used as first-line therapy unless the client is allergic to one of these drugs. Typically, antibiotic therapy continues for 10 days to 2 weeks.

Antibiotics may be administered orally or by the single large-dose method described in Chapter 34. In severe cases of acute pyelonephritis, intravenous antibiotics may be administered. With oral therapy, the client must understand that completing the full course of antibiotic therapy is important to prevent recurrence of the infection. Recurrent infections are commonly treated with long-term prophylactic antibiotic therapy. Additional pharmacologic therapy may be needed to correct any predisposing factors.

RELIEVE PAIN. Analgesic or urinary antiseptic medications can be prescribed to reduce discomfort. Antibiotics quickly reduce discomfort as well.

CHRONIC PYELONEPHRITIS

The desired outcome of medical management is prevention of further renal damage. If bacteria are found, appropriate antibiotics are given, as in acute pyelonephritis. Chronic pyelonephritis tends to be less painful. Above all, hypertension must be controlled. Additional intervention depends on the degree of renal failure that has already occurred. Although high fluid intake may be advisable in acute pyelonephritis, it may be contraindicated in chronic pyelonephritis if the degree of renal dysfunction is significant.

INHIBIT BACTERIAL GROWTH. Antibiotics specific to the bacteria present are given to treat chronic pyelonephritis (see Chapter 34 and Acute Pyelonephritis).

CONTROL HYPERTENSION. Renal damage can cause hypertension, which can cause further renal damage. Thus, it is important to control the client's blood pressure. Reduction of dietary sodium and pharmacologic therapy may be indicated. Management of hypertension is discussed in Chapters 34 and 52.

Nursing Management of the Medical Client

ASSESSMENT

Assessment of the client with pyelonephritis begins with a thorough history and physical examination, with close attention to the presence of risk factors, previous urinary tract infections, hypertension, and CVA tenderness. Look for evidence of pyelonephritis.

DIAGNOSIS, OUTCOMES, INTERVENTIONS

Risk for Fluid Volume Deficit. A common diagnosis is *Risk for Fluid Volume Deficit related to fever, nausea, vomiting, and possible diarrhea.*

Outcomes. The client will remain free from fluid volume deficit, as evidenced by balanced intake and output, maintenance of adequate hydration, and an absence of signs or symptoms of dehydration.

Interventions. Prepare the client for the diagnostic tests and probable antibiotic therapy. Clients with severe nausea and vomiting may require intravenous fluids. Keep in mind that overhydration may dilute antimicrobials, diminishing their effectiveness. See Chapter 34 on the nursing care of the client with cystitis.

Pain. Another common diagnosis is *Pain related to an inflammatory process in the kidney and possible colic.*

Outcomes. The client will report no pain or will report that pain is controlled.

Interventions. Medications can be given to control pain caused by calculi. CVA tenderness should decrease as the antibiotics control the infection. Medication for nausea can be given as needed with antipyretics for high fevers. Adequate treatment of the infection quickly reverses the dysuria, pyuria, and frequency. Urinary analgesics (see Chapter 34) can also help the client with these problems. Fluid intake of 3 to 4 L/day is recommended. This fluid helps to dilute the urine and to reduce irritation and burning. The continual flow of urine serves to prevent stasis and discourage multiplication of bacteria in the urinary tract.

Altered Health Maintenance. Client teaching is important to promote self-care and prevent recurrent infections. Write the diagnosis *Altered Health Maintenance related to prevention of recurrent infections.*

Outcomes. The client will understand how to prevent recurrent infections, as evidenced by the client's statements and no recurrence of infection.

Interventions. The preventive measures for acute and chronic pyelonephritis are similar to those for cystitis (see Chapter 34). It is important to prevent permanent renal damage. Make sure that the client can recognize the manifestations of a urinary tract infection and knows to seek prompt medical attention when they occur.

When the acute infection subsides, instruct the client to continue follow-up care. This care includes completing the full course of antibiotic therapy and having repeated urine cultures. Also, teach ways to prevent further infections in the urinary tract, including ensuring a high fluid intake (see Chapter 34).

It is vital that the client return for follow-up urine cultures and possibly other diagnostic tests if the cause of the pyelonephritis is not clear. Emphasize that follow-up cultures are important because bacteriuria may be present but may produce no manifestations. Advise the client to report any manifestations of recurrence immediately so that retreatment can begin.

EVALUATION

The infection should subside with adequate antibiotic treatment. Successful management results in reduced pain and negative findings on follow-up urine cultures. The client must also be made aware of the cause of this infection and ways to prevent further infections (see Chapter 34).

Self-Care

The focus of client self-care is to maintain high levels of fluid intake and prevent recurrence of infection. If manifestations arise, the client must report them promptly and begin treatment to prevent further renal damage.

Modification for Elderly Clients

In older clients, the kidneys may be less able to recover from a severe infection. Antibiotic therapy should be monitored closely because older adults may vary in their sensitivity and response to the medication. Older adults may also have altered blood levels of antibiotics because renal perfusion decreases with age, reducing the kidney's ability to excrete drugs.

RENAL CANDIDIASIS

Bacteria cause most cases of pyelonephritis, but the incidence of renal candidiasis, a fungal infection, is increasing. Primary renal candidiasis is most common in women with diabetes mellitus. Clinical manifestations include ureteral obstruction secondary to a bezoar (tangled hyphae or clumps of yeast cells); progressive oliguria, sometimes alternating with episodic diuresis; ureteral colic; passing tissue or stone-like material; pyuria; and progressive renal failure. Diagnosis is based on the presence of fungi in several properly collected urine cultures; the presence of serum *Candida* precipitins; and selected radiologic findings, such as hydronephrosis, caliceal erosion, and filling defects called fungus balls.

Amphotericin B and flucytosine are the keys to medical management, although these medications require careful administration and monitoring of dosage to prevent nephrotoxicity. In clients with severe disease, surgery or nephrectomy may be needed to remove the obstruction.

RENAL TUBERCULOSIS

Tuberculosis of the kidney, which affects men more than women, occurs when the causative organism, *Mycobacterium tuberculosis*, reaches the kidney via the bloodstream from another source in the body, usually the lungs. In the kidney, the organism may become dormant for many years. By the time it again becomes active, the original infection is often well healed. Frequently, the primary tubercular site is asymptomatic, which makes it difficult to identify renal tuberculosis on the basis of history.

Clinical Manifestations

The clinical course of renal tuberculosis is generally indolent, and clinical manifestations often do not become evident until the later stages of the disease. Early disease involves the renal cortex or medulla. Tissue destruction extends in all directions, eventually eroding into a calix at the tip of the papilla and progressing to rupture into the renal pelvis. When the infection reaches the pelvis, it spreads along the mucosa. The causative organisms then have full access to the rest of the kidney and can move down the urinary tract and infect any of the urinary organs. If untreated, this destructive process continues to form large, caseating masses that coalesce and destroy kidney tissue. X-ray examination at this time shows a moth-eaten appearance of the kidneys.

Organisms that reach the lower urinary tract usually cause fibrosis, stricture formation, and destruction of the ureterovesical valve. If these processes result in stenosis (narrowing) of the ureter, reducing the exit for pus and urine from the infected kidney, renal destruction accelerates. Descending tubercle bacilli may also lodge in the male reproductive organs, causing reduced function.

When renal tuberculosis becomes evident, assessment findings are often nonspecific. Renal manifestations may be preceded by general malaise, weight loss, low-grade fever, and night sweats, but these are not as frequent as with pulmonary tuberculosis. Manifestations of cystitis, as described in Chapter 34, commonly form the client's chief complaint. Flank pain may be present, and hematuria and pyuria are common. Males frequently have evidence of epididymitis.

Growth of *M. tuberculosis* in a culture of the urine confirms the diagnosis. Culture specimens are collected on at least three successive mornings. Because tubercle bacilli are shed intermittently, three to 12 negative cultures are needed to rule out active renal tuberculosis.

Outcome Management

▪ Medical Management

Chemotherapy with antitubercular agents has reduced the need for surgical intervention. Therapy that combines several medications (rifampin, ethambutol, isoniazid, and pyridoxine, for example, or streptomycin, cycloserine, and sodium para-aminosalicylate) is the most common intervention. Because tubercle bacilli divide slowly, the medications are usually given in a single daily dose. If side effects develop, the day's dose may be divided. See Chapter 62 for further information on antitubercular medications.

▪ Nursing Management of the Medical Client

During the acute phase, nursing interventions involve assisting with diagnostic procedures, protecting against the spread of causative organisms, providing relief of manifestations, and assisting the client with the medication regimen. Because tuberculosis arouses a great deal of fear and a feeling of social isolation, expect your nursing diagnoses to include fear and anxiety for the client as well as for significant others. Help the client discuss and work through feelings. Listen to the client's concerns, and make a referral for additional counseling if necessary.

▪ Surgical Management

Surgical intervention includes total or partial nephrectomy (discussed later) or cutaneous ureterostomy (see Chapter 34). Permanent urinary diversion may be necessary if strictures are severe or bladder damage is irreparable (see Chapter 34). Indications for surgery include persistent infection that fails to respond to chemotherapy, intractable pain, hemorrhage, uncontrollable hypertension, renal malignancy, and progressive strictures.

If surgery is needed, perioperative nursing intervention is similar to that for any client having major surgery (see Chapter 15).

▪ Self-Care

Renal tuberculosis is a prolonged illness that requires long-term care and support. Because the client is usually seen on an outpatient basis, instruction in self-care is important in maintaining and restoring health. One of the biggest challenges with clients recovering from renal tuberculosis is ensuring that they continue with the prescribed medical and nursing regimens, particularly when they begin to feel better. Help the client understand the need for continuing medication therapy and continuing follow-up examinations.

Explain the importance of maintaining general good health, such as proper nutrition, adequate rest, and good hygiene. Work in partnership with the client during recovery, and give the client positive feedback for taking medications regularly, if appropriate. If the client is not taking medications, help develop strategies that facilitate willingness to take medications.

RENAL ABSCESS

A renal abscess (renal carbuncle) is a localized infection in the cortex of the kidney. It can form when smaller infectious foci or microabscesses combine in the renal parenchyma. It is usually secondary to urinary tract infection with a species of Enterobacter and is often complicated by renal calculi and obstruction. Organisms from extrarenal sites may also cause this infectious process. For example, many clients report a history of recent cutaneous furuncles (boils).

Clients with renal abscess typically have high fever and moderate to severe pain. The pain is usually constant and located in the upper abdomen or the costovertebral area; it sometimes resembles renal colic. Unlike the findings in pyelonephritis, the urine is usually sterile because the abscess does not reach into the urinary collecting system. Other manifestations of this infectious process include weakness, anorexia, weight loss, night sweats, and leukocytosis.

Medical and nursing interventions for renal abscess resemble those for acute pyelonephritis. Aggressive antibiotic therapy is usually successful. Needle aspiration of the abscess may be done for culture and sensitivity studies, which help identify appropriate antimicrobial therapy. Surgical incision and drainage of the abscess are sometimes necessary. If incision and drainage are performed, nursing intervention expands to include postoperative care of the incision. A drain is left in place for some time.

PERINEPHRIC ABSCESS

A perinephric abscess involves the fatty tissue surrounding the kidney. It may be an extension of a renal infectious process (most common), or the organism may have spread in the bloodstream from an extrarenal site. The abscess may spread in several directions, extending to the peritoneal cavity, chest, or skin.

Assessment findings are the same as for a renal abscess—fever, tenderness, flank or loin pain, and other manifestations of sepsis—with the possible addition of swelling over the site.

Medical and nursing interventions are almost identical to those for renal abscess. Appropriate antibiotics are administered and symptomatic interventions undertaken. Because of the nature of a perinephric abscess, incising and draining are more likely than with a renal abscess. After this surgical procedure, there may be profuse drainage from the wound; frequent dressing changes and nursing interventions are required to prevent or treat skin excoriation.

HYDRONEPHROSIS

Hydronephrosis is distention of the renal pelvis and calices caused by an obstruction of normal urine flow. Urine production continues, and the urine is trapped proximal to the obstruction. Causes of occlusion include calculus, tumor, scar tissue, congenital structural defects, and a kink in the ureter.

Whatever the cause, the accumulating urine exerts pressure on the renal pelvis wall. At low to moderate pressures, the kidney may dilate with no obvious loss of function. Over time, sustained or intermittent high pressure causes irreversible nephron destruction. In addition to pressure-related problems, pyelonephritis is always a risk because of urinary stasis.

Outcome Management

■ Medical Management

Treatment aims to relieve the obstruction and prevent infection. Depending on the location of the obstruction, it may involve placement of a ureteral catheter or stent above the point of obstruction. Typically, surgery is required (see Chapter 34) to relieve the obstruction and restore adequate drainage of the urinary system.

Removal of the obstruction results in sudden release of the pressure on the renal parenchyma caused by the trapped urine, which leads to diuresis. Thus, postobstructive diuresis occurs and can lead to fluid and electrolyte imbalances, including dehydration. The kidney gradually begins to concentrate urine appropriately.

■ Nursing Management of the Medical Client
ASSESSMENT

Assessment of a client with hydronephrosis includes monitoring for the presence, location, intensity, and character of pain. Monitor urine output, and report manifestations of renal failure (oliguria, anorexia, lethargy), hematuria, and dysuria. Reduced urine output could indicate obstruction. Palpate the client's bladder to assess for any manifestations of distention. The kidneys, if palpated, may be tender.

DIAGNOSIS, OUTCOMES, INTERVENTIONS

Risk for Fluid Volume Deficit. *Risk for Fluid Volume Deficit related to increased urine output* is the most important nursing problem. Because of the dangers involved in postobstruction diuresis, it is crucial to monitor the client closely after an obstruction is released.

Outcomes. The client will remain free of a fluid volume deficit, as evidenced by balanced intake and output, maintenance of adequate hydration, and no manifestations of dehydration.

Interventions. Make frequent assessments, including hourly outputs; daily weights; vital signs every 30 minutes for the first 4 hours and then every 2 hours; urine for specific gravity, albumin, and glucose; and edema. Make periodic serum electrolyte and glucose determinations as well. Consider the expected presence of severe fatigue caused by urinary losses and the need for frequent observation. Fluid management during this period is crucial; hourly fluid replacement is based on the previous hour's output.

EVALUATION

The client with hydronephrosis must understand the importance of fluid balance, the need to monitor urinary output, and the need to report any changes in condition. Specific evaluation criteria will vary depending on the cause of obstruction.

■ Surgical Management

Surgery is commonly required to relieve the obstruction causing hydronephrosis. Management of the surgical client is discussed under urolithiasis in Chapter 34.

■ Self-Care

Clients who have had hydronephrosis should watch for signs of infection and obstruction, such as pain and reduced urine output. Avoiding urinary tract infections is important in preventing pyelonephritis and preserving renal function (see Chapter 34).

RENAL CANCER

Benign kidney tumors are rare. Classifications include lymphangioma, lipoma, medullary fibroma, adenoma, leiomyoma, and oncocytoma. When large benign tumors occur, it is relatively impossible to distinguish them from a malignant tumor by x-ray examination.

At least 85% of all renal tumors are malignant, and approximately 12,000 people die of kidney cancer each year. The tumors are most common in people between ages 50 and 70. They affect men more than women. Approximately 31,200 new cases of renal cancer were expected to be diagnosed in the United States in the year 2000.[2]

Etiology and Risk Factors

The exact cause of renal tumors is unknown. Some links have been established between renal cancer and tobacco, lead, cadmium, and phosphates. A genetic link has also been postulated.

Because of the possible association between smoking and renal cancer, one means of avoiding renal cancer may be to quit or not start smoking; avoiding exposure to chemicals such as lead, phosphate, and cadmium may also prevent some renal cancers. However, the cause of many renal cancers is not established and prevention may not be possible.

After surgery, most people have difficulty in dealing with cancer and the risk of recurrence. If nephrectomy is required, clients are often concerned about living with only one kidney. Assure them that one kidney can meet the body's needs but that care should be taken to protect that kidney. The care includes preventing injuries and infections, controlling blood pressure if necessary, and maintaining overall health and well-being by getting adequate nutrition, rest, and so on.

Pathophysiology

Renal cell carcinoma, or adenocarcinoma, is the most common tumor type; it accounts for 90% of all kidney neoplasms. Tumor growth begins in the renal cortex and usually continues for some time before it produces manifestations. The tumor can grow very large and tends to compress the adjacent renal parenchyma rather than infiltrate it. The tumor, usually avascular, tends to surround blood vessels and constrict them. The lungs and mediastinum are the most frequent metastatic sites of occurrence. Liver, bone, skin, spleen, renal vein, and brain are other common sites.

Other types of renal cancer include (1) nephroblastoma, (2) sarcoma, and (3) epithelial tumors in the renal pelvis.

Nephroblastoma, or Wilms' tumor, is primarily a childhood disease, although it occasionally occurs in adults. The prognosis for adults is worse than for children, with some sources reporting only a 25% survival rate.

Sarcoma is infrequent and typically arises in the renal capsule.

Most tumors of the renal pelvis are primarily urothelial in origin and include three tissue types: transitional cell, squamous cell, and adenocarcinoma.

Spontaneous regression of renal adenocarcinoma reportedly occurs in fewer than 1% of all cases. Most of these regressions occur after nephrectomy and involve metastatic areas. Authorities consider these episodes as more evidence that the disease is associated with immunologic or hormonal factors.

Clinical Manifestations

Manifestations of renal malignancies vary, and tumor growth may advance significantly before the disease is discovered. It is not uncommon for the client to have clinical manifestations apparently unrelated to renal disease. Frequently, a palpable abdominal mass found during a routine physical examination arouses the first suspicion. The average time between the onset of hematuria and the onset of pain is 9 months, and that between initial pain and diagnosis is 14 months. Extrarenal manifestations are commonly found before a diagnosis of renal cancer is confirmed. As many as 35% of clients have metastasis when the final diagnosis of a renal neoplasm is made.

The common triad of manifestations consists of hematuria, flank pain, and a palpable abdominal or flank mass. The hematuria is usually gross and intermittent, which helps explain the client's delay in seeking medical advice. The clinical picture also contains a combination of the following usual findings: fever, weight loss and cachexia, fatigue, hypertension, amyloidosis, thrombophlebitis, anemia, erythrocytosis, hypercalcemia, abnormal serum liver profile, and an elevated erythrocyte sedimentation rate (ESR). Less frequent findings include peripheral neuropathy, inferior vena cava obstruction, priapism, and varicocele. Hydronephrosis may occur if the tumor obstructs the ureteropelvic junction. The incidence of pulmonary embolus as a presenting manifestation may be higher than previously thought because of the high rate of vena cava and renal vein involvement. Plasma erythropoietin, renin, and chorionic gonadotropin levels are elevated, and prostaglandin production increases in renal cell carcinoma.

Several diagnostic tests help confirm a diagnosis of renal cancer. IVP is probably the most helpful in identifying a space-occupying lesion. Ultrasonography helps differentiate a cyst from a solid mass. Other noninvasive procedures include CT scan, nephrotomography, and radioisotope studies. Arteriography is used to evaluate the renal vascular system. Renal biopsy, usually done percutaneously, provides definitive data about the lesion.

Outcome Management

Staging of the tumor helps delineate the appropriate treatment and can suggest the client's prognosis (Fig. 35–1). Five-year survival rates for stage I are about 65%; for stage II, about 40%; 10-year rates drop to 40% and 35%, respectively. Five-year survivals are rare in stages III and IV.

▮ Medical Management

RADIATION THERAPY

Radiation may be used as an adjunct with chemotherapy and surgery. Irradiation is most useful in preoperative preparation of the tumor. It is sometimes also used postoperatively to destroy residual or recurrent tumor cells, treat lymphatic involvement, and treat metastatic sites, such as bones, palliatively.

CHEMOTHERAPY

Clinical investigators continue to search for an effective chemotherapeutic regimen. Medroxyprogesterone and testosterone have been used as hormonal therapy, but their

FIGURE 35–1 Staging system for renal carcinoma. Stage I tumor is confined within the renal capsule. Stage II tumor extends beyond the renal capsule to invade local perinephric fat but has no metastasis. Stage III tumor extends into the renal vein or involves local lymphatics. Stage IV tumor has metastasized to other parts of the body.

effectiveness has been limited. Vinblastine seems to be the most effective single agent, with response rates of 25%. Combination regimens seem to increase toxic effects without improving response rates. Many agents are being studied, but renal cancer cells seem insensitive to chemotherapeutic or hormonal agents, possibly because of their slow growth rate.

IMMUNOTHERAPY

Immunotherapy holds some promise in the treatment of renal cancer. Stimulants of the immune system have led to some positive results as long as the tumor is not too large and the immunosuppression not too severe. There has also been some response to natural and recombinant interferon-alfa. Interleukin-2 has been approved by the Food and Drug Administration for treating renal carcinoma.

■ Nursing Management of the Medical Client

Nursing management of the client with renal cancer must include general aspects of care for any cancer (see Chapters 18 and 19).

■ Surgical Management

NEPHRECTOMY

For renal cell carcinoma, the surgical procedure of choice is generally radical nephrectomy, which includes removal of the kidney, the adrenal gland, and perinephric fat with the retroperitoneal lymphatics. Several surgical approaches can be used to remove the diseased kidney. Transabdominal and thoracoabdominal approaches are

preferred to secure the renal artery and vein and to prevent the spread of malignant cells.

A retroperitoneal approach is also possible. An incision of 6 to 10 inches is made, usually in the flank area; muscle layers are divided; and tissues are excised. The renal artery and vein are clamped and cut, and the ureter is dissected. When the tumor is in the renal pelvis, a nephroureterectomy is usually performed because of a tendency for transitional cell cancer to "seed" down the ureter into the bladder. With nephroureterectomy, a cuff of the adjacent bladder is removed.

Lymphadenectomy remains controversial. Even in advanced cases, when the prognosis is poor, nephrectomy may be done to relieve pain and hematuria.

If the neoplastic disease is bilateral or if there is a solitary functioning kidney, a partial nephrectomy may be done on at least one kidney, leaving enough renal tissue to support life without long-term dialysis. If partial nephrectomy is not possible in either instance, the entire kidney is removed and the client is given dialysis. These clients may be candidates for renal transplantation, but they are usually maintained with dialysis for about a year to watch for recurrence of the disease.

Although open nephrectomy tends to be the procedure of choice for many urologists, laparoscopic nephrectomy is being performed in a number of centers with considerable success. Four small incisions are made, through fewer muscle layers. A special laparoscope is inserted through one of the incisions, and laparoscopy instruments are placed in the others. Carbon dioxide is passed through a tube in one incision to inflate the abdominal cavity, which enables the surgeon to see the organs and provides room for manipulation of instruments. At the end of the procedure, the kidney is removed through a small 2- to 3-inch incision below the navel.

The surgical procedure tends to be longer (6.9 versus 2.2 hours), but clients undergoing the laparoscopic procedure require fewer analgesics, resume oral intake earlier, are discharged home earlier, and return to work sooner than those undergoing open surgery. Increasingly, even removal of a kidney for organ donation is being performed laparoscopically.

INDICATIONS. Nephrectomy or heminephrectomy is indicated with tumors of the kidney. Other treatments are not successful.

CONTRAINDICATIONS. As with any surgery, nephrectomy is contraindicated in clients with systemic or respiratory infections. General health must be satisfactory to withstand anesthesia, blood loss, and surgical stress. Any metabolic and systemic disorders should be stabilized before surgery.

COMPLICATIONS. Because the kidney is a very vascular organ, the risk of hemorrhage is high. Renal artery embolization of the affected kidney may be done to obstruct the tumor's blood supply and reduce its vascularity, thereby reducing the risk of hemorrhage. Embolization is usually accomplished by occluding the renal artery using an absorbable gelatin sponge (Gelfoam), metal coil, barium, subcutaneous fat, isobutyl-2-cyanoacrylate, absolute ethanol, or a balloon. This procedure may also be performed to control hemorrhage in an inoperable kidney. In addition, some researchers believe that embolization may stimulate an immune response against the dying cancer cells.

Other possible complications include those associated with any major surgery, such as atelectasis, pneumonia, thromboembolism, and infection of the surgical wound.

OUTCOMES. Nephrectomy reduces pain and hematuria caused by the tumor. The hospital stay is typically 4 to 6 days, with a return to work in 4 to 8 weeks. With laparoscopic nephrectomy, hospitalization is reduced and return to work after 2 to 4 weeks is not uncommon. Living with one kidney has few, if any, negative effects. Long-term outcomes, however, depend on the stage of the cancer.

■ Nursing Management of the Surgical Client

PREOPERATIVE CARE

Preoperative preparation of the client having renal surgery includes the general guidelines described in Chapter 15. Increase fluid intake, if indicated, to ensure adequate excretion of waste products before surgery. Give emotional support because the client may be anxious, not only about the surgery but also about postoperative renal function and possible recurrence of the disease. If the remaining kidney functions adequately, assure the client that this kidney can fully meet the body's needs.

POSTOPERATIVE CARE
ASSESSMENT

Postoperatively, monitor the client's vital signs frequently and watch for any manifestations of bleeding or hemorrhage. Bleeding may be through the incision or internal.

Surgically induced or spontaneous pneumothorax occurs occasionally after nephrectomy; monitor for this complication by assessing for sudden shortness of breath and loss of breath sounds on the affected side.

DIAGNOSIS, OUTCOMES, INTERVENTIONS

Risk for Injury: Postoperative Complications. The nursing diagnoses are likely to include *Risk for Injury: Postoperative complications related to surgical procedure.* Although postoperative care is similar to that for laparotomy, one of the biggest challenges is reestablishing effective breathing patterns. Deep breathing and coughing are difficult because the incision is very close to the diaphragm. Also, assuming the jackknife position on the surgical table increases pain and soreness in the thoracic region, limiting respiratory excursion. Paralytic ileus is a common problem. Urine output must be maintained.

Outcomes. The client will maintain normal respiratory excursion and have no additional breath sounds and no signs of atelectasis or infection. There will be normal bowel sounds within 2 to 3 days. Urine output will be at least ½ ml/kg/hr.

Interventions. Liberal use of narcotics (including patient-controlled analgesia) to relieve pain and external mechanical support of the chest and abdomen with pillows or hands help the client to perform deep-breathing and coughing exercises more effectively. An incentive spirometer provides immediate feedback about the effectiveness of deep breathing.

Other interventions include carefully assessing the client's urine output and gastrointestinal status postoperatively and beginning oral intake only after adequate bowel function has resumed. Total urine output from all urine collection tubes should total ½ ml/kg/hr. Notify the physician of lesser amounts. Other wound drainage tubes also need to be monitored. Early ambulation is indicated.

Pain. A diagnosis of *Acute Pain related to surgery* is common because the nephrectomy incision is extensive and causes significant discomfort. Muscle pain may develop from the prolonged position maintained during surgery.

Outcomes. Pain will be controlled, as indicated by the client's reports of reduced discomfort as well as by nonverbal indications of reduced discomfort, particularly during movement.

Interventions. The pain may be relieved by narcotic analgesics (including the use of patient-controlled analgesia) and proper positioning. Epidural fentanyl or morphine sulfate can provide effective analgesia.

Anxiety. People with cancer and people undergoing surgery experience anxiety because of uncertainty about the future. A diagnosis of *Anxiety related to disease and surgery* is probable.

Outcomes. Ideally, the client will report having the information needed to reduce uncertainty and will report that the information reduced anxiety.

Interventions. To help reduce feelings of anxiety, continue to keep the client and significant others informed about the progress made. Encourage them to express their concerns and to talk with one another. This need for support continues throughout the follow-up period.

EVALUATION

The client should be able to resume regular activities within 6 to 8 weeks after surgery. Long-term survival is dependent upon the stage of cancer diagnosed.

■ Self-Care

With shorter hospitalizations, clients who have undergone nephrectomy may require home care and support. Clients are weakened by surgery and possibly by other treatments. Activity should increase gradually; typically, 6 weeks must elapse before clients are ready to return to work or lift more than 10 pounds.

Concern about recurrence of the cancer is common. The American Cancer Society and other support groups may by helpful in the client's adjustment to cancer. People with one kidney can lead normal lives. There is, however, a need to protect the remaining kidney by prevention of infection and trauma.

TUBULOINTERSTITIAL DISEASE

Traditionally, the term "interstitial nephritis" has been applied to renal disease characterized by the presence of inflammatory cells in the spaces between the renal tubules. However, not all disease processes included in this classification are inflammatory. Therefore, the term *tubulointerstitial disease* is being advocated for this category of renal disorders.

Tubulointerstitial diseases are commonly classified as either acute or chronic. The acute form usually represents an allergic reaction and has a rapid onset. Assessment findings are typically related to tubular injury. Manifestations often include fever, skin rash, eosinophilia, oliguric renal failure, and occasionally gross hematuria. The disease may progress along any of three courses:

- Complete recovery
- Rapid progression to renal failure and death
- Movement to the chronic form

Although corticosteroids are commonly prescribed, their value is unclear. Treatment is similar to that for acute renal failure.

Chronic tubulointerstitial disease is characterized by progressive interstitial fibrosis and usually chronic inflammatory cell infiltration with tubular atrophy. In the terminal stages, the altered renal vasculature and renal structure make the disease virtually indistinguishable from chronic pyelonephritis.

Morphologic findings in tubulointerstitial disease include interstitial edema, cellular infiltration of the interstitium, tubular cellular atrophy and flattening, and interstitial fibrosis. As the disease progresses, renal involvement extends beyond the tubules to progressive fibrosis of Bowman's capsule with secondary involvement of the glomeruli.

Potential causes of this pathologic process are many:

- Acute pyelonephritis
- Septicemia
- Analgesic abuse, especially with phenacetin, aspirin, and acetaminophen
- Immunologic mechanisms, for example, renal allograft, systemic lupus erythematosus, and Sjögren's syndrome
- Heavy metal toxicity
- Drug toxicity
- Hypercalcemia
- Hypocalcemia

In addition, several medication hypersensitivities may contribute. The medications involved include rifampin, penicillin and its analogs, sulfonamides, cephalosporins, allopurinol, captopril, cimetidine, azathioprine, phenytoin, thiazide, lithium, NSAIDs, and possibly furosemide.

An early manifestation of tubulointerstitial disease is a sudden, unexplained decrease in renal function that may be mild to severe. Specifically, there may be inability to concentrate urine, salt wasting, and poor acidification of the urine leading to metabolic acidosis. Finding a variety of urine sediment abnormalities is also common. Because glucose, uric acid, phosphates, amino acids, and bicarbonate are not effectively reabsorbed in the tubules, they appear in the urine. Severe bicarbonaturia is an indicator of renal tubular acidosis. Proteinuria is less severe than with other renal disease. Systemic hypertension is a common finding.

GLOMERULONEPHRITIS

Glomerulonephritis encompasses a variety of diseases, most of which are caused by an immunologic reaction that results in proliferative and inflammatory changes in glomerular structure. Glomerulonephritis can be acute or chronic. It is usually manifested by either a nephrotic syndrome or a nephritic syndrome. Percutaneous renal biopsy is typically used to identify the type of glomerulonephritis, and the findings assist in planning interventions and determining the prognosis.

■ NEPHROTIC SYNDROME

Nephrotic syndrome is a set of clinical manifestations caused by protein wasting secondary to diffuse glomerular damage. Manifestations include proteinuria (>3.5 g/day), hypoalbuminemia, and edema. Abnormal permeability of the glomerular basement membrane (especially to albumin) results in loss of protein in the urine. The resulting hypoalbuminemia alters oncotic pressure in the vascular tree, and fluid moves into the interstitial spaces, causing edema. This movement stimulates plasma renin activity and augments aldosterone production; as a result, the kidney retains sodium and water, thus adding to the accumulation of extracellular fluid.

Hyperlipidemia usually occurs as well, probably because of increased hepatic lipoprotein synthesis in response to decreased serum albumin. Depending on the degree of renal failure, some level of normocytic anemia is common.

The causes of nephrotic syndrome are numerous. Besides glomerulonephritis, certain systemic disorders can cause it, such as diabetes mellitus, systemic lupus erythematosus (SLE), amyloidosis, hepatitis B, syphilis, carcinoma, leukemia, infectious disease, and preeclampsia. Other predisposing factors include:

- Allergic reactions
- Reactions to such drugs as penicillamine, anticonvulsants, probenecid, captopril, gold salts, heroin, and NSAIDs
- Renal vein thrombosis
- Sickle cell disease
- Heart failure

Potential complications of nephrotic syndrome include the effects of extracellular fluid accumulation and the progressive development of renal failure. The client may also experience severe hypovolemia, thromboembolism, secondary aldosteronism, abnormal thyroid function, osteomalacia, and increased susceptibility to infections.

Usually, edema is the client's chief problem. Although its onset may be insidious, it becomes massive. The client's skin typically takes on a characteristic waxy pallor, resulting from the edema rather than anemia. Other manifestations include anorexia, malaise, irritability, and abnormal or absent menses. Large amounts of protein appear in the client's urine along with granular and epithelial cell casts and fat bodies; proteinuria may account for losses of 4 to 30 g/day. Some hematuria may be present. Serum albumin concentrations may drop as low as 1.0 to 2.5 g/dl.

The primary aim of treatment for nephrotic syndrome is to heal the leaking glomerular basement membrane, stop the loss of protein in the client's urine, and break the cycle of edema. Interventions typically include maintaining the client's fluid and electrolyte balance, reducing inflammation, preventing thrombosis, and minimizing protein loss.

MAINTAIN FLUID AND ELECTROLYTE BALANCE. Unless the client is hyponatremic, fluids are not usually restricted. The client's fluid balance should, however, be carefully monitored via daily weights, girth measurements, and intake and output determinations. These data are important because weight loss may represent true tissue loss involving protein rather than fluid.

Loop diuretics (i.e., those that work on the loop of Henle), such as furosemide (Lasix), are typically prescribed. Plasma volume expanders, such as albumin, plasma, and dextran, may be administered to raise the oncotic pressure in the vascular tree. The increased pressure pulls fluid from the extracellular spaces, making it available for kidney filtration. Diuresis in older clients must be handled with particular caution because of their reduced ability to tolerate sudden shifts in intravascular volume.

Because the kidneys have a reduced capacity to excrete sodium, mild sodium restriction is usually instituted. The diet should be as palatable as possible, however, because the client must consume adequate protein and calories. Potassium may also be restricted as serum potassium levels rise.

Because edema disrupts cellular nutrition, the client is at increased risk for skin breakdown. Thus, skin care is vital. Interventions include good hygiene, massage, position changes, and possibly special mattresses. Use research-based tools to assess the client's risk of breakdown (see Chapter 16).

REDUCE INFLAMMATION. Steroid therapy helps some clients, depending on the cause of disease. Cytotoxic agents such as cyclophosphamide and chlorambucil, indomethacin, anticoagulants, and antiplatelet agents may be used as well.

PREVENT THROMBOSIS. Because clients with nephrotic syndrome are vulnerable to renal vein thrombosis, some are given long-term anticoagulation therapy. Teach such clients how to monitor for hemorrhage, and encourage them to carry identification that lists the drugs they take.

MINIMIZE PROTEIN LOSS. For clients with nephrotic syndrome, most physicians recommend a protein intake of 1.0 to 1.5 g/kg/day with more than 35 kcal/kg/day to prevent further protein breakdown. Twenty-four-hour urine collections are used to measure urinary protein losses and monitor the success of treatment. Treatment to reduce inflammation ultimately reduces protein loss.

An important nursing role is to help the client with nephrotic syndrome maintain health and cope with the illness. Teach the client to take prescribed medications regularly, follow the prescribed diet, and report changes in health status, such as increasing edema, reduced urine output, weight gain, respiratory distress, and signs of infection. Explain that the amount of exercise allowed is based, at least in part, on the severity of the edema. Bed rest is imposed only during severe edema. As the fluid level moves toward normal, the client is allowed more activity. Other important areas of teaching include nutrition, prevention of infection, and methods of careful self-assessment.

■ NEPHRITIC SYNDROME

Nephritic syndrome refers to a set of clinical manifestations that include hematuria and at least one of the following: oliguria (urine output < 400 ml/24 hours), hypertension, elevated blood urea nitrogen (BUN), or decreased GFR. Nephritic syndrome is common with many types of glomerulonephritis, including immunoglobulin A (IgA) nephropathy and Henoch-Schönlein purpura. Treatment includes management of the underlying disease (usually through immunosuppressive drugs, as noted later) and symptomatic treatment of blood pressure and uremia.

TYPES OF GLOMERULONEPHRITIS

There are many types of glomerulonephritis, most of which involve either nephrotic syndrome or nephritic syndrome. The diagnosis of the specific type can be made by assessment of clinical manifestations and through renal biopsy. Box 35–2 presents a classification system based on

---

BOX 35–2   Classification of Glomerulonephritis Based on Etiology

Primary Glomerulonephritis—Immune Response to Pathogens

- Acute glomerulonephritis
- Postinfectious glomerulonephritis
- Group A beta-hemolytic streptococcus
- Other infectious conditions such as cytomegalovirus infection, measles, mumps, staphylococcus, or pneumococcal bacteremia
- Infectious glomerulonephritis
- Membranoproliferative glomerulonephritis
- Rapidly progressive glomerulonephritis
- Idiopathic membranous glomerulonephritis
- Immunoglobulin A (IgA) nephropathy
- Chronic glomerulonephritis
- Lipoid nephrosis
- Focal glomerular sclerosis

Secondary Glomerulonephritis—Related to Systemic Disease

- Goodpasture's syndrome
- Hemolytic-uremic syndrome
- Henoch-Schönlein purpura
- Polyarteritis
- Progressive systemic sclerosis
- Systemic lupus erythematosus
- Wegener's granulomatosis
- Thrombocytopenic purpura
- Postpartum renal failure

TABLE 35–1	TYPES OF GLOMERULONEPHRITIS: ONSET, FINDINGS, AND PROGNOSIS		
Type	**Onset**	**Diagnostic Findings**	**Prognosis**
Poststreptococcal glomerulo-nephritis	1 to 3 weeks after beta-hemo-lytic streptococcal infection of throat or skin Nephritic syndrome	Underlying infection Elevated antistreptolysin O titer Microscopic urinalysis, urine with many casts	Variable Complete recovery to end-stage renal disease
Membranoproliferative glo-merulonephritis	Nephrotic syndrome some-times preceded by a strepto-coccal infection	Proteinuria Hematuria (microscopic or gross)	Gradual progressive chronic renal failure
Rapidly progressive glomeru-lonephritis	Nephritic syndrome Sudden May follow antigen or infec-tion Peak ages 40–60 yr	Hematuria Edema Hypertension Proteinuria Oliguria Acidosis	Progresses to renal failure within weeks or months
Idiopathic membranous glo-merulonephritis	Insidious Peak ages 40–70 yr Unknown antigen	Asymptomatic proteinuria or nephrotic syndrome	Mixed: 25% have spontaneous remission, 25% have renal failure, 25% have persistent proteinuria, 25% have dete-riorating renal function
Immunoglobulin A (IgA) nephropathy (also called Berger's disease)	Most frequent in young adults Nephritic syndrome	Hematuria Red blood cell casts on micro-scopic urinalysis	Usually progresses slowly over 10–20 yrs. A small proportion progress to renal failure.
Lipoid nephrosis (also called minimal change glomerulo-nephritis)	Nephrotic syndrome	Found on biopsy	Generally good May be relapses and sponta-neous remission
Focal glomerular sclerosis	Peaks between ages 30 and 50 yr Nephrotic syndrome	Found on biopsy May be few symptoms	Poor, although rate of deterio-ration varies widely Recurs after transplantation
Membranous glomerulo-nephritis	Commonly secondary to drug therapy toxins or systemic autoimmune disease Nephrotic syndrome Insidious onset	Heavy proteinuria	Variable 30% have spontaneous remis-sion
Hemolytic-uremic syndrome	Follows infection with *Esche-richia coli* (01571 H7 sero-type) History of eating undercooked hamburger Children and older adults par-ticularly vulnerable	Hemorrhagic manifestations, such as bleeding and bruising Purpura manifestations, such as acute renal failure, he-molytic anemia, and throm-bocytopenia	Recovery rate 95% but may leave residual renal damage

etiology. Table 35–1 describes the onset, diagnostic find-ings, and prognosis for various types of glomerulonephritis.

Pathophysiology

Glomerulonephritis is an immunologic disorder that causes inflammation and increased cells in the glomeru-lus. Because the primary function of the glomerulus is to filter blood, most cases result when antigen-antibody complexes produced by an infection elsewhere in the body become trapped in the glomerulus. This entrapment causes inflammatory damage and impedes glomerular function, reducing the glomerular membrane's capacity for selective permeability. The source of the antigens may

be either *exogenous* (e.g., after streptococcal infection) or *endogenous* (as in systemic lupus erythematosus). Evi-dence also indicates that some antigen-antibody com-plexes may form in the kidney itself.

Glomerulonephritis may also result from antibodies af-fixed to the glomerular basement membrane. For exam-ple, Goodpasture's syndrome involves pulmonary hemor-rhage and glomerulonephritis.

The primary pathologic processes in glomerulonephri-tis, lipoid nephrosis, and focal glomerular sclerosis are proliferation and inflammation. However, lipoid nephrosis and focal glomerular sclerosis are characterized by degen-eration. Figure 35–2 depicts the pathophysiologic mecha-nisms of glomerulonephritis.

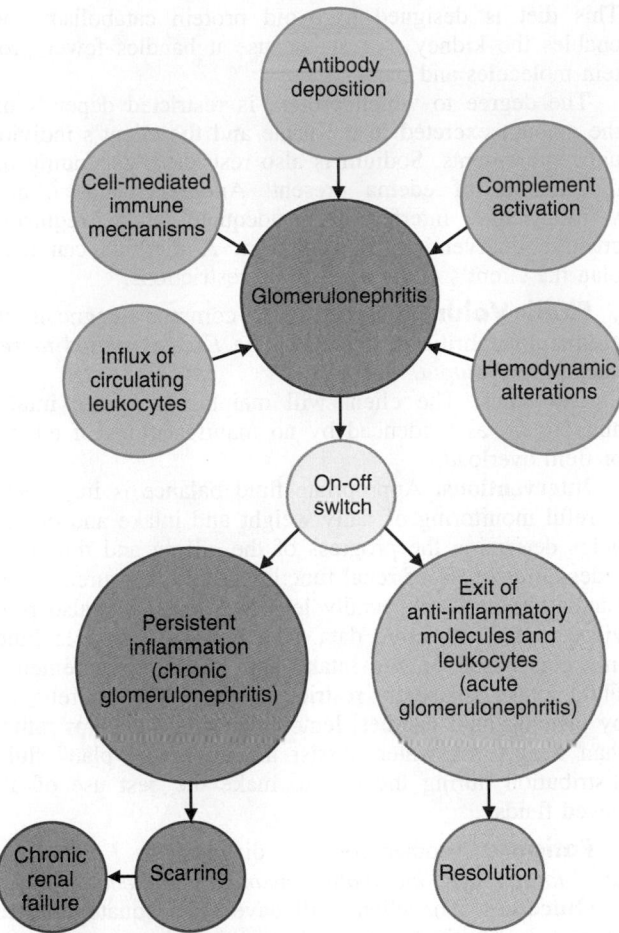

FIGURE 35–2 Pathophysiologic mechanism of glomerulonephritis.

Clinical Manifestations

Acute glomerulonephritis may develop insidiously or suddenly, varying considerably with the pathophysiology involved. Classic manifestations of sudden onset include hematuria with red blood cell casts and proteinuria. Fever, chills, weakness, pallor, anorexia, nausea, and vomiting may be present. Generalized edema, particularly facial and periorbital swelling, is a typical finding. The client may have ascites, pleural effusion, and heart failure.

The client is likely to have a headache and moderate to severe hypertension. Visual acuity may be reduced because of retinal edema. Abdominal or flank pain may develop, probably because of kidney edema and distention of the renal capsule. Oliguria, even anuria, may be present for several days; the longer it persists, the more irreversible the kidney damage. In contrast, the disease may be so mild that the client reports only vague weakness, anorexia, and lethargy.

Acute glomerulonephritis can become a fulminant process, proceeding quickly to uremia or chronic glomerulonephritis. Most clients, however, start to recover within 14 days. Most clinical manifestations disappear within several weeks, although hematuria and proteinuria may be present for longer periods. If complete recovery does not occur within 2 years, it probably will not occur at all.

Some clinicians use the term *subacute glomerulonephritis* to describe disease persisting more than 6 to 8 weeks. Although most of the manifestations of the acute disease have disappeared, the client is still at high risk for exacerbation of glomerulonephritis. The term *latent glomerulonephritis* refers to an asymptomatic condition characterized by significant albumin levels and casts in the urine for more than 1 year after acute onset. These findings indicate continued but slow parenchymal changes.

Most types of glomerulonephritis can progress to a chronic state. Sometimes, glomerulonephritis is first seen as a chronic process. Chronic glomerulonephritis progresses over an extended period, often as long as 30 years. When it progresses to end-stage renal failure, dialysis must begin or the client will die.

As the glomeruli and tubules are destroyed by the pathologic process, the kidneys shrink and become severely contracted. Fibrous and scar tissue replaces functioning renal tissue. Sclerosis of renal blood vessels also occurs. The destruction rates vary.

Common manifestations include malaise, weight loss, edema, increasing irritability and mental cloudiness, a metallic taste in the mouth, polyuria and nocturia resulting from the kidney's inability to concentrate urine, headache, dizziness, and digestive disturbances. As the disease progresses, these manifestations intensify, and the client may experience respiratory difficulty and angina.

The cardinal manifestation of this disease is hypertension. It is not uncommon for the client to experience such complications as nosebleed, manifestations of arteriosclerosis, cardiomegaly, and hemorrhage into the kidneys, lungs, retina, or cerebrum. Edema increases as heart failure becomes more severe and the serum albumin decreases. Examination of the eyegrounds shows vascular changes and edema of the discs. Urinalysis shows a fixed specific gravity, small amounts of proteinuria except during exacerbation, casts, WBCs, renal tubular cells, and consistent hematuria. Anemia tends to be severe.

Examining the urine usually provides the information necessary for a diagnosis of glomerulonephritis (see Chapter 32). Gross hematuria and proteinuria are the cardinal findings. The client's urine, which may be scant, usually has a dark, smoky, cola-colored, or red-brown hue. The proteinuria produces a persistent and excessive foam. The urine may have a low pH and a specific gravity in the midnormal to high-normal range if there is enough renal damage to affect the kidneys' ability to concentrate.

Other studies may assist in the diagnosis as well. Serum urea nitrogen and creatinine levels may be elevated, and creatinine clearance rates may be decreased. C-reactive proteins and antistreptolysin O titer are usually elevated in poststreptococcal glomerulonephritis, and the serum complement level is low in many forms of glomerulonephritis. Hematocrit and hemoglobin studies may indicate anemia, particularly if renal failure is imminent.

Outcome Management

Medical Management

Medical intervention aims to eliminate antigens, to alter the client's immune balance, and to inhibit or alleviate inflammation to prevent further renal damage and improve kidney function. Although some clients may require initial hospitalization, treatment is typically on an outpatient basis.

REDUCE INFLAMMATION

Plasmapheresis has been used in some research protocols to reduce the number of antigens in certain types of glomerulonephritis, including rapidly progressive glomerulonephritis. This intervention is usually administered in conjunction with corticosteroids and immunosuppressive agents (azathioprine, cyclophosphamide). The technique is designed to remove the specific circulating antibody or mediators of the inflammatory response. Large volumes of the client's plasma are cyclically removed and replaced with fresh frozen plasma through a continuous-flow blood cell separator.

Antibiotic therapy (such as penicillin for streptococcal organisms) is used to treat poststreptococcal glomerulonephritis. It is also used prophylactically after streptococcal infections to prevent further damage.

MAINTAIN FLUID AND ELECTROLYTE BALANCE

Volume overload and hypertension are treated with diuretics, antihypertensives, and restriction of dietary sodium and water. Common complications of fluid overload include heart failure with pulmonary edema and increased intracranial pressure. Renal failure may develop (see Chapter 36). Appropriate monitoring is essential and should include vital signs, intake and output, and weight. Recognizing complications early facilitates prompt medical intervention.

◼ Nursing Management of the Medical Client

ASSESSMENT

For any client with suspected glomerulonephritis, take a comprehensive history that includes upper respiratory tract infection (such as strep throat), skin infections, scarlet fever, or a history of glomerulonephritis. Also question the client about systemic disorders that might be present, such as SLE, scleroderma, amyloidosis, and hypertension. Any recent invasive procedures should also be noted.

Physical examination may reveal ascites, pleural effusion, and manifestations of heart failure with pulmonary edema. Examine the urine closely for color, amount, and abnormal substances. In particular, microscopic analysis of the urine can be a valuable diagnostic tool with glomerulonephritis; urinary casts are commonly seen under high magnification (see Chapter 32). Check the client's vital signs closely, especially blood pressure.

DIAGNOSIS, OUTCOMES, INTERVENTIONS

Altered Nutrition: Less Than Body Requirements. If the client has a reduced appetite or an aversion to food, the diagnosis *Altered Nutrition: Less than body requirements related to anorexia and increased metabolic demands* is appropriate.

Outcomes. The client will maintain adequate nutritional intake, as evidenced by no weight loss, absence of a negative nitrogen balance, and normal electrolytes.

Interventions. It is important to protect the kidneys while they are recovering their function. The prescribed diet is likely to be high in calories and low in protein.

This diet is designed to avoid protein catabolism and enables the kidney to rest because it handles fewer protein molecules and metabolites.

The degree to which protein is restricted depends on the amount excreted in the urine and the client's individual requirements. Sodium is also restricted, depending on the amount of edema present. Anorexia, nausea, and vomiting may interfere with adequate intake, requiring creative intervention on your part. A dietitian can help plan the client's diet around these restrictions.

Fluid Volume Excess. A common diagnosis in glomerulonephritis is *Fluid Volume Excess related to reduced urine output.*

Outcomes. The client will maintain balanced intake and output, as evidenced by no manifestations of edema or fluid overload.

Interventions. Appropriate fluid balance is important. Careful monitoring of daily weight and intake and output helps determine the progress of the edema and thus provides an estimate of renal function. Daily measurement of edematous parts (especially legs and abdomen) also provides useful, objective data. The client's allowable fluid intake is based on the intake and output measurements. Fluid intake is usually restricted. Thirst may be relieved by offering hard candies, lemon slices, or ice chips rather than a glass of water. Assist the client to "plan" fluid distribution during the day to make the best use of allowed fluids.

Fatigue. Another common diagnosis is *Fatigue related to increased metabolic demands and anemia.*

Outcomes. The client will have an adequate balance of rest and activity, as evidenced by absence of complaints of fatigue.

Interventions. Rest is essential—both physical and emotional. As mentioned, activity level correlates directly with the amount of hematuria and proteinuria. Exercise also increases catabolic activity. The allowable amount of activity depends on the results of serial urinalyses. Bed rest interspersed with periods of limited activity may continue for several weeks to months. Therefore, the client may need help in arranging personal matters, such as family, home, job, finances, and community responsibilities.

Encourage the client to talk about any fears or concerns, and, if necessary, help the client deal with the emotional reactions expected during a long-term illness with a questionable prognosis. Only after handling these problems can the client rest emotionally. Appropriate diversionary activities may help the client cope with prolonged physical immobility.

Risk for Impaired Skin Integrity. A typical diagnosis is *Risk for Impaired Skin Integrity related to edema.*

Outcomes. The client will remain free of skin breakdown, as evidenced by continued intact skin.

Interventions. Edema interferes with cellular nutrition, which makes the client more susceptible to skin breakdown. Take precautions to prevent this complication. Interventions include good hygiene, massage, and position changes as well as other prophylactic measures, such as mattress devices. Use research-based tools to assess the client's risk of breakdown (see Chapter 16).

Risk for Infection. Another diagnosis after immunosuppressive therapy is *Risk for Infection related to altered immune response secondary to treatment.*

Outcomes. The client will remain free of infection, as evidenced by normal temperature and an absence of local or systemic manifestations of infection.

Interventions. Glomerulonephritis markedly diminishes a client's natural defenses to infection, especially to streptococcal organisms. Immunosuppressives and corticosteroids further reduce host resistance. Although isolation is not necessary, take care to protect the client from people with obvious infectious processes. General supportive measures help boost the client's defense mechanisms. Client teaching should involve appropriate ways to avoid infections, especially respiratory and urinary tract infections.

EVALUATION

The client must be able to understand the condition and the reasons for limitations, including dietary and fluid restrictions. Stress the importance of follow-up treatments to minimize the risk of recurrence.

■ Self-Care

Clients with glomerulonephritis are followed as outpatients, often for many years. Self-care activities should include regular follow-up, recommended medications and dietary restrictions, and monitoring for changes in condition. It is vital that blood pressure be controlled to prevent further renal damage; many clients learn to monitor their own blood pressure at home. Because the disease may progress to renal failure, there are numerous quality-of-life issues, as discussed in Chapter 36.

■ Modification for Elderly Clients

The older client is at greater risk for renal damage because of the pre-existing effects of age on the kidneys. The older client is also more likely to have concurrent chronic diseases—such as hypertension and diabetes—that may have affected the kidneys, although treatment is the same.

Renal Trauma

Serious kidney injury is relatively rare because of the protection afforded by the rib cage, the heavy muscles of the back, and the tough capsule surrounding the kidney. Traffic accidents and falls in which the client lands on the abdomen, flank, or back are the most common cause of injury, usually from blunt trauma. Kidney lacerations can result from fractures of the spine and ribs as well as penetrating injuries from bullets and knives.

Pathophysiology

Five categories of traumatic injury can affect the kidney:

- Contusion with intrarenal hemorrhage
- Minor laceration (rupture with subcapsular hemorrhage)
- Major laceration (rupture into the renal pelvis)
- "Fractured" kidney (shattered rupture)
- Vascular (pedicle) injury, which damages renal blood supply (Fig. 35-3)

In a contusion, a hematoma develops and remains confined within the renal parenchyma. Rupture of the kidney may cause hemorrhage between the capsular walls; bleeding may or may not reach into the renal pelvis. A shattered or fractured kidney causes hemorrhage throughout the renal tissue. The pedicle holds the renal artery and other vital circulatory and nervous system connections to the kidney. Injury to the pedicle may jeopardize the life of the kidney and may occur with or without intrarenal hemorrhage.

Clinical Manifestations

The type of injury the client has suffered gives the first real key to identifying renal trauma. Commonly, the client has multiple serious injuries, and renal trauma may not be immediately apparent. Hematuria (gross or microscopic) is a cardinal manifestation and is found in about 80% of cases. However, serious renal injury can occur without hemorrhage and clear urine does not automatically rule out renal trauma. Other findings include shock, flank pain, and a palpable mass in the affected flank area or over the 11th or 12th rib. Paralytic ileus may also occur. You may see bruises over the client's flank and lower back secondary to retroperitoneal hemorrhage, a development known as Grey Turner's sign. A KUB film, IVP, retrograde pyelography, renal scan, ultrasonography, CT scan, and renal arteriography all help confirm the type and degree of kidney injury.

Contusion   Minor laceration   Major laceration   "Fractured" kidney   Vascular injury

FIGURE 35-3 Categories of renal trauma.

Complications

In addition to the immediate problems of hemorrhage and loss of functioning renal tissue, kidney trauma makes the client highly susceptible to a number of other problems. Even in closed injuries, there is a high risk of sepsis leading to kidney and perinephric abscesses. Secondary hemorrhage is not uncommon. Other complications include hypertension resulting from fibrosis and ischemic kidney, renal artery thrombosis, arteriovenous aneurysms, fistula formation from extravasation of urine, urinomas, and pseudocysts.

Outcome Management

Whether conservative or surgical treatment should be used for renal trauma is controversial. Most physicians agree that kidney contusion calls for conservative treatment. Other minor injuries, such as small subcapsular hematomas and minor lacerations without extravasation, may also be better followed conservatively.

Clients with major injuries (e.g., renal fracture, parenchymal injury with major arterial occlusion, avulsion injuries, tears in the renal artery or vein, and parenchymal lacerations with extending perirenal hematomas or urinary extravasation) may require surgical exploration. Possible indications include continued moderate to severe hemorrhage and continued urinary extravasation. Urinary extravasation itself is not a definite reason for surgery because sterile urine usually resolves or is encapsulated spontaneously. However, it sometimes produces a severe tissue reaction and causes fistula formation. The pocket of extrarenal urine may also become obstructive.

■ Medical Management

Medical management, which primarily involves waiting and watching, is possible because the retroperitoneal space allows tamponade. In the absence of other injuries, a client with microscopic hematuria and normal findings on IVP may be observed on an ambulatory basis with careful instructions about activity restrictions and the need for adequate hydration. If there is gross hematuria, bed rest is required until the urine clears. Serial observations of the urine, hematocrit, and vital signs are made to watch the progress of the hemorrhage. Sequential urine specimens may be collected to compare current and previous urine color and turbidity.

Even if replacement fluids are not needed, a prophylactic intravenous line may be established, and a type and crossmatch for blood may be done. If a hematoma is present or IVP shows urine extravasation, the client may receive antibiotics to prevent sepsis. The physician prescribes blood transfusions if the hematocrit is low. After the urine clears, the client can be more active. After discharge, the client needs follow-up blood pressure checks and IVP studies to rule out secondary hypertension and anatomic changes in the renal system.

■ Nursing Management of the Medical Client

Nursing management of the client with renal trauma varies considerably, depending on extent of injury. The goals of nursing care are to prevent further bleeding and injury and to alleviate the client's anxiety.

ASSESSMENT

Assessment includes checking for tenderness at the CVA. Watch for bleeding, which may occur as hematuria or may be internal, depending on the nature of the injury. Assess the client's vital signs for evidence of shock. Make serial observations of urine, hematocrit, and vital signs to watch the progress of hemorrhage. Sequential urine specimens may be collected to compare current and previous urine color and turbidity.

DIAGNOSIS, OUTCOMES, INTERVENTIONS

Risk for Injury: Hemorrhage. The goals of nursing after renal trauma are related to monitoring for shock and minimizing the risk of further bleeding. For this reason, the nursing diagnosis is *Risk for Injury: Hemorrhage related to blood loss, further injury, and hypovolemia.*

Outcomes. The client will not experience shock, and bleeding will stop, as evidenced by a decrease in hematuria, pain, or other bleeding.

Interventions. Nursing interventions during conservative treatment center on monitoring urinary elimination patterns and helping the client to cope and comply with the medical regimen. If there is gross hematuria, bed rest is required until the urine clears. Monitoring includes assessment of vital signs as well as intake and output. Notify the physician if urine output drops below ½ ml/kg/hr. Because bed rest can cause problems with bowel elimination and adequate fluid intake, circulation, and respiratory function, take appropriate measures to minimize the risk of these complications (passive exercise, for example). A client with microscopic hematuria and normal IVP results who is observed on an ambulatory basis should be given careful instructions about activity restrictions and the need for adequate hydration.

Anxiety. Renal trauma can cause considerable anxiety over the possible loss of renal function and possible shock. Hence, a nursing diagnosis of *Anxiety related to injury* is highly likely.

Outcomes. The client will report less anxiety and will have the information needed to understand the situation and prognosis.

Interventions. Nursing care related to anxiety involves providing information about the plan of care, including activity restrictions. The client is concerned about the progress, and you may be in a position to facilitate communication between the patient and other members of the health care team.

EVALUATION

It is expected that the client will have no further bleeding or injury and that renal function will be maintained, whether monitoring is done on an outpatient basis or in an acute care setting. With limited activity, most clients can be managed at home unless surgical intervention is required.

■ Surgical Management

The greatest diversity of opinion concerns proper handling of the renal damage discovered during exploration. When the other kidney is functioning effectively, some physicians recommend free use of nephrectomy to avoid later sequelae, whereas others believe that the goal should be salvaging maximal renal function. The latter group advocates giving the conservative approach a fair trial and, if surgery is necessary, attempting to repair the kidney before deciding to remove it. With renal vascular injury, fewer than half of kidneys can be salvaged if the injury is 18 hours old; there is virtually no chance of renal recovery after 24 hours.

Renal hemorrhage may be controlled by injection of an autologous clot into the secondary arteries supplying the bleeding site. Blood is drawn from the client and allowed to clot. The clot is then injected angiographically. Because normal endothelium has a strong clot-lysing effect, the clot disappears from the normal adjacent vasculature after several hours and affects only the damaged portion.

If kidney repair is attempted rather than nephrectomy, the surgical procedure is designed to debride devitalized tissue, achieve hemostasis, establish a watertight seal of the collecting system, approximate the renal parenchymal edges, and drain the renal fossa.

Two surgical techniques improve the outcome of repair:

- *Extracorporeal,* or *bench, surgery* allows the kidney to be removed from the body for better visualization and manipulation of the organ during the repair process; the kidney is returned by autotransplantation. During its time outside the body, the kidney is maintained by hypothermia or by a perfusate mechanically pulsed through it.
- The *slush technique,* in which the kidney is immersed in iced saline slush, slows the metabolism and oxygen requirement of the renal tissue, allowing longer intraoperative ischemic times. This technique causes some systemic hypothermia, but it is not significant. Pedicle vascular injury may also be repaired.

If either technique fails, nephrectomy is necessary.

■ Nursing Management of the Surgical Client

Nursing management of the client undergoing surgery for renal trauma is similar to that for other surgical procedures on the kidney (see nephrectomy in this chapter).

■ Self-Care

The client being observed on an ambulatory basis requires an appropriate teaching plan covering health maintenance activities and the need for a follow-up program. The client should promptly report any change in condition or recurrence of bleeding or pain to the physician. Strenuous activity should be avoided for several weeks or more, depending on the extent of the injury. The client must also maintain adequate hydration.

RENAL VASCULAR ABNORMALITIES

The kidneys depend on adequate blood circulation to nourish tissues and provide blood for filtration so that they can perform their intended functions. Anything that interferes with the normal circulatory flow significantly reduces renal function.

RENAL ARTERY DISEASE

Etiology and Risk Factors

Ninety per cent of all renal artery disease is caused by atherosclerosis or fibromuscular dysplasia. Atherosclerosis affects males more often than females and usually involves the proximal third of the artery. Health promotion activities are the same as those for atherosclerosis as discussed with circulatory and cardiac disorders. Fibromuscular dysplasia is an alternating stenosis and dilation; arteriographic studies demonstrate a "string-of-beads" appearance of the artery. This condition affects females four to five times as often as males. Because the cause is unknown, there are no health promotion actions.

There are several other, less common, causes of renal artery disease. Cancer may obstruct the vessels. Embolism or thrombosis can cause acute obstruction. Trauma, as described earlier, can interrupt blood flow. The renal artery may be purposely occluded to produce a "medical nephrectomy" or total renal infarction; the occlusion may be done preoperatively in the case of renal adenocarcinoma or to control proteinuria or hypertension. Shredded Gelfoam may be used, or a liquid substance that polymerizes instantly when it comes in contact with blood may be injected into the renal artery. A dissecting aneurysm in the renal artery may also interrupt renal circulation.

Pathophysiology

The end result of any of these conditions, if severe enough, is reduced renal blood flow. The reduced flow causes renal parenchymal ischemia and, finally, renal atrophy. The role of renal artery disease in renovascular hypertension is also well documented, and hypertension alone may indicate treatment of the condition.

Clinical Manifestations

Because of the kidney's compensatory mechanisms, the gradual development of renal artery stenosis from atherosclerosis and cancer may give rise to very few manifestations, at least until the resulting hypertension and decreasing renal function become evident. Acute obstruction makes itself known relatively quickly, however. Manifestations of this sudden episode include flank pain over the affected kidney or abdominal pain and fever. Atrial dysrhythmias are a frequent finding; however, because they commonly alternate with periods of normal sinus rhythm, this manifestation can be missed. Urinalysis may be normal, and blood chemistry profiles may show elevated aspartate aminotransferase and lactic dehydrogenase. IVP shows a nonfunctioning kidney, and a renal scan shows no arterial blood flow.

In response to reduced renal circulation, collateral circulation helps preserve the kidney if sufficient development takes place before total obstruction. Collateral circulation, in addition to a marked reduction in filtration, renal work, and oxygen requirements, allows the kidney to tolerate ischemic periods for up to several weeks. In acute total occlusion, a normal kidney can remain viable for about 2 hours before infarction and tissue necrosis begin.

Outcome Management

■ Surgical Management

Treatment of the ischemic kidney usually involves surgical revascularization. Arterial endarterectomy may be done with follow-up anticoagulant or antiplatelet therapy. In the technique known as *percutaneous transluminal renal angioplasty* (PTRA), the vessel is cleared with a balloon catheter. If it cannot be recanalized, a renal artery resection with end-to-end anastomosis or an aortorenal bypass graft procedure may be performed.

PERCUTANEOUS TRANSLUMINAL RENAL ANGIOPLASTY

In clients undergoing PTRA, a balloon-tipped catheter is inserted, usually through the femoral artery, and threaded under radiologic guidance to the obstructed renal artery. The physician inflates the balloon and pulls it through the obstructed area, stretching it and increasing the size of the arterial lumen. A stent may be placed at the site of occlusion to maintain the size of the lumen, prevent restenosis, and minimize the risk of abrupt vessel reclosure. If a stent is placed, antiplatelet agents or anticoagulants may be prescribed to minimize the risk of acute thrombosis.

INDICATIONS. Renal artery angioplasty is usually the first intervention for renovascular hypertension. If angioplasty is unsuccessful or if the condition recurs, more invasive surgical approaches are considered.

CONTRAINDICATIONS. Angioplasty may be contraindicated if there is previous damage to the femoral artery or severely impaired circulation to the limb.

COMPLICATIONS. Renal artery angioplasty is considered a relatively safe procedure. The overall complication rate is about 10%. The most common complications include renal artery dissection, renal artery thrombosis or occlusion, segmental renal infarction, and hematoma formation or puncture trauma.

OUTCOMES. About one third of clients with renovascular hypertension do not respond to this therapy. A significant number are cured, and about half improve significantly. The treatment can be repeated if necessary. Clients usually return home in 24 to 48 hours.

■ Nursing Management of the Surgical Client

PREOPERATIVE CARE

Because the length of stay is limited for most clients undergoing PTRA, it is a challenge to coordinate their care during the diagnostic and intervention phases of treatment. Typically, diagnostic tests such as angiograms and blood work are completed during the week before the procedure. Teaching about angioplasty and discharge instructions must be provided in a short time period.

POSTOPERATIVE CARE

Care after PTRA is similar to other care after any angioplasty. Just after the procedure, vital signs are monitored every 15 minutes for 1 hour, every 30 minutes for 2 hours, hourly for 3 hours, and then regularly according to the established protocol. Check the dressing at these times for manifestations of bleeding or hematoma formation, and check peripheral pulses to assess circulation in the affected limb. Bed rest for up to 24 hours may be ordered.

In the longer term, the client's blood pressure should be monitored because hypertension can indicate recurrence of the lesion. Control of hypertension is crucial to preserving renal function.

After renal artery bypass graft surgery, nursing care is similar to other care after any kidney surgery, such as nephrectomy (see earlier). However, in the postoperative period after an aortorenal bypass graft procedure, the client may experience an initial exacerbation of hypertension. Its cause is unclear, but it is thought to be related to systemic vasoconstriction secondary to general anesthesia and intraoperative hypothermia, severe pain, or transient renin secretion caused by clamping the aorta and manipulating the kidney. This episode usually lasts no more than 48 hours, but it can be significant and may require medical intervention. You must monitor blood pressure frequently.

RENAL VEIN DISEASE

The primary pathologic process involving the renal vein is thrombosis. Obstruction of venous drainage increases interstitial pressure, which reduces renal function. Findings include severe lumbar pain, renal enlargement, proteinuria, and hematuria. If the obstruction is bilateral, oliguria and azotemia occur. Contributing factors include diabetic nephropathy, chronic glomerulonephritis, and renal amyloidosis.

Kidney survival depends largely on the development of collateral circulation before the vessel is fully occluded. Embolectomy or ligation of the renal veins may be done, and anticoagulants may be prescribed. Intravenous streptokinase is used to lyse the occluding clot. If enough renal damage has occurred, nephrectomy is an option.

CONGENITAL DISORDERS

Renal congenital anomalies usually involve abnormalities in the number, position, form, size, or structure of the kidneys. Blood supply may be abnormal, although malformations that significantly affect renal function are rare. Anomalies of the ureteropelvic junction usually obstruct at that point and result in hydronephrosis. Typically, this situation is discovered and treated during childhood.

ANOMALIES INVOLVING KIDNEY NUMBER AND POSITION

Renal agenesis is the absence of one or both kidneys. Having only one kidney presents no difficulty if this kidney functions adequately. A client can live normally with one properly functioning kidney, as kidney donors aptly demonstrate. Bilateral agenesis, however, is fatal. Even in unilateral agenesis, the functioning kidney is at high risk for development of additional anomalies.

Supernumerary kidneys (more than two kidneys) are usually asymptomatic and are discovered during IVP. The extra ureter enters either the ipsilateral ureter or the bladder.

Ectopic, or malpositioned, kidneys are usually found in the pelvis, although thoracic kidneys have been docu-

FIGURE 35-4 Horseshoe kidney.

mented. Problems associated with this anomaly include respiratory difficulties, pain caused by pressure on nerves or surrounding structures, and difficulty in childbirth.

Occasionally, one kidney may be across the midline, so that both kidneys are on the same side. This condition usually remains undiscovered until infection or obstruction indicates a need for x-ray examination.

ANOMALIES INVOLVING KIDNEY FORM AND SIZE

Anomalies of kidney form and size include aplasia, hypoplasia, dysplasia, and *horseshoe kidney*. Aplastic kidneys are small and contracted and contain no functioning renal tissue. Renal hypoplasia produces miniature kidneys with some functioning tissue. Although clinically this condition may be asymptomatic, it may cause hypertension and recurrent urinary tract infection.

Horseshoe kidney results when two kidneys are joined into a single organ whose shape somewhat resembles that of a horseshoe (Fig. 35-4). The kidneys are connected, usually at the lower poles, by an isthmus of tissue. Because the developmental error interferes with normal ascent and medial rotation, the kidney is usually located in the lower lumbar region with its pelvis facing anteriorly. Although clients with horseshoe kidney may be asymtomatic, they are susceptible to hydronephrosis, infection secondary to ureteropelvic junction obstruction, and calculus formation.

ANOMALIES INVOLVING CYSTIC DISEASE

Cystic disease in renal tissue can range from a simple, solitary fluid-filled mass to almost complete replacement of renal structures by cystic tissue. A simple renal cyst commonly originates superficially in the renal parenchyma. It grows slowly and usually produces no manifestations until adulthood, when it may cause heaviness and pain in the abdomen and become a palpable mass. Arriv-

ing at a diagnosis may be complicated because renal cysts closely resemble malignant tumors; naturally, differentiation between the two is vital. As long as a simple renal cyst remains asymptomatic, intervention usually is unnecessary. If intervention is necessary, the cyst may be aspirated with a needle or a partial nephrectomy may be performed to remove it.

■ POLYCYSTIC KIDNEYS

Polycystic disease of the kidney is a hereditary disorder in which grape-like cysts containing serous fluid, blood, or urine replace normal kidney tissue (Fig. 35-5). The condition may develop at any age.

Infantile polycystic kidney disease is inherited as an autosomal recessive trait, and both parents must have carried the gene. It is a rare disorder that affects both kidneys and often the liver. In an infant, the disease usually causes death within days. Milder forms of the disease do not appear until childhood.

Adult polycystic disease accounts for about 10% of the clients receiving dialysis or transplantation. It is inherited as an autosomal dominant trait. It usually appears after age 40 years, although it may begin as early as age 20 or as late as age 80. There are diverse manifestations; the most common are dull, aching lumbar or flank pain, which may be colicky, and hematuria. Other common findings are proteinuria, palpable kidney masses, pyuria, calculi, and uremia (see Chapter 32). Early in the disease, the ability to concentrate urine decreases. Hypertension develops along with cardiac enlargement and heart failure.

Polycystic liver disease occurs in about one third of cases, and cystic lesions are sometimes found in the thyroid, lung, pancreas, spleen, ovary, testis, epididymis, uterus, and bladder. Cerebral aneurysms occur in about 2% of clients with polycystic kidney disease.

The cystic kidney can become so enlarged that it causes severe pressure on other organs, with production of additional extrarenal manifestations. The ultimate result of this disease is chronic renal failure (see Chapter 36). As the disease slowly progresses, renal nephrons are de-

FIGURE 35-5 Polycystic kidney disease.

stroyed, renal function deteriorates, and uremia ultimately results. The mean duration of polycystic kidney disease from onset of manifestations to development of uremia varies a great deal and may be 15 to 30 years or more.

Because there is no known way to arrest the progress of the destructive cysts, conservative medical treatment is designed to preserve kidney function. Urinary tract infection is the most common complication because of the distorted renal architecture; chronic infection may occur if resistant bacteria develop. Aggressive control of hypertension is essential.

Unlike clients with decreasing creatinine clearance rates caused by other kidney diseases, those with polycystic kidney disease seem to waste rather than retain sodium. Thus, they need an increased sodium and water intake. When end-stage renal disease develops, dialysis or renal transplantation is required. Nursing interventions for clients with renal failure are discussed in Chapter 36.

Genetic counseling is advisable because of the hereditary nature of the disease—especially if the disease is diagnosed during childbearing years. However, because the disease typically appears after the childbearing period, the likelihood of transmitting the disease to another generation is high. Therefore, counseling the extended family is essential when the disease has been identified.

■ ADULT-ONSET MEDULLARY CYSTIC DISEASE

Adult-onset medullary cystic disease, sometimes called *uremic sponge kidney* or *medullary polycystic disease*, is also an autosomal dominant disorder. It is similar to polycystic disease in all aspects except that it progresses to uremia rapidly after its onset in the teenage years or in one's 20s. Hemodialysis and renal transplantation are likely to be required.

■ MEDULLARY SPONGE KIDNEY

Medullary sponge kidney is a cystic disorder in which spaces are produced at the apex of the renal pyramids. Onset peaks during adolescence or between ages 30 and 40 years. Infection, calculi, pain, and hematuria are potential complications. Renal function usually remains adequate unless the client has uncontrolled infection or calculi.

OTHER HEREDITARY RENAL DISORDERS

Other hereditary renal disorders include some types of chronic nephritis (such as Alport's disease), congenital nephrotic syndrome, distal renal tubular acidosis, idiopathic hypercalciuria, and nephrotic diabetes insipidus. Many of these conditions are fatal during childhood, but some persist into adulthood and are discussed in the appropriate parts of this text.

CONCLUSIONS

Renal disorders are highly complex. You must have a clear understanding of the structure and function of the renal system to care for clients with these conditions. The outcomes of successful treatment include preservation of renal function.

THINKING CRITICALLY

1. **A 35-year-old newlywed woman enters the emergency department with acute abdominal pain and a temperature of 101.8° F. Her abdomen is distended, and she has not had a bowel movement today, even though she is usually regular. The abdominal pain is diffuse and on the right side. She has no rebound tenderness and no pain at McBurney's point. Her WBC count is 15,000/mm³. What problems other than appendicitis might she be experiencing? What other assessments should be made?**

Factors to Consider. What type of renal problem might she be experiencing? What teaching would she need when the diagnosis is made? What medication might be prescribed and why? What follow-up is needed?

2. **L. S. is a 22-year-old male college student with a diagnosis of acute glomerulonephritis. Three weeks ago, he received oral antibiotic therapy for strep throat. He is scheduled for a renal biopsy to confirm a diagnosis of acute poststreptococcal glomerulonephritis. What other diagnostic assessments should be made? What is the expected course of treatment?**

Factors to Consider. What teaching does this client need when the diagnosis is confirmed? What medication might be prescribed, and how will it be delivered? What follow-up is needed?

3. **C. H. is a 68-year-old retired mail carrier who lives with his wife. They spend 6 months living in their midwestern home state and spend the winter months in Arizona. The client is admitted with a diagnosis of suspected renal cell carcinoma. Diagnostic tests confirm the diagnosis. What surgical procedure will be scheduled? What nursing interventions are associated with this procedure?**

Factors to Consider. What diagnostic tests were used to confirm the diagnosis of renal carcinoma? What tests will be used to determine whether radiation, chemotherapy, and immunotherapy are needed? Describe the postoperative assessments you should make for pain management, vital signs, surgical dressings, drainage tubes, and urine output. If Mr. and Mrs. H. plan to drive to Arizona a month after surgery, what should you discuss with them about their travel plans?

BIBLIOGRAPHY

1. Ambrus, J., & Nagaraja, N. (1997). Immunologic aspects of renal disease. *Journal of the American Medical Association, 278*(22), 1938–1945.
2. American Cancer Society. (2000). *Cancer facts and figures—2000.* Atlanta: Author.
3. Bennett, J. C., & Plum, F. (Eds.). (1996). *Cecil textbook of medicine* (20th ed.). Philadelphia: W. B. Saunders.
4. Breisch, A. J., & Perez, J. A. (1995). The cardiovascular clinical nurse specialist as case manager during endovascular revascularization of renal artery stenosis. *Journal of Vascular Nursing, 13*(1), 14–20.
5. Brenner, B. M. (Ed.). (1996). *Brenner and Rector's the kidney* (5th ed.). Philadelphia: W. B. Saunders.

6. Burrows-Hudson, S. (Ed.). (1999). *Standards and guidelines of clinical practice for nephrology nursing.* Pitman, NJ: American Nephrology Nurses Association.
7. Chow, W., et al. (1999). Rising incidence of renal cell cancer in the United States. *Journal of the American Medical Association, 281*(17), 1628–1631.
8. Clark, P. (1999). 13-year experience with percutaneous management of upper tract transitional cell carcinoma. *Journal of Urology, 161,* 772–776.
9. Diamond, G. L., & Zalups, R. K. (1998). Understanding renal toxicity of heavy metals. *Toxicology and Pathology, 26*(1), 92–103.
10. Dickson, C. (1995). Treatment of renal carcinoma. *Nursing Times, 91*(34), 29–31.
11. Eggena, P. (1996). *Renal physiology.* Rensselaerville, NY: Novateur Medmedia.
12. Fong, K. Y., et al. (1998). Systemic lupus erythematosus: Initial manifestations and clinical features after 10 years of disease. *Annals of the Academy of Medicine, Singapore, 26*(3), 278–281.
13. Gill, I. (1995). Advances in urological laparoscopy. *Journal of Urology, 154*(10), 1275–1294.
14. Glassock, R. J. (1998). *Current therapy in nephrology and hypertension* (4th ed.). St. Louis: Mosby–Year Book.
15. Gunnarsson, I., et al. (1997). Occurrence of anti-C1q antibodies in IgA nephropathy. *Nephrology Dialysis and Transplantation, 12*(11), 2263–2268.
16. Guyton, A. C., & Hall, J. E. (1996). *Textbook of medical physiology* (9th ed.). Philadelphia: W. B. Saunders.
17. Guyton, A., & Hall, J. (1997). *Human physiology and mechanisms of disease* (6th ed.). Philadelphia: W. B. Saunders.
18. Hansen, M. (1998). *Pathophysiology: Foundations of disease and clinical intervention.* Philadelphia: W. B. Saunders.
19. Hiller, J., et al. (1997). Functional advantages of laparoscopic live donor nephrectomy versus open nephrectomy. *Journal of Transplant Coordination, 7*(3), 134–140.
20. Hinman, F. (1998). *Atlas of urologic surgery* (2nd ed.). Philadelphia: W. B. Saunders.
21. Hricik, D., Chung-Park, M., & Sedor, J. (1998). Glomerulonephritis. *New England Journal of Medicine, 339*(13), 888–899.
22. Karlowicz, K. A. (Ed.). (1995). *Urologic nursing: Principles and practice.* Philadelphia: W. B. Saunders.
23. Koeppen, B. M., & Stanton, B. A. (1997). *Renal physiology* (2nd ed.). St. Louis: Mosby–Year Book.
24. Krivak, L. (1995). Laparoscopic transperitoneal nephrectomy. *Canadian Operating Room Nursing Journal, 13*(2), 21–24.
25. Lancaster, L. E. (Ed.). (1995). *Core curriculum for nephrology nursing* (3rd ed.). Pitman, NJ: American Nephrology Nurses Association.
26. Levine, D. Z. (Ed.). (1997). *Caring for the renal patient* (3rd ed.). Philadelphia: W. B. Saunders.
27. Loeb, W. F. (1998). The measurement of renal injury. *Toxicology and Pathology, 26*(1), 26–28.
28. Lubkin, I. (1998). *Chronic illness: Impact and interventions* (4th ed.). Boston: Jones & Bartlett.
29. Mansi, M. K., & Alkhudair, W. K. (1997). Conservative management with percutaneous intervention of major blunt renal injuries. *American Journal of Emergency Medicine, 15*(7), 663–637.
30. Massry, S. G., & Glassock, R. J. (Eds.). (1995). *Massry and Glassock's textbook of nephrology* (3rd ed.). Baltimore: Williams & Wilkins.
31. Matthews, L. A., & Spirnak, J. P. (1995). The nonoperative approach to major blunt renal trauma. *Seminars in Urology, 13*(1), 77–82.
32. McCarthy, S., & McMullen, M. M. (1997). Autosomal dominant polycystic kidney disease: Pathophysiology and treatment. *ANNA Journal, 24*(1), 45–56.
33. McCorkle, R., et al. (1996). *Cancer nursing: A comprehensive textbook* (2nd ed.). Philadelphia: W. B. Saunders.
34. McDougall, E., & Clayman, R. (1994). Advances in laparoscopic urology. Part I: History and development of procedures. *Urology, 43*(4), 420–426.
35. McKinney, B. (1996). When this rare cancer strikes . . . renal cell carcinoma. *RN, 59*(12), 36–41, 51.
36. McKinney, B. (1998). Softening the edge of radical nephrectomy. *Nursing 98, 28*(7), 32hn1–32hn4.
37. Moody, F. (1999). *Atlas of ambulatory surgery.* Philadelphia: W. B. Saunders.
38. Morey, A. F., & McAninch, J. W. R. (1996). Renal trauma: Principles of evaluation and management. *Trauma Quarterly, 13*(1), 79–94.
39. Motzer, R., Bander, N., & Nanus, D. (1996). Renal cell carcinoma. *New England Journal of Medicine, 335*(12), 865–874.
40. Muehlbauer, P. (1998). Are you prepared for interleukin-2? *RN, 68*(2), 34–39.
41. Ritchie, W. (1999). Interferon and survival in metastatic renal carcinoma: Early results of a randomized controlled trial. *Lancet, 353,* 14–17.
42. Sansevero, A. C. (1997). Dehydration in the elderly: Strategies for prevention and management. *Nurse Practitioner, 22*(4), 41–42, 51–52, 54–57.
43. Schrier, R. W. (Ed.). (1995). *Manual of nephrology.* Boston: Little, Brown.
44. Schrier, R. W. (1997). *Renal and electrolyte disorders* (5th ed.). Boston, Little, Brown.
45. Schrier, R. W., & Gottschalk, C. W. (Eds.). (1997). *Diseases of the kidney* (6th ed.). Boston: Little, Brown.
46. Segal, S. (1996). Nursing rounds: Radical nephrectomy. *Nurse Practitioner, 96*(7), 37.
47. Staudenherz, A., et al. (1999). Is there a diagnostic role for bone scanning of patients with a high pretest probability for metastatic renal cell carcinoma? *Cancer, 85,* 153–155.
48. Stone, J., Wyman, J., & Salisbury, S. (1999). *Clinical gerontological nursing: A guide to advanced practice* (2nd ed.). Philadelphia: W. B. Saunders.
49. Tanagho, E. A., & McAninch, J. W. (1995). *Smith's general urology* (14th ed.). Norwalk, CT: Appleton & Lange.
50. Thumboo, J., et al. (1998). Clinical predictors of nephritis in systemic lupus erythematosus. *Annals of the Academy of Medicine, Singapore, 27*(1), 16–20.
51. Valtin, H., & Schafer, J. A. (1995). *Renal function: Mechanisms preserving fluid and solute balance in health* (3rd ed.). Boston: Little, Brown.
52. Vander, A. (1995). *Renal physiology* (5th ed.). New York: McGraw-Hill.
53. Walsh, P., et al. (1998). *Campbell's urology* (7th ed.). Philadelphia: W. B. Saunders.

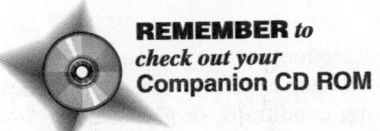

CHAPTER 36

Management of Clients with Renal Failure

Anita E. Molzahn

NURSING OUTCOMES CLASSIFICATION (NOC)
for Nursing Diagnoses—Clients with Renal Failure

Altered Nutrition: Less Than Body Requirements
Nutritional Status
Nutritional Status: Food and Fluid Intake
Anxiety
Anxiety Control
Coping
Constipation
Bowel Elimination
Hydration
Fatigue
Activity Tolerance
Endurance
Energy Conservation
Nutritional Status: Energy
Fluid Volume Deficit
Electrolyte and Acid-Base Balance
Fluid Balance
Hydration
Fluid Volume Excess
Electrolyte and Acid-Base Balance

Fluid Balance
Hydration
Risk for Impaired Skin Integrity
Dialysis Access Integrity
Nutritional Status: Biochemical Measures
Risk Control
Risk Detection
Self-Mutilation Restraint
Tissue Integrity: Skin & Mucous Membranes
Tissue Perfusion: Peripheral
Risk for Ineffective Breathing Pattern
Respiratory Status: Ventilation
Risk for Ineffective Family Coping: Compromised
Family Coping
Family Normalization
Risk for Ineffective Individual Coping
Coping
Decision-Making
Role Performance

Risk for Ineffective Management of Therapeutic Regimen: Families
Family Functioning
Family Health Status
Family Participation in Professional Care
Risk for Ineffective Management of Therapeutic Regimen: Individuals
Family Functioning
Family Health Status
Family Participation in Professional Care
Risk for Infection
Dialysis Access Integrity
Immune Status
Risk Control
Risk Detection
Tissue Integrity: Skin and Mucous Membranes
Risk for Injury
Risk Control
Risk Detection
Symptom Control

A disruption in renal function impairs the body's ability to maintain fluid, electrolyte, and acid-base balance. Reduced renal function interferes with erythropoietin and prostaglandin synthesis. Insulin degradation and the renin-angiotensin-aldosterone system are also affected by decreased renal function.

The diseases and problems that cause renal failure are described in Chapter 35. This chapter identifies common manifestations of acute and chronic renal failure and outlines treatments used to replace or restore renal function, such as dialysis and transplantation. For clients and families, psychosocial needs may arise from the physiologic problems caused by renal failure. You have a key role in helping to promote quality of life and rehabilitation for these clients.

UREMIC SYNDROME

The terms uremia, uremic syndrome, and renal failure are used synonymously. *Uremia* literally means "urine in the blood." This term and the term *uremic syndrome* describe a set of manifestations that result from loss of renal function. This loss may be of sudden onset or may develop over a long period. It may be self-limiting or irreversible. Sudden loss of kidney function, as occurs with damage from trauma, shock, toxins, or acute glomerulonephritis, brings on uremia rapidly and usually causes severe deterioration of the client's condition. Gradual loss of kidney function over an extended period may occur with glomerulonephritis, hypertension, chronic pyelonephritis, and other diseases.

Because the kidneys perform a wide variety of functions, the effects of uremia occur not only in the kidneys but also in other organ systems. Because of the time involved, chronic renal failure causes more degenerative changes throughout the body than acute uremia does. However, both types of renal failure have many of the same consequences. Unless the process can be halted or replacement therapy initiated, coma, seizures, and death result.

ACUTE RENAL FAILURE

Acute renal failure (ARF) refers to the abrupt loss of kidney function. Over a period of hours to a few days, the glomerular filtration rate (GFR) drops. Serum creatinine and urea nitrogen rise. A healthy adult who eats a normal diet needs a minimum urine output of about 400 ml over 24 hours to excrete the body's waste products through the kidneys. An amount lower than this indicates a decreased GFR. *Oliguria* refers to daily outputs of urine between 100 and 400 ml; *anuria* refers to urine output of less than 100 ml.

Etiology and Risk Factors

There are many possible causes of ARF, the most common of which are hypotension and prerenal hypovolemia. The etiologic mechanism of these disorders is discussed in Chapter 35.

CLASSIFICATION

The numerous causes of ARF can be categorized into three major areas: prerenal, renal, and postrenal (Fig. 36–1).

Prerenal Causes

Prerenal causes of ARF are those that interfere with renal perfusion. The kidneys depend on adequate delivery of blood to be filtered by the glomeruli. Therefore, reduced renal blood flow lowers the GFR and can lead to ARF. Conditions that contribute to decreased renal blood flow include the following:

- Circulatory volume depletion, as may occur with diarrhea, vomiting, hemorrhage, excessive use of diuretics, burns, renal salt-wasting conditions, or glycosuria
- Volume shifts, as from third-space sequestration of fluid, vasodilation, or gram-negative sepsis
- Decreased cardiac output, as during cardiac pump failure, pericardial tamponade, or acute pulmonary embolism
- Decreased peripheral vascular resistance, as from spinal anesthesia, septic shock, or anaphylaxis
- Vascular obstruction, such as bilateral renal artery occlusion or dissecting aneurysm

Intrarenal Causes

Intrarenal (or renal) causes of ARF involve parenchymal changes caused by disease or nephrotoxic substances. Acute tubular necrosis is the most common intrarenal cause of ARF and accounts for about 75% of cases. This destruction of the tubular epithelial cells results from impaired renal perfusion or direct damage by nephrotoxins. In addition to the nephrotoxins described in Chapter 35, acute tubular necrosis may be caused by heme pigments, such as myoglobin and hemoglobin, which are liberated from damaged muscle tissue. This release may result from trauma (rhabdomyolysis), such as surgery, crush injury, and electric shock, or from nontraumatic conditions, such as severe muscle exertion, genetic conditions (such as diabetes mellitus or malignant hyperthermia), infectious disease, metabolic conditions (such as hypokalemia, phosphatemia, or heat stroke), and rejection of a transplanted kidney.

Other intrarenal causes of ARF include glomerulonephritis; microvascular and large vascular lesions, as in hemolytic-uremic syndrome; thrombosis; vasculitis; scleroderma; trauma; atherosclerosis; tumor invasion; and cortical necrosis, which is caused by prolonged vasospasm of the cortical blood vessels.

Postrenal Causes

Postrenal causes of ARF arise from an obstruction in the urinary tract, anywhere from the tubules to the urethral meatus. Common sources of obstruction include prostatic

FIGURE 36–1 Causes of acute renal failure: prerenal, intrarenal, and postrenal.

PRERENAL FAILURE

Circulating volume depletion
Volume shifts
Decreased cardiac output
Decreased peripheral
   vascular resistance
Renal vascular obstruction

INTRARENAL FAILURE

Acute tubular necrosis
Trauma
Severe muscle exertion
Certain genetic conditions
Infectious disease
Metabolic disorders
Glomerulonephritis
Vascular lesions

POSTRENAL FAILURE

Obstruction
Spinal cord injury
Pelvic trauma

hypertrophy, calculi, invading tumors, surgical accidents, ureteral or urethral strictures or stenosis, and retroperitoneal fibrosis. Spinal cord injury may lead to decreased bladder emptying and a functional obstruction.

GENERAL CONSIDERATIONS

In management of the client with ARF, it is important to determine whether the disorder originates from prerenal, intrarenal, or postrenal causes before intervention begins. Appropriate interventions require determining the cause of the disorder.

One health promotion strategy is to teach clients about the risks of nephrotoxic agents identified in Chapter 35. Other health promotion and health maintenance actions include monitoring of vital signs and urine output and early identification and reversal of hypotension and hypovolemia, the two causes of ARF associated with the highest mortality rates. Prevention of urinary obstruction is another health promotion and maintenance action.

Pathophysiology

The pathogenesis of ARF is not clear. One hypothesis is that the damaged tubules cannot conserve sodium normally, which activates the renin-angiotensin-aldosterone system. The effect is to redistribute the renal vascular supply by increasing the tone of both the afferent and efferent arterioles. The resulting ischemia may cause an increase in vasopressin, cellular swelling, inhibition of prostaglandin synthesis, and further stimulation of the renin-angiotensin system. The reduced blood flow decreases glomerular pressure, GFR, and tubular flow; thus, oliguria occurs.

Another theory is that cellular and protein debris in the tubule obstruct the lumen, which raises the intratubular pressure. The increasing oncotic pressure opposes filtration pressure until glomerular filtration stops. A biochemical theory claims that decreased renal blood flow leads to decreased oxygen delivery to the proximal tubules; this causes a reduction in cellular adenosine triphosphate, which increases cytosolic and mitochondrial calcium concentrations. The result of this process is cell death and tubular necrosis. Vasomotor nephropathy, which causes spasms of peritubular capillaries, may result in tubular damage. Other possible pathogenic mechanisms include leakage of filtered urine through damaged tubules back into the peritubular capillaries and chemical or morphologic changes in the basement membrane of the glomerular capillary, which decrease nephron filtration. The reversibility of this mechanism depends on the level of destruction of the basement membrane.

Clinical Manifestations

The clinical course of ARF is marked by several phases. The onset (or initiating) phase covers the period from the precipitating event to the development of renal manifestations. Manifestations may begin immediately or up to a week after the precipitating event. The oliguric-anuric (or nonoliguric) phase lasts 1 to 8 weeks. The longer this phase, the poorer the prognosis. Dialysis may be required during the oliguric-anuric phase.

A gradual or abrupt return to glomerular filtration and leveling of the blood urea nitrogen (BUN) signal the diuretic phase. Urine output may be 1000 to 2000 ml/day, which may lead to dehydration; 25% of the deaths from ARF occur during this phase.

The recovery phase lasts 3 to 12 months. During this time, the client commonly returns to an activity level similar to that before the onset of the illness. Mild tubular abnormalities, including glycosuria and decreased concentrating ability, may continue for years, and the client is continually at risk for fluid and electrolyte imbalance, especially during times of stress.

The effects of ARF are widespread. The major consequences include the following:

- Fluid and electrolyte imbalances (fluid overload or depletion, hyperkalemia, hyponatremia, hypocalcemia, and hypermagnesemia)
- Acidosis
- Increased susceptibility to secondary infections
- Anemia
- Platelet dysfunction
- Gastrointestinal complications (anorexia, nausea, vomiting, diarrhea or constipation, and stomatitis)
- Increased incidence of pericarditis
- Uremic encephalopathy characterized by apathy, defective recent memory, episodic obtundation, dysarthria, tremors, convulsions, and coma
- Impaired wound healing

Other manifestations are usually a result of these sequelae. The most common overall manifestation of ARF is alteration of the expected urine output. Usually, oliguria or anuria is found, but polyuric ARF accounts for 30% of the cases. There are two varieties of ARF: nonoliguric and oliguric.

NONOLIGURIC RENAL FAILURE

Although nonoliguric, or polyuric, ARF is being recognized more often, its status remains controversial. It may be an independent entity, or it may be a phase of oliguric ARF.

Clients with nonoliguric renal failure may excrete as much as 2 L/day, and this must be recognized as a possible sign of ARF. The urine produced is dilute and nearly isosmolar, reflected in a low urine specific gravity indicating that not all nephrons have stopped filtering. Hypertension and tachypnea, with manifestations of fluid overload, are comonly found. The client may also demonstrate manifestations of extracellular fluid depletion, such as dry mucous membranes, poor skin turgor, and orthostatic hypotension. Nonoliguric renal failure is usually associated with less morbidity and mortality than the oliguric form, probably because of the lesser degree and shorter duration of azotemia.

OLIGURIC RENAL FAILURE

In oliguric ARF, urine production usually falls below 400 ml/day. However, the aging kidney normally loses its concentrating ability, and renal function becomes more susceptible to insult. Therefore, an older client may have had oliguria even at urine volumes of 600 to 700 ml/day.

The clinical manifestations of oliguric ARF depend on the cause. In prerenal failure, assessment findings are quite diverse, depending on the underlying condition. The client commonly has a history of a precipitating event, such as hemorrhage or cardiac insult. The urine has a high specific gravity and osmolarity, and there is little or no proteinuria. Urine sediment is usually normal, although it may contain a few hyaline and granular casts. There is very little urinary sodium excretion. The BUN-creatinine ratio is significantly elevated, reaching levels between 10:1 and 40:1.

Systemic manifestations of intrinsic renal failure may include edema, weight gain, hemoptysis resulting from elevated left ventricular end-diastolic pressure, weakness from anemia, and hypertension. The urine has a fixed specific gravity, a high sodium concentration, and definite proteinuria. The client with glomerulonephritis has hematuria and red blood cell and hemoglobin casts. Acute tubular necrosis causes muddy brown granular casts. If there has been significant tissue damage, expect elevated levels of serum creatinine, phosphokinase, and potassium.

Urine produced in postrenal failure may have fixed specific gravity and elevated sodium concentration with little or no proteinuria. Urine sediment is generally normal. The most definitive manifestations are those indicating obstruction, as described with calculi and neoplasms. Wide fluctuations between anuria and polyuria may indicate intermittent urinary tract obstruction.

Urinalysis and determinations of urine specific gravity and sodium levels, serum creatinine, and urea nitrogen are common diagnostic tests for ARF. The amount of urine in relation to intake is also important in formulating the diagnosis. To measure the exact urine output or to obtain a specimen for culture and sensitivity, the client may need to be catheterized one time only (with a straight catheter).

Prognosis

The mortality rate in ARF may be as high as 50%; the highest mortality rates occur when failure is caused by trauma or surgery. The lowest mortality rate is in ARF caused by nephrotoxic substances (see Chapter 35). When obstruction or glomerulonephritis is the cause, the mortality rate is low.

Outcome Management

■ Medical Management

PREVENT ACUTE RENAL FAILURE
The medical management of ARF is largely based on preventing and treating its effects. As with any disease process, prevention is the primary intervention. Attaining and maintaining adequate hydration and diuresis in high-risk clients is crucial, as is the prevention of contributing factors.

Once ARF has developed, prompt recognition and action facilitate restoration of optimal renal function. Correction of the underlying condition, such as hydration for a client with hypovolemic shock, may be all that is necessary in ARF caused by prerenal disorders. Postrenal causes must be rectified. In the meantime, the sequelae of ARF require specific intervention.

MAINTAIN FLUID AND ELECTROLYTE BALANCE
In ARF, maintenance of fluid and electrolyte balance is key to survival. Imbalances are common and pose significant challenges to the clinician.

Fluid replacement must be done carefully to avoid fluid overload. Fluid replacement volumes are usually calculated on the basis of some fraction of the previous day's urine output plus an amount (commonly 400 ml) to account for the usual insensible losses that occur during a 24-hour period. Amounts lost in other ways, such as vomiting and diarrhea, are added to the daily allotment. Unless the client is receiving total parenteral nutrition (TPN), some physicians use a daily weight loss of 0.2 to 0.5 kg/day as a measure of the success of the fluid replacement program. This amount represents the usual daily weight loss through catabolism and loss of lean body mass.

Diuretic therapy may be used cautiously. Furosemide and mannitol are the drugs used most often, but furosemide can be nephrotoxic, increasing the risk of further renal damage. It is also important to avoid dehydration, and fluids should be replaced as needed to maintain adequate blood flow to the kidneys.

Electrolyte replacement is based primarily on urine and serum electrolyte concentrations. Hyperkalemia is probably the most dangerous imbalance because of its contribution to cardiac arrhythmias and arrest. In addition to the kidney's inability to excrete potassium, this electrolyte is released in greater quantities from the body cells when acidosis is present and is further increased by rapid tissue catabolism.

Electrocardiographic monitors are commonly used to check for effects of hypokalemia or hyperkalemia. Cation exchange resins may be administered orally or rectally to facilitate excretion of potassium through the gastrointestinal tract. Sorbitol, an osmotic cathartic, is given with cation exchange resins to induce a diarrhea to eliminate the potassium ions that were exchanged for sodium ions in the resins. Sorbitol can be given orally, as an enema, or by nasogastric tube. Potassium-containing foods and medications should be avoided. In an emergency, administration of 50% glucose and regular insulin, with sodium bicarbonate if necessary, can temporarily prevent cardiac arrest by moving potassium into the cells and reducing serum potassium levels.

Hyponatremia usually results from dilution rather than true lack of sodium. Therefore, intervention is a matter of proper fluid replacement (i.e., fluid restriction and self-correction).

Because magnesium is normally excreted by the kidneys, it can accumulate in renal failure. Dark green vegetables, unrefined grains, seeds, nuts, legumes, and antacids and osmotic laxatives containing magnesium should be avoided because they increase serum magnesium levels.

Metabolic acidosis usually results from the accumulation of acid waste products. Sodium bicarbonate, sodium lactate, or sodium acetate may be used in the short term to correct this condition. Dialysis is usually used for severe acidosis.

Low doses (1 to 5 μg/kg/min) of dopamine hydrochloride (Intropin) may be given to activate dopamine receptors in the kidney. Dopamine, a sympathomimetic, can dilate renal blood vessels, which improves renal function, increases urine flow, and increases sodium excretion to improve renal function.

REPLACE RENAL FUNCTION
Dialysis (detailed later in the chapter) is frequently required for treatment of ARF. Indications for dialysis include:

- Significant volume overload
- Uncontrolled hyperkalemia or acidosis
- Progressive uremia, as evidenced by rising BUN and creatinine concentrations
- Altered central nervous system function
- Pericarditis

There are some special considerations for dialysis of clients with ARF. First, heparin is generally decreased to reduce the risk of bleeding. Because hypotension is common, clients must be carefully monitored and replacement fluids provided as appropriate.

For clients with ARF, continuous renal replacement therapy (CRRT) has benefits. There are several types of CRRT, including (1) continuous arteriovenous hemofiltration (CAVH), (2) continuous venovenous hemofiltration (CVVH), (3) continuous venovenous hemodialysis (CVVHD), (4) continuous arteriovenous ultrafiltration (CAVU), and (5) slow continuous ultrafiltration (SCUF). In essence, these methods involve removal of plasma water and dissolved contents from the client's blood across a membrane. In contrast, in dialysis, particles are removed by diffusion. Slow continuous removal of waste products and water through CRRT is less stressful to the client than shorter, more efficient dialysis treatments.

PREVENT INFECTIONS

Secondary infections are a significant cause of death in clients with ARF. The client must be monitored carefully for infectious processes; if these occur, they should be treated aggressively. Except to monitor urine output during ARF, indwelling urethral catheters are usually avoided because of their great potential for introducing infection. If a catheter is placed, meticulous catheter care is essential.

MONITOR THE CLIENT

Treatment of ARF may take place in an intensive care unit or other critical care unit, depending on the cause. Much of the care consists of physiologic monitoring and assessment. In addition to monitoring fluid and electrolyte balance, you should monitor the progression of manifestations associated with renal failure. Pericarditis occurs in as many as 18% of clients with renal failure. Assessment findings include pleuritic pain (which may subside when the client assumes an upright position), pericardial friction rub, tachycardia, and fever. Treatment usually starts with steroids or nonsteroidal anti-inflammatory drugs (NSAIDs). Pericardiocentesis and pericardiectomy may be necessary if cardiac function is compromised.

Other problems call for relief of manifestations. The rising BUN decreases the seizure threshold, resulting in a rise in the number of seizures. These seizures may be relieved by intravenous phenytoin or phenobarbital. Anemia is treated by transfusions or the use of recombinant erythropoietin. Erythropoietin is a hormone produced by the kidney that stimulates red blood cell production. Erythropoietin is used in chronic renal failure, but its use in ARF has not been studied extensively. Bleeding tendencies may be minimized by correcting vitamin K deficiencies as well as by lowering the serum BUN level, because BUN interferes with platelet aggregation.

MAINTAIN NUTRITIONAL STATUS

Proper nutrition is crucial. A high-calorie, low-protein diet is usually prescribed. The diet may also be low in sodium, magnesium, phosphate, and potassium. The protein must be of high biologic value (complete), containing the essential amino acids to reduce nitrogenous waste products. Adequate carbohydrate intake reverses the process of gluconeogenesis. During the acute phases, intake should be 135 to 150 nonprotein kilocalories (kcal) for each 6.25 g of protein ingested; this ratio is considered adequate for preventing protein catabolism. Liquid supplements, low in potassium, may also be used. If oral intake is not sufficient to meet requirements, tube feedings or total parenteral nutrition, including lipids, may be instituted.

■ Nursing Management of the Medical Client
ASSESSMENT

Carefully monitor any client with risk factors for ARF. In fact, it is important to assess fluid balance in any hospitalized or seriously injured client. Because hypovolemia is a common cause, assess the client closely for this problem. When the diagnosis is ARF, carefully assess for such complications as pleural effusion, pericarditis, acidosis, and uremia. See the Case Study on acute renal failure.

DIAGNOSIS, OUTCOMES, INTERVENTIONS
Fluid Volume Deficit or Fluid Volume Excess. A common diagnosis in ARF is *Fluid Volume Deficit related to fluid loss from a variety of causes.* Another common nursing diagnosis is *Fluid Volume Excess related to inability of the kidneys to produce urine secondary to ARF.*

Outcomes. The client will not have fluid volume deficit and ARF; if ARF does occur, fluid volume excess will not develop or it will be managed with dialysis or CRRT, as evidenced by a return to balanced intake and output (I & O).

Interventions. Careful monitoring of fluid balance indicators is crucial to the management of ARF. Accurate intake and output measurements guide the fluid replacement regimen. Compare these values, and look for 24- to 48-hour trends. Check the client's vital signs (including postural blood pressures and apical pulses), skin turgor, and mucous membranes about every 4 hours, depending on the severity of the illness. Carefully obtain daily weights using the same scale at the same time of day. Obtain blood pressure measurements via an arterial line, if one is in place.

Urine specific gravity, usually an indication of fluid balance, may not be useful with intrinsic renal disease. Abnormalities in heart sounds, breath sounds, and mental status may indicate the presence of fluid and electrolyte imbalances.

When the physician has determined the client's fluid allotment, make sure that intake amounts for each shift are followed. This means carefully monitoring fluid intake to ensure that the prescribed amount is taken. Often, this amount represents a significant fluid restriction for the client, which causes a problem with thirst. Help the client stay within the prescribed restriction with careful oral hygiene and judicious use of ice chips, lip ointments, and appropriate diversionary activities. Placing the allotted water in a spray bottle may help to spread out the amount

Acute Renal Failure and Abdominal Aortic Aneurysm Resection

Mr. Carlson is a 70-year-old retired farmer who is brought in by squad to a small rural hospital complaining of boring abdominal pain that radiates through to the back. A CT scan of the abdomen reveals a dissecting abdominal aneurysm. Mr. Carlson is subsequently flown to an urban hospital for emergency resection of the aneurysm. Complications encountered in surgery require that the aorta be cross-clamped for a number of hours. Multiple blood products are administered to replace those lost through hemorrhage. Mr. Carlson is admitted to the surgical intensive care unit for postoperative care and monitoring.

Initial Postoperative Orders

Routine postoperative vital sign monitoring
Monitor urine output every 1 hour and call if less than ½ ml/kg/hr
5% dextrose in 0.2% normal saline (D_5¼ NS) at 150 ml/hr
Cefazolin sodium (Ancef) 1 g IV every 6 hours
Morphine sulfate 1 to 4 mg IV every 1 hour as needed (prn) for pain
Check metabolic chemistry panel and CBC in AM
Turn, cough, and deep-breathe every 2 hours
Incentive spirometer every 1 hour while awake
NG tube to low intermittent suction, irrigate prn

Nursing Admission Assessment

Mr. Carlson is groggy but easily arousable. His wife of 45 years is at his bedside. She relates that Mr. Carlson expressly told her not to let them keep him alive if anything "bad" should happen. She reports that her husband previously had been in good health and was enjoying his retirement and their grandchildren. He was a coffee drinker but did not use tobacco.

Nursing Physical Assessment

Height: 6 ft
Weight: 175 lb (79.5 kg)
Vital signs: BP, 100/50; TPR, 96.8, 112, 14
LOC: groggy but arousable
EENT: PERLA
Cardiac: sinus tachycardia, S_1 and S_2 readily audible without rubs or murmurs
Pulmonary: breath sounds diminished throughout
Abdominal: NG tube in place and draining small amounts of brown drainage. Large abdominal dressing in place. Abdomen flat; bowel tones absent
Genitourinary: Foley catheter in place draining clear straw-colored urine
Peripheral pulses: 2/2, without edema noted

Throughout the night, Mr. Carlson's urine output dropped and the color changed to dark amber. By 6 AM Mr. Carlson was averaging 30 to 40 ml/hr. He was cooperating well with turning and had received morphine on an hourly basis which was controlling his pain. His dressings remain dry and intact and the NG drainage had changed to golden bile colored liquid. Mr. Carlson's abdomen remains flat and without bowel sounds. The AM laboratory specimens were drawn as ordered, revealing the following pertinent values:

AM Laboratory Values

RBCs: 3.0 million/mm³
Hb: 10.0 g/dl
Hct: 30%
WBCs: 13,000/mm³
Sodium: 145 mEq/L
Chloride: 105 mEq/L
Potassium: 4.8 mEq/L
Creatinine: 2.6 mg/dl
BUN: 47 mg/dl

Consider the pathophysiologic causes of the abnormalities noted in the AM laboratory values. In the next 48 hours. Mr. Carlson's urine output continued to dwindle and his potassium, creatinine, and BUN continued to rise. Mr. Carlson has become increasingly confused and the doctors have turned to Mrs. Carlson to give consent for various treatments. Mr. Carlson's surgeon ordered a nephrology consultation, and the decision has been made to start hemodialysis. A dopamine infusion has been started at the renal perfusion dosage, and intravenous steroid therapy has been initiated. Consider Mr. Carlson's wishes to have no heroic measures.

Dialysis is performed in Mr. Carlson's room every day for the first 3 days and then every other day for the next week. Mr. Carlson's urine output increases, and his blood and urine chemistry values reflect return of marginal renal function. Furosemide (Lasix) at 80 mg twice a day is instituted, and hemodialysis is discontinued. Mr. Carlson is transferred to a medical surgical nursing unit. Mr. Carlson's bowel tones have returned, but he reports a lack of appetite and that food tastes "funny." Mr. Carlson's medications have been converted to oral dosages. It is expected that he will be discharged to his home in his wife's care tomorrow.

Discharge and Post-treatment Considerations

Average length of stay for abdominal aortic aneurysm repair without complications, 5.7 days; with complications, 12.4 days
Complete discharge teaching (including diet, wound care, medications, activity, and follow-up appointments)
Community referral: nutrition and postoperative care support to home nursing service

Questions to Be Considered

1. Compare and contrast the ethical considerations related to treatment options for clients with acute renal failure

and for those with chronic renal failure. Discuss the nurse's role in assisting clients and families with resolution of ethical dilemmas regarding treatment options.

2. Discuss the nutritional and fluid replacement considerations necessary for a postoperative client who develops acute renal failure. Identify nutritional and fluid replacement considerations that are necessary for clients receiving diuretic therapy.

3. Compare and contrast the causes, clinical manifestations, and management of acute renal failure versus chronic renal failure. Identify nursing care and monitoring of the catheters or arteriovenous fistulas used for the various types of dialysis.

4. Identify the nursing measures used to monitor client's fluid and electrolyte status (i.e., fluid balance, sodium, potassium, calcium, chloride, magnesium, and phosphorus).

5. Discuss the nursing measures used to prevent secondary infections for clients with acute renal failure. Identify the factors that place these clients at greater risk for secondary infections.

6. Compare and contrast hemodialysis and peritoneal dialysis. Identify factors that made Mr. Carlson ineligible for peritoneal dialysis.

7. Identify classes of drugs that may be nephrotoxic. Discuss the rationale and implications for the use of these drugs for patients with renal failure.

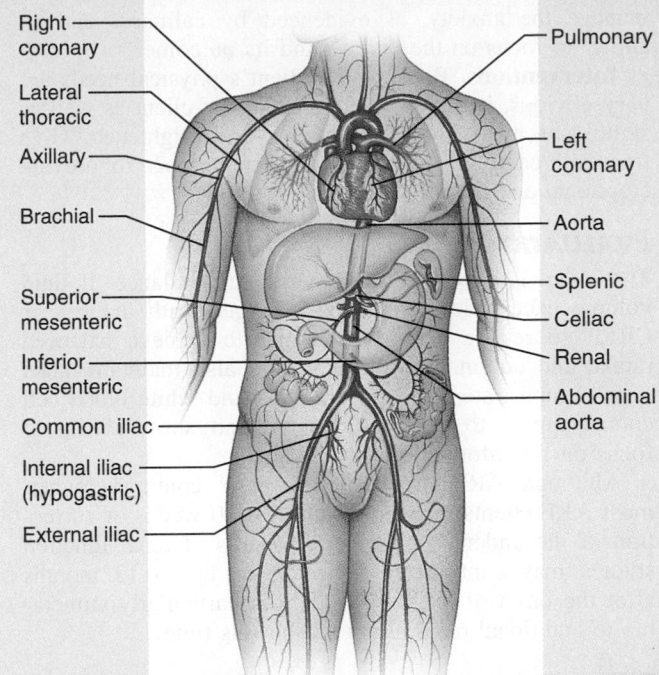

● Major arteries of the chest and abdomen. (Modified from Thibodeau, G. A., & Patton, K. T. [1999]. *Anatomy and physiology* [3rd ed.]. St. Louis, Mosby–Year Book. Illustrated by Barbara Cousins.)

BP, blood pressure; BUN, blood urea nitrogen; CBC, complete blood count; CT, computed tomography; EENT, eyes-ears-nose-throat; Hb, hemoglobin; Hct, hematocrit; IV, intravenous; LOC, level of consciousness; NG, nasogastric; prn, as needed; PERLA, pupils equal and reactive to light and accommodation; RBCs, red blood cells; TPR, temperature, pulse, respirations; WBCs, white blood cells.

taken. Fluid from foods must be taken into account as well. To conserve fluids for the client, administer medications with meals, if possible.

Altered Nutrition: Less Than Body Requirements.
Another common diagnosis for clients with this disorder is *Altered Nutrition: Less Than Body Requirements related to anorexia and altered metabolic state secondary to renal failure.*

Outcomes. The client will maintain adequate nutrition, as evidenced by sufficient intake to prevent protein catabolism and laboratory values within safe levels.

Interventions. A client with renal failure commonly experiences anorexia, nausea, stomatitis, and taste changes. These, combined with a generally less palatable diet, make adequate nutrition a challenge for nurse and client. Work with the client to plan a diet that is most acceptable. The therapeutic dietitian is a good resource.

Provide a pleasant environment at mealtime. Preparing foods in an attractive manner and presenting them in small amounts may help. Medications to alleviate the discomfort of nausea and stomatitis may be useful. Enteral or parenteral nutrition may be instituted if the client's nutritional status cannot be maintained with oral intake.

Risk for Impaired Skin Integrity.
You may need to use the diagnosis *Risk for Impaired Skin Integrity related to poor cellular nutrition and edema.*

Outcomes. The client will not develop impaired skin integrity, as evidenced by intact skin.

Interventions. The poor systemic nutrition and edema that accompany renal failure may cause skin breakdown. Meticulous skin care, frequent turning, and special mattresses are important. Range-of-motion exercises facilitate movement and increase circulation.

Risk for Infection.
Acute or chronic renal failure makes clients more susceptible to infection, resulting in a diagnosis of *Risk for Infection related to lowered resistance.*

Outcomes. The client will not develop infection, as evidenced by normal vital signs, a normal white blood cell count, and no outward manifestations of infection.

Interventions. The client with ARF is immunocompromised and very susceptible to secondary infection, a stress that the kidneys cannot handle. Nursing intervention must be designed to prevent infection in the usual high-risk sites (e.g., respiratory tract, wounds, central catheters, and mouth). Urethral catheters are avoided if possible. If they must be used, provide meticulous catheter care. Also, be alert to early manifestations of infection so that aggressive medical treatment may be instituted.

Anxiety.
Inevitably, the client will experience *Anxiety related to unknown outcome of disease process.*

Outcomes. The client will demonstrate an ability to

manage the anxiety, as evidenced by calmness and an ability to focus on the disease and its outcome.

Interventions. Because the client's physical needs are very obvious, it is easy to forget that the client as well as significant others will be anxious and frightened. Give frequent, careful explanations, and remember to provide emotional and psychological support.

EVALUATION

The client is expected to maintain fluid balance. If fluid volume excess develops, it is managed with dialysis or CRRT to reduce body weight and to achieve balanced intake and output. The client should also maintain intact skin, demonstrate normal vital signs and white blood cell count, appear to be less anxious, and show ability to focus on the information provided.

Although ARF manifestations may continue longer, most ARF clients recover within 4 to 10 weeks of correction of the underlying problem. Results of renal function studies may continue to improve for up to 12 months after the onset of ARF. The client is particularly vulnerable to additional renal injury during this time.

▊ Self-Care

It is important for the client to understand the implications of ARF and the importance of following the therapeutic regimen. The client and significant others have to understand which manifestations might indicate further renal damage or chronic renal failure (CRF). The client must be closely observed by a nephrologist for at least a year after ARF is reversed so that deterioration of renal function can be monitored. The client and significant others require knowledge of renal failure and an understanding of the possible need for ongoing treatment.

▊ Modifications for Elderly Clients

Older clients are at increased risk for ARF because of reduced cardiac contractile function, vascular compliance, renal plasma flow, and renal mass. The older adult has more difficulty maintaining a homeostatic fluid balance. The ability to retain sodium declines with age, as does the ability to concentrate urine. Older clients are also more likely to have pre-existing renal damage from such diseases as hypertension, diabetes, and benign prostatic hypertrophy in men. Therefore, dosages of medications that are nephrotoxic or excreted by the kidney may need to be adjusted.

CHRONIC RENAL FAILURE

Chronic, or irreversible, renal failure is a progressive reduction of functioning renal tissue such that the remaining kidney mass can no longer maintain the body's internal environment. CRF can develop insidiously over many years, or it may result from an episode of ARF from which the client has not recovered.

The incidence of CRF varies widely by state and country. In the United States, the incidence is 268 new cases per million population. According to the U.S. Renal Data System, at the end of 1997, more than 300,000 people were being treated for CRF or end-stage renal disease (ESRD). More than 191,000 people were receiving hemodialysis and 86,000 people had functioning renal transplants.[45]

Etiology and Risk Factors

The causes of CRF are numerous. Chapter 35 discussed various injuries and disease processes that may end in renal failure. Chronic glomerulonephritis, ARF, polycystic kidney disease, obstruction, repeated episodes of pyelonephritis, and nephrotoxins are examples of causes. Systemic diseases, such as diabetes mellitus, hypertension, lupus erythematosus, polyarteritis, sickle cell disease, and amyloidosis, may produce CRF. Diabetes is the leading cause and accounts for more than 30% of clients who receive dialysis. Hypertension is the second leading cause of CRF.

To reduce the risk of CRF, the client should be closely observed and should receive adequate treatment to control or slow the progress of these problems before they progress to ESRD. Some conditions, such as lupus and diabetes, can progress to renal failure despite close treatment.

Pathophysiology

The pathogenesis of CRF involves deterioration and destruction of nephrons with progressive loss of renal function. As the total GFR falls and clearance is reduced, the serum urea nitrogen and creatinine levels rise. Remaining functioning nephrons hypertrophy, as they are required to filter a larger load of solutes. A consequence is that the kidneys lose their ability to concentrate urine adequately. In an attempt to continue excreting the solutes, a large volume of dilute urine may be passed, which makes the client susceptible to fluid depletion. The tubules gradually lose their ability to reabsorb electrolytes. Occasionally, the result is salt wasting, in which the urine contains large amounts of sodium, which leads to more polyuria.

As renal damage advances and the number of functioning nephrons declines, the total GFR decreases further. Thus, the body becomes unable to rid itself of excess water, salt, and other waste products through the kidneys. When the GFR is less than 10 to 20 ml/min, the effect of uremic toxins on the body becomes evident. If the disease is not treated by dialysis or transplantation, the outcome of CRF is uremia and death.

Clinical Manifestations

The clinical manifestations of the early stages of renal failure depend on the disease process and contributing factors. As the destruction of nephrons progresses to ESRD, the manifestations become similar and are described as uremic syndrome. The clinical course of irreversible renal disease and uremic syndrome follows a pattern:

- *Reduced renal reserve* refers to the state in which BUN is high-normal but the client has no clinical manifestations. Normal functioning is evident as long as the client is not exposed to unusual physiologic or psychosocial stress.

- *Renal insufficiency* reflects a more advanced pathologic process with mild azotemia when the client is receiving a general diet. Impaired urine concentration, nocturia (excessive urination at night), and mild anemia are common findings. Renal function is easily impaired by stress.
- *Renal failure* is indicated by severe azotemia, acidosis, impaired urine dilution, severe anemia, and a number of electrolyte imbalances, such as hypernatremia, hyperkalemia, and hyperphosphatemia.
- *ESRD* is characterized by two groups of clinical manifestations: deranged excretory and regulatory mechanisms and a distinctive grouping of gastrointestinal, cardiovascular, neuromuscular, hematologic, integumentary, skeletal, and hormonal manifestations. The kidneys can no longer maintain homeostasis.

The clinical manifestations of CRF are present throughout the body. No organ system is spared. Renal alterations (described previously) include the kidney's inability to concentrate urine and regulate electrolyte excretion. Polyuria progresses to anuria, and the client loses normal diurnal patterns of voiding. In addition, all normal functions of the kidney, such as regulation of acid-base balance, regulation of blood pressure, synthesis of 1,25-dihydroxycholecalciferol, biogenesis of erythropoietin, degradation of insulin, and synthesis of prostaglandins, become curtailed and are eventually lost.

See the algorithm Understanding Chronic Renal Failure and Its Treatment.

ELECTROLYTE IMBALANCES

Electrolyte balance may be upset by impaired excretion and utilization in the kidney. Although many clients maintain a normal serum sodium level, the salt-wasting properties of some failing kidneys, in addition to vomiting and diarrhea, may cause hyponatremia. Apparent hyponatremia may be a dilutional effect of water retention. Late in the disease, salt and water retention often contributes to hypertension and heart failure.

Because the kidneys are efficient at excreting potassium, potassium levels usually remain within normal limits until late in the disease. However, hyperkalemia then becomes a challenging problem. Catabolism, potassium-containing medications, trauma, blood transfusions, and acidosis contribute to potassium excess.

Several mechanisms contribute to hypocalcemia. Conversion of 25-hydroxycholecalciferol to 1,25-dihydroxycholecalciferol (necessary to absorb calcium) is decreased, which results in reduced intestinal absorption of calcium. At the same time, phosphate is not excreted, which causes hyperphosphatemia. Because calcium and phosphate are inversely related, a high phosphate level results in a reduced calcium level. This combination stimulates the parathyroid glands to secrete parathyroid hormone in an attempt to facilitate phosphate excretion and raise the serum calcium level by resorbing calcium from bone. Osteomalacia, osteitis fibrosa, and osteosclerosis are commonly seen in clients with CRF as a result of these metabolic alterations in calcium, phosphorus, parathyroid hormone, and vitamin D. In some clients, hypercalcemia

may develop because of persistent secretion of parathyroid hormone.

Mildly elevated serum magnesium levels are found early in the disease. Magnesium does not usually reach a dangerous level unless the client is receiving magnesium-containing laxatives or antacids.

METABOLIC CHANGES

In advancing renal failure, BUN and serum creatinine rise as waste products of protein metabolism accumulate in the blood. The serum creatinine level is the most accurate measure of renal function. The normal ratio of BUN to creatinine is 10:1, and it remains the same as both the creatinine and BUN rise.

The proteinuria accompanying renal disease and sometimes inadequate dietary intake of proteins cause hypoproteinemia, which lowers the intravascular oncotic pressure. Serum uric acid is often high but is not commonly associated with manifestations of gout.

Carbohydrate intolerance results from impaired insulin production and metabolism. Four mechanisms are responsible:

- Peripheral insulin antagonism
- Impaired insulin secretion
- A prolonged insulin half-life, which is directly related to kidney malfunction
- Abnormalities in circulating insulin

Therefore, special care is needed in adjustment of insulin doses for clients with diabetes mellitus complicated by renal failure. Even short-acting regular insulin functions as a longer-acting insulin, resulting in a need for lower dosages or fewer injections per day. Serum glucose levels must be monitored closely.

Elevated triglycerides are found almost universally. This type IV hyperlipidemia is thought to be caused by increased production of lipids by the liver in response to elevated blood glucose and insulin levels. At the same time, assimilation of lipids in the peripheral tissues appears to be reduced, possibly because of the blockage of lipoprotein lipase activity. This contributes to a secondary complication of cardiovascular disease.

Metabolic acidosis occurs because of the kidney's inability to excrete hydrogen ions. Decreased reabsorption of sodium bicarbonate and decreased formation of dihydrogen phosphate and ammonia contribute to this problem. Acidosis accentuates hyperkalemia and the reabsorption of calcium from the bones.

Pericarditis is usually related to the accumulation of uremic toxins, rarely to infection. Manifestations include pericardial pain (often relieved by an upright position), tachycardia, pleural friction rub, and fever. The condition may progress to pericardial effusion and cardiac tamponade, a life-threatening complication.

HEMATOLOGIC CHANGES

The primary hematologic effect of renal failure is anemia, usually normochromic and normocytic. It occurs because the kidneys are unable to produce erythropoietin, a hormone necessary for red blood cell production. If it is left untreated, hematocrit levels can drop below 20%. Frequently, the fatigue, weakness, and cold intolerance accompanying the anemia lead to a diagnosis of renal failure.

Understanding Chronic Renal Failure and Its Treatment

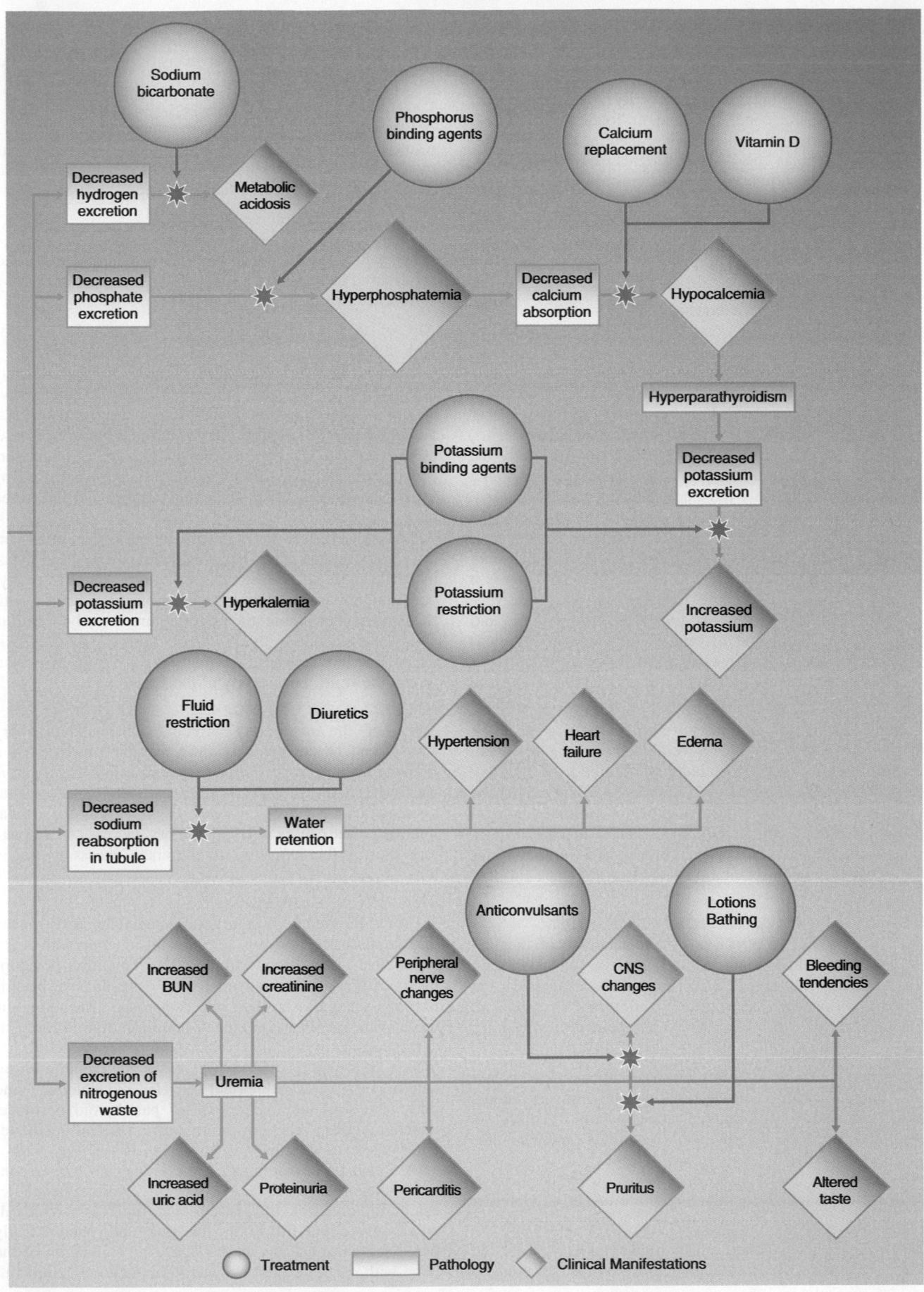

Treatment ⬤   Pathology ▭   Clinical Manifestations ◇

■ BUN, blood urea nitrogen; CNS, central nervous system.

The mild anemia found in the early stages is usually due to reduced production of the hormone, erythropoietin, which results in decreased production of red blood cells. Later, hemolysis, gastrointestinal losses, and clotting abnormalities contribute to the severity of the condition. Occasionally, the client has iron or folate depletion because of nutritional deficiencies. Bleeding tendencies become apparent as the disease progresses. Platelet abnormalities are the primary defect responsible for bleeding in the uremic client. The accumulation of uremic toxins interferes with platelet adhesiveness.

GASTROINTESTINAL CHANGES

The entire gastrointestinal system is affected. Transient anorexia, nausea, and vomiting are almost universal. Clients often experience a constant bitter, metallic, or salty taste, and their breath commonly smells fetid, fishy, or ammonia-like. Stomatitis, parotitis, and gingivitis are common problems because of poor oral hygiene and the formation of ammonia from salivary urea. Accumulations of gastrin (from increased secretion of gastric acid) may be a major cause of ulcer disease. Esophagitis, gastritis, colitis, gastrointestinal bleeding, and diarrhea may be present. Serum amylase levels may be increased, although they do not necessarily indicate pancreatitis.

Constipation is a common problem. It often results from phosphate-binding agents; restriction of fluids and high-fiber foods, many of which are rich in potassium and phosphorus; and decreased activity. Constipation is a particular challenge because many of the usual interventions to prevent it (i.e., adding fruits, vegetables, and grains to the diet) and to treat it (e.g., magnesium-containing laxatives) are contraindicated for a client with renal failure.

IMMUNOLOGIC CHANGES

Impairment of the immune system makes the client more susceptible to infection. Several factors are involved, including depression of humoral antibody formation, suppression of delayed hypersensitivity, and decreased chemotactic function of the leukocytes. Immunosuppression is an important part of the medical management of renal diseases such as glomerulonephritis. Immunosuppression after transplantation is discussed later in this chapter.

CHANGES IN MEDICATION METABOLISM

CRF has a serious effect on the metabolism of medications. The uremic client is at high risk for medication toxicity because of the effect of renal changes on the pharmacokinetics (absorption, distribution, metabolism, and excretion) of otherwise therapeutic medications. There are three main causes of this toxicity:

- A high plasma level of the medication caused by low serum albumin, decreased binding sites, impaired renal excretion, or impaired hepatic metabolism of the drug
- Increased sensitivity to the medication because of uremia-induced changes in the target organ
- A metabolic load due to administration of the medication; for example, hypoalbuminemia means less protein available for binding

Various tables and formulas are available to help guide dosage decisions. Remember, medication dosages must be altered and the usual dosage ranges are not safe for a client with CRF. Assess the client carefully for toxic reactions. Keep in mind that many medications, particularly water-soluble ones, are removed by dialysis.

CARDIOVASCULAR CHANGES

Between 50% and 65% of deaths that occur during CRF result from cardiovascular complications. The most common clinical manifestation is hypertension (which may also be the cause of renal failure), produced through:

- Mechanisms of volume overload
- Stimulation of the renin-angiotensin system
- Sympathetically mediated vasoconstriction; for example, increased levels of dopamine β-hydroxylase
- Absence of prostaglandins

Any of the many systemic complications of prolonged high blood pressure may be found.

The effects of volume overload on the heart are seen, including left ventricular hypertrophy and congestive heart failure. Heart failure may also result from anemia, vascular access, complications of coronary artery disease, electrolyte imbalance, acidosis, myocardial calcification, and thiamine depletion. Dysrhythmias may be caused by hyperkalemia, acidosis, hypermagnesemia, and decreased coronary perfusion.

Atherosclerosis is accelerated because of abnormal carbohydrate and lipid metabolism; impaired fibrinolysis, which leads to the development of microemboli; and hyperparathyroidism. Arterial calcifications have been identified, the ankles being the most common early location. Other sites include the abdominal aorta, feet, pelvis, hands, and wrists. These vascular calcifications also occur within the heart, particularly at the mitral valve.

RESPIRATORY CHANGES

Some of the respiratory effects, such as pulmonary edema, can be attributed to fluid overload. Pleuritis is a frequent finding, especially when pericarditis develops. A characteristic condition called *uremic lung* is a type of pneumonitis that responds well to fluid removal. Metabolic acidosis causes a compensatory increase in respiratory rate as the lungs try to eliminate excess hydrogen ions.

MUSCULOSKELETAL CHANGES

The musculoskeletal system is affected fairly early in the disease process, and up to 90% of clients with CRF experience renal osteodystrophy. This condition develops insidiously and takes several forms: osteomalacia, osteitis fibrosa, osteoporosis, and osteosclerosis. The etiologic mechanism involves the kidney-bone-parathyroid and calcium-phosphate-vitamin D connections. As the GFR decreases, phosphate excretion decreases and calcium elimination increases. Abnormal levels of calcium and phosphate stimulate the release of parathyroid hormone, which mobilizes calcium from the bones and facilitates phosphate excretion.

As renal failure progresses, the kidney no longer converts vitamin D to its active form, 1,25-dihydroxycholecalciferol. The lack of this substance interferes with calcium absorption from the intestine and paradoxically facilitates phosphate retention. Thus, mineralization of the bone with calcium and phosphate is impaired. Demineralization of the bone frees more calcium and phosphorus into the blood. As the disease progresses, the parathyroid gland may become unresponsive to the normal feedback system and continue to produce parathyroid hormone, accelerating renal osteodystrophy. Partial parathyroidectomy is the treatment of choice when hypercalcemia and high plasma levels of parathyroid hormone cannot be controlled with medication.

In addition to bone demineralization, this process leads to deposition of calcium in subcutaneous, vascular, and visceral tissues throughout the body. In advanced stages, joint pain is severe. The client may also report diffuse and generalized bone and muscle pain. Bone deformities and frequent fractures are common. In children, bones fail to calcify, causing growth retardation. Tissue calcifications may be lethal if they develop in vital tissues, such as cerebral, coronary, or pulmonary vessels.

Some clients complain of muscle cramps. These may result from osmolar changes in the body fluids or sometimes hypocalcemia.

INTEGUMENTARY CHANGES

Integumentary problems are particularly uncomfortable for some clients with CRF. The skin is also often very dry because of atrophy of the sweat glands. Severe and intractable pruritus may result from secondary hyperparathyroidism and calcium deposits in the skin. Pruritus can lead to excoriated skin because of continued scratching.

Several color changes affecting the skin are found in clients with renal failure. A bleeding tendency often results in increased braising, petechiae, and purpura. These do not usually cause problems themselves, but their presence may be alarming to the client. The pallor of anemia is evident. The cause of retained urochrome pigments, making the skin orange-green or gray in color, is not clear.

Hair is brittle and tends to fall out; nails are thin and brittle as well. Characteristic red bands that develop on the nails are called Muercke's lines. Another nail pattern that has been observed is a "half-and-half" nail, with the proximal half normally white and the distal portion brown.

NEUROLOGIC CHANGES

Although dialysis has reduced the incidence of neurologic changes, some clients experience these problems early in the disease process. Peripheral neuropathy causes many manifestations, such as burning feet, inability to find a comfortable position for the legs and feet (restless legs syndrome), gait changes, footdrop, and paraplegia. These manifestations move up the legs and may extend to include the arms. Initially, it is primarily a problem of the sensory system; however, if left untreated, it may progress to the motor system. Nerve conduction becomes slower, and deep tendon reflexes and vibratory sense are diminished.

Central nervous system involvement is demonstrated through forgetfulness, inability to concentrate, short attention span, impaired reasoning ability and judgment, impaired cognitive functioning, increased nervous irritability, nystagmus, twitching, dysarthria, seizures, central nervous system depression, and coma. Involvement of the cranial nerves may alter any of the senses. Hearing threshold levels show a high-frequency deficit early in the disease, and hearing progressively deteriorates. Uremic amaurosis is the sudden onset of bilateral blindness, which seems to be reversed in hours to days. The eyes often contain calcium salts, which give them an irritated appearance.

REPRODUCTIVE CHANGES

Reproductive system changes can be alarming. Women commonly experience menstrual irregularities, particularly amenorrhea (absence of menstrual periods), and infertility. However, some women with CRF have conceived and had successful term pregnancies. Men commonly report impotence of both physiologic and psychological causes. They may also experience testicular atrophy, oligospermia (decreased sperm count), and reduced sperm motility. Both sexes report decreased libido, possibly from both physiologic and psychological factors.

ENDOCRINE CHANGES

CRF also affects the endocrine system, such as the insulin utilization and parathyroid function discussed already. Pituitary hormones, such as growth hormone and prolactin, may be increased in some people. The levels of luteinizing hormone and follicle-stimulating hormone vary greatly from client to client. Thyroid-stimulating hormone is usually normal, but it may show a blunted response to thyrotropin-releasing hormone; this commonly results in hypothyroidism.

PSYCHOSOCIAL CHANGES

Psychosocial changes probably result from both the physiologic alterations and the extreme stress experienced by a client who has a chronic, life-threatening disease. Common stressors include feelings of powerlessness and lack of control over the illness and treatment, intrusive therapy, restrictions imposed by the medical regimen, changes in body image, and changes in sexuality.

Clients commonly suffer from role reversal, loss or reduction of work, financial strain, and many lifestyle changes. Scheduling dialysis can create many difficulties. The client's self-concept and body image may be altered, leading to further problems with work and relationships.

People cope with these stressors in various ways, and not all coping strategies are positive. They can range from obtaining support from family and friends and seeking more information about the condition to depression and thoughts of suicide. Indeed, helping a client cope with psychosocial changes will be one of the hardest nursing challenges you face.

PROGNOSIS

The survival rate of people with CRF has improved with the advent and improvement of dialysis and transplantation. At 1 year after dialysis begins, the survival rate is about 79%. After 5 years, it drops to 33%.[16, 45]

Outcome Management

■ Medical Management

Conservative intervention does not cure CRF, but it may slow the progress of the disease. Eventually, most clients need renal replacement therapy. However, even successful dialysis and transplantation do not preclude the potential for death from complications of renal failure or its treatment.

After correcting contributing factors, control of blood pressure and fluid and dietary adjustments are the mainstays of conservative intervention for a client with CRF. The five goals of medical management are:

- To preserve renal function
- To delay the need for dialysis or transplantation as long as feasible
- To alleviate extrarenal manifestations as much as possible
- To improve body chemistry values
- To provide an optimal quality of life for the client and significant others

PRESERVE RENAL FUNCTION AND DELAY DIALYSIS

Preservation of renal function can delay the need for dialysis therapy. It can be accomplished by controlling the disease process (see Chapter 35), by controlling blood pressure, and by reducing dietary protein intake and catabolism.

CRF commonly causes hypertension, which accelerates kidney damage. Good blood pressure control helps to preserve renal function. Blood pressure can be controlled through diet, weight control, and medications (see Chapters 35 and 52).

Specific adjustments of dietary elements often depend on the results of the client's blood chemistry studies. Although there is some debate over whether and how to restrict proteins, keeping the daily intake of protein of high biologic value below 50 g may slow the progression of renal failure. Generally, recommendations range from no restriction other than avoiding high-protein fad diets to a restriction to 1 g/kg/day. This protein must be of high biologic value so that the essential amino acids can be used more efficiently with less nitrogenous waste. This restriction of proteins also limits accumulation of acid, potassium, and phosphate.

It is also important to provide adequate nonprotein calories to prevent or reduce catabolism. One recommendation is a carbohydrate and fat intake of 40 to 50 kcal/kg/day. As the renal disease progresses, the client's ability and willingness to take in adequate nutrition diminish and the challenge becomes not only to maintain appropriate intake of nonprotein calories but also to satisfy protein needs. In these instances, elemental diets, enteral feedings, or TPN may be used instead of or in addition to regular food intake.

ALLEVIATE EXTRARENAL MANIFESTATIONS

Pruritus can be very annoying. Many interventions have been tried, including topical emollients and lotions, antihistamines, intravenous lidocaine, and ultraviolet B light, but relief has been inconsistent and usually temporary. Subtotal parathyroidectomy has sometimes helped, but there have been reports of recurrence. Effective dialysis seems to relieve the manifestations for many clients.

Neurologic manifestations require safety measures to protect the client from injury. Anticonvulsants and sedatives may be used. Phenothiazines are potentiated by uremia and should be avoided. The rise of uremic toxins causes a reduction in cognitive functioning, and patience is required in explaining things to the client.

The hematologic changes can also be treated medically. Therapy with epoetin alfa three times a week helps to stimulate the production of red blood cells. Supplemental iron, vitamin B_{12}, and folic acid are usually administered as well.

IMPROVE BODY CHEMISTRY

The client's body chemistry can be improved through dialysis, medications, and diet. Dialysis removes excess water and nitrogenous wastes, reducing the manifestations of renal failure. Dialysis can be used temporarily if the client has ARF or as a permanent, life-sustaining treatment if the client has CRF. In the latter case, dialysis must continue for the rest of the client's life unless a successful kidney transplantation is performed.

Dialysis is also used to control uremia and to physically prepare the client to receive a transplanted kidney. Dialysis is usually necessary to keep the client alive until a suitable donor kidney is found. If the transplanted kidney does not immediately function adequately, dialysis may help prevent uremia until the kidney begins functioning sufficiently.

The four basic goals of dialysis therapy are:

- To remove the end products of protein metabolism, such as urea and creatinine, from the blood
- To maintain a safe concentration of serum electrolytes
- To correct acidosis and replenish the blood's bicarbonate levels
- To remove excess fluid from the blood

Principles of ultrafiltration and diffusion are used to accomplish the goals of dialysis. *Ultrafiltration* refers to removal of fluid from the blood using either osmotic or hydrostatic pressure to produce the necessary gradient. *Diffusion* is the passage of particles (ions) from an area of high concentration to an area of low concentration. Both processes occur across a semipermeable membrane with pores large enough to allow certain particles (such as urea, creatinine, and electrolytes) to pass through but too small to allow the passage of larger particles (such as protein and red blood cells). When the two solutions are separated by a semipermeable membrane, solute particles move toward the solution of lower concentration. Simultaneously, water moves toward the solution of higher solute concentration.

Solute particles and water can move freely across the membrane in either direction between the blood and the dialysate. Thus, if the blood has a higher concentration of urea, creatinine, and certain electrolytes than does the prepared dialysate solution, these particles move into the dialysate solution, lowering the level in the blood. If the blood is deficient in a substance, such as bicarbonate, the higher concentration of this substance in the dialysate causes it to move into the blood, raising the blood level.

There are two types of dialysis: *peritoneal dialysis* and *hemodialysis*. The semipermeable membrane in the dialyzer or "artificial kidney" used is either the peritoneal membrane (for peritoneal dialysis) or an artificial membrane (for hemodialysis). The blood and a specially prepared electrolyte solution, called the *dialysate*, are placed in compartments on opposite sides of the membrane. The tendency is always toward equalization of the concentrations of the two solutions.

Peritoneal Dialysis

Peritoneal dialysis involves repeated cycles of instilling dialysate into the peritoneal cavity, allowing time for substance exchange, and then removing the dialysate. The procedure is useful for both ARF and CRF and for fluid and electrolyte imbalances. It has been used to treat overdoses of drugs and toxins, but because its clearance is much slower than that with hemodialysis, it may not be satisfactory for this purpose.

One of the primary advantages of peritoneal dialysis is its relative ease, which allows it to be used in community health care facilities without all the sophisticated equipment needed for hemodialysis. It can be easily managed at home and commonly allows the client more independence and mobility than hemodialysis does.

Peritoneal dialysis is typically used for clients with severe cardiovascular disease, especially those whose problems would be worsened by the rapid changes in urea, glucose, electrolytes, and fluid volume that occur during hemodialysis. Some physicians prescribe peritoneal dialysis for diabetic clients to reduce the risk of retinal hemorrhage associated with the heparin used during hemodialysis and because good blood glucose control can be achieved by adding insulin to the dialysate. Peritoneal dialysis is the dialysis treatment of choice for children because it seems to have less effect on growth.

Contraindications to peritoneal dialysis include hypercatabolism, in which peritoneal dialysis cannot adequately clear uremic toxins, and poor condition of the peritoneal membrane because of adhesions or scarring. Relative contraindications to peritoneal dialysis include obesity, a history of ruptured diverticula, abdominal disease, respiratory disease, recurrent episodes of peritonitis, abdominal malignancies, severe vascular disease, back problems (because the increased weight of fluid may increase back strain), and extensive abdominal surgery with drains or tubes that may increase the risk of infection.

TYPES OF PERITONEAL DIALYSIS. Several types of peritoneal dialysis are in use today. The most common are continuous ambulatory and automated peritoneal dialysis.

Continuous Ambulatory Peritoneal Dialysis (CAPD). In the continuous type of peritoneal dialysis, 1.5 to 3.0 L of dialysate is instilled into the abdomen and left in place for a prescribed period of time. The empty dialysate bag is folded up and carried in a pouch or pocket until it is time to drain the dialysate. The bag is then unfolded and placed lower than the insertion site so that the fluid drains by gravity flow. When full, the bag is changed and new dialysate is instilled into the abdomen as the process continues.

Another version of this procedure is the disconnect system. With this system, the client removes the empty dialysate bag after inflow and attaches a protective cap to the dialysis catheter. A new sterile bag is used for each drainage and infusion, which eliminates the need to wear the tubing and bag between exchanges.

CAPD usually uses four dialysis cycles every 24 hours, including an 8-hour dwell overnight. There are two major advantages. First, because there is no need for machinery, electricity, or a water source, the client can go about almost any desired activity during dialysis. Second, because the continuous exchange process closely resembles normal renal function, the body more easily maintains homeostasis, allowing fewer dietary and fluid restrictions. For management of diabetic clients, insulin can be added to the dialysate.

See Bridge to Home Health Care.

Automated Peritoneal Dialysis. Automated peritoneal dialysis necessitates use of a peritoneal cycling machine. This method can be performed as continuous cyclic, intermittent, or nightly intermittent peritoneal dialysis.

Continuous cyclic peritoneal dialysis. In this variation, there are usually three cycles at night and one cycle with an 8-hour dwell in the morning. The advantage of this procedure is that the peritoneal catheter is opened only for the on-and-off procedures, which reduces the risk of infection. Another advantage is that the client does not require exchanges at work or school.

Intermittent peritoneal dialysis. This is not a continuous dialysis procedure. Instead, dialysis is performed for 10 to 14 hours, three to four times a week, by the same peritoneal cycling machine as in continuous cyclic peritoneal dialysis. Hospitalized clients may be dialyzed for 24 to 48 hours at a time if they are catabolic and require additional dialysis time.

Nightly intermittent peritoneal dialysis. Dialysis is performed for 8 to 12 hours each night with no daytime dwells.

PERITONEAL DIALYSIS PROCEDURES. Several steps are involved.

Peritoneal Catheter Insertion. For a client who needs peritoneal dialysis, one of several types of soft catheters is inserted through the abdominal wall and into the peritoneal cavity. Usually, the catheter is inserted in the operating room, with the client under local anesthesia, although it may be inserted at the client's bedside. The client is medicated before the procedure to provide relaxation and to reduce discomfort.

The preferred insertion site is 3 to 5 cm below the umbilicus, an area that is relatively avascular and has relatively low fascial resistance. Figure 36–2 illustrates three types of peritoneal catheters. The Tenckhoff catheter has two polyester (Dacron) felt cuffs bonded to the catheter. Over a period of 1 to 2 weeks, there is an ingrowth of fibroblasts and blood vessels into the cuffs, which fix the catheter in place and provide an effective barrier against dialysate leakage and bacterial invasion. Note in Figure 36–2 that a subcutaneous tunnel is created for the catheter to reduce direct bacterial invasion into the peritoneum. The other catheters illustrated have cuffs to provide stability.

Dialysate. The dialysate is usually allowed to run into the peritoneal cavity by gravity flow. It is warmed slightly to avoid chilling the client and to dilate the peritoneal blood vessels, thus facilitating substance exchange. In an adult 2 L is usually instilled, although smaller amounts may be needed at first until the client adjusts. Throughout the procedure, care must be taken to prevent air from entering the peritoneal cavity.

The *dwell time* is the period during which the dialysate is left in the peritoneal cavity. In intermittent peritoneal dialysis, equilibrium between the dialysate and the body fluids usually occurs within 15 to 30 minutes, with the maximum exchange during the first 5 minutes. Therefore, the solution is typically left in place 30 to 45 minutes for manual dialysis or 10 to 20 minutes when an automatic

BRIDGE TO HOME HEALTH CARE

Living with Peritoneal Dialysis

When you admit clients to home health services who have end-stage renal disease, are starting peritoneal dialysis, and have Medicare benefits, you will be collaborating with physicians and the staff of the peritoneal dialysis unit. The unit staff is the designated provider of total services, including nursing services. Clinic nurses can and do make limited visits; a peritoneal dialysis nurse is on 24-hour call.

You are involved when clients need Medicare-reimbursed services in addition to dialysis treatments. While you provide care, it is important to discuss what the life of your client and the client's family was like before the recent hospitalization, what they know about dialysis, and how long they expect the client to receive dialysis. Share both physical and psychosocial information with the other health care team members to help clients and their families consider their options and adapt their lifestyles and home to the requirements of peritoneal dialysis.

Hospitals have sophisticated equipment readily available and are treatment oriented. When clients return home, home health nurses can suggest ways to improve the quality of daily life and decrease the focus on technology. For example, the nurse may suggest an alternative way to hang the bags for the dialysis solution, such as hooking the bag on a hanger and a door frame or using a floor-style plant hanger rather than a pole for intravenous solutions. When clients have continuous ambulatory peritoneal dialysis (CAPD), the solution runs for 4 to 10 hours four times per day. Because no machinery, electricity, or water source is required, clients can go about most of their daily activities. Clients have fewer dietary and fluid restrictions, and they maintain better ho-

meostasis. When clients have ambulatory peritoneal dialysis (APD), the solution dwells for 4 to 10 hours before being changed four times per day. Often a dwell time of 8 hours is used during the daytime with three shorter cycles being completed during the night. Clients have less freedom to move about and go about daily activities. Although APD requires a peritoneal cycling machine, it can be scheduled as a continuous, intermittent, or nightly procedure.

Instruct clients and their families to watch for untoward manifestations. A drop in blood pressure can cause dizziness or faintness, and elevated blood pressure can cause headaches. Fluid overload can cause shortness of breath. If clients experience any of these manifestations, they should notify the nurse or physician immediately.

When assessing psychosocial issues, the home health nurse should identify barriers to care and determine how much responsibility clients can assume for self-care and how much assistance they need. If clients feel depressed or lack confidence, they may not follow instructions involving the dialysis procedure, their diet and fluid intake, or their medications. The nurse needs to offer support and allow the client and family members to ask questions and verbalize concerns. The entire dialysis process might involve much more than clients and family had expected. Suggest involving friends or neighbors who can be taught about peritoneal dialysis and become part of the client's and family's support system. Discuss other appropriate community resources such as spiritual and financial counselors. Provide information about resources and support groups available through the National Kidney Foundation (1-800-622-9010) or the American Kidney Fund (1-800-638-8299).

Shawnda M. Braun, RN, *Case Manager, Allied Health Alternatives, Inc., Faribault, Minnesota*

cycler is used. The fluid is then allowed to run out through the catheter by gravity. In continuous ambulatory and automated peritoneal dialysis procedures, the dwell time is prolonged to 4 to 8 hours with a solution that allows continuous exchange and better clearance of certain elements.

Cycles. The number of dialysis cycles depends on the normalization of body fluids and blood chemistries, as indicated by laboratory studies. Peritoneal clearance is influenced by several factors, including the size of the membrane area, blood flow to the peritoneum, and alterations in the permeability of the peritoneal membrane.

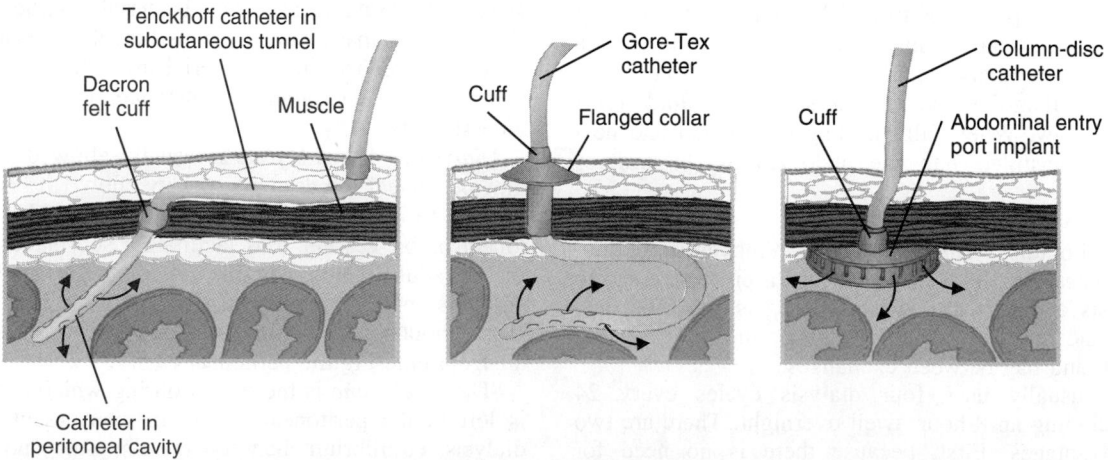

FIGURE 36–2 Three types of peritoneal dialysis catheters. The Tenckhoff catheter has two polyester (Dacron) felt cuffs that hold the catheter in place and prevent dialysate leakage and bacterial invasion; a subcutaneous tunnel also helps to prevent infection. The Gore-Tex catheter has a Dacron cuff above a flanged collar. The column-disc catheter has a cuff and a large abdominal entry port implant.

COMPLICATIONS OF PERITONEAL DIALYSIS. Although peritoneal dialysis is considered a safe procedure, a number of complications can be attributed to it.

Peritonitis. Peritonitis is the major concern; therefore, meticulous aseptic technique must be maintained during handling of the catheter, tubing, and dialysate solution. Bacteria may enter the peritoneal cavity through contaminated dialysis fluid, a contaminated catheter lumen, or the catheter insertion site.

Clinical evidence of peritonitis includes fever, rebound abdominal tenderness, nausea, malaise, and a cloudy dialysate output. Laboratory tests routinely used to diagnose peritonitis include white blood cell counts with differential, culture, and sensitivity and Gram's stain of the peritoneal fluid. Peritonitis is the diagnosis when the dialysate white blood cell count is above 100/mm^3 and neutrophils are above 50%. The causative organism does not always grow in routine cultures, but Gram's stain is positive in up to 40% of the samples.

If peritonitis develops, appropriate antibiotics are added to the dialysate; in addition, systemic antibiotics may be used.

Catheter-Related Complications. Catheter problems include displacement and obstruction. Obstruction may be due to malposition, adherence of the catheter tip to the omentum, or infection. Constipation can reduce catheter flow, possibly because peristalsis facilitates outflow. A bisacodyl suppository may be used prophylactically even if the client is not constipated. Fluid leakage may indicate improper catheter function, incomplete healing of the insertion site, or excessive instillation.

Especially in the early stages, it is sometimes necessary to use small-volume instillations. Bloody effluent is usually insignificant and disappears spontaneously. Heparin may be added to the dialysate to prevent fibrin clot formation in a new catheter or after treatment for peritonitis. Also be aware of the possibility of bowel perforation, which is most likely to occur in cachectic (profoundly ill and malnourished) clients or those who have abdominal adhesions. Fecal material returned in the dialysate or massive diarrhea after instillation may also signal perforation. Bladder perforation can also occur if the bladder has not been emptied before catheter insertion.

Dialysis-Related Complications. Pain during dialysis may result from rapid instillation, incorrect dialysate pH or temperature, dialysate accumulation under the diaphragm, or excessive suction during outflow. Some pain is expected in the early stages but should disappear after 1 to 2 weeks. Low back pain may develop with continuous dialysis procedures because the abdominal weight affects posture; appropriate exercises help relieve this problem. Hernia may occur. Systemic cardiovascular and neurologic effects are usually the result of fluid and electrolyte imbalances. Especially during small-volume exchanges, a significant amount of dialysate fluid may be absorbed by the body.

Hypotension may result from too rapid removal of fluid. Overhydration, from insufficient fluid removal, may be manifested as heart failure and pulmonary edema. Hypoalbuminemia leading to hypovolemia often occurs because the peritoneal membrane allows the passage of albumin, as much as 100 g/day if the client is infected. It is especially a problem if dietary intake of protein is poor,

the client is infected, or dialysis treatment is used for several consecutive days. Hyperglycemia may occur in diabetic clients as a result of absorption of glucose from the dialysate and electrolyte changes. These clients require extra insulin. Respiratory difficulties may occur during dwell time because of pressure on the diaphragm. Weight gain may occur because of the high concentration of glucose in the dialysate.

OUTCOMES. Long-term outcomes associated with peritoneal dialysis are considered good. The treatment is usually effective for years. However, scarring of the peritoneum and repeated infections may require a change to hemodialysis.

Hemodialysis

Hemodialysis is used for clients with acute or irreversible renal failure and fluid and electrolyte imbalances. It is usually the treatment of choice when toxic agents, such as barbiturates after an overdose, need to be removed from the body quickly.

HISTORICAL OVERVIEW. The first artificial kidney was developed in 1943 in The Netherlands. In 1960, the first successful treatment of clients with CRF was reported. In the early years, although the technology was available, the exorbitant cost and lack of equipment required a stringent selection process in choosing clients for hemodialysis. Clients were screened on the basis of their motivation, intelligence, emotional stability, and rehabilitative potential. In essence, it had to be decided who among the many potential candidates would best be able to cope with the program and who would make the biggest contribution to society.

In 1972, an amendment to the Social Security Act required that anyone with CRF be able to have any lifesaving treatment needed. In 1973, Medicare took over the financial responsibility for many clients receiving hemodialysis. Thus, availability of this treatment for clients with end-stage renal failure has become more prevalent. Generally, self-selection is the only criterion used now. As a result, the population receiving hemodialysis now represents a wide cross-section of age, rehabilitative potential, and socioeconomic status. There continue to be problems with selection of appropriate candidates, when to start, and when and how to stop. With the reduction in available health care dollars, the problems associated with selection criteria will only increase.

HEMODIALYSIS PROCEDURE. In hemodialysis, the client's toxin-laden blood is diverted into a dialyzer, cleaned, and then returned to the client (Fig. 36–3). While the blood is in the dialyzer, a mechanical proportioning pump causes dialysis fluid to flow on the other side of the membrane (Fig. 36–4). Toxins diffuse across the membrane from the blood to the dialysate. Strict asepsis must be maintained throughout the procedure.

One of the vital aspects of hemodialysis is the establishment and maintenance of adequate blood access. Without it, hemodialysis cannot be done. The major routes of access are external arteriovenous shunts and subclavian catheters for acute dialysis and internal arteriovenous fistulas and grafts for chronic dialysis.

The external arteriovenous shunt requires surgical placement of two rubber-like silicone (Silastic) cannulas into the forearm or leg. The two cannulas are connected

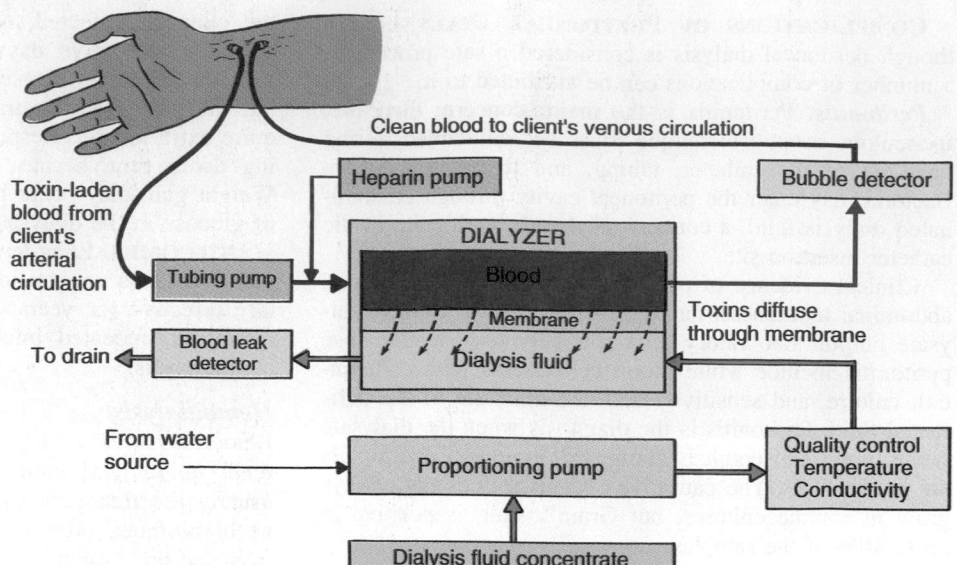

FIGURE 36–3 Typical hemodialysis system. Toxin-laden blood from the client diffuses across the membrane within the dialyzer into the dialysis fluid. Clean blood is returned to the client.

to form a U shape. Blood flows from the client's artery through the shunt into the vein.

When the client is to be connected to the hemodialyzer, a tube leading to the membrane compartment is connected to the arterial cannula. Blood then fills the membrane compartment and flows back to the client by way of a tube connected to the venous cannula. When dialysis is completed, the arterial cannula is clamped. Once the blood in the membrane compartment has been returned to the body, the venous cannula is clamped and the ends of the two cannulas are reattached to form their U. This access can be created quickly and thus is particularly suitable when dialysis must be started immediately.

FIGURE 36–4 A client undergoing outpatient hemodialysis. (Reprinted with permission from Althin Medical, Inc., Miami Lakes, FL.)

Infection at the insertion site and clotting are complications that often necessitate moving the cannula sites. Other problems that occur with shunts are accidental dislodgment, hemorrhage, and skin erosion.

The internal arteriovenous fistula is the access of choice for clients receiving chronic dialysis. The fistula is created through a surgical procedure in which an artery in the arm is anastomosed to a vein in an end-to-side, side-to-side, side-to-end, or end-to-end fashion (Fig. 36–5A). The result is an opening or fistula between a large artery and a large vein. The flow of arterial blood into the venous system causes the veins to become engorged (Fig. 36–5B). These fistulae require up to 6 weeks to mature before they can be used, which makes this approach inappropriate for immediate hemodialysis. Peritoneal dialysis or large venous access catheters may be used while the fistula is maturing. External arteriovenous shunts are rarely used.

The internal arteriovenous graft is used primarily for chronic dialysis. In this approach, an artificial graft made of water-repellent fabric (Gore-Tex) or a bovine carotid artery is used to create an artificial vein for blood flow. The graft is used in clients who do not have adequate blood vessels for surgical creation of a fistula. One end of the artificial graft is anastomosed to an artery, tunneled under the skin, and anastomosed to a vein. The graft can be used 2 weeks after insertion. Complications include clotting, aneurysms, and infection.

Once the fistula graft is placed and ready for use, two 15- or 16-gauge needles are placed in the access at each dialysis treatment (Fig. 36–5C). A pump pulls arterial blood out by way of the fistula and into the hemodialyzer. Blood returns to the client by a tube connected to the other needle. Alternatively, single-needle dialysis may be used. With this device, only one puncture is required each time, but there may be significant recirculation of dialyzed blood, meaning that clearance rates are decreased. Internal arteriovenous grafts may cause hand swelling or ischemia (steal syndrome), carpal tunnel syndrome, hemorrhage, thrombosis, and aneurysms. Besides the arm, the subclavian, thigh, and ankle areas may be used as sites for hemodialysis access.

Subclavian, jugular, and femoral catheters can be inserted at the bedside for vascular access or surgically placed in the operating room. Double-lumen catheters are usually used to provide access for both removal and return of blood. These catheters are usually a temporary source of vascular access and must be replaced frequently to prevent infection. Strict aseptic technique must be used during insertion, and dressing changes are usually performed by a limited number of trained nurses. Thrombosis and infection are the most common complications.

DIALYZERS. Several types of dialyzers are available, including flat plate and hollow fiber mold devices. Choice of a particular system is mostly a matter of preference. There are differences in urea and creatinine clearance rates as well as ultrafiltration rates. Many centers that perform chronic dialysis now reprocess and disinfect the unit and reuse it for the same client to reduce costs. The dialysate solution is altered to fit the client's need.

HEMODIALYSIS SCHEDULES. Hemodialysis as a treatment for CRF must be continued intermittently for the client's lifetime unless successful kidney transplantation is performed. A typical schedule is 3 to 4 hours of treatment 3 days per week. This schedule varies with the size of the client, the type of dialyzer used, the rate of blood flow, the personal preference of the client, and other factors.

THERAPEUTIC EFFECTS OF HEMODIALYSIS. The overall therapeutic effects of hemodialysis are to (1) clear waste products from the body; (2) restore fluid, electrolyte, and acid-base balances; and (3) reverse some of the untoward manifestations of irreversible renal failure. Success is varied. Excess fluid, potassium, urea nitrogen, and acid ions are removed but only temporarily; between dialyses, these elements build up again. Nutritionally, carbohydrate intolerance is usually reduced. Amino acids, protein, glucose, and water-soluble vitamins are lost. Anemia generally worsens because of blood loss associated with the therapy. The predialysis causative factors are still present, and additional losses occur during dialysis because of blood sampling, residual blood left in the dialyzer, and bleeding secondary to anticoagulation during dialysis. Serum iron stores are also further depleted.

Hyperlipidemia (elevated serum lipid levels) seems to increase and is associated with accelerated atherosclerosis. Renal osteodystrophy usually improves, and this can be further enhanced by adding calcium to the dialysate. Pruritus may occur for reasons not yet understood. Men who have maintenance dialysis often have low testosterone levels and develop gynecomastia, which is usually transient. Many other sexual manifestations of uremia are reversed after a period of adaptation.

The usual effect of hemodialysis on serum concentration of medications is increased clearance, which is therapeutic in the case of overdose. Dosage schedules are

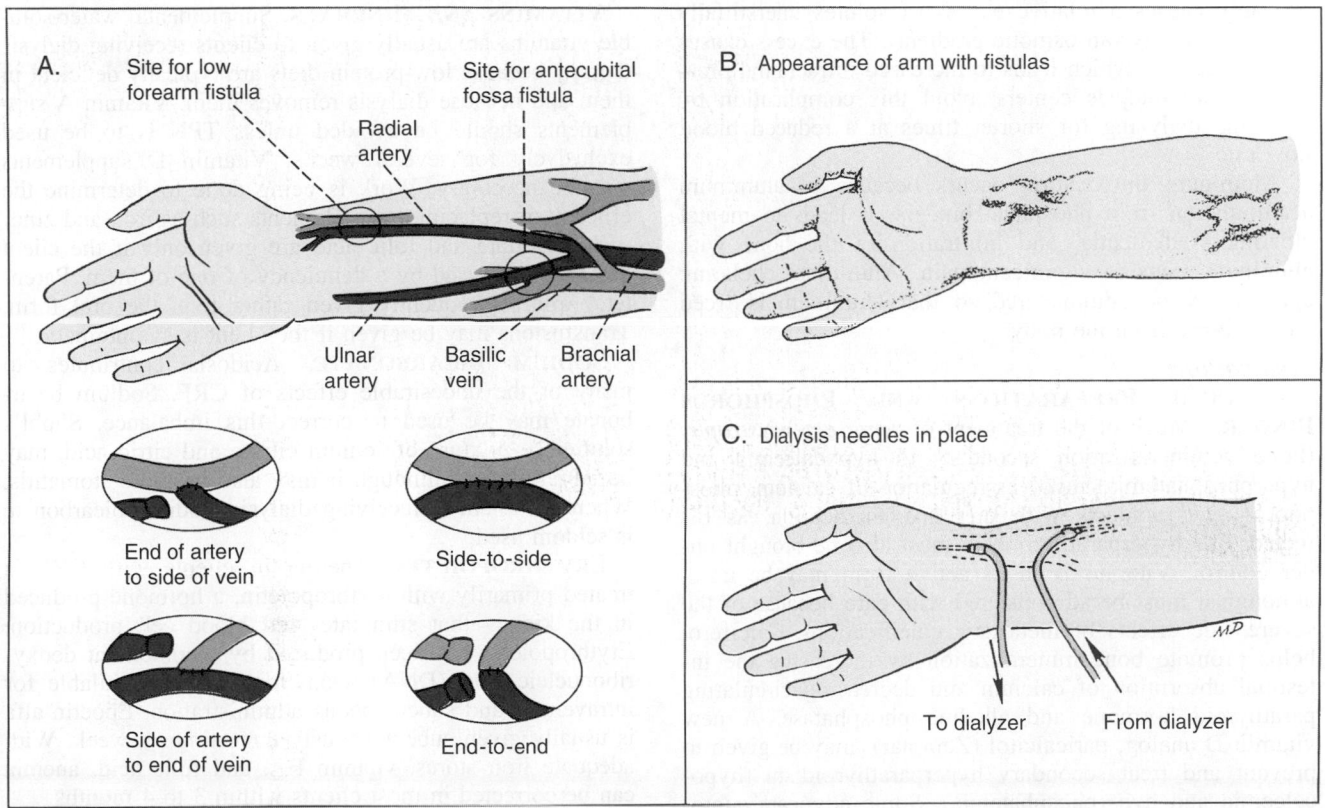

FIGURE 36-5 Internal arteriovenous fistula. Surgical creation of an arteriovenous anastomosis provides easy access to blood for hemodialysis. This method reduces the risk of infection and makes external shunts unnecessary except during hemodialysis. The internal fistula must be created 2 to 6 weeks before it can be used. In this illustration, arteries, not veins, are toned. *A,* Types of fistulas. *B,* Appearance of arm with fistulas. *C,* Dialysis needles in place.

altered to prevent, as much as possible, loss of medications through dialysis. Supplemental doses may be necessary to maintain therapeutic levels of certain medications.

COMPLICATIONS OF LONG-TERM HEMODIALYSIS. In addition to its therapeutic effects, chronic hemodialysis can cause a number of complications:

- Technical problems, such as blood leaks, overheating of the dialysate solution, insufficient loss of fluid, improper concentration of salts in the dialysate, and clotting
- Hypotension or hypertension
- Cardiac dysrhythmias from potassium imbalance
- Air embolus
- Hemorrhage resulting from heparinization with particular concern for subdural, retroperitoneal, pericardial, and intraocular bleeding
- Restless legs syndrome
- Pyrogenic reactions

Gastrointestinal ulcer disease is often complicated by hemorrhage. Muscle cramps may occur as a result of hyponatremia or hyposmolality and too rapid removal of fluid. Infection is a significant complication, with hepatitis B being a significant risk. Frequent infectious processes include local access infection, bacteremia, and infectious endocarditis.

Dialysis disequilibrium syndrome can occur, particularly during the client's first few dialysis episodes. It is characterized by mental confusion, deterioration of the level of consciousness, headache, and seizures. It may last for several days. Rapid solute removal from the blood probably causes a relative excess of solutes interstitially or intracellularly (an osmotic gradient). The excess causes cerebral edema, which leads to increased intracranial pressure. Many dialysis centers avoid this complication by first-time dialyzing for shorter times at a reduced blood flow rate.

Aluminum intoxication occurs because of aluminum accumulation from phosphate binders. It leads to mental cloudiness, dementia, and infiltration of the bone with aluminum, causing significant pain. Aluminum chelating agents may be administered so that aluminum is freed and dialyzed from the body.

Medications

CALCIUM PREPARATIONS AND PHOSPHORUS BINDERS. Much of the treatment of *renal osteodystrophy* (bone demineralization secondary to hypocalcemia and hyperphosphatemia) involves regulation of calcium, phosphorus, and acidosis with diet and medication, as directed. The hyperparathyroidism must also be brought under control. Vitamin D in its active form may be used, although it must be administered with care because of the severe side effects of metastatic calcifications. Calciferol helps promote bone mineralization by increasing the intestinal absorption of calcium and decreasing circulating parathyroid hormone and alkaline phosphatase. A new vitamin D analog, paricalcitol (Zemplar), may be given to prevent and treat secondary hyperparathyroidism (hypocalcemia and hyperphosphatemia). Some advocate subtotal parathyroidectomy if all other methods fail.

Phosphorus intake is usually limited to less than 1000 mg/day. To improve excretion of phosphorus, the client is given calcium-based phosphate binders such as calcium acetate or calcium carbonate. Aluminum-based antacids such as Alu-Cap, Amphojel, and Basaljel were formerly used to bind phosphorus so that it could be excreted in the feces. These medications are seldom used now because they increase the risk of dementia related to excessive absorption of aluminum.

ANTIHYPERTENSIVE AGENTS. Fluid regulation and sodium regulation are the major interventions in heart failure. Other cardiovascular manifestations are managed in much the same way as for clients without CRF, but diuretics are not used except in the early stages of conservative management. Hypertension must be aggressively controlled with stronger medications such as angiotensin-converting enzyme inhibitors and calcium-channel blockers. Antihypertensive drugs are administered as necessary in relation to renal function and nephrotic response.

DIURETICS. Diuretics may be used early to stimulate excretion of water by the kidneys. The appearance of edema indicates fluid overload, but some physicians prefer to have a little end-of-the-day edema so that it is more evident that fluid depletion is not a danger. Thirst is not a reliable indicator; if thirst were used as a guide, fluid overload would be inevitable. As renal failure progresses, diuretics are not effective and it usually becomes necessary to restrict fluid intake. Although authorities differ in the exact amounts, daily fluid allowances may be 400 to 1000 ml plus measured output. Diuretics are not given before dialysis because of potential problems with hypotension. Antihypertensive medications are also often withheld until after dialysis.

VITAMINS AND MINERALS. Supplemental water-soluble vitamins are usually given to clients receiving dialysis therapy because low-protein diets are typically deficient in them and because dialysis removes them. Vitamin A supplements should be avoided unless TPN is to be used exclusively for several weeks. Vitamin D supplements may be necessary. Work is being done to determine the efficacy of replacing trace elements such as iron and zinc.

Iron sulfate and folic acid are given only if the client has anemia caused by a deficiency of one of them. Parenteral iron is frequently given rather than the oral form. Transfusions may be given if the client is symptomatic.

SODIUM BICARBONATE. Acidosis contributes to many of the undesirable effects of CRF. Sodium bicarbonate may be used to correct this imbalance. Shohl's solution, a mixture of sodium citrate and citric acid, may be administered, although it may also promote stomatitis. When the client is receiving dialysis, sodium bicarbonate is seldom used.

ERYTHROPOIETIN. Anemia in clients with CRF is treated primarily with erythropoietin, a hormone produced in the kidney that stimulates red blood cell production. Erythropoietin has been produced by recombinant deoxyribonucleic acid (DNA) technology and is available for intravenous and subcutaneous administration. Epoetin alfa is usually given subcutaneously three times a week. With adequate iron stores, vitamin B_{12}, and folic acid, anemia can be corrected in most clients within 3 to 4 months.

Diet

Dietary adjustment is dictated by many components of CRF, including accumulation of nitrogenous waste products, impaired excretion of electrolytes, vitamin deficiencies, and continued catabolism. The wasting syndrome is a major problem. The client with renal failure constantly loses body weight, muscle mass, and adipose tissue.

Dietary intake of electrolytes may be encouraged or restricted. The regulation of sodium is a delicate matter. At times the kidneys waste salt, and sodium intake must be encouraged to replace it. More frequently, however, the kidneys retain sodium. Some believe that there should be moderate restriction with careful monitoring of urinary sodium excretion as a guideline. Serial monitoring of fluid status also gives important information about sodium needs. Many regimens are used.

Potassium is frequently restricted. Clients must be reminded not to use salt substitutes because they contain potassium chloride. When hyperkalemia becomes evident, restriction of potassium in food and fluids is instituted. In an emergency situation, when the serum potassium is above 7.0 mEq/L, the client may receive intravenous glucose (50% dextrose in water, $D_{50}W$) and insulin; oral or rectal sodium polystyrene sulfonate (Kayexalate), which is a cation exchange resin; or both. Dissolving the resin in ginger ale helps to prevent it from sticking to the client's teeth and helps to mask its gritty texture. Sorbitol is usually given with the resin to avoid constipation and counteract the sodium retention that can occur. Dialysis is also effective in removing potassium from the blood.

If serum calcium levels are low, adequate calcium intake is important. Dietary sources may be supplemented with calcium carbonate, calcium lactate, or calcium gluconate. Supplements are definitely needed for clients receiving dialysis therapy. If serum calcium levels are high, however, dietary restriction may be recommended. Phosphorus is restricted. In addition, calcium carbonate may be used to reduce phosphorus levels further. Finally, mild magnesium restriction may be imposed.

PROMOTE QUALITY OF LIFE

Renal failure and its therapies significantly affect the quality of life of the client and family members. As noted earlier, there are numerous stressors and life changes. Much of the care required by clients receiving chronic peritoneal dialysis and hemodialysis and their significant others concerns the psychosocial aspects of dialysis.

Clients receiving maintenance dialysis often have ambivalent feelings. They realize that dialysis therapy is their tie to life, but the many restrictions and lifestyle changes it imposes make continuation of the program extremely difficult. Clients often report that they feel in limbo between the worlds of life and death.

The process of adaptation to loss is part of adjustment. It is not uncommon for clients to feel grateful and optimistic at the start of dialysis treatments. Usually, they have felt ill for some time, and they view the intervention as a route to survival and feeling well again. It takes a few days or weeks for them to realize fully the permanent place of dialysis in their lives. Depression during this period is expected. The suicide rate among clients receiving dialysis has been estimated as 100 times that of the general population.

Common psychosocial problems include changes in body image, dependence on technology, and uncertainty regarding the future. The client's own feelings of weakness and illness and the presence of the arteriovenous fistula and dialysis equipment are constant reminders that the client is no longer a "whole person." These clients often play one of three roles:

- Professional client, in which all of life revolves around the dialysis
- Rebel, in which the client acts noncompliant or mischievous
- Adult, in which the client uses appropriate coping skills and is able to focus outward

Relationships with relatives and friends, job, and community roles and responsibilities are probably altered. The client's normal need for independence is continually threatened by dependence on the dialysis equipment and care providers. This is especially true of adolescents and young adults. Other emotional problems include the need for identity, safety, control of the environment, love, esteem, and communication. The stress on marital relationships and significant others is extreme.

Research suggests that the quality of life of people with ESRD is influenced positively by transplantation, erythropoietin therapy, social support, a positive outlook on life, and the ability to function (including work and activities of daily living). Providing an optimal quality of life involves a concerted effort by all members of the health care team with the client and family members as active partners. Many dialysis facilities have established active rehabilitation programs. Elements of these programs include education, exercise, encouragement, employment, and evaluation.[12, 26, 27]

■ Nursing Management of the Medical Client

ASSESSMENT

When a client is thought to have CRF, take a complete history and look closely for risk factors. Question the client about past and present medications, diet and weight changes, energy levels and unexplained fatigue, and the pattern of urinary elimination.

Assess the client for the multiple effects of CRF on all body systems, such as the presence of cardiovascular or respiratory abnormalities, neurologic changes, gastrointestinal problems, or skin changes.

Assess the client's understanding of CRF, the diagnostic tests that will be done, and the possible treatment regimens. Evaluate the client's level of anxiety and ability to cope. Involve the family in the assessment to determine their ability to cope with the disease and treatments.

When a client has CRF, the client, significant others, the nephrologist, and the nephrology nurse discuss the use of dialysis and decide which type best meets the client's needs. If the client is to receive dialysis, assess the client's and significant others' understanding of the treatment regimen and the client's ability to cope with the treatment regimen. The family's ability to cope and their ability to support the client are also vital.

When the client begins peritoneal dialysis, the first assessment is for infection. Inspect the insertion site carefully for redness or other problems. Carefully assess the drained dialysate or effluent for cloudiness, fibrin streaks, or blood. Monitor the client's vital signs and weight closely.

If the client is undergoing hemodialysis, the first assessment is for the patency of the venous access site. In a patent arteriovenous fistula or graft, a "thrill" or vibrating sensation should be palpable and a bruit should be audible with a stethoscope. It is vital that this site be assessed for possible occlusion or, if it is an external site, for infection. Also ascertain the client's understanding of the access site and its care.

DIAGNOSIS, OUTCOMES, INTERVENTIONS

Fluid Volume Deficit or Fluid Volume Excess.
As with all renal disorders, a common diagnosis is *Fluid Volume Deficit or Fluid Volume Excess related to impaired renal function, fluid shifts between dialysate and blood, and blood loss during hemodialysis.*

Outcomes. Neither a fluid volume deficit nor an excess will occur, as evidenced by the absence of edema or dehydration.

Interventions

Monitor Fluid Volume Status. A fluid volume deficit or overload is a serious problem. The current fluid status must be known and fluid intake carefully regulated in keeping with it. Monitor the client's fluid status by observing daily weights, orthostatic blood pressure, skin turgor, and mucous membrane moistness and by meticulous intake and output comparisons.

Give written instructions to outpatients that explain how to weigh themselves properly and how to interpret the relationship of daily weight loss or gain to their need for sodium and water. Help the client understand that vomiting, diarrhea, and working or playing in a hot environment may cause excessive fluid loss and must be prevented or controlled. Teach the client how to take his or her blood pressure and record it daily.

Follow Fluid Restrictions. When the fluid allowance for the day has been determined, help the client follow the recommendation. Fluid restrictions are difficult for most clients. Offer suggestions about reducing thirst and moistening lips with lip balms, frequent oral hygiene, and taking ice chips or spray bottles rather than drinking. Spread out fluid intake over a longer period of time. If intravenous fluids are used, carefully attend to them to ensure proper administration rates. Water may be restricted so that the client can drink more nutritious liquids, such as apple juice, cranberry juice, or milk.

Monitor Fluid Status During Dialysis. During dialysis, carefully monitor the client's vital signs, including postural blood pressure, pulse, weight, and intake and output. Watch for hypovolemia and retention of dialysate. The amount of desired fluid loss may be ordered by the dialysis physician. Alternatively, a "dry" or "ideal" weight is established and you select appropriate solutions to remove additional fluid.

If fluid does not drain properly during peritoneal dialysis, check the system for kinks or other obstructions. Inform the physician about fluid accumulations that exceed the limit set in the dialysis orders. If the client is undergoing hemodialysis, hypotension and excess fluid removal are risks; monitor carefully.

Altered Nutrition: Less Than Body Requirements.
Yet another common diagnosis in CRF is *Altered Nutrition: Less Than Body Requirements, related to anorexia and nausea.*

Outcomes. The client will maintain adequate nutrition, as evidenced by maintenance of weight without loss of muscle mass.

Interventions. Dietary management is vital to the conservative management of CRF. Anorexia results from many of the manifestations of irreversible renal failure, emotional depression, and a frequently unpalatable diet. Thus, a major nursing challenge is to help the client take in adequate nutrition while minimizing uremic toxicity. This problem grows as the disease progresses, and the client may develop an aversion to meat and other sources of protein.

To help stimulate the client's appetite, take measures to relieve nausea and vomiting, stomatitis, and other gastrointestinal manifestations. Diet counseling is essential. Teaching aids (such as those in Fig. 36–6) may be helpful. Arrange for dietary consultation if possible. The client needs to know how to translate the dietary regimen into a palatable, understandable food program. Help the client select and prepare foods and learn where to obtain special foods if necessary. Exercise may also improve appetite.

Constipation.
The treatment of CRF leads to the predictable diagnosis of *Constipation related to medications, fluid and dietary restrictions, and decreased activity level.*

Outcomes. The client will remain free of constipation, as evidenced by a bowel movement at least every other day.

Interventions. Constipation is a major problem for clients with CRF. Because of fluid restrictions, inability to eat most high-fiber foods, and limited activity, it is difficult to use customary measures for preventing constipation. Phosphate-binding agents contribute to the problem as well.

Bran, which is not rich in potassium or phosphorus, can be used. Stool softeners are often administered regularly, although care should be taken to avoid those that contain calcium and sodium. If necessary, bulk laxatives (such as psyllium hydrophilic mucilloid) may be given. The recommended amount of fluid should be taken with the powder and subtracted from the day's fluid allotment.

Stimulant and lubricant laxatives should be used only if necessary, especially compounds containing magnesium or phosphorus, such as sodium biphosphate–sodium phosphate (Fleet) enemas. If none of these measures is effective, small-volume, gentle stimulant enemas may be used sparingly, but large-volume enemas should be avoided because of possible fluid and saline absorption. Clients with renal failure are at risk for diverticular disease because of the constipation and straining.

Fatigue.
Physiologic alterations can ensure a diagnosis of *Fatigue related to anemia and altered metabolic state.*

Outcomes. The client will have a balance of rest and activity, as evidenced by the client's statement of decreased fatigue.

Interventions. Rest is important to any client whose body is under a great deal of stress. Encourage frequent naps. Insomnia is frequently a problem, and you may

TIPS ON PROTEIN INTAKE

THERE ARE TWO DIFFERENT TYPES OF PROTEIN

One is called animal or high biological protein, which contains ALL essential amino acids.

The other kind is vegetable or low biological protein, which contains SOME amino acids.

THE HEMODIALYSIS AND THE PERITONEAL MEMBRANE ARE NOT SELECTIVE, WHICH MEANS THAT VITAL AMINO ACIDS AND VITAMINS AS WELL AS UNWANTED WASTES ARE REMOVED

If you are on HEMODIALYSIS, you should aim for **1.2 grams of protein per kg of body weight.** E.g., if you weigh 65 kg (143 lb), your protein intake should be about 78 grams per day.

If you are on PERITONEAL DIALYSIS, you should aim for **1.3 grams of protein per kg of body weight.** E.g., if you weigh 70 kg (154 lb), your protein intake should be about 91 grams per day.

EXAMPLES OF PROTEIN SOURCES

3.5 oz. of extra lean ground beef has 24 grams of protein, while rib eye has 28 grams of protein.

Half of a chicken breast (3.5 oz.) has 29 grams of protein. Turkey light meat (3.5 oz) has 30 grams of protein.

One can of Ensure has 13 grams of protein, while 1 scoop of Promod has 5 grams and one egg has 6 grams of protein.

15 large cooked shrimp have 17 grams of protein. A 3 oz. can of white tuna in water has 22 grams of protein.

One cup of milk has 8 grams of protein, while ½ cup of regular tofu has 10 grams and one slice of white bread has 2 grams of protein.

One cup of cooked corn, peas, potato, pasta or rice has about 4 grams of protein.

FIGURE 36–6 Renal teaching aids: Tips on Protein Intake. (Modified from Darlene Michl, Sidney, British Columbia.)

need to make suggestions about how to solve this problem (as by observing a presleep quiet time and establishing a presleep routine). Assessment in a sleep center may be helpful.

Hypnotics and sedatives must be used cautiously because they may alter mentation and may be metabolized differently by a client with renal failure. The client also needs to establish and maintain an appropriate exercise program. Anemia should be treated with iron and erythropoietin therapy to increase energy levels.

Risk for Impaired Skin Integrity. Edema and skin changes create a *Risk for Impaired Skin Integrity related to edema, dry skin, and pruritus.*

Outcomes. The client will not develop impaired skin integrity, as evidenced by intact skin.

Interventions. Dry skin is a common problem. Use of soap may need to be eliminated. Because of the increased risk of secondary infection, however, the client's skin still needs to be kept clean. Moisturizing oils in the bath water or applied directly to the skin help to correct dryness. Avoid any products that contain alcohol or perfumes; they increase dryness and pruritus. If edema is present, avoid sustained pressure on the area. The potential for skin breakdown is particularly acute in clients with diabetes. Observe for poor circulation and areas of breakdown or infection.

Risk for Ineffective Individual and Family Coping. An important diagnosis is *Risk for Ineffective Individual and Family Coping related to chronic illness, uncertain future for the client, role reversal, and effects of long-term dialysis.*

Outcomes. The client and family will cope with the client's chronic illness and future deterioration, as evidenced by acceptance of the client's problems and ability to support the client. The client and family will cope effectively with the effects of long-term dialysis, as evidenced by the client's level of activity, feelings of self-worth, and participation in dialysis treatment.

Interventions

Involve in Decision-Making. Assistance for the client and significant others must begin before dialysis is started. A client with CRF faces a future of continued deterioration but with an unknown course and timetable. In addition, the disease itself produces behavioral manifestations that contribute to the client's susceptibility to stress.

Many such clients must make important decisions about the choice of treatment modes at a time when they do not feel well. It is often difficult for the client to voice concerns about discontinuing dialysis, and it may be difficult for care providers and families to accept the client's decision to stop treatment and choose death instead. For these reasons, you need to assess how the client handled change and stress before the illness began. The client and significant others need to be actively involved in the care planning process because they will be living with the disease for many years.

Provide Support. The client and significant others will have many questions about such issues as family functioning, job or school demands, dependence, and sex. The client may experience reduced self-esteem. Significant others commonly report a decline in their quality of life that correlates directly with changes in the client's quality of life. Encourage the client and significant others to discuss their feelings and concerns, together and individually, using therapeutic communication techniques. Support groups and peer counseling programs are often helpful.

Offer Home Dialysis. About 15% of all clients who receive dialysis do so at home. The cost of this type of program is less than that of in-center dialysis, and it usually improves the client's quality of life. Home dialysis offers the client more access to significant others and greater feelings of independence and control. However, this type of treatment also produces stress on personal relationships, especially on the person who becomes the "dialysis helper" during home hemodialysis. Some spouses have voiced concern about lack of free time and increased responsibility; others see it as an opportunity to give something back to their spouse or loved one. Some states have funding available to pay for a non–family member to serve as dialysis helper. In some instances, this may reduce tension and improve the quality of life for the family.

Clients for home dialysis programs must be selected carefully. Criteria might include stability of relationships, psychological stability, financial support, and lack of severe physical complications. A successful program requires care providers who are advocates of home dialysis, a good training program, and good support services, possibly including nursing, medical, and social services; provision of supplies; equipment maintenance; dietary counseling; home visits; and retraining as necessary.

Risk for Ineffective Management of Therapeutic Regimen: Individuals and Families.

There is *Risk for Ineffective Management of Therapeutic Regimen: Individuals and Families related to lack of knowledge of the disease process and treatment.*

Outcomes. The client will understand the disease process and treatment regimen as evidenced by ability to describe the disease and treatment and participate in the treatment regimen.

Interventions

Provide Information. Teaching is a crucial part of the nursing management plan. Most of the time, the client is observed on an outpatient basis and is responsible for following the recommended treatment regimen. The client and significant others must know about normal renal function and how the disease has altered it, the details of the management protocol and how to follow it, a number of self-assessment skills as described earlier, and when to seek professional consultation for possible complications. Teaching aids are available from many sources, such as the National Kidney Foundation, the National Association of Patients on Hemodialysis and Transplantation, various corporations, and the Internet. The American Nephrology Nurses Association regularly publishes a directory of educational resources.[2]

Explain Dialysis. The client and significant others need to know about dialysis and how to work with its ramifications. With peritoneal dialysis, most clients continue the treatment mode in their homes; hence, their knowledge needs to be complete and detailed. They participate in a complete training program so that they can handle the entire dialysis process independently.

Continuous monitoring during hemodialysis provides vital information about the progress of the treatment and allows early diagnosis of potential complications. There should be a well-organized plan for observing and recording vital signs, dialysate composition and temperature, and functioning of the entire dialysis system and blood flow. The client should also be alert to early manifestations of potential complications, as listed earlier. The nurse often serves as case manager and coordinates the services provided by the nephrology team, which includes the physician, nurses, social worker, and dietitian.

Reduce Anxiety. Although clients with renal disease must learn about their disorder, they may not always be ready to learn. Anxiety itself interferes with learning. In addition, the disease interferes with normal cognitive functioning; memory deficits and a short attention span may require simple presentations and frequent repetition of information. Retained learning must be continually evaluated.

Significant others may be especially frustrated during teaching sessions by the client's inability to grasp the concepts being presented. The client may seem out of touch with reality. Significant others need reassurance that this is an effect of the disease and that the client will become more capable of learning, especially after institution of dialysis.

Risk for Infection.
Indwelling catheters carry a high *Risk for Infection related to the presence of an indwelling peritoneal catheter and instillation of dialysate or related to venipuncture and connection of tubing during hemodialysis.*

Outcomes. The client will remain free of infection, as evidenced by a normal white blood cell count, absence of fever, and clear dialysate.

Interventions. Because peritonitis is the main complication of peritoneal dialysis, strict aseptic technique must be used throughout the procedure. Masks are worn by the nurse and client when the peritoneal dialysis circuit is opened. Gloves are worn by anyone touching the catheter during all connection and disconnection procedures. The catheter is soaked before and after these procedures in a povidone-iodine solution. Dressing changes around the catheter site are performed according to the specific unit protocol. Be sure dressings are kept dry at all times.

With hemodialysis, use strict aseptic technique during venipuncture and when attaching the tubing and solution.

Risk for Ineffective Breathing Pattern.
Peritoneal dialysis also creates a *Risk for Ineffective Breathing Pattern related to pressure from dialysate.*

Outcomes. The client will have an effective breathing pattern, as evidenced by an absence of shortness of breath.

Interventions. Because dialysate presses on the diaphragm, its full excursion may be reduced and an immobilized client may be at risk for respiratory problems. Encourage the client to cough and deep-breathe regularly. Keep the client in the semi-Fowler position to ease breathing. Also, remind the client to stay alert for early manifestations of compromised respiratory function.

Risk for Injury. Trauma and complications associated with the vascular access for hemodialysis may occur, leading to the diagnosis *Risk for Injury related to trauma to hemodialysis venous access site.*

Outcomes. The client will not experience injury to the venous access site, as evidenced by continued patency of the site.

Interventions. Careful attention to the access site—to prevent infection and clotting—is important to its life expectancy. A dressing is used to protect cannulas and subclavian catheters from infection. The access site must also be protected from trauma that could cause clotting, bleeding, or physical disruption of the site. For example, warn the client against wearing tight sleeves or carrying a purse over the access site. The limb that contains the access site should not be used to take blood pressure or to draw blood.

Between dialysis periods, the skin over the fistula or graft requires only routine care with soap and water. The site of a fistula should be carefully assessed. To assess patency, palpate over the fistula for a thrill and auscultate for a bruit at regular intervals. The client must also learn to assess the access site for patency.

EVALUATION

The client is expected to improve physically and mentally when dialysis begins. The client's weight and blood pressure should begin to stabilize if dietary and fluid restrictions are followed and as fluid balance stabilizes.

Normal electrolyte and albumin levels reflect adequate nutrition and compliance with diet. The client should report regular, normal bowel movements. The client should report less fatigue and increased energy and activity as hematocrit values approach normal levels. Skin should remain intact.

The client should understand and adapt to the treatment regimen and be successfully maintained with peritoneal dialysis or hemodialysis. Clients receiving peritoneal dialysis (and some receiving hemodialysis) should be able to demonstrate successful performance of the dialysis procedure and care of the vascular access site or peritoneal catheter. They should remain free from complications associated with dialysis. As long as venous or peritoneal access can be maintained, the client can be managed with dialysis until transplantation (if the client is a candidate) is completed, the client elects to stop dialysis, or other complications result in death.

Significant others should cope with the client's chronic illness and dialysis, show acceptance of problems, support the client, and report improved satisfaction with their own quality of life. The family and significant others should assist the client with treatment as needed.

■ Self-Care

Clients must comply with dietary and fluid intake modifications and take prescribed medications as ordered. They must monitor and record weight and blood pressure daily and care for the venous access or peritoneal catheter as ordered. Noncompliance with the regimen leads to com-

plications. The client or family must perform dialysis at home or keep scheduled dialysis appointments.

■ Modifications for Elderly Clients

The types of dialysis for older clients are evaluated on the basis of the presence of other chronic disorders that would limit the ability to comply with any treatment.

Older clients may have had multiple abdominal surgical procedures with the development of adhesions that limit the usefulness of peritoneal dialysis. They are more likely to have pre-existing cardiovascular problems that may limit the usefulness of many venous access sites.

■ Surgical Management

RENAL TRANSPLANTATION

INDICATIONS. Renal transplantation is the surgical implantation of a human kidney from a compatible donor in a recipient. This procedure is performed as an intervention in irreversible kidney failure. The kidney is surgically placed extraperitoneally in the iliac fossa. The renal artery is anastomosed to the recipient's hypogastric internal or external iliac artery (occasionally the aorta) and the renal vein to the recipient's iliac vein (Fig. 36–7). Usually, the kidney begins to function immediately.

Selection of a transplant recipient is based on careful evaluation of the client's medical, immunologic, and psychosocial status (see Chapter 80). Usually, a recipient is younger than age 70, has an estimated life expectancy of 2 years or more, and is expected to have an improved quality of life after transplantation. Conservative management and dialysis should have made the client's state as nontoxic as possible. Bilateral nephrectomy may be performed before the transplantation procedure for persistent or active bacterial pyelonephritis, uncontrolled renin-mediated hypertension, polycystic kidneys, or rapidly progressive glomerulonephritis.

Successful transplantation prolongs life and markedly improves its quality. The client is freed from the restrictions of dialysis and from the reversible manifestations of uremia.

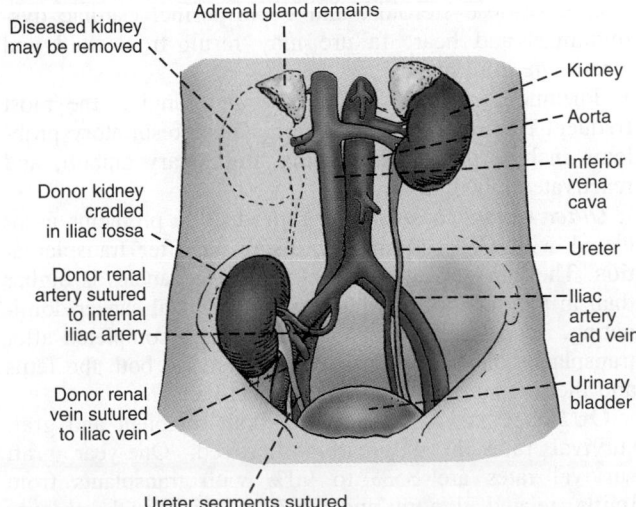

FIGURE 36–7 Transplanted kidney placement in the right iliac fossa.

Because graft survival rates are higher, the most desirable source of kidneys for transplantation is a living related donor who matches the client closely. Willing family members are evaluated for physical and mental health and screened for ABO blood group, tissue-specific antigen, and human leukocyte antigen histocompatibility (see Chapter 80). Consideration has been given to transplanting kidneys from emotionally related donors, such as friends or spouses. Nevertheless, most transplanted kidneys are cadaver organs.

CONTRAINDICATIONS. Infection and active malignancy are the only absolute contraindications to transplantation. Some physical conditions markedly increase the risk for the client, however, primarily because long-term immunosuppressive medications are necessary to avoid graft rejection. Clients with liver disease, psychological disorders, advanced atherosclerosis, hypertension, respiratory disease, and gastrointestinal bleeding need particular consideration. The primary factor limiting the number of transplantations done is the availability of kidneys.

COMPLICATIONS. Major complications of transplantation, such as graft rejection (and antirejection therapy), infection, skin and gastrointestinal problems, and other complications, are discussed in Chapter 80.

Graft Rejection. The manifestations of renal transplant rejection include fever, graft tenderness at the site of the transplanted kidney, anemia, and malaise.

Urinary Tract Complications. Several complications may occur in the urinary tract. Although it is rare, spontaneous rupture of the kidney may occur because of rejection or ischemic damage. Leaking of urine from the ureter-bladder anastomosis causes the development of a urinoma, which eventually puts pressure on the kidney and ureter, reducing renal function. Long-term uremia and steroid therapy may predispose the client to ureteral, bladder, or caliceal-cutaneous fistulas. Other urinary tract complications include ureteral, bladder, or pelvic leaks; obstruction; reflux; and lymphoceles.

Cardiopulmonary Complications. Hypertension occurs in 50% to 60% of adult recipients and may be caused by renal artery stenosis, acute tubular necrosis, acute and chronic graft rejection, hydronephrosis, hyperaldosteronism, large-dose steroids, and cyclosporine. Cardiac dysrhythmias and heart failure may result from fluid and electrolyte imbalances.

Pneumonia caused by bacteria and fungi is the most frequent respiratory complication. Other respiratory problems include pulmonary edema, pulmonary emboli, and reactivated tuberculosis.

Other Complications. The reproductive problems associated with CRF commonly disappear after transplantation. The incidence of gynecologic malignancies is higher than in the general population, with cervical cancer dominating. Successful pregnancies have been completed after transplantation, although there is a risk for both the fetus and the mother with a transplanted kidney.

OUTCOMES. Over the years, both recipient and graft survival rates have greatly improved. One-year graft survival rates are 85% to 90% with transplants from living related donors and 75% to 80% with cadaver kidneys. The overall mortality rate 2 years after transplantation is about 10%.[21] This represents a dramatic decrease; two decades ago, the 2-year survival was 40% to 50%.

In particular, the decrease in the death rate related to infection in the first 2 years after transplantation has been dramatic. Advances in immunosuppressive therapy and the treatment of infectious diseases have contributed to the overall improvement. Cardiovascular problems remain the leading cause of death in the late transplantation period. Myocardial infarction, stroke, and heart failure are the primary causes of death.

■ Nursing Management of the Surgical Client

PREOPERATIVE CARE

Before kidney transplantation, assess the client's understanding of the procedure and follow-up regimen. Also, assess the client's ability to cope with a complex medication regimen after transplantation. The client needs to understand the transplantation and therapeutic regimen. Preoperative preparation of both the living donor and the recipient includes all aspects of general preoperative care as outlined in Chapter 15.

POSTOPERATIVE CARE

Assessment for renal transplant recipients is similar to that for most other postoperative clients (see Chapter 15), with the exception of the focus on renal function. Give particular attention to fluid balance, and carefully monitor intake and output (every 30 to 60 minutes) and weight (daily). To monitor renal function and maintain electrolyte balance, obtain serial laboratory determinations of hemoglobin, hematocrit, BUN, creatinine, electrolytes, white blood cell count, and platelets. Auscultate the kidney regularly to check for bruits, which might indicate stenosis. Monitoring of vital signs is key, because even a slight temperature increase may indicate an infection.

The function of the transplanted kidney is a primary concern after surgery. A kidney from a cadaver may not function immediately, and the client may be maintained with hemodialysis until it functions adequately. Postoperatively, manage intravenous fluids carefully; the amount of fluid infused is typically based on the previous hour's output. A high urine output is usually desired. The additional care required by the recipient is related to potential complications. Care of the client with a transplant is discussed in more detail in Chapter 80.

Psychologically, the client must be helped to incorporate the new kidney as a part of the whole being. Provide education and counseling to enhance changes in lifestyle that promote health-seeking behaviors and compliance with transplantation medications. If the graft fails, expect the client to feel anger, hostility, guilt, and a helplessness-hopelessness syndrome. Relatives and friends may mirror these feelings. Role changes that were well established during the chronic illness may lead to problems, as with the family member who no longer feels needed as the caregiver. Likewise, the client may have difficulty giving up the sick role.

■ Self-Care

Failure to follow the prescribed regimen is a major problem after transplantation, and your knowledge and creativity are needed to help the client follow the recommended regimen. Many clients—particularly adolescents—miss doses of their immunosuppressive medications (see Chapter 80). This practice contributes to early loss of renal function and possible graft loss.

Clients may be reluctant to take medications for many reasons. For some, the side effects disrupt their lives. Others may believe that they no longer need the medications because they are stable. Economic concerns also need to be addressed. Immunosuppressive medications, particularly cyclosporine, are expensive. Currently, Medicare covers payment of these drugs for up to 48 months after transplantation. After that time, other sources of funding need to be explored to ensure compliance with medications. Work with the client to provide needed information and to develop strategies that fit the client's lifestyle.

Overall, transplantation offers clients with CRF a much better quality of life than does dialysis therapy. Renal function returns, and many of the clinical manifestations of CRF disappear. Complications do occur, and care must be taken to prevent graft loss. Renal transplant recipients are monitored regularly at transplantation clinics. The visits become less frequent as renal function stabilizes and time passes. Blood tests are taken regularly to monitor serum creatinine levels and cyclosporine levels. Every transplantation center has protocols for routine follow-up tests.

Modifications for Elderly Clients

One of the major modifications for older clients may be fewer options available for treatment. Renal transplantation is not routinely done for elderly clients. Clients older than 60 years are evaluated on an individual basis; clients as old as 75 years of age have had successful transplantations. One problem for elderly clients is that a less effective immune system in conjunction with immunosuppressants can lead to further complications.

CONCLUSIONS

Caring for the client with renal failure involves many challenges. There are numerous physical and psychosocial manifestations associated with renal disease and its treatment. The nurse can significantly impact the client's quality of life through the provision of education, encouragement, promotion of exercise, and ongoing assessment of the client and family as well as evaluation of programs offering treatment for end-stage renal disease. The nurse, in collaboration with the multidisciplinary team, can facilitate positive outcomes.

THINKING CRITICALLY

1. You are caring for a 74-year-old man 1 day after coronary artery bypass surgery. His urine output is about 15 ml/hr. He has a long history of hypertension (controlled), and his blood pressure usually ranges from 180 to 190 over 90 to 100 mm Hg. His blood pressure since surgery has ranged from 120 to 130 over 70 to 76 mm Hg. His serum sodium concentration is 145

mEq/L and potassium is 4.9 mEq/L. His skin turgor is poor, and mucous membranes are dry. What is your first assessment and action?

Factors to Consider. What has his intake been since surgery? What are the possible causes of his low blood pressure, increased electrolytes, and decreased urine output? If he has renal failure, what is the probable cause? What other assessments should you make?

2. You are caring for a 60-year-old woman with diabetes, hypertension, and chronic renal failure. She has had hemodialysis for over a year and has decided that she no longer wants to continue living this way. She has informed her physician and family that she no longer wishes to continue dialysis. Her family is trying to persuade her that she should go for her next treatment. She asks you your opinion, "Would you want to live this way?" How would you respond? How would you ensure that she is making the right decision?

Factors to Consider. What is the client's cognitive and emotional status? How have the client and her family members coped with the illness and its treatment? Given the information you have, what is her prognosis? Do people have the right to refuse life-sustaining therapy? Knowing that health care resources are finite, what is the best use of resources for all members of society?

BIBLIOGRAPHY

1. Abuelo, J. G. (Ed.). (1995). *Renal failure: Diagnosis and treatment.* Norwell, MA: Kluwer.
2. American Nephrology Nurses Association. (1997). 1997 educational resource directory. *ANNA Journal, 24*(4), 427–440.
3. Arnold, R. M. (Ed.). (1995). *Procuring organs for transplant: The debate over non–heart-beating cadaver protocols.* Baltimore: Johns Hopkins University Press.
4. Bach, F. H., & Auchincloss, H., Jr. (1995). *Transplantation immunology.* New York: Wiley-Liss.
5. Badzek, L., Hines, S. C., & Moss, A. H. (1998). Inadequate self-care knowledge among elderly hemodialysis patients: Assessing its prevalence and potential causes. *ANNA Journal, 25*(3), 293–300.
6. Bennett, J. C., & Plum, F. (Eds.). (1996). *Cecil textbook of medicine* (20th ed.). Philadelphia: W. B. Saunders.
7. Binik, Y. M., & Mah, K. (1994). Sexuality and end-stage renal disease: Research and clinical recommendations. *Advances in Renal Replacement Therapy, 1*(3), 198–209.
8. Brenner, B. M. (Ed.). (1996). *Brenner and Rector's the kidney* (5th ed.). Philadelphia: W. B. Saunders.
9. Burrows-Hudson, S. (Ed.). (1999). *Standards and guidelines of clinical practice for nephrology nursing.* Pitman, NJ: American Nephrology Nurses Association.
10. Busson, M., et al. (1995). Analysis of cadaver donor criteria on the kidney transplant survival rate in 5,129 transplantations. *Journal of Urology, 154*(2, Pt. 1), 356–360.
11. Corbett, J., & Ross, K. (1998). Neoral: The new cyclosporine. *ANNA Journal, 25*(1), 71–72.
12. Crampton, K., et al. (1998). Renal rehabilitation programs: Keys to success. *ANNA Journal, 25*(2), 248–251.
13. Flye, M. W. (Ed.). (1995). *Atlas of organ transplantation.* Philadelphia: W. B. Saunders.
14. Glassock, R. J. (1998). *Current therapy in nephrology and hypertension* (4th ed.). St. Louis: Mosby–Year Book.
15. Guyton, A. C., & Hall, J. E. (1996). *Textbook of medical physiology* (6th ed.). Philadelphia: W. B. Saunders.

16. Health Care Financing Administration. (1998, October). HCFA research report provides ESRD facility data. *Contemporary Dialysis and Nephrology, 19*(10), 18.

17. Headley, C. M. (1998). Hungry bone syndrome following parathyroidectomy. *ANNA Journal, 25*(3), 283–292.

18. Headley, C. M. (1998). Osteitis fibrosa: Treatment trends. *ANNA Journal, 25*(1), 21–30.

19. Horsburgh, M. E., Rice, V. H., & Matuk, L. (1998). Sense of coherence and life satisfaction: Patient and spousal adaptation to home dialysis. *ANNA Journal, 25*(2), 219–230.

20. Jacobs, C., et al. (1996). *Replacement of renal function by dialysis.* Norwell, MA: Kluwer.

21. Karlowicz, K. A. (Ed.). (1995). *Urologic nursing: Principles and practice.* Philadelphia: W. B. Saunders.

22. Kinzer, C. L. (1998). Warfarin sodium (Coumadin) anticoagulant therapy for vascular access patency. *ANNA Journal, 25*(2), 195–209.

23. Koeppen, B. M., & Stanton, B. A. (1997). *Renal physiology* (2nd ed.). St. Louis: Mosby–Year Book.

24. Lancaster, L. E. (Ed.). (1995). *Core curriculum for nephrology nursing* (2nd ed.). Pitman, NJ: American Nephrology Nurses Association.

25. Lev, E. L., & Owen, S. V. (1998). A prospective study of adjustment to hemodialysis. *ANNA Journal, 25*(1), 495–506.

26. Levine, D. Z. (Ed.). (1997). *Caring for the renal patient* (3rd ed.). Philadelphia: W. B. Saunders.

27. Life Options Rehabilitation Advisory Council. (1997). *Building quality of life: A practical guide to renal rehabilitation.* San Francisco: Amgen.

28. Long, J. M., et al. (1998). Medication compliance and the older hemodialysis patient. *ANNA Journal, 25*(1), 43–56.

29. Massry, S. G., & Glassock, R. J. (Eds.). (1995). *Massry and Glassock's textbook of nephrology* (3rd ed.). Baltimore: Williams & Wilkins.

30. Molzahn, A. E., & Kikuchi, J. F. (1998). Reported quality of life of children and adolescents with parents on dialysis. *ANNA Journal, 25*(6), 411–418.

31. Molzahn, A. E., Northcott, H. C., & Dossetor, J. B. (1997). Quality of life of individuals with end stage renal disease: Perceptions of patients, nurses, and physicians. *ANNA Journal, 24*(3), 325–336.

32. Neyhart, C. D. (1998). Contraception in ESRD and immunosuppression for the pregnant transplant patient. *ANNA Journal, 25*(3), 345–348.

33. Nolan, M. T., & Augustine, S. M. (Eds.). (1995). *Transplantation nursing: Acute and long-term management.* Norwalk, CT: Appleton & Lange.

34. Parker, J. (Ed.). (1998). *Contemporary nephrology nursing.* Pitman, NJ: American Nephrology Nurses Association.

35. Parker, K. P. (1997). Sleep and dialysis: A research-based review of the literature. *ANNA Journal, 24*(6), 626–639.

36. Redman, B. K., Hill, M. N., & Fry, S. T. (1997). Ethical conflicts reported by certified nephrology nurses practicing in dialysis settings. *ANNA Journal, 24*(1), 23–34.

37. Richbourg, M. J. (1997). Vision screening in older adults on dialysis: Do nephrology nurses have a role? *ANNA Journal, 24*(3), 541–544, 549.

38. Rodriguez, D., & Lewis, S. L. (1997). Nutritional management of patients with acute renal failure. *ANNA Journal, 24*(2), 232–241.

39. Rogers, A. E. (1997). Nursing management of sleep disorders. Part 1: Assessment. *ANNA Journal, 24*(6), 666–671.

40. Rogers, A. E. (1997). Nursing management of sleep disorders. Part 2: Behavioral interventions. *ANNA Journal, 24*(6), 672–675.

41. Schlatter, S., & Ferrans, C. E. (1998). Teaching program effects on high phosphorus levels in patients receiving hemodialysis. *ANNA Journal, 25*(1), 31–42.

42. Schrier, R. W. (Ed.). (1995). *Manual of nephrology.* Boston: Little, Brown.

43. Schrier, R. W., & Gottschalk, C. W. (Eds.). (1997). *Diseases of the kidney* (6th ed.). Boston: Little, Brown.

44. Wicks, M., et al. (1997). Subjective burden and quality of life in family caregivers of patients with end stage renal disease. *ANNA Journal, 24*(5), 527–540.

45. United States Renal Data System. (1999). *Annual data report.* Washington, DC: United States Department of Health and Human Services, Health Care Financing Administration, Bureau of Data Management and Strategy.

Sexuality and Reproductive Disorders

Anatomy and Physiology Review: The Reproductive Systems

37 Assessment of the Reproductive System

38 Management of Men with Reproductive Disorders

39 Management of Women with Reproductive Disorders

40 Management of Clients with Breast Disorders

41 Management of Clients with Sexually Transmitted Disorders

Anatomy and Physiology Review
The Reproductive Systems
Robert G. Carroll

The human reproductive system is specialized for the production and joining of *germ cells*—the ovum, or egg (female) and the sperm (male). The female reproductive system is also specialized to nurture and protect the fertilized ovum during the 9-month gestation period. Gonadal development begins in utero, but maturation of the reproductive system *(puberty)* is delayed until adolescence. At 45 to 60 years of age, fertility gradually decreases, ending at *menopause* (permanent cessation of menstruation) in women.

GONADAL DEVELOPMENT

The *gonads* are the sex glands of the female *(ovaries)* and male *(testes)*. Their primary function is to form germ cells, which have half the normal number of chromosomes. The ovaries produce ova; the testes produce spermatozoa (sperm).

Gonadal development begins during the 5th week of fetal life, and gonadal differentiation occurs in the 7th and 8th weeks of gestation. Human chorionic gonadotropin (HCG) is released from the placenta, stimulating the ovaries to release estradiol and progesterone and the testes to release testosterone. In males, the Wolffian ducts develop into the epididymis, vas deferens, and seminal vesicles, and the Müllerian ducts regress. In females, the Wolffian ducts regress and the Müllerian ducts develop into fallopian tubes, uterus, and upper vagina. The external genitalia—the glans penis and scrotum—are complete in boys by 14 weeks of gestation. The clitoris, labia majora, and labia minora are complete in girls by 11 weeks of gestation.

FEMALE REPRODUCTIVE SYSTEM

GENITAL STRUCTURES

■ EXTERNAL STRUCTURES

The female reproductive organs consist of both external and internal structures. The external structures, collectively termed the *vulva* or *pudendum,* play a role in sexual stimulation and provide a barrier to protect the body from foreign materials (Fig. U8–1A). External female genital structures consist of the mons pubis, labia majora and minora, clitoris, vestibular bulbs, and vestibule (Table U8–1). The *perineum* is the area posterior to the vestibule, between it and the anus.

The *hymen,* a fold of mucous membrane that is sometimes present, partially covers the opening to the vagina. In the past, the presence or absence of a hymen was used as proof of a woman's virginity or sexual activity. However, the hymen may be ruptured in various ways (e.g.,

during exercise, sexual activity, surgery, vaginal examination, tampon insertion). Pregnancy has even been known to occur with an intact hymen.

■ INTERNAL STRUCTURES

The internal female genital structures produce and release the reproductive cell or ovum, transport ova to the potential site of fertilization, and provide an appropriate environment for the implantation, growth, and delivery of the fetus (see Table U8–1).

Ovaries are the female gonads, producing both the female germ cell (ovum) and hormones (estrogen and progesterone). Normally two ovaries are located in the pelvis, one on either side of the uterus and below the fallopian (uterine) tubes (Fig. U8–1B). The ovaries are contained in the posterior surfaces of the broad ligaments. They are also supported by the suspensory ligament (to the side of the pelvis) and by the utero-ovarian ligament (to the uterus). In young females, ovaries are smooth; with age, they become pitted.

Ova, in various stages of development in addition to their surrounding tissue, make up the *ovarian follicles.* Each follicle contains a developing ovum; it grows and matures in the stroma, close to an abundant blood and lymphatic supply. A mature follicle (a mature ovum and its surrounding tissues) is an endocrine gland secreting estrogen hormones (see Estrogens). At birth, several hundred thousand follicles, each containing an oocyte or end-stage ovum, are present. They decrease in number as puberty (the onset of functional reproductive capability) approaches, and they gradually disappear around menopause.

The *corpus luteum* is a glandular body that produces the hormones progesterone and estrogen. It develops from a graafian follicle after ovulation (see Secretory Phase).

Two *fallopian tubes* connect the uterus to the ovaries and are the usual site of fertilization (Fig. U8–1C). They convey the ovum to the uterus. Each fallopian tube is about 10 cm long.

The *uterus* is located in the pelvic cavity slightly below and between the fallopian tubes, almost at a right angle to the vagina. The normal uterus is movable in all directions, but maintains its normal position in the body cavity through the action of various ligaments and the pelvic floor. The cardinal (lateral cervical) ligaments run between the pelvic wall and the cervix and vagina and provide the most support. If these ligaments are weak, the uterus is likely to prolapse (drop) into the vagina.

The uterus has three functional layers: (1) the *parametrium,* the thin peritoneal and fascial covering of the uterus; (2) the *myometrium* (bulk of the uterus), a muscular layer composed of three layers, mainly of involuntary

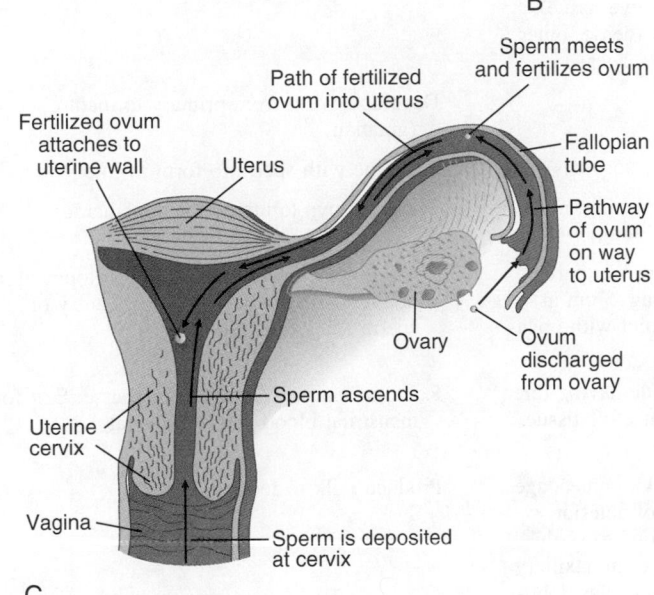

FIGURE U8–1 *A,* Anatomic landmarks of external female genitalia. *B,* Midsagittal section of the female pelvis. *C,* Pathways of sperm and ovum in the female reproductive organs. (Modified from Miller, B. F., & Keane, C. B. [1992]. *Encyclopedia and dictionary of medicine, nursing and allied health* [5th ed., p. 1085]. Philadelphia: W. B. Saunders.)

muscles; and (3) the *endometrium,* the mucous membrane lining the inner surface of the uterus. The superior two thirds of the endometrium responds cyclically to hormones. A fertilized ovum implants in the endometrium. When the ovum is not fertilized, the endometrial lining is shed (see Menstruation).

The *vagina* is a musculomembranous canal connecting the uterus with the external genitalia. The mucosa of the inner surface of the vaginal wall folds over in small ridges (rugae) extending laterally upward. This rugal pattern adds to the vagina's elasticity, making it very distensible. The rectum is posterior to its lower two thirds. The vagina's smooth rugal pattern and elasticity diminish during the menopausal and postmenopausal years. The vagina can easily become infected from urethral or rectal secretions.

■ **PELVIC BLOOD SUPPLY, INNERVATION, AND LYMPHATIC DRAINAGE**

BLOOD SUPPLY

The most important *blood supply* to the external genitalia comes from the internal iliac (hypogastric) artery. This artery branches to supply the pelvic floor, pelvic walls, and pelvic viscera. The principal vessels supplying the internal genitalia are the *uterine arteries,* from the internal iliac artery, and the *ovarian arteries,* which stem directly from the aorta. The uterine artery provides a rich vascular bed to the uterus, and anastomoses the arterial supply to the vagina (vaginal arteries). The ovarian artery supplies blood to the ovaries, fallopian tubes, and body of the uterus. Venous drainage roughly parallels the arterial supply.

TABLE U8–1	FEMALE REPRODUCTIVE STRUCTURES AND THEIR FUNCTIONS	
Structure	**Description**	**Function**
Vulva		Vulva protects the body from foreign materials and plays a role in sexual stimulation
Mons pubis	Rounded pad of flesh over symphysis pubis; hair-covered after puberty	
Labia majora	Two elongated folds of tissue separated by a cleft	
Labia minora	Two thin folds of tissue between labia majora and vaginal opening; they divide and unite to form the hood-like prepuce of the clitoris	
Clitoris	Homologous to penis	
Vestibular bulbs	Two sacculated collections of veins; homologous to corpus spongiosum	
Vestibule of vagina	Almond-shaped space, consisting of delicate mucous membranes, between labia minora; bounded anteriorly by clitoris and posteriorly by fourchette	Provides opening for urethra, vagina, and two ducts of Bartholin's glands
Bartholin's glands	Two mucus-secreting glands	Help to lubricate tissues during intercourse
Ovaries	Two almond-sized glands consisting (outer to inner layers) of surface germinal epithelium, tunica albuginea (dense connective tissue), and stroma. Stroma has cortex (dense, outer layer) and medulla (loose inner layer).	Produce ova for fertilization, synthesize and secrete estrogens and progesterone
Ovarian follicle	Ovum plus surrounding tissue	Develops ovum from primary to mature (graafian)
Ovum	Female reproductive cell (23 chromosomes)	Combine with sperm to form zygote
Fallopian tubes	Thin-walled tubes with serosal covering, muscular layer, and ciliated mucous lining	Transport ova to uterus for implantation
Uterus	Pear-shaped, hollow muscular organ in pelvic cavity (2–5 cm thick, 5 cm long, 5 cm at widest to 2 cm at narrowest point with opening to vagina (cervix)	Environment for implantation, development, and delivery of fetus; cervix allows entry of sperm for fertilization
Vagina	Canal between uterus and vestibule having three layers: epithelium, fibrous connective tissue, and muscular layer	Route of entry for sexual intercourse. Exit for menstrual blood and birth canal
Breasts	Modified sebaceous glands and skin appendages lying within superficial fascia of anterior chest wall (vertically from second to sixth rib, horizontally from sternum to midaxillary line). Parenchyma consists of ductular, lobular, and acinar epithelial structures; stroma is made of fibrous and fatty tissue.	Produce milk to feed infants

INNERVATION

Both the sympathetic and parasympathetic autonomic nervous systems provide innervation to the pelvic structures. Sexual arousal is controlled by the parasympathetic dilatation of blood vessels in the vestibular bulbs and clitoris. The uterine myometrium is innervated only by the sympathetic nerve fibers. The perineum is supplied principally by the pudendal nerve.

LYMPHATIC DRAINAGE

The pelvic *lymphatics* are a rich network of superficial and deep systems that roughly parallel the blood supply. The intermingling of the pelvic lymphatics and blood vessels is significant for the potential spread of cancer.

THE BREASTS

■ FEMALE BREASTS

Structures of the Breast

Breasts play an important role in our culture. Because breasts are visible, their size and shape are often mistakenly viewed as a measure of sexuality, femininity, and attractiveness. However, breasts are a secondary sexual characteristic; that is, reproduction can occur without them. The physiologic function of female breasts is secretion of milk to feed infants. An average nonlactating breast weighs between 150 and 250 g, and a lactating breast weighs 400 to 500 g.

The *parenchyma* of a breast consists of ductular, lobular, and acinar epithelial structures. The stroma of a breast is made of fibrous and fatty tissue. The upper lateral quadrant of the breast, which is mostly glandular, is the most common site of tumor occurrence. A breast consists of 12 to 20 *lobes,* subdivided into *lobules,* made up of acini. Breast lobes are arranged like the spokes of a wheel around the nipple. Each lobe is drained by a duct, 12 to 20 of which open independently on the surface of the nipple.

The *nipple,* located at the fourth intercostal space, is surrounded by a circular pigmented area called the *areola.* Estrogen increases pigmentation of the areola at any age. The areolar epithelium contains some small hairs and sebaceous glands, sweat glands, and accessory mammary glands. The sebaceous glands (Montgomery's glands) enlarge to lubricate the nipple during pregnancy and lactation.

BLOOD SUPPLY
The two main sources of the breast's blood supply are the lateral mammary artery and the lateral thoracic artery. These arteries form an extensive network of anastomoses. The main veins follow the arterial pattern.

LYMPHATIC DRAINAGE
Lymphatic pathways generally follow the pathways of the veins. There are three types of lymphatic drainage of the breast (Fig. U8–2):

- Cutaneous or superficial lymphatic drainage from the skin
- Areolar lymphatic drainage from the areola and nipple
- Glandular lymphatic drainage from deep glandular tissue

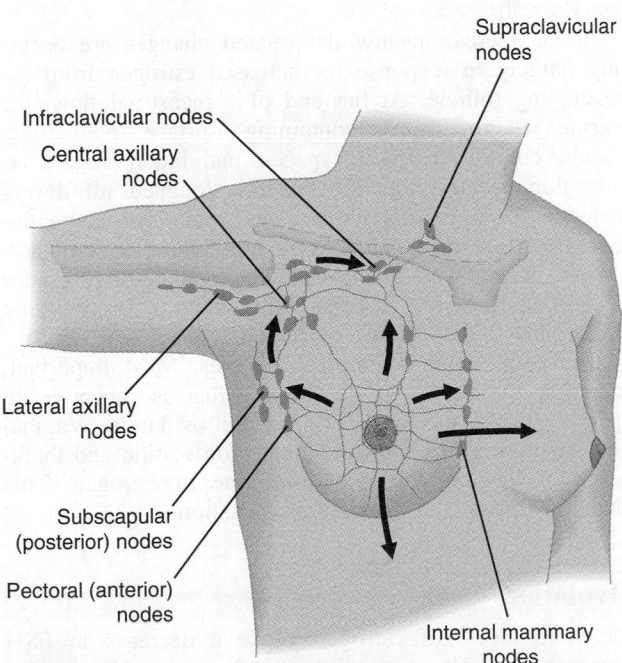

FIGURE U8–2 Routes of lymphatic drainage from the breast. These routes are very important in the spread of breast cancer.

Lymphatic drainage pathways and lymph nodes are important in the prognosis and treatment of breast cancer (see Chapter 40). The nerve supply is derived from the anterior and lateral branches of the fourth to sixth intercostal nerves.

Functions of the Breast
The physiologic changes that affect the breast are:

- Growth and development
- The menstrual cycle
- Pregnancy and lactation

Estrogen and progesterone act synergistically with the pituitary growth hormones prolactin and corticotropin to produce breast development and function. Breast development usually occurs between 9 and 16 years of age and takes 4 to 5 years. Estrogen is responsible for the growth of the breast and periductal stroma. Progesterone promotes the development of lobular and acinar structures.

After menopause, the ovaries stop producing estrogen and progesterone. Estrogen is then produced by the adrenals through stimulation from the anterior pituitary. During this life stage, there is a continuous involution of the breast with loss of glandular elements and tissue atrophy.

During pregnancy, estrogen, progesterone, and pituitary hormones increase, increasing breast vascularity and the permeability and dilation of breast lymphatics. When pregnancy ends, prolactin initiates lactation. Prolactin and corticoptropin help maintain lactation. The "letting down" (flow) of milk is a complex response involving a mother's subjective response and the mechanical stimulation of suckling. Suckling releases the pituitary hormone oxytocin into the bloodstream. This causes the mammary acini to contract and release milk into the duct system.

■ MALE BREASTS
The male breast is similar to that of a preadolescent girl. It contains a few ducts surrounded by connective tissue. Estrogen can cause a man's breast to enlarge (*gynecomastia*) (see Chapter 83). Accumulation of fat in obese men can also make the breasts appear large.

FEMALE REPRODUCTION
■ ROLE OF HORMONES
Under control of the hypothalamic releasing factors and anterior pituitary FSH and LH, the ovaries manufacture estrogens and progestins. These hormones accomplish the following functions:

- Stimulate sexual desire
- Interact with the hypothalamic-pituitary unit and the uterus for (1) ovarian changes (follicular development, ovulation, corpus luteum formation), (2) pregnancy (implantation of a fertilized ovum), or (3) menstruation
- Exert additional effects elsewhere in the body

Estrogens
Estrogens (female sex hormones) produce cyclic changes in the uterine endothelium and vaginal epithelium. Estrogens are steroids that are secreted in both males and

females by the adrenal cortex and in females by the ovary (main source) and placenta. Natural estrogens include estradiol, estrone, and estriol. Estrogens in low doses may be used therapeutically as a replacement hormone during menopause.

The main effects of estrogenic stimulation on the body occur at puberty and include breast growth (fatty tissue deposition, pigmentation), fat deposition in the vulva, pubic and axillary hair growth, bony pelvis growth and broadening, closure of the epiphyseal plates of long bones, vaginal epithelial changes, and general growth. The effects of hormones on menstruation are discussed later.

It is not known precisely how the trophic actions of estrogen interact with other endocrine systems. Thus, whether estrogen replacement should be given during menopause is under investigation. Osteoporosis (increased bone porosity) is associated with estrogen deficiency in adult women.

Progesterone

Progesterone is a steroid hormone that helps prepare the endometrium to receive and implant the fertilized ovum; it also promotes development of the placenta (a spongy structure in the uterus that provides nourishment for a developing fetus) and the mammary glands.

Progesterone is used therapeutically to treat threatened abortion and such menstrual problems as dysmenorrhea or amenorrhea. It is secreted from the placenta and the corpus luteum under control of the anterior pituitary hormone luteinizing hormone (LH). Progesterone plays a minor role in sodium and water balance. It also influences nitrogen balance, breast function, and body temperature during the menstrual cycle, raising body temperature by 1° F in the postovulatory phase of the cycle.

■ MENARCHE

The beginning of menstrual life (menarche) is a biologic, psychological, and social milestone. Psychosocial support, education about the physical changes that are happening, and knowledge about self-care are essential to a young woman at this stage of life.

The average age for menarche in the United States is now 12.8 years. Menarche is preceded by characteristic body changes (such as breast development) that occur between ages 9 and 16 years.

The age at which menarche occurs is affected by genetic factors. Menarche may be delayed by poor nutrition, high levels of exercise (athletes or dancers), and several medical conditions, such as diabetes mellitus, congenital heart disease, and ulcerative colitis. Early menarche may occur with other conditions, such as hypothyroidism, central nervous system (CNS) tumors, and head trauma. Girls usually show an increase in height of only 2 to 3 inches after the onset of menstruation.

Early menstrual cycles are often irregular and anovulatory (not preceded by ovulation and discharge of an ovum). Although menstrual cycles may not be regular for several years, the woman is still potentially fertile.

■ MENSTRUAL CYCLE

The menstrual cycle is a complex set of recurrent changes in the uterus, ovaries, cervix, and vagina. The cycle consists of:

- Proliferation
- Secretion
- Premenstrual phases

■ MENSTRUATION

Each phase is characterized by specific histologic changes in the endometrium. The length of the menstrual cycle is calculated from the first day of menstrual flow. The cycle generally runs about 25 to 32 days but can vary from month to month, even in the same woman.

The menstrual cycle depends on interactions between the CNS, anterior pituitary, ovaries, and uterus. Variations in the length of the proliferative phase (which ends with ovulation) typically cause a change in the length of the entire cycle. Environmental influences, climatic changes, emotionally traumatic experiences, stress, or acute or chronic illness also may affect the menstrual cycle.

Proliferative Phase

The proliferative phase of the menstrual cycle depends on the ratio of follicle-stimulating hormone (FSH) to LH. In the ovary, after menstrual flow has begun, primary follicles (containing oocytes, or primitive ova) and follicular cells begin to develop under the influence of FSH from the anterior pituitary gland (Fig. U8–3). The thecal (stromal) cells surrounding ova produce estrogens. The increased level of estrogen signals the pituitary to inhibit FSH production and to stimulate secretion of LH. Acting together, the two pituitary hormones then stimulate further estrogen production. Estrogens further inhibit FSH release from the anterior pituitary. LH becomes dominant, stimulating maturation of the follicle.

About 2 days before ovulation, a graafian follicle reaches full maturity and the remaining primary follicles degenerate. Ovulation occurs when the graafian follicle migrates to the ovary's cortex and ruptures through the ovary's wall.

In the uterus, meanwhile, related changes are occurring, largely in response to increased estrogen from the developing follicle. At the end of a menstrual flow, the uterine endometrium (containing surface epithelium, glands, connective tissue, spaces, and blood vessels) is very thin because much of it has sloughed off during menstrual flow. Estrogen stimulates creation of new endometrial surface layer and uterine epithelium. It stimulates growth of glands and stroma. The epithelium becomes thicker and more vascular. Endometrial proliferation peaks about 2 days before ovulation.

The cervix also undergoes changes. Most important, secretion of mucus, a clear fluid that is receptive to sperm, greatly increases just before ovulation. Vaginal changes during this phase include proliferation and thickening of the vaginal epithelium due to estrogen. This change is greatest at the time of ovulation.

Ovulation

Increased levels of estrogen cause a decrease in FSH secretion, allowing a flood of LH to occur. Over a 24-hour period, this process causes the thecal and granulosa cells lining the follicle to hypertrophy and proliferate.

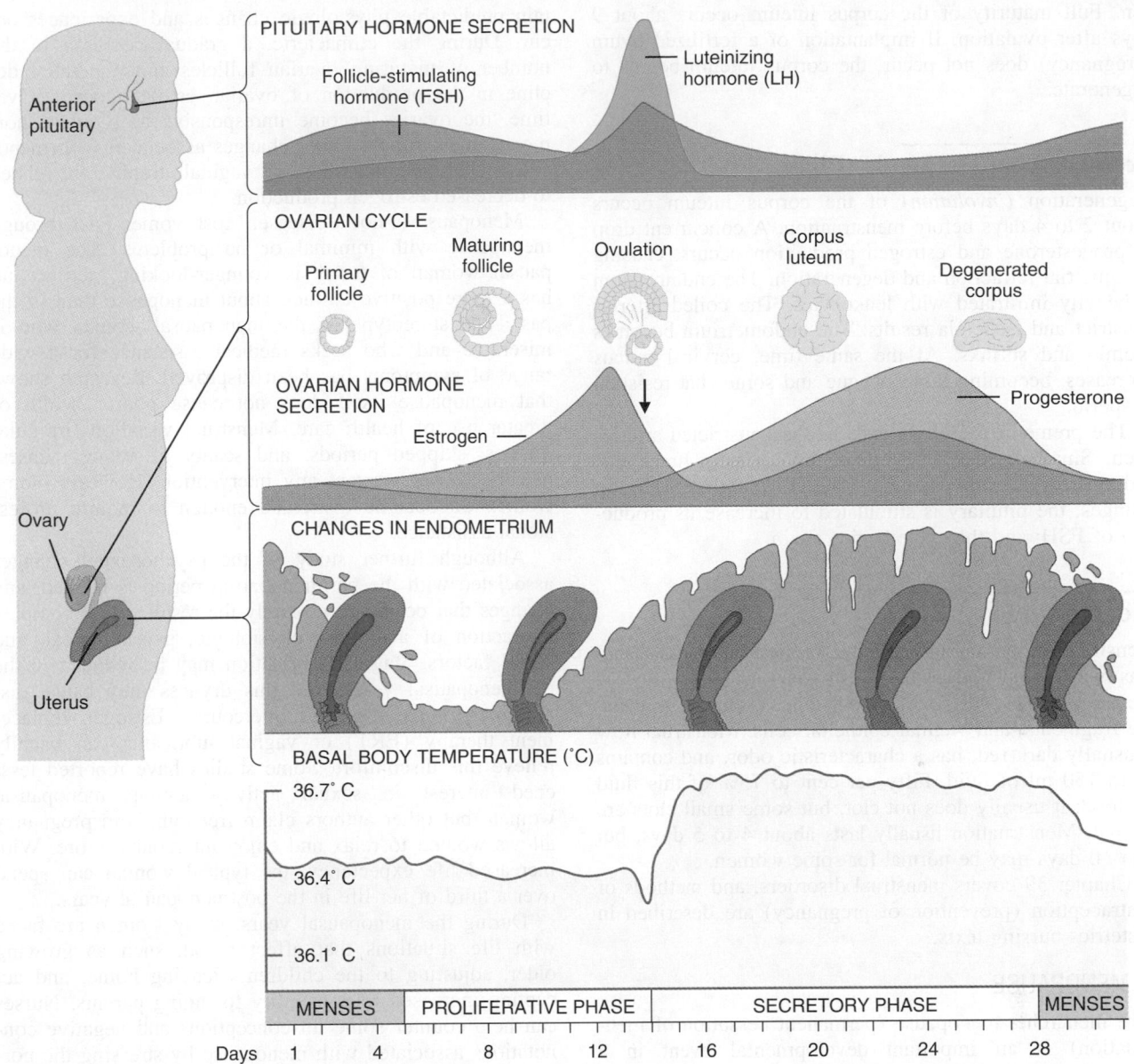

PITUITARY HORMONE SECRETION

Follicle-stimulating hormone (FSH)

Luteinizing hormone (LH)

OVARIAN CYCLE

Primary follicle

Maturing follicle

Ovulation

Corpus luteum

Degenerated corpus

OVARIAN HORMONE SECRETION

Estrogen

Progesterone

CHANGES IN ENDOMETRIUM

BASAL BODY TEMPERATURE (°C)

36.7° C

36.4° C

36.1° C

MENSES | PROLIFERATIVE PHASE | SECRETORY PHASE | MENSES

Days 1 4 8 12 16 20 24 28

Anterior pituitary

Ovary

Uterus

FIGURE U8–3 Menstrual (uterine) cycle. Note hormonal control of the menstrual cycle and the effects on ovaries *(center)* and endometrium *(bottom).*

When ovulation occurs, the ovarian follicle collapses and estrogen production temporarily drops.

At ovulation, the graafian follicle breaks through the ovary's wall and passes into the abdominal cavity. Some hemorrhage occurs into the center of the ruptured follicle, where a clot quickly forms. This may produce a transient abdominal pain *(mittelschmerz).*

Once in the abdominal cavity, the graafian follicle is usually picked up by the fimbriated ends of the fallopian tube and is slowly transported to the uterus. Unless it is fertilized, it eventually passes out of the body with the menstrual flow.

Ovulation occurs 12 to 15 days before the onset of the next menstrual period. It is almost impossible to determine exactly when ovulation will occur, even if one counted from the first day of the preceding menstrual period.

Secretory (Luteal) Phase

During the secretory phase (lasting 10 to 14 days), progesterone and estrogen promote marked changes in the endometrium. Connective tissue hypertrophies. The arteries coil and become tortuous. The glands become larger and more tortuous and abundantly secrete a substance containing glycogen. The endometrium becomes edematous, compact, and thickened. Development peaks 7 to 8 days after ovulation. This is the most favorable time for implantation of a fertilized ovum.

In the ovary after ovulation, the corpus luteum (yellow body) develops within the ruptured ovarian follicle. First, the clot that developed in response to follicular hemorrhage is replaced with yellowish luteal cells containing lipids. These cells eventually form the *corpus luteum,* an endocrine body that secretes progesterone and some estrogen. Full maturity of the corpus luteum occurs about 9 days after ovulation. If implantation of a fertilized ovum (pregnancy) does not occur, the corpus luteum begins to degenerate.

Premenstrual (Ischemic) Phase

Degeneration *(involution)* of the corpus luteum occurs about 2 to 4 days before menstruation. A concurrent drop in progesterone and estrogen production occurs, causing endometrial retraction and degeneration. The endometrium is heavily infiltrated with leukocytes. The coiled arteries constrict and ischemia results. The endometrium becomes anemic and shrinks. At the same time, cervical mucus decreases, becoming more opaque and somewhat resistant to sperm.

The premenstrual phase ends as the constricted arteries open. Small patches of necrotic endometrium break off, and menstrual flow begins. The LH and FSH ratio changes; the pituitary is stimulated to increase its production of FSH; and the cycle begins again.

Menstruation

Menstruation, commonly called a "period" or *menses,* begins with the withdrawal of estrogen and progesterone. Menstrual flow consists of blood, mucus, endometrial tissue fragments, and vaginal epithelial cells. Menstrual flow is usually dark red, has a characteristic odor, and contains 60 to 150 ml of fluid. Fifty per cent to 75% of this fluid is blood; it usually does not clot, but some small clots are normal. Menstruation usually lasts about 4 to 5 days, but 1 to 10 days may be normal for some women.

Chapter 39 covers menstrual disorders, and methods of contraception (prevention of pregnancy) are described in obstetrics nursing texts.

■ MENOPAUSE

Like menarche, menopause (permanent cessation of menstruation) is an important developmental event in a woman's life, having physical, psychological, and social implications for the woman. Menopause is one event of a complex biologic aging sequence of the *climacteric,* or *perimenopausal,* period. This period lasts about 15 to 20 years (ages 40 to 60); during this time, the body makes the transition from fertility to infertility. Menopause usually occurs between the ages of 48 and 54, but it may occur as early as age 35. The average age at menopause appears to be increasing in industrialized countries.

Menstrual cessation may be abrupt, but usually it occurs over 1 to 2 years. Periodic menstrual flow gradually lessens, occurs less frequently, and becomes irregular. Anovulatory cycles are common, and occasional episodes of profuse bleeding may be interspersed with episodes of scant bleeding. Menopause is said to have occurred when there have been no menstrual periods for 12 consecutive months. Because unplanned pregnancy may occur during the premenopausal period, sexually active women should use contraception for at least 6 months after menses have ceased. Any spontaneous uterine bleeding after menopause is abnormal and should be investigated.

Although the cause of menopause is not known, cer-

tain predictable physiologic changes and experiences occur. During the climacteric, a gradual decrease in the number of maturing ovarian follicles and a parallel decline in the production of ovarian estrogen occur. Over time, the ovaries become unresponsive to pituitary hormones and atrophy. Other changes associated with menopause, such as hot flashes and vaginal atrophy, are related to decreased estrogen production.

Menopause is not a disease. Most women pass through menopause with minimal or no problems. The menopausal woman of today is younger-looking, active, and has a more positive attitude about menopause than in the past. The stereotype of the menopausal woman who is miserable and who seeks medical assistance for a wide range of symptoms has been disproved. Research shows that menopause itself does not cause poorer health or greater use of health care. Menstrual variation (irregular menses, skipped periods, and scanty or heavy menses) usually do not warrant any intervention. However, some women do become distressed enough to require professional assistance.

Although further study of the psychosexual changes associated with the perimenopausal period is needed, any changes that occur are probably the result of the complex interaction of anatomic, physiologic, psychological, and social factors. Vaginal lubrication may be reduced in the perimenopausal years, and this dryness may cause discomfort or bleeding with intercourse. Estrogen replacement therapy (ERT) or vaginal lubricants can usually relieve this discomfort. Some studies have reported lessened interest in sexual activity among menopausal women, but other authors claim freedom from pregnancy allows women to relax and enjoy intercourse more. With increased life expectancy, the typical woman can spend over a third of her life in the postmenopausal years.

During the menopausal years, many women are faced with life situations that affect mood, such as growing older, adjusting to the children's leaving home, and accepting increased responsibility for aging parents. Nurses can help counter some misconceptions and negative connotations associated with menopause by stressing the normal and positive aspects of the experience, clarifying misconceptions about menopause, and differentiating the physiologic manifestations of menopause from midlife developmental changes.

MALE REPRODUCTIVE SYSTEM

STRUCTURES

The male reproductive organs consist of paired *testicles,* lying within the scrotum; epididymides; seminal ducts; spermatic cords; seminal vesicles; ejaculatory ducts; bulbourethral (Cowper's) glands; the prostate gland; and the penis (Table U8–2 and Fig. U8–4). The penis and scrotum are external, visible genitalia, whereas the other structures are internal. The male perineum is the external area between the scrotum and the anus.

■ PENIS AND RELATED STRUCTURES

The *penis* is both a sexual organ (organ of copulation) and an organ for urination. This cylindrical, pendulous

TABLE U8–2	MALE REPRODUCTIVE STRUCTURES AND THEIR FUNCTIONS	
Structure	**Description**	**Function**
Penis	Erectile tissue arranged in three columns, each enclosed in a fascial sheath (tunica albuginea): two lateral columns (corpora cavernosa) and a median column (corpus spongiosum) that contains the urethra. All are surrounded by a thick, fibrous envelope (Buck's fascia)	Ejects semen for fertilization; excretes urine
Bulbourethral (Cowper's) glands	Two small glands above the corpus spongiosum; homologous to Bartholin's glands	Enhances lubrication during intercourse
Scrotum	Double pouch of muscular contractile tissue between the root of the penis and the perineum. It is bisected by a ridge. Each half contains a testicle and epididymis, and part of a spermatic cord made up of nerves, testicular vessels (spermatic artery, vein, lymph vessels), and vas deferens	Provides protective environment for production of sperm
Testicles	Two smooth, solid, ovoid structures (4 cm × 2 to 2.5 cm) with outer coat of inelastic fibrous tunica albuginea. Lobules in testicles contain tubules composed of germ cells (develop into sperm) and Sertoli cells (support spermatogenesis). Between the tubules are Leydig cells (source of testosterone)	Produce testosterone and sperm
Sperm	Germ cell with flattened, broad, oval head with a nucleus, protoplasmic middle piece or neck, and a hair-like tail (flagellum); has 23 chromosomes	Fertilizes ovum
Epididymis	Small oblong structure consisting of a convoluted tube 3.96 to 6.1 m long; attaches to upper end of testicle	Transports sperm
Vas deferens	Smooth muscle tube about 46 cm long	Stores and transmits sperm from testicles
Prostate gland	Partly muscular, partly glandular structure posterior to the symphysis pubis; urethra and ejaculatory ducts pass through it	Contributes to liquefaction of semen
Seminal vesicles	Two sac-like structures 5 cm long; they connect to the vas deferens	Secretions contribute to sperm nutrition and activation

structure suspends from its attachment to the pubic arch. The skin of the penis is dark, hairless, thin, and loose (permitting considerable distention).

The portion of the penis between its end or head and its attachment to the pubic bone is the *shaft*. In males, the urethra's external opening *(meatus or orifice)* is in the glans *(glans penis)*, the cone-shaped end or head of the penis. The glans is the conical expansion of the corpus spongiosum. The expanded posterior border of the glans is the *corona*. At its junction with the shaft is the *coronal sulcus*. A flap of movable skin *(foreskin or prepuce)* covers the glans. *Smegma* is a cheesy, thick, odoriferous secretion of sloughed-off epithelial cells that collects under the prepuce. (In females, smegma is the secretion of the apocrine glands of the clitoris together with epithelial cells.)

The penis is homologous to the female clitoris. Usually, the penis is flaccid, but, when stimulated (physically or during sexual excitement), it becomes rigid. An *erection* occurs when the corpora cavernosa fill with blood.

The tissue becomes congested (hyperemic) with blood. Following *orgasm* (climax of sexual excitement) and *ejaculation* (emission of semen), the blood leaves. An erect penis may differ in size from a flaccid penis. Penis size, however, does not physically influence sexual pleasure. The secretion of the *bulbourethral (Cowper's) glands* forms part of the semen.

SCROTUM AND TESTES

The *scrotum* is a double pouch hanging from the root of the penis. It is separated into halves internally by muscular contractile tissue *(tunica dartos)* and externally by a *raphe* (ridge) that runs over the scrotum from the root of the penis to the anus. Each half of the scrotum contains (1) a testicle with its epididymis and (2) part of a spermatic cord held together by spermatic fascia.

The *vas deferens (ductus deferens, seminal duct)* is the testicle's excretory duct. It is the continuation of the epididymis and it conveys sperm from the testicle to the prostatic urethra (from the epididymis to the ejaculatory

FIGURE U8–4 Midsagittal section of the male pelvis and external genitalia.

duct). The *ejaculatory duct* then conveys semen to the urethra.

The *spermatic cord* goes through the inguinal canal, and the vas deferens continues into the abdominal cavity. It passes behind the bladder, anterior to the rectum, to join the duct of the seminal vesicle, becoming the ejaculatory duct. The spermatic cord is movable for protection from trauma and facilitates optimal production of mature, functional sperm.

Testicles produce the male hormone *(testosterone)* and the male reproductive cells *(sperm).* Many lobules, separated by septa, divide a testicle. Each lobule contains one to three seminiferous tubules where sperm are produced. There are 600 to 1200 seminiferous tubules (90% of the mature testis) in each testicle. Between the seminiferous tubules are interstitial cells called *Leydig cells,* the source of testosterone, the male hormone. The lobules of the testicles lead to straight ducts that join a plexus, from which efferent ducts lead to the epididymis.

The *epididymis* rests on and beside the posterior surface of the testicle. Its head caps the upper end of the testicle and its tail becomes continuous with the vas deferens, which joins other vessels to form the spermatic cord. The head of the epididymis contains 12 to 20 testicular efferent ducts.

■ **SPERM**

Sperm are mature male sex or germ cells that develop after puberty. Resembling tadpoles, sperm propel them-

selves by hair-like tails like *flagella.* A normal sperm has a flattened, broad, oval head with a nucleus. A middle piece or protoplasmic neck connects to the tail. During fertilization, the sperm's head pierces an ovum. The sperm's tail is lost when fusion of two cells occurs. Sperm are produced in the seminiferous tubules of the testicles. Sperm develop in great quantities from spermatids (spermoblasts) and are stored in the vas deferens.

■ **PROSTATE GLAND AND RELATED STRUCTURES**

The prostate gland surrounds the neck of the male urinary bladder and urethra. In childhood the prostate is small, but during puberty it grows to the size of a chestnut. The adult prostate gland lies like a flattened cone in the pelvis, about 2 cm posterior to the symphysis pubis. In a normal adult man, the prostate weighs 15 to 20 g and is 4 to 6 cm long. The prostate is inverted, so that its apex is inferior, and it is suspended by the urogenital diaphragm. The base of the prostate is superior and at the bladder neck, anterior to the rectum. A firm fibrous capsule, containing smooth muscle fibers in its inner layer, encloses the prostate. The bladder overlies the prostate's basal surface.

The posterior surface of the prostate is in close contact with the rectal wall. This is the surface of the prostate that is available for digital examination.

The portion of the urethra that passes through the prostate is called the *prostatic urethra.* Prostatic muscle fibers encircle the urethra and separate the prostate's glandular tissue.

The *seminal vesicles* are sac-like structures whose secretion, a component of *semen* (seminal fluid, or ejaculate), may contribute to sperm nutrition and activation. They lie behind the bladder and connect to the vas deferens on each side.

MALE SEXUAL DEVELOPMENT AND FUNCTION

Development of the male genitalia requires two hormones: (1) müllerian duct inhibitory factor, secreted by *Sertoli cells,* and (2) testosterone, secreted by Leydig cells (see gonadal development earlier). Germ cells develop into spermatozoa, and Sertoli cells support spermatogenesis.

The hypothalamus and pituitary gland regulate testicular function. The hypothalamus secretes gonadotropin-releasing hormone (GnRH) in a pulsatile fashion. GnRH stimulates the anterior pituitary gland to produce LH and FSH. LH stimulates Leydig cells to produce testosterone, which modulates the secretion of GnRH and therefore LH through negative feedback to the hypothalamus and pituitary gland. FSH and testosterone stimulate Sertoli cells and germ cells to start and complete spermatogenesis. *Inhibin,* released from Sertoli cells, provides a negative feedback on FSH release by the anterior pituitary.

Testosterone is the primary androgen secreted by the testis. The testis also secretes androstenedione and estradiol. Estradiol may be important for skeletal maturation in the male.

■ SPERMATOGENESIS

Spermatogenesis is the process of sperm production and development that occurs within the seminiferous tubules during active sex life. It begins at puberty as a result of stimulation by the gonadotropic hormones from the anterior pituitary.

Spermatogonia are the germinal epithelial cells found in the outer border of the tubular epithelium. These cells are continually formed to replenish themselves while a portion continue to develop into sperm. During the first stage of spermatogenesis, the spermatogonia divide and migrate toward the Sertoli cells. The spermatogonia penetrate the membranes of Sertoli cells and become enveloped within the cytoplasm of these cells. The spermatogonia continue this close relationship with Sertoli cells throughout their development.

During the 24 days when it is in contact with Sertoli cells, the spermatogonium changes and enlarges to form a primary *spermatocyte.* After this development, the spermatocyte splits into two secondary spermatocytes, each with only 23 chromosomes. After 2 to 3 days, the spermatocytes undergo a second division to form four *spermatids,* again with 23 chromosomes. The sperm that eventually fertilizes the female ovum contains half the genetic material; the ovum contains the other half.

The period of spermatogenesis from germinal cell to sperm takes about 74 days. During this time, the spermatocytes lose some cytoplasm, the chromatin material of the head reorganizes to form a compact head, and the remaining cytoplasm and cell membranes collect at one end of the cell to form the tail of the sperm.

■ ROLE OF HORMONES

Testosterone is essential to the growth and division of the germinal cells that form the sperm. LH stimulates Leydig cells to secrete testosterone. FSH stimulates Sertoli cells to promote spermatogenesis. Estrogens, formed from testosterone when Sertoli cells are stimulated by FSH, appear to be essential in spermatogenesis. Growth hormone (GH) promotes early division of spermatogonia.

■ MATURATION IN THE EPIDIDYMIS

After the sperm are formed in the seminiferous tubules, they spend several days passing through the epididymis. After about 24 hours in the epididymis, they become motile and capable of fertilization (i.e., they are mature).

Sperm are stored in small amounts in the epididymis but are mainly stored in the vas deferens and the ampulla of the vas deferens. With low levels of sexual activity, the sperm can be stored there up to a month, maintaining their motility and fertility. When sexual activity is frequent, sperm may be stored only a few days.

■ PROSTATIC FLUID

The prostate gland secretes a milky fluid that forms part of the semen. This fluid aids the passage of sperm and helps keep them alive, supplying them with food, if needed. Prostatic secretion is manufactured in a network of branching glands embedded in muscle within the prostate. This muscle contracts during ejaculation, and prostatic secretions are ejected through the ejaculatory ducts into the urethra.

■ SEMEN

Semen is a viscid, thick, opalescent secretion discharged by males through the urethra at the climax of sexual excitement or orgasm. It contains sperm and other secretions. About 10% of the semen is composed of sperm and fluid from the vas deferens, with about 60% made up of fluid from the seminal vesicles. The remaining 30% is composed of prostatic fluid and small amounts of mucoid secretion from the bulbourethral glands.

Semen is slightly alkaline, with a pH of about 7.5. The prostatic fluid contains a clotting enzyme, causing the fibrinogen of the seminal vesicle fluid to form a weak coagulum. This coagulum holds the semen near the uterine cervix. The coagulum dissolves in about 15 to 30 minutes, at which time the sperm become highly motile. The sperm can live within the vagina for 24 to 48 hours after ejaculation.

CONCLUSIONS

The human reproductive system is tremendously complex, and reproductive and sexual characteristics can have a great physical and emotional impact on our lives from conception. Changes initiated at the fetal stage cause differentiation between male and female. Sexual maturation, starting between the ages of 9 and 13 years, alters both external and internal structures. A thorough knowledge of the structure and function of the female and male reproductive systems is important so that the nurse will be able to provide safe, effective care for clients with associated problems. The nurse must be sensitive to the delicate nature of reproductive problems because many disorders affect sexuality.

BIBLIOGRAPHY

1. Fauci, A. S., et al. (1998). *Harrison's principles of internal medicine* (14th ed.). New York: McGraw-Hill.
2. Guyton, A. C., & Hall, J. E. (1996). *Textbook of medical physiology* (9th ed.). Philadelphia: W. B. Saunders.
3. Silverthorn, D. (1998). *Human physiology.* Upper Saddle River, NJ: Prentice Hall.

37

Assessment of the Reproductive System

Rhonda Holloway

Your ability to assess the reproductive system competently and compassionately is important to your clients on both physical and psychosocial levels. To perform this task well, you will need a combination of sound assessment skills and a nonjudgmental attitude that is both professional and empathic.

Because of the close association between the reproductive, urinary, and bowel elimination systems, you must be prepared for some overlap in their assessment (see also Chapter 32.) You also must be prepared for some difficulty in discussing reproductive and elimination topics. Many clients are uncomfortable talking about them. Language and semantic barriers may interfere with communication as well, in part because of the many words and slang terms used to describe reproductive anatomy, function, and problems. Educational or cultural barriers also can inhibit a client from discussing a problem. Remain sensitive and nonjudgmental, and do your best to put the client at ease.

Clients have the right to be informed and to actively participate in decisions about their health. A supportive, respectful attitude on your part promotes comfort, cooperation, and participation in health care. Be alert to sexist attitudes in yourself and the health care system, either of which may lead to ignored health complaints, unnecessary or inappropriate prescriptions, and unneeded procedures. Be an advocate, and positively influence the client's perception of health care and the importance of health maintenance.

Especially when assessing the reproductive system, provide privacy and create an environment conducive to the expression of feelings. Encourage the client to voice concerns and ask questions. Assess the client's understanding of health care information, and explore what the client perceives as needs and problems. You may need to repeat information, especially if the client is anxious or feeling stressed, for example, during a pelvic or prostate examination. Provide a sensitive, humane orientation to reproductive health care. Teaching and counseling promote health maintenance.

Besides providing a history and physical examination, an adequate reproductive assessment should include an in-depth review of the client's lifestyle, health habits, self-perception, body image, and developmental stage along with cultural, religious, socioeconomic, and educational factors. These factors influence the client's health and health-seeking behaviors. Throughout your assessment, you will find that a respect for others' values facilitates effective care. Cultural or ethnic background, socioeconomic status, and sexual preference should never limit a client's access to, or quality of, health care.

THE FEMALE REPRODUCTIVE SYSTEM

Many women receive most, if not all, of their primary health care from obstetric and gynecologic health care providers—not only for gynecologic conditions but also for general health. An annual gynecologic examination provides opportunity to discuss health maintenance activities. For example, during a client's health visit for a Papanicolaou (Pap) smear, take the opportunity to teach breast self-examination and discuss risk factors associated with gynecologic cancer and heart disease. Explain developmental changes (e.g., adolescence, menarche, or menopause) and menstrual hygiene and symptom management. Discuss lifestyle factors that affect health maintenance, such as diet, exercise, adequate sleep and rest, stress management, cessation of smoking, and general risk factor identification. If appropriate, provide information about protection against sexually transmitted diseases (STDs).

After establishing rapport, perform a comprehensive gynecologic nursing assessment appropriate to the situation. (For a review of a comprehensive history and psychosocial assessment, see Chapter 9). Follow the health history with a systematic physical examination. Diagnostic tests may be ordered, some of which you will perform. The resulting data are the basis for nursing intervention.

HISTORY

The health history for the female reproductive system includes data related to the genitals, the reproductive system, the breasts, and the woman's overall health status. Conduct the interview in private while the woman is clothed to maintain her level of comfort.

■ BIOGRAPHICAL AND DEMOGRAPHIC DATA

Biographical and demographic data can help to establish the client's health risk status. The incidence of some gynecologic cancers is higher in certain age groups. For example, the risk of breast cancer rises with age. Ethnicity may also be a risk factor for certain gynecologic cancers, such as cancer of the cervix. Because controversy exists about the influence of environmental factors in the development of reproductive disorders, the client's living and working environments may prove to be important.

■ CURRENT HEALTH: THE CHIEF COMPLAINT

Ask the client to describe her reason for seeking gynecologic care. Be alert to the possible nature of the problem as well as to the level of the woman's understanding of the problem. This information will direct the health history interview and your health teaching. If the client's visit is for a specific problem rather than for a routine examination, ask her to relate the history of the problem and conduct a symptom analysis (see Chapter 9).

■ PAST HEALTH HISTORY

To investigate the client's past health history, review her childhood and infectious illnesses, major illnesses and hospitalizations, medications, and allergies.

Childhood and Infectious Diseases

The most serious childhood infectious illness that may affect a woman of childbearing age is *rubella*. Maternal rubella during the first trimester increases fetal risk for congenital disorders. Ask the client if she has had rubella or has immunity to it. If she is contemplating pregnancy, suggest that a rubella titer be drawn to determine her immunity status. If the titer is negative, indicating that immunity is lacking, encourage the woman to be vaccinated. Advise the newly immunized woman to avoid pregnancy for at least 3 months. A pregnant woman should not be vaccinated.

Ask the client about her history of STDs and STD exposure. Many of these diseases, left unrecognized or untreated, can damage the reproductive system, particularly the fallopian tubes. The result may be problems with fertility and achieving pregnancy.

Major Illnesses and Hospitalizations

Ask about major illnesses. For instance, diabetes is associated with increased maternal and fetal morbidity and mortality. Pregnancy and oral contraceptive use are also linked with higher morbidity and mortality rates in women who have a history of cardiovascular disease, such as angina, hypertension, and thrombophlebitis. Anemia can result from menstrual disorders, such as dysfunctional uterine bleeding. Hypothyroidism and hyperthyroidism can affect the menstrual cycle, as can other endocrine disorders.

Urinary tract disorders can interfere with sexual function. Women who have migraine headaches or seizure disorders may need to avoid oral contraceptives because of the increased risk of migraines and seizures associated with their use. Oral contraceptives, pregnancy, dietary changes, or a high-fat diet may worsen cholecystitis. Hepatitis and other liver disorders contraindicate estrogen use because of its route of metabolism. Estrogens are usually contraindicated in women who have had breast cancer or cancers of the reproductive tract.

Ask about surgery involving the reproductive system. Specific surgical procedures include dilation and curettage (D&C), tubal ligation, cryosurgery or cryotherapy, cystocele and rectocele repair, hysterectomy, oophorectomy, salpingectomy and salpingotomy. Inquire about interrupted pregnancies, including both elective and spontaneous abortions.

Medications

Collect a complete medication history, including prescription and over-the-counter medications, vitamin and mineral supplements, and recreational or illegal substances. Contraceptive medications can include oral contraceptive pills, medroxyprogesterone injections, and vaginal preparations. Ask about episodic medications, such as those used for premenstrual syndrome (PMS) and menstrual discomforts (e.g., diuretics), and the use of herbal or other "natural" substances. These may include:

- Black cohosh (*Cimicifuga racemosa*) for menstrual irregularity, PMS, and menopausal problems
- Chamomile (*Martricaria recutita, Chamaemelum nobile*) for menstrual cramps
- Chaste tree (*Vitex agnuscastus*) for PMS and menopausal problems and possibly for mastalgia
- Evening primrose (*Oenothera biennis*) for PMS
- Feverfew (*Tanacetum parthenium*) for menstrual problems
- Sage (*Salvia officinalis*) for menstrual irregularity
- Soybeans and other legumes for their phytoestrogens that may help prevent breast cancer

Ask specifically about hormone replacement therapy (including estrogen, progesterone, thyroid hormones, and corticosteroids). Recreational or illegal substances, such as alcohol, amphetamines, barbiturates, marijuana, and hallucinogens, may affect sexual behavior and risk status for exposure to an STD, among other problems.

Allergies

Ask the client about all allergies, including allergic reactions. Antibiotics are used to treat genitourinary infections. Latex and rubber are used in contraceptive devices such as condoms, cervical caps, and diaphragms, some of which are used in conjunction with spermicides. Some intrauterine contraceptive devices contain copper. Allergies to these substances eliminate their use for contraception. Use vinyl gloves instead of latex while examining the client, if necessary.

■ GYNECOLOGIC HISTORY

A gynecologic history includes questions about breasts, menstruation, contraceptives, sexual practices, obstetric problems, genitourinary problems, and reproductive health practices. For a menopausal or older woman or a woman who has had a hysterectomy, ask only the appropriate questions.

Breast History

Ask the client about breast pain or tenderness and its occurrence in relation to the menstrual cycle. Many women experience breast tenderness before menstruation in relation to hormonal changes. Ask whether the woman has had or currently has breast lumps or masses. If a lump is present, ask the woman to describe its location, onset, and size and whether it is painful. Determine whether the lump has changed shape, size, consistency, or degree of tenderness since it was first noticed. Does the lump change during the menstrual cycle? Because the breasts become more firm and cystic during the luteal phase, the best time to perform breast palpation is 7 to 10 days after onset of menses.

Ask about any nipple discharge, which would be abnormal in women who are not pregnant or lactating. If discharge is present, determine the color, consistency, amount, and odor.

Ask whether the woman performs a monthly breast self-examination (BSE). Ask about frequency of examination and the technique used so that you can decide whether the client needs a review of the procedure and supervised practice. Note whether the woman includes the axillary nodes in the BSE (see Chapter 2.)

Finally, ask whether there is a history of breast cancer in the client's blood-related female relatives, including mother, sisters, maternal grandmother, or maternal aunts. Breast cancer in these relatives indicates an increased risk of breast cancer for the client.

Menstrual History

Ask the woman at what age she started menstruating. Determine the first day of her last menstrual period. Ask the number of days per cycle and the regularity of cycles. Assessing the amount of menstrual flow is difficult. Knowing whether more than one pad or tampon per hour becomes saturated helps to determine whether the flow is unusually profuse. Are there clots in the flow? How long does the menstrual period last?

Does the woman experience pain during menstruation? If so, have her describe the pain, its duration, whether it occurs with every cycle, and what she uses for relief. Does she experience midcycle bleeding, spotting, or pain. Are there any moliminal (premenstrual discomfort) manifestations? Are there any menopausal manifestations, including menstrual cycle changes?

Contraceptive History

Document the current contraceptive method (if any), satisfaction with the method, duration of use, any contraceptive problems, and any desire to change methods. Ask about previous contraceptive methods, problems encountered, and reason for discontinuation. Provide contraceptive information if appropriate. For a woman of reproductive age who is not sterilized and who is heterosexually active, determine whether she wants to become pregnant.

Sexual History

Obtain a sexual history using a direct approach and terms the woman understands. The purpose of a sexual history is to identify sexual problems and to give the woman an opportunity to ask questions or express concerns (Table 37–1). To help put the client at ease, explain why you are asking for this information and assure her that it will be kept confidential.

Begin with general questions about whether the woman is satisfied and comfortable with her current sexual activity. A nonjudgmental approach is essential; make no assumptions about anything, including the sex or number of partners. Follow up on any concerns or issues she raises. Of particular importance are difficulties or concerns she may have. Be alert for any risk-taking behaviors, including those that put her at risk of STDs. See Chapter 9 for further information on sexuality assessment.

Obstetric History

If the woman is in her childbearing years, ask if she thinks she may be pregnant. (Pregnancy may contraindicate mammography or other radiologic studies as well as certain medications.) If the woman has been pregnant, obtain information about each pregnancy, including the delivery and postpartum period. Document details of any difficulties or complications (physical or psychosocial). Record any spontaneous or planned abortions. If the woman has never been pregnant, ask whether children were or are desired. If the woman has relinquished a child for adoption, explore the circumstance and her feelings about it. See Chapter 9 for detailed questions to assess the obstetric history.

Genitourinary History

Ask about previous problems with genitourinary infections and vaginitis. Determine whether the woman has had a previous pelvic infection or STD, treatment, or complications. Determine whether the woman experiences urinary or fecal incontinence and the circumstances surrounding the incontinence. (Chapter 34 discusses urinary incontinence, and Chapter 33 discusses fecal incontinence.)

Reproductive Health Practices

Seek information about menstrual, sexual, and gynecologic hygiene, including douching. Ask about the frequency of gynecologic examinations. If appropriate, ask the client whether she uses protection against STDs and unwanted pregnancy.

■ FAMILY HEALTH HISTORY

A family history of diabetes, cardiovascular disease, or cancer of a reproductive organ may indicate a higher risk for development of those diseases. If the woman's mother received diethylstilbestrol (DES) while pregnant with the client, the woman may be at risk for reproductive tract cancer or structural and functional abnormalities.

■ PSYCHOSOCIAL HISTORY

Occupation and Environment

Ask the woman about any exposures to hazards encountered at work, including toxins or radiation. Many sub-

TABLE 37-1	**SEXUAL HEALTH ASSESSMENT**

Sexual health assessment may include consideration of the client's current

  Knowledge about sexuality
  Attitudes about sexuality and toward sexual partner(s)
  Level of comfort and feelings of adequacy regarding own sexuality
  Concerns about sexuality of significant others
  Perception of own sex role and that of sexual partner(s)
  Sexual self-concept as a female or male
  Fears and anxiety about intimacy and other aspects of sexuality
  Self-perception of own body (body image)
  Ability to function sexually (e.g., to obtain an erection and control ejaculation, to please sexual partner, to achieve pain-free
    orgasm, to reproduce, to obtain adequate contraception, to obtain sufficient vaginal lubrication, to give and receive effective
    sexual stimulation and pleasure)
  Typical sexual patterns and activities (e.g., partner choice [female, male, spouse, extramarital, multiple, single, same partner,
    different partners], frequency of sexual activity, type of sexual activity [vaginal, anal, oral, masturbation], partner satisfaction,
    self-satisfaction)
  Level of interest in sexual activity (sex drive)
  Level of satisfaction regarding current sexual opportunity and activity
  Physical health problems affecting sexuality (e.g., menstrual problems, pregnancy, medication, surgery [colostomy, surgical
    amputation, recent heart surgery or brain surgery], paralysis, illness [hypertension, diabetes, recent myocardial infarction,
    cerebral vascular accident, injury [recent spinal cord injury, recent head injury, burns, traumatic amputations], sexually
    transmitted disease, genitourinary problems)

Sexual History

There is no single approach to taking a sexual health history. Information obtained may relate to historical (past) information
  about the following:

BOTH FEMALES AND MALES
  Pregnancies (information about unplanned pregnancies)
  Fertility management
  Genitourinary problems
  Sexually transmitted disease
  Sexual abuse (e.g., incest, rape, pedophilia, battering)
  Relationship-partner history (e.g., number of sexual partners, sexual orientation [bisexual, homosexual, heterosexual])
  First experience of sexual activity
  Early sexual development and influences
  Adolescent sexual experiences
  Sexual techniques used (e.g., masturbation, intercourse ([oral, vaginal, anal])
  Role models for sexuality (e.g., peers, parents, guardians, famous people, advertising models)
  Spiritual-philosophical models influencing the client's sexuality

FEMALES
  History specific to menstruation, abortion, pregnancy

MALES
  History specific to impotence, nocturnal emissions

stances can affect overall health status generally and reproductive function specifically.

Habits

Ask whether the client smokes cigarettes. Smoking is associated with an increase in morbidity, especially when used in conjunction with oral contraceptives, and also may be related to an earlier than normal onset of menopause. Note the use of alcohol and recreational drugs, habits that increase risk of acquiring STDs.

Domestic Violence

In private, ascertain whether the woman is a victim of domestic violence. Ask every client about violence in her life. Explain that the same question is asked of all women

and that she is not being singled out. (She might assume that you ask the question because of her race, nationality, or socioeconomic status.) Clients frequently deny domestic violence many times before acknowledging it; consequently, repeated questioning in a variety of ways may help determine whether the client is a victim. Be alert to physical and behavioral manifestations that are inconsistent with the explanation of their cause. Also be aware of an overprotective significant other. This is also a good time to educate women about options available should violence be or become a problem.

Psychosocial Factors

Because the genital organs and their reproductive capacity have symbolic significance for many women, problems in this area can affect a woman's sexuality and sense of femininity. Gynecologic problems may be associated with changes in self-concept, body image, personal identity, and role performance. Reproductive capabilities, the expression of sexuality, and sexual activities may be affected. In short, gynecologic disorders may result in psychological consequences. For this reason, psychological assessment is especially important. A woman's outward reaction to gynecologic problems does not necessarily correspond with either her inner experience or the seriousness of the condition.

Be sensitive when interviewing and examining a woman. Do not insist on information that she is hesitant to reveal. The woman herself may not understand her responses. Empathic listening is supportive and may lessen the stress the woman feels.

The woman may express fear because of a suspected unhealthy change in the genitals or of unwanted pregnancy. She may feel anxious and embarrassed before undergoing a pelvic examination. Many women consider the pelvic examination unpleasant despite its minimal risk of injury or physical pain. Other feelings that may be expressed include humiliation, guilt, or anger. Deep, powerful feelings may prevent women from seeking gynecologic care. Intrusive gynecologic procedures may evoke memories or strong reactions in women who have experienced sexual abuse or assault. The opportunity to express and discuss feelings with a nurse skilled in therapeutic communication may help these women cope more effectively and follow through with appropriate care. A therapeutic conversation can provide opportunities for clarifying a woman's misconceptions about her diagnosis, proposed treatment, and preventive care. Many women have never received accurate information about reproductive problems.

■ REVIEW OF SYSTEMS

Review the client's physical health history, proceeding from head to toe. Note especially (1) cardiovascular disorders (hypertension, angina [pain], myocardial infarction [MI], thrombophlebitis), (2) endocrine disorders (hypothyroidism, hyperthyroidism), (3) disorders of the pituitary gland, (4) liver disorders, and (5) cholecystitis. Ask about problems involving the urinary tract and reproductive system, such as urinary tract infection, urinary incontinence, vaginitis, and any bleeding disorders associated with menstruation (e.g., amenorrhea, dysmenorrhea, breakthrough bleeding, menorrhagia, or postcoital bleeding). Detailed questions for the review of systems are found in Chapter 9.

PHYSICAL EXAMINATION

Elements of a standard gynecologic examination can vary slightly but usually include the following physical assessment and laboratory data:

- Vital signs (temperature, pulse, respiration, blood pressure)
- Height
- Weight
- Hematocrit (or complete blood count)
- Urinalysis
- Pelvic examination and Pap smear

- Physical assessment of skin, heart, lungs, breasts and axillae, thyroid, and abdomen
- Periodically, lipid profile and thyroid-stimulating hormone (TSH) level
- As appropriate for age and history, colorectal sigmoidoscopy, fecal occult blood testing, and mammography

If unusual or abnormal findings are obtained during the gynecologic history or physical examination, additional data must be sought.

■ BREASTS AND AXILLAE

Examination of the breasts and axillae is an important part of the gynecologic examination. Good lighting is essential. Some examiners complete this portion of the examination before assessing the anterior lungs and heart. Because the breasts are sensitive and closely associated with sexuality, some examiners delay this portion until there has been more hands-on interaction with the client during assessment of the lungs and heart. Others integrate assessments so that the client is sitting for those portions of the heart, lungs, breasts, and axillae examination before being helped to a supine position for the remaining portions. Any sequence is acceptable as long as you are thorough, you maintain the client's privacy, and the client can tolerate the position changes. Instruct the client in BSE while examining the breasts. (See Chapter 2.)

Ask the client when her last menstrual period began. Breasts are usually tender the week before onset of menses and least tender the week after menses has ceased. If the client reports that one breast is tender, begin palpation with the opposite breast. Thorough examination requires exposure of both breasts for comparison.

Inspection

Begin breast inspection while the client is seated with her arms at her sides. Ask her to raise her hands over her head. Finally, ask her to press her hands firmly on her hips or together to tighten the pectoral muscles. Examine women who have large or pendulous breasts while they bend at the waist and face forward with the breast hanging down (Fig. 37–1). In all positions, inspect the breasts for symmetry, size, shape, contour, and skin characteristics, including the vascular pattern.

Breasts are symmetrical, although it is not unusual for one breast to be slightly larger than the other. The breasts should hang evenly between the third and fourth ribs with the nipples about level with the fourth intercostal space when the client sits with her arms at her sides. With aging and loss of tissue elasticity, the breasts hang lower, especially after pregnancy and breast-feeding. The contour is even. Dimpling (retraction), masses, or surface flattening are abnormal. Skin color is the same as that of the abdomen. *Striae* (stretch marks from rapid skin stretching) may be present; recent striae are reddened and become paler with time. Venous patterns, if noticeable, should be symmetrical. Local areas of hyperpigmentation or edema should be absent.

Ask the client to raise her arms over her head while you examine the lateral and undersurfaces of each breast. Contraction of the pectoral muscles exaggerates signs of retraction or skin flattening. Note areas of redness or excoriation from poorly fitting brassieres. The breasts

FIGURE 37-1 Positions for breast examination. *A,* Arms at side. *B,* Hands raised over head. For tightening pectoral muscles, the examiner asks the client to press hands firmly on hips (*C*) or to press hands together (*D*). *E,* Breasts may also be examined with the woman leaning forward at the waist, allowing the breasts to hang down.

should elevate evenly so that the areolae remain at the same level. Then ask the client to put her hands on her hips and press inward firmly while you repeat the inspection for masses, retraction, or skin flattening.

Inspect the areolae and nipples for size, shape, contour, symmetry, surface characteristics, and masses or lesions. Areolae are pink in fair-skinned women and darker in dark-skinned women. Slight asymmetry is common, but the nipples should point in symmetrical directions. Masses or lesions are abnormal. Montgomery's tubercles may be prominent around the nipple, which is normal. The nipples are round or oval, equal in size, of the same color, soft, and smooth. If one or both nipples are inverted, ask whether this is a recent occurrence or has been present for a while and how long. Recent nipple inversion is abnormal, and the client should be referred to an appropriate health care provider for follow-up. Rashes, crusts, or discharge should be absent unless the client is in the late stages of pregnancy, when colostrum (a yellowish fluid) may leak from the nipples.

Inspect the axillae for rashes, masses, and areas of unusual pigmentation, which should be absent. Axillary hair should be present unless the client removes it.

Palpation

Palpation of axillae is usually done while the client is seated; breast palpation is facilitated with the client supine. For clients who have large and pendulous breasts or

a history of breast masses or cancer or who are at increased risk for breast cancer, the breasts should be palpated in both positions.

Palpation of the axillae includes examination of five sets of lymph nodes (Fig. 37-2). Encourage the client to relax her arm; this relaxes the chest muscles and eases palpation. Begin by palpating the edge of the pectoralis major muscle along the anterior axillary line, using a bimanual technique if necessary, to examine the pectoral (anterior) nodes. Then reach high up into the axilla at the midaxillary line to palpate the midaxillary (central) nodes against the ribs and serratus anterior. Palpate the subscapular (posterior) nodes along the posterior axillary fold along the anterior edge of the latissimus dorsi. Palpate the brachial (lateral) nodes along the humerus in the upper inner arm.

Last, palpate the infraclavicular area. The supraclavicular nodes, which also receive lymphatic drainage from the breasts, are usually examined with the neck nodes. All the nodes should be nonpalpable, although detection of one or two small, nontender, mobile central nodes is often a normal finding. Abnormal findings include firm, fixed nodes that may or may not be tender. If nodes are palpated, note the number of nodes felt, their location, size, shape, mobility, tenderness, and consistency.

Conduct breast palpation systematically to examine all breast tissue, including the tail of Spence in the upper outer quadrant. Any one of several approaches may be used as long as each portion of the breasts, areolae, and

FIGURE 37-2 Assessment of axillary lymph nodes. *A,* Location of the groups of nodes examined. *B,* Pectoral (anterior) nodes. *C,* Midaxillary (central) nodes. *D,* Subscapular (posterior nodes). *E,* Brachial (lateral) nodes. *F,* Infraclavicular (subclavicular) nodes. Axillary nodes are also palpated for male clients.

nipples is palpated. The breast and areola may be palpated in concentric circles, in a wheel-and-spokes pattern, or back and forth from superior to inferior. When the client is sitting, you may prefer to use a bimanual technique, especially if the breasts are large. When the client is supine, place a small folded towel under her shoulder to enhance breast flattening against the chest wall. Have her place her arm behind her head. Slide your fingers along the tissue using a rotary motion to press the breast against the chest wall. Your fingers remain in contact with the skin surface. The firm, curved ridge along the inferior breast is the inframammary ridge.

Breast consistency varies from firm and elastic in young women to stringy and nodular in older women. If the client reports a mass, begin palpation with the unaffected breast so that you have a basis for comparison. Pay particular attention to the upper outer quadrant and tail of Spence, where most of the glandular tissue is located and 50% of breast lesions are found. There should be no masses or local areas of warmth. If you feel a lump or mass, note its characteristics. Include the exact location (and the position the client is in for the palpation), using the areola for a reference point. Note size, shape, contour, consistency, mobility, tenderness, and discreteness. Visualize the breast as having four quadrants plus the tail; the location of lesions can be diagramed in the written record. See the feature *Physical Assessment Findings in the Healthy Adult* for a recording example.

Palpate the areola and nipple gently. Compress the nipple between your thumb and index finger. There

PHYSICAL ASSESSMENT FINDINGS IN THE HEALTHY ADULT

Female Reproductive System

Inspection

Breasts and Axillae: Breasts symmetrical, full, rounded, smooth in all positions, without dimpling, retractions, or masses. Faint, even vascular pattern and striae noted. Nipples everted, areolae even. Axillae even color, without masses or rash.

Genitalia: Pubic hair distribution varies with stage of sexual development; clean, coarse. Labia majora covered with pubic hair in adult women; may gape open slightly. Labia minora pink, smooth. Clitoris midline, smooth. Urethral meatus pink, discharge absent. Vaginal orifice clean, without bulges. Vaginal walls intact, pink, glistening, rugae present; discharge, bulges, and masses absent. Cervix round with os round or oval in nulliparous women and slit-like in parous women; discharge absent.

Palpation

Breasts and Axillae: Breasts firm without masses, lumps, local areas of warmth, or tenderness. Nipples without discharge. Axillae smooth, nodes nonpalpable.

Genitalia: Pelvic floor musculature firm. Skene's glands without discharge or tenderness. Bartholin's glands without masses or tenderness. No bulges in vaginal wall with straining. Uterus anteverted, firm, smooth, mobile, nontender, without masses. Ovaries oval, firm, movable, nontender.

should be no discharge. Nipple erection and wrinkling with manipulation are normal.

■ PELVIS

Women often find pelvic examinations embarrassing, humiliating, and anxiety-provoking, especially if they are performed roughly or in a perfunctory and hurried manner. Insensitive professional treatment produces fear, humiliation, submission, and low self-esteem. Meet the client, and interview her before she disrobes in the examining room. Memories of an uncomfortable or otherwise unpleasant pelvic examination may make women avoid future examinations and neglect gynecologic health care.

Put the woman at ease before and during the pelvic examination. Promote comfort by being nonjudgmental, relaxed, and competent. Explain your actions before proceeding. Avoid quick movements, because they may cause the client to tense her muscles, which results in greater discomfort. Enhance comfort with gentleness, privacy, keeping the woman warm, warming hands and instruments, using a lubricant to ease insertion during invasive maneuvers, and cleaning the perineum after the examination. Protect the woman's dignity, and communicate with her before, during, and after the examination. Use a mirror during the examination to show the woman her anatomic structures, if she desires, to facilitate the learning process.

A pelvic examination is less dreaded when a woman can participate and learn while retaining a sense of power and self-control. Encourage questions and expression of concerns, feelings, and wishes. Some women are afraid that the examiner will detect their sexual "secrets" from a pelvic examination. Provide these clients with a sense of control over self-disclosure so that they do not feel you are prying or able to "read their past."

Remain professional, and avoid actions or remarks that may be misconstrued by the client as demeaning or sexually provocative. For example, use a firm touch instead of gentle stroking. Be aware that the client may become sexually stimulated; alter the sequence of the examination, if necessary, but continue in a professional manner. Some facilities mandate that a female assistant be present when an examiner performs a pelvic examination to both comfort the client and discourage accusations of sexual impropriety.

Preparation

Instruct the woman not to douche, have intercourse, or use any vaginal products for 2 to 3 days before a pelvic examination. If a Pap smear is to be obtained, the woman should not be menstruating. Just before the examination, ask the woman to empty her bladder and bowels to to enhance comfort and accuracy. If necessary, collect a urine specimen at this time.

Ask the woman to remove enough clothing to allow examination of the abdomen and perineum. If a breast examination is planned, request that the woman disrobe completely and have her put on a gown. Ask about previous experiences with pelvic examinations, and acknowledge any feelings the woman may have. If this is the client's first examination, explain the procedure fully and

show her how the speculum works. All women should be told which examinations are to be performed. Tell the woman when and where she will be touched to help her avoid tensing up, which produces discomfort.

Equipment

The following equipment is used during a pelvic examination:

- Vaginal speculum of an appropriate size
- Materials for obtaining smears and culture specimens for cytologic and microbiologic tests, including sterile cotton-tipped swabs, vaginal spatulas (wooden or plastic) or cytology brush, glass slides and coverslips, cytology fixative, culture plates, and enzyme immunoassay kits for *Chlamydia* and gonorrhea screening
- Adequate, adjustable light source
- Water-soluble lubricant
- Appropriately sized examination gloves (vinyl if the client is latex-sensitive).

Long forceps and cotton balls may be used after smears and specimens have been obtained to clean the cervix or vaginal areas so that any suspected areas may be examined more easily. Have biopsy equipment available in case the examination reveals that a biopsy is necessary.

Position

Help the client to assume a dorsal recumbent or lithotomy position, and keep her draped until it is time for the examination. In the lithotomy position, the buttocks should be aligned with the end of the table. The client may not have to put her feet into stirrups if only the external genitalia are examined. Help the client to flex and abduct her hips and knees with her arms at her sides or crossed over the chest. Adjust the stirrups to accommodate the woman's height.

The lithotomy position, with the perineum exposed, may be uncomfortable and embarrassing. Do not keep a woman exposed any longer than necessary. Elevate the client's head on a small pillow to aid abdominal muscle relaxation and facilitate the examination. Low back pain or a hip deformity may contraindicate this position; an alternative position, such as Sims, might be necessary (see Fig. 10–6), or an assistant can help the client abduct one or both legs. There must be an adjustable light source. Wear nonsterile, disposable examining gloves (latex or vinyl).

External Genitalia

Inspect the external genitalia and perineum (Fig. 37–3A). Assess secondary sexual characteristics, such as pubic hair distribution and developmental stage of external genitalia, during examination of the external genitalia and rectum while these areas are uncovered. Before touching the client's perineum, place one hand on the client's thigh to avoid startling her.

The mons pubis is a mound of tissue superior to the labia. In adults, it is usually covered by pubic hair distributed as an inverse triangle over the mons, anterior

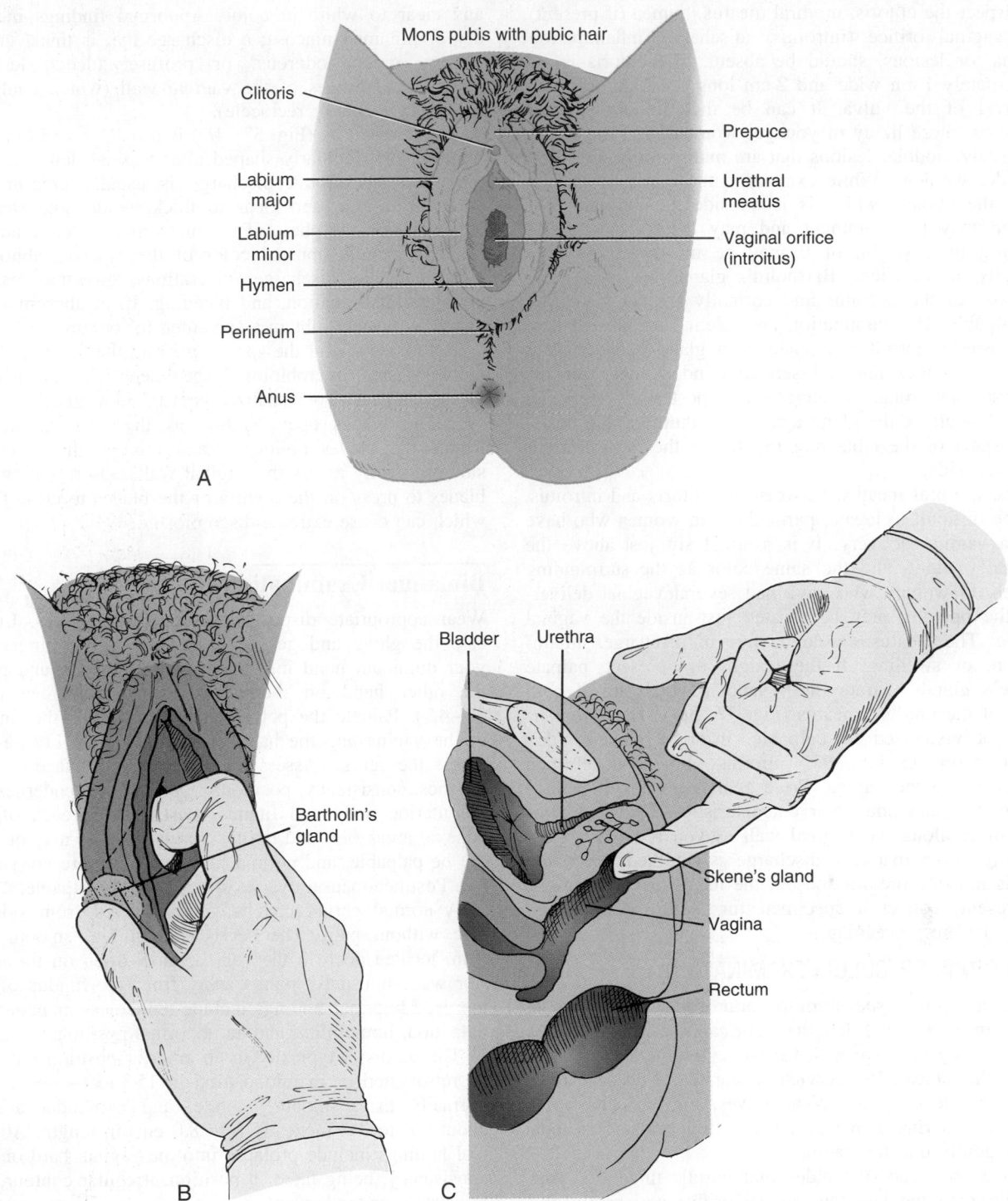

FIGURE 37-3 *A*, Anatomy of the female perineum and external genitalia. *B*, Palpation of Bartholin's glands. *C*, Palpation of Skene's glands.

perineum, and medial aspects of the upper thighs. Inspect the hair for nits and the skin for parasites, irritation, inflammation, edema, and lesions. An offensive odor should not be present. Any discharge should be scanty and clear to white in color.

Perineal skin is slightly darker than the rest of the body. The labia majora are symmetrical, rounded, and full. If the client has had a previous vaginal delivery, the labia majora gape slightly and the labia minora are evi-

dent. After menopause, the labia majora slowly atrophy. They should be free of edema, inflammation, and lesions. The labia minora are thinner than the labia majora, and one side may be larger than the other side. Gently separate the labia to inspect the vulva and remaining external structures. Place the thumb and index finger of your nondominant hand inside the labia minora, and retract the tissues laterally. Maintain a firm hold to avoid unnecessary manipulation of sensitive tissues.

Inspect the clitoris, urethral meatus, hymen (if present), and vaginal orifice (introitus); discharge, inflammation, edema, or lesions, should be absent. The clitoris is approximately 1 cm wide and 2 cm long, the same color as the rest of the vulva. It can be the site of syphilitic chancres (more likely in younger women), and the site of dry, scaly, nodular lesions that are malignant (more likely in older women). While examining the introitus, also inspect the hymen, which is just inside the introitus. The hymen may be prominent and may restrict the vaginal opening in a virgin, or it may be mostly absent in a sexually active client. Bartholin's glands are found near the base of the introitus and normally are not visualized or palpable. If inflammation and edema are present near the posterior introitus, palpate each gland between your thumb and index finger. Insert your index finger into the introitus, and rotate it laterally and posteriorly (see Fig. 37–3B). Palpate the gland against the thumb at the posterior aspect of the labia majora. Repeat the maneuver for the other side.

The urethral meatus, between the clitoris and introitus, can be difficult to locate, particularly in women who have had a vaginal delivery. It is a small slit just above the vaginal opening and the same color as the surrounding tissues. In women who have had several vaginal deliveries, the opening may be located just inside the vaginal orifice. The meatus should be free of discharge, inflammation, or swelling. If these signs are present, palpate Skene's glands (paraurethral glands), which are at both sides of the urethral meatus (Fig. 37–3C). They are usually not visualized or palpable. Insert a gloved index finger palm up into the introitus and about 1 inch (2.5 cm) into the vagina. Press gently upward to palpate the glands, and note their characteristics. Draw your index finger along the vaginal wall as you remove it from the vagina so that any discharge is "milked" from the glands into the urethra and out the meatus. If a discharge is present, collect a specimen for culture and change gloves before proceeding.

■ VAGINAL SPECULUM EXAMINATION

Select a vaginal speculum of appropriate size; specula differ in width and length. Lubricants cannot be used because they interfere with various cytologic studies, such as the Pap smear. If a cervical smear is not needed, use a water-soluble lubricant. Wear gloves, and insert the speculum, either rinsed in warm water or lubricated as indicated, gently into the vagina.

To do so, place the index and middle fingers of your nondominant hand in the vaginal orifice and gently pull posteriorly. Insert the closed speculum at a 45-degree angle, with the tip pointing downward into the vaginal orifice over your fingers (Fig. 37–4A). Withdraw your fingers while slowly rotating the speculum downward into the vagina until the handle is in a vertical position and the blades are fully inserted (Fig. 37–4B). Open the blades to observe the vaginal walls and cervix (Fig. 37–4C and D). You may need to make several gentle attempts to correctly position the cervix between the blades of the speculum. Offer the woman a mirror if she wants to see her cervix.

Vaginal mucous membranes are moist and pink, without discharge. If a discharge is present, it should be thin and clear to white in color. Abnormal findings include dry or inflamed mucosa; a discharge that is thick, curdy, yellow, green, odorous, or profuse; ulcers; lesions; masses; and bulges of the vaginal wall (which could be from a cystocele or rectocele).

The cervical os (Fig. 37–4D) is usually round but may be a slit or irregularly shaped after vaginal delivery. It is pink and smooth. A discharge is usually present that varies from thin and clear to thick, white, and stringy, depending on the phase of the menstrual cycle. Abnormal findings include unusual color of the mucosa, abnormal consistency of discharge, ulcerations, growths, masses, nodules, inflammation, and bleeding. If an abnormal discharge is present, obtain a specimen for culture.

Before removing the speculum from the vagina, obtain cytologic and microbiologic specimens, if indicated, as discussed later. To visualize the vaginal walls, leave the speculum blades open slightly as they are withdrawn. Rotate the blades obliquely, and remove the speculum slowly to fully assess the vaginal walls. Do not allow the blades to press on the urethra or the blades to close fully, which can cause extreme discomfort.

Bimanual Examination

Wear appropriate disposable examination gloves. Lubricate the glove and gently insert one or two fingers of your dominant hand into the vagina, palm up, and place the other hand on the client's lower abdomen (Fig. 37–4E). Palpate the pelvic contents between the fingers in the vagina and the hand on the abdomen. Locate and assess the cervix. Assess the size, shape, surface characteristics, consistency, position, mobility, and tenderness of the uterine body and fundus. Last, palpate each of the adnexal areas (left and right). Normal ovaries may or may not be palpable, and normal fallopian tubes are not palpable. Postmenopausal ovaries should not be palpable.

A normal cervix can be gently moved from side to side without pain. The cervix should feel smooth and firm, located deep in the vagina, most often on the anterior wall. It usually points away from the fundus of the uterus. Abnormal findings include tenderness or pain with palpation, immobility, and an abnormal position.

The uterus is typically in an anterior position but may be retroverted or in midposition in 15% of women. It is normally firm, smooth, mobile, and nontender and is about 2⅛ to 3⅛ inches (5.5 to 8.0 cm) in length. Abnormal findings include prolapse into the vagina, hard or soft consistency, being fixed in position, irregular contour, enlargement, or tenderness.

A normal ovary is 4 to 6 cm in diameter and feels smooth, firm, and oval. Slight tenderness on palpation is normal, but extreme tenderness, pain, or masses are not.

Withdraw your hand, palm up, halfway from the vaginal orifice, and assess the integrity of the pelvic floor musculature. Ask the client to contract her pelvic floor muscles as if trying to stop the flow of urine. The muscles will constrict around your fingers with more tone in a nulliparous client than in a client who has had a vaginal delivery. Next, ask the client to bear down as if straining to void. Feel for bulging of the vaginal walls pressing down against the introitus. If the anterior wall of the vagina bulges, the client probably has a *cystocele* (pro-

FIGURE 37–4 Pelvic examination and insertion of the vaginal speculum. *A,* The speculum blades are turned obliquely, and any pressure is directed downward onto the perineum. *B,* After full insertion, the blades are rotated to a horizontal position. *C,* Squeezing the speculum handles opens the blades. *D,* A full view of the cervix and cervical os. *E,* The bimanual examination. The abdominal hand presses the pelvic organs to be palpated toward the intravaginal hand.

lapse of the urinary bladder). A posterior vaginal wall bulge is often the result of a *rectocele* (rectal wall prolapse). Both of these are common in multiparous or obese clients.

Rectovaginal Examination

Insert your lubricated middle finger into the rectum and the index finger into the vagina (Fig. 37–5) to assess the rectal tissues for abnormalities, such as hemorrhoids (see Chapter 32). Ask the woman to bear down in order to ease insertion of your finger into the rectum. Rectal examination also confirms uterine position. If the uterus is retroverted, palpate the body and fundus. Reassess the adnexal areas, and palpate the rectovaginal septum and cul-de-sac. Normal pelvic organs can be palpated through the posterior cul-de-sac. Abnormal masses or normal ovaries are often felt in the cul-de-sac.

Assess anal sphincter tone and the rectal wall, which should be smooth. Assess the rectovaginal wall, which should be smooth, firm, and resilient (see Chapter 32). If the uterus is retroverted, it may be felt through the rectovaginal wall. The cervix feels smooth, round, firm, and movable without tenderness. Do not mistake the cervix or a vaginal tampon (if one is left in place) for a rectal mass.

If a stool specimen is needed for occult blood testing, obtain it at this time. When the examination is completed, help the client sit up and offer her tissues or wipes to clean the perineum.

If it has been well performed, a vaginal examination in women who have no pathologic conditions usually causes no or minimal discomfort. Some discomfort may occur during palpation of the ovaries during the bimanual and rectal examinations. Acknowledge this, and help the

FIGURE 37–5 Rectovaginal examination. The examiner combines bimanual and rectal examination by inserting the index finger in the woman's vagina and the middle finger in the rectum.

woman relax by asking her to bear down during the rectal examination and to breathe deeply through her mouth during palpation of the ovary. After completing the examination, give instructions and conduct appropriate health teaching.

Sometimes abnormal cervical or vaginal tissue, a mass, or other problem is discovered during a pelvic examination. Colposcopy or biopsy of the abnormal tissue may be performed. Further examination under anesthesia may be necessary for exploration of a mass or unexplained tenderness. A pelvic examination is conducted before various other gynecologic tests (such as a Pap smear, colposcopy, hysterosalpingogram) and before surgery (such as laparoscopy or laparotomy).

DIAGNOSTIC TESTS
■ GYNECOLOGIC STUDIES

Laboratory Studies

The most common gynecologic laboratory studies are the Pap smear, wet smear, and cervical culture. The woman should not be menstruating at the time specimens are collected. Instruct her to avoid douching or using vaginal hygiene sprays or deodorants for at least 24 hours before a test.

PAPANICOLAOU SMEAR
Cytology is examination of the structure, function, pathology, and chemistry of the cell (Fig. 37–6). In gynecology, the most common cytologic test is the Pap smear, named after George Papanicolaou, the physician who devised it. The Pap smear identifies preinvasive and inva-

sive cervical cancer. A new technique that improves the quality of Pap smears is the ThinPrep Pap test. Cells are collected and processed in such a way that a thinner layer of cells can be examined on the slide. Clinical trials have demonstrated improved detection of precancerous cervical cells using the ThinPrep Pap test compared with the conventional Pap smear.

PROCEDURE
The principle of the Pap test is based on the fact that both normal and abnormal cells are shed from the uterine and cervical linings and pass into their secretions. When a cytologic smear of these secretions is examined under a microscope, early cellular changes may be detected before disease becomes clinically apparent. The Pap test is up to 95% accurate in the diagnosis of early cervical carcinoma provided, of course, that correct sampling and handling techniques are used. It is only about 40% accurate in detecting endometrial carcinoma.

Specimens for the Pap test consist of a small amount of secretions taken from the endocervix and exocervix (Fig. 37–6B and C). With the conventional Pap test, these secretions are smeared separately on clean, dry slides or may be placed on one slide divided into sections (Fig. 37–6E). The slides are marked with "C" for cervix and "E" for endocervix. Immediately after the smears are made on the slides, they are fixed with either a commercial spray or solution. The secretions must be fixed before they dry. Cells in the specimen may be distorted if they dry or are contaminated with lubricant, which makes accurate reading difficult or impossible. With the ThinPrep test, the collected secretions are placed in a small bottle of preservative.

A Pap smear is usually painless. The American Cancer Society (ACS) recommends that women who are or have been sexually active or who have reached age 18 years should have annual Pap tests and pelvic examinations. After a woman has had three or more consecutive normal annual examinations, the Pap smear may be performed less often at the discretion of the health care provider. Many health care providers, however, continue to recommend annual examinations. The Pap test should be continued after menopause. Vaginal smears are obtained for Pap smear in women who have had a hysterectomy with removal of the cervix (see Chapter 39). Secretions are obtained from the vaginal pool, located in the posterior fornix (Fig. 37–6D).

In the past, reported findings were classified numerically. Descriptive reports are preferred because they are more useful in clinical decision-making. Reports either classify findings as normal or describe more fully the cellular changes seen. Specific infections may also be identified, and hormonal assessment may be done.

An abnormal Pap smear does not always mean malignancy. There is about a 5% false-positive or false-negative rate for the Pap test, and this rate is much higher if the specimen has been incorrectly collected or handled. However, having an abnormal Pap smear can be a frightening experience. Careful interpretation of cytologic findings is very important. The woman needs an opportunity to ask questions, to discuss concerns and feelings, and to participate in follow-up care planning.

If the cervix appears abnormal to the naked eye during

A. SPECIMEN COLLECTION EQUIPMENT

ThinPrep

Vaginal speculum

Normal saline

KOH

SALINE

Cervical broom

Cervical spatula

Long-handled cotton swabs

Glass slides with coverslips

Agar plate

Labels and pencil

FIXA

Chlamydia tests

Fixative

E. SLIDE PREPARATION

NAME Turner, H
DATE 9/12/92
AREA Endocerv
ID # 03 9127

Smear specimen evenly on glass slide. Add drop of KOH or saline and cover with cover glass. Label with name, date, area of sample, identification number.

F. GONOCOCCAL CULTURE

HOPPER, J
9/3/92
Cervical
03 3946

Obtain endocervical specimen with swab. Smear in Z pattern on agar plate. Cover and label as above.

B. ENDOCERVICAL SPECIMEN

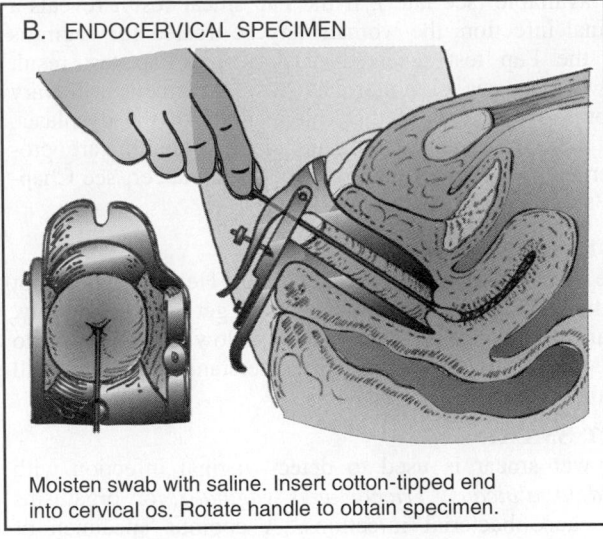

Moisten swab with saline. Insert cotton-tipped end into cervical os. Rotate handle to obtain specimen.

C. EXOCERVICAL SPECIMEN

Insert Ayre spatula with longer tip in cervical os. Rotate end of spatula around cervical opening.

D. CUL-DE-SAC   POOL SPECIMEN

Insert saline-moistened swab into cul-de-sac pool to obtain specimen.

FIGURE 37–6 *A–F,* Collection of cervical cytocology specimens.

the examination, colposcopy may be done at that time if it is available (see later). If the Pap smear result reveals a vaginal infection, the woman may be treated for vaginitis and the Pap test repeated later. If the Pap test result shows dysplasia or abnormal tissue, treatment will vary according to extent of the lesion, grade of the dysplasia, and preference of the woman and her health care provider. For more information on cervical cancer, see Chapter 39.

POSTPROCEDURE CARE
Care is minimal following a Pap test. Help the client out of the stirrups, and tell her not to get up too rapidly. Clean off any excess lubricant, or allow the client to do so. Make sure that the client understands how she will get the results of her Pap test.

WET SMEAR
The wet smear is used to detect vaginal infection with *Candida albicans, Trichomonas vaginalis,* or organisms that cause bacterial infections. A copious specimen of discharge from the vaginal vault is obtained with a cotton-tipped swab and placed in about 1 ml of warm normal saline to check for *T. vaginalis* and clue cells (indicative of bacterial vaginosis). A second specimen can be placed in about 1 ml of potassium hydroxide to check for *C. albicans.* Both specimens are mixed to produce a suspension and then placed on a glass slide with a coverslip for microscopic examination (Fig. 37–6*E*).

CERVICAL CULTURE
A cervical culture or antigen detection test can be done to detect infection with *Neisseria gonorrhoeae* or *Chlamydia trachomatis.* A cotton-tipped swab is rotated in the endocervical canal and placed in the appropriate culturette tube or rolled in a Z pattern onto a culture medium, depending on the organism. The culture medium should be at room temperature before inoculation with the specimen (Figs. 37–6*B* and *F*). Because of the asymptomatic nature of these infections, sexually active women are often tested routinely during regular examinations.

Radiography

Computed tomography (CT) and magnetic resonance imaging (MRI) are modalities in which images of the pelvic organs are obtained in the assessment of reproductive and urologic disorders. (see Chapters 11 and 32). There is no special preparation for CT scan or MRI unless a contrast agent (dye) is given. Pregnancy and morbid obesity contraindicate both tests. Ask the woman whether she has an intrauterine device in place, the presence of which may contraindicate MRI.

Ultrasonography

An ultrasound study of the uterus and adnexae requires a full bladder. Obtain an informed consent. No other special preparation is needed (see Chapter 11).

When performed with a vaginal probe, an ultrasound examination enhances the view of the adnexae. This technique is used to evaluate ovarian cancer and cysts and ovaries that have been stimulated with fertility-enhancing drugs. For this approach, the bladder must be empty to promote comfort. The woman inserts the vaginal probe

(sheathed in a protective, lubricated cover). Once the probe is inserted, the technician maneuvers it to obtain the best images. Inform the woman to expect the technician to manipulate the probe.

Endoscopy

Endoscopic procedures for assessing the female reproductive system include colposcopy, hysteroscopy, and laparoscopy.

COLPOSCOPY
Colposcopy involves the use of stereoscopic binocular microscope (colposcope) to examine the cervical epithelium, vagina, and vulva (Fig. 37–7). It is indicated for all women whose Pap smears show dysplasia. It also may be used to examine suspected lesions in the lower genital tract.

Explain to the woman that the procedure is similar to a pelvic examination and that, when the speculum is in place, a special microscope is used to look at the cervix. Colposcopy increases diagnostic accuracy and reduces the need for biopsy. The procedure is safe and painless, and it can be performed in pregnant women.

Help the woman into the lithotomy position. The cervix is exposed with a vaginal speculum. A solution of 3% acetic acid (common household vinegar) is applied to the cervix to remove mucus and cellular debris and to slightly dehydrate the cells. The cervix and upper vagina are then inspected with the colposcope. Biopsy is usually performed at this time if a lesion is present and can easily be done without the use of anesthesia. Cervical biopsy is avoided on pregnant women. (See discussion of cervical biopsy in this chapter.)

HYSTEROSCOPY
During a hysteroscopic examination, the intrauterine cavity is directly viewed through an endoscope called a hysteroscope (Fig. 37–8). Hysteroscopes have a fiberoptic lighting system and use 5% glucose in water, highly viscous dextran solutions, or carbon dioxide as the uterine-distending medium. After an anesthetic agent is administered, the hysteroscope is passed into the uterus via the vagina. The uterine cavity is distended and may be rinsed to clear away blood and debris that would obstruct vision. In addition to direct visualization of the uterine cavity, directed biopsies and resections of endometrial abnormalities can be done. The hysteroscope can also be used to deliver a laser beam into the uterus for therapeutic procedures.

Hysteroscopy may be used for (1) ruling out organic causes in abnormal uterine or postmenopausal bleeding, (2) examining suspected leiomyomas or polyps, (3) removing an intrauterine device with a missing string, (4) evaluating infertility, and (5) performing surgical techniques for uterine abnormalities. It is contraindicated if the client has acute pelvic inflammatory disease, recurrent chronic upper genital tract infection, recent uterine perforation, or suspected or known cervical malignancy. It also is contraindicated in pregnancy.

Explain the procedure to the client, and obtain an informed consent. Position the client in the lithotomy position, as for a pelvic examination. Complications of the procedure may include bleeding, uterine perforation,

View

Colposcope

Beam of
light

Vaginal
speculum

FIGURE 37–7 A colposcope is used to evaluate clients with an abnormal Papanicolaou smear and a grossly normal cervix. (From Hacker, N. F., & Moore, J. G. [1998]. *Essentials of obstetrics and gynecology* [3rd ed.]. Philadelphia: W. B. Saunders.)

infection, and rarely, bowel injuries. The woman may have referred shoulder pain if carbon dioxide was introduced into the pelvic cavity during the procedure; it usually resolves within 24 hours. Monitor the client's vital signs, and assess pain levels and location carefully.

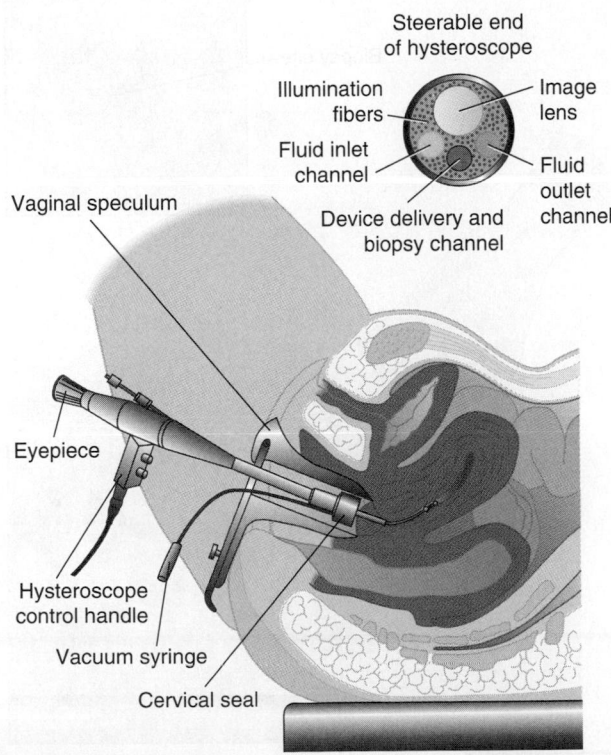

Steerable end
of hysteroscope

Illumination
fibers

Image
lens

Fluid inlet
channel

Fluid
outlet
channel

Device delivery and
biopsy channel

Vaginal speculum

Eyepiece

Hysteroscope
control handle

Vacuum syringe

Cervical seal

FIGURE 37–8 Hysteroscopy.

LAPAROSCOPY

A laparoscope, a common diagnostic and therapeutic tool (Fig. 37–9), is a telescope with an illuminated optical system. It is inserted into the abdomen through a small incision in or near the umbilicus to visualize abdominal and pelvic organs. Laparoscopy is a safe, convenient procedure that can be performed in hospitals, offices, or clinics equipped for outpatient surgery. The postprocedure recovery period is short, and the scar is small.

Laparoscopy may be performed diagnostically for conditions such as pelvic pain, pelvic masses, infertility, suspected ectopic pregnancy, and endometriosis. It also may be performed therapeutically for such procedures as tubal ligation, lysis of adhesions, treatment of endometriosis, drainage and removal of cysts, and for laparoscopic-assisted hysterectomy.

The main contraindication to laparoscopy is serious cardiac or pulmonary disease, although severe obesity may preclude its use. Previous lower abdominal surgery is not a contraindication, but it should be considered.

To prepare a client for laparoscopy, explain the procedure and inform the client how she can expect to feel afterward. Tell her to take nothing by mouth past midnight on the night before the procedure. Someone else should drive her to the health care facility because she should not drive after the procedure. Suggest that she wear loose-fitting clothes because it will be easier to dress after discharge. Typically, women who have laparoscopy in a same-day surgery setting can go home 2 to 4 hours after the procedure.

After laparoscopy, take the client's vital signs every 15 minutes for the first hour or until they are stable. If local anesthesia has been used, the woman can have fluids and a light snack as soon as she wants. After general anesthesia, the woman may have fluids and a light snack as soon as she is fully awake and has no nausea.

FIGURE 37–9 Laparoscopy.

Explain that she may experience mild-to-moderate transient shoulder pain or a feeling of bloating as a result of the carbon dioxide or nitrous oxide that was used to distend the abdomen, separate the organs, and allow better visualization during the procedure. The discomfort usually lasts only a few hours and may be relieved by positioning or mild analgesics. The woman may also experience mild incisional pain or abdominal cramping for the first few hours or days after the procedure, which is usually relieved by rest.

If general anesthesia was used, the client might have a sore throat from intubation. Soreness should disappear within 48 hours.

Teach her how to keep the incision clean and dry. After it heals, the scar will be barely noticeable. Sexual intercourse can be resumed within a week or less.

Biopsy

CERVICAL BIOPSY

Cervical biopsy is performed to rule out malignancies. A specimen of the cervical lesion that has been identified with the naked eye or with colposcopic magnification is usually obtained in the outpatient setting with little or no anesthesia. A solution of 3% acetic acid can be applied to the cervix to identify areas suspected to be dysplasia, metaplasia, or malignancy. These areas undergo a color change and appear white after acetic acid is applied.

When colposcopy cannot identify an abnormal lesion on the cervix or vagina, Schiller's test may be performed. Lugol's iodine solution is applied to the vagina and cervix. Normal tissue takes up the stain and appears as a homogeneous mahogany-brown color. Usually, abnormal tissue does not take stain as well and may appear light yellow instead. This is a positive finding and can indicate areas necessitating biopsy. A biopsy may be done when a cervical lesion is first noted, or it may be delayed until about 1 week after the menstrual period, when the cervix is least vascular. Multiple biopsy specimens are usually obtained at specific sites with biopsy forceps (Fig. 37–10). Hemostasis is achieved with topical application of Monsel's solution or silver nitrate. For ruling out

FIGURE 37–10 Cervical biopsy.

disease in the endocervical canal, endocervical curettage may be performed.

Before a cervical biopsy, explain the purpose of the test and obtain the client's informed consent. The test is usually not done while the client is menstruating. The lithotomy position is assumed.

After a cervical biopsy, allow the client to rest for a short time before she goes home. Although she may note a small amount of blood-tinged vaginal discharge or the mustard and blackish discharge from the Monsel's solution, tell her to report any excessive bleeding immediately. Advise her to abstain from vaginal sexual activity and to avoid tampons and douching until the bleeding has completely stopped, in order to achieve hemostasis, to lessen trauma, and to promote healing.

ENDOMETRIAL BIOPSY

An endometrial tissue sample is obtained for histologic study through the technique of endometrial biopsy. Tissue may be analyzed for endometrial cancer, dysfunctional uterine bleeding, and occasionally, for infertility. The biopsy is performed after bimanual examination of the uterus. Because the biopsy procedure may result in cramping, the woman may receive a nonsteroidal anti-inflammatory drug, a paracervical block, or both to relieve the discomfort.

The cervix is dilated under sterile conditions, and a uterine sound is inserted to measure the depth of the uterine cavity. An aspirating instrument is passed into the uterus, and a small amount of tissue is removed from the endometrium for examination (Fig. 37–11).

Explain the purpose of the test and the procedure, including the use of an anesthetic block. Obtain an informed consent. Position the client as for a pelvic examination.

If cramping persists after the procedure, administer analgesics as ordered or apply heat to the lower abdomen.

■ BREAST STUDIES

Laboratory Studies

No laboratory tests can screen for breast cancer. Some progress has been made in identifying biologic tumor

FIGURE 37–11 *A,* Endometrial sampling devices for uterine cancer screening. Endometrial curets range in size, composition (stainless steel, plastic), and flexibility (rigid, semirigid, flexible) and may be used with a vacuum collection syringe or with an irrigation system and suction syringe. The uterus is sounded for position and depth to determine the size of the curet to be used. Loosened cells collected in the syringe are transferred to a specimen jar with fixative for cytopathologic examination. (Courtesy of Milex Products, Inc.) *B,* Endometrial uterine lavage using sterile normal saline and negative pressure. *Arrows* indicate the flow of the irrigating solution and collection of the specimen. Fluid does not enter the fallopian tubes. A plug at the cervical os helps maintain negative pressure within the uterus. (From Boone, M. I., et al. [1984]. Uterine cancer screening by the family physician. *American Family Physician, 30,* 157.)

markers for breast cancer that detect metastatic disease. Elevations in carcinoembryonic antigen (CEA), alkaline phosphatase, ferritin, and gamma-glutamyltransferase seem to be associated with the recurrence of breast cancer. Other possible tumor markers that have been studied include C-reactive protein, acid glycoprotein, sialyltransferase, the urinary hydroxyproline-creatinine ratio, and gross cystic disease fluid protein.

Radiography

Various techniques have been tried to identify early-stage breast cancer in women accurately and safely when assessment indicates breast lesions. Such techniques are also important in finding an effective method to screen women without clinically apparent manifestations. At present, only mammography has been shown to be useful for widespread screening. While ultrasonography is not specific enough to identify lesions suggestive of cancer, it does differentiate cystic from solid lesions. Other methods of testing are being investigated.

Mammography

A mammogram is a soft tissue radiographic breast examination used to detect small invasive and noninvasive tumors and benign lesions. Two common methods of obtaining mammograms are *film-screen mammography* (Fig. 37–12) and *xeromammography* (Fig. 37–13). The film-screen method uses x-ray film. Xeromammography produces an electrostatic image on plastic-coated paper. Each

FIGURE 37–12 Mammography, a technique for obtaining an x-ray image of the breast, is the most reliable mechanical method of detecting a breast cancer before it can be felt. This technique is also used to help diagnose breast cancer.

technique has strengths and limitations and involves acceptably low radiation doses.

Common questions and possible answers about mammography include the following:

1. *How often should I have a screening mammogram?* Use the ACS or National Cancer Institute (NCI) guidelines for the age and risk group.
2. *What is the cost?* Prices vary. Inquire at the facility where the mammogram will be performed. Tell the client that while it is worthwhile to compare prices, ensure that the facility meets the necessary quality standards.
3. *How much time is involved?* About 15 to 30 minutes. Results are usually available within 1 to 21 days, depending on the facility.
4. *What preparation is required?* The woman should not wear any body powder, creams, or deodorant on the torso the day of the procedure.
5. *Is there pain?* Discomfort may be experienced because of the compression needed to obtain the best image. Some women find it helpful to schedule a mammogram for the week after the end of their menses, when the breasts are less tender. Women who have tender breasts may take a nonsteroidal anti-inflammatory drug, if not contraindicated, about 30 minutes before the procedure.
6. *Is there a risk in the exposure to the radiation?* Both methods of mammography use the smallest dose possible. The long-term effects of an annual mammogram are considered to be harmless.

During a mammogram, the woman disrobes from the waist up and her gown is separated to expose one breast at a time. The breast is placed between an x-ray plate and a compression paddle that is adjusted so the breast is compressed between the two plates to obtain the best image possible. Usually, two views of each breast are taken from different angles. Cranial-caudal and oblique views are most common.

Mammography can identify some breast cancers before they are palpable. The Breast Cancer Detection Demonstration Project included 280,000 participants who were followed up by mammogram for at least 5 years. Mammography alone detected 41.6% of the cancers—an impressively high rate in the diagnosis of small cancers.[18]

Indications for mammography include:

- Diagnosis of potentially curable cancer and follow-up after treatment
- Evaluation of questionable breast masses or other abnormal physical findings to help determine whether and where a biopsy should be performed
- Detection of breast cancer in a woman with metastatic cancer if the primary site is unknown
- Routine screening

Some controversy exists about the age at which to begin routine screening mammograms. The ACS recommends a baseline mammogram for all women by age 40 and mammography screening of asymptomatic women ages 40 to 49 at intervals of 1 to 2 years and annually over age 50.[1] The NCI no longer recommends routine screening of women under age 50 years. Until there is further evidence, the decision when to begin may be

FIGURE 37-13 A xeromammogram, performed before a planned biopsy of a palpable mass that proved to be benign (*small arrow*), revealed the presence of a hidden cancerous lesion (*large arrow*). (From Lippman, M. E., et al. [1988]. *Diagnosis and management of breast cancer.* Philadelphia: W. B. Saunders.)

made on an individual basis, with the woman and her health care provider together evaluating her risk for breast cancer as well as the possible risks and benefits of the screening test. A woman who is at high risk for breast cancer should follow the recommendations of her health care provider.

Ultrasonography

An ultrasound study of the breast involves scanning with an automated whole breast scanner and a hand-held real-time sector scanner. Ultrasonography is useful in determining the consistency of breast masses and differentiating cystic (fluid-filled) from solid lesions; however, it cannot differentiate solid benign from solid cancerous lesions. Ultrasound is useful in confirming the fluid consistency of cystic-appearing lesions seen on a mammogram. It is also useful in guiding fine-needle aspiration of cysts and other breast masses. No special preparation is needed, and the procedure is painless; no radiation risk is involved.

Biopsy

Biopsy is essential to the diagnosis of breast cancer. No treatment should be undertaken without an unequivocal histologic diagnosis of cancer. A *core needle biopsy* and a *fine-needle aspiration* (FNA) biopsy may be performed with local anesthesia during an office visit.

Core needle biopsy, a simple procedure, takes just a few minutes. After the site is cleaned and prepared with povidone-iodine, a small core of tissue is obtained with a special needle (e.g., Vim-Silverman). The core of tissue removed is placed in formalin and sent to the pathologist for histologic diagnosis. Occasionally, a suture is needed to close the skin.

With a fine-needle aspiration biopsy, a needle and syringe are used to aspirate cells from a breast mass or fluid from a cyst. The cells are fixed on a slide (as in a Pap smear), and a cytologic diagnosis is made. Mammography is used to guide the needle for aspiration of nonpalpable lesions. The cytologic examination is useful for confirming the diagnosis of clinical and mammographic findings of fibroadenoma (a fibrocystic condition), intramammary lymph nodes, fat necrosis, subareolar papillomatosis, chronic subareolar abscess, and cancer. If the cytologic findings suggest that the specimen is acellular or that only blood and adipose cells are present, a biopsy or further evaluation is needed to rule out breast cancer.

Both fine-needle aspiration and core needle biopsy involve taking only a small amount of cells and tissue from a lesion. Because false-negative results are possible, an *open biopsy* may still need to be performed.

Incisional or *excisional* open biopsies are usually performed in an operating room or a minor surgical suite with the use of local anesthetic or intravenous (IV) sedation. About 35% of clients who require an open biopsy for a breast lesion have a malignancy. Excisional biopsy involves removal of the entire palpable mass, incisional biopsy only a portion of the mass. In both cases, the tissue removed is sent to the pathologist for histologic assessment. The incision is closed with sutures, and a dressing (sometimes a pressure dressing) is placed over the site. Typically, the dressing is in place for 24 to 48 hours before it is removed.

Percutaneous needle localization determines the area for an open biopsy if a mass is very small, for example, those detected by a mammogram alone. The lesion is localized in the radiology department. A thin needle is passed into the area in question that has been identified by mammography. A second mammogram confirms the position of the lesion. The needle is secured in place with tape, and the woman is taken to the operating room, where an open biopsy is immediately performed. Frozen section examination may be done for rapid diagnosis.

Before a breast biopsy, explain the purpose of the biopsy to the client and obtain her consent. Restrict food and fluids if IV sedation is to be used. Discuss the postprocedure self-care activities that the client should follow. Most women fear that the biopsy will result in a finding of cancer; some clients may ask about what will happen if cancer is found (see Chapter 40).

After the biopsy, instruct the woman to report any bleeding, swelling, or evidence of infection. After a needle biopsy, normal activity can be resumed as soon as it is comfortable to do so. Vigorous activity should be avoided for 1 to 2 weeks after an open biopsy. The woman may find it more comfortable to wear a supportive brassiere 24 hours a day until the site is healed, as long as the wires and elastic do not rub on the incision.

THE MALE REPRODUCTIVE SYSTEM

Disorders of the male reproductive and urinary tract (which is closely associated with the reproductive tract) occur in men of all ages. Assessing these disorders requires expertise in conducting the health history interview and physical examination. Be sensitive and tactful because many men are uncomfortable discussing issues associated with these disorders. Discuss lifestyle factors that affect health maintenance, such as diet, exercise, adequate sleep and rest, stress management, smoking cessation, and individual risk factor identification. If appropriate, provide information about protection against STDs. Explain what is involved in the physical examination, use easily understood terms, and discuss any diagnostic tests that may be indicated.

HISTORY

A complete health history, including sexual and reproductive systems, and physical examination are necessary for men experiencing reproductive disorders. History-taking provides an opportunity to:

- Allow men to express sensitive concerns
- Identify and dispel myths and misinformation
- Teach health information
- Offer referrals
- Facilitate further communication

The following discussion addresses the major risk factors pertinent to men's reproductive health history.

■ BIOGRAPHICAL AND DEMOGRAPHIC DATA

Review the client's biographical and demographic data to determine his health risk status. Age, race, and occupation all have health risk implications. Men over age 50 years may have benign prostatic hypertrophy (BPH), an enlargement of the prostate gland. Men younger than age 40, who have manifestations that resemble those of BPH, are more likely to have prostatitis. African American men and those over age 40 are at increased risk for adenocarcinoma of the prostate. Younger men, particularly those between ages 25 and 35, have a higher incidence of testicular cancer. Occupations and activities that involve prolonged, strenuous lifting or straining can provoke hernias. Exposure to some chemicals and pesticides may be linked to fertility and reproductive disorders.

■ CURRENT HEALTH: THE CHIEF COMPLAINT

The client may present with problems related to the genitourinary or reproductive system or to sexuality. A chief complaint may include the following areas:

- Systemic disturbances, such as weight loss, fever, and malaise
- Voiding disturbances, such as frequency, polyuria, oliguria, nocturia, pyuria, enuresis, dysuria, urgency, or incontinence
- Disturbances in urine characteristics, such as hematuria and pyuria
- Gastrointestinal disturbances, such as nausea, vomiting, anorexia, abdominal discomfort, constipation, or diarrhea
- Reproductive disturbances, infertility, history of STDs, genital lesions, or genital discharge in self and partner; genital trauma
- Sexual functioning (whether the client is sexually active or celibate), such as changes in libido; changes in erectile ability; decreased ejaculatory ability; gynecomastia (breast enlargement); and the effects of disability, chronic disease, trauma, surgery, or treatment

For each reported manifestation, conduct a symptom analysis (see Chapter 9).

■ PAST HEALTH HISTORY

Significant health history for the male reproductive system includes childhood and infectious diseases, immunizations, major illnesses and hospitalizations, medications, and allergies.

Childhood and Infectious Diseases

The most significant childhood infectious illness to affect male fertility is mumps. Its occurrence in young men is associated with sterility. Ask whether the client has ever had mumps or been immunized against it. Question the client also about the presence of cryptorchidism at birth and the age at which the testicles descended or were brought down surgically.

Major Illnesses and Hospitalizations

Ask about major illnesses, such as diabetes, hypertension, cerebrovascular accident (CVA), and MI. Men who have diabetes commonly have problems with potency related to the accompanying neurologic and vascular changes. Hypertension and CVA can cause impotence related to physiological or psychological factors. Impotence may also occur in men who have had an MI because they may fear having another episode as a result of sexual excitement and activity.

Urinary tract disorders can interfere with sexual functioning because of the close proximity of anatomic structures. Endocrine disorders can also affect sexual performance. Be alert to the man's concerns and fears, remain nonjudgmental, and offer the support of counseling and referral to peer groups established for this purpose.

Ask the client about any previous surgery involving the reproductive system, such as herniorrhaphy, vasectomy, prostatectomy, varicocelectomy, orchiopexy, and testicular torsion repair.

Medications

Obtain a complete medication history for prescription, over-the-counter, and recreational drugs; nutritional supplements; and herbal remedies. Some medications prescribed for hypertension (e.g., methyldopa, clonidine, guanethidine, and hydralazine) may cause impotence. Tranquilizers can interfere with sexual performance. Other medications can decrease sperm count and motility. Recreational drugs (e.g., marijuana and hallucinogens) that alter behavior can also affect physiologic reproductive function and may raise the risk of STDs. Herbs frequently used to treat reproductive disorders include saw palmetto (*Seronoa repens*) for BPH and yohimbe (*Pausinystalia yohimbe*) for erectile dysfunction and impotence.

Allergies

Ask the client about any allergies to antibiotics, rubber, or latex. Male genitourinary disorders are often treated with antibiotics, and latex and rubber are found in condoms as well as in examination gloves commonly worn during the physical examination. If the man is allergic to latex, wear vinyl gloves.

■ SEXUAL AND REPRODUCTIVE HISTORY

A sexual and reproductive history includes questions about breasts, contraceptives, sexual practices, genitourinary problems, and reproductive health practices (see Chapter 9).

Breast History

Collect data about the breasts and axillae. Ask about breast pain, masses, skin changes, and nipple discharge. Ask whether the man has noticed any changes in breast tissue, such as enlargement. *Gynecomastia* can occur in obese or older men and as a side effect of some medications. Ask whether the client performs BSE, similar to the technique taught to women.

Contraceptive History

Document the man's current contraceptive method (if any), his satisfaction with the method, the effect of contraception on sexual function, and any desire to change methods. Has the man used contraceptive methods previously? If so, did any problems lead to their discontinuation?

Sexual History

Inquire about the client's patterns of sexual relationships. Can the man relate the total number of sexual partners he has had and the frequency of sexual activity? Multiple partners and contacts increase the client's risk of STDs. Does the man use condoms during sexual intercourse? Does he have homosexual or bisexual relationships, both of which increase the risk of human immunodeficiency virus (HIV) infection.

Does the client have any sexual concerns, such as an inability to attain or maintain an erection? If so, does this problem occur frequently or occasionally? Is the client able to discuss sexual concerns with his partner? Have he and his partner developed ways to cope with or adjust to disturbances in sexual function? If sexual dysfunction exists, does the client want a referral to, or consultation with, a sex counselor?

Throughout the interview, ask questions directly. Phrase questions in a neutral, nonjudgmental way. This interview technique helps preserve dignity and self-esteem instead of fostering guilt or shame. Chapter 9 provides further information on sexuality assessment.

Genitourinary History

Ask about past problems with genitourinary infections, such as prostatitis. Determine whether the client has had a previous pelvic examination. Does he have such problems as urinary incontinence, dribbling, hesitancy, a weak urinary stream, or other manifestations? Chapter 32 describes assessment of the urinary system.

Reproductive Health Practices

Inquire about sexual and reproductive hygiene. How often does the man examine his breasts and testes? (See Chapter 2.) Does he protect himself against STDs? Chapter 9 discusses health risk management.

■ FAMILY HEALTH HISTORY

Ask whether the client has a family history of infertility, diabetes, hypertension, CVAs, or endocrine disorders. As with women whose mothers took DES during pregnancy, men who have been exposed to DES in utero are at increased risk for congenital anomalies, including structural defects of the genitourinary system and reduced semen levels.

■ PSYCHOSOCIAL HISTORY

Assess the client's occupation, environment, habits, and psychosocial factors.

Occupation and Environment

Determine the client's type of work and recreational activities to identify any exposure to chemicals, pesticides, heat, heavy metals, hormones, and radiation. These materials can directly affect the number and integrity of sperm and the quality of germinal tissue.

Habits

Assess the client's use of caffeine, alcohol, tobacco, and recreational drugs, including marijuana. These substances may affect the sperm count, contribute to impotence, decrease libido, or encourage risk-taking behaviors. Physical and recreational sports can put the client at risk for genital trauma if protective gear is not used.

Psychosocial Factors

Review the following subjects when conducting a health history interview with a man who has a reproductive disturbance. You may not be able to obtain detailed information in each of these areas, but the outline should help you to view each man and his significant others as individuals and to avoid stereotypical and, possibly, judgmental nursing care. Note:

1. *Self-concept.* How has the client's health affected how he feels about himself? How do his partner and significant others feel about him? What is his

posture, dress, grooming? What is his emotional response? What is his mood? His tone?

2. *Role relationships.* Who are the important people in this client's life? Who accompanied him to the health care facility? Who is his most significant other? How is he able to carry out his various social roles (partner, husband, friend, father, worker)? How has his health affected his economic situation and his partner or significant others?

3. *Communication.* How does the client communicate, both verbally and nonverbally, with you and his significant others? Does he maintain eye contact? Does he use gestures or touch? How does he speak (volume, tone, vocabulary, repetition)?

4. *Value system.* What values, opinions, and beliefs does the client hold? What is his predominant lifestyle? What is his cultural or subcultural background?

5. *Coping and stress tolerance.* Who supports and nurtures the client? Does he experience intimacy with anyone? How connected is the client with significant others? What supports and resources does he have? How does he spend his leisure time? To what extent does he engage in physical activity or exercise?

6. *Cognitive-perceptual.* How does the client use words? Can he read? What is his level of comprehension? What is his major source of information about reproductive health?

■ REVIEW OF SYSTEMS

Ask about diabetes, hypertension, CVA, angina, MI, endocrine disorders, renal disorders, and urinary tract problems. Detailed questions for the review of systems may be found in Chapter 9.

PHYSICAL EXAMINATION

Skillful history-taking helps to establish a therapeutic relationship that facilitates physical examination. Many men find physical examination of the reproductive system stressful and embarassing. Some men may view the genitals as private or unclean.

Help the client become more comfortable by sharing normal findings while you proceed. Explain each step. Increase the client's comfort by maintaining eye contact, proceeding in an unhurried manner, and involving the client in self-examination. Occasionally, a man will have an erection during an examination. A kind, professional manner and a firm, yet gentle touch lessen this possibility. If the man does have an erection, explain that this is normal and does not have sexual connotation.

The physical examination focuses on findings that may be associated with reproductive or sexual disorders. These may include the following disorders:

- Inflammatory, such as enlarged, tender, movable, or fixed lymph nodes in the inguinal region
- Endocrine and genetic, including indications of such conditions as Cushing's syndrome or acromegaly, hair distribution, and gynecomastia
- Neurologic, including a gross neurologic examination of the legs

- Vascular, including the femoral and pedal pulses
- Traumatic, such as a hernia

Follow an orderly sequence for the physical examination, and teach the client how to perform similar self-examinations regularly. The male breasts and axillae are included here as part of the reproductive system examination.

■ BREASTS AND AXILLAE

Examine the client's breasts and axillary nodes. Although the incidence of breast cancer in men is low, it can occur because men have glandular tissue beneath each nipple.

Inspect and palpate the breasts and axillae while the man is sitting, following the same guidelines as for the female breast examination. The male breast is flat and symmetrical, without nodules, edema, or ulceration. One-sided (unilateral) breast enlargement that persists beyond puberty is abnormal. Palpation reveals a small, flat disc of glandular tissue under the areola. There should be no masses or discharge. Axillary nodes should be nonpalpable (see Fig. 37-2).

■ EXTERNAL GENITALIA

The client's urinary bladder should be empty. The client may be supine or lying on his side with his legs spread slightly for the first portion of the genital examination; ask him to stand during the assessment for inguinal herniation. Alternatively, the client might stand for the entire examination of the genitals while you remain seated. Because the male urethra is the common conduit for both urine and semen, examination of the male reproductive tract also includes assessment of the urinary system. Wear nonsterile, disposable examining gloves.

Inspect the external genitalia and perineum (Fig. 37-14), observing the pubic hair and skin. You must be familiar with normal growth and development of the male genitalia. Observe general appearance and body build. Note the hair distribution. Pubic hair distribution in men is triangular, with hair covering the symphysis pubis, base of the penis, and inner aspects of the thighs. Hair distribution may also spread toward the umbilicus in a diamond pattern. Inspect hair for nits and the skin for parasites, rashes, excoriation, and lesions. Masses, lesions, edema, and offensive odors should be absent. Scrotal skin is darker than other skin surfaces and is loose and wrinkled.

The penis includes the penile shaft, prepuce (foreskin), glans, and urethral meatus (Fig. 37-15). Inspect and palpate these structures for lesions, nodules, swelling, inflammation, atrophy, and discharge. Penile skin in a flaccid penis is wrinkled. The foreskin, if present, covers the glans. The foreskin is absent in a circumcised client. Instruct the client to retract the foreskin to expose the glans, which is easily accomplished. You may see a small amount of cheesy, thick, white, odoriferous *smegma* between the glans and the foreskin; it is normal. If other discharge is noted, obtain a specimen for culture. The area between the glans and foreskin is a common site of venereal lesions. The area is normally free of lesions; if any are present, palpate them for tenderness, size, shape, and consistency, then change gloves before proceeding.

Next, inspect the urethral meatus, located at the tip of the penis. It looks like a slit. Malposition of the meatus

FIGURE 37–14 *A,* Male genitourinary anatomy. *B,* Anatomy of male inguinal structures. *C,* Palpation to detect an indirect hernia.

Dorsal
vein

Coronal
ridge

Glans
penis

Scrotum

Urethral
meatus

Dorsal
vein

Foreskin
(prepuce)

Urethral
meatus

A

B

FIGURE 37–15 Appearance of a circumcised (*A*) and an uncircumcised (*B*) penis.

on either the underside of the penile shaft (*hypospadias*) or upper side (*epispadias*) is usually a congenital condition. The meatus is pink and without ulcers, scars, inflammation, or discharge. Gently compress the glans between your thumb and index finger to open the meatus, and inspect for discharge. If the client reports a urethral discharge, ask the client to compress the penis from base to tip between his thumb and fingers in an attempt to express a discharge. If one appears, obtain a specimen for culture or microscopic examination. You may need to change gloves again before continuing with the examination.

Palpate the penile shaft gently between your thumb and first two fingers. It is smooth and semi-firm, and the skin should move easily over underlying structures. The normal penis is free of nodules, thickened or hard areas, and tenderness.

Inspect the scrotum and palpate for symmetry, size, shape, and swelling. Size and shape vary among individuals. The scrotum has a right and a left half, each containing a testis, epididymis, and vas deferens. The left testis hangs lower than the right. Scrotal size varies with ambient temperature; cold results in contraction, warmth in relaxation. Ask the client to hold the penis to one side and then the other and to lift the scrotum up for inspection. The skin should be loose, without tension. The testes are ovoid, about 4/5 × 1 3/5 inches (2 × 4 cm). On palpation, they are normally smooth, firm, and rubbery, without nodules, masses, or tenderness. Older clients have smaller, less firm testes.

In younger, adolescent males, note whether both testes are present in the scrotum. Testes may temporarily migrate from being touched during examination or being exposed to cold air. They may be palpable later in the examination, when the client is more relaxed. If a testis is not apparent, palpate the femoral and inguinal area. If the client has an undescended testis, refer him to an appropriate health care provider. A small (pea-sized), hard lump located on either the anterior or lateral aspect of a testis suggests a malignancy; again, refer the client for follow-up. Compare testes bilaterally for similarity.

Palpate each epididymis between your thumb and index finger. The epididymis is located on the superior

aspect of the testis and extends down the posterior surface. It feels soft, resilient, and tender. Swelling and hardness are abnormal. The vas deferens (spermatic cord) begins at the superior, lateral aspect of the testis. It is differentiated from the epididymis by its firmer, tubular feel. Compare findings bilaterally. Palpate the vas deferens along its length toward the inguinal canal. Note any thickening or asymmetry, which is abnormal.

If you find swelling, nodules, or other abnormalities during the scrotal examination, perform transillumination of the scrotum (Fig. 37–16). Darken the room, and shine a flashlight through the scrotum from behind the mass. A scrotum filled with serous fluid will transilluminate as a

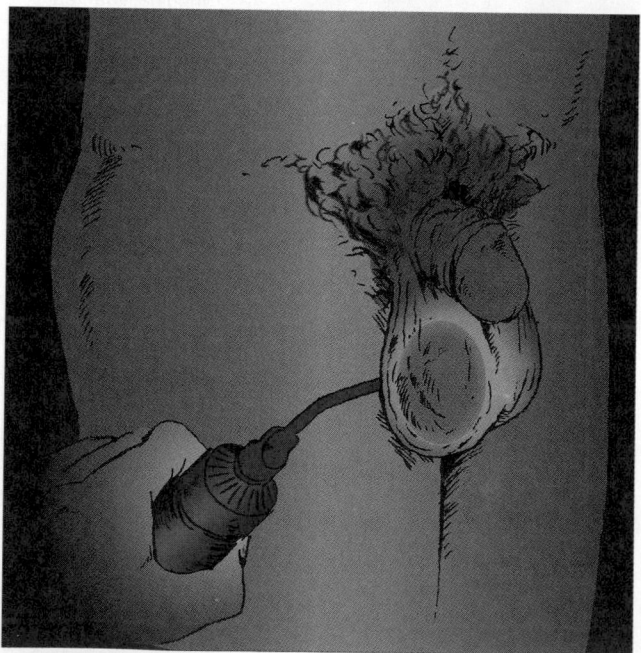

FIGURE 37–16 Transillumination of the scrotum. In a darkened room, place a strong, lighted flashlight or transilluminator next to the scrotum, as shown. Light normally passes through the scrotum (transillumination), but this does not occur with testicular tumor. A hydrocele shines red.

red glow. More solid lesions, such as a hematoma or mass, do not transilluminate and may be seen as a dark shadow. Record the characteristics of the abnormality, including whether it transilluminates.

While the client is standing, examine for an inguinal *hernia* (a prolapse or protrusion of a loop of intestine through the inguinal wall or canal). Inspect the inguinal areas for bulges while the client stands quietly and again after he bears down and strains, as though attempting a bowel movement. Bulges should be absent.

A *direct* inguinal hernia enters the inguinal canal behind the external ring because of a weakened abdominal wall; it does not pass through the inguinal canal. Assess for a direct hernia by gently inserting an index finger into the loose scrotal skin over the external inguinal ring; the finger does not enter to the external ring. Use the left index finger to palpate the client's right side and the right finger for the client's left side while the client faces you. Instruct the client to bear down while you feel for a bulge, which should be absent.

An *indirect* inguinal hernia enters the inguinal canal through the internal ring and can remain in the canal or pass down through the external ring and into the scrotum. To palpate for an indirect hernia, gently invaginate the scrotal skin with the index or little finger, following the vas deferens to where it passes into the external ring (Fig. 37–14C). Ask the client to flex the knee on that same side to help relax the muscles so that the finger can be inserted through the external ring and into the inguinal canal. Advance the palpating finger as far as possible, and instruct the client to bear down while you feel for a tissue mass touching the finger. The mass retreats up the canal when the client relaxes.

A *femoral* hernia, which is more common in women, occurs inferiorly and more laterally compared with an inguinal hernia; it often has the appearance of an enlarged inguinal lymph node. Palpate the inguinal area directly for a femoral hernia while the client is relaxed and again after instructing him to bear down. A palpable mass should be absent.

■ PROSTATE

After examining the anterior genitalia, assess the anus, rectum, and prostate gland. A rectal-prostatic examination should be performed annually in men over age 40 years to look for signs of an STD, changes in the size and consistency of the prostate gland, and evidence of a tumor or acute or chronic infection. Emphasize the importance of regular examinations as the best way to detect prostatic cancer for effective treatment.

Just before the examination, ask the client to empty his bladder, and collect a urine specimen at this time if one is needed. Explain that an empty bladder makes the examination more comfortable and more accurate. Also explain that it is normal to experience sensations of having to urinate or defecate during the examination.

Two possible positions for the client during the rectal examination are the knee-chest position, with the buttocks elevated, or bending over from the hip, with elbows placed either on the knees or on the examining table. (Positions are discussed in Chapter 10, and the anal and rectal examination is discussed in Chapter 32.)

Wear gloves, and apply water-soluble lubricant to the examining finger. Place your dominant hand on the client's hip to stabilize his position and to reassure him. Gently spread his buttocks with the nondominant hand. Observe the perineum and perianal areas for lesions, hemorrhoids, inflammation, or discoloration. Ask the client to bear down. Explain that this helps relax the anal sphincter and makes it easier to insert the examining finger.

Insert the ball of the finger toward the anterior wall of the rectum. The normal prostate is located 2 to 5 cm beyond the anal sphincter along the anterior wall of the rectum. It is normally about 4 cm long and 5 cm wide (Fig. 37–17A and B). The prostate is shaped like a doughnut wrapped around the neck of the urethra (Fig. 37–17C). Only the posterior and lateral lobes can be felt through the rectal wall (Fig. 37–17D and E). The lateral lobes should be symmetrical. A normal prostate feels smooth, rubbery, and firm, somewhat like the base of the thumb. In a man with BPH, the prostate feels larger than normal, with a firmer consistency, like that of the chin. Tenderness and bogginess (like the cheek of the face) may indicate acute or chronic prostatitis. Carcinoma feels like a stone or hard nodule, that is, a circumscribed area of induration. Any induration is abnormal. The seminal vesicles (superior and lateral to the prostate) are normally nonpalpable.

Prostatic massage may be indicated even when the client is asymptomatic to aid in the detection of prostatitis. Roll the pad of your index finger across the prostate gland, starting laterally and superiorly and moving toward the midline of the prostate (Fig. 37–17F). Then strip (or "milk") the area of the seminal vesicles, starting laterally and superiorly, toward the midline (Fig. 37–17G). Send the resulting meatal secretions for microscopic examination. A large number of pus cells suggests prostatitis. Staining may identify acid-fast organisms. Cultures may be needed to identify organisms such as gonococcal, chlamydial, or tubercous bacilli. If a culture is required, the glans of the penis must be cleaned and the bladder emptied to clear the urethra before prostatic massage. Collect meatal secretions in sterile culture media.

Withdraw your finger from the rectum, and observe for stool on the glove. Feces, if present, are normally brown. Mucus or blood and black, tarry, light-tan, or gray stools are abnormal. Test the stool sample for occult (hidden) blood, which should be absent (see Chapter 32). If you suspect an STD, obtain a rectal swab for culture. Wipe the perianal area, and inform the client that the examination is completed. See the Physical Assessment feature for an example of a recorded examination of the male reproductive tract.

DIAGNOSTIC TESTS

Various diagnostic tests may be done to assess for disorders of the male reproductive system. Men and their significant others are often anxious about diagnostic tests. You can help to reduce anxiety by giving careful explanations before and during the tests. It is much less frightening if a client knows what to expect and what is included in the process. Sedation or pain relief may be required before a test. An informed consent may be necessary. Physiologic preparations may be required, such as fasting or an enema. During the test, tell the client what

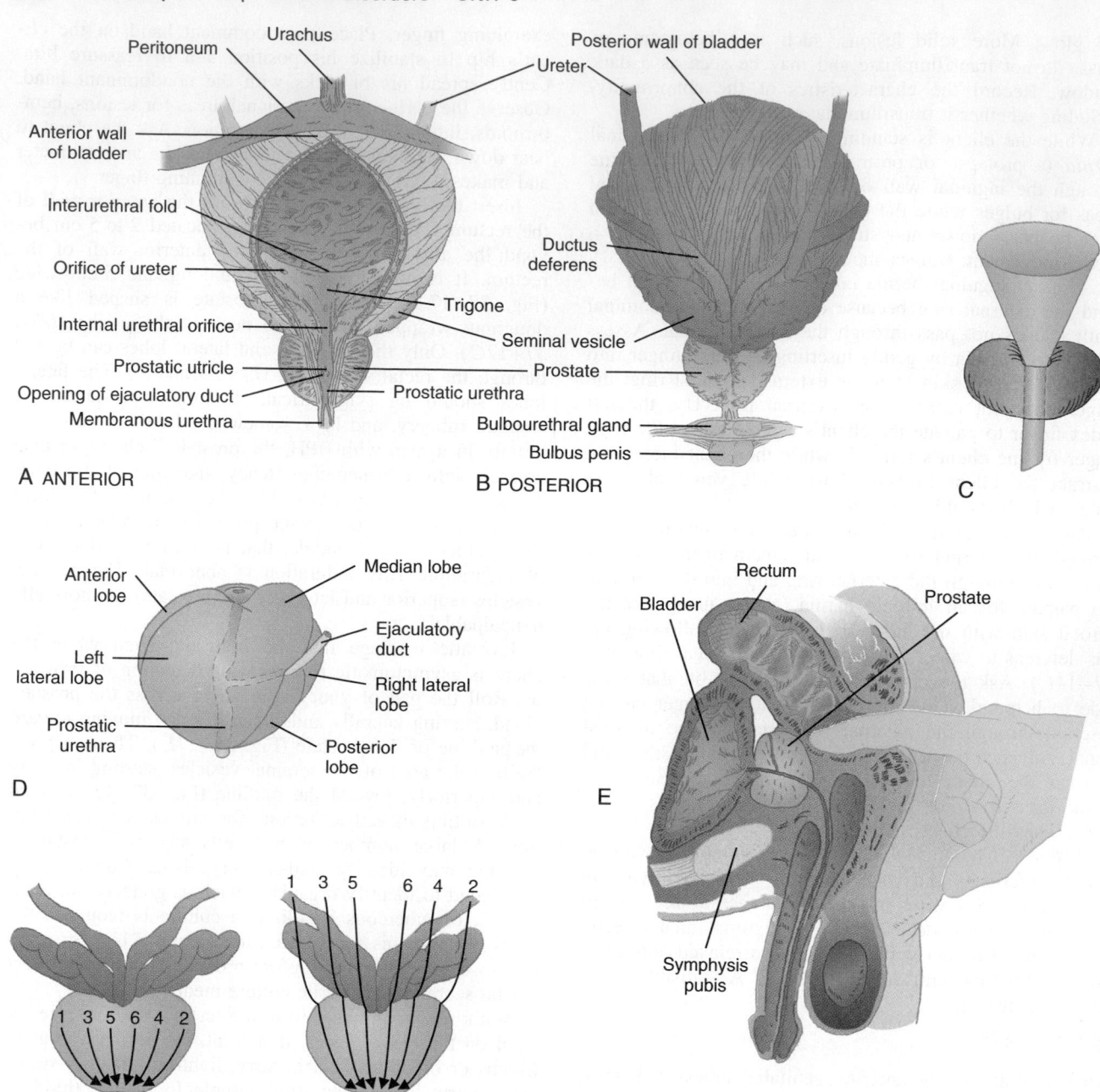

FIGURE 37–17 Rectal-prostatic assessment. *A* and *B,* Anterior and posterior views of the prostate gland. *C,* Diagrammatic representation of the anatomic position of the prostate gland. The gland surrounds the urethra rather like a doughnut wrapped around the outlet of a funnel. *D,* Posterior and lateral lobes of the prostate. *E,* Rectal examination. Insert a gloved index finger into the anus while the client is bearing down. Palpate all surfaces. *F,* Prostatic massage. Roll the pad of the index finger across the prostate, starting laterally and superiorly and moving toward the midline of the prostate. *G,* Seminal vesicles and prostatic massage. Use the same technique as for prostatic massage, but extend the finger over the area of the seminal vesicles.

is happening. Help him maintain the required positions. Observe him during and after the test for adverse reactions, such as pain, excessive anxiety, pallor, or nausea.

■ LABORATORY STUDIES

Blood Studies

PROSTATE-SPECIFIC ANTIGEN
Prostate cancer screening has been revolutionized by the prostate-specific antigen (PSA) assay. PSA, a substance found in prostatic fluid, aids the liquifaction of semen. PSA serum levels in men without prostate cancer are very low. The PSA level increases with age, and some controversy exists over the normal level. A level of 4.0 ng/ml or higher may be normal only for men over age 65, with a lower level being normal for younger men. Prostatic massage or rectal examination within 48 hours before the assay can cause elevated PSA levels. The PSA test has largely replaced the measurement of serum acid phosphatase as a screening tool for prostate cancer.

PHYSICAL ASSESSMENT FINDINGS IN THE HEALTHY ADULT

Male Reproductive System

Inspection

Breasts and Axillae: Breasts symmetrical, smooth in all positions, without retractions or masses. Vascular pattern and striae absent. Nipples everted and areolae even. Axillae even color, without masses or rash.

Penis: Penis size and shape vary among individuals. Foreskin may or may not be present. Head of penis slightly rounded without discharge (if client is circumcised). Smegma under the foreskin (normal if client is uncircumcised). Urinary meatus at the tip of the head of the penis, free of discharge or drainage. Shaft smooth.

Scrotum: Scrotal size and shape vary normally. Hangs below the penis with the left side lower than the right. Scrotal skin thin and rugose. Sparse hair on the scrotum. Transillumination shows no masses or areas of thickness.

Inguinal-Femoral Area: Coarse hair covers symphysis pubis, inner thighs, extending toward umbilicus. No bulges over the inguinal or femoral area, either at rest or with coughing or straining.

Palpation

Breasts and Axillae: Breasts firm without masses, lumps, local areas of warmth, or tenderness. Nipples even, without discharge. Axillae smooth, nodes nonpalpable.

Penis: Masses along the penile shaft and head of the penis absent. Firm, nontender.

Testis: Two testicles present, smooth, oval, and similar in consistency. Mobile and equal in size. Slight tenderness with palpation.

Epididymis: Present at the posterior of the scrotum (found in the anterolateral or anterior area of the testis in a small percentage of men). No tenderness.

Vas Deferens: Cord-like, mobile, smooth, and nontender. No masses.

Inguinal Canal: No bulge or mass in inguinal canal either at rest or with straining.

To further clarify the meaning of the PSA level, there are two additional tests: (1) PSA *density* (PSAD) and (2) PSA *velocity* (PSAV). PSA density relates PSA level to prostate size. PSA velocity involves the rate of change in PSA level over time. The PSA density test is combined with transrectal ultrasonography to determine the volume of the prostate. Clients who have PSA density levels less than 0.10 ng/ml are considered unlikely to have significant prostate cancer. As PSA levels rise, however, the presence of cancer cells is more likely. Clients who have a PSA velocity that rises more than 0.7 ng/ml per yr or that increases 20% or more a year are considered at high risk of having prostate cancer.

ALKALINE PHOSPHATASE

Alkaline phosphatase is present ubiquitously and is particularly associated with a variety of bone diseases. It is used as a diagnostic test in men with prostate cancer as a measure of possible bone metastasis. With higher levels in clients with known prostate cancer, the probability of bone metastasis is higher. However, many medications can artificially raise or lower the level.

Semen Examination

Semen testing is used to evaluate fertility. One to three samples of semen, collected at intervals of 2 to 4 weeks, are examined to accommodate for normal variations. To provide an adequate sample, the client should abstain from ejaculation for 2 to 5 days before the test. Prolonged abstinence may decrease sperm quality and motility, whereas more frequent ejaculations reduce sperm concentration and volume.

In the laboratory or office, the client masturbates into a clean, dry specimen container. Ordinary condoms or coitus interruptus is not an appropriate method because contamination or loss of the specimen is likely. If the client must collect the specimen outside the laboratory or office, the specimen should be kept at room temperature and brought to the laboratory within 30 minutes of collection.

Sperm analysis is used to assess infertility and to evaluate the effectiveness of a vasectomy. Tests for infertility include a sperm count, morphology, and motility along with semen pH, viscosity, appearance, and volume. If abnormalities are found, further analysis for the presence of antibodies can also be performed. If the test is being done to evaluate the effectiveness of a vasectomy, the presence or absence of sperm is sufficient.

Secretion Analysis

Secretions from the throat, penis, and anus or lesions from the oral, pharyngeal, and perineal areas may be examined for microorganisms. A sterile, cotton-tipped applicator is placed on or in the affected area, and the specimen is transferred to a sterile tube or slide. Be careful not to touch any other surface with the applicator.

■ RADIOGRAPHY

CT scanning and MRI are used to assess male reproductive and urologic disorders. Procedures include clinical staging of testicular and prostate cancers and imaging of pelvic organs for epididymitis, hydrocele, spermatocele, scrotal hernia, or testicular torsion and infarction. Chapter 11 covers these diagnostic procedures.

■ ULTRASONOGRAPHY

A transrectal approach is used in prostatic ultrasonography. The rectum must be free of feces. Help the client into a left lateral Sims' position. After a rectal examination, a well-lubricated transducer is inserted. The probe is covered with a water-filled condom to enhance sound wave transmission; a full bladder may also improve sound transmission. The examiner moves the probe along the prostate to complete the scan. Tell the client that some discomfort may be felt with probe insertion and manipulation. Once the probe has been removed, there should be no further discomfort.

■ RADIONUCLIDE IMAGING

Radioisotope scans may be used to assess testicular abnormalities, such as torsion, epididymitis, abscess, tumors, hydroceles, varicoceles, and spermatoceles. A radioactive substance is administered intravenously, and several scans are taken. Before a scan is taken, ask the client whether he has any history of allergies.

■ CYSTOSCOPY

Cystoscopy is indispensable for assessing and treating prostate and urologic problems. It is used to determine the cause of urinary manifestations, such as those related to prostatic hypertrophy, and to obtain specimens, such as in a transurethral prostatic biopsy. Cystoscopy may be done in a urologist's office or in an operating room before surgery. Inspection of the bladder interior includes looking for trabeculation, diverticula, and bladder neck contracture and checking the size and contours of the prostatic lobes. Chapter 32 describes the procedure and client care in detail.

■ URODYNAMIC ASSESSMENT

Urodynamic studies measure pressure from the bladder or urethra, urinary flow, and striated muscle activity. Common tests include uroflometry, cystometrography, electromyography, and a urethral pressure profile. They are useful in determining the cause of frequency and decreased urinary stream in men (as from prostatic obstruction). Chapter 32 describes urodynamic testing in detail.

■ PROSTATIC BIOPSY

Areas of the prostate that suggest a problem are assessed by biopsy after abnormal findings in PSA level, transrectal ultrasonography, or digital rectal examination. Biopsy of the prostate allows cytologic examination for the presence of cancer. The tissue may be obtained by a transurethral, transrectal, or perineal approach. The client must understand the approach to be used, the preparation, and the procedure for it. Obtain an informed consent. Physical preparation often includes an enema for the transrectal or perineal approach. The client must void before the procedure.

For the *transurethral* approach, place the client in the lithotomy position. Local anesthesia is used. The biopsy tissue is removed through transurethral endoscopy. Even though direct visual guidance is used in this approach, malignant tissue may be missed. This is partly because prostate cancer commonly begins in the posterior lobe, making it more difficult to obtain a specimen by this approach.

For the *perineal* approach, the lithotomy position is usually used; a jackknife position is an alternative. After the perineal area is cleaned and anesthetized, one or more biopsies are taken. This approach allows direct access to the posterior lobe of the prostate. Direct pressure is applied to the area. If there is no bleeding, a sterile dressing is applied.

For a *transrectal* approach, place the client in Sims' position. A rectal examination is performed to identify any hard nodules. The biopsy is performed with the examiner's finger as a guide. Some think that this approach is inappropriate because malignant cells from the nodule may be seeded into the rectal mucosa.

After the procedure, monitor the client's vital signs at regular intervals to detect signs of hemorrhage. If a transurethral approach was used, some hematuria is normal, although frank bleeding should be reported. The client must be able to void after the procedure. With the perineal approach, carefully assess the dressing for blood. After a transrectal approach, monitor for bleeding or infection.

PREVENTION OF MALE REPRODUCTIVE PROBLEMS

Primary prevention (preventing a problem before it occurs) includes genetic counseling, immunization against infectious diseases, good nutrition, careful genital hygiene, the use of condoms to prevent STDs, knowing one's partner, avoiding multiple sex partners, and avoiding sexual intercourse (oral, anal, or genital) with a person who has genital lesions.

Secondary prevention (detecting and treating a problem early) includes screening activities, such as serum PSA levels in men over age 50 and testicular self-examination (TSE). See Chapter 2 for discussion of BSE and TSE.

Tertiary prevention (avoiding complications and rehabilitation) is health care provided for clients experiencing acute and chronic disorders. For example, teaching perineal exercises after a prostatectomy helps men regain urinary control.

CONCLUSIONS

Assessment of the female and male reproductive systems requires knowledge of the physiologic and psychological implications associated with reproductive disorders. Exhibit a concerned, caring attitude when assessing any client with a reproductive disorder because these disorders are laden with psychosocial overtones. Assess the client in a thorough but matter-of-fact manner to put the client at ease and to expedite a complete assessment.

BIBLIOGRAPHY

1. American Cancer Society (1997). *Special touch: A personal plan of action for breast health.* Publication No. 97-500M-No. 2095-CC. Atlanta: Author.
2. American Cancer Society. (1997). *Guidelines for the early detection of cancer.* Publication No. 97-700M-No. 2070-CC. Atlanta: Author.
3. American Cancer Society. (1999). *Cancer facts and figures, 1999.* Publication No. 99-300M-No. 5008.99). Atlanta: Author.
4. Bickley, L. S. (1999). *Bates' guide to physical examination and history taking* (7th ed.). Philadelphia: J. B. Lippincott.
5. Benign Prostatic Hyperplasia Guideline Panel. (1994). *Benign prostatic hyperplasia: Clinical practice guideline.* AHCPR Publication No. 94-0583. Rockville, MD: Agency for Health Care Policy and Research, Public Health Service, U.S. Department of Health and Human Services.
6. Benign Prostatic Hyperplasia Guideline Panel. (1994). *Benign prostatic hyperplasia: Diagnosis and treatment.* AHCPR Publication No. 94-0582. Rockville, MD: Agency for Health Care Policy and Research, Public Health Service, U.S. Department of Health and Human Services.
7. Benign Prostatic Hyperplasia Guideline Panel. (1994). *Benign prostatic hyperplasia: Patient guide.* AHCPR Publication No. 94-0584. Rockville, MD: Agency for Health Care Policy and Research, Public Health Service, U.S. Department of Health and Human Services.

8. Bobak, I. M., & Jensen, M. D. (1997). *Maternity and women's health care* (6th ed.). St. Louis: Mosby–Year Book.

9. Grimes, J., & Burns, E. (1996). *Health assessment in nursing practice* (4th ed.). Boston: Little, Brown.

10. Hacker, N. F., & Moore, J. G. (1998). *Essentials of obstetrics and gynecology* (3rd ed.). Philadelphia: W. B. Saunders.

11. Jarvis, C. (2000). *Physical examination and health assessment* (3rd ed.). Philadelphia: W. B. Saunders.

12. Karlowicz, K. A. (Ed.). (1995). *Urologic nursing: Principles and practice.* Philadelphia: W. B. Saunders.

13. Kee, J. L. (1999). *Laboratory and diagnostic tests with nursing implications* (5th ed.). Stamford, CT: Appleton & Lange.

14. Kirby, R., & Christmas, T. (1997). *Benign prostatic hypertrophy* (2nd ed.). Chicago: Mosby International.

15. Mashburn, J., & Scharbo-DeHaan, M. (1997). A clinician's guide to Pap smear interpretation. *The Nurse Practitioner, 22*(4), 115–143.

16. McCorkle, R., et al. (1996). *Cancer nursing: A comprehensive textbook.* Philadelphia: W. B. Saunders.

17. Reeder, S., Mattin, L., & Koniak-Griffin, D. (1997). *Maternity nursing* (18th ed.). Philadelphia: J. B. Lippincott.

18. Seidman, H., et al. (1987). Survival experience in the breast cancer detection demonstration project. *CA: A Cancer Journal for Clinicians, 37*(5), 258–291.

19. Smith, D. R. (1996). *General urology* (14th ed.). Norwalk, CT: Appleton & Lange.

20. Star, W., Lommel, L., & Shannon, M. (Ed.). (1998). *Women's Primary Health Care Protocols for Practice.* Washington, DC: American Nurses Publishing.

21. Weber, E. S. (1997). Questions and answers about breast cancer diagnosis. *American Journal of Nursing, 97*(10), 34–38.

22. Youngkin, E. Q., & Davis, M. S. (1998). *Women's health* (2nd ed.). Stamford, CT: Appleton & Lange.

CHAPTER 38

Management of Men with Reproductive Disorders

Patricia McCallig Bates

NURSING OUTCOMES CLASSIFICATION (NOC) for Nursing Diagnoses—Men with Reproductive Disorders

Altered Urinary Elimination
Urinary Continence
Urinary Elimination
Ineffective Management of Therapeutic Regimen (Individuals)
Compliance Behavior
Knowledge: Treatment Regimen
Participation: Health Care Decisions
Treatment Behavior: Illness or Injury

Pain
Comfort Level
Pain Control
Pain: Disruptive Effects
Pain Level
Risk for Injury: Postoperative Complications
Circulation Status
Electrolyte and Acid/Base Balance
Fluid Balance

Risk Control
Risk Detection
Safety Status: Physical Injury
Symptom Control
Tissue Perfusion: Abdominal Organs
Tissue Perfusion: Peripheral
Urinary Continence
Urinary Elimination
Vital Signs Status

Today, men are more actively involved in health maintenance. This is evidenced by their increased interest in fitness and exercise, increased attainment of lifestyle factors related to fitness (such as smoking cessation), and increased participation in childbirth and parenting. As men learn to express their interest in general health maintenance, you can extend these interests to reproductive and urinary health maintenance. Often, knowledge about risk factors, preventive measures, and improved disease management encourages men to make changes in lifestyles and attitudes and to see health care providers for counsel or early detection of reproductive disorders.

Reproductive and genital disorders are significant, and their incidence is being increasingly recognized. Because the male urinary and reproductive systems involve the same structures, men may have mixed problems. Men are often reluctant to ask for help because they see such problems as a potential threat to their sexuality and are embarrassed to talk about them. Some men may also fear negative reactions from their health care providers because of their age or sexual preference.

Because of this reluctance to seek help, skillful therapeutic interaction is essential to help men express their concerns. Sensitivity to fear and embarrassment, respect for privacy and confidentiality, careful history-taking, and addressing information needs help put these clients at ease. When the client allows, partners should be brought into management plan discussions because most reproductive and genital disorders affect relationships.

Statements such as "Many men are concerned about how this problem will affect their sex lives," "It is common to worry about how your partner might feel about this problem," and "What are some of your concerns?" may help the client begin to talk about his concerns.

Giving men permission to express their feelings and their health-related concerns draws them and their significant others into the process of health care. Having topic-related brochures visible may provide the impetus for a man to ask questions.

PROSTATE DISORDERS

BENIGN PROSTATIC HYPERPLASIA

The prostate is the genital organ most commonly affected by benign and malignant neoplasms. Enlargement of the prostate gland with aging is called *benign prostatic hypertrophy* or *hyperplasia* (BPH). Hyperplasia (an increase in the number of cells) is the more acceptable term. BPH becomes a disorder when enlargement obstructs the urinary channel and causes changes in the urinary tract with associated manifestations.

Prostatic enlargement eventually occurs in 80% of men. By age 50, about 50% of men have some degree of BPH. The incidence is increased in African American men and is lower in Asians.

Etiology and Risk Factors

The exact cause of BPH is not known. Because BPH is a universal disorder in older men, several theories concerning the cause have been examined. Diet, effects of chronic inflammation, socioeconomic factors, heredity, race, body build, and sexual activity have been investigated, but no significant relationships have been found. It is thought that hormonal alteration is responsible. Testicular androgen appears to be the hormone suspected as the cause. BPH rarely occurs in men who are castrated or who have permanent hypogonadism before puberty or in early adulthood.

Because aging is the major risk factor for the development of BPH, little can be done for health promotion and prevention. Dietary factors have been examined, and it has been concluded that lycopene in cooked tomatoes and in green and yellow vegetables and other elements of the traditional Japanese diet appear to provide some protection against BPH. Early detection can lead to early treatment, which can prevent complications related to urinary obstruction. Men should be encouraged to discuss changes in urinary patterns and to have a digital rectal examination (DRE) annually if they are older than 40 years of age.

Pathophysiology

Benign prostatic enlargement refers to an abnormal increase in the number of normal cells (hyperplasia) in the prostate along with increased contraction of the smooth muscle elements of the prostatic stroma. These processes are often referred to as *static* and *dynamic* processes in the development of BPH. Many theories have been postulated, but the pathophysiology may be complex and is not clearly understood.

The pituitary secretes luteinizing hormone (LH) in response to changes in serum levels of LH, testosterone, and luteinizing hormone–releasing hormone (LHRH) produced by the hypothalamus. LH causes the testes to produce testosterone, which combines with an enzyme in the prostate, 5α-reductase, to form dihydrotestosterone (DHT). DHT influences prostatic cellular production. Simultaneously, alpha-adrenergic receptors in the smooth muscle of the prostate, along with the smooth muscle of the bladder neck and rhabdosphincter, cause contraction. This muscle contraction may cause enough resistance to restrict urine flow.

In response to increasing *bladder outlet obstruction* (BOO), urinary tract changes occur (Fig. 38–1). Urine remains in the bladder after urination. The detrusor muscle compensates by thickening to increase pressure against the outlet's resistance to empty the bladder. When it can no longer compensate, trabeculation (banding of fibromuscular tissue that appears thick in some places and thinner in others) and bladder diverticula (outpouchings in

---

ALTERNATIVE THERAPY

Benign Prostatic Hyperplasia

Benign prostatic hyperplasia (BPH) is a common problem in men after 50 years of age. Enlargement of prostatic tissue often leads to a variety of manifestations, including urinary frequency, hesitancy in voiding, decreased force of urine flow and postvoid dribbling. For many years, an herb known as saw palmetto (the fruit of the scrub palm *Serenoa repens* which grows on the southeastern Atlantic coast) has been used to treat this condition.

Saw palmetto seems to be effective in a number of ways. It appears to block the conversion of testosterone to 5α-dihydrotestosterone (DHT) by the enzyme 5α-reductase. It is DHT that stimulates growth of prostatic tissue. The herb apparently also has an anti-inflammatory effect that, when combined with the anti-androgenic effect, helps to reduce manifestations of BPH.[2] In one review,[3] saw palmetto produced similar positive benefits as the drug finasteride with fewer side effects.

The German Commission E monograph on saw palmetto recommends a daily dosage of 1 to 2 g of the berry, or 320 mg of a lipophilic extract.[1] The latter amount is necessary for proper extraction of the active constituents, which cannot be extracted in water. The herb does not shrink the prostate but only relieves the manifestations associated with BPH.[1]

Another herb, stinging nettle root (*Urtica dioica* L. or *U. urens* L.) has also been effective.[1, 2] Unlike saw palmetto, the root of stinging nettle may be prepared as a tea because the active ingredients appear to be water-soluble. To date, however, less research is available regarding this plant for the treatment of BPH.

References

1. Blumenthal, M. (1998). *The complete German Commission E monographs.* Austin, TX: American Botanical Council.
2. Tyler, V. (1994). *Herbs of choice.* Binghamtom, NY: Pharmaceutical Products Press.
3. Wilt, T. J., et al. (1998). Saw palmetto extracts for treatment of benign prostatic hyperplasia: A systematic review. *Journal of the American Medical Association, 280,* 1604–1609.

James Higgy Lerner, RN, LAc, *Private practice of acupuncture, traditional Oriental medicine, and biofeedback*

---

the bladder wall) may occur. Diverticula may retain urine, causing infection and stones.

Compensation and decompensation can also cause reflux (backflow of urine past the ureterovesical junction [UVJ]) and upper urinary tract infection (UTI). "Fishhooking" of the ureters is common (i.e., ureters looping downward like a fishhook as they enter the bladder). Compensation and decompensation processes may also occur in the ureter and kidney, causing conditions of hydroureter and hydronephrosis. Eventually, the renal parenchyma atrophies, resulting in irreversible loss of kidney function.

Clinical Manifestations

BPH usually develops slowly and may persist in a silent state without creating a major problem. As a man becomes older, he may assume that increasing frequency of

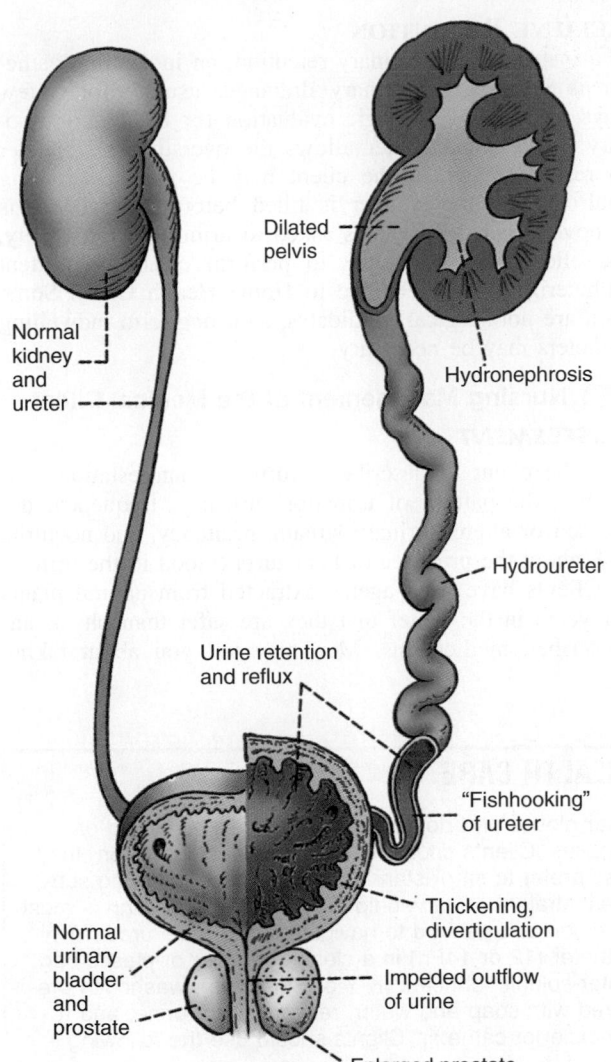

FIGURE 38–1 Complications of benign prostatic enlargement. *Left,* Normal kidney, ureter, bladder, and prostate. *Right,* Potential complications.

Labels in figure:
- Dilated pelvis
- Normal kidney and ureter
- Hydronephrosis
- Hydroureter
- Urine retention and reflux
- "Fishhooking" of ureter
- Thickening, diverticulation
- Normal urinary bladder and prostate
- Impeded outflow of urine
- Enlarged prostate

urination is part of aging. He may wait until he is bothered by retention before seeking medical care. Acute urinary retention in the client with BPH is often precipitated by cold weather, alcoholic beverages, infection, a delay in voiding, or bed rest. Some medications, such as decongestants, anticholinergics, and antidepressants, may also precipitate retention.

The severity of manifestations caused by BPH varies and is not related to the size of the enlargement. For example, a man with mild BPH may have strong stromal resistance and may experience severe bladder outlet obstruction. Another man may have enlargement of a median lobe of the prostate that grows up toward the bladder. This type of enlargement would not be detected by rectal examination. He, too, may experience moderate to severe bladder outlet obstruction. In contrast, another man may have a very large prostate with minimal manifestations.

History-taking includes specific questions about the size and force of the urine stream, hesitancy, need to strain, frequency, intermittency, urgency, nocturia (excessive urination at night), incomplete emptying, and urinary leakage. The American Urological Association's International Prostate Symptom Score Index (IPSS) is a short questionnaire commonly used by urologists to assess the client's opinion about the severity of these manifestations. The client scores manifestations from "not at all" to "almost always." The client also rates his quality of life from "delighted" to "terrible." The IPSS may also be used to evaluate treatment effectiveness.

A digital rectal examination is performed to evaluate size and tissue consistency and to rule out nodules or a tender, boggy prostate. Urinalysis, urine culture, blood tests for kidney function, and a *prostate-specific antigen* (PSA) test may be done to exclude accompanying urologic diseases. Chemistry panels, such as electrolyte, liver function, and blood coagulation studies, may be added if surgery is being considered.

Uroflowmetry is used to estimate the pattern and force of voiding. A man starts this test with a full bladder, voids into a specific toilet or container, and empties his bladder to the best of his ability. Residual urine is determined after the urine flow either by catheterization or by ultrasonography. A normal urine flow is considered to be 20 to 25 ml/second, but the figure may be lower for older men. BPH may cause decreased flow and a long, weak flow pattern with evidence of starts and stops or strained voiding. Depending on the severity of the client's manifestations and general medical condition, cystourethroscopy, intravenous pyelography (IVP), or urodynamic studies may be done.

Outcome Management

◼ Medical Management

Medical management has become a common initial approach for BPH because it is noninvasive and can be effective. "Watchful waiting" is a relatively new approach to BPH, particularly for the client who has few or mild manifestations. Periodic reassessment is necessary to reassess the severity of manifestations and to detect developing complications. Treatment is instituted if significant changes occur.

Definitive treatment is aimed at prostatic muscle relaxation or at androgen deprivation, which slows growth of the prostate and reduces its size. Relief of lower urinary tract manifestations is the subjective tool used to evaluate the effectiveness of treatment.

SLOW PROSTATE GROWTH

Finasteride (Proscar), a 5α-reductase inhibitor, blocks the conversion of testosterone to DHT and thus reduces BPH. Because finasteride is metabolized mostly in the liver, liver function tests are important before therapy is started. Side effects include a decrease in ejaculatory semen, decreased libido, and *erectile dysfunction* (inability to achieve or maintain an erection), although the latter two effects occur in only about 1% to 5% of men taking this drug. Finasteride may have to be taken for 6 to 12 months before any improvement in lower urinary tract manifestations occurs. Finasteride lowers the level of PSA (a glycoprotein) and can mask the occurrence of prostate cancer. Because finasteride can cause abnormal development of a male fetus, pregnant women should not come in contact with the semen of a man taking this drug.

Antiandrogens and LHRH antagonists (testosterone-ablating agents), agents used to treat prostate cancer, have been tried in the treatment of BPH, but side effects outweigh the benefits for most men. Side effects include loss of libido, hot flashes, gynecomastia (breast enlargement), and impotence. These agents are used on occasion.

Relax Prostate Muscle

Alpha-adrenergic blocking medications act on receptors in prostatic muscle tissue and seem to be effective in reducing manifestations. This group of drugs includes terazosin (Hytrin), phenoxybenzamine (Dibenzyline), prazosin (Minipress), doxazosin (Cardura), and tamsulosin (Flomax). The major side effects are orthostatic hypotension, dizziness, and tachycardia. Dry mouth, nasal congestion, palpitations, blurred vision, headache, and fatigue may also occur. Clients are started at a lower dose, which is increased if the medication is tolerated. Clients should not adjust the dosage without permission of the physician because serious cardiovascular consequences can occur. Several weeks of treatment may be necessary before improvement of lower urinary tract manifestations can be evaluated.

Relieve Retention

If a man has acute urinary retention, an indwelling catheter is inserted for urinary drainage, usually for a few days, before any urologic evaluation for BPH. A temporary indwelling catheter allows the overstretched bladder to rest, after which the client may be given a voiding trial; that is, the bladder is filled before the catheter is removed, and the client is asked to urinate. Alternatively, the client may be taught to perform clean intermittent catheterization (see Bridge to Home Health Care). Some men are not surgical candidates, and long-term indwelling catheters may be necessary.

◼ Nursing Management of the Medical Client

ASSESSMENT

Ask the client to describe all urinary manifestations, including the pattern of urination, urgency, frequency, decreased or altered urinary stream, hesitancy, and nocturia. Ask about the presence of hematuria (blood in the urine).

Clients have used agents extracted from natural plants for years in the belief that they are safer than physician-prescribed medications. Men may tell you about taking

BRIDGE TO HOME HEALTH CARE

Intermittent Self-Catheterization for Men

Intermittent self-catheterization is indicated for transient or persistent urinary retention. Retention occurs when clients are unable to empty their bladders completely as a result of neurologic conditions such as spinal cord injury, multiple sclerosis, or brain injury. An obstructive condition such as an enlarged prostate is another common cause of retention. The amount of residual urine that clients retain can vary greatly.

When intermittent self-catheterization is used to manage urinary retention, an indwelling catheter is not needed and the risk of infection is decreased. The procedure can be used as a temporary measure, for example, for the development of temporary bladder atony after bladder surgery. Before self-catheterization is selected for long-term management, a thorough assessment should be completed and noninvasive methods should have been attempted without success.

To use intermittent self-catheterization successfully, clients should have sufficient manual dexterity and cognitive ability, and they should follow guidelines. Because they must not overfill their bladders, it is essential that clients be motivated to catheterize four or five times daily. The goal is to obtain a quantity of urine that does not exceed 500 ml per catheterization. Most physicians recommend a moderate daily fluid intake. They tell clients to establish a consistent plan that includes the time and amount of their intake so that they do not overfill their bladders. It is also important that clients understand that poor or inconsistent technique increases the risk of complications. Infection is the most frequently occurring complication; persistent overfilling of the bladder can cause ureterovesical reflux with subsequent renal damage.

Clean self-catheterization is acceptable in the home setting. Using clean technique implies that clients do not wear gloves and do not need to use a sterile field or supplies. Clients should use a comfortable position; they may prefer to sit or stand. They need the following supplies: straight or curved-tip Tiemann (the Tiemann is most common and desired to navigate in the male urethra) catheter (12 or 14Fr.) in a clean container or plastic bag, water-soluble lubricant (K-Y or Surgilube) prepared with soap and water, washcloth prepared with soap and water, receptacle for urine, and receptacle for catheter. Clients should use the following procedure:

1. Wash hands and gather equipment. (Storing all equipment in one easy-to-carry container simplifies the procedure.)
2. Assume desired position. If sitting on bed, place plastic under a towel to protect bedding.
3. Retract foreskin if present, and wash tip of penis thoroughly with soap and water.
4. Remove catheter from container and lubricate first 4 to 6 inches with lubricant; place other end over receptacle or toilet to catch urine.
5. Hold penis at right angles to the body, keeping foreskin retracted.
6. Insert catheter 7 to 10 inches into penis or until urine flows; then insert one more inch.
7. Allow catheter to drain while pressing down with abdominal muscles to promote complete emptying.
8. After drainage is complete, gently withdraw catheter.
9. Wash and dry area.
10. Wash catheter in warm soapy water, rinse with clear water, shake dry (to eliminate excess water in lumen), and dry outside with paper towel. Place in a plastic bag for storage. (Use catheters for 2 to 4 weeks; then discard.)
11. Wash hands.

Eleanor M. Stockbridge, CRRN, MS, FNP, *Community Nurse Case Manager, Poudre Valley Health System, Fort Collins, Colorado* saw palmetto, *Serenoa repens, Echinacea,* or pollen to lessen BPH manifestations.

DIAGNOSIS, OUTCOMES, INTERVENTIONS

Ineffective Management of Therapeutic Regimen (Individuals). The nurse has a major teaching role to help the client avoid *Ineffective Management of Therapeutic Regimen related to lack of understanding of disease, manifestations, and medical treatments.*

Outcomes. The client will understand disease, manifestations, and medical treatment, as evidenced by client statements, increased fluid intake, and ability to follow medication regimen.

Interventions

Provide Teaching About BPH. Men often have only a vague understanding of what an enlarged prostate is, much less where the gland lies. Many men fear they have prostate cancer or that BPH is a precursor of prostate cancer. Beliefs about treatment affecting their sexual functioning are also a concern. Show the client and significant other a picture of the reproductive organs and prostate, and explain the effects of enlargement on urine excretion.

Encourage Fluids. Many clients limit their fluid intake to combat the manifestations of BPH. Explain that concentrated urine acts as an irritant to the bladder. Caffeine, alcohol, acidic juices, and spicy foods may also irritate the bladder and should be avoided. Clients increase their risk of UTI with limited fluid intake. Unless it is otherwise contraindicated, the client should maintain an intake of at least 2000 ml/day to prevent UTI.

Explain Medications. If medications are being used to treat BPH, men need a thorough explanation of how the medications work, their side effects, and precautions. Warn the client to increase dosage only under the physician's orders because more medication may not help manifestations and may cause serious cardiovascular problems. Encourage clients to be patient, as effects of medication on the prostate may take time. Discourage clients from taking medications that contain alpha-adrenergic agonists, such as cold medicines and diet pills, because they can cause a man with BPH to experience acute urinary retention.

Altered Urinary Elimination. The client with BPH usually experiences manifestations such as frequency, urgency, hesitancy, change in stream, incontinence, retention, and nocturia. Write the nursing diagnosis as *Altered Urinary Elimination related to increasing urethral occlusion.*

Outcomes. The client will remain free of manifestations of BPH or those manifestations will decrease with treatment, as evidenced by absence of frequency, urgency, hesitancy, change in stream, incontinence, retention, or nocturia.

Interventions

Catheterize. When the client has urinary difficulties, such as obstruction, urinary retention, or diminished renal function, some form of catheterization may be necessary. Table 38–1 shows various types of urethral catheters, and the Bridge to Home Health Care feature explains intermittent self-catheterization for men. Never force a urinary catheter. If it cannot be inserted with gentle pressure, notify a urologist, who may need special instruments to get the catheter past the obstruction. Bladder spasms are common with indwelling catheters. If bladder discomfort and leakage are significant, medications can be ordered to reduce them (see Chapter 34). Clean the meatus several times a day with water and mild soap.

Monitor Urine Output. If an indwelling catheter is placed for acute retention, observe the client for hourly urinary output (should be at least ½ ml/kg/hr), hematuria, and shock caused by postobstructive diuresis. Hematuria can occur because of the sudden release of pressure on the blood vessels supplying the bladder. Postobstructive diuresis means increased urine output caused by inability of the renal tubules to absorb water and electrolytes after prolonged urinary obstruction. It is usually self-limiting but can cause sodium depletion in some clients, which leads to vascular collapse and death if not detected and treated.

EVALUATION

The client should be able to manage the manifestations of the disease and to take the medication appropriately. Clients should also continue follow-up so that the usefulness of the medical treatment can be assessed. Surgical intervention may be needed if medical management fails.

■ Surgical Management

Surgery is indicated for severe obstruction, recurrent UTIs, hematuria, bladder stones, changes in the upper urinary tract, or severe discomfort and inconvenience of the client. The part of the gland causing the obstruction is removed in a procedure called a *prostatectomy.* The term prostatectomy is a misnomer because the procedure is actually removal of new tissue growth. The true prostate and fibrous capsule are not removed. Figure 38–2 illustrates various surgical approaches. The method used depends on the size of the prostate and the general health of the client.

Regrowth of prostate tissue after prostatectomy for BPH may require a second operation, but this is rare. Prostate cancer may still develop because the total prostate is not removed. These clients need the same follow-up as other men who have not had prostate surgery.

OPERATIVE TECHNIQUE

Transurethral Resection

Transurethral resection of the prostate (TURP) is the most widely used of all prostatic surgical techniques. Newer surgical procedures are also used for treating BPH, but TURP is still the "gold standard" with which they are compared. TURP is especially suitable for men who have relatively small prostatic enlargements or are poor surgical risks. No incision is made.

A resectoscope is inserted through the urethra (Fig. 38–2A). The surgeon is able to visualize the inside of the bladder by inserting a telescope through the resectoscope. A movable loop is inserted through the resectoscope that cuts tissue and coagulates bleeding vessels with high-frequency electric current. (A cold-punch resectoscope that punches out tissue, piece by piece, with a circular knife blade is rarely used today.)

In a new procedure, transurethral electrovaporization of the prostate (the Vapor-Trode procedure), an electrova-

Text continued on page 954

Name	Appearance	Purpose or Use	Remarks
URINARY CATHETERS			
1. Nélaton red rubber urethral catheter		One-time, immediate drainage of the bladder; used when indwelling catheter is not needed	Blunt, round-tip straight catheter with one eye
2. Robinson red rubber urethral catheter		Same as No. 1	Round, hollow-tip straight catheter with two eyes
3. Councill red rubber urethral catheter (5-ml balloon)		Used when passage of a filiform or guide wire is required	Hole at tip
4. Tiemann coudé red rubber urethral catheter		Used when a catheter must be negotiated through a urethral, prostatic, or bladder neck blockage	Curved, olive-tip catheter with two eyes

5. Indwelling Foley urethral catheter		Used when a catheter must be retained in the bladder for continuous drainage	Various French sizes of catheters with 5- or 30-ml balloon
6. Three-way Foley urethral catheter		Used when irrigation of a retention catheter may be needed (e.g., after transurethral resection of the prostate)	Various French sizes of catheters with 5- or 30-ml balloon and a third port for irrigation
7. Coudé round-tip Foley urethral catheter		Used when retention catheter must be passed through urethral, prostatic, or bladder neck blockage	Curved tip; various French sizes of catheters with 5- or 30-ml balloon
8. Double-balloon Foley urethral catheter		Used when bladder drainage and pressure on a resected area must be accomplished simultaneously	

Table continued on following page

TABLE 38–1   UROLOGIC INSTRUMENTS MOST COMMONLY ENCOUNTERED IN A CLINICAL SETTING *Continued*

Name	Appearance	Purpose or Use	Remarks
9. Malecot catheter		Sometimes used to drain and irrigate continent reservoirs; for temporary or continuous suprapubic drainage	Self-retaining winged catheter; design may have two or four wings; Stamey type used for suprapubic puncture
10. Otis bougie à boule		Catheter-like device used to dilate urethra; used to calibrate urethral passage	Olive tip; usually available in even sizes from 8 to 40 F
11. Walther sound. *A,* Dilator. *B,* Tapered dilator		Metal instrument used to dilate female urethra	Tapers toward handle
12. Béniqué sound		Used to dilate male urethra	Curve in tip is more pronounced than in other sounds
13. LeFort sound		Often used to dilate severe (usually trauma-induced) urethral strictures in males	Threaded tip for attachment of woven filiform

14. Catheter stylet or guide

Stiff wire inserted into a channel catheter to make it rigid for easier insertion into the urethra

Another type of guide is the filiform guide wire; has threads at the end to attach filiforms to aid in inserting a Councill catheter

15. Filiforms (*A*) and followers (*B*)

Used to establish access to the urinary bladder when urethral abnormalities exist or to dilate urethral strictures

Filiform is small and has different shaped tips; follower attaches to end of filiform once entry to bladder has been established; available in variety of French sizes

From Karlowicz, K. A. (Ed.). (1995). *Urologic nursing: Principles and practice* (p. 660). Philadelphia: W. B. Saunders.

A. TRANSURETHRAL   B. SUPRAPUBIC

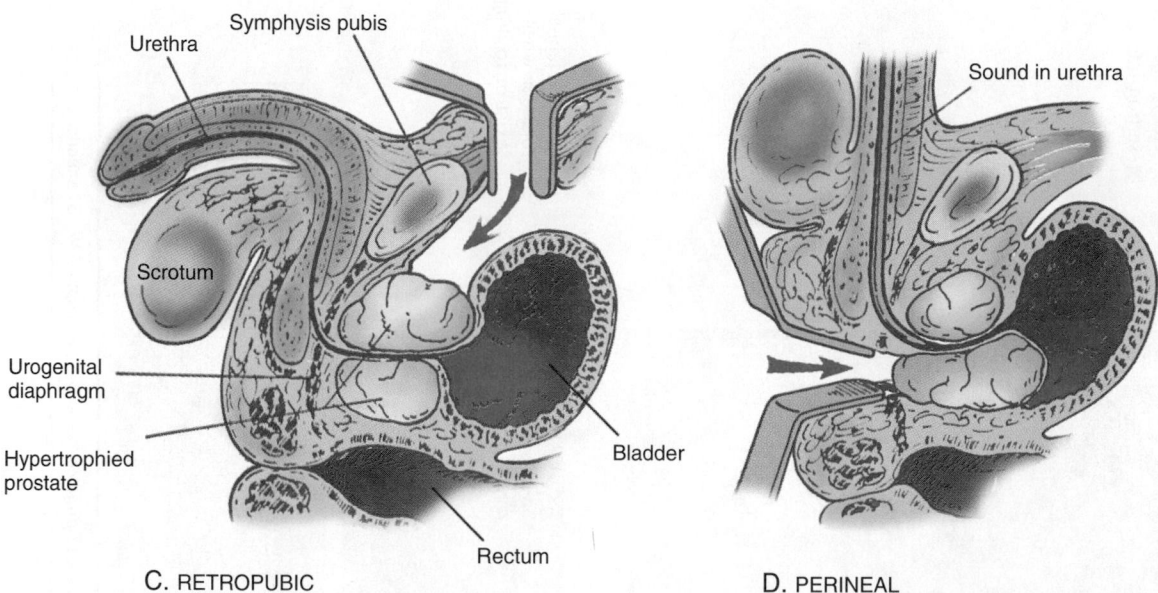

C. RETROPUBIC   D. PERINEAL

FIGURE 38–2 Surgical approaches to the prostate. *A,* Transurethral resection of the prostate (TURP) is a closed method of treatment; no incision is made, and the hyperplastic prostate tissue is removed through a resectoscope (like a cystoscope), which is inserted through the urethra. *B,* Suprapubic (transvesical) prostatectomy is an open method of treatment in which the hyperplastic prostatic tissue is enucleated through the anterior walls of the abdomen and bladder. *C,* Retropubic (extravesical) prostatectomy is an open method of treatment; a low abdominal incision is made between the pubic arch and the bladder. *D,* Perineal prostatectomy is an open method of treatment involving an incision between the anus and the scrotum.

porization ball or bar is inserted through the resectoscope. The ball or bar is attached to an electrocautery power source. Tissue vaporization requires electric power of 200 to 300 watts, compared with the 80 to 150 watts used to cauterize blood vessels during TURP.

Irrigating fluid can be passed into and out of the area through the scope; debris falls back into the bladder and is washed out. Closed-system, sterile gravity irrigation is used with an isotonic fluid solution. Water is never used because it is hypotonic, is absorbed into the bloodstream, and can precipitate hyponatremia, hypervolemia, hemolysis, and acute renal failure. Normal saline is also not used

because of the risk of conductivity injuries. Surgery must be completed within about 60 to 90 minutes to avoid excessive blood loss and absorption of irrigating fluid. Bleeding is common after this procedure; constant or intermittent irrigation may be required.

Suprapubic Prostatectomy

Suprapubic prostatectomy is a surgical approach that involves a lower abdominal incision (Fig. 38–2B). It may be the operation of choice when (1) the prostate is too large to be resected transurethrally; (2) a large, pedunculated middle prostatic lobe or later lobes are present; (3) a bladder abnormality needs correction; or (4) an abdominal surgical exploration is necessary. An incision is made into the bladder, and the enlarged tissue is enucleated by blunt dissection. Both suprapubic and urethral catheters are inserted. Bladder abnormalities can be treated concurrently with this procedure, and complete tissue removal is facilitated; however, hemostasis can be difficult to achieve.

The client may experience more bladder spasms, urinary leakage into the abdominal wound around the suprapubic catheter, and a relatively prolonged and uncomfortable convalescence. Incontinence and *erectile dysfunction* (impotence) can occur after this procedure.

Retropubic Prostatectomy

In the retropubic prostatectomy (Fig. 38-2C), the surgeon approaches the prostate through a low abdominal incision without entry into the bladder. This is the operation of choice when the prostate is very large and a severe urethral stricture is present. Advantages include direct visualization of the prostate and direct hemostasis in the prostatic fossa. Disadvantages are that associated bladder problems cannot be treated and osteitis pubis (pubic bone inflammation) may occur.

Perineal Prostatectomy

An incision is made into the perineum between the anus and the scrotum (see Fig. 38-2D). This operation is rarely used for treating BPH because of the great potential for erectile dysfunction. The client must be in a lithotomy position, which is contraindicated for people with severe arthritis or cardiopulmonary disease. Other complications include rectourethral fistula, UTIs, epididymitis, and urinary retention.

Transurethral Incision of the Prostate

Transurethral incision of the prostate (TUIP) is an option for men with a small prostate that is causing outlet obstruction. Incisions are made into the prostatic tissue to enlarge the lumen of the prostatic urethra. This procedure is associated with relatively few postoperative complica-

tions and can be performed with local anesthesia for high-risk clients. High client satisfaction has also been reported with this procedure; many clients report no change in ejaculation, which makes this an excellent procedure for younger men with a small prostate gland.

Transurethral Balloon Dilation of the Prostate

Transurethral balloon dilation of the prostate has become a popular technique (Fig. 38-3). The concept of dilating the prostate is not new—sounds, bougies, and other dilators have been used in the past—but use of the balloon is fairly new. The procedure is actually not surgical, but it is invasive.

A small catheter is inserted into the urethra. The balloon is positioned within the prostatic urethra and is inflated for 15 minutes. This measure applies pressure to the enlarged gland, which causes the prostatic urethra to dilate. Care is taken to ensure that the balloon does not migrate downward, which can damage the sphincter, or upward into the bladder, which can negate the effect of the procedure.

The client has a urethral catheter at least overnight. There is no blood loss, and postprocedure complications are few. There are two major concerns: (1) the duration of effectiveness of the procedure and (2) the possibility that prostate cancer will be missed because no tissue is removed. Manifestations may return in as little as 3 months, but some clients have gone without manifestations for more than 3 years.

Transurethral Ultrasound-Guided Laser Incision of the Prostate

Transurethral ultrasound-guided laser incision of the prostate (TULIP) is a newer procedure in which a laser is used to make the incision into the prostate. The procedure causes minimal blood loss, no irrigation is necessary, and the client does not need a catheter after surgery. This procedure is usually done in an ambulatory or outpatient setting.

FIGURE 38-3 Balloon dilation of the prostate. (After Dowd, J. B., & Smith, J. J. [1990]. Balloon dilation of the prostate. *Urologic Clinics of North America, 17*[3], 673.)

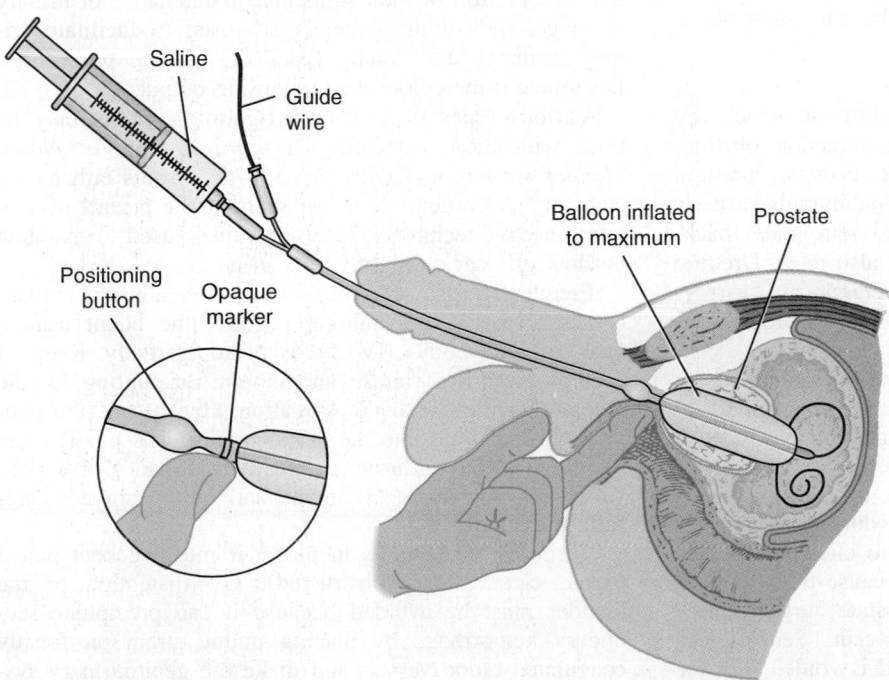

Saline

Guide wire

Positioning button

Opaque marker

Balloon inflated to maximum

Prostate

Visual Laser Ablation of the Prostate

Visual laser ablation of the prostate (VLAP) has become more successful since the development of right-angle laser fibers. Neodymium–yttrium aluminum garnet (YAG) is the medium that produces the energy to destroy tissue through a special endoscope. Sloughing of tissue may be delayed, but blood loss is minimal. Dysuria (painful urination) and the need for longer catheterization have been noted.

Hyperthermia and Thermal Therapy

Hyperthermia and thermal therapies are new procedures. Hyperthermia refers to administration of temperatures below 45° C; thermal therapy refers to administration of higher temperatures. Microwave, radiofrequency, or high-intensity ultrasound waves are used to heat prostate tissue. Microwave hyperthermia is delivered via a rectal probe over four to 10 treatments. Each treatment lasts about 60 minutes. Transurethral thermal therapy is showing more promising short-term results, but postprocedure urinary retention and urinary discomfort are significant side effects.

The transurethral needle ablation (TUNA) system uses radiofrequency energy to destroy prostatic tissue. All of these procedures are performed without anesthesia on an outpatient basis. The ultimate efficacy of these approaches has not been determined.

Prostatic Stent

Prostatic stent insertion, another new treatment, at first was used for clients who were extremely poor operative risks. The mesh-like tube (a coil-shaped device has also been used) can be inserted through an endoscope into the prostatic urethra, where it holds the urethra open mechanically. Over time, usually about 3 to 6 months, epithelial cells grow over the stent, which is permanent in most cases. Irritative voiding problems seem to be common but subside within several months. The stents have had to be removed when they migrate, become encrusted or infected, or cause persistent perineal discomfort. To prevent complications, clients should be cautioned not to be catheterized through the stent for 3 months after stent placement.

COMPLICATIONS

Complications after treatment, depending on which approach is used, may include bleeding, infection, obstruction, accidental displacement of the catheter, urethral stricture, bladder neck contracture, epididymitis, urinary incontinence, erectile dysfunction, and retrograde (backward) ejaculation. Manifestations may also recur. Urethral strictures and bladder neck contractures are usually treated with dilation. If this is ineffective, urethroplasty is a surgical option.

Persistent incontinence after prostate operations occurs in 2% to 4% of clients. Clients who have bladder instability along with obstruction preoperatively may need a year to attain complete urinary control.

Erectile dysfunction occurs in 5% to 10% of clients and only when nerves are damaged during surgery for prostate resection. Of major concern to clients is the occurrence of retrograde ejaculation. Because the verumontanum is destroyed during most prostate surgery, antegrade (forward) ejaculation cannot occur. Semen goes into the bladder during ejaculation and is voided with the next urination. The urine is cloudy. This effect is harmless, and the ability to have an erection or experience orgasm is not affected.

OUTCOMES

It is expected that the client will achieve significant improvement in manifestations without complications. Although many of these procedures are completed in an outpatient setting, the full benefits of the procedure may not be known for several weeks or months.

■ Nursing Management of the Surgical Client

PREOPERATIVE CARE

Assess the client's ability to empty his bladder. The bladder should be palpated for distention. If the client cannot void, a urethral catheter may have to be placed. Clients receiving anticoagulants should have stopped taking them, as ordered, before the procedure. Careful preoperative assessment in both physical and psychosocial areas is important. Assess the client's knowledge about the surgery and its outcomes.

You may be able to lessen the client's fear and anxiety by taking a nursing history and giving appropriate explanations. Respond to the concerns of the client and significant others with empathic listening, accurate information, and ongoing support. Restating the explanations given by the surgeon and anesthetist when securing informed consent may be necessary because stressed clients frequently forget what they have been told.

Informed consent requires that the man understand the risks (e.g., possible sexual dysfunction, including erectile dysfunction; retrograde ejaculation; and infertility) and short-term and long-term benefits (e.g., relief of urinary manifestations and arrested reduction of renal function). It is important for the client to receive honest answers to questions concerning sexuality and reproduction.

POSTOPERATIVE CARE
ASSESSMENT

Immediately after surgery, your major task is postoperative observation of vital signs and maintenance of urinary drainage. Indwelling catheters are used to facilitate urinary drainage after many types of prostate procedures. Document urine color when recording output.

Various types of catheter irrigation systems may be used with these catheters. Closed irrigation, or *closed bladder irrigation* (CBI) (Fig. 38–4), permits either constant or intermittent irrigation without the hazard of violating aseptic technique. Isotonic fluid is used to maintain outflow of clear or slightly pink urine.

Frequently assess drainage from the catheter. Urinary catheters should be draining because the client usually receives intravenous (IV) fluids postoperatively. Keep an accurate record of intake and output, accounting for the amount instilled with the irrigation. Because of the constant flow of fluid into the drainage bag, it is possible for the client to have a urine output of less than ½ ml/kg/hr, which may be missed if intake and output are not carefully measured.

While the catheter is in place, it must be kept patent (open, clear, and unobstructed). Overdistention of the bladder must be avoided because it can precipitate secondary hemorrhage by placing undue strain on freshly coagulated blood vessels and make the genitourinary sys-

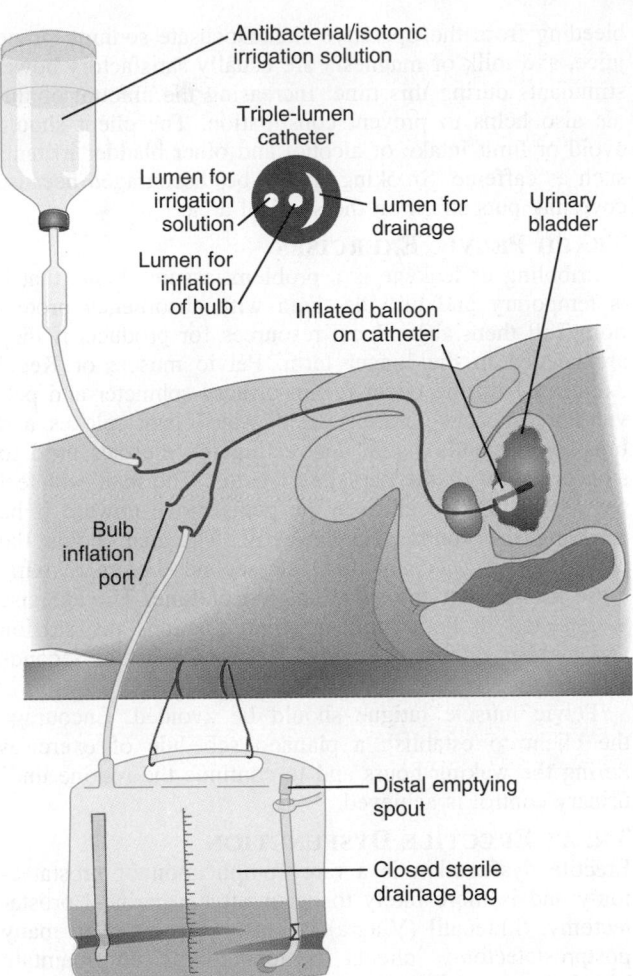

Antibacterial/isotonic irrigation solution

Triple-lumen catheter

Lumen for irrigation solution

Lumen for drainage

Urinary bladder

Lumen for inflation of bulb

Inflated balloon on catheter

Bulb inflation port

Distal emptying spout

Closed sterile drainage bag

FIGURE 38–4 A closed bladder irrigation system.

tem more prone to infection. Proper positioning of the catheter and drainage system is important to maintain good drainage and prevent obstruction of the system. Blood clots, prostatic debris, mucus plugs, kinked tubing, or catheter displacement may obstruct urinary flow. Assess catheter patency frequently to make sure the catheter is draining.

DIAGNOSIS, OUTCOMES, INTERVENTIONS

Risk for Injury. A common problem after all procedures is *Risk for Injury related to presence of urinary catheters, hematuria, irrigation, or suprapubic drains.*

Outcomes. The client will not experience hemorrhage, as evidenced by absence of gross bleeding, infection, catheter obstruction, and water intoxication and maintenance of urine output of at least ½ ml/kg per hour.

Interventions

Maintain Irrigation. Closed bladder irrigation decreases the development of obstruction. If obstruction is suspected, manual (hand) irrigation may be necessary. After prostatectomy for BPH, at least 60 ml of irrigant must be used, with some force, to dislodge and evacuate blood clots and other debris. If there is resistance to the introduction of irrigating fluid into the catheter or if there is no return of irrigating fluid, *do not force the fluid.* Notify the surgeon immediately. If a catheter cannot be cleared, it may have

to be removed and a new one inserted. In such cases, the surgeon usually performs this procedure.

Catheters and the procedures themselves cause increased urethral mucus production. Practice good meatal care. Keep the penis and meatal area clean by washing them with soap and water at least twice a day. Antibacterial ointments were formerly used, but they are no more effective than cleansing. Antibacterial soaps or antiseptics may dry out skin.

Monitor for Bleeding. Some hematuria is usual for several days after surgery. However, frank bleeding, arterial or venous, may occur during the first day after surgery. Arterial blood is bright red, has numerous clots, and is viscous. Blood pressure may fall, and emergency surgical intervention may become necessary. Venous bleeding in the prostatic area may be controlled by increasing the pressure (adding fluid) in the balloon end of the urethral catheter, pulling the catheter tightly to move the balloon into the prostatic fossa, and taping or using a Velcro device (self-fastening tape) to secure the catheter to the thigh (called *applying traction*). Traction is left in place for 24 hours or more and is released by the physician when the bleeding has stopped. The surgeon can also remove fluid slowly from the balloon as the bleeding decreases.

Prevent Catheter Dislodgment. The client may be confused immediately after surgery or may forget he has a catheter and accidentally pull out the catheter. Show him how to get in and out of the bed or chair without pulling on the catheter. Remind the client that he has a tube in his bladder through his penis or abdomen (whichever it is), and instruct him not to touch it. A displaced or removed urinary catheter after prostatic surgery is painful and disrupts recovery. Securing the catheter with a wide catheter holder, tape, or stockinette may be necessary. If the client does pull the catheter out, notify the surgeon immediately.

Prevent Infection. Observe the client carefully for local or systemic indications of infection. Handle catheters, drainage apparatus, and urine collection carefully to avoid introducing microorganisms into the urinary tract. Maintain a closed urinary drainage system unless manual irrigation is absolutely required. Encourage increased fluid intake, ambulation, and deep-breathing exercises.

Wound drains are usually removed earlier than suprapubic catheters. Keep skin around drain and catheter sites clean, dry, and protected. Observe for redness, edema, or infection.

The suprapubic catheter is left in place until voiding function has returned. When the client is voiding well, the suprapubic catheter can be removed. Expect urinary leakage from the suprapubic catheter site, mostly on the day the catheter is removed, until the wound is completely healed. Frequent dressing changes are necessary at first. If a suprapubic catheter is removed before the client has returned to normal voiding, the wound may not heal properly, leading to fistula formation.

Monitor for Retention. The length of time urethral catheters are left in place varies according to the surgeon's preference, the client's recovery, and the type of surgery. After a urethral catheter is removed (and after a transurethral resection), monitor the client closely for manifestations of urinary retention or difficulty.

Manage Temporary Incontinence. Advise the client that irritative manifestations such as frequency, urgency, leakage, and dysuria are natural until complete healing occurs. Keep reminding him that these problems are temporary and may take some time to resolve. Be understanding of the man's feelings, and keep him dry without embarrassing him. Absorbency products may be needed temporarily. They vary in size, shape, and absorbency capacities. Pelvic muscle exercises may help to reduce this problem. Additional surgery is sometimes required for persistent incontinence.

Pain. A common nursing diagnosis is *Pain related to surgery and bladder spasms.*

Outcomes. The client's pain will be under control, as evidenced by the client's report.

Interventions. Pain control after surgery is discussed in Chapters 15 and 23. Bladder spasms frequently occur after prostate procedures. Be sure that the drainage system is not obstructed, because obstruction as well as bladder irritation causes bladder spasms. Antispasmodic medications, such as belladonna and opium suppositories, propantheline bromide (Pro-Banthine) or oxybutynin (Ditropan), may be prescribed. They may cause complications, however. Clients with severe cardiac disease or glaucoma should not receive these agents. Since antispasmodic drugs can cause constipation and straining at stool can precipitate bleeding from the operative site, stool softeners such as docusate sodium (Colace) are often given.

EVALUATION

It is expected that the client will be discharged without complications and resume regular activities within 4 to 6 weeks. Depending on the procedure performed, some clients return home the same day. The client who has undergone TURP is usually discharged about 2 to 3 days after the operation. Clients who had open procedures are discharged after 4 to 6 days. Voiding of urine improves, and complications such as urgency, frequency, and dribbling end within 3 months.

▣ Self-Care

PROVIDE TEACHING

In addition to teaching the client verbally, give him written materials to take home after discharge. If applicable, review catheter and wound management. Clients who go home with a catheter have leg bags for day use and a Foley bag for use at night.

Some activities are limited after prostatectomy. The surgeon's orders should be followed regarding heavy lifting, strenuous activity, prolonged sitting, sexual activity, and driving or riding in an automobile. Because prolonged sitting increases intra-abdominal pressure and may precipitate bleeding, the man should avoid sitting except during meals. Clients should avoid driving an automobile or taking prolonged automobile rides until at least 2 weeks after surgery, when the risk of bleeding lessens. Strenuous exercise is also contraindicated for 4 to 6 weeks.

PREVENT INJURY

Advise the client not to strain during defecation for at least 6 weeks after surgery, because this can lead to bleeding from the operative site. Docusate sodium, prune juice, and milk of magnesia are usually satisfactory bowel stimulants during this time. Increasing the amount of fluids also helps to prevent constipation. The client should avoid or limit intake of alcohol and other bladder irritants such as caffeine. Smoking should be discouraged because coughing puts strain on the surgical area.

TEACH PELVIC EXERCISES

If dribbling or leakage is a problem, assure clients that it is temporary and provide them with absorbency protection. Tell them about local resources for products if they are needed in the longer term. Pelvic muscle or Kegel exercises help the client regain urinary sphincter and pelvic floor muscle control. Briefly, the client relaxes and breathes normally while contracting the muscles used to stop urination or the passage of flatus. The man will feel the rectum tighten and see the penis move upward if he is doing the contraction correctly. The man holds the contraction for a count of a few seconds before relaxing these muscles for the same amount of time. The exercise is repeated in both number of contractions per session and number of sessions per day. The number of seconds a contraction is held can also be increased.

Pelvic muscle fatigue should be avoided. Encourage the client to establish a planned schedule of exercises during the waking hours and to continue the routine until urinary control is achieved.

TREAT ERECTILE DYSFUNCTION

Erectile dysfunction is a rare complication of prostatectomy and is more likely to occur after a perineal prostatectomy. Sildenafil (Viagra) is now being given to many postprostatectomy clients postoperatively to maintain blood flow to the corpora cavernosa during the recovery period. As a result, fewer men are experiencing erectile dysfunction.

Information and supportive care of the significant other are extremely important. Referral for sexual counseling may be helpful. The man needs to know that he can still please a partner and that lovemaking techniques other than intercourse may be necessary. The couple may need information about alternatives to intercourse, such as cuddling, stroking, or manual or oral stimulation to orgasm. Vacuum erection devices, intracorporeal injections, and intraurethral or oral medications are also topics that sexual counselors can discuss. A penile implant may be considered (see Erectile Dysfunction later).

ARRANGE FOLLOW-UP

Be sure the client knows when and where to reach the surgeon and how to get in touch with health care professionals if he has concerns. He should especially report any elevated temperature, unusual bleeding, signs of wound infection or UTI, and obstructed urinary flow. He should know the date and time of his follow-up appointment with the surgeon.

PROSTATE CANCER

Prostate cancer is the most common cancer among men and the second most common cause of cancer death among men in the United States. The American Cancer Society has estimated that 180,400 new cases of prostate cancer would be diagnosed in the United States in the year 2000.[1] The risk for development of prostate cancer increases with age, and the disease typically occurs in men at age 50 years and older. Younger men tend to have more aggressive disease. African American men have a higher rate of prostate cancer. The diagnosis of prostate cancer is more common today because of the development of better screening tools.

Etiology and Risk Factors

The cause of prostate cancer is unknown, but epidemiologic studies suggest several associated factors. BPH does not lead to the development of prostate cancer.

Men with a family history of prostate cancer are at greater risk. Research has identified a gene on the X chromosome that appears more often in men with prostate cancer who have strong family histories. The gene, called human prostate cancer on the X chromosome (*HPCX*), is in the early stages of investigation.

Because the risk of prostate cancer increases with age, it may be associated with the hormonal shifts that accompany aging. It is rarely found in men younger than 40 years of age. Occult prostate cancer has been demonstrated at autopsy in 95% of men older than 90 years who died of other causes.

Diet may also be a factor. Asians have a lower rate of prostate cancer, but the rate is increased in those who move to the United States. High fat consumption (typical of American diets) can alter cholesterol and steroid metabolism, which may increase the risk of cancer. Green and yellow vegetables (typical of Japanese diets) and lycopene in cooked tomatoes may have a protective effect against prostate cancer. Some studies have postulated that a vitamin D deficiency may play a role. People who received more sunlight exposure had a lower incidence of and lower death rate from prostate cancer.

Occupational and environmental exposure to carcinogens may be risk factors. A higher incidence of prostate cancer is found in men living in urban areas. Occupations linked to higher rates of prostate cancer include employment in fertilizer, textile, and rubber industries and work with batteries containing cadmium.

Sexually transmitted virus-like organisms have been found in prostate cancer tissue, suggesting that viruses may be associated with the disease. High levels of testosterone have also been linked to development of prostate cancer.

Questions have arisen regarding a relationship between vasectomy and the development of prostate cancer, although the National Institutes of Health (NIH) has concluded that a relationship could not be proved. The NIH recommended further study but suggested no change in practice for providing vasectomies. The NIH also recommended that prostate cancer screening be the same for men who have and have not had vasectomies.

It is hoped that late prostatic cancer will become rare as increasing emphasis is placed on early diagnosis through routine rectal examinations, rectal ultrasound studies, measurements of PSA, and prompt intervention.

Except for diet, not much has been discovered in relation to prevention of prostate cancer. Reducing saturated fats and increasing the intake of lycopene (found in tomatoes) seem to reduce the incidence of the disease. Other dietary ingredients being investigated are genistin and diadzien (found in soy products), selenium, and vitamin E.

Health maintenance activities include annual digital rectal examinations and determination of serum PSA levels for early detection. Health restoration includes teaching pelvic muscle exercises to improve return of urinary control in postoperative clients and sexual counseling after radical perineal prostatectomy.

Pathophysiology

Prostate tumors are usually adenocarcinomas that begin in the periphery of the posterior lobe of the gland, whereas BPH occurs centrally and the gland is large by the time it restricts urination. The tumor may appear as normal prostatic tissue, which delays diagnosis. Typically, such lesions grow slowly and remain confined to the prostatic capsule, and if they occur late in life, the client may die of other causes. Sometimes, however, the tumor grows rapidly and metastasis has occurred by the time a diagnosis is made.

When prostate cancer metastasizes (spreads), it does so mainly through direct extension to the bladder neck and seminal vesicles. Other spread occurs through lymphatic and hematogenous routes. Obturator and iliac nodes are commonly positive. With advanced disease, metastasis to the bone is common, as is spread to the lungs and liver.

Clinical Manifestations

Men with prostate cancer commonly have no manifestations. Manifestations are usually related to other prostate conditions such as BPH and prostatitis. Early diagnosis through PSA measurement and digital rectal examination is essential. These tests are recommended for men between 50 and 70 years of age and younger men if they are African American or have a family history of the disease. The benefit of PSA screening after a man is 70 years old with a life expectancy of less than 10 years is questionable.

PSA, a glycoprotein produced by the prostate gland, may be elevated in men with prostate conditions. The detection rate of PSA screening for prostate cancer is about 55%. Normal PSA levels are below 4.0 ng/ml, but some variation is allowed for age and other conditions. A PSA level below 4.0 ng/ml is of concern if there is a rapid rise (i.e., 2.0 to 3.5). A hard nodule, asymmetry, or induration felt on digital rectal examination raises the suspicion of malignancy.

Other specialized tests that may be performed when PSA levels and digital rectal examination findings are normal but prostate cancer is suspected measure *prostate-specific antigen density* (PSAD) and *free PSA*. These tests seem to be more useful as part of the screening process when the PSA value is moderately elevated (4 to 10 ng/ml).

- The PSAD is calculated by dividing the PSA by the prostatic volume, as determined on ultrasonography. Men with PSAD scores above 0.15 are more likely to have cancer than men with lower PSAD scores.
- Free PSA is PSA that is not bound to proteins in the blood. Prostate cancer cells secrete more bound PSA than normal or noncancerous cells. Therefore, a lower ratio of free PSA to total PSA suggests prostate cancer and the need for further tests.

If the PSA is elevated or an abnormal prostate is felt, or both, the client undergoes a transrectal prostate biopsy with ultrasound imaging. The client must not take aspirin-containing medications or anticoagulants for several days before prostate biopsy in order to prevent bleeding at the biopsy sites. Premedication with diazepam or similar medications should be offered.

A probe is inserted into the rectum so that the prostate can be visualized and measured. Small cores of tissue are taken from different areas of the prostate for pathologic examination. Ultrasound visualization cannot confirm the presence or absence of cancer; it helps guide the needle to selected areas. The client and physician wait for the pathology report. Complications include bleeding, infection, and a missed cancer. Biopsies are also performed by a transperineal approach in some institutions.

Prostate cancer is graded according to the differentiation of tumor cells. Differentiation is directly related to the cancer's aggressiveness. *Well-differentiated* cancer cells differ only slightly from normal cells and tend to grow slowly. *Poorly differentiated* cancer is characterized by very abnormal, disorganized cells that tend to grow more rapidly. A Gleason score on a scale of 1 to 5 is given to the tissues examined on the basis of primary and secondary tumor patterns. The Gleason score is the sum of two grades assigned to the different areas:

- Well differentiated, a score of 2 to 4
- Moderately well differentiated, a score of 5 to 7
- Poorly differentiated, a score of 8 to 10

A premalignant condition that may appear on a prostate pathology report is *prostatic intraepithelial neoplasia* (PIN). Close surveillance is necessary and may include repeated prostate biopsies throughout the gland.

If prostate cancer is found, additional tests are ordered to stage the cancer and to determine how far it has spread. Staging is done through bone scans, computed tomography (CT), or magnetic resonance imaging (MRI). Two main classification systems are used to stage prostate cancer: the Whitmore-Jewett A-B-C-D system and the tumor, nodes, and metastasis (TNM) system. These classifications are outlined in Box 38–1.

BOX 38–1   Staging and Grading of Prostate Tumors

Stage A: Tumor Microscopic (T1 N0 M0)
A1: Microscopic focus
A2: Diffuse

Stage B: Tumor Macroscopic (T1–2 N0 M0)
B1: One lobe involved, nodule ≤ 1.5 cm
B2: Both lobes involved, nodule ≥ 1.5 cm

Stage C: Tumor Extracapsular (T3 N0 M0)
C1: Localized, nodule ≤ 70 g
C2: Pelvic sidewall fixation, nodule ≥ 70 g

Stage D: Metastatic Disease (T4, N1–3, M)
D1: Confined to pelvis
D2: Extrapelvic

A specific imaging scan can be used to locate metastases of prostate cancer in soft tissue. Capromab pendetide (ProstaScint) targets prostate-specific membrane antigen (PSMA), which is found in prostate cancer cells. Two sessions 4 days apart are required. The ProstaScint scan is especially useful in finding "skipped" metastases (i.e., abdominal lymph node involvement without pelvic lymph node involvement), but it is expensive.

Outcome Management

Nursing Management of Clients Undergoing Diagnosis

PROVIDE SUPPORT
Men with prostate cancer and their significant others need ongoing sensitive support and accurate information to make the difficult decisions required of them. Their concerns are considerable and may include the choices of available treatments, fear of death, anxiety about residual disability and illness, feelings of loss of control, and the possible effects of the illness on people in their social network and in their marriage. After diagnosis, prostate cancer can affect their masculinity and self-esteem. Depression and fatigue are common after many treatments for prostate cancer.

SUGGEST RESOURCES
Increased awareness of prostate cancer has led to the development of many resources, including books, articles, and Internet Web sites in the public sector. Local and national prostate cancer support groups have organized. Information is also available from the American Cancer Society (Man to Man program), the American Foundation for Urologic Disease in Baltimore (800-242-2383), and US TOO International in Hinsdale, Ill. (800-808-7866).

Be sure to include the client's partner or spouse in planning care at the time of diagnosis and when the client is choosing treatment as well as when he is adapting to the treatment. The partner usually takes on essential support responsibilities when the client is gathering information and coping with the disease and treatments.

Surgical Management

RADICAL PROSTATECTOMY
Radical prostatectomy is the treatment of choice for cancer confined within the prostate if the client is in good enough health to undergo surgery and has a life expectancy of 10 to 15 years. Radical surgery involves removing the entire prostate gland (rather than just enucleation), the outer capsule, the seminal vesicles, sections of the vas deferens, adjacent lymph nodes, and portions of the bladder neck. Bilateral prostatic lymph node dissection (BPLND) is not done as much today in health care institutions, especially when PSA values and Gleason scores are low. Laparoscopic lymph node dissection is performed when required.

Surgical approaches include retropubic (see Fig. 38–2C) and perineal (see Fig. 38–2D) approaches. Radical retropubic surgery is the procedure most commonly performed. Today techniques are used to preserve the neurovascular bundles, which reduces the consequences of permanent erectile dysfunction or incontinence. Bladder neck contracture occurs in about 5% of clients.

In some institutions, radical perineal prostatectomy is an alternative approach. The rates of seminal vesicle and rectal injury are higher, but the incidence of incontinence and erectile dysfunction is about the same when surgeons are experienced with the two techniques. After this procedure, less blood is lost during surgery and less postoperative pain occurs.

CRYOSURGICAL ABLATION

In cryosurgical ablation of the prostate, the surgeon uses guided transrectal ultrasonography to insert cryoprobes into desired areas of the prostate to freeze and thereby destroy the tissue. A warming tube in the urethra keeps the urethra from freezing. Cryosurgery may be an option for clients with localized cancer and other serious medical conditions that preclude them as candidates for radical surgery. Although the technique is less invasive and causes less pain and bleeding than radical surgery, it is considered investigational.

▮ Nursing Management of the Surgical Client

PREVENT INJURY

The physical nursing care for the client with prostatic cancer is essentially the same as that for clients undergoing other major surgery (see Chapter 15) and similar to that for the client undergoing surgery for BPH. A few special exceptions are observed:

1. The catheter stays in at least 2 to 3 weeks after the surgery while the anastomosis of bladder and urethra heals.
2. Securing the catheter to prevent accidental removal is imperative.
3. Enemas and rectal thermometers are avoided in most hospitals and used with extreme caution in others.

A midline lower incision is closed with staples and drains are in place when a retropubic approach is used. Regularly observe drainage, and change or reinforce dressings as ordered. If a perineal approach is used, aseptic technique is especially important because of the high possibility of infection in a wound close to the anal area. Sitz baths or heat lamps may be ordered to facilitate perineal wound healing. A double-tailed T binder, mesh pants, or scrotal support may be used to secure perineal dressings.

PROVIDE SUPPORT

The psychosocial and emotional care of these clients differs from care of clients with BPH because issues such as cancer and sexual image must be addressed. Thoughts of postoperative self-care at home are overwhelming. Both the client and significant other need detailed instructions, much reassurance, and resources for supplies and advice should concerns surface at home. Sildenafil (Viagra) is given to many clients after prostatectomy to maintain blood flow to the corpora cavernosa during recovery. As a result, fewer men are experiencing erectile dysfunction.

▮ Medical Management

Medical management of prostate cancer is approached in several ways: radiation, hormonal manipulation, watchful waiting, and, sometimes, chemotherapy. One of these approaches is always chosen for cancer that has spread outside the prostate. Controversy exists regarding the most effective management of prostate cancer.

Watchful waiting is a reasonable choice only when a client has a very low-grade, low-stage prostate cancer. Many physicians add the criterion that life expectancy should be less than 10 years. Mortality in older clients is often due to other causes. Routine follow-up and PSA determinations are very important. If there are changes in the digital rectal examination or PSA elevation, treatment should be initiated.

DECREASE TUMOR GROWTH

RADIATION THERAPY. Radiation therapy is an alternative choice for cancer confined to the prostate. Treatment can be in the form of external beam radiation, interstitial seed implantation, or a combination of both methods. Radiation therapy can be used to reduce bone pain when prostate cancer has metastasized. Strontium 89 (Metastron) and samarium 153 lexidronam (Quadramet) are radioactive agents that are injected to help control pain related to bone metastases. Men usually begin to notice a reduction in pain 10 to 20 days after the injection. Pain reduction lasts for 4 to 15 months but usually only about 6 months. If pain returns, the injection can be repeated every 3 months with no limit on the number of injections given.

External beam radiation is administered to the prostate and surrounding tissue daily for several weeks (see Chapter 19).

In the technique of interstitial seed implantation (*brachytherapy*), special needles are used to insert radioactive isotopes directly into the prostate. Because the radioactive focus of the seeds is more controlled than in external beam radiation, surrounding tissues are usually not as affected. Radioactive palladium, iodine, or gold seeds are used for this procedure. The long half-life of these seeds allows delivery of an effective radiation dose for 1 year. Temporary irritative and obstructive voiding manifestations are common after implantation.

HORMONAL THERAPY. Hormonal manipulation blocks androgen (testosterone) production and includes a selection or combination of bilateral orchiectomy, estrogens, gonadotropin-releasing hormone analogs, and antiandrogens. The greatest amount of androgen is produced in the testicles, and small amounts are produced in the adrenal glands.

Orchiectomy (removal of testicles) is a minor surgical procedure that removes the source of androgen. Local anesthesia is usually used. Because the procedure is irreversible, the psychological impact on a man is great. Most men want medications to control their prostate cancer.

Estrogen. Estrogen (diethylstilbestrol) suppresses the release of pituitary gonadotropin and reduces serum testosterone levels. Side effects can be serious and include edema, myocardial infarction, cerebrovascular accident, hypertension, thrombophlebitis, and pulmonary embolism. Gynecomastia and abdominal discomfort are other side effects.

Gonadotropin-Releasing Hormone (GnRH) Analogs. GnRH analogs, commonly called luteinizing hormone–releasing hormone (LHRH) agonists, stimulate and then suppress pituitary gonadotropins, which interferes with androgen production in the testicles. Leuprolide (Lupron) and goserelin acetate (Zoladex) are injected every 1 to 4 months, depending on the time-released dosage. Hot flashes, erectile dysfunction, loss of libido, and minor weight gain caused by water retention are common side effects. The client with metastasis and bone pain may experience an initial increase in pain or voiding manifestations.

Antiandrogens. Antiandrogens such as flutamide (Eulexin) and bicalutamide (Casodex) block androgens produced by the adrenal glands. These medications are often combined with LHRH therapy. Gynecomastia, diarrhea, and erectile dysfunction are common side effects. Finasteride is also used.

Intermittent Hormonal Therapy. Use of intermittent hormonal therapy is a newer concept for control of disease and prevention of hormonal side effects or resistance to hormonal treatment. It is being investigated as a safe alternative to continuous hormonal therapy for prostate cancer.

CHEMOTHERAPY. Chemotherapy is used for palliation (alleviation of manifestations) when prostate cancer is hormone-resistant. Chemotherapeutic agents may be given singly or in combination, depending on protocols. Examples of agents sometimes used are cyclophosphamide (Cytoxan), fluorouracil, estramustine phosphate (Emcyt), doxorubicin (Adriamycin), and mitomycin (Mutamycin), taxol, and VP-16 or etoposide (Etopophos). Mitoxantrone (Novantrone) is a chemotherapeutic drug used in combination with corticosteroids to relieve pain in hormone-resistant prostate cancer. This treatment is often successful after just one dose.

■ Nursing Management of the Medical Client

PROVIDE EDUCATION

Nursing care depends on the type of medical therapy. Explain how treatments help prostate cancer, their side effects, and expected outcomes. Repetitive explanations are often necessary because clients must absorb much information and make decisions during a period when they may be in a state of shock. Provide information in a variety of formats, and include telephone numbers to be called when the client or partner has questions.

EXPLAIN SIDE EFFECTS

Common side effects of external beam radiation to the pelvic area include irritable voiding problems, diarrhea, and dermatitis. If a client is undergoing brachytherapy, specific safety precautions should be followed. These entail how close family members can be to the client for the first week after therapy and how to retrieve and return expelled seeds.

Clients receiving hormonal manipulation therapy must comply with medication directions in order to maintain therapeutic blood levels. Clients need a great deal of support to help them cope with erectile dysfunction and hot flashes. With all approaches used for hormonal manipulation, the importance of follow-up cannot be overstressed.

PROVIDE SUPPORT

Encourage men with prostate cancer and their significant others to attend relevant support groups or to subscribe to publications by organizations mentioned earlier. The best ways for clients to control fear and to keep a positive

attitude are to learn as much as they can about treatments and to meet other men with prostate cancer. A health care provider who specializes in erectile dysfunction can best counsel a couple about ways to achieve sexual satisfaction.

RELIEVE PAIN

When a client has metastases, assess pain levels (see Chapter 23) as well as activities of daily living. Keeping a pain diary is useful for the client's and provider's awareness. Men tend to be stoic about pain and may have misconceptions about taking narcotics. Carefully explain that addiction and decreasing drug effectiveness are not problems when cancer pain is being treated. Better pain control helps a man stay active and in control of his life.

PROSTATITIS

Prostatitis (inflammation of the prostate gland) is a common and often perplexing problem. As many as 50% of men experience manifestations of prostatitis in their lifetime. Traditionally, prostatitis is categorized as acute bacterial prostatitis, chronic bacterial prostatitis, nonbacterial prostatitis, or prostatodynia (painful prostate without a cause). Nonbacterial prostatitis is the most common form of the disease.

Etiology and Risk Factors

Gram-negative bacteria such as *Escherichia coli, Klebsiella,* and *Enterobacter* are the usual cause of acute and chronic prostate infections. *Enterococcus,* a gram-positive organism, can also cause chronic prostate infection. Other organisms, such as *Chlamydia, Ureaplasma,* gonococci, and cytomegalovirus, are less common causes. It has also been proposed that nonbacterial prostatitis is an autoimmune disease.

Factors predisposing to chronic prostatitis are those that cause prostatic congestion, such as perineal trauma, excess alcohol intake, and certain sexual practices. Inadequately treated acute prostatitis may also predispose to chronic prostatitis. Muscle spasms in the prostate and bladder neck are believed to be the cause of prostatodynia, which occurs more frequently in younger and middle-aged men.

Pathophysiology

Routes of infection (Fig. 38–5) include urethral ascent, descent from the urinary bladder or kidneys, direct extension or lymphatogenous spread from the rectum, and hematogenous spread.

Marked inflammation occurs in acute prostatitis. Small abscesses or spread to the periprostatic space can occur if the condition is untreated. Repeated bouts of acute prostatitis may cause fibrosis within the gland and can be confused with prostate cancer on digital rectal examination. Small calculi (stones) commonly form in the prostate after chronic infections and are rarely significant.

Clinical Manifestations

The client's manifestations depend on the type of prostatitis he has. The client with acute bacterial prostatitis presents with abrupt onset of urinary urgency, frequency,

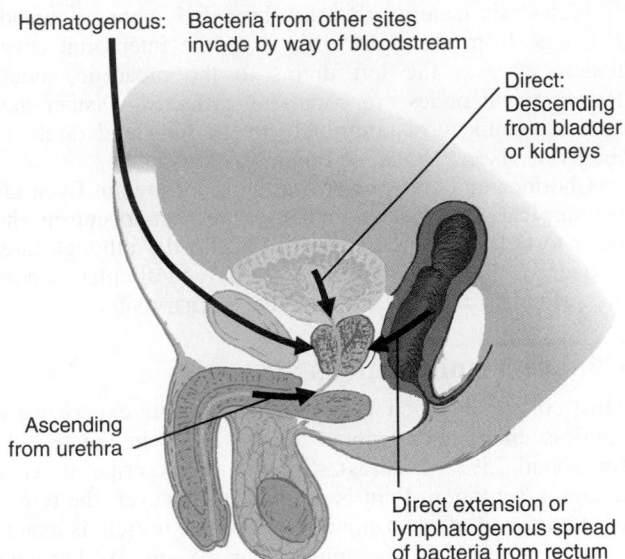

Hematogenous: Bacteria from other sites
invade by way of bloodstream

Direct:
Descending
from bladder
or kidneys

Ascending
from urethra

Direct extension or
lymphatogenous spread
of bacteria from rectum

FIGURE 38–5 Postulated pathways of infection to the prostate gland.

nocturia, and dysuria, and he may have urinary retention. Fever, chills, and malaise are present, and the client complains of low back and perineal pain. He appears quite ill and may be experiencing nausea and vomiting. The prostate is extremely tender and boggy when examined. Prostate massage (expression of prostate secretions via digital rectal examination) is usually not performed because it is painful to the client and can precipitate bacteremia. Urine is usually infected.

Manifestations may or may not be present in chronic bacterial prostatitis. Episodes of urinary infection may occur intermittently. Asymptomatic bacteriuria may be an incidental finding in some clients. Usually, voiding problems and pain are mild to moderate and rectal examination is normal or shows slight tenderness. Microscopic examinations of expressed prostatic secretions (EPSs) along with segmented urine cultures help to differentiate this condition from nonbacterial prostatitis, urethritis, and prostatodynia.

It is best if the client has a full bladder when segmented urine specimens are collected. The technique is as follows:

1. The client washes the glans and retracts the foreskin (if uncircumcised). He keeps the foreskin retracted throughout the entire urine collection procedure.
2. He voids about the first 10 ml of urine into a sterile container. This is the urethral specimen and is labeled VB1.
3. He then voids about another 200 ml of urine, and a specimen is obtained. This is the bladder specimen and is labeled VB2.
4. The client stops voiding after the second specimen, and a prostatic massage is performed to obtain prostatic secretions. This specimen is labeled EPS.
5. The client voids about another 10 ml. This specimen has prostatic secretions mixed in it and is labeled VB3.

All specimens are checked for the presence of white blood cells (WBCs) and are sent for culture analysis. If the VB1 and VB2 specimens have greater bacterial colony counts, urethritis and bladder infection, respectively, are the diagnoses. If the EPS and VB3 specimens have significantly greater colony counts, the diagnosis is bacterial prostatitis.

The manifestations of nonbacterial prostatitis are similar to those of chronic prostatitis. WBCs are found in the EPS, but no organism is found on culture analysis. Digital rectal examination findings are normal.

Men with prostatodynia complain of similar manifestations, but they have no history of UTI and have normal segmented urine specimens and EPS. Fever is never present. Pelvic and perineal pain is the major complaint.

Outcome Management

Medical Management

REDUCE INFLAMMATION
Clients with *acute* bacterial prostatitis may be so ill that they need hospitalization and IV antibiotics. Practically all antibiotics diffuse into the prostate when it is inflamed. Quinolones are the drugs of choice. Levofloxacin (Levaquin) is a newer quinolone drug that has less bacterial resistance potential than other drugs in this class. An alternative antibiotic is sulfamethoxazole-trimethoprim (Bactrim). Transurethral instrumentation is avoided unless absolutely necessary for urinary retention. The client should have at least 4 weeks of antibiotic therapy to eradicate the infection completely and to prevent chronic prostatitis.

The same antibiotics are used for *chronic* bacterial prostatitis because they can penetrate the noninflamed gland. Doxycycline (Vibramycin) is also used for both chronic and nonbacterial prostatitis. Clients with chronic bacterial prostatitis are treated longer with antibiotics, usually 3 months, and often given lower suppressive doses.

Because no bacteria are found in nonbacterial prostatitis, doxycycline may be ordered for 2 weeks to see whether there is any improvement in manifestations. It is not continued if there is no improvement.

Clients with prostatodynia are treated with alpha-blockers. Nonsteroidal anti-inflammatory drugs (NSAIDs), hot sitz baths, and regular sexual activity (ejaculation) may be ordered as adjunctive treatment.

Surgery may be considered for the client with chronic bacterial prostatitis when medical therapy does not improve manifestations that affect the man's quality of life; however, surgery is rarely performed because of the potential for surgical complications.

Nursing Management of the Medical Client

In all cases of prostatitis, rest, increased fluids, and analgesics are important. Sometimes alcohol or spicy foods exacerbate (worsen) manifestations. Be aware of manifestations of bacteremia. Constipation can be a painful problem for clients with prostatitis. Often, stool softeners are ordered.

The client may be uncomfortable, frustrated, and fearful that the manifestations will never go away or may lead to something more serious than infection. He may have sexual or fertility concerns or may believe that the infection can be sexually transmitted. Clients need much reassurance and teaching. They should understand the importance of complying with the total treatment course and know the side effects of prescribed medications. Clients should also be taught that increasing sexual activity or masturbation may help decrease prostatic gland congestion.

TESTICULAR AND SCROTAL DISORDERS

TESTICULAR CANCER

Testicular cancer is the most common and serious solid tumor cancer in men between the ages of 15 and 35 years. It rarely occurs in men younger than age 15 or older than age 40. In broad perspective, it is rare, with approximately 3.7 cases per 100,000 cases diagnosed in the United States and European countries each year. In many cases it is curable, sometimes even in an advanced stage.

Testicular cancer is less common in African American and Asian men. The incidence is about the same in Hispanic men as in white men. In Israel, the rate is three times higher in Jewish men than non-Jewish men. Testicular cancer is about twice as frequent in high socioeconomic groups.

Etiology and Risk Factors

The cause of testicular cancer is unknown. Family history, exogenous estrogen, and cryptorchidism (undescended testicles) are known risk factors. Cryptorchidism is the major risk factor. Surgery (orchiopexy) is recommended soon after birth, but it does not completely eliminate the risk of cancer.

The male offspring of women who used estrogen in the form of diethylstilbestrol (DES) during the first trimester of pregnancy (called *DES sons*) or who were exposed to estrogen-progestin combinations frequently used in diagnostic tests to confirm pregnancy are at greater risk for testicular cancer. Between 1940 and 1970, DES was given to pregnant women who had a high risk of spontaneous abortion. DES sons also have an increased risk of genitourinary abnormalities such as micropenis, meatal stenosis, varicocele, hypoplastic testicles, infertility, and abnormal semen.

Children with an undescended testicle should be closely observed. Men 15 to 45 years of age should practice monthly testicular self-examination (TSE) (see Chapter 37). Men at high risk for testicular cancer should see a physician for yearly examinations. Early detection can lead to early diagnosis and cure.

Pathophysiology

Most testicular cancers (90% to 95%) are germinal cell tumors, such as seminoma (about 30% to 40% of all tumors), embryonal carcinoma (about 20%), teratocarcinoma, or choriocarcinoma. Seminomas generally carry a favorable prognosis (about a 90% 5-year survival rate) because they are usually localized, metastasize late, and are radiosensitive.

Nongerminal tumors make up the remainder of testicular tumors and are classified as either interstitial cell tumors or testicular adenomas. They arise from interstitial cells or cells that compose the fibrous and vascular networks. They are usually benign.

Metastasis occurs primarily through lymphatic spread. Drainage from the right testis is to the interaortal caval nodes, whereas the left drains to the preaortic nodes. Retroperineal nodes are commonly affected. Distant metastasis occurs most commonly to the lung and rarely to the liver, viscera, bone, or brain.

Choriocarcinoma spreads via the bloodstream. Even after surgical removal, testicular cancer can occur in the other testicle. Carcinoma in situ (localized), although rare, frequently involves both testes. Rarely, testicular tumors are secondary to cancers in another primary site.

Clinical Manifestations

Most commonly, men with testicular tumors experience a painless enlargement, noted as heaviness, in the testicle (in about 75% of cases). Some men describe it as a dragging sensation. Pain is rarely felt; however, the tumor is often found after an injury because the testicle is examined as a result of the injury (Fig. 38–6). A thorough description of family and birth histories and manifestations is the first step in assessment.

Assessment findings suggesting metastasis to the retroperitoneal lymph nodes include back pain, vague abdominal pain, nausea and vomiting, bowel and bladder changes, anorexia, and weight loss. If the lungs are involved, manifestations may include cough, dyspnea, and hemoptysis.

The next step is physical examination of the scrotum and testicles, in which the health care provider determines the location and size of any nodule. If there is a nodule, a light may be held against the scrotum to see whether it is transilluminated (to see whether light passes through). Whereas cysts and hydroceles are transilluminated, tumors and hernias are not.

Ultrasonography of the testes follows. If tumor is suspected, chest x-ray studies and CT scans are ordered to detect metastases. An IVP may be ordered to detect urinary tract involvement.

Tumor usually asymptomatic. Found on testicular self-examination.

Scrotal discomfort may result from hemorrhage within tumor.

Pain is not usually elicited by squeezing. However, some men have testicular pain.

Testis does not transilluminate.

Testis may be irregular or ovoid.

Hydrocele or hematocele may develop.

Painless enlargement or heaviness of testicle.

FIGURE 38–6 Some characteristics of tumors of the testes.

Blood tests are ordered. Alpha-fetoprotein (AFP), beta human chorionic gonadotropin (beta-HCG), and lactic acid dehydrogenase (LDH) are the tumor markers used to detect testicular cancer. Elevated AFP is not seen in clients with testicular seminomas. Beta-HCG can be elevated in either seminomas or nonseminomas and, when elevated, may cause gynecomastia in men with testicular cancer. LDH is often elevated in germinal testicular cancers because of the cancer's cell activity, and this elevation also suggests metastasis because LDH is produced in the liver, kidney, and brain.

Testicular cancer is verified by inguinal exploration. If a definite mass is not found, a frozen biopsy may be done. If there is still suspicion, a radical orchiectomy is performed. The testis, epididymis, and vas deferens are removed. The spermatic cord is ligated just inside the internal inguinal ring to prevent seeding of the cancer. Any testicular mass is considered malignant until proved otherwise.

Staging testicular tumors helps to guess at prognosis and to determine treatment options. Testicular tumors are staged as follows:

Stage I_a: Tumor confined to testicle (T1 N0 M0)

Stage I: Metastasis to para-aortic or iliac nodes (T1 N1 M0)

Stage II: Tumor spread to retroperitoneal nodes but disease limited to below the diaphragm (T23, N2, M0)

Stage III: Tumor above the diaphragm or spread to body organs (usually the lungs) T4, N3–4, M+)

Outcome Management

■ Surgical Management

Radical orchiectomy, performed to diagnose testicular cancer, is also the primary treatment. *Retroperitoneal lymph node dissection* (RPLND) may be done when there is lymph node involvement. The primary use of this procedure is controversial in advanced-stage cancer because treatment with chemotherapy for nonseminomas is very successful. Impotence rates are high after RPLND because many of the autonomic nerves necessary for ejaculation are located in this area. RPLND is performed when testicular cancer is embryonal because this type of cancer metastasizes rapidly.

In other types of testicular cancer, surgeons who perform RPLND believe that it limits the amount of chemotherapy needed. This approach may be used as an adjunct to chemotherapy when only a partial response is achieved. A thoracoabdominal or transabdominal incision is made, and modified dissection techniques are used. The newest approach is a *laparoscopic node dissection.* A smaller incision and fewer complications (especially retrograde ejaculation) result after laparoscopic surgery.

■ Nursing Management of the Surgical Client

Clients undergoing radical orchiectomy usually require a short hospital stay and experience few complications. The scrotal area is tender and slightly swollen after surgery. Ice bags are applied to the scrotum, and a scrotal support is worn when the client is ambulating. Teach the client self-care strategies and how to monitor for the development of complications. Provide written instructions, a resource he can call should questions or concerns arise, and

a follow-up appointment with the surgeon. The client needs to be aware that testicular cancer can recur in the other testicle, and he should know how to do testicular self-examination.

If the client undergoes RPLND, hospitalization is longer, depending on the approach used. Counseling about potential infertility problems and sperm banking takes place before the procedure.

Postoperatively, the client must be monitored closely for possible problems associated with major abdominal surgery. The client requires adequate pain control to comply with ambulation and vigorous coughing and deep breathing to prevent respiratory complications. Anxiety and fear about cancer, sexuality, quality of life, and life expectancy are issues that must frequently be addressed. Be sure that follow-up appointments are made with the surgeon and oncologist for further treatment if appropriate.

■ Medical Management

Medical management follows radical orchiectomy during the treatment of testicular cancer. A period of close follow-up and observation is necessary to detect recurrence and plan future care.

DESTROY CANCER CELLS

RADIATION THERAPY. Low-grade seminomas are particularly radiosensitive. The perineum and pelvis are irradiated, as are the mediastinal and supraclavicular nodes if peritoneal nodes are positive for cancer. Side effects include common complications associated with pelvic radiation: irritable bowel and bladder problems, skin reactions, fatigue, nausea, and anorexia. Radiation may also cause temporary or permanent infertility. Side effects are usually minimal because the dose and number of treatments required are low. Almost 95% of clients with low-stage seminomas survive more than 5 years.

CHEMOTHERAPY. Nonseminomatous tumors are not radiosensitive, and they and high-grade seminomas are therefore treated with chemotherapy. The major agent used is cisplatin in combination with vinblastine and bleomycin. Cisplatin in combination with other agents dramatically increases the long-term survival rate for men with testicular cancer. These agents, in combination with a variety of others, have been used to treat metastatic disease or refractory tumors with some success. (Complications of these chemotherapeutic agents are covered in Chapter 19.) Cisplatin has nephrotoxic effects, bleomycin causes pneumonitis, and vinblastine causes peripheral neuropathy.

■ Nursing Management of the Medical Client

During assessment of a man born between 1940 and 1971, ask whether his mother took any medication during pregnancy to prevent pregnancy or miscarriage. If he appears at particular risk but does not know these details, it may be necessary to obtain the mother's medical history. Information and referral are available through DES Action, Long Island Jewish-Hillside Medical Center, New Hyde Park, NY 11040.

Supportive nursing care for these young men is important during both diagnosis and treatment. Be aware of the threat to sexuality that this condition and its treatment pose to young men. Chapter 19 reviews the care of clients undergoing chemotherapy and radiation therapy.

TESTICULAR TORSION

Testicular torsion (Fig. 38–7A) occurs when a testicle is mobile and the spermatic cord twists, cutting off the blood supply. It is the most common testicular disorder in children. It can occur at any age but is most usual at puberty, and about 30% of cases occur in men in their 20s. Manifestations usually arise suddenly, with acute scrotal swelling and severe pain as blood supply to the testicles is interrupted.

If testicular torsion is suspected, a testicular scan and Doppler ultrasonography are performed to assess the blood supply. Torsion causes a decrease (blood supply would be increased with epididymitis).

Testicular torsion is an emergency requiring immediate surgical intervention. The spermatic cord is untwisted and the testicle immobilized by suturing it to the scrotum (orchiopexy). Without prompt surgery, the testicle may atrophy or develop an abscess. If the testicle is necrotic, it is removed. Because there is a risk that the other testicle will be prone to torsion, it is also affixed to the scrotum at the time of surgery.

ORCHITIS

Orchitis is a rare, acute testicular inflammation. It may be associated with trauma or an infection elsewhere in the body, such as mumps, pneumonia, tuberculosis, and syphilis. Mumps orchitis, which occurs in about 30% of men who develop mumps after puberty, is usually bilateral.

Assessment reveals edematous and extremely tender testicles, reddened scrotal skin, fever, and prostration. Treatment includes bed rest, scrotal support, local heat to the scrotum, and medications for pain relief, fever, and infection. An acute phase may last about a week. Permanent sterility may occur if both testicles are affected, whereas decreased fertility may result if only one is affected.

EPIDIDYMITIS

Epididymitis is more common than orchitis. Infections in the urethra, prostate, or bladder can spread along the vas deferens; infections also spread through the lymphatic and vascular systems. Bladder outlet obstruction can cause reflux of infected urine. Epididymitis can occur as a complication related to urethral instrumentation, such as catheterization or instrumentation in transurethral surgeries, but its frequency has decreased since prophylactic antibiotics have been prescribed after such procedures. Sexually transmitted organisms frequently cause the condition in younger men, and urinary pathogens cause epididymitis in older men. Trauma is a noninfectious cause.

Epididymitis is almost always unilateral. Early in the disease, a client has local pain and swelling. As epididymitis progresses, the testicle becomes involved (epididymo-orchitis), the entire scrotum becomes reddened and painful, and an inflammatory hydrocele can occur. After the acute phase, fibrosis and occlusion may result, with subsequent sterility. Recurrences are common when other conditions are unresolved. Treatment is the same as for orchitis.

HYDROCELE, HEMATOCELE, AND SPERMATOCELE

Hydrocele (Fig. 38–7B) is a painless collection of clear, yellow fluid in the scrotum caused by an opening between the peritoneum and the tunica vaginalis or by an imbalance in production and reabsorption of fluid within the tunica vaginalis. The soft intrascrotal mass is translucent to light. Often, if the hydrocele is due to a communication with the peritoneum, it decreases in size when the man lies down. If constant discomfort, embarrassment, or impaired circulation occurs, aspiration or surgical drainage may be performed. Hydroceles can conceal a testicular tumor or inguinal hernia.

A hematocele is a collection of blood in the tunica vaginalis caused by trauma. Hematoceles are less likely than hydroceles to be transilluminated on light examination. They require only drainage.

A spermatocele is a cystic dilation of part of the epididymis that contains a milky fluid and dead spermatozoa. It is painless, and surgery is usually not required.

VARICOCELE

Varicocele (Fig. 38–7C) is a dilation and varicosity of the pampiniform plexus (the network of veins supplying

A   Testicular torsion   B   Hydrocele   C   Varicocele

FIGURE 38–7 Disturbances of the testicles.

the testicles) within the scrotum. They usually arise slowly. Ninety per cent of varicoceles are left-sided because the left spermatic vein enters the renal vein at a 90-degree angle, causing back-pressure. Pain may be relieved by masturbation or sexual intercourse. Varicoceles are found in 19% to 41% of men who are evaluated for infertility. A right-sided varicocele suggests tumor or retroperitoneal fibrosis.

On palpation, with the man standing, a varicocele feels like a mass of tortuous veins above and posterior to the testicle. When the man lies down, the mass abates. Treatment includes the use of a scrotal support. Surgery is performed if there is severe pain or if the varicocele is thought to contribute to infertility.

VASECTOMY (ELECTIVE STERILIZATION)

A vasectomy is an elective surgical procedure to ensure a permanent method of contraception. It is sometimes performed after a prostatectomy to prevent retrograde epididymitis. The surgery is usually performed in the urologist's office or in an outpatient setting with the use of local anesthesia. The procedure, performed through a small incision in the scrotum, involves cutting out a segment of the vas deferens, ligating the ends, and tucking them into different tissue planes to prevent reanastomosis (Fig. 38–8).

Slight pain, swelling, and bruising occur postoperatively, but discomfort is controlled with ice, a mild analgesic such as acetaminophen (aspirin is avoided to prevent bleeding), and rest for a few days. A scrotal support also increases client comfort. The client can resume heavy lifting and sexual intercourse about a week after surgery. The client must continue to practice other means of birth control until the follow-up semen analysis shows azoospermia (absence of sperm), because live sperm are left in the ampulla of vas deferens. Bleeding, infection, and mild chronic pain (rare) are complications that can occur after vasectomy.

The client must consider vasectomy a permanent means of contraception. Vasovasostomy, which is a surgical reversal of a vasectomy, can be done; however, it is expensive and fertility is not guaranteed.

FIGURE 38–8 Vasectomy.

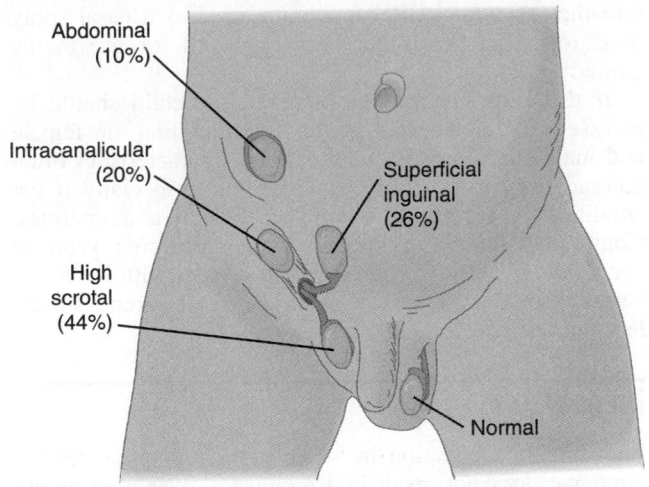

FIGURE 38–9 Undescended or mispositioned testis (cryptorchidism).

UNDESCENDED OR MISPOSITIONED TESTICLES

The most common congenital testicular condition is that of mispositioned undescended testes (cryptorchidism) (Fig. 38–9). Testes normally descend from the abdomen into the scrotum before birth, but sometimes they do not. One or both testicles may be arrested in the abdomen, inguinal canal (canalicular), low pelvis, or high scrotum. An ectopic testicle descends to the wrong area outside the normal path of decent (e.g., perineum). A retractile testicle descends into the scrotum but pulls back into the inguinal canal because of a hyperactive cremasteric reflex. Complete absence of a testicle may also occur.

Undescended testicles occur in about 4% of full-term male infants and are more common in premature infants. Many resolve by the first year of life. Inguinal hernias and torsion commonly occur with undescended testicles.

Cryptorchidism is associated with infertility. High body temperature, endocrine understimulation, and an abnormal epididymis that seems to accompany an undescended testicle cause changes that prevent normal fertility in the future. The incidence of testicular cancer is high in men with undescended testes if the condition is not corrected before puberty. A man with an undescended testicle has a 1 in 80 chance of testicular cancer development. Correction, however, does not guarantee prevention.

Treatment, which is surgical, is performed when the child is between 9 and 12 months old, and certainly by 18 months, not only to allow time for spontaneous descent but also to decrease the risk of total infertility and testicular cancer. An inguinal incision is used so that additional repair (i.e., hernia repair or excision of connective tissue bands) or orchiectomy (should the testicle look abnormal) can be done.

Retractile testes usually descend and stay in the scrotum by puberty, but surgery is not required. HCG has sometimes been used to promote passage of the testicle into the scrotum. LHRH is administered as a nasal spray in Europe, but it has not been approved for use in the United States.

If the cryptorchidism is bilateral, the child should be assessed for intersexuality (an intermingling of female and male characteristics with external characteristics often contradictory to internal characteristics), especially if the condition is associated with other genital abnormalities. Continuous follow-up through the childbearing years is necessary to detect malignancy and to deal with infertility issues, should they arise. Clients and their parents should learn how to do testicular self-examination.

INFERTILITY

Infertility is a situation in which regular, unprotected intercourse does not result in a pregnancy over a 12-month period. Infertility affects 20% to 35% of couples in the United States who are trying to have children, and requests for infertility services are increasing rapidly.

A male factor contributes partially or totally to the couple's inability to conceive in about 50% of the cases. However, it is best that the two partners be treated together. Minimal fertility (subfertility) in one partner can be offset by strong fertility in the other. If both partners are minimally fertile, infertility is more likely. Awareness of these statistics alerts health care professionals to clients who may have concerns about infertility but who have difficulty expressing them. Male factors for infertility are discussed in this chapter.

Etiology and Risk Factors

Pretesticular (hormonal) causes involve endocrine dysfunction and account for approximately 3% to 25% of cases. Examples are pituitary and adrenal tumors, thyroid disorders, diabetes, and cirrhosis.

Testicular causes are most common. Varicoceles are found in 19% to 41% of infertility cases. Other testicular causes include congenital abnormalities, torsion, genitourinary infection, trauma, and exposure to substances known to interfere with spermatogenesis (sperm formation). Cryptorchidism is directly related to infertility.

Post-testicular causes include congenital blockage of the vas deferens and other malformations of structures distal to the testes. Epididymitis, emotional factors, surgical procedures that cause retrograde ejaculation, and some medical conditions such as renal disease or paraplegia are additional causes.

Infection of the prostate, epididymis, or testicle can affect fertility. The mumps virus attacks the testicle in 5% to 37% of adults who acquire the infection. Of these men, 16% to 65% have bilateral involvement. Although rare in the Western world, tuberculosis is a genital infection seen in other countries and in immigrants to the United States.

Whether testicular trauma and infertility are related is a matter of controversy. The formation of anti-sperm antibodies is one theory. Some surgical procedures cause retrograde ejaculation.

Chemicals, drugs, and other substances that affect spermatogenesis are called gonadotoxins (e.g., heavy use of alcohol, marijuana, and anabolic steroids). Many medications, including allopurinol, cimetidine, nitrofurantoin,

sulfasalazine, and chemotherapeutic drugs, have been related to infertility. Alpha-adrenergic blockers and ganglion blockers may cause retrograde ejaculation and may thus be a secondary cause of inability to conceive. Exposure to agricultural, industrial, and warfare agents is an increasing concern. Lead, Agent Orange (a herbicide used as a defoliant in Vietnam), and some pesticides affect fertility. Tobacco smoke has been investigated as a cause of infertility, but a clear link has not been established; data suggest that smoking may be involved in subfertility. Radiation and hyperthermia also affect fertility.

Problems with intercourse are responsible for infertility in about 5% of couples. These include erectile dysfunction, premature ejaculation, unfavorable timing or frequency of intercourse, excessive masturbation, and aberrant sexual behaviors. Many water-soluble lubricants used during intercourse can be toxic to sperm.

Pathophysiology

The pathophysiologic mechanisms involved in infertility vary, and the problem is often a complex one. Hormonal imbalance between the hypothalamus, pituitary gland, and testicles can interfere with the production and maturation of sperm. Hypoxia of the testicle and elevated scrotal temperature cause germ cell damage. Seminal WBCs present in genitourinary infections are believed to release bioactive cytokines that affect spermatogenesis.

Some viruses and bacteria directly destroy cells or cause enough inflammation to cause tissue necrosis. Sexually transmitted diseases, particularly gonorrhea and infection with Chlamydia trachomatis, may account for cases of infertility because they can cause testicular atrophy, but a clear relationship has not been proved. Immune responses may prevent the formation of normal sperm. Gonadotoxins can decrease the number of sperm, decrease motility (the forward movement of sperm), or cause abnormal morphology. Congenital factors and trauma can impair patency of the ductal system that extends from the testicles through the prostate.

Clinical Manifestations

Assessment of infertility includes obtaining a detailed occupational, sexual, medical, and reproductive history and conducting a thorough physical examination. During an examination, the presence of testicles and their size, varicocele or other scrotal and penile abnormalities, and secondary sex characteristics are noted. A prostate massage and specimens of secretions may be obtained for culture to check for infection. A postejaculatory urine specimen may also be checked for the presence of sperm, suggesting retrograde ejaculation.

Semen analysis is performed on more than one specimen. Semen volume and viscosity, number and concentration of sperm, motility, and morphology are analyzed. The presence of WBCs or agglutination of sperm is noted. A normal semen analysis would show the following values:

- Semen volume, 1.5 to 5.0 ml
- Concentration, >20 million sperm/ml
- Total sperm count, >50 to 60 million
- Motility, ≥60% grade 2 or higher (on a scale of 1 to 4)
- Morphology, ≥60% normal

Motility refers to the forward movement of sperm; *morphology* refers to sperm form and size. Normally, sperm have one head and one tail. Abnormal sperm may be immature, may have misshapen heads, or may have two tails. Some infertility specialists consider slightly lower percentages for sperm count, motility, and morphology to be adequate when evaluating semen quality. Other more specific tests may be done to evaluate semen, such as checking for viscosity, coagulation, and the presence of fructose.

Serum endocrine studies are conducted to assess testosterone, prolactin, LH, and follicle-stimulating hormone (FSH). For example, if testosterone levels are normal, nonhormonal causes are pursued. If testosterone levels and prolactin levels are low but LH levels are high, primary testicular disease may be suspected. If FSH levels are high, spermatogenesis is probably arrested. If FSH levels are normal, *azoospermia* (absence of sperm) or *oligospermia* (scarcity of sperm) is probably caused by obstruction in the post-testicular ducts, which may be corrected by microsurgery.

If anatomic abnormalities are suspected, imaging techniques such as Doppler ultrasonography, MRI, cavernosography, and color flow Doppler imaging are ordered. A testicular biopsy may be performed if sperm are absent or scarce along with normal hormone levels. Clients are carefully selected for such studies because the tests are costly and, when invasive, may cause testicular damage.

Outcome Management

■ Medical Management

PRETESTICULAR CAUSES

Treatment of male infertility with pretesticular causes varies. No treatment is available for primary testicular failure or hypogonadism. Testosterone may be prescribed to correct low testosterone levels. A testosterone patch is applied directly to the scrotum (Testoderm) or to the torso or extremities (Androderm). Scrotal skin is five times more permeable, and there is concern about too much absorption and side effects. With both transdermal methods, skin irritation or contact dermatitis is experienced in about 9% of clients. Testosterone is contraindicated for men with prostate cancer or severe bladder outlet obstruction. Hyperprolactinemia may be treated by surgical removal of a pituitary tumor or by administration of bromocriptine (Parlodel).

Treatment of male sexual dysfunction is discussed under Erectile Dysfunction. For oligospermia caused by excessive frequency of ejaculation, recommend that the couple have intercourse only once every 36 hours during the woman's periovulatory period, because it takes 24 hours for a normal sperm count to be generated after ejaculation.

TESTICULAR CAUSES

Treatment of male infertility with testicular causes also varies. Instruct the client to avoid factors that depress spermatogenesis such as heat, drugs, alcohol, and marijuana. He should keep the testicles cool by avoiding hot baths and tight clothing or by using a commercially prepared, water-dampened scrotal cooling device; keeping the testes cool appears to improve the sperm count. Advise the client to maintain good nutrition. Medications such as HCG or testosterone (Depo-Testosterone) are sometimes prescribed as hormonal treatments. Nonhormonal therapy may consists of kallikrein, steroids, indomethacin, arginine, zinc, or vitamins. Varicocele is treated surgically.

POST-TESTICULAR CAUSES

Treatment of male infertility with post-testicular causes involves correcting ejaculatory abnormalities and obstruction. Ejaculatory abnormalities may be corrected by the split-ejaculate technique. The first half of the ejaculate contains more sperm than the second half. The first half may be used for artificial insemination or may be deposited in the vagina during intercourse, followed by withdrawal of the penis. Absence of ejaculation or retrograde (backward) ejaculation may be treated with drugs such as ephedrine, imipramine, or antihistamines. When the client experiences retrograde ejaculation, artificial insemination may be performed using sperm from urine obtained by centrifugation. Obstructive infertility is treated by surgery.

Appropriate antimicrobial drugs are used to treat genitourinary infections. Male infertility with immunologic causes may be treated with steroids and artificial insemination of sperm that have been washed to remove antibodies contained in the sperm.

■ Nursing Management of the Medical Client

PROVIDE SUPPORT

The client and his partner are often highly emotional in the diagnostic phase, and your sensitivity can ease their concerns somewhat. Both may need help and support to express their feelings and concerns about infertility. Failure to conceive may make several demands on the couple, threatening their individual self-concepts, sex roles, relationship, and sexual interaction. Guilt and blame about previous sexual activity, sexually transmitted diseases (STDs), or abortion may come between them. Some men find masturbation (necessary to obtain a semen sample) difficult for personal, cultural, or religious reasons. Many men do not know what chemicals they have been exposed to at the workplace or elsewhere. Fear and anxiety may be lessened during your assessment and teaching sessions. This provides you with the opportunity to support, respond to questions, and explain diagnostic and treatment procedures. Emphasize the need for consistent follow-up to evaluate progress.

Referral for counseling or support groups, or both, for infertile couples may be appropriate. A nationally known support group in the United States is RESOLVE (Department P, Box 474, Belmont, MA 02178).

PROVIDE EDUCATION

Because thorough and complete fertility assessment is expensive and can be ineffective, the client needs to understand the testing and the reasons for the various examinations. Explain fully how to collect a specimen for sperm analysis so that results are accurate. Written as well as verbal instructions are important because anxiety levels may be high. The man should refrain from sexual activity for 3 days before collecting a semen sample and should take the specimen immediately (within 1 hour) to the laboratory for analysis. Masturbation is the preferred method because some semen is lost during intercourse. Condoms and lubricants may make the sperm immotile. The specimen should be kept close to the body to maintain normal temperature. Two to three interval specimens are required for evaluation because results can vary. Ensure that the client understands the medical regimen suggested and the importance of following it closely.

PREVENT INFERTILITY

If possible, it is more effective to prevent infertility than to treat it. Clients who want to conceive at present or in the future can try to prevent infertility by:

1. Avoiding gonadotoxins, as discussed earlier.
2. Decreasing exposure to occupational and environmental hazards.
3. Keeping the scrotum cool by avoiding excessive heat, hot baths, and tight clothing.
4. Avoiding transmission of STDs by limiting the number of sexual partners and by using condoms.
5. Developing effective means of stress reduction.
6. Eating a well-balanced, nutritious diet.

PENILE DISORDERS

PHIMOSIS

Phimosis occurs when the penile foreskin (prepuce) is constricted at the opening, making retraction difficult or impossible. The condition can be congenital or a result of inflammation, infection, or local trauma. It is not usually painful, but it can lead to obstructive uropathy if it is severe enough. Prolonged phimosis, caused by chronic inflammation and irritation, predisposes to penile cancer. Assessment reveals edema, erythema, tenderness, and purulent discharge. Intervention includes controlling infection with local treatment and broad-spectrum antimicrobial drugs.

Effective genital hygiene is essential to prevent acquired penile disorders. In uncircumcised males, the man cleans the penis by pulling the foreskin back gently and washing the area with a washcloth (Fig. 38–10). This technique should be done daily to eliminate the normally accumulated smegma, and the foreskin should be returned to its normal position.

Routine *circumcision* (surgical removal of the foreskin) of male infants has not been considered medically necessary by the American Academy of Pediatrics and other health professionals and health organizations. Some parents have religious or cultural reasons for continuing the practice of circumcision. The operation may be indicated for clients with penile infection, phimosis, or paraphimosis. The rate of penile cancer is almost nil in circumcised men. The procedure should be done with the client under general anesthesia. Potential risks include excessive bleeding, infection, and penile trauma.

PARAPHIMOSIS

Paraphimosis (Fig. 38–11) occurs when a tight foreskin, once retracted, cannot be returned to its normal position. This sometimes happens after rigorous cleaning, masturbation, sexual intercourse, catheter insertion, or cystos-

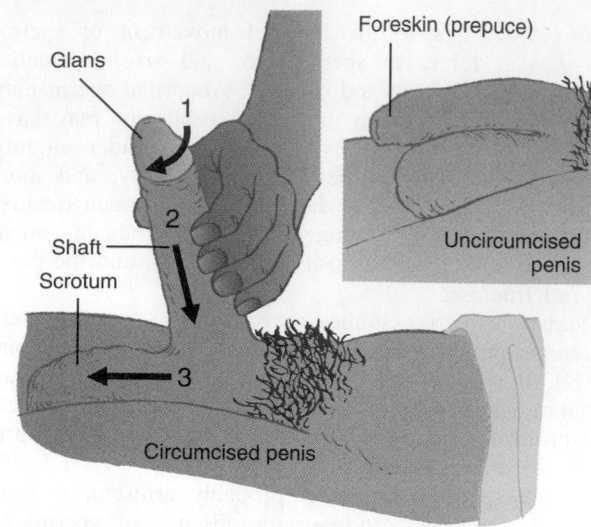

FIGURE 38–10 A circumcised penis and an uncircumcised penis. The foreskin of an uncircumcised penis should retract easily. During physical examination, ask the man to retract his foreskin himself. Effective genital hygiene is essential to prevent acquired penile problems. Many men have never been taught how to do this. *1,* Begin washing at the tip of the penis. For an uncircumcised penis, gently retract the foreskin and wash. *2,* Proceed down the penis shaft toward the body. *3,* Next wash the scrotum. Wash the anal area last.

copy if the foreskin is not returned to its normal position. Circulation is thus impeded, and the glans swells rapidly. It is painful and edema is common. The foreskin can be gently compressed either manually or with an elastic wrap. The client can then attempt manual reduction by gently pulling the foreskin. Surgical incision of the foreskin with local anesthesia may be necessary if the condition does not resolve.

POSTHITIS AND BALANITIS

Posthitis (foreskin inflammation) and balanitis (inflammation of the glans penis and the mucous membrane beneath it) (Fig. 38–12) are caused by irritation and invasion of microorganisms. Good hygiene and thorough drying of the penis are recommended. It is important to assess for diabetes, which predisposes the client to secondary infection. Antibiotics may help control local infection. Circumcision may be necessary.

FIGURE 38–11 Paraphimosis.

FIGURE 38–12 Posthitis and balanitis.

URETHRITIS

Urethritis, an acute urethral inflammation, is discussed under STDs and urinary disorders (see Chapters 34 and 41). It is mentioned throughout this chapter because it predisposes to other genitourinary disorders.

URETHRAL STRICTURE

Urethral stricture is caused by urethral scarring or narrowing. It may be congenital or caused by untreated or severe urethritis or urethral injury (including urologic instrumentation, e.g., cystoscopy). Manifestations are caused by obstruction: small-caliber urinary stream, hyperdistended bladder, infection, fever, and dysuria. Urethral strictures are released surgically by urethral dilation or urethroplasty. See Chapter 34 for further information.

EPISPADIAS

Epispadias (Fig. 38–13A) is a rare congenital condition in which the urethral meatus opens dorsally on top of the penis, proximal to the glans, most commonly at the abdominal-penile junction. Surgery is required to correct urinary incontinence and to return the urethra to a normal position in the penis.

HYPOSPADIAS

Hypospadias (Fig. 38–13B) is a congenital condition in which the urethral meatus opens on the ventral side of the penis. Common locations include the glans penis, penile shaft, penoscrotal junction, and perineum. *Chordee* (curvature of the penis) is often associated with hypospadias. Hypospadias occurs in about two to eight per thousand live male births.

Early assessment of internal reproductive organ development is necessary to confirm the child's sex. For psychological reasons, hypospadias should be repaired before the child starts school. It is important to ask about this condition when taking the history.

PEYRONIE'S DISEASE

Fibrous plaques develop in the connective tissue in Peyronie's disease, usually near the dorsal midline of the penile shaft in middle-aged and older men. Although the etiologic mechanism is unknown, one theory is that the disease is caused by an abnormal fibrotic reaction to trauma. The disease has two phases: acute and chronic. Pain is more likely during the initial phase, and plaques begin to develop. This phase can last about 1 to 1½ years. Pain usually subsides during the chronic phase, but fibrosis is increased.

Diagnosis may be made during history-taking, although men usually seek a physician because of concern about penile lumps (fear of cancer), painful erection, or erectile dysfunction. The man may have penile curvature on erection, painful erection, and unsatisfactory vaginal penetration. Peyronie's disease is often associated with Dupuytren's contracture of the hand tendons.

Some cases improve spontaneously. Reassure the client that this is not a malignant condition and does not lead to development of cancer. If a client is not having discomfort and has soft plaques and minimal curvature, the physician may advise waiting several months before instituting therapy. Medical treatment includes vitamin E,

A EPISPADIAS

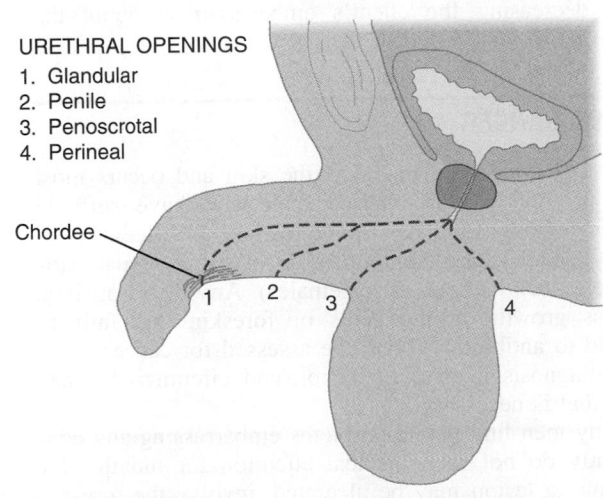

B HYPOSPADIAS

FIGURE 38–13 Epispadias *(A)* and hypospadias *(B)*.

para-aminobenzoic acid, tamoxifen, and colchicine. Intralesional injections, local radiation, and ultrasonography have also been used. Surgical correction is necessary when previous treatments have failed and the client is unable to perform sexually.

PRIAPISM

Priapism is a prolonged, persistent penile erection without sexual desire. It can last hours or even days and may be very painful. The condition is sometimes associated with leukemia or sickle cell anemia. Self-injection of medications (mainly papaverine) to treat impotence is the other common cause. It may also result from some medications, such as anticoagulants, alcohol, phenothiazines, alpha-adrenergic blockers, and marijuana.

Two major types of priapism have been defined according to a physiology-based system. *High-flow* arterial priapism, the less common type, usually occurs after trauma and is less painful. *Low-flow* veno-occlusive priapism, the more common form, is an emergency situation and is extremely painful.

In the client with low-flow priapism, circulation to the penis is compromised, predisposing to ischemia and permanent erectile dysfunction. The client may also be unable to void. Treatment in most cases consists of aspiration of blood from the penis followed by serial intracavernosal injections of phenylephrine.

Low-flow priapism must be resolved within 24 hours to prevent penile ischemia, gangrene, fibrosis, and erectile dysfunction. If the more conservative treatments are unsuccessful, more invasive therapy is required to prevent permanent damage. Surgical treatment is designed to drain the congested blood from the corpora cavernosa.

High-flow priapism can often be treated with ice and compression. If these measures are not successful, the client may require selective embolization or ligation of the traumatized artery.

Be sensitive to the embarrassing nature of this problem. Men are often reluctant to admit that this problem has occurred and yet may be in severe pain. Be understanding, and try to make the client comfortable while decreasing the client's embarrassment about the problem.

PENILE CANCER

Penile cancer is rare. It affects the skin and occurs most often in older, uncircumcised men who have suffered chronic irritation and have poor hygiene practices. Associated genital cancer sometimes develops in sexual partners (e.g., cervical cancer in females). Any dry, wart-like, painless growth on the penis or foreskin that fails to respond to antibiotics should be assessed for cancer. If an early diagnosis is made, excision and circumcision may be all that is necessary.

Many men find penile problems embarrassing and consequently do not seek medical attention for months. By this time, a lesion may be ulcerated, involve the foreskin and penile shaft, and have metastasized to the inguinal nodes. Penile shaft resection or sometimes penectomy and dissection of enlarged inguinal nodes may be necessary.

PENILE AND SCROTAL INJURIES

Although fairly protected, the penis and scrotum can sustain various injuries. *Nonpenetrating* injuries result from sudden force, such as a straddle injury or penile fracture during intercourse. Underlying structures can be bruised or ruptured. Items placed around the penis that strangulate may also cause significant tissue damage. *Penetrating* injuries usually involve knife or gunshot wounds but also include self-emasculation attempts and amputation. The male genitalia can also be injured by radiation, chemical or electrical burns, and avulsion (from accidents caused by working with machinery).

Hemorrhage is immediate, whether microscopic or obvious. Pain and edema accompany bleeding. Minor hemorrhage is controlled by ice packs, bed rest, analgesia, and scrotal elevation. Direct compression and pressure dressings may be needed if bleeding is worse. For penile injury, a retrograde urethrogram is obtained to rule out urethral injury. If the urethra is intact, an indwelling catheter is inserted. If bleeding from the penis is noted, urethral disruption is assumed and instrumentation is contraindicated. For scrotal injury, scrotal ultrasonography is performed.

Surgery is necessary to drain a hematoma, to debride necrotic tissue, or to repair damage, including reanastomosis if appropriate. Microsurgical techniques are used. Postoperative antibiotics are given, and catheterization continues until penile injuries are healed. Often, further operations are required for repair of strictures, skin grafting, or reconstruction. If scrotal skin is avulsed, the remaining scrotal skin is usually replaced over the scrotal organs; scrotal skin regenerates. When this is not possible, surgeons may perform skin grafts and temporarily reimplant the testes into subcutaneous thigh pouches. These clients need professional approaches and much explanation and reassurance to reduce anxiety. If the client has sustained self-inflicted injuries, psychological referral is part of the care.

When the urinary tract is disrupted, urine can escape into the peritoneum, scrotum, or penile tissue, thus creating an emergency condition. Assessment reveals discoloration of tissue, shock, and fever. Emergency intervention includes alternative drainage of urine (urethral or suprapubic catheter) and drainage of the tissues with a Penrose drain.

ERECTILE DYSFUNCTION

Since the 1980s, erectile dysfunction (impotence) has received more attention and there are more choices for treatment. Erectile dysfunction is defined as inability to achieve or maintain an erection, but other problems may contribute, such as decreased libido and ejaculatory or orgasmic difficulties. Men now living in their 70s and beyond want to stay sexually active. In most cultures, sexual performance is a measure of manhood. Erectile dysfunction was once thought to be psychogenic in origin, but physiologic causes are found in more than 50% of the cases.

Etiology and Risk Factors

Both psychological and physiologic factors may contribute to erectile dysfunction, such as performance anxiety, stress and fatigue, low self-esteem, depression, and changes in a relationship. After experiencing failure once, a man may be so anxious that he "fails" again and again, worsening the problem. Stress caused by psychological factors can increase catecholamine levels and can block sympathetic response, causing a physiologic dysfunction.

True psychogenic erectile dysfunction is distinguished by the following:

- Normal and sustained erection during foreplay but loss of erection at the moment of intromission (penetration)
- Normal erection with some sexual partners but not with others
- Normal erection with masturbation but not with partners
- Sudden onset of total impotence in a man younger than 40 years of age
- Alternating periods of normal function and total impotence

Physiologic causes include diseases, interruption related to surgery, anatomic abnormalities, and medications or substance abuse. Erectile dysfunction may be partial or total. Vascular conditions, such as arteriosclerotic changes, trauma to the penile blood supply, hypertension, stroke, diabetes mellitus, sickle cell anemia, leukemia, Hodgkin's disease, and aortic aneurysms, are common causes. Neurologic causes include interference with sympathetic or parasympathetic innervation, degenerative diseases, and spinal cord injury. Endocrine disorders that lower testosterone also cause erectile dysfunction. Peyronie's disease, prostatitis, and prolonged priapism are genitourinary causes.

Congenital anomalies of the penis, chordee, and a short penis are anatomic factors. Surgical disruption may occur during radical prostatectomy, pelvic lymph node dissection, radical cystectomy, and, of course, bilateral orchiectomy. Numerous medications can affect erection, libido, orgasm, and ejaculation, but erectile problems do not always arise in men who take the medications. Recreational drugs, alcohol, and smoking also cause erectile dysfunction.

Pathophysiology

A normal erection requires desire, sensual stimulation, release of LH, arterial engorgement of the corpora cavernosa (and venous constriction), and an intact nervous system from the brain to the penile nerves. Anything that interferes with this process can cause erectile dysfunction.

Clinical Manifestations

A detailed medical and sexual history is the first step in determining the cause of erectile dysfunction. A limited physical examination is performed to rule out obvious genitourinary causes. Laboratory tests may include determinations of serum testosterone, LH, FSH, and prolactin levels and thyroid function. Increased prolactin blocks testosterone effectiveness and decreases the desire for sexual activity. Both hyperthyroidism and hypothyroidism may cause erectile dysfunction, usually affecting libido.

When erectile function is normal, men have involuntary erections during times of deep sleep when rapid eye movement (REM) occurs. Nocturnal penile tumescence (NPT) studies help to determine the presence of these erections; some tests can evaluate the quality. The least expensive test employs a snap gauge device with pressure bands wrapped around the penis. The bands break at increasing pressures during nocturnal erections. NPT monitors can also be used to evaluate several nocturnal erections during a night's sleep. A special monitor, called a Rigiscan, records nocturnal erections and their quality (duration, rigidity, and changes in circumference of the penile shaft during each erection). Other tests include penile Doppler ultrasonography, penile angiography, and dynamic infusion cavernosometry (DICC). DICC provides information about arterial inflow, cavernous sinoid compliance, and venous leakage.

Outcome Management

▮▮ Medical Management

CORRECT PSYCHOLOGICAL PROBLEMS

Sometimes just giving accurate information about normal sexual function, alternative sexual activity, and dispelling myths is all that is necessary for a client to deal with erectile dysfunction. Myths about sexual activity greatly influence outcome success. Behavioral modification techniques (the best known were developed by Masters and Johnson in the 1960s) may be used when psychogenic causes are determined. Psychologists and sexual therapists may use psychometric testing, including the Minnesota Multiphasic Personality Inventory (MMPI), the Derogatis Sexual Function Inventory, or the Walker Sex Form, to assess psychological functioning.

CORRECT PHYSIOLOGIC PROBLEMS

When physiologic causes are involved, several approaches may be used. Medications used for diseases may need to be changed or habits (use of recreational drugs or alcohol and smoking) eliminated. Medical conditions causing erectile dysfunction need to be treated if possible. Low testosterone levels, once treated by intramuscular injection of testosterone, is now more commonly treated with testosterone dermal patches that can be placed on several areas of the body. Testosterone can increase libido but does not necessarily help erectile dysfunction. Administration of testosterone is contraindicated for men with prostate cancer and those with normal testosterone production (suppresses natural production).

STIMULATE ERECTION

MEDICATIONS. Yohimbe, an adrenergic blocking medication, may cause vasodilation in the corpora cavernosa. It is usually ordered three times a day. It can cause side effects such as fluid retention, nausea, orthostatic hypotension, and diaphoresis or may not be effective at all.

Intracavernosal vasodilating drugs such as papaverine, phentolamine, and prostaglandin E_1 (PGE$_1$) can be injected. Combinations of these drugs may be given in a single injection. Because pain, bruising, or fibrosis at the injection site and priapism are possible side effects, it is recommended that injections be given not more than two or three times per week.

Intraurethral instillation of an alprostadil (PGE$_1$) pellet has been successful. This approach eliminates injection of the penis, but the technique must be accurately performed in order to achieve the erection. This can be a good approach for a client who is obese or has problems with dexterity or vision. The dosage varies from 125 to 1000 μg and can be given no more than twice in a 24-hour period. Side effects are the same as described before; intraurethral pain and minor bleeding may occur. PGE$_1$ administration is contraindicated if penile anatomy is abnormal or the client has urethritis.

Sildenafil (Viagra), an oral agent, is the newest medication for treatment of erectile dysfunction. It inhibits an enzyme in the corpora cavernosa that chemically ends the erection. This drug does not produce the erection; direct penile stimulation is required to release nitric oxide in the penile nerves, which activates another enzyme to relax the corporeal blood vessels. Side effects may include headache, a flush feeling, dyspepsia, nasal congestion, and a color tinge or other mild visual disturbances. Sildenafil is contraindicated for any client taking nitrates in any form. Caution must be observed when men are taking alpha-adrenergic blockers or have a peptic ulcer. The dosage is usually 25 to 100 mg taken no more than once a day.

VACUUM ERECTION DEVICES. Vacuum erection devices are legitimate medically prescribed pumps that mechanically achieve an erection. A cylinder is placed over the penis and a pump is used to create vacuum suction, thus drawing blood into the corpora cavernosa. When an erection is achieved, a compression ring is applied to the base of the penis and the cylinder is removed for intercourse. The ring must be removed within about 30 minutes to prevent tissue damage caused by interrupted circulation. Bruising and cold penile skin as well as lack of spontaneity are minor problems that may result. Priapism can also occur.

■ Nursing Management of the Medical Client

PROVIDE SUPPORT
A sensitive, caring approach is vital for nurses who work with these clients because embarrassment may cause many men to avoid treatment. Just knowing that erectile dysfunction is common and treatment alternatives are available can be reassuring to the client. Involve the sexual partner when the client permits. Erectile dysfunction is a "couple" problem.

PROVIDE EDUCATION
Teach the client about normal erectile physiology, factors that interfere, and how different approaches correct the problem. Inform the client about public or community resources. If medication is used, explain how to administer the medication and caution the client to follow directions as prescribed and not to use the medication more often then directed. Some men erroneously believe that if a little does work, more would be better.

The client who must use intracorporeal injections needs to know how to draw up medication into a syringe, cleanse the site, inject the medication, and safely dispose of equipment. He should know that bruising may occur. Injections should be given at the 2 o'clock or 10 o'clock position, and sites should be rotated to minimize fibrotic changes. Intraurethral pellets require using the applicator correctly, careful insertion, and waiting about 10 minutes for an erection to occur. Standing or walking during this time and stimulation are important.

■ Surgical Management

Surgical management of erectile dysfunction includes implantation of a penile prosthesis, revascularization procedures, and incision of Peyronie's plaques. Penile prostheses are the most common if medical therapy is not effective and if the client is a good surgical candidate.

PENILE PROSTHESIS
There are two basic categories of penile prostheses (Fig. 38–14):

1. *Inflatable* prostheses come in one-piece, two-piece, and three-piece units that are hydraulic devices. In the one-piece prosthesis, the reservoir, pump, and cylinders fit within the penis. Two-piece units have a reservoir-pump system within the scrotum. The reservoir on the three-piece devices is implanted in the abdominal cavity and the pump is implanted in the scrotum.
2. *Semi-rigid* prostheses can be malleable, with spring-like mechanisms that help make the penis more erect for intercourse, or mechanical, with cable strands in the device that can be bent to make the penis more erect.

Ice and penile or scrotal elevations are used postoperatively to minimize swelling. Pain should be well controlled with medication. Sexual activity can usually be resumed 6 to 8 weeks after surgery when healing is complete and pain is controlled. Infection, extrusion of the prosthesis, and mechanical failure are some of the complications after surgery.

REVASCULARIZATION
Revascularization surgical procedures attempt to restore circulation to the corpora cavernosa. Techniques involve reanastomosis, angioplasty, endarterectomy, and grafts. Venous ligation is used to treat penile vein incompetence. Over time, collateral veins form and "leakage" recurs.

■ Nursing Management of the Surgical Client

Care of the client having surgery for erectile dysfunction is the same as that of any surgical client. Penile circulation and dressing should be observed consistently as ordered. Encourage the client to use pain medication before the pain becomes severe. All clients are given antibiotics before and after surgery. The client is taught preoperatively how to use the prosthesis and cautioned not to use it before healing has occurred. These men need a great deal of emotional support because of secrecy with friends, emotional issues with partners, and sometimes doubt about the decision to have surgery related to pain.

FIGURE 38-14 Penile prostheses. *A*, Mark II (two-piece inflatable penile prosthesis). *B*, Mark II prosthesis erect and flaccid. *C*, Alpha I (three-piece inflatable penile prosthesis). *D*, Alpha 1 prosthesis erect and flaccid. (Courtesy of Mentor, Santa Barbara, CA.)

CONCLUSIONS

Male genital and reproductive disorders can be complex problems for the client and the nurse. The client often finds that these disorders threaten sexuality and sexual function or normal urinary elimination. These effects may be physiologic, but complex psychosocial problems also arise.

Prostate disorders are among the most common problems experienced by clients throughout their lifetime. Cancers of the male reproductive tract can be life-threatening, but if they are detected early, they can be cured or at least controlled for long periods. Problems such as erectile dysfunction and infertility directly affect both partners, who experience the diagnostic and treatment phases together. The nurse acts as a caregiver, educator, support, and resource person.

THINKING CRITICALLY

1. **Your client underwent a laser-assisted TURP yesterday. Closed bladder irrigation is being used, and his urine is dark to bright red with multiple clots. He is complaining of intense cramping pain in the lower abdomen. What further assessments should you make? What could be causing the cramping pain? What nursing action should you take?**

Factors to Consider. Is the dark to bright red urinary output normal at this stage? What does the nature of the client's pain tell you about its likely cause?

2. **A young man in his early 20s is given a diagnosis of testicular cancer, and he is very concerned about the treatment's effects on his ability to**

perform sexually and to father children. What issues should you discuss with him?

Factors to Consider. What impact might a bilateral orchiectomy or a radical lymph node dissection have on erectile function and fertility? What might be the effect of a unilateral orchiectomy? What options for fathering children are important to consider before the client undergoes treatment?

BIBLIOGRAPHY

1. American Cancer Society. (2000). *Cancer facts and figures.* Atlanta: Author.
2. Anderson, P., et al. (1998). Prostate disease patients: Planning services to meet their coping needs. *Urologic Nursing, 18*(3), 195–197.
3. Bartkiw, T., Kraetschmer, N., & Trachtenberg, J. (1997). Understanding microwave therapy as a treatment option for benign prostatic hyperplasia. *Urologic Nursing, 17*(2), 53–57.
4. Bates, P. (1997). Clinical conversation: Intraurethral alprostadil (MUSE). *Urologic Nursing, 17*(4), 159–161.
5. Benign Prostatic Hyperplasia Guideline Panel. (1994). *Benign prostatic hyperplasia: Clinical practice guideline* (Agency for Health Care Policy and Research Publication No. 94-0583). Rockville, MD: U.S. Department of Health and Human Services.
6. Benign Prostatic Hyperplasia Guideline Panel. (1994). *Benign prostatic hyperplasia: Diagnosis and treatment* (Agency for Health Care Policy and Research Publication No. 94-0582). Rockville, MD: U.S. Department of Health and Human Services.
7. Benign Prostatic Hyperplasia Guideline Panel. (1994). *Benign prostatic hyperplasia: Patient guide* (Agency for Health Care Policy and Research Publication No. 94-0584). Rockville, MD: U.S. Department of Health and Human Services.
8. Bosl, G., & Motzer, R. (1997). Testicular germ-cell cancer. *New England Journal of Medicine, 337*(4), 242–253.
9. Bruce, R., Waid, T., & Lucas, B. (1997). Understanding postobstructive diuresis. *Contemporary Urology, 9*(6), 53–66.
10. Catalona, W., Smith, D., & Ornstein, D. (1997). Prostate cancer detection in men with serum PSA concentrations of 2.6 to 4.9 ng/ml and benign prostate examination. *Journal of the American Medical Association, 277*(18), 1452–1455.
11. Chin-A-Loy, S., & Fernsler, J. (1998). Self-transcendence in older men attending a prostate cancer support group. *Cancer Nursing, 21*(5), 358–363.
12. Colpo, L. (1998). Evaluation, treatment, and management of erectile dysfunction: An overview. *Urologic Nursing, 18*(2), 100–106.
13. D'Amico, A., et al. (1998). Biochemical outcome after radical prostatectomy, external beam radiation therapy, or interstitial radiation therapy for clinically localized prostate cancer. *Journal of the American Medical Association, 280*(11), 969–974.
14. Ebersole, M. (1996). Hormonal administration in prostate cancer: A caring approach. *Urologic Nursing, 16*(1), 23–26.
15. Elder, J., & Shapiro, E. (1998). Undescended testes. *Family Urology, 3*(1), 13–16.
16. Fox, S., et al. (1999). Male genitourinary cancer sexuality questionnaire. *Urologic Nursing, 19*(2), 101–107.
17. Gallo, M., & Fallon, P. (1996). Evaluation of a pelvic floor treatment plan for patients undergoing radical prostatectomy. *Urologic Nursing, 16*(1), 9–13.
18. Gordon, S., et al. (1997). When the dx is penile cancer. *RN, 60*(3), 41–45.
19. Gray, M. (1992). *Genitourinary disorders.* St. Louis: Mosby–Year Book.
20. Gray, M., & Allensworth, D. (1997). Medical management of benign prostatic hyperplasia. *Urologic Nursing, 17*(4), 137–141.
21. Gray, M., & Allensworth, D. (1999). Electrovaporization of the prostate: Initial experiences and nursing management. *Urologic Nursing, 19*(1), 25–31.
22. Gregoire, I. (1995). Pharmacologic erection program: An alternative solution for the man with erectile dysfunction. *Urologic Nursing, 15*(1), 10–13.
23. Gregoire, I., Kalogeropoulis, D., & Corcos, J. (1997). The effectiveness of a professionally led support group for men with prostate cancer. *Urology Nursing, 17*(2), 58–66.
24. Hanson, K., & Lieber, M. (1996). Role of a urology nurse in evaluating patients with prostatism. *Urologic Nursing, 16*(3), 108.
25. Harris, J. (1997). The prevalence of impotence after radical prostatectomy. *Urologic Nursing, 17*(4), 142–145.
26. Heyman, E., & Rosner, T. (1996). Prostate cancer: An intimate view from patients and wives. *Urologic Nursing, 16*(2), 37–44.
27. Hinman, F. (1998). *Atlas of urologic surgery* (2nd ed.). Philadelphia: W. B. Saunders.
28. Intili, H., & Nier, D. (1998). Self-esteem and depression in men who present with erectile dysfunction. *Urologic Nursing, 18*(3), 185–187.
29. Intili, H. (1998). Impotence and perceived partner support. *Urologic Nursing, 18*(4), 279–280, 287.
30. Karlowicz, K. A. (Ed.). (1995). *Urologic nursing: Principles and practice.* Philadelphia: W. B. Saunders.
31. Keetch, D. W., & Andriole, G. L. (1996). Prostate cancer screening: What are physicians to do? What have we learned? *Monographs in Urology, 17*(3), 31–48.
32. Kennedy, W., Huff, D., & Snyder, H. (1998). The value of testis biopsies in cryptorchidism. *Contemporary Urology, 10*(4), 46–57.
33. Kletscher, B., & Osterling, J. (1995). Prostatic stents: Current prospectives for the management of BPH. *Urologic Clinics of North America, 22,* 423–430.
34. Laumann, E., Paik, A., & Rosen, R. (1999). Sexual dysfunction in the United States: Prevalence and predictors. *Journal of the American Medical Association, 281*(6), 537–544.
35. Lipshultz, L. (1996). Is semen quality declining? *Contemporary Urology, 8*(9), 50–62.
36. Lipshultz, L. (1997). Medical therapies for erectile dysfunction. *Contemporary Urology, 9*(12), 34–45.
37. Lipshultz, L., & Meacham, R. (1998). Male infertility: Causes and management. *Family Urology, 3*(2), 19–22.
38. Lipski, B., Garcia, R., & Brawer, M. (1996). Prostatic intraepithelial neoplasia: Significance and management. *Seminars in Urologic Oncology, 14*(3), 149–155.
39. Maffeo, R. (1997). Managing testicular cancer. *Nursing, 27*(5), 32hn6–32hn8.
40. Moody, F. (1999). *Atlas of ambulatory surgery.* Philadelphia: W. B. Saunders.
41. Moore, K., & Estey, A. (1999). The early postoperative concerns of men after radical prostatectomy. *Journal of Advanced Nursing, 29*(5), 1121–1129.
42. Moore, R., Partin, A., & Marshall, F. (1997). LPLND or mini-lap for lymphadenectomy. *Contemporary Urology, 9*(4), 39–50.
43. Moul, J. (1998). Pelvic muscle rehabilitation in males following prostatectomy. *Urologic Nursing, 18*(4), 296–301.
44. Moul, J., & Lipo, D. (1999). Prostate cancer in the late 1990s: Hormone refractory disease options. *Urologic Nursing, 19*(2), 125–132.
45. Newton, M., & Kosier, J. (1998). Nonsteroidal anti-androgens: Role in treating advanced prostate cancer. *Urologic Nursing, 18*(1), 56–57, 83.
46. Ortega, A., & Cunha, B. (1997). The perplexing nature of prostatitis. *Contemporary Urology, 9*(5), 73–80.
47. Padma-Nathan, H. (1997). The future of pharmacological management of impotence. *Family Urology, 2*(1), 13–15.
48. Partin, A., et al. (1997). Combination of prostate-specific antigen, clinical stage, and Gleason score to predict pathological stage of localized prostate cancer. *Journal of the American Medical Association, 277*(18), 1445–1451.
49. Pound, C., et al. (1999). Natural history of progression after PSA elevation following radical prostatectomy. *Journal of the American Medical Association, 281*(17),1591–1597.
50. Prostate Health Council of the American Foundation for Urologic Disease. (1998). Survey on BPH awareness. Baltimore: Author.
51. Raper, J. (1995). Priapism: Causes and treatment. *Urologic Nursing, 15*(3), 75–79.
52. Ross, S. (1995). Getting beyond chronic nonbacterial prostatitis. *Urologic Nursing, 15*(2), 61–63.
53. Sabiston, D. (Ed.). (1997). *Textbook of surgery* (15th ed.). Philadelphia: W. B. Saunders.
54. Shipley, W., et al. (1999). Radiation therapy for clinically localized prostate cancer: A multi-institutional pooled analysis. *Journal of the American Medical Association, 281*(17), 1598–1604.
55. Sprouse, D. (1994). Fertility issues and anejaculation. *Urologic Nursing, 14*(2), 62–65.

56. Sprouse, D. O. (1995). Sexual rehabilitation of the prostate cancer patient. *Cancer Supplement, 75*(7), 1954–1956.

57. Stamey, T., et al. (1999). Biological determinants of cancer progression in men with prostate cancer. *Journal of the American Medical Association, 281*(15), 1395–1400.

58. Thompson, I., et al. (1995). Chemoprevention of prostate cancer. *Seminars in Urology, 23*(2), 122–129.

59. Tingen, M., et al. (1998). Perceived benefits: A predictor of participation in prostate cancer screening. *Cancer Nursing, 21*(5), 349–357.

60. Walsh, P., et al. (Eds.). (1998). *Campbell's urology* (7th ed.). Philadelphia: W. B. Saunders.

61. Watt, E., & Lillibridge, J. (1998). Time of day urinary catheters are removed. *Urologic Nursing, 18*(1), 23–25.

62. Witt, T., et al. (1998). Saw palmetto extracts for treatment of benign prostatic hyperplasia. *Journal of the American Medical Association, 280*(18), 1604–1608.

63. Witte, M., & Morton, R. (1997). Prostate cancer in high-risk groups: Searching for explanations. *Contemporary Urology, 6*(7), 52–63.

64. Zaccagnini, M. (1999). Prostate cancer. *American Journal of Nursing, 99*(4), 34–35.

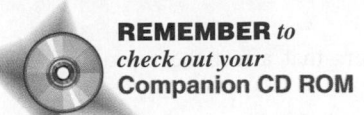

CHAPTER 39

Management of Women with Reproductive Disorders

Francie Bernier

NURSING OUTCOMES CLASSIFICATION (NOC)
for Nursing Diagnoses—Women with Reproductive Disorders

Constipation
Bowel Elimination
Hydration
Risk for Dysfunctional Grieving
Concentration
Coping
Family Coping
Grief Resolution

Psychosocial Adjustment: Life Change
Role Performance
Risk for Infection
Immune Status
Knowledge: Infection Control
Risk Control
Risk Control: Sexually Transmitted
    Diseases

Risk Detection
Tissue Integrity: Skin and Mucous
    Membranes
Treatment Behavior: Illness or Injury
Wound Healing: Primary Intention
Wound Healing: Secondary Intention

The major themes of all gynecologic disorders are sexuality and self-concept, including body image and self-esteem. Any disorder of the reproductive tract may lead to changes in sexual functioning or sexual identity. Change in sexual habits, such as abstinence from sexual activities or use of different positioning during vaginal intercourse, can be related to this diagnosis as well. The disorders and their treatments have the potential to change a woman's perceived or actual body structure, possibly leading to shame, embarrassment, and other negative emotions.

Alterations in sexuality and body image have a major effect on some women's feminine identity. Even in the 19th century, the common medical view was that the reproductive organs dominated a woman's body. Some aspects of this view, which reduces women's identity to the functioning of their body parts, persist in our culture today.

Contraception is a major health issue in various religious groups. Many religions, such as the Church of Jesus Christ of Latter-Day Saints (Mormons), the Roman Catholic Church, some Orthodox Jewish groups, and Baha'i, encourage followers to be fruitful and multiply. Sterilization and abortion are opposed by religious doctrine in many groups.

This chapter incorporates material written for the fifth edition by Elizabeth Carlson.

MENSTRUAL DISORDERS

CULTURAL INFLUENCES

Attitudes toward menstruation are often culturally based, and adolescent girls may be taught a variety of folk beliefs and practices at the time of puberty. Among Hispanic Americans, for example, menstruating females are not permitted to walk barefooted, wash their hair, or take showers or baths. Some Hispanic Americans believe that sour or iced foods cause menstrual blood to coagulate. Some Puerto Rican women have been taught that drinking lemon or pineapple juice will increase menstrual cramping. The nurse should be aware of these beliefs and respect cultural practices.

Some Arab women who practice Islam, such as Palestinians, Lebanese, Jordanians and Saudi Arabians, and some African women have ethnoreligious prohibitions and duties during and after menstruation. In Islam, blood is considered to be unclean (*najis*). The blood of menstruation, as well as blood lost during childbirth, renders the woman ritually impure. In Islamic legal language, the term used for menstruation is *hayz* and the menstruating woman is called *ha'iz*. Because one must be in a pure state in order to pray, the *ha'iz* are forbidden to perform certain acts of worship, such as touch the Koran, enter a mosque, pray, and participate in certain feasts. During the menstrual period, sexual intercourse is forbidden for both men and women. When the menstrual flow stops, the woman performs *ghusl*, a washing ritual to purify herself.

In the Navajo culture, a ceremony called the *kinaalda* announces the achievement of menarche (beginning of menstruation). Although fertility was the goal of the ceremony in the past, the most common reason for the *kinaalda* today is educational, to equip the girl to participate in society as an adult female. Menstruating Navajo women may not look at sand painting, enter a ceremonial *hogan*, attend or lead a sing, or join in the dancing that occurs at certain ceremonies.

In various cultures, menstruating women may be subject to restrictions on work and physical activities as well as rules related to the disposal of menstrual fluid and the proper disposal of sanitary napkins. Attitudes toward intercourse during menstruation are variable. Many religions also require or encourage women to engage in certain practices during and after menstruation. It is easy to understand why reproductive disorders can have such far-reaching effects on women.

REACTIONS TO MANIFESTATIONS

Women may experience some menstrual problems during their 30 or more years of menstruating. They tend to seek professional help for obvious abnormalities, such as excessive and irregular vaginal bleeding; however, they may not bring other menstrual problems to the attention of health care providers.

Women react to menstrual problems individually. Although some promptly seek health care, others do not, for various reasons. For example, one woman may hesitate and may be unable to discuss menstruation. She may view the subject as a personal and intimate problem that should be kept private. Another woman may have low self-esteem or may have been told that problems are to be expected. Therefore, she may dismiss her own complaints as unimportant or may not seek help, expecting the problems will disappear in time. Others may desire a relief of manifestations or may fear that the treatment will be worse than the problem. It is not uncommon for menstrual problems to remain undetected unless the nurse is skillful and sensitive in assessment. The nurse may identify a menstrual problem during a discussion of contraception or other needs. Some of the most common menstrual problems are dysmenorrhea (painful menstruation), premenstrual syndrome (PMS), and abnormal uterine bleeding.

DYSMENORRHEA

Dysmenorrhea is estimated to affect 30% to 75% of women. *Primary* dysmenorrhea is believed to be caused by either a prostaglandin excess or an increased sensitivity to prostaglandins with no underlying pathologic pelvic disorders. Prostaglandins are hormone-like secretions which cause smooth muscle contraction. *Secondary* dysmenorrhea begins with an underlying disease condition.

Etiology and Risk Factors

There are no preventive measures for dysmenorrhea, which has a variety of causes. The causes can be grouped according to five factors that affect the reproductive system in various ways:

- Elevated levels of uterine prostaglandins
- Endocrine factors
- Myometrial factors
- Biochemical factors
- Psychosocial factors

Secondary dysmenorrhea is suspected when pain is concentrated in a specific area, is unilateral, or begins after age 20 years. It may be caused by:

- Pelvic inflammatory disease (PID)
- Endometriosis
- Adenomyosis (invasion of uterine myometrium by endometrial tissue) (see Anatomy and Physiology Review at the beginning of this unit)
- Uterine prolapse
- Uterine myomas
- Polyps

Pathophysiology

Prostaglandin synthesis at the time of menstruation appears to produce strong myometrial contractions. The severe muscle spasms constrict blood vessels supplying the uterus, causing ischemia and pain. The excess prostaglandins in smooth muscle also help explain the presence of gastrointestinal (GI) manifestations, headache, and other manifestations.

Clinical Manifestations

Primary dysmenorrhea characteristically begins 1 to 2 months after menarche (onset of menses) in conjunction with ovulatory cycles. Generally, it increases in severity over several years with a decline when the woman reaches her mid-20s. Primary dysmenorrhea often decreases significantly after childbirth.

The discomfort of primary dysmenorrhea commonly begins 1 to 2 days before the onset of menstrual flow. The more severe discomfort is usually experienced during the first 24 hours of flow and typically subsides by the second day. More than half of the women experiencing dysmenorrhea also have systemic manifestations, such as nausea and vomiting, diarrhea, syncope, headache, and back pain.

Diagnosis is based on a thorough history, including medications used for symptomatic relief. A physical examination is performed to rule out underlying pathologic causes of dysmenorrhea.

Outcome Management

▆ Medical Management

The current approach to primary dysmenorrhea emphasizes prevention and education. For women with mild manifestations who want to avoid medication, nonpharmacologic remedies might be effective. For example, biofeedback, Therapeutic Touch, or acupuncture might be helpful. Nutritional measures include decreasing the intake of sodium and increasing the intake of vitamin B_6, calcium, magnesium, and protein.

ADMINISTER ORAL CONTRACEPTIVES

If contraception as well as relief of dysmenorrhea is desired, combination oral contraceptives may relieve menstrual pain. The combination inhibits ovulation, resulting in decreased endometrial prostaglandin production and a concurrent reduction of uterine activity. For the woman with a contraceptive *intrauterine device* (IUD), removal of the IUD may lead to relief. Another form of contraception may be desired.

PROMOTE EXERCISE

Exercise, such as aerobic exercise and swimming, has also been used as a remedy for dysmenorrhea. Exercise increases blood flow of beta-endorphins, the body's endogenous opiates, making them available for pain relief. The exact mechanism responsible for pain relief is not known.

ADMINISTER PROSTAGLANDIN SYNTHESIS INHIBITORS

Prostaglandin synthesis inhibitors (antiprostaglandin agents) may provide relief by decreasing prostaglandin activity, even in the presence of ovulatory cycles. Some commonly prescribed medications in this group are ibuprofen (Motrin), mefenamic acid (Ponstel), indomethacin (Indocin), and naproxen (Naprosyn). Ibuprofen (Advil) and naproxen (Aleve) are available as nonprescription drugs in lower doses, which makes them easy to obtain.

These medications may have GI side effects. Other possible side effects are sodium and water retention, rashes, and potential allergic reactions. For maximum effectiveness, the medications should be administered either before or at the onset of menses. Sometimes a client may have to try several prostaglandin synthesis inhibitors to find the one with maximum effectiveness for her.

Treatment of secondary dysmenorrhea is directed toward the underlying cause, such as endometriosis or PID (see later). Antiprostaglandin agents may provide some relief.

■ Nursing Management of the Medical Client

Education and supportive reassurance are important nursing interventions for clients with primary dysmenorrhea. Provide information about the mechanisms involved in dysmenorrhea and the actions and possible side effects of any prescribed medications. Assess the client's general health status. Encourage adequate nutrition, decreased caffeine intake, and appropriate rest, sleep, and exercise. Assess stress, which may increase manifestations, and explore methods of stress management.

PREMENSTRUAL SYNDROME

Premenstrual syndrome is defined as a combination of emotional and physical manifestations that occur cyclically in the female before menstruation and regress or disappear during menstruation. PMS is somatic (a physical syndrome), not psychic, in origin. It is a complex mechanism involving not only the endocrine system but the autonomic and central nervous systems as well. A predominant alteration is the retention of body fluids.

The incidence of PMS is difficult to determine because of its variable manifestations and the lack of a clear understanding about the syndrome. PMS manifestations peak in women 30 to 40 years old. Variable reports in the literature indicate that 20% to 60% of all women experience some form of PMS.

Etiology and Risk Factors

The cause of PMS is unclear. However, neuroendocrine mechanisms appear to be involved. It is not clear whether PMS is a single syndrome or a group of separate disorders. Some suggested causes of PMS are as follows:

- Estrogen-progesterone imbalance, especially in estrogen excess and a progesterone deficiency, or estrogen deficiency at time of manifestations
- Interaction among estrogen, progesterone, and aldosterone
- Excess of prolactin, hypothyroidism, or hypoglycemia
- Dietary factors, such as deficiency of vitamin B_6, magnesium, or both
- Lifestyle factors, such as increased stress and poor diet

Health promotion and health maintenance activities include good nutrition, vitamin and mineral supplements, stress management, exercise, and rest.

Clinical Manifestations

Typically, manifestations of PMS appear during the last few premenstrual days and are relieved suddenly with full menstrual flow. However, manifestations may begin with ovulation and may not be relieved until during or toward the end of menses. Characteristically, manifestations gradually worsen until menses begin.

Various manifestations are attributable to PMS, including altered emotional states, behavioral changes, somatic problems, changes in appetite, and motor effects. Different sets of manifestations are experienced by individual women. Emotional manifestations may include tension, depression, irritability, hostility, insomnia, loneliness, a tendency to cry easily, and indecision. Forgetfulness and mental confusion may occur. Psychosis and suicidal tendencies are rare.

Somatic problems are headache, breast tenderness and abdominal bloating, peripheral edema, joint pain and backache, hives, constipation, and exacerbation of pre-existing conditions, such as migraine and herpes. Because PMS manifestations usually do not occur during the menstrual flow, women may not associate them with the menstrual cycle.

To date, there is no objective method of diagnosing PMS. The diagnosis is usually made by documenting the cyclic nature of the manifestations on a menstrual calendar. A diary of manifestations and menstrual periods is an essential part of the assessment when PMS is suspected. Manifestations must occur for a minimum of three menstrual cycles. The diagnosis is confirmed according to the timing of manifestations rather than on the presence of particular manifestations.

Outcome Management

■ Medical Management

RELIEVE MANIFESTATIONS

VITAMINS AND MINERALS. Daily intake of vitamin B_6 and elimination of caffeine have improved some premenstrual manifestations. Nonprescription over-the-counter medications include calcium, vitamins A and C, magnesium, and trace elements. Essential fatty acid supplements are often recommended.

MEDICATIONS. Prescription medications commonly include oral spironolactone (Aldactone), progesterone, oral contraceptives, and anti-anxiety agents.

Spironolactone is a synthetic steroid aldosterone antagonist that inhibits the physiologic effect of aldosterone on the distal renal tubules. It is commonly used to treat the edema associated with excessive aldosterone secretion.

Progesterone may relieve physiologic and psychological manifestations. Bromocriptine (Parlodel) reduces serum prolactin concentrations by inhibiting prolactin release from the anterior pituitary gland. It has been used successfully to reduce breast pain in some cases of PMS.

Sedatives and analgesics, including antiprostaglandin agents, are often prescribed. Antidepressants may be prescribed for severe PMS.

See Alternative Therapy feature, p. 1009.

■ Nursing Management of the Medical Client

Nurses are in a key position to help women identify and cope with PMS when it is present. Clients who are in poor physical condition may be particularly susceptible to premenstrual difficulties. Thus, the nursing assessment includes general lifestyle, sleep and dietary habits, and overall health maintenance.

PROVIDE EDUCATION
Once the diagnosis of PMS is confirmed, the client needs accurate information about the syndrome and reassurance about the physiologic basis of the manifestations. Women often benefit from the opportunity to talk about their feelings and experiences with PMS, especially because of the confusion and misconceptions surrounding the syndrome. Instructions on how to take medications, if ordered, are important.

ENCOURAGE LIFESTYLE MODIFICATIONS
Suggested dietary modifications include reducing intake of salt and refined carbohydrates. Eating small, frequent meals to stabilize blood glucose levels can decrease fatigue, irritability, and craving. A calcium intake of at least 1000 mg/day may also decrease manifestations. Other vitamins and minerals have already been discussed along with medical management.

It may also be helpful to reduce alcohol and caffeine intake and to stop smoking. Give careful attention to stress management and reduction.

Weight reduction, if applicable, may decrease manifestations. Daily exercise (such as aerobics, jogging, or swimming) has been recommended to improve circulation, reduce stress, and promote a sense of well-being.

IMPROVE COPING
Another major nursing responsibility is helping the client and her significant others cope with the manifestations of PMS. Keep in mind the client's particular lifestyle and preferences. For example, a reallocation of responsibilities within the family might help to reduce her stress. If the client prefers to retain her current responsibilities, explain how she might manage them in ways that minimize stress.

Support groups or educational sessions may be helpful

as well. These sessions can serve as a forum for sharing information, providing mutual support, and discussing feelings. You can help form such a group if none exist in the area.

ABNORMAL UTERINE BLEEDING

Abnormal uterine bleeding encompasses a wide variety of menstrual disorders, such as lack of menstrual flow and irregular or excessive uterine bleeding. Changes in menstrual patterns can create anxiety in any woman. Associated manifestations disrupt activities of daily living. Sometimes abnormal uterine bleeding indicates an underlying pathologic disease. The term *dysfunctional uterine bleeding* refers to abnormal uterine bleeding for which no organic cause can be found through the usual assessment techniques. The presence of abnormal uterine bleeding necessitates careful assessment by a qualified health care provider.

■ AMENORRHEA

Amenorrhea means the absence of menses. *Primary* amenorrhea occurs if a woman has not begun to menstruate by the age of 16. *Secondary* amenorrhea is the absence of menses for 6 months in a woman who previously had regular cyclic bleeding or 12 months in a woman with a history of irregular bleeding.

Etiology and Risk Factors

There are many causes of amenorrhea, and they may appear alone or in combination (Fig. 39–1).

Clinical Manifestations

Results of the physical examination are usually normal. Laboratory tests and on occasion, endometrial biopsy may be used to identify and treat amenorrhea.

Outcome Management

■ Medical Management

Treatment depends on the woman's needs and the cause of the amenorrhea. Particularly important are her wishes regarding childbearing. If pregnancy is not desired at this time, progesterone may be prescribed. If pregnancy is desired, ovulation induction with clomiphene citrate (Clomid) may be undertaken.

■ Nursing Management of the Medical Client
RULE OUT PREGNANCY
The absence of spontaneous menstrual flow in a female older than 16 years requires careful assessment, including history and physical examination. Pregnancy also must be ruled out for any woman of childbearing age experiencing secondary amenorrhea. Ask about the presence of manifestations of pregnancy, such as breast tenderness, nausea, urinary frequency, weight gain, fatigue, and changes in food tolerance. Even if the client has been consistently using birth control, pregnancy must be considered.

PRIMARY AMENORRHEA		SECONDARY AMENORRHEA
	HYPOTHALAMUS	Anorexia nervosa Weight loss Strenuous exercise Pseudocyesis Systemic disease Post-pill amenorrhea Tumor
Anorexia nervosa Strenuous exercise Isolated GnRH deficiency Congenital defects Tumor	PITUITARY	
Prolactinoma Hyperprolactinemia Hypopituitarism		Prolactinoma Hyperprolactinemia
Hypothyroidism	THYROID	Hypothyroidism Hyperthyroidism
Congenital adrenal hyperplasia Adenomas/carcinoma	ADRENAL	Congenital adrenal hyperplasia Adenomas/carcinoma Cushing's disease Ectopic ACTH
Ovarian failure Polycystic ovary disease 17-Hydroxylase deficiency	OVARIAN	Ovarian failure Resistant ovary syndrome Tumors
Vaginal agenesis Transverse vaginal septum Imperforate hymen Testicular feminization	EXTRAUTERINE UTERINE VAGINAL	Ectopic pregnancy
		Intrauterine pregnancy Trophoblastic disease Uterine synechiae

FIGURE 39–1 Causes of amenorrhea. GnRH, gonadotropin-releasing hormone; ACTH, adrenocorticotropin-releasing hormone.

Young girls may deny having had sexual intercourse (penile penetration), but may admit, on careful questioning, that they have engaged in sexual play involving ejaculation between the thighs or near the introitus (opening into the vagina). Pregnancy can result from the migration of sperm in these situations, and a pregnancy test is necessary. If the pregnancy test result is positive, an ultrasound study should be performed to determine fetal size and to confirm estimated date of confinement (EDC). Additionally, if the test result is positive, the client should be offered appropriate opportunity to discuss her wishes about continuing or terminating the pregnancy.

PROVIDE TEACHING

Teaching opportunities are an important part of nursing care. Depending on the cause of amenorrhea, the client may need help in reducing energy drain from excessive physical activity and in controlling stress. Assess her general health, and help her plan and make changes as indicated.

■ MENORRHAGIA

The term *menorrhagia* means excessive vaginal bleeding at normal intervals.

Etiology and Risk Factors

There are a number of causes of menorrhagia, including:

- Anovulatory menstrual cycles
- Uterine fibroids and adenomyosis
- Anatomic lesions
- Spontaneous abortion
- Inflammatory processes (e.g., endometritis and salpingitis)
- Blood dyscrasias (disordered cellular elements)
- Hypothyroidism
- Use of an IUD
- Endometrial carcinoma
- Medications (e.g., anticoagulants)

Clinical Manifestations

Assessing the amount of blood loss can be difficult. Many women are unable to give a reliable history of blood loss. Asking the client to compare the number of pads or tampons used during the abnormal period with the number used during a normal cycle is a way of determining abnormality. Significant blood loss may be considered if the client is changing her pad or tampon every 1 to 2 hours. Because this information may not be adequate, a hematocrit or hemoglobin measurement may be performed to check for anemia.

Another test for significant uterine bleeding is transvaginal uterine ultrasound, which may reveal an increased thickness of the endometrium indicating abnormal tissue growth.

Outcome Management

Medical Management

Medical management may involve prescription of (1) estrogens and progestins, alone or in combination, (2) oral contraceptives, or (3) antifibrinolytic agents, depending on which factors are thought to be associated with the bleeding.

Surgical Management

An endometrial biopsy may be performed to determine the cause of uterine bleeding. A tiny amount of uterine tissue is removed and is sent to the pathologist for evaluation. The specimen is analyzed for hormone effects on the tissues and for any irregular or abnormal tissue growth. Often, the tissue demonstrates abnormal tissue proliferation that responds to hormone therapy.

Outpatient endometrial ablation (removal) is used to permanently stop uterine bleeding. A laser fiber is inserted into the uterus through a hysteroscope (an endoscope used to examine the cervix and uterus), and the laser beam is directed at destroying the endometrium. The destroyed tissue is then removed by irrigation of the uterus with saline. Sterility caused by uterine scarring is a likely consequence of the procedure.

Nursing Management of the Surgical Client

Other than an explanation of biopsy and the obtaining of informed consent for the procedure, no preoperative care is required before an endometrial biopsy, although emotional support is indicated. For an ablation, preoperative care includes having the client restrict food and fluid intake for anesthesia. The client is placed in the lithotomy position for this procedure.

Postoperatively, a perineal pad is in place. The pad should be checked and changed frequently. There may also be vaginal packing, which is usually removed within 24 hours.

During the first few hours, monitor vital signs and assess for excessive vaginal bleeding. Assess the client's ability to urinate. Urination may be difficult, especially if vaginal packing is exerting pressure on the urethra. Report excess bleeding, inability to void, or excessive pain. The client usually experiences only minimal uterine cramping postoperatively. Mild analgesics, such as acetaminophen and codeine (Tylenol No. 3) usually relieve any discomfort. The client should avoid aspirin for the first 24 to 48 hours to prevent excessive bleeding.

Follow-up instructions are as follows:

1. Avoid strenuous activity for about 1 week.
2. Do not douche or engage in vaginal or rectal intercourse until your physician judges that healing is complete.
3. Expect a small amount of pinkish vaginal discharge, followed by a dark red or dark brown discharge, during the healing process.
4. Subsequent menstrual periods may or may not be affected. Your next menses may not occur, may be on schedule, or may vary from the usual time.
5. Call your physician if any complications such as excessive bleeding (more than one pad per hour), excessive pain, or temperature elevation of greater than 100° F occur.
6. Return for a follow-up appointment.

■ METRORRHAGIA

Metrorrhagia (vaginal bleeding between menses) may occur as spotting or outright bleeding. Possible causes include ectopic pregnancy, spotting with ovulation, cervical polyps, breakthrough bleeding with oral contraceptives, and those listed for menorrhagia.

Pregnancy, as well as the presence of malignant or nonmalignant cells or hormonal or physical abnormalities, needs to be ruled out or treated appropriately. Anemia caused by excessive blood loss should be treated. For breakthrough bleeding in conjunction with the use of oral contraceptives or *hormone replacement therapy* (HRT), assess the length of time the hormones have been given, how long the bleeding has been present, and the amount of bleeding the client is experiencing in order to suggest any change in oral contraceptive or HRT dosing.

MENOPAUSE

Physiologic menopause (cessation of menstruation) is discussed in the Anatomy and Physiology Review.

■ SURGICAL MENOPAUSE

Menopause may be induced at any age by surgical removal of the ovaries, ablation with chemicals, or pelvic irradiation. *Hysterectomy* is the removal of only the uterus, not the ovaries, and does not usually cause surgical menopause. On occasion, the surgical intervention may have menopausal manifestations. In these instances, it is possible that blood vessels supplying the ovaries have been injured. The resulting loss of blood supply causes the ovaries to atrophy. Another possible cause is the hormone imbalance produced by removal of the uterus and its loss as a hormone receptor.

■ PERIMENOPAUSAL CHANGES

A wide variety of physical and psychosocial manifestations have been attributed to the perimenopausal period, but the only manifestations due to menopause itself (not the associated changes that are due to aging or stressful life events) are vasomotor instability, menstrual irregularities, and vaginal changes. A positive clinical manifestation is a follicle-stimulating hormone (FSH) level greater than 40 mIu/ml, indicating the intense attempt of the pituitary gland to stimulate the ovaries to produce estrogen, with the subsequent low serum estradiol level.

VASOMOTOR INSTABILITY. Manifestations of vasomotor instability, such as "hot flashes," night sweats, and the occasional palpitations and dizziness associated with menopause, appear to be caused by hormonal changes.

Hot flashes are sudden involuntary waves of heat that begin in the upper chest or neck and proceed up the face and head. These sensations last from a few seconds to an hour and are exacerbated by anything that increases heat production in the body. A hot flash may or may not be accompanied by a *hot flush*, which consists of a measurable change in skin temperature, a visible pink to bright red change in the skin, and perspiration.

A *night sweat* is a hot flash with or without a hot flush that occurs in the night, is accompanied by perspiration, which can be profuse, and is often followed by chills. Voda[37] describes the following types of hot flashes:

1. *Mild hot flash.* A warm feeling, often so fleeting it is barely noticeable. May or may not be accompanied by dampness and slight flushing.
2. *Moderate hot flash.* A warm to extremely warm feeling, that lasts longer and is more noticeable than a mild hot flash. Often accompanied by sweat and sometimes by flushing.
3. *Severe hot flash.* An intense or extremely hot feeling, usually accompanied by profuse and very uncomfortable sweating or flushing. The thermal discomfort of a severe hot flash may lead a woman to stop her activity at the time of the hot flash and to seek relief by using a fan, showering, removing or changing clothes, or lying down. Other bodily sensations associated with a severe hot flash are feelings of waves of heat, dizziness, a feeling of suffocation, inability to concentrate, and chest pain.

Generally, the manifestations of the hot flash occur about 45 seconds before the hot flush. In perimenopausal women, the reported incidence of the hot flash varies from 68% to 92%. There is a great variance in both the quantitative and qualitative aspects of women's experiences of hot flashes. Women in other cultures do not all report experiencing hot flashes; thus, the hot flash may not be a universal manifestation, or it may not be culturally acceptable for women to discuss menopausal manifestations.

ATROPHIC VAGINITIS AND OTHER CHANGES. The vaginal mucous membrane is especially responsive to low estrogen levels. When these levels remain low both during and following menopause, the vaginal walls become thinner and drier, with greater sensitivity and susceptibility to infection. These changes lead to the manifestations of atrophic vaginitis in menopausal women. Other manifestations are vaginal irritation, burning, pruritus, increased leukorrhea (vaginal discharge), bleeding, and dyspareunia (difficult or painful intercourse).

Vaginal epithelium loses its elasticity and subcutaneous fat after menopause. Pubic hair may become thinner. As the epidermal layer thins, the labia minora flatten and become flush with the labia majora. Other urogenital changes may be related to the loss of the estrogen-rich mucosal layer of the urethra and urethral atrophy associated with a higher incidence of cystitis and urethritis. In addition, these manifestations may also be confused with a urinary tract infection (UTI) or vaginitis.[4]

The pubococcygeus muscles tend to lose their tone, and stress urinary incontinence (see Chapter 34) also may occur. In addition, manifestations of urge incontinence, such as urgency, frequency and urine loss, may increase and may be confused with persistent UTI.

Some women experience difficulty sleeping. Others have backache, joint pain, and other manifestations of osteoporosis (a skeletal disorder characterized by the loss of bone mass and bone calcium). The calcium loss leads to an increased predisposition to bone collapse or fracture. Estrogen has been clinically proven to inhibit bone breakdown and loss. A decrease or absence of estrogen in conjunction with other risk factors may lead to osteoporosis.

Many myths abound about the occurrence of depression at the time of menopause, but no relationship between depression and menopause has been demonstrated. Some women appear to complain of depression or emotional changes at menopause more than at any other time in their lives. A woman's experience of menopause is affected not only by hormonal changes but also by her life circumstances and relationships. Psychosocial stress at the time of menopause, however, may affect menopausal manifestations.

Outcome Management

▪ Medical Management

REPLACE HORMONES
Hormone replacement therapy (estrogen plus progesterone) may be part of the medical management of perimenopausal, menopausal, and postmenopausal manifestations. Women must be informed of the advantages and risks of HRT so that they can make informed decisions about treatment. Some studies of the benefits and risks of the long-term use of HRT have demonstrated a decrease in incidence of cardiovascular disease, osteoporosis, Alzheimer's disease, and urogenital dysfunction.

It is often difficult for women to decide to begin and continue HRT because of conflicting information and fears related to a rise in the incidence of breast and uterine cancer associated with the treatment. Some researchers have claimed that the risk of breast cancer actually decreases with HRT, although further study is necessary to support this claim. HRT alleviates vasomotor instability, vaginal and urinary tract atrophy, and dyspareunia. It is also a preventive measure against osteoporosis and, possibly, cardiovascular disease.

In the middle to late 1970s, evidence of an association between *estrogen replacement therapy* (ERT) and endometrial cancer was discovered. In subsequent years, this association has been studied extensively. Today, estrogen is given with a progestational agent to simulate normal endometrial tissue. The progestin provides a protective effect against endometrial cancer. *Unopposed ERT* (estrogen without progestin) is no longer recommended for a woman with an intact uterus. It is generally accepted that estrogens should not be given to women with the following features:

- Known or suspected breast or uterine cancer or any estrogen-dependent cancer (or a strong family history of the same)
- Undiagnosed abnormal uterine bleeding
- Previous or present thrombophlebitis
- Acute liver disease
- Risk factors such as obesity, varicosities, hypertension, and heavy smoking, which become even more significant when they occur in combination
- Additional risk factors related to uterine fibromyomas,

severe varicose veins, chronic hepatic dysfunction, and diabetes mellitus, which require thorough assessment before estrogen is prescribed

The use of ERT or HRT should be individualized according to the client's needs and wishes, individual manifestations, and risks. The risk for women with fibrocystic breast disease is unclear, but careful assessment must be made. Risks should be assessed for endometrial cancer, osteoporosis, cardiovascular disease, and breast cancer. Both ERT and HRT are effective against perimenopausal hot flashes, atrophic vaginitis, and urinary tract changes. Unless otherwise indicated, HRT or ERT should be considered lifelong replacement therapy. Dosage may decrease with the client's age. Some recent research suggests that hormone replacement therapy be taken for only 5 years.

Both ERT and HRT decrease the risk of osteoporosis. The optimal duration of therapy for osteoporosis prevention is not known but is considered lifelong. Raloxifene (Evista) is a medication that prevents osteoporosis and may provide cardioprotective effects without increasing cancer risk. The possible cardioprotective effects of ERT, HRT, and raloxifene are being investigated. Hormone therapy is considered replacement of female hormones and should be discussed as such with the client before it is started.

If a client opts for ERT or HRT, she should be monitored for the development of breast cancer or any complication with annual breast examinations and mammography. Women must receive adequate education regarding the risk factors and anticipated effects of HRT as well as signals of impending problems it may cause.

Treatment regimens vary for estrogen-progesterone combinations. In some cases, estrogens may be used for 25 days each month or continually, whereas progesterones may be prescribed for 10 to 14 days a month. A low-dose continuous progesterone therapy may be given along with continuous ERT. The advantage of continuous combined therapy is the elimination of withdrawal bleeding. Bleeding usually ceases in about 4 months.

Side effects of high-dose progesterone therapy include bloating, depression, acne, breast tenderness, and premenstrual tension; however, these effects can generally be lessened by adjusting the dose, as with continuous therapy, or lengthening the duration of therapy. Side effects of progesterone may unfavorably alter the ratio of high-density-lipoprotein (HDL) and low-density-lipoprotein (LDL) cholesterol. Therefore, unopposed estrogen has been recommended for the client whose uterus has been surgically removed.

Transdermal estrogen patches are an alternative when oral estrogens cannot be tolerated or when the hepatic effects of estrogen (increased secretion of renin substrate causing hypertension and increased clotting factors as a result of liver stimulation) are a problem.

Vaginal estrogen is indicated for any woman experiencing urogenital manifestations of menopause (e.g., atrophic vaginitis, incontinence, and vaginal dryness). Vaginal estrogen can be delivered in continuous dosing, such as in a vaginal ring that is changed every 3 months. A small amount of vaginal cream, 0.5 to 1 g, can be inserted into the vagina at bedtime, several times per week.

■ Nursing Management of the Medical Client

PROVIDE EDUCATION

Nurses have a unique role in providing education for women undergoing menopause and their partners or significant others. The role involves providing support, education, and assistance in moving through this normal life experience as comfortably as possible. Accurate information about menopause and what to expect can be helpful and reassuring. Provide educational information about the risks and benefits of estrogen therapy.

To help clients cope with the minor discomforts of menopause, you may recommend the following self-care advice:

1. *Relief of vaginal dryness.* Intercourse and masturbation aid circulation and keep tissues flexible; use water-soluble vaginal lubricants as often as needed. Topical estrogen cream or other vaginal estrogen preparations eliminate manifestations.
2. *Prevention of osteoporosis.* Take part in weight-bearing exercises; increase calcium intake; stop smoking; reduce alcohol and caffeine intake.
3. *Prevention of UTIs.* Increase fluid intake (six to eight glasses of water per day; attempt to void every 2 to 3 hours; maintain good perineal hygiene; wear cotton underwear.
4. *Pelvic relaxation.* Perform Kegel (pelvic floor) exercises to increase muscle tone (see later and Chapter 34); lose weight if appropriate.

Remind women experiencing menopause of the value of good health habits. Balanced nutrition and adequate sleep and rest are important. Phytoestrogens (plant estrogens), found in soy products, flaxseed oil, nuts, and brown rice, have a very mild estrogenic effect that may reduce vaginal dryness. Exercising at least three to four times per week for 45 minutes improves bone and cardiovascular health.

See Alternative Therapy feature, p. 1009.

POSTMENOPAUSAL BLEEDING

Postmenopausal bleeding (vaginal bleeding occurring after menopause) is a manifestation, not a diagnosis (Fig. 39–2). Careful assessment is necessary because it may be a manifestation of many conditions of the lower reproductive tract: atrophic vaginitis, cervical polyps, uterine fibroids, endometrial hyperplasia, cervical erosion, and uterine or cervical cancer.

PELVIC INFLAMMATORY DISEASE

The term *pelvic inflammatory disease* refers to ascending pelvic infection that involves the upper genital tract.

Etiology and Risk Factors

Chlamydia trachomatis, gonococci, staphylococci, streptococci, and other pus-producing (pyogenic) organisms commonly cause PID. A common risk factor is an untreated bacterial infection. Most of these infections are sexually transmitted. The lack of condom use increases the risk of passing the bacteria between partners.

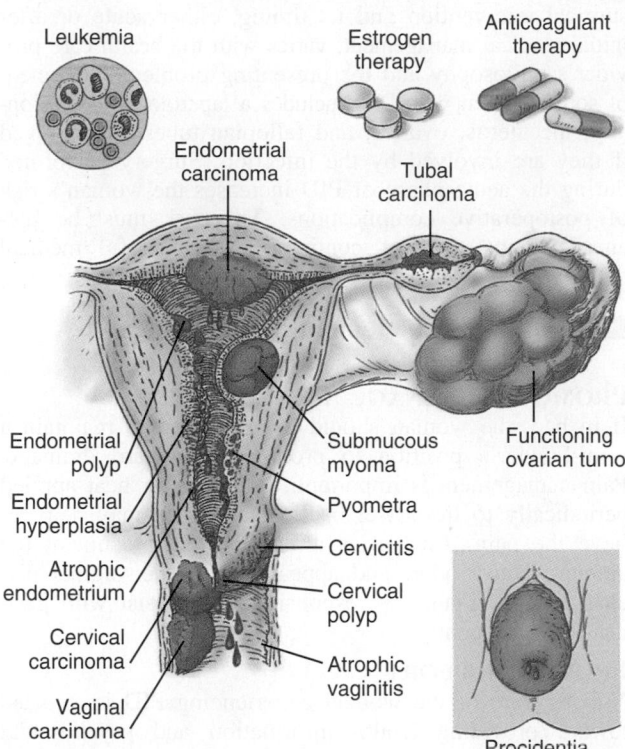

FIGURE 39–2 Causes of postmenopausal bleeding.

Health promotion actions are to advise clients to avoid (1) unprotected intercourse, (2) sex with multiple partners, especially with use of an IUD, (3) IUD for birth control, and (4) douches. To maintain health, clients should seek treatment immediately when manifestations of PID appear and if a sexual partner has a sexually transmitted disease (STD).

Health restoration activities include advising clients to complete the full course of medications used to treat a PID and to follow health promotion recommendations to prevent reinfection.

Pathophysiology

Once an infection is in the upper genital tract, the bacteria may travel along several routes (Fig. 39–3). Tuberculosis (TB), a rare cause of PID, travels through the blood and affects the fallopian tubes and sometimes the ovaries, uterus, and pelvic peritoneum. The woman's excreta are contaminated until the antituberculin medications have taken effect.

C. trachomatis and gonococcal and staphylococcal organisms spread along the uterine endometrium to the fallopian tubes, where an acute *salpingitis* (inflammation of the fallopian tubes) occurs. The tubes become partially occluded and may drain pus, leukocytes, and other debris into the pelvic cavity, causing pelvic peritonitis, or the material may form a pocket around the ovary, causing a tubo-ovarian abscess.

Streptococci spread similarly, but they tend to travel via the uterine or cervical lymphatics across the parametrium to the tubes or ovaries. Pelvic cellulitis and occasional thrombophlebitis of the major pelvic veins with additional risk of the development of emboli may occur.

Another route of infection is from the pelvic cavity itself. Organisms such as *Escherichia coli* may be extruded from a ruptured bowel, causing peritonitis.

Although septic shock and other complications may appear, the most common is a pelvic abscess.

More than 50% of women with a history of PID have difficulty becoming pregnant or experience an ectopic pregnancy after the infection has cleared. These problems are due to scarring by the inflammatory process and subsequent closing and scarring of the fallopian tubes.

Clinical Manifestations

PID may be "silent" (asymptomatic), especially in the early stage. Clinical manifestations of PID include malaise, fever, chills, anorexia, nausea and vomiting, aching and tachycardia. In addition, the woman usually experiences acute, sharp, severe aching pain on both sides of the abdomen or pelvis. Pain is worsened by urination or defecation and may be accompanied by a heavy, purulent, and, possibly, odorous discharge. Occasionally, vaginal bleeding occurs. The rapidity of onset of PID depends on (1) the virulence (degree of severity) of the infecting organism, (2) the status of the client's pelvic organs, and (3) the client's general health.

Other helpful clues to PID are obtained from the history. A history of acute lower genital tract infection is significant. Other data, including a thorough sexual history, are important. A history of contraceptive use is established because the presence of an IUD correlates with a higher incidence of PID.

The long-term sequelae of untreated, silent PID may be detected when attempts to achieve a pregnancy have proved unsuccessful. During a clinical evaluation of the client, routine screening tests, such as cultures, may yield

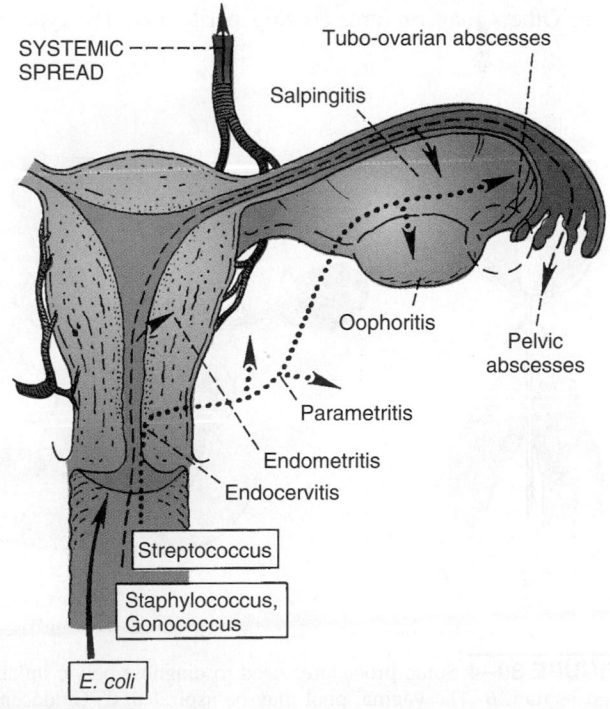

FIGURE 39–3 Routes of spread of pelvic inflammatory disease.

positive results. The usual laboratory tests for infection, including multiple cultures (Fig. 39–4), are performed. Some practitioners perform a culture of any evident drainage and obtain specimens from various sites, such as the cervix, vagina, and urethra. Additional specimens from the vagina and the adjacent structures may be obtained to evaluate for bacterial infection of the genital tract. If multiple organisms are found, several types of antibiotics may be necessary to treat the infection.

Histologic examination of endometrial biopsy specimens, colposcopy (examination with use of a large color-filtering, magnifying instrument), or ultrasonography to identify an abscess may also be used in the diagnosis of PID.

Outcome Management

■ Medical Management

ELIMINATE CAUSATIVE ORGANISM
Most clients with PID are treated as outpatients, receiving antibiotics appropriate to the specific organism causing the infection. They are cautioned to avoid sexual activity, douching, and other activities that might enhance the infectious process. With improvement, the client should return to the clinic in a week for reevaluation of status. Advise the client being treated at home for PID to return sooner if her condition deteriorates or if manifestations increase.

Hospitalization may be necessary for a client with PID who is acutely ill. During hospitalization, antibiotics are administered in maximal doses if the cause of PID is bacterial; PID resulting from TB is treated with antituberculosis medications. Treatment with medication is aimed at removing or destroying the causative organism.

■ Surgical Management

Some abscesses must be removed by surgical intervention. Others may rupture, causing peritonitis. The type of surgical intervention and its timing, either acute or after initial medical management, varies with the health care provider's philosophy and the presenting problem. Treatment of some women with PID includes a laparotomy. Occasionally, the uterus, ovaries, and fallopian tubes are removed if they are involved by the infection. Surgery performed during the acute phase of PID increases the woman's risk of postoperative complications. This risk must be balanced against that of continuing unsuccessful medical therapy, which often leads to chronic PID.

■ Nursing Management of the Medical-Surgical Client

PROMOTE DRAINAGE AND COMFORT
If in bed, the woman should be instructed to maintain a semi-Fowler's position to promote downward drainage. Pain management is important. Sitz baths or heat applied periodically to the lower back or abdomen may help relieve the pain. Analgesics are also used. Document the amount, color, odor, and appearance of the vaginal discharge. It is a nursing responsibility to assist with perineal care frequently.

PROVIDE SUPPORT
Nursing care of the woman experiencing PID is directed toward providing health information and psychosocial support to the client and her significant others. Because PID is often caused by STDs, there may be guilt feelings and emotional stress within the relationship. Usually, the woman's sexual partner requires treatment whether symptomatic or not.

Some women are infertile after PID. This loss of fertility may be difficult for the client and her significant other to accept. Plan and provide time for the expression of such feelings.

PROVIDE EDUCATION
Education is important for the client with PID. Women with PID can benefit from factual discussion about the

FIGURE 39–4 Some procedures used to diagnose pelvic inflammatory disease. *A*, Swabs may be obtained from the cervix, urethra, and rectum. *B*, The vaginal pool may be aspirated. *C*, Culdocentesis may be performed. Gram's stains of cervical secretions show gram-negative intracellular diplococci. Cultures are placed on Thayer-Martin medium. Negative stains and cultures do not rule out gonococcal disease.

infection, recognizing the manifestations of recurrences, and general hygienic and sexual measures to help prevent new infections. The client should be instructed to wash the perineal area regularly with soap and water, to wipe the perineum from front to back after elimination, to change tampons and pads several times a day during menses, and to wash hands before and after changing tampons or pads.

Balanced nutrition, adequate rest, sleep, and exercise can improve general health and reduce the risk of infection. Inform clients when sexual activity can be resumed, how to ensure the safety of sexual encounters, and when other restrictions can be lifted.

CHRONIC PELVIC INFLAMMATORY DISEASE

Chronic PID can occur if the acute phase of the illness does not respond to treatment or if treatment is inadequate. Clinical manifestations of chronic PID include chronic pelvic discomfort, menstrual disturbances or dysfunctional uterine bleeding, constipation, malaise, and periodic return of acute manifestations. Sterility, one of the more serious complications, results from destruction of part of the fallopian tubes and loss of their patency (their being wide open).

Treatment of chronic PID is aimed at removing the offending organism and improving the client's general health. If treatment is unsuccessful, surgical removal of the pelvic organs may be necessary.

UTERINE DISORDERS

ENDOMETRIOSIS

Endometriosis is an abnormal condition in which *endometrium*, the tissue that normally lines the uterus, is located in internal sites other than in the uterus. Endometriosis most commonly affects women in their mid-30s. It occasionally occurs in women younger than 20 years of age. There is a familial predisposition, and the highest incidence is in white women who are nulliparous (have not given birth).

Etiology and Risk Factors

The cause of endometriosis is unknown, although a few theories have been proposed, for instance:

1. *Retrograde menstruation theory.* Menstrual secretions flow backward through the fallopian tubes and deposit particles of viable endometrial tissue outside the uterine cavity. Spread then occurs as endometrial tissue reproduces itself, a process called *metaplasia*.
2. *Vascular and lymphatic dissemination theory.* Spread (metastasis) of endometrial tissue occurs through the lymphatic and vascular systems to locations outside the uterus. This may explain some of the distant sites of metastasis, such as the lungs and kidneys.

Pathophysiology

Although the abnormally located endometrial tissue is usually confined to the pelvic cavity, it may be found in other areas. The most common sites are the ovary and the dependent portion of the pelvic peritoneum. Rarely, tissue may lie outside the pelvis, such as in surgical scars, lungs, and extremities. Possible sites are shown in Figure 39–5.

Regardless of the site, this misplaced endometrial tissue responds to hormonal stimulation and bleeds, producing a variety of manifestations. Scarring and inflammation occur at these extrauterine sites. Repeated episodes of intraperitoneal bleeding, due to hormonal stimulation of the endometrial tissue, cause adhesions. Scarring and adhesions cause the organs and peritoneal surface to become fixed to each other.

Because endometrial tissue is hormone-dependent, the tissue usually atrophies with the normal ovarian regression associated with menopause; it also regresses during pregnancy.

Infertility is a major complication of endometriosis. Usually, the infertility is due to scarring, leading to obstruction of the fallopian tubes.

Clinical Manifestations

Manifestations of endometriosis relate more to the *site* than to the *extent* of disease present. Pain is the most characteristic manifestation; however, about 25% of women with this condition are asymptomatic. Pain typically begins before the menstrual period, lasting for the duration of menstruation and sometimes for several days afterward. The intensity of pain is not correlated with the extent of endometriosis. Pain usually reaches its peak just before the onset of menstrual flow and during the first 1 or 2 days of the menstrual period. The pain may be located in several areas, making the diagnosis more difficult to confirm. Unfortunately, some health care providers may view some women with endometriosis as having psychosomatic complaints and drug-seeking behaviors.

Other manifestations of endometriosis are dyspareunia, menstrual irregularities, and infertility in the absence of tubal obstruction. When the condition occurs inside the ovary, it can produce a "chocolate" cyst, or *endometrioma*. Severe pain is associated with the presence or rupture of this cyst. Implants of endometrium on the ureters may cause obstruction. Rectal implants may be associated with bleeding, diarrhea, or obstruction. Bowel involvement may cause painful defecation.

The diagnosis is generally made from the history, a pelvic examination, and observation of lesions either by laparoscopic examination or pelvic surgery. Direct observation of lesions is necessary for a definitive diagnosis.

Outcome Management

� Medical Management

Appropriate treatment of endometriosis depends on the client's manifestations, age, number of children (parity), and extent of disease. When manifestations and extent of disease are mild, the client is given support, information, and coping strategies for pain management. Mild analgesics may be helpful. If manifestations become severe or the disease progresses, additional treatment is generally necessary.

A. SITES OF ENDOMETRIOSIS   B. LYMPHATICS

FIGURE 39–5 Endometriosis. *A*, Sites of endometriosis. The locations most frequently affected are the ovaries and the dependent pelvic peritoneum. However, many other sites may be involved. *B*, Pelvic and lymph nodes are important.

REDUCE MANIFESTATIONS

Medication may inhibit endometriosis enough to allow pregnancy or, at least, relieve manifestations. Hormonal intervention includes inducing a *pseudopregnancy* (false pregnancy) with oral contraceptives, progesterone, or both. During the course of this treatment, progestins cause the endometrial implants to slough off. Thus, theoretically, the endometrial tissue no longer functions in abnormal sites. This type of treatment is not successful in all women.

The other hormonal treatment is to induce *ovarian suppression* or *pseudomenopause* (false menopause). Danazol (Danocrine) is an antigonadotropin testosterone derivative that inhibits gonadotropin release, causing ovarian suppression and regression of endometriosis. The medication provides rapid and safe relief of manifestations. Side effects may include acne, hirsutism (excess hair), weight gain, decreased breast size, hot flashes, and vaginal dryness.

Leuprolide (Lupron), a synthetic analog of luteinizing hormone (LH), reduces endometrial pain and lesions. The client can administer it herself monthly in an intramuscular (IM) injection or daily in a subcutaneous (SC) injection. This medication also carries associated menopausal side effects.

Nafarelin (Synarel) acts as a synthetic analog of gonadotropin-releasing hormone (GnRH). Lesions are reduced because endometrial lesions are sensitive to ovarian hormones. It is administered intranasally twice a day and may create menopausal side effects.

Hormonal treatments are very expensive, costing from $100 to more than $300 per month.

Surgical Management

Exploratory or therapeutic surgery directed at endometriosis may make pregnancy possible. Conservative surgi-

cal intervention involves restoring normal anatomy and removing or destroying endometriotic foci. A carbon dioxide laser may be used to vaporize adhesions and endometrial implants. Even if the client claims that pregnancy is not desirable at this time, conservative surgery should be considered.

More radical surgery involves removing the uterus, as many implants as possible, and, possibly, the ovaries. This procedures has wide-reaching consequences for affecting sexuality, cardiovascular health, and the risk of osteoporosis unless HRT is also given. This surgical intervention is used only when other measures have failed and the client does not wish to preserve fertility. It causes surgically induced menopause and permanent sterility.

Controversy exists about the use of HRT after such an extensive surgical procedure. The client with a history of endometriosis who undergoes surgically induced menopause may be at risk for induction of additional growth of endometrial implants if she is given some form of HRT after the procedure, particularly in the first few months postoperatively. Conservative surgery is effective for most women. More radical surgery is almost completely effective.

Nursing Management of the Medical-Surgical Client

Nursing care of the woman with endometriosis is individualized and depends on (1) severity of manifestations, (2) extent of disease, (3) age, and (4) childbearing status. Nursing care consists of support during the diagnostic process as the client considers the various treatment options.

Nursing interventions should include discussion of information about the nature of endometriosis, its treatment, and ways to cope with the manifestations. Yoga and relaxation techniques may provide relief. If infertility is an issue, provide information and support in decision-making in this area as well.

Surgical management is similar to that discussed for abdominal hysterectomy, tubal ligation, or laparoscopy (see later).

BENIGN UTERINE TUMORS (LEIOMYOMAS)

Leiomyomas are the most common tumors of the female genital tract. They occur in more than 20% to 30% of all women during the menstrual years. The incidence is two to three times greater in African American women than in white women. Leiomyomas are more common in women approaching menopause.

Leiomyomas are known by various names related to the tissue involved such as fibroids, fibromas, fibromyomas, fibroleiomyomas, myomas, and fiber balls. Leiomyomas are composed mainly of muscle and fibrous connective tissue.

Etiology and Risk Factors

The cause of leiomyomas is unknown. Their growth seems to be related to estrogen stimulation because the fibroids often enlarge with pregnancy and shrink with menopause. A leiomyoma begins as a simple proliferation of smooth muscle cells. It has been suggested that this type of proliferation is stimulated by physical or mechanical means and may occur at points of maximal stress within the myometrium. Because there are many points of stress within the uterus resulting from contractions, fibroids are often multiple (Fig. 39–6).

Pathophysiology

Leiomyomas develop from the uterine myometrium. Growth is usually associated with proliferation of the

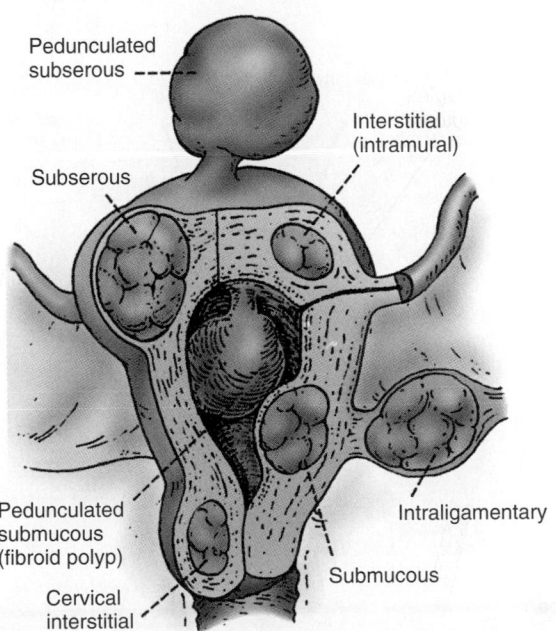

Pedunculated subserous

Interstitial (intramural)

Subserous

Pedunculated submucous (fibroid polyp)

Intraligamentary

Submucous

Cervical interstitial

FIGURE 39–6 Some sites of leiomyomas (fibroids). Uterine leiomyomas, depending on their location and size, may interfere with passage of sperm and implantation of a fertilized ovum.

smooth muscle cells. Estrogen and other hormones influence growth of the muscle cells. Manifestations usually decrease after menopause.

Classification

Leiomyomas may be classified according to their location (those occurring in the uterine body are most common; see Fig. 39–6):

1. *Intramural.* Found in the uterine wall, surrounded by myometrium. Clinical manifestations include increased uterine size, vaginal bleeding between menses, and dysmenorrhea.
2. *Submucosal.* Located directly under the endometrium, involving the endometrial cavity. May become pedunculated (grow on a stalk). Clinical manifestations include prolonged vaginal bleeding and cramps, and the tumor may be seen protruding through the cervix.
3. *Subserosal.* Found on the outer surface (under the serosa) of the uterus. Tends to become pedunculated, to wander (see later), and to be multiple and large. Clinical manifestations include backache, constipation, and bladder problems.
4. *Wandering or parasitic.* A pedunculated leiomyoma that twists on its pedicle, breaks off, then attaches to other tissues, particularly the omentum.
5. *Intraligamentary.* Implants on the pelvic ligaments. May displace the uterus or involve the ureters.
6. *Cervical.* Occur infrequently and may obstruct the cervical canal.

Clinical Manifestations

Frequently, leiomyomas are asymptomatic. Manifestations relate to tumor size, location, and number. Additionally, abnormal bleeding, often resulting in hypermenorrhea (excessive uterine bleeding), is frequently related to the fibroid's hormone dependence.

Manifestations vary widely and occur in about half of clients with leiomyomas. When present, manifestations often relate to the size, location, and number of leiomyomas. The onset of manifestations most commonly occurs in a client's late 40s and early 50s, just before menopause. Once menopause begins, manifestations often cease. It is rare for manifestations to begin after menopause, when leiomyomas tend to regress with decreasing estrogen stimulation. If new manifestations develop during these years, other diagnoses, such as cancer, need to be ruled out.

The most common clinical manifestation is abnormal uterine bleeding, which may be excessive in either amount or duration. Additionally, it may accompanied by anemia, with manifestations of tiredness, weakness, and lethargy. Dysmenorrhea and a sense of pelvic pressure are often present. Urinary frequency is common when the tumor presses on the bladder. Urinary retention also may occur when bladder function is compromised by tumor size. Constipation, hydroureter (abnormal distention of ureter with urine), hydronephrosis (distention of kidney due to abnormal accumulation of urine in the kidney pelvis), abdominal pain, and dyspareunia are less common manifestations.

Occasionally, the client may have vaginal discharge, which may be foul or water-tinged and blood-tinged. Abdominal pressure occurs if the leiomyoma is large enough to cause abdominal distention. The tumor may be palpable. Also, the client may experience sterility or have a history of one or more spontaneous abortions.

A characteristic history, confirmed by findings of abdominal and pelvic examinations, usually establishes the diagnosis. Ultrasonography may demonstrate an abnormal uterine shape. Various disorders, such as cancer and a problem pregnancy, must be ruled out before treatment is planned.

Outcome Management

■ Medical Management

A plan of treatment for leiomyomas depends on manifestations, age of the client, location and size of the tumors, onset of complications, and client's desire to preserve fertility. Leiomyomas can be assessed every 6 months by a practitioner if the client is not pregnant; if there is no excessive bleeding or pressure on the bladder, bowel, or ureters; and if the tumor is not rapidly growing.

GnRH analogs (see Endometriosis earlier) may be administered to reduce size and inhibit growth of tumors. Malignant degeneration is rare. A rapid increase in the size of the leiomyoma, as indicated by manifestations or detected on examination, should be thoroughly evaluated, and aggressive therapy should be considered.

■ Surgical Management

Surgical treatment may involve cutting off the blood supply to the fibroid or *myomectomy* (removal of a tumor without removal of the uterus). Both procedures preserve the reproductive organs and reproductive capability. However, because of the increased risk that additional leiomyomas may develop later, a hysterectomy may be the preferred procedure.

HYSTERECTOMY

INDICATIONS. Three types of hysterectomy may be performed:

Total hysterectomy—removal of the uterus and cervix. Can be performed either abdominally or vaginally.

Total hysterectomy with bilateral salpingo-oophorectomy (TAH-BSO)—removal of uterus, cervix, fallopian tubes, and ovaries. Can be performed vaginally or abdominally (Fig. 39–7).

Radical hysterectomy—same as a TAH-BSO plus removal of the lymph nodes, upper third of the vagina, and parametrium. Usually performed if a malignant tumor is found.

CONTRAINDICATIONS. The only contraindication to hysterectomy is any health condition that prevents surgery.

COMPLICATIONS. Hemorrhage and infection are the primary complications.

OUTCOMES. It is expected that the client will return home in 2 to 4 days and resume regular activities within 4 to 6 weeks, depending on the type of hysterectomy performed. Pain, abnormal bleeding, and anemia, if present, will cease. For all procedures except myomectomy, menstruation ends.

■ Nursing Management of the Surgical Client

PREOPERATIVE CARE

The client seeks medical help because of some form of abnormal uterine bleeding, dyspareunia, or pelvic pain. Obtain a thorough history from the client, especially if there are complaints of irregular bleeding. It is also important to assess the client's knowledge of her condition and the surgery. Listen carefully for any questions she has about sexuality after treatment.

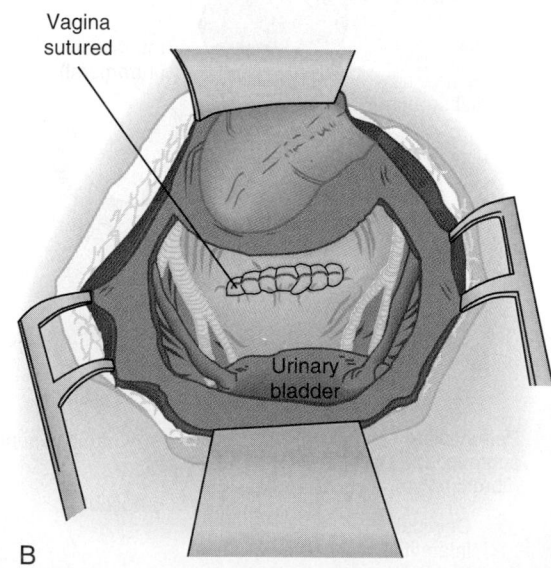

FIGURE 39–7 Total abdominal hysterectomy with salpingo-oophorectomy. *A,* The uterus with attached uterine tubes and ovaries is lifted out after it has been freed from the ligaments holding it. *B,* After the specimen has been removed en masse, the vagina is sutured closed.

REDUCE PAIN. Before surgery is performed, the client can be taught ways to reduce pain associated with intercourse, such as assuming positions in which leiomyomas are not pressed on during intercourse and using water-soluble lubricants. Pain medications can be used for severe pain. Sometimes, sitz baths or the application of heat to the lower abdomen may be helpful.

PROVIDE EDUCATION. The client undergoing a hysterectomy has many learning needs. Frequently, a woman undergoing gynecologic surgery needs help understanding the problem and the proposed operation. She needs to understand her options and the differences among the procedures proposed.

If a hysterectomy is planned, inform the client about the loss of fertility. If the ovaries are to be removed in conjunction with the hysterectomy, discuss surgical menopause and HRT. Some women are relieved that the operation will remove the risk of unwanted pregnancy and monthly menstrual manifestations.

Discuss how sexual intercourse may change after a hysterectomy. Although the client's ability to achieve orgasm should not change, the vagina will be shortened and there may be scar tissue.

The client whose ovaries are removed may complain of a decrease in *libido* (sexual desire). This is due to the loss of testosterone that is normally produced by the ovaries. HRT may include a small daily dose of testosterone. Tell the client that once healing has occurred, intercourse should be pain-free. Answer any questions asked, and encourage the client and her significant other to express their feelings and concerns about sexuality.

POSTOPERATIVE CARE
ASSESSMENT

Perform the usual postoperative assessments. Evaluation of psychological manifestations is also important.

The proximity of the bladder to the female reproductive organs increases the risk of urinary problems, which must be monitored postoperatively. A Foley catheter is usually inserted at the time of surgery to prevent bladder distention and injury during surgery; the catheter is often left in place for 24 hours postoperatively. Potential postoperative problems related to the placement of a Foley catheter are UTI and temporary urinary retention due to voiding dysfunction.

Assess GI function by listening for bowel sounds, noting distention and seeing whether the abdomen is soft or firm. Passing of flatus (bowel gas) indicates the return of GI function. After an abdominal hysterectomy, assess the abdominal incision for bleeding and intactness.

Assess vaginal bleeding. One saturated pad should be necessary in 4 hours after abdominal or vaginal hysterectomy. Excessive bleeding should be considered if one sanitary napkin is saturated in one hour or less.

DIAGNOSIS, OUTCOMES, INTERVENTIONS
Risk for Dysfunctional Grieving. Some women experience grief about their loss of the female reproductive organs, making *Risk for Dysfunctional Grieving related to loss of reproductive capacity and perceived loss of femininity* an appropriate nursing diagnosis for a client undergoing hysterectomy.

Outcomes. The client can be expected to go through a grieving process over her loss after hysterectomy and may express her feelings about the loss.

Interventions. When reproductive ability is lost, the client may undergo a grief response. It is important for the nurse to understand the grieving process and to be able to help the woman understand that this response is normal. Some women experience relief rather than grief. Support normal grieving, including temporary denial, which is a part of the grieving process. If the client continues to experience grief beyond the normal degree or time expected, she may require counseling.

Risk for Infection. During surgery for a hysterectomy, a Foley catheter is inserted, leading to the nursing diagnosis *Risk for Infection related to surgical intervention and presence of a urinary catheter.*

Outcomes. The client will remain free of infection, or will report any infection immediately for proper diagnosis and treatment.

Interventions
Prevent Urinary Infection. When a Foley catheter is in place, instruct the client to keep the urinary drainage catheter below the level of the bladder, drink at least 2 to 4 L of liquid daily, and report any urinary pain or discomfort. Check the urinary drainage system closely for leaks and kinks in the system, provide complete perineal care every shift, and report any change in color or odor of the urine. When a Foley catheter is discontinued, monitor the client for the first void. Voiding frequently in small amounts, inability to void, and bladder distention or hematuria should be reported to the physician.

Prevent Retention. Often, a suprapubic catheter is placed instead of a Foley catheter. This allows the client to clamp the catheter and attempt to void as soon as she is ambulatory. If the suprapubic area becomes distended when the catheter is clamped and the client is unable to void, the suprapubic catheter can be opened and drained. Using a suprapubic catheter avoids the need for recatheterization of a client who cannot void.

Constipation. Because of bowel manipulation during surgery, the nursing diagnosis *Constipation related to bowel manipulation during surgery* is appropriate.

Outcomes. The client will not become constipated, and bowel distention will be treated, as evidenced by return to a normal bowel pattern and absence of abdominal distention.

Interventions
Promote Peristalsis. Pain and discomfort after abdominal hysterectomy usually center on the incision and postoperative gas pains. After abdominal hysterectomy, GI functioning returns slowly. Uncomfortable gas pains are often experienced during the early postoperative period. Early, frequent ambulation helps to improve GI function. If gas pains persist, a small enema may be prescribed to facilitate peristalsis and to prevent constipation. Continue to encourage frequent ambulation to facilitate the return of normal GI functioning. Drinking warm fluids may encourage the return of peristalsis.

EVALUATION

It is expected that the client will recover from a hysterectomy without complications. She can return to normal activities within 4 to 6 weeks without permanent problems.

Self-Care

The client should understand the type of surgery she has had and the follow-up needed. If she has had a myomectomy, pregnancy is still an option. She must continue to have routine gynecologic examinations and to use birth control measures until her physician judges that she can attempt a pregnancy. If she has undergone TAH-BSO, discuss menopause and HRT with her. Discharge teaching should also include the following instructions:

1. Eat a well-balanced diet, drink six to eight glasses of water daily, and get plenty of rest.
2. Avoid heavy lifting for about 6 weeks, to prevent straining on the abdominal muscles and surgical sites.
3. Avoid activities that increase pelvic congestion, such as aerobic activity, horseback riding, and prolonged standing. Optimal circulation is necessary to promote healing of pelvic tissues.
4. Avoid vaginal and rectal intercourse and douching until healing is complete, usually in about 6 weeks. These activities can interfere with healing of the vaginal cuff or other healing tissues and can introduce infection.
5. Report any fresh bleeding and any abnormal vaginal discharge to the surgeon.
6. Return for follow-up care as requested by the surgeon.

ENDOMETRIAL (UTERINE) CANCER

Endometrial cancer is the most common malignancy of the female genital reproductive system. In 2000, it was estimated that 36,100 new cases of uterine cancer would be diagnosed in the United States. The 5-year survival rate is 95% if the cancer is discovered at an early stage and 64% if the cancer is identified at a regional stage.[1]

Etiology and Risk Factors

Endometrial cancer is thought to be related to overstimulation of the endometrium from excessive circulating estrogen. Common sources of excessive estrogen are successive anovulatory menstrual cycles and unopposed ERT (estrogen without progestin) in a woman who still has her uterus. Other factors are history of pelvic radiation, other reproductive cancer, family history, history of diabetes or hypertension, obesity, and hyperestrogenism (early menarche, late menopause, dysfunctional uterine bleeding, delayed onset of ovulation).

Health promotion actions include advising overweight women to lose weight and use of HRT (estrogen and progestin) or raloxifene (Evista) instead of estrogen therapy. Health maintenance actions are to advise women to have yearly pelvic examinations even after menopause, ensure that high-risk women undergo endometrial biopsy at regular intervals, and inform the client to have post-menopausal bleeding assessed.

Pathophysiology

In women with endometrial cancer, the cell type is usually adenocarcinoma, a tumor that involves the glands. This relatively slow-growing tumor metastasizes late in its course and tends to spread slowly to other organs. Most commonly, the carcinoma invades the uterus, causing uterine enlargement. The cancerous process may extend along the endometrial surface to the cervix or fallopian tubes and ovaries. It can spread to other peritoneal structures, including the lymphatics and blood vessels. It can then spread to the vagina, through the lymphatics to other areas, and, occasionally, to distant sites such as the brain and lungs.

Clinical Manifestations

Because there is no practical, accurate method of screening for endometrial cancer, the cancer is usually discovered after the first manifestations appear. The most significant manifestation is some type of abnormal uterine bleeding, especially in the postmenopausal woman. Other manifestations relate to invasion, metastasis to other organs, or both (Fig. 39–8).

A diagnosis of endometrial cancer is usually established by pelvic examination and pathologic analysis of an endometrial biopsy specimen. Women at high risk may undergo endometrial biopsy at each annual or biannual pelvic examination. An endovaginal ultrasound study of the endometrium may be used to detect a thickened endometrium, or a hysteroscope (a small intrauterine instrument that visualizes uterine contents) with biopsy may be used to assist in the diagnosis.

Outcome Management

Surgical Management

Endometrial cancer is generally treated with surgery, radiation, or a combination. Early endometrial cancer is sur-

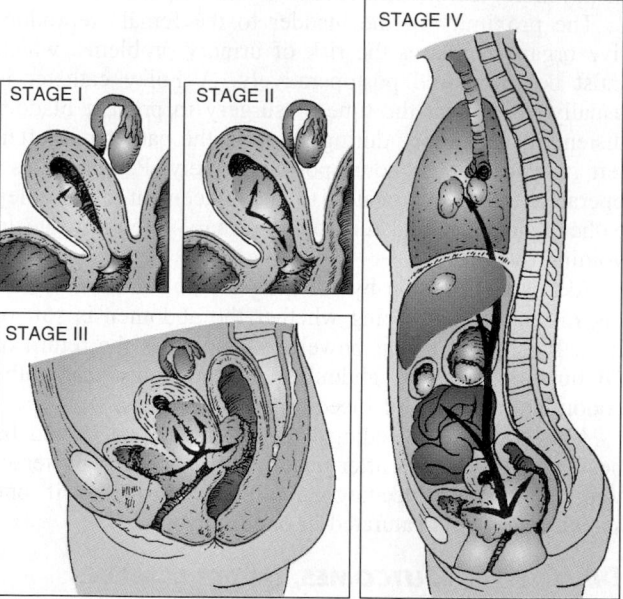

FIGURE 39–8 Staging uterine cancer. *Stage 1,* The tumor is confined to the uterine corpus. *Stage 2,* The cancer has also invaded the cervix. *Stage 3,* The cancer has spread beyond the uterus but remains confined to the pelvis, such as in the bladder or rectum. *Stage 4,* Highest level of invasiveness since the cancer has spread beyond the pelvis, causing metastatic disease and large masses, such as in the liver or lungs.

gically treated with a TAH-BSO. Surgery may be preceded or followed by irradiation, either external of internal. Surgical management is the same as for benign uterine tumors (leiomyomas).

■ Medical Management

External irradiation is discussed in Chapter 19. If intracavity (internal) radiation therapy (IRT) or brachytherapy is selected, an applicator is placed through the vagina into the uterus with the use of anesthesia. Correct placement is verified by x-ray study, and the client is taken to a hospital room. A radiologist places a radioactive isotope in the applicator, which remains for 1 to 3 days.

Precancerous endometrial changes may be treated with the hormone progesterone. Chemotherapy and hormonal therapy with tamoxifen (Nolvadex) are used to treat late stages of endometrial cancer.

■ Nursing Management of the Medical-Surgical Client

Nursing care of the surgical client is the same as described for the client with benign uterine tumors (leiomyomas).

While the radioactive implants are in place, the client is strictly isolated in a private room. She must remain at bed rest, with the head of the bed flat or elevated no more than 20 degrees. Movement is restricted except for deep breathing and leg exercises. A Foley catheter is inserted to prevent dislodgment of the implants, and the client is given a low-residue diet to prevent bowel movements, which may dislodge the implant. Increased fluid intake, to prevent urinary stasis, is encouraged. You may also administer antiemetics, broad-spectrum antibiotics, sedatives, analgesics, antidiarrheal medications, and heparin (to prevent thrombophlebitis).

Radiation precautions are enforced while a radioactive implant is in place. Pregnant nurses or female nurses attempting to become pregnant must not be assigned to care for such a client. Organize care so that you spend minimal time at the client's bedside. Give care from as far away as possible, behind lead shields when possible. Visitors should keep visits brief. Radiation therapy is detailed in Chapter 19.

The high dose of radiation may cause vaginal shrinkage, because exposure thins the vaginal epithelium and reduces vaginal lubrication. It may also cause vaginal adhesions and stenosis. Such changes can make vaginal sexual activities uncomfortable or painful. Vaginal penetration, with water-soluble lubrication as needed, during the course of irradiation and in subsequent months minimizes the possibility of vaginal stenosis and contracture. Depending on personal preference, vaginal penetration and dilation can be accomplished with the woman's own fingers, a vaginal dilator, or her sexual partner's fingers or penis. Vaginal dilators can be used for 10 minutes per day with water-soluble lubricants until sexual activity is resumed in 2 to 6 weeks. Support for the woman experiencing body image changes is extremely important.

CERVICAL CANCER

The incidence of invasive cervical cancer has steadily decreased over the years, whereas that of cervical carci-

noma in situ (localized) has risen. The decrease is largely attributed to the prevalence of screening with the Papanicolaou test (Pap smear). About 12,800 new cases of invasive cervical cancer were expected to have been diagnosed in 2000, with approximately 4600 cervical cancer deaths expected.[1] The incidence in African American and Native American women is nearly twice as high as in white women. Spanish-speaking women younger than 39 years are the least likely to have Pap smears.

Etiology and Risk Factors

The exact cause of cervical cancer is unknown, although chronic irritation is often present prior to diagnosis of cervical cancer. There is a strong relationship between the presence of the human papillomavirus (HPV), types 16 and 18, and cervical intraepithelial neoplasia (CIN). CIN has increasingly progressed to carcinoma in situ and invasive cervical cancer. Other risk factors are:

- Having multiple sexual partners or a partner who has had multiple sexual partners
- Early age of first intercourse
- Smoking tobacco
- Low socioeconomic status
- Untreated chronic cervicitis
- STDs
- Having a sexual partner with a history of penile or prostate cancer

Health promotion actions involve instructing clients (1) to avoid and to seek early treatment of vaginal or cervical infection, (2) to limit the number of sexual partners, and (3) to use condoms to limit the transmission of STDs and HPV. Yearly Pap smears for high-risk women is a health maintenance activity. After three or more consecutive annual examinations with normal results of Pap smears, the client with average risk may undergo Papanicolaou testing less frequently, at the discretion of the health care provider. Pap smears are important because cervical carcinoma in situ is potentially 100% curable.

Pathophysiology

Cervical dysplasia (an abnormal alteration in cell structure), the earliest premalignant change noted in cervical epithelium, is now further divided into several levels:

- Mild dysplasia, or CIN 1
- Moderate dysplasia, or CIN 2
- Severe dysplasia, or CIN 3
- Carcinoma in situ

Potentially, all women with carcinoma in situ and 91% of women with nonmetastatic disease can be cured. Five to 10 years may elapse between the preinvasive and invasive stages of cervical cancer. Most cervical cancers are of the squamous cell type. Squamous cell carcinoma usually begins at the squamocolumnar junction, near the external end of the cervix. The spread of squamous cell cervical cancer occurs first by direct extension to the vaginal mucosa, the lower uterine segment, parametrium, pelvic wall, bladder, and bowel. Distant metastasis occurs mainly through lymphatic spread, with some spread occurring through the circulatory system to the liver, lungs, or bones.

On occasion, cervical adenocarcinomas occur, but they are more difficult to identify. Adenocarcinoma generally involves the endocervical glands.

Clinical Manifestations

There are no early indications of carcinoma in situ or early cervical cancer. An abnormal Pap smear result, however, indicates the need for further assessment. Abnormal Pap smear results may be followed by HPV deoxyribonucleic acid (DNA) testing to confirm malignancy or repeating of the Pap smear. Another effective diagnostic test involves swabbing the cervix with vinegar; a flashlight then illuminates abnormal cells.

Assessment findings in late stages of cancer include the presence of vaginal discharge and bleeding, especially after intercourse. Metrorrhagia, postmenopausal bleeding, and *polymenorrhea* (increased frequency of menstrual bleeding) may be present. Early bleeding also may occur as spotting or contact bleeding from cervical trauma secondary to sexual intercourse or douching. This early minimal bleeding increases in amount and duration as the cancer progresses.

Vaginal discharge, which is normally watery, becomes dark and foul-smelling as the disease advances. With infection of the neoplastic area, the discharge becomes more profuse and malodorous. Concurrent bleeding makes this condition more unpleasant.

Other assessment findings that develop as the disease progresses relate to the areas involved in the malignant process. They include (1) pressure on the bowel, bladder, or both, (2) bladder irritation, (3) rectal discharge, (4) manifestations of ureteral obstruction, and (5) heavy, aching abdominal pain. Fistulae may form as the malignancy erodes through the walls of adjacent organs.

Pain is another late manifestation. It usually becomes a difficult problem with the onset of *cachexia*, or general wasting syndrome. This syndrome often accompanies the terminal stage of cervical cancer.

PAP SMEAR

The Pap smear is the primary diagnostic tool for cervical cancer. Further assessment of an abnormal Pap smear result typically includes repetition of cytologic and pelvic examinations. Colposcopic examination can often locate lesions for biopsy. Biopsy specimens are collected with the aid of a colposcope. After the cervix is wiped clean of any mucus or discharge, acetic acid is placed on it. The practitioner views the cervix through the colposcope, looking for abnormalities of color and cell formation. Tiny biopsy specimens are collected from any areas under suspicion. Colposcopy is an office procedure that causes mild discomfort.

COLD CONIZATION

Occasionally, biopsy specimens may be obtained by cold conization, a procedure that may be performed when colposcopic examination is not considered adequate and a larger specimen is necessary. A cone-shaped section of the cervix is obtained with a scalpel. This procedure enables more tissue to be provided for analysis, thus increasing the chances of identifying an area of invasive carcinoma or carcinoma in situ. The procedure is particularly helpful if areas such as the endocervical glands are involved and are not readily visualized.

Sometimes analysis of the tissue removed during a cold conization demonstrates that a wide area of normal tissue surrounds an excised malignancy. When this situation occurs, conization serves not only serves as the diagnostic procedure but may also be the only treatment needed. This procedure allows the woman to maintain reproductive capacity. Cautery (burning of abnormal cervical tissue) or *cryosurgery* (freezing of cervical tissue) may be performed instead of cold conization.

LOOP ELECTROCAUTERY EXCISION PROCEDURE

A loop electrocautery excision procedure (LEEP) is the newest and most common procedure. A LEEP is performed to excise the cervical areas causing concern. Once the clinician has identified the lesions with colposcopy, a paracervical nerve block is administered for anesthesia, and the lesion or lesions are totally removed by a low-voltage diathermy loop (an electrical current causing burning). There is less risk with this procedure because it is performed in the ambulatory setting without general anesthesia.

Outcome Management

◼ Medical Management

Irradiation is used as primary therapy for early cervical cancer. It is usually curative, but it induces menopause. Intracavity radiation has been described previously (see uterine cancer), and external irradiation is discussed in Chapter 19. In 1999, cancer experts recommended a change in the treatment of advanced surgical cancer, urging that chemotherapy be added to the standard treatment using irradiation.

Treatment of clients with cervical cancer during pregnancy varies, depending on the stage of the cancer, the duration of the pregnancy, and the client's wish to preserve fertility. A client can usually complete the pregnancy if CIN or carcinoma in situ is diagnosed. She may then be treated with cold conization or a LEEP 2 to 3 months post partum if she desires further childbearing. If a pregnant woman has invasive cervical carcinoma, however, abortion is recommended up to 24 weeks into the pregnancy. After 24 weeks, therapy is delayed until the fetus is viable (28 to 32 weeks), and a cesarean section is performed. The client may then be treated with either hysterectomy or irradiation in the postpartum period.

◼ Nursing Management of the Medical Client

PREVENT COMPLICATIONS

For the care of a client with radiation implants, see uterine cancer earlier; external radiation is covered in Chapter 19.

PREVENT RECURRENCE

All clients who have been treated conservatively for cervical cancer need information about recurrence. Encourage clients who have been treated for cervical cancer to have frequent health examinations to identify manifestations of recurrence of the cancer. Pelvic examinations and Pap smears should be scheduled every 3 months for the first 2 years, as advised by the physician.

Surgical Management

Treatment may range from cryosurgery, conization, laser therapy, or LEEP for localized tumors to a radical hysterectomy for invasive cancer:

1. *Cryosurgery* is the local freezing of abnormal cells and tissues with volatile gases such a nitrous oxide or carbon dioxide. Cell death results from dehydration and cell membrane destruction; dead tissue then sloughs off with a heavy discharge for 2 to 3 weeks.
2. *Conization* is the removal of a small cone of tissue with a sharp instrument (see earlier).
3. *Laser therapy* or *LEEP* (see earlier) may also be performed to remove abnormal tissue. Laser therapy causes a burn of the tissues, leading to an increase in sloughing discharge for several weeks. There may also be minimal bleeding.

A total abdominal hysterectomy can be used to treat carcinoma in situ in women who have finished childbearing or to treat invasive cancer. *Pelvic exenteration* (Fig. 39–9), an extremely radical procedure, is performed if the cancer has spread. This procedure involves removal of all pelvic organs, including the uterus, fallopian tubes, ovaries, vagina, bladder, rectum, and colon. In addition, an ileal conduit and ileostomy may be performed if removal of the bladder or colon is indicated.

Nursing Management of the Surgical Client

For care of the client with a hysterectomy, see benign uterine tumors (leiomyomas). For care of the client with an ileal conduit, see Chapter 34. For care of the client with a colostomy or ileostomy, see Chapter 33.

CRYOSURGERY, LASER THERAPY, LEEP

EXPLAIN PROCEDURE. Nursing preparation of a client for cryosurgery, laser therapy, or a LEEP involves informing the client that a surgical incision will not be made. Explain that the procedure is performed with a vaginal speculum in place, as during a routine pelvic examination. During treatment, a few clients experience headaches, dizziness, flushing, and some cramping.

PROVIDE SUPPORT. During the procedure, provide psychological support by (1) staying with the client, (2) informing her of what is to be done, (3) talking with her, listening to her, and facilitating her expression of concerns, (4) continuing to acknowledge her presence during

A   Normal anatomy

B   Anterior exenteration

FIGURE 39–9 Pelvic exenteration. *A*, Natural pelvic structures. *B*, Anterior exenteration: formation of the ileal conduit. *C*, Posterior exenteration: formation of colostomy. *D*, Total exenteration: formation of both ileal conduit and colostomy.

C   Posterior exenteration

D   Total exenteration

the procedure rather than excluding her, and (5) allowing her to retain as much self-control as possible. For example, tell her what she can do during the procedure to help it move along quickly and smoothly.

PROMOTE COMFORT. Assess the client's discomfort during the procedure. A mild analgesic may be prescribed for pain following the procedure. Discuss how she can help manage postprocedure discomfort, such as performing slow, deep breathing. Tell the client what to expect afterward; mild cramping may continue for several days.

ENCOURAGE PERINEAL HYGIENE. A clear, watery discharge usually occurs for up to several weeks. This is followed by a malodorous discharge containing debris from the sloughing of dead cells. If the discharge continues longer than 8 weeks, an infection is suspected.

Meticulous perineal hygiene minimizes the risk of infection and makes the client more comfortable. Healing takes about 6 weeks. The client should take showers during this time, avoiding tub and sitz baths.

RADICAL HYSTERECTOMY

After a radical hysterectomy, the vagina is shortened and the trigone region of the bladder and the sigmoid colon may adhere to the vaginal apex. This may cause dyspareunia, the pain of which may be felt deep in the pelvis. Recommend that during penile penetration the client keep her thighs adducted and use her thumb and index finger at the vaginal opening to encircle the shaft of the penis, providing some extra length to the vagina.

Despite vigorous treatment, some women with cervical cancer become terminally ill (see Chapter 22 for end-of-life care) In this situation, the goals of care change and are directed toward physiologic and psychosocial comfort. Pain relief (see Chapter 23) may be accomplished through use of narcotic analgesics. Palliative irradiation may also be used as a pain relief measure in some cases.

▮ Modifications for Elderly Clients

In older clients, cervical cancer may be treated with less invasive methods. The older client undergoing internal irradiation treatments should be monitored closely after treatment for development of fistulae.

UROGENITAL DISPLACEMENT AND PROLAPSE

Urogenital displacement and prolapse occur with relaxation and descent of the pelvic organs adjacent to the vagina. This is a common problem found in menopausal women. The organs that descend with urogenital displacement and then prolapse are the urethra, bladder, uterus, vaginal apex if the uterus has been removed, bowel, and rectum.

Surgery has been very successful in reducing prolapse. However, some women who are poor surgical candidates or who choose not to proceed with a surgical intervention may elect a nonsurgical approach, such as using a vaginal support device known as a *pessary* (a device to hold the organs in correct position) or increasing the pelvic floor support with Kegel exercises.

Etiology and Risk Factors

Menopause causes a decrease in circulating estrogens. With a decrease of estrogen, the supporting structures of the pelvic floor lose their elasticity and ability to support, causing relaxation and prolapse of the urogenital organs.

Additional factors that put a woman at risk for development of prolapse are multiparity, childbirth trauma, chronic straining, and inability to maintain the perineal musculature. The occurrence of prolapse has decreased with improved obstetric care. Better preparation of women for labor and the rare use of forceps during delivery have helped. Help prevent prolapse by encouraging pregnant clients to seek qualified obstetric care and instructing them to perform Kegel exercises before and after delivery.

▮ CYSTOCELE AND URETHROCELE

A *cystocele* involves a descent of the urinary bladder because of weakened pelvic floor muscles; it is seen as a protrusion of the anterior part of the vaginal wall (Fig. 39–10A and B). A *urethrocele* (prolapse of the urethra) often accompanies a cystocele as the bladder descends into the vagina. Urinary difficulties caused by the cystocele and urethrocele include incontinence, urinary tract infections, and urinary retention. Additionally, the client may complain of vaginal pressure with or without pelvic discomfort.

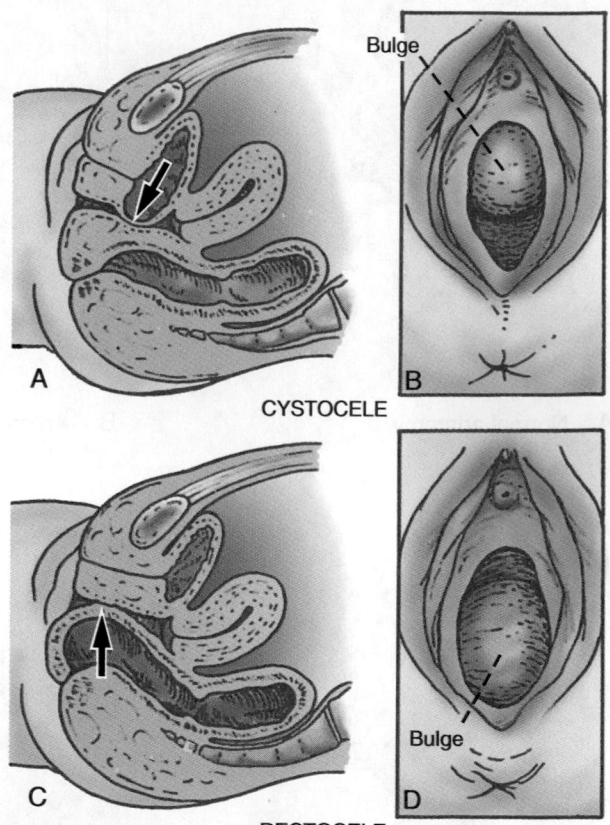

CYSTOCELE

RECTOCELE

FIGURE 39–10 *A,* Cystocele. Note the bulging of the anterior vaginal wall. The urinary bladder is displaced downward. *B,* The cystocele pushes the anterior vaginal wall downward into the vagina. *C,* Rectocele. *D,* Note the bulging of the posterior vaginal wall.

RECTOCELE AND ENTEROCELE

A *rectocele* is the protrusion of the vaginal wall musculature that supports the rectum (Fig. 39–10C and D). A rectocele can produce constipation, incomplete emptying of the rectum, fecal incontinence, and rectal or vaginal pressure. To completely empty the rectum, some women find it necessary to support the posterior wall of the vagina with a finger while having a bowel movement.

An *enterocele* is the descent of the bowel and protrusion of the upper portion of the posterior wall of the vagina. It often accompanies a rectocele and is usually without manifestations when it is seen alone.

VAGINAL OR UTERINE PROLAPSE

Vaginal or uterine prolapse is the descent of the uterus into the vagina (Fig. 39–11). The associated manifestations are increasing vaginal pressure, dyspareunia, and backache. As the prolapse descends through the vagina, there may be bleeding from irritation and ulcerations on the prolapsing cervix.

Clinical Manifestations

Manifestations of displacement and prolapse often depend on the level of descent and clinical signs. Some clients present with significant descent but have no manifestations. Clinically, prolapse should be assessed by the level of the descent. The grading scale is as follows[29]:

Grade 0: No descent
Grade 1: Descent half way between the ischial spines and the hymenal ring
Grade 2: Descent to the hymenal ring
Grade 3: Descent halfway beyond the hymenal ring
Grade 4: Descent fully outside the hymenal ring

Outcome Management

Surgical Management

Treatment of prolapse depends on the extent of prolapse and the client's health status. The most effective treatment is reconstructive surgery. A vaginal pessary may be used if surgery is not desired or the health status of the client is less than optimal.

The cystocele is often corrected by a procedure called an *anterior colporrhaphy;* an additional procedure called a *Burch colposuspension* may be included if a urethrocele is present (see Chapter 34). The rectocele is usually corrected with a *posterior repair.* The accompanying enterocele is often corrected at the same time by one of various enterocele reconstructive procedures. Hence, an anterior and posterior (A & P repair) involves both procedures.

A hysterectomy may be performed at the same time as the reconstructive surgery if the client does not want to preserve fertility and if the uterus has descended into the vagina. The hysterectomy is performed by way of incisions through the vaginal wall into the pelvic cavity and supportive structures. The uterus is removed from its supporting broad, round, and uterosacral ligaments. The supporting ligaments are then attached to the vaginal cuff to maintain vaginal length.

Nursing Management of the Surgical Client

PREVENT BLADDER DISTENTION

During the operation and for at least the first 24 hours afterward, the bladder is kept decompressed. If a Foley catheter is placed, it is usually removed as soon as the client is ambulatory. When the catheter is removed, the client must be taught to keep her bladder empty by voiding every 2 hours to avoid placing pressure along the suture line. If a suprapubic catheter is placed, bladder retraining is begun once the client is ambulatory.

MONITOR BLEEDING

Postoperatively, monitor the client closely for excessive vaginal bleeding. There is normally a small to moderate amount of frank vaginal bleeding. If heavy vaginal bleeding is accompanied by a rapidly distending, rigid abdomen, referred shoulder pain, and indications of shock, immediate surgery may be indicated. Other times of potential bleeding are the 4th, 9th, 14th, and 21st days after surgery as sutures dissolve. If vaginal packing, a drain, or both are in place, the surgeon usually removes them after 24 to 48 hours.

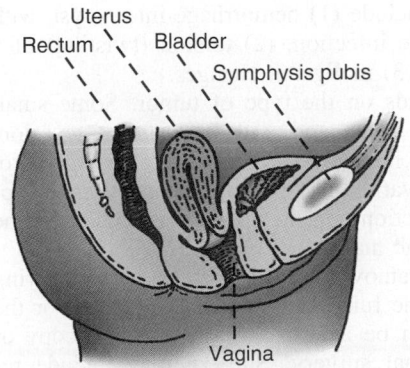

Uterus
Rectum
Bladder
Symphysis pubis
Vagina

FIRST-DEGREE PROLAPSE

SECOND-DEGREE PROLAPSE

THIRD-DEGREE PROLAPSE

FIGURE 39–11 Uterine prolapse.

Medical Management

The vaginal pessary has been used more successfully over the last few years as an alternative to surgery or as a comfort measure during the wait for surgery. This device holds the prolapsing vaginal organs in the correct position. Pessaries come in different sizes and styles. A well-fit pessary should be comfortable. Therefore, for proper compliance, the client should not experience any discomfort from the pessary during activities. She should be able to void normally with the pessary in place and should be comfortable inserting and removing it.

Nursing Management of the Medical Client

TEACH PELVIC FLOOR (KEGEL) EXERCISES

Mild manifestations may be relieved by pelvis-strengthening Kegel exercises. These exercises may be prescribed to help a client achieve pubococcygeal muscle control. Instruct the client to practice alternately tightening and relaxing her rectal and vaginal muscles. She tightens these muscles as if she were trying to hold back a bowel movement or a stream of urine. She holds this tightened position for a few seconds and then relaxes the muscles. Over time, she should hold the contraction for a longer period. Kegel exercises can be performed frequently during the day, whenever the clients thinks of them, or for a specified number of times two or three times a day.

TEACH PESSARY CARE

Because a pessary has the potential to irritate the vaginal mucosa, instruct the client to remove the device daily and to reinsert it after cleaning it with a mild, unscented soap and water.

Follow-up care is important. Within 2 weeks after fitting and insertion of the pessary, the client needs professional reassessment. At that time, the clinician performs a pelvic examination to assess the vaginal mucosa for irritation. The pessary may be changed or removed as indicated. Estrogen cream is often inserted into the vagina at bedtime two times a week in an effort to maintain tissue integrity.

If a pessary is left in place too long, it may erode the tissues and adhere to the mucosa. It is important for the client to understand the need for follow-up care. Most clients can care for a pessary without assistance, but some clients with poor manual dexterity need help with its removal and cleaning.

POLYPS

Polyps are pedunculated tumors arising from the mucosa and extending into the opening of a body cavity. Genital polyps occur primarily in the uterus and cervix (Fig. 39–12). Uterine polyps may cause hypermenorrhea, intermenstrual bleeding, and postmenopausal bleeding. They occasionally undergo malignant changes, particularly in postmenopausal women. Cervical polyps may bleed after vaginal intercourse and are susceptible to infection.

If polyps are asymptomatic, they may simply be monitored. Because cervical polyps have a pedicle, they are easily removed by ligation. This procedure is usually performed in the physician's office. Uterine polyps are not easily removed because of their location within the uterus. Uterine polyps do not usually need to be removed

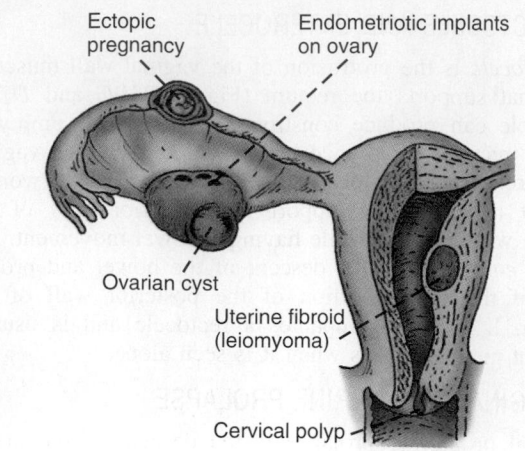

FIGURE 39–12 Common sites of some common benign gynecologic lesions.

unless they become symptomatic; if they must be removed, hysteroscopy is usually performed.

OVARIAN DISORDERS

BENIGN OVARIAN TUMORS

Benign ovarian tumors are either solid or cystic. Ovarian tumors are often asymptomatic until they are large enough to cause discomfort associated with pressure; this characteristic makes their early detection difficult. Typical manifestations associated with pressure are constipation, urinary frequency, a full feeling in the abdomen, vague pelvic aching and sensations of heaviness, painful defecation, and dyspareunia. Acute pain may be experienced during menses or with rupture. With an increasing growth, the client's abdominal girth increases, and her clothes may not fit as well. Generally, the client is unable to become pregnant.

Late and rare manifestations of a benign tumor include marked abdominal distention with dyspnea, peripheral edema, and anorexia. Pelvic pain may be present as a later manifestation if the ovarian tumor is growing rapidly. If the tumor produces hormones, menstrual irregularities and masculinizing or feminizing effects may be seen.

Complications include (1) hemorrhage into a cyst, with rupture and possible infection, (2) torsion (twisting) of a cystic pedicle, and (3) malignant changes.

Treatment depends on the type of tumor. Some small cystic masses can be treated with ovarian suppression, which is usually achieved with the use of birth control pills. Placing the ovaries in a pseudopregnancy state suppresses ovarian function and, in most cases, decreases the size of ovarian cystic masses.

Tumors can be removed surgically if they are growing rapidly or disrupt the function of the pelvic organs or the ovary. Removal can be achieved through laparoscopy or with open abdominal surgery. Surgery may include removal of (1) only the tumor, (2) the tumor and the ovary or ovaries, or (3) the tumor, both ovaries and tubes, and the uterus. The type of nursing care needed depends on the extent of surgery performed.

Ovarian cysts are physiologic tumors of ovaries. They are common and may or may not have manifestations. When manifestations do occur, the women may experience pelvic pain that is often worse on one side, pressure in the lower abdomen, backache, and menstrual irregularities.

A client with an ovarian cyst may be monitored for a month or two to determine whether the cyst might regress without intervention. If the cyst does not regress but is small, oral contraceptive therapy may provide a noninvasive therapy. Explain the treatment plan and condition to the client, and provide information about follow-up health care appointments and how to seek emergency care if needed.

A *follicular cyst* is caused by an unruptured follicle at the time of ovulation. It is often asymptomatic and frequently disappears without intervention. Sometimes, however, a cyst continues to enlarge as a result of hormone stimulation. Oral contraceptive therapy may be used if the cyst is small. Surgical intervention is required if the cyst increases in size and does not respond to medical management.

Corpus luteum cysts form when the corpus luteum fails to regress after discharging the ovum. Oral contraceptive therapy may be helpful for small cysts. However, surgical excision of the corpus luteum may be necessary. The remainder of the ovary can usually be saved.

OVARIAN CANCER

Ovarian cancer, although not the highest in incidence among reproductive tumors, is the leading cause of death from genital reproductive malignancies. The death rates have risen over time, probably because of a lack of early detection methods. An estimated 23,100 new cases of ovarian cancer were expected to have been detected in the United States in 2000, with 14,000 deaths.[1] White women show higher rates of ovarian cancer than African American women do.

Etiology and Risk Factors

The cause of ovarian cancer is unknown. Risk factors include:

- Age above 40 years
- Family history of ovarian or breast cancer (mutations in *BRCA1* or *BRCA2* genes have been observed in families)
- Family history of hereditary nonpolyposis colorectal cancer (HNPCC)
- Nulliparity
- History of infertility
- History of dysmenorrhea
- Use of ovulation-stimulating medications (a high number of ovulations increases the chances that a tumor suppressor gene called p53 can be mutated)

Pregnancy and the use of oral contraceptives appear to reduce the risk of ovarian cancer.

Health promotion factors include telling clients that ovarian cancer may be prevented by anything that interrupts constant ovulatory cycles, such as more than one full-term pregnancy, oral contraceptive use, breast-feed-

ing, and bilateral oophorectomy. Health maintenance activities include routine pelvic examinations, determinations of CA-125 antigen levels in high-risk women, and performance of transvaginal ultrasound combined with bimanual pelvic examination and Doppler studies for lesions in question. Prophylactic mastectomy and oophorectomy may be performed in women with *BRCA1* or *BRCA2* mutations as a way of increasing life expectancy.

Pathophysiology

Most ovarian cancers are epithelial tumors, although some are adenocarcinomas. Ovarian cancer tends to grow and spread silently until manifestations of pelvic pressure on adjacent organs or abdominal distention cause the woman to seek medical care. When these pressure-related manifestations finally appear, the malignancy has usually spread to the fallopian tubes, uterus, and ligaments. Ovarian cancer often spreads to the other ovary and associated structures. The cancer may invade bowel surfaces, the omentum, liver, and other organs. When the pelvic blood vessels become involved, distant metastasis occurs. The usual routes of spread are lymphatic spread, hematogenous spread (through blood), local extension, and peritoneal seeding.

Clinical Manifestations

Clinical manifestations of ovarian cancer include (1) abdominal distention with increasing abdominal girth, (2) urinary frequency and urgency, (3) pleural effusion, (4) malnutrition with weight loss, (5) pain from pressure caused by the growing tumor and the effects of urinary or bowel obstruction, (6) constipation, (7) ascites with dyspnea, and (8) ultimately, general severe pain. Indications of ovarian cancer do not typically appear until the malignancy is well established, which is often not until it has spread. Unfortunately, unless the malignancy is diagnosed early, when it is most likely asymptomatic, most affected clients eventually have terminal cancer.

Identification of a pelvic mass by palpation is usually the first assessment finding. However, detecting such a mass may be difficult in a woman who is obese or who cannot relax during the examination. Palpation of the ovary in postmenopausal women should always be considered an abnormal finding and should be followed up with pelvic sonogram to rule out abnormalities.

When an ovarian mass is suspected, a complete evaluation is performed. This includes an intravenous pyelogram (IVP), computed tomography (CT) scan, and, possibly, a barium enema study. Ultrasonography can determine whether the mass is solid or cystic. Generally, after the evaluation, exploratory surgery is performed to directly visualize the ovaries, obtain biopsy specimens of the adjacent structures, and perform a resection if the mass is malignant.

A serum CA-125 determination may be performed to be used as a tumor marker to track tumor growth and regression. This test should not be the only one used to determine the presence of ovarian cancer because it can give false-positive and false-negative results.

A new diagnostic blood test may soon be available that measures levels of a chemical in the body called lysophosphatidic acid (LPA), which stimulates the growth of ovarian cancer cells. Elevated levels of LPA would indicate that a woman has ovarian cancer. This test is more precise than CA-125 measurement. Further research is needed before the LPA test becomes readily available.[41]

Outcome Management

Surgical Management

The extent of an ovarian malignancy is determined by exploratory surgery. Ovarian cancer is usually treated aggressively. A young woman with a borderline malignancy may be treated conservatively with a TAH-BSO. The surgery of choice is a TAH-BSO, partial or complete omentectomy, and removal of all visible tumor. The less residual tumor left, the better the prognosis.

Some women with ovarian cancer recover following treatment. Oncologists may recommend a second-look laparotomy in women who are clinically free of disease and who have received chemotherapy for 6 to 24 months to aid in the decision whether to continue treatment. During this procedure, multiple biopsy specimens are collected and analyzed to determine the presence or absence of residual tumor.

Medical Management

Adjuvant therapy varies with the stage of the disease. With stage I ovarian cancer, women typically receive irradiation or chemotherapy after surgery to destroy cancer cells that may have spread into the abdominal cavity. Systemic chemotherapy may be administered (see Chapter 19). Women with stage II or higher ovarian cancers typically receive the same treatment as those with stage I disease, with the inclusion of pelvic and, possibly, abdominal radiation.

Nursing Management of the Medical-Surgical Client

For the nursing care of the client who has undergone TAH-BSO, see earlier in this chapter; for care of the client with ovarian cancer, see Chapter 19.

VAGINAL DISORDERS

VAGINAL DISCHARGE AND PRURITUS

The female reproductive tract maintains its integrity through various natural defense mechanisms. Inflammation and infection occur when organisms disrupt or overcome these natural defenses. The resulting manifestations, although usually not life-threatening, can be uncomfortable and annoying. Vaginal discharge and itching are among the most common problems women mention to health care providers.

All women have normal, nonbloody, asymptomatic vaginal discharge called *leukorrhea*. This discharge, secreted by the endocervical glands, is a clear or white exudate that keeps vaginal mucous membranes moist and clear. As this exudate passes through the vagina, it may become cloudy and acquire a slight odor as desquamated epithelial cells, leukocytes, and normal vaginal flora are added.

The amount of vaginal discharge often varies in relation to the menstrual cycle. It is greatest at ovulation and just before menses. Pregnancy, sexual stimulation, and oral contraceptives tend to increase the discharge. Changes in the amount, color, character, or odor of vaginal discharge may indicate a problem.

Some women view normal vaginal discharge and odor as offensive and go to great lengths to eliminate it. However, use of douches or vaginal deodorants may disrupt the normal vaginal bacterial flora, causing vaginal irritation and infection. The consensus in the medical literature holds that periodic douching is unnecessary. There is evidence that douching may actually be detrimental. Douching washes away protective mucus and normal bacterial flora of the vagina and may cause overgrowth of undesirable bacteria and yeast.

The most common causes of vaginal discharge and irritation are (1) vaginal infections, (2) parasites, such as pinworms, (3) STDs (see Chapter 41), and (4) mechanical or allergic irritants. An example of a mechanical irritant is a tampon left in place too long. Some forms of contraceptive creams or foams may be allergenic irritants for some clients.

Most inflammatory and infectious vaginal problems are accompanied by pathologic vaginal discharge, which may be copious, malodorous, and abnormal in color. The discharge frequently causes itching, irritation, and redness of the vulva and surrounding areas. It may be accompanied by burning and frequency of urination, anal discomfort, and pain in the lower abdominal region.

VAGINITIS

Vaginitis is inflammation of the vagina, a common problem experienced by most women at some time in their life. Causes of vaginitis include change in normal vaginal flora, change in vaginal pH, and invasion of the vagina by virulent organisms. These conditions can be caused by congestion of the pelvic organs, mechanical irritation, vaginal infection, overmedication with antibiotics, long-term steroid therapy, uncontrolled diabetes, and acquired immunodeficiency syndrome (AIDS). Candidiasis (*Candida albicans* infection) is one of the most common causes of vaginitis. Health promotion actions related to vaginitis are described in the accompanying Client Education Guide: Preventing Vaginitis

The vagina is a cavity with a normal protective population of flora, including various bacteria. The adult vagina is normally acidic because of lactic acid formed from the glycogen in desquamating vaginal epithelium. Normal vaginal function depends on a delicate balance between hormones and bacteria. Disturbance of this balance can precipitate infection.

Vaginitis is characterized by a change in vaginal discharge. It may become profuse, odorous, and purulent. The diagnosis is confirmed by a speculum examination and microscopic examination of the discharge. Specimens may be obtained for culture if manifestations indicate an STD or bacterial infection. As a result of edema and tenderness in the vagina, the examination may be painful and must be performed as gently as possible. Some bleeding may occur during and after the examination. Inform the client beforehand about the potential for pain and possible bleeding from the intrusion of the examination.

Vaginitis can be a stubborn, discouraging problem. Early, vigorous treatment may be necessary to prevent chronicity. Treatment is aimed at correcting the cause of the vaginitis. Attention must be given to the client's overall health.

TOXIC SHOCK SYNDROME

Toxic shock syndrome (TSS) is an acute condition caused by the toxin of a local infection with *Staphylococcus aureus*, which can develop into a systemic infection. It usually occurs in women who are menstruating and are using tampons or who have chronic vaginal infections.

TSS begins suddenly with a high fever, vomiting, and severe, watery diarrhea. Within 48 hours, a characteristic rash and hypotensive shock develop. Once the diagnosis is confirmed, antistaphylococcal antibiotics and fluid replacement therapy are begun.

Advise women to change tampons several times daily or to alternate tampons with sanitary napkins and to practice good hand-washing techniques to prevent development of TSS. If a vaginal sponge or diaphragm is used for contraception, it should be removed within 24 (diaphragm) to 30 (vaginal sponge) hours after intercourse. The diaphragm should not be used during menstruation.

ATROPHIC VAGINITIS

Atrophic vaginitis occurs in postmenopausal women. Atrophic, thin, vaginal mucosa and increased watery alkaline vaginal discharge provide an environment conducive to invasion by pyogenic bacteria. Assessment findings include a discharge with or without a bloody tinge, a vaginal burning sensation, itching of the vagina and vulva, and dyspareunia. If secondary infection is present, vulvar excoriation and burning with urination often occur. Long-

term use of estrogen cream is the usual medical treatment. If a secondary infection is present, therapy with an appropriate antibiotic is added.

VAGINAL FISTULAE

Vaginal fistulae are abnormal tube-like passages from the vagina to the bladder *(vesicovaginal)*, rectum *(rectovaginal)*, or urethra *(urethrovaginal)* (Fig. 39–13). Fistula formation is an extremely distressing problem in the genitourinary tract.

Etiology and Risk Factors

Fistulae may be congenital or may result from injury or surgery. About 10% of all fistulae occur in the female reproductive area. Vaginal fistulae may occur because of the spread of a malignant lesion, after irradiation for cancer, as a result of inflammatory disease, and after a prolonged, difficult labor and traumatic delivery.

Clinical Manifestations

Urine or flatus and feces leak into the vagina. Vaginal and vulval tissues become excoriated and irritated. Chronic urinary tract infection may result. Rectovaginal fistulas may cause an offensive, particularly unpleasant odor. The client experiences wetness and a sensation of feeling unclean.

In addition to their unpleasant physical manifestations, vaginal fistulae produce severely distressing psychosocial problems. Clients often become social recluses. Fistulae greatly disrupt intimate relationships and social activities. Clients often do not seek professional health care until the problem becomes severe. Even then, they may be embarrassed and reluctant to discuss it.

A simple diagnostic test is the instillation of methylene blue dye into the bladder or rectum via Foley catheter and placement of a tampon in the vagina. The woman is asked to walk and perform exertional exercise for a short while. The tampon is then removed and evaluated for color and absorption. The test is considered positive if blue dye is found on the tampon. A *fistulogram* (injection of dye into the vagina) can be performed to assess the location and extent of the fistula.

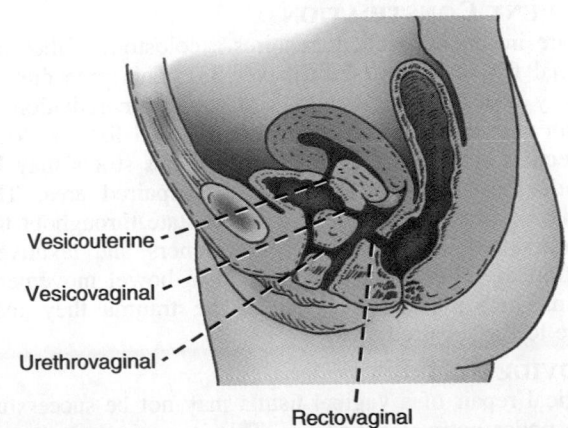

Vesicouterine

Vesicovaginal

Urethrovaginal

Rectovaginal

FIGURE 39–13 Locations of main types of vaginal fistulas.

Outcome Management

■ Medical-Surgical Management

The diagnosis and treatment of a vaginal fistula may be difficult. Treatment varies with the fistula's location, extent, and cause and the client's general health. Occasionally, a fistula heals spontaneously. Medical management is used first to treat infection because surgical management is rarely successful, especially when an infection is present. The client must be in optimal physical condition before surgery is attempted.

On occasion, a temporary colostomy may be necessary to treat a rectovaginal fistula (see Chapter 33), and a suprapubic catheter must be inserted to prevent bladder distention after a repair of a vesicovaginal fistula. Excision of either of these fistulae is difficult with a high rate of recurrence.

■ Nursing Management of the Medical-Surgical Client

An accepting attitude of health professionals to a client with a vaginal fistula is essential to help her comfortably accept and follow through with needed treatments. Help the client to minimize the manifestations and care for herself.

PREVENT INFECTION

Some clients unadvisedly restrict their fluid intake in an attempt to decrease the drainage. This action may actually increase the size of the fistula and raise the chance of infection. Make sure the woman understands the importance of increasing her fluid intake to reduce the risk of infection. Perineal hygiene measures may include cleansing the perineum every 4 hours, taking sitz baths, and changing perineal pads frequently.

If surgery is used to repair the fistula, care is directed at avoiding physical stress on the repaired area and preventing infection. A Foley or suprapubic catheter is used after a vesicovaginal or urethrovaginal fistulectomy to drain the urinary bladder. Careful attention is necessary to keep the catheter patent and draining. Provide and encourage enough fluid intake so that internal catheter irrigation is accomplished. It is a nursing responsibility to monitor the catheter for patency. If the catheter becomes obstructed, the increased bladder pressure could adversely affect the surgical sites and cause the fistula to reopen.

PREVENT CONSTIPATION

In rare instances, a client requires a colostomy following vaginal fistula repair (see Chapter 33). This procedure is usually necessary for fistulas resulting from radiation or Crohn's disease and for postoperative rectal fistulas. After corrective bowel surgery, the client's first stools may be liquid. This prevents stress on the repaired area. The stools may be maintained in a liquid state throughout the postoperative period with stool softeners and laxatives. Caution the client not to strain with a bowel movement. Enemas are avoided because of the trauma they may cause to the repaired area.

PROVIDE SUPPORT

Surgical repair of a vaginal fistula may not be successful, even under optimal conditions. This is particularly true if a client has extensive tissue damage from tumors or irra-

diation. Supportive nursing care is extremely important for women experiencing this distressing disorder and for their significant others as well.

VAGINAL CANCER

Primary invasive vaginal cancer is a rare lesion, typically occurring in women over 50 years old. However, it is seen in younger women whose mothers took diethylstilbestrol (DES) during pregnancy. DES was widely prescribed in the United States from 1940 to 1970 for threatened miscarriage and other high-risk pregnancy problems. Among women who have not been exposed to DES, vaginal cancer is rare in African Americans and almost nonexistent in Jews.

Etiology and Risk Factors

The risk factor for vaginal (clear cell) cancer is maternal ingestion of DES. Other potential causes of vaginal cancer are (1) exposure to the drug in utero in girls and women between menarche and age 30 (adenocarcinoma), (2) repeated pregnancies, (3) a history of STD, herpes virus, or HPV, (4) prior irradiation, (5) immunosuppressive therapy, and (6) significant irritation due to a poorly fitting pessary. Leukoplakia and leukorrhea are often associated with vaginal cancer.

Pathophysiology

The staging of vaginal cancer is similar to that used for other pelvic malignancies. The primary lesion and involvement of adjacent structures are considered. Primary invasive cancer tends to involve the anterior or posterior vaginal walls, or both. Complications may involve the urinary bladder or bowel, as in fistula formation.

Despite active treatment, the prognosis for vaginal cancer is generally poor. The overall cure rate reported by the American Cancer Society is about 35%. Half of women with vaginal cancer die within 18 months of diagnosis.[1] Low survival rates are due to the rarity of the cancer (2100 cases per year in the United States), which makes it difficult to identify, the typically advanced stage of the cancer when it is diagnosed, and the difficulty in treating this cancer with radiation or surgery because of the proximity of important structures.

Clinical Manifestations

Indications of vaginal cancer include foul vaginal discharge, painless vaginal bleeding, pruritus, pain (not associated with bleeding), and the presence of a vaginal mass or lesion. Urinary bladder manifestations, such as pain and frequency, may occur if a vaginal mass compresses the bladder.

Women exposed to DES in utero should receive careful examination of the cervix, along with cytologic examination of the cervix and any questionable area in the vagina. Colposcopy may be used to identify areas to be sampled for biopsy. During pelvic examination, Lugol's solution may be applied to any vaginal areas that appear abnormal. Lack of staining identifies suspect areas. Unfortunately, the lesions of vaginal cancer are often well advanced before manifestations appear. Earlier lesions might be missed during pelvic examination.

Outcome Management

■ Medical Management

The usual treatment for vaginal cancer is either external or intravaginal radiation therapy or, less often, surgery. External radiation therapy is used for all stages of vaginal cancer. Internal radiation is generally used only in the earlier stages. The difficulty of applying radiation to the vagina without causing harm to the bladder and rectum has led some physicians to prefer surgical intervention.

■ Surgical Management

For earlier stages, radical hysterectomy, lymphadenectomy, and vaginectomy are performed. *Partial vaginectomy* refers to removal of the upper third to half of the vagina as part of the procedure in a radical hysterectomy. Pelvic exenteration is used in more advanced cancer if the bladder or rectum is involved; it is also indicated in a client with recurrent metastases.

■ Nursing Management of the Medical-Surgical Client

During assessment, ask young women born between 1940 and 1970 about medications their mothers may have taken during pregnancy. All those whose mothers took DES when pregnant with them should have a gynecologic examination at least twice yearly beginning at menarche, or at age 14, whichever comes first.

PROVIDE SUPPORT
Vaginal surgery may be anxiety-promoting and frightening. Ostomies (see Chapters 33 and 34) also may need to be performed, adding to the client's fears and problems.

DISCUSS SEXUALITY
Sexuality is an important nursing consideration in the care of women with vaginal cancer. Postoperatively, vaginal sexual activity is not possible unless vaginal reconstruction has been performed. Vaginal sex may be difficult after surgery or radiation therapy because of changes in the size and shape of the vagina. Assess the client's previous sexual history and her self-esteem to identify possible problems. Create a therapeutic environment that allows her to feel comfortable discussing sexual concerns.

Discuss the potential impact of the disease process and treatment on sexuality, as appropriate. Potential problems include fatigue, pain, dyspareunia, decreased libido, and altered body image. If a partial vaginectomy is performed, the client can probably still enjoy normal vaginal sexual activity, using large amounts of lubricant and modified positioning, because the vaginal tissue will stretch.

PROMOTE REST
To help the client cope with fatigue and pain, suggest that she schedule sexual activity after resting. Also, schedule pain medication so that the peak of action coincides with sexual activity. A warm bath, a back rub, alternate positioning, or relaxation techniques might also help. Advise the client to use a water-soluble lubricant

during intercourse and, perhaps, a vaginal dilator at other times to prevent vaginal fibrosis and tightening.

VULVAR DISORDERS

VULVITIS

Vulvitis (inflammation of the vulva) is caused by direct irritation of vulvar tissues or by direct extension of irritation from the vagina to the vulva that results in itching. Risk factors associated with vulvitis include skin disorders, inflammatory problems, infection, allergies, postmenopausal atrophy and dryness, uncontrolled diabetes, pediculosis, scabies, cancer, incontinence, and poor perineal hygiene.

Medical treatment is based on the specific cause of the condition. Itching, the most common manifestation associated with vulvitis, can be severe. A local or systemic antipruritic or antihistamine agent, such as hydrocortisone cream, diphenhydramine hydrochloride (Benadryl), or hydroxyzine hydrochloride (Atarax), may be given to relieve the itching.

Teach the client the following measures to relieve itching:

1. Apply cold compresses.
2. Wear light, nonrestrictive clothing, including well-washed and well-rinsed cotton underpants. Synthetic underpants tend to keep the vulvar area warm and moist.
3. Avoid feminine hygiene sprays.
4. Apply prescribed hydrocortisone ointment or anesthetic sprays.
5. Keep the vulva clean and dry. Clean after elimination by washing the vulva with very mild soap and water; wiping with toilet tissue or a washcloth from front to back; rinsing and drying the area well; and applying cornstarch to maintain dryness.

VULVAR CANCER

Vulvar cancer is found mainly in women older than 50 years of age. It accounts for about 3400 cases of female genital carcinoma each year in the United States.[1]

Etiology and Risk Factors

Vulvar disorders (e.g., lichen sclerosus, previously called kraurosis vulvae or atrophic leukoplakia, and diabetic vulvitis) increase the risk of vulvar cancer. Contracting certain STDs, such as HPV, also raises the risk.

Pathophysiology

Vulvar cancer arises from skin, urethra, glands, or subcutaneous tissues. Approximately 90% to 95% of vulvar cancers are squamous cell carcinoma. The remaining 5% to 10% are adenocarcinoma, Paget's disease, malignant melanoma, or sarcoma.

Vulvar cancer grows slowly and remains localized for a long time. Most lesions are located in the labia, primarily the labia majora. Some are on the clitoris. Local spread may occur to the urethra, vagina, anus, and rectum. Lymphatic spread is to the inguinal, femoral, pelvic, and finally, periaortic nodes. The usual causes of death from widespread vulvar cancer are distant metastasis, urethral obstruction, infection, uremia, and hemorrhage.

The prognosis is poor with vulvar invasive lesions. Five-year survival rates for clients who have undergone vulvectomy and lymphadenectomy are approximately 65%. Recurrence as well as distant metastasis may appear in the first 2 years. When lesions are diagnosed in an advanced stage with node involvement, the survival rate is only 8% to 10%.

Clinical Manifestations

Lichen sclerosus is characterized by thickened gray patches of epithelium scattered over the vulva and perineum. Cracked areas in these patches provide an ideal medium for infection, which causes the tissues to ulcerate and macerate. Eventually, these areas may become malignant.

Secondary infection is characterized by a bright red, smooth, almost transparent vulvar epithelium. Lichen sclerosus is most common in postmenopausal women. With its progression, the vulvar tissues shrink and constrict the vaginal opening.

Initially, lichen sclerosus causes itching and soreness or pain but may be asymptomatic. Clinical manifestations of early vulvar cancer include pruritus, minimal vulval soreness, dyspareunia, and tissue irritation with some bleeding. The potential seriousness of these relatively mild problems may not be appreciated by women or their health care providers because the manifestations are similar to those of nonmalignant vulvar lesions. As the vulvar cancer progresses, clinical manifestations of vulvar edema and pelvic lymphadenopathy develop. Secondary infection may cause a foul-smelling discharge. Biopsy of the affected area confirms the diagnosis.

Outcome Management

■ Medical Management

When lichen sclerosus is present, a biopsy to rule out cancer is indicated. Infection is treated with an appropriate systemic or topical antibiotic, steroid creams, and hormone cream. Other manifestations are treated symptomatically.

Irradiation and chemotherapy are used less often than surgical therapy. Irradiation is not generally used because the involved tissues do not tolerate it well. Chemotherapy is typically not given unless metastasis has occurred. The agent of choice is then selected according to the extent of metastasis.

■ Nursing Management of the Medical Client

Nursing management of the client with lichen sclerosus is mainly supportive care throughout the diagnostic period. Itching can be treated symptomatically with antipruritic creams such as hydrocortisone.

■ Surgical Management

A vulvectomy is performed to remove abnormal tissue through procedures such as a skinning technique, local wide excision, or a simple or radical vulvectomy. A laser may be used in conjunction with these procedures to destroy specific abnormal tissue.

A *simple vulvectomy* involves removal of the labia majora, labia minora, and sometimes the glans clitoris. Occasionally, the perineal area is also removed, requiring plastic surgery to cover the vulvar area. However, extensive surgery is avoided if the client's condition allows a simpler procedure.

A *radical vulvectomy* (Fig. 39–14) consists of excision of tissue from the anus to a few centimeters below the symphysis pubis (skin, labia majora, labia minora, and clitoris). Bilateral dissection of groin lymph nodes, such as the superficial groin and deep inguinal, femoral, iliac, hypogastric, and obturator nodes, also may be performed.

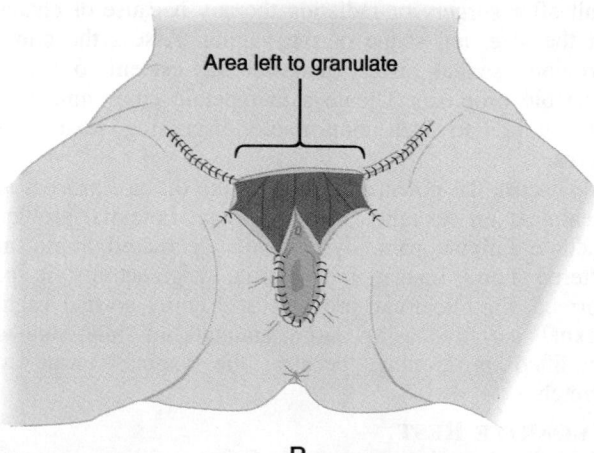

A   B

FIGURE 39–14 Radical vulvectomy. *A,* Area to be excised and line of incision *(dashed line).* The vulvar skin, underlying subcutaneous tissue and muscles, and regional lymph nodes are excised. If the anus is involved, the incision also continues around it. Inguinal and femoral lymph nodes are resected en bloc. *B,* Completed surgery. Perineal skin is approximated to the vagina, and a large area is left open to heal gradually by filling in with granulation tissue. A simple vulvectomy (not shown) does not remove the lymph nodes. Hence, the incision does not extend into the groin.

Full recovery is possible but may take 6 months or longer. Wound infections and delayed wound healing may lead to numerous problems. The long recovery and potential complications further impair the client's body image.

■ Nursing Management of the Surgical Client

PREOPERATIVE CARE

For a woman experiencing vulvar surgery, psychosocial support is especially important and should begin preoperatively. Some problems you might anticipate are fear of disfigurement, grief over the loss of a body part, fear of death, and sexual concerns.

Preoperative preparation is similar to that for other gynecologic procedures. The client scheduled for a vulvectomy must understand what the surgery entails, know what preoperative procedures will be performed, and have an idea of what to expect in the postoperative period. See the Client Education Guide: Recovering from Radical Vulvectomy.

POSTOPERATIVE CARE

The client undergoing a radical vulvectomy is susceptible to many postoperative complications because of the extensive nature of the operation. In addition to routine postoperative care, a suction device (e.g., Hemovac), tubes, or drain must be placed in the incision to remove drainage and to reduce the risk of infection. Carefully monitor the amount of bleeding. A bed cradle is helpful in keeping bed linens away from the incision.

CLIENT EDUCATION GUIDE

Recovering from Radical Vulvectomy

Client Instructions

- Avoid strenuous exercise involving the legs and pelvis.
- Gradually resume normal physical activities.
- Resume sexual activity, if desired, when the surgeon indicates. If intercourse is resumed, top or side positions are preferable to avoid direct pressure on the operative area. Water-soluble lubricants can be used for comfort.
- Take showers rather than tub baths. Showers reduce the likelihood of postoperative wound infection. Gentle, thorough washing of the genital area is important. Wipe gently from front to back after bowel movements and urinating. Do not douche without permission from the surgeon.
- Notify the surgeon if any of the following problems occurs:
  - Perineal pain unrelieved by prescribed medication
  - Foul-smelling perineal discharge
  - Heavy perineal bleeding or clots
  - Foul odor from the incision
  - Change in color of the incision (especially manifestations of decreased circulation)
  - Swelling of the groin or genital area
  - Frequent urination, urinating in small amounts, or discomfort or burning on urination
  - Temperature of 100° F (37.8° C) or higher
  - Pain, tenderness, or redness in the calves

PREVENT THROMBOPHLEBITIS. The client wears antiembolism or sequential compression stockings to prevent leg edema and thrombophlebitis, which constitutes a postoperative and a long-term problem. Keep the legs elevated as much as possible. Resuming ambulation postoperatively as early as possible helps to decrease leg edema and thrombophlebitis. The client should perform leg exercises to prevent circulatory problems. Teach the client to avoid sitting with the legs dependent, standing, and crossing the legs. A low-dose anticoagulant, such as heparin, warfarin (Coumadin), or aspirin, may be used prophylactically (as prevention) to reduce the risk of phlebitis and subsequent pulmonary embolism.

Lower extremity lymphedema can cause a change in clothing size and an upsetting change in appearance. In addition, some clients have difficulty sitting for long periods, making activities such as long automobile trips difficult.

PREVENT INFECTION. Prevent infection in the incisional area through frequent dressing changes, perineal care or sitz baths after voiding and bowel movements, and meticulous wound care. A Foley catheter is usually in place for 7 to 14 days or until healing is adequate. If the catheter is removed, carefully monitor urination with supportive care to prevent infection and voiding dysfunction. Additionally, it is important to monitor bowel movements. Once healing has occurred, the client may require reconstructive surgery.

PROVIDE SUPPORT. Psychosocially, a vulvectomy may be a devastating experience for a woman because of its direct effect on the external genitalia. The surgery, especially a radical vulvectomy, may compromise the client's physical integrity and her sense of wholeness. Some important issues for a woman are fear of recurrence and metastasis, disfigurement, concern about future sexual activity, and fear of her partner's rejection.

Nursing care involves helping the woman redefine her self-image to include the physical changes of vulvectomy. Try to create an environment in which she can express her feelings. Provide opportunities for her to mourn the loss and its effect on her sexuality. Encourage her to resume her normal activities as soon as possible to reinforce her feelings of self-worth.

Stress in social relationships is common after this radical surgery. The client and her significant other may benefit from counseling aimed at developing healthy coping skills.

The effect of a vulvectomy on female sexuality has not been well described. The disfigurement secondary to the surgery can lead to body image distortion, which affects sexual functioning. Physical changes, such as removal of the clitoris, result in loss of the ability to experience orgasm. The client may experience loss of sensation within the vagina. Also, stenosis of the introitus may follow surgery, making intercourse painful or difficult; this can have a major impact on sexuality. If stenosis occurs, it can be treated with vaginal dilators. If dilation is unsuccessful, plastic surgery should be considered.

Sexual counseling should be considered for all women undergoing vulvectomy and their partners. Assist the client and her sexual partner by communicating openly with them, answering their questions, explaining structural vulvar changes, and suggesting alternative forms of sexual arousal for the client.

PROMOTE VOIDING. Some women experience unpredictable voiding difficulties following a radical vulvectomy. A client may present with complaints of incontinence, retention, or a dysfunctional voiding pattern (see Chapter 34).

BARTHOLINITIS

Inflammation of Bartholin's glands can be caused by various organisms, including gonococci, streptococci, staphylococci, and *E. coli*. The infection involves the duct of the gland, producing edema and, eventually, obstruction. Because the inflamed gland cannot drain, it swells, and an abscess forms. Cellulitis develops in the surrounding tissues, producing more pain and systemic manifestations. The abscess may rupture spontaneously or may require incision and drainage.

After the acute episode, occlusion of the duct by fibrosis and scarring causes retention of secretions and dilation of the duct. It then becomes a palpable, mobile cyst, which usually is not painful. Manifestations, which relate to the size of the cyst, include dyspareunia and pain on walking.

Systemic antibiotics specific for the causative organism are prescribed. Local heat with hot packs or sitz baths may help promote drainage. Surgery may be necessary, such as an incision and drainage or removal of the gland if cancer is suspected or for repeated infections with abscess formation.

FEMALE GENITAL MUTILATION

Female genital mutilation (FGM), often called *female circumcision*, is a medically unnecessary surgical modification of the female genitalia practiced in several African, Asian and Middle Eastern countries. It may be seen in female immigrants from these areas. The procedure is performed on girls between ages 4 and 12 years old. Globally, FGM is estimated to affect 130 million girls and women, with approximately 2 million new FGM procedures performed yearly. About 120,000 immigrants to the United States between 1991 and 1995 originated from countries in which FGM is practiced.[24]

There are four major types, and types 1 and 2 are performed in 85% of cases[24]:

Type 1, Sunna: excision of the clitoral prepuce only, or *clitoridectomy* (partial or complete removal of the clitoris).
Type 2, Excision: removal of prepuce and clitoris along with adjoining parts of labia minora.
Type 3, Infibulation: removal of parts described in type 2 and parts of interior labia majora. The raw surfaces of the two sides of the vulva are then sutured together, obliterating the introitus. A small opening is left to allow for urine and menstrual flow.
Type 4, Other: burning of instead of cutting of the clitoris, stretching labia minora to enhance sexual pleasure, or making cuts into the vagina.

Etiology and Risk Factors

The FGM procedure originated from the belief that women are highly sexual and promiscuous. Type 3 FGM is performed to isolate women from sexual desires and temptation. Other factors are (1) religious influences, (2) promotion of social and political cohesion, (3) distinguishing chaste from adulterous women, (4) distinguishing indigenous from non-indigenous women, and (5) economic benefits for the father are additional reasons. Some practitioners of FGM believe that removal of the external genitalia makes the woman cleaner and more sexually attractive. Others believe that the clitoris generates additional excitement for the male, leading to early ejaculation, so that removal of the clitoris limits sexual excitement for both sexes. Still others believe that FGM after childbirth ensures fidelity in a marriage. Finally, some ethnic groups believe that the clitoris can kill a child if it touches the child's head during birth.

The decision to perform FGM is left to mothers, grandmothers, and elderly women. The rationale for disfavoring the practice includes marriage complications, labor complications, psychosexual beliefs, abandonment because of sterility, and the effects of the traumatic experience. Despite these problems, many ethnic groups, including men and women, continue to support the practice of FGM even while living in the United States.

Clinical Manifestations

Complications from FGM include:

- High infant mortality rate
- Hemorrhage, shock, and death during the procedure
- Keloid formation
- Chronic vaginal and pelvic infections
- Acute urinary retention
- Recurrent urinary tract infections
- Urolithiasis
- Urinary, rectal, and vaginal fistulas
- Damage to the urethra
- Prolonged labor and problems with delivery
- Psychological trauma

Clinical manifestations of these complications may lead the woman to seek health care.

Outcome Management

Management of the client with FGM is directed toward relief of clinical manifestations related to the complications. Some of these conditions have been discussed earlier in this chapter and in Chapter 34. To enable childbirth, a cesarean section or *deinfibulation* (opening of the incisional area anteriorly) may be required.

When caring for a woman with FGM, remain sensitive and nonjudgmental to gain her confidence and establish a trusting, therapeutic relationship. Teach her about the complications of the procedure; this issue is extremely important if she has daughters, who may be at risk for FGM. Unresolved grief and low self-esteem after the trauma of the experience or sterility caused by chronic PID may require supportive intervention or counseling.

Health care providers must act as advocates for women and girls affected by FGM by increasing professional and public awareness of the practice and its existence in the United States. Report FGM involving a girl younger than 18 years, because it is considered child abuse.

ALTERNATIVE THERAPY

Female Reproductive System: Premenstrual Syndrome and Menopause

Premenstrual Disorders

For the 20% to 50% of women who suffer from premenstrual tension or premenstrual syndrome (PMS) at some point in their lives, nutrient and herbal remedies may also be helpful. One review of vitamin B_6 in treating PMS found that although many studies were not of good quality, thus warranting further research, vitamin B_6 at doses up to 100 mg/day appeared to be helpful in treating PMS and premenstrual depression.[11]

Even more effective than vitamin B_6, in a comparison trial, was the herb chaste tree berry (*Vitex agnus-castus*). Several studies have found chaste tree berry beneficial in treating PMS.[7] Although more side effects were seen in the chaste tree berry group than in the vitamin B_6 group, no serious side effects were observed.

As with the treatment of menopausal manifestations, Chinese herbs are commonly used in treating PMS.[3] Aside from anecdotal reports, however, there is a lack of controlled studies using these therapies.

Menopause

Although a normal, natural and asymptomatic process for many women, menopause can be an uncomfortable transition time for others. There seem to be cultural and geographic differences in menopausal manifestations reported around the world, perhaps in part related to dietary variations. Some have suggested that there has been a "medicalization" of menopause, a focus on "the change" as a pathologic condition requiring treatment rather than as a normal healthy process.[9]

Chinese herbal therapies are widely used by practitioners of Asian (Oriental) medicine for treating the manifestations of perimenopause and menopause. Although such use is detailed in the Asian medical literature, Western research in this area remains inconclusive. Interestingly, in Japan the main manifestation reported by perimenopausal women is stiffness of the neck and shoulders, with hot flashes low on the report list of manifestations.

The herb black cohosh (*Cimicifuga racemosa*), originally used by native Americans, has been extensively studied in Europe in more than 1700 clients, over 3 to 6 months, showing benefits in treating hot flashes, sweating, and sleep disturbances related to menopause.[5] Such preparations of black cohosh have been used for more than 40 years in Europe. More recently, black cohosh has been combined with St. John's wort for concomitant treatment of depressive manifestations during menopause and to enhance its effect for clients with sleep disturbances.[8]

Phytoestrogens (plant hormones) have been studied for their potential effects in treatment of menopausal manifestations and for their longer-term effects in preventing both heart disease and osteoporosis. Phytoestrogens from soy products have been studied extensively, and it is speculated that intake of soy products in Asia may account for differences in menopausal manifestations reported there compared to the West. Phytoestrogens may help as many as two thirds of women with hot flashes, although there is little evidence that they help with vaginal dryness, another complaint of menopausal women.[4] Soy products have been shown to reduce total and low-density lipoprotein cholesterol levels, to lower diastolic blood pressure, and to decrease the severity of vasomotor manifestations.[10] In rat studies, soy isoflavones have conserved bone. Research in postmenopausal women has been limited but has shown small, positive effects only in lumbar vertebrae.[2]

The importance of lifestyle factors in the prevention of heart disease and osteoporosis is well known. With newer evidence for antioxidant vitamins in the prevention of heart disease and calcium for delaying osteoporosis, women have a number of choices of treatment of menopausal symptoms and of longer-term prevention of osteoporosis and heart disease.[1, 6]

References

1. Adams, A. K., Wermuth, E. O., & McBride, P. E. (1999). Antioxidant vitamins and the prevention of coronary heart disease. *American Family Physician, 60,* 895–904.
2. Anderson, J. J., & Garner, S. C. (1998). Phytoestrogens and bone. *Baillieres Clinical Endocrinology and Metabolism, 12,* 543–557.
3. Bensky, D., & Barolet, R. (1990). *Chinese herbal medicine-formulas and strategies.* Seattle: Eastland Press.
4. Eden, J. (1998). Phytoestrogens and the menopause. *Baillieres Clinical Endocrinology and Metabolism, 12,* 581–587.
5. Foster, S. (1999). Black cohosh: *Cimicifuga racemosa,* A literature review. *HerbalGram, 45,* 35–49.
6. Keller, C., Fullerton, J., & Mobley, C. (1999). Supplemental and complementary alternatives to hormone replacement therapy. *Journal of the American Academy of Nurse-Practitioners, 11(5),* 187–198.
7. Klepser, T., & Nisly, N. (1999). Chaste tree berry for premenstrual syndrome. *Alternative Medicine Alert, 2,* 64–67.
8. Liske, E., Gerhard, I., & Wustenberg, P. (1997). Phytocombination alleviates psychovegetative disorders. *TW Gynakologie, 10,* 172–175.
9. Locke, M. (1993). *Encounters with aging: Mythologies of menopause in Japan and North America.* Berkeley, CA: University of California Press.
10. Washburn, S., et al. (1999). Effect of soy protein supplementation on serum lipoproteins, blood pressure, and menopausal symptoms in perimenopausal women. *Menopause, 6,* 7–13.
11. Wyatt, K. M., et al. (1999). Efficacy of vitamin B_6 in the treatment of premenstrual syndrome: Systematic review. *British Medical Journal, 318,* 1375–1381.

James Higgy Lerner, RN, LAc, *Private practice of acupuncture, traditional Oriental medicine, and biofeedback*

CONCLUSIONS

Female reproductive disorders can occur throughout a woman's life. These problems range from menstrual disorders to life-threatening malignancies. Nurses can provide much of the needed education to help clients become more aware of preventive measures. The physical and psychosocial care of these clients is important. The skillful and empathic nurse can assist the woman through what is often an extremely distressing diagnosis and treatment.

Nurses who need more information on reproductive issues should consult a women's health (obstetrics and gynecology) textbook. Information on contraception, tubal ligation, abortion, and other issues can be found there.

THINKING CRITICALLY

1. The client, a 52-year-old woman, comes into the clinic stating, "I can't put up with it any longer!" Her last menstrual period was 4 months ago, and she has had severe hot flashes and night sweats for almost 6 months with no abatement. Vaginal intercourse has become so painful that she and her husband have refrained from sexual activity for 3 months. She states that the night sweats are so bad that she has had very few nights of uninterrupted sleep.

Factors to Consider. What are your priorities for her care? What interventions might be used?

2. A 38-year-old woman enters the clinic with a complaint of acute, sharp, severe bilateral pelvic pain. She has a temperature of 102.2° F, a pulse rate of 100 beats/min, a respiratory rate of 20 breaths/min, and chills. Her cervical culture shows gonococcal infection. She uses oral contraceptives for birth control.

Factors to Consider. Besides teaching her about antibiotic medication, what is your priority in caring for her, and what interventions are necessary?

3. The client, a 61-year-old woman, had a TAH-BSO 2 days ago for early endometrial cancer. Her Foley catheter was removed yesterday. Her temperature is 101.1° F, her pulse rate is 96 beats/min, and her respiratory rate is 16 breaths/min. Her blood pressure is 128/74 mm Hg. She complains of flank pain and urinary hesitancy. Her urine output for the past 4 hours is 120 ml, which is the total from three separate voidings. Her urine is cloudy and has a slightly foul odor.

Factors to Consider. What is your priority, and what interventions are needed?

BIBLIOGRAPHY

1. American Cancer Society. (2000). *Cancer facts and figures.* Atlanta: Author.
2. Avis, N. E., & McKinlay, S. M. (1995). The Massachusetts Women's Health Study: An epidemiologic investigation of the menopause. *Journal of the American Medical Women's Association, 50*(2), 45–49.
3. Baker, V., & Deppe, G. (1997). *Management of perioperative complications in gynecology.* Philadelphia: W. B. Saunders.
4. Bernier, F., & Jenkins, P. (1997). The role of vaginal estrogen in the treatment of urogenital dysfunction in postmenopausal women. *Urologic Nursing, 17*(3), 92–95.
5. Bobak, I. M., & Jensen, M. D. (1997). *Maternity and women's health care* (6th ed.). St. Louis: Mosby–Year Book.
6. Compston, J., & Marsh, M. (1999). *HRT and the menopause: Current therapy.* London: Martin Dunitz.
7. Cunningham, G., & Williams, J. (1997). *Williams' obstetrics* (20th ed.). Stamford, CT: Appleton & Lange.
8. DiSaia, P., & Creasman, W. (1997). *Clinical gynecologic oncology.* St. Louis: Mosby–Year Book.
9. Fogey, C. I., & Woods, N. F. (Eds.). (1995). *Women's health care: A comprehensive handbook.* Thousand Oaks, CA: Sage Publications.
10. Fontana, P. (1998). Endometrial cancer, cervical cancer, and the adnexal mass. In B. Agar (Ed.), *Primary Care: Oncology, 25*(2), 433–458.
11. Griffith, C. (1997). *Gynecologic oncology.* London: Mosby-Wolfe.
12. Hansen, M. (1998). *Pathophysiology: Foundations of disease and clinical intervention.* Philadelphia: W. B. Saunders.
13. Hopkins, W., Perez, C., & Young, R. (1997). *Principles and practice of gynecologic oncology* (2nd ed.). Philadelphia: Lippincott-Raven.
14. Howell, D. (1999). *The unofficial guide to coping with menopause.* New York: Macmillan.
15. Hulley, S., et al. (1998). Randomized trial of estrogen plus progestin for secondary prevention of coronary heart disease in postmenopausal women. *Journal of the American Medical Association, 280*(7), 605–613.
16. Kolander, C., Ballard, D., & Chandler, C. (1999). *Contemporary women's health: Issues for today and the future.* Boston: WCB McGraw-Hill.
17. Lichtman, R. (1996). Perimenopausal and postmenopausal hormone replacement therapy: I. An update of the literature on benefits and risks. *Journal of Nurse-Midwifery, 41*(1), 3–28.
18. Manos, M., et al. (1999). Identifying women with cervical neoplasia using human papillomavirus DNA testing for equivocal Papanicolaou results. *Journal of the American Medical Association, 281*(17), 1605–1610.
19. McCorkle, R., et al. (1996). *Cancer nursing: A comprehensive text* (2nd ed.). Philadelphia: W. B. Saunders.
20. Mills, D. (1999). *Endometriosis: A key to healing through nutrition.* Boston: Shaftesbury Dorset.
21. Mishell, D., et al. (1997). *Comprehensive gynecology.* (3rd ed.). St. Louis: Mosby–Year Book.
22. Mogus, M. (1997). Pelvic floor surgery? *RN, 67*(4), 36–41.
23. Moody, F. (1999). *Atlas of ambulatory surgery.* Philadelphia: W. B. Saunders.
24. Morris, R. (1999). Female genital mutilation: Perspectives, risks and complications. *Urologic Nursing, 19*(1), 13–19.
25. Ozols, R. (Ed.). (1998). *Gynecologic oncology.* Boston: Kluwer Academic Publishers.
26. Raz, S. (1996). *Female urology* (2nd ed.). Philadelphia: W. B. Saunders.
27. Sabiston, D. (1997). *Textbook of surgery: The biological basis of modern surgical practice* (15th ed.). Philadelphia: W. B. Saunders.
28. Schrag, D., et al. (1997). Decision analysis: Effects of prophylactic mastectomy and oophorectomy on life expectancy among women with *BRCA1* or *BRCA2* mutations. *New England Journal of Medicine, 336*(20), 1565–1471.
29. Schull, B. (1996). Initial evaluation and physical examination. In L. Brubaker & T. Sacharides (Eds.), *The female pelvic floor* (pp. 41–49). Philadelphia: F. A. Davis.
30. Selleck, C. (1997). Identifying and treating bacterial vaginosis. *American Journal of Nursing, 97*(9), 16AAA–16DDD.
31. Seltzer, V., & Pearse, W. H. (Eds.). (1995). *Women's primary health care.* New York: McGraw-Hill.
32. Shurpin, K. (1997). Ovarian cancer. *American Journal of Nursing, 97*(4), 34–35.
33. Smith, A., & Hughes, P. (1998). The estrogen dilemma. *American Journal of Nursing, 98*(4), 17–20.
34. Smith-Bindman, R., et al. (1998). Endovaginal ultrasound to exclude endometrial cancer and other endometrial abnormalities. *Journal of the American Medical Association, 280*(17), 1510–1517.
35. Star, W. L., Lommel, L. L., & Shannon, M. T. (Eds.). (1995). *Women's primary health care: Protocols for practice.* Washington, D.C.: American Nurses Publication.
36. Teaffy, N. (1999). *Perimenopause: Preparing for the change: A guide to the early stages of menopause and beyond* (2nd ed.). Rocklin, CA: Prima.
37. Voda, A. M. (1994). Risks and benefits associated with hormonal and surgical therapies for healthy midlife women. *Western Journal of Nursing Research, 16*(5), 507–523.
38. Walsh, B., et al. (1998). Effects of raloxifene on serum lipids and coagulation factors in healthy postmenopausal women. *Journal of the American Medical Association, 279*(18), 1445–1451.
39. World Congress on Endometriosis. (1998). *Understanding and managing endometriosis: Advances in research and practice*: Proceedings of the Sixth World Congress on Endometriosis, June 30–July 4, 1998. Quebec City, Canada: Author.
40. Wright, S., et al. (1995). Short-term Lupron or danazol therapy for pelvic endometriosis. *Fertility and Sterility, 63*(3), 504–507.
41. Xu, Y., et al. (1998). Lysophosphatidic acid as a potential biomarker for ovarian and other gynecologic cancers. *Journal of the American Medical Association, 280*(8), 719–723.

CHAPTER 40

Management of Clients with Breast Disorders

Michelle Goodman
Stephanie Mellon-Reppen

NURSING OUTCOMES CLASSIFICATION (NOC)
for Nursing Diagnoses—Clients with Breast Disorders

Altered Nutrition: Less Than Body Requirements
Nutritional Status: Food and Fluid Intake
Nutritional Status: Nutrient Intake
Body Image Disturbance
Grief Resolution
Psychosocial Adjustment: Life Change
Self-Care: Activities of Daily Living (ADL)
Self-Esteem
Effective Management of Therapeutic Regimen and Knowledge Deficit
Decision-Making
Family Participation in Professional Care
Knowledge: Diet

Knowledge: Disease Process
Knowledge: Medication
Knowledge: Treatment Regimen
Knowledge: Treatment Procedures
Participation: Health Care Decisions
Risk for Impaired Skin Integrity
Tissue Integrity: Skin and Mucous Membranes
Treatment Behavior: Illness or Injury
Wound Healing: Primary Intention or Secondary Intention
Risk for Ineffective Individual Coping and Risk for Ineffective Family Coping
Caregiver Emotional Support

Coping
Decision-Making
Family Coping
Family Normalization
Family Participation in Professional Care
Information Processing
Role Performance
Social Support
Risk for Injury
Symptom Control

A woman who finds a breast lump or other breast problem will probably first suspect cancer, even though eight of 10 lumps are benign. Despite many misconceptions regarding the etiology of breast cancer, public awareness about this health threat has grown dramatically. In the past, the subject was avoided, or if information was shared, it was often inaccurate. Now breast cancer is openly discussed, and information about this topic is frequently presented in mass media. With the recent media focus on breast cancer awareness and early detection, the public is becoming more aware of the role that breast self-examination, clinical examination, and especially routine mammograms have in the early detection of a breast mass.

Nurses have a responsibility to teach the public about breast lesions and cancer, to correct misconceptions, and to provide accurate information concerning normal breasts and breast disease, detection, and treatment. Facts about the disease, treatment, and prognosis need to be shared openly with all members of society, particularly the underserved. If women understand the importance of early detection and treatment, they are more likely to have regular mammograms and less likely to delay seeking medical care when an abnormality is found. Delay in seeking medical care is often due to (1) fear that the problem is cancer and (2) lack of knowledge that breast cancer can be curable if caught early.

BREAST CANCER IN WOMEN

Breast cancer is the most common malignancy in women in the United States and is second only to lung cancer as a cause of cancer death.[1] The incidence of breast cancer in the United States has been increasing gradually for the past 30 years. In 2000, the number of new cases of breast cancer diagnosed in the United States was estimated at 182,800, with 40,800 deaths caused by the disease.[1] At age 85, a woman's risk for breast cancer is one in eight, depending on where she lives. The highest incidence of breast cancer is found in the United States and Europe.

Before 1990, there had been little evidence of any decrease in the United States age-standardized death rate from breast cancer. Currently, breast cancer mortality appears to be declining among white women but increasing among African American women, especially those who are premenopausal. (Breast cancer in men is rare and is discussed later in this chapter.) The decrease in mortality may be ascribed to the combined benefits of early detection and better treatment (particularly with adjuvant chemotherapy and tamoxifen) during the 1980s.[28, 39] The increase in early diagnosis due to mammography and the generally increased awareness of breast cancer among women and their physicians have resulted in detection of smaller tumors, which are more likely to be localized and to be treated successfully.[10]

Probably the most important encouragement to breast cancer detection has been the discovery that screening mammography reduces breast cancer deaths by 30%.[2, 32] The Breast and Cervical Cancer Mortality Act of 1990 was enacted to ensure that underinsured or uninsured women receive mammograms and appropriate treatment services.[3] Women need to understand the importance of mammography in detecting breast cancers while the tumors are small. Likewise, they should understand that the treatment is less toxic and more effective for all modalities used when the disease is detected early, even before the tumor is palpable. With regard to surgery, less tissue is removed when the tumor is small; therefore, better cosmesis is possible. With irradiation of a smaller volume of diseased tissue, cure is more likely and a lower dose is needed for cure by radiation therapy. With adjuvant treatment, a small tumor burden means that systemic therapy may not be needed; if it is needed, drug treatment will be more successful. Smaller tumors also mean less regional node involvement and fewer complications associated with axillary node dissection.[25]

Nurses need to provide current and accurate information concerning the latest approaches to breast cancer treatment and related complications. Encouraging the client to participate in research, if appropriate, is especially important, so that critical questions regarding breast cancer therapy can be addressed. Clients and their families are required to make many difficult decisions. The nurse can be especially helpful by ensuring that the client understands treatment options and by providing clarification when appropriate.

Etiology and Risk Factors

The cause of breast cancer is not known. Many women are anxious about their risk for breast cancer, and many tend to overestimate their risk. Although genetic, hormonal, or biochemical factors are likely to be involved, 70% of women with breast cancer had no known risk factors.

AGE AND ETHNICITY
All women are at risk for breast cancer, and the most important single risk factor is age. Risk increases with age, although the rate of increase slows after menopause. The annual incidence of breast cancer in American women 80 to 85 years of age is 15 times higher than that in women 30 to 35 years of age. African American women under age 50 years have a higher age-specific incidence of breast cancer than that in Caucasian women.

Edwards and colleagues, in their examination of the impact of race on survival in breast cancer, found that not only are African American women less likely to be cured than their non-African American counterparts, but they also survive for a shorter time until death from breast cancer.[20] Even when matched for tumor stage, they are more at risk for micrometastatic disease and early death.

It is not clear whether these findings are related to tumor biology, host response, or variability in treatment. Psychosocial and socioeconomic factors have a major role in governing access to medical care. Uninsured clients and those insured by Medicaid present with more advanced disease, have a higher risk of death, and have lessened survival compared with privately insured clients.[20]

Breast cancer incidence among Hispanic women living in North America is only 40% to 50% as great as that among non-Hispanic white women. Asian women born in Asia have a very low lifetime risk of breast cancer, but their daughters born in North America have the same lifetime risk of breast cancer as for American white women.[3]

OVARIAN AND HORMONAL FUNCTION
Early menarche (first menses) and late menopause (cessation of menses) lead to an increased total lifetime number of ovulatory menstrual cycles and a corresponding 30% to 50% increase in breast cancer risk. The woman who experiences natural menopause before age 45 years has a risk for breast cancer that is half that of the woman whose menopause occurs after age 55 years.[2] Likewise, oophorectomy before a woman reaches menopause lowers her risk of breast cancer by approximately two thirds. Both nulliparity (no births) and age over 30 years at first live birth are associated with a nearly doubled risk of subsequent breast cancer.[48] The use of hormone replacement therapy (HRT) has also demonstrated a small but significant increase in risk for breast cancer in women who used it for more than 10 years. The Women's Health Initiative study, which includes women who are randomized to receive hormones or placebo, should ultimately answer the question of the effect of other hormonal factors. Definitive findings are expected to be available in the year 2005.

At present there is no convincing evidence that oral contraceptive use affects the risk of breast cancer. The question is difficult to address because the oral contraceptives in use today are vastly different (in that dosages are much lower) from those used 15 and 20 years ago. Even if oral contraceptives influence the incidence of breast cancer, it would be only of historical interest because the drugs used years ago are not comparable to those used today.

BENIGN BREAST DISEASE
Benign breast disease is not more common in women with other risk factors for breast cancer. Nonproliferative lesions (such as cysts, duct ectasia, mild hyperplasia, and fibroadenoma) do not increase the risk of breast cancer; however, cellular atypia or atypical hyperplasia (a proliferative disease) is an example of a histologic change associated with a higher risk. Sclerosing adenosis increases the risk of breast cancer by approximately 70%.[2] Nearly 40% of women with a family history of breast cancer and atypical hyperplasia subsequently have breast cancer.

FAMILY HISTORY
Family history is one of the known risk factors for breast cancer. Breast cancer due to the inheritance of a specific germline mutation from either maternal or paternal relatives is rare. In fact, the breast cancer susceptibility gene *BRCA1* and *BRCA2* and the p53 tumor suppressor gene have been identified in fewer than 10% of all women

with breast cancer. Certain populations have a higher incidence of *BRCA* mutations than the general population (e.g., native Icelanders and Ashkenazi Jews).[8]

Depending on the familial context, the lifetime risk of breast cancer, ovarian cancer, or both associated with carrying a mutation ranges from 50% to 85%.[2, 8] Families with several affected first-degree relatives and clients with early-onset disease have been found to harbor mutations at a higher frequency. Women who have the *BRCA2* mutation tend to have early-onset (before age 50) breast cancer but not ovarian cancer. Identification of the *BRCA1* gene makes it possible to identify women who have a 90% to 95% lifetime likelihood of developing breast cancer (with a 70% risk of breast cancer by age 60).[8] Tests for these mutations exist, and research efforts to develop comprehensive genetic screening and counseling programs are ongoing.

ENVIRONMENTAL AND DIETARY FACTORS

An increased incidence of breast cancer has been reported in women who received mantle radiation for the treatment of Hodgkin's disease, particularly if they were younger than 20 years of age.[14] The latency period is between 10 and 25 years. The disease in this group typically presents more aggressively, with a high rate of nodal involvement and bilaterality. It is for this reason that all persons who receive mantle radiation for Hodgkin's disease, especially those treated prior to age 20, receive a regular mammography follow-up examination in order to detect these lesions early.[14]

Alcohol intake is the best-established dietary risk factor for breast cancer in epidemiologic studies. The positive correlation of alcohol intake with breast cancer risk has been established, and it appears that moderate alcohol intake (two drinks per day) increases the risk of breast cancer by altering estrogen metabolism.[30]

As is commonly observed, Japanese women living in Japan have a very low incidence of breast cancer. When they move to the United States, their risk for breast cancer approximates that of native white women within one generation. In a large study involving nearly 338,000 women, there was no apparent correlation between breast cancer risk and dietary intake of fat.[30] If fat intake is relevant to breast cancer, it is probably early in life, perhaps at adolescence. Epidemiologic evidence does not support any substantial increase in breast cancer risk associated with caffeine consumption.

Nurses have a unique role in fostering health promotion and in teaching women about breast cancer as well as in identifying a woman's individual risk for breast cancer. Because most women—especially those with any family history of breast cancer—greatly overestimate their risk for breast cancer, it is helpful to instruct women about the known risk factors and, as indicated, provide support to lessen some of their fears (Table 40–1). Counseling, with appropriate referrals when required, should always accompany specific recommendations for clients with significant risks.

HEALTH PROMOTION ACTIVITIES

Although no known agent or practice guarantees that a woman will remain free of breast cancer, methods are

TABLE 40–1	BREAST CANCER RISK ASSESSMENT AND RECOMMENDATIONS	
	Recommendations	
Risk Factors	**Low Risk** (<15%*)	**Moderate to High Risk** (15%–>30%*)
Gender: Women are affected far more often than men, in a ratio of 99:1	Mammogram: Baseline at age 35; every other year ages 40–50; every year after age 50	Mammogram: Baseline at age 30; frequency of subsequent mammograms depends on findings and on recommendations of radiologist
Age: Risk increases with age	Clinical breast examination every year	Clinical breast examination every 6 months
Place of birth: North America; northern Europe	Breast self-examination every month	Breast self-examination every month
Socioeconomic status: High		For known *BRCA1* or *BRCA2* mutation carriers, possible prophylactic mastectomy, prophylactic oophorectomy, or both after childbearing.
Age at first full-term pregnancy: Older than 30 years		
Menstrual history: Early menarche; late menopause		
Health history: History of breast cancer; diagnosis of atypical hyperplasia; exposure to radiation		
Family history: Mother or sister with history of breast cancer; any first-degree relative with breast cancer; *BRCA1* gene carrier		

*Lifetime cumulative risk.

under investigation that may alter the risk and therefore can be considered health promotion activities.

Chemoprevention

Chemoprevention is the use of a drug to prevent the development of a certain malignancy. Two agents have been found to decrease the risk of breast cancer: tamoxifen (Nolvadex) and raloxifene (Evista).

Tamoxifen is an agent commonly used in clients who have breast tumors with receptors for estrogen. Fisher and colleagues[22] looked at tamoxifen and its role in decreasing the incidence of breast cancer in high-risk clients. In this study, 13,388 high-risk women were randomized to receive either placebo or tamoxifen 20 mg/day. Tamoxifen reduced the risk of invasive breast cancer by 49% overall; however, endometrial cancer developed in twice as many women in the tamoxifen group as in the placebo group. In another study, 7705 women with osteoporosis were randomized to receive either placebo or raloxifene.[13] Through a period of 33 months, nearly twice as many invasive breast cancers were seen in the placebo group as in the raloxifene group.

In contrast to the tamoxifen trial, there was no increase in the incidence of endometrial cancer in women who received raloxifene. Because raloxifene has never been compared with tamoxifen as a chemopreventive agent and has not been studied in women at high risk for breast cancer, the National Surgical Adjuvant Breast Project (NSABP) is conducting a double-blind study that will compare these two drugs in 22,000 high-risk women. Tamoxifen is currently the more widely used of the two drugs; it costs approximately $75 in the United States for a month's supply and is covered by most insurance plans.

Prophylactic Mastectomy

The only other measure that may predictably prevent the occurrence of breast cancer and be considered a method of health promotion is prophylactic mastectomy. All of the breast tissue is removed in a woman who does not have evidence of breast cancer. Women who may benefit from this procedure are those who have a strong family history of breast cancer, a history of breast cancer in the other breast, a history of atypical hyperplasia on repeated surgical biopsies, or presence of a mutated *BRCA1* or *BRCA2* gene.

Lifestyle Changes

Women can also be encouraged to make changes in lifestyle to lower their potential risk for breast cancer. For instance, they can decrease their consumption of alcohol. Although a moderate decrease in dietary fat intake does not reduce appear to reduce the risk of breast cancer, decreasing fat intake to 20% of dietary calories is a worthwhile goal.[30]

Exercise may have an indirect role in the prevention of breast cancer. Exercise leads to a decrease in body fat, thereby reducing the amount of free estrogen stored in body fat. Hence, it is another health promotion activity.

HEALTH MAINTENANCE ACTIVITIES

Health maintenance involves optimal screening and early detection of breast cancer. Regardless of the method used, regular and careful physical examination is the key to identifying asymptomatic cancerous lesions. When combined with mammography, physical examination decreases

mortality, especially in women over age 50. According to the National Cancer Advisory Board (NCAB), a committee that advises and consults with the director of the National Cancer Institute (NCI), data presented at the Consensus Development Conference showed that regular screening mammography of average-risk women in their 40s reduces deaths from breast cancer by about 17% to 24%.[10, 46] On the basis of this finding, the NCAB recommended to the NCI that women between the ages of 40 and 49 years have screening mammograms every 1 to 2 years if they are at average risk for breast cancer.

For women 50 years and older, a mammogram is recommended every 1 to 2 years regardless of risk. However, the American Cancer Society, the American College of Radiology, and the American College of Obstetrics and Gynecology recommend a mammogram every 1 to 2 years for women between ages 40 and 50 and then annually after the age of 50. In addition, the American Cancer Society advises that a baseline mammogram be obtained between ages 35 and 40.

The currently available data do not warrant a universal recommendation for mammography for all women in their 40s. The decision to have a screening mammogram in the absence of risk factors in this age group is based on the woman's personal wishes and the recommendation of her primary health care provider. Cost is an important issue in the use of mammography screening in younger women; the cost of screening younger women may approach $1 billion annually.

Once a mammogram reveals an area suggestive of cancer, an ultrasound study is a useful complement to diagnostic mammography as a means for distinguishing cystic from solid masses. For women with particularly dense breasts or with implants, magnetic resonance imaging (MRI) scanning and digital mammography provide improved sensitivity. It is hoped that better mammography technology, including digitized radiography, routine use of magnified views, and greater skill in interpretation, combined with MRI and positron emission tomography (PET) scanning will make it possible to identify breast cancers at an earlier stage.

Health care professionals and health care advocates have for many years promoted breast self-examination (BSE) as a key component of early cancer detection because most breast cancers are detected by the woman herself, usually after the mass has grown to the size of 2.5 cm or larger. The only reason the cancer is detected then is that the mass is large enough to be felt. A better goal would be to detect the cancer while it is still small, before it can be felt (Fig. 40–1). The only way to do this is by regular mammography and physical examination by a trained clinician (see Chapter 37). BSE has not been proven to save lives or to increase survival. There is insufficient evidence to recommend for or against the teaching of BSE.[24] Of course, teaching a woman to examine her breasts is an important strategy for increasing her awareness of the risk of breast cancer. See Chapter 37 for a discussion of BSE.

HEALTH RESTORATION ACTIVITIES

Arm exercises and positioning after surgery to prevent lymphedema, obtaining a prosthesis, and breast reconstruction are health restoration activities. If lymphedema

FIGURE 40–1 *A,* Screening mammogram of a 56-year-old woman with a strong family history of breast cancer, right mediolateral oblique view. The mammogram shows a small, irregular, nonpalpable mass *(arrow)*, which was highly suggestive of malignancy. *B,* The left mediolateral oblique view shows a normal breast.

develops despite exercises and positioning, referral to a physical therapist or specialized nurse for lymphedema management is recommended.

Pathophysiology

Breast cancers are malignant tumors that typically begin in the ductal-lobular epithelial cells of the breast and spread via the lymphatic system to the axillary lymph nodes. The tumor may then metastasize to distant regions of the body, including lungs, liver, bone, and brain. The finding of breast cancer in the axillary lymph nodes is an indicator of the tumor's ability for potential distant spread and is not merely contiguous growth into the adjacent region of the breast. Most primary breast cancers are adenocarcinomas located in the upper outer quadrant of the breast (Fig. 40–2).

CARCINOMA IN SITU

Malignant-appearing cells confined to the ductal or lobular units without permeation of the basement membrane are considered to represent carcinoma in situ. *Ductal car-* *cinoma in situ* (DCIS) is considered a precursor of infiltrating carcinoma. Pathologists classify DCIS as high-intermediate-grade or low-grade according to the growth pattern of cells occupying the ducts, their nuclear features, mitotic activity, presence of necrosis, and type of microcalcifications. Low-grade DCIS tends to be the most common and is typically multifocal; high-grade DCIS is second in prevalence and tends to be architecturally contiguous and associated with prominent microcalcifications. High-grade DCIS tends to be estrogen receptor–negative, shows increased expression for human epidermal growth factor receptor (HER-2)/Neu protein (c-erbB2), and has a mutated p53 tumor suppressor gene.

Ipsilateral (affecting the same side) invasive carcinoma develops within 10 years in approximately 30% of cases of DCIS. Left untreated, intraductal carcinoma will be transformed into invasive ductal carcinoma.

Lobular carcinoma in situ (LCIS) is characterized by a solid proliferation of atypical cells expanding lobular units. In contrast to DCIS, LCIS is usually found incidentally and is not typically associated with microcalcifica-

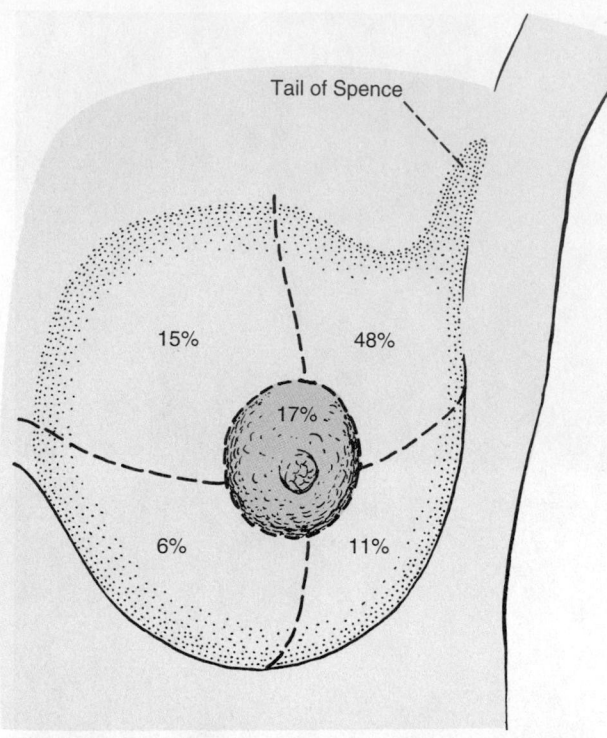

Tail of Spence

15%   48%

17%

6%   11%

FIGURE 40-2 Frequency of occurrence of breast cancer according to location. The highest occurrence is in the upper outer quadrant and in the tail of Spence.

tions. LCIS has a lower tendency to develop into infiltrating carcinoma.

INVASIVE BREAST CANCER

The majority of breast cancers (75%) are infiltrating ductal carcinomas. They typically metastasize to regional lymph nodes and beyond. Lobular carcinomas account for about 5% to 10% of cases and usually present as a generalized thickening. Tumor types that are associated with a favorable prognosis include tubular (accounting for 2% of cases), medullary (5% to 7%), and mucinous (colloid) carcinoma (3%). These histologic types tend to have low-grade histology, positive estrogen and progesterone receptors status, diploid deoxyribonucleic acid (DNA) content, low S phase fraction (discussed later under Prognosis and Defining Extent of Disease), and no oncogenic markers. Tumors with poor clinical prognosis are those associated with high-grade histology and dermal lymphatic invasion designated as "inflammatory carcinoma." Inflammatory breast cancer is characterized by skin redness and induration. Edema and warmth are other common associated findings. Frequently, palpable axillary and supraclavicular nodes and distant metastases are involved.

Clinical Manifestations

Most breast cancers present as painless, nontender, hard, irregularly shaped, nonmobile masses. About 60% of cancers are somewhat movable, 40% have regular borders by palpation, and 40% can feel soft or cystic. Even when no mass is present, other physical findings, such as nipple discharge, induration, and dimpling, can suggest malignancy. Heat and erythema of the breast skin may be related to inflammation but may also indicate inflamma-

tory carcinoma. Skin edema is characteristic of malignant disease. The edema is due to the invasion and obstruction of dermal lymphatics by the tumor. If a tumor is suspected on the basis of the physical findings, a diagnostic mammogram is indicated.

RADIOGRAPHIC FINDINGS

Additional diagnostic films of the affected breast, as well as localized compression and magnification views, increase the specificity of identifying the abnormality. Digital mammography and computer-assisted diagnosis (CAD) may be useful to evaluate the lesion, because these tests allow more variations in exposure and show the differences in tissue contrast more clearly. CAD utilizes a software program to target lesions suspected to be malignant. The specificity of the image is enhanced by on-screen evaluation that allows manipulation of contrast, which improves detection.

FINE-NEEDLE ASPIRATION

Fine-needle aspiration (FNA) is performed on an outpatient basis. The purpose is to determine whether a solid lump is a cyst or to confirm a clinically apparent diagnosis. If the mass turns out to be a cyst, the lump should disappear after the aspiration. If a lump is solid, a cytologic specimen may be obtained by making several passes into the lesion to retrieve small cell samples; this technique can reduce the incidence of false-negative results. If the FNA results are negative and the physician suspects cancer from the clinical findings, excisional biopsy (open) is indicated.

STEREOTACTIC NEEDLE-GUIDED BIOPSY

Stereotactic needle-guided biopsy (SNB) is used mainly to target and identify nonpalpable lesions in the breast that have been detected with mammography. The basic goal is to immobilize the breast from fixed horizontal and vertical coordinates to calculate the exact position of the lesion within a three-dimensional field. SNB permits biopsy diagnosis of benign disease without the trauma or scarring of an open biopsy.

OPEN BIOPSY

Excisional or open biopsy is chosen when the lesion is determined to be solid and indeterminate in nature, when results of cytologic or histologic analysis are insufficient, or when the clinical or mammographic findings suggest malignancy. A wire-localized biopsy procedure similar to the stereotactic method can be used; the aim of this procedure is to assist the surgeon in locating the nonpalpable lesion for the purpose of excisional biopsy and to minimize the volume of tissue removed to avoid unnecessary deformity.

Prognosis and Defining Extent of Disease

Once a diagnosis of cancer is made, the cancer needs to be evaluated further to determine the most appropriate therapy. For example, if breast-conserving surgery (lumpectomy) is being considered, the presence of microcalcifications would need to be evaluated further to determine whether the disease in the breast is multifocal.

The tumor is staged according to the extent of local, regional, and distant spread. *Staging* permits an accurate definition of the extent of the disease and therefore a more accurate prognosis. The American Joint Committee on Cancer (AJCC) staging system for breast cancer is based on the tumor-node-metastasis (TNM) system, presented in Table 40–2. Prognosis for breast cancer is associated primarily with the extent of disease at detection. The tumor staging is based on (1) the size of the primary tumor; (2) whether it extends to the chest wall or skin; (3) the presence of axillary lymph nodes; (4) whether they are matted, fixed, or mobile; and (5) the presence of distant metastases (Fig. 40–3). The 5-year survival rate for breast cancer based on stage of disease is presented in Table 40–3.

Prognostic factors are used to determine prognosis or the natural history of breast cancer. At present, only pathologic lymph node status, tumor size, estrogen and proges-terone receptor status, histologic grade, and histopathology are considered to be independent prognostic indicators and therefore appropriate to consider in determining therapy and prognosis. Another factor that is often taken into consideration is the DNA content of the tumor. *DNA ploidy* refers to the degree of multiplication of chromosome sets. *Diploid* and *euploid* signify an exact multiple of the haploid number of chromosomes. *Aneuploid* indicates a deviation from an exact multiple of the haploid number and a poorer prognosis. The S phase index identifies the percentage of tumor cells in S phase (start of DNA synthesis) of the cell growth cycle. The higher the percentage of cells in S phase, the more aggressive the cancer.

TABLE 40–2   TNM STAGING SYSTEM FOR BREAST CANCER

Primary Tumor (T)

TX	Primary tumor cannot be assessed
T0	No evidence of primary tumor
Tis	Carcinoma in situ: intraductal carcinoma, lobular carcinoma in situ, or Paget's disease of the nipple with no tumor
T1	Tumor 2 cm or less in greatest dimension
T1mic	Microinvasion 0.1 cm or less in greatest dimension
T1a	Tumor more than 0.1 cm but not more than 0.5 cm in greatest dimension
T1b	Tumor more than 0.5 cm but not more than 1 cm in greatest dimension
T1c	Tumor more than 1 cm but not more than 2 cm in greatest dimension
T2	Tumor more than 2 cm but not more than 5 cm in greatest dimension
T3	Tumor more than 5 cm is greatest dimension
T4	Tumor of any size with direct extension to (a) chest wall or (b) skin, only as described below
T4a	Extension to chest wall
T4b	Edema (including peau d'orange) or ulceration of the skin of the breast or satellite skin nodules confined to the same breast
T4c	Both T4a and T4b
T4d	Inflammatory carcinoma

Regional Lymph Nodes (N)

NX	Regional lymph nodes cannot be assessed (e.g., previously removed)
N0	No regional lymph node metastasis
N1	Metastasis to movable ipsilateral axillary lymph node(s)
N2	Metastasis to ipsilateral axillary lymph node(s) fixed to one another or to other structures
N3	Metastasis to ipsilateral internal mammary lymph node(s)

Distant Metastasis (M)

MX	Distant metastasis cannot be assessed
M0	No distant metastasis
M1	Distant metastasis (includes metastasis to ipsilateral supraclavicular lymph node[s])

Stage Grouping

Stage	T	N	M
0	Tis	N0	M0
I	T1*	N0	M0
IIA	T0	N1	M0
	T1*	N1†	M0
	T2	N0	M0
IIB	T2	N1	M0
	T3	N0	M0
IIIA	T0	N2	M0
	T1†	N2	M0
	T2	N2	M0
	T3	N1	M0
	T3	N2	M0
IIIB	T4	Any N	M0
	Any T	N3	M0
IV	Any T	Any N	M1

*T1 includes T1mic.
†The prognosis for patients with N1a cancers is similar to that for patients with N0 cancers.
Adapted, with permission, from Fleming I. D., Cooper J. S., Henson D. E., et al. (Eds). *AJCC Cancer staging manual* (5th ed.). Philadelphia, Lippincott-Raven, 1997.

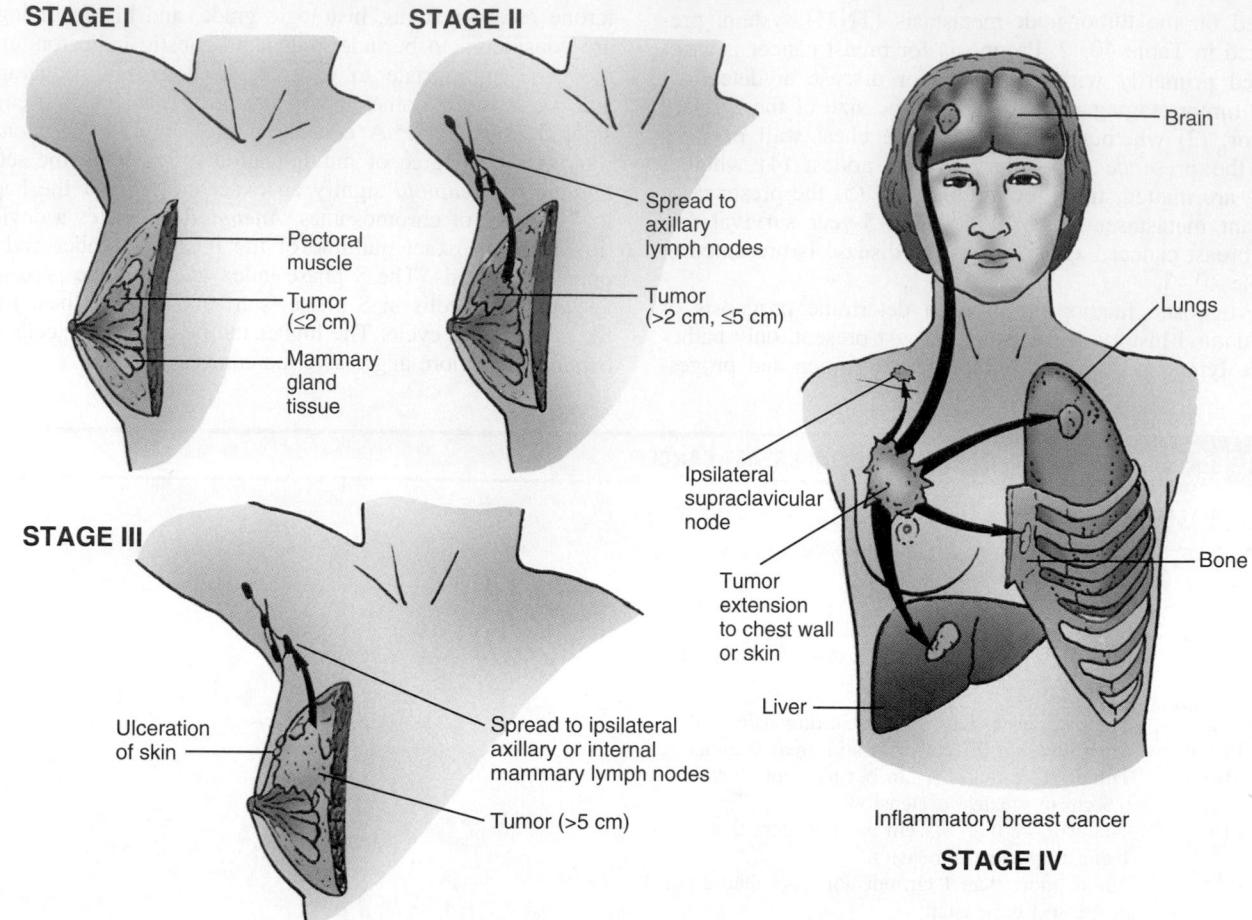

STAGE I

Pectoral muscle
Tumor (≤2 cm)
Mammary gland tissue

STAGE II

Spread to axillary lymph nodes
Tumor (>2 cm, ≤5 cm)

STAGE III

Ulceration of skin
Spread to ipsilateral axillary or internal mammary lymph nodes
Tumor (>5 cm)

Brain
Lungs
Ipsilateral supraclavicular node
Bone
Tumor extension to chest wall or skin
Liver

Inflammatory breast cancer
STAGE IV

FIGURE 40–3 Clinincal staging of breast cancer. *Stage I,* Tumor 2 cm or less in diameter and confined to the breast. *Stage II,* Tumor up to 5 cm, or early metastasis to axillary lymph nodes. *Stage III,* Tumor larger than 5 cm with involvement of the ipsilateral axillary or internal mammary lymph nodes. *Stage IV,* Distant metastasis, such as to brain, bone, or liver; ipsilateral supraclavicular lymph node; skin and/or extension to chest wall; or inflammatory breast cancer.

The tumor is generally graded to determine the degree of differentiation and therefore prognosis. Tumors are classified as *well differentiated* (grade I), *moderately well differentiated* (grade II), or *poorly differentiated* (grade III) according to the degree of anaplasia observed. Other factors identified on the pathology report include nucleus size and shape, presence or absence of mitotic figures, and degree of tubule formation. Dermal lymphatic invasion and microvascular invasion may also be predictive of metastatic disease.

Although the prognostic significance of HER-2/Neu protein (c-erbB2) remains under investigation, it appears that overexpression of this protein in the primary tumor correlates with less favorable prognostic indicators and may be predictive of response to chemotherapy, especially paclitaxel (Taxol). Post-chemotherapy c-erbB2 levels are also a prognostic indicator of disease-free survival.[4] Steroid receptor status is an accepted predictive factor for response to endocrine therapies. If the tumor is determined to be estrogen receptor–positive and progesterone receptor–positive, antiestrogen therapy would be an appropriate therapeutic option with or without chemotherapy.

Tumor markers are not considered useful preoperatively when adjuvant therapy for cure is planned. Tumor markers are assessed as part of the work-up of advanced disease and generally have significance only in a woman with metastatic disease. Carcinoembryonic antigen (CEA), CA-125, and CA 15-3 are substances that are produced by the tumor and are present in the serum of the woman with breast cancer. A tumor marker would be expected to be present only in metastatic disease, in which case it is assessed on a monthly basis to monitor response to therapy.

TABLE 40–3	FIVE-YEAR SURVIVAL RATE FOR BREAST CANCER BY STAGE
Stage	**5-Year Survival (% of Patients)**
0	99
I	92
IIA	82
IIB	65
IIIA	47
IIIB	44
IV	14

Data from Surveillance Epidemiology End Results (SEER), National Cancer Institute, *http://www.seer.ims.nci.nih.gov.*, April 25, 2000.

Pretreatment assessment also includes a metastatic work-up to determine extent of disease. Tests are selected according to the clinical presentation and the likelihood of metastatic disease. A chest x-ray film and a bone scan are possible useful baseline studies. A bone scan is usually not indicated unless the client has invasive breast cancer that is at least stage II or III. Only 30% to 60% of clients with a true-positive bone scan have increased alkaline phosphatase levels, and only 20% of clients with elevated alkaline phosphatase levels are disease-free. If the bone scan is abnormal, then radiographs of the affected sites are necessary to confirm metastatic disease and to exclude a benign etiologic mechanism.

A complete metabolic panel and physical examination will detect any liver dysfunction and may identify the need for a liver scan. The liver scan is usually not done unless there is reason to suspect that the disease has spread or except in the presence of stage III disease. When metastatic disease is strongly suspected, an MRI study or a computed tomography (CT) scan may be ordered to further define and measure the extent of disease. A PET scan is not usually indicated unless results of the MRI or CT scan are indeterminate and metastatic disease is strongly suspected. PET may also be used to determine whether a sentinel node biopsy is appropriate.

Outcome Management

In the past, management of the client with breast cancer typically included a modified radical or a radical mastectomy. Postoperatively, the surgeon would assure the woman that all the cancer was removed, and that would be the end of her treatment. Today the management approach to localized breast cancer is much more complicated, because much more is known about the systemic nature of breast cancer and the need for local control as well as appropriate adjuvant therapy. Historically, it was believed that cancer spread locally to the lymph nodes in an orderly, defined manner. If this were true, radical mastectomy should eliminate the disease. It is now known that breast cancer does not spread in an orderly manner and that cancer cells metastasize through the bloodstream and lymphatic system to other tissues and organs such as skin, regional lymph nodes, or more distant sites, including bone, lung, liver, and brain. Because breast cancer is now considered a systemic disease, less radical, more breast-conserving surgical procedures are done in combination with radiation therapy, hormonal therapy, or chemotherapy.

Soon after a biopsy-proven diagnosis of breast cancer, the client should consult with a team of interdisciplinary consultants who are part of a comprehensive breast center, before deciding on the definitive approach to management of her breast cancer. Most insurance companies encourage this consultation because there are numerous approaches to the management of breast cancer and an interdisciplinary approach is not only most advantageous for the client but also most efficient and cost-effective. The interdisciplinary team generally includes a medical oncologist, a radiation oncologist, and a surgical oncologist. An oncology nurse practitioner, a nutritionist, and a psycho-oncologist are also vital members of the team, because many clients have questions concerning quality of life, how to maintain nutrition, and ways to promote communication among family members. Another advantage to evaluation at a comprehensive breast center is that such centers usually have the most advanced diagnostic tools, offer the most current research protocols, and can provide a comprehensive breast cancer risk assessment, genetic evaluation, and appropriate counseling.

■ PRIMARY BREAST CANCER

Carcinoma in situ (meaning that it has not invaded the tissue of origin) is becoming more of an issue in local control of breast cancer, owing to the success of mammography in detecting these small cancers. DCIS is generally managed by local excision with or without radiation. The risk of local recurrence following breast-sparing surgery is approximately 10% at 10 years. Whether radiation therapy is necessary for all clients is uncertain. The addition of tamoxifen as therapeutic as well as prophylactic treatment following local treatment is gaining acceptance. Obviously, women require scheduled diagnostic follow-up mammograms along with physician examination every 6 to 12 months.

LCIS is considered a risk factor for breast cancer rather than a precursor lesion. Because of the bilateral multifocal nature of LCIS, options for management range from careful observation and mammography at 6- to 12-month intervals to bilateral prophylactic mastectomy—options that for many women appear either too conservative or too extreme. The physician-nurse team needs to explain the options carefully and permit time for the client to understand her risks and choices for management.

The management of localized invasive breast cancer has changed dramatically since the mid-1980s. Approximately 30% of women with breast cancer are now managed with breast-conserving surgery. Many more women are candidates for this procedure, but unfortunately surgeons are reluctant to change, and research takes many years and thousands of clients to prove that one form of therapy is superior to another. However, several studies have indicated that breast-conserving treatments, consisting of the removal of the primary tumor by some form of lumpectomy with or without irradiation to the breast, may result in survival that is equal to that of more extensive procedures, including mastectomy and modified radical mastectomy.[34, 35] Similarly, the addition of radiation therapy to mastectomy does not improve 10-year survival rates and is not indicated if the surgical margins are clear and if no other factors place the client at high risk for local recurrence.

At the time of the initial consultation, a plan of care is devised and the goal of therapy is determined. It is crucial to identify clients at substantial risk for recurrence because they do benefit from systemic therapy. Likewise, in a woman with a tumor smaller than 1 cm with no evidence of axillary node involvement, there is little justification for adjuvant chemotherapy. When the tumor is larger than 1 cm and there is evidence of axillary lymph node involvement, other parameters are assessed, such as estrogen receptor status and measures of tumor growth rate. These help determine not only the need for adjuvant chemotherapy but also whether a doxorubicin-containing regimen is appropriate.

For example, tumors with a high proportion of cells in the S phase of cell division are associated with a greater risk of relapse, and chemotherapy offers a greater survival benefit. Cancers that lack either estrogen or progesterone receptors are more likely to recur than those that are estrogen receptor–positive and progesterone receptor–positive. Tumors with a poor nuclear grade have a higher degree of recurrence than tumors with a good nuclear grade.

Tumors that overexpress HER-2/Neu protein (c-erbB2) or that have a mutated p53 gene have a poor prognosis. Tumors that overexpress HER-2/Neu protein are more likely to respond to higher doses of doxorubicin. (The presence of c-erbB2 is determined at the time of surgery and usually appears on the pathology report.) HER-2/Neu status (positive or negative) is usually considered in therapeutic decisions about the use of a doxorubicin- or taxane-containing regimen.

Surgical Management

The extent of the surgical intervention is determined by the clinical presentation and by the possibility of resecting the tumor with clean margins. The goal today is to preserve the breast, because there is no evidence that a mastectomy is more beneficial than lumpectomy plus radiation therapy. However, because of size or the multifocal or multicentric extent of disease, a mastectomy may be necessary to provide adequate tumor removal.

BREAST-PRESERVING PROCEDURES

INDICATIONS. Breast-preserving procedures are selected for stage I and stage II breast cancers. Such conservative surgical approaches may be appropriate, depending on the size of the primary tumor. Clients with small invasive cancers generally require a wide local excision under local or general anesthesia for partial mastectomy involving removal of the tumor plus a 1- to 2-cm margin of normal tissue (lumpectomy). A variation of the procedure is the quadrantectomy (removal of the quadrant of the breast in which the cancer is located).

Radiation therapy is begun once healing is confirmed, provided that the client is not receiving a doxorubicin- or taxane-containing regimen. If the individual is to receive either of these two chemotherapeutic agents plus radiation, then the radiation therapy commences 3 weeks after the last course of chemotherapy. If the client is to receive methotrexate (Mexate) and 5-fluorouracil (5-FU) with or without cyclophosphamide (Cytoxan), the radiotherapy may begin with the chemotherapy, may be sandwiched in after the third course and continue for 5 to 6 weeks, or may begin a few weeks after the last course of chemotherapy.

CONTRAINDICATIONS. Breast-conserving surgery is not performed when women cannot tolerate irradiation because of pregnancy or pre-existing rheumatic disorders, such as arthritis, lupus, and scleroderma. Other contraindications are extensive intraductal involvement requiring a wide incision, the presence of two cancers simultaneously in the same breast, diffuse malignant microcalcifications throughout the breast, and large, aggressive tumors. Client preference for a complete breast removal, client fear of radiation burns or other cancer development following irradiation, and inability to travel to and from a

radiation therapy facility are additional contraindications.

COMPLICATIONS. Although rare, infection, cellulitis, hematoma, and, less commonly, lymphedema may occur after the surgery.

OUTCOMES. After breast-conserving surgery with radiation therapy or chemotherapy or both, the the client will remain free of cancer and its recurrence.

MASTECTOMY

INDICATIONS. Mastectomy is the treatment of choice when the following apply:

- The tumor involves the nipple-areola complex
- The tumor is larger than 7 cm
- The tumor exhibits extensive intraductal disease involving multiple quadrants of the breast
- The woman cannot comply with daily radiation therapy

A *modified radical mastectomy* is an en bloc removal of the breast, axillary lymph nodes, and overlying skin, with the muscles left intact. Owing to more sophisticated diagnostic techniques that detect breast cancers of a smaller size and at an earlier stage, this procedure is done much less frequently now than 10 years ago. In a *total* or *simple* prophylactic *mastectomy,* used most commonly to prevent cancer in high-risk women, breast tissue and some skin are removed.

CONTRAINDICATIONS. Although not contraindicated for treatment of small tumors, mastectomy is usually not used for stage I and stage II tumors unless the client prefers this approach.

COMPLICATIONS. Possible complications of breast surgery include lymphedema, infection, seroma, hematoma, and cellulitis. Because clients are often discharged from the hospital within a few days of surgery, they should be taught to report any unusual manifestations early. Any evidence of infection, such as fever, chills, or an area of redness or inflammation along the incision line, should be reported to the physician. Any increase in drainage, foul odor, or separation at the incision site should be reported immediately.

OUTCOMES. After surgery and adjuvant chemotherapy or radiation therapy, the client will remain free of cancer and its recurrence. If a cancer-free state cannot be achieved, the focus is on promoting quality of life for the client. See Guide to Clinical Pathway.

AXILLARY DISSECTION

The role of axillary dissection is in transition. In women with clinically negative node disease and a primary tumor that is 1 to 2 cm in size, a node dissection is probably not necessary.[2] When more extensive surgery is required (e.g., if disease is multicentric or the primary tumor is larger than 5 cm), a mastectomy and axillary dissection are done using two incisions. Except when it is necessary to remove obvious tumor, the axillary dissection is not a therapeutic procedure but, rather, is a diagnostic procedure. The number of axillary nodes involved has in the past helped to determine the need for chemotherapy as well as whether more aggressive therapy is required. Information regarding nodal status is also valuable in determining prognosis and eligibility for research protocols and high-dose chemotherapy regimens.

Recognizing that most women with breast cancer benefit from adjuvant chemotherapy, hormonal therapy, or

GUIDE TO CLINICAL PATHWAY

Mastectomy

The woman having mastectomy expects to be hospitalized only 24 hours, and nursing care must therefore be very organized to meet all the goals. In addition to the usual postoperative care, the client is taught the care of her incisions and how to strip the drainage tubes, empty drains, and record the amount of drainage. The operative arm is elevated to reduce edema, and use of the arm is limited to allow for incisional healing. Because the client is going home in the morning, ambulation the night of surgery is important.

The CareMap focuses on education. Teach the client and family how to care for the incision, begin exercising the arm, and recognize the manifestations of infection. Some clients do not know their cancer diagnosis, yet the use of "Reach to Recovery" is discussed. Because of the fear of cancer, it is important to develop a therapeutic relationship with the client. Even after only a few hours of nursing care, the client may be comfortable enough to discuss fears and concerns with you. Needs may be modified upon discharge from the hospital, with additional referrals based on these fears or concerns.

The CareMap is reprinted with permission from Baptist Health System.

Helen Andrews, BSN, RN, *Care Manager, Alegent Health Bergan Mercy Medical Center, Omaha, Nebraska,* and
Linda R. Haddick, MSN, RN, *Clinical Nurse Specialist, Alegent Health Home Care & Hospice, Omaha, Nebraska*

---

both, some authorities claim that it is no longer necessary to determine the status of the axillary lymph nodes in clients with breast cancer. However, the lymph node status in clients with early breast cancer remains the most powerful predictor of recurrence and survival. The 5-year survival rate for clients with nodal metastasis is about 40% less than that for clients who are free of nodal disease. Further, nearly a third of clients with clinically negative nodes are found to have pathologically involved nodes. Information obtained from pathologic examination of axillary lymph nodes frequently changes the adjuvant therapy plan for women with nonpalpable axillary lymph nodes.[16]

In some cases, axillary node dissection is not necessary because its findings would not affect the choice of therapy. For example, a client presenting with a large primary cancer or evidence of metastatic disease that requires extensive surgery does not need an axillary dissection, nor does a client undergoing mastectomy for a tumor greater than 5 cm or a client in whom the surgical margins are positive for residual tumor. In both of these cases, the risk of local recurrence is sufficiently high to warrant the use of post-mastectomy radiotherapy to the chest wall and supraclavicular areas. Women who have four or more positive axillary lymph nodes also are at increased risk for local recurrence; chest wall and supraclavicular radiotherapy is usually considered even though it is not certain that prophylactic chest wall radiotherapy would improve overall survival.

SENTINEL NODE BIOPSY

Nodal assessment may be conducted using the sentinel node biopsy, a diagnostic test to determine the status of regional lymph nodes. The sentinel node is the first lymph node to receive lymphatic drainage from a tumor. The node can be detected by injection of a blue dye or radioactive colloid around the primary tumor, which travels to and identifies the first draining (sentinel) node. The sentinel lymph node can reveal whether there are lymphatic metastases, making extensive axillary dissection obsolete.[36]

The procedure is technically challenging. Although it is still undergoing clinical investigation, the possibility that this procedure may replace axillary dissection and reduce the potential for lymphedema is encouraging.[33]

Nursing Management of the Surgical Client

PREOPERATIVE CARE

ASSESSMENT

The preoperative time, before the biopsy for breast cancer and before a woman knows whether she has cancer in her breast or not, is extremely stressful, constituting a psychological emergency. To put off the biopsy for more than just a few days is often impossible for the woman once a cancer is suspected. Once the diagnosis is established, the woman can return to the routines of her life, or if the biopsy result is positive, she can begin to mobilize her resources to determine the next step. Initially, the woman may be in shock and perhaps even denial, because her decision to undergo the biopsy procedure may have been based largely on her recognition that 8 out of 10 breast masses are benign. A few days are often needed for her to recover from the diagnosis of cancer before beginning the consultation process.

Most women do not sign a consent for an immediate surgical resection or mastectomy upon evidence of a positive biopsy result. Generally, women are given ample time to evaluate the options for management once the diagnosis is confirmed. Most authorities recommend that definitive surgery be performed within 2 weeks of the biopsy, but some women need more time to sort through the copious literature before deciding on a course of treatment. Physicians are required to present the risks and benefits of each of the numerous treatment options for breast cancer and to allow the woman to choose her course of treatment. The options include (1) mastectomy alone, (2) mastectomy with immediate reconstruction, and (3) breast-preserving treatment. Because there is no absolute right answer for many women, each option must be fully considered. Every woman with breast cancer deserves time to deliberate and to participate actively in the decision-making process. Because the possibilities for treatment may be overwhelming, it is appropriate to refer the woman to a comprehensive breast center in which all disciplines are available to address her concerns regarding therapy.

The plan for treatment, which may include surgery, radiation therapy, chemotherapy, hormone therapy, and/or biologic immunomodulation therapy, is laid out before treatment is begun. In addition, clients should be offered a research protocol if there is one for which they are eligible. Be familiar with these multimodality protocols

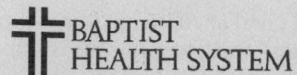

BAPTIST
HEALTH SYSTEM

MASTECTOMY CAREMAP

(Addressograph)

	Pre-Admit/Pre-Op Date: _____	INITIAL Met	Not Met	Day of Surgery Date: _____	INITIAL Met	Not Met
General Safety:	Home activity			Bed rails up x 2 Fall precautions Call light within reach Post sign in room: **NO BP/IV IN R/L ARM**		
Activity	Ad Lib			1. OOB/BRP with assistance 2. Limited use of arm on affected side		
	Goal:			**Goal:** Tolerates ambulation		
Dietary: Consult Date/Time Completed _____	NPO at MN day prior to surgery			1. Clear liquid post-op 2. Reg/Home diet for dinner		
	Goal: Verbalizes understanding of NPO after MN			**Goal:** Tolerates > 50% of diet		
Respiratory: Consult Date/Time Completed _____	Incentive Spirometer Instruction **Goal:** Pt. verbalizes and is able to demonstrate use of Incentive Spirometer			Incentive Spirometer q2H WA **Goal:** Lungs clear to auscultation		
Rehab: Consult Date/Time Completed _____	Goal:			Goal:		
Discharge Planning: Consult Date/Time Completed _____	1. Assess for D/C needs and support system 2. SWS for HHC if indicated 3. Notify Case Management Dept. for anticipated D/C delays			1. SWS for HHC if indicated 2. Notify Case Mgmt Dept. for anticipated D/C delays		
	Goal: Potential D/C needs identified			**Goal:** Potential D/C needs identified		
Nursing: Consult Date/Time Completed _____	1. Pre-op & Post-op Instructions 2. Consult Anesthesia for pre-op assessment and instruction 3. Have pt. sign appropriate consents 4. Notify Reach to Recovery (American Cancer Society) 5. SCD Hose (Order for day of surgery) if ordered 6. Have pt. view Mastectomy Video 7. Provide written handouts for pre-op/post-op instruction 8. Instruct in technique of emptying, measuring and recording JP drainage 9. Review hospital plan of care with patient and family 10. Review Patient/Family CareMap and give copy to patient 11. Evaluate pre-op emotional status regarding surgery			1. Give pt. Mastectomy Information Bag & review contents with pt./family 2. Show Mastectomy Video if not viewed in PAT 3. No BP/IV in affected arm 4. Empty and record JP drainage 5. Keep drains stripped and compressed 6. Keep affected arm up on pillow 7. Notify MD for excessive JP drainage 8. Apply SCD Hose while in bed (if ordered pre-op). D/C when up ambulating 9. Encourage to Turn, Cough & Deep Breathe q 2 H while in bed 10. Review expectations of care progress with pt./family		
	Goal: Pt./Family verbalizes understanding of pre-op & post-op care			**Goal:** Pt./Family verbalizes understanding of drain and arm care **Goal:** No lymphadema		
Tests:	Labs as ordered					
	Goal: MD notified of any abnormal results			Goal:		
Other:				Consult Chaplain if needed		
	Goal:			**Goal:** Pt. able to verbalize fears and concerns regarding surgery		

MASTECTOMY CAREMAP

G-99-5137-2 PG REV. 8/17/99

for treating breast cancer. It is an enormous challenge to help clients understand and feel confident in their decisions regarding therapy. To be knowledgeable about the client's options for therapy, make every effort to be present for the initial discussion between the physicians and the client and family. Then clarify any misconceptions the client and family members may have, and reinforce what they have been told regarding the therapy.

DIAGNOSIS, OUTCOMES, INTERVENTIONS

Knowledge Deficit. The nursing diagnosis may be expressed as *Knowledge Deficit related to inexperience*

BAPTIST HEALTH SYSTEM

MASTECTOMY CAREMAP

(Addressograph)

	Post-Op Day 1 (D/C Day) Date: _____	INITIAL Met	Not Met	Date: _____	INITIAL Met	Not Met
General Safety:	Bed rails up x 2 Fall precautions Call light within reach Post sign in room: **NO BP/IV IN R/L ARM**			Bed rails up x 2 Fall precautions Call light within reach Post sign in room: **NO BP/IV IN R/L ARM**		
Activity	1. Up ad lib 2. Limited use of affected arm (Do not raise arm above shoulder level					
	Goal: Tolerates ambulation **Goal:** Verbalizes understanding of limited use of affected arm	___	___	**Goal:**	___	___
Dietary: Consult Date/Time Completed _____	Regular or Home diet					
	Goal: Tolerates > 50% of diet	___	___	**Goal:**	___	___
Respiratory: Consult Date/Time Completed _____	Incentive Spirometer q 2-4 WA					
	Goal: Lungs clear to ausculatation	___	___	**Goal:**	___	___
Rehab: Consult Date/Time Completed _____						
	Goal:	___	___	**Goal:**	___	___
Discharge Planning: Consult Date/Time Completed _____	1. Assess for D/C needs and support system 2. SWS for HHC if indicated 3. Notify Case Management Dept. for anticipated D/C delays					
	Goal: Potential D/C needs identified	___	___	**Goal:**	___	___
Nursing: Consult Date/Time Completed _____	1. Notify Reach to Recovery if not done pre-op 2. Ensure pt. has Mastectomy Information Bag and Mastectomy Video 3. Instruct pt./caregiver in emptying, measuring & recording JP drainage 4. Review Mastectomy Discharge Instructions and give copy to pt. 5. No BP/IV in affected arm 6. Empty & record JP drainage & keep drains stripped and compressed 7. Notify MD for excessive drainage 8. Keep affected arm up on pillow					
	Goal: Pt. has viewed and has copy of Mastectomy Video **Goal:** Pt. has received Mastectomy Information Bag **Goal:** Pt./Caregiver demonstrates ability to empty, measure and record JP drainage **Goal:** Pt. verbalizes understanding & has copy of Mastectomy Discharge Instructions **Goal:** Pt. verbalizes understanding of bringing drainage record to MD on first post-op visit **Goal:** Pt. has prescription for pain meds prior to discharge **Goal:** Pt. verbalizes understanding of when to follow-up with MD **Goal:** Pt./Caregiver verbalizes understanding of rehab exercises & has copy of instructions **Goal:** Pt./Caregiver verbalizes understanding of signs & symptoms to report to MD **Goal:** Pt. has been contacted or visited by Reach to Recovery Volunteer prior to discharge	___ ___ ___ ___ ___ ___ ___ ___ ___ ___	___ ___ ___ ___ ___ ___ ___ ___ ___ ___	**Goal:**	___	___
Tests:	Labs as ordered					
	Goal: MD notified of any abnormal results	___	___	**Goal:**	___	___
Other:						
	Goal:	___	___	**Goal:**	___	___

MASTECTOMY CAREMAP

G-99-5137-3 PG REV. 8/17/99

and new information regarding available options for treatment.

Outcomes. The client will understand the available treatment options, as evidenced by her questions and statements concerning options and her ability to explain her choice.

Interventions

Explain Options. The woman should receive information about recommendations and treatment options before surgery or treatment is initiated. The nurse can help women understand treatment options.[2, 9, 35]

Initiate Teaching Plan. Because the typical hospital

stay for a modified radical mastectomy or lumpectomy and axillary node dissection surgery is 1 to 3 days, preoperative teaching is done on an outpatient basis, usually in the physician's office. Give clients written instructions regarding postoperative care, including wound care and hand and arm care.

Nursing assessment provides data about knowledge deficits for use in formulating a teaching plan. This plan includes preoperative activities, explanations of surgery, postoperative care, discharge planning, and a discussion of any limitations the woman may have as a result of surgery. Encourage the woman to question her physicians about lymph node dissection versus lymph node sampling. Alert her to the possibility of radiation therapy modification in order to preserve the lymphatics and minimize underlying tissue scarring.[29, 41] Because the woman's anxiety level may be so high that she cannot remember new information, it is important to provide written as well as oral instructions. Give instructions in the presence of a family member. Because clients are discharged early postoperatively, they also need emergency phone numbers and instructions regarding whom to call if they have a question or a problem after discharge. Evaluate the client's and family members' learning, and repeat information as often as is necessary.

Risk for Ineffective Individual Coping and Risk for Ineffective Family Coping.
The nursing diagnosis may be expressed as *Ineffective Individual Coping and Ineffective Family Coping related to diagnosis of cancer and surgical changes in breast.*

Outcomes. The client will cope with the diagnosis of cancer and surgical changes in the breast, as evidenced by her statement of acceptance and decisions about treatment. Family members will also cope effectively, as evidenced by support given to the client.

Interventions. Preoperatively or before any treatment, assess the client's and significant others' coping ability and concerns. Do not rush the assessment. Identify the coping mechanisms usually used by the client and her significant others. Are there any potentially disabling coping patterns? Use this information as the basis of support. The woman may fear pain, mutilation, death, loss of control, and the hospital environment. Use these findings to establish a plan of care to help the client use positive, growth-producing coping and to avoid disabling coping.[9, 11]

EVALUATION

For a positive outcome, the client will be adequately prepared for surgery and its outcomes. Recovery from the surgical procedure is usually uncomplicated. Delayed grieving, even for months following mastectomy, is not uncommon, because intellectually the woman knows the surgery is necessary and because her grief is overshadowed at first by fear of dying.

POSTOPERATIVE CARE
ASSESSMENT

Assess the client's psychological reaction to the surgery. Also, inspect the wound and drains, assess for the presence of clinical manifestations of infection and pain, and perform routine postoperative assessments as discussed in Chapter 15.

DIAGNOSIS, OUTCOMES, INTERVENTIONS

Body Image Disturbance. A nursing diagnosis of *Body Image Disturbance related to impending changes in breast and sexuality* may be appropriate.

Outcomes. The client will begin to exhibit her presurgical or baseline positive body image, as evidenced by wearing usual make-up and using her own nightgown or other feminine attire after surgery.

Interventions

Initiate Referral. Because the hospital stay is usually only 1 to 3 days, there may be little opportunity for the woman to express her usual feelings regarding her femininity and the manner in which she might display a positive adaptation to her surgery. In this case, it is appropriate merely to ask the woman if she feels that she or family members might benefit from a consultation with the psycho-oncologist, social worker, or sex therapist. Ask if she would like to talk to someone who has had a similar surgical procedure, possibly someone from the American Cancer Society's Reach for Recovery program. (See the Case Study: Breast Cancer with Mastectomy.)

Assess Coping Strategies. Women who undergo surgery for breast cancer experience a sense of loss—changes in life routines, social interactions, self-concept, and body image—and fear of death. Recovery during the postoperative period after mastectomy requires a great deal of energy. Fatigue is a persistent complaint for 6 months or more after surgery. A client's usual coping strategies may not be effective. Not everyone perceives or handles stress in the same way. Displacement, projection, denial, hope, prayer, meditation, stoicism, fatalism, and any combination of these reactions may be used as coping mechanisms. Clients who have surgically lost a breast may adapt in the same way as they would to any loss.

Encourage Self-Care Activities. Effective postoperative care is essential for successful psychosocial and physical rehabilitation. During the 1- to 3-day hospital stay, the focus of nursing care is on recovery from surgery and anesthesia as well as on discharge planning for self-care postoperative management. The client's self-image improves with self-care activities.

Explain Possible Body Image Concerns After Discharge. The full impact of losing a breast or having breast cancer may not be felt until a while after the client goes home. Many women are surprised by events such as the amount of pain and discomfort, marked fatigue, slow incision healing, and arm swelling. Ordinary motions, such as shifting to a comfortable position in bed, may be difficult and painful. As time passes, however, the woman and her significant others reorganize and restructure their lives. During this time, the woman resumes her role in society. Important changes in this role may be necessary. Individual women cope differently; feelings of sexual inadequacy, poor body image, and loss of a sense of femininity are common. Because body image is further altered by weight gain and alopecia if the woman is undergoing chemotherapy, she should be encouraged to purchase a wig and other hair coverings prior to hair loss. Fatigue, decreased libido, and periods of depression are common in women receiving chemotherapy and radiation therapy.

Discuss Strategies to Improve Body Image. Gradually the woman will decide whether to conceal her incision from significant others or let it be seen. The incision may be camouflaged for a woman by an appropriately fitted brassiere or a special bathing suit or evening dress, but doubts and fears about her attractiveness may affect even the most secure woman. You can offer understanding and facilitate communication between the client and significant others. The woman may wish to talk with other breast cancer survivors who have faced similar problems due to breast cancer. Breast cancer support groups may also be beneficial, but, they should be composed of women in similar stages of illness. A woman who is undergoing adjuvant therapy for curative breast cancer, for example, may be overwhelmed and frightened by the discussions and concerns of women with advanced metastatic breast cancer.

Risk for Impaired Skin Integrity. The nursing diagnosis may be expressed as *Risk for Impaired Skin Integrity related to surgery or radiation therapy.*

Outcomes. The client will remain free of impairment in skin integrity after surgery or radiation therapy, as evidenced by healing skin without redness, infection, hematoma formation, or breakdown.

Interventions

Provide and Explain Dressing and Drain Care. Postoperatively, a pressure dressing is usually used initially. Explain that a drain, connected to gentle suction, prevents blood or serum collection in the operative space after a modified radical mastectomy or axillary node dissection. Instruct the woman about emptying the drain and recording the amount of drainage. Advise her to notify the physician if the drain becomes plugged or dislodged or shows any sign of infection or if frank bleeding develops.

When changing the dressing, gently encourage the woman to look at the incision. Seeing the incision for the first time is often difficult, but the nurse's matter-of-fact approach can help. In future dressing changes, teach methods of cleaning the incision at home and of watching for manifestations of infection.

Prevent Skin Complications Following Radiation Therapy. During radiation therapy, scaling, flaking, dryness, itching, erythema, hair loss, rash, or dry desquamation of the involved skin may occur. Careful treatment of the skin is important in minimizing the skin effects of radiation therapy. Instruct women not to wash the area with soap but to rinse it with water only. No lotion or powder is to be put on the skin that overlies the radiation port. If the area under the arm becomes reddened because of friction, moisture, or radiation damage, place a soft, clean gauze pad between skinfolds to prevent skin breakdown.

Risk for Injury. The nursing diagnosis may be expressed as *Risk for Injury related to increased risk of infection and lymphedema secondary to axillary node dissection.*

Outcomes. The client will not experience injury, as evidenced by absence of infection or lymphedema.

Interventions

Arm edema (e.g., lymphedema) occurs less commonly today owing to the performance of less extensive mastectomy procedures and less extensive axillary dissection. Lymphedema results from insufficient transport of water and protein from the skin and subcutaneous tissue because of an inadequate development or eradication of lymphatic vessels. Lymphedema following axillary dissection has been reported in as many as 70% of cases, although probably a more accurate estimate of the average occurrence of lymphedema as a significant consequence of local therapy for breast cancer is 20% in the United States and Europe.[2] Clearly, the major risk for lymphedema exists when complete axillary dissection with stripping of the axillary vein and nodal irradiation is combined with mastectomy.

Older age, obesity, and lifting of heavy objects such as grocery bags and suitcases are also thought to increase the risk of lymphedema. Arm edema, stiffness, pain, and numbness have been reported in 40% to 50% of clients approximately 1 month after beginning radiation therapy to the axilla.[32] Lymphedema occurring years after surgery or radiation therapy is generally the result of infection, inflammation, or recurrent tumor.

Prevent Lymphedema. In the early postoperative period, encourage arm exercises, described in the Client Education Guide: Postmastectomy Exercises; elevate the arm on a pillow so that the elbow is level with the heart and the hand rests just higher than the elbow. The goal is to promote lymphatic drainage and prevent infection.

Administer Antibiotics for Infection. If a woman complains of redness, swelling, and a generalized area of warmth on the affected arm with or without fever, she should be examined for possible infection in the hand or arm. If an infection is present, the woman may need to be admitted to the hospital for intravenous antibiotics to treat the infection. Such infections can occur from a slight cut on the hand, and though they may seem innocuous, they pose a serious threat to these clients.

Minimize Lymphedema. Wearing an elastic bandage or a custom-fitted pressure-gradient elastic sleeve may be helpful in the months following surgery if lymphedema is present. Some women feel that wearing a sleeve while they are on an airplane minimizes swelling due to pressure changes in the airplane, although no studies have confirmed the efficacy of this practice.

Emphasize that it is important to prevent lymphedema. Once lymphedema occurs, it is more likely to occur again and be progressive. This is because the tissue, like a balloon, is a potential space that, once expanded, will expand again to that size and beyond at the least provocation.

Available treatments include application of compression garments, intermittent pneumatic compression, and massage by a trained physiotherapist.[45] Clients can obtain more information from the National Breast Cancer Coalition, the International Society of Lymphology, and the Oncology Nursing Society.

EVALUATION

The client who has undergone breast surgery for cancer will be discharged from the hospital 24 to 72 hours postoperatively. The surgical wounds may be healed within 4 weeks. Regaining complete use of the affected arm and shoulder may take as long as 6 weeks to several months, depending on the extent of the surgical procedure, rate of healing, compliance with exercises, and the degree of postoperative complications.

Breast Cancer with Mastectomy

Samantha Guern is a 33-year-old African American who presents to a free health care clinic with complaints of a painless rash on her left breast. She indicates that she does not perform breast self-examination and has not noticed any pain or tenderness in either breast. A mammogram is ordered, and Samantha is informed that a follow-up ultrasound examination and biopsy of the lump may be necessary. Samantha is tearful and asks: "How will I pay for these tests? What if you find something awful?!" Consider appropriate responses that the nurse might make.

The mammogram reveals a 3.5-cm solid lesion in the left breast. A follow-up ultrasound examination confirms that this is a solid lesion. A fine-needle aspiration of the lesion is performed, and the pathology report confirms the diagnosis of poorly differentiated breast cancer. A chest radiograph and bone scan are subsequently ordered. Results indicate no gross indications of metastasis at this time.

Samantha is referred to an oncologist to receive consultation about her treatment options. Because Samantha's lesion is a stage III carcinoma, she is advised to consider a modified radical mastectomy with a possible stem cell transplant procedure after the mastectomy. Samantha also meets with a social worker to determine whether there are any financial or other entitlements for which she would be eligible. In addition, the social worker assists Samantha in drafting a medical power of attorney that would provide the father of her children with authority to make decisions for her if necessary. Samantha is relieved to find that she qualifies for Medicaid.

Samantha's mastectomy is scheduled for the following day. Consider the behaviors that Samantha would exhibit that indicate she has been properly educated and prepared for the procedure.

Nursing History

Samantha is alert and cooperative. Samantha reports that she works full-time for a small local business that does not offer health benefits and that she has three school-aged children. Samantha is not married and mentions that occasionally the father of her three children stays at their house. She denies any known health problems, stating, "When you're a single parent and don't have health insurance, you can't afford to be sick." She says she has no allergies. Samantha indicates that she drinks iced tea and caffeinated sodas but states that she does not use alcohol, tobacco, or any other controlled substances. Samantha states that one of her mother's sisters had breast cancer and that she is not aware of any other cancer history in her family. Samantha's current method of birth control is a Depo-Provera injection, which she receives at the clinic every 3 months. Consider factors that place Samantha at risk for breast cancer.

Nursing Preoperative Physical Assessment

Height: 5'8" Weight 130 lb (59.1 kg)
Vital Signs: BP 140/90, TPR 98.6, 84, 22
LOC: Alert and cooperative
EENT: WNL

Cardiac: Heart tones are regular. S_1 and S_2 are readily audible with no murmurs or rubs noted; *nontender walnut-sized lump noted in upper outer quadrant of left breast during auscultation of heart tones.*
Pulmonary: Lung sounds are clear bilaterally.
Abdominal: Abdomen is flat and nontender with normal, active bowel tones.
Genitourinary: Deferred
Peripheral pulses: 2/2, without edema

Samantha returns to the nursing unit from the recovery room. Her initial postoperative treatment orders include the following:

Meds: Cefazolin 1 gm IVPB every 6 hours
Morphine by PCA pump with basal rate of 1 mg per hour and 1 mg available per patient demand with a 15-minute lockout; no 4-hour limit is specified
Compazine 25-mg suppository PR every 6 hours as needed for nausea
Percocet 1 or 2 tabs every 4 to 6 hours as needed for less severe pain
D_5/½NS with 20 mEq KCl at 150 ml/hr
Clear liquids this evening progressing to DAT
Routine postoperative vital signs
Dangle patient this PM and to chair as tolerated in AM
No blood pressures, IV lines, or venous laboratory draws in patient's left arm
Call physician for urine output of less than 1 ml/kg/hr
Empty and record drain outputs every 4 hours
Reinforce dressings as needed

Samantha progresses satisfactorily and is scheduled for hospital discharge tomorrow. The surgical drains will be left in place after discharge.

Discharge Criteria

Average LOS: 2.1 days without complications, 2.9 days with complications
Initiate "Reach to Recovery" referral. What other community referrals would you make? Why?
Initiate instructions for home care and follow-up appointments with surgeon and oncologist.

Questions to Be Considered

1. A home health nurse is scheduled to visit Samantha to empty the surgical drains and to assess her ability to perform this procedure herself. What information should be taught and what behaviors might Samantha display that would indicate her ability or inability to empty her own drains?

2. Discuss the usual postoperative treatment course for a client with a stage III carcinoma considering a stem cell transplant procedure. Compare these treatment options with those for a client with a stage I or II carcinoma. What are the risks and benefits of each treatment option? What side effects might be expected by the client?

3. Three weeks postoperatively, Samantha returns to the clinic and reports that she is concerned about the recurrent swelling in her left arm and hand. Explain the physiologic basis for the swelling. What instructions should the nurse give Samantha to aid in reducing this problem?
4. Compare and contrast bone marrow transplantation and stem cell transplantation in the treatment of malignant breast cancer. What are the risks and benefits of transplant procedures for breast cancer clients?
5. Impaired body image is a concern for mastectomy clients. Outline the nursing interventions that could be

used to assist the client to improve her body image. What behaviors would indicate that a client is successfully coping with her altered body image? Discuss the options that Samantha would have, if she elected to have breast reconstruction completed.

BP, blood pressure; D₅, 5% dextrose; DAT, diet as tolerated; EENT, eye-ear-nose-throat; IV, intravenous; IVPB, intravenous-piggyback; KCl, potassium chloride; LOC, level of consciousness; LOS, length of stay; NS, normal saline; PCA, patient-controlled analgesia; PR, per rectum (rectally); TPR, temperature-pulse-respirations; WNL, within normal limits.

CLIENT EDUCATION GUIDE

POSTMASTECTOMY EXERCISES:

When to Begin	Purpose	Exercises: Perform Exercises 5–10 Times Each, Three Times a Day
Postoperative days 1–5	Prevent and/or reduce swelling	▪ Position arm against your side in a relaxed position. Elbow should be level with your heart, and the wrist just above the elbow when resting. ▪ Rotate wrist in a circular fashion. ▪ Touch fingers to shoulder and extend arm fully.
After drains are removed	Promote muscle movement without stretching	▪ While standing, brace yourself with your other arm and bend over slightly, allowing your affected arm to hang freely. Swing the arm in small circles and gradually increase in size. Make 10 circles—rest—repeat in the opposite direction. ▪ Swing arm forward and back as far as you can without pulling on the incision. ▪ While standing, bend over slightly and swing arms across the chest in each direction. ▪ While sitting in a chair, rest both arms at your side. Shrug both shoulders, then relax. ▪ While sitting or standing, pull shoulders back, bring the shoulder blades together.
After sutures are removed	To stretch and regain full range of motion. To gain mobility of your shoulder, you must move it in *all* directions, several times a day	▪ While lying in bed with arm extended, raise arm over your head and extend backwards. ▪ While lying in bed, grasp a cane or short pole with both hands across your lap. Extend arms straight up and over your head and return. ▪ Repeat, rotating the cane clockwise and then counterclockwise while over your head. ▪ While standing, extend arm straight over your head and down. ▪ Extend your elbow out from your side at a 90° angle—hold it for 10 seconds—relax. ▪ Extend your arm straight out from your side even with your shoulder—extend arm straight up toward the ceiling. ▪ Stand at arm's length facing a wall. Extend arms so your fingertips touch the wall. Creep fingers up the side of the wall, stepping forward as necessary. Repeat the procedure going down the wall—keep arms extended. ▪ Stand sideways to the wall. Extend arm out so fingers touch the wall. Creep up the wall a little more each day. ▪ Use hand and arm normally.
After 6 weeks	To strengthen arm and shoulder and to regain total use of arm and shoulder	▪ Begin water aerobics. ▪ Begin overall fitness program. ▪ Begin aerobics, Jazzercise, or other resistive exercises. ▪ Avoid using weights, as these may increase arm edema and subsequent swelling.

■ **Self-Care**

To promote self-care, the client will need to learn about postoperative arm exercises, postoperative care, and care of the breast prosthesis. A referral to Reach for Recovery may also be helpful.

TEACH ARM EXERCISES

In the early postoperative period (days 1 and 2), encourage the client to focus on the elbow, wrist, and hand of the affected side. The client performs active elbow flexion and extension, gently squeezes a soft rubber ball, and does deep breathing to facilitate lymph flow. Shoulder shrugs and active range of motion, including flexion and abduction, can be added on the second postoperative day. Encourage self-care activities (e.g., feeding, combing hair, washing face) and other activities that use the arm, with care taken not to abduct the arm or to raise the arm or elbow above shoulder height until the drains are removed.

Approximately 10 days after surgery, the client can begin active assisted range of motion exercises (see Client Education Guide: Postmastectomy Exercises). Tell the client to do these exercises at least twice a day as tolerated. Provide pain medication 30 minutes before exercises to permit the client to perform exercises without pain. Women who do not carry out these exercises as instructed are at greater risk for lymphedema and loss of shoulder joint mobility. (Arrangements for a physical therapist to assist with range of motion and strengthening exercises may need to be made at the same time surgery is planned because of the shortened hospital stay.) Always provide written and oral instructions about arm precautions after axillary node dissection, as shown in the Client Education Guide for arm care.

REFER TO REACH FOR RECOVERY

The Reach for Recovery program of the American Cancer Society is a rehabilitation program for breast cancer survivors, specifically those who have had breast surgery. This program is designed to help women meet common psychosocial, physical, and cosmetic needs. With authorization of the physician and the client's permission, volunteers from this program visit the hospital or the home and give the woman information and help, including:

1. A kit, ball, book, rope, and temporary soft cotton prosthesis for women who have had a mastectomy
2. Instruction sheet for and demonstration of postoperative axillary node dissection exercises
3. Discussion of brassiere comfort, various breast prostheses, clothing adjustments, and personal problems as appropriate

PROVIDE BREAST PROSTHESIS

Women who have had a mastectomy may wear a temporary lightweight prosthesis immediately after the sutures and drains are removed. This may facilitate adjustment to the loss of the breast. A soft cotton breast form may be supplied by the Reach for Recovery visitor; cotton padding inserted into a pocket sewn into a lightweight brassiere is also a good temporary substitute. A permanent prosthesis should not be purchased until the wound has healed completely because the contours of the incision site may change. Cocoa butter may be rubbed into the

---

CLIENT EDUCATION GUIDE

Arm Care After Axillary Lymph Node Dissection

Because you have had an axillary node dissection, the affected arm may swell and is less able to fight infection. Use your arm normally, following these recommendations.

Avoid burns while cooking or smoking.
Wear a long-length oven mitt.
Do not reach into a hot oven with this arm.
Do not hold a cigarette in the affected hand.
Avoid sunburn and insect bites.
Wear long-sleeved shirts and gloves.
Use sunscreen.
Use insect repellent to avoid bites and stings.
Avoid cuts, pinpricks, and scratches.
Wear gloves when gardening.
Do not work near thorny plants or dig with your hands.
Use a thimble when sewing.
Use an electric razor with a narrow head for underarm shaving to reduce the risk of nicks or scratches.
Never cut or pick at cuticles; use hand cream or lotion.
Wash cuts promptly; treat them with antibacterial medication and cover them with sterile dressing, and check often for redness, soreness, pus, or other manifestations of infection.
Avoid strong detergents, harsh chemicals, and abrasive compounds.
Wear protective gloves while doing dishes and cleaning.
Avoid other trauma.
Have all injections, vaccinations, blood samples, and blood pressure tests done on the other arm whenever possible.
Wear a medical identification tag that cautions against test injections or blood pressure readings on the affected arm.
Carry your handbag and other heavy objects on the other arm.
Wear watch or jewelry loosely, if at all, on the operated arm.
Avoid elastic cuffs on blouses and nightgowns.
Use a lanolin hand cream a few times each day.
Wear an elastic sleeve if recommended by your physician.
Contact your physician if the arm or hand becomes red, is swollen, or feels hot; in the meantime, try to keep your arm over your head and periodically pump your fist.

Adapted from National Cancer Institute. (1987). *After breast cancer: A guide to follow-up care* (NIH Publication No. 87–2400). Washington, DC: Author.

---

incision once healing has occurred to help soften the scar and prevent scar contracture.

Because breast prostheses are expensive and not very comfortable, many women choose breast reconstruction. If a woman chooses to have a prosthesis, even temporarily while considering breast reconstruction, she should choose one that is appropriate for her. A breast prosthesis may be purchased in foundation departments in most large stores or at medical-surgical supply stores that sell durable medical equipment. Most of these stores have experienced sales associates to help women obtain the proper fit. Most private and government insurance plans pay for at least the first breast prosthesis and brassiere, provided that a written prescription from the physician accompanies the receipt. Many plans also pay for yearly replacements.

■ BREAST RECONSTRUCTION

Many women have feelings of loss, depression, and alterations in body image after mastectomy. Breast reconstruction is an accepted component of the treatment plan. In the 1990s, improvements were made to surgical prostheses and surgical techniques, helping women become more confident in their choice to have reconstructive surgery and retain their self-confidence and body image, thereby enhancing their quality of life. The goal for clients having reconstructive surgery is to "feel whole again." This includes appearing "normal" in a bathing suit as well as in the nude.

The only contraindications to breast reconstruction are the client's need for chest wall irradiation and the physical inability to withstand additional surgery due to a co-morbid condition. Breast reconstruction is not contraindicated by a woman's age, her need for adjuvant chemotherapy, a poor prognosis, or even the presence of metastatic disease. The timing of the breast reconstruction may be immediate (at the time of the mastectomy) or delayed, even until years after mastectomy. When adjuvant chemotherapy is planned, the surgeon may prefer to wait until the chemotherapy is completed to begin reconstructing the breast.

Several surgical techniques can be used to reconstruct the breast mound and nipple-areola complex. The choice of technique is based upon the client's wishes, the amount of tissue available, and whether the woman has had radiation therapy in the past. The simplest method of reconstruction involves the insertion of an implant into a pocket of skin purposely left by the surgeon. This approach is best for women with small or moderate-size breasts, in whom the implant is of a size similar to the remaining breast. Other methods of reconstruction include the following.

TISSUE EXPANDERS

A tissue expander is a deflated silicone envelope that is inserted under the chest muscles and expanded slowly over 6 to 8 weeks by adding 60 to 200 ml of saline per week via a remote percutaneous injection port. When the skin overlying the breast mound is sufficiently overinflated to accommodate the implant comfortably, the expander is removed and the implant is inserted. Many times the expanded implant is expanded to become the permanent implant.

TRANSVERSE RECTUS ABDOMINIS MUSCLE FLAP

The transverse rectus abdominis muscle (TRAM) flap procedure is commonly referred to as the "tummy tuck." A low transverse elliptical incision is made, and abdominal muscle and fat are tunneled under the abdominal skin to the mastectomy site. Tissue viability and perfusion are retained by the superior epigastric vessel. The tissue can also be transferred as a free flap. The donor site in the abdomen is closed as for a modified abdominoplasty (Fig. 40-4). Contraindications to the TRAM flap are the presence of abdominal scars and inadequate abdominal tissue.

LATISSIMUS DORSI MUSCLE FLAP

The latissimus dorsi muscle, a large fan-shaped muscle beneath the scapula, is used when inadequate skin is available at the mastectomy site. It is considered an expendable muscle because alternative muscle groups are able to adduct the humerus and rotate the shoulder posteriorly. An ellipse of skin along with the latissimus dorsi muscle is tunneled through the axilla and rotated onto the mastectomy site. The viability of the tissue is maintained through the thoracodorsal vessels (Fig. 40-5).

FIGURE 40-4 Breast reconstruction using transverse rectus abdominis myocutaneous flaps. *A,* Preoperative appearance. *B,* Postoperative appearance.

FIGURE 40–5 An ideal result of reconstructive surgery using a latissimus dorsi myocutaneous flap and an implant. *A,* Preoperative appearance. *B,* Postoperative appearance. A subpectoral implant is used in the right breast for symmetry.

GLUTEAL MUSCLE FREE FLAPS

A much less common form of breast construction involves the use of the gluteus muscle. The muscle and overlying skin are lifted from their bed and connected to the chest wall using an operating microscope.

NIPPLE-AREOLA RECONSTRUCTION

Some women elect also to have the nipple-areola reconstructed. To achieve symmetry, nipple reconstruction should be delayed for several months following breast reconstruction. During the healing process, the contour of the reconstructed breast may change as the incisions heal and edema subsides. Areola can be reconstructed with a tattoo or by nipple sharing. The dark tissue of the areola is most commonly reconstructed by tattooing. Nipple projection is constructed with a skate flap (Fig. 40–6). Many years ago, the nipple was removed from the breast before amputation and stored ("banked") on the inner thigh. This procedure is no longer performed because of the risk of cancer spread.

◼ Nursing Management of the Client with Breast Reconstruction

PREOPERATIVE CARE

Preoperatively, the nurse reinforces the physician's instructions regarding the goals of reconstruction and any postoperative care needs. It is important that the client have realistic expectations of the outcome of the surgery. The client may be shown pictures of reconstructed breasts to familiarize her with what can be achieved. The client may express anger, disbelief, and fear related to the surgery, especially if the reconstruction is being combined with a mastectomy for a known carcinoma. Many women will at the same time express relief that the cancer surgery is being done and the cancer is being removed. Some will find comfort in discussing their feelings of disbelief at this time. Periods of depression are normal.

Encourage clients to express their feelings and fears with family members and to seek assistance from the psycho-oncology service or chaplain should this be appropriate. Assess risks for anesthesia-related problems and operative blood loss prior to surgery. Advise any client who smokes cigarettes to stop, because smoking compromises flap and skin circulation.

POSTOPERATIVE CARE

In addition to providing the postoperative nursing care required by any person having surgery, after reconstructive breast surgery you will assess the flap or breast area for color, temperature, and capillary refill. If any area appears dusky and congested with blood, the flap may be suffering from venous obstruction. A flap that is pale is not receiving blood and may be experiencing arterial constriction. Whenever circulation or perfusion is in question, notify the physician immediately. The success of this surgical procedure is directly dependent on astute nursing assessment and proper physician notification of complications. Laser Doppler flow may be used to monitor skin perfusion after free flap transfer.

Inform a woman with a recent subpectoral implant that initially the implant feels very firm and is higher on the chest than a normal breast. Over time, the muscle stretches, allowing the implant to drop and soften. Women with subpectoral implants do not wear bras, because the implant needs to move into the pocket created in the chest wall. Women who undergo other types of surgery may return from the operating room wearing a bra to support the breasts. A front-closing support bra without underwires is preferred. Wearing a bra also helps some women feel more normal, encouraging a return to

FIGURE 40–6 Nipple-areola reconstruction.

wellness. Psychosocial readjustment to breast reconstruction, including incorporation of the reconstructed breast into the woman's body image, usually occurs 3 to 4 months after surgery.

■ Medical Management

ELIMINATE OR PREVENT SPREAD OF CANCER

After surgery or instead of surgery, it may be possible to prevent further extension of cancer or to completely eliminate the cancer cells by using radiation therapy, chemotherapy, and/or hormonal therapy modalities.

Radiation Therapy

Radiation therapy is used in breast cancer treatment as follows:

- The breast and underlying chest wall are irradiated after lumpectomy or quadrantectomy as adjuvant therapy for stage I or II breast cancer.
- Women who are poor surgical candidates because of health problems such as heart disease typically receive radiation therapy to the affected breast.
- The chest wall is irradiated if it is involved or for local control after mastectomy with positive margins.
- The axilla is irradiated in women at high risk for axillary metastases who are poor surgical candidates for axillary dissection or who have gross disease that was not surgically excised.
- The supraclavicular region is irradiated if positive axillary nodes are found.
- Additional areas are irradiated for management of metastatic disease to the brain, bone, or skin.

Radiation in combination with lumpectomy or quadrantectomy is an accepted treatment for early-stage breast cancer. An axillary dissection or a sentinel node biopsy is usually done for staging purposes. Radiation therapy, when used to treat micrometastatic disease following mastectomy, successfully reduces the risk of local recurrence and therefore of distant metastases. The utility of radiation therapy following mastectomy or modified radical mastectomy comes into question when the client is also receiving adjuvant chemotherapy, tamoxifen, or both. Although it may decrease local recurrence, the addition of radiation therapy does not influence survival unless there is microscopic disease in the margins. Therefore, the use of postoperative radiation therapy is not indicated in clients with negative axillary nodes except when there is evidence of disease at the deep margins of the tumor.[2] Where axillary nodes are positive, radiation therapy is useful to reduce the likelihood of local recurrence and to improve survival.

When chemotherapy is given with radiation therapy, the radiotherapy may be given concomitantly or sandwiched with the chemotherapy, or given sequentially after completion of the chemotherapy. Concomitant therapy results in a greater incidence of skin reactions than has been reported with sequential treatment. The only situation in which radiation therapy might be given prior to chemotherapy is in a case in which there are negative axillary nodes (and therefore low risk for distant disease) and positive surgical margins, when the risk for local recurrence is great. The real risk to women with breast cancer is that it is a systemic disease. Therefore, chemo-

therapy is critically important to eradicate any micrometastatic disease wherever it may be, including the chest.

Radiation therapy can be administered through an external beam or via iridium implants. For external beam irradiation, the radiation is administered on an outpatient basis 5 days a week for 5 to 6 weeks to the entire breast (and possibly the lymphatics), usually with a boost to the tumor bed. The total dose of radiation is approximately 5000 rad. Regional lymph nodes may be treated if they have not been removed.

Interstitial implant therapy using iridium^{192} (^{192}Ir) is an in-hospital procedure. The insertion of the iridium implant may be done using local anesthesia. Stainless steel guide needles are threaded through the tumor area at 1-cm intervals. Flexible plastic tubes are inserted in the guide needles. The guide needles are then removed, leaving the tube in place. Strands of radioactive iridium seeds are threaded through each tube (Fig. 40–7). The seeds, at 1-cm intervals, form a grid with those above and below to cover the tissues evenly with radiation.

At the end of the insertion procedure, a button is attached to the end of the tubes and the ends are crimped and cut to prevent the seeds from falling out. An x-ray film confirms the implant's location. The implant usually must remain in place for 2 or 3 days. The procedure is mildly uncomfortable. The woman is able to be up and about in her room. Radiation precautions related to time, distance, and shielding are maintained (see Chapter 19). Because of the excellent results from breast reconstruction, most women opt for complete tumor removal rather than the use of implants, which potentially leave residual disease behind.

Side effects of radiation therapy to the breast include:

- Temporary skin changes such as itching, dryness, tenderness, redness, swelling, and/or dry desquamation
- Moist desquamation, especially in skinfolds
- Fatigue
- Dry throat may occur owing to radiation scatter, especially if the supraclavicular area is irradiated
- Pneumonitis (rare); may present as a dry cough and dyspnea; a result of inflammatory changes in the irradiated underlying lung
- Arm edema (rare), occurring more commonly with axillary irradiation
- Increased susceptibility to rib fracture in the irradiated field
- Difficulty in obtaining optimal doses of chemotherapy in women receiving chemotherapy concurrently with radiation therapy because of the effect of radiation on bone marrow

Radiation therapy can be emotionally taxing and physically fatiguing. Nursing support is needed during the 5- to 7-week treatment period. Women receiving radiation therapy have many of the same fears as those having a mastectomy: fear of death, fear of mutilation, and feelings of sexual inadequacy. These are compounded by the stress of daily treatment and the fatigue that occurs with coping with a chronic illness, often while recovering from the side effects of chemotherapy.

Systemic Chemotherapy

LOCALIZED BREAST CANCER. Adjuvant systemic chemotherapy for early stage I and stage II breast cancer gener-

A   B

FIGURE 40–7 Radiation therapy is given via an external beam (*A*) or iridium implants (*B*).

ally follows local surgical intervention and includes combinations of cyclophosphamide (Cytoxan), doxorubicin (Adriamycin), methotrexate (Mexate), 5-fluorouracil (5-FU), paclitaxel (Taxol), and docetaxel (Taxotere), with or without tamoxifen (Nolvadex). Six cycles of cyclophosphamide, methotrexate, and 5-fluorouracil (CMF) and four cycles of doxorubicin and cyclophosphamide with methotrexate, 5-fluorouracil, or leucovorin (Wellcovorin) all are standard adjuvant (curative) therapy for breast cancer.

For the most part, clients are divided into three groups: those who have no involved axillary lymph nodes, those with one to three involved nodes, and those with four or more involved nodes. Adjuvant systemic therapy is usually not given to women whose tumors are 0.5 cm or less in greatest diameter and without lymph node involvement. Clients whose tumors are larger than 0.5 cm but less than 1.0 cm and without lymph node involvement may be divided into those with a low risk of recurrence and those who have unfavorable prognostic features that warrant consideration of adjuvant therapy. Unfavorable prognostic features include lymphatic invasion, high S phase fraction, high nuclear and histologic grades, and HER-2–positive status.

Clients with lymph node involvement or with tumors larger than 1.0 cm in diameter are appropriate candidates for adjuvant systemic therapy. Cytotoxic chemotherapy using CMF or a regimen of cyclophosphamide, doxorubicin, and 5-FU (CAF) is appropriate for women younger than 50 years of age (or premenopausal) and for those 50 years of age or older (or postmenopausal) with hormone receptor–negative tumors.

For women who are 50 years of age or older and have receptor-positive tumors, tamoxifen therapy for 5 years is recommended. The addition of tamoxifen therapy significantly improves the 10-year survival for this population.[18]

The benefit of the addition of tamoxifen therapy to chemotherapy is less clear for women younger than 50 years of age and those with hormone receptor–positive tumors. The addition of chemotherapy to tamoxifen therapy for women 50 years of age or older with hormone receptor–positive, pathologic stage II cancers is somewhat controversial.

The decision to use tamoxifen with or without chemotherapy in women with estrogen receptor–positive disease should be based on the absolute magnitude of risk reduction expected with the systemic therapy and the individual client's willingness to experience toxicity in order to achieve that incremental risk reduction. Obviously, for women with estrogen receptor–negative disease, the choice is for adjuvant chemotherapy. A meta-analysis has shown that combination chemotherapy on the average produces an absolute improvement of 7% to 11% in 10-year survival for women younger than 50 years of age and of 2% to 3% for those aged 50 to 69.[18]

Because there is little agreement about optimal chemotherapy regimens, it is particularly difficult for clients to choose their treatment. For some, the decision is based on whether they will lose their hair and be finished after four injections over 9 weeks, or perhaps whether they will keep their hair but take treatment that lasts for 6 months and requires 12 visits to complete.

In some instances, the physician may recommend primary, induction, or "neoadjuvant" chemotherapy (i.e., given before surgery). Primary chemotherapy is beneficial because the physician can evaluate response to chemotherapy directly, which is impossible once the cancer is removed. Therefore, the physician can know whether the choice of chemotherapy is optimal. In addition, the tumor may actually shrink so much that the disease may be "downstaged," permitting a breast-preserving procedure.

Because induction therapy is given promptly after a diagnosis of breast cancer, the treatment of potential micrometastases, without delays related to surgery, theoretically could result in higher cure rates.[7]

However, although preoperative chemotherapy was as effective as postoperative chemotherapy NB, the results have not demonstrated higher cure rates or influenced survival for stage I and II breast cancers. It does, however, offer the opportunity to observe the biologic response of the tumor to the effects of chemotherapy.[5, 21] When given to clients with inflammatory breast cancer, primary chemotherapy permits shrinkage of the tumor and possible mastectomy, whereas without prior chemotherapy, it might not have been possible to obtain clear surgical margins.

ADVANCED LOCALIZED BREAST CANCER. When a client has more extensive (stage III) yet curable disease, her options and decisions for therapy are even more difficult and controversial. Women with unfavorable stage IIIA or IIIB breast cancers generally require a more aggressive management approach. Affected women typically have larger tumors (>5 cm), direct invasion of the skin of the breast or the chest wall, or fixed or matted axillary lymphadenopathy. Usually, these women undergo preoperative chemotherapy, with or without hormone therapy, followed by surgery and radiotherapy. An alternative approach involves the use of high-dose combination chemotherapy, followed by an additional combination of agents that are also active in breast cancer. The concept is to minimize the risk of drug resistance and to attempt to kill cells before they have an opportunity to mutate to resistance. The addition of paclitaxel every three weeks for four cycles following the standard doxorubicin (Adriamycin) and cyclophosphamide regimen every three weeks for four cycles for women with node-positive breast cancer is associated with increased relapse-free survival.[26]

Other adjuvant treatments under investigation include the combination of paclitaxel and the monoclonal antibody trastuzumab (Herceptin). When these two agents are combined, there appears to be significant synergy without increased toxicity.[44] HER-2 is overexpressed in 25% to 30% of human breast cancers and indicates a worse prognosis in clients who have positive axillary lymph nodes. Despite the association of HER-2 overexpression with poor prognosis, a clinical response to taxanes was three times more likely to occur in HER-2–positive clients than in HER-2–negative clients.[4, 43]

A multicenter research trial combining trastuzumab, doxorubicin, and cyclophosphamide with paclitaxel is being proposed by the NCI. All women with stage III breast cancer who enter the research study would receive all four drugs plus dexrazoxane (Zinecard)—a drug to prevent cardiac damage, included because all four drugs are associated with cardiac toxicity. Once the chemotherapy treatment is complete, the women would then be randomized either to continue trastuzumab for a year or to have no further chemotherapy.[27]

Dose intensification requiring the use of colony-stimulating factors or autologous hematopoietic support is not considered standard therapy in adjuvant breast cancer. Research conducted by the National Surgical Adjuvant Breast Project included two randomized trials (NSABP B22 and NSABP B25) of dose intensification, and neither one to date has demonstrated that higher doses of drug given in a compressed time period are superior to standard dosing of the same drugs (doxorubicin and cyclophosphamide).[23] Furthermore, the toxicity associated with dose intensification is significant.[15] Although pilot trials of autologous bone marrow transplant procedures for women with multiple positive nodes have shown some success, more research is needed to demonstrate the efficacy of bone marrow transplantation in breast cancer.

▪ Nursing Management of the Medical Client
ASSESSMENT
Nursing management of the woman receiving chemotherapy for breast cancer centers on her need for information and instructions regarding self-care procedures. Because in most cases the woman undergoes her breast surgery in the hospital and goes home 1 to 3 days later, there is often little time to discuss her concerns regarding chemotherapy and radiation therapy. Even though the client does not start these treatments until complete healing has taken place (usually 3 to 4 weeks after surgery), the nurse has an important role in providing the client and family members with information regarding the side effects of chemotherapy and radiation therapy. In planning care, be sure to consider the emotional, social, cognitive, spiritual, and physical impact of the diagnosis and treatment on the woman and her family.

DIAGNOSIS, OUTCOMES, INTERVENTIONS
Effective Management of Therapeutic Regimen. The nursing diagnosis may be expressed as *Effective Management of Therapeutic Regimen related to chemotherapy and radiation therapy.*

Outcomes. The client will understand the purpose and goals of chemotherapy and radiation therapy as evidenced by her statements concerning the necessity for treatment and possible side effects associated with that treatment.

Interventions
Teach About Radiation Therapy. Teaching is a major role of the nurse who is caring for clients receiving radiation therapy.

Include in the teaching plan instructions regarding skin care, sun protection, and management of fatigue. If the client is receiving chemotherapy concurrently, there is heightened risk for infection due to neutropenia. Therefore, instruct clients to report any evidence of infection. Monitor blood counts on a weekly basis. Tell the client that written materials, including the booklet *Radiation Therapy and You,* are available from the NCI free of charge by calling 1-800-4-CANCER. See Chapter 19 for further information on radiation therapy.

Teach About Chemotherapy. Nurses are responsible for teaching clients about the side effects of chemotherapy. The booklet *Chemotherapy and You* (also available free of charge from the NCI) explains the purpose of chemotherapy and possible side effects. Once the regimen is selected, discuss side effects. Teach the client the names of the drugs, how the drugs are given, expected side effects and their management, preventive measures, and complications that need to be reported to the physician or nurse (e.g., infection, fever, bruising, bleeding, mouth sores).

You should vary the teaching plan, depending on the drug regimen selected, because the side effects are different for each of the drugs. For example, not all chemotherapy agents cause hair loss. Women receiving methotrexate and 5-FU will not experience hair loss, whereas women receiving doxorubicin and cyclophosphamide will have complete hair loss at 2½ weeks after their first injection. Cyclophosphamide taken orally for 14 days and methotrexate and 5-FU given by injection twice a month will cause a gradual thinning of the hair, but generally the woman can get by without a wig, especially if her hair is kept short. Methotrexate and 5-FU can cause diarrhea and stomatitis, which may interrupt therapy. Advise women taking cyclophosphamide by mouth for the 14-day regimen to drink eight glasses of water a day to prevent hemorrhagic cystitis.

Altered Nutrition: Less Than Body Requirements. The nursing diagnosis may be expressed as *Altered Nutrition: Less Than Body Requirements related to nausea, vomiting, and stomatitis secondary to chemotherapy.*

Outcomes. The client will maintain adequate nutrition, as evidenced by absence of nausea and vomiting, control of stomatitis, intake of adequate calories daily, and no or minimal weight loss.

Interventions. Nausea, vomiting, anorexia, stomatitis, and taste change are common side effects of chemotherapy agents. Some drugs, specifically doxorubicin and methotrexate, will cause stomatitis 4 to 5 days after the injection.

Provide Oral Hygiene. To minimize the severity of the stomatitis, the client is instructed to perform oral hygiene three to four times a day and to rinse with baking soda and water to maintain a basic environment in the oral cavity. Bacteria thrive in an acid environment. If a client experiences any mouth soreness, she should suck on ice during injection of the chemotherapy agent. This simple form of cryotherapy helps to minimize exposure of the oral cavity to the irritating effects of chemotherapy agents.

Prevent Nausea and Vomiting. Nausea and vomiting are usually preventable when antiemetic medications are taken on a schedule rather than just as needed. A combination of a dopamine antagonist, a serotonin antagonist, and a steroid is usually adequate to prevent nausea and vomiting from chemotherapy. Because chemotherapy slows colonic transit time, clients often experience epigastric distress and bloating after administration of these agents. In addition, the serotonin antagonists can be constipating. For these reasons, encourage clients to eat lightly, taking primarily liquids for the 3 days following chemotherapy. Drugs such as metoclopramide (Reglan) or cisapride (Propulsid) are useful to enhance gastric emptying and to reduce bloating. Most women who receive chemotherapy for breast cancer do not lose weight; in fact, they gain weight. Women receiving CMF therapy may gain between 15 and 25 pounds during their therapy. Counsel clients to control their weight and to watch what they are eating.

EVALUATION

Many factors affect the duration of the chemotherapy regimen. Some considerations are:

- Whether the chemotherapy is adjuvant
- Stage at which the breast cancer was diagnosed
- Co-morbidities
- Whether the disease remains stable during chemotherapy

■ Self-Care

TEACH ABOUT FOLLOW-UP SURVEILLANCE

The highest risk factor for breast cancer is a history of breast cancer. Therefore, instruct clients that they require follow-up cancer surveillance for the rest of their lives. Most women are emotional and apprehensive after completing their adjuvant therapy. For the most part, they are happy to be finished but nervous that they are no longer receiving any therapy to oppose the cancer. If they are receiving tamoxifen, remind them that it is treatment for their cancer as well as a medicine to help prevent breast cancer. Women express fear that the cancer will come back, and many wonder whether they could ever endure chemotherapy again if the disease did come back. It is important to acknowledge and discuss the fact that they will worry and feel afraid, so that they can realize that such feelings are normal.

Explain that the physical examination by the physician every 3 to 4 months is designed to detect any problem early and that they should make every effort to keep their appointments. The surveillance schedule involves a physical examination every 3 to 4 months for 3 years, every 6 months for 2 years, and then once a year. A mammogram and a chest film (optional) are obtained every 12 months. Routine chemistry screening is done every year. For women on tamoxifen who still have their uterus, a pelvic examination is done every year.

Routine liver, bone, and brain scans are not indicated as surveillance tests for recurrent disease.[42] Until research determines that early institution of therapy is critical to the outcome, the goal of surveillance is to detect the disease just as the disease begins to be symptomatic.[2]

PROMOTE ACCEPTANCE OF BODY IMAGE

For the woman who has had a mastectomy (a less common procedure today), acceptance of the change in body image takes time. Evaluate adaptation to this loss by asking the woman how she feels about the loss and whether she thinks it would be helpful to see a social worker or psycho-oncologist to discuss strategies for coping. Adaptation and acceptance of the loss may be evident by her ability to discuss plans for a permanent prosthesis or by her questions regarding breast reconstruction. Do not insist that a woman look at her incision; she needs to wait until she is ready. A woman's reluctance to look at the incision is in no way evidence of inability to accept her loss.

Inform women of outside resources that can help them adapt to the changes imposed by the disease. For example, breast cancer support groups and other resources are designed to help the woman and her significant other learn to cope. Information about where to buy a prosthesis and a wig is helpful. Even having the telephone number and name of a person who can help with a wig or prosthesis can make a difficult time more bearable.

■ LOCAL RECURRENCE

Nearly 80% of local recurrences appear within 5 years of mastectomy.[2] Local recurrence after mastectomy generally presents as an isolated nodule in or under the skin of the chest wall, usually near the mastectomy scar. Breast reconstruction does not interfere with early detection of a local recurrence. A complete staging work-up is conducted to define the extent of recurrence. Wide local excision and radiation therapy have been the standard form of local treatment for clients with local recurrence after mastectomy. Hormone therapy is appropriate if the tumor is estrogen receptor–positive, or chemotherapy is recommended in view of the very high risk for distant metastases. The goal of therapy is control of local and distant disease.

Local recurrence after breast-preserving surgery and radiation therapy carries a better prognosis than that associated with local recurrence after mastectomy. Mastectomy is the standard form of therapy for local recurrence, provided that there is no evidence of supraclavicular node involvement or distant metastases. After a mastectomy, many women have breast reconstruction with a myocutaneous flap, which is psychologically important but also improves healing.

■ METASTATIC BREAST CANCER

■ Medical Management

DETERMINE EXTENT OF DISEASE

Despite adjuvant therapy, after varying periods of disease-free survival, nearly half of clients who have received treatment for apparently localized breast cancer develop metastatic disease. The majority of cases occur within 2 years of definitive surgery, but several initial breast cancer recurrences occur more than 5 years after initial therapy.[34] In general, the clinical course and presentation of metastatic disease are variable in terms of growth rate and responsiveness to systemic therapy. As a result of the heterogeneous nature of breast cancer, the disease may present as aggressive visceral disease in multiple organs, as a small skin recurrence such as in a supraclavicular lymph node, or as metastatic bone disease.

Selection of therapy depends on the extent of disease and whether any visceral organs are involved. The goal of therapy is control of disease and optimal palliation with prolongation of life and minimal disruption of the woman's lifestyle and quality of life. Life expectancy after breast cancer recurrence is variable. If disease recurs in the liver, most women die within 3 years of the recurrence. Others with disease in bone or skin may survive for many years. Women with more aggressive disease tend to be *premenopausal,* with estrogen receptor–negative, HER2–positive disease that recurs in liver or lung. Women with less aggressive disease tend to be *postmenopausal,* with estrogen receptor–positive disease that is HER-2–negative and recurs in bone and skin.

All clients with suspected metastatic disease undergo a metastatic work-up to determine the extent of disease. Typically, a physical examination, serum chemistry profiles, a complete blood count, chest radiograph, and a bone scan are obtained initially. If the client has clinical manifestations associated with organ dysfunction, a CT scan of the area is appropriate. A CT scan or MRI study of the chest, abdomen, or pelvis may also be done if the client is being considered for a research protocol. Serum markers include CEA, CA-125, and CA 15-3. Serum markers that are elevated are monitored monthly to evaluate response to therapy.

PREVENT FURTHER EXTENSION OF CANCER

Once extent of disease is determined, an overall therapeutic approach is established based on the client's age, disease-free interval, hormone receptor status, and location and extent of disease. For older women with limited and non–life threatening disease, no significant manifestations of disease, and estrogen receptor–positive tumors, hormone therapy is the initial treatment of choice. If the disease involves liver or lung or if the tumor is estrogen receptor–negative, the choice of treatment is chemotherapy, with or without trastuzumab if the tumor is HER-2–positive. Radiation therapy is instituted only if the disease is symptomatic.

The basic philosophy of management of the woman with metastatic breast cancer is to use all therapies to their fullest worth, but not to the point of toxicity, when the treatment becomes worse than the disease. A treatment that creates a stable condition is still a worthwhile treatment. Treatments are not abandoned until their utility is fully spent. The emphasis is on the need for therapeutic options.

Endocrine Therapy

As stated earlier, when a woman is known to have breast cancer, her tissue sample is tested for the presence of estrogen and progesterone receptors. Estrogen and progesterone receptor assays are performed using radioimmunoassay and immunohistochemical techniques. The more strongly estrogen receptor–positive the tumor, the more likely it is that the disease will respond to hormone therapies. Yet although more than 60% of human breast cancers are estrogen receptor–positive, no more than two thirds of them will respond to endocrine therapy.

Hormone therapies are generally classified as *ablative* (removal of the hormone) or *additive* (addition of a hormone changes the hormonal environment sufficiently to affect tumor growth). The response rates for all hormonal manipulations are basically similar. Women who have a response to one hormonal intervention often have a response to a second after the first becomes ineffective.

In general, the least toxic intervention is chosen first. Once the disease is no longer controlled with a specific approach, the next least toxic agent is selected, and so forth. With the exception of tamoxifen, which is an antiestrogen, hormone therapies are reserved for women with metastatic disease. There is no therapeutic benefit to combining hormone therapies. It is generally accepted practice to continue each therapy for as long as it provides benefit before instituting other therapy. Even withdrawing a hormone manipulation may result in a therapeutic response.

Antiestrogens

If the woman has not previously received tamoxifen, it is typically the first hormonal agent given because of its limited toxicity. Tamoxifen works in premenopausal women, but it is more active in the absence of ovarian function and is therefore especially effective in postmenopausal women. Tamoxifen is a partial estrogen agonist that has mixed estrogenic and antiestrogenic properties; it has a favorable effect on cardiac status and opposes calcium loss as women age. Side effects include nausea, hot flashes, weight gain, menstrual irregularities, and thromboembolic events in 1% to 2% of cases. The risk of endometrial cancer is minimal (2 cases per 1000 women annually in postmenopausal women).[12] Other antiestrogens include toremifene (Fareston), raloxifene, and long-acting ICI 182,780 (Faslodex).

Ablative Endocrine Procedures

Ablative endocrine procedures have been replaced by specific, well-tolerated hormone treatments. In premenopausal women, it is possible to administer goserelin (Zoladex), a luteinizing hormone–releasing hormone (LHRH) agonist that causes a medical oophorectomy. Injections are given every 1 to 3 months depending on the preparation. The only difference between surgical oophorectomy and medical oophorectomy is that results with surgical intervention are immediate and permanent.

For women in whom initial hormone ablation therapy fails, administration of either megestrol acetate (Megace) or an aromatase inhibitor is an option. Aromatase inhibitors prevent the peripheral conversion or aromatization of other steroids (namely, androgens to estrogen), primarily in body fat. The efficacy of aromatase inhibitors is limited to postmenopausal women. In clinical trials it appears that anastrozole (Arimidex) and letrozole (Femura) as aromatase inhibitors are associated not only with less toxicity but also with greater efficacy and even survival than have been reported for megestrol acetate.[40]

Chemotherapy

Eventually, all hormone-responsive tumors become refractory to hormone manipulation, and chemotherapy becomes the treatment of choice. The selection of combination chemotherapy again is guided by the toxicity of the regimen and the extent of disease. A doxorubicin-containing regimen is usually selected if the client has lung or liver disease, because the response is usually prompt and durable. CMF is also a good option and is somewhat less toxic. The taxanes with or without trastuzumab are excellent options, as is vinorelbine (Navelbine). All of these drugs and drug combinations are options for the woman with metastatic disease, and each offers some degree of response and tumor control.

For the most part, metastatic breast cancer is considered an incurable disease. However, long-term responses have been seen with aggressive high-dose chemotherapy regimens, including autologous stem cell transplantation. This latter procedure involves having the woman donate her own bone marrow, either through bone marrow aspiration or through peripheral stem cell pheresis. The client then is given very-high-dose chemotherapy, followed by reinfusion of her own marrow or stem cells after the chemotherapy has destroyed her own marrow. Further information on bone marrow transplantation can be found in Chapter 78. These high-dose therapies are associated with increased expense and toxicity of therapy.[6]

Another important option for treatment in women with bone metastases is a bisphosphonate added to the chemotherapeutic or hormonal therapy regimen. Pamidronate (Aredia) and clodronate (Ostac) not only reduce pain and incidence of complications but also help the bone to heal and prolong survival of the client without complications associated with bone metastases. Pamidronate is given intravenously over 2 hours every month. Adjuvant clodro-nate therapy has been shown to decrease the risk of bone metastases.[17, 40]

BREAST CANCER IN MEN

Breast cancer in men is rare, with approximately 1400 new cases diagnosed and nearly 400 deaths due to breast cancer each year.[1] The average age at onset is about 60 years (10 years older than the average for women). Factors associated with an increased risk of breast cancer in men include:

- A first-degree male or female relative with breast cancer
- Presence of the *BRCA2* gene
- Klinefelter's syndrome
- Hepatic schistosomiasis
- Exposure to ionizing radiation

Breast cancer in men tends to be identified at a more advanced stage, possibly because of the unexpected nature of the disease and the fact that the mass is usually painless and located beneath the nipple-areola complex. Generally, the mass is detected when it becomes large, ulcerates, or becomes fixed to underlying muscle. Assessment findings indicating male breast cancer include a painless lump beneath the areola or, more often, nipple discharge, retraction, crusting, or ulceration.

Biopsy is necessary for diagnosis of male breast cancer. The most common histologic type is infiltrating ductal carcinoma. Most male breast cancers are estrogen receptor–positive and respond to endocrine therapy. Staging of disease is the same as for women. Axillary dissection is done to determine nodal status and prognosis.

A modified radical mastectomy is usually required to obtain clear margins. Radiation therapy may be indicated, depending on the size of the primary tumor. Chemotherapy, usually a doxorubicin-containing regimen, is administered as adjuvant therapy and followed by radiation. Tamoxifen therapy is appropriate for adjuvant therapy. In the presence of metastatic disease, an LHRH agonist (goserelin) is appropriate hormonal manipulation and takes the place of orchiectomy. The pattern of metastasis is similar to that of female breast cancer.

BENIGN BREAST DISEASE

Most women have a profound underlying fear of breast cancer. For some women the fear is so great that they are immobilized, and ignore the problem altogether. This is why some women who see a physician because of a lump, pain, or nipple discharge present with breast cancer at an advanced stage. Mastalgia, or breast pain, is frequently linked emotionally to the fear of breast cancer. Become sensitive to the emotional aspects associated with breast problems, take clients' fears seriously, provide reassurance through discussion, and perform appropriate evaluation.

The basic techniques of breast evaluation consist of:

- A breast-oriented medical history, including the woman's age, menstrual history, family and personal history of breast cancer, last mammogram, and current or past history of hormone therapy

- Clinical breast examination
- Mammography
- FNA of a persistent palpable mass

■ FIBROCYSTIC BREASTS

Fibrocystic breasts are the most frequently occurring pathologic problem in the female breast.[35] The exact cause is unknown, although some evidence indicates hormonal imbalance and even high caffeine consumption may be associated with it. The fibrocystic condition typically improves during pregnancy and lactation. It occurs during the reproductive years and disappears with menopause.

Typical fibrocystic lesions are fluid-filled cysts that are round, well circumscribed, and movable. Depending on the amount of fluid in the cyst, the cyst may feel soft or hard. Assessment findings may include nodularity and tenderness. Pain is common, and the cysts frequently increase in size premenstrually. Cysts are generally aspirated rather than undergo surgical biopsy. If there is any question, however, a biopsy is done. A biopsy is necessary if the cyst keeps recurring after being aspirated. Fibrocystic disease is considered a risk factor for breast cancer when it is accompanied by cellular proliferation and atypia.

■ HYPERPLASIA AND ATYPICAL HYPERPLASIA

Ductal hyperplasia is found in 20% of all breast biopsy specimens.[35] Atypical lobular hyperplasia is found in 1% of breast biopsy specimens. The diagnosis of hyperplasia and atypical hyperplasia can be confirmed only by pathologic examination of breast tissue from a biopsy. The presence of hyperplasia or atypical hyperplasia indicates an increased risk for breast cancer.

■ FIBROADENOMA

Fibroadenoma is a common breast tumor that usually occurs in young women, most frequently between ages 15 and 30 years.[35] This tumor is generally a nontender, round, firm, or rubbery mass 1 to 3 cm in diameter. Movability of the adenoma in the breast tissues is one of its most distinctive characteristics. Fibroadenomas are readily diagnosed by FNA cytology.

■ PAPILLOMA

Intraductal papillomas are lesions growing in the terminal portion of a duct (solitary) or throughout the duct system of a sector of breast (multiple or intraductal). Papillomas typically occur in women in their 40s. Solitary intraductal papillomas are usually not precancerous. Multiple papillomas may occasionally be cancerous. Intraductal papilloma is usually identified as a serous, serosanguineous, or bloody discharge from the nipple. Often, no mass is palpable, although a small soft tumor in a central or periareolar portion of the breast is usually present. Examination by FNA or excision is necessary to determine whether the lesion is benign or malignant.

■ DUCT ECTASIA

Duct ectasia, a disease of ducts in the subareolar zone, occurs in aging breasts, usually in perimenopausal or postmenopausal women. Manifestations may include a palpable dilated duct; a thick, sticky nipple discharge; and burning pain, itching, and inflammation. There appears to be no association with cancer. However, biopsy is performed because on physical examination it is difficult to differentiate duct ectasia from cancer.

■ MASTODYNIA AND MASTALGIA

Mastodynia and mastalgia refer to breast pain. Breast pain is the most common breast complaint. Pain is not usually associated with breast cancer. Many women have cyclic premenstrual mastodynia. Women with cyclic premenstrual mastodynia usually have lumpy breast (nodularity) and pain for the week before menses. After any other problems have been ruled out, treatment is symptomatic. Wearing a well-fitting brassiere for support, particularly during jogging and other bouncing exercise, may be helpful. Decreasing caffeine intake may also be helpful.

■ GYNECOMASTIA

Gynecomastia (hypertrophy of one or both male breasts) is common at puberty and in older men. The hormonal mechanism causing gynecomastia is not well understood, although several drugs, an increase in estrogen levels, tumors, and thyroid and hepatic problems may contribute. Usually the situation is temporary. If the gynecomastia causes severe psychosocial trauma, reduction mammoplasty can be performed, or antiestrogen (tamoxifen) or synthetic androgen (danazol [Danocrine]) medications may be administered.

MAMMAPLASTY

Mammaplasty is the surgical revision in the size or shape of the breast. It is often performed electively for cosmetic reasons to enlarge or reduce breast size.

■ BREAST AUGMENTATION

Clients seeking breast augmentation are often young women who have had chronic feelings of inadequacy and self-consciousness because of small or undeveloped breasts. Some clients are mature women who have postpartum breast atrophy. Current prostheses are durable, seamless, silicone rubber envelopes filled with saline. The prosthesis is inserted beneath existing breast tissue or the pectoralis muscle (called subpectoral placement) through an inframammary (under the breast), transaxillary (through the axilla), or periareolar (around the nipple) incision (Fig. 40–8).

Thorough preoperative breast assessment is essential to rule out breast cancer. Mammography is generally not recommended in women younger than 35 years of age unless they have a positive family history of cancer or a suspicious lump. Surgery is performed on an outpatient basis. Nurses provide teaching and support, mostly over the telephone.

Early complications of breast augmentation include changes in breast or nipple sensation, hematoma (collection of clotted blood), infection, or leakage from the prosthesis. The most frequent complication is capsule formation (development of fibrous sacs of scar tissue enclosing the implant), followed by contracture of the scar. These complications cause excessive breast firmness and distortion of the breast into a hard, round ball. Possible causes of capsular contracture include infection and formation of a seroma (a collection of serosanguineous fluid) or hema-

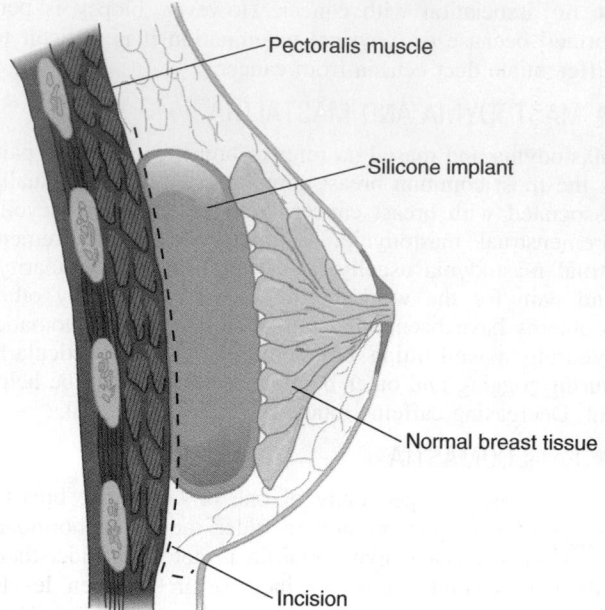

Pectoralis muscle

Silicone implant

Normal breast tissue

Incision

FIGURE 40–8 Augmentation mammaplasty is achieved by insertion of a saline-filled implant beneath normal breast tissue or beneath the pectoral muscle. An inframammary approach is illustrated. Before beginning the retromammary dissection, the surgeon creates a subcutaneous flap. The incision is represented by a *dashed line.*

toma. The basic problem in these processes is that the body's defense mechanisms respond to the prosthesis as a foreign body, and scar tissue forms around the prosthesis to wall it off. Capsule formation is usually treated with open (surgical) capsulotomy. Open capsulotomy, performed under general anesthesia, involves incising the capsule.

Breast massage may be prescribed postoperatively with smooth-walled implants or after capsulotomy to reduce capsule formation. Breast massage typically begins post-

operatively according to the surgeon's instructions. Teach the woman to push each breast up, to the side, and toward the middle of the chest, supporting the breast in each position for a count of 10. Discharge instructions usually include the following:

- To reduce edema, maintain a head-elevated position for a week when in bed.
- To reduce hematoma formation, get plenty of rest for a week (no excessive activity, take it easy).
- To avoid moving the pectoralis muscle and irritating the surgical site, do not raise the arms above the head for 3 weeks (e.g., while washing or brushing hair), do not play golf or tennis or swim for 6 weeks, sleep on the back and not on the stomach or sides, and be careful when closing car doors.
- Because of their anticoagulant effect, do not use aspirin or aspirin-containing compounds.
- Notify the physician if bleeding occurs or if a fever with temperature higher than 37.6° C (99.6° F) develops.

■ REDUCTION MAMMAPLASTY

Reduction mammaplasty surgically reduces the size of large, pendulous breasts. Women usually seek such surgery to reduce the physical and psychosocial discomforts of large breasts, such as back pain, the presence of bra strap indentations in the shoulders, inability to wear normal clothing styles, intertriginous dermatitis (skin breakdown under large breasts), and distress from others' comments about breast size.

Excess breast tissue is removed through incisions under the breast (Fig. 40–9). The nipple is transposed on a pedicle of tissue or grafted onto the newly formed breast. A possible complication is loss of blood supply to the nipple-areola complex. Any duskiness or pallor around the nipple-areola complex should be reported to the physician. Altered sensation and the inability to perform breast-feeding are common findings after this procedure.

FIGURE 40–9 Reduction mammaplasty, in which breasts are surgically reduced. Excess breast tissue is removed, and the breast is recontoured. The nipple is relocated (e.g., moved higher) on a pedicle of tissue. The pedicle supplies the nipple with blood until new blood vessels form.

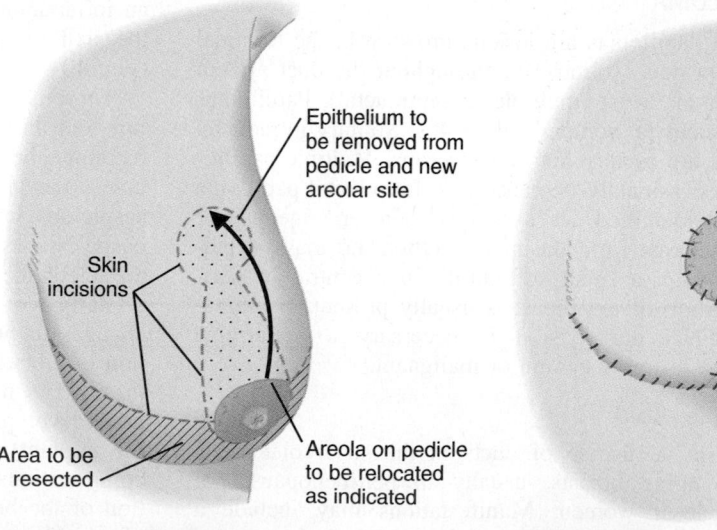

Epithelium to be removed from pedicle and new areolar site

Skin incisions

Area to be resected

Areola on pedicle to be relocated as indicated

PENDULOUS BREAST BEFORE SURGERY

SAME BREAST AFTER RECONTOURING

■ MASTOPEXY

Mastopexy is the correction of mammary ptosis (drooping), to achieve an improved breast contour and position. Mastopexy may be performed with subcutaneous mastectomy or on normal breasts to improve contour. Postoperative care is similar to that with other types of breast surgery.

CONCLUSIONS

Diseases of the breast are usually benign conditions that occur throughout the life cycle. Breast cancer, however, has greatly increased in incidence over the last 30 years. The nurse has a vital role in teaching clients early detection methods so that breast cancer can be detected at a curable stage.

All diseases of the breast potentially pose problems in body image and sexuality. Even benign fibrocystic disease can cause breast tenderness and possibly interfere with sexual functioning. Breast cancer and the possibility of mastectomy as treatment can be extremely threatening to a woman's body image. The nurse can help the client cope with these potential threats and successfully adapt to any changes that occur.

CRITICALLY THINKING

1. The pathology report of your client's breast biopsy reads: "8 mm invasive ductal carcinoma, invasive carcinoma to the margins, estrogen receptor– and progesterone receptor–positive." The client is considering further treatment and asks you what her options are. How would you respond?

Factors to Consider. What treatment options might the client have? What interventions might be required?

2. **Your client has come to the surgery clinic 10 days after a modified radical mastectomy. The breast incision line is clean and intact. A Jackson-Pratt drain is sutured in place in the axilla. The skin around the drain is clean and intact. Drainage is serosanguineous, and the client has recorded 25 ml and 20 ml, respectively, of drainage per 24 hours for the last 2 days. The client looks at the incision and the drain and asks questions while you examine her incision and drainage site. She asks when the drain will come out, when she can drive her car, when she can shower and resume her normal activities, and when she can be fitted for a prosthesis. What would you tell her? What else should you assess? What medical and nursing care does this client need during her appointment? What other teaching needs does she have?**

Factors to Consider. Think about what structures are removed as part of the modified radical mastectomy. What are the functions of these structures? What functional limitations can be expected to affect the client's self-care needs? Consider the client's needs in this immediate postoperative period, in a few months, and over the long term.

3. **Two years ago, your client's stage II cancer of the right breast was treated with a quadrantectomy (margins negative), axillary lymph node dissection (8 of 19 nodes positive), radiation therapy of the chest and axilla, and six courses of CAF (Cytoxan [cyclophosphamide], Adriamycin [doxorubicin], 5-fluorouracil) chemotherapy. Today, she presents with pain, tingling, and swelling of her right hand and arm. She states that although she noticed intermittent problems with slight swelling over the past 6 months, it has become severe over the past 2 weeks and is affecting her ability to work as a court stenographer. What further information should you assess? What are your priority interventions?**

Factors to Consider. What do pain, tingling, and swelling of the hand and arm suggest in a client who has undergone lymph node dissection? Should a referral to a physical therapist for lymphedema management be made?

REFERENCES

1. American Cancer Society. (2000). *Cancer facts and figures.* Atlanta: Author.
2. Abeloff, M., et al. (2000). Breast. In M. Abeloff, et al. (Eds.), *Clinical oncology* (2nd ed., pp. 2051–2159). New York: Churchill Livingstone.
3. Anonymous. (1998). Use of cervical and breast cancer screening among women with and without functional limitations—United States, 1994–1995. *Morbidity and Mortality Weekly Report, 47*(40), 853–856.
4. Baselga, J. B., et al. (1997). HER2 overexpression and paclitaxel sensitivity in breast cancer: Therapeutic implications. *Oncology, 11*(3), 43–48.
5. Bear, H. D. (1998). Indications for neoadjuvant chemotherapy for breast cancer. *Seminars in Oncology, 25*(2), 3–12.
6. Bezwoda, W. R., Seymour, L., & Dansey, R. D. (1995). High-dose chemotherapy with hematopoietic rescue as primary treatment for metastatic breast cancer: A randomized trial. *Journal of Clinical Oncology, 13,* 2483–2489.
7. Brenin, D. R., & Morrow, M. (1998). Breast-conserving surgery in the neoadjuvant setting. *Seminars in Oncology, 25*(2), 13–18.
8. Brody, L. C., & Biesecker, B. B. (1998). Breast cancer susceptibility genes. *BRCA1* and *BRCA2. Medicine, 77*(3), 208–226.
9. Chapman, D., & Goodman, M. (1997). Breast cancer. In S. Groenwald, et al. (Eds.), *Cancer nursing principles and practice* (4th ed., pp. 916–979). Boston: Jones & Bartlett.
10. Chu, K. C., et al. (1996). Recent trends in U.S. breast cancer incidence, survival, and mortality rates. *Journal of the National Cancer Institute, 88*(4), 1571–1579.
11. Cohen, M. Z., Kahn, D. L., & Steeves, R. H. (1998). Beyond body image: The experience of breast cancer. *Oncology Nursing Forum, 25*(5), 835–841.
12. Cuenca, R. E., Giachino, J., Arredondo, M. A., et al.(1996). Endometrial carcinoma associated with breast carcinoma: Low incidence with tamoxifen use. *Cancer, 77,* 2058–2063.
13. Cummings, S. R., et al. (1999). The effect of raloxifene on risk of breast cancer in post menopausal women: Results from the Multiple Outcomes of Raloxifene (MORE) trial. *Journal of the American Medical Association, 281,* 3, 2189–2197.
14. Cutuli, B., et al. (1996). Breast cancer after treatment for Hodgkin's disease. Analysis of clinical and pathological characteristics in 54 cases [Abstract]. *Proceedings of the Annual Meeting of the American Society of Clinical Oncology, 15,* A1299.
15. Decillis, A. (1997). Acute myeloid leukemia (AML) and myelodysplastic syndrome (MDS) in NSABP B-25: An update (Abstract). *Proceedings of the Annual Meeting of the American Society of Clinical Oncology, 16*;130a.
16. Dees, E. C., et al. (1997). Does information from axillary dissection change treatment in clinically node-negative patients with breast cancer? An algorithm for assessment of impact of axillary dissection. *Annals of Surgery, 226,* 279–286.

17. Diel, I. J. (1998). Reduction in new metastases in breast cancer with adjuvant clodronate treatment. *New England Journal of Medicine, 339,* 357.

18. Early Breast Cancer Trialists' Collaborative Group. (1998). Tamoxifen for early breast cancer: An overview of the randomized trials. *Lancet, 351,* 1451–1467.

19. Early Breast Cancer Trialists' Collaborative Group. (1998). Polychemotherapy for early breast cancer: An overview of randomized trials. *Lancet, 352,* 930–942.

20. Edwards, M. J., et al. (1998). Infiltrating ductal carcinoma of the breast: The survival impact of race. *Journal of Clinical Oncology, 16*(8), 2693–2699.

21. Fisher, B., Bryant, J., & Wolmark, N. (1998). Effective preoperative chemotherapy on the outcome of women with operable breast cancer. *Journal of Clinical Oncology, 16*(8), 2672–2685.

22. Fisher, B., et al. (1998). Tamoxifen for prevention of breast cancer. Report of the National Surgical Adjuvant Breast and Bowel Project: Project P-1 Study. *Journal of the National Cancer Institute, 90,* 1371–1388.

23. Fisher, B. (1997). Increased intensification and total dose of cyclophosphamide in a doxorubicin-cyclophosphamide regimen for the treatment of primary breast cancer: Finding from the National Surgical Adjuvant Breast and Bowel Project B-22. *Journal of Clinical Oncology, 15,* 1858–1863.

24. Frykberg, E. R. (1996). Screening mammography in women under fifty years of age. *Breast, 2,* 221–225.

25. Heimann, R., & Hellman, S. (1998). Aging, progression, and phenotype in breast cancer. *Journal of Clinical Oncology, 16*(8), 2686–2692.

26. Henderson, I. C. (1998). Improved disease-free survival (DFS) and overall survival (OS) from the addition of sequential paclitaxel (T) but not from the escalation of doxorubicin (A) dose level in the adjuvant chemotherapy of patients (pts) with node-positive primary breast cancer (BC) (Abstract). *Proceedings of the Annual Meeting of the American Society of Clinical Oncology, 17,* 101a.

27. Herceptin raises its sights beyond advanced breast cancer. (1998). *Journal of the National Cancer Institute, 90*(2), 882–883.

28. Hortobagyi, G. N. (1998). Treatment of breast cancer. *New England Journal of Medicine, 339* (14), 974–984.

29. Humble, C. A. (1995). Lymphedema: Incidence, pathophysiology, management, and nursing care. *Oncology Nursing Forum, 22*(10), 1503–1509.

30. Hunter, D., & Willett, W. C. (1996). Nutrition and breast cancer. *Cancer Causes and Control, 7,* 56–68.

31. Hunter, D., et al. (1996). Cohort studies of fat intake and the risk of breast cancer: A pooled analysis. *New England Journal of Medicine, 334,* 356.

32. Knobf, M. T. (1996). Breast cancer. In R. McCorkle, et al. (Eds.) *Cancer nursing: A comprehensive textbook* (2nd ed., pp. 547–610). Philadelphia: W. B. Saunders.

33. Krag, D., et al. (1998). The sentinel node in breast cancer. *New England Journal of Medicine, 339*(14), 941–946.

34. Lippman, M. E. (1998). Breast cancer. In A. S. Fauci, et al. (Eds.), *Principles of Internal Medicine* (14th ed., pp. 562–568). New York: McGraw-Hill.

35. Marchant, D. J. (1997). *Breast disease.* Philadelphia: W. B. Saunders.

36. McMasters, K. M., et al. (1998). Sentinel-lymph node biopsy for breast cancer—not yet the standard of care. *New England Journal of Medicine, 339*(14), 990–995.

37. Mehta, R. R., et al. (1998). Plasma c-erbB-2 levels in breast cancer patients: Prognostic significance in predicting response to chemotherapy. *Journal of Clinical Oncology, 16*(7), 2409–2416.

38. Parker, S. L., et al. (1997). Cancer statistics. *CA: A Cancer Journal for Clinicians, 47*(1), 5–27.

39. Peto, R. (1996). Five years of tamoxifen—or more? *Journal of the National Cancer Institute, 88*(24), 1791–1793.

40. Powles, T. J. (1998) Oral clodronate reduces the incidence of bone metastasis in patients with operable breast cancer (Abstract). *Proceedings of the American Society of Clinical Oncology, 17,* 123a.

41. Price, J., & Purtell, J. R. (1997). Prevention and treatment of lymphedema after breast cancer. *American Journal of Nursing, 97*(9), 34–37.

42. American Society of Clinical Oncology. Recommended breast cancer surveillance guidelines. (1997). *Journal of Clinical Oncology, 15,* 2149–2156.

43. Seidman, A. D., et al. (1997). Paclitaxel for breast cancer: The Memorial Sloan-Kettering Cancer Center experience. *Oncology, 11*(3), 20–28.

44. Slamon, D., et al. (1998). Addition of Herceptin to first-line chemotherapy for HER2 overexpressing metastatic breast cancer markedly increases anticancer activity: A randomized multinational controlled phase III trial [Abstract]. *Proceedings of the American Society of Clinical Oncology, 17,* 98a.

45. Smith, J. (1998). The practice of venipuncture in lymphedema. *European Journal of Cancer Care, 7*(2), 97–98.

46. Tabar, L. (1996). Breast-cancer screening with mammography in women aged 40–49 years. *International Journal of Cancer, 68,* 693–699.

47. Thomas, D. B., et al. (1997). Randomized trial of breast self-examination in Shanghai: Methodology and preliminary results. *Journal of the National Cancer Institute, 89,* 335–340.

48. Vogel, V. G. (1996). Assessing women's potential risk of developing breast cancer. *Preventive Medicine, 10*(10), 1451–1463.

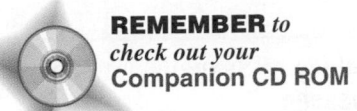

REMEMBER *to*
check out your
Companion CD ROM

C H A P T E R

41

Management of Clients with Sexually Transmitted Diseases

Meg Blair

NURSING OUTCOMES CLASSIFICATION (NOC)
for Nursing Diagnoses—Clients with Sexually Transmitted Diseases

Altered Health Maintenance	Knowledge: Treatment Regimen	Anxiety
Health Belief: Perceived Resources	Participation: Health Care Decisions	Anxiety Control
Health Promoting Behavior	Psychosocial Adjustment: Life Changes	Coping
Health Seeking Behavior	Risk Detection	Impulse Control
Knowledge: Health Behaviors	Self-Direction of Care	Social Interaction Skills
Knowledge: Health Promotion	Social Support	
Knowledge: Health Resources	Treatment Behavior: Illness or Injury	

SEXUALLY TRANSMITTED DISEASES: AN OVERVIEW

The term *sexually transmitted disease* (STD) refers to any infection contracted primarily through sexual activities or contact. *STD* has replaced the older term *venereal disease* (VD), which referred to diseases transmitted only by sexual intercourse. STD is also known as sexually transmitted infection (STI). More than 50 organisms are known to spread through sexual activity. The five most widely known STDs are chlamydial infection, gonorrhea, syphilis, genital herpes, and genital warts (see later). Other infections are chancroid, lymphogranuloma venereum, granuloma inguinale, trichomoniasis, acquired immunodeficiency syndrome (AIDS), and some enteric and ectoparasitic infections. The number of STDs is increasing as new agents are implicated in the sexual transmission of disease.

STDs share the following characteristics:

1. STDs can be transmitted by any sexual activity between opposite-sex or same-sex partners (not only vaginal-penile sex but also oral and anal sex).
2. Having one STD confers no immunity against future reinfection with that STD or with any other STD (except, possibly, for hepatitis B).
3. Sexual partners of infected clients need to be assessed for treatment (see individual diseases for specific recommendations).
4. STDs affect people from all socioeconomic classes, cultures, ethnicities, and age groups.
5. Women bear a disproportionate number of the effects of STDs.
6. Frustration, anger, anxiety, fear, shame, and guilt are emotions commonly associated with an STD diagnosis.
7. STDs frequently coexist in the same client (for example, a client may have both chlamydial infection and gonorrhea).

The last fact may be responsible for some treatment failures. Current treatment guidelines for STDs are available in the United States from the Centers for Disease Control and Prevention (CDC) in Atlanta.

STDs are a very serious public health problem. Recognized since the beginning of recorded history, these diseases are associated with substantial morbidity and, in some cases, mortality. The incidence of STDs continues to increase worldwide, and infections are becoming more severe. STDs also facilitate the development of human immunodeficiency virus (HIV) infection and AIDS. Thus, the scope of the health problem they create is increasing

This chapter incorporates material written for the fifth edition by Patricia E. Downing.

rather than decreasing. It is a matter of public concern that treatments for STDs be safe, inexpensive, and effective.

Except for the common cold and influenza, STDs are the most prevalent communicable diseases in the United States, which has the highest STD rate in the industrialized world. Most sources describe STD rates as epidemic. Symptomatic STDs are diagnosed in more than 13 million people in this country annually, not including HIV infection and AIDS, and 86% of affected people are between 15 and 29 years of age. Another 40 million people are infected with human papillomavirus (HPV), which causes genital warts. It is estimated that 50% of all Americans will have had an STD by age 30 years. Although AIDS is probably the best publicized and most dangerous, the most common STDs are chlamydial infection, gonorrhea, genital herpes, genital warts, and syphilis.

Official national incidence statistics for STDs are published by the CDC and by local health authorities, but the actual incidence is unknown. Accurate statistics are difficult to compile for a number of reasons. Statistics reflect the accuracy of case reporting, and reporting is not mandatory for all STDs. Rates for some STDs, such as genital herpes and genital warts, are based on estimates derived from local studies and physician reports. These estimates are thought to be low. Even rates developed from mandatory case reporting are believed to be low.

The costs of STDs are staggering, both in medical expense and in emotional suffering. Up to $10 billion a year is spent to treat STDs and their sequelae (consequences), including at least $1 billion a year to treat subsequent infertility. These figures, like statistics, can be misleading. For instance, women, who are two times more likely to be infected with an STD than men, are less likely to receive treatment, often because the STD is asymptomatic. Also, STDs can lead to infertility. The cost of treating infertility due to STDs is an indirect cost of the STD. Many couples in lower socioeconomic classes cannot afford infertility treatments. Hence, infertility services are used most often by middle-class and upper-class couples. The true cost of STDs that result in infertility cannot be accurately estimated.

Etiology and Risk Factors

STDs can be caused by bacteria, viruses, protozoa, fungi, and ectoparasites (Box 41–1). Anyone who engages in intimate physical contact can contract and transmit an STD. Many health care providers do not always acknowledge that fact, especially in regard to middle-class, upper-class, or older clients. Although younger people have the highest rates for STDs (86%), all age groups are at risk. The fetus or neonate can be infected across the placenta or during vaginal birth. Infants and children can be infected through child abuse. Older adults can be infected or can experience residual sequelae from infections contracted earlier in their lives. When a client complains of manifestations that might be those of an STD, STDs should always be part of the differential diagnosis.

The worldwide increase in the incidence of STDs is a result of many factors. STDs due to antibiotic-resistant strains of bacteria have become more common. For exam-

---

BOX 41–1 Etiology of Sexually Transmitted Diseases

STDs Caused by Bacteria

Gonorrhea
Chlamydial infection
Syphilis
Bacterial vaginosis
Nongonococcal urethritis
Chancroid
Lymphogranuloma venereum
Granuloma inguinale
Sexually transmitted enteric infections

STDs Caused by Viruses

Acquired immunodeficiency syndrome (AIDS)
Genital herpes
Genital warts
Hepatitis B
Hepatitis A
Hepatitis C (possible sexual transmission)

STD Caused by Protozoa

Trichomoniasis

STD Caused by Fungi

Vulvovaginal candidiasis

STDs Caused by Ectoparasites

Scabies
Pediculosis pubis

---

ple, the incidence of gonorrhea has risen since the evolution of penicillinase-producing *Neisseria gonorrhoeae*. The use of intrauterine devices (IUDs) and oral contraceptives may lower women's resistance to infection and facilitate transmission of STDs. Women may not think to use an infection barrier *in addition to* effective contraception. Sterilized women often do not use condoms.

Lack of knowledge also plays a role in the incidence of STDs. Clients may find it difficult to obtain accurate information, even from health professionals. Politics and religion continue to affect the controversy over sex education in schools. Accurate information about sex and STDs is not always presented in a manner designed to appeal to, and therefore influence the behavior of, young people.

Specific risk factors for acquiring STDs are:

- Intravenous (IV) drug use
- Other substance abuse
- High-risk sexual activity (use of prostitutes, multiple or casual sexual partners, sex with IV drug users and infected people, unprotected sex, exchanging sex for money or drugs)
- Younger age
- Younger age at *sexarche* (the beginning of sexual activity)

- Inner city residence
- Poverty
- Poor nutrition
- Poor hygiene

The young are particularly at risk; immaturity of the immune system, cervical differences, peer group pressure, and the belief that they are invincible all combine to make young people particularly susceptible to STDs. Many people have a cavalier attitude about infection and illness in general because of the advances that have been made in antimicrobial therapy. Many people think any infection can now be easily cured, and thus they do not consider STDs to be serious diseases with possible complications.

According to the CDC, STD prevention and health promotion should focus on five major concepts:

- Education
- Detection of active disease (including asymptomatic infections)
- Effective diagnosis and treatment
- Evaluation and treatment of sexual partners
- Pre-exposure vaccination if available

Sex education in schools, risk-reduction counseling, promotion of safer sex, and an open, accepting attitude from health professionals can increase knowledge levels. Health professionals must be comfortable asking clients about sexual activity and practices and must provide information in a way that does not "turn off" the client or cause embarrassment.

Health maintenance consists of:

- Screening high-risk people
- Maintaining a high index of suspicion for asymptomatic infections
- Providing accurate, timely diagnosis and treatment
- Performing follow-up after treatment when indicated
- Reporting cases of STDs
- Identifying and treating sexual partners of clients with STDs

Health restoration includes measures to reverse the effects of disease, such as infertility (see Chapters 38 and 39). Although some STDs can be passed nonsexually, most are transmitted sexually because the causative organisms thrive in a warm, dark, moist environment within the body and survive only very briefly outside that environment. Therefore, their transmission requires intimate contact. Prevention and control must concentrate on breaking the chain of sexual transmission of disease.

Pathophysiology

An STD occurs when an individual is infected by an organism through sexual contact. Some STDs remain localized; others spread and become systemic. Some STDs are seen in an acute episode; others are chronic illnesses. See discussions of specific STDs for more detailed information.

Clinical Manifestations

Clinical manifestations vary among the STDs and depend on the organism involved and the location of the infection (local or systemic). Diseases may be grouped according to their primary manifestation (e.g., those that cause vaginal discharge). Diagnostic testing is individualized for each condition. See specific STDs for more detailed information.

Outcome Management

Medical Management

Medical management focuses on eradicating the offending organism, if possible, or managing a chronic condition. Table 41–1 provides a concise overview.

Nursing Management of the Medical Client

Nursing outcomes are similar to medical outcomes. The following discussion of nursing care can be generalized to all STDs. Specific details are provided in the discussion of each STD.

ASSESSMENT

A thorough nursing assessment consists of (1) general health assessment and examination, (2) sexual history, preference, and practices, (3) previous history of STDs, (4) specific complaints (60% to 80% of STDs are asymptomatic), (5) genital hygienic practices (douching), (6) contraceptive history, and (7) infection barriers used. A holistic approach also includes lifestyle, nutrition, stress, and sexuality. High-risk clients should be screened for STDs regardless of whether manifestations are present at the time of a visit to a health care provider. Never assume that a client is not sexually active and at risk, and make sure that the client understands questions exactly.

Nurses need to know about the variety of sexual activities, their effect on transmission of STDs, and the common manifestations for which to assess. Examine your own attitudes about sexuality and sexual behavior. Separate your personal views of morality from appropriate nursing activities. Judgmental attitudes may deter clients from seeking care and may interfere with therapeutic professional relationships. Bias and prejudice can be communicated in obvious and subtle ways that make the client feel uncomfortable, judged, and discounted. A prejudiced health professional cannot provide comprehensive care. An accepting attitude may ensure treatment and prevent disease transmission.

STDs are associated with a social stigma. Ashamed, many clients try to keep the diagnosis secret. Many relate STDs with low social status and immorality, and many have misconceptions and fears about the dangers of STDs. Other problems may surface with discovery of an STD. For example, a newly infected client may be angry at the responsible sexual partner or may hesitate to identify or inform the sexual partner or partners about the STD. When a marital or committed relationship is involved, questions about infidelity or infertility may arise.

Clients can seek treatment from various sources: health department STD clinics, physician offices, Planned Parenthood clinics, and other community-based clinics. Such clinics frequently deal with STDs and have staff especially sensitive to the needs of clients with STDs. Strict confidentiality is essential. It is especially, but not exclusively, important to gay men and lesbians, who may be at

TABLE 41–1	TREATMENT OF COMMON SEXUALLY TRANSMITTED DISEASES (STDs)			
Condition (Causative Organism)	**Diagnostic Methods**	**Manifestations**	**Treatment**	**Management of Sexual Partner**

Gonorrhea (*Neisseria gonorrhoeae*)	Smear
	Culture
		Incubation period: 3–8 days
		Female
		  Asymptomatic or thick, purulent vaginal discharge
		  Genital irritation
		  Urinary symptoms
		  Pelvic pain (PID)
		  May be asymptomatic
		Male
		  Urethral discharge
		  Urinary manifestations
		  Scrotal pain (epididymitis)
		  Perineal pain (prostatitis)
		Either sex
		  Pharyngeal infection
		  Conjunctivitis
		Disseminated infection
		  Bacteremia
		  Arthritis-dermatitis syndrome
			Ceftriaxone, IM once
			or
			Cefixime, PO once
			or
			Ciprofloxacin, PO once
			or
			Ofloxacin, PO once
			plus
			Doxycycline, PO for 7 days
			or
			Azithromycin, once
			
			Ceftriaxone, IM or IV q 24 hours; continue for 24–48 hours after improvement then switch to PO to complete 1 full week of treatment
				Treat if sexual contact occurred in last 60 days
				or
				Treat *most recent* partner

Chlamydial infection (*Chlamydia trachomatis*)	Culture
	Antigen-antibody
	DFA, ELISA
		Incubation period: 7–21 days
		Female
		  Asymptomatic or pelvic pain (PID)
		Male
		  Asymptomatic or mild dysuria
		  White or clear urethral discharge
		  Scrotal pain
			Azithromycin, PO once
			or
			Eythromycin ethylsuccinate, PO for 7 days or doxycycline bid for 7 days
			or
			Ofloxacin, PO for 7 days
				Treat if sexual contact occurred in last 60 days

Syphilis (*Treponema pallidum*)	Dark-field microscopy
	Serology
	  Nonspecific (e.g., VDRL test)
	  Specific (e.g., FTA-ABS test)
		Incubation period: 10–90 days
		Primary stage
		  Painless chancre at site of exposure
		  Regional lymphadenopathy
		Secondary stage
		  Maculopapular rash
		  Generalized lymphadenopathy
		  Mucous patches
		  Condylomata lata
		  Fever, malaise
		  Alopecia
		Latent stage
		  Asymptomatic
		Tertiary stage
		  Cardiovascular changes
		Neurosyphilis
		  Central nervous system changes
			Primary, secondary, and early latent stages
			Benzathine penicillin G, IM once
			Late latent stage and tertiary stage
			Benzathine penicillin G, IM weekly for 3 weeks
			Neurosyphilis
			Aqueous penicillin G, IV q 4 h for 10–14 days
			or
			Procaine penicillin, IM daily for 10–14 days
			plus
			Probenecid, PO for 10–14 days
				See CDC guidelines

TABLE 41–1 TREATMENT OF COMMON SEXUALLY TRANSMITTED DISEASES (STDs) *Continued*

Condition (Causative Organism)	Diagnostic Methods	Manifestations	Treatment	Management of Sexual Partner
Genital herpes	Culture Pap smear Visual examination	Incubation period: 3–7 days *Acute phase* Paresthesia/burning Painful genital ulcers Fever/chills/muscle pain *Latent phase* Asymptomatic	*Initial episode* Acyclovir, PO for 7–10 days *or* Famciclovir *or* valacyclovir, PO for 7–10 days	All contacts should be evaluated and treated if symptomatic
Genital warts, human papillomavirus	Pap smear Colposcopy Biopsy	Incubation period: 1–2 months Single or multiple genital or anal warts	Topical podophyllin or podofilox *or* Topical trichloroacetic acid *or* Cryotherapy *or* Electrocautery *or* CO_2 laser *or* Surgical excision	All contacts should be evaluated and treated if symptomatic Female partners need Pap smear at diagnosis and at least annually

The CDC considers the following diseases reportable: gonorrhea; syphilis; chlamydial infection; chancroid; granuloma inguinale; lymphoma inguinale; and acquired immunodeficiency syndrome (AIDS). However, laws vary from state to state. Nurses working with clients who have STDs should know their state's reporting requirements.

bid, twice a day; CDC, Centers for Disease Control and Prevention; CO_2, carbon dioxide; DFA, direct fluorescent antibody; ELISA, enzyme-linked immunosorbent assay; FTA-ABS, fluorescent treponemal antibody absorption tests; IM, intramuscularly; IV, intravenously; Pap, Papanicolaou; PID, pelvic inflammatory disease; PO, orally; VDRL, Venereal Disease Research Laboratory.

risk for discrimination if their sexual orientation is disclosed.

DIAGNOSIS, OUTCOMES, INTERVENTIONS

Altered Health Maintenance. The client with an STD needs to improve health behaviors, which makes *Altered Health Maintenance related to lack of understanding of the causes, treatments, and prevention of STDs* the priority nursing diagnosis.

Outcomes. The client will understand the cause, treatment, and prevention of specific STDs, as evidenced by client's statements, the client's avoidance of STDs, successful treatment of an STD, and, if possible, the absence of recurrence of the STD.

Interventions

Teach About STDs. Provide accurate, factual information about the transmission, prevention, and treatment of STDs (see the Client Education Guide on STDs). Myths about STDs abound; for example, many people erroneously believe that oral contraceptives protect them against STDs. Promote the use of condoms in conjunction with nonbarrier contraceptives, even though clients regard using two methods as difficult. Teaching methods should consider religious and cultural concerns. Include the following topics in teaching sessions about STDs:

1. Name, nature, and seriousness of the condition
2. Mode of transmission
   a. Any sexual activity can spread STDs, not just intercourse.
   b. High-risk activities include new or multiple partners.
3. Actions the client should take to prevent the spread of infection to others

CLIENT EDUCATION GUIDE

Sexually Transmitted Diseases

Treatment will not protect you from getting this disease again. Having a sexually transmitted disease (STD) will not keep you from getting the same disease again or from getting another STD. You must take precautions and use a condom with every sexual encounter to avoid getting STDs.

It is best to wait until you and your sexual partner have finished all your medications before you resume sexual activity. If you wait, you will not be in danger of spreading the infection to your sexual partner or, possibly, of getting the disease again yourself. If you feel that you cannot wait, be sure to use barrier protection, such as a condom.

We would like to see you again if (1) the manifestations do not go away after you have finished your medication, (2) the manifestations return, or (3) you think you may have been exposed to another infection. Be sure to call us if you have any questions.

For women: You should have yearly gynecologic examinations. Along with the Pap smear, ask your doctor to check for STDs. You may have an STD even if you do not have any manifestations.

a. Always use a new latex condom for each sexual act (male and female condoms are available).
b. Finish all the medication given to you.
c. Ensure that your partner is evaluated and treated if needed.
d. Do not have sex until you and your partner have been treated.
e. Do not have sex if you or your partner have any manifestations of an STD.

4. Incubation periods
5. Manifestations of infection
6. Asymptomatic problems
7. When and how to seek treatment
   a. Be sure the client understands the difference between Papanicolaou (Pap) smears and STD examinations; both are not always done at the same time.
8. Treatment methods
   a. Teach client about medication or other treatments.
9. Follow-up care (when and how to obtain it)
10. Consequences of not completing treatment
    a. Infertility
    b. Chronic abdominal pain
    c. Higher risk of ectopic pregnancy or spontaneous abortion
11. Risks and consequences of recurrent infections
    a. STDs increase the risk of acquiring AIDS

Teach Condom Use. The latex condom (called a *rubber* in lay terms) is the most effective mechanical barrier to STDs and its use by sexually active people who are at risk should be promoted. Sexually active men and women should learn to use condoms properly, effectively, and consistently.

There are several barriers to the use of condoms by sexually active people. Women may not believe that they are empowered to make healthy choices. Condoms require male cooperation; unfortunately, many women are in relationships defined by an imbalance of power in which they believe they cannot insist on condom use. Some studies have shown that the fear of losing a sexual partner is greater for some women than the fear of contracting an STD, even AIDS. Condoms may not be acceptable to some clients for religious, social, cultural, or ethnic reasons.

Condom failure is primarily due to improper or inconsistent use rather than to product defect. The Client Education Guide on how to use a condom provides instructions for correct condom use.

Use Therapeutic Communication. When caring for clients with STDs, you obtain privileged or private information and provide instruction about these diseases. Both activities require sensitivity and skillful interaction. You need to be very adept in interpersonal communication to help clients seeking counsel or treatment for STD. Such clients need encouragement, support, and accurate information.

Identify Resources. Nurses play a pivotal role in identifying community and national resources available to clients. Most public health agencies have STD education, prevention, and treatment programs that are open to the public. Clients can also obtain information anonymously from the National STD Hotline (1-800-227-8922) or the National HIV/AIDS Hotline (1-800-342-AIDS).

Anxiety. The client with an STD often experiences a great deal of uncertainty, which makes *Anxiety related to threat to biologic integrity and threat to self-concept* an important nursing diagnosis.

CLIENT EDUCATION GUIDE

How to Use a Condom

Client Instructions

Before Intercourse

- Talk to your partner about using condoms *before* you begin to have sex.
- Decide that you will have sex *only* with a condom.
- Before you have sex, practice using a condom.
- Keep condoms in a handy place.

To Use a Male Condom

- Use a *new latex* condom *each time* you have sex. Do not use natural membrane condoms.

  - Put the condom on before your genitals touch your partner's genitals.
  - Place a spermicide with nonoxynol 9 inside the condom, unless you or your partner is allergic to it. You can buy spermicides in a drug store without a prescription.
  - Place the rolled-up condom on the head of the erect penis.
  - Pinch the end of condom to create a little space to catch what is ejaculated.

  - Unroll the condom until your fingers reach the base of the penis. The condom should unroll easily. If it doesn't, replace it with a new one.
  - Right after ejaculation, hold the condom firmly at the base of the penis and withdraw the penis from the vagina before the erection goes away.
  - Throw the condom away in a safe place. *Never* reuse a condom.

- If you use a lubricant, use only a water-soluble lubricant. Never use oil-based lubricants such as petroleum jelly, baby oil, cooking oil, or shortening, which would destroy the condom.

To Use a Female Condom

- Squeeze the inner ring of the pouch between your fingers, and insert it into the vagina.
- Advance the inner ring until the ring is just behind the pubic bone.
- Leave 1 inch (2.25 cm) of the pouch's open end (the outer ring) outside the vagina.
- Immediately after ejaculation, twist the outer ring and gently pull out the pouch.
- Throw the condom away. *Never* reuse a condom.

Adapted from The American College of Obstetricians and Gynecologists (1995). *ACOG patient education: Gonorrhea and chlamydia* (Pamphlet AP071). Washington, DC: Author.

Outcomes. The client will experience a decrease in anxiety, as evidenced by verbal statements, showing acceptance of the condition, and demonstrating appropriate coping methods.

Interventions

Provide Support. STDs can threaten a client's self-concept and pose potential physical problems, such as infertility and fetal damage. The client may express guilt, apprehension, and fear of rejection. Help the client reduce anxiety by being warm and supportive, facilitating the expression of feelings, and encouraging effective coping strategies.

Help with Problem-Solving. Assist the client with learning and problem-solving once anxiety is reduced. Role-playing and practicing negotiation skills may help a woman become more assertive in being able to ensure her sexual health.

EVALUATION

It is expected that the STD will be succesfully treated and, if possible, eradicated. The client will be able to state the cause, manifestations, treatment, and prevention of STDs and to remain free of STDs.

DISEASES CHARACTERIZED BY URETHRITIS OR CERVICITIS

CHLAMYDIAL INFECTIONS

Chlamydial infection is the nation's most common bacterial STD (see Table 41-1). The number of new cases per year is estimated to be at least 4 million.

Etiology and Risk Factors

The causative organism, *Chlamydia trachomatis,* is a nonmotile, gram-negative bacterium. This organism is the most common cause of what was previously diagnosed as nonspecific vaginitis in women and of nongonococcal urethritis (NGU) in men.

C. trachomatis is always transmitted by intimate sexual contact. Women usually acquire the infection during intercourse with an infected man. Homosexual males can also transmit the infection through oral-anal contact or anal penetration. The infection does not cross the placenta, but passage through the birth canal of an infected mother can cause conjunctivitis and pneumonia in a newborn.

Pathophysiology

Chlamydial infection is known as "the great sterilizer." Undetected and untreated cases can progress to have serious, irreversible consequences. *C. trachomatis* causes inflammation that leads to scarring and ulceration of involved tissue. In women, the infection can extend to the endometrium and salpinx (fallopian tube); the major consequence is salpingitis (inflammation of the fallopian tubes) with subsequent infertility or high risk of ectopic (tubal) pregnancy. Secondary extension to the peritoneum can cause *pelvic inflammatory disease* (PID) (see Chapter 39). In men, the infection can cause a urethral stricture that may extend to the *epididymis.* Sterility can result from the ensuing epididymitis. A serious systemic complication more common in men is Reiter's syndrome, which consists of urethritis, polyarthritis, and conjunctivitis.

Clinical Manifestations

Chlamydial infections primarily affect the cervix, urethra, and rectum. In most cases, the infection is asymptomatic for an extended period. When present, manifestations closely resemble those of gonorrhea but are less severe. In women, the primary site of infection is the endocervix. The cervix becomes edematous and produces a yellow, mucopurulent vaginal discharge. This discharge may be accompanied by spotting at menstrual midcycle or with sexual intercourse. *C. trachomatis* also causes urethritis with dysuria (painful or difficult urination) and urinary frequency in women. One study found that in 65% of women who had urinary manifestations and negative urine culture results, results of culture for *C. trachomatis* were positive. Involvement of Bartholin's duct produces a purulent discharge.

In males, the chief manifestation is urethritis with dysuria (painful and difficult urination) and clear to mucopurulent discharge. In both sexes, proctitis (rectal inflammation) and pharyngitis (inflammation of the pharynx) may develop with rectal and orogenital contact.

Because chlamydial infection may produce few or no manifestations, clients tend not to seek medical treatment and the diagnosis is difficult and often missed. Because chlamydial and gonorrheal infections often coexist, diagnostic tests are recommended for both when either condition is suspected. Presumptive treatment for chlamydial infection in clients being treated for gonorrhea is appropriate, particularly when testing for *C. trachomatis* is not performed.

The definitive test for the fast and accurate diagnosis of chlamydial infection has yet to be developed. The best and most sensitive diagnostic test is tissue culture of cellular material from the urethra, endocervix, or rectum. This test, however, is expensive and technically difficult.

Rapid nonculture detection tests performed on urogenital secretions are readily available, including direct fluorescent antibody (DFA), microscopy and enzyme-linked immunosorbent assay (ELISA), and monoclonal antigen-antibody tests to detect *C. trachomatis* antigens. Although less accurate than cultures, these tests are more convenient, less expensive, and quicker. For men who refuse insertion of a cotton applicator 2 to 4 cm into the urethra to obtain an adequate specimen of urogenital secretions, the ELISA test can be used to detect *C. trachomatis* antigen in the initial 10 to 20 ml of voided urine. These tests are recommended for screening of asymptomatic, high-risk clients in whom chlamydial infection might otherwise go undetected. Priority groups for testing are (1) high-risk pregnant women, (2) adolescents, and (3) women aged 20 to 24 years who have new or multiple sexual partners or who do not use condoms routinely. Many sources also recommend testing any woman with a history of infertility, ectopic pregnancies, or spontaneous abortions.

Outcome Management

■ Medical Management

ERADICATE DISEASE AND MANIFESTATIONS

The treatment of choice for chlamydial infection is doxy-cycline (Vibramycin) given orally for 7 days or one dose of azithromycin (Zithromax). To prevent salpingitis and other serious sequelae, it is imperative that treatment be aggressive and started early and that the entire course of antibiotics be completed. Antichlamydial therapy is almost always effective; therefore, test of cure is not necessary unless manifestations persist or reinfection is suspected.

All partners with whom the client has had sexual contact within 60 days before diagnosis should be examined and treated. When the client's last sexual contact occurred more than 60 days before diagnosis, the last partner should be treated. If testing for chlamydial infection is not available, treatment is often prescribed on the basis of clinical diagnosis only or as co-treatment for gonorrhea. The Bridge to Home Health Care provides information on teaching clients about STDs in a holistic, sensitive manner.

■ Nursing Management of the Medical Client

ERADICATE DISEASE AND MANIFESTATIONS

Instruct clients about the greater risk of infection with multiple sexual partners and inform them of the serious danger of sterility, particularly for women. Infected clients should scrupulously avoid all sexual activity until both partners are cured, and they should use condoms thereafter.

To increase the efficacy of doxycycline, advise clients to space the pills equally throughout each 24-hour period and to avoid iron, dairy products, and antacids during treatment. Clients should report manifestations of superinfection (such as yeast infection, thrush).

GONORRHEA

Gonorrhea (also known as *clap, white, drips, strain,* and *dose* in lay terms) can be divided into two categories: local and disseminated. *Local infection* can involve the mucosal surfaces of the cervix, urethra, and rectum; vestibular glands; pharynx; or conjunctiva. *Systemic infection (disseminated gonococcal infection)* involves bacteremia

---

BRIDGE TO HOME HEALTH CARE

Teaching About Sexually Transmitted Infections

When you are working with people who have sexually transmitted infections, it is important to consider the whole person in relation to their history and development. The infection may be symptomatic of an underlying pattern of risk behavior, such as chemical or alcohol use; such patterns impair your clients' judgment. Adolescents may believe that they are invincible to the risks of these behavior patterns.

Unless you, as the nurse, address the underlying cause of risk behaviors and your clients take action, the chance of recurrent infection remains unchanged. Talk about testing even when manifestations are not present, especially if your client changes partners. The most prevalent sexually transmitted organism, *Chlamydia trachomatis,* is easily transmitted and may not produce manifestations that make intercourse painful or prompt people to seek treatment. If chlamydial infection is detected early in asymptomatic clients, transmission and future problems with infertility can be prevented. Women can be tested easily when they have their Pap smear. When your client has one infection, be alert to the possibility of others. The risk of reinfection continues if the client's partner is not treated at the same time.

Become informed about community resources that offer testing for sexually transmitted infections and contraceptive care. As part of your health education, help clients identify needed resources. Many young adults are uninsured. Adolescents do not want the charges for tests to appear on their parents' bills. Often, community clinics provide testing and treatments at reduced rates and ensure confidentiality for adolescents and young adults. A list of community clinics can be obtained from your state's public health department.

The concept of safer sex is an important focus of preventive education. The only sure protection is a monogamous relationship with a low-risk partner, one who has not used intravenous drugs and has not had previous partners. Although it is advisable to use condoms, they can also give a false sense of security. Genital herpes and warts can be spread to the partner if the lesions are on the perineum and not covered by condoms. Condoms can also break or slip off. Provide information about the correct use of condoms. Instruct clients that irritation from condom latex and spermicides may produce vaginitis that appears to be an infection in sensitive individuals. The irritation increases tissue vulnerability to infection.

Teaching about sexually transmitted infections should include:

- Anticipatory guidance to reduce high-risk behaviors
- Manifestations of infection and consequences of transmission and untreated infection
- Facts about incidence and risk to help clients make informed decisions
- Community resources that offer low-cost, confidential testing and treatment of infections
- Responsibility to inform others who may be exposed to the infection
- Pamphlets about sexually transmitted infections
- Anatomic illustrations and models

As nurses, we can help prevent unnecessary human suffering, birth defects, preterm labor, loss of fertility, premature death, and costly treatments if we provide education and facilitate access to early diagnosis and treatment.

Susan Flannigan, RNC, ANP, MPH, *Adult Nurse Practitioner, Fairview Lakes Medical Center, Chisago City, Minnesota* with polyarthritis, dermatitis, endocarditis, and meningitis. Systemic infection is more common in women.

Etiology and Risk Factors

Gonorrhea is one of the most prevalent STDs in the United States; more than 600,000 new cases are reported each year. It is widely believed that the incidence of gonorrhea is underreported and that the actual number of cases is much greater. Teenagers and young adults are at highest risk. Most cases of gonorrhea occur in people age 15 to 29 years, with the highest rate in those age 20 to 24 years.

Pathophysiology

Gonorrhea is caused by the gram-negative diplococcus *Neisseria gonorrhoeae*. The causative organism does not survive long outside the body. Gonorrhea, therefore, is almost always transmitted by direct sexual contact. The few rare exceptions are infection in infants, who can contract gonorrhea during vaginal birth, and infection of medical personnel through broken skin.

Clinical Manifestations

The endocervical canal is the primary site of gonorrheal infection in women. In most women, the urethra is also infected. Infection can also involve the vestibular glands and anus. The vagina is resistant to the infection in adulthood but not before puberty. The disease may be asymptomatic in women. There is a large *carrier population* (people who carry the organism and have no manifestations but can transmit the disease) for gonorrhea. Manifestations of gonorrhea include (1) heavy, yellow-green, purulent vaginal discharge, (2) cervical erythema, (3) a red, swollen, sore vulva, (4) abnormal menstrual bleeding, and (5) dysuria and urinary frequency.

The most common complication of gonorrhea in women is salpingitis, which can progress to PID. Both PID and salpingitis can produce infertility secondary to scarring and occlusion of the fallopian tubes. The first recognizable manifestations of gonorrhea in women may arise from PID.

Manifestations of gonorrhea are usually evident earlier in men than in women. The infection is principally one of the anterior urethra that produces a purulent discharge, dysuria, and urinary frequency. Complications include epididymitis and prostatitis, but these are not common with early and complete antibiotic therapy.

In addition to the gender-specific manifestations, both men and women may have conjunctivitis or pharyngitis due to orogenital contact or proctitis from anal contact.

Disseminated infection, the most serious form of gonorrhea, results from gonococcal bacteremia and is often manifested by septic arthritis, skin lesions, asymmetrical arthralgias, and tenosynovitis (inflammation of the tendon and synovial membrane). Rarely, hepatic adhesions (Fitz-Hugh–Curtis syndrome), endocarditis, or meningitis may occur.

Diagnosis of gonorrhea is made through history, physical examination, identification of the gonococcus on a smear, and culture of the exudate from infected areas. Culture with selective culture media remains the cornerstone of diagnosis.

Outcome Management

▇ Medical Management

ERADICATE DISEASE AND MANIFESTATIONS

All sexually active women in high-risk groups should be screened for gonorrhea on a regular basis. All clients in whom gonorrhea is detected should also be tested for chlamydial infection.

Gonorrhea is treated aggressively with antibiotics. Before the advent of resistant organisms, penicillin was the treatment of choice. The current recommended regimen for uncomplicated gonorrhea is a single intramuscular (IM) dose of ceftriaxone (Rocephin), or a single oral dose of cefixime (Suprax), ciprofloxacin (Cipro), or ofloxacin (Floxin). Any of these single doses is followed by oral doxycycline (Vibramycin) for 7 days for the presumptive treatment of co-infection with *C. trachomatis* (chlamydial infection commonly coexists with gonorrhea). A single IM injection of spectinomycin (Trobicin) plus oral doxycycline can be used for clients who cannot tolerate ceftriaxone.

For clients with disseminated gonococcal infection, the recommended regimen is administration of ceftriaxone, given IM or IV every 24 hours and continued 24 to 48 hours after improvement begins, followed by cefixime or ciprofloxacin, given orally for a full week.

After therapy for uncomplicated gonorrhea is completed, a follow-up examination and culture are not necessary. Treatment failure following combined ceftriaxone-doxycycline therapy is rare. Manifestations that persist after treatment should be evaluated with a follow-up culture. Any gonococcal organisms appearing on the second culture should be tested for antibiotic sensitivity to identify possible resistant organisms.

▇ Nursing Management of the Medical Client

ERADICATE DISEASE AND MANIFESTATIONS

Discuss the importance of identifying and treating all sexual partners, as there seems to be a reservoir population of asymptomatic men. Recurrence due to reinfection may indicate the need for improved client education and sexual partner referral.

Warn pregnant clients of the danger of infecting their newborns during delivery. Clients receiving treatment for gonorrhea must understand the importance of taking the *complete* course of prescribed medication. Common side effects of treatment are pain at the injection site and yeast infection. Clients should understand that because of its long half-life, azithromycin is given only once.

Investigation of the client's sexual contacts is essential for the prevention and control of gonorrhea. All sexual partners who were exposed to the client's gonorrhea within the 60 days before the diagnosis should undergo examination, culture, and presumptive treatment. Reporting sexual contacts can be difficult and frightening for an infected client. Ask for contact information in a positive, non-threatening, sensitive way during the initial treatment visit.

DISEASES CHARACTERIZED BY ULCERATIONS

SYPHILIS

Syphilis (lay terms are *bad blood, lues, pox,* and *syph*) is a systemic, highly infectious STD (see Table 41–1). It became less prevalent after the advent of penicillin, but the disease has not been eradicated. The incidence of syphilis has been rising since about 1960, and it is one of the most commonly reported communicable diseases in the United States.

Etiology and Risk Factors

Syphilis is caused by the delicate motile (self-moving) spirochete *Treponema pallidum.* Although *T. pallidum* cannot survive long outside the body, syphilis is highly infectious. Sexual transmission of *T. pallidum* occurs only when the mucocutaneous lesions of primary and secondary syphilis are present. Adolescents, young adults, African American men, and homosexual men are at greatest risk.

Pathophysiology

T. pallidum enters the body through intact mucous membranes or abraded skin, almost exclusively by direct sexual contact. After entry, the organisms multiply locally and disseminate systemically through the bloodstream and lymphatics. The infection can also be passed transplacentally from an untreated pregnant woman to her fetus during any stage of the disease (*congenital syphilis*).

In rare instances, syphilis has been contracted through nonsexual personal contact, accidental inoculation, or blood transfusion from a syphilitic donor. Syphilis can progress to irreversible blindness, mental illness, paralysis, heart disease, and death.

Clinical Manifestations

STAGES

Syphilis is characterized by well-defined sequential stages that occur over years: primary, secondary, latent (early latent and late latent), and late or tertiary.

PRIMARY STAGE. The principal manifestation of primary syphilis is the appearance of a genital chancre. A *chancre* is an oval ulcer with a raised firm border that does not bleed readily and is painless unless infected (Fig. 41–1). The chancre develops at the site of inoculation, usually the genitalia, anus, or mouth. Most commonly, a single chancre occurs about 4 weeks after initial infection. Chancres in women often remain unnoticed. Lymphadenopathy may occur as lymph glands near the chancre become enlarged. Nodes are painless, firm, and discrete. If untreated, a chancre heals spontaneously in 4 to 6 weeks, leaving a thin, atrophic scar.

SECONDARY STAGE. If the primary disease is untreated, secondary syphilis develops 6 to 8 weeks after infection. Indications of the second stage are:

1. *Generalized rash.* Typically, a maculopapular and nonpruritic rash appears on the palms of the hands and soles of the feet (few other diseases cause a rash in these locations).

FIGURE 41–1 Ulcer of primary syphilis. (Courtesy of Dr. Rodney M. S. Basler.)

2. *Generalized, nontender, discrete lymphadenopathy.*
3. *Mucous patches.* Gray, superficial patches occur on the mucous membranes in the mouth and may be accompanied by a sore throat.
4. *Condylomata lata.* Broad-based, flat papules, these lesions usually can be easily distinguished from the typical narrow-based, pedunculated growth of condylomata acuminata (genital warts). Condylomata lata may develop in warm, moist body areas—most commonly on the labia or anus or at the corners of the mouth. They are highly contagious.
5. *General flu-like manifestations,* including nausea, anorexia, constipation, headache, muscle, joint, and bone pain, and a chronically elevated temperature.
6. *Patchy hair loss* from eyebrows and scalp (alopecia).

Secondary stage manifestations usually disappear after 2 to 6 weeks. A latency period then begins.

LATENT STAGE. The latent stage of syphilis typically produces no manifestations. *Latent syphilis* is defined as that period after infection with *T. pallidum* when a client is seroreactive (with a positive blood test) but shows no other evidence of disease. During this stage, syphilis is noninfectious except via transplacental spread or blood transfusion. Syphilis is not transmitted by sexual contact during the latent phase unless a secondary syphilitic mucocutaneous skin lesion reoccurs during early latent syphilis. Latent syphilis usually occurs 1 to 2 years after the primary lesion and can last as long as 50 years. About 66% of infected clients remain in this stage without further problems.

TERTIARY STAGE. In 1 to 35 years after the primary infection, about 33% of clients with untreated syphilis experience devastating, irreversible complications, such as chronic bone and joint inflammation, cardiovascular problems (for example, valvular involvement, aneurysms), granulomatous lesions (*gummas*) on any part of the body, and ophthalmic, auditory, and central nervous system problems. This stage, although not infectious, may be terminal if untreated (see Chapter 69 for manifestations of neurosyphilis [syphilis affecting the central nervous system]).

DIAGNOSIS

The diagnosis of syphilis is based on health assessment and various direct and indirect laboratory studies. A *direct test* identifies the causative organism; an *indirect test* identifies antibodies of the causative agent. *T. pallidum* cannot be grown in culture. Primary or secondary stage lesions can be scraped and the causative organism identified directly with dark-field microscopy or DFA testing. Dark-field examination must be done by an expert, because other spirochetes closely resembling *T. pallidum* are present in oral and genital mucosa. This test confirms a diagnosis of syphilis in the primary stage (when other tests are generally negative) and the secondary stage.

Serologic tests for syphilis are indirect tests that detect antibodies. These antibodies are not present in the serum until 4 weeks *after* the appearance of the chancre. Such tests include:

- The Venereal Disease Research Laboratory (VDRL)
- Rapid plasma reagin (RPR), which uses an antigen to detect the antibody relatively specific for *T. pallidum*
- Fluorescent treponemal antibody absorption (FTA-ABS) tests

The VDRL test for nonspecific antibodies is the most commonly used screening test. Results are negative in the early primary stage, before antibodies to *T. pallidum* are formed and are present in the circulation. Results may be falsely positive if the VDRL test is performed during the early stages of several common viral illnesses (mumps, measles, hepatitis, chickenpox, infectious mononucleosis). Results are given as "nonreactive," "borderline," "weakly reactive," or "reactive." Reactive and weakly reactive results are considered to be positive.

The FTA-ABS serologic test is more specific because it measures antibodies specific to *T. pallidum*. It is used when the VDRL result is positive but the diagnosis of syphilis is still uncertain. In clients who have mononucleosis or systemic lupus erythematosus, a false-positive test result is possible. The FTA-ABS test result usually becomes positive 3 to 4 weeks after infection. Once positive, FTA-ABS test results usually remain positive for the client's life, regardless of treatment or cure. Cerebrospinal fluid may be examined for characteristic findings in late neurosyphilis.

Syphilis often coexists with other infections. The CDC recommends that all clients with syphilis be counseled on the risks of HIV infection and AIDS and encouraged to undergo HIV testing.

Outcome Management

■ Medical Management

ERADICATE DISEASE AND MANFESTATIONS

Parenteral penicillin remains the treatment of choice for all stages of syphilis; however, the structural changes present in late syphilis are irreversible despite successful treatment. The dosage schedule and length of therapy are determined by the stage of the disease and current guidelines for treatment. For primary, secondary, and early latent syphilis, the treatment of choice is benzathine penicillin G, given IM in one dose. Late latent syphilis is treated with three weekly penicillin injections. Neuro-syphilis is treated with IV aqueous crystalline penicillin G.

Use of penicillin to treat syphilis in clients with penicillin allergy is a complicated issue. Clients who are pregnant or noncompliant with therapy or who have neuro-syphilis should undergo desensitization and treatment with penicillin. Desensitization guidelines are available from the CDC. For nonpregnant clients who are allergic to penicillin, oral doxycycline or tetracycline for 2 weeks may be given, but they are not as effective as penicillin.

Treatment failure can occur with any given regimen. Compliance is often a problem. Clients should be reexamined clinically and evaluated with serologic testing at 6, 12, and 24 months after treatment. No definitive criteria for cure exist. With successful treatment, ideally, no evidence of disease should be present and serial serologic test values should decline.

Treating sexual partners is also a complex issue; treatment is best guided by information available from the CDC. All people who have had sexual contact with the client who has primary syphilis must be identified and evaluated. Most practitioners treat sexual contacts as if they have primary syphilis whether or not they show evidence of infection.

■ Nursing Management of the Medical Client

ERADICATE DISEASE AND MANIFESTATIONS

A client with syphilis needs information and psychosocial support to deal with this complex illness. Individualize health teaching to meet the client's particular needs and psychosocial situation. A diagnosis of syphilis can be frightening and difficult to accept.

Clients with primary or secondary syphilis should abstain from sexual contact for at least 1 month after treatment. Adequate treatment should be curative, but reinfection is possible and can be detected with clinical examinations and monitoring of serologic test values. Proper follow-up, although essential, is time-consuming and difficult. Many clients do not understand the severe consequences of not obtaining adequate treatment.

GENITAL HERPES

Genital herpes is a recurrent, systemic viral infection (see Table 41–1). Although recognized for centuries, genital herpes has received renewed attention because of its epidemic incidence. Now one of the most common STDs (45 million cases in the United States), it is the most frequent cause of genital ulceration. Its peak incidence is among adolescents and young adults.

Etiology and Risk Factors

Caused by herpes simplex virus (HSV) type 2, the infection is closely related to other herpes infections, such as the classic cold sore caused by HSV type 1. HSV type 1 infection is mainly nongenital, occurring above the waist (often on the lips or nose). HSV type 2 infection occurs primarily below the waist as a sexually transmitted genital infection. It is possible for HSV type 1 to cause genital infections and for HSV type 2 to cause oral lesions (Fig. 41–2).

FIGURE 41–2 Typical herpes vesicles. (Courtesy of Dr. Rodney M. S. Basler.)

Pathophysiology

The HSV organism is present in the exudate of the lesion. Herpes can be transmitted while a lesion is present and for 10 days after a lesion has healed. Genital herpes is usually transmitted by direct contact with the exudate during sexual activity, but transmission is possible by *fomites* (objects that can harbor pathogenic microorganisms), such as towels used by an infected person. Many cases of genital herpes are acquired from people who do not know they have an infection or who are asymptomatic at the time of sexual contact. Newborns can be infected during vaginal delivery when active genital lesions are present. Birth by cesarean section prevents this transmission.

Clinical Manifestations

Many people with HSV type 2 infection have mild or unrecognized disease. Manifestations of genital herpes usually occur 3 to 7 days after contact. Initially, a burning sensation (paresthesia) is noted at the site of inoculation. Next, numerous small vesicles with an erythematous border form painful, shallow ulcers that then crust and heal with a scar in about 2 to 4 weeks.

The major problem with HSV is recurrence. Up to 75% of clients have a recurrent infection within 1 year of the first episode. The virus is believed to lie dormant in the body, probably in nerve ganglions, until it is activated, at which point another episode of genital herpes, with characteristic lesions, occurs. Stress, infection, trauma, menses, or sexual activity may trigger recurrent episodes.

Characteristically, recurrent genital herpes causes local, but not systemic, manifestations. Prodromal (pre-onset) manifestations of a burning sensation may occur before the vesicles erupt. The vesicles tend to reappear at the sites of previous infection, but they can involve new sites. Manifestations are similar to, but usually less severe than, those in the primary infection. Vesicles rupture in 24 to 48 hours, and the syndrome generally lasts 7 to 10 days.

Potential complications of HSV infections include disseminated infections, meningitis, and transverse myelitis.

Women are at risk for spontaneous abortion, and it has been suggested that HSV type 2 predisposes to carcinoma of the cervix.

A diagnosis of genital herpes is often made visually. The diagnosis is confirmed by a viral culture, direct immunofluorescence staining, or antigen detection testing of the vesicular exudate. A Pap smear can also be performed; the presence of multinucleated giant cells in the Pap smear, with or without inclusion bodies, is characteristic of a herpes infection.

Outcome Management

▮ Medical Management

REDUCE MANIFESTATIONS

Genital herpes is a chronic disease without a cure. Management is geared toward preventing or lessening occurrences and giving palliative care. The recommended treatment for an acute primary infection is acyclovir (Zovirax), an antiviral agent, taken orally for 7 to 10 days. Episodic recurrences are treated with acyclovir, valacyclovir (Valtrex), or famciclovir (Famvir) taken for 5 days.

Clients with frequent recurrences (six or more episodes in 1 year) take daily suppressive therapy. Daily acyclovir taken for 4 months to 3 years may prevent or reduce the frequency and severity of recurrence in most clients. After 1 year, the acyclovir should be discontinued to assess the need for continued suppressive therapy. If genital herpes recurs, daily therapy is resumed.

Severe disease is treated with IV acyclovir for 5 to 7 days.

▮ Nursing Management of the Medical Client

PREVENT REINFECTION

When the vesicles of herpes rupture, they release a highly contagious exudate. Clients as well as health care personnel must observe strict medical asepsis in the presence of HSV infection. Clients should wash their hands thoroughly after any contact with the herpetic lesions to avoid *autoinoculation* (spread of the disease to another part of their own bodies). HSV infections of the eye are particularly serious. Advise infected clients to have separate towels and other personal items and to avoid touching their eyes. Clients should use condoms during latent periods because the possible risk of transmission exists even when lesions are not present. Women should have annual pelvic examinations and Pap smears because of the association of HSV with cervical cancer.

PROVIDE SUPPORT

Coping with genital herpes may cause tremendous psychosocial stress. Although recurrence cannot always be predicted, nurses can help clients identify possible triggers. Reappearance of the disease can significantly affect sexual activity. Support groups may help clients deal with the anger, guilt, and shame that many commonly feel. Stress reduction techniques may be helpful. Sexual partners should be offered counseling, evaluation, and treatment if needed.

RELIEVE PAIN

The pain of herpes lesions is problematic. Palliative measures include (1) keeping the involved area clean and dry,

(2) wearing loose-fitting, nonsynthetic undergarments, and (3) using sitz baths, cooling applications, and analgesic medications, such as aspirin, for pain relief.

Clients should understand that acyclovir does not cure HSV infection or prevent its spread. Clients should begin oral suppressive therapy when they first recognize the prodromal sensations or first become symptomatic. Topical acyclovir ointment should be applied with a glove and should never be put in or around the eyes.

CHANCROID

Chancroid is a highly contagious infection caused by the gram-negative bacillus *Haemophilus ducreyi*. The initial papules or pustules produce multiple painful, irregular, and deep genital ulcers, often accompanied by tender inguinal lymphadenopathy (Fig. 41–3). Although chancroid is more common in the tropics, the incidence is endemic in many areas of the United States. Chancroid is well established as a cofactor for HIV transmission. There is a high rate of HIV infection in clients with chancroid.

Definitive diagnosis requires the culture of *H. ducreyi*. It is difficult to isolate the organism, and culture of *H. ducreyi* is not widely available. A probable diagnosis may be made if the client has one or more painful genital ulcers and regional lymphadenopathy (especially tender inguinal adenopathy) without clinical or serologic evidence of syphilis or genital herpes. People with whom the client has had sexual contact within 10 days before the onset of manifestations should be examined and treated. Clients with chancroid should also be tested for HIV infection, HSV infection, and syphilis.

Recommended treatment is oral azithromycin or ceftriaxone given IM in a single dose; alternatively, ciprofloxacin or erythromycin may be given orally.

LYMPHOGRANULOMA VENEREUM

Lymphogranuloma venereum is a systemic infection that is rare in the United States. It is caused by certain strains of *C. trachomatis*. The primary lesion is a small, painless papule on the glans penis or the vaginal mucosa that heals spontaneously and may go unnoticed.

FIGURE 41–3 Chancroid lesions. (Courtesy of Dr. Rodney M. S. Basler.)

The most common clinical manifestations are markedly tender, enlarged, and inflamed inguinal lymph nodes (*buboes*), which are usually unilateral and appear 2 to 6 weeks after the primary lesion. Eventually, draining ulcerations, scarring, lymphatic obstruction, and marked external genital deformity may occur. Rectal fibrosis and strictures are late sequelae.

Definitive diagnosis is made with a positive culture for *C. trachomatis*. Recommended therapy is doxycycline, given orally for 21 days. Oral erythromycin is an alternative.

GRANULOMA INGUINALE

Granuloma inguinale (donovanosis) is a chronic infection endemic in some tropical and developing areas but rare in the United States. It is caused by the small gram-negative bacillus *Calymmatobacterium granulomatis*.

Granuloma inguinale is characterized by genital and perianal papular lesions without lymphadenopathy. These become painless, gradually enlarging, ulcerating granulomatous lesions that cause tissue destruction that is difficult to differentiate from cancer. The lesions are highly vascular, bleed easily, and have a beefy-red appearance. Diagnosis is made by microscopic identification of Donovan's bodies (inclusion bodies of the causative organism) in a smear taken from edge scrapings of the lesion.

Treatment consists of a long course of an antibiotic such as trimethoprim-sulfamethoxazole or doxycycline. Relapses can occur despite adequate treatment. IV aminoglycosides are given for infections that do not improve with first-line antibiotics. All partners who have had sexual contact with an infected client within 60 days before diagnosis need evaluation and treatment.

INFECTION WITH HUMAN PAPILLOMAVIRUS

GENITAL WARTS (CONDYLOMATA ACUMINATA)

Etiology and Risk Factors

Genital warts, the fourth most common STD, are caused by HPV; they are usually transmitted by sexual contact (see Table 41–1). Factors that may favor their development include HIV, pregnancy, smoking, drug or alcohol use, poor nutrition, and fatigue.

Pathophysiology

More than 20 types of HPV affect the genital tract. The natural history of HPV is complex and poorly understood. Infection with certain strains of HPV is strongly associated with carcinomas of the genitals, including the cervix.

Clinical Manifestations

Genital warts are benign growths that typically occur in multiple, painless clusters on the vulva, vagina, cervix, perineum, anorectal area, urethral meatus, or glans penis 1 to 2 months after exposure (Fig. 41–4). Oral, pharyngeal, and laryngeal lesions can also occur. HPV can cause

FIGURE 41–4 Genital warts (condylomata acuminata). (Courtesy of Dr. Rodney M. S. Basler.)

laryngeal papillomatosis in infants born to mothers with vaginal warts.

Diagnosis is typically made visually. Subclinical (asymptomatic or not visible) warts can be identified through Pap smear and colposcopy (examination of vagina and cervical tissues with a scope containing a magnifying lens) of the cervix. Biopsy of lesions may be performed to differentiate warts from carcinoma or condylomata lata of the secondary stage of syphilis.

Outcome Management

▪ Medical Management

REMOVE VISIBLE WARTS

There is no cure for genital warts. A variety of chemical, mechanical, and ablative techniques are used for visible lesions, but no specific antiviral therapy for the HPV is available. Treatment varies according to the site and severity of the warts and is also guided by client preference. Treatment is more successful if the warts are small and have been present for less than a year.

TOPICAL THERAPY. The most common pharmacologic treatment is podophyllin in compound tincture of benzoin or trichloroacetic acid (TCA) applied topically to the warts *only*. Treatments are repeated weekly until all the lesions have disappeared and the skin is healed. Podophyllin is contraindicated during pregnancy because of its *abortifacient* (abortion-causing) properties.

Topical podofilox is the only agent approved for self-application by clients at home. For safe application, the client must be able to see and reach the warts easily. Podofilox is also contraindicated during pregnancy. If warts persist, other modes of therapy should be considered.

OTHER TREATMENT. Warts can be treated with cryotherapy using liquid nitrogen or a cryoprobe. Carbon di-

oxide lasers, electrocautery, and simple surgical excision can be used on extensive warts. The antiviral drug interferon has also been used, but it is expensive and is associated with a high rate of adverse side effects. Remember, genital warts are not cured, and recurrence is very common.

It is not necessary to evaluate and treat sexual partners of clients with genital warts, since treatment is not effective in eradicating the disease or its spread. Female partners should be referred for a Pap smear, and all sexual partners should be offered the opportunity to be examined and tested for other STDs.

▪ Nursing Management of the Medical Client

Inform clients with genital warts that no cure exists. Clients must be warned that they are at increased risk for genital malignancy. HPV infections are strongly associated with cancer of the cervix and vulva in women and squamous cell carcinoma of the penis in men. All women with genital warts should receive a Pap smear *at least* every year and, when indicated, cervical colposcopy and biopsy. Encourage condom use. Improved detection and treatment of HPV infection in men may be important to prevent genital carcinoma in women.

DISEASES CHARACTERIZED BY VAGINAL DISCHARGE

Infections manifested by vaginal discharge include trichomoniasis and vaginitis (bacterial and yeast). Though occasionally transmitted sexually, candidiasis (vaginal yeast infection) is generally not considered an STD. Recurrent vaginal yeast infections are a common manifestation of HIV infection in women (see Chapter 39 for discussion of vaginitis).

TRICHOMONIASIS

Etiology and Risk Factors

Trichomoniasis is a protozoal infection causing vulvovaginitis. Although not life-threatening, the incidence is very high worldwide and the disease remains a major health problem. Often asymptomatic, trichomoniasis affects 3 million people annually, and its role in PID and infertility may be greatly underestimated.

Pathophysiology

Trichomoniasis is caused by the anaerobic, flagellated, parasitic protozoan *Trichomonas vaginalis*. The organism is almost always transmitted sexually. *T. vaginalis* prefers an alkaline environment (pH 6 to 7), and alterations in the vaginal *flora* (the usual bacteria and fungi) make a woman more susceptible to infection. Trichomoniasis can be very resistant to treatment, and recurrence is common.

Clinical Manifestations

Manifestations may be minor, especially in men. In women, manifestations include a copious, malodorous, yellow-green vaginal discharge. This is irritating to the vulva and causes severe itching, burning, and excoriation and maceration of the vulvar tissues. Occasionally, the cervix is covered with punctate (point-like) hemorrhages ("strawberry cervix"). The vaginal mucosa appears reddened and slightly edematous. Some women experience dyspareunia (pain during sexual intercourse).

If trichomoniasis extends to the urethra, urinary frequency and burning with urination may occur. This is the most common manifestation in a man. Anal involvement may also occur, either asymptomatically or with a slight discharge. Bladder and anal involvement are more common when the infection has become chronic.

The diagnosis can be made immediately in the health care facility after a fresh, warm specimen of vaginal exudate in a saline wet mount is examined under a microscope and the highly motile organisms are identified. Cultures are an option but are rarely necessary. A wet mount is obtained by placing a drop of vaginal exudate on a glass slide, mixing in a drop of saline, and covering it with a cover slide. The vaginal speculum used to obtain the exudate must be inserted without lubrication to avoid destroying the organism. If possible, instruct the client not to douche before the vaginal examination.

Outcome Management

■ Medical Management

ERADICATE DISEASE AND MANIFESTATIONS
The preferred treatment of trichomoniasis is a single oral dose of metronidazole (Flagyl) with simultaneous treatment of all sexual partners for a cure. Metronidazole should not be taken during the first trimester of pregnancy because it may adversely affect fetal development. *T. vaginalis* does not affect the fetus. Single-dose metronidazole therapy is usually curative, but recurrence is common.

Instruct clients to seek prompt treatment if manifestations return. Metronidazole may be given in a 7-day regimen for recurrent infection.

■ Nursing Management of the Medical Client

Advise clients taking metronidazole not to drink alcoholic beverages, because doing so might cause nausea, vomiting, and headaches. This prohibition includes all alcohol-containing products, such as cough syrup. Emphasize the importance of good perineal hygiene.

Treatment should continue through the client's menstrual period because the vagina is more alkaline during this time and a flare-up is more likely to occur. Metronidazole can be taken without regard to meals. Advise clients that urine may turn dark, reddish brown.

BACTERIAL VAGINOSIS

Bacterial vaginosis (BV), formerly known as nonspecific or *Gardnerella* vaginitis, is a common condition in adults.

Etiology and Risk Factors

Bacterial vaginosis is linked to sexual activity, although not all cases are caused by sexual activity.

Pathophysiology

Like the organisms responsible for vulvovaginal *Candida* (yeast) infections, the causative bacteria are found in the normal vagina. The infection is thought to be caused by the overgrowth of a number of different organisms, including *Gardnerella vaginalis* and vaginal anaerobes. Overgrowth may occur when the normal flora and pH of the vagina are altered.

Clinical Manifestations

The vulvovaginitis produced by bacterial vaginosis is mild or asymptomatic. The main manifestation is a mild to moderate, malodorous vaginal discharge. The discharge is usually thin, watery, and grayish white and tends to adhere to the vaginal wall. The odor is described as "fishy," and is often more noticeable after sexual intercourse. Manifestations are almost always confined to the vulvovaginal area. Mild vaginal burning and irritation may occur, but redness and pruritus are not common.

Evaluation is mainly by physical examination of the vagina, microscopic examination of the discharge, and determination of the pH of the discharge. The diagnosis is determined by the presence of at least three of the following manifestations:

- A homogeneous gray or white discharge that adheres to the vaginal wall
- Vaginal fluid pH higher than 4.5 (normal pH is 4.0 to 4.5)
- Positive result of the "whiff" test—a fishy odor elicited when potassium hydroxide (KOH) is added to the vaginal fluid
- Presence of *clue cells* (desquamated vaginal epithelial cells characteristically stippled by the adherence of coccobacilli to their surfaces) on either a saline wet mount or a Gram's stain of vaginal fluid

Outcome Management

■ Medical Management

The recommended treatment of bacterial vaginosis in nonpregnant women is metronidazole (Flagyl), given orally for 7 days. Single-dose regimens can be used to improve compliance, but they are less effective than the 7-day regimen. Pregnant women are treated with lower doses of metronidazole to minimize exposure to the fetus. Alternative treatment includes metronidazole in a high, single dose, clindamycin orally, or metronidazole vaginal gel (data are limited on metronidazole gel use during pregnancy).

■ Nursing Management of the Medical Client

BV is not necessarily transmitted sexually, though its occurrence is associated with sexual activity. Treatment of male partners is recommended only with recurrent or resistant infection. Recurrence is common.

ACQUIRED IMMUNODEFICIENCY SYNDROME

AIDS is a viral STD that has reached epidemic proportions worldwide. HIV infection has had an effect on the transmission of STDs, and vice versa. People with AIDS are more susceptible to other STDs. These coexistent STDs require more aggressive therapy and tend to recur. Conversely, people infected with an STD, especially those with genital ulcerations, are more susceptible to AIDS. On the positive side, national campaigns to prevent and control the transmission of HIV have had a beneficial effect on the incidence of some STDs (e.g., reduced incidence of hepatitis B in the homosexual population). AIDS is discussed in Chapter 79.

VACCINE-PREVENTABLE DISEASES

Vaccines for STDs are receiving attention as possible strategies for control of STDs. Currently, vaccines are available for hepatitis B and hepatitis A. Trials are under way for vaccines against other STDs.

HEPATITIS A AND HEPATITIS B

Sexual contact is the most frequently reported mode of transmission for the hepatitis B virus (HBV) (30% to 60% of all cases), although blood-borne and perinatal transmission also occur. Clients at high risk for sexually transmitted hepatitis B are (1) heterosexuals with multiple sexual partners, (2) sexual partners of IV drug users, and (3) homosexual men. Sexually transmitted hepatitis B has decreased dramatically in the homosexual population, probably as a result of the modification of high-risk sexual behaviors to prevent AIDS.

Hepatitis A is caused by a virus shed in the stool. The virus is also found in serum and saliva. Risk factors for hepatitis A include (1) sexual contact with people who have the virus, (2) homosexual activity, and (3) IV drug abuse or sexual contact with an IV drug user. Vaccination is recommended for gay and bisexual men and for sexual partners of IV drug users if a local outbreak occurs within this population. See Chapter 47 for further discussion of hepatitis A and B.

DISEASES CAUSED BY INFESTATIONS

PEDICULOSIS PUBIS AND SCABIES

Cutaneous infestation with pubic lice (pediculosis pubis) or mites (scabies) results either from close physical contact with an infected person or from contact with contaminated objects of an infected person, such as linens and clothing. Because sexual transmission is possible, these conditions are included in any list of STDs. For further discussion, see Chapter 49.

SEXUALLY TRANSMITTED ENTERIC INFECTIONS

Gastroenteritis caused by enteric pathogens are typically acquired from food or water contaminated with fecal matter. Since the mid-1970s, it has been recognized that these pathogens can also be transmitted by oral and anal sexual contact. Sexually transmitted enteric infections include shigellosis, salmonellosis, amebiasis, and giardiasis.

Homosexual men are at highest risk for these infections. See Chapter 33 for discussion of gastroenteritis.

MANAGEMENT OF CLIENTS REPORTING SEXUAL ASSAULT

Victims of sexual assault need immense support from health care professionals, a discussion of which is beyond the scope of this chapter. Regarding STDs, a sexual assault victim needs an immediate physical examination, including tests for pregnancy, gonorrhea, chlamydial infection, trichomoniasis, HIV, hepatitis A and B, and syphilis. Follow-up testing should be repeated in 2 weeks; syphilis and HIV testing should also be repeated at 6, 12, and 24 months. Prophylaxis for HIV infection is described in Chapter 79.

CONCLUSIONS

STDs are more prevalent now than ever before. This phenomenon is attributable to many factors. The improper and indiscriminate use of antibiotics has produced a number of resistant organisms. Sexual activity, especially among adolescents and young adults, has increased. Many STDs are asymptomatic and go undetected. As a nurse, you are in a unique position to help clients salvage or restore their sexual health and have an ever-increasing responsibility and role in the prevention, early detection, and treatment of STDs.

THINKING CRITICALLY

1. **A 20-year-old unmarried man comes to a walk-in STD clinic with a purulent urethral discharge. The diagnosis is uncomplicated gonorrhea. The client has no known allergies. He is sexually active with multiple partners. He gives a temporary address. What are the priorities of care? What are the priority interventions?**

Factors to Consider. What effect would the client's status as a walk-in client have on your planning? Consider the fact that gonorrhea often leads to PID in women. What effect would the client's temporary address have on your planning and need for identification of partners? What diseases are likely to coexist with gonorrhea?

2. **Your client is a 65-year-old widowed woman who comes for treatment of acute, symptomatic genital herpes. Her male sexual contact told her when their sexual relationship began that he had a history of genital herpes but that, because he had no active lesions, there was no risk of her becoming infected. She is humiliated by having contracted herpes and tells you that she feels dirty and contaminated. She also states that she "knows nothing" about condoms, and, furthermore, that she "wouldn't be caught dead buying them." What are the goals of her care? What interventions might be used?**

Factors to Consider. How accurate is the client's knowledge about the transmission of genital herpes? What are the client's psychosocial needs? What obstacles to buying condoms can you identify, and how will you help this client control her sexual health?

3. A 25-year-old monogamous woman seeks outpatient treatment for the irritating, malodorous vaginal discharge of trichomoniasis. She has had trichomoniasis before, and metronidazole (Flagyl) was prescribed. What interventions should the care of this client include?

Factors to Consider. Knowing that metronidazole is usually curative, consider what might have caused the client's recurrence.

BIBLIOGRAPHY

1. Able, E., Hilton, P., & Miller, I. (1996). Sexual risk behavior among urban women of childbearing age: Implications for clinical practice. *Journal of American Academy of Nurse Practitioners, 8*(3), 115–124.
2. Borchardt, K., & Noble, M. (Eds.). (1997). *Sexually transmitted diseases: Epidemiology, pathology, diagnosis, and treatment.* Boca Raton, FL: CRC Press.
3. Buzby, M. (1996). Viral hepatitis: A sexually transmitted disease? *Nurse Practitioner Forum, 7*(1), 10–15.
4. Carson, S. (1997). Human papillomatous virus infection update: Impact on women's health. *Nurse Practitioner: American Journal of Primary Health Care, 22*(4), 24–5, 28, 30, 35–37.
5. Centers for Disease Control and Prevention. (1998). 1998 guidelines for treatment of sexually transmitted diseases. *Morbidity and Mortality Weekly Report (Suppl.), 47*(RR-1), 1–116.
6. Dienstag, J. L. (1997). Sexual and perinatal transmission of hepatitis C. *Hepatology, 26*(3, suppl. 1), 66S–70S.
7. Ferreira, N. (1997). Sexually transmitted *Chlamydia trachomatis. Nurse Practitioner Forum, 8*(2), 70–76.
8. Fleming, D., et al. (1997). Herpes simplex virus type 2 in the United States, 1976–1994. *New England Journal of Medicine, 337,* 1105–1111.
9. Ford, K., & Norris, A. E. (1996). Sexually transmitted diseases: Experience and risk factors among urban low income, African American and Hispanic youth. *Ethnicity and Health, 1*(2), 175–184.
10. Fugate, K. A., & McClusky, M. M. (1996). The impact of sexually transmitted diseases on fertility. *Infertility and Reproductive Medicine Clinics of North America, 7,* 521–534.
11. Gorbach, S., Bartlett, J., & Blacklow, N. (1998). *Infectious diseases* (2nd ed.). Philadelphia: W. B. Saunders.
12. Gunn, R., et al. (1998). The changing paradigm of sexually transmitted disease control in the era of managed health care. *JAMA, 279,* 680–684.
13. Hiltabiddle, S. J. (1996). Adolescent condom use, the health belief model, and the prevention of sexually transmitted disease. *Journal of Obstetric, Gynecologic, and Neonatal Nursing, 25,* 61–66.
14. Jackson, S., & Soper, D. (1997). Sexually transmitted diseases in pregnancy. *Obstetrics and Gynecology Clinics of North America, 24,* 631–644.
15. Kenney, J., Reinholtz, C., & Angelini, P. (1998). Sexual abuse, sex before age 16, and high-risk behaviors of young females with sexually transmitted diseases. *Journal of Obstetric, Gynecologic, and Neonatal Nursing, 27,* 54–63.
16. Lappa, S., Coleman, M.T., & Moscicki, A. B. (1998). Managing sexually transmitted diseases in adolescents. *Primary Care, 25*(1), 71–110.
17. O'Connell, M. (1996). The effect of birth control methods on sexually transmitted disease/HIV risk. *Journal of Obstetric, Gynecologic, and Neonatal Nursing, 25,* 476–480.
18. Pagana, K., & Pagana, T. (1998). *Mosby's diagnostic and laboratory test reference.* St. Louis: Mosby–Year Book.
19. Roe, V., & Gudi, A. (1997). Pharmacological management of sexually transmitted diseases. *Journal of Nurse-Midwifery, 42,* 275–289.
20. Rooney, G., & Robinson, A. (1997). Look out for the hidden STD. *The Practitioner, 241,* 372–382.
21. Sharts-Hopko, N. (1997). STDs in women: What you need to know. *American Journal of Nursing, 97*(4), 46–55.
22. Skidmore-Roth, L. (1998). *Mosby's drug guide for nurses.* St. Louis: Mosby–Year Book.
23. Urban, M., Coury-Doniger, P., & Reichman, R. (1997). Results of a screening program for *Chlamydia trachomatis* infection in men attending a sexually transmitted diseases clinic. *Sexually Transmitted Diseases, 24,* 587–592.

Metabolic Disorders

Anatomy and Physiology Review: The Metabolic Systems

42 Assessment of the Endocrine and Metabolic Systems

43 Management of Clients with Thyroid and Parathyroid Disorders

44 Management of Clients with Adrenal and Pituitary Disorders

45 Management of Clients with Diabetes Mellitus

46 Management of Clients with Exocrine Pancreatic and Biliary Disorders

47 Management of Clients with Hepatic Disorders

Anatomy and Physiology Review
The Metabolic Systems
Robert G. Carroll

Metabolism depends on the availability of fuel (glucose and fatty acids), oxygen, and the balance of *anabolic* (building) against *catabolic* (break-down) processes. The regulation of this balance is dynamic and is one function of the endocrine and neuroendocrine systems. Metabolic processes affect all cells of the body, and whole-body metabolic regulation involves numerous endocrine structures, the liver, muscle, and fat cells.

Endocrine secretions, together with the nervous system, coordinate the balance of metabolism, reproduction, water and electrolyte balance, and nutrient absorption. Metabolism is closely regulated by thyroid hormone, with some influence exerted by cortisol and epinephrine. Growth and development are regulated by growth hormone (also called somatotropin), with thyroid hormone, insulin-like growth factors, and the sex hormones providing significant effects. Plasma glucose is closely regulated by insulin, with glucagon and the metabolic hormones cortisol, growth hormone, and epinephrine having a role. Endocrine agents involved in water and electrolyte balance, nutrient absorption, and reproduction are described in Units 6 and 8.

The liver and pancreas have both endocrine and exocrine roles. The exocrine secretions assist the digestion and absorption of the diet (see Unit 6). The endocrine role is tied closely to metabolism, particularly the regulation of plasma glucose. Plasma glucose represents the balance of glucose absorption from the diet, movement into and out of storage pools, new glucose synthesis from amino acids *(gluconeogenesis),* and, finally, glucose consumption by the tissues. The liver plays a central role in these processes and is a good point to begin the discussion of metabolism.

STRUCTURE OF THE METABOLIC SYSTEMS

LIVER

The liver is the largest gland in the body, representing about 2.5% of body weight. It lies in the upper right quadrant of the abdomen, just below the diaphragm. The rib cage encloses the liver except for the lower margin. The lungs extend over the liver's upper portion. The lower portion of the liver provides a "roof" for the stomach and intestines. A peritoneal covering blankets most of the liver and also the adjacent gallbladder. The liver divides at the falciform ligament into two major lobes, right and left (Fig. U9–1). These two lobes, in turn, divide into superior and inferior portions of the posterior, anterior, medial, and lateral segments.

Liver blood flow represents about 20% of the cardiac output, about 1 L/min. The hepatic artery supplies the liver with about one third of its blood, and the portal vein supplies the other two thirds (see *inset,* Fig. U9–1). The hepatic artery carries oxygenated blood; the portal vein carries deoxygenated blood. The superior and inferior mesenteric veins and the splenic vein, which receive blood from the pancreas, spleen, stomach, intestines, and gallbladder, join to form the portal vein. The portal vein carries nutrients, metabolites, and toxins from the digestive organs to the liver for processing, detoxification, or assimilation. Blood pressure in the hepatic sinuses is low; hence, any process elevating central venous pressure causes liver engorgement. Similarly, any process impeding blood flow through the liver causes engorgement of vessels draining the digestive organs. The liver is an important reservoir for blood, with contraction of the hepatic venules and veins moving about 500 ml into the circulation.

The functional unit of the liver is the *lobule,* and the *hepatocyte* is the major cell. Hepatocytes are arranged in a hub-like fashion around a central vein. One side of the polyhedral hepatocyte faces the *hepatic sinusoids* (the capillary system of the liver); another faces the bile canaliculi. As incoming blood from the portal vein and the hepatic artery enters the sinusoids and passes through the liver lobules, many substances are exchanged between the blood and the hepatocytes. Lymphatic ducts drain excess interstitial fluid. Bile is formed in the hepatocytes, is secreted into the *bile canaliculi,* and travels through bile ductules to the gallbladder. Endothelial and *Kupffer's cells* form the walls of the sinusoids.

Kupffer's cells are an important part of the mononuclear phagocyte system (formerly, the reticuloendothelial system). This system is so effective that fewer than 1% of the bacteria entering the portal system from the intestine pass through the liver. After leaving the sinusoids, blood flows into the central vein, the hepatic veins, and the inferior vena cava.

ENDOCRINE SYSTEM

The endocrine glands are distributed throughout the body. *Endocrine* tissues *(endo,* within) secrete a compound (hormone) that is carried by the blood to act on a target tissue. This is in contrast to *exocrine (exo,* outside) tissues, which secrete across an epithelium, such as sweat and pancreatic peptidases (the lumen of the gastrointestinal [GI] tract is "outside" the body), and *paracrine (para,* around) cells, whose secretions do not need to be transported in the blood to reach their target tissue.

Hormones are generally classified on the basis of molecular structure as follows:

1. *Steroids.* Steroids are derived from cholesterol, and are consequently poorly soluble in water. After secretion, steroids are transported in the blood by

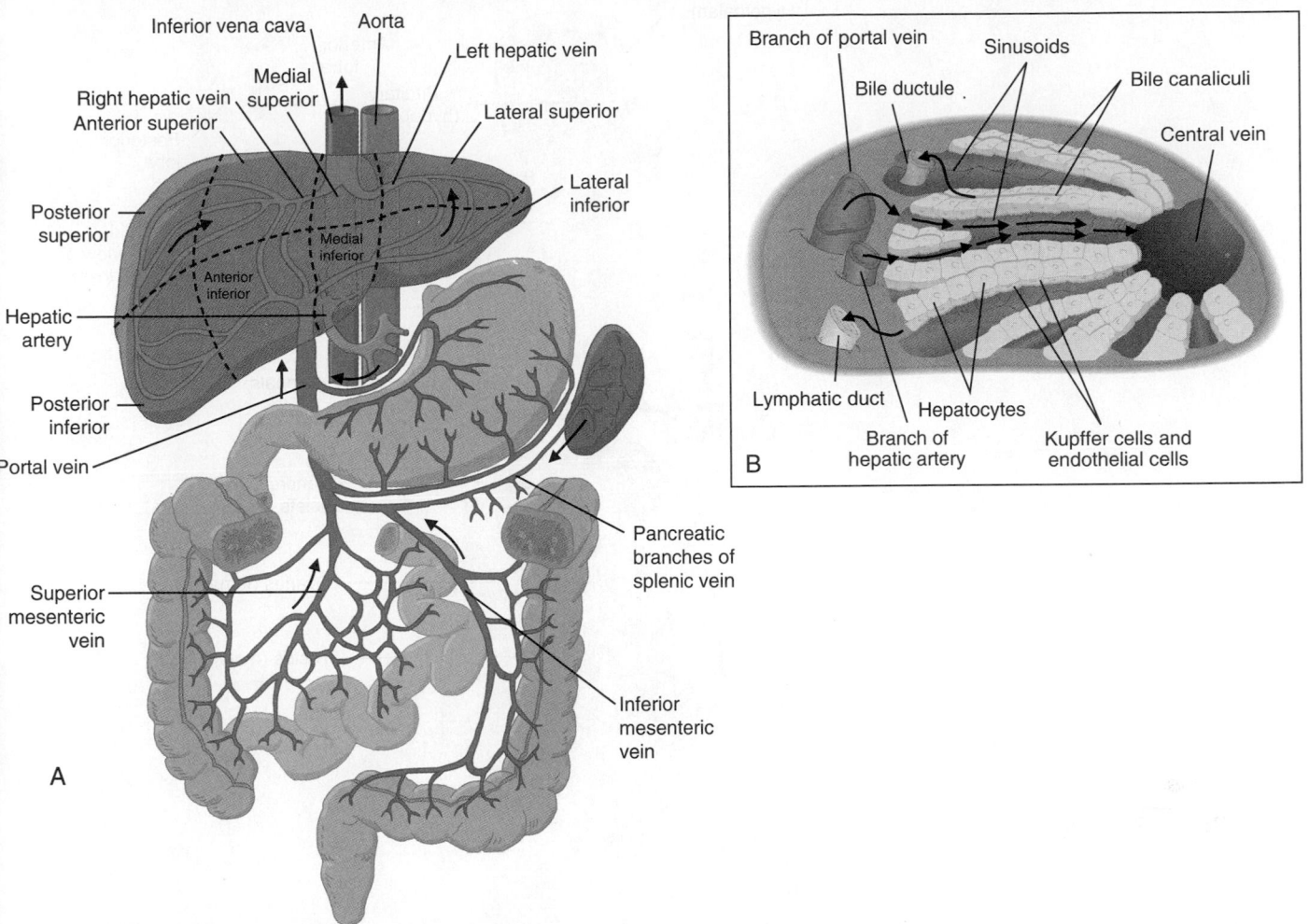

FIGURE U9–1 The liver and vascular drainages. Blood enters the liver from the hepatic artery, and the hepatic portal vein supplies the liver with blood from the digestive organs. *Inset,* Liver lobule. Blood from the hepatic artery and portal vein is processed by the hepatocytes as it flows through the sinusoids into the central vein. Lymphatics and bile ducts leave the liver through separate pathways.

carrier proteins. Steroids diffuse across the cell membrane of the target tissue, bind to a cytoplasmic-binding protein, and the steroid-binding protein complex enters the nucleus where it alters deoxyribonucleic acid (DNA) transcription. There is usually a time lag of minutes to hours before steroids exert their effects.

2. *Peptides. Proteins* and *polypeptides* are synthesized in the endoplasmic reticulum of the endocrine tissue and are secreted in vesicles. After transport in the blood, they bind to cell membrane receptors on the target tissues and activate either second messenger systems or ion channels. Peptide hormones generally have rapid response times.

3. *Amino acid derivatives.* The derivatives of tyrosine include thyroid hormone and the catecholamines epinephrine, norepinephrine, and dopamine. Thyroid hormone alters DNA synthesis through a pathway similar to that for steroids, but the catecholamines bind cell membrane receptors, similar to the mechanism of peptides.

The major endocrine organs described in this review include the pituitary, the thyroid, the parathyroid, the pan-

creas, the adrenal, and, to a lesser extent, the gonads (Fig. U9–2). Other organs have important endocrine secretions, including the kidney (renin and erythropoietin), the heart (atrial natriuretic peptide), and the placenta of a pregnant female (human chorionic gonadotropin [HCG], estrogen, progesterone, and the growth hormone somatomammotropin). See Units 7, 8, and 12.

Hypothalamus and Pituitary Gland

The pituitary gland *(hypophysis)* is a small (1 g) extension on the dorsal surface of the hypothalamus, connected to the hypothalamus by the hypophyseal stalk (Fig. U9–3). The pituitary has three histologically distinct sections, two of which secrete hormones in humans:

1. The *anterior pituitary (adenohypophysis)* is glandular tissue, containing a variety of secretory cell types.

2. The *posterior pituitary (neurohypophysis)* is neural tissue, containing glia cells and terminal axons from cells of the hypothalamus.

3. The *pars intermedia* is a vestigial remnant in humans, with little physiologic significance.

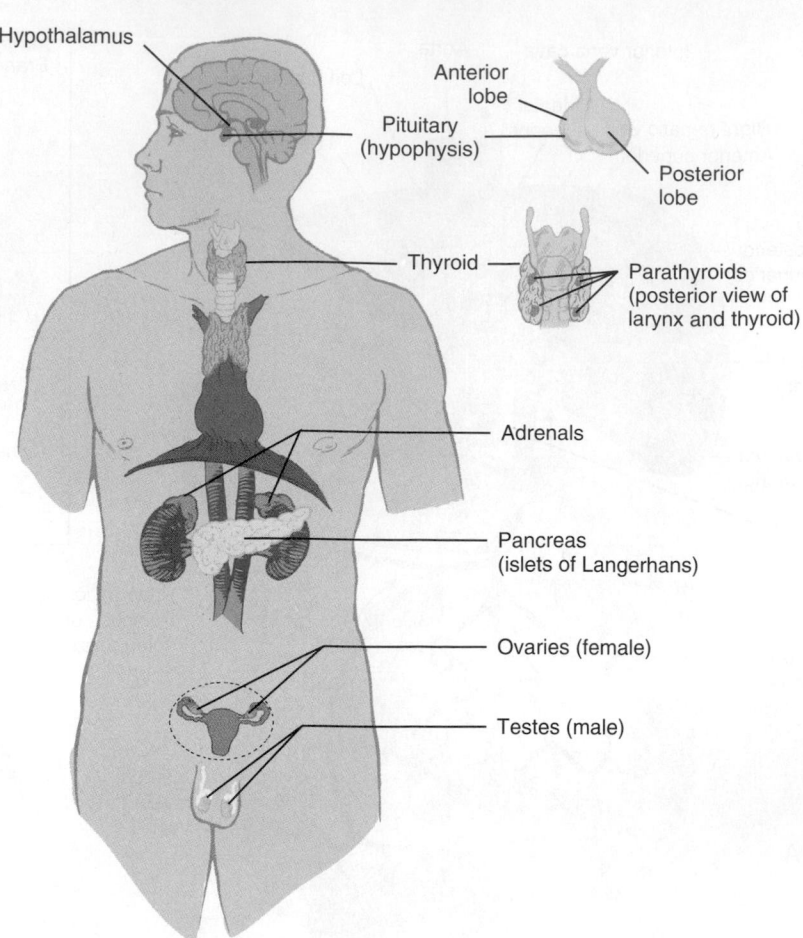

FIGURE U9–2 Organs of the endocrine system.

The hypothalamus lies dorsal to the pituitary gland and regulates secretion of both the anterior and the posterior pituitary hormones. The hypophyseal stalk has two distinct pathways leading from the hypothalamus to the pituitary.

The *neural stalk* contains axons originating in the hypothalamus that terminate in the posterior pituitary. Cell bodies are in the supraoptic and paraventricular nuclei, and axons terminate in the posterior pituitary, where the synaptic terminals secrete hormones, rather than make synaptic connections with another neuron.

The *hypothalamo-hypophyseal portal system* provides a vascular connection between the median eminence of the hypothalamus and the anterior pituitary. Arterial blood enters the capillaries of the hypothalamus. Blood flows through portal vessels in the hypophyseal stalk, before entering a second set of capillaries (sinuses) in the anterior pituitary. Blood then exits the anterior pituitary and joins with other venous drainages. This vascular supply ensures that releasing and inhibiting hormones secreted in the median eminence of the hypothalamus remain concentrated until delivered to the target cells of the anterior pituitary.

The *anterior pituitary* is the end organ for growth hormone and prolactin secretion. The other anterior pituitary hormones act on endocrine target organs to stimulate the release of additional hormones. In the *posterior pituitary* are glia-like cells, which support and nourish the nerve endings. Oxytocin and antidiuretic hormone (ADH) are synthesized in the hypothalamus and transported to the posterior pituitary gland for secretion.

Thyroid and Parathyroid

The thyroid gland is located in the neck, just below the cricoid cartilage, somewhat H-shaped (Fig. U9–4). The right and left lateral lobes lie on either side of the trachea. The lobes are connected by a thin mass of tissue (the *isthmus*), which stretches over the surface of the trachea. Each lobe is composed of irregularly shaped lobules, which consist of a multitude of tiny sacs (follicles) filled with a jelly-like, iodine-containing substance called *colloid* (see *inset,* Fig. U9–4). The main component of colloid is thyroglobulin—the storage form of the hormone thyroxine. The *parathyroid glands* are four small glands near, attached to, or embedded in the thyroid gland.

Endocrine Pancreas

The pancreas (see Fig. U9–2) contains islets of Langerhans, which secrete three hormones that regulate blood glucose: (1) *alpha* cells secrete *glucagons,* (2) *beta* cells secrete *insulin,* and (3) *delta* cells secrete *somatostatin,* identical to the growth hormone inhibitory hormone secreted by the hypothalamus. The close proximity of these

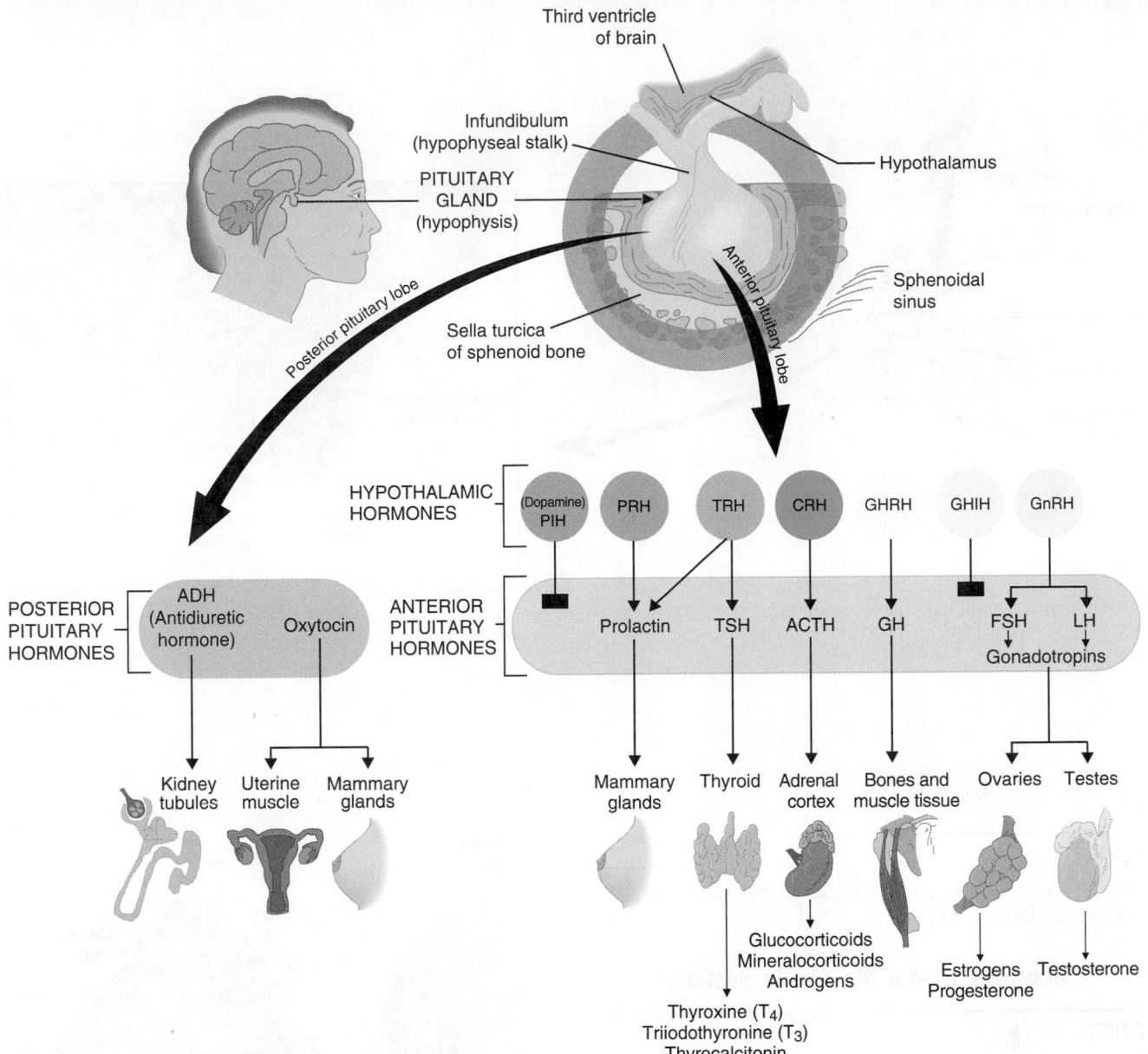

FIGURE U9–3 Hypothalamus, pituitary gland, and target tissues. The pituitary gland is suspended from the hypothalamus by the infundibular or hypophyseal stalk. Hormones released from the hypothalamus travel in a portal vascular system to the anterior pituitary gland, where they stimulate (or inhibit) the release of anterior pituitary hormones. Posterior pituitary hormones are synthesized in the hypothalamus and are released from axons in the posterior pituitary gland.

cells within the islets allows a coordinated paracrine regulation of pancreatic secretion, as insulin inhibits glucagon release, and somatostatin inhibits both insulin and glucagon release.

Adrenal Glands

The adrenal glands are paired endocrine organs situated at the superior poles of the kidneys. The adrenal gland is divided into an outer cortex and an inner medulla (Fig. U9–5). The *cortex* has three zones. The outer *zona glomerulosa* secretes the mineralocorticoids aldosterone and corticosterone. The inner *zona fasciculata* and *zona reticularis* secrete the glucocorticoids cortisol and

corticosterone as well as androgen sex hormones. Corticosterone and deoxycorticosterone are secreted in small amounts and exert both glucocorticoid and mineralocorticoid effects. Adrenal cortical hormones are steroids formed from a cholesterol nucleus. Deficits in synthetic enzymes often lead to overproduction of other adrenal hormones. Stimuli that enhance adrenal cortical secretions also cause hypertrophy of the appropriate cortical zones.

The *adrenal medulla* functions as a postganglionic sympathetic nerve, secreting the catecholamines epinephrine and norepinephrine. About 80% of the basal (resting) catecholamine secretion is epinephrine, but this ratio varies with adrenal stimulation.

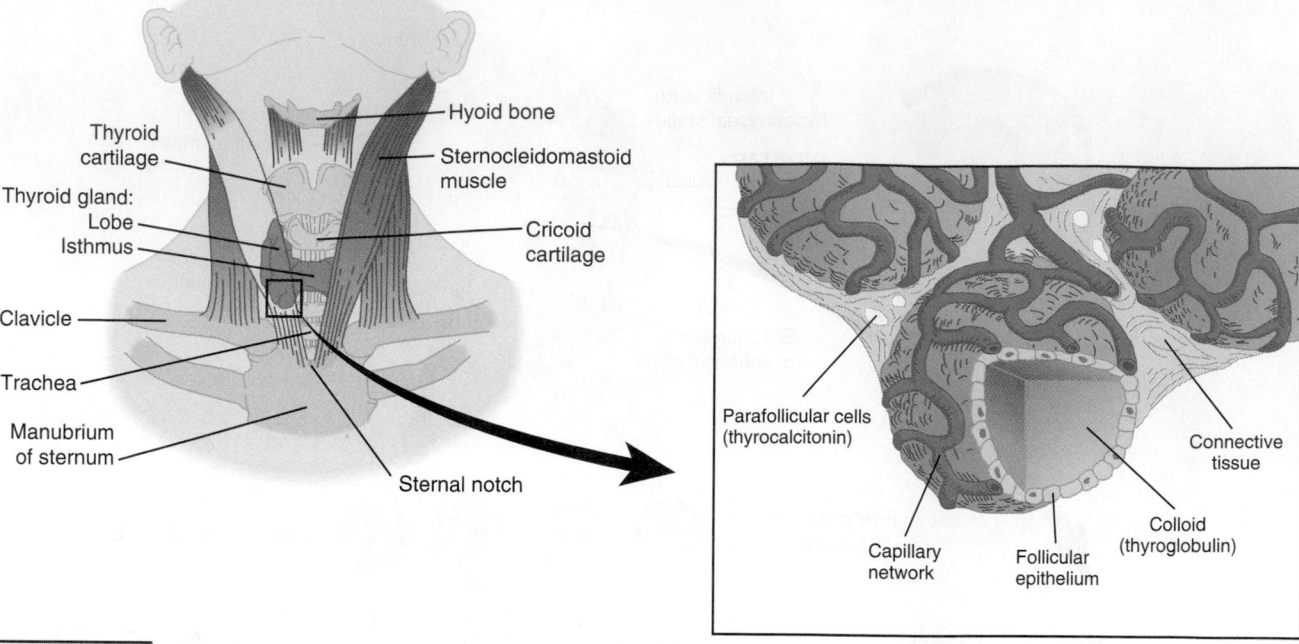

FIGURE U9–4 Gross and microscopic *(inset)* anatomy of the thyroid gland.

Gonads

The structure of the gonads (ovaries and testes) is covered in the Unit 8 review.

Functions of the Metabolic Systems

LIVER

The liver plays a central role in the regulation of metabolic substrates, glucose, and fatty acids. Additionally, hepatic synthesis provides most of the proteins circulating in the plasma.

The liver is the major storage organ for *glycogen,* a polymer of glucose. In addition to storage, the liver converts glucose to glycogen *(glycogenesis),* breaks down glycogen into glucose *(glycogenolysis),* and forms glucose from other sugars (galactose and fructose) or amino acids *(gluconeogenesis).* The regulation of these processes is discussed later.

The major functions of the liver in relation to fat metabolism are as follows:

- Oxidation of fatty acids for energy
- Formation of most lipoproteins
- Synthesis of cholesterol and phospholipids
- Synthesis of fat from proteins and carbohydrates

The liver provides energy from fats by splitting them into glycerol and fatty acids; when the fatty acids are oxidized, tremendous amounts of energy are released.

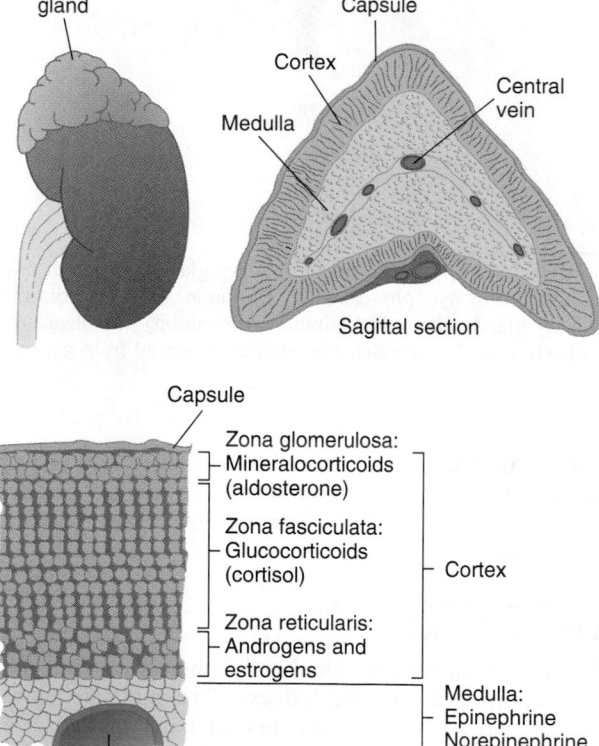

FIGURE U9–5 Gross and microscopic anatomy of the adrenal gland.

Most of the cholesterol synthesized in the liver is converted into bile salts; the remainder is transported in the lipoproteins throughout the body. Phospholipids are also synthesized in the liver and transported in lipoproteins. The cholesterol and phospholipids help form cell membranes and intracellular structures and are involved in cellular function.

The primary functions of the liver in relation to protein metabolism are as follows:

- Deamination of amino acids
- Formation of urea for removal of ammonia from the body
- Formation of plasma proteins
- Biotransformation of hormones, drugs, and other substances

Degradation is the process of excess amino acid catabolism. This process begins in the liver with deamination, the removal of amino groups ($-NH_2$). Ammonia (NH_3), which results from deamination, is converted into urea by the liver and is excreted by the kidneys and intestines. Ammonia can also be formed in the intestines by bacterial action. In severe liver disease or damage, ammonia that is normally converted to urea by the liver accumulates to dangerously high levels in the blood. As a result, a severe toxic state *(hepatic encephalopathy)* develops.

The liver also synthesizes plasma proteins, such as albumin, prothrombin, fibrinogen, and clotting proteins (factors V, VI, VII, IX, and X). Albumin is essential for maintaining plasma oncotic pressure, while the other proteins contribute to blood clotting. Plasma oncotic pressure prevents intravascular fluid from moving out into the extravascular spaces, where it manifests as *ascites* and varying degrees of peripheral edema. Vitamin K, a fat-soluble vitamin, must be present for synthesis of several clotting proteins. Assimilation of vitamin K depends on the presence of bile in the intestine. Gamma globulins are the only plasma proteins not synthesized by the liver.

The liver primarily detoxifies and biotransforms hormones, drugs, and other chemicals. Some substances are deactivated by deamination, hydroxylation, oxidation, or reduction. Through conjugation, other substances become soluble in water, resulting in their excretion through the bile and, therefore, in feces or urine.

Clients with compromised liver function are at high risk for untoward reactions to many medications, all opiates, and many chemicals. The two major problems that result are prolonged action and increased potency of the substance.

ENDOCRINE SYSTEM

Regulation of endocrine secretions is generally by a negative feedback loop, linking the hormone to a response, to another hormone, or to glucose of some other plasma compound. Endocrine agents also have significant trophic effects on the target tissues, with high hormone levels often causing hypertrophy, and inadequate hormone levels causing atrophy, of the target tissues. Regulation of endocrine systems is often integrated with the nervous system. When the distinction between endocrine and nervous systems is blurred, the system is described as the *neuroendocrine system.*

Hypothalamus and Pituitary Gland

The hypothalamus regulates secretion of anterior and posterior pituitary hormones. Five hypothalamic-releasing hormones and two hypothalamic inhibitory hormones regulate secretion of the six anterior pituitary hormones (see Fig. U9–3).

GROWTH HORMONE (SOMATOTROPIN)
The anterior pituitary is the end organ for secretion of growth hormone, which exerts several effects:

- Stimulates growth in almost all body tissues, causing both an increase in cell size *(hypertrophy)* and an increase in cell number *(hyperplasia)*
- Diverts amino acids into protein synthesis *(anabolism)* and decreases protein breakdown *(catabolism)*
- Enhances use of free fatty acids as metabolic substrates, which depletes body fat stores
- Increases plasma glucose levels but protects amino acid pools (see later)

Insulin has an important permissive, or facilitatory, role in growth hormone–mediated growth. It enhances the entry of both glucose and amino acids into cells. Growth hormone exerts some of its effects through an intermediary, the somatomedins, or insulin-like growth factors.

Growth hormone secretion is enhanced by various stressful and normal stimuli, including starvation, chronic protein deficiency, hypoglycemia, low plasma levels of free fatty acids, exercise, and the first hours of sleep. Hypothalamic secretion of growth hormone releasing and inhibitory hormones is the primary regulator of growth hormone release.

PROLACTIN
The hypothalamus is the end organ for prolactin secretion. Hypothalamic control of prolactin is unique, in that the normal control of prolactin release is hypothalamic prolactin inhibitory hormone. Consequently, interruption of the hypothalamo-hypophyseal portal system increases pituitary prolactin release. Prolactin-releasing hormone is important in the suckling reflex (see review, Unit 8).

ANTIDIURETIC HORMONE AND OXYTOCIN
Nerve endings in the *posterior pituitary* secrete oxytocin and antidiuretic hormone (ADH), also known as *vasopressin.* Oxytocin, formed primarily in the paraventricular nucleus of the hypothalamus, promotes uterine contraction during parturition, causing expression of milk ("letdown") following suckling (see Unit 8). ADH is formed primarily in the supraoptic nucleus and is released by increases in plasma osmolarity or by low blood pressure. Stress and trauma can also promote ADH release. The mechanism of ADH control of water and electrolyte balance is discussed in Unit 7.

Thyroid Gland

Thyroid hormone is a conglomerate of three (T_3) or four (T_4) iodinated tyrosine residues. Tri-iodothyronine (T_3) and thyroxine (T_4) together are called thyroid hormone. Thyroid hormone is lipid-soluble, and 99% of thyroid hormone in the plasma is bound to thyroid-binding globulin. Of the two thyroid hormones, T_3 has the most rapid effect on target tissues, requiring 3 days for peak effect; T_4 (the more common) requires 11 days for peak effect.

Thyroid hormone has several functions:

- Increases metabolism, enhancing carbohydrate consumption and increasing the size and density of mitochondria.
- Assists in acclimatization to cold environments by increasing metabolic rate (heat production is a by-product of metabolism)
- Increases DNA translation and transcription
- Increases protein synthesis but also has protein catabolic effects
- Promotes growth and is required for normal growth in children.

Finally, thyroid hormone has a permissive effect to increase other endocrine secretions.

Thyroid hormone is formed in epithelium-lined follicles that contain the glycoprotein thyroglobulin. Thyroglobulin can contain five to six thyroid hormone molecules. Dietary iodine is required for thyroid hormone synthesis. Iodine is oxidized within the follicles, and binds a tyrosine residue (T_1) of thyroglobulin. Iodinated tyrosines are coupled while still part of the thyroglobulin molecule, forming T_3 and T_4. The mature hormone is released by digestion of thyroglobulin, with recycling of unused iodine, T_1, and T_2.

Release of thyroid hormone is regulated by negative feedback by T_4 on thyroid-stimulating hormone (TSH) release at the anterior pituitary. TSH stimulates proteolysis of thyroglobulin, releasing T_3 and T_4. TSH also stimulates iodine uptake by the thyroid for new thyroid hormone synthesis, increasing the activity of thyroid gland cells and increasing thyroid hormone synthesis. TSH release is controlled by the hypothalamic tripeptide thyrotropin-releasing hormone (TRH). Cold exposure is a potent stimulus for TRH release, but the feedback loop for the effect of temperature on TRH is not yet established.

Parathyroid Glands

The endocrine secretion of the parathyroid glands is the polypeptide parathyroid hormone (PTH). A fall in serum calcium levels causes release of PTH: PTH acts on bone, GI tract, and kidneys to increase circulating plasma calcium levels, an action coordinated with vitamin D and calcitonin (see later).

Endocrine Pancreas

The islets of Langerhans of the pancreas secrete three hormones that regulate blood glucose: (1) insulin, (2) glucagon, and (3) somatostatin.

INSULIN

Insulin is a small protein derived successively from a preprohormone and a prohormone. Insulin circulates as a free hormone, has a short plasma half-life of about 6 minutes, and is cleared from the plasma primarily by the liver and kidneys. Insulin binds to receptors on the surface of target tissues and enhances glucose transport across the membrane. Insulin decreases blood glucose by

enhancing uptake, use, and storage of glucose in hepatic, muscle, and adipose tissues (see later). Insulin enhances amino acid transport into cells; it acts synergistically with growth hormone to promote cell hypertrophy and hyperplasia.

Note that the brain is refractory to insulin and must use glucose for a metabolic substrate. Because the brain glucose transporter has a much higher glucose affinity than the insulin-sensitive transporter, only a severe decline in the blood glucose level can lead to hypoglycemic shock.

Insulin is released after ingestion and absorption of carbohydrates. The initial phase, from release of stored insulin, peaks in 5 minutes. A delayed phase, from synthesis of new insulin, persists until blood glucose returns to fasting levels. The ability of insulin to control plasma glucose levels is the basis of the glucose tolerance test (GTT). In the absence of insulin, fats are used as metabolic substrates. The incomplete oxidation of fatty acids results in the ketoacidosis that is characteristic of untreated diabetes mellitus. The lack of insulin elevates blood glucose, causing an osmotic diuresis (see Unit 7 review). Finally, the lack of insulin promotes protein catabolism and inhibits growth.

GLUCAGON

Glucagon is an extremely potent hormone that is released when blood glucose levels drop below 90 mg/dl. Glucagon acts on the liver to elevate plasma glucose, an action opposite that of insulin (see later). The second messenger for glucagon is cyclic adenosine monophosphate (cAMP); it allows excessively high glucagon levels to affect other tissues (enhancing cardiac contractility, enhancing bile secretion, and inhibiting gastric acid secretion). Protein ingestion enhances glucagon release as well as insulin release. This simultaneous secretion of insulin and glucagon allow cells to use and store glucose without severely decreasing plasma glucose levels. Glucagon is also released during exercise and helps prevent hypoglycemia despite enhanced glucose use by muscle.

SOMATOSTATIN

Somatostatin is a small polypeptide with a short (2-minute) half-life; it has many inhibitory actions. Somatostatin is released after ingestion of a meal and inhibits release of both insulin and glucagon. The net action of somatostatin is to delay nutrient absorption by the GI tract, thus prolonging the duration of intestinal food absorption after a meal.

Adrenal Glands

ADRENAL CORTEX

ALDOSTERONE. The primary mineralocorticoid secreted by the adrenal cortex is aldosterone. About 50% of aldosterone is free in the plasma; the remainder is bound. Aldosterone is degraded in the liver and is excreted in the urine and feces as a glucuronide or sulfate. Infusion of aldosterone causes a drop in plasma potassium levels by increasing renal excretion of potassium. Plasma potassium concentration is the primary regulator of aldosterone release through a negative feedback control mechanism. Angiotensin II can also promote aldosterone synthesis and release, and adrenocorticotropic hormone (ACTH) has a permissive role in aldosterone production and secretion.

CORTISOL. The primary glucocorticoid secreted by the adrenal cortex is cortisol. Following secretion, 94% of cortisol is bound in the plasma to transcortin, a cortisol-binding globulin, and 6% is free. Cortisol is degraded in the liver and is excreted in the urine and feces as a glucuronide or sulfate. Cortisol is a potent metabolic regulatory hormone, increasing plasma glucose and promoting use of alternate metabolic substrates for energy (see later). Cortisol stimulates appetite, which leads to central deposition of fat in some central adipose tissues despite the use of fat from peripheral tissues (see clinical description of Cushing's syndrome). Cortisol's metabolic changes assist the transition to nonglucose support of metabolism in starvation.

Cortisol release is regulated by a hypothalamus-pituitary-adrenal cascade. The hypothalamus secretes corticotropin-releasing hormone (CRH), which is carried by the hypothalamo-hypophyseal portal system to the anterior pituitary gland, where it stimulates ACTH release. ACTH travels in the blood to the adrenal gland, where it promotes conversion of cholesterol to pregnenolone, the rate-limiting step in adrenal glucocorticoid and androgen secretion. Because of a common synthetic pathway, pituitary ACTH also stimulates adrenal androgen production.

ACTH release coincides with the release of other compounds formed from the same pre-prohormone. These include (1) melanocyte-stimulating hormone (which stimulates pigment production in epidermal cells), (2) beta-lipotropin (which may stimulate aldosterone release), and (3) the opiate beta-endorphin.

Cortisol is generally described as a stress hormone. Painful stimuli promote release of CRH from the hypothalamus. Emotional stress generated in the limbic system also promotes hypothalamic release of CRH. Cortisol has significant anti-inflammatory effects, retarding the development and enhancing the resolution of the inflammatory response. Glucocorticoid secretion exhibits a strong diurnal rhythm, found to be highest in the early morning and lowest in the late evening.

ADRENAL MEDULLA

The adrenal medulla secretes the catecholamines epinephrine and norepinephrine, whose actions mimic those of the sympathetic nervous system but have a longer duration. Epinephrine has strong beta-adrenergic effects and is a potent stimulator of heart rate and contractility. Epinephrine has strong metabolic effects and increases metabolic rate by up to 100%. These effects include increasing metabolic substrates in the plasma by lipolysis and glycogenolysis (see later).

Gonads

The sex hormones have important trophic and metabolic effects. The synthetic pathways for estrogens and androgens share many common precursors with each other and with the adrenal cortical steroids. Consequently, sex hormones originate predominantly from the gonads but are secreted in lower amounts from the adrenal glands.

Androgens, primarily testosterone, have a potent anabolic action. Testosterone is controlled by the hypothalamic-pituitary axis, and gonadotropin-releasing hormone (GnRH) and luteinizing hormone (LH) act on the Leydig cells of the testes to promote testosterone synthesis and release. The reproductive significance of testosterone is discussed in Unit 8. A secondary effect of testosterone is to promote protein synthesis as well as the musculoskeletal growth that accompanies puberty.

In the female, LH also stimulates androgen production in the ovarian thecal cells, but the aromatase of the ovarian granulose cells converts the androgens into the estrogen estradiol. The puberty-related increase in musculoskeletal growth and onset of menstruation are a result of increases in the cyclic release of estrogen and progesterone (see Unit 8).

METABOLIC SUBSTRATES

Plasma Glucose

Glucose is the primary metabolic substrate for the body. The plasma glucose level is normally about 100 mg/dL in both the fed and fasted states. Glucose entry into most cells is insulin-dependent. The notable exception is in the brain; cerebral glucose utilization is independent of insulin and requires a plasma glucose level of only 60 mg/dL—levels below this will disrupt brain function.

Plasma glucose represents the balance between glucose absorption from the diet, movement into and out of storage pools, and utilization by the tissues. Glucose storage pools include glycogen, the glycerol component of fat, and amino acids. Although only insulin acts to decrease plasma glucose levels, the hormones glucagon, cortisol, growth hormone, and epinephrine all can elevate plasma glucose levels. This multiple endocrine control allows protection of one or more glucose storage pools (Fig. U9–6). For example, glucagon mobilizes all storage pools, resulting in increased plasma glucose. Growth hormone prevents gluconeogenesis but increases glucose by the other mechanisms. Cortisol preserves glycogen and fat stores in the center of the body but mobilizes all other glucose pools, including gluconeogenesis. Epinephrine mobilizes fat and glycogen pools.

After a meal, excess plasma glucose is moved into storage, facilitated by insulin. During periods of fasting, glucose is moved from the storage pools, first from glycogen, then from fats, and—if the fast is sufficiently long—from the amino acid pools.

Plasma Amino Acids

Plasma amino acid levels are not controlled by a tight negative feedback mechanism. Ingestion of a protein-rich meal, however, increases both insulin and growth hormone levels. Growth hormone alone enhances cellular uptake of amino acids and preserves amino acid stores (by blocking gluconeogenesis) when insulin is not elevated. When insulin is elevated, the combined action of growth hormone and insulin greatly enhances uptake of amino acids.

Plasma Free Fatty Acids

Free fatty acids are the baseline metabolic substrate and are used unless insulin shifts metabolism to glucose as a metabolic fuel. The heart in particular can oxidize free

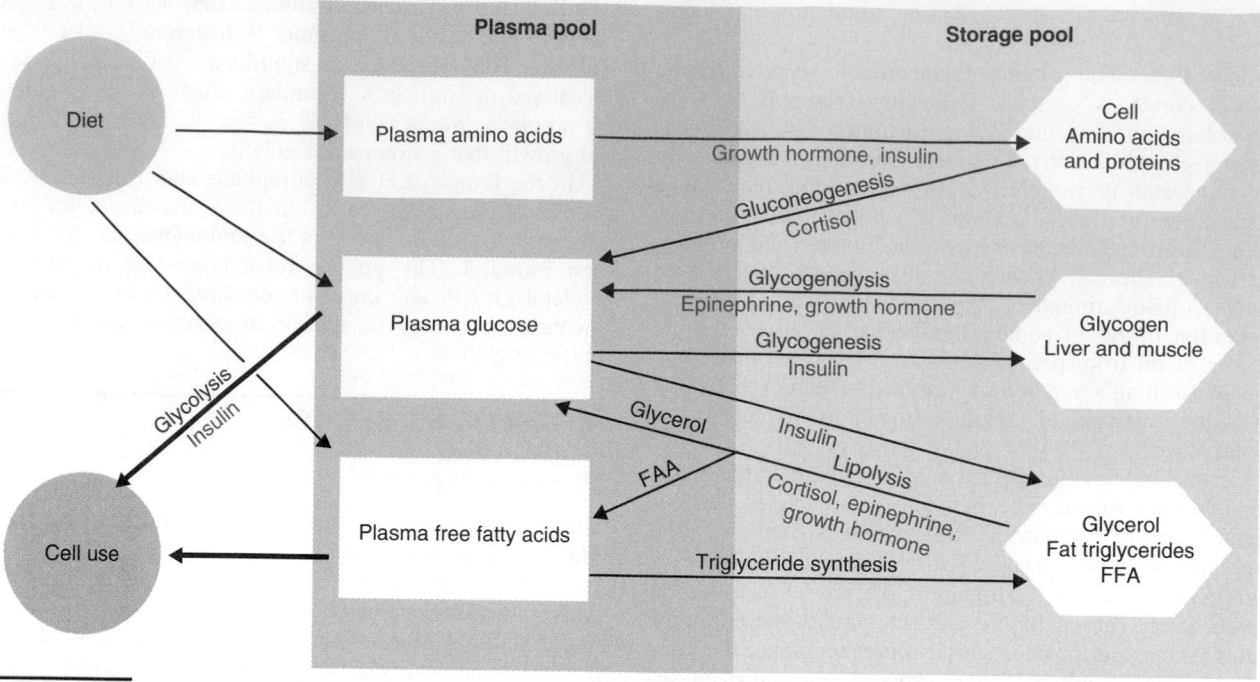

FIGURE U9–6 Regulation of metabolic substrates. Cells consume glucose or fatty acids to support metabolism. Plasma glucose is regulated by multiple endocrine mechanisms, which act primarily on the movement into and out of storage pools. Glucose is stored if the plasma glucose level is above 110 mg/dL; glucose is mobilized from storage pools if the plasma glucose level is below 90 mg/dL. FFA, free fatty acid.

fatty acids and thus is not as dependent on glucose as a metabolic substrate as the remainder of the body is. In the American diet, food is ingested with sufficient frequency that insulin levels are high, and glucose is normally used as the metabolic fuel. When metabolized, fatty acids are incompletely oxidized, however, with ketone bodies produced as a metabolic by-product.

Plasma levels of free fatty acids are not controlled by a tight negative feedback mechanism. A drop in plasma glucose levels, however, causes the release of epinephrine, cortisol, and growth hormone, all of which promote lipolysis. This results in the movement of fatty acids from the storage pool in fat cells into the plasma pool, providing an alternative substrate for metabolism when glucose availability is limited.

Plasma Calcium

The plasma calcium level (Ca^{2+}) is tightly regulated around 9.4 mg/dl, with a normal range of 9 to 10 mg/dl. About 40% of plasma Ca^{2+} is tightly bound to plasma proteins, and an additional 10% is combined in nonionized salts with citrate and phosphate. About 5 mg/dl (50%) of plasma Ca^{2+} is free.

More than 99% of calcium within the body is stored in bone, most of it combined with phosphate in hydroxyapatite crystals. Regulation of plasma calcium levels involves balancing dietary absorption, renal excretion, and exchange between the plasma and storage areas. PTH and Vitamin D$_3$ are the major regulators of plasma calcium, with a minor role for the hormone calcitonin.

Infusion of PTH results in elevated plasma calcium levels and decreased plasma phosphate levels. The in-

crease in plasma calcium occurs by enhancing dietary calcium absorption (via vitamin D$_3$), by decreasing renal calcium excretion, and by mobilizing calcium from the bone storage pools. Plasma calcium is the primary regulator of PTH release. PTH synthesis and release are stimulated by a drop in plasma calcium and helps regulate calcium levels during pregnancy and lactation.

Dietary absorption of calcium requires activated vitamin D. Vitamin D can be absorbed from the diet or synthesized through ultraviolet (sun) light action on 7-dehydrocholesterol. Vitamin D is then converted successively in liver and kidney to 1-25-hydroxcholecalciferol, the active form.

Calcitonin is a polypeptide secreted by the parafollicular C cells of the thyroid gland. While infusion of calcitonin decreases the plasma calcium concentration, its role in regulating plasma calcium levels is minor.

Alterations in plasma calcium levels produce physiologic changes. Hypocalcemia increases neuronal excitability. Motor neurons exhibit spontaneous depolarizations, leading to tetanic muscular contractions. The hand is particularly susceptible, resulting in carpopedal spasm. Hypercalcemia depresses neuronal and muscle activity.

EFFECTS OF AGING

With aging, the functions of the liver, biliary system, and exocrine pancreas all begin to deteriorate. In the liver, the number and size of hepatic cells is reduced, leading to a decreased weight and mass. Fibrotic tissue also increases, leading to a decrease in protein synthesis, liver enzymes, and cholesterol synthesis. The decrease in enzyme activity diminishes the liver's ability to detoxify drugs and increases the risk of toxic levels of a variety of medications in older adults.

The pancreas is also affected by the process of aging, with calcification of the pancreatic vessels, and by changes in the size of the ducts through distention and dilation. These changes lead to decreased production of lipase, resulting in reduced fat absorption and digestion. Older people also may experience a decreased absorption of fat-soluble vitamins and an increase of fat excreted through the feces (steatorrhea).

CONCLUSIONS

Metabolic regulation is a complex body function, involving the gastrointestinal tract, liver, muscle, and fat tissues.

The multiple endocrine systems that regulate the availability of metabolic fuels reflect the essential role of glucose and fatty acids in survival. The process is complicated by the fact that the body must cope both with periods of excess nutrients (after a meal) and with prolonged fasting.

BIBLIOGRAPHY

1. Guyton, A. C., & Hall, J. (1996). *Textbook of medical physiology* (9th ed.). Philadelphia: W. B. Saunders.
2. Kacsoh, B. (2000). *Endocrine physiology.* New York: McGraw-Hill.
3. McPhee, S. J., et al. (2000). *Pathophysiology of disease* (3rd ed.) New York: McGraw-Hill.
4. Silverthorn, D. (1998). *Human physiology.* Upper Saddle River, NJ: Prentice-Hall.

CHAPTER

42

Assessment of the Endocrine and Metabolic Systems

Dianne Smolen

Clients with endocrine or metabolic system disorders may have specific complaints such as nausea, diarrhea, or fatigue. These same clients may also have vague, intermittent, generalized manifestations. Because of the different functions of the endocrine glands and the organs of metabolism, there is no single, uniform assessment for clients with endocrine or metabolic disorders. Assessment of clients with such disorders includes a complete health history, physical examination, and diagnostic tests. It is important to perform a complete assessment and analyze the data related to the client's current and past health history.

HISTORY

During the health history interview, help the client place the recalled experiences and manifestations in a time sequence. Linking events and clinical manifestations aids the diagnostic process.

■ BIOGRAPHICAL AND DEMOGRAPHIC DATA

Note biographical and demographic data, such as the client's age, sex, ethnic background, and geographical residence. Some disorders, such as gallbladder disease, diabetes mellitus, and hepatitis, are associated with age or sex as well as where a person lives. For example, as a person ages, fewer hormones and metabolic secretions may be produced or their effect on target organs may diminish.

■ CURRENT HEALTH

Chief Complaint

Thorough investigation of the client's chief complaint is necessary for accurate assessment. Like gastrointestinal manifestations, the manifestations of endocrine and metabolic disorders may be ambiguous with a puzzling origin. Indicate the onset, duration, intensity, and characteristics of manifestations and any alterations in growth patterns, especially changes in weight, height, or hand, foot, or head size.

Symptom Analysis

For purposes of discussion, common manifestations related to the endocrine and metabolic systems are grouped by body system as follows (see Chapter 9):

GASTROINTESTINAL MANIFESTATIONS

- An enlarged, red tongue (*glossitis*)? May be present in clients with diabetes mellitus.
- Weight gain or loss or changes in appetite? These manifestations may be an indication of an endocrine or metabolic disorder. For example, increased eating but loss of weight may indicate hyperthyroidism; gaining weight may suggest hypothyroidism. Excessive appetite (*polyphagia*) may be indicative of diabetes mellitus.
- Excessive thirst (*polydipsia*)? May indicate diabetes mellitus.
- Abdominal pain? Right upper quadrant discomfort suggests gallbladder or liver disorders.
- Nausea or vomiting? Occurs in 70% of clients with pancreatitis.
- Anorexia? Especially prevalent in liver disorders.
- Fatty food intolerance? May be indicative of pancreatic or biliary tract disease.
- Excessive eructation (belching or *aerophagia*)? Suggests gallbladder disease. Heartburn (*pyrosis*)? May be a manifestation of cholecystitis or refluxed acid or bile.
- Disturbed bowel pattern, such as diarrhea (dark-colored, tarry stools)? May be caused by hyperthyroidism or a biliary tract problem.
- Constipation? May indicate hypothyroidism or a biliary disorder. Clay-colored stools or *acholic* (without bilirubin) stools? May occur briefly in viral hepatitis; common in obstructive jaundice.
- Fatty, foul-smelling stools (*steatorrhea*)? May occur with chronic pancreatitis or after gastric surgery; partially the result of rapid gastric emptying, which prevents adequate mixing with pancreatic and biliary secretions.

NEUROLOGIC MANIFESTATIONS

- Weakness? Generalized or localized? May indicate late manifestations of diabetes mellitus.

- Mild depression? May be a manifestation of pancreatic cancer or an endocrine disorder.
- Changes in mental status or mood (increased irritability)? Extreme alterations in consciousness, such as coma, may occur in uncontrolled diabetes mellitus.
- Emotional lability? Alterations in consciousness? These manifestations may indicate liver or endocrine disorders.
- Drowsiness? A change in mental status and neurologic manifestations can signal the development of hepatic encephalopathy or uncontrolled diabetes mellitus.
- Pain? If radiating to the back, it can be a manifestation of a pancreatic, gallbladder, or biliary tract disorder.
- Tremors? If uncontrolled, can indicate hyperthyroidism.
- Loss of sensation, especially in hands or feet? Suggests diabetes mellitus.

GENITOURINARY AND REPRODUCTIVE MANIFESTATIONS

- Dark yellow or tea-colored urine? Indicates impaired excretion of bilirubin caused by hepatocellular disease.
- Frequent urination (*polyuria*)? May be indicative of diabetes mellitus.
- Menstrual cycle irregularities (including amenorrhea)? Loss of libido? Loss or premature development of secondary sex characteristics? Impotence or infertility? These sexual changes are characteristics of endocrine disorders.
- Renal problems? Calcium stone formation may be caused by hyperparathyroidism (because calcium is resorbed from bone).

INTEGUMENTARY MANIFESTATIONS AND CHANGES IN APPEARANCE

- Red, noninflammatory blisters and erosions on dorsum (back) of hands? Commonly demonstrated in clients infected with hepatitis C virus.
- Jaundiced skin? Causes include viral hepatitis, cirrhosis, and obstructive or cholestatic liver disease.
- Unexplained puncture holes? May be the route of entry for hepatitis (type B or C) or other pathogens.
- Spider angiomas? Petechiae? Dilated abdominal veins? May indicate hepatic cirrhosis.
- Skin lesions that do not heal? May indicate pancreatic dysfunction (see Chapter 45).
- Hyperpigmentation or hypopigmentation? Addison's disease, caused by chronic adrenocortical insufficiency, causes excessive pigmentation of skin; areas of hypopigmentation (*vitiligo*) may indicate other endocrine disorders.
- Hard, nonpitting edema? Occurs in adult hypothyroidism (*myxedema*).
- Delayed healing? May indicate diabetes mellitus.
- Changes in hands, head, feet, and face? Acromegaly produces enlargement of the head, hands, and feet and coarsening of facial features. Adrenocortical hyperfunction (Cushing's syndrome)? Is manifested in moon facies, thin extremities, and truncal obesity.
- Growth delayed? Stunted (*dwarfism*)? Excessive (*gigantism*)? Inappropriate (*acromegaly*)? All may indicate a pituitary or other type of endocrine disorder.
- Changes in hair? Distribution, amount, or texture? Excessive hair (*hirsutism*) may indicate ovarian or adrenocortical disorders; loss of pubic and ancillary hair may

indicate a pituitary problem; dry, brittle hair may indicate hypothyroidism; and soft, silky hair may indicate hyperthyroidism.

OPHTHALMIC MANIFESTATIONS

- Bulging eyes (*exophthalmos*)? Characteristic of hyperthyroidism.
- Diminished or blurred vision? Visual problems may be caused by diabetes mellitus; visual loss may be caused by a pituitary tumor.

CARDIOVASCULAR MANIFESTATIONS

- Nosebleeds or bruising easily? Hemorrhoids? *Ascites* (fluid accumulation in peritoneal cavity)? Edema of limbs? All may be indicative of a hepatic disorder in which fluid overload results from the liver's improper functioning and metabolism of hormones, such as aldosterone and antidiuretic hormone (ADH).
- Changes in vital signs? Hyperthyroidism may cause elevation of body temperature and pulse rate.
- Hypertension? May be caused by an adrenal tumor (e.g., pheochromocytoma). Insufficient secretion of ADH from the pituitary gland can cause dehydration; oversecretion can cause excessive retention of body water.
- Increased heart rate and flushing? May occur in hyperthyroidism and in pheochromocytoma.
- Kussmaul's respiration (deep, rapid breathing)? A direct result of diabetic ketoacidosis.

OTHER MANIFESTATIONS

- Yellow sclerae? Suggests biliary obstruction.
- Fever? May indicate an acute gallbladder, pancreas, or liver problem.
- Intolerance of alcohol or medications? Fatigue? Malaise? All occur with hepatitis or endocrine disorders.
- Dehydration? May indicate insufficient levels of ADH.
- Bone or joint pain? Hyperparathyroidism may cause calcium to be reabsorbed from bone and contribute to bone pain, fracture, or both. Adrenal insufficiency (Cushing's syndrome) may produce a rapid breakdown of bone.
- Muscle cramps? Tetany? May result from inadequate secretion of parathyroid hormone (PTH).

■ PAST HEALTH HISTORY

Childhood and Infectious Diseases

Ask the client and family members about any episodes of endocrine or metabolic disorders the client may have experienced as a child or an adolescent. For example, did the client have any growth patterns that were different from those of other members of the family? Did these changes in body size occur after physical maturation?

Have there been any changes in head circumference or size of the hands or feet? For instance, has the client needed to buy hats, gloves, rings, or shoes in a larger size?

Ask the client about changes in the amount and distribution of hair, such as increased facial hair (women), decreased hair (men), or changes in pubic or axillary hair (both men and women). Has the client had any episodes of excessive thirst and urination? In addition, ask female clients about their menstrual history, pregnancies, or fertility problems.

Immunization Status

Inquire about the client's immunization status. Did the client receive the routine childhood vaccinations (see Chapter 9)? Were the vaccinations given when the client was an infant or later in life? Was a tetanus shot received recently? Has the client been immunized against hepatitis A or B or ever received post-exposure immunization for hepatitis A?

Major Illnesses, Hospitalizations, and Operations

Ask the client to identify any illnesses or injuries to the head or neck. Is there a history of head trauma, such as a forceful blow? Trauma can lead to hypopituitarism. Has the client been hospitalized for surgery to the head or neck? Does the client have a history of surgery, chemotherapy, or radiation therapy to the head or neck? Ask about diagnosis or treatment for related disorders, such as primary brain or spinal cord tumors, metastatic tumors, meningitis, brain infarctions, diabetes mellitus, diabetes insipidus, hypertension, and goiter.

Have the client describe any past problems with jaundice, hepatitis, abdominal pain, gallbladder disease, anemia, or changes in bowel elimination, such as diarrhea, clay-colored stools, or melena. Has the client ever been hospitalized for any of these disorders or ever had surgery of the liver or gallbladder?

Have diagnostic procedures, such as a gallbladder x-ray study, liver biopsy, or ultrasound examination of the gallbladder ever been performed? Has the client ever received a transfusion of blood or blood products?

Procedures Causing Skin or Membrane Disruption

Has the client had recent blood tests, transfusions of blood products, dental procedures, ear or other body piercing, tattooing, or any intravenous injection with a potentially contaminated needle? Note such procedures in an assessment, because breaks in the skin may be the route of entry for hepatitis virus (type B or C) or other pathogens.

Medications

Ask specifically about the use of hormones and steroids, including name, dose, and duration of use. Does the client have a history of taking anabolic steroids? Ask specifically about medications the client is currently taking or has taken previously, including over-the-counter drugs. Many drugs and chemicals are potentially hepatotoxic, such as alcohol, gold compounds, mercury, phosphorus, anabolic steroids, acetaminophen, isoniazid, halothane, sulfonamides, arsenic, thiazide diuretics, zidovudine (azidothymidine [AZT]), and anticancer drugs, such as methotrexate. Other medications to ask about are oral contraceptives, anesthetic agents, and antipsychotic agents.

Ask about the use of alternative therapies, such as herbal medicines. Herbal medicines used in the treatment of non–insulin-dependent diabetes include aloe vera juice, beans (*Phaseolus* species), bitter gourd, karela (*Mo-*

mordica charantia), black tea (*Camellia sinensis*), fenugreek (*Trigonella foenum-graecum*), gumar (*Gymnema sylvestre*), macadamia nut, and Madagascar periwinkle (*Catharanthus roseus*). Effects of these herbs include lowering of blood pressure (fenugreek), a boosting of insulin production (gumar), and increased use of available insulin (black tea).

Kelp (*Fucus vesiculosus*) may help with weight loss in hypothyroid disorders. Milk thistle (*Silybum marianum*) is used for treatment and prophylaxis of chronic hepatotoxicity, inflammatory liver disorders, and certain types of cirrhosis.

Allergies

Ask the client about known allergies to food or medications. Specifically ask about reactions to iodine. Iodine is contained in contrast media used in some diagnostic studies of the metabolic system.

■ FAMILY HEALTH HISTORY

When assessing a client with an endocrine or metabolic disorder, inquire about the family history. A number of endocrine disorders are inherited or tend to run in families. Has any family member had problems similar to those of the client? Disorders to inquire about include growth and development problems, obesity, goiter, hypothyroidism or hyperthyroidism, hypertension, low blood pressure (hypotension), diabetes mellitus, diabetes insipidus, autoimmune diseases (Addison's disease), and problems with the adrenal glands (e.g., pheochromocytoma).

Ask the client whether any family members have had cancer (especially of the bowel, liver, or pancreas), jaundice, bleeding disorders, hepatitis, nutritional deficiencies, alcoholism, obesity, pancreatic disease, or gallbladder disease. A history of these disorders in family members increases the risk of their development in the client.

■ PSYCHOSOCIAL HISTORY

Assessment of the psychosocial history and lifestyle patterns provides data about the client's physical and psychological status. Inquire about the client's occupation, environment, and habits.

Occupation, Geographical Location, and Environment

Because *stress* can increase the severity of disorders such as diabetes mellitus, ask about the client's stress tolerance and coping patterns. Stress can be either *physiologic* (caused by illness) or *emotional*. Ask about job-related stressors, such as amount of time spent on the job both in the work setting and at home. Do strained interpersonal relationships at work contribute to increased stress levels? Does the client have opportunities to retreat from the workplace and to engage in recreational activities?

Ask about the home environment and family interpersonal relationships and obligations. What support systems are available to the client? Does the client report effective current coping strategies? If possible, ask family members to corroborate or to help identify behavior changes.

Ask about the client's occupation and work environment. Are there any factors that are known to cause liver damage? For example, heavy metals such as mercury and lead, anesthetic agents such as nitrous oxide, and chemicals such as carbon tetrachloride and certain pesticides are known hepatotoxins. Does the client engage in activities that increase the risk of exposure to substances that cause hepatitis or pancreatitis? Ask about the following:

- Any close contact with hazardous waste
- Travel in areas where hepatitis or pancreatitis is endemic
- Eating raw or steamed shellfish (oysters, clams, scallops) from polluted water
- Swimming or bathing in polluted water
- Any known contact with hepatitis-infected animals or people
- Ingestion of mushrooms that have not been purchased in a store

Exercise, Nutrition, and Habits

When assessing the client for endocrine or metabolic disorders, also consider other aspects of lifestyle and coping. Ask the client about exercise, food intake, sleep and rest patterns and about the use of alcohol, illicit drugs, or tobacco products. Ask about usual patterns as well as any alteration in patterns. Related to food intake, investigate the following:

- Food preferences
- Daily intake of proteins, carbohydrates, fats, and sodium
- Changes in eating patterns, including onset of changes
- Meal preparation (by whom, style of preparation)
- Recent development of food intolerances

In the case of a chronic condition such as diabetes mellitus, careful control is crucial to prevent complications. Diet and physical activity are important in the management of both type 1 and type 2 diabetes (see Chapter 45). One type, non–insulin-dependent diabetes mellitus, can often be prevented through diet and physical activity. According to *Healthy People 2000*, the goal of the Public Health Service is to "reduce diabetes-related deaths to no more than 34 per 100,000 people (an 11% decrease)."[12] You have an important role in helping clients adjust to chronic conditions such as diabetes mellitus or liver disease by assisting them to adopt health-seeking behaviors related to diet, exercise, and necessary medication.

Carefully explore the client's use of alcohol and other mind-altering substances. Pay attention to alcohol use patterns, because alcoholism often accompanies liver and pancreatic disease causing fatty infiltration of the liver.

Be alert to whether the client provides confusing or conflicting data. Is the client's behavior altered in any way as the assessment proceeds? For example, does the client become angry, silent, or tearful? If significant others are present, do they corroborate the client's account? The client who does not acknowledge a substance abuse problem may not provide reliable information about usage. The client who takes illicit drugs may be unwilling to describe drug use patterns. If you suspect that the client's history is unreliable, ask significant others to provide additional information. (Chapter 24 discusses alcoholism and other drug use.)

■ REVIEW OF SYSTEMS

If an endocrine or metabolic disorder is suspected, a careful review of systems (ROS) is important because endocrine and metabolic disorders can affect multiple systems. During this review, ask about the gastrointestinal, genitourinary, integumentary, cardiovascular, and neurologic systems and mental status (see Chief Complaint and Symptom Analysis). Specifically, inquire about jaundice, pruritus (itching), abdominal swelling indicating edema or ascites (fluid-filled abdomen), dark-colored urine, clay-colored stools, bleeding tendencies (purpura), spider angiomas (spider nevi or telangiectasia), fatigue, excessive thirst, excessive urination, and weight loss or weight gain. Detailed questions for the review of systems may be found in Chapter 9, Box 9–2.

PHYSICAL EXAMINATION

Physical assessment of endocrine or metabolic (liver, biliary, or pancreatic) dysfunction involves careful examination of the entire body and is integrated throughout the interaction with the client. Specifically, the assessment covers general health and nutritional status along with the skin, head, neck, thorax, abdomen, upper and lower extremities, and genitalia. Examine all body systems in a systematic manner from head to toe (see Chapter 10) using inspection, auscultation, percussion, and palpation.

Before the examination, ask the client to point to any painful area; examine that area last. As stated earlier, hepatic or biliary pain is often located in the right upper quadrant (Fig. 42–1). Pain that is dull and difficult to localize or describe may arise from an organ (viscera). Somatic pain is sharp, piercing, and easy to localize, and it arises from nerve endings in the peritoneum.

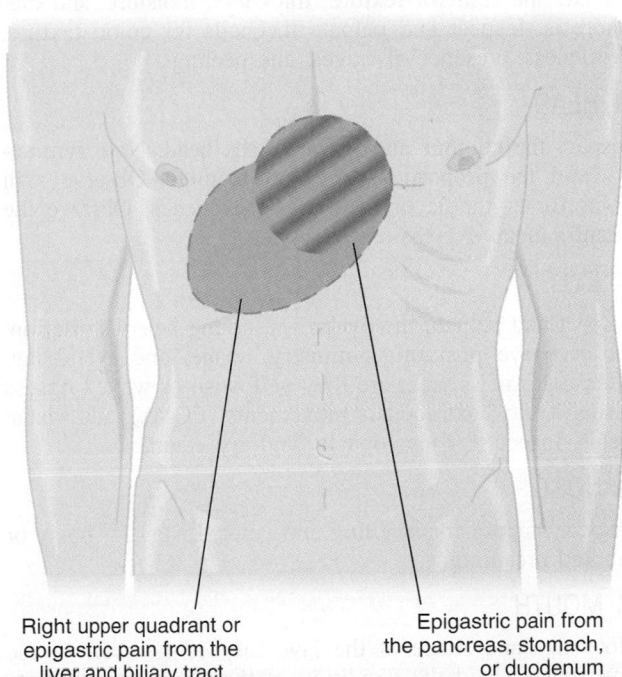

Right upper quadrant or epigastric pain from the liver and biliary tract

Epigastric pain from the pancreas, stomach, or duodenum

FIGURE 42–1 Location of abdominal pain with hepatic, biliary, or pancreatic disorders.

■ GENERAL APPEARANCE AND NUTRITIONAL STATUS

Begin by assessing the client's general appearance and health status. Is the client alert and responding appropriately to questions? Observe the client's mood, level of consciousness (orientation, alertness), verbal and nonverbal behavior, memory, affect, and speech patterns. Note any anxiety or nervousness, depression, apathy, or anger.

Does the client appear acutely or chronically ill? Question the client's use of alcohol and other substances. Because handwriting deteriorates with diminishing liver function, obtain a handwriting sample for subsequent comparison should the client have progressive hepatocellular damage (see Chapter 47).

Assess nutritional status. Weigh the client, and determine the amount of subcutaneous fat and muscular development. Obesity may accompany gallbladder disease. Ask whether the client has a pattern of right upper quadrant pain after eating certain high-fat foods (e.g., nuts, chocolate). Clients with a history of substance abuse or cirrhosis may be malnourished. Observe the client's state of dress, growth and development, and body size. Chapter 28 describes the assessment of nutrition.

■ VITAL SIGNS

Measure and assess vital signs. Temperature is elevated in hyperthyroidism or may be low-normal or below normal in hypothyroidism. Observe respirations for altered rate and rhythm. Blood pressure alterations include hypotension, hypertension, widening pulse pressure, and orthostatic changes in the pulse rate.

■ INTEGUMENT

Observe hair texture and distribution over body surfaces. Note brittleness or loss of hair (alopecia). Inspect the skin for color, pigmentation, striae, ecchymoses, or mottling. Palpate the skin for texture, thickness, moisture, and diaphoresis. Inspect and palpate the nails for color, texture, brittleness, presence of ridges, and peeling.

■ HEAD

Inspect the contour and shape of the head. Note symmetry and the proportion of facial features. Observe skin color for erythema or rash over the cheeks. Observe the client's facial expression for anxiety.

■ EYES

Inspect and palpate the eyebrows, noting hair distribution. Observe eye position, symmetry, shape, and eyelid lag. Note color of sclerae: are they yellowish or white? Assess visual acuity, extraocular movements (EOMs), and visual fields. Inspect for lens opacity and eye edema.

■ NOSE

Inspect mucosa for swelling and color. Listen for noisy or labored breathing.

■ MOUTH

Note size and shape of the jaw. Inspect the color of the oral mucosa and the condition of the client's teeth. Note malocclusion. Observe tongue size and activity for fasciculations.

■ NECK

Listen to the client's voice for hoarseness or huskiness. Note clarity, pitch, and volume of speech. Ask the client to swallow, and observe for difficulty in swallowing or pain; repeat this maneuver with the client's neck in a hyperextended position. Inspect the neck for symmetry, alignment, thickness, or bulging over the thyroid gland, and examine the midline position of the trachea. Observe for scars related to thyroidectomy, trauma, or other neck surgery. Note presence of hyperpigmentation.

Observe for forceful pulsations over the carotid arteries. Palpate the thyroid gland unless it is noticeably enlarged; vigorous palpation can stimulate release of thyroid hormone, which increases the risk of precipitating a thyroid crisis in a client with thyroid hyperplasia. If the thyroid gland is enlarged, auscultate the lobes for bruits.

The thyroid gland may be palpated by means of an anterior or posterior approach (Fig. 42–2). In both approaches, gently run a finger down the anterior part of the neck, locating the thyroid and cricoid cartilages and the isthmus of the thyroid gland. The isthmus feels soft and compressible compared with the firmer cartilage ring just superior to it. Ask the client to swallow while you palpate the isthmus. It should rise in the neck and should not be enlarged. Figure 42–2 explains the anterior and posterior approaches for palpating the lobes of the thyroid gland. The thyroid gland is normally nonpalpable. If it is palpable, note the texture of the gland because it is usually smooth and firm, without lumps, roughness, hardness, asymmetry, or tenderness (see the Physical Assessment Findings feature).

■ EXTREMITIES

Examine the arms and legs for size, shape, and symmetry, and check their proportionality to the trunk. The distance from the symphysis pubis to the heel is usually about half of the body's total height. Note peripheral edema. Palpate and note peripheral pulse amplitude (see Chapter 10). Assess deep tendon reflexes, and observe their relaxation time (see Chapter 67).

Upper Extremities

Ask the client to extend the hands with palms down; observe for fine tremors and for reddened palms (palmar erythema). Inspect for thenar wasting, Dupuytren's contracture, and nail clubbing (see Chapter 59). Note the size of the client's hands in proportion to the rest of the body. Assess grip strength and muscle strength of the fingers and arms (see Chapter 25).

Lower Extremities

Note the color and distribution of hair. Assess the size of the client's feet in proportion to the rest of the body. Inspect for corns and calluses. Separate the toes, and observe for deformities and skin changes, such as thickening, fissures, and nail thickening. Palpate and note pedal pulses (see Chapter 10). Assess leg muscles for weakness (see Chapter 25).

Thyroid
cartilage

Cricoid
cartilage

Isthmus of
the thyroid

Lobe of the
thyroid

Trachea

Sternocleidomastoid
muscle

Thyroid
gland

Left
sternocleidomastoid
muscle

A   Posterior approach

B   Anterior approach

FIGURE 42–2 Palpation of the thyroid. *A,* Posterior approach. Stand behind the client. Ask the client to lower the chin to relax the neck muscles, and tilt the head slightly to the right. To examine the right lobe of the thyroid, use the fingers of your left hand to displace the trachea slightly to the right. This moves the thyroid laterally. You can then palpate between the trachea and the sternocleidomastoid for the right lobe with the fingers of your right hand. Ask the client to swallow while you palpate; doing so causes the gland to rise in the neck. Repeat for the left lobe by reversing your hand placement and positioning the client toward the left. Projection of the thyroid can be enhanced by having the client drink water. *B,* Anterior approach. Stand in front of the client. To palpate the thyroid gland's right lobe, flex the client's head toward the right to relax the neck muscles on that side. Use the fingers of your right hand to displace the trachea slightly to the client's right. Then ask the client to swallow while you palpate the right lobe of the thyroid with the fingers of your left hand. Repeat for the left lobe. You can also assess for thyroid enlargement by palpating deep on each side of the sternocleidomastoid muscle.

■ THORAX

In males, inspect for gynecomastia (breast enlargement), which can develop because of decreased metabolism of estrogen when the liver is dysfunctional. Auscultate for extra heart sounds, such as a systolic murmur (see Chapter 54).

PHYSICAL ASSESSMENT FINDINGS IN THE HEALTHY ADULT*

Thyroid Gland

Inspection

The thyroid gland is not normally seen on inspection.

Palpation

The gland rises and falls with swallowing. Isthmus at midline, soft. Right lobe slightly larger than the left lobe. Texture rubbery without nodules. Nontender.

Auscultation

No bruits heard over either lobe.

---

* Findings for the metabolic system are found in Chapter 28 as part of the abdominal assessment.

■ ABDOMEN

Assessment of the abdomen includes inspection, auscultation, percussion, and palpation. Table 42–1 summarizes the key points of a physical examination for endocrine and metabolic disorders.

Inspection

Note areas of hyperpigmentation, such as in scars or striae. Observe the client for manifestations of pain during light palpation; examine painful areas last. Characteristics of ascites include a distended abdomen with tight and glistening skin, bulging flanks, and prominent abdominal veins. Measure abdominal girth if ascites is present. Ascites may account for recent rapid onset of weight gain with accompanying loss of muscle mass.

Auscultation

Auscultation for possible hepatic or biliary problems is performed by gently placing a warmed stethoscope on the right upper quadrant while the client is supine. Note whether a soft hum is heard during both the systolic and diastolic components of the heartbeat. A *hum* indicates increased collateral circulation between the portal and systemic venous systems, as might occur in hepatic cirrhosis.

TABLE 42-1	KEY POINTS OF A PHYSICAL EXAMINATION: ENDOCRINE AND METABOLIC DISORDERS	
Steps	**Normal or Common Findings**	**Significant or Abnormal Findings**
Inspection		
Note:		
Color of skin	Same as or lighter than other areas	Redness, cyanosis, jaundice, lesions, ecchymosis, needle marks, or hematomas
Eyes	White sclerae	Sclerae: yellow tint
Symmetry, contour, shape of abdomen	Flat, rounded abdomen	Distended, asymmetrical, masses
Surface of abdomen	Smooth	Tight, shiny; engorged, prominent veins, spider angiomas
Rectal area	No dilated veins (hemorrhoids)	Presence of distended veins (hemorrhoids)
General nutritional state Weigh Observe for ascites	Adequate for height and build	Obesity or malnutrition
Auscultation Place stethoscope (warmed) over right upper quadrant. Listen for vascular sounds or friction rubs	No venous hums No friction rubs	Venous hum with both diastolic and systolic components
Percussion *Abdomen:* Note percussion sounds in four quadrants	Tympany over abdomen, bladder, intestines, and aorta, and dull over liver, spleen, pancreas, kidneys, and uterus	Dullness over enlarged organs; indicates need for further assessment for ascites
Liver: Span. Percuss upward from below client's umbilicus on the right midclavicular line (MCL), until dullness is heard. Mark this point. Percuss downward from lung resonance in right MCL to dullness and measure distance between two marks. Note if tender, soft, or firm, smooth or nodular	Liver span is 6–12 cm. No tenderness Slightly tender, soft, smooth surface	Liver span is greater than 12 cm Nodular, more than slightly tender, hard
Spleen: Note size. Percuss downward in left posterior axillary line, beginning with lung resonance until dullness is heard	Dullness between ribs 6 and 10	Dullness extends above sixth rib or covers large area—indicates enlargement
Palpation Use palmar surface of extended fingers		
Liver: Palpate lightly on right side and then palpate deeply	No tenderness, pain, masses	Tenderness, rigidity, nodules, enlarged
Spleen: Note: If spleen can be percussed, it is best not to palpate it. Palpate lightly on left side, distal to MCL	No tenderness, pain, masses	Tenderness, rigidity, nodules, enlarged
ADAPTATIONS FOR OLDER ADULTS		
Inspection Contour	Sagging and rounded because of loss of muscle tone and accumulation of fat	
Palpation Note liver span and borders	Span may be shortened but border more easily palpated	Right upper quadrant or epigastric pain from the liver and biliary tract Epigastric pain from pancreas, stomach, or duodenum

Listen for a *friction rub* (a grating sound heard with respiratory ventilation). A friction rub suggests inflammation of the peritoneal surface of an organ, as from a liver tumor, chlamydial or gonococcal perihepatitis, or recent liver biopsy.

If a systolic *bruit* (swishing sound indicating vascular turbulence) accompanies a hepatic friction rub, carcinoma of the liver is suspected.

Percussion

Percuss the abdomen, especially the liver and spleen. Assess liver size by percussing the span of the liver at the right midclavicular line (RMCL) and the midsternal line (MSL). Begin by percussing in the right midclavicular line either superior or inferior to the estimated borders of the liver. Superiorly, begin at the third intercostal space (ICS) over lung resonance; percuss down the thorax until the sound changes to dull. Mark this level on the skin with a pen. Inferiorly, start over a tympanic area and percuss upward until the sound changes to dull. Also mark this with the pen.

At the midsternal line, percuss upward from above the umbilicus from tympany to dull. Mark where the sound changes. Superiorly, percuss down the sternum until the percussion note changes; mark this too. Measure the distance between each set of marks.

At the right midclavicular line, the liver span ranges from 6 to 12 cm (2½ to 5 inches); at the midsternal line, it ranges from 4 to 8 cm (1½ to 3 inches). The lower border of the liver at the right midclavicular line is usually at the right costal margin, and the upper border is between the fifth and seventh intercostal spaces.

Liver size varies with body size. Measurements larger than the norms indicate liver enlargement. Ask the client to take a deep breath and hold it while you percuss the lower liver border in the right midclavicular line again. With deep inspiration, the pressure of the diaphragm causes the liver to descend lower into the abdomen. The distance of liver descent is marked and measured and ranges from 2 to 3 cm (~1 inch). Use the marked level of liver descent as a guide for later palpation of the liver.

Spleen size may be determined by percussion, particularly if the spleen is enlarged. The spleen is located by percussion as a small area of dullness just posterior to the left midaxillary line (LMAL) between the sixth and 10th ribs. It normally has a span of approximately 7 cm (2½ to 3 inches). If the spleen enlarges, the area of dullness shifts inferiorly below the 10th rib and anteriorly toward or beyond the left anterior axillary line (LAAL).

Percussion is also used to assess for ascites in the abdomen by observing for a *fluid wave*. This infrequently performed maneuver is an advanced physical assessment technique because of the potential difficulty in detecting a fluid wave. A more common method of assessment for ascites is to measure changes in abdominal girth and weight gain over time. Another advanced assessment technique to detect ascites is the *test for shifting dullness,* described in Chapter 32.

The *fluid wave test* is performed while the client is supine. Two nurses participate. One nurse places the edges of the hands on the client's abdominal midline to stabilize the abdominal wall. The second nurse places one hand on one side of the client's abdomen while briskly tapping the opposite side of the abdomen with the other hand. The second nurse feels for the movement of a fluid wave against the palpating hand opposite the side percussed.

Palpation

Use palpation initially to assess for muscle guarding or tenderness. Observe the client for facial grimaces, tensing, or other indications of discomfort. Next, perform deep palpation to evaluate tenderness, indicating possible inflammation. Light and deep palpation techniques are discussed in Chapter 10.

Because the peritoneum is often involved, evaluate for localized peritoneal irritation. Press the abdomen firmly at a point away from any tender area, and quickly remove the examining hand. Severe pain accompanies this maneuver when inflammation is present, indicating *rebound tenderness.*

Perform *liver palpation* standing at the client's right side. Use one of two bimanual techniques:

First technique. Place your left hand under the client's right posterior thorax over the 11th and 12th ribs, and push the thorax upward. Place the right hand below the right costal margin at the previously marked level of liver descent, as determined by percussion. Point your fingers upward toward the costal margin, then gently push up and in as the client takes a deep breath using the abdominal muscles. As the client inhales, feel for the liver's edge to slip over the finger tips as it descends. If the liver's edge is felt, it should feel firm, sharp, smooth, and regular. Palpate at several points medially and laterally to assess the edge along its inferior border.

Second technique. Place the right hand below the right costal margin as described. Superimpose the left hand on the right hand. Perform the remainder of the maneuver as described earlier.

The liver is difficult to palpate in clients who are obese or tense or who have taut abdominal muscles because they are physically fit. Abnormal findings include a hard, nodular feel to the liver and more than minimal tenderness as perceived by the client. If extreme ascites is present, the liver edge is nonpalpable.

Spleen palpation is an advanced physical assessment technique. If percussion has shown that the spleen is enlarged, the nurse does not usually palpate it because of the possibility of rupture. If no enlargement is noted on percussion, perform spleen palpation in a manner similar to that for the liver; however, perform the technique on the left side of the abdomen below the costal margin. Ask the client to turn onto the right side, allowing gravity to bring the spleen forward and down, closer to the abdominal wall. Place your left hand behind the client's left posterior rib cage, and push forward while palpating with the right hand. The spleen is normally nonpalpable. Congestion caused by portal hypertension results in enlargement of the spleen and is a common finding in cirrhosis.

Blunt (fist) percussion is used to determine organ tenderness over the liver. This maneuver is performed after all other abdominal assessment techniques are completed to avoid producing discomfort in the presence of organ tenderness. When assessing for *liver tenderness*, use *only* indirect fist percussion over the costal margin at the right midclavicular line to avoid trauma to the liver. This maneuver is also known as a *liver tap*. For comparison, perform indirect fist percussion over the left costal margin at the midclavicular line (Chapter 10 explains blunt percussion). Tell the client what is going to be done to avoid a reaction of surprise that may be misinterpreted as tenderness. Note the client's reaction to the blows.

Record physical findings for the liver and spleen as part of the abdominal examination. Chapter 28 includes a recording of a normal abdominal physical assessment.

GENITALIA AND RECTUM

Observe the pattern of pubic hair distribution, particularly in women. A diamond-shaped (male) pattern is indicative of a masculinizing tumor. Note the size of the testes in male clients and the clitoris in female clients for comparison with expected norms. The remainder of endocrine assessment consists of diagnostic studies, since the only endocrine glands accessible to physical examination are the thyroid and gonads (see Chapter 37).

Inspect the rectal area for dilated veins (hemorrhoids). These may be present in cirrhosis with portal hypertension.

MODIFICATIONS FOR OLDER ADULTS

When assessing the older adult client for possible endocrine or metabolic disorders, remember to divide the physical assessment into several parts to avoid fatigue. Allow adequate time for the physical examination so that the information needed is clearly communicated to the client.

When inspecting the abdomen, note the contour and color. A rounded, sagging abdomen is a normal finding because of the tendency for fat to accumulate in the lower abdomen and hips and for the abdominal muscles to weaken. Note any areas of tenderness or discomfort because old age may blunt the manifestations of pain caused by peritoneal inflammation, for example (see Table 42–1).

DIAGNOSTIC TESTS

A client with an endocrine dysfunction may need several general types of diagnostic tests. Blood levels of various hormones specific to the endocrine glands are measured. Some hormones are measured for specific levels; others, such as thyroid hormone, are measured according to how well they combine with plasma proteins or radioactive iodine.

The client may be anxious about the tests and the possible results. In many cases, endocrine disorders have been misdiagnosed for years because of the nonspecific manifestations of the disorders. After the correct diagnosis is made, the client and family may need help coping with ongoing care.

Similarly, a client with a metabolic dysfunction (exocrine pancreas, liver, or biliary tract) frequently requires multiple diagnostic measures. No single laboratory test,

radiographic study, or surgical procedure yields sufficient data to confirm a diagnosis or establish the degree of malfunction. Foster a sense of self-worth and understanding in the client during repeated diagnostic procedures. Such a sense promotes cooperation and reduces the fatigue and anxiety that frequently accompany these evaluations.

In the discussion that follows, common diagnostic tests of endocrine function are identified according to specific endocrine organs: pancreas, thyroid, adrenal, and pituitary, after which diagnostic tests involving organs of metabolism (exocrine pancreas, liver, biliary tract, and gallbladder) are discussed.

ENDOCRINE FUNCTION STUDIES

Laboratory Studies

A more detailed presentation of laboratory tests for specific endocrine disorders may be found in the chapters on these disorders.

Tests of Pancreatic Function

Diagnostic assessment of pancreatic endocrine function is related to blood glucose levels. Elevated fasting blood glucose is usually the first indication of hyperglycemia. Glycosylated hemoglobin (HbA1c), or glycohemoglobin, is a measure of the average blood glucose over 3 months and can be obtained in the nonfasting state. A more detailed presentation of diagnostic tests related to diabetes appears in Chapter 45.

Tests of Thyroid Function

Several tests are available to assess thyroid function. A brief overview of the most common diagnostic tests follows.

SERUM THYROXINE AND TRIIODOTHYRONINE
Radioimmunoassay can be used to measure serum concentrations of thyroxine (T_4) and triiodothyronine (T_3).

T_4 is transported in the blood largely bound to thyroxine-binding globulin and is an effective indicator of thyroid function; conditions that affect thyroid-binding globulin levels alter the serum T_4 concentration. Hyperthyroidism, viral hepatitis, pregnancy, and oral contraceptives increase serum T_4; hypothyroidism, strenuous exercise, heparin, and lithium decrease serum T_4.

T_3 (like T_4) circulates in the bloodstream, attached to plasma proteins and to erythrocytes. However, T_3 binds far more readily to plasma proteins than to erythrocytes. T_3 binds to erythrocytes only when plasma protein binding sites are limited.

Analysis of T_3 and T_4 concentrations has largely replaced the older technique of estimating basal metabolic rate (BMR). BMR is calculated by measuring the amount of oxygen the body consumes when in a state of complete mental and physical relaxation.

T_3 RESIN UPTAKE
If thyroid function is below normal or if serum protein levels are high, resin uptake of T_3 is depressed. If thyroid function is above normal or serum protein levels are low, resin uptake of T_3 is elevated. T_3 resin uptake is one test

used to measure thyroid function but should not be the only one.

RADIOIODINE UPTAKE AND EXCRETION TEST

The body cannot distinguish between radiolabeled ("tagged") iodine and nonradiolabeled iodine. Consequently, the thyroid takes up radioactive iodine (RAIU) and processes it just as it does regular iodine. ^{131}I has been used for measuring thyroid function, but ^{123}I is preferable because it allows the use of a lower radiation dose.[30] Radioiodine is excreted in the urine just as is ordinary iodine. A scintillation scanner is used to measure the amount of radioactive iodine present in the thyroid 24 hours after administration of a radioiodine isotope preparation. The laboratory may measure the client's urine output of radioactive iodine after the test.

Many factors can distort findings. Before the procedure, therefore, question the client about the following, and inform the physician if the client answers "yes" to any of these questions.

- Have you taken any iodine-containing medications within the last 30 days?
- Are you taking estrogens that can cause a false elevation?
- Have you undergone x-ray studies of the gallbladder, ureters, bronchi, fallopian tubes, or heart within the last 10 years?
- Within the last 2 weeks, have you principally eaten seafood? (Seafood is so rich in iodine that ^{131}I uptake can show a falsely low reading.)

SERUM THYROID-STIMULATING HORMONE CONCENTRATION

Measurement of the basal serum thyroid-stimulating hormone (TSH) concentration is useful in the diagnosis of both advanced and subclinical hypothyroidism. In one stage of hypothyroidism, the thyroid gland compensates for a functional abnormality that impairs the ability to synthesize hormones and hypersecretes TSH. In thyrotoxic states, the serum TSH concentration is almost always low or undetectable.

THYROTROPIN-RELEASING HORMONE STIMULATION TEST

Thyrotropin-releasing hormone (TRH) is released from the hypothalamus, and it normally stimulates release of TSH from the pituitary. During the TRH stimulation test, people with thyroid disorders are given TRH intravenously. A rise in TSH levels indicates that the pituitary is functioning normally. TSH levels do not rise in the presence of hyperthyroidism or when the pituitary cells that secrete TSH are diseased.

SERUM CHOLESTEROL

The serum cholesterol level may be elevated in primary hypothyroidism, which may explain why this condition is accompanied by a marked tendency toward atherosclerosis. People with hyperthyroidism usually have a lower serum cholesterol level. Serum cholesterol is not a specific test of thyroid function, however, because its levels are influenced by many factors other than thyroid hormone levels.

ANTITHYROID ANTIBODY TESTS

Many thyroid disorders are presumed to have an autoimmune basis, such as Hashimoto's thyroiditis, some types of myxedema, and Graves' disease (a form of hyperthyroidism). Serologic tests may be performed to determine whether the client's blood contains antithyroid antibodies.

ACHILLES TENDON REFLEXES

The Achilles tendon reflex test measures the amplitude and duration of the ankle jerk with a special instrument, which is used to tap the strong tendon at the back of the heel. Clients with hyperthyroidism may demonstrate a more rapid tendon reflex. Clients with an underactive thyroid gland or diabetes mellitus and pregnant women have slower reflexes and prolonged relaxation times. Chapter 67 covers tendon reflex testing.

Tests of Adrenal Function

Adrenal function tests may be used to evaluate medullary and cortical hormones. Adrenocortical hormones include cortisol (glucocorticoid), aldosterone (mineral corticoid), and small amounts of sex hormones (androgens). Adrenal medullary hormones include epinephrine and norepinephrine (catecholamines).

CORTISOL SUPPRESSION TEST

Cortisol is secreted in a diurnal pattern, and levels are assessed at 8 AM and 8 PM. A cortisol suppression test involves the suppression of pituitary ACTH with dexamethasone. Normally, after administration of dexamethasone, 24-hour levels of ketosteroid in the urine drop by 50%. Dexamethasone can also be given at midnight and serum cortisol then assessed at 8 AM. In clients with increased adrenocortical stimulation, no decrease is seen in ketosteroid production in urine or in serum levels of cortisol.

ALDOSTERONE LEVELS

Plasma levels of aldosterone, angiotensin II, and renin can be measured at any time. Plasma levels of aldosterone can be increased by giving potassium, restricting sodium, or having the client assume an upright position. Plasma levels of aldosterone can be decreased by infusion of saline.

SERUM ADRENOCORTICOTROPIC HORMONE

Serum levels of ACTH can be assessed after infusion of synthetic ACTH. Urine levels of ketosteroid would be expected to rise to 25 mg in 24 hours; plasma levels of cortisol should rise to 10 to 40 μg/dl. Urine levels of ketosteroid can be measured with 24-hour urine specimens. *Ketosteroids* are metabolites of the hormones produced by the adrenal cortex. A preservative is required for the collection bottle. If the client has an indwelling catheter, the urinary drainage bag is emptied frequently and the urine is refrigerated. Collection of 24-hour urine specimens is explained in Chapter 11.

URINARY CATECHOLAMINES

Adrenal medullary function can be assessed through urine levels of catecholamines and their metabolites (vanillylmandelic acid [VMA]). A 24-hour urine sample is collected and assayed. Adrenal medullary secretion can be suppressed by administration of ganglionic blocking agents, which normally decrease the urine levels of catecholamines. In clients with pheochromocytoma (a tumor of the adrenal medulla), ganglionic blocking agents have a negligible effect in controlling blood pressure. An older assessment test for pheochromocytoma, which involved blood pressure manipulation, is rarely performed today.

RADIOGRAPHY

The adrenal cortex can be assessed for tumors by x-ray study, computed tomography (CT), and magnetic resonance imaging (MRI) (see Chapter 11).

Tests of Pituitary Function

RADIOGRAPHY

The structure of the pituitary gland can be assessed by skull x-ray study, CT, or MRI. Tumors of the pituitary may be visualized with these studies (see Chapter 11).

HORMONE ASSAYS

Hormonal disorders caused by malfunction of the pituitary gland can lead to a wide variety of clinical manifestations, depending on which hormone is involved. Growth hormone (GH) and ADH are discussed here.

GROWTH HORMONE LEVELS. GH is secreted in a diurnal pattern, and its level can be assayed. In a determination of basal levels, the blood sample is usually drawn in the morning after the client has had nothing by mouth (*nil per os*, NPO) for 8 to 10 hours. Usual levels for males are less than 5 ng/ml; for females, less than 10 ng/ml. GH can be stimulated by administration of (1) levodopa (500 mg, orally), (2) insulin (0.05 to 0.3 unit/kg, intravenously), or (3) bromocriptine (5 mg, orally). After the stimulus, blood is drawn at intervals for up to 120 minutes. GH levels usually peak 60 minutes after stimulation.

DEHYDRATION TESTS. Absence of ADH leads to diabetes insipidus. A dehydration test is used to confirm the diagnosis of diabetes insipidus. Fluids are withheld long enough to result in stable hourly urinary osmolalities (4 to 18 hours). During this time, the client's vital signs, urine output, and urine specific gravity are assessed hourly. Hypovolemic shock can develop from dehydration. After the third hour of stable urinary osmolality, the client is given vasopressin as 5 units aqueous arginine vasopressin or 1 μg desmopressin by subcutaneous injection or 10 μg desmopressin by nasal spray.[19] A client without diabetes insipidus responds with decreased urine output and increased urine osmolality. A client with diabetes insipidus cannot respond and continues to produce high volumes of dilute urine (low osmolality).

■ METABOLIC FUNCTION STUDIES

Laboratory Studies

The most common laboratory tests for metabolic function (liver, biliary, and exocrine pancreas) include those used to measure levels of serum enzymes, proteins, antigens, antibodies, fats, and bleeding and clotting factors and related urine and stool studies (Table 42–2). Details on hepatitis virus infection are presented in Chapter 47.

Tests of All Metabolic Organ Functions

LIVER, GALLBLADDER, BILIARY TRACT, AND PANCREAS

ULTRASONOGRAPHY. Ultrasonographic examination provides valuable diagnostic information about liver, pancreatic, and biliary tract conditions. The technique is rapid, and little or no preparation is required. Depending on the area to be examined, the client may or may not fast before the procedure. Reassure the client that the test is painless and safe. There are no specific precautions or observations after ultrasonography. See Chapter 11 for a discussion of ultrasonography.

RADIOGRAPHY. Many procedures used to diagnose disorders of the liver, pancreas, and biliary tract involve the use of x-rays. Plain x-ray films of the abdomen may show diaphragm elevation caused by hepatic enlargement or calcification in the abdominal organs. Upper or lower gastrointestinal series using barium contrast medium also provide important information about the accessory organs of digestion (i.e., liver, gallbladder, and pancreas). One such test of the pancreas, hypotonic duodenography, requires insertion of barium sulfate and air into the duodenum via a catheter passed through the client's nose to the duodenum. Spot x-ray films are taken to detect pancreatic and duodenal diseases (i.e., tumor at the head of the pancreas or a stricture caused by chronic pancreatitis).

Radiologic studies with iodinated contrast media permit visualization of tubes and vessels. Before any of these procedures are performed, question the client about known hypersensitivity to iodine (see Chapter 11).

Computed Tomography. CT is used to identify and evaluate liver, biliary tract, gallbladder, and pancreatic disorders. It is useful for distinguishing cysts or tumors and differentiating obstructive from nonobstructive jaundice (Fig. 42–3). The client is instructed to fast, except for water, for 8 to 12 hours before the test. See Chapter 11 for a more detailed discussion of CT.

Angiography. Angiography allows visualization of the hepatic, biliary, and pancreatic arterial vessels after administration of contrast medium. It is used to identify abnormalities of vascular structure and function, observe masses, and note bleeding sites in the pancreas, spleen, and portal system. To inject the contrast medium, the examiner usually introduces a needle into the femoral artery. Next, the needle is exchanged for a catheter, which is then passed into the celiac artery or one of its branches (superior mesenteric or hepatic). After contrast medium injection, rapid sequence filming is done. See Chapter 11 for additional details.

Preprocedure care

Explain the purpose of the examination to the client. The client usually takes nothing by mouth for 6 to 8 hours before the test. Ask the client about any use of medications that might lead to bleeding, such as anticoagulants or nonsteroidal anti-inflammatory drugs (NSAIDs). These medications should be stopped up to a week before the test. Bleeding or clotting tests are usually ordered before the test. Remind the client that it is necessary to lie very still during the examination. Explain that there may be a sensation of pressure during introduction of the catheter. Assess the pulses distal to the insertion site for comparison with pulses afterward.

Postprocedure care

After angiography, assess the needle insertion site for manifestations of bleeding. Clients with liver conditions often have concurrent clotting disorders, which may lead to a hematoma. Assess the pulses below the level of

TABLE 42–2	**LABORATORY TESTS OF LIVER, BILIARY, AND PANCREATIC FUNCTION**

Measurement	Normal Value*	Procedure	Interpretation
		EXOCRINE PANCREATIC ASSESSMENT	
Serum amylase with isoenzymes	60–160 Somogyi U/dl	Blood drawn 1–2 hr after eating, preferably while no IV solutions are infusing	Pancreatic digestive enzyme released with breakdown of acinar cells; serum levels increase with acute and chronic pancreatitis, obstruction of pancreatic duct, acute alcoholic intoxication, and diabetes mellitus; elevations not directly correlated with severity; decreased with advanced chronic necrosis of liver and chronic alcoholism; amylase test measures both pancreatic and salivary amylase; pancreatic isoamylase is a more specific test
Urine amylase	4–37 U/dl/24 hr	2- or 24-hr urine collection bottle must have a preservative. Specimens collected after initial voiding	Urine levels elevated longer with pancreatitis
Serum lipase	14–280 mU/ml 20–180 IU/L	Blood drawn after client NPO except for water for 8–12 hr	Lipase aids in digesting fats and is increased in acute and chronic pancreatitis, early-stage cancer of pancreas, and obstruction of pancreatic duct; decreased in late cancer of pancreas and hepatitis
Pancreatic function		Oral bentiromide given after overnight fast; urine is collected for 6 hr	Pancreatic chymotrypsin splits bentiromide; para-aminobenzoic acid (PABA), a breakdown product, is excreted in urine; less PABA is excreted with pancreatic insufficiency
		LIVER ASSESSMENT	
Serum bilirubin Direct (conjugated) Indirect (unconjugated) Total	0.1–0.3 mg/dl 0.2–0.8 mg/dl 0.1–1.2 mg/dl	Blood drawn after client NPO after midnight except for water; protect sample from ultraviolet light or sunlight	Direct bilirubin increased with biliary obstruction, causing conjugated fraction to accumulate in plasma Indirect bilirubin increased with excessive erythrocyte hemolysis Total bilirubin measures direct and indirect levels together
Urine bilirubin	0–0.02 mg/dl	Urine collection (urine appears smoky or tea colored); protect from light	Urine bilirubin measures conjugated bilirubin only; increased with biliary obstruction
Urine urobilinogen	Random: 0.3–3.5 mg/dl 24-hr: 0.05–2.5 mg/24 hr	2- or 24-hr afternoon collection placed in brown refrigerated bottle with sodium carbonate preservative	Urine urobilinogen decreased with biliary obstruction or liver damage; increased with erythrocyte hemolysis and certain drugs (e.g., sulfonamides) and liver, toxic, or infectious hepatitis
Fecal urobilinogen	75–275 EU/100 g	Entire stool specimen to laboratory	Fecal urobilinogen decreased with biliary obstruction; increased in erythrocyte hemolysis
Serum cholesterol	150–240 mg/dl <200 mg/dl desired	Blood drawn after low-cholesterol diet for 12 hr	Elevated when excretion blocked by bile duct obstruction, diabetes mellitus, and pancreatitis; may be decreased in chronic liver disease, hyperthyroidism, and adrenal hormone excess (Cushing's syndrome)

Table continues on following page

TABLE 42–2 **LABORATORY TESTS OF LIVER, BILIARY, AND PANCREATIC FUNCTION** *Continued*

Measurement	Normal Value*	Procedure	Interpretation
Liver enzyme tests†			
Aspartate aminotransferase (AST)	0–35 U/L	Blood drawn without special preparation	Serum AST, ALT, and LDH released from damaged liver, heart, kidney, and muscle cells; prolonged elevation in liver disease may be first indicator of chronic active hepatitis; a rapid drop may signal liver failure
Alanine aminotransferase (ALT)	5–35 U/ml (Frankel)		
Lactate dehydrogenase (LDH) isoenzyme	100–190 IU/L		
Alkaline phosphatase (ALP) and isoenzyme	20–90 U/L at 30° C		Elevated in biliary obstruction; produced by cells lining the biliary tract; this enzyme is also found in bone, intestine, and placenta
Serum 5'-nucleotidase	<17 U/L		Enzyme located mainly in liver and liver disease confirmed if ALP and this enzyme both elevated
Serum γ-glutamyltransferase (GGT)	4–23 IU/L (male) 3–13 IU/L (female)		Enzyme located primarily in liver and kidney; elevation of GGT and ALP significant indication of liver disorders
Leucine aminopeptidase (LAP)	8–22 mU/ml		Elevated in liver disease. LAP frequently ordered with 5'-NT and LAP tests to confirm liver disease
Protein metabolism			
Total protein	6.0–8.2 g/dl	Blood drawn without special preparation	Impaired protein synthesis or utilization caused by chronic liver disease, pancreatic insufficiency (albumin, α- and β-globulins); γ-globulins produced by B lymphocytes, not liver
Serum albumin	3.5–5.0 g/dl		
Serum globulin includes α_1, α_2, β, γ	2.1–4.2 g/dl		
A/G (albumin/globulin) ratio	1.0–2.0 g/dl		Decrease in the ratio may indicate chronic liver disease
Plasma ammonia	15–45 g/dl	Blood drawn after client NPO except for water for 8–12 hr before the test. Blood must be iced and tested immediately	Reduced synthesis of urea from body ammonia in severe hepatocellular damage produces elevated blood ammonia
Hemostatic function			
Prothrombin time (PT)	11–15 sec or 70%–100%	Blood drawn without special preparation	Increase in PT may occur in liver disease. Assesses function of extrinsic pathway in clotting process (factors I, II, V, VII, X). PT prolonged with (1) decreased synthesis of prothrombin because of liver cell damage or (2) decreased vitamin K absorption because of bile duct obstruction. Vitamin K necessary for liver to synthesize prothrombin
Platelets	150,000–400,000 μl (mean = 250,000 μl)		May fall in liver disease (cirrhosis, chronic active hepatitis), anemias, leukemias. Elevated in trauma, metastatic carcinoma TB
Metabolism of foreign substances			
Bromsulphalein (BSP) excretion	<5% retention in 1 hr	Control blood specimen (or sample) taken after fasting for 12 hr; BSP given, blood drawn at intervals	Dye retained with diminished hepatocellular ability to remove it from blood and excrete it; test is infrequently used

TABLE 42-2	LABORATORY TESTS OF LIVER, BILIARY, AND PANCREATIC FUNCTION *Continued*		
Measurement	**Normal Value***	**Procedure**	**Interpretation**
Antigens and antibodies			
Hepatitis antigens and antibodies	Negative for antigens. Positive or negative for antibodies, depending on history	Blood drawn without special preparation	Antigens indicate hepatitis, antibodies indicate past or present hepatitis or immunization (hepatitis B)
Antimicrobial antibody (AMA)	Negative at 1:5 Positive at >1:160		Test done to differentiate between biliary cirrhosis and other liver diseases
Alpha-fetoprotein (AFP), antigen associated with cancer	<10 ng/ml		AFP is synthesized by fetus but not by healthy adult; AFP level >1000 ng/ml usually indicates hepatocellular carcinoma

*Normal values may differ significantly between laboratories.
†Trends in elevation are of particular importance in predicting the rapidity with which the liver is failing. If levels rise, fall, then rise again, liver failure may be occurring.
A, albumin; AFP, alpha-fetoprotein; ALP, alkaline phosphatase; ALT, alanine aminotransferase; AMA, antimicrobial antibody; AST, aspartate aminotransferase; BSP, Bromsulphalein (sulfobromophthalein sodium); EU = Ehrlich units; G, globulin; GGT, gamma-glutamyltransferase; IV, intravenous; LAP, leucine aminopeptidase; LDH, lactate dehydrogenase; NPO, *nil per os* (nothing by mouth); 5'-NT, 5'-nucleotidase; PABA, para-aminobenzoic acid; PT, prothrombin time; TB, tuberculosis.
Data from Kee, J. L. (1998). *Laboratory and diagnostic tests with nursing implications.* (5th ed.). Stamford, CT: Appleton & Lange.

catheter insertion and compare with the preprocedure baseline findings.

RADIONUCLIDE IMAGING. Radionuclide imaging with technetium 99m dimethylacetanilide (hepato-iminodiacetic acid [HIDA], diethyl-iminodiacetic acid [DIDA], and diisopropyl-iminodiacetic acid [DISIDA]) involves intravenous infusion of gamma-emitting isotopes. After infusion, a scintillation detector is passed over the abdomen. This procedure is used to investigate biliary obstruction and indicates whether a tumor or abscess is present in the liver, gallbladder, or pancreas. Useful isotopes include colloidal gold (^{198}Au), gallium (^{67}Ga), technetium (^{99}Tc), and selenium (^{75}Se). ^{67}Ga accumulates in inflamed tissue. ^{99}Tc is used to evaluate liver, gallbladder, and biliary tract function. ^{75}Se is useful for identifying pancreatic abnormalities.

Tests of Specific Metabolic Organ Functions

LIVER

PERITONEOSCOPY. Insertion of a peritoneoscope through an abdominal stab wound permits direct visualization of the liver and peritoneum. Visualization of structural changes aids in the diagnosis of cirrhosis and cancer. During peritoneoscopy, the examiner may take photographs and perform a biopsy. Peritoneoscopy is relatively safe and simple.

Contraindications include infections of the abdominal cavity, clotting disorders, or intestinal obstruction. In addition, the client must be able to cooperate throughout the procedure. Obesity and ascites interfere with test results.

Preprocedure care

To prepare a client for peritoneoscopy:

- Check that written consent has been obtained.
- Check the laboratory record to make certain the client has normal or adequate clotting factors. If not, inform the physician.

FIGURE 42-3 Computed tomographic scan of chronic pancreatitis. Pancreatic atrophy and a dilated pancreatic duct (*arrow*) are present, but there is no evidence of pancreatic calcification. (From Moss, A. A., et al. [1983]. *Computed tomography of the body.* Philadelphia: W. B. Saunders.)

- Check the client and health care record for contraindications to preprocedural medications.
- Inquire whether the client is sensitive to local anesthetics.
- Prepare the skin, and administer preprocedural medication when appropriate.
- Instruct the client to take nothing by mouth and to empty the bowel and bladder just before the procedure begins.
- Provide adequate teaching before and during the actual procedure.
- Explain to the client that it may be difficult to breathe when air is placed in the abdominal cavity.
- Instruct the client to elevate the abdominal wall by holding the breath to protect major organs during needle insertion.

Postprocedure care

When peritoneoscopy includes liver biopsy, bed rest for 24 hours follows the procedure (see discussion of liver biopsy later in this chapter). If biopsy is not performed, the client resumes activity after recovery from the effects of the medication. Complications are uncommon and are more often related to biopsy. Possible complications after peritoneoscopy are pneumothorax, subcutaneous emphysema, air embolism, bile peritonitis, perforation of a hollow organ, and shoulder or abdominal pain.

PORTAL PRESSURE MEASUREMENTS. Measurements of portal pressure and flow help to (1) diagnose portal hypertension, (2) indicate the severity of portal hypertension, and (3) guide decisions about appropriate intervention, which may include surgery. Also, the indirect calculation of sinusoid pressure helps determine the location of an obstruction in the liver and thus identify the underlying disorder. Normal portal pressure is 5 to 10 mm Hg. Portal hypertension is present when the wedged venous pressure is more than 5 mm Hg higher than the inferior vena cava pressure.[8]

The major portal pressure measurements are:

- *Wedged hepatic venous pressure* (WHVP). The portal pressure is obtained indirectly by percutaneous hepatic vein catheterization. The examiner uses either an arm vein or a femoral vein.
- *Umbilical vein catheterization.* This procedure allows direct measurement of portal pressure.
- *Splenic pulp manometry.* During manometry, the examiner places a needle between two of the lower ribs and inserts a manometer into the spleen. Instruct the client to hold the breath during needle insertion and passage.

Preprocedure care

Portal pressure measurements are minor surgical procedures that are performed in the operating room or a special studies laboratory. In many instances, the surgeon may concurrently inject a contrast agent. These measures require standard preoperative and postoperative care (see Chapter 16).

Postprocedure care

Observe for bleeding or pneumothorax. Assess the incision site for hematoma formation. Other nursing care is the same as for the client after liver biopsy (see next).

BIOPSY. Biopsy is the single most valuable diagnostic study because it is often the determining factor for the final diagnosis. It involves removal of a sample of living tissue for analysis. Biopsies may be open or closed procedures.

An *open biopsy* necessitates a general anesthetic and a major abdominal incision. A client may have an open biopsy at the time of a concurrent operative procedure. An advantage of the open biopsy is that the surgeon can observe the entire liver, identify grossly altered tissue, and remove the biopsy specimen for study.

A *closed biopsy*, or percutaneous liver biopsy, is performed to aspirate a core of tissue via needle for histologic study. The biopsy is usually a "blind" procedure (Menghini's technique) performed under local anesthesia using a transpleural or subcostal approach. The primary limitation of Menghini's technique is that the surgeon cannot see where the needle is going. Needle biopsy of the liver is indicated for unexplained hepatomegaly, hepatosplenomegaly, cholestasis (stoppage of bile secretion), persistently abnormal liver function tests, or suspected primary or metastatic liver tumor.

Contraindications to percutaneous liver biopsy are severe thrombocytopenia, local infection of the lung base, prolonged prothrombin time, peritonitis, massive ascites, an uncooperative client, and extrahepatic obstructive jaundice, especially with an enlarged gallbladder. The client with cancer or amyloidosis is at increased risk for postprocedure hemorrhage. If the client is unable to remain still and cooperative during the procedure, the surgeon can accidentally puncture another organ.

Procedure

The liver biopsy procedure may be performed at the bedside, in a procedure room, or in a gastrointestinal unit using a local anesthetic. Sedation and analgesia, such as with diazepam or midazolam, may be given to help allay the client's fears and make the client more comfortable. Place the client either in the supine or left lateral position with the right arm elevated. Less frequently, you may ask the client to assume a prone position. During insertion of the needle, have the client exhale and then hold the breath on expiration for 5 to 10 seconds to avoid puncture of the diaphragm (Fig. 42–4).

When the purpose of liver biopsy is to assess a focal lesion or abnormality, the blind procedure has definite limitations. The chance of inserting the needle into the wrong part of the liver and missing the lesion is great. With the use of concurrent ultrasonography, however, the physician can view the entire procedure and thus guide the needle. Guided biopsy allows better localization of a focal lesion or abnormality.

Fine-needle aspiration biopsy, often performed when a questionable area of the liver is localized, helps to confirm malignancy. This approach is ideal when only a few cells are necessary for cytologic study. The risks of fine-needle aspiration biopsy are far less than those of a guided regular biopsy because the tissue sample is much smaller. This procedure greatly reduces any risk of tumor metastasis along the needle track.

There are few contraindications to the guided regular or fine-needle aspiration biopsy procedures. Clients with impaired coagulation associated with liver disease, however, may not be appropriate candidates for the closed procedure. When biopsy is indicated for these clients, a

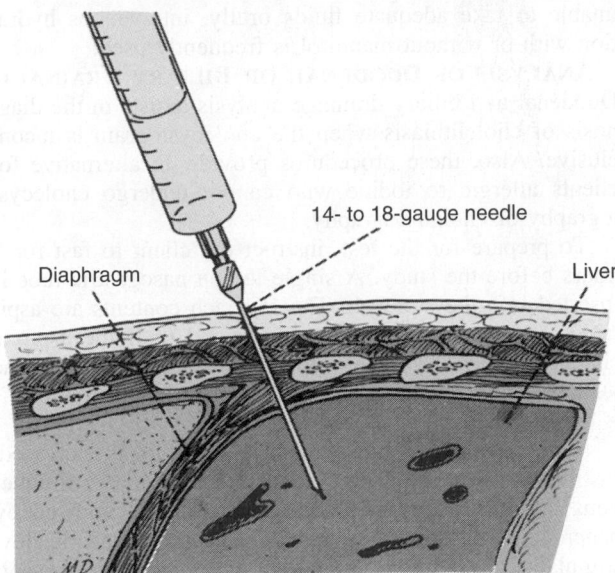

14- to 18-gauge needle

Diaphragm

Liver

MD

FIGURE 42–4 Percutaneous liver biopsy requires the client's cooperation. The client must be able to lie quietly and hold his or her breath after exhaling.

"plugged" biopsy procedure minimizes the risk of hemorrhage. This procedure allows injection of absorbable gelatin material on withdrawal of the biopsy needle. The gelatin material applies pressure to the bleeding site and closes the potential track. The client must be able to hold the breath for up to 15 seconds.

Preprocedure care

At least 2 weeks before a liver biopsy, the client must refrain from ingesting aspirin, NSAIDs, or anticoagulants. In addition, blood clotting tests (i.e., prothrombin time, bleeding time, partial thromboplastin time, platelet count, and hematocrit) are done beforehand.

Before the procedure is begun, the client fasts for at least 6 hours. Check the client's chart for the coagulation profile results; also check that the client has signed a consent form. Explain the procedure, including its purpose, insertion of an intravenous line during the procedure, and positioning during and after the procedure. When a client is informed about the procedure, the recovery period is smoother and less anxiety-producing than when no information is given. Emotional support is important to decrease apprehension and to help the client feel more in control.

Postprocedure care

After percutaneous liver biopsy, perform the following nursing assessments and interventions:

- Monitor vital signs every 15 minutes for 2 hours, every 30 minutes for 2 hours, and every 60 minutes for 4 hours.
- Assess for tachycardia and decreasing blood pressure, which may indicate hemorrhage.
- Check the puncture site by monitoring the dressing, palpating the surrounding area for crepitus, and observing for hematoma formation.
- Observe for pain in the right upper quadrant of the abdomen caused by a subcapsular accumulation of

blood or bile or at the right shoulder as a result of blood on the undersurface of the diaphragm.
- Beginning 2 hours after the procedure, elevate the head of the bed 30 degrees. Two hours later, elevate it to 45 degrees. Maintain the client with bed rest for 24 hours after the procedure. Lying on the right side for the first 1 to 2 hours decreases the risk of hemorrhage and bile leakage.
- Administer postprocedure medications on an individual basis, depending on the client's physical status.
- Give vitamin K if prescribed.
- Assess respiratory status for manifestations of dyspnea.

Inherent risks of the biopsy procedure include hemorrhage and puncture of adjacent organs or structures. Hemorrhage, the most serious complication, may result from penetration of the arterial tree or a distended vein radicle during the first 24 hours after the biopsy procedure. The risk of hemorrhage is increased if vascular channels are distended or if the client breathes during needle insertion into the liver. Puncture of a lung can cause pneumothorax.

A large (14- to 18-gauge) biopsy needle can penetrate a dilated intrahepatic duct in a client with obstructive jaundice. Bile leakage and resultant peritonitis can develop. Bile peritonitis is treated with surgical decompression. Cross-contamination may occur after puncture of an adjacent organ. Clients with potentially effusive conditions (e.g., ascites, chronic lung disease) in addition to liver abnormality are at great risk for cross-contamination.

GALLBLADDER, BILIARY TRACT, AND PANCREAS

ORAL CHOLECYSTOGRAPHY (GALLBLADDER SERIES). Cholecystography is an x-ray test for gallbladder or cystic duct disease. Oral cholecystography (OCG) has been the standard examination for gallstones for almost 50 years but has been largely replaced by ultrasonography. Oral cholecystography is still useful for selecting clients for noninvasive treatment of gallstone disease, such as by lithotripsy or bile acid dissolution therapy. Oral cholecystography is useful in accurate identification of gallstones (90% to 95%)[10] and in assessing the patency of the cystic duct and gallbladder emptying function.

Procedure

During the test, radiography permits visualization of the gallbladder. When contraction of the gallbladder is desirable, the client consumes a high-fat meal during the procedure. After oral cholecystography, some people experience burning on urination because of the presence of the dye in the urine. Forcing fluids decreases this problem.

Poor or no visualization of the gallbladder indicates gallbladder disease, presumably because biliary obstruction prevents passage of the dye. Occasionally, stones can be visualized as shadows within the opaque medium. The test results are accurate only when gastrointestinal and liver function allows absorption and conjugation of the dye.

Preprocedure care

The evening before the examination, the client ingests a radiopaque dye according to the fat content of the evening meal. The client who has a regular or low-fat dinner may receive ipodate sodium. After a high-fat dinner, the client must be given iopanoic acid. These dyes contain iodine. Observe the client for allergic reactions even when the health history reveals no known allergies to iodine. Possible hypersensitive reactions include nausea and vomiting, diarrhea, abdominal pain, rash, and anaphylaxis. If diarrhea develops, the radiopaque dye may not be absorbed, resulting in nonvisualization of the gallbladder.

Conjugation of the dye occurs in the liver. Be aware that these dyes are potentially toxic to the liver and kidneys, especially in clients with pre-existing hepatic or renal failure. After excretion of the opaque medium into the bile, the gallbladder concentrates the contrast medium.

Postprocedure care
The client can eat after the examination. There is no other specific postprocedure care.

CHOLANGIOGRAPHY. Cholangiography or cholangiopancreatography allows visualization of the bile ducts. After administration of an organic iodine dye (iodipamide meglumine), x-ray filming begins. There are four types of cholangiography:

- *Intravenous cholangiography* is used for common bile duct visualization. The radiopaque dye burns intensely upon injection.
- *Percutaneous transhepatic cholangiography* involves injecting the dye directly into the ductal system through the skin via a long, slender needle.
- *Endoscopic retrograde cholangiopancreatography* (ERCP). After a local anesthetic solution is sprayed on the back of the throat, a fiberoptic endoscope is passed through the mouth to the papilla of Vater in the duodenum. The examiner passes a catheter into the common bile duct and, possibly, the pancreatic duct that allows injection of contrast material into pancreatic and biliary systems. The biliary tract and the pancreatic duct are observed for possible strictures, stones, cysts, or tumors.
- *T-tube cholangiography* involves injecting dye into a pre-existing bile drainage tube.

In all four types of cholangiography, failure of the opaque dye to pass through the bile ducts provides evidence of duct obstruction.

Preprocedure care
Explain the procedure to the client and significant others. Check that written consent has been obtained. Ask whether the client has had a history of allergies to iodine or contrast dye. If so, inform the physician. Explain that there may be a flushing sensation when the contrast medium is injected. Food and fluids may be restricted for 8 hours.

Obtain baseline vital signs. Administer sedatives as prescribed.

Postprocedure care
Check vital signs as ordered by the physician. A rising temperature may indicate an infection. Monitor skin color for signs of jaundice, which may indicate a disease process or the result of injury. The client should be monitored for an allergic reaction for 24 hours after the procedure. Warn the client that there may be some discomfort with urination while the dye is excreted. Also, to prevent renal damage, instruct the client to drink ample amounts of fluid after administration of the dye. If the client is

unable to take adequate fluids orally, intravenous hydration with or without mannitol is frequently used.

ANALYSIS OF DUODENAL OR BILIARY DRAINAGE. Duodenal and biliary drainage analysis assists in the diagnosis of cholelithiasis when the cholecystogram is inconclusive. Also, these procedures provide an alternative for clients allergic to iodine who cannot undergo cholecystography or cholangiography.

To prepare for the test, instruct the client to fast for 8 hours before the study. A single-lumen nasogastric tube is inserted into the stomach. The stomach contents are aspirated, and the tube is slowly advanced until the aspirate changes to clear, golden, and alkaline. At this point, the tube is in the duodenum and clear golden bile ("A bile") is collected.

Next, the flow of bile into the duodenum is increased. Instillation of magnesium sulfate into the tube or intravenous administration of secretin (sometimes followed by pancreozymin) stimulates bile flow. After these bile flow stimulants are administered, it should be possible to aspirate 30 to 60 ml of concentrated bile ("B bile") from the duodenum. Bile can also be collected through an endoscope.

Collected fluid is sent to the laboratory to be analyzed for volume and bicarbonate, enzyme, and bile content. Disproportions in the bile and pancreatic juice fractions indicate obstruction in the bile or pancreatic duct. The presence of cholesterol crystals indicates lithiasis.

Other Metabolic Function Tests

PARACENTESIS. Paracentesis (peritoneal tap) is used to (1) extract fluid accumulations in the peritoneum (ascites), (2) relieve intra-abdominal tension, which can impair the client's respiratory status, or (3) obtain fluid for culture. After cleaning of the skin and infiltration with a local anesthetic, the physician, using sterile technique, inserts a long aspirating needle with a syringe to collect a fluid specimen. To drain ascitic fluid (if desired), the physician aseptically inserts a trocar through a small stab wound below the umbilicus. This procedure allows fluid (usually several liters) to drain slowly through a catheter into a collection bottle.

Preprocedure care
The nurse actively participates in the procedure, which usually takes place at the bedside. Obtain written permission before the procedure begins, and explain the purpose and steps involved. Ask the client to void immediately before the procedure to decrease the risk of bladder puncture. Have the client sit upright on the edge of the bed with the feet resting on a stool and the back well supported.

Postprocedure care
The major complication of paracentesis is *hypovolemia* and shock secondary to fluid drainage from the peritoneum, the resulting fluid shift from intravascular to interstitial space, and the sudden change in intra-abdominal pressure on the vessels. This fluid shift is exacerbated by hypoalbuminemia.

Assess vital signs and peripheral circulation every few minutes during and immediately after paracentesis. Observe for hypovolemic shock: pallor, tachycardia, decreased blood pressure, oliguria, and dyspnea.

Hepatic encephalopathy, caused by reduced tissue perfusion, is another complication resulting from drainage of ascitic fluid. Because ascitic fluid contains a high concentration of protein, the physician may prescribe albumin infusions for 24 hours after paracentesis to compensate for protein losses. Potassium depletion may also occur after multiple paracentesis procedures. Infection, peritonitis, and bleeding related to vessel trauma occasionally complicate paracentesis.

Carefully assess for abdominal pain after paracentesis. In addition, monitor the puncture site for persistent leakage of ascitic drainage.

CONCLUSIONS

Once you have gained a thorough knowledge of the structure and function of the endocrine and metabolic organs, you must examine the diagnostic assessment of these organs. Systematic assessment of the client with possible disorders of the endocrine and metabolic organs can lead to prompt diagnosis and treatment. You can facilitate the diagnostic process by adequately preparing the client for diagnostic procedures and by assisting with or collecting assessment data.

BIBLIOGRAPHY

1. Banks, P. A. (1998). Acute and chronic pancreatitis. In M. Feldman, B. F. Scharschmidt, & M. H. Sleisenger (Eds.), *Gastrointestinal and liver disease* (Vol. 1, 6th ed.). Philadelphia: W. B. Saunders.
2. Bates, B. (1995). *A guide to physical examination and history taking* (6th ed.). Philadelphia: J. B. Lippincott.
3. Bilhartz, L. E., & Horton, J. D. (1998). Gallstone disease and its complications. In M. Feldman, B. F. Scharschmidt, & M. H. Sleisenger (Eds.), *Gastrointestinal and liver disease* (Vol. 1, 6th ed.). Philadelphia: W. B. Saunders.
4. Birch, C. (1997). Caring for people with endocrine disorders. In J. Luckmann (Ed.), *Saunders manual of nursing care.* Philadelphia: W. B. Saunders.
5. Ebersol, P., & Hess, P. (1998). *Toward healthy aging: Human needs and nursing response* (5th ed.). St. Louis: Mosby–Year Book.
6. Ferri, F. F. (1995). *The care of the medical patient* (3rd ed.). St. Louis: Mosby–Year Book.
7. Friedman, L. S. (1995). Liver, biliary tract, pancreas. In L. M. Tierney, S. J. McPhee, & M. A. Papadakis (Eds.), *Current medical diagnosis and treatment* (34th ed.). Norwalk, CT: Appleton & Lange.
8. Friedman, S. L. (1998). Cirrhosis of the liver and its major sequelae. In J. C. Bennett & F. Plum (Eds.), *Cecil textbook of medicine* (20th ed.). Philadelphia: W. B. Saunders.
9. Ganong, W. F. (1997). *Review of medical physiology* (18th ed.). Norwalk, CT: Appleton & Lange.
10. Greensberger, N. J., & Isselbacher, K. J. (1998). Diseases of the gallbladder and bile ducts. In A. S. Fauci et al. (Eds.), *Harrison's principles of internal medicine* (14th ed., pp. 1725–1736). New York: McGraw-Hill.
11. Guyton, A. C., & Hall, J. E. (1996). *Textbook of medical physiology* (9th ed.). Philadelphia: W. B. Saunders.
12. *Healthy people 2000: National Health Promotion and Disease Prevention Objectives.* (1990). Washington, DC: U.S. Public Health Service.
13. Jarvis, C. (2000). *Physical examination and health assessment* (3rd ed.). Philadelphia: W. B. Saunders.
14. Kee, J. L. (1999). *Laboratory and diagnostic tests with nursing implications* (5th ed.). Stamford, CT: Appleton & Lange.
15. McCance, K., & Heuther, S. (1994). *Pathophysiology: The biological basis for disease in adults and children* (2nd ed.). St. Louis: Mosby–Year Book.
16. Melillo, K. D. (1993). Interpretation of abnormal laboratory values in older adults: Part II. *Journal of Gerontological Nursing, 19*(2), 35–40.
17. Melillo, K. D. (1993). Interpretation of laboratory values in older adults. *Nurse Practitioner, 18*(7), 59–67.
18. Mirowski, G. W. & Berger, T. G. (1998). Oral and cutaneous manifestations of gastrointestinal disease. In M. Feldman, B. F. Scharschmidt, & M. H. Sleisenger (Eds.), *Gastrointestinal and liver disease* (Vol. 1, 6th ed.). Philadelphia: W. B. Saunders.
19. Moses, A. M., & Streeten, D. H. P. (1998). Disorders of the neurohypophysis. In A. S. Fauci et al. (Eds.), *Harrison's principles of internal medicine* (14th ed., pp. 2003–2011). New York: McGraw-Hill.
20. Murray, W. J., & Gabel, T. L. (1998, May). *What about herbal medicine?* Unpublished manuscript, University of Nebraska Medical Center, Omaha.
21. Niedzwick, L., & Stringer, C. (1994). Liver biopsy and nursing intervention. *Gastroenterology Nursing, 17*(1), 17–19.
22. Ober, K. P. (1996). Work-up of endocrine abnormalities. *Hospital Medicine, 32*(10), 15–25.
23. Podolsky, D. K., & Isselbacher, K. J. (1998). Evaluation of liver function. In A. S. Fauci et al. (Eds.), *Harrison's principles of internal medicine* (13th ed., pp. 1663–1667). New York: McGraw-Hill.
24. Price, S., & Wilson, L. (Eds.). (1994). *Pathophysiology* (4th ed.). St. Louis: Mosby–Year Book.
25. Seidel, H. M., et al. (1995). *Mosby's guide to physical examination* (3rd ed.). St. Louis: Mosby–Year Book.
26. Sommers, M. S., & Johnson, S. A. (1997). *Davis's manual of nursing therapeutics for disease and disorders.* Philadelphia: F. A. Davis.
27. Swearingen, P. L. (1994). *Manual of medical-surgical nursing care* (3rd ed., pp. 380–481). St. Louis: Mosby–Year Book.
28. Swearingen, P. L. (1995). *Mosby's medical-surgical nursing* (2nd ed.). St. Louis: Mosby–Year Book.
29. Treseler, K. M. (1995). *Clinical laboratory and diagnostic tests* (3rd ed.). Norwalk, CT: Appleton & Lange.
30. Wartofsky, L. (1998). Diseases of the thyroid. In A. S. Fauci, et al. (Eds.), *Harrison's principles of internal medicine* (14th ed., pp. 2012–2034). New York: McGraw-Hill.
31. Wilson, J., & Foster, D. (1992). *Williams textbook of endocrinology* (8th ed.). Philadelphia: W. B. Saunders.

Management of Clients with Thyroid and Parathyroid Disorders

Anne Larson

NURSING OUTCOMES CLASSIFICATION (NOC)
for Nursing Diagnoses—Clients with Thyroid and Parathyroid Disorders

Activity Intolerance	Urinary Elimination	Social Interaction Skills
Activity Intolerance	**Constipation**	Social Involvement
Endurance	Bowel Elimination	**Risk for Impaired Skin Integrity**
Energy Conservation	Hydration	Fluid Balance
Self-Care: Activities of Daily Living	Medication Response	Immobility Consequences: Physiologic
Altered Nutrition: Less than Body	Mobility Level	Nutritional Status
Requirements	**Decreased Cardiac Output**	Risk Control
Nutritional Status	Cardiac Pump Effectiveness	Risk Detection
Nutritional Status: Food and Fluid Intake	Circulation Status	Thermoregulation
Nutritional Status: Nutrient Intake	Tissue Perfusion: Peripheral	Tissue Integrity: Skin and Mucous
Altered Nutrition: More than Body	Vital Signs Status	Membranes
Requirements	**Hyperthermia**	Tissue Perfusion: Peripheral
Nutritional Status: Food and Fluid Intake	Thermoregulation	**Risk for Injury**
Nutritional Status: Nutrient Intake	Vital Signs Status	Knowledge: Personal Safety
Weight Control	**Hypothermia**	Neurological Status
Altered Urinary Elimination	Thermoregulation	Risk Control
Knowledge: Disease Process	Vital Signs Status	Risk Control: Visual Impairment
Symptom Control	**Impaired Social Interaction**	Risk Detection
Symptom Severity	Role Performance	Symptom Control

THYROID DISORDERS

Many terms describe normal and abnormal states of thyroid function. *Euthyroidism* means that the thyroid gland is functioning normally. Like other endocrine disorders, the two primary thyroid disorders are related to increased secretion (*hyperthyroidism*) and decreased secretion (*hypothyroidism*) of the gland's hormones. Such alterations in thyroid hormone (TH) secretion result in increased or decreased rates of metabolic function, heat production, and oxygen consumption. In addition, a third disorder is related to enlargement of the thyroid gland. These enlargements are called *goiters*.

This chapter incorporates material written for the fifth edition by Carol Birch.

GOITER

Enlargement of the thyroid gland may be seen with both hyperthyroidism and hypothyroidism. It generally results from lack of iodine, inflammation, or benign or malignant tumors. Enlargement may also appear in hyperthyroidism, especially Graves' disease, in which the client typically has exophthalmos as well.

Etiology and Risk Factors

There are two major forms of simple goiter: endemic and sporadic.

Endemic goiter is caused principally by nutritional iodine deficiency. It tends to occur in goiter "belts," geographical areas characterized by soil and water that are deficient in iodine. Major goiter belts in the United States are the Midwest, Northwest, and Great Lakes regions. Iodine is readily available in regions with access to salt water and also through consumption of seafood. Hence, goiters are less common in coastal areas.

Endemic goiter typically occurs in fall and winter months and is twice as prevalent in women as in men. Also, because the need for TH is particularly great during growth spurts, pregnancy, and lactation, goiter commonly develops in adolescents, pregnant women, and nursing mothers living in iodine-deficient regions.

Sporadic goiter is not restricted to any geographical area. Major causes include:

- Genetic defects resulting in faulty iodine metabolism
- Ingestion of large amounts of nutritional *goitrogens* (goiter-producing agents that inhibit thyroxine [T_4] production), such as rutabagas, cabbage, soybeans, peanuts, peaches, peas, strawberries, spinach, and radishes, all of which contain goitrogenic glycosides
- Ingestion of medicinal goitrogens, for example, adrenergic antagonists, glucocorticoids, dopamine, methimazole, lithium, iodinated radiographic contrast agents, phenytoin, rifampin, carbamazepine, propylthiouracil (PTU), and thiocarbamides (aminothiazole, tolbutamide)

Health promotion practices include ingestion of iodized salt and avoidance of goitrogens. Health maintenance or restoration interventions include teaching about the use of iodized salt.

Pathophysiology

If a person's diet lacks sufficient iodine or if production of thyroid hormones is suppressed for any other reason, the thyroid enlarges in an attempt to compensate for hormonal deficiency. Under these circumstances, goiter is essentially an adaptation to a deficiency of thyroid hormones. Enlargement of the gland also occurs in response to increased pituitary secretion of thyroid-stimulating hormone (TSH). TSH stimulates the thyroid to secrete more T_4 when blood T_4 levels are low. Eventually, the gland may become so large that it compresses structures in the neck and chest, causing respiratory problems and dysphagia.

Clinical Manifestations

Diagnosis of simple goiter is confirmed by history, clinical findings, and laboratory tests (Fig. 43–1). The client is often euthyroid because the gland enlarges enough to produce normal amounts of T_4. Needle biopsy of the goiter may be indicated to rule out malignancy.

Outcome Management

■ Medical Management

When enlargement is a compensatory reaction to iodine deficiency and consequent suppression of T_4 secretion, the client can be treated with preparations of iodine and thyroid hormones. Either a strong iodine solution (Lugol's solution) or saturated solution of potassium iodide (SSKI) drops can be administered. Iodine reduces the size and vascularity of the enlarged gland. The availability of io-

FIGURE 43–1 Massive thyroid enlargement caused by diffuse toxic goiter. *A,* Front view. *B,* Side view. (From Swartz, M. H., [1998]. *Textbook of physical diagnosis* [3rd ed.]. Philadelphia: W. B. Saunders.)

dized salt and thyroid hormones has made replacement therapy with iodine obsolete in the United States.

The client's diet should also be higher in iodine. The client may switch to iodized salt. Dietary goitrogens (e.g., turnips, soybeans, rutabagas, and, to a lesser degree, seafood, green leafy vegetables, carrots, and peanuts) should be avoided.

Endemic goiter can be prevented altogether by the use of iodized salt. Adults require at least 50 mg of iodine per day. However, 200 to 300 mg/day is considered the minimum adequate intake needed to prevent goiter. Iodized salt, used in the United States since 1924, contains 1 part iodine to 100,000 parts of salt. Thus, the average person, who ingests about 6.2 g of salt a day, is also taking 474 mg of iodine daily if the salt is iodized.

Many clients do not understand the need for iodized salt as a goiter preventative. Some believe that any additive to food or water is harmful and, therefore, avoid iodized salt. These two problems, along with the fact that many modern foods are processed with cheaper non-iodized salt, contribute to the potential for development of simple goiter. Nurses need to educate the public about the importance of iodized salt.

Surgical Management

Surgery is indicated for a goiter that is very large, does not respond to treatment, or is putting too much pressure on other structures in the neck. Surgery is discussed in detail under Hyperthyroidism.

HYPOTHYROIDISM

Hypothyroidism is a deficiency of TH resulting in slowed body metabolism, decreased heat production, and decreased oxygen consumption by the tissues. The underactivity of the thyroid gland may result from primary thyroid dysfunction or be secondary to anterior pituitary dysfunction.

The term hypothyroidism is not synonymous with m*yxedema* (mucinous edema), a complication of hypothyroidism characterized by a generalized hypometabolic state. *Myxedema coma* is a life-threatening condition in which all body systems are severely compromised by the hypometabolic state.

The frequency of hypothyroidism depends on the population being studied. The incidence of overt hypothyroidism is one to two in 1000 people in community surveys and five to 20 in 1000 clients seeking medical care.

Hypothyroidism affects women more than men (about 4:1). Although hypothyroidism may be congenital (cretinism) and therefore present at birth, the highest incidence is in adults between 30 and 65 years of age. About 95% of all people with hypothyroidism have the *primary* form of the disease. *Central hypothyroidism* resulting from pituitary or hypothalamic disease accounts for fewer than 10% of cases. Myxedema is most commonly identified in postmenopausal, hypothyroid women in their 60s.

Etiology and Risk Factors

Primary hypothyroidism may be caused by:

- Congenital defects of the thyroid (cretinism)
- Defective hormone synthesis
- Iodine deficiency (prenatal and postnatal)
- Antithyroid drugs
- Surgery or treatment with radioactive agents for hyperthyroidism
- Chronic inflammatory (autoimmune) diseases such as Hashimoto's disease, amyloidosis, and sarcoidosis

Hashimoto's disease is the most common type of autoimmune hypothyroidism. In primary hypothyroidism, TH levels are low and TSH levels are elevated, indicating that the pituitary is attempting to stimulate the secretion of thyroid hormones and the thyroid is not responding.

Secondary hypothyroidism develops when there is insufficient stimulation of a normal thyroid gland; consequently, TSH levels are decreased. This condition may start as a malfunction of the pituitary or hypothalamus. It may also be caused by peripheral resistance to TH. When this occurs, both TSH and TH levels are low in the serum.

Tertiary or *central hypothyroidism* can develop if the hypothalamus cannot produce thyroid-releasing hormone (TRH) and subsequently does not stimulate the pituitary to secrete TSH. It may be due to a tumor or other destructive lesion in the hypothalamic region. When this occurs, both TSH and TH levels are again low in the serum.

Subclinical hypothyroidism is defined as hypothyroidism that is diagnosed with an elevated TSH level but a normal to low-normal T_4 level. Manifestations resemble those of mild hypothyroidism with subtle cardiac defects, especially in clients with pre-existing cardiac disease. Subclinical hypothyroidism is found in 20 to 120 of 1000 persons in the community. The causes are the same as those of primary hypothyroidism. Its prevalence increases

with age. Low-dose levothyroxine sodium (Synthroid) is effective for relief of manifestations and improvement in cardiac function and lipid profile.

Use of iodized salt and avoidance of goitrogens are health promotion activities. Health restoration practices involve lifelong hormone replacement.

Pathophysiology

The thyroid gland needs iodine to synthesize and secrete thyroid hormones: T_4, triiodothyronine (T_3), and thyrocalcitonin (calcitonin). Production of thyroid hormones depends on secretion of TSH from the anterior pituitary and ingestion of adequate protein and iodine. The hypothalamus regulates the pituitary secretion of TSH via a negative feedback system.

Decreased levels of thyroid hormones lead to overall slowing of the basal metabolic rate. This slowing of all body processes leads to achlorhydria (decreased secretion of hydrochloric acid in the stomach), decreased gastrointestinal tract motility, bradycardia, slowed neurologic functioning, and a decrease in heat production resulting in a decreased basal body temperature.

The most important changes caused by reduced levels of thyroid hormones are those affecting lipid metabolism. The reduction in thyroid hormones causes an increase in serum cholesterol and triglyceride levels and an increase in arteriosclerosis and coronary heart disease in clients with hypothyroidism.

Because thyroid hormones play a role in the production of red blood cells, people with hypothyroidism also show evidence of anemia, with possible vitamin B_{12} and folate deficiency.

Myxedema, a mucinous edema, is caused by accumulation of hydrophilic proteoglycans in the interstitial spaces. The cause of this problem remains unclear.

Clinical Manifestations

The manifestations of hypothyroidism depend on whether it is mild or complicated by myxedema or myxedema coma.

MILD HYPOTHYROIDISM

Clients with mild hypothyroidism (the most common form) may be asymptomatic or may experience vague manifestations so ordinary as to escape detection. For example, clients may experience sensitivity to cold, lethargy, dry skin or hair, forgetfulness, depression, and some weight gain (Table 43–1).

The client's physical appearance changes. Often, obesity develops, features become coarse, hair becomes dry and sparse, and the skin feels dry, flaky, and inelastic. In addition, clients with hypothyroidism are sensitive to cold because of a decreased metabolic rate and a decreased basal body temperature. The client's ability to sweat also diminishes. Constipation and fecal impaction related to slowed peristaltic action and lack of normal physical activity are serious problems. Also, there is increased susceptibility to infection.

Vital sign changes may be minimal: the heart rate is normal or slow; blood pressure may be normal, or both systolic and diastolic pressures may be slightly elevated; temperature may be normal to subnormal; and respiratory

TABLE 43–1	MANIFESTATIONS OF HYPOTHYROIDISM AND HYPERTHYROIDISM	
System	**Hypothyroidism**	**Hyperthyroidism**
Cardiovascular	↓ HR + ↓ SV: ↓ CO ↓ Myocardial O_2 demand ↑ Peripheral vascular resistance Possible hypertension Hyperlipidemia Hypercholesterolemia Distant heart sounds	↑ HR + ↑ SV: ↑ CO ↑ O_2 consumption Systolic BP ↑ 10–15 mm Hg Diastolic BP ↑ 10–15 mm Hg Palpitations Rapid, bounding pulse Possible heart failure, edema
Hematologic	Normocytic, normochromic anemia Macrocytic anemia (pernicious) Easy bruising	No specific changes
Respiratory	Reduced hypoxic drive Hypercapnic ventilatory drive Respiratory muscle weakness Possible CO_2 retention on arterial blood gas tests Dyspnea	↑ Respiratory rate and depth Shortness of breath
Renal	Fluid retention ↓ Urinary output ↑ Total body water Dilutional hyponatremia ↓ Production of erythropoietin	Fluid retention ↓ Output
Gastrointestinal	↓ Peristalsis Anorexia Possible weight gain Constipation ↓ Protein metabolism ↑ Serum lipids Delayed glucose uptake ↓ Glucose absorption	↑ Peristalsis ↑ Appetite Weight loss Diarrhea ↑ Use of adipose and protein stores ↓ Serum lipids ↑ Gastrointestinal secretions Vomiting, abdominal pain
Musculoskeletal	Transient pain Muscle cramps and stiffness Slow movements ↑ Bone density ↓ Bone formation and resorption	Negative nitrogen balance Malnutrition Fatigue Muscle weakness Proximal muscle wasting Incoordination caused by tremors
Integumentary	Dry, coarse, scaly skin Hair that falls out Thick, brittle nails Expressionless face Periorbital edema Thick, puffy skin: face and pretibial areas Cold intolerance	Profuse sweating Moist skin Flushed, warm skin Hair: fine, soft, straight, possible hair loss Heat intolerance
Endocrine	Normal to enlarged thyroid	Thyroid usually enlarged Bruit over thyroid
Neurologic	↓ Deep tendon reflexes Muscle sluggishness Fatigue, somnolence Slow, deliberate speech Apathy, depression, paranoia Impaired short-term memory Lethargy	↑ Deep tendon reflexes Fine tremors Nervousness, restlessness Emotional instability: anxiety, worry, paranoia
Reproductive	Females: menorrhagia, anovulation, irregular menses, decreased libido Males: decreased libido, impotence	Females: amenorrhea, irregular menses, ↓ fertility, ↑ tendency for spontaneous abortion Males: impotence, decreased libido ↓ Sexual development prepuberty
Other	Myxedema	Exophthalmos

BP, blood pressure; CO, cardiac output; CO_2, carbon dioxide; HR, heart rate; O_2, oxygen; SV, stroke volume.

rate and rhythm may be affected by goiter size and degree of respiratory distress.

As the degree of hypothyroidism worsens, the thyroid may enlarge (goiter) in an attempt to produce enough T_4.

Typically, clients seek medical advice when the goiter grows large enough to distort the appearance of the neck. They may also experience respiratory distress and dysphagia if the goiter is very large.

MYXEDEMA

Myxedema may develop in clients with undiagnosed or undertreated hypothyroidism who experience stress. Stressors include infection, drugs (phenothiazines, barbiturates, narcotics, anesthetics), respiratory failure, heart failure, cerebral vascular accident, trauma, prolonged exposure to cold, metabolic disturbances, surgery, and seizures.

Myxedema is characterized by a dry, waxy type of swelling with abnormal deposits of mucin in the skin and other tissues. The edema is of the nonpitting type and is common in the pretibial and facial areas (Fig. 43–2).

Myxedema is most commonly diagnosed in hypothyroid women in their 60s. Untreated myxedema has been associated with severe atherosclerosis and has been attributed to the increase in serum cholesterol concentrations, particularity low-density lipoproteins. TH replacement improves these changes.

MYXEDEMA COMA

The major complication of hypothyroidism is myxedema coma, an extremely rare condition with a mortality rate approaching 100%. Myxedema coma is characterized by a drastic decrease in metabolic rate, hypoventilation leading to respiratory acidosis, hypothermia, and hypotension. Complicating conditions include hyponatremia, hypercalcemia, secondary adrenal insufficiency, hypoglycemia, and water intoxication. Myxedema coma may be brought on by stress—as from surgery or infection—or by noncompliance with thyroid treatment.

Diagnostic tests for hypothyroidism confirm the clinical picture of hypometabolism and depressed thyroid activity (Table 43–2). The serum TSH level is elevated in primary hypothyroidism. Radioactive iodide uptake is decreased in hypothyroidism.

Clients with myxedema may also have hypercholesterolemia, hyperlipidemia, and proteinemia as a result of T_4 changes in the synthesis, mobilization, and degradation of serum lipids. Elevated lipid levels may contribute to the later development of cardiac problems. Dilutional hyponatremia may develop as a result of the marked impairment of water excretion because of decreased delivery of sodium and volume to the distal renal tubules associated with decreased renal blood flow. Elevated creatine phosphokinase, aspartate aminotransferase, and lactate dehydrogenase may also develop secondary to altered metabolism.

Outcome Management

Hypothyroidism is rarely a primary diagnosis. Usually, the diagnosis is made after the development of another medical problem. Clients with hypothyroidism are typically managed on an outpatient basis with TH replacement. Treatment is an ongoing, lifelong process. Clients with myxedema or myxedema coma are managed as a medical emergency.

■ Medical Management

MYXEDEMA AND MYXEDEMA COMA

The desired outcome of the medical management of myxedema coma is to reverse the condition to save the client's life. Supportive measures begin immediately and include maintaining a patent airway, giving oxygen, and replacing fluids intravenously. The client is kept warm, and vital signs are closely monitored until the client begins to recover. Vasopressors are used to maintain tissue perfusion.

Levothyroxine sodium is given intravenously with glucose and corticosteroids. When administering TH to a client with myxedema heart disease, assess the client carefully for angina, dyspnea, or orthopnea. The event that precipitated the coma (surgery, infection, noncompliance) must be evaluated and treated as well.

The desired outcomes of the medical management of hypothyroidism are to correct TH deficiency, reverse manifestations, and prevent further cardiac and arterial damage.

CORRECT THYROID HORMONE DEFICIENCY. For hypothyroidism to be reversed permanently, the client must usually take TH for life. Levothyroxine sodium is the principal form of replacement therapy. Dosages vary with age, the severity of the hypothyroidism, general medical condition (particularly cardiovascular disorders), and the client's response to medical treatment at the initiation of TH therapy. Children and older adults receive smaller doses.

Clients who respond to TH therapy receive a maintenance dose of T_4 daily for life. Pharmacologic goitrogens are replaced by drugs that do not interfere with TH function. The drug of choice for thyroid replacement is levothyroxine sodium, which is converted in the body to both T_4 and T_3 (Table 43–3). Desiccated thyroid and liothyronine sodium (Cytomel), once commonly used in replacement therapy, are now used infrequently because of problems with fluctuating plasma levels and side effects.

FIGURE 43–2 Typical facial appearance of myxedematous client. (From Jacob, S. W. [1982]. *Structure and function in man* [5th ed.] Philadelphia: W. B. Saunders.)

| TABLE 43–2 | **DIAGNOSTIC TESTS FOR THYROID DISORDERS*** | | |

Test	Description	Nursing Notes	Indications
THYROID FUNCTION TESTS			
Thyroid-stimulating hormone (TSH) assay	TSH controls triiodothyronine (T_3) and thyroxine (T_4) release; TSH released from anterior pituitary	None	↑: Hypofunction of thyroid gland; primary hypothyroidism ↓: Pituitary disorders; hyperthyroidism; high dosages of dopamine or corticosteroids
Radioactive iodine uptake	Used to determine the metabolic activity of the thyroid gland by measuring absorption of ^{131}I in thyroid	Client education: radioactive dose is small and harmless Contraindicated in pregnancy Drugs that may elevate results: barbiturates, estrogen, lithium, phenothiazines Seafood may elevate results Drugs that may decrease results: Lugol's solution, saturated solution of potassium iodide (SSKI), antithyroid, cortisone, aspirin, antihistamines 24-hr urine collection begins after oral tracer dose given Thyroid scanned after 24 hr	↑: Hyperthyroidism, thyroiditis, liver cirrhosis; urine: hypothyroidism ↓: Hypothyroidism; urine: hyperthyroidism
Thyroid antibodies	Measures the presence of antibodies produced by body; may cause inflammation and destruction of thyroid gland	Note if client receiving oral contraceptives because they may elevate titers	↑: Thyroiditis
Free thyroxine (FT_4) concentration	FT_4 is metabolically active form of thyroxine	Results may be inaccurate with high estrogen levels or low serum protein levels	↑: Hyperthyroidism ↓: Hypothyroidism
Thyroxine (T_4)	A direct measurement of total amount of T_4 present in blood	Fasting is recommended Note on laboratory slip if client is taking thyroid supplements; levels can be increased by pregnancy or oral contraceptives	↑: Hyperthyroidism Normal– ↓: Hypothyroidism
Triiodothyronine (T_3) radioimmunoassay	Measures small amount of potent thyroid hormones; T_3 is active form of thyroid hormone	Same as T_4	↑: Hyperthyroidism, pregnancy, oral contraceptives Normal– ↓: Hypothyroidism, hypoprotein conditions
T_3 resin uptake (T_3 RU)	Measures T_3 that is protein bound	None	↑: Hyperthyroidism, low serum protein levels ↓: High serum protein, hypothyroidism
Thyroid-binding globulins (TBGs)	Measures T_4 that is protein bound	None	↑: Hyperthyroidism, low serum protein ↓: High serum protein, hypothyroidism
Thyroid-releasing hormone (TRH)	TRH influences TSH release	None	↑: Hypothyroidism ↓: Hyperthyroidism

TABLE 43-2	DIAGNOSTIC TESTS FOR THYROID DISORDERS* *Continued*

Test	Description	Nursing Notes	Indications
DIAGNOSTIC IMAGING STUDIES			
Thyroid scan	Injection of radioactive isotopes used to identify thyroid gland	No preparation Radioactive iodine taken orally; dose is harmless Scanning done 24 hr later Be aware of contraindications such as potassium iodide, Lugol's solution, seafood intake, thyroid medications	Cold nodules: cancer Hot nodules: benign
Ultrasonography	Identifies presence, size, and location of gland and nodules; differentiates solid tumors from fluid-filled cysts	No preparation necessary Remind clients that they will not be radioactive Provide client education to alleviate anxiety	
Thyroid scan	Injection of radioactive isotopes used to identify thyroid gland	No preparation Radioactive iodine taken orally; dose is harmless Scanning done 24 hr later Be aware of contraindications such as potassium iodide, Lugol's solution, seafood intake, thyroid medications	Cold nodules: cancer Hot nodules: benign
Magnetic resonance imaging	Used to visualize gland size, location, identify abnormalities	Test cannot be done in clients with metal implants (such as pacemakers, arthroplasties, skull plates) Assess for allergy to contrast media Inquire about claustrophobia	
Computed tomography	Identifies location and structure of gland	Client education Noninvasive Contrast media may be used; note allergy history	
OTHER PROCEDURES USED TO DIAGNOSE ENDOCRINE DISORDERS			
Fine-needle aspiration	Provides sample of cells for histologic studies; usually used as thyroid biopsy	Client education for short, relatively pain-free procedure Observe site for swelling and bleeding	Benign or malignant

*The following drugs affect thyroid function test results: amiodarone hydrochloride (HCl) (Cordarone), corticosteroids, cough medicine (with iodine), dopamine HCl (Dopastat, Intropin), estrogens., lithium carbonate (Eskalith, Lithane, Lithobid), phenytoin (Dilantin), salicylates.
    Data from Malarkey, L. M., & McMorrow, M. E. (1996). *Nurses' manual of laboratory tests and diagnostic procedures.* Philadelphia: W. B. Saunders.

REVERSE MANIFESTATIONS. Clients with hypothyroidism of long duration notice an improvement in manifestations within 2 to 3 weeks of starting medication; however, hoarseness, anemia, and changes in hair and skin may take many months to resolve.

PREVENT CARDIAC COMPLICATIONS. A client with cardiac complications starts with a small dose of TH. Large doses may precipitate heart failure or myocardial infarction by increasing body metabolism, myocardial oxygen requirements, and, consequently, the workload of the heart.

▪ Nursing Management of the Medical Client with Myxedema

ASSESSMENT

Observe the client for the physical manifestations of myxedema, such as periorbital and facial edema, a blank facial expression, a thick tongue, and generalized slowing of all muscle movement. The client's vital signs are also affected and must be monitored closely. The client is hypothermic. Depressed respirations precipitate respiratory acidosis. Alterations in heart rate and blood pressure follow.

| TABLE 43–3 | NURSING IMPLICATIONS FOR MEDICATIONS USED TO TREAT THYROID DISORDERS |

Class	Action	Therapeutic Outcomes	Adverse Outcomes	Dosing
HYPERTHYROID MEDICATIONS (ANTITHYROID DRUGS)				
Propylthiouracil (PTU)	Temporarily inhibits thyroid hormone synthesis	Thyroid hormone level returns to normal; resting heart rate less than 100 beats per minute	Use carefully in combination with any drug that causes agranulocytosis Monitor blood counts for agranulocytosis Observe for signs of hypothyroidism	100–150 mg PO tid Give orally every 8 hr around the clock Urge continued compliance because response is slow
Radioactive iodine (^{131}I)	Antithyroid drug that destroys thyroid tissue; used to treat hyperthyroidism; may be used to treat thyroid cancer	Thyroid hormone level decreases	Monitor for evidence of local irritation from irradiation concentration in the neck	4–10 mCi PO for hyperthyroidism, 50–150 mCi for thyroid cancer Stop all antithyroid medications 1 week before giving ^{131}I Monitor thyroid function closely Give on an empty stomach Institute radiation precautions for body secretions for 3 days after ingestion Tell client to avoid close, prolonged contact with children for 1 week; should also sleep alone for 1 week Client should not resume antithyroid medications for 6 weeks
HYPOTHYROID MEDICATIONS				
Levothyroxine sodium (Synthroid, Levothroid, Levoxine)	Thyroid replacement medication (T_4) used to treat hypothyroidism	Thyroid hormone level returns to normal range; signs and symptoms of decreased thyroid hormones resolve	Watch for adverse effects early in treatment Toxicity may last for weeks with overdose Monitor for improvement of manifestions Serum levels may be decreased when client is also taking aluminum hydroxide antacid Monitor pulse, blood pressure, and thyroid function	Initial low dose daily increased until response to 0.1–0.2 mg/day in hypothyroidism (less in older clients); 0.2–0.5 mg IV in myxedema coma Give a single dose in AM Watch for adverse effects early in treatment Stress need for lifetime replacement Smaller doses required for older clients

DIAGNOSIS, OUTCOMES, INTERVENTIONS

Decreased Cardiac Output. The client with myxedema is susceptible to severe arteriosclerotic heart disease and other cardiac abnormalities, leading to the nursing diagnosis *Decreased Cardiac Output related to sustained bradycardia, resulting in edema and decreased urine output.*

Outcomes. The client will maintain a normal cardiac output and will remain free of heart failure, as evidenced by normal heart rate, evidence of normal perfusion, absence of edema, and urine output of at least ½ ml/kg/hr.

Interventions. As the client proceeds with hormone replacement therapy, the edema and puffiness start to lessen. Continue to monitor the client's intake and output, which will become more balanced. Urinary output should increase significantly during thyroid therapy. Monitor the client's weight daily.

To help prevent further strain on the already overburdened heart, help the client conserve energy. For example, always help the client turn in bed. If any new cardiac manifestations occur, notify the physician immediately. Do not give TH until the physician has reappraised the client's condition.

When administering thyroid preparations, assess the client carefully for manifestations of thyrotoxicosis, such as tachycardia, increased appetite, diarrhea, sweating, agitation, tremor, palpitations, and shortness of breath. If any of these manifestations develop during thyroid therapy, notify the physician at once so that the dosage can be reduced.

Hypothermia. A client with severe myxedema has a very low metabolic rate, leading to an important nursing diagnosis of *Hypothermia related to slowed metabolic rate resulting in subnormal body temperature.*

Outcomes. The client's body temperature will return to normal.

Interventions. Provide the client with a comfortable, warm environment. Remember that hypothyroidism sharply increases sensitivity to cold. If necessary, supply extra clothing and warm blankets. Encourage the client to dress warmly and avoid extreme cold whenever possible. In cases of severe hypothermia, a warming blanket may be necessary.

Risk for Injury: Myxedema Coma. A client with acute hypothyroidism is susceptible to development of myxedema coma, leading to the nursing diagnosis *Risk for Injury: Myxedema coma related to hypersensitivity to anesthetics, sedatives, and narcotics secondary to decreased metabolic rate.*

Outcomes. The client will not receive the usual doses of anesthetics, sedatives, and narcotics so that development of myxedema coma will be prevented and the client will not be injured.

Interventions. The client should not receive sedatives unless it is absolutely necessary. If a sedative or narcotic must be given, administer no more than one-third to one-half the usual dose. Then assess the client carefully for respiratory depression or a decreased level of consciousness.

Risk for Impaired Skin Integrity. A client with myxedema is very susceptible to skin breakdown, leading to the nursing diagnosis *Risk for Impaired Skin Integrity related to edema and dryness secondary to infiltration of fluid into interstitial spaces.*

Outcomes. The client's skin will remain intact, as evidenced by absence of injury and resolution of edema.

Interventions. Monitor the sacrum, coccyx, elbows, scapulae, and other pressure points for redness or tissue breakdown. Remember that edematous tissues are more susceptible to pressure ulcers. Have a strict turning schedule for the client, and use a pressure reduction mattress.

EVALUATION

It is expected that after successful treatment the client will demonstrate no evidence of heart failure, edema, or skin impairment; temperature and urine output will be normal; and there will be no further evidence of myxedema. After the client is out of danger and alert, long-term management begins (see next).

■ Nursing Management of the Medical Client with Hypothyroidism

ASSESSMENT

Carefully assess the client for manifestations of hypothyroidism. Obtain a careful history; look for evidence of decreased metabolic function, such as weight gain, excessive sleeping, and generalized fatigue. The Critical Monitoring feature on Hypothyroidism lists other manifestations of decreased metabolic functions. Take a thorough diet history, looking particularly at the intake of iodine. Does the client take any goitrogenic substances or reside in a goiter belt?

Ask the client about other medical conditions that might be present, such as a history of hyperthyroidism treated with surgery or radioactive iodine, both of which predispose to hypothyroidism. Does the client use any medication that might lead to hypothyroidism? Lithium, aminoglutethimide, sodium or potassium perchlorate, and cobalt can slow thyroid metabolism.

DIAGNOSIS, OUTCOMES, INTERVENTIONS

Altered Nutrition: More than Body Requirements. The slowed metabolic rate places a hypothyroid client at risk for weight gain, leading to the nursing diagnosis *Altered Nutrition: More than Body Requirements related to a slowed metabolic rate resulting in weight gain.*

Outcomes. The client will return to normal weight, as evidenced by loss of at least 2 pounds weekly.

Interventions. When the client begins taking thyroid medication, the activity level and decreased edema commonly result in a significant initial weight loss without any change in diet. Typically, however, appetite also increases as the medication begins to work. Therefore, teach the client to maintain a low-calorie diet until weight stabilizes at the ideal body weight. The client should gain more energy as the TH level returns to normal, allowing an increase in activity to help in weight loss.

Activity Intolerance. A client with hypothyroidism usually feels fatigued, which commonly leads to the nursing diagnosis *Activity Intolerance related to weakness and*

CRITICAL MONITORING

Hypothyroidism

These manifestations should be monitored in a client who is thought to have a diagnosis of hypothyroidism. Serum laboratory tests confirm the diagnosis:

- Lethargy, depression
- Sensitivity to cold, weight gain; later, an enlarged thyroid
- Dry skin
- Normal to subnormal temperature
- Normal to slow pulse
- Normal respiratory rate unless affected by goiter size
- Normal to slight elevation of blood pressure
- Augmentation of heart failure

apathy secondary to a decreased metabolic rate and re-sulting in an increased heart rate and shortness of breath with activity.

Outcomes. The client will develop increased tolerance for activity, as evidenced by a return to pre-illness activity levels.

Interventions. While the client still has hypothyroidism, energy levels are decreased and the client tires easily. Usually, the result is a decreased activity level. When TH replacement begins, the client returns to a level of physical and mental activity that should gradually improve with hormone therapy.

Constipation. A client with hypothyroidism has decreased gastrointestinal motility, leading to the nursing diagnosis *Constipation related to decreased peristalsis secondary to slowed metabolic rate and activity intolerance, resulting in decreased frequency of stools and painful defecation.*

Outcomes. The client will experience a return to a normal pre-illness bowel pattern, as evidenced by a bowel movement at least every other day.

Interventions. Implement measures to prevent constipation and fecal impaction. As the hypothyroidism is reversed and cardiac status improves, encourage more activity. Advise the client to drink six to eight glasses of water every day and to eat foods high in fiber, such as fresh fruits, vegetables, and grains. If these measures are ineffective, a stool softener or cathartic may be indicated.

EVALUATION

Once hypothyroidism has been diagnosed and replacement therapy begun, it is expected that the condition will be reversed over 3 to 12 weeks. A maintenance dosage of TH replacement is determined. If reversal of the condition does not continue, the client must be assessed for compliance with the therapeutic regimen.

■ Self-Care

Hypothyroidism is a lifelong disease that must be managed with the client's full participation. The client should understand the pharmacologic regimen, nutrition, and follow-up required to control the condition.

To promote self-care, focus your teaching on the client's need to understand the manifestations of hyperthyroidism and hypothyroidism, to follow the medication regimen and diet, and to seek medical attention appropriately. Evaluate the client's level of knowledge about the disorder and the importance of taking TH daily for life. Develop and implement a teaching plan based on the client's particular needs. Also, provide a written list (such as the one in the Client Education Guide) of the manifestations of thyroid deficiency or excess. Instruct the client on how to monitor pulse rate. Instruct the client and significant others to telephone the physician if those manifestations develop.

Monitor the client's weight weekly. Physical manifestations of hypothyroidism should decrease over 3 to 12 weeks as TH levels increase. Emphasize the need for iodized salt. Advise the client to drink sufficient fluids, increase physical activity, and eat a high-fiber diet to prevent constipation. Remind the client to have TH levels checked routinely until they stabilize and then at regular intervals to be sure that they remain normal.

■ Modification for Elderly Clients

Subclinical hypothyroidism refers to a combination of elevated TSH levels, normal T_3 and free thyroxine (FT_4) levels, and no clinical manifestations. Subclinical hypothyroidism occurs in up to 15% of postmenopausal women. The most common causes of are, in order of frequency, autoimmune thyroiditis, Hashimoto's disease, previous thyroid surgery or treatment with radioactive agents, and non-compliance with prescribed T_4 replacements.

CLIENT EDUCATION GUIDE

Thyroid Supplements

The usual initial dosage in adults is 0.025 to 0.1 mg by mouth (PO) per day, increased by 0.05 to 0.1 mg PO every 1 to 4 weeks until the desired response is achieved. The maintenance dose is 0.1 to 0.4 mg/day.

- Take your medication at the same time every day to maintain appropriate levels in your blood. Morning is preferred to prevent insomnia.
- Check your pulse rate, and tell your physician if it is over 100. Side effects may result from your dosage and your sensitivity.

  - Central nervous system effects include nervousness, insomnia, and tremor.
  - Cardiovascular effects may include tachycardia, palpitations, dysrhythmias, angina pectoris, hypertension, and worsening of pre-existing cardiac conditions, such as heart failure.
  - Gastrointestinal effects may include an increase in appetite, nausea, and diarrhea.
  - Other side effects resemble the manifestations of hyperthyroidism: headache, leg cramps, weight loss, heat intolerance, sweating, fever, and menstrual irregularities.

- Do not take a thyroid supplement if you have had a heart attack, thyrotoxicosis, or untreated adrenal insufficiency.
- Use these drugs with caution if you have angina pectoris (chest pain), other cardiovascular disorders, renal insufficiency or failure, or poor circulation.
- Tell your physician right away if you experience angina or manifestations of hyperthyroidism (suggesting overdose or exacerbated or difficult-to-control cardiac disease).
- Notify your other physicians or health care providers that you are taking a thyroid supplement, which will alter your thyroid function test results.
- Thyroid supplements prolong the prothrombin time, a measure of the speed at which your blood clots. Therefore, if you are taking blood thinners, you will need a smaller dose.
- Notify your physician immediately if you are pregnant or plan to become pregnant so that your dose can be adjusted accordingly.

Medical treatment is not indicated for clients who have no manifestations. Clients with generalized complaints may benefit from small doses of T_4, which indicates that their condition was symptomatic rather than subclinical. Remember, a principal hazard in giving T_4 to an elderly client is the development of ischemic heart disease, as evidenced by angina. The response to therapy and serum levels must be observed closely. The client's pulse should be monitored daily.

The difficulty in diagnosing hypothyroidism in older adults is that the manifestations are usually vague and generic to other disease processes. Hypothyroidism must be considered in the differential diagnosis of a variety of conditions affecting older people.

HYPERTHYROIDISM

Hyperthyroidism (excessive secretion of TH) is a highly preventable endocrine disorder. Like most thyroid conditions, it is a disorder predominantly affecting women (in a female-to-male ratio of 4:1), especially women between ages 20 and 40 years.

Etiology and Risk Factors

Hyperthyroidism may be due to overfunctioning of the entire gland or, less commonly, to single or multiple functioning adenomas of thyroid cancer. Overtreatment of myxedema with TH may also result in hyperthyroidism.

The most common form of hyperthyroidism is Graves' disease (toxic, diffuse goiter), which has three principal hallmarks: hyperthyroidism, thyroid gland enlargement (goiter), and exophthalmos (abnormal protrusion of the eyes). Graves' disease is an autoimmune disorder mediated by immunoglobulin G (IgG) antibody that binds to and activates TSH receptors on the surface of the thyroid cells.

Other causes of hyperthyroidism include toxic nodular goiter, toxic adenoma (benign), thyroid carcinoma, subacute and chronic thyroiditis, ingestion of TH, and ingestion of amiodarone hydrochloride for atrial fibrillation. Health maintenance and restoration activities include monitoring TH levels if TH replacement is given, removal of thyroid tumors, and administration of antithyroid medications.

Pathophysiology

Graves' disease may be due to excessive stimulation of the adrenergic nervous system or excessive levels of circulating TH.

Hyperthyroidism is characterized by loss of the normal regulatory controls of TH secretion. Because the action of TH on the body is stimulatory, hypermetabolism results, with increased sympathetic nervous system activity. Excessive amounts of TH stimulate the cardiac system and increase the number of beta-adrenergic receptors, leading to tachycardia and increased cardiac output, stroke volume, adrenergic responsiveness, and peripheral blood flow. Metabolism increases greatly, leading to a negative nitrogen balance, lipid depletion, and a state of nutritional deficiency and weight loss.

Hyperthyroidism also results in altered secretion and metabolism of hypothalamic, pituitary, and gonadal hormones. If hyperthyroidism occurs before puberty, sexual development is delayed in both sexes. After puberty, it results in diminished libido in both men and women. Women also have menstrual irregularities and decreased fertility.

Clinical Manifestations

Because hyperthyroidism is caused by excessive secretion of TH, the clinical picture of Graves' disease is, in many ways, opposite to that of hypothyroidism. Assessment reveals a client who appears extremely agitated and irritable, with a hand tremor at rest. Despite a ravenous appetite, weight loss occurs as a result of the quickened metabolism. Because of the high levels of circulating TH, the client's body processes "speed up." As described in the Critical Monitoring feature called Hyperthyroidism, manifestations include loose bowel movements, heat intolerance, profuse diaphoresis (perspiration), tachycardia, and incoordination related to tremor. The skin becomes warm, smooth, and moist because of accelerated circulation to the tissues. Hair appears thin and soft.

Moreover, the client's emotions are adversely affected by the turbulent activity within the body. Moods may be cyclic, ranging from mild euphoria to extreme hyperactivity to delirium. The excessive hyperactivity in turn leads to extreme fatigue and depression, again followed by episodes of overactivity. As a result of the client's chaotic emotional state, interpersonal relationships may deteriorate, further accentuating the emotional disturbance.

Goiter, the second characteristic of Graves' disease, is due to hyperplasia and hypertrophy of the thyroid cells. The gland may grow to three or four times its normal size. Cellular overgrowth results in the release of excessive amounts of TH into the blood.

Exophthalmos is the third major manifestation of Graves' disease. The cause of the ophthalmologic changes in Graves' disease seems to be autoimmunity against retro-orbital tissues. The client who develops exophthalmos has protruding eyes and a fixed stare caused by accumulation of fluid in the fat pads and muscles that lie behind the eyeballs (Fig. 43–3). Because the eyes are surrounded by unyielding bone, edema forces them forward out of their sockets, producing the typical facies of exophthalmos. In severe cases, clients may be unable to

---

CRITICAL MONITORING

Hyperthyroidism

These manifestations should be monitored in a client who is thought to have a diagnosis of hyperthyroidism.

- Anxiety, short attention span, irritability
- Heat intolerance, unintentional weight loss
- Warm, moist skin
- Increased temperature
- Increased pulse
- Increased blood pressure
- Fatigue and weakness
- Augmentation of other disorders, such as atrial fibrillation, heart failure, angina pectoris (chest pain), paranoia, and anxiety

FIGURE 43–3 Extreme exophthalmos in hyperthyroidism. Because the eyes are surrounded by unyielding bone, fluid accumulation in the fat pads and muscles behind the eyeballs causes protruding eyes and a fixed stare in the client with exophthalmos. Without intervention, the client with severe exophthalmos may be unable to close the eyelids and may develop corneal ulceration or infection. Eventually, this can result in total loss of vision. (From Scheie, H. G. [1997]. *Textbook of ophthalmology* [9th ed.] Philadelphia: W. B. Saunders.)

close their eyelids and must have their lids taped shut to protect the eyes. Without intervention, severe exophthalmos can progress to corneal ulceration or infection and loss of vision. In some cases, exophthalmos is not reversed by intervention. It may actually worsen with radioactive iodine therapy.

The diagnosis of Graves' disease is confirmed on the basis of the client's often striking physical appearance (enlarged neck, protruding eyes, agitated expression); the manifestations of agitation, restlessness, and weight loss; and laboratory findings. Serum TH levels are usually all elevated, although they are occasionally within the normal range (so-called euthyroid Graves' disease). Serum cholesterol levels are usually depressed. See Table 43–2 for the usual laboratory findings.

Complications

The three major complications of Graves' disease are exophthalmos, heart disease, and thyroid storm (thyroid crisis, thyrotoxicosis).

EXOPHTHALMOS
Exophthalmos develops as a result of proptosis, lid retraction, muscle swelling, and tissue edema from a prolonged hyperthyroid condition. Manifestations may include a gritty sensation in the eye, photophobia, lacrimation, inflammatory changes, and dyslogia.

Unlike the manifestations of goiter and hyperthyroidism, exophthalmos does not necessarily regress with therapy. Diuretics may alleviate some of the periorbital edema. Glucocorticoids such as prednisone are given in large doses to reduce inflammation of the periorbital tissues. Unfortunately, steroids produce many undesirable side effects, including acute psychoses. Estrogen therapy is occasionally of value in postmenopausal women. Methylcellulose eye drops, 14% four times daily, help reduce eye irritation. Radiation therapy to the retro-orbital tissues may help in severe cases. Surgical decompression of the orbits may be performed when all other measures fail to correct exophthalmos. This procedure may save the client's vision when eye changes are severe.

A number of general nursing interventions also help to reduce eye discomfort and prevent corneal ulceration and infection. Instruct a client with exophthalmos to wear dark eyeglasses. Warn the client to avoid getting dust or dirt in the eyes. If the eyelids cannot be closed easily or at all, have the client wear a sleeping mask (available in drug stores) or lightly tape the eyes shut with nonallergic tape. Elevate the head of the bed at night, and have the client restrict salt intake to relieve edema.

HEART DISEASE
Heart disease poses a serious threat. Tachycardia almost always accompanies thyrotoxicosis, and atrial fibrillation may also appear. Heart failure is found among older clients with long-standing thyrotoxicosis. Propranolol is the drug of choice but is contraindicated if asthma or heart failure is a pre-existing condition. The treatment of these cardiac complications is covered in Unit 12.

THYROID STORM (THYROTOXICOSIS)
Thyroid storm (thyrotoxicosis) is a potentially fatal, acute episode of thyroid overactivity characterized by high fever, severe tachycardia, delirium, dehydration, and extreme irritability. Thanks to modern intervention techniques, this once common problem seldom develops today. Factors that may precipitate a thyroid storm include undiagnosed or untreated hyperthyroidism, infection, thyroid ablation, metabolic catastrophes, surgery, trauma, labor and delivery, myocardial infarction, pulmonary embolus, medication overdosage, or inadequate preparation for thyroid surgery.

A client with thyrotoxicosis may have an increase in clotting factor VIII. Despite this increase, the hyperthyroid client has increased sensitivity to coumarin derivatives because of the accelerated metabolic clearance of the vitamin K–dependent clotting factors. Thyroid storm is a clinical diagnosis; no laboratory tests differentiate hyperthyroidism from thyroid storm in general.

Outcome Management

■ Medical Management

The desired outcomes of medical management for clients with Graves' disease are to curtail the excessive secretion of TH and to prevent and treat complications. Choice of intervention is based on age, goiter size, and whether other health problems exist. The three major forms of therapy are antithyroid medication, radioiodine therapy, and surgery.

CURTAIL EXCESSIVE SECRETION OF THYROID HORMONE
ANTITHYROID MEDICATION THERAPY. Antithyroid medication is recommended for clients younger than 18 years of age and for pregnant women (see Table 43–3). The major medications used to control hyperthyroidism include iodide, propylthiouracil, and methimazole (Tapazole). Adrenergic blocking agents may be administered as adjunctive therapy.

Propylthiouracil is the most commonly used antithyroid medication. It corrects hyperthyroidism by impairing TH synthesis. With the usual dosage regimen, propylthiouracil ameliorates Graves' disease within 4 to 8 weeks. However, several months may pass before manifestations completely abate. When euthyroid, the client is given a maintenance dose of propylthiouracil, usually three times daily. Although an ideal medication in many ways, propylthiouracil causes significant side effects in about 9% of people who use it.

The most serious toxic effect is agranulocytosis (see Chapter 75). A white blood cell (WBC) count should be obtained before initial administration of the medication. Instruct the client to report a sore throat, fever, or rash immediately so that further WBC tests can be performed and the client's condition evaluated. Less severe adverse reactions include mild allergies (rash and pruritus). Rarely does hepatitis or drug fever develop.

Methimazole blocks the action of TH in the body. Unfortunately, it produces agranulocytosis in a small percentage of people.

Iodine therapy is prescribed for two reasons: (1) to reduce the vascularity of the thyroid gland before subtotal or total thyroidectomy and (2) to treat thyroid storm. Iodine preparations act temporarily to prevent release of TH into the circulation by increasing the amount of TH stored in the gland. The stored TH is eventually released back into the circulation, however, once again producing hyperthyroidism. For this reason, iodine preparations are usually given only for 10 to 14 days before surgery. If iodine is given for a longer period or if it is given alone (not in combination with propylthiouracil), the thyroid gland may "escape" before thyroidectomy. Escape of the thyroid means that the iodine is no longer capable of maintaining TH storage. As a result, TH floods the circulation, and hyperthyroidism becomes more severe than before.

The iodine medication of choice is potassium iodide. Lugol's solution is also used but is more expensive than potassium iodide and tends to inactivate antithyroid preparations in the bowel.

RADIOIODINE THERAPY. Therapy with radioactive iodine (^{131}I) is prescribed mainly for middle-aged and older clients. This intervention offers many advantages: it is economical, is simple to administer, and can be prescribed on an outpatient basis, as described in the accompanying Case Study. Radiotherapy is contraindicated for pregnant women and is rarely used for children.

The rationale behind ^{131}I therapy for Graves' disease is simple. The thyroid gland is unable to distinguish between regular iodine atoms and radioiodine atoms. Consequently, when the client receives a dose of ^{131}I, the thyroid gland picks up the radioiodine and concentrates it just as it would regular iodine. As a result, the cells that concentrate ^{131}I to make T_4 are destroyed by the local irradiation, TH secretion diminishes, and the manifestations of hyperthyroidism and goiter disappear. However, because radioiodine destroys thyroid cells, one of the major possible complications of ^{131}I therapy is hypothyroidism. Therefore, assess for manifestations of hypothyroidism after ^{131}I therapy.

^{131}I is dissolved in water and administered orally. The dosage is determined both by the size of the gland and by the thyroid's uptake of a tracer dose of radioiodine. After receiving the radioiodine, the client may go home unless the dosage is extremely large. In the latter case, the client must be placed in isolation for several days to prevent radioactive contamination.

The manifestations of hyperthyroidism usually subside within 6 to 12 weeks after ^{131}I administration. Because of the delay in achieving a therapeutic response with ^{131}I, concurrent treatment with beta-adrenergic blockers may be desirable. Sometimes resistant clients require a second or, in rare instances, a third dose of radioiodine.

The client who becomes euthyroid still needs regular medical examinations because hypothyroidism may develop several years after radiotherapy. Clients who become hypothyroid require lifelong hormone replacement with thyroid preparations.

PREVENT AND TREAT COMPLICATIONS

ADRENERGIC BLOCKING AGENTS. Adrenergic blocking agents are sometimes given as adjunctive therapy to control the activity of the sympathetic nervous system. There is now evidence that these agents are of great benefit to the "hyperthyroid heart," which has increased sensitivity to catecholamines and an increased number of beta-adrenergic receptor sites. Therefore, these agents help lessen distressing manifestations such as palpitations and tachycardia. Tremor and nervousness may also be alleviated by adrenergic blocking agents. These medications include propranolol and reserpine. Treatment of Graves' hyperthyroidism may involve a long delay (weeks to months) between the start of therapy and substantial improvement or resolution of manifestations.

DIETARY THERAPY. The client with hyperthyroidism needs a high-calorie, high-protein diet to compensate for the hypermetabolic state. A diet of 4000 to 5000 calories with high protein levels may be necessary to prevent a negative nitrogen balance and weight loss.

TREATING THYROID STORM. Because thyroid storm is an emergency, heroic intervention is needed for control. The high fever is treated with hypothermia blankets; dehydration is reversed with intravenous fluids. Management of thyroid storm involves suppressing hormone release, inhibiting hormone synthesis, blocking conversion of T_4 to the more active T_3, inhibiting the effects of TH on body tissues, and treating the precipitating cause, if known.

Blockade of TH release is usually achieved by oral administration of iodides, such as potassium iodide. Sodium iodide may be given intravenously. Glucocorticoid, dexamethasone, and propylthiouracil are also commonly used oral drugs. Beta-blockers are given to decrease the effects of sympathetic nervous system stimulation and to treat tachycardia.

■ Nursing Management of the Medical Client

ASSESSMENT

Begin your assessment by obtaining a complete history. By asking questions concerning weight, appetite, activity, heat intolerance, and bowel activity, you can assess for the presence of typical manifestations of hyperthyroidism. Also ask about mood alterations. Mood swings, irritability, decreased attention span, and manic behavior may be experienced by the client with hyperthyroidism. Because the client may not be aware of some of the mood changes, consider questioning significant others about changes in the client's behavior.

Hyperthyroidism and Postmenopausal Osteoporosis

Mrs. Gonzales is a 55-year-old Hispanic woman who presents at a free clinic for migrant farm workers. She is dressed in a lightweight sundress and sandals despite outdoor temperatures around 50° F. Mrs. Gonzales complains of pounding in her chest and shortness of breath without exertion. She relates that she has lost 20 pounds in the last 6 weeks even though she has been eating more than usual. A thyroxine (T_4) level determined at the clinic is twice the normal value. The nurse practitioner has arranged for additional outpatient diagnostic studies.

Selected Outpatient Laboratory Values for Mrs. Gonzales

Red blood cells: 3.8 million/mm^3
Hemoglobin, 11.8g/dl
Hematocrit: 35%
White blood cells: 9000/mm^3
Glucose: 90 mg/dl
Thyroxine: 20 mg/dl
Thyroid-stimulating hormone: 0 mIU/ml
^{131}I (radioactive iodine) uptake: 50% in 2 hr without evidence of malignancy
Calcium: 10 mg/dl

Nursing Assessment

Mrs. Gonzales reports that she has worked in the fields all her life. She met her husband in California while they were picking grapes 40 years ago. They have three children, who are married and work in the fields. She does not see them often, however, because they cannot always work in the same area. Mrs. Gonzales was born in Mexico. She speaks fluent Spanish and only a few words of English. She is concerned about how she and her husband will pay for her treatment.

Mrs. Gonzales reports that she went through "the change of life" 14 years ago. She cannot afford hormone replacement therapy. Mrs. Gonzales denies a family history of cancer, heart disease, or diabetes mellitus.

Nursing Physical Examination

Height: 5 ft 5 inches. Weight: 105 lb (47.7 kg)
Vital signs: Blood pressure (BP) 160/94; temperature, pulse, and respirations (TPR) 99.6, 126, 24
Level of consciousness: Awake, alert, restless
Eyes, ears, nose, throat: pupils equal, round, reactive to light and accommodation (PERRLA), increased tears, photophobia, exophthalmos, goiter
Cardiac: Tachycardia, regular rate and rhythm, palpitations
Pulmonary: Lungs clear bilaterally
Abdominal: Soft, nontender, with hyperactive bowel sounds
Genitourinary: Within normal limits
Peripheral pulses: 4/4, with slight pretibial and pedal edema

Initial Outpatient Treatment Plan

Medications: Propranolol (Inderal) 20 mg PO tid
Propylthiouracil (PTU) 100 mg PO tid
Artificial tears or other over-the-counter (OTC) eyedrops as needed; arrange for sample medications if possible)
Diet: As tolerated, no added salt
Activity: As tolerated; monitor heart rate; call if pulse 160 BPM at rest
Other: Call if there is difficulty swallowing or breathing or other signs of enlarging goiter; return to clinic in 2 weeks

On the basis of the diagnostic work-up, Mrs. Gonzales will have radioactive iodine therapy. At her return visit, her T_4 level is within normal limits. She reports that she has not had any more pounding in her chest. Her resting heart rate at the clinic is 84 BPM.

Review of her diet history reveals an average daily intake of about 2000 to 2500 calories consisting largely of tortillas, beans, and the foods currently being harvested in the fields. She reports that she does not drink milk or eat cheese because they cause bloating and diarrhea.

Mrs. Gonzales receives the prescribed dose of radioactive iodine orally and is instructed to return in 30 days for laboratory work and to call if any problems develop.

Discharge and Post-treatment Considerations

1. Average length of stay (LOS): outpatient only
2. Complete post-treatment instruction
3. Coordinate health benefits with department of social services

Questions to Be Considered

1. What influence would Mrs. Gonzales' use of the Spanish language have on her treatment plan? Identify implications for formal nursing education preparation.
2. How might Mrs. Gonzales' care differ from that of a person with health care benefits? Discuss ethical considerations that may affect the allocation of scarce health care resources.
3. Compare and contrast the manifestations of menopause and hyperthyroidism. Discuss the implications for diagnosis and treatment.
4. Discuss the pathophysiology of the relationship between the pituitary gland and the thyroid gland. How is this manifested in Mrs. Gonzales' case?
5. Discuss the management of Mrs. Gonzales' diet before and after radioactive iodine treatment. Include cultural and economic factors in your discussion. In addition, consider the implications of Mrs. Gonzales being postmenopausal and having lactose intolerance.
6. Discuss the nursing implications and client teaching aspects associated with Mrs. Gonzales' prescription medications before radioactive iodine treatment. Identify potential OTC drug contraindications in the pretreatment period. Discuss medication requirements and related client teaching after radioactive iodine treatment.

DIAGNOSIS, OUTCOMES, INTERVENTIONS

Altered Nutrition: Less than Body Requirements.
A client with hyperthyroidism is hypermetabolic, leading to the nursing diagnosis *Altered Nutrition: Less than Body Requirements related to accelerated metabolic rate resulting in weight loss and decreased energy levels.*

Outcomes. The client's weight loss will end, as evidenced by an ability to consume sufficient calories to return to ideal body weight.

Interventions. Provide the client with a well-balanced, high-calorie diet. Clients with Graves' disease are usually extremely hungry because of the increased metabolism. Six full meals a day may be needed to satisfy their appetite. Despite unusually large meals, however, clients may lose weight rapidly; they are also usually in a state of negative nitrogen balance. Therefore, encourage the client to eat foods that are nutritious and contain ample amounts of protein, carbohydrates, fats, and minerals. Discourage foods that increase peristalsis and thus result in diarrhea, such as highly seasoned, bulky, or fibrous foods.

The client should be weighed daily, and weight losses of more than 4.4 pounds (2 kg) should be reported. If the client continues to appear malnourished despite an ample diet, supplemental vitamins, particularly vitamin B complex, may be needed.

Activity Intolerance.
Another nursing diagnosis related to the client's hypermetabolic state is *Activity Intolerance related to exhaustion secondary to accelerated metabolic rate resulting in inability to perform activity without shortness of breath and significant increases in heart rate.*

Outcomes. The client will engage in a normal level of activity, as evidenced by ability to maintain a proper balance of rest and activity to prevent exhaustion.

Interventions. Provide the client with an environment that is restful both mentally and physically. It is a challenge to help hyperthyroid clients relax. Assign the client to a private room to promote rest and to prevent the client from disturbing others through hyperactivity and restlessness.

Risk for Injury.
Many ocular problems can develop in a client with hyperthyroidism. Therefore, an important nursing diagnosis for this client is *Risk for Injury: Corneal ulcerations, infection, and possible blindness related to inability to close the eyelids secondary to exophthalmos.*

Outcomes. The client will not experience corneal ulceration, infection, or blindness, as evidenced by no further development of exophthalmos.

Interventions. Treatment should be started as soon as possible after the diagnosis is made so that exophthalmos —a potentially permanent condition—can be avoided. The client should use artificial tears and eye patches as needed to prevent irritation if exophthalmos has already developed. When treatment has begun, the exophthalmos should not increase; however, it may not diminish quickly or at all.

Hyperthermia.
A client with hyperthyroidism is in a hypermetabolic state, leading to the nursing diagnosis *Hyperthermia related to accelerated metabolic rate resulting in fever, diaphoresis, and reported heat intolerance.*

Outcomes. The client will not exhibit hyperthermia, as evidenced by a return to normal body temperature.

Interventions. Tell the client to stay in a cool environment. Use only a lightweight sheet for the top cover, and give the client light, loose pajamas. The client who is diaphoretic may need fresh bed sheets and clothes frequently. Encourage the client not to overexert because doing so raises the body temperature and metabolic rate.

Impaired Social Interaction.
A client with hyperthyroidism is hyperactive, possibly leading to the nursing diagnosis *Impaired Social Interaction related to extreme agitation, hyperactivity, and mood swings resulting in inability to relate effectively with others.*

Outcomes. The client will not suffer from impaired social interaction, as evidenced by ability to interact without difficulty and without agitation, hyperactivity, or mood swings.

Interventions. Explain to significant others that any bizarre, difficult behavior is likely to be temporary and should improve steadily with intervention. Maintain a quiet, understanding manner when caring for a client with Graves' disease. Accept the irritation and emotional outbursts as normal expressions of the disease.

Incorporate occupational therapy into care planning. The occupational therapist may be able to provide simple activities designed to distract the client from the disorder (such as putting together a puzzle with large pieces, molding clay, or watching television). For a very restless client, discuss with the physician the need for a sedative such as diazepam (Valium) or possibly an adrenergic blocking agent.

EVALUATION

The client with Graves' disease should recover from the hyperthyroidism without difficulty when the medication regimen has begun.

■ Surgical Management

THYROIDECTOMY

Surgery for hyperthyroidism has been performed since the early 1880s. Thyroidectomy (removal of the thyroid gland) may be total or partial. *Total* thyroidectomy is performed to remove thyroid cancer. Clients who undergo this operation must take thyroid hormones permanently. *Subtotal* thyroidectomy is performed to correct hyperthyroidism and extreme cases of simple goiter. About five sixths of the gland is removed. Because one sixth of the functioning gland is left intact, hormone replacements may not be necessary.

INDICATIONS AND CONTRAINDICATIONS. Ideally, clients selected are young and free from any condition that makes them poor operative risks (such as diabetes, heart disease, renal disease, or drug allergies).

Preoperative preparation for a subtotal thyroidectomy is extremely important. The client must be euthyroid before the operation, if possible. Preoperative care for a client with Graves' disease includes administration of antithyroid drugs to suppress secretion of thyroid hormones and iodine preparations to reduce the size and vascularity of the organ, thereby diminishing the chance of hemorrhage (see Medical Management). The client should be adequately rested, at optimal weight, and in good health before entering the operating room. Adequate preoperative preparation may take as long as 2 to 3 months.

TABLE 43–4 POSTOPERATIVE ORDERS, RATIONALES, AND ASSOCIATED NURSING INTERVENTIONS AFTER THYROIDECTOMY

Postoperative Order	Rationale	Associated Nursing Interventions
Take vital signs every 15 min until stable; then every hour for next 24 hr.	After thyroidectomy, hemorrhage and respiratory obstruction may develop. Elevated pulse and hypotension indicate hemorrhage and shock. Dyspnea, stridulous respirations, and retraction of neck tissues indicate respiratory obstruction.	Check dressing after checking vital signs. Observe for bleeding at front, sides, and back of neck. Examine back of neck and shoulders for bleeding because blood tends to drain posteriorly. Check dressing for tightness; uncomfortable tautness may indicate bleeding into tissues. Loosen dressing and call surgeon immediately.
Use semi-Fowler position when client conscious unless client is hypotensive. Support head and neck with pillows and sandbags. Ambulation on day 2 as tolerated.	Immobilization of head and neck is essential to prevent flexion and hyperextension of neck with resultant strain on suture line. Semi-Fowler position used for comfort.	Place sandbags on either side of head for immobilization and good alignment. Warn client not to extend or hyperextend neck; reassure client that sandbags will prevent moving head too much. Gently rub back of neck to relieve tension. Support client's head and neck when moving or changing position.
Give fluids by mouth as tolerated. If nausea or vomiting, notify surgeon. Start soft diet on afternoon of day 2.	Give intravenous fluids if nausea or vomiting. Otherwise, start oral fluids as soon as client is fully conscious.	Maintain intake and output record for 2–3 days. Assess for difficulty swallowing. Normally this problem lasts for only 1–2 days postoperatively. Weigh client once a full diet is started; weight lost during early postoperative period should be regained.
Give meperidine (Demerol) or morphine sulfate every 1–2 hr as needed for pain in throat area.	Meperidine and morphine sulfate are both used during early postoperative period to relieve pain and promote rest.	Do not give narcotics if client has respirations below 12/min or respiratory congestion. Consult physician for further orders.
Cough and deep-breathe every hour. Suction mouth and trachea if necessary.	Pooling of mucous secretions in trachea, bronchi, and lungs causes respiratory obstruction with resultant atelectasis and pneumonia. Secretions must be raised to prevent respiratory complications.	Instruct client to cough and deep-breathe as taught during preoperative period. If client cannot raise secretions, gently suction mouth and trachea. Do not oversedate clients with profuse respiratory secretions; given narcotics judiciously.
Have tracheostomy set, endotracheal tube, laryngoscope, and oxygen on hand.	Acute respiratory obstruction due to hemorrhage, edema of glottis, laryngeal nerve damage, or tetany is an emergency. Equipment for establishing an airway and administering oxygen must be available for immediate use.	Continuously assess for manifestations of airway obstruction, such as increasing restlessness, tachycardia, apprehension, cyanosis, stridulous respiration, and retraction of neck tissues. Report any of these manifestations to the surgeon immediately.
Give continuous mist inhalation until chest is clear.	Humidification of air promotes easier breathing and helps to liquefy mucous secretions.	Keep doors closed so that moist air is retained in room.
Take temperature every 4 hr for 24 hr, then routinely.	One of the first manifestations of thyroid storm is elevated temperature.	Carefully assess for manifestations of thyroid storm: elevated temperature, extreme restlessness, agitation, and tachycardia. Report any elevation over 100° F (37.7° C) rectally or 99° F (32.2° C) orally.
Assess client for hypocalcemia and monitor calcium, magnesium, and phosphorus.	Inadvertent removal or devascularization of the parathyroid glands can cause postoperative hypoparathyroidism.	Mild hypocalcemia can be asymptomatic. Severe hypocalcemia can produce circumoral paresthesias, positive Chvostek's or Trousseau's sign. Administer calcium supplements for hypocalcemic levels.

Postoperative orders, rationales, and associated nursing interventions after thyroidectomy are presented in Table 43–4.

COMPLICATIONS. Besides the usual complications of any surgery, which include hemorrhage and infection, the client after thyroidectomy is at risk for thyroid storm, tetany, respiratory obstruction, laryngeal edema, and vocal cord injury. If the client is not euthyroid, the risk of intraoperative or postoperative thyroid storm is greatly increased.

Although uncommon, respiratory obstruction may result from swelling related to the surgical site. Rarely, vocal cord paralysis may result from nerve damage. Hypoparathyroidism may result from inadvertent removal of parathyroid gland tissue. The parathyroid glands lie just behind the lobes of the thyroid and are commonly disturbed and sometimes inadvertently removed during surgery. Careful postoperative monitoring of neurologic irritability and serum calcium levels is performed for this reason.

OUTCOMES. Surgical treatment is effective in most people with Graves' disease. A small percentage remain hyperthyroid, and hypothyroidism develops in some.

Nursing Management of the Surgical Client

ASSESSMENT

Assess the client for typical manifestations of Graves' disease. A hypermetabolic state may be obvious from apparent weight loss, and exophthalmos may be obvious as well. Also, question the client about visual difficulties, fatigue, weakness, tremors, and insomnia, as outlined in the earlier Critical Monitoring feature on Hyperthyroidism.

DIAGNOSIS, OUTCOMES, INTERVENTIONS

Risk for Injury: Thyroid Storm, Hypocalcemia, or Hemorrhage. The client undergoing a thyroidectomy should be euthyroid preoperatively. Thus, an important nursing diagnosis is *Risk for Injury: Thyroid storm, hypocalcemia, or hemorrhage related to surgical procedure and not being in a euthyroid state.*

Outcomes. Thyroid storm, hypocalcemia, or hemorrhage will be prevented or will be detected early and the client protected from injury.

Interventions

Promote Preoperative Euthyroid State. The client must be carefully prepared for a thyroidectomy to avoid complications (such as thyroid storm and hemorrhage). Outcomes of successful preparation for thyroid surgery are as follows:

- The client is euthyroid before entering the operating room. Tests of thyroid function are within normal limits.
- Manifestations of thyrotoxicosis are greatly diminished or absent. The client appears rested and relaxed.
- Weight and nutritional status are normal; any weight lost earlier has been regained.
- Cardiac problems are under control, pulse rate is normal, and preoperative electrocardiograms show no dangerous dysrhythmias.

To help meet these outcomes, antithyroid drugs, iodine preparations, bed rest, a nutritious diet, and supplemental vitamins are prescribed. Cardiac monitoring is maintained. Thorough preparation may take months. When good health has been restored, however, the client can undergo surgery with confidence that the operation will be successful and the manifestations alleviated.

Provide Postoperative Care. The immediate desired outcomes of postoperative care after thyroidectomy are to maintain airway patency, minimize strain on the suture line, relieve discomfort related to the sore throat and tracheal irritation, prevent pooling of respiratory secretions, prevent or relieve complications, and monitor for decreased parathyroid function.

Monitor for Postoperative Complications. Assemble the needed equipment at the bedside before the client returns from surgery. The equipment includes a blood pressure cuff and stethoscope, additional pillows, oxygen, suction equipment, intubation supplies, and a tracheostomy set. Ampules of calcium gluconate should be on hand in the medicine room or on the emergency cart.

As noted earlier, major complications after thyroidectomy may include:

- Respiratory obstruction caused by edema of the glottis, bilateral laryngeal nerve damage, or tracheal compression from hemorrhage
- Hemorrhage
- Weakness and hoarseness of the voice from trauma or damage to one laryngeal nerve
- Hypocalcemia and tetany from accidental removal of one or more parathyroid glands
- Thyroid storm (if the client is not euthyroid preoperatively)

Promote Voice Rest. Temporary hoarseness and voice weakness may occur if there has been unilateral injury to the recurrent laryngeal nerve during surgery. To assess the voice, ask the client's name after full recovery from the anesthesia. Have the client speak every 30 to 60 minutes thereafter, and carefully note any voice changes. If hoarseness or voice weakness is present, reassure the client that the problem will probably subside in a few days. Discourage unnecessary talking to minimize hoarseness.

Monitor and Treat Hypocalcemia. Muscle twitching and hyperirritability of the nervous system may indicate hypocalcemic tetany. Hypocalcemia can develop after thyroidectomy if the parathyroid glands are accidentally removed during surgery. Manifestations may develop 1 to 7 days after surgery. Monitor the client for Chvostek's (facial nerve irritability) and Trousseau's (carpal spasm) signs; report positive responses to the physician immediately. Also, if the client develops numbness and tingling around the mouth, fingertips, or toes; muscle spasms; or twitching, call the physician immediately. Make sure calcium gluconate ampules are available at the bedside and that the client has a patent intravenous line.

EVALUATION

The client should be discharged within several days of surgery without difficulty. The wound should heal within about 6 weeks without infection.

Self-Care

Hyperthyroidism is a chronic disease that must be managed with the client's full participation. When the immediate postoperative period and its dangers have passed, turn your attention to teaching. Several important areas should be included.

NECK EXERCISES. First, teach the client how to support the weight of the head and neck when sitting up in bed. Show the client how to place the hands at the back of the head when flexing the neck or moving. The client will probably be able to perform this maneuver by the first postoperative day.

Second, as the wound heals (about the 2nd to 4th postoperative day), demonstrate range-of-motion exercises to prevent contractures. With the surgeon's permission, teach the client to flex the head forward and laterally, to hyperextend the neck, and to turn the head from side to side. Have the client perform these exercises several times every day.

MEDICATIONS. If a total thyroidectomy has been performed, explain self-administration of thyroid medications (see the Client Education Guide earlier). Teach the client the medication regimen and the need for lifelong replacement therapy.

FOLLOW-UP MONITORING. Make an appointment for the clinic or physician's office after discharge. Serum thyroid levels must be determined to monitor treatment. Emphasize that the client who has had a thyroidectomy must see a physician at least twice yearly to avert possible complications (e.g., hypothyroidism, hypoparathyroidism, or recurrent hyperthyroidism) related to hormonal replacement. TH levels must be measured at regular intervals until the replacement medication is adjusted to a maintenance dose. The client should then see the physician twice a year for examinations.

PROMOTE WOUND HEALING. Teach the client how to care for the incision when it has healed by using lanolin cream to soften the wound and minimize the scar.

■ Modification for Elderly Clients

Hyperthyroidism in older adults accounts for 10% to 15% of all thyrotoxic clients. Some clients present with typical manifestations of hyperthyroidism, especially when the diagnosis is Graves' disease. However, hyperthyroidism in older people is also notorious for atypical or minimal manifestations. It is often overlooked because the manifestations are not the usual ones.

Indeed, manifestations are commonly attributed to aging. Weight loss, lack of ocular findings, and normal-sized thyroid glands are commonly found on assessment. Many clients actually appear apathetic instead of hyperactive. Cardiovascular abnormalities, such as heart failure, atrial dysrhythmias (usually digoxin resistant), and various degrees of heart block may be caused by hyperthyroidism. If the cardiac condition is pre-existing, it may be exacerbated by hyperthyroidism. Relative lack of tachycardia has been documented; about 40% of elderly clients have heart rates under 100 beats per minute (BPM).

The diagnosis of hyperthyroidism is established by appropriate laboratory tests. It is usual to find elevated T_4 and suppressed TSH levels. Hyperthyroidism in elderly clients is treated with radioactive iodine.

THYROIDITIS

Thyroiditis (inflammation of the thyroid gland) appears in three basic forms:

- Acute suppurative
- Subacute thyroiditis, either granulomatous (painful or de Quervain's thyroiditis) or lymphocytic (silent or painless thyroiditis)
- Chronic thyroiditis, also known as Hashimoto's disease

Etiology and Risk Factors

Acute suppurative thyroiditis is an uncommon inflammatory disease usually caused by bacterial invasion in the

form of an abscess of the thyroid gland. *Streptococcus pyogenes, Staphylococcus aureus*, and *Pneumococcus pneumoniae* are the most common etiologic agents. Acute thyroiditis is more common in females. Usually, it affects women between 20 and 40 years of age, although it also occurs in children and older people. Most affected clients have a pre-existing thyroid disorder.

Subacute granulomatous thyroiditis is a self-limiting inflammatory condition. No etiologic agent has been identified, although the condition may be viral in origin and commonly follows a respiratory infection. Autoimmune abnormalities have been described. There also appears to be a genetic predisposition to the development of both subacute granulomatous and lymphocytic thyroiditis. Of people with subacute granulomatous thyroiditis, 80% are women between 40 and 50 years old.

Chronic thyroiditis (Hashimoto's disease) is the most common form of thyroiditis. It is more prevalent in women than men and usually occurs between ages 20 and 50 years. Hashimoto's disease is a long-term inflammatory disorder. It is most commonly caused by autoimmune destruction of the thyroid gland. Genetic predisposition also plays a role in its causation.

Pathophysiology

Acute thyroiditis is a state of acute infection and inflammation. Usually, one lobe of the thyroid is more affected than the other. Follicular destruction, cell infiltration, and colloid depletion occur. Microabscesses form.

Subacute thyroiditis has three phases:

Phase 1: The condition begins with a 3- to 4-week prodromal viral illness. Fever and malaise precede the sudden onset of a tender goiter. The thyroid gland may become two to three times its normal size. Mild hyperthyroidism may be present because of sudden release of thyroid hormones into the circulation as a result of the inflammation and destruction of the thyroid gland.

Phase 2: Mild hypothyroidism develops because of incomplete recovery of the injured gland and exhaustion of stored thyroid hormones. Relapse may occur. Hypothyroidism is rarely permanent.

Phase 3: The recovery phase may begin 2 to 4 months after onset.

Hashimoto's disease is manifested by an enlarged thyroid gland that may produce hypothyroid manifestations if the gland is destroyed by the autoimmune system. A euthyroid state may prevail if the gland is not destroyed.

Clinical Manifestations

Manifestations of acute thyroiditis include abrupt onset of unilateral anterior neck pain with possible radiation to the ear or mandible on the affected side. Fever, diaphoresis, and other manifestations of bacterial toxicity may also be present.

Subacute granulomatous thyroiditis is usually painful, whereas subacute lymphocytic thyroiditis is usually painless. Assessment data may include characteristic anterior, unilateral neck pain that may have an abrupt onset, usually after a respiratory infection or viral episode. Radiation to the ear on the ipsilateral side may occur. There may be manifestations of viral infection, such as myalgia, low-grade fever, lassitude, and sore throat. About 50% of clients present with thyrotoxicosis.

Subacute lymphocytic thyroiditis is characterized by occasional hyperthyroidism and a painless goiter. The goiter is firm, diffuse, and mildly enlarged.

Manifestations of chronic thyroiditis include painless, asymmetrical enlargement of the gland, which causes pressure on the surrounding structures and can lead to dysphagia and respiratory distress. Most clients are euthyroid, about 20% are hypothyroid, and less than 5% are hyperthyroid.

The diagnosis of thyroiditis may be confirmed by evaluation of serum T_3, FT_4, ^{131}I uptake, TSH, erythrocyte sedimentation rate, and thyroid antibodies. See Table 43–5 for the results of these tests. Clients with acute thyroiditis are typically euthyroid according to laboratory tests.

For subacute granulomatous thyroiditis, laboratory findings reveal hyperthyroidism in approximately 50% of clients. With subacute lymphocytic thyroiditis, laboratory diagnosis includes decreased radioactive iodine uptake, elevated T_3 and T_4, and frequently positive thyroid antibodies.

In chronic thyroiditis, immune antibodies are usually positive. Other thyroid function levels may be normal, increased, or decreased.

Outcome Management

■ Medical Management

Acute thyroiditis usually responds to parenteral antibiotic therapy. Treatment of subacute granulomatous thyroiditis is supportive. Therapy may include salicylates, nonsteroidal anti-inflammatory agents (NSAIDs), and oral glucocorticoids such as prednisone. The desired outcome of treatment in subacute lymphocytic thyroiditis is to provide relief of manifestations of hyperthyroidism with beta-adrenergic blocking agents. Antithyroid medications are not indicated.

The course of Hashimoto's disease varies. Some clients experience spontaneous remission, whereas others remain stable for years. In about one third of cases, hypothyroidism develops from gradual atrophy of the gland. Intervention is intended to reduce the size of the gland and correct any thyroid function abnormalities. Immunologic tests are not useful in monitoring these clients.

■ Surgical Management

Clients with acute thyroiditis that does not respond to medical treatment may require incision and drainage of the affected gland. Depending on the size of the thyroid area to be incised and concurrent medical problems, the procedure may be done in the physician's office or during a short stay in the hospital. A fine-needle biopsy may be performed to rule out malignancy in chronic thyroiditis.

■ Nursing Management of the Medical-Surgical Client

Nursing care of a client with thyroiditis is usually supportive until the diagnosis is made. Then, as with other thyroid disorders, care revolves around helping the client learn correct medication administration. If surgery is necessary, care is the same as discussed earlier.

Discharge teaching focuses on ensuring that the client understands the medication and how to take it. Thyroid function is monitored at regular intervals after client discharge for development of hyperthyroidism or hypothyroidism and for testing the effectiveness of medication.

THYROID CANCER

The incidence of thyroid cancer is rising. One reason may be the maturation of people exposed to low-dose radiation early in life. Thyroid cancer accounts for 3 to 4 new cases per 100,000 population per year in the United States and about 1% of cancer deaths. The ratio of females to males is 4:1. Its incidence peaks during the 60s, but it may arise from infancy to old age. Mortality is lowest in the young if the cancer is well differentiated.

Etiology and Risk Factors

Benign adenomas are usually not dangerous, although they occasionally grow large enough to cause respiratory problems by pressing against the trachea. Malignant transformation sometimes occurs, and the benign nodules become cancerous. Also, malignant transformation of benign nodules can apparently follow prolonged stimulation of the thyroid gland by TSH. Other risk factors include genetic predisposition, a family history of thyroid or other endocrine cancer, and a history of thyroid cancer.

TABLE 43–5	DIAGNOSTIC TESTS FOR THYROIDITIS		
Test	Acute Thyroiditis	Subacute Thyroiditis	Chronic Hashimoto's or Lymphocytic Thyroiditis
Serum triiodothyronine	Normal–low	↑ at first; ↓ later	↑ or ↓
Free thyroxine	Normal–low	↑ at first; ↓ later	↑ or ↓
Radioactive iodine uptake	Low in about 40%	Low	Low or high-normal
Thyroid-stimulating hormone	↓	↓ at first; ↑ later	↑ or ↓
Erythrocyte sedimentation rate	NA	↑ ↑	NA
Thyroid antibodies	NA	Not detected	↑

NA, not applicable.
Adapted from Luckmann, J. (Ed.) (1997). *Saunders manual of nursing care.* Philadelphia: W. B. Saunders.

Pathophysiology

There are four major types of thyroid cancer:

- Papillary adenocarcinoma
- Follicular adenocarcinoma
- Medullary carcinoma
- Anaplastic carcinoma

These cancers vary in their characteristics, interventions, and prognoses (Table 43–6). Benign adenomas and malignant thyroid tumors constitute the third most common cause of thyroid enlargement, with hypothyroidism and hyperthyroidism being the two most common causes. Like other benign tumors, most thyroid adenomas are usually well encapsulated and, as a result, do not spread or extend into other tissues.

Clinical Manifestations

The major manifestation of thyroid cancer is the appearance of a hard, irregular, painless nodule in an enlarged thyroid gland. The nodule itself is typically solitary, rapidly enlarging, and "cold" (it does not take up radioactive iodine) in contrast to benign adenomas, which may take up radioactive iodine. The examiner can make this determination by giving a tracer dose of ^{131}I and performing a thyroid scan 24 hours later to assess ^{131}I uptake by any nodules. "Hot" nodules absorb more isotope than normal tissue and are usually benign.

If the tumor has metastasized, the lymph nodes are sometimes palpable. In long-standing cases, the client may have respiratory difficulty and dysphagia (difficulty swallowing) resulting from the enlarged thyroid pressing against neck structures. The diagnosis of thyroid cancer is confirmed by fine-needle aspiration biopsy.

Outcome Management

▬ Medical Management

Without prompt, aggressive therapy, a client with thyroid cancer risks death. Chemotherapy, ^{131}I, external radiation, or TSH suppressive therapy may be used for metastasis, as discussed earlier. A client with a benign nodule is likely to undergo long-term suppression therapy with levothyroxine. The desired outcome is to suppress serum TSH without causing hypothyroidism.

TABLE 43–6	TYPES OF THYROID CANCER: INCIDENCE, CHARACTERISTICS, INTERVENTION, AND PROGNOSIS			
Type	**Incidence**	**Characteristics**	**Intervention**	**Prognosis**
Papillary adeno-carcinoma	Constitutes 75% of thyroid cancers Affects clients in all age groups	Slow-growing firm tumor Palpable nodule Spreads to regional nodes in about half of cases Radiation-related thyroid cancer with 10- to 20-year latency period	Total or near-total thyroidectomy Others recommend lobectomy and isthmectomy	Excellent if cancer restricted to thyroid gland Lymph node metastasis is common Surgery usually curative
Follicular adeno-carcinoma	Constitutes 15% of thyroid cancers Mainly affects clients 50 and older	Slow-growing nodule with about 15% metastasis to regional nodes at diagnosis Associated with radiation, iodine deficiency, edemic goiter, thyrotoxicosis	Total or near-total thyroidectomy Aggressive radioactive iodine therapy for metastases	Good but inferior to that of papillary adenocarcinoma 5-yr survival is 60%–90% Lymph node metastasis is uncommon Distant metastasis is common
Medullary thyroid carcinoma	Constitutes 5%–10% of thyroid cancers Mainly affects clients of all age groups Disease is familial in 20% of all clients	Growth rate is moderate Tends to secrete adreno-corticotropic hormone, serotonin Metastases to surrounding structures at diagnosis in 50% Associated with multiple endocrine neoplasia	Total or near-total thyroidectomy Radioactive iodine to ablate the gland	Lymph node and distant metastases are common 5-yr survival is 70%–80%
Anaplastic carcinoma (nondifferentiated)	Constitutes 5%–15% of thyroid cancers Mainly affects clients between ages 60 and 70	Highly malignant Grows rapidly Local and widespread metastasis within 1 yr	Combination of thyroidectomy, external radiation therapy, chemotherapy, and tracheostomy as needed Aggressive therapy is palliative at best	Grave; mean survival, 6.2 mo; 10-yr survival, 1%

From Baker, K., & Feldman, J. (1993). Thyroid cancer: A review. *Oncology Nursing Forum, 20*(1), 95–104.

■ Surgical Management

Treatment usually includes removal of all or part of the thyroid. Neck resection may be done for metastases to the neck. (Thyroid surgery has been covered earlier.) As with a thyroidectomy for noncancerous lesions, the major postoperative complications are respiratory distress, recurrent laryngeal damage, hemorrhage, and hypoparathyroidism.

■ Nursing Management of the Medical-Surgical Client

Nursing care of the client with thyroid cancer is similar to the care of any client undergoing a thyroidectomy. The client also needs the support and teaching that a client with cancer requires. If the client is to have chemotherapy, additional teaching is needed.

If the client has undergone a total thyroidectomy, replacement of thyroid hormones is necessary. Discharge teaching focuses on ensuring that the client understands the medication and how to take it. Home health needs reflect those of any client after thyroidectomy or receiving chemotherapy or radiation therapy. The client should be checked at regular intervals for recurrence, and thyroid function should be monitored.

PARATHYROID DISORDERS

HYPERPARATHYROIDISM

Hyperparathyroidism, a disorder caused by overactivity of one or more of the parathyroid glands, is classified as primary, secondary, or tertiary. It usually occurs in clients older than age 60 and affects women twice as often as men. It is not related to age in clients with renal failure. The overall incidence of hyperparathyroidism is 27 per 100,000.

Etiology and Risk Factors

Primary hyperparathyroidism develops when the normal regulatory relationship between serum calcium levels and parathyroid hormone (PTH) secretion is interrupted. The interruption occurs when an adenoma or hyperplasia of the gland exists without an identifying injury.

Secondary hyperparathyroidism occurs when the glands are hyperplastic because of malfunction of another organ system. It is usually the result of renal failure but may also occur with osteogenesis imperfecta, Paget's disease, multiple myeloma, or carcinoma with bone metastasis.

Tertiary hyperparathyroidism occurs when PTH production is irrepressible (autonomous) in clients with normal or low serum calcium levels.

Pathophysiology

The normal function of PTH is to increase bone resorption, thereby maintaining the proper balance of calcium and phosphorus ions in the blood (see Chapter 42). Excessive circulating PTH leads to bone damage, hypercalcemia, and kidney damage.

PRIMARY HYPERPARATHYROIDISM

The severity of hypercalcemia reflects the quantity of hyperfunctioning parathyroid tissue. Excessive PTH stimulates transport of calcium into the blood from the intestine, kidneys, and bone. Nephrolithiasis is secondary to calcium phosphate kidney stones and deposition of calcium in the soft tissues of the kidney. Pyelonephritis may complicate the nephrolithiasis. Bone resorption related to hypercalcemia may develop.

Myopathy is a common condition characterized by neuropathic atrophy and proximal muscle weakness. Hypercalcemia can stimulate hypergastrinemia, abdominal pain, and peptic ulcer disease. Pancreatitis is also influenced by high calcium levels.

SECONDARY HYPERPARATHYROIDISM

Chronic renal failure and hyperphosphatemia cause secondary hyperparathyroidism. As the glomerular filtration rate (GFR) decreases in chronic renal failure, serum phosphorus levels rise. This increase causes the serum calcium level to fall. PTH secretion is stimulated. This increase decreases renal tubular absorption of phosphorus, causing serum phosphorus levels to return to normal. As the GFR continues to decrease, PTH is secreted in increased amounts in order to decrease tubular reabsorption of phosphorus and maintain serum phosphorus at or close to normal limits.

Clinical Manifestations

Some clients with hyperparathyroidism may be asymptomatic. Others have myriad manifestations arising from the skeletal disease, renal involvement, gastrointestinal tract disorders, and neurologic abnormalities, as outlined in the Critical Monitoring feature Hyperparathyroidism and Hypoparathyroidism and in Figure 43–4.

Manifestations of bone disease range from backache, joint pain, and bone pain to pathologic fractures of the spine, ribs, and long bones. In long-standing cases, assessment reveals deformity and bending of the bones. Osteitis fibrosa with superperiosteal resorption or bone cysts, arthritis, or radiologic osteoporosis may be diagnosed.

Manifestations of renal involvement include polyuria and polydipsia; the appearance of sand, gravel, or stones

---

CRITICAL MONITORING

Hyperparathyroidism and Hypoparathyroidism

These manifestations should be monitored in a client who is thought to have a diagnosis of hyperparathyroidism or hypoparathyroidism.

Hyperparathyroidism	Hypoparathyroidism
Increased bone resorption	Decreased bone resorption
Elevated serum calcium levels	Depressed serum calcium levels
Depressed serum phosphate levels	Elevated serum phosphate levels
Hypercalciuria and hyperphosphaturia	Hypocalciuria and hypophosphaturia
Decreased neuromuscular irritability	Increased neuromuscular activity, which may progress to tetany

FIGURE 43–4 Clinical manifestations of primary hyperparathyroidism. (Adapted from Strewler, G. J., & Rosenblatt, M. (1995). *Mineral metabolism.* In P. Felig, J. D. Baxter, & L. A. Frohman [Eds.], *Endocrinology and metabolism* [3rd ed., pp. 1407–1499]. New York: McGraw-Hill.)

(calculi) in the urine; azotemia; and hypertension resulting from renal damage. Without intervention, renal insufficiency may progress to fatal renal hypertension and uremia.

Hypercalcemia produces mainly gastrointestinal manifestations, such as thirst, nausea, anorexia, constipation, ileus, and abdominal pain. Decreased neuromuscular irritability is also common. Often, clients have a history of peptic ulcer or gastrointestinal bleeding. Assessment may also reveal psychiatric manifestations. Listlessness, depression, and paranoia are sometimes associated with high levels of serum calcium. Finally, calcification may form in the eyes, impairing vision.

Major complications include the manifestations associated with hypercalcemia and those associated with treatment, such as dehydration, hypocalcemia, and gastrointestinal problems.

The diagnosis of hyperparathyroidism mainly rests on laboratory and x-ray findings (Table 43–7). Serum calcium levels are elevated, serum phosphate levels are depressed, and both urine calcium and phosphorus levels are high. In addition, alkaline phosphatase is elevated in the 25% of clients who have associated bone disease. Clients with skeletal damage have the following characteristic x-ray findings: diffuse demineralization of bones, bone cysts, subperiosteal bone resorption, and loss of the lamina dura around the teeth. Ultrasonography or magnetic resonance imaging (MRI) may be used for preoperative localization of the parathyroid glands.

Outcome Management

▰ Medical Management

The desired outcomes of the medical treatment of hyperparathyroidism include lowering severely elevated cal-

cium levels and long-term management of hypercalcemia with drugs to increase bone resorption of calcium.

LOWER ELEVATED CALCIUM LEVELS. Serum calcium levels are lowered by hydration and calciuria. Hydration may be achieved with an infusion of normal saline solution. Normal saline is the fluid of choice because it both expands the volume and acts in the kidney to inhibit the resorption of calcium. Furosemide (Lasix), a loop diuretic, may also be used to promote calciuria after rehydration has occurred. Thiazide diuretics are not used because they promote calcium retention in the kidneys. A client with hypercalcemia should have a diet low in calcium and vitamin D.

ANTIRESORPTION AGENTS. Drugs that inhibit bone resorption include plicamycin (Mithracin), gallium nitrate (Ganite), phosphates, and calcitonin (Table 43–8). Plicamycin is a chemotherapeutic drug that is effective in lowering serum calcium levels. The hypocalcemic effect occurs after 24 hours and lasts for about 1 to 2 weeks. The dose is about one-tenth that used for cancer treatment, and the adverse effects are proportionally lower.

Gallium nitrate, a newer drug, is now being used more often because it has even fewer side effects. Glucocorticoids may be used to reduce hypercalcemia by decreasing gastrointestinal absorption of calcium. Etidronate (Didronel) or calcitonin may be used to decrease the release of calcium by bones.

▰ Nursing Management of the Medical Client

ASSESSMENT

There are no obvious manifestations of hyperparathyroidism and the resultant hypercalcemia. Elicit a good history from the client to see whether any risk factors are present. The client may exhibit psychological changes,

| TABLE 43-7 | DIAGNOSTIC TESTS OF PARATHYROID FUNCTION: PURPOSE, PROCEDURE, NORMAL RANGE, AND INTERPRETATION OF ABNORMAL FINDINGS |

Test	Purpose	Procedure	Normal Range	Interpretation of Abnormal Findings	Remarks
Total serum calcium	Measures amount of ionized and non-ionized calcium in serum	Venous blood to laboratory	4.8–5.2 mEq/L or 8–11 mg/dl	Elevated in hyperparathyroidism; depressed in hypoparathyroidism, tetany, rickets, nephrosis, and osteomalacia	Normally 50% of total serum calcium is ionized; the amount of ionized calcium available decreases in alkalosis
Qualitative urinary calcium (Sulkowitch test)	Measures roughly amount of calcium in urine; used as quick method for diagnosis if tetany is due to hypoparathyroidism	Collect urine specimen and send to laboratory	Fine white precipitate should form when Sulkowitch reagent is added to urine specimen	Absent or decreased density of precipitate indicates low serum calcium and hypoparathyroidism	Medications that elevate serum calcium levels include vitamin D, parathyroid infection, and dihydrotachysterol
Quantitative urinary calcium (calcium deprivation test)	Measures exact amount of calcium in 24-hr urine specimen	Collect 24-hr urine specimen and send to laboratory	75–175 mg calcium per 24 hr	Elevated in hyperparathyroidism; depressed in hypoparathyroidism	Foods high in calcium include milk, cheese, molasses, turnip greens, and dandelion greens
Serum phosphorus	Measures amount of inorganic phosphorus in serum	Venous blood to laboratory	1.3–1.75 mEq/L (2.5–4.5 mg/dl) in adults	Depressed in hypoparathyroidism, uremia, and alkalosis; elevated in hyperparathyroidism, rickets, and osteomalacia	There is an inverse relationship between serum calcium and serum phosphorus
Serum alkaline phosphatase	Measures amount of alkaline phosphatase in serum; aids in diagnosing bone and liver disorders	Venous blood to laboratory	2.0–5.0 Bodansky units	Elevated in hyperparathyroidism, osteomalacia, rickets, healing fractures, and pregnancy and after ingestion of large amounts of vitamin D	Alkaline phosphatase is an enzyme normally present in small amounts in serum; medications causing false elevations of alkaline phosphatase levels include allopurinol, some androgens, colchicine, erythromycin, methyldopa, some oral contraceptives, procainamide, and tolbutamide
Parathyroid hormone (PTH) radioimmunoassay	Measures level of PTH in serum	Venous blood to laboratory	Depends on serum calcium level	High concentrations indicate hyperparathyroidism	When evaluated in conjunction with serum calcium levels, this is the most specific test for hyperparathyroidism

such as lethargy, drowsiness, memory loss, and emotional lability, all manifestations seen in hypercalcemia.

DIAGNOSIS, OUTCOMES, INTERVENTIONS

Risk for Injury. The client with hyperparathyroidism is at great risk for injury, leading to the nursing diagnosis *Risk for Injury related to demineralization of bones resulting in pathologic fractures.*

Outcomes. The client will remain free from injury, as evidenced by absence of pathologic fractures or hypercalcemia.

Interventions

Prevent Fractures. Protect the client from accidents. If bone involvement exists, pathologic fractures may develop from even small bumps or minor falls. Keep the client's bed in the low position and use the side rails. If the client is weak or has joint or skeletal disease, help with ambulation.

Assist with Activities. If the client suffered from severe osteoporosis or pathologic fractures, some assistance may be required at home. The client may need a visiting nurse to help assess the home situation and to make recommen-

TABLE 43-8	DRUGS USED TO TREAT HYPERCALCEMIA			
Class	**Action**	**Therapeutic Outcome**	**Adverse Outcome**	**Dosing**
Loop diuretic (furosemide)	Promotes renal excretion of calcium	Improved muscle tone and coordination Relief of nausea, vomiting, and anorexia Decreased serum calcium	Monitor intake and output, blood pressure and pulse Watch serum calcium level closely and monitor for numbness, tingling, and other signs of decreased calcium	Up to 100 mg IV Give with 0.9% sodium chloride
Chemotherapeutic agent (plicamycin)	Inhibits bone resorption and lowers serum calcium level	Therapeutic effect in hypercalcemia may not be seen for 24–48 hr and may last 3–15 days Improve muscle tone and coordination Improved appetite and decreased nausea and vomiting	Monitor serum electrolytes, liver enzymes, and BUN and creatinine Monitor platelet count and watch for bleeding Watch for sudden drop in serum calcium; check closely for signs of hypocalcemia	25 mg IV daily for 1–4 days Give antiemetics before administration to reduce nausea
Electrolyte modifier (etidronate disodium)	Decreases release of calcium from bones	Decreased serum calcium May take months for onset of improved muscle tone and coordination and improved appetite	Diarrhea, nausea, bone pain; protect from fractures Elevated serum phosphate; monitor for increased serum phosphate Tell client that onset of therapeutic effect may take several months Monitor renal function	5 mg/kg PO daily as single dose 2 hr before meals, up to dose of 20 mg/kg Do not administer with food or antacids Do not give for more than 6 months continuously; stop, then restart after 3 months
Hormone (calcitonin)	Used in secondary hyperparathyroidism as a phosphate-binding agent and nutritional supplement to the low-phosphate diet; prescribed to decrease acidosis	Decreased serum calcium Improved appetite Improved muscle tone and coordination	Monitor for numbness, tingling, and other signs of hypocalcemia Monitor serum phosphate Warn client about transient facial flushing	4–8 IU/kg SC daily or two to three times a week (salmon) or 0.5 mg two to three times a week (human) or as a nasal spray daily Administer at bedtime to decrease nausea and vomiting Treatment may last for 6 months

BUN, blood urea nitrogen; IV, intravenously; PO, orally; SC, subcutaneously.

dations on how safety might be enhanced. The home should be cleared of articles that can increase the risk of falling, such as throw rugs. The client may also need assistive devices, such as a railing in the bathroom, a bedside commode, or a walker.

Altered Urinary Elimination. The development of urinary lithiasis in clients with hyperparathyroidism may lead to the nursing diagnosis *Altered Urinary Elimination related to renal involvement secondary to hypercalcemia and hyperphosphaturia resulting in urolithiasis, painful urination, hematuria, and spasms.*

Outcomes. The client will resume a normal urinary output, as evidenced by urine production of ½ ml/kg/hr without development of stones.

Interventions
Encourage Fluids. The client should consume at least 3000 ml of fluid a day. Dehydration is dangerous in clients with hyperparathyroidism because it increases the serum calcium level and promotes the formation of renal stones.

Prevent Urolithiasis. Cranberry juice or prune juice may help make the urine more acidic. Acidification helps prevent renal stone formation, because calcium is more soluble in acidic urine than in alkaline urine.

Strain Urine of Stones. If a kidney stone is present, strain all urine to detect gravel and stones. Save any specimens of abnormal urine for the physician to examine and for laboratory analysis. Also, observe the urine for blood and assess the client for renal colic (see Chapter 34).

Altered Nutrition: Less Than Body Requirements.

The client is likely to experience nutritional problems, suggesting the nursing diagnosis *Altered Nutrition: Less than Body Requirements related to anorexia and nausea resulting in decreased food intake and weight loss.*

Outcomes. The client will have an adequate intake, as evidenced by absence of nausea and return to or maintenance of ideal body weight.

Interventions. Encourage a low-calcium diet to correct hypercalcemia. Explain that abstaining from milk and milk products may help alleviate some of the distressing gastrointestinal manifestations. A client who has peptic ulcers needs to take antacids or histamine receptor antagonists. Help the client create a diet that is high enough in calories without dairy products. If necessary, have a dietitian see the client to help with meal planning.

Constipation.

A client with hyperparathyroidism is susceptible to bowel problems, leading to the nursing diagnosis *Constipation related to adverse effects of hypercalcemia on the gastrointestinal tract resulting in decreased frequency of stools and painful defecation.*

Outcomes. The client will maintain a normal bowel pattern, as evidenced by a daily, soft, formed bowel movement.

Interventions. Work to prevent constipation and fecal impaction resulting from hypercalcemia. Help the client stay as active as the extent of bone disease allows. Increase fluid intake and the amount of fiber in the diet. The client should drink at least six to eight glasses of water a day unless contraindicated. If constipation continues despite these measures, obtain an order for a stool softener or laxative.

EVALUATION

Depending on the cause of the hypercalcemia, medical management may be able to control primary hypercalcemia. If it does not, surgery may be required. If the condition is secondary to renal failure, the management is more chronic in nature.

■ Surgical Management

PARATHYROIDECTOMY

INDICATIONS. Definitive treatment of primary hyperparathyroidism is surgical removal of the gland or glands causing hypersecretion of PTH. Usually, only the diseased parathyroid glands are resected. If all four glands are hyperplastic, however, three and one-half glands are removed. Fortunately, one half of a parathyroid gland is usually sufficient to maintain normal levels of circulating PTH.

Autotransplantation of the parathyroid glands is a useful modality for the management of certain forms of hyperparathyroidism and radical neck surgery. After partial

parathyroidectomy, it is possible to transplant the remaining healthy parathyroid tissue to a safer location, such as the brachioradial muscle of the forearm. Reexploration of the neck in the future may cause laryngeal nerve damage and influence complications of the original surgery. Transplantation procedures take some time to come to full effect. In the meantime, the client must supplement the diet with calcium and vitamin D to prevent hypoparathyroidism and hypocalcemia.

If hyperparathyroidism is surgically treated early in its course, the chance of total recovery is good. Bone pain may disappear within 3 days after removal of parathyroid tissue, and bone lesions may heal completely. Unfortunately, serious renal disease might not be reversible by parathyroid surgery.

COMPLICATIONS. The complications after parathyroidectomy are similar to those following thyroidectomy and rarely occur. Hypocalcemia is a potentially life-threatening complication even if some parathyroid glands are left untouched because edema reduces their function. The client may also experience respiratory distress related to either hemorrhage or recurrent laryngeal nerve damage.

OUTCOMES. The cure rate for primary hyperparathyroidism after surgical removal is greater than 95%. This high success rate is directly related to the experience of the surgeon and adequate exploration of the neck.

■ Nursing Management of the Surgical Client

ASSESSMENT

The client undergoing surgery may have long-standing hyperparathyroidism and thus should be assessed for complications of the disease. Renal function should be carefully assessed preoperatively.

DIAGNOSIS, OUTCOMES, INTERVENTIONS

Risk for Injury. The client undergoing surgery for hyperparathyroidism is at risk for a number of complications. An important nursing diagnosis is *Risk for Injury related to preoperative drug sensitivities and postoperative complications.*

Outcomes. The client will not suffer injury, as evidenced by the absence of medication reactions preoperatively and by the absence of respiratory distress, hemorrhage, and hypocalcemia postoperatively.

Interventions

Administer Digitalis. If the client is receiving digitalis, administer this medication with extreme caution. Clients with hypercalcemia are hypersensitive to digitalis, and toxic manifestations may develop quickly.

Monitor for Postoperative Complications. During the postoperative period, new problems arise, some of which are the reverse of those found preoperatively. During the immediate postoperative period, nursing care is similar to that after thyroidectomy; that is, assess the client carefully for hemorrhage, airway obstruction, injury to the recurrent laryngeal nerve, and tetany. Also watch for manifestations of hormonal imbalance.

Mild tetany resulting from a drop in the serum calcium level is expected after removal of parathyroid tissue. Typically, the uncomfortable tingling of the hands and around the mouth that follows parathyroid resection is temporary.

If it persists or is severe, however, calcium gluconate is administered intravenously.

Prevent Osteoporosis. Clients with bone disease require additional therapy after surgery. Removal of the parathyroid glands reduces bone resorption, and because bone rebuilding proceeds at a rapid rate, the client may experience the "hungry bones" syndrome. This is characterized by hypocalcemia and severe tetany resulting from the rapid utilization of calcium by the bones.

To prevent low serum calcium levels resulting from bone recalcification, instruct the client to eat foods high in calcium. Tetany is treated with injections of calcium gluconate. To maintain adequate calcium levels, the client usually takes oral calcium preparations for months until the skeletal tissues have been rebuilt. Finally, encourage ambulation as soon as possible after surgery, because weight-bearing speeds the recalcification process.

EVALUATION

If hypercalcemia remains unrelieved by medical management, surgery is usually therapeutic. If a partial parathyroidectomy is unsuccessful, the remaining gland may need to be transplanted to the forearm to reduce absorption of the hormone. This measure usually eliminates the problem. As long as the client is closely observed in the immediate postoperative period, complications of hypocalcemia are usually controllable.

■ Modification for Elderly Clients

Hyperparathyroidism in older adults is an overlooked disease. It is estimated that 1 of 1000 men and 2 of 1000 women older than 60 years of age experience hyperparathyroidism. This disease often goes undiagnosed in older people because manifestations in the early stages are subtle and attributed to old age, depression, or anxiety. The manifestations intensify as the serum calcium level continues to rise and other physiologic and functional changes occur. Laboratory diagnosis is the same as for a younger client, but treatment may be complicated by medical problems and medication.

HYPOPARATHYROIDISM

Hyposecretion of the parathyroid glands produces the reverse syndrome of hyperparathyroidism. That is, serum calcium levels are abnormally low, serum phosphate levels are abnormally high, and pronounced neuromuscular irritability (tetany) may develop.

Hypoparathyroidism is diagnosed in women more often than men. The incidence is related to thyroid surgery. The incidence of temporary hypoparathyroidism after total thyroidectomy ranges from 6.9% to 25%. The incidence after subtotal thyroidectomy is 1.6% to 9.0%.

Etiology and Risk Factors

The causes of hypoparathyroidism are either *iatrogenic* (treatment-induced) or *idiopathic* (without a specific cause). Iatrogenic causes include accidental removal of the parathyroid glands during thyroidectomy, infarction of the parathyroid glands because of an inadequate blood supply to the glands during surgery, and strangulation of one or more of the glands by postoperative scar tissue. Health maintenance actions include monitoring of PTH, calcium, and phosphorus levels. Calcium supplements are required for life to prevent tetany.

Idiopathic hypoparathyroidism, like Graves' disease and Hashimoto's disease, may be an autoimmune disorder with a genetic basis. It is far less common than the iatrogenic form. *Pseudohypoparathyroidism* (Albright's hereditary osteodystrophy) is an inherited form of hypoparathyroidism involving lack of end-organ responsiveness to PTH.

Pathophysiology

PTH normally acts to increase bone resorption, which maintains proper serum calcium levels. The hormone also regulates phosphate clearance by the renal tubules, thereby maintaining the correct inverse balance between serum calcium and serum phosphate. Consequently, when parathyroid secretion is reduced, bone resorption slows, serum calcium levels fall, and severe neuromuscular irritability develops. Somewhat paradoxically, calcifications form in various organs, such as the eyes and basal ganglia. Also, without sufficient PTH, fewer phosphorus ions are secreted by the distal tubules of the kidney, renal excretion of phosphate falls, and serum phosphate levels rise.

The client may fully recover from the effects of hypoparathyroidism if the condition is diagnosed early, before serious complications begin. Unfortunately, cataracts and brain calcification, once formed, are irreversible.

Clinical Manifestations

The manifestations of hypoparathyroidism result mainly from low serum calcium levels. Manifestations are always more severe in clients with an elevated serum pH (alkalosis) of any cause (such as hyperventilation or ingestion of antacids). They worsen because, when the pH of the blood rises, the amount of ionized calcium drops, although total serum calcium remains the same. With less ionized calcium available to the body, the manifestations resulting from hypocalcemia become more severe until the alkalosis is corrected.

ACUTE HYPOPARATHYROIDISM

Acute hypoparathyroidism is caused by accidental damage to parathyroid tissues during thyroidectomy. It is characterized by greatly increased neuromuscular irritability, which results in tetany. Clients with tetany experience painful muscle spasms, irritability, grimacing, tingling of the fingers, laryngospasm, and dysrhythmias. Assessment also reveals Chvostek's and Trousseau's signs. In some cases, tetany is so severe that a tracheostomy is required to correct acute respiratory obstruction secondary to laryngospasm.

CHRONIC HYPOPARATHYROIDISM

Chronic hypoparathyroidism is usually idiopathic, resulting in lethargy; thin, patchy hair; brittle nails; dry, scaly skin; and personality changes. Ectopic or unexpected calcification may appear in the eyes and basal ganglia. Thus, cataracts and permanent brain damage, accompanied by psychosis or convulsions, may develop. In addition, severe persistent hypocalcemia adversely affects the heart, causing dysrhythmias and eventual cardiac failure.

The diagnosis of hypoparathyroidism is based on the following physical examination findings related to hypocalcemia:

- Presence of Chvostek's sign (spasms of facial muscles after a tap over the facial nerve, signifying facial hyperirritability)
- Presence of Trousseau's sign (spasms of the wrist and hand after compression of the upper arm, as by a blood pressure cuff)
- Hyperactive deep tendon reflexes (DTRs)
- Circumoral paresthesia
- Numbness and tingling of fingers

The diagnosis of hypoparathyroidism also stems from these findings:

- Laboratory findings showing low calcium, low PTH, high phosphorus, decreased urine calcium
- Radiographic studies of the skull or computed tomography (CT) of the head showing areas of calcification
- Ophthalmic examination revealing calcification of the ocular lens, which may lead to cataract formation

Complications

If treatment is not started rapidly in acute hypoparathyroidism, death can result from the respiratory obstruction secondary to tetany and laryngospasms. In chronic hypoparathyroidism, the complications are calcifications in the eye and basal ganglia that can occur if treatment is delayed.

Outcome Management

■ Medical Management

Acute hypoparathyroidism (with its major manifestation of acute tetany) is a life-threatening disorder. The desired outcomes of emergency care are to elevate serum calcium levels as rapidly as possible, to prevent or treat seizures, and to control laryngeal spasm and consequent respiratory obstruction.

For clients with chronic hypoparathyroidism, the desired outcome of intervention is to restore the serum calcium level to normal concentrations. The calcium level is increased more gradually than in acute hypoparathyroidism.

ELEVATE SERUM CALCIUM

CALCIUM GLUCONATE. In clients with acute hypoparathyroidism, in order to elevate serum calcium levels quickly, the physician prescribes 10% calcium gluconate solution in an intravenous infusion. While administering the calcium gluconate, instruct the client to inhale carbon dioxide by breathing into a paper bag. Carbon dioxide inhalation causes a mild metabolic acidosis, which elevates the amount of ionized calcium in the blood.

ORAL CALCIUM REPLACEMENTS. When the condition has stabilized and the dangers of tetany have passed, the client is given oral calcium salts to maintain normal serum calcium levels. The desired outcome of therapy for chronic hypoparathyroidism is to keep the client asymptomatic with a serum calcium level of about 8.5 to 9.2 mg/dl. The client is given oral calcium salts (calcium gluconate, calcium lactate, or calcium carbonate).

VITAMIN D. The client is given vitamin D in addition to calcium supplements to maintain serum calcium levels. Commercially available forms of vitamin D include ergocalciferol (vitamin D_2) and dihydrotachysterol (Hytakerol). Although ergocalciferol is a more reliable and less expensive drug than dihydrotachysterol or dihydroxycholecalciferol, all three forms of vitamin D are effective in correcting hypocalcemia. They are available as either tablets or oily liquids. Aluminum hydroxide gel (Amphojel) is also prescribed.

PARATHYROID HORMONE. The ideal treatment of this PTH-deficient condition is replacement of the absent hormone. A pure form of PTH has now been synthesized and is available.

HIGH-CALCIUM, LOW-PHOSPHATE DIET. A client with hypoparathyroidism should receive a diet high in calcium but low in phosphorus. Again, vitamin D is needed to maintain serum calcium levels, and clients should be encouraged to select foods or supplements enriched with vitamin D.

ADDRESS SEIZURES AND LARYNGEAL SPASM

Tetany and laryngeal spasms may occur suddenly and without warning in patients at risk for acute hypoparathyroidism. Calcium gluconate should be readily available at the bedside, and in many cases an order is left to have a tracheotomy tray available at the bedside.

■ Nursing Management of the Medical Client

ASSESSMENT

Carefully assess the client at risk for acute hypoparathyroidism (e.g., the post-thyroidectomy client) for development of hypocalcemia. Question the client about any numbness or tingling around the mouth or in the fingertips or toes. Check for Chvostek's and Trousseau's signs. In addition, assess for any manifestation of respiratory distress secondary to laryngospasm.

In a client with chronic hypoparathyroidism, assess for obvious physical changes, such as dry skin and hair. Also assess for a Parkinson-like syndrome or cataracts. Assess the teeth because pits may encircle them, indicating enamel hypoplasia.

DIAGNOSIS, OUTCOMES, INTERVENTIONS

Risk for Injury: Muscle Tetany. A client with hypoparathyroidism is susceptible to hypocalcemia, which can lead to the nursing diagnosis *Risk for Injury: Muscle tetany related to decreased serum calcium levels.*

Outcomes. The client will remain free from injury, as evidenced by a return of calcium levels to normal range, a normal respiratory rate, and blood gases within normal limits.

Interventions
Prevent Respiratory Arrest. When caring for a client with severe hypoparathyroidism, always be prepared for laryngeal spasm and respiratory obstruction. Have an endotracheal tube, laryngoscope, and tracheostomy set available when caring for a client with acute tetany.

Monitor and Prevent Tetany. When a client is at risk for sudden hypocalcemia, as after thyroidectomy, an ampule of intravenous calcium carbonate is usually kept at the bedside for immediate use if necessary. When the intravenous tubing is removed, it is sometimes capped so that rapid venous access is available. Sometimes clients are encouraged to take in a ready source of calcium carbonate, such as Tums.

EVALUATION

If the hypocalcemia is transient after a thyroidectomy, it usually resolves as edema decreases. If it is chronic, the client is usually able to manage the therapeutic regimen with minimal difficulty.

◼ Self-Care

Because hypoparathyroidism can be a chronic condition, the client must be able to provide self-care. Teaching is important for the client with chronic hypoparathyroidism because this client requires lifelong medication and dietary modification.

MEDICATIONS

When teaching the client about take-home medications, make sure the client knows that all forms of vitamin D, except dihydroxycholecalciferol, are slowly assimilated by the body. Therefore, it may take a week or longer for the manifestations to improve.

DIET MODIFICATIONS

Teach the client about a diet high in calcium but low in phosphorus. Remind the client to omit cheese and milk products, which have a high phosphorus content. Explain that calcium supplements may be obtained in either tablet or solution form, depending on preference. Oral calcium administration is usually discontinued when the client responds to vitamin D preparations.

Emphasize the importance of lifelong medical care for the client with chronic hypoparathyroidism. Instruct the client to have serum calcium levels checked by a physician at least three times a year. Normal blood serum calcium levels must be maintained to prevent complications. If hypercalcemia or hypocalcemia develops, the physician will adjust the treatment regimen to correct the imbalance.

CONCLUSIONS

You must make careful assessments of clients with thyroid or parathyroid disorders. These disorders can be controlled and the manifestations reversed if they are discovered in a timely manner and prompt and proper treatment is begun. You are an important resource for these clients, who require considerable education. You are also responsible for closely monitoring any client who needs surgery for either the thyroid or parathyroid gland. The client is particularly vulnerable during this postoperative period, and high-level nursing surveillance and intervention facilitate successful recovery.

THINKING CRITICALLY

1. A 64-year-old man comes to the clinic with a 6-month history of progressive fatigue, weakness, and dyspnea. On further questioning, you find that he has had an unintentional weight loss of 30 pounds despite an increased appetite.

   Your physical examination reveals an alert and oriented man who looks his stated age. He is somewhat anxious. His attention span is short, and you must repeat many questions. His heart rate is 118 BPM; blood pressure, 154/98 mm Hg; temperature, 101 °F; the skin is warm and moist; deep tendon reflexes are hyperactive. What are priorities for care?

   Factors to Consider. What additional subjective and objective data should you collect to confirm a diagnosis? What medication might be started after the diagnosis is made?

2. The client is a woman with a long history of chronic renal failure. She receives dialysis three times a week. She is currently hospitalized for a complicated pneumonia. Upon reviewing her laboratory values, you note that her serum calcium level is 6.8 mg/dl. What are the implications for care?

   Factors to Consider. What is the relationship of calcium metabolism to renal function? What are the dangers associated with this serum calcium level? What treatments should be initiated to treat this and what should be done to prevent recurrence?

3. A middle-aged woman comes to the clinic with manifestations of weight gain, lethargy, fatigue, and severe constipation. After diagnostic evaluation, the client is given Synthroid, 0.1 mg, for hypothyroidism. What general information should you give the client about hypothyroidism? About the medication?

   Factors to Consider. What should you teach about the expected therapeutic response to this medication? About side effects? How often are blood studies required for the client being treated with thyroid medications?

BIBLIOGRAPHY

1. Angelucci, P. A. (1995). Caring for patients with hypothyroidism. *Nursing, 25*(5), 60–61.
2. Behnia, M. & Gharib, B. (1996). Primary care diagnosis of thyroid disease. *Hospital Practice, 31*(6), 121–134.
3. Burrow, G. N. (1995). The thyroid: Nodules and neoplasm. In P. Felig, J. D. Baxter, & L. A. Frohman (Eds.), *Endocrinology and metabolism* (3rd ed., pp. 521–549). New York: McGraw-Hill.
4. Corbett, J. V. (1999). *Laboratory tests and diagnostic procedures* (5th ed.). Norwalk, CT: Appleton & Lange.
5. Daylan, C. M. & Daniels, G. H. (1996). Chronic autoimmune thyroiditis. *New England Journal of Medicine, 335*(2), 89–105.
6. DeGroot, L. (Ed.). (1995). *Endocrinology* (3rd ed.). Philadelphia: W. B. Saunders.
7. Dunn, J. (1996). Seven deadly sins in confronting endemic iodine deficiency, and how to avoid them. *Journal of Clinical Endocrinology and Metabolism, 81*(4),1332–1335.
8. Facts and Comparisons Staff. (1999). *Drug facts and comparisons* (2nd ed.). St. Louis: Facts & Comparisons.
9. Fitzpatrick, L., & Arnold, A. (1995). Hypoparathyroidism. In P. Felig, J. D. Baxter, & L. A. Frohman (Eds.), *Endocrinology and metabolism* (3rd ed., pp. 1123–1135). New York: McGraw-Hill.
10. Frohman, L. A. (1995). Diseases of the anterior pituitary. In P. Felig, J. D. Baxter, & L. A. Frohman (Eds.), *Endocrinology and metabolism* (3rd ed., pp. 289–369). New York: McGraw-Hill.

11. Gambert, S. R. (1995). Hyperthyroidism in the elderly. *Clinics in Geriatric Medicine, 11*(2), 181–188.

12. Goldsmith, C. (1999). Clinical snapshot. Hypothyroidism. *American Journal of Nursing, 99*(6), 42–43.

13. Heitman, B., & Irizarry, A. (1995). Hypothyroidism: Common complaints, perplexing diagnosis. *Nurse Practitioner, 20*(3), 54–60.

14. Hubener, J., Arnold, A., & Potts, J. (1995). Hyperparathyroidism. In L. DeGroot (Ed.), *Endocrinology* (3rd ed., pp. 1044–1060). Philadelphia: W. B. Saunders.

15. Jankowski, C. B. (1996). Irradiating the thyroid: How to protect yourself and others. *American Journal of Nursing, 96*(10), 50–54.

16. Kennedy, L. W. & Caro, J. F. (1996). The ABCs of managing hyperthyroidism in the older patient. *Geriatrics, 51*(5), 22–24, 27, 31, 32.

17. Lehne, R. (1998). *Pharmacology for nursing care* (3rd ed.). Philadelphia: W. B. Saunders.

18. Loriaux, G. C. (1996). Endocrine assessment: Red flags for those on the front lines. *Nursing Clinics of North America, 31*(4), 695–714.

19. McKenzie, J. M., & Zakarija, M. (1995). Hyperthyroidism. In L. DeGroot (Ed.), *Endocrinology* (3rd ed., pp. 676–711). Philadelphia: W. B. Saunders.

20. McMorrow, M. E. (1996). Myxedema coma: Do you recognize the clues to this rare complication of hypothyroidism? *American Journal of Nursing, 96*(10), 55.

21. Miller, W. L., & Tyrrell, J. B. (1995). Adrenal cortex. In P. Felig, J. D. Baxter, & L. A. Frohman (Eds.), *Endocrinology and metabolism* (3rd ed., pp. 521–549). New York: McGraw-Hill.

22. Molitch, M. E. (1995). Neuroendocrinology. In P. Felig, J. D. Baxter, & L. A. Frohman (Eds.), *Endocrinology and metabolism* (3rd ed., pp. 221–275). New York: McGraw-Hill.

23. Pagana, K., & Pagana, T. (1997). *Diagnostic testing and nursing implications* (4th ed.). St. Louis: Mosby–Year Book.

24. Robertson, G. (1995). Posterior pituitary. In P. Felig, J. D. Baxter, & L. A. Frohman (Eds.), *Endocrinology and metabolism* (3rd ed., pp. 385–423). New York: McGraw-Hill.

25. Rusterholtz, A. (1996). Interpretation of diagnostic laboratory tests in selected endocrine disorders. *Nursing Clinics of North America, 31*(4), 715–724.

26. Singer, P., et al. (1995). Treatment guidelines for patients with hyperthyroidism and hypothyroidism. *Journal of the American Medical Association, 273*(10), 808–813.

27. Strief, M. M., & Pachucki-Hyde, L. C. (1996). Management of the patient with thyroid disease. *Nursing Clinics of North America, 31*(4), 779–796.

28. Strewler, G. J., & Rosenblatt, M. (1995). Mineral metabolism. In P. Felig, J. D. Baxter, & L. A. Frohman (Eds.), *Endocrinology and metabolism* (3rd ed., pp, 1407–1499). New York: McGraw-Hill.

29. Trivalle, C., et al. (1996). Differences in the signs and symptoms of hyperthyroidism in older and younger patients. *Journal of the American Geriatric Society, 44*(1), 50–53.

30. Tunbridge, W. M. G., & Caldwell, G. (1996). The epidemiology of thyroid diseases. In L. E. Braverman & R. O. Utiger (Eds.), *Werner & Ingbar's the thyroid: A fundamental and clinical text* (7th ed.). Philadelphia: J. B. Lippincott.

31. U.S. Public Health Service. (1996). Put prevention into practice: Thyroid function. *Journal of the American Academy of Nurse Practitioners, 8*(10), 495–496.

32. Utiger, R. (1995). Hypothyroidism. In L. DeGroot (Ed.), *Endocrinology* (3rd ed., pp. 753–768). Philadelphia: W. B. Saunders.

33. Utiger, R. D. (1995). The thyroid: Physiology, thyrotoxicosis, hypothyroidism and the painful thyroid. In P. Felig, J. D. Baxter, & L. A. Frohman (Eds.), *Endocrinology and metabolism* (3rd ed., pp. 435–509). New York: McGraw-Hill.

34. Wartofsky, L. (1995). The thyroid gland. In K. L. Becker, et al. (Eds.), *Principles and practice of endocrinology and metabolism* (2nd ed). Philadelphia: J. B. Lippincott.

35. Young, J. (1999). Actionstat: Thyroid storm. *Nursing, 29*(8), 33.

REMEMBER *to*
check out your
Companion CD ROM

CHAPTER

44

Management of Clients with Adrenal and Pituitary Disorders

Anne Larson

NURSING OUTCOMES CLASSIFICATION (NOC)
for Nursing Diagnoses—Clients with Adrenal and Pituitary Disorders

Activity Intolerance
Activity Tolerance
Endurance
Energy Conservation
Self-Care: Activities of Daily Living (ADL)
Self-Care: Instrumental Activities of Daily Living (IADL)
Altered Thought Processes
Cognitive Ability
Cognitive Orientation
Concentration
Decision-Making
Distorted Thought Control
Identity
Information Processing
Memory
Neurological Status: Consciousness
Knowledge Deficit
Knowledge: Diet
Knowledge: Disease Process
Knowledge: Energy Conservation
Knowledge: Health Behaviors
Knowledge: Health Resources

Knowledge: Illness Care
Knowledge: Infection Control
Knowledge: Medication
Knowledge: Personal Safety
Knowledge: Prescribed Activity
Knowledge: Treatment Procedures
Knowledge: Treatment Regimen
Pain
Comfort Level
Pain Control
Pain: Disruptive Effects
Pain Level
Risk for Impaired Skin Integrity
Immobility Consequences: Physiologic
Nutritional Status
Risk Control
Risk Detection
Tissue Integrity: Skin and Mucous Membranes
Tissue Perfusion: Peripheral
Wound Healing: Primary Intention
Risk for Infection
Immune Status

Knowledge: Infection Control
Nutritional Status
Risk Control
Risk Detection
Tissue Integrity: Skin and Mucous Membranes
Treatment Behavior: Illness or Injury
Wound Healing: Primary Intention
Risk for Injury
Circulation Status
Knowledge: Personal Safety
Neurologic Status
Risk Control
Risk Detection
Safety Behavior: Fall Prevention
Safety Behavior: Home Physical Environment
Safety Behavior: Personal
Safety Status: Physical Injury
Symptom Control
Vital Signs Status

ADRENOCORTICAL DISORDERS

Glandular hypofunction and hyperfunction characterize the major disorders of the adrenal cortex. Underactivity of the adrenal cortex results in a deficiency of glucocorticoids, mineralocorticoids, and adrenal androgens. The person with adrenal hypofunction is a prime candidate for injury, knowledge deficit, and feelings of powerlessness. Overactivity of the adrenal cortex results in excessive

production of glucocorticoids, mineralocorticoids, and androgens or estrogens. The person with adrenal hyperfunction needs to focus on preventing injury and infection, acquiring effective coping mechanisms, and learning about the disease process.

ADRENAL INSUFFICIENCY

Hypofunction of the adrenal cortex can originate from a disorder in the adrenal gland itself (primary adrenal insufficiency), or it may result from hypofunction of the pituitary-hypothalamic unit (secondary adrenal insufficiency).

This chapter incorporates material written for the fifth edition by Carol Birch.

PRIMARY ADRENAL INSUFFICIENCY

Commonly known as *Addison's disease,* primary adrenal insufficiency results from idiopathic atrophy or destruction of the adrenal glands by an autoimmune process or other disease. Thomas Addison first described this disorder in 1849.

Etiology and Risk Factors

Primary adrenal insufficiency is caused by hypofunction of the adrenal glands. It is a rare disorder, and its incidence and prevalence in the United States are unknown. An autoimmune process accounts for 75% of primary adrenal insufficiency. It is commonly seen in people with acquired immunodeficiency syndrome (AIDS). Tuberculosis is the cause in about 20% of cases of Addison's disease. Adrenal metastasis from the lung, breast, gastrointestinal tract, melanoma, or lymphoma may also cause primary adrenal insufficiency. Additional causes include bilateral adrenalectomy and hemorrhagic infarction with necrosis of the adrenal gland.

Risk factors for primary adrenal insufficiency include (1) a history of other endocrine disorders, (2) taking glucocorticoids for more than 3 weeks with sudden cessation, (3) taking glucocorticoids more than once every other day, (4) adrenalectomy, and (5) tuberculosis.

Health promotion and health maintenance activities for clients receiving glucocorticoids include instruction on the risks and benefits of this therapy and instruction on the proper means of withdrawing glucocorticoids. Health maintenance activities for those receiving long-term steroid therapy include education about the need for supplemental steroids to prevent acute adrenal insufficiency and having parenteral steroids available for use when the client is unable to take oral steroids. Health restoration activities include ensuring that the client is mindful of the need for follow-up with the physician to monitor steroid levels.

Pathophysiology

Autoimmunity is the most common cause of adrenal insuffciency. Lymphocytic infiltration of the adrenal cortex is the characteristic feature. Addison's disease is frequently accompanied by other immune disorders. Gradual destruction leads to chronic adrenal insufficiency. Continued loss of cortical tissue accompanies a deficiency of mineralocorticoids as well as glucocorticoids. Adrenocortical hypofunction results in decreased levels of mineralocorticoids (aldosterone), glucocorticoids (cortisol), and androgens (Fig. 44–1).

Clinical Manifestations

The onset of Addison's disease is usually insidious. The client experiences mild fatigue, languor, irritability, weight loss, nausea, vomiting, and postural hypotension, usually weeks or months before the diagnosis is confirmed. As the disorder progresses, manifestations intensify. By then, the client has lost more than 90% of both adrenal cortices (Table 44–1).

Diagnosis of Addison's disease depends primarily on

FIGURE 44–1 Effects of Addison's disease. *Dashed arrows* show feedback mechanisms. ACTH, adrenocorticotropic hormone; Na, sodium; K, potassium; CRH, corticotropin-releasing hormone.

blood and urine hormonal assays (Table 44–2). Primary adrenal insufficiency is characterized by a low cortisol production rate and a high plasma adrenocorticotropic hormone (ACTH) concentration.

Other diagnostic tests may be ordered to evaluate the effects of hypofunction of the adrenals on the body: (1) serum electrolytes (especially hyponatremia and hyperkalemia in primary adrenal insufficiency and hyponatremia alone in secondary disease); (2) blood glucose; (3) complete blood count (to assess for anemia); (4) x-ray studies, computed tomography (CT); and (5) magnetic resonance imaging (MRI) of the adrenals and pituitary.

Outcome Management

Addisonian crisis is an emergent condition requiring careful monitoring in the critical care unit. Thereafter, the rate of recovery is client-specific. Normally, Addison's disease can be managed on an outpatient basis if the client is compliant and receives proper self-care instructions.

▮ Medical Management

ADDISONIAN CRISIS

Addisonian crisis, or *acute adrenal insufficiency,* may occur when the client has been under stress without appropriate hormone replacement. Stressors include pregnancy, surgery, infection, states of dehydration or anorexia, fever, and emotional upheaval. Manifestations are related to the degree of hormone deficiency and electrolyte imbal-

TABLE 44–1	ADRENAL HORMONES: FUNCTION AND CONSEQUENCES OF DYSFUNCTION		
Hormone	**Usual Function**	**Insufficient State: Addison's Disease**	**Excess State: Cushing's Syndrome**
MINERALOCORTICOIDS			
Aldosterone Stimulated by adrenocorticotropic hormone (ACTH) production Major control is renin-angiotensin system	Promotes retention of Na⁺ (and water) in kidney	More than 90% of the adrenal gland is destroyed before the clinical picture of *adrenal insufficiency* emerges Increased excretion of Na⁺ and water influences dehydration, hyponatremia, orthostatic hypotension, ↓ urine output, ↓ cardiac output, weight loss, salt craving, acidosis, circulatory collapse, shock	Increased retention of Na⁺ and water results in edema, weight gain, hypertension, augmentation of cardiac problems such as left ventricular hypertrophy, congestive heart failure
GLUCOCORTICOIDS			
Cortisol Regulated by ACTH release from anterior pituitary	Promotes gluconeogenesis Maintains plasma glucose level Promotes appetite Causes release of epinephrine from adrenal medulla Assists in adaptation to stress by ↑ gluconeogenesis releasing an anti-inflammatory response; augmenting release of catecholamines (epinephrine, norepinephrine) to increase blood pressure	Decreased gluconeogenesis causes depleted liver glycogen stores manifested by hypoglycemia, weakness, fatigue, anorexia, weight loss, vomiting, mental confusion, emotional disturbances (mild neurosis to depression) Inadequate release of epinephrine produces hypoglycemia, hypotension Lowers resistance to stress and produces a "hyperresponse" to stressors: hypoglycemia, hypotension, hyperthermia	Increased circulating cortisol causes memory loss, poor concentration, depression, euphoria, anxiety, sleep disorders Increased susceptibility to infection and suppression of inflammatory response: vulnerability to infections, poor response to infectious process, poor wound healing
ACTH release controls cortisol secretion	ACTH regulates melanocyte-stimulating hormone (MSH)	Stimulates an increase in MSH: increases skin and mucous membrane pigmentation, especially in fingers, toes, and sun-exposed body parts (skin appears bronzed)	No effect
ANDROGENS			
Regulated by ACTH release from anterior pituitary		Females: oligomenorrhea or amenorrhea, decrease in body hair Males: no manifestations in males because testes produce adequate quantities of sex hormone	Females: acne, thinning of scalp hair, excessive growth of body and facial hair in male pattern (hirsutism), menstrual irregularities, infertility common Males: decreased libido, impotence

ance and include sudden penetrating pain in the back, abdomen, or legs; depressed or changed mentation; volume depletion; hypotension; loss of consciousness; and shock.

CORRECT FLUID AND ELECTROLYTE IMBALANCES. The overall desired outcome of treatment is prevention of the morbidity and mortality associated with the addisonian crisis. Untreated, addisonian crisis is fatal. The cause of the crisis must be determined and treated immediately. Hypotension and electrolyte imbalance need to be corrected quickly. Rapid rehydration is essential. An isotonic solution usually corrects the volume depletion, salt depletion, and hypotension. The client may also need oxygen, vasopressors, or volume expanders. Sodium polystyrene sulfonate (Kayexalate) may be administered orally or as an enema in combination with sorbitol. Kayexalate is a resin that releases sodium ions in exchange for potassium ions.

TABLE 44-2	DIAGNOSTIC TESTS OF ADRENOCORTICAL FUNCTION		
Test	**Purpose**	**Nursing Notes**	**Interpretation**
Cortisol level with dexamethasone suppression test	Evaluates function of adrenal cortex	Give dexamethasone before phlebotomy to suppress diurnal formation of adrenocorticotropic hormone (ACTH) Give 1 mg dexamethasone at 11 PM to suppress ACTH formation in time for 8 AM phlebotomy and later at 8 PM; estrogen therapy can falsely increase results	↑ Pituitary tumor, Cushing's syndrome or disease, hyperplasia of adrenal cortex (benign or malignant) ↓ Addison's disease
Cortisol plasma levels	Evaluates function of adrenal cortex	Plasma cortisol levels have diurnal effect: levels higher in AM than PM Fasting prephlebotomy 2 hrs of supine activity are necessary before test because activity increases cortisol level Estrogens increase level Aldactone (spironolactone) can cause false-positives	↑ Pregnancy, recent physical activity, obesity, Cushing's disease or syndrome ↓ Addison's disease
17-Hydroxysteroids (Porter-Silber reaction)	Measures metabolites of glucocorticoids and aldosterone	24-hr urine collection to be kept on ice Many drugs can invalidate results	↑ Cushing's disease or syndrome; ACTH administration; nonadrenal ACTH-producing tumor ↓ Addison's disease or exogenous steroid suppression
Cosyntropin test	Diagnoses adrenal insufficiency with ACTH stimulation	Give ACTH IV; 45 min later, obtain serum cortisol level	↑ Normal ↓ Dysfunction of hypothalamic-pituitary axis Secondary adrenal insufficiency
Computed tomography (CT) or magnetic resonance imaging (MRI) of adrenals	Identifies and locates adrenal glands	No preparation except client education	Small, atrophied glands = autoimmune adrenal insufficiency Bilateral enlarged glands = hemorrhage (with areas of high density), neoplasm
Rapid ACTH stimulation		Give cosyntropin IV; obtain plasma cortisol and aldosterone level at baseline + 30 min	↓ Cortisol and aldosterone = primary adrenal insufficiency
17-Ketosteroids	Measures steroid metabolites from adrenal cortex and testes (does not include testosterone)	24-hr urine test; keep collection cold; may need preservative Many drugs make test invalid	↑ Tumors of adrenal cortex or testes, Cushing's syndrome ↓ Hypofunction of adrenal, or in clients with removal of testes or ovaries

CORRECT HYPOGLYCEMIA. Hypoglycemia must be evaluated and corrected with intravenous (IV) glucose (5% dextrose [D_5] solution IV or IV glucose push bolus).

REPLACE STEROIDS. Hydrocortisone at 100 mg is administered as an IV bolus followed by 100 mg IV every 8 hours for 24 hours. The IV hydrocortisone is tapered as the client's status dictates. Oral hydrocortisone is initiated.

ADDISON'S DISEASE
Addison's disease was once fatal within months. Today, with the availability of synthetic corticosteroids (Table

TABLE 44-2	DIAGNOSTIC TESTS OF ADRENOCORTICAL FUNCTION *Continued*

Test	Purpose	Nursing Notes	Interpretation
Aldosterone	Measures mineralocorticoid production	Client to be supine 2 hr before phlebotomy ↑ Aldosterone can cause ↑ extracellular fluid Oral contraceptive, sodium restriction, and potassium may ↑ level	↑ Primary or secondary hyperaldosteronism, severe liver dysfunction ↓ Addison's disease (may be undetectable or ↓ in Addison's)
Urinary cortisol level	Measures cortisol, not metabolites		↑ Adrenal hyperfunction, Cushing's syndrome ↓ Not necessarily adrenal hypofunction
Renin level	Measures renin, an enzyme produced by juxtaglomerular apparatus in response to decreased blood flow to kidneys	Client in supine position Results high in AM Note sodium content in diet on laboratory slip The following medications interfere with results: diuretics, estrogens, oral contraceptives, antihypertensives	↑ Hypertension, upright position with phlebotomy ↓ High-sodium diet
Plasma ACTH or serum corticotropin	Tests anterior pituitary function as it may cause Cushing's syndrome, Addison's disease	Fasting sample Stress may artificially increase results	↑ Cushing's syndrome caused by bilateral adrenal hyperplasia or ectopic ACTH-producing tumors; Addison's disease (primary adrenal insufficiency) caused by adrenal gland failure, surgical removal of adrenals, adrenal suppression with long-term exogenous steroid supply ↓ Secondary adrenal insufficiency caused by hypopituitarism; cushingoid client may have adrenal adenoma as cause of hyperfunction
Captopril test	Rules out renal artery stenosis	Nuclear medicine captopril renal scan done first to evaluate resting glomerular filtration rate (GFR); captopril administered PO; GFR reevaluated after captopril	↓ GFR renal artery stenosis same ↑ GFR after captopril: negative for renal artery stenosis
Corticotropin-releasing hormone (CRH) stimulation	Measures CRH from hypothalamus to pituitary necessary to stimulate ACTH and cortisol release	Give CRH IV; measure plasma ACTH and cortisol at baseline and after 15, 30, and 60 min	↑ ACTH and cortisol indicate primary adrenal insufficiency ↓ ACTH and cortisol indicate pituitary or hypothalamic dysfunction, secondary adrenal insufficiency

44–3), clients with Addison's disease can live normal, active lives, provided they receive adequate glucocorticoid replacement. Use corticosteroids with caution. Table 44–4 shows the adverse consequences of administering corticosteroids in selected disorders. Carefully assess clients for manifestations of hypercortisolism, which can

result from excessive long-term cortisol therapy. Most clients receive glucocorticoid and mineralocorticoid replacement.

Osteoporosis is a complication that may develop with excessive use of glucocorticosteroids because the protein matrix in the bones is broken down and therefore

| TABLE 44-3 | NURSING IMPLICATIONS OF CORTICOSTEROIDS | | | |

Class	Action	Therapeutic Outcomes	Adverse Outcomes	Dosing
GLUCOCORTICOIDS				
Long-acting (dexamethasone, Decadron)	Inhibits inflammation Suppresses cell-mediated immune response	Inflammation and allergic responses are reduced	Monitor for infection (use good handwashing) Monitor for hypocalcemia	Take with food or milk Do not stop abruptly
Intermediate-acting (methylprednisolone, Medrol)	Inhibits inflammation Suppresses cell-mediated immune response	Adrenal crisis is averted Muscle strength returns Blood pressure normalizes	Monitor for heartburn Monitor for signs and symptoms of hypercortisolism	Give with food or milk Give as single dose before 9 AM Do not stop abruptly
Short-acting (hydrocortisone, Hydrocortone)	Inhibits inflammation Suppresses cell-mediated immune response	Adrenal crisis is averted Muscle strength returns Blood pressure normalizes	Monitor for heartburn Monitor for signs and symptoms of increased cortical effects, insomnia, mood swings, increased hunger Protect from infection (use good handwashing)	Give oral dose with food or milk Give as single dose before 9 AM Have client wear Medic-Alert bracelet Tell client not to stop drug abruptly
MINERALOCORTICOIDS				
Fludrocortisone (Florinef)	Increases retention of sodium and therefore water	Postural hypotension diminishes	Monitor for edema Monitor for hypokalemia Monitor intake and output Monitor daily weights	Give with food or milk Do not stop abruptly

calcium cannot be retained. Closely observe clients with other medical problems that may be worsened with steroid use.

Nursing Management of the Medical Client

ADDISONIAN CRISIS

ASSESSMENT

Monitor the client's vital signs closely while the disease is being diagnosed. Check the pulse carefully, at least

TABLE 44-4	CONSEQUENCES OF CORTICOSTEROID USE IN SELECTED DISORDERS*
Disorder	**Consequence**
Diabetes mellitus	Augments hyperglycemia
Inflammatory bowel disorders	Fluid retention may exacerbate peristalsis
Hypertension	Contributes to fluid retention
Congestive heart failure	Contributes to fluid retention
Renal insufficiency	Worsens fluid retention

* Corticosteroids are contraindicated in clients with viral, fungal, or tubercular infections.

every 4 hours. Take orthostatic blood pressure (BP) readings and pulses. Report drops in BP or orthostatic changes.

As rehydration occurs and electrolyte imbalances are corrected, assess increased physical vitality and emotional well-being. Assess bone prominences for pressure ulcers in immobilized clients. With therapy, listlessness and exhaustion should gradually disappear.

Monitor for exposure to cold and infections. Immediately inform the physician if evidence of infection develops, such as a sore throat or burning on urination. Remember, a client with Addison's disease cannot tolerate stress. Infection imposes additional stress on the body, and cortisol levels need to be higher during infectious illnesses.

Carefully assess for manifestations of sodium and potassium imbalance (see Chapter 13). Obtain daily weights for objective measurement of fluid gain or loss. If steroid replacement therapy is inadequate, sodium loss and potassium retention continue uncorrected. If the steroid dosage is too high, excessive amounts of sodium and water are retained and potassium excretion is high.

DIAGNOSIS, OUTCOMES, INTERVENTIONS

Risk for Injury: Addisonian Crisis. The client must be diligent in self-care, or the diagnosis may be *Risk for Injury: Addisonian crisis related to adrenal insufficiency.*

Outcomes. The client will not exhibit injury, as evidenced by absence of hypotension, shock, or other manifestations of acute adrenal insufficiency.

Interventions

Monitor for Manifestations of Crisis. Addisonian crisis usually develops over 24 to 48 hours. Closely monitor for sudden profound weakness; severe abdominal, back, and leg pain; hyperpyrexia (although this may be suppressed by steroids) followed by hypothermia; hypotension associated with high cardiac output, normal wedge pressure, and low systemic resistance; coma; renal shutdown; and death.

An adrenal crisis is a medical emergency that must be treated rapidly and vigorously. The three major desired outcomes of intervention are (1) reversal of shock, (2) restoration of blood circulation (the client usually has a deficit of at least 20% of extracellular fluid volume), and (3) replenishment with essential steroids.

Correct Fluid, Electrolyte, Steroid Imbalances. Immediately on admission, 1000 ml of normal saline with water-soluble glucocorticoid (hydrocortisone phosphate or hydrocortisone sodium succinate) added is rapidly infused. The dosage of the prescribed glucocorticoid is gradually reduced. It is administered intramuscularly (IM) or IV every 8 hours on days 1 and 2 of the crisis and gradually reduced thereafter. Hypoglycemia is controlled by a glucose infusion, either an IV bolus or IV drip as part of rehydration. Hyperkalemia is controlled or corrected with Kayexalate. The precipitating event must be corrected. Plasma, oxygen, and vasopressor medications may be indicated.

Throughout the emergency period, monitor BP, administer IV infusion and medications, monitor hourly urine output, report oliguria (a manifestation of shock), and minimize exposure to emotional and physical stress. Observe for manifestations of glucocorticoid overdose and overhydration, such as generalized edema from fluid retention, hypertension, flaccid paralysis from hypokalemia, psychosis, and loss of consciousness. Also evaluate electrolytes for hyperkalemia, hyponatremia, and hypoglycemia, and correlate these findings with the client's manifestations.

With rapid, efficient intervention, addisonian crisis usually resolves within 12 hours. The client's condition stabilizes, and the convalescent period begins. When the client can tolerate food and fluids by mouth, steroid replacement can be administered orally.

Prevent Future Crises. After the immediate crisis is over, help the client avoid further development of adrenal insufficiency. Obtain a medical identification (Medic-Alert) bracelet and an emergency kit before discharge from the hospital. Instruct the client to carry these items at all times. The client's name and diagnosis should appear on the identification bracelet, and a wallet card should state that the client receives daily hydrocortisone and that the medication must be administered by injection in an emergency.

Dexamethasone can be kept in a prepared syringe in an emergency kit with sterile alcohol wipes for cleaning the injection site. The kit should also contain written information about the client's diagnosis, prescribed drugs, dosage schedules, and emergency phone numbers, including the physician's name and phone number.

Adrenal insufficiency is a potentially life-threatening condition, but when properly recognized and treated, it has little or no effect on life span. There are no dietary or activity restrictions.

EVALUATION

The outcome of treatment for addisonian crisis is easily evaluated, usually within 12 hours of treatment. By this time, the client should no longer exhibit any manifestations of addisonian crisis or death would have occurred.

■ Self-Care

Management of Addison's disease takes place in the community with regular medical follow-up of the client's status. Hence, the focus of management is on self-care. Carefully assess the client's ability to understand and perform self-care. The client needs extensive instruction in self-care activities to achieve independence. Appropriate outcomes for the client with Addison's disease are that the client's weight remains stable, vital signs and cortisol levels remain within normal limits, and the client states that fatigue has decreased.

STEROID REPLACEMENT

The client must learn how to take steroids correctly. Provide the client and significant others with written instructions on self-administration of steroids. (The client and significant others should have demonstrated their ability to prepare and administer injections.) The client needs to know the following information:

- Actions of prescribed hormones (hydrocortisone, fludrocortisone)
- Importance of taking medications daily, without fail, exactly as prescribed
- Principles of self-administration of oral medications (e.g., the client must check the label on the bottle before taking the medication and documenting medications taken and their side effects)
- Manifestations of overdosage and underdosage
- Importance of hydrocortisone self-injection when unable to tolerate oral medication (because of nausea and vomiting) and during times of acute stress (motor vehicle accident, trauma) because the body is unable to provide the needed additional glucocorticoid coverage
- Need for an IM self-injection kit to be available at all times
- Need for a Medic-Alert bracelet showing the diagnosis and the need for cortisol replacement
- Need for the client to call a health care provider if questions arise after discharge from the medical center

Emphasize that the client who takes glucocorticoids must call the physician to obtain a dosage increase when experiencing stressful situations (e.g., emotional upheavals, dental extractions, minor surgery, upper respiratory infections). The general rule is to double the glucocorticoid dosage for up to 1 week, depending on manifestations, and then resume normal dosage. In addition, temporary mineralocorticoid dosage is reduced by 50% to avoid excessive salt retention and hypertension. Encourage the client to consult the physician for dose adjustment. The medication must be administered IM when nausea and vomiting prevent oral administration.

FOLLOW-UP MONITORING

Remind clients to keep semiannual appointments with the physician, even when their health is good and self-medication is proceeding smoothly. As with diabetes mellitus, the control of Addison's disease is a lifelong responsibility.

■ Modification for Elderly Clients

Adrenal diseases are uncommon in older people. The effects of normal aging on the adrenals are unclear. It appears, however, that ACTH and cortisol production remains constant throughout life. Elderly people may be more sensitive to the side effects of steroid therapy because these problems (e.g., osteoporosis, hypertension, diabetes) already exist.

SECONDARY ADRENAL INSUFFICIENCY

Secondary adrenal insufficiency results from dysfunction of the hypothalamic-pituitary-adrenal (HPA) axis (Fig. 44–2). The most common cause is chronic treatment with glucocorticoids for nonendocrine uses. Other causes include:

- Hypopituitarism resulting in decreased ACTH secretion by the pituitary gland, which causes decreased secretion of cortisol and androgens by the adrenal gland
- Pituitary tumor or infarction
- Radiation
- Suppression of hypothalamic-pituitary secretion of ACTH related to hypercortisolism caused by either exogenous administration of corticosteroids or oversecretion of corticosteroids by an adrenal tumor (in both cases, the adrenal glands atrophy and become filled with lipids)

Secondary adrenal insufficiency is characterized by low cortisol production and low plasma ACTH. Because circulating levels of corticosteroids remain high, these clients do not experience manifestations of adrenocortical insufficiency unless steroid therapy is discontinued suddenly or the tumor is resected. If corticosteroid therapy is tapered gradually, with the dosage reduced each day, adrenal gland function usually returns to normal.

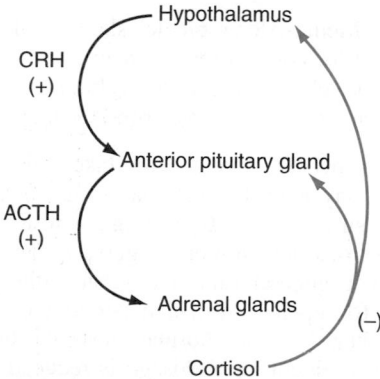

FIGURE 44–2 The hypothalamic-pituitary-adrenal (HPA) axis, demonstrating stimulation and feedback between the hypothalamus, anterior pituitary, and adrenal glands. ACTH, adrenocorticotropic hormone; CRH, corticotropin-releasing hormone.

Assessment reveals that clients with secondary adrenal insufficiency experience cortisol deficiency. Aldosterone continues to be secreted in sufficient amounts. Treatment involves administering glucocorticoids, as in Addison's disease. Mineralocorticoid replacement is unnecessary. Instruct the client to wear an emergency identification bracelet and to carry an emergency kit for hydrocortisone injection in case of an adrenal crisis.

ADRENOCORTICAL HYPERFUNCTION

Hyperfunction of the adrenal cortex can result in excessive production of glucocorticoids, mineralocorticoids, and androgens. Major conditions of adrenocortical hyperfunction are hypercortisolism (glucocorticoid excess) and primary aldosteronism (aldosterone excess).

HYPERCORTISOLISM

Hypercortisolism (Cushing's syndrome) was first described by Harvey Cushing in 1932. It results from overactivity of the adrenal gland, with consequent hypersecretion of glucocorticoids. Cushing's syndrome is relatively rare, and its incidence is unknown. It occurs mainly in women ages 20 to 40 years; however, it can occur up to age 60.

Etiology and Risk Factors

Iatrogenic hypercortisolism (resulting from medical interventions) accounts for most cases because of the frequent therapeutic use of high-dose glucocorticoids. Hypersecretion of cortisol can be caused by a cortisol-secreting adrenal tumor or adrenal hyperplasia, resulting from overproduction of ACTH. Adrenal tumors are responsible for about 30% of cases of Cushing's syndromes. Most (85%) are benign, but 15% are malignant. There are two sources of excessive ACTH secretion:

- Pituitary hypersecretion and pituitary tumors, which cause about 70% of cases of Cushing's syndrome. These usually benign tumors are either small basophil adenomas or large chromophobe adenomas. Pituitary hypersecretion of ACTH that results in glucocorticoid excess is called *Cushing's disease.*
- Ectopic secretion of ACTH (or *ectopic ACTH syndrome*). ACTH-secreting tumors located outside the pituitary gland are a rare cause of Cushing's syndrome. Oat cell carcinoma of the lung, pancreatic islet cell carcinoma, and carcinoid tumors of the lung, gut, thymus, and ovary are the tumors that most frequently cause ectopic ACTH syndrome.

Iatrogenic Cushing's syndrome, another form of the disorder, results from exogenous (originating outside the body; e.g., taking supplemental medication) administration of synthetic glucocorticoids in supraphysiologic amounts. Thus, educating clients to avoid unnecessary use of exogenous steroids is an important health promotion activity. Health maintenance activities include (1) educating clients who are at risk for manifestations of Cushing's syndrome; (2) treating clinical manifestations of hypernatremia, hypokalemia, hyperglycemia, and hypertension;

and (3) teaching clients about adrenalectomy and steroid replacement. Health restoration activities include making sure that clients understand the importance of surgery, lifelong steroid replacement, and recognizing disease complications that may have already developed (such as osteoporosis or "buffalo hump," a fat pad on the neck).

Pathophysiology

When Cushing's syndrome develops, the normal function of the glucocorticoids becomes exaggerated and the classic picture of the syndrome emerges (Fig. 44–3). This exaggerated physiologic action of glucocorticoids appears as follows:

- Persistent hyperglycemia (or "steroid diabetes").
- Protein tissue wasting, which results in muscle wasting and weakness; capillary fragility, which results in ecchymosis; and osteoporosis from bone matrix wasting. Osteoporosis can become so severe that even mild trauma can cause fractures. Compression fractures can develop in the osteoporotic spine, leading to kyphosis and loss of height.
- Potassium depletion, leading to hypokalemia, dysrhythmias, muscle weakness, and renal disorders.
- Sodium and water retention, which causes edema and hypertension.
- Hypertension, which eventually predisposes the client to

left ventricular hypertrophy, heart failure, and cerebrovascular accidents.

- Abnormal fat distribution (in conjunction with edema), which results in a moon-shaped face, a dorsocervical fat pad on the neck (buffalo hump), and truncal obesity with slender limbs. Also, pink and purple striae appear on the breasts, axillary areas, abdomen, and legs because of thinning of the skin. Striking changes in appearance occur after the development and cure of Cushing's syndrome. Old photographs can be useful in showing changes over time.
- Increased susceptibility to infection and lowered resistance to stress increase vulnerability to microorganisms of all types. Because of suppression of the inflammatory response, people with Cushing's syndrome show few manifestations of infection. They also demonstrate poor wound healing.
- Possible increased production of androgens can cause virilism (masculine characteristics) in women. Manifestations of virilism include acne, thinning of scalp hair, and hirsutism (excessive bodily and facial hair in a male pattern).
- Mental changes include memory loss, poor concentration and cognition, euphoria, and depression. Sometimes a condition called "steroid psychosis" develops. Depression can predispose the client to suicidal thoughts. About 80% of the clients meet the criteria for a major affective disorder: 50% with unipolar depression, 30% with bipolar illness.

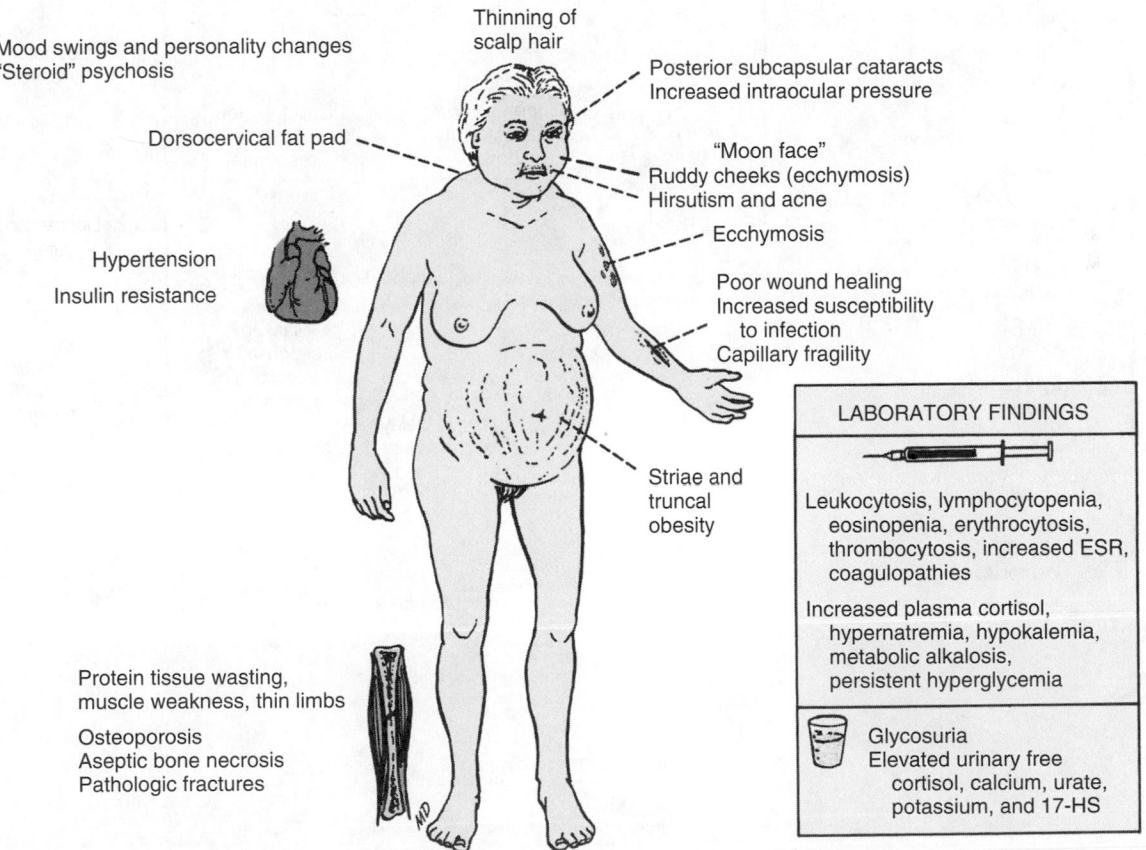

FIGURE 44–3 Assessment data for Cushing's syndrome. *Inset,* Laboratory findings. ESR, erythrocyte sedimentation rate; 17-HS, 17-hydroxysteroid.

Understanding Hypercortisolism (Cushing's Disease) and Its Treatment

■ ACTH, adrenocorticotropic hormone.

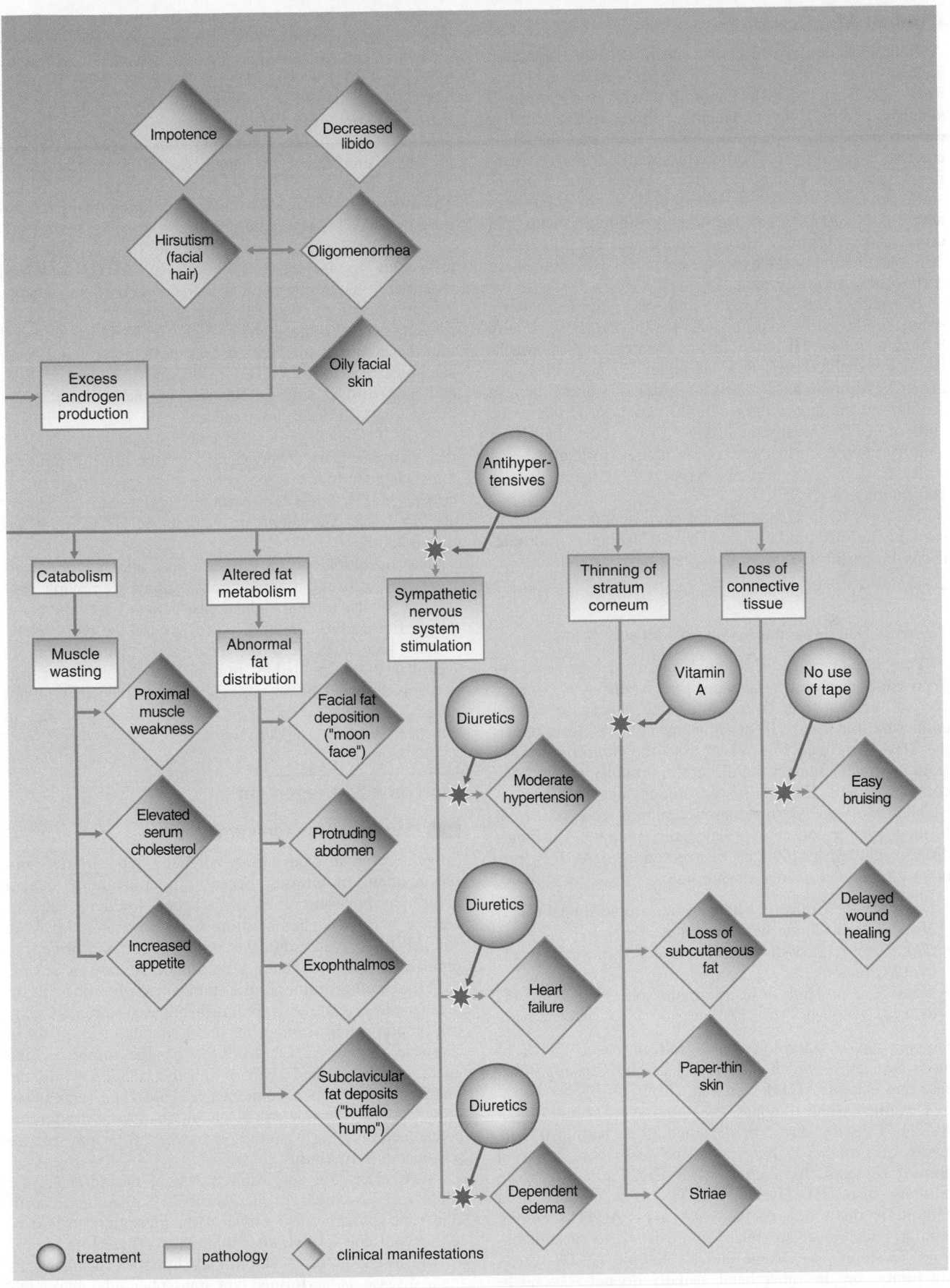

treatment   pathology   clinical manifestations

Clinical Manifestations

Although clients have a classic cushingoid appearance, it is important to perform diagnostic studies for confirmation (see Table 44–2). Laboratory tests for Cushing's syndrome reflect hyperglycemia, fluid and electrolyte disturbances, and immunosuppressive responses that characterize excessive glucocorticoid secretion. Thus, in Cushing's syndrome glucose tolerance decreases and glucosuria appears. The white blood cell count often rises above 10,000/mm³, but the total eosinophil count can drop below 50/mm³. Also, lymphocytes can fall below 20%. Both urinary 17-hydroxysteroid (17-HS) and blood cortisol levels are elevated.

Normally, plasma cortisol follows a diurnal pattern, rising in the early morning (10 to 25 mg/dl), gradually falling to below 10 mg/dl in the evening, and approaching undetectable levels near midnight. Clients with Cushing's syndrome have elevated plasma cortisol levels throughout the day without diurnal variation. Urinary free cortisol (UFC) measurement is used as a screening test to identify elevated urinary excretion of free cortisol. Clients with Cushing's syndrome have UFC levels above 100 mg/day.

The *overnight* dexamethasone suppression test is often used in the differential diagnosis of Cushing's syndrome. It can be performed on an outpatient basis as follows:

- *Day 1:* Administer dexamethasone, 1 mg orally (PO) at 11 PM.
- *Day 2:* Determine plasma cortisol level at 8 AM.

The normal range is below 5 mg/dl. Severe stress or depression can cause false-positive results (i.e., plasma cortisol greater than 5 mg/dl despite otherwise normal endocrine function). If dexamethasone fails to suppress the HPA axis (see Fig. 44–2) and the morning cortisol level is greater than 5 mg/dl, an abnormality of feedback compatible with Cushing's syndrome is suggested.

The *standard* dexamethasone suppression test (performed over 6 consecutive days) differentiates Cushing's disease (caused by pituitary oversecretion of ACTH) from other causes of Cushing's syndrome:

- *Days 1 to 6:* Collect 24-hour urine sample for UFC.
- *Days 1 to 2:* Obtain baseline value.
- *Days 3 to 4:* Low-dose dexamethasone test: 0.5 mg PO every 6 hours.
- *Days 5 to 6:* High-dose dexamethasone test: 2 mg PO every 6 hours.

Suppression is interpreted as a fall in basal 17-HS of more than 50%, which is compatible with Cushing's disease and ectopic ACTH secretion.

Dexamethasone suppresses pituitary secretion of ACTH. Thus, by day 2 of dexamethasone administration, levels of urinary 17-HS should be less than 2 mg in normal subjects. In a client with Cushing's disease (a pituitary disorder), levels of 17-HS drop because of a pathologic disruption of the HPA axis. ACTH-secreting pituitary adenomas are relatively resistant to dexamethasone. Cushing's syndrome and an ectopic ACTH-secreting tumor, on the other hand, usually do not respond to dexamethasone (i.e., levels of 17-HS do not decrease).

In the plasma ACTH test, low ACTH levels point to an adrenal tumor as the cause of hypercortisolism. Overproduction of cortisol by the adrenal tumor provides negative feedback to the pituitary gland, which responds by reducing ACTH release. The high cortisol level also provides feedback to the hypothalamus, which reduces release of corticotropin-releasing hormone.

An ectopic ACTH-producing tumor usually yields a normal or elevated ACTH level. ACTH production by the tumor is independent of pituitary production of ACTH. Thus, despite negative feedback to the hypothalamic-pituitary unit, ACTH levels remain high.

The inferior petrosal sinus sampling test is a radiologic test used to isolate the source of ACTH secretion (whether it is in the pituitary gland and, if so, where). The left and right petrosal sinuses carry blood from the pituitary gland to the jugular veins. Catheters are threaded into the inferior petrosal sinus via the femoral veins. With sampling of serum ACTH levels drawn from the right and left petrosal sinuses, the side of the pituitary gland producing ACTH can be identified.

If ACTH levels from the petrosal sinuses are greater than this one from a peripheral site (the arm), a pituitary tumor is identified as the source of hypercortisolism. If central ACTH levels (petrosal) and peripheral ACTH levels (arm) are equivalent, an ectopic ACTH-secreting tumor is likely.

The development of this test has allowed neurosurgeons to perform a hemihypophysectomy, removing only the half of the pituitary gland that contains the microadenoma. Before the availability of this test, the entire gland usually had to be removed because of the difficulty in localizing these "invisible" tumors. An adrenal CT scan is performed to detect an adrenal mass in the right or left adrenal gland. Contrast dye is used, when possible, to enhance the clarity of the scan.

Outcome Management

■ Surgical Management

Surgical removal of even one adrenal gland requires careful inpatient monitoring because the remaining adrenal gland may have atrophied and stopped producing adrenocortical hormones. For Cushing's syndrome caused by an adrenal tumor, an adrenalectomy can be performed to remove the gland containing the tumor. In case of ectopic ACTH-secreting tumors, the tumor can be difficult to localize. If no source is found, a bilateral adrenalectomy can be performed to interrupt the production of cortisol in response to the ACTH produced by the tumor, or the client can be treated with antiglucocorticoids while the search for the tumor continues. Laparoscopic adrenalectomy is being evaluated as an alternative to traditional adrenalectomy. Early studies indicate that it may reduce postoperative morbidity.[27, 31]

After successful surgical removal of the adrenals, the client receives lifelong glucocorticoid and mineralocorticoid replacement. Most physical manifestations of Cushing's syndrome resolve after bilateral adrenalectomy.

The resection of most pituitary tumors causing Cushing's disease is performed via transsphenoidal hypophysectomy (see Chapter 69). Occasionally, large or anatomically complex tumors are excised via a transfrontal approach (see discussion of hypophysectomy). A surgical cure rate of 85% to 90% has been documented. Because the HPA axis has been suppressed, adrenal insufficiency develops postoperatively. The axis takes 12 to 24 months to recover. Replacement steroids are indicated during this time.

■ Nursing Management of the Surgical Client

PREOPERATIVE CARE
ASSESSMENT

Begin by obtaining a careful history from a client with possible Cushing's syndrome. The client may exhibit the characteristic clinical manifestations identified previously. Support the client during the diagnostic phase of care. At this point, there is often a great deal of uncertainty about the cause of the disorder. Explain to the client why these tests must be performed before treatment can be started.

During the preoperative phase, the client with Cushing's syndrome requires expert nursing assessment and care. The crucial problems of hypertension, edema, possible heart disease, diabetes mellitus, increased susceptibility to infection, decreased resistance to stress, and emotional lability (tendency toward frequent mood changes) or instability must all be assessed and brought under control before surgery.

DIAGNOSIS, OUTCOMES, INTERVENTIONS

Risk for Injury: Fractures, Hypertension, or Diabetes. Until the diagnosis is made and the problem treated, the client is at *Risk for Injury: Fractures, Hypertension, or Diabetes related to osteoporosis, sodium and water retention, or the presence of an insulin antagonist, respectively.*

Outcomes. Injury will not occur, as evidenced by absence of fractures. The client will not have hypertension, hyperglycemia, or diabetes.

Interventions
Prevent Injury. Protect the client from falls and accidents. Clients with Cushing's syndrome have osteoporosis and tend to develop fractures even with mild trauma. Keep the bed in its lowest position, and raise the side rails for protection. Assist clients with ambulation to avoid falls.

Monitor for Hypertension and Diabetes. Monitor vital signs at frequent intervals. Assess the client carefully for evidence of severe hypertension, such as elevated BP, headache, failing vision, irritability, and dyspnea. Check for postural hypotension (but have the client change position slowly to avoid injury from a sudden drop in BP).

Obtain the client's weight daily in a consistent manner. If sodium intake is reduced, edema and weight should diminish. Obtain daily blood glucose levels via finger stick. Positive results may indicate diabetes mellitus (steroid diabetes) caused by the insulin antagonist action of the excessive cortisol.

Knowledge Deficit. A typical nursing diagnosis for the client undergoing surgery to correct adrenocortical excess is *Knowledge Deficit regarding the disease, surgery, and proper diet related to no previous instruction and new diagnosis resulting in anxiety, misinformation, and questions.*

Outcomes. The client will understand the disease, the surgery planned, and the importance of a proper diet, as evidenced by statements of understanding and choice of a proper diet.

Interventions
Explain Disease and Treatment. It is important for clients to understand their condition and the proposed treatment. Give clients an opportunity to ask questions about the treatment, and assess their understanding of it.

Provide Adequate Nutrition. Encourage a diet low in calories, carbohydrates, and sodium but with ample protein and potassium. Such a diet promotes weight loss, reduction of edema and hypertension, control of hypokalemia, and rebuilding of wasted tissue. The client with diabetes mellitus or gastric ulcers requires a special diet.

EVALUATION

It is expected that clients will have minimal complications or have appropriate management of complications before surgery so that they can undergo the adrenalectomy successfully. The client will be able to explain the desired outcome of surgical intervention, possible complications, and related treatment. A glucocorticoid preparation will be given on the morning of surgery to prevent adrenal insufficiency during the procedure.

POSTOPERATIVE CARE
ASSESSMENT

Routine postoperative monitoring of the incision and special assessments for manifestations of shock, addisonian crisis, and renal shutdown are required. Assess the client's ability to perform self-care and to manage the disease for the remainder of his or her life. The client's current level of knowledge must be assessed and a teaching plan carefully developed.

DIAGNOSIS, OUTCOMES, INTERVENTIONS

Risk for Injury. After surgery, the client may have *Risk for Injury related to complications of the surgical procedure.*

Outcomes. Injury will not occur or will be detected early, as evidenced by absence of shock, hemorrhage, infection, or addisonian crisis.

Interventions. On the morning of surgery, administer a glucocorticoid preparation IM or IV as prescribed. A water-soluble cortisol preparation (diluted in an IV infusion) may be given throughout the surgery. Cortisol protects against the development of acute adrenal insufficiency during the adrenalectomy. Even if the surgeon plans to remove only one adrenal gland, temporary glucocorticoid support may be needed until the remaining adrenal gland begins to secrete sufficient cortisol. Because of the excessive secretion of cortisol by the tumorous gland, the healthy gland can atrophy and needs time to readjust.

During the immediate postoperative phase, major desired outcomes are prevention of shock and infection, maintenance of adequate cortisol levels, and control of pain and incisional discomfort. Observe for manifestations of shock related to hemorrhage (hypotension and a rapid, weak pulse). Document vital signs every 15 minutes. Measure urine and record hourly output, observing for oliguria, a manifestation of shock and renal shutdown. Administer IV fluids, pressor amines, and corticosteroids as prescribed.

The manifestations of addisonian crisis resemble those of shock. Closely assess the client for this complication, and administer IV cortisol in high doses until the manifestations subside. The client will require increased amounts of steroids until the remaining adrenal gland returns to a normal level of functioning and the stress associated with the treatment subsides.

Risk for Infection. The client receiving steroid replacement will be at *Risk for Infection related to lowered resistance to stress and compromised immune response.*

Outcomes. Infection will not develop or will be detected early, as evidenced by absence of leukocytosis, fever, and other manifestations of infections.

Interventions. After surgery, encourage the client to cough, turn, and deep-breathe to prevent respiratory infections. Employ meticulous sterile technique with wound care to prevent infection. Paralytic ileus is less common because the flank approach is usually used.

Protect the client from exposure to infectious organisms. Isolate the client from health care personnel and significant others who have contagious disorders. Wash your hands meticulously before contact with the client.

Because glucocorticoids suppress immune and inflammatory reactions, a client with Cushing's syndrome may have only mild manifestations of even a severe infection. The white blood cell count does not show significant elevation in immunosuppressed clients. A slight elevation in body temperature may indicate the presence of a severe infection.

Activity Intolerance. A client receiving steroids may exhibit *Activity Intolerance related to fatigue and muscle weakness from protein wasting, persistent hyperglycemia (and possible diabetes mellitus), and potassium depletion resulting in an inability to maintain a normal activity level without increased heart rate or shortness of breath.*

Outcomes. The client will be able to balance rest and activity.

Interventions. Promote mental and physical rest for the client with Cushing's syndrome. Minimize stress and confusion so that the client can achieve maximal periods of rest.

Risk for Impaired Skin Integrity. A client receiving steroids is at *Risk for Impaired Skin Integrity related to tissue catabolism (thinning of skin), loss of connective tissue, and edema secondary to sodium and water retention.*

Outcomes. The client will maintain intact skin.

Interventions. Monitor the client's skin meticulously for breakdown. The client is extremely susceptible to breakdown from tissue catabolism. Avoid using tape or other irritants that may tear or excoriate the skin.

Altered Thought Processes. The client may exhibit *Altered Thought Processes (memory loss, cognitive impairment, mood swings, euphoria, or depression) related to increased levels of glucocorticoids and ACTH, resulting in an inability to make decisions and remember.*

Outcomes. The client will not have memory loss, cognitive impairment, or mood swings, or these manifestations will be minimized.

Interventions. Anticipate mood swings. Clients may become easily upset by changes in their appearance caused by the disease and may also become alarmed by bizarre feelings and emotions. Reassure clients that appearance and moods should gradually return to normal after treatment unless steroid replacement is necessary. If clients need steroid therapy, some side effects will continue.

EVALUATION

If the surgical management of Cushing's disease is successful, neither injury related to the surgery nor addisonian crisis will develop. If complications do occur, desired outcomes may be related to successful management of the complications, such as control of hemorrhage, prevention of shock, and control of addisonian crisis.

Appropriate outcomes also include the control of side effects of the steroid therapy. Because these cannot be completely avoided, the client's ability to control them is an appropriate area to evaluate. The client should be able to differentiate complications from the side effects of medications.

■ Medical Management

Usually, a client with primary adrenal hyperplasia is treated surgically as an inpatient. Medical management is reserved for clients with inoperable tumors or metastatic tumors that warrant palliative care (Table 44–5). The outcome, therefore, is related to achieving comfort versus cure. Medical management options include radiation therapy and administration of adrenal blocking agents or ACTH-reducing agents to decrease the effects of the adrenal hyperplasia.

RADIATION THERAPY. Radiation therapy can be used to treat primary pituitary tumors and other ACTH-secreting adenomas. Radiation can be applied to the pituitary gland either internally or externally. Internally, the radiation is applied through a transsphenoidal implant. Radiation must be used with care because of the proximity of the optic nerve. Radiation is not always effective in even palliative treatment of tumors and may destroy normal tissue. For ACTH-secreting adenomas, such as lung tumors, palliation is possible. Radiation therapy is commonly used concurrently with surgical or pharmacologic management to enhance its effectiveness and reduce long-term side effects.

ADRENAL BLOCKING AGENTS. Medications that interfere with ACTH production or adrenal hormone synthesis are available. Mitotane (Lysodren) is a cytotoxic antihormonal agent that inhibits corticosteroid synthesis without destroying cortical cells. Aminoglutethimide (Cytadren) and trilostane (Modrastane) are other cytotoxic agents that block the synthesis of glucocorticoids and adrenal steroids.

ACTH-REDUCING AGENTS. Cyproheptadine (Periactin), bromocriptine, or somatostatin is used to treat hypersecretion caused by pituitary abnormalities and resulting in increased ACTH levels. These agents appear to interfere with ACTH production, thereby reducing the effect on the adrenals.

TABLE 44-5	THERAPIES FOR CUSHING'S SYNDROME, CUSHING'S DISEASE, AND ECTOPIC ACTH SYNDROME		
Condition	**Responsible Lesion**	**Therapies**	**Remarks**
Cushing's syndrome	Adrenal tumor (benign or malignant)	Adrenalectomy	Adrenalectomy for benign unilateral tumor; usually curative Bilateral adrenalectomy must be followed by lifelong administration of corticosteroids
	Adrenal carcinoma with widespread metastases	Surgery and chemotherapy (mitotane)	Chemotherapy largely unsuccessful
Cushing's disease	Pituitary tumor (or unidentified lesion) that secretes excessive amounts of ACTH	Microsurgical resection of pituitary adenoma	Pituitary surgery successful in 95% of cases
		Irradiation of pituitary gland	Irradiation successful in 75% of cases; therapeutic effects not apparent for months after initiation of therapy
		Total bilateral adrenalectomy (corrects adrenal hyperplasia caused by excessive ACTH stimulation)	Total bilateral adrenalectomy must be followed by lifelong replacement therapy with glucocorticoid and mineralocorticoid
Ectopic ACTH syndrome	Extra-adrenal malignant tumor	Surgical removal of ectopic malignant tumor; chemotherapy used to control hypercortisolism and promote remission in clients with inoperable cancer	Surgery rarely successful because metastasis usually occurs before diagnosis; chemotherapy purely palliative

ACTH, adrenocorticotropic hormone.

Self-Care

The client with a bilateral adrenalectomy needs to learn self-care, because lifelong glucocorticoid replacement is essential. If only one adrenal gland has been removed, daily cortisol replacement continues until the remaining gland functions normally (usually after 6 to 12 months). Before discharge, the client and significant others need instruction on self-administration of replacement hormones (hydrocortisone). They should successfully demonstrate the injection technique before discharge. The client should also be able to repeat and comply with instructions and to remain free from addisonian crisis or adrenal insufficiency.

Modifications for Elderly Clients

Older clients may exhibit excessive manifestations of Cushing's syndrome because these clients may already have osteoporosis, hypertension, and diabetes. Older clients are also more susceptible to the side effects of steroid replacement therapy.

HYPERALDOSTERONISM

Aldosterone is the most powerful of the mineralocorticoids. Its primary role is to conserve sodium, and it also promotes potassium excretion. The incidence of primary hyperaldosteronism in the hypertensive population is unknown, affecting approximately 1%. It affects women twice as often as men and appears most frequently in the middle-aged.

Etiology and Risk Factors

Primary hyperaldosteronism refers to hypersecretion of aldosterone resulting from an adrenal lesion, which is usually benign. The disease, which produces secondary hypertension, hypokalemia (in most), and hypernatremia, is also known as *Conn's syndrome.*

Secondary hyperaldosteronism results from a variety of conditions that cause overproduction of aldosterone. These conditions include sodium-wasting renal disease, laxative or diuretic abuse, dehydration, cirrhosis with ascites, heart failure, and a decrease in intravascular volume. Hypertension is uncommon.

There are no particular risk factors for primary hyperaldosteronism. Risk factors for secondary hyperaldosteronism include chronic heart failure, cirrhosis with ascites, nephrotic syndrome, and hypertension caused by destructive renal artery disease. Health promotion measures, therefore, are successful treatment and control of the causative disease process. The more successfully these factors are controlled, the less secondary hyperaldosteronism is present.

Pathophysiology

Aldosterone affects tubular reabsorption of sodium and water and excretion of potassium and hydrogen ions in the renal tubular epithelial cells (Fig. 44–4). These effects lead to the development of hypernatremia, hypervolemia, hypokalemia, and metabolic alkalosis. With hypervolemia and hypernatremia, BP increases, often to very high levels, and renin production is suppressed. The hypertension can lead to cerebral infarcts and renal damage.

Secondary hyperaldosteronism is a result of continuous secretion of aldosterone secondary to high levels of angiotensin II, resulting from high plasma renin activity. Decreased renal perfusion of a variety of causes is the underlying mechanism.

Clinical Manifestations

Clients with primary hyperaldosteronism may be asymptomatic, but incidental findings include hypertension, hypernatremia, and hypokalemia. Without intervention, all of the complications of chronic hypertension, such as visual disturbances, heart failure, renal damage, and cerebrovascular accident, may occur. Unfortunately, the renal complications resulting from long-term hypertension tend to be progressive. Therefore, clients with primary hyperaldosteronism need to be identified and treated early in the course of the disease.

Hypokalemia results from excessive urinary excretion of potassium ions. This problem, in turn, causes muscle weakness, paralysis, or cardiac dysrhythmias, because potassium loss reduces normal neuromuscular irritability. In addition, excessive potassium excretion results in polyuria. The large urinary output leads to polydipsia (excessive thirst). Finally, hypokalemia leads to metabolic alkalosis because of shifting of hydrogen ions into the cells in exchange for potassium and exchange of hydrogen ions in the tubular cells for sodium ions from the tubular urine. Metabolic alkalosis causes a decrease in ionized calcium levels, which can result in tetany and respiratory suppression.

Despite sodium retention, clients with hyperaldosteronism rarely develop overt edema. Although extracellular fluid increases moderately, excessive water is normally excreted in the urine with potassium ions. Over time, the kidneys tend to adjust physiologically to excessive secretion of aldosterone, and water excretion reaches an equilibrium with sodium intake. The kidneys' eventual "escape" from the sodium-retaining and water-retaining action of aldosterone is sometimes called the *escape phenomenon.*

The diagnosis of primary hyperaldosteronism is based on low serum potassium levels, alkalosis, and elevated urinary or plasma aldosterone levels with low plasma renin levels (elevated in secondary hyperaldosteronism). In addition, radiographic studies may reveal cardiac hypertrophy resulting from chronic hypertension. Radionuclide scanning techniques using radiolabeled iodocholesterol allow visualization of the tumors.

Outcome Management

▪ Surgical Management

Surgery is the treatment of choice for the client with primary hyperaldosteronism. A unilateral or bilateral adrenalectomy must be performed. A client undergoing a unilateral adrenalectomy may need temporary replacement of glucocorticoids. A client who requires a bilateral adrenalectomy needs permanent replacement (see Addison's Disease). Clients usually receive glucocorticoids preoperatively to prevent adrenal hypofunction. In two thirds of the cases, removal of the aldosterone-secreting tumor completely resolves the hypertension, hypokalemia, and hypernatremia. Most clients have normal BP readings by the third postoperative month.

▪ Nursing Management of the Surgical Client

Help prepare the client for the diagnostic assessment so that the diagnosis of hyperaldosteronism can be achieved rapidly and the treatment performed before permanent damage occurs. Administer prescribed medications, and closely monitor the client for hypertension or renal damage. Preoperative and postoperative management is the same as that described for hypercortisolism.

Discharge planning must include client education about a low-sodium diet, medications, and manifestations of hypokalemia if the client is to be medically treated. The client should also understand the disease process and manifestations.

▪ Medical Management

A client who cannot be treated surgically may receive spironolactone (Aldactone) to increase sodium excretion and to treat the hypertension and hypokalemia. Hypertension may take 4 to 8 weeks to correct. Potassium levels should be carefully monitored for the development of

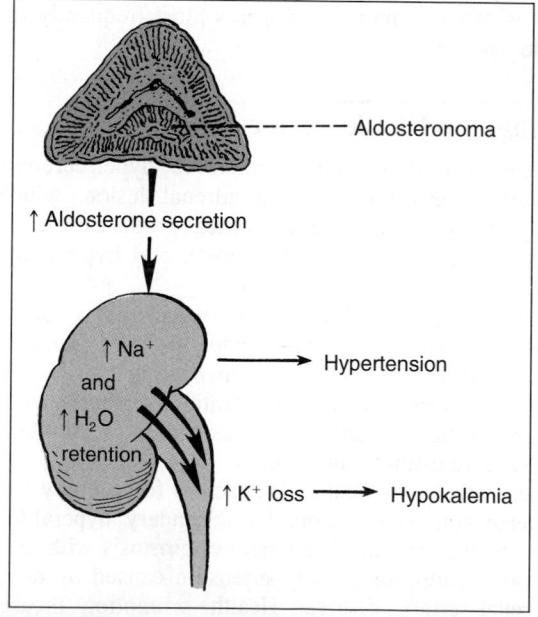

FIGURE 44–4 Effects of primary aldosteronism. Excessive aldosterone secretion causes increased sodium (Na^+) and water (H_2O) retention and increased excretion of potassium (K^+).

Labels in figure: Aldosteronoma; ↑ Aldosterone secretion; ↑Na^+ and ↑H_2O retention; Hypertension; ↑K^+ loss → Hypokalemia hyperkalemia, especially if the client has been receiving potassium supplements or a high-potassium diet (Box 44–1). Amiloride is the drug of choice for clients who cannot tolerate spironolactone.

■ Nursing Management of the Medical Client

Assess the client's ability to manage the complex therapeutic regimen. Plan and implement a teaching program for self-care.

ADRENOMEDULLARY DISORDERS

Two important tumors occur in the adrenal medulla: *pheochromocytoma,* a tumor that causes hyperactivity of the gland, and *neuroblastoma,* a malignant tumor made up of cells resembling a neuroblast. For a complete description of neuroblastoma, an important tumor in children, consult a pediatric textbook.

PHEOCHROMOCYTOMA

A pheochromocytoma is a catecholamine-secreting tumor of the chromaffin cells of the sympathetic nervous system that is usually found in the adrenal medulla. Pheochromocytomas are rare. In autopsy series, the incidence of pheochromocytoma is 0.1% in clients with diastolic hypertension. The condition is equally common in women and men. Although the disease can occur at any age, it is most common in middle age and rarely occurs after age 60 years.

Etiology and Risk Factors

The cause of pheochromocytomas is unknown. In some cases, they appear to have a familial basis. They often occur together with neuroectodermal diseases and with multiple endocrine neoplasia type IIA. There are no known risk factors for pheochromocytoma.

Pathophysiology

Usually weighing less than 200 g, a pheochromocytoma is composed of chromaffin cells, so named (Latin *affinis,*

affinitas, affinity) because these cells stain brownish yellow with chromic salts. In 85% to 95% of cases, pheochromocytomas arise within the adrenal medulla. Occasionally, however, they develop from the chromaffin tissues found in the sympathetic paraganglia. Pheochromocytomas are typically benign; fewer than 10% are malignant. Because of the excessive amounts of epinephrine and norepinephrine they secrete, they can produce severe manifestations and even death (Table 44–6).

Once a pheochromocytoma is diagnosed, certain risk

TABLE 44–6	THE EFFECTS OF EPINEPHRINE AND NOREPINEPHRINE	
Epinephrine	**Norepinephrine**	
CARDIOVASCULAR SYSTEM		
Constricts superficial blood vessels; in small doses, dilates muscle, brain, and coronary vessels, thus shunting blood supply to organs; essential for "fight or flight"	Constricts blood vessels (especially peripheral), causing increased peripheral resistance	
Raises blood pressure	Raises blood pressure greatly	
Increases cardiac output	Decreases cardiac output because of increased peripheral resistance	
Increases pulse dramatically	Increases pulse moderately	
Constricts spleen, shunting stored red blood cells into general circulation		
Increases coagulability of blood		
RESPIRATORY SYSTEM		
Increases rate and depth of respirations		
Dilates bronchi		
NERVOUS SYSTEM		
Stimulates central nervous system, increasing alertness and producing a feeling of fright, excitation, and impending doom		
Dilates pupils	Dilates pupils	
Inhibits gastrointestinal tract	Inhibits gastrointestinal tract	
METABOLISM		
Increases nonesterified fatty acid level of blood	Increases nonesterified fatty acid level of blood	
Promotes conversion of glycogen to glucose		
Increases body metabolism	Increases body metabolism slightly	

Data from DeGroot, L. (Ed.). (1995). *Endocrinology* (3rd ed.). Philadelphia: W. B. Saunders.

factors are known to influence catecholamine release. Catecholamine release occurs with various frequencies and intensities and is called a *paroxysm*. Risk factors that may stimulate a paroxysm include:

- Smoking
- Micturition (voiding reflex)
- Activities that displace abdominal organs, such as bending, exercising, straining, vigorous palpation of the abdomen, and pregnancy
- Certain drugs, such as histamines, anesthetics, atropine, opiates, fentanyl, steroids, and glucagon

Without early intervention, the client is at risk for cerebral hemorrhage and cardiac failure. If a pheochromocytoma is discovered early in its development, it can usually be removed surgically.

Clinical Manifestations

A client with pheochromocytoma may present with manifestations of diabetes mellitus (elevated blood glucose and glucosuria), hypertension (elevated BP, headaches), hyperthyroidism (increased metabolic rate, diaphoresis, agitation, rapid pulse, palpitations, emotional outbursts), and psychoneurosis (emotional instability).

Hypertension is the principal manifestation of pheochromocytoma and can be persistent, fluctuating, intermittent, or paroxysmal (rapid onset and abrupt cessation). Typically, the client has episodes of high BP accompanied by pounding headaches. Other manifestations of sympathetic overactivity include sweating, apprehension, palpitations, nausea, and vomiting. Excessive release of catecholamines also results in excessive conversion of glycogen into glucose in the liver. Consequently, hyperglycemia and glucosuria occur during attacks. Such manifestations can develop spontaneously or may be precipitated by emotional stress, physical exertion, or change in body position.

Acute attacks may be associated with profuse diaphoresis (perspiration), dilated pupils, and cold extremities. Severe hypertension can precipitate a cerebrovascular accident or sudden blindness.

Because pheochromocytoma is curable, early and accurate diagnosis is essential. Current methods of diagnosis include the following:

1. *History and physical examination.* The client may describe symptomatic attacks over weeks, months, or even years. The BP may change with exertion or emotional upset. In long-standing cases, complications of intractable hypertension (such as visual disturbances), manifestations of heart disease (dyspnea, edema), and manifestations of kidney damage (albuminuria, proteinuria, and increased blood urea nitrogen) can coexist.

2. *Chemical tests* of urinary catecholamines and their metabolites (metanephrines and vanillylmandelic acid [VMA]) and of plasma catecholamine concentrations. Assays of catecholamines are performed on single-voided urine specimens, 2- to 4-hour specimens, and 24-hour urine specimens. The normal range of urinary catecholamines is up to 14 mg per 100 ml of urine, with higher levels occurring in clients with pheochromocytoma. Assays of urinary VMA levels are performed only on 24-hour urine specimens. Advise the client to avoid tea, chocolate, vanilla, and all fruits for at least 2 days before urine collection begins, and remind the client not to take any medications for 2 to 3 days before the test. Normally, the amount of VMA is less than 7 mg in 24 hours. Urinary VMA levels increase in clients with pheochromocytoma. Plasma catecholamine concentrations are also determined.

3. *Direct assay* of catecholamines (epinephrine and norepinephrine) in the blood. The normal ranges of catecholamines in the blood are epinephrine, 0.02 to 0.2 mg/L, and norepinephrine, 0.1 to 0.5 mg/L.

4. *X-ray imaging.* Various radiographic techniques, such as CT and MRI, can help confirm and identify adrenomedullary tumor location.

5. *Nonspecific laboratory tests.* In the presence of pheochromocytoma, the basal metabolic rate increases, blood glucose rises to abnormal levels, and glycosuria can occur.

Outcome Management

▇ Surgical Management

ADRENALECTOMY

INDICATIONS. The primary treatment of a pheochromocytoma is surgical removal of one or both adrenal glands, depending on whether the tumor is unilateral or bilateral. The procedure is the same as that described for Cushing's syndrome.

CONTRAINDICATIONS. The presence of complications of pheochromocytoma may make the client a poor surgical risk. Ideally, surgery is performed before complications develop. However, high BP and vascular complications may necessitate treatment before surgery can take place. Alpha-adrenergic blocking agents, such as phentolamine (Regitine), can be used in an IV bolus or IV drip for hypertensive crisis. Oral phenoxybenzamine (Dibenzyline) is used at least 7 days preoperatively to control BP, reduce manifestations, and eliminate paroxysms before surgical removal of the affected gland.

Complications associated with pheochromocytoma that may delay surgery include hypertensive retinopathy, hypertensive nephropathy, myocarditis, increased platelet aggregation, cerebrovascular accident, and heart failure. Death may result from myocardial infarction, cerebrovascular accident, dysrhythmias, irreversible shock, renal failure, or dissecting aortic aneurysm.

COMPLICATIONS. The surgical procedure for pheochromocytoma is not without danger. There are two serious hazards. First, excessive discharge of pressor hormones during induction of anesthesia or manipulation of the tumor can cause extreme rises in BP and cardiac dysrhythmias. Second, after resection of the tumor, BP can fall precipitously.

OUTCOMES. Surgical removal of the pheochromocytoma can be curative in most cases, if the growth is discovered before cardiovascular damage becomes permanent. Some clients may receive less medication at discharge after surgery. Lifelong steroid replacement must be initiated after a bilateral adrenalectomy.

Nursing Management of the Surgical Client

PREOPERATIVE CARE

ASSESSMENT

Assess and control the client's BP preoperatively. Closely monitor the client for the development of stressful episodes before treatment has begun. Evaluate the client's neurologic status in case the client has a stroke because of the extremely elevated BP.

DIAGNOSIS, OUTCOMES, INTERVENTIONS

Risk for Injury. The client with a pheochromocytoma is at great risk for injury preoperatively. Write the nursing diagnosis *Risk for Injury related to excessive release of epinephrine and norepinephrine preoperatively.*

Outcomes. Injury will not occur or will be detected early, as evidenced by absence of hypertensive episodes and cardiovascular or cerebral damage.

Interventions. During the preoperative phase, the desired outcome of treatment is preventing attacks of acute paroxysmal hypertension, thereby lowering the risk of further damage to the cardiovascular system. Important nursing interventions include (1) promoting rest and relief from stress; (2) administering prescribed sedatives; (3) providing a diet high in vitamins, minerals, and calories; (4) prohibiting beverages containing caffeine, such as coffee, tea, and colas; and (5) monitoring vital signs. In most cases, the physician prescribes an alpha-adrenergic blocking agent, such as phenoxybenzamine.

POSTOPERATIVE CARE

ASSESSMENT

The first 24 to 48 hours after surgery is a critical period demanding vigilant nursing assessment. After surgery, the client should be closely monitored for adrenal insufficiency, hypotension, hemorrhage, and shock. Urine output and BP are assessed hourly.

DIAGNOSIS, OUTCOMES, INTERVENTIONS

Risk for Injury. The client is at increased risk for such problems as hypotension postoperatively. Write the nursing diagnosis as *Risk for Injury related to postoperative hypotension, hemorrhage, and shock.*

Outcomes. Injury will not occur or will be detected early, as evidenced by a normotensive state and an absence of hemorrhage, shock, or addisonian crisis.

Interventions

Monitor and Prevent Shock. During the immediate postoperative period, observe for manifestations of shock and hemorrhage. After removal of the tumor, profound shock can develop as catecholamine levels drop. Hypotension can persist for 24 to 48 hours. Hemorrhage can occur because of the high vascularity of the adrenal glands. To prevent postoperative shock, do the following:

1. Give IV fluids as prescribed, such as blood, plasma, dextran, or glucose in water to maintain blood volume.
2. Administer IV pressors as prescribed at a rate sufficient to maintain BP within a safe range. Check BP as often as necessary to titrate the medication.
3. Carefully measure hourly urinary output. If the client voids less than ½ ml/kg/hr, notify the physician.

Oliguria can signify impending shock and consequent renal shutdown.

4. Assess the client for manifestations of hemorrhage. Check the dressing every half-hour for bloody drainage. If the client is bleeding internally, an abdominal hematoma can develop, resulting in paralytic ileus or nonmechanical bowel obstruction (see Chapter 33). Manifestations of paralytic ileus include abdominal pain, distention, severe nausea, vomiting, and diminished or absent bowel sounds.
5. If cortical tissue has been resected during surgery, assess the client closely for manifestations of adrenal insufficiency (see Addisonian Crisis). If both adrenal glands have been removed, the client must receive cortisol replacement for life.

Pain. Postoperatively, the client must be monitored for *Pain related to surgery, headache, and other manifestations of pheochromocytoma resulting in verbal reports of pain and guarding behaviors.*

Outcomes. The client will not have pain, as evidenced by the client's statements, normotensive state, and an absence of pained expressions.

Interventions. When administering medication for incisional pain, monitor BP frequently. Although narcotics, particularly meperidine, produce hypotension as a side effect, withholding pain medication can also lead to hypotension (or even hypertension) and severe pain. It is important to control the pain so that the client's level of stress decreases.

EVALUATION

It is expected that the client will have no complications postoperatively or that complications that occur will be managed successfully so that the client is discharged within 4 to 5 days postoperatively. Self-care outcomes are evaluated by the client's ability to manage steroid replacement after surgery. Although side effects of steroids cannot be avoided, there are ways to minimize them, and the client's ability to control these and avoid complications can be evaluated.

Self-Care

After a bilateral adrenalectomy, the client must learn self-care measures. When the critical postoperative period is over, most clients experience an uneventful convalescence. A client who will be self-administering corticosteroids needs instruction concerning the administration and side effects (see Addison's Disease).

Modification for Elderly Clients

Damage related to hypertensive episodes associated with the pheochromocytoma tends to affect older clients, whose cardiovascular and cerebrovascular systems may be weak and thus susceptible to damage by elevated BP.

ANTERIOR PITUITARY DISORDERS

Disorders of the pituitary gland occur most frequently in the anterior lobe (Table 44–7; see also Fig. 44–2). Major causes of pituitary disease include functioning tumors, nonfunctioning tumors, pituitary infarction, genetic disor-

TABLE 44-7	PITUITARY HORMONES				
Name	Releasing Factor	Target Cells	Response	Increased Level	Decreased Level
ANTERIOR PITUITARY					
GH	GHRH	Bone, muscle	Stimulates growth; promotes active transport of amino acids into cell and influences lipid, CHO, and Ca^{2+} metabolism	Child: gigantism (before epiphyseal closure); child grows very tall. Adult: acromegaly (after epiphyseal closure); bones increase in thickness; increase in soft tissue growth	Child: dwarfism Adult: lethargy, increased weight, loss of reproductive function, premature aging
ACTH	CRH	Adrenal cortex	Stimulates adrenal gland secretion of mineralocorticoids and glucocorticoids	Cushing's disease: increased amounts of cortisol and aldosterone	Addison's disease: decreased cortisol and aldosterone, increased MSH
TSH	TRH	Thyroid	Stimulates thyroid to increase secretion of thyroxine (controls rate of most chemical reactions in body)	Goiter; increased BMR; decreased weight; increased cardiac output, HR, and BP; increased cerebration; fine muscle tremors	Reduced thyroid activity; decreased BMR; increased weight; decreased cardiac output, HR, and BP; decreased cerebration; somnolence
Prolactin		Breast	Stimulates breast to lactate	Amenorrhea	Too little milk
FSH	LHRH	Ovaries, testes	Stimulates growth of ovaries and sperm		Late puberty
LH	LHRH	Ovaries, testes	Stimulates growth of follicles and increased secretion of estrogen and progesterone; increases testosterone secretion in the male	Excess testosterone, menstrual cycle disturbance	Amenorrhea; diminished progesterone and testosterone
POSTERIOR PITUITARY					
Oxytocin	Labor, sucking	Uterus, breasts	Stimulates uterus to contract at childbirth; stimulates lactation	Precipitates childbirth, excess milk	Prolonged childbirth, diminished milk
ADH (vasopressin)	Dehydration	Arterioles, distal renal tubule	Vasoconstricts arterioles to increase arterial pressure; increases water reabsorption in distal tubules, stimulates smooth muscle of gastrointestinal tract	Increased BP, decreased urinary output, edema	Diabetes insipidus, dilute urine, increased urinary volume

ACTH, adrenocorticotropic hormone; ADH, antidiuretic hormone; BP, blood pressure; BMR, basal metabolic rate; CHO, carbohydrate; CRH, corticotropin-releasing hormone; FSH, follicle-stimulating hormone; GH, growth hormone; GHRH, growth hormone–releasing hormone; HR, heart rate; LH, luteinizing hormone; LHRH, luteinizing hormone–releasing hormone; MSH, melanocyte-stimulating hormone; TRH, thyrotropin-releasing hormone; TSH, thyroid-stimulating hormone.

Data from DeGroot, L. (Ed.). (1995). *Endocrinology* (3rd ed.). Philadelphia: W. B. Saunders.

ders, and trauma. The three principal pathologic consequences of pituitary disorders are (1) hyperpituitarism, (2) hypopituitarism, and (3) local compression of brain tissue by expanding tumor masses.

HYPERPITUITARISM AND HYPERPROLACTINEMIA

Etiology and Risk Factors

Hyperpituitarism is defined as oversecretion of one or more of the hormones secreted by the pituitary gland. It is caused primarily by a hormone-secreting pituitary tumor, typically a benign adenoma. Syndromes associated with hyperpituitarism are Cushing's syndrome, acromegaly, amenorrhea, galactorrhea, hyperthyroidism, and, rarely, hypergonadism in the male.

Pathophysiology

Prolactin and growth hormone are the hormones most commonly overproduced by adenomas. They lead to hyperprolactinemia and acromegaly (Fig. 44–5), respectively. Increased amounts of growth hormone lead to rapid growth of all body tissues. This increased growth leads to gigantism (Fig. 44–6) if it occurs before closure of the epiphysis and acromegaly if it occurs after epiphyseal closure.

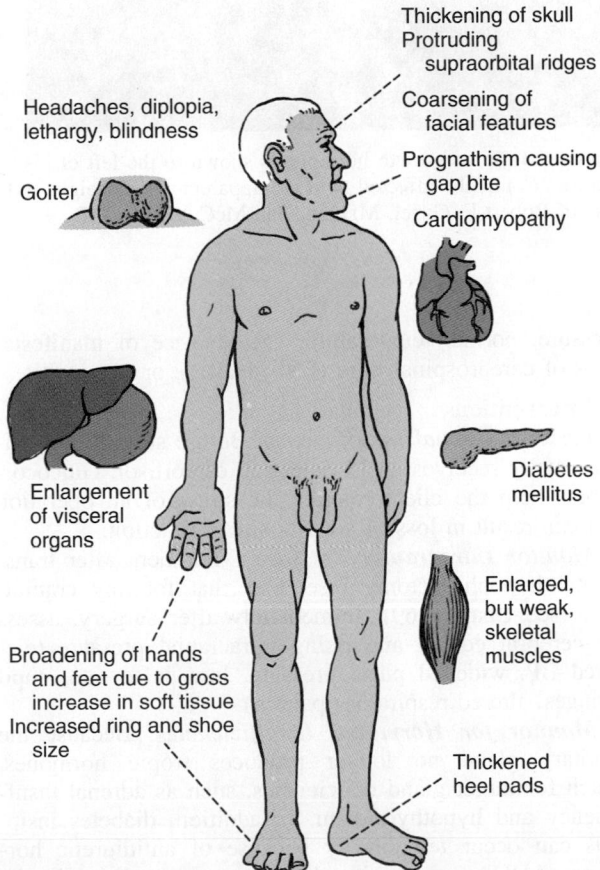

Headaches, diplopia, lethargy, blindness

Goiter

Enlargement of visceral organs

Broadening of hands and feet due to gross increase in soft tissue Increased ring and shoe size

Thickening of skull
Protruding supraorbital ridges

Coarsening of facial features

Prognathism causing gap bite

Cardiomyopathy

Diabetes mellitus

Enlarged, but weak, skeletal muscles

Thickened heel pads

FIGURE 44–5 Assessment data for acromegaly.

Clinical Manifestations

Pituitary tumors produce both systemic and local effects. Systemic effects include excessive or abnormal growth patterns related to overproduction of growth hormone, abnormal milk secretion (galactorrhea), and overstimulation of one or more of the target glands, resulting in release of excessive thyroid, sex, or adrenocortical hormones.

Locally, pituitary tumors produce manifestations because the bony cranium that houses the tumor cannot expand to accommodate a growing mass. Local manifestations include visual field abnormalities resulting from pressure on the optic chiasm, headaches, and somnolence. See Table 44–8 for additional information related to hyperprolactinemia and acromegaly.

Outcome Management

■ Surgical Management

A client with a pituitary tumor must have the tumor resected. A variety of approaches can be used to remove a pituitary tumor. Usually, a transsphenoidal hypophysectomy is performed (see Chapter 69).

■ Nursing Management of the Surgical Client

ASSESSMENT

Most clients are frightened by the prospect of having the pituitary gland removed. Provide the client and significant others with emotional support and comfort throughout the preoperative period.

The initial manifestations are vague; therefore, the client may have seen many physicians and may have had multiple examinations and tests while seeking a diagnosis. The client and family may be fearful, skeptical, or relieved with the final diagnosis of pituitary tumor. Assess the client's reaction to the diagnosis, expectations for the surgery, educational needs related to the diagnosis and treatment plan, and available support network after discharge.

Physical assessment includes baseline vital signs and weight as well as neurologic assessment. The client should also have a preoperative eye examination by an ophthalmologist. These findings are essential to establish a baseline for postoperative comparison. To perform the neurologic assessment, check the following:

- Pupil equality and reactivity to light
- Handgrip for strength, equality, and ability to release on command
- Level of consciousness
- Orientation to time, place, person, and location
- Appropriate response to stimuli
- Visual acuity and visual fields

DIAGNOSIS, OUTCOMES, INTERVENTIONS

Knowledge Deficit. Preoperatively, the client must to be taught about the surgery and its implications. A typical nursing diagnosis would be *Knowledge Deficit: Surgery and possible outcomes related to lack of instruction resulting in anxiety, misinformation, and questions.*

FIGURE 44–6 Primary gigantism. *A,* a 22-year-old man with gigantism due to excess growth hormone is shown to the left of his identical twin. The increased height (*A*), enlarged hand (*B*), and enlarged foot (*C*) of the affected twin are apparent. Their height and features began to diverge at the age of approximately 13 years. (Courtesy of Robert F. Gagel, MD, and Ian McCutcheon, MD, University of Texas M.D. Anderson Cancer Center, Houston, TX.)

Outcomes. The client will understand the planned surgery and possible outcomes as evidenced by his or her statements, questions, and ability to describe the procedure and outcomes.

Interventions. Explain the surgery to the client in detail, along with potential outcomes of surgical treatment. Use drawings of the brain to explain the transsphenoidal approach. Prepare the client for the presence of an indwelling urinary catheter, IV lines, and any other lines or monitors that may be needed after surgery. Tell the client that vital signs will be monitored closely after surgery. Preoperative preparation also includes coaching the client in deep-breathing exercises and assisting in keeping records of intake and output.

Risk for Injury. A typical postoperative nursing diagnosis would be *Risk for Injury related to postoperative complications.*

Outcomes. Injury will not result from surgery as evidenced by absence of addisonian crisis, balanced intake and output, no manifestations of increased intracranial

pressure, normal temperature, and absence of manifestations of cerebrospinal fluid (CSF) leakage or meningitis.

Interventions

Prevent Adrenal Insufficiency. Before surgery, the client usually receives an IV injection of cortisol. Glucocorticoids help the client tolerate the stress of an operation that can result in loss of adrenocortical function.

Monitor Intracranial Pressure. Treatment after transfrontal hypophysectomy resembles that for any craniotomy (see Chapter 69). Immediately after surgery, assess for cerebral edema and rising intracranial pressure (elevated BP, widened pulse pressure, low pulse rate, pupil changes, altered respiratory pattern).

Monitor for Hormonal Insufficiencies. Because the pituitary gland no longer produces tropic hormones, watch for target gland deficiencies, such as adrenal insufficiency and hypothyroidism. In addition, diabetes insipidus can occur temporarily because of antidiuretic hormone (ADH, vasopressin) deficiency, as outlined in the accompanying Critical Monitoring feature. This deficiency

TABLE 44-8   HYPERPROLACTINEMIA AND ACROMEGALY IN HYPERPITUITARISM

	Hyperprolactinemia	Acromegaly
Hormone secreted	Excessive prolactin (PRL) causes prolactinoma	Excessive growth hormone (GH)
Risk factors	Hyperprolactinemia; estrogen therapy; oral contraceptive use; pregnancy may increase tumor size and dysfunction	None
Etiology	Pregnancy; hypothalamic-pituitary disorders; hypothyroidism; drug ingestion (estrogen or oral contraception)	Anterior pituitary adenoma; abnormal hypothalamic function (rare)
Pathophysiology	PRL-producing tumors deliver excess PRL systemically	GH-producing adenomas deliver excess GH systemically, leading to rapid growth in other body tissues (with exception of the CNS) causing organomegaly; increase in tumor size within confined space can result in destruction of entire pituitary and cause hypopituitarism
Clinical manifestations related to hormone oversecretion	Abnormal lactation (galactorrhea) in nonlactating breast; amenorrhea; decreased vaginal lubrication; decreased libido in men; impotence; depression; anxiety; headache; visual loss	Local overgrowth of bone: skull and mandible; soft tissue overgrowth; lethargy; weight gain; paresthesias; glucose intolerance; coarse facial features; irregular or absent menses; enlargement of hands and feet over 1-10 yr; depression; headache; visual field impairment; osteoarthritis; paresthesias; impotence
Complications related to tumor growth	Headaches; visual disturbances affecting cranial nerves III, IV, VI; hypopituitarism; infertility; decreased bone growth	Hypopituitarism; neoplasms of gastrointestinal tract; increased mortality secondary to cardiovascular atherosclerosis, cerebral atherosclerosis, congestive heart failure, respiratory disease, hypertension, diabetes mellitus
Pharmacologic intervention	Bromocriptine is treatment of choice; bromocriptine can reduce PRL levels in 90% of clients; adverse reactions may contribute to noncompliance: nausea, headaches, dizziness, nasal stuffiness, hypotension, depression	Somatostatin analog octreotide is very effective in reducing GH levels; pharmacologic treatment may cause cholelithiasis; bromocriptine is effective in 60%-80% of clients
Surgical intervention	Transsphenoidal microsurgery; complications: residual tissue may produce elevated hormone levels, visual loss, diabetes insipidus, postoperative infection	Transsphenoidal microsurgery is treatment of choice; complications: same as in hyperprolactinemia
Radiation treatment	May decrease adenoma, but local complications are common because of tissue scarring and impairment of anterior pituitary function (hypopituitarism)	Produces slower decline of GH levels, implying higher morbidity related to atherosclerotic disease, respiratory disease, hypertension, diabetes mellitus, and gastrointestinal cancer; hypopituitarism
Diagnosis	Measurement of GH, ACTH, FSH, LH, PRL, testosterone, gonadotropins; thyroid function tests (T_3, T_4, FT_4, TSH); liver function tests (LDH, CPK, AST, alkaline phosphatase), coagulation studies; kidney function tests (serum creatinine, BUN, 24-hr urine collection for protein, creatinine clearance, GFR); urinalysis; pregnancy testing; CT or MRI for pituitary adenoma localization	Radioimmunoassay or enzyme-linked immunosorbent assay for GH level; serum GH level; insulin-like growth factor; CT scan or MRI for pituitary edema localization; oral GTT may demonstrate hyperglycemia; usually, GTT suppresses normal GH release 1-2 hr after ingestion, but in acromegaly the GH level remains elevated

ACTH, adrenocorticotropic hormone; AST, aspartate aminotransferase; BUN, blood urea nitrogen; CNS, central nervous system; CPK, creatine phosphokinase; CT, computed tomography; FSH, follicle-stimulating hormone; FT_4, free thyroxine; GFR, glomerular filtration rate, GH, growth hormone; GTT, glucose tolerance test; LDH, lactate dehydrogenase; LH, luteinizing hormone; MRI, magnetic resonance imaging; PRL, prolactin; TSH, thyroid-stimulating hormone; T_3, triiodothyronine; T_4, thyroxine.

is related to surgical manipulation. Maintain strict documentation of intake and output. Notify the physician if urine output is above 200 ml/hr with a specific gravity below 1.005.

Monitor for Meningitis. Assess the client carefully for meningitis, a potential complication of surgery. Report any temperature elevation, severe headache, irritability, or nuchal rigidity.

Provide Oral Hygiene. The client who has undergone transsphenoidal hypophysectomy requires frequent oral hygiene with a gauze sponge; the lips should be lubricated with petroleum jelly. The client should not brush the teeth for 2 weeks after surgery.

Monitor for CSF Drainage. The nasal packing is usually removed in 2 to 5 days. After its removal, observe the client for rhinorrhea, which can indicate a CSF leak.

CRITICAL MONITORING

Does Your Client Have an Antidiuretic Hormone (ADH) Imbalance?

	Diabetes Insipidus	Syndrome of Inappropriate Secretion of Antidiuretic Hormone
ADH	↓	↑
Urine output	↑	↓
Urine osmolality	↓	↑
Urine specific gravity	↓	Value insignificant
Serum Na⁺	↑	↓
Urine Na⁺	↓	↑
Plasma osmolality	↑	↓
Daily weights	↓	Sudden ↑ (without edema)
Mentation changes	Related to electrolyte imbalance and hypotension	Related to degree of hyponatremia

Have the client report frequent postnasal drainage. Collect any serous drainage, and test it for the presence of CSF (see Chapter 67) or send it to the laboratory for analysis. It is possible for the muscle or fat graft to dislodge, causing a CSF leak. Instruct the client to avoid sneezing, coughing, and bending over from the waist to avoid disrupting the graft.

EVALUATION

Appropriate outcomes after a hypophysectomy include the absence of postoperative complications and the client's ability to manage lifetime hormone replacement. If complications occur, appropriate outcomes are that these are controlled without permanent problems.

■ Self-Care

After a hypophysectomy, the client must take replacement hormones for life. Instruct the client to avoid gastric irritation by taking cortisone with milk, food, or an antacid. Advise the client to notify the physician about gastritis, tarry stools, or frank blood in the stools. Some clients may also require thyroid or sex hormone replacement. In addition, some need vasopressin replacement to treat *diabetes insipidus*. As a result of deficient ADH, clients may experience polyuria (large urine output) and low urine specific gravity readings. Diabetes insipidus is usually transient after surgery but can persist, indicating the need for chronic hormone replacement.

SEXUAL DISTURBANCES

Excess secretion of gonadotropic hormones, such as luteinizing hormone (LH) and follicle-stimulating hormone (FSH), from pituitary tumors can produce sexual precocity in children. Excess prolactin secretion can cause amenorrhea or galactorrhea (excessive flow of milk) in women. Physicians consider surgical removal the treatment of choice for radiologically demonstrable tumors.

Clients with increased prolactin secretion and no radiologic or neurologic evidence of a pituitary tumor often respond to bromocriptine, an ergot-like compound. Cli-

ents with prolactinomas can be successfully treated with bromocriptine. A dopamine agonist, bromocriptine inhibits prolactin secretion. Surgery is no longer the treatment of choice in most cases.

HYPOPITUITARISM

In contrast to hyperpituitarism, hypopituitarism is a deficiency of one or more of the hormones produced by the anterior lobe of the pituitary. When both the anterior and posterior lobes fail to secrete hormones, the condition is called *panhypopituitarism*. Hypopituitarism and panhypopituitarism are rare disorders.

Etiology and Risk Factors

The nine most important causes of hypopituitarism are known as the "nine Is":

- Invasion (most common)—pituitary tumors, central nervous system tumors, carotid aneurysm
- Infarction—postpartum necrosis (Sheehan's syndrome), pituitary apoplexy
- Infiltration—sarcoidosis, hemochromatosis
- Injury—head trauma, child abuse
- Immunologic—lymphocytic hypophysitis
- Iatrogenic—surgery, radiation therapy
- Infectious—mycoses, tuberculosis, syphilis
- Idiopathic—familial
- Isolated—deficiency of an anterior pituitary hormone, such as growth hormone, LH, FSH, thyroid-stimulating hormone (TSH), ACTH–lipotropic pituitary hormone (ACTH-LPH), or prolactin

Clinical Manifestations

The pituitary gland has enormous functional reserve; therefore, manifestations of hypopituitarism usually do not appear until 75% of the pituitary has been obliterated by tumor or thrombosis. Manifestations depend on age of onset as well as the hormones that are deficient. The onset of hypopituitarism is usually gradual. The classic course of progressive hypopituitarism is an initial loss of growth hormone and gonadotropin, followed by deficiencies of TSH, then ACTH, and finally prolactin.

Specific disorders resulting from pituitary hyposecretion include:

- *Short stature.* Severely stunted growth results from either a congenital lack of growth hormone or the development of a space-occupying intracranial tumor, meningitis, or brain injury during early childhood.
- *Sexual and reproductive disorders.* Deficiencies of the gonadotropins (LH and FSH) can produce sterility, diminished sex drive, and decreased secondary sex characteristics. Decreased FSH and LH lead to infertility and amenorrhea, diminished spermatogenesis, and testicular atrophy.
- *Hypothyroidism.* Because the synthesis of thyroid hormone depends on TSH, therapeutic ablation or pathologic destruction of the pituitary gland causes hypothyroidism unless the client receives thyroid hormone (see Chapter 43).
- *Secondary adrenocortical insufficiency.* Adrenal insufficiency can follow diminished synthesis of ACTH by the pituitary gland, which, in turn, causes diminished secretion of adrenocortical hormones by the adrenal cortex (see Fig. 44–2).
- *Prolactin deficiency.* This deficiency is indicated by absence of lactation in the postpartum woman.

Diagnosis of growth hormone deficiency rests on the inability of stimulating agents—such as levodopa, arginine, and insulin—to increase plasma growth hormone levels. ACTH levels can be measured to diagnose secondary adrenal insufficiency. Cortisol levels are low in both primary and secondary hypothyroidism; however, when it is a primary deficiency, ACTH levels are high. In a client with secondary hypopituitarism, ACTH levels are low. Low serum thyroid hormone levels, together with low serum TSH levels, establish the diagnosis of hypothyroidism. Sexual and reproductive disorders are diagnosed by low levels of sex steroids and low levels of plasma FSH and LH. Skull x-ray studies may reveal enlargement of the sella turcica, erosion of the sphenoid bone, or calcification of a suprasellar mass. CT or MRI may provide an enhanced view of an x-ray finding.

Outcome Management

Treatment of hypopituitarism involves removal, if possible, of the causative factor (such as a tumor) and permanent replacement of the hormones secreted by the target organs.

■ Medical Management

Injections of human growth hormone successfully treat growth hormone deficiency. Previously, human growth hormone was scarce and available for only a few clients. Now it is produced by recombinant deoxyribonucleic acid (DNA) technology and is readily available. Medications prescribed to replace hormones include corticosteroids to correct secondary adrenocortical insufficiency, thyroid hormone to treat myxedema, and sex hormones to correct hypogonadism.

Assessment of the client with hypopituitarism focuses on target organs that depend on pituitary secretions (see specific disorders such as Addison's disease and hypothyroidism). Nursing interventions are also directed at problems resulting from deficiency at the target organ. See the appropriate secretions for specific interventions.

POSTERIOR LOBE (NEUROHYPOPHYSEAL) DISORDERS

Unlike the adenohypophysis, the neurohypophysis is rarely destroyed by disease. Even if the posterior lobe becomes damaged or is surgically destroyed with the anterior lobe, hormonal deficiencies usually do not develop because the hypothalamus continues to synthesize oxytocin and ADH. If the hypothalamus suffers damage, however, deficiencies of oxytocin and ADH develop even if the neurohypophysis is healthy and intact.

The major disorder of the posterior lobe is ADH deficiency, also known as diabetes insipidus (Fig. 44–7). Excessive ADH causes a condition called the *syndrome of inappropriate antidiuretic hormone* (SIADH), which can occur with lung cancer, head injuries, cranial surgery, pituitary tumors, encephalitis, poliomyelitis, and myxedema. Table 44–9 compares diabetes insipidus and SIADH.

GONADAL DISORDERS

Testicular dysfunction can be primary, a disorder of testicular function, or secondary to a disorder of hypothalamic-pituitary function. Primary testis dysfunction can involve the seminiferous tubules (germ cells or Sertoli's cells), Leydig's cells, or both. Germ cell abnormalities cause infertility by disrupting spermatogenesis. Secondary sexual development and virilization are normal because testosterone production is not interrupted. When Leydig cell function is impaired, testosterone production falls, and virilization is impaired.

Causes of primary hypogonadism include genetic defects, malnutrition, trauma, infection, renal failure, radiation, chemotherapy, and environmental toxins (such as lead or alcohol). The cause, however, is usually unknown. Klinefelter's syndrome, caused by a chromosomal anomaly with a 47,XXY chromosome constitution, is an example of a genetic disorder causing primary testicular failure.

Secondary testicular dysfunction is frequently referred to as *hypogonadotropic hypogonadism* and results from inadequate secretion of gonadotropins. This complication leads to infertility and hypoandrogenism. The extent of LH and FSH deficiency and the age of onset determine clinical manifestations. Prepubertal hypogonadism leads to eunuchoid body proportions (resulting from deficiency in male hormones), small testes, and lack of virilization.

Causes of secondary hypogonadism include hypothalamic or pituitary tumors, trauma, degenerative lesions, and radiation. Kallmann's syndrome, involving a deficiency of gonadotropin-releasing hormone (GRH) production by the hypothalamus, is an example of congenital secondary testicular dysfunction. People with Kallmann's syndrome do not mature normally because of gonadotro-

TABLE 44–9 COMPARISON OF DIABETES INSIPIDUS AND SYNDROME OF INAPPROPRIATE SECRETION OF ANTIDIURETIC HORMONE

	Diabetes Insipidus (DI)	Syndrome of Inappropriate Secretion of Antidiuretic Hormone (SIADH)
Definition	A deficiency of antidiuretic hormone (ADH, vasopressin) results in inability to conserve water	Excessive amounts of ADH secreted from posterior pituitary and other ectopic sources
Incidence	Unknown; DI idiopathic in about 30% of all clients with DI; tumors can be related to 25% of DI cases; head injury accounts for 16%; cranial surgery for 20% of DI cases	Approximately 80% of clients with small cell carcinoma have evidence of impaired ability to excrete water secondary to ectopic production of vasopressin
Etiology	Central CI or neurogenic DI: CNS interruption of anatomic integrity of posterior pituitary; localized or generalized edema from head trauma, vascular lesions, centrally acting drugs, or CNS infections may also cause central DI; ADH synthesis or release is affected; may be transient or permanent Complete DI occurs when there is disruption of hypophyseal tract and a complete absence of ADH Nephrogenic DI: rare hereditary disorder; acquired structural or functional change in kidney occurs; ADH produced normally, but distal and collecting tubules cannot respond Idiopathic DI	Ectopic production of vasopressin by malignancy is most common cause (degree of vasopressin impairment is relative to extent of malignant disease); see Risk factors below
Risk factors	Head injury, neurosurgery, hypothalamic tumors, pituitary tumors, brain infections or inflammation; drugs that inhibit vasopressin release: ethanol, glucocorticoids, adrenergic agents, phenytoin, narcotic antagonists, lithium	Vasopressin overuse (from DI); malignant conditions that may contain ectopic sources of vasopressin-like hormone: bronchogenic carcinoma; lymphoma of duodenum, brain, bladder; pancreatic cancer; prostatic cancer; increased intracranial pressure secondary to infectious processes or brain trauma; infectious processes—viral or bacterial pneumonia; drugs that may stimulate vasopressin release: vincristine, cyclophosphamide, thiazides, phenothiazides, carbamazepine, vinblastine, cisplatin, oxytocin; endocrine disorders: adrenal insufficiency, myxedema, anterior pituitary insufficiency; analgesics; vomiting
Pathophysiology: normally ADH increases kidneys' permeability to water to promote water reabsorption and decrease urine output; ADH is normally released in response to: ↑ serum osmolality and ↓ extracellular volume	With ADH deficiency: permeability of water is diminished resulting in excretion of large volumes of hypotonic fluid Three patterns may develop: (1) transient DI—abrupt onset within first few days after neurosurgery, resolves within several days; (2) permanent DI (prolonged DI)—abrupt and early onset, persists for several weeks or forever, usually occurs after damage to hypothalamus or neurohypophyseal stalk; (3) triphasic DI—immediate postinjury increase in urine volume with decrease in urine osmolality lasting 4–5 days; interphase occurs over next 5–7 days when urine volume decreases to normal and is followed by a permanent phase of polyuria	Key features of ADH excess: (1) water retention, (2) hyponatremia, (3) hypo-osmolality; a continual release of ADH causes water retention from renal tubules and collecting ducts; extracellular fluid volume increases with dilutional hyponatremia; hyponatremia suppresses renin and aldosterone secretions causing a decrease in proximal tubule reabsorption of Na^+
Physical examination	Integumentary: dry, cool skin, dry mucous membranes Cardiovascular: tachycardia Physical manifestations related to specific electrolyte imbalance	Physical manifestations related to hyponatremia: decreased deep tendon reflexes, fatigue, headache, anorexia, nausea, decreased mental status, seizures, coma Physical manifestations related to fluid volume excess: weight gain without edema, jugular venous distention, tachycardia, tachypnea, rales

TABLE 44–9	COMPARISON OF DIABETES INSIPIDUS AND SYNDROME OF INAPPROPRIATE SECRETION OF ANTIDIURETIC HORMONE *Continued*

	Diabetes Insipidus (DI)	Syndrome of Inappropriate Secretion of Antidiuretic Hormone (SIADH)
Clinical manifestations	Genitourinary: polyuria—a few liters to 18 L/day; clear urine; urinary frequency; nocturia Gastrointestinal: weight loss; polydipsia (if thirst mechanism intact) Integumentary: dry skin and mucous membranes Neurologic: mentation changes as electrolyte imbalance and hypotension worsen	Related to degree of hyponatremia: confusion, lethargy, irritability, seizures, coma Gastrointestinal: decreased motility with anorexia, nausea, vomiting; abrupt weight gain *without edema* of 5%–10%
Complications	Electrolyte imbalance; hypovolemia; hypotension; shock	Seizures; coma; permanent brain damage; disease processes already in progress may be complicated
Diagnosis	Urine: output—a few liters to 18 L/day; specific gravity 1.005; osmolality <200 mOsm/kg H_2O Plasma osmolality ↑ secondary to hypovolemia and dehydration Serum Na^+ ↑ secondary to hypovolemia and dehydration Serum osmolality >290 mOsm/kg H_2O Serum Na^+ ↓ secondary to volume depletion Water deprivation study: positive results Hypertonic saline test: positive for DI if there is little or no ↑ in plasma ADH levels	Serum Na^+ ↓; urine Na^+ ↑; blood urea nitrogen ↑; serum osmolality ↓; urine osmolality ↑; absence of hypotension, hypovolemia, or edematous states; water load test: positive for SIADH, abnormal water excretion; serum Na^+ remains ↓; serum osmolality remains ↓; urine osmolality remains ↑
Surgical management	Hypophysectomy to remove posterior pituitary tumor	None
Medical management	IV fluids; ADH replacement with DDAVP (desmopressin) IV, SQ, or intranasal; nasal solution bid is drug of choice; onset of action is 1 hr, 6–24 hr duration; Pitressin tannate in oil is given IM; aqueous Pitressin is used for acute, transient form of DI	Hypertonic IV fluids to correct hyponatremia; sodium restriction; diuretics to correct low plasma osmolality; monitor urine electrolyte loss; replace electrolyte loss; demeclocycline to facilitate free water clearance; treat the underlying cause
Nursing management	1. Know which clients are at risk 2. Monitor intake and output 3. Monitor for excessive thirst or urination 4. Assess serum and urine values: ↓ specific gravity, ↓ urine osmolality, ↑ serum osmolality, are early indicators of DI 5. Observe effects of DI on concurrent medical and surgical disorders 6. Client and family teaching	1. Know which clients are at risk 2. Monitor appropriate urine and serum laboratory tests 3. Assess for manifestations of hyponatremia by evaluating neurologic status 4. Monitor daily weights and intake and output 5. Observe for changes in concurrent disorders 6. Administer demeclocycline as ordered to interfere with ADH action; monitor for possible nephrotoxicity 7. Monitor for hypernatremia with fluid overcorrection 8. Client and family teaching
Prognosis	Excellent if there is compliance with vasopressin therapy	Dependent on cause and sodium level and serum osmolality; poor for client with bronchogenic carcinoma; seizures and coma contribute to chronic brain dysfunction

pin deficiency. Midline defects, such as cleft lip or palate, color blindness, anosmia, and ataxia, are common findings in these people.

CONCLUSIONS

Adrenal, pituitary, and gonadal disorders are not common but are extremely complex and diverse. Obtaining a thorough understanding of the adrenal, pituitary, and gonadal anatomy and physiology can help you care for clients with these disorders. Most of these conditions (such as hypopituitarism) are acute and affect many body systems, whereas others become chronic and lead to a wide variety of other problems, such as Addison's disease. Teaching is vital to the care of these clients; understand these conditions so that appropriate teaching plans can be initiated.

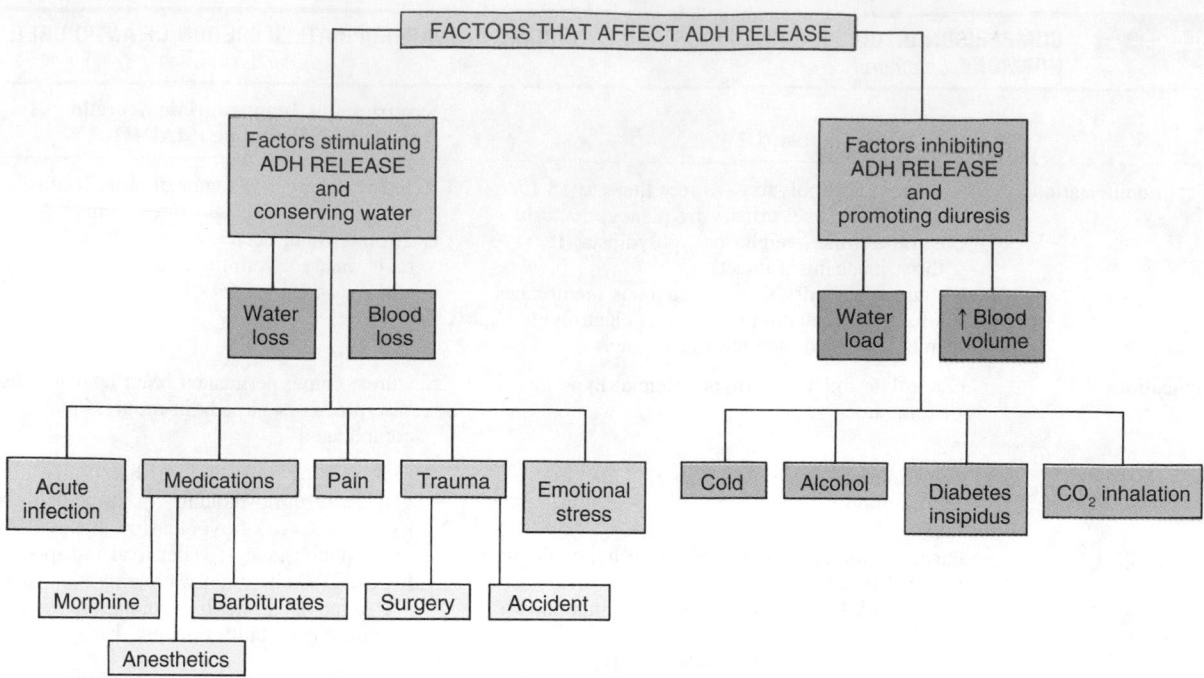

FIGURE 44–7 Factors that stimulate and inhibit the release of antidiuretic hormone (ADH). CO_2, carbon dioxide.

THINKING CRITICALLY

1. **The client is a woman with a 9-year history of Addison's disease. Normally, she takes her prescribed doses of a glucocorticoid (dexamethasone [Decadron]) and a mineralocorticoid (fludrocortisone [Florinef]) without fail. She is 29 years old and is otherwise in good health. The client stayed home from work today because she began to experience nausea, vomiting, diarrhea, and fever with diaphoresis. Because of the nausea and vomiting, she did not take her medications. When her husband returned home at 5:30 PM, he found her unconscious. What events led to the client's unconsciousness? How might missing her medications have affected the client?**

Factors to Consider. What acute disorder do the nausea, vomiting, diarrhea, and fever suggest? How might they affect a person with Addison's disease?

2. **A 50-year-old woman has been taking glucocorticoids for 10 years for asthma. She is admitted to the hospital for sudden onset of severe low back pain. What factors may have contributed to her back pain?**

Factors to Consider. What are the potential long-term effects of oral glucocorticoid therapy? What are their manifestations?

3. **A 23-year-old man is admitted for a head injury related to an automobile accident. While doing your hourly checks, you note that his urine output has been 800 ml since the last check. Over the next 3 hours, the client excretes an additional 3000 ml of very clear urine. His blood pressure has dropped, and urine specific gravity**

is less than 1.005. What are your priorities for care?

Factors to Consider. Is the urine output within normal limits? How might his urine output be related to his head injury?

BIBLIOGRAPHY

1. Anonymous. (1998). A quick check of the endocrine system. *Nursing, 28*(7), 32cc12–32cc13.
2. Bianco, C. (1996). Diabetes insipidus: Your role in managing this multifaceted disease. *American Journal of Nursing, 96*(8), 30–31.
3. Birch, C. (1997). Caring for people with endocrine disorders. In J. Luckmann (Ed.). *Saunders manual of nursing care.* Philadelphia: W. B. Saunders.
4. Clayton, L., & Dilley, K. B. (1998). Cushing's syndrome: Here's how to recognize and treat the manifestations of excess corticoids. *American Journal of Nursing, 98*(7), 40–41.
5. Coskeran, P. (1999). Management and treatment of patients with acromegaly. *Nursing Times, 95*(13), 50–52.
6. Cryer, P. (1995). Diseases of the sympathochromaffin system. In P. Felig, J. D. Baxter, & L. A. Frohman (Eds.), *Endocrinology and metabolism* (3rd ed., pp. 713–748). New York: McGraw-Hill.
7. Davies, P. (1996). Caring for patients with diabetes insipidus. *Nursing, 26*(5), 62–63.
8. Davis-Martin, S. (1996). Pearls for practice: Disorders of the adrenal glands. *Journal of the American Academy of Nurse Practitioners, 8*(7), 323–326.
9. DeJong, M. J. (1998). Hyponatremia: A life-threatening complication of the widely used thiazide diuretics. *American Journal of Nursing, 98*(12), 36.
10. Edwards, C. (1995). Primary mineralocorticoid excess syndromes. In L. DeGroot (Ed.), *Endocrinology* (3rd ed., pp. 1775–1803). Philadelphia: W. B. Saunders.
11. Eisenberg, A., & Redick, E. (1999). Caring for a patient after resection of pituitary adenoma. *Critical Care, 29*(12), 32cc1–2, 32cc4–6.
12. Eisenberg, A., & Redick, E. (1998). Preventing complications. Transsphenoidal resection of pituitary adenoma: Using a critical pathway. *Dimensions of Critical Care Nursing, 17*(6), 306–312.
13. Frohman, L. A. (1996). Acromegaly: What constitutes optimal ther-

apy? *Journal of Clinical Endocrinology and Metabolism, 8*(2), 443–445.

14. Go, H., et al. (1995). Laparoscopic adrenalectomy for Cushing's syndrome: Comparison with primary hyperaldosteronism. *Surgery, 117*(1), 11–17.

15. Greenspan, F., & Strewler, G. (Eds.). (1997). Basic and clinical endocrinology (5th ed.). Stamford, CT: Appleton & Lange.

16. Gumowski, J., & Loughran, M. (1996). Diseases of the adrenal gland. *Nursing Clinics of North America, 31*(4), 747–768.

17. Huether, S., & Tomky, D. (1998). Alterations of hormonal regulations. In K. McCance & S. Huether (Eds.), *Pathophysiology: The biologic basis for disease in adults and children* (3rd ed., pp. 656–706). St. Louis: Mosby–Year Book.

18. Jenkins, P. J., et al. (1995). The long term outcome after adrenalectomy and prophylactic pituitary radiotherapy in adrenocorticotropin-dependent Cushing's syndrome. *Journal of Clinical Endocrinology and Metabolism, 80*(1), 165–171.

19. Kee, J., & Hayes, E. (1997). *Pharmacology: A nursing process approach* (2nd ed.). Philadelphia: W. B. Saunders.

20. Keiser, H. (1995). Pheochromocytoma and related tumors. In L. DeGroot (Ed.), *Endocrinology* (3rd ed., pp. 1853–1877). Philadelphia: W. B. Saunders.

21. Loriaux, T. C. (1996). Endocrine assessment: Red flags for those on the front lines. *Nursing Clinics of North America, 31*(4), 695–714.

22. Loriaux, D. L., & McDonald, W. J. (1995). Adrenal insufficiency. In L. DeGroot (Ed.), *Endocrinology* (3rd ed., pp. 1731–1740). Philadelphia: W. B. Saunders.

23. McEwen, D. R. (1995). Transsphenoidal adenomectomy. *AORN Journal, 61*(2), 321–337.

24. Miller, W., & Tyrell, J. B. (1995). The adrenal cortex. In P. Felig, J. D. Baxter, & L. A. Frohman (Eds.), *Endocrinology and metabolism* (pp. 555–711). New York: McGraw-Hill.

25. Molitch, M. (1999). Advances in the management of pituitary tumors. *Endocrinology and Metabolism Clinics of North America, 28*(1), 1–240.

26. Nieman, L., & Cutler, G. B. (1995). Cushing's syndrome. In L. DeGroot (Ed.), *Endocrinology* (3rd ed., pp. 1741–1769). Philadelphia: W. B. Saunders.

27. O'Donnell, M. (1997). Addisonian crisis: Overexertion brought this patient's adrenal insufficiency to light. *American Journal of Nursing, 97*(3), 41.

28. Oekler, W. (1996). Adrenal insufficiency. *New England Journal of Medicine, 335*(16), 1206–1212.

29. Romeo, J. H. (1996). Hyper- and hypofunction in the anterior pituitary. *Nursing Clinics of North America, 31*(4), 769–778.

30. Rusterholtz., A. (1996). Interpretation of diagnostic laboratory tests in selected endocrine disorders. *Nursing Clinics of North America, 31*(4), 715–724.

31. Utiger, R. D. (1997). Treatment and retreatment of Cushing's disease. *New England Journal of Medicine, 336*(3), 215–217.

32. Werbel, S., & Ober, K. P. (1995). Pheochromocytoma. *Medical Clinics of North America, 79*(1), 131–153.

33. Winger, J. M., & Hornick, T. (1996). Age-associated changes in the endocrine system. *Nursing Clinics of North America, 31*(4), 827–844.

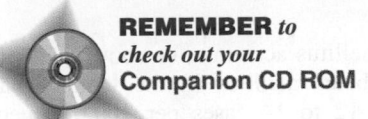

C H A P T E R

45

Management of Clients with Diabetes Mellitus

James A. Fain

NURSING OUTCOMES CLASSIFICATION (NOC)
for Nursing Diagnoses — Clients with Diabetes Mellitus

Altered Health Maintenance		Risk for Ineffective Management of
Health Belief: Perceived Resources	Knowledge: Treatment Regimen	Therapeutic Regimen (Individuals)
Health Promoting Behavior	Participation: Health Care Decisions	Compliance Behavior
Health Seeking Behavior	Psychosocial Adjustment: Life Change	Knowledge: Disease Process
Knowledge: Health Behaviors	Risk Detection	Knowledge: Treatment Regimen
Knowledge: Health Promotion	Self-Direction of Care	Participation: Health Care Decisions
Knowledge: Health Resources	Social Support	Treatment Behavior: Illness or Injury
	Treatment Behavior: Injury or Illness	

Diabetes mellitus is a chronic systemic disease characterized by either a deficiency of insulin or a decreased ability of the body to use insulin. Diabetes mellitus is sometimes referred to as "high sugars" by both clients and health care providers. The notion of associating sugar with diabetes is appropriate because the passage of large amounts of sugar-laden urine is characteristic of poorly controlled diabetes. However, high levels of blood glucose are only one component of the pathologic process and clinical manifestations associated with diabetes mellitus. Diabetes mellitus can be associated with serious complications, but people with diabetes can take preventive measures to reduce the likelihood of such occurrences.

In 1979, The National Diabetes Data Group[33] (NDDG) developed criteria for the classification and diagnosis of diabetes. In 1997, the Expert Committee on the Diagnosis and Classification of Diabetes Mellitus[23] proposed changes to the original NDDG classification scheme. Such changes were supported by the American Diabetes Association (ADA) and the National Institute of Diabetes and Digestive and Kidney Diseases (NIDDK). Previously, diabetes was classified as either insulin-dependent diabetes mellitus (IDDM) or non–insulin-dependent diabetes mellitus (NIDDM). With the use of insulin therapy commonplace with both types of diabetes, IDDM is now referred to as type 1 diabetes, and NIDDM is referred to as type 2 diabetes. The ADA also recommended using Arabic numerals—type 1 and type 2—rather than Roman numerals in referring to the two types of diabetes.[23]

Type 1 diabetes is characterized by destruction of pancreatic beta cells, usually leading to absolute insulin deficiency. Type 1 diabetes affects 10% of people who have diabetes, and it can develop at any age; usually, however, it is diagnosed before the age of 30 years. The most common form of diabetes, type 2, affects 90% to 95% of people who have diabetes and usually is diagnosed after age 40. Type 2 diabetes is more common among older adults and certain ethnic populations.

Clients who do not have type 1 or type 2 diabetes may nevertheless be classified as having impaired glucose tolerance, also known as *impaired fasting glucose*. This new diagnostic category is defined by fasting glucose levels above 110 mg/dl (milligrams per deciliter), but below 126 mg/dl. These glucose values are higher than the level considered normal but lower than the level diagnostic of diabetes.[23] It is estimated that 11% of the population has impaired fasting glucose.

Diabetes may also result from other disorders or treatments. Genetic defects in the beta cells can lead to the development of diabetes. Several hormones, such as growth hormone, cortisol, glucagon, and epinephrine, antagonize or counteract insulin. Excess amounts of these hormones—as in acromegaly, Cushing's syndrome, glucagonoma, and pheochromocytoma—cause diabetes. In addition, certain drugs, such as glucocorticoids and thiazides, and infections may cause diabetes. Such types of secondary diabetes account for 1% to 2% of all diagnosed cases of diabetes.

Gestational diabetes mellitus is a diagnosis of diabetes mellitus that applies only to women in whom glucose intolerance develops or is first discovered during pregnancy. Gestational diabetes develops in 2% to 5% of all

---

This chapter incorporates material written for the fifth edition by Carol Birch and Kerry H. Greear.

pregnant women but disappears when the pregnancy is over. It occurs more frequently in African Americans, Hispanic Americans, Native Americans, and women with a family history of diabetes, and obesity is also a risk factor. See Box 45–1 for an overview of the types of diabetes mellitus.[19, 21]

Diabetes mellitus is a significant public health concern in the United States. About 16 million people (5.9% of the population) have diabetes, nearly half of whom do not yet know they have it. Some 3.2 million of affected people are 65 years of age or older. Diabetes imposes a heavy economic burden on the United States each year. It is estimated that more than $100 billion in direct and indirect costs (such as disability, work loss, and premature death) are attributed to diabetes mellitus.[13]

Diabetes is the seventh leading cause of death in the United States, with more than 180,000 deaths attributable to the disease in 1995. Even when it does not kill, diabetes can cause major disabilities. For example, diabetes mellitus is the single greatest contributor to the number of cases of blindness in adults, end-stage renal failure, and nontraumatic amputations. Diabetes is the leading cause of new cases of blindness in adults 20 to 74 years of age. It is also the leading cause of end-stage renal disease, accounting for about 40% of new cases. In 1995, about 98,000 people with diabetes underwent dialysis or kidney transplantation. Likewise, more than half of leg amputations are performed among people with diabetes. From 1993 to 1995, about 67,000 amputations were performed each year.[20] The increasing burden of diabetes is alarming, but the good news is that much of the burden of this major public health problem can be prevented by early detection, improved delivery of care, and better education for diabetes self-management.

BOX 45–1 Types of Diabetes Mellitus and Abnormal Glucose Metabolism

Diabetes Mellitus

1. Type 1 diabetes
2. Type 2 diabetes
3. Causes of secondary diabetes
   a. Genetic defects
   b. Diseases of the pancreas (such as pancreatitis, neoplasia, trauma/pancreatectomy)
   c. Endocrinopathies (such as acromegaly, Cushing's syndrome, pheochromocytoma, hyperthyroidism)
   d. Drug/chemical-induced (as from glucocorticoids, thyroid hormone, diazoxide, thiazides, phenytoin sodium [Dilantin], nicotinic acid)
   e. Infections (such as congenital rubella, cytomegalovirus infection)
   f. Genetic syndromes associated with diabetes (such as Down syndrome, Klinefelter's syndrome, Huntington's chorea)
4. Gestational diabetes mellitus

Impaired Glucose Tolerance

1. Impaired fasting glucose

Adapted from American Diabetes Association. (1997). Report of the Expert Committee on the Diagnosis and Classification of Diabetes Mellitus. *Diabetes Care, 20*(7), 1183–1197.

Type 1 diabetes mellitus accounts for about 10% of all known cases of diabetes mellitus in the United States. Annual incidence is 12 to 14 cases per 100,000 people younger than 20 years, with a prevalence of 1 case per 500 people younger than 16 years. It is one of the most common childhood diseases, being three to four times more common than such chronic childhood diseases as cystic fibrosis, juvenile rheumatoid arthritis and leukemia, and 10 times more common than nephrotic syndrome or muscular dystrophy. The incidence of type 1 diabetes mellitus in males is similar to that in females, and the condition is more common in African Americans, Hispanic Americans, Asian Americans, and Native Americans than in whites.[13] Risk factors are less well defined for type 1 diabetes than for type 2 diabetes.

Type 2 diabetes mellitus accounts for about 90% to 95% of all known cases of diabetes mellitus in the United States. About 8 million Americans have this type of diabetes, but an almost equal number of cases are undiagnosed. Type 2 diabetes is present, on average, for about 6.5 years before its clinical identification and treatment. The prevalence is markedly higher in Native Americans, African Americans, and Hispanic Americans, as well as in older and obese people.[13]

Etiology and Risk Factors

TYPE 1 DIABETES MELLITUS

Type 1 diabetes, previously called IDDM or *juvenile-onset diabetes,* is inherited as a heterogeneous, multigenic trait. Identical twins have a risk of 25% to 50% of inheriting the disease, whereas siblings have a 6% risk and offspring a 5% risk. Despite this strong familial influence, 90% of people in whom type 1 diabetes develops do not have a first-degree relative with diabetes. An association also exists between type 1 diabetes and several human leukocyte antigens (HLAs). Environmental factors such as viruses appear to trigger an autoimmune process that destroys beta cells. Islet cell antibodies (ICAs) then appear, increasing in amount over months to years as beta cells are destroyed.[37] Fasting *hyperglycemia* (elevated blood glucose level) occurs when 80% to 90% of beta cell mass has been destroyed.

Identification of ICAs has made it possible to detect type 1 diabetes mellitus in its preclinical stage. Autoantibodies directed against insulin are found in 20% to 60% of clients with type 1 diabetes prior to initiation of exogenous insulin therapy. The combination of large amounts of ICAs, presence of insulin autoantibodies, and decreased first-phase insulin secretion (representing insulin stored in beta cells) can predict the onset of type 1 diabetes mellitus within 5 years.[37]

There are no known health promotion activities to prevent type 1 diabetes mellitus; however, regular exercise and adherence to the prescribed diet may limit the development of complications. Health maintenance activities involve:

- Maintaining blood glucose at levels as normal as possible
- Preventing hypoglycemia and hyperglycemia with stress, illness, or exercise by closely monitoring blood glucose levels and taking early action; performing daily foot care

- Preventing complications of diabetes mellitus by removing or treating coexisting risk factors such as smoking, hypertension, hyperlipidemia, and use of nephrotoxic drugs.

Health restoration actions include:

- Prompt treatment of foot abrasions or infections
- Follow-up visits to assess for complications of diabetes and to reinforce learning needs
- Yearly funduscopic examinations by an ophthalmologist with treatment as needed
- Treatment of coexisting risk factors as described previously

TYPE 2 DIABETES MELLITUS

Type 2 diabetes mellitus, previously called NIDDM or *adult-onset diabetes,* also appears to be a heterogeneous disorder involving both genetic and environmental factors. It is not associated with HLA tissue types, and circulating ICAs are rarely present. Heredity plays a major role in the expression of type 2 diabetes. It is more common in identical twins (58% to 75% incidence) than in the general population. Obesity is also a major risk factor; 85% of all people with type 2 diabetes are obese. It is unclear whether impaired tissue (liver and muscle) sensitivity to insulin or impaired insulin secretion is the primary defect in this type of diabetes.[37] In addition, the prevalence of coronary artery disease in people with type 2 diabetes is twice that in the non-diabetic population, and cardiovascular and total mortality rates are two-fold to three-fold greater than in non-diabetic people.[41]

Cases have been documented of families in which type 2 diabetes is present in all age groups and in which an autosomal dominant inheritance has been established. This form of diabetes is referred to as *maturity-onset diabetes of the young* (MODY).

Health promotion actions for type 2 diabetes mellitus include:

- Eating habits based on the "Food Guide Pyramid" (as noted later on)[40]
- Avoidance of foods high in refined sugars and saturated fats
- Maintaining ideal body weight, starting in childhood
- Exercising regularly
- Returning to pre-pregnancy weight or ideal body weight post partum

Health maintenance activities involve:

- Screening high-risk people, such as those with first-degree relatives who have type 2 diabetes, those who are obese, members of high-risk racial groups, people over age 40 with any other risk factor, people with hypertension or hyperlipidemia, clients with previous impaired glucose tolerance, women with previous gestational diabetes mellitus or those who have had a baby weighing more than 9 pounds, and people with a history of recurrent infections
- Performing periodic assessments to determine the client's learning needs and to assess glycemic control
- Using strategies shown to reduce complications of diabetes by removing or treating coexisting risk factors such as smoking, hypertension, hyperlipidemia, and use of nephrotoxic drugs
- Performing daily foot care

- Preventing hypoglycemia or hyperglycemia by closely monitoring blood glucose levels and taking early action

Health restoration actions include:

- Teach diet and exercise programs to reduce obesity
- Prompt treatment of foot abrasions or infections
- Follow-up visits to assess for complications of diabetes and reinforce learning needs
- Yearly funduscopic examinations by an ophthalmologist with treatment as needed
- Treatment of previously described risk factors
- Control of angina and peripheral vascular disease

Pathophysiology

TYPE 1 DIABETES MELLITUS

The development of type 1 diabetes mellitus can be broken down into five stages:

Stage 1: genetic predisposition
Stage 2: environmental trigger
Stage 3: active autoimmunity
Stage 4: progressive beta cell destruction
Stage 5: overt diabetes mellitus

Type 1 diabetes mellitus does not develop in all people who have a genetic predisposition. Of those in whom gene markers (DR3 or DR4 HLA) indicate risk, diabetes ultimately develops in fewer than 1%. Environmental triggers have long been suspected in type 1 diabetes. Incidence is increased in both spring and fall, and onset is often coincidental with epidemics of various viral diseases. Active autoimmunity is directed against the beta cells of the pancreas and their products. ICAs and insulin antibodies serve to progressively decrease the effective circulating insulin level.

This slow, progressive insult to the beta cells and endogenous insulin molecules can result in an abrupt onset of diabetes. Hyperglycemia can result from acute illness or stress (see the Case Study), which increases insulin demand beyond the reserves of the damaged beta cell mass. When the acute illness or stress resolves, the client may revert to a compensated state of variable duration in which the pancreas once again manages to produce adequate amounts of insulin. This compensated state, referred to as the *honeymoon period,* typically lasts for 3 to 12 months. The process ends when the diminishing beta cell mass cannot produce enough insulin to sustain life. The client then becomes dependent on exogenous insulin (produced outside the body) administration to survive.[32, 37]

TYPE 2 DIABETES MELLITUS

The pathogenesis of type 2 diabetes mellitus differs significantly from that of type 1. A limited beta cell response to hyperglycemia appears to be a major factor in its development. Beta cells chronically exposed to high blood levels of glucose become progressively less efficient when responding to further glucose elevations. This phenomenon, termed *desensitization,* is reversible by normalizing glucose levels. The ratio of *proinsulin* (a precursor to insulin) to insulin secreted also increases.[37]

A second pathophysiologic process in type 2 diabetes mellitus is resistance to the biologic activity of insulin in both the liver and peripheral tissues. This state is known as *insulin resistance.* People with type 2 diabetes have a

Understanding Diabetes Mellitus and Its Treatment

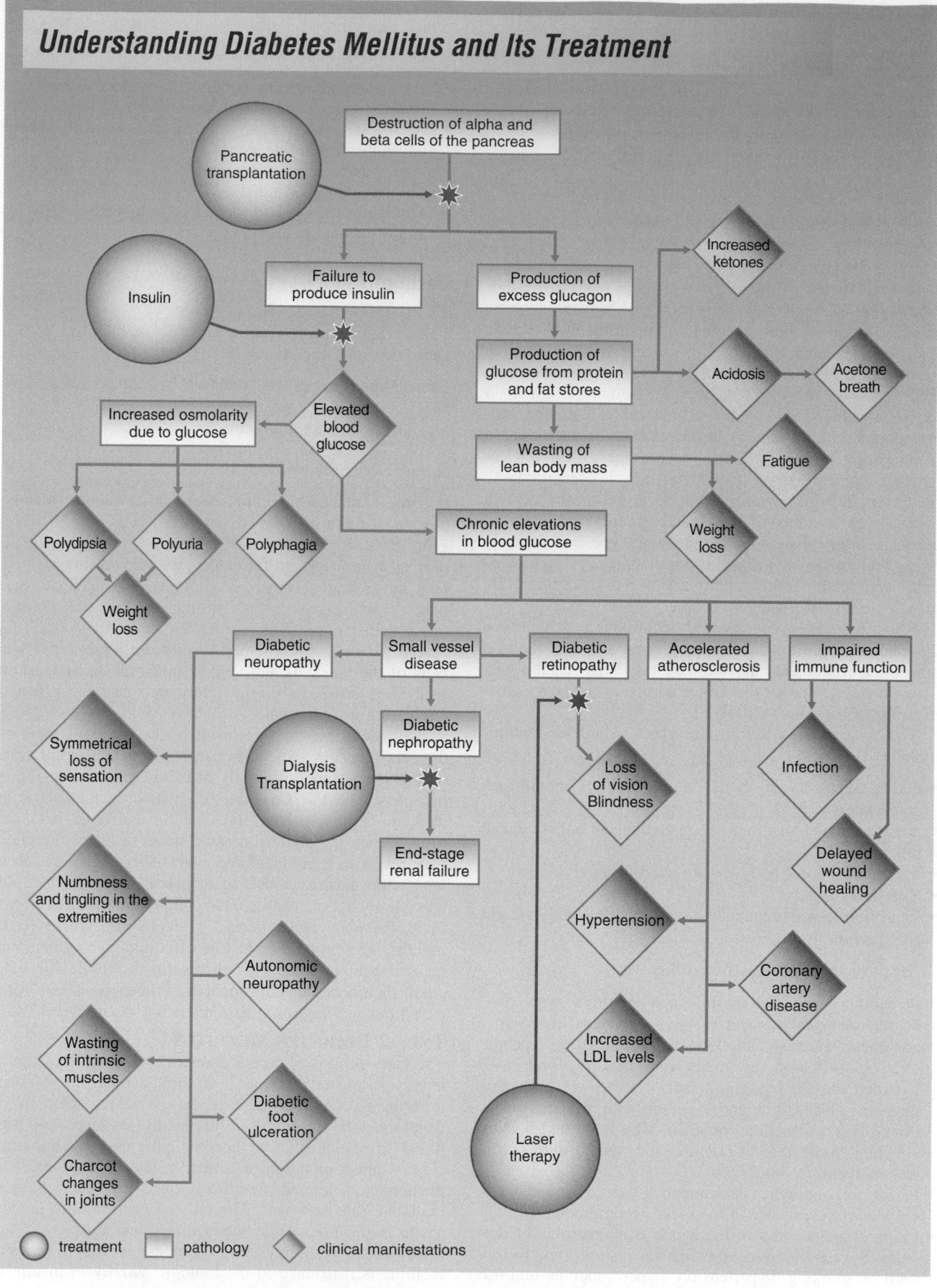

treatment pathology clinical manifestations

Diabetes and Pneumonia

Ms. Washington is a 44-year-old black woman who has been sick for the past week. She has been treated with erythromycin (E-Mycin) 500 mg q 6 h and phenylpropanolamine-guaifensin (Entex LA) q 12 h as an outpatient after being seen in the clinic for a persistent cough, loss of voice, chest pain from coughing, fever, chills, and mild nausea without vomiting. She now reports that she has been coughing sputum that is brown to green, with small amounts of red blood present. Ms. Washington is also complaining of left shoulder pain of 3 days' duration, fatigue, sinus pressure, congestion, fullness in the ears, and postnasal drainage. She also reports frequent urination without dysuria or urgency and feeling thirsty all the time.

Her history is significant for gestational diabetes 11 years ago, at which time she administered her own insulin injections. At this time, she is being admitted for failed treatment of pneumonia and control of new-onset diabetes. Consider whether Ms. Washington has type 1 or type 2 diabetes mellitus and the effect of that type of diabetes on her treatment plan and future complications.

● Ms. Washington's chest x-ray shows thickened bronchioles and left lower-lobe infiltrates. The cardiac silhouette is normal.

Admission Laboratory Values	
RBC count	3.7 million/mm³
Hb	10.5 g/dl
Hct	31%
WBC count	15,600/mm³
Neutrophils	81%
BUN	5 mg/dl
Creatinine	0.7 mg/dl
Cholesterol	176 mg/dl
Triglycerides	134 mg/dl
Potassium	5.3 mEq/L
Chloride	96 mEq/L
Sodium	139 mEq/L
Glucose	335 mg/dl

Nursing Admission Assessment

Ms. Washington is a single mother of an 11-year-old son. She works from 6 AM to 2 PM at a fast food restaurant 6 days a week, where she stands at the counter. She reports that the benefits of the job are medical insurance and the free food for herself and discounted food for her son when he stops for breakfast on his way to school. Her father died of diabetes complicated by heart disease, and her mother died of diabetes complicated by stroke. She admits to smoking one pack of cigarettes a day for 20 years and denies use of alcohol. However, she reports drinking 1 gallon of bottled fruit juice daily.

Nursing Physical Examination

Height: 5'7" Weight: 192 lb
 (87.3 kg)
Vital signs: BP = 144/94
 TPR = 100.8, 78, 18
Level of consciousness: Alert and cooperative

EENT: Nasal mucosa unremarkable, yellow-green drainage on pharynx.
Cardiac: Regular rate and rhythm without gallop or murmur
Pulmonary: Decreased breath sounds at bases, with the left greater than the right; wheezes and rhonchi noted at the left lower lobe; increased tactile fremitus
Abdominal: Soft and nontender with active bowel tones
Genitourinary: Reports vaginal itching and white "clumpy" discharge
Peripheral pulses: 3/3, without edema

Initial Treatment Plan

Medications

Cefazolin (Ancef) 1 g IV q 8 h
Triamcinolone acetonide (Kenaject-40) 40 mg IM now
Human insulin (Humulin) NPH 20 U SC AM, 10 U SC PM; sliding-scale insulin AC and HS: Humulin regular SC according to serum glucose level:
<150 mg/dl: 0 units
151–250 mg/dl: 3 units
251–350 mg/dl: 6 units
>350 mg/dl: call physician

Saline flush IV lock bid and after medications
 What effect, if any, would the admission medication orders have on Ms. Washington's blood glucose?

Diet: 1200-calorie ADA; develop a sample 24-hour diet plan for Ms. Washington
Activity: As tolerated

Case Study continued on following page

Respiratory treatments: Albuterol (Ventolin) 2.5 mg in 3 ml NS aerosol qid; incentive spirometer q 2 h while awake

Diagnostic tests: Blood glucose levels qid AC and HS; repeat complete blood count, electrolytes, chest x-ray in AM

At 11:00 AM on day 2, Ms. Washington's serum glucose level is 265 mg/dl. How much insulin will she require?

Over the next 3 days, Ms. Washington's blood glucose levels stabilize. Her physician adds 10 U Humulin regular to her routine AM insulin dose and 5 U Humulin regular to her routine PM insulin dose and discontinues the orders for sliding-scale insulin. Metformin (Glucophage) is initiated at 500 mg PO bid with meals. The physician writes an order for the client to continue monitoring blood glucose levels with a glucometer qid. Yesterday, her fluid intake was 1980 ml, and her urinary output was 1575 ml. She remains on her 1200-calorie ADA diet, but says that she would like a hamburger and French fries. Yesterday, the nurse discovered several candy bars in the drawer of Ms. Washington's bedside table.

Ms. Washington no longer complains of sinus pressure or postnasal drainage. Her cough remains productive of small amounts of white, thick sputum. Lung sounds remain diminished, but clear after coughing. She is able to raise her incentive spirometer measurement to 1500 ml. Her antibiotic has been changed to clarithromycin (Biaxin) 500 mg bid with food × 10 days. The physician has also ordered miconazole (Monistat) vaginal cream daily. What instructions would you give Ms. Washington about administration of the vaginal cream?

Most recent laboratory values reveal a potassium of 4.0 mEq/L, chloride of 100 mEq/L, and sodium of 139 mEq/L. Her fasting blood sugar this AM was 95 mg/dl, and the WBC count was 10 × 10⁹/L.

The physician is planning to discharge her tomorrow.

Discharge Criteria

- Average length of stay: 5.5 days without complications; 8.4 days with complications.
- Initiate diabetes instruction for survival, home care, and improved lifestyle. Consider differences in discharge planning between chronic illnesses, such as diabetes, and episodic or acute illnesses, such as sinusitis.
- Complete community referrals. What referrals would you make? Why?

Questions to Be Considered

1. In the progress notes, Ms. Washington's physician reports a shift to the left in her WBC count. What does this mean? Discuss the relationship between diabetes mellitus and susceptibility to infection and response to treatment. What influence do infections exert over control of diabetes mellitus?

2. How would the physician's decision to prescribe mixed-dose insulin and metformin (Glucophage) influence the triangle of control (diet, exercise, pharmacologic agents)? What are the benefits? What are the risks?

3. What influence did her socioeconomic status, race, and heredity have on Ms. Washington's development of diabetes mellitus? What continuing influence will these factors play in her regulation of the diabetes? What effect will her current employment probably have on Ms. Washington's compliance with, and ability to financially afford, diet, foot care, glucose monitoring, and exercise?

4. Describe the pathophysiologic basis for the change in Ms. Washington's potassium levels and her development of polyuria, polydipsia, polyphagia, and weight loss.

5. Ms. Washington's employer telephones the nurses' station and states: "Ms. Washington has informed me that she will be unable to return to work for 10 days. Is this true?" How would you respond? What are the ethical considerations you should make in formulating your response?

6. Ten days after discharge, Ms. Washington complains of fever, nausea, vomiting, and diarrhea. What directions would you give?

AC, at meals; ADA, American Diabetes Association; BP, blood pressure; EENT, eye, ear, nose, throat; Hb, hemoglobin; Hct, hematocrit; IM, intramuscular; NS, normal saline; RBC, red blood cell; SC, subcutaneous; TPR, temperature, pulse, respirations; WBC, white blood cell.

---

decreased sensitivity to glucose levels, which results in continued hepatic glucose production, even with high plasma glucose levels. This is coupled with an inability of muscle and fat tissues to increase glucose uptake. The mechanism causing peripheral insulin resistance is not clear; however, it appears to occur after insulin binds to a receptor on the cell surface (Fig. 45–1).

Insulin is a building (anabolic) hormone. Without insulin, three major metabolic problems occur: (1) decreased glucose utilization, (2) increased fat mobilization, and (3) increased protein utilization. (See the algorithm called Understanding Diabetes Mellitus and Its Treatment), p. 1152.)

Decreased Glucose Utilization

In diabetes, cells that require insulin as a carrier for glucose can take in only about 25% of the glucose they require for fuel. Nerve tissues, erythrocytes, and the cells of the intestines, liver, and kidney tubules do not require insulin for glucose transport. Skeletal and cardiac muscles and adipose tissues do. Without adequate amounts of insulin, much of the ingested glucose cannot be used.

With inadequate amounts of insulin, blood glucose levels rise. This elevation continues because the liver cannot store glucose as glycogen without sufficient insulin levels. In an attempt to restore balance and return blood glucose levels to normal, the kidney excretes the excess glucose. Glucose appears in the urine (*glucosuria*). Glucose excreted in the urine acts as an osmotic diuretic and causes excretion of increased amounts of water, resulting in fluid volume deficit.[37]

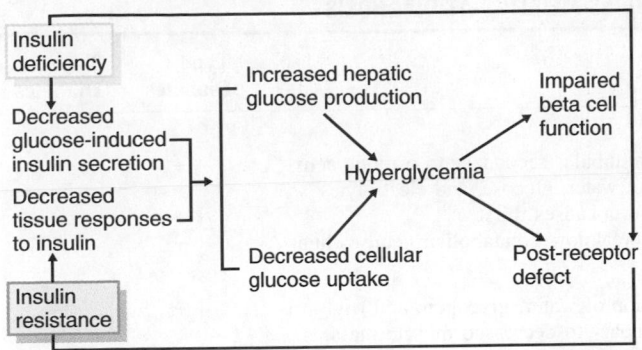

FIGURE 45–1 Relationship between insulin resistance and insulin secretion in type 2 diabetes mellitus. (Modified from American Diabetes Association [1998]. *Medical management of non-insulin dependent (type 2) diabetes* [4th ed., p. 18]. Alexandria, VA: Author.)

Increased Fat Mobilization

In type 1 diabetes and occasionally with severe stress in type 2 diabetes, the body turns to fat stores for energy production when glucose is unavailable. Fat metabolism causes breakdown products called *ketones* to form. Ketones accumulate in the blood and are excreted through the kidneys and lungs. Ketone levels can be measured in the blood and urine; high levels can serve as an indicator of uncontrolled diabetes.

Ketones interfere with the body's acid-base balance by producing hydrogen ions. The pH can fall, and metabolic acidosis (discussed later) can develop. In addition, when ketones are excreted, sodium is also eliminated, resulting in sodium depletion and further acidosis. The excretion of ketones also increases osmotic pressure, leading to increased fluid loss. Also, when fats are the primary source of energy, body lipid levels can rise to five times normal, leading to increased atherosclerosis.[37]

Increased Protein Utilization

Lack of insulin leads to protein wasting. In healthy people, proteins are constantly being broken down and rebuilt. In people with type 1 diabetes, without insulin to stimulate protein synthesis, the balance is altered, which leads to increased catabolism (destruction). Amino acids are converted to glucose in the liver, further elevating glucose levels. If this condition goes untreated, clients with type 1 diabetes appear emaciated. The pathophysiologic processes of diabetes continue, leading to many acute and chronic complications, as discussed later in the chapter.[37, 41]

Clinical Manifestations

Hyperglycemia, the medical term for an elevated blood glucose level, leads to common clinical manifestations associated with diabetes. In type 1 diabetes, the onset is sudden, with diabetic ketoacidosis being the first indication of the disease. In contrast, type 2 diabetes may develop so gradually that some affected people notice few or no manifestations for a number of years. Clients may initially complain of chronic problems, as from peripheral neuropathy (nerve damage in hands and feet). Other times, the diagnosis of type 2 diabetes may be made by a routine laboratory test in clients who have no manifestations.

The classic clinical manifestations of diabetes are increased frequency of urination (*polyuria*), increased thirst and fluid intake (*polydipsia*), and, as the disease progresses, weight loss despite increased hunger and food intake (*polyphagia*). These clinical manifestations are caused by hyperglycemia and the accompanying spillover of excess glucose in the urine. See Tables 45–1 and 45–2 for other common manifestations.

DIAGNOSIS OF DIABETES MELLITUS

Physical examination, medical history, and laboratory tests are employed to evaluate clients with diabetes. Clinical manifestations suggest the presence of diabetes, but laboratory tests are needed to make a definitive diagnosis.

FASTING BLOOD GLUCOSE. Diabetes is diagnosed by measuring blood glucose levels. The fasting blood glucose level is normally less than 110 mg/dl. The diagnosis of diabetes can be made when a client's fasting blood glucose level is above 125 mg/dl. Values between 110 and 125 mg/dl indicate impaired fasting glucose. Critical values in adults are those less than 60 mg/dl or more than 500 mg/dl (see Box 45–2).

A fasting blood glucose sample is drawn when the client has not ingested any nutrients other than water for 8 to 12 hours. This sample generally reflects glucose from hepatic production. If the client is receiving a dextrose IV solution, the results of the test must be analyzed with that variable in mind. In clients who are known to have diabetes, food and insulin are withheld until after the specimen is obtained. The fasting blood glucose gives the best indication of overall glucose homeostasis.

RANDOM BLOOD GLUCOSE. A blood sample for determination of glucose level may be drawn at any time and requires no client preparation. Results should be within normal limits for both non-diabetic and diabetic clients with good control of their blood glucose. Elevated blood glucose levels may occur after meals, after stressful events, if the sample was drawn from above an intravenous (IV) site, or in cases of diabetes. Table 45–3 lists conditions and medications that can cause hyperglycemia or *hypoglycemia* (decreased blood glucose level).

POSTPRANDIAL BLOOD GLUCOSE. Postprandial (after a meal) blood glucose samples are drawn 2 hours after a standard meal and reflect the efficiency of insulin-mediated glucose uptake by peripheral tissues. Normally, blood glucose should return to fasting levels within 2 hours. In older adults, levels are higher, typically rising by 5 to 10 mg/dl per decade after age 50 years because of the normal decline in glucose tolerance associated with aging. Smoking and drinking coffee can lead to falsely elevated values at 2 hours, whereas strenuous exercise can lead to falsely decreased values.

GLYCOSYLATED HEMOGLOBIN. Glucose normally attaches itself to the hemoglobin molecule on a red blood cell. Once attached, it cannot dissociate. Therefore, the higher the blood glucose levels, the higher the levels of glycosylated hemoglobin (HbA_{1C}). The results of this test show the average blood glucose level over the previous 3 months. It is therefore useful in evaluating long-term glycemic control. HbA_{1C} samples can be drawn at any time during the day. Conditions that increase erythrocyte turnover, such as bleeding, pregnancy, or asplenia (absence of

TABLE 45-1   SELECTED CLINICAL MANIFESTATIONS OF DIABETES MELLITUS AT DIAGNOSIS

Clinical Manifestation	Pathophysiologic Basis	Type 1 Diabetes	Type 2 Diabetes
Cardinal manifestations			
Polyuria* (frequent urination)	Water not reabsorbed from renal tubules secondary to osmotic activity of glucose; leads to loss of water, glucose, and electrolytes	+ +	+
Polydipsia* (excessive thirst)	Dehydration secondary to polyuria causes thirst	+ +	+
Polyphagia* (excessive hunger)	Starvation secondary to tissue breakdown (catabolism) causes hunger	+ +	+
Weight loss*	Initial loss secondary to depletion of water, glycogen, and triglyceride stores; chronic loss secondary to decreased muscle mass as amino acids are diverted to form glucose and ketone bodies	+ +	−
Recurrent blurred vision	Secondary to chronic exposure of ocular lens and retina to hyperosmolar fluids	+	+ +
Pruritus, skin infections, vaginitis	Bacterial and fungal infections of the skin seem to be more common; research conflicting	+	+ +
Ketonuria	When glucose cannot be used for energy in insulin-dependent cells, fatty acids are used for energy; fatty acids are broken down into ketones in the blood and excreted by the kidneys; in type 2 diabetes, sufficient insulin is present to depress excessive use of fatty acids, but not enough to permit use of glucose	+ +	−
Weakness and fatigue, dizziness	Decreased plasma volume leads to postural hypotension; potassium loss and protein catabolism contribute to weakness	+ +	+
Often asymptomatic	The body can "adapt" to a slow rise in blood glucose to a greater extent than it can to a rapid rise	−	+ +

* Often referred to as *classic manifestations* of diabetes.
+, sometimes seen; + +, usually seen; −, not usually seen.

TABLE 45-2   DISTINGUISHING FEATURES OF TYPE 1 AND TYPE 2 DIABETES MELLITUS

Feature	Type 1	Type 2
Synonyms	Insulin-dependent diabetes mellitus (IDDM), juvenile diabetes, labile or brittle diabetes	Non–insulin-dependent diabetes mellitus (NIDDM), adult or maturity-onset diabetes, mild diabetes
Age at onset	Usually occurs before age 30 years, but may occur at any age	Usually occurs after age 30 years, but can occur in children
Incidence	~10%	~90%
Type of onset	Usually abrupt, with rapid onset of hyperglycemia	Insidious, may be asymptomatic or mildly asymptomatic; body adapts to slow onset of hyperglycemia
Endogenous insulin production	Little or none	Below normal, normal, or above normal
Body weight at onset	Ideal body weight or thin	85% of clients are obese; may be of ideal body weight
Ketosis	Prone to ketosis, usually present at onset, frequently present during poor control	Resistant to ketosis, can occur with infection or stress
Manifestations	Polyuria, polydipsia, polyphagia, fatigue	Frequently none, may be mild manifestations of hyperglycemia
Dietary management	Essential	Essential
Exercise management	Essential	Essential
Exogenous insulin administration	Dependent on insulin for survival	20% to 30% of clients may require insulin
Oral hypoglycemic agents	Not effective	Effective
Teaching needs	At diagnosis and ongoing	At diagnosis and ongoing

BOX 45–2 Screening and Diagnosis Guidelines for Diabetes Mellitus

Guidelines for Testing for Diabetes

- Testing for diabetes should be considered in all persons at age 45. If results are normal, test should be repeated at 3-year intervals.
- Testing should be considered at a younger age or performed more often for clients with the following risk factors:
  - Obesity (>120% of desirable body weight or a body mass index above 27 kg/m²)
  - Diabetes in a first-degree relative
  - Racial predisposition (as in African American, Hispanic, Native American populations)
  - In women, giving birth to a baby weighing more than 9 lb or a history of gestational diabetes
  - Hypertension (blood pressure > 140/90 mm Hg)
  - A high-density lipoprotein level < 35 mg/dl or triglyceride level > 250 mg/dl
  - On previous testing, impaired glucose tolerance or impaired fasting glucose

Guidelines for Diagnosis of Diabetes Mellitus

- Manifestations of diabetes plus random plasma glucose concentration above 200 mg/dl (11.1 mmol/L). *Random* is defined as any time of day without regard to time since last meal. Classic manifestations include polyuria, polydipsia, and unexplained weight loss.

OR

- Fasting plasma glucose level above 126 mg/dl (7.0 mmol/L). Fasting is defined as no caloric intake for at least 8 hours.

OR

- A 2-hour postprandial glucose level above 200 mg/dl during an oral glucose tolerance test. This test should be performed using a glucose load containing the equivalent of 75 g of anhydrous glucose dissolved in water.

Plasma Glucose Values

Fasting plasma glucose	<110 mg/dl	Normal fasting glucose
	110–126 mg/dl	Impaired fasting glucose
	>126 mg/dl	Diagnosis of diabetes
Oral glucose tolerance test, 2 hours after eating	<140 mg/dl	Normal glucose tolerance
	140–200 mg/dl	Impaired glucose intolerance
	>200 mg/dl	Diagnosis of diabetes

Adapted from American Diabetes Association. (1997). Report of the Expert Committee on the Diagnosis and Classification of Diabetes Mellitus. *Diabetes Care, 20*(7), 1183–1197.

sylated albumin (fructosamine) represents the average blood glucose over the previous 7 to 10 days. This measurement is useful when short-term determinations of average blood glucose are desired. The reliability and clinical applicability continue to be evaluated.

CONNECTING PEPTIDE. When the proinsulin produced by pancreatic beta cells is broken apart by an enzyme, two products are formed: insulin and connecting peptide, commonly called *C-peptide.* Because C-peptide and insulin are formed in equal amounts, this test indicates the amount of endogenous insulin production. Clients with type 1 diabetes usually have no or low concentrations of C-peptide. Clients with type 2 diabetes tend to have normal or elevated levels.

ORAL GLUCOSE TOLERANCE TEST. The oral glucose tolerance test is often unnecessary for the diagnosis of diabetes mellitus, especially if the client's fasting blood glucose is above 140 mg/dL. Bed rest, infection, trauma, medications, and stress can alter the test results.

TABLE 45–3 SELECTIVE FACTORS CONTRIBUTING TO HYPOGLYCEMIA AND HYPERGLYCEMIA

Predisposing Factors	Associated Medications
HYPOGLYCEMIA	
Too much insulin	Insulin
Erratic absorption of insulin	Salicylates/NSAIDs
Sudden increase in activity	Sulfonamides
Starvation	Beta-blockers
Alcohol ingestion	Sulfonylureas (oral hypoglycemic agents)
Age >60 years	
Acute illness	Allopurinol
Cerebrovascular accident	Dicumarol
Heart failure	Haloperidol
Decreased kidney function	Anticholinergic antagonists
Gastroparesis	Monoamine oxidase inhibitors
Abnormal liver function	Para-aminobenzoic acid
Hypopituitarism	Dextropropoxyphene
Adrenocortical insufficiency	Clofibrate
	Imipramine
	Histamine H_2-receptor antagonists
HYPERGLYCEMIA	
Inadequate insulin	Diuretics, especially thiazides
Infection	Beta-blockers
Inactivity	Diphenylhydantoin
Obesity	Glucocorticoids
Intravenous dextrose	Lithium
Diabetes	Phenothiazines
Emotional stress	Progestins
Physical stress	Levothyroxine
Liver disease	NSAIDs
Hyperthyroidism	Epinephrine
Lack of oral hypoglycemic agents	Tricyclic antidepressants
Decreased muscle mass	Oral contraceptives
Chronic pancreatitis	Rifampin
	Nicotinic acid
	Isoniazid

NSAID, nonsteroidal anti-inflammatory drug.

the spleen as after splenectomy), will lead to falsely low HbA_{1C} concentrations. High aspirin doses, alcohol ingestion, uremia, elevated hemoglobin levels, and heparin therapy can cause falsely elevated levels of HbA_{1C}. Normal values are 6% to 7%.[24]

GLYCOSYLATED ALBUMIN. Glucose also attaches to proteins, primarily albumin. The concentration of glyco-

This test is not usually recommended in hospitalized clients.

The client needs a diet that offers at least 150 g of carbohydrate per day for 3 days before the test. A sample is drawn to test fasting blood glucose, and the client is given 75 g of glucose in water to drink. Blood samples are taken at intervals afterward (such as at 1 and 2 hours). The client cannot consume any food or fluid other than water between the glucose load ingestion and the end of the test. Diagnosis of diabetes mellitus or impaired glucose tolerance after the glucose tolerance test is dependent on fasting and follow-up glucose levels. The oral glucose load and levels diagnostic of diabetes are different for the pregnant client undergoing testing for gestational diabetes mellitus.[24]

KETONURIA. Urine levels of ketones can be tested by clients, as well as by laboratories, by use of dip-strips. The presence of ketones in the urine (a condition called *ketonuria*) indicates that the body is using fat as a major source of energy, which may result in ketoacidosis. All clients with diabetes should test their urine for ketones during acute illness or stress, when blood glucose levels are consistently elevated, and when they are pregnant or have evidence of ketoacidosis (such as nausea, vomiting, or abdominal pain). The presence of ketones in the urine of a nonfasting client with type 2 diabetes is also a major cause for concern.

PROTEINURIA. A routine urinalysis tests the sample for protein. The presence of protein in the urine (called *proteinuria*) is a manifestation of nephropathy. Testing the urine for microalbuminuria shows early nephropathy, long before it would be evident on routine urinalysis.

SELF-MONITORING OF BLOOD GLUCOSE

The development of devices that enable diabetic clients to monitor their own blood glucose levels has revolutionized diabetes care. These machines use reagent strips or a photometer, or both, and produce a digital readout of blood glucose values. Some have memory chips. Self-monitoring of blood glucose is recommended for all clients with diabetes, but it is required for people with type 1 diabetes, people with type 2 diabetes who need insulin, highly motivated clients with type 2 diabetes, women with gestational diabetes, clients who use insulin pumps, and clients whose diabetes is in poor control. These tests must be performed with extreme care and accuracy, because the results are used to adjust insulin, manage exercise, and monitor dietary management of diabetes. Most devices have a process by which the client can verify accuracy by using control samples. This method of testing is not used to diagnose diabetes, but it is instrumental in managing diabetes.

Self-monitoring of blood glucose levels uses whole blood, whereas laboratories use serum or plasma for glucose determinations. Values obtained with these monitoring methods are not equal. Glucose levels in whole blood are about 12% to 15% lower than those in plasma because glucose is not distributed in hemoglobin. To compare self-monitored levels and laboratory levels of glucose, divide the serum or plasma level by 1.12, which represents the 12% difference between the two. The results of self-monitoring should fall within 15% to 20% of the laboratory results.

Several noninvasive methods of measuring blood glucose levels are being developed and tested. Infrared radiation spectroscopy, polarized light rotation, and the use of minimally invasive devices that analyze interstitial fluid from the skin are some of the methods under active study.

Outcome Management

▬ Medical Management

The desired outcomes with medical management for clients with diabetes include restoring and maintaining blood glucose levels to as near normal as possible by balancing diet, exercise, and the use of oral hypoglycemic agents or insulin.[9, 27, 42] In general, when diabetes is successfully managed, clients avoid the complications of hyperglycemia and hypoglycemia. Unfortunately, complications may develop in some clients with diabetes despite their vigorous efforts to carefully control the disease.[12]

Initial as well as ongoing client education is vital in helping the client manage this chronic condition. Interventions must be individualized to the client's goals, age, lifestyle, nutritional needs, maturation, activity level, occupation, type of diabetes, and ability to independently perform the skills required by the management plan. Incorporation of psychosocial aspects into the overall plan is vital.[16]

REGULATE BLOOD GLUCOSE
Promote Proper Nutrition

Dietary management is an essential component of diabetes care and management. The general goal of dietary management is to help diabetic clients improve metabolic control by making changes in nutrition habits. Specific goals include (1) improving blood glucose and lipid levels, (2) providing consistency in day-to-day food intake (in type 1 diabetes), (3) facilitating weight management (in type 2 diabetes), and (4) providing adequate nutrition for all stages of life and with coexisting medical conditions.[9]

Achieving nutrition-related goals requires a team approach that includes the client. Effective self-management requires an individualized approach, taking into account the client's personal lifestyle and diabetes management goals. A nutritional assessment is used to determine the nutrition prescription on the basis of what the client with diabetes is able and willing to do. Glucose levels (self-monitored), lipid levels, blood pressure, and renal status are all essential aspects of nutrition-related management.

Promote Regular Physical Activity

A program of planned exercise is a crucial part of the treatment plan for a diabetic client. Exercise lowers blood glucose by increasing carbohydrate metabolism, fosters weight reduction and maintenance, increases insulin sensitivity, increases high-density lipoprotein (HDL) levels, decreases triglyceride levels, lowers blood pressure, and reduces stress and tension.[3, 27]

The primary side effect of acute exercise is hypoglycemia (low glucose level). Occasionally, hyperglycemia (elevated glucose level) and ketosis can occur in clients with type 1 diabetes. Hypoglycemia is a significant risk for clients who exercise while taking insulin or oral hypoglycemics. Adjustments are sometimes needed to prevent hypoglycemia in the client taking insulin, because hepatic glucose production is blocked or partially inhibited by exogenous insulin. For example, a reduction in short-acting insulin of 30% to 50% can decrease the risk of hypoglycemia. Clients who use meal planning and exercise alone to control type 2 diabetes are not at risk for hypoglycemia when exercising.

Administer Medications

ORAL ANTIDIABETES AGENTS. Five chemical classes of oral antidiabetes agents are available in the United States for the management of diabetes (Table 45–4):

- Sulfonylureas (oral hypoglycemic agents)
- Meglitinides (oral hypoglycemic agents)
- Biguanides (insulin sensitizers)
- Thiazolidinediones (also insulin sensitizers)
- Alpha-glucosidase inhibitors

Pharmacologic interventions should be considered when the client cannot achieve normal or near-normal plasma glucose levels with nutrition and exercise therapies.[42]

Oral hypoglycemic agents are effective in people with type 2 diabetes after nutrition and exercise therapy have failed. About 35% of clients with type 2 diabetes take oral hypoglycemic agents. The client most likely to respond well to oral antidiabetes agents is one who first has diabetes after age 40, has had diabetes for less than 5 years, is of normal weight or obese, and either has never received insulin or has well-controlled diabetes with less than 40 units of insulin per day. Indications for these agents are (1) random blood glucose levels less than 300 mg/dl, (2) fasting blood glucose level less than 250 mg/dl, (3) and inadequate control after exercise and diet therapies.

INSULIN THERAPY. Clients with type 1 diabetes do not produce enough insulin to sustain life. They depend on exogenous insulin administration on a daily basis. In contrast, clients with type 2 diabetes are not dependent on exogenous insulin for survival. They may need supplemental insulin for adequate glucose control, especially in times of stress or illness.

Insulin Types. Before 1991, insulin was classified by species (beef, pork, and human) and duration of action (short-, intermediate-, and long-acting). Most clients who require insulin therapy now receive human insulin produced by recombinant deoxyribonucleic acid (DNA) technology (Table 45–5).[42] Compared with animal insulins, human insulin peaks more precisely and predictably, has a shorter duration of action, and has reduced antigenicity (ability to produce antigen response), and it does not cause lipoatrophy (loss of subcutaneous fat) or lipodystrophy (fat metabolism disturbance leading to loss of subcutaneous fat) at the injection site.

Insulin works to lower blood glucose by promoting the transport of glucose into cells, and by inhibiting the conversion of glycogen and amino acids to glucose. The type and species of the insulin used, injection technique, site of injection, level of insulin antibodies, and individual client response all can affect the onset, peak, and duration of action of insulin. Insulin injected into the abdomen is absorbed fastest, with less rapid-absorption after injection into the arm and leg, respectively. Insulin inhal-

ers are being developed and may replace the syringes used for insulin injection. The normal secretory pattern of endogenous insulins follows a basal-level secretion, with increased production in response to an incoming carbohydrate load. In clients with type 1 diabetes, the goal is to mimic this increase with injections of exogenous insulin.

Humalog, an insulin analog, was released in 1996. Its action and potency as a hypoglycemic agent are the same as for human regular insulin, but the onset of action is immediate after subcutaneous injection, with a duration of action of about 2 hours. Humalog should be taken immediately before eating. Humalog is approved only for subcutaneous injection or continuous insulin infusion pump use. Humalog provides many benefits in achieving glucose control and may ultimately prevent or delay diabetes-related complications. Remind clients that because Humalog works so quickly, hypoglycemia can develop rapidly if they do not consume adequate calories immediately after injection.

Insulin Dosage. Insulin therapy should be individualized. For a client with newly diagnosed diabetes, a simple regimen with fixed doses may be used at first. The starting dose of insulin is 0.5 unit/kg/day. Two thirds of the dose is commonly given in the morning, one third in the evening. The health care team works to adjust the numbers and timing of injections to smooth out normal patterns. Then the dose can be increased. Algorithms are detailed guidelines to help clients self-adjust the daily insulin dose, based on self-monitored blood glucose levels, food intake, exercise, and departures from normal routine (such as added stress or illness). These guidelines use a prospective (predictive) approach to blood glucose control.[5, 42]

Insulin dosage varies greatly (Fig. 45–2). In determining it, the health care team must consider both the client's requirements and the client's response to the insulin. After initial stabilization, the team helps the client learn how to make adjustments in insulin doses, timing, food intake, and exercise. Unexplained fluctuations in blood glucose often occur. The team needs to help the client feel confident in his or her ability to control the diabetes.

Insulin Pump Therapy. Small portable pumps for the continuous administration of regular insulin are sometimes used (Fig. 45–3). The small pump, worn externally, injects insulin subcutaneously into the abdomen through an indwelling needle site that is usually changed daily. Insulin is normally infused at a low basal rate (a rate that matches the client's basal metabolic needs), with additional infusion of larger amounts (boluses) of insulin before meals.

Insulin pumps commonly improve blood glucose control by means of continuous subcutaneous insulin infusion. However, they do not have a built-in feedback mechanism for monitoring blood glucose levels. To benefit from use of an insulin pump, the client must comply with dietary requirements and usually must deliver the correct premeal bolus of insulin. The client must also monitor blood glucose levels four to six times a day and make decisions about dosages by using problem-solving skills.[1] Complications from use of insulin pumps include infection at the injection site, hypoglycemia from pump malfunction or mistakes in calculating the insulin dosage,

TABLE 45–4   **NURSING IMPLICATIONS FOR ORAL ANTIDIABETIC MEDICATIONS**

Class with Example Drug	Action(s)	Therapeutic Outcomes	Adverse Outcomes	Dosing
FIRST-GENERATION SULFONYLUREAS				
Chlorpropamide (Diabinese) Includes short-acting, intermediate-acting, and long-acting drugs	Stimulates beta cells of pancreas to secrete insulin Mild diuretic	Control of type 2 diabetes mellitus with blood glucose levels within preset parameters*	Monitor for hypoglycemia and hyperglycemia Monitor for hyponatremia in elderly May cause photosensitivity Monitor for weight gain, gastrointestinal and hematologic defects Increased risk of hyperglycemia with infection, fever, surgery, trauma, injury	Take 1–3 times/day with meals Avoid alcohol as it may result in hypoglycemia Allopurinol, clofibrate, aspirin, anticoagulants, anticonvulsants, beta-blockers may enhance action of drug and lead to hypoglycemia Caffeine, nicotine, glucocorticoids, NSAIDs, oral contraceptives, cough and cold medicines, thiazide diuretics, barbiturates, thyroid hormone, and phenothiazines may decrease action of drug and lead to hyperglycemia Women should avoid if pregnant or breast-feeding
SECOND-GENERATION SULFONYLUREAS				
Glipizide (Glucotrol)	Increases tissue response to insulin (insulin sensitizer); decreases glucose production by liver; stimulates beta cells to secrete insulin Mild diuretic	Control of type 2 diabetes mellitus with blood glucose levels within preset parameters*	Monitor for adverse outcomes similar to those seen with first-generation sulfonylureas	Take 1–2 times/day 30 minutes before breakfast (and evening meal if 2 times/day) Avoid alcohol and medications as described with first-generation sulfonylureas Women should avoid if pregnant or breast-feeding
BIGUANIDES				
Metformin (Glucophage)	Increases tissue response to insulin (insulin sensitizer); decreases hepatic production of glucose; decreases absorption of glucose from small intestine; decreases triglyceride and low-density lipoprotein levels	Control of type 2 diabetes mellitus with blood glucose levels within preset parameters* Decreases amount of insulin needed by type 2 diabetics who use insulin (research shows moderate decrease in insulin needed for type 1 diabetics, but no FDA approval for use in type 1 diabetics)	Monitor for lactic acidosis Hypoglycemia and hyperglycemia not seen because drug does not stimulate beta cells to produce insulin; clients taking other antidiabetic drugs, however, may experience these effects Long-term use results in decreased absorption of amino acids, vitamin B_{12}, folic acid May cause metallic taste at start of therapy	Take 1–3 times/day with or before meals; often given with sulfonylureas or insulin Hold for 24 hours before and after contrast media containing iodine Alcohol, Histamine H_2-receptor antagonists, calcium-channel blockers, and diuretics may increase effect of drug and result in hypoglycemia Avoid in pregnancy, during breast-feeding, in kidney or liver disease Decreases half-life of furosemide

TABLE 45-4	NURSING IMPLICATIONS FOR ORAL ANTIDIABETIC MEDICATIONS *Continued*				
Class with Example Drug	**Action(s)**	**Therapeutic Outcomes**	**Adverse Outcomes**	**Dosing**
ALPHA-GLUCOSIDASE INHIBITORS				
Acarbose (Precose)	Delays digestion of complex carbohydrates and certain sugars, so blunts peak of blood glucose and insulin levels after meals	Control of type 2 diabetes mellitus with blood glucose levels within preset parameters*	Monitor for gastrointestinal effects of flatulence, diarrhea, distension Monitor liver function studies every 3 months Does not cause hypoglycemia, but blood sugar can become so low that client becomes hypoglycemic	Take 3 times/day before meal or with first bite Give with sulfonylurea or metformin, but watch for hypoglycemia Calcium-channel blocker, estrogen, oral contraceptives, thyroid hormone, thiazide diuretics may decrease action of drug and result in hyperglycemia
MEGLITINIDES				
Repaglinide (Prandin)	Stimulates insulin secretion via closing or inhibition of ATP-sensitive K⁺ channels in beta cells	Control of type 2 diabetes mellitus with blood glucose levels within preset parameters*	Monitor for hypoglycemia Monitor for hyperglycemia if infection, fever, trauma, or surgery Monitor for upper respiratory infections, which occur more frequently	Take 30 minutes before or with meals 1–3 times/day Given most often with metformin If dose is missed, skip it and take next dose with next meal; skip dose if meal is skipped Calcium-channel blockers, diuretics, beta-blockers, oral contraceptives, estrogen, thyroid hormone may decrease action of drug and result in hyperglycemia
THIAZOLIDINEDIONES				
Rosiglitazone (Avandia)	Increases insulin action at receptors and postreceptor level in hepatic and peripheral tissue (decreases insulin resistance) Decreases triglycerides	Control of type 2 diabetes mellitus with blood glucose levels within preset parameters* Decrease insulin dosage for type 1 and type 2 diabetes if >30 units of insulin/day (dosage may be decreased 10–25%)	Monitor for hypoglycemia in client taking insulin or sulfonylurea	Take once a day before breakfast Avoid cholestyramine because it will decrease drug absorption and lead to hyperglycemia May lead to pregnancy by decreasing effect of oral contraceptives Usually given with sulfonylurea or insulin

*Preset parameters are generally considered to be fasting blood glucose level of 70–130 mg/dl; 2-hour postprandial blood glucose level of <160 mg/dl; glycosylated hemoglobin (HbA₁C) of <7.0.

NSAIDs, nonsteroidal anti-inflammatory drugs.

and diabetic ketoacidosis from injecting too little insulin to meet regular or increased metabolic needs.

At the start of insulin pump therapy, the client must be supervised carefully in either an inpatient or an outpatient setting. During this time, the clinician adjusts the pump for basal and bolus doses before meals, according to the client's usual diet and exercise regimen and previous insulin requirements. Researchers are trying to produce an implantable pump that not only administers insulin but also monitors blood glucose levels, much as a normal pancreas does.

INTENSIVE DIABETES THERAPY. In 1983, the NIDDK launched a 10-year, randomized clinical trial to assess the safety and determine the benefits of intensive

TABLE 45-5	TYPES OF HUMAN INSULIN AND COMPARATIVE ACTIONS				
			Action (h)*		
Action	**Preparation**	**Appearance**	*Onset*	*Peak*	*Duration*
Short-acting	Humalog (insulin lispro injection)	Clear	Immediate	0.5–1.5	2–4
	Regular	Clear	½–1	2–3	3–6
Intermediate-acting	NPH	Cloudy	2–4	4–10	10–16
	Lente	Cloudy	3–4	4–12	12–18
	Premixed (70% NPH, 30% regular)	Cloudy	½–1	Two peaks: 3–4, 8–12	16–24
Long-acting	Ultralente	Cloudy	6–10	None	18–20

* Absorption rates may vary by 20%–40% from day to day in any one client.

diabetes therapy. The most comprehensive diabetes study ever conducted, it compared the effects of two different treatment methods on the long-term development of diabetes complications—specifically, eye, kidney, and nerve disease.[22]

Twenty-nine medical centers in the United States and Canada enrolled 1441 people in the study; 52% were men and 48% were women. The average age at entry was 27 years. To participate in the study, volunteers had to be 13 to 19 years old; to have had type 1 diabetes for at least 1 year but no more than 15 years; to have no manifestations or only early manifestations of diabetic complications; and to be taking no more than two insulin injections a day. After being invited to participate in the study, clients were randomly assigned to either an intensive treatment group or a conventional treatment group.

Clients in the intensive treatment group learned to adjust their insulin doses to keep their blood glucose levels as close to normal as possible. Treatment included three or more insulin injections a day or the use of an insulin pump, self-monitoring of blood glucose levels four or more times a day, a special diet, an initial hospital stay, and weekly to monthly clinic visits. Clients in the conventional treatment group followed a regimen used by most people with type 1 diabetes: insulin injections once or twice a day, daily self-monitoring of blood glucose, and clinic visits every 3 months. Researchers monitored clients in both groups for signs of diabetic eye disease (retinopathy) as well as kidney (nephropathy) and nerve (neuropathy) disease.

Results of the trial indicated that intensive therapy delayed the onset or slowed the progression of chronic complications of diabetes by 35% to more than 70%. The risk of hypoglycemia was three times higher in the intensive treatment group than in the conventional treatment group. However, the risk of hypoglycemia was believed to be greatly outweighed by the reduction in microvascular and neurologic complications. On the basis of these results, it is recommended that clients with type 1 diabetes receive closely monitored intensive regimens. However, intensive therapy should be implemented with caution in clients who have repeated severe hypoglycemia or an unawareness of hypoglycemia.

With the intensive therapy approach, the client must be willing to monitor blood glucose levels four to six times a day and take three to five insulin injections a day. Throughout the initiating period of intensive therapy, the clinician must assess the client's knowledge of the meal plan, monitoring techniques, management goals, and manifestations of and interventions for hyperglycemia and hypoglycemia. The client also needs to be made aware of the extra financial and emotional burdens of this approach. The family and significant others need to be involved in the teaching process. Finally, the client needs to know that neither protocol is guaranteed to prevent long-term complications.[35]

COMBINATION THERAPY. *Combination therapy* is defined as the use of two or more oral antidiabetes agents or an oral agent combined with insulin. The advantage is that because the various groups of oral agents have different sites and mechanisms of action, they can complement and even augment each other.

In some clients with type 2 diabetes (mostly non-obese clients) in whom sulfonylurea agents alone failed to normalize blood glucose levels, insulin therapy has been required to achieve metabolic control very early in the course of disease. In these clients, daily insulin dosage is markedly higher than in clients with type 1 diabetes. This is attributed to insulin resistance. Because sulfonylurea agents enhance the effect of endogenous insulin by reducing insulin resistance, it has been thought that combining insulin therapy with sulfonylureas may be effective. One prescribed regimen is an injection of an intermediate-acting insulin at bedtime with daytime coverage by a sulfonylurea. This regimen is commonly called BIDS (*b*edtime *i*nsulin with *d*aytime *s*ulfonylurea).[38]

Nursing Management of the Medical Client

Diabetes self-management is the responsibility of clients and their families. The client with diabetes must be empowered to accept self-management and to become the focus of the team approach to treatment. Physiologic treatment of manifestations is neither the means nor the end of responsibility in dealing with a chronic disease like diabetes. Clients require consistent follow-up, updating, and reinforcement. Assessment of the client's level of acceptance of personal responsibility is necessary. This guides the practitioner to appropriate teaching and behavioral techniques to encourage a higher level of acceptance on the client's part.

Because of the multidisciplinary nature of the treatment, a team approach is recommended in managing cli-

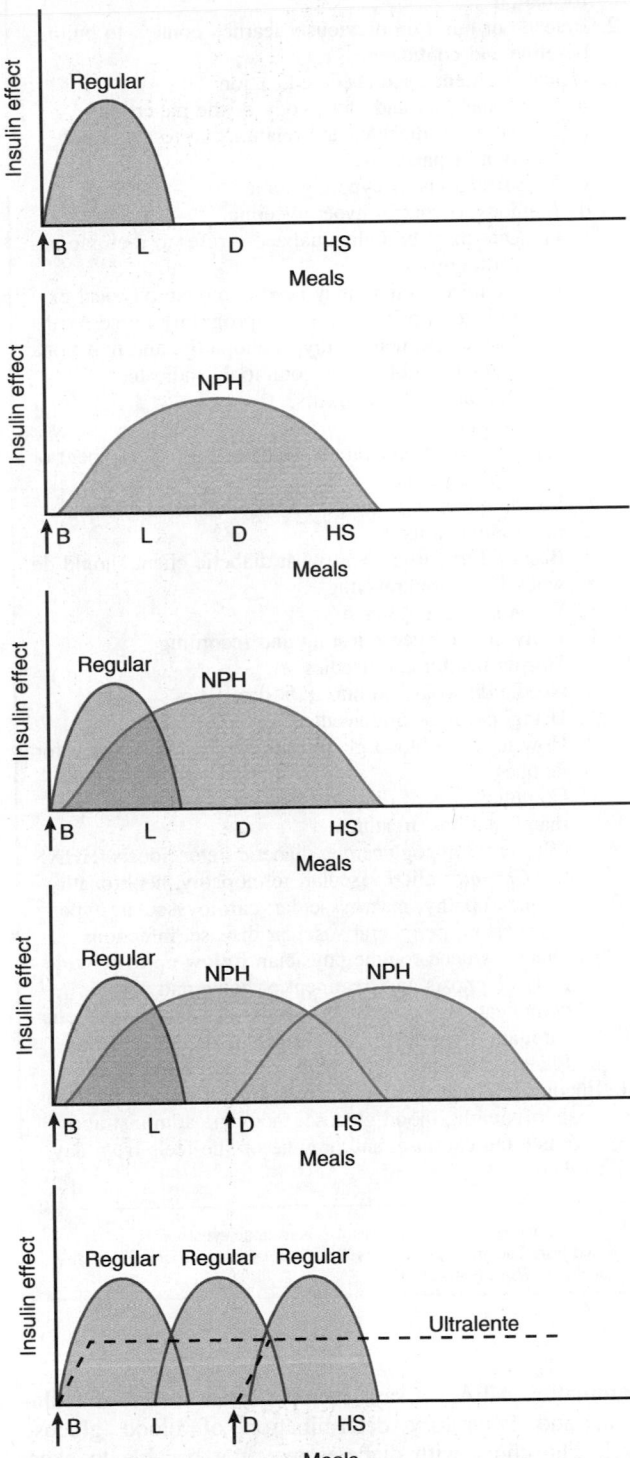

FIGURE 45–2 Insulin regimens. Only a few of a variety of possible regimens are shown here. Some clients require only one injection per day, whereas others may require split mixed doses (such as mixtures of NPH or Ultralente and regular insulin) or several doses of the same type of insulin (such as NPH insulin). Insulin regimens must be individualized for each client. B, breakfast; L, lunch; D, dinner; HS, bedtime.

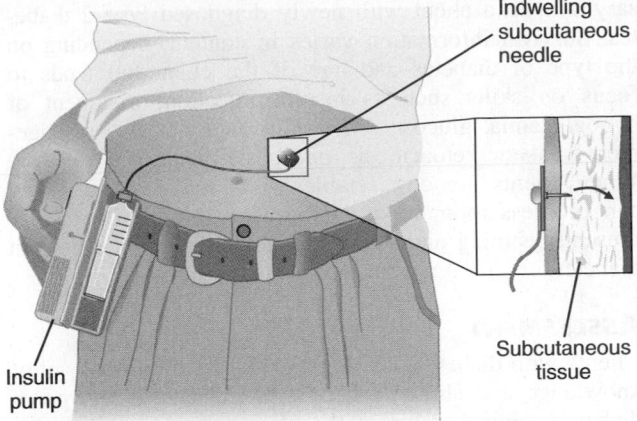

FIGURE 45–3 Insulin pumps are worn externally and connected to an indwelling subcutaneous needle, usually inserted in the abdomen.

ents with diabetes. This approach is particularly appropriate for client education when learners must acquire knowledge and skills from a variety of disciplines. Crucial members of the health care team include, whenever possible, a nurse, a dietitian, and a physician as the core members. Depending on need and availability, other members may include a psychologist, a social worker, a pharmacist, an exercise physiologist, and a podiatrist. Team meetings are planned to share information gained from individual client assessments and to develop a plan of action to respond to the client's clinical and educational priorities. The integration of various roles within the team strengthens the communication essential to client self-management.

There are two approaches to diabetes education[14, 15, 25]:

- The *compliance-based approach* is intended to improve client adherence to the treatment recommendations of health care professionals. It is based on the assumption that health care professionals are diabetes care experts and that in general, clients should comply with their recommendations regarding diabetes self-management.
- In the *empowerment-based approach,* the primary purpose of diabetes education is to prepare clients to make informed decisions about their own diabetes care. This approach assumes that most clients with diabetes are responsible for making important and complex decisions.

Few members of the health care team use one approach all the time to the exclusion of the other approach. Indeed, many health care professionals use some combination of the two approaches based on their own values and understanding of the purposes of education. For example, clients with newly diagnosed diabetes may wish to have the health care team make most of the decisions until they become familiar with the costs and benefits of various options in diabetes self-management.

Survival education includes the crucial information necessary to meet the client's immediate survival needs. These vary widely from client to client. For example, insulin injection is a survival skill for a client with newly diagnosed type 1 diabetes but is unlikely to be a necessary skill in a client with newly diagnosed type 2 diabetes. Survival information varies in content, depending on the type of diabetes and age of the client but tends to focus on skills such as insulin injection, treatment of hypoglycemia, glucose self-monitoring, sick-day management, diabetic ketoacidosis, and basic dietary information. When clients are comfortable with survival skills, they can progress to more in-depth information.[28] Box 45–3 presents learning and teaching guidelines for clients with diabetes.

ASSESSMENT

Clients with diabetes must be closely assessed for level of knowledge and ability to perform self-care. The type of diabetes, clinical status of the client, and plans for treatment are also important assessments. Ask clients if they take any vitamin, mineral, or herbal supplements, whether to decrease blood glucose levels or for other purposes. Chromium and garlic may lower blood glucose and cholesterol levels, and magnesium may increase insulin sensitivity. Blueberries, especially European bilberries, may also decrease blood glucose levels. Niacin may impair glucose tolerance.

DIAGNOSIS, OUTCOMES, INTERVENTIONS

Altered Health Maintenance. The client with diabetes must be able to perform self-care to keep the condition well controlled, leading to the nursing diagnosis *Altered Health Maintenance related to lack of knowledge about diabetes mellitus, lack of knowledge about exercise regimen for diabetes management, and lack of knowledge about dietary management of diabetes mellitus.*

Outcomes. The client will relate the basic pathophysiologic mechanism of diabetes mellitus, explain the need for exercise and diet in the treatment, and list the clinical manifestations of acute and chronic complications. The client will plan an exercise program to maintain blood glucose levels at preset levels and will identify strategies to monitor for and prevent complications associated with exercise.

The client will state the relationship of dietary management to blood glucose control, and will choose foods that meet caloric needs and offer a well-balanced diet. The client will recognize the times at which it is necessary to substitute a food to maintain blood glucose control. The client will discuss with the health care team difficulties seen in compliance with plans for diet, maintain blood glucose levels within preset parameters, and maintain weight within preset parameters.

Interventions

Explain the Pathophysiology of Diabetes. You or a diabetes educator should explain to the client and family the basic pathophysiologic mechanism of diabetes and how the disorder is managed. Sometimes the information is given through classes or by videotape. The client should also receive some form of written information to reinforce the material. Also, the client should be monitored for denial or anger about the diagnosis as part of a coping response.

Plan an Exercise Program. Clients with diabetes must consult the clinician before starting an exercise program. Pre-exercise screening may include a history, physical

---

BOX 45–3 **Learning and Teaching Guidelines for Clients with Diabetes**

1. Assess knowledge about diabetes mellitus, correct misinformation
2. Reteach or build on previously learned content to build baseline and confidence
3. General content for diabetic education
   a. Basic anatomy and physiology of the pancreas
   b. Definition of diabetes and relationship to abnormal function of pancreas
   c. Manifestations of hyperglycemia
   d. Methods to control hyperglycemia
      (1) Diet must be individualized—refer to dietitian accordingly
      (2) Exercise—client may need complete physical examination prior to exercise program to assess cardiac status, neuropathy, retinopathy, and nutritional needs (weight loss is commonly indicated)
      (3) Oral antidiabetic agents
      (4) Insulin
      (5) Recognize precipitating factors for development of hyperglycemia
   e. Insulin education: how/when/why/where to give insulin combinations
   f. Basic information about what diabetic client should do when ill and/or traveling
   g. When to call physician
   h. Daily blood glucose testing and recording
   i. Storing insulin and needles
   j. Needle disposal and universal precautions
   k. Using and recycling needles
   l. How to use a blood glucose monitor and test urine for ketones
   m. Complications of diabetes mellitus—definition, cause, manifestations, treatment
      (1) *Acute:* hypoglycemia, diabetic ketoacidosis, HHNS
      (2) *Chronic:* microvascular: retinopathy, nephropathy, neuropathy; macrovascular: cardiovascular, hypertension, peripheral vascular disease, infections
   n. Diabetics need routine physician follow-up to provide early diagnosis and treatment of acute and chronic complications, evaluation of present means of diabetic care, and treatment of coexisting medical disorders
   o. Identify available community and family resources
4. Encourage client to keep written goals and diary outlining goals of weight, blood glucose, medicine administration, and diet and exercise, and how he or she feels from day to day.

HHNS, hyperglycemic, hyperosmolar, nonketotic syndrome.
Adapted from Luckmann, J. (Ed.). (1995). *Saunders manual of nursing care.* Philadelphia: W. B. Saunders.

---

examination, HbA_{1C} assay, exercise stress test, foot evaluation, and laboratory determination of blood glucose level. The client with diabetes may not be able to exercise intensely to achieve a calculated heart rate because of a pre-existing cardiac condition, advanced age, or joint problems. The client should be helped to choose an exercise regimen and to set reasonable goals, because any increase in activity level is beneficial. Walking is usually well tolerated. Using a stationary bicycle or swimming is possible for clients with foot problems.

Clients with diabetes must start any new activity at a well-tolerated intensity level and duration, with gradual (over a period of weeks or months) increases in intensity and duration until preset exercise goals are reached. Exercise should include warm-up and cool-down periods before and after the activity. It is best to exercise at the same time of day, if possible. Because regular exercise is very important, have the client plan an alternative activity in case environmental or other factors make the usual exercise difficult. Unplanned exercise can be dangerous for clients taking insulin or oral hypoglycemic agents. During periods of exercise, the muscles are stimulated to take up glucose. Therefore, blood glucose levels can fall abruptly.[27]

Prevent Complications from Exercise. Clients should make sure they are adequately hydrated before starting exercise. They should eat 15 to 30 g of carbohydrate before exercise if the blood glucose level is less than 100 mg/dl and should carry a carbohydrate snack as well as their diabetes identification. If blood glucose is 100 to 150 mg/dl, the client may exercise and have a snack later. If blood glucose is greater than 250 mg/dl and the client has not just eaten, ketone levels should be checked. Clients with glucose at this level should wait to exercise, because vigorous activity can raise blood glucose levels by releasing stored glycogen. Alcohol and beta-blockers should be avoided because they may increase the risk of hypoglycemia or hyperglycemia.[27]

Plan Nutrition Therapy to Achieve Target Blood Glucose. A balanced nutritional plan is important for all clients, whether or not they have diabetes. Emphasize to the client and family members that they are not eating a "diabetic diet" but, rather, are following a balanced meal plan. Adherence to nutrition principles is one of the most challenging aspects of diabetes management. It requires a team effort. For an effective plan, assessment of the person's present eating patterns, knowledge of a healthy eating plan, and willingness and ability to modify patterns and nutritional needs is vital. Specific nutritional information should include the following[9]:

- Appetite
- Food allergies
- Ethnic and cultural influence on food habits
- Ability to obtain and prepare food (including financial ability)
- Community resources currently used
- Amount and type of physical activity
- Chronic disease requiring dietary modification
- Gastrointestinal disease
- Vitamin, mineral, or food supplements used
- Weight patterns
- Current eating patterns
- Dietary concerns of client
- Dental and oral health
- Medications with nutritional implications

The results of this assessment form a personal profile used to arrive at individualized goals. As a member of the health care team, you must have a knowledge base of both nutritional assessment and appropriate interventions.

Basic nutritional assessment includes anthropometric measures, biochemical tests, physical assessment, and dietary evaluation. No single parameter can measure the client's nutritional status or determine problems or needs. Figure 45–4 shows how assessment fits into the total nutritional plan for the collaborative management of diabetes. After the assessment, individualized goals are determined. Nutritional assessment and the client's understanding that optimal nutrition can lead to reduction of risk factors for chronic health problems and improve overall health constitute the starting point for goal selection.

For example, if the client has type 2 diabetes and is obese, emphasize that nutritional changes can help to lower blood glucose levels, decrease lipid levels, and lower blood pressure as well as help in losing weight. Weight loss also appears to increase insulin sensitivity and to normalize liver glucose production. The client should understand that dietary treatment is the best and initial treatment. If nutritional status does not improve, glucose-lowering medications, insulin, lipid-lowering agents, or antihypertensives may be required.

A standard "diabetic diet" is no longer prescribed for all clients with diabetes; instead, many dietary options exist (Table 45–6). Basically, the client with diabetes should strive to follow the Dietary Guidelines for Americans (the "Food Guide Pyramid") issued by the U.S. Department of Agriculture (USDA) and U.S. Department of Health and Human Services (USDHHS) in 1992 for current recommended nutritional guidelines.[40]

Calories. Caloric restrictions, especially for people with lifelong obesity, may be perceived negatively. Obesity is a complex interaction between genetic and environmental factors. The most successful approach to weight reduction is unclear, but you should understand caloric restriction, regular exercise, behavior modification, and peer and professional support. Moderate caloric reduction is described as a reduction of 250 to 500 calories per day less than usual. Reduction of fat calories may be a good initial modification. Regular exercise (three to five times weekly) enhances weight loss and is a predictor for successful weight maintenance.[9]

Protein. In general, Americans with and without diabetes consume more protein than needed to meet nutritional

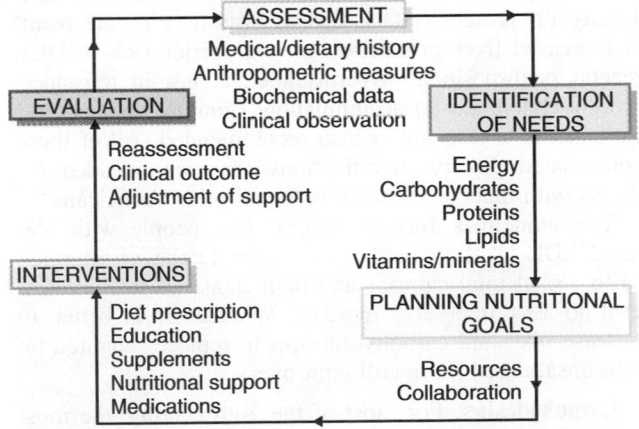

FIGURE 45–4 Assessment as part of the total nutritional plan for the collaborative management of diabetes. (Redrawn from Groth, K. [1995]. Nutritional alterations in critical illness. In L. C. Copstead [Ed.], *Perspectives on pathophysiology* [p. 1124]. Philadelphia: W. B. Saunders.)

TABLE 45–6	CURRENTLY RECOMMENDED NUTRITIONAL GUIDELINES FOR THE CLIENT WITH DIABETES MELLITUS
Calories	Sufficient to achieve and maintain reasonable weight
Protein	Adequate to ensure maintenance of body protein stores; people with diabetes have the same protein requirements as for non-diabetic people; in general 10%–20% of the total daily calories should come from protein (equal to ~0.8 g/kg/day)
Fats	Less than 30% of calories should be from fat, with less than 10% of that from saturated fat sources; if individualized risk factors indicate elevated VLDL and LDL levels, total calories from saturated fat may be reduced to 7%; cholesterol intake should be limited to 300 mg/day or less
Carbohydrates	50% to 60% of total calories should be from carbohydrates; simple and complex sugars do not differ appreciably in their ability to worsen hyperglycemia
Fiber	Clients with diabetes are urged to consume 20–35 g of fiber per day, which is the same as the recommendation for all Americans

LDL, low-density lipoprotein; VLDL, very-low-density lipoprotein.

needs. Protein should be incorporated into the diet through a variety of foods. Very-low-calorie diets are often deficient in protein and may result in accelerated protein breakdown. High protein intake increases renal workload and glomerular filtration rate. Some studies in people with diabetes indicate that lowering protein intake may delay progression of nephropathy. At present, the lower end of the recommended scale for protein intake (about 10% of daily calories) is sufficiently restricted and is recommended for clients with nephropathy. In certain cases, protein requirements vary from the adult recommended daily allowance; this is true for infants, children, adolescents, and pregnant women.[9]

Fat. The USDA national food consumption surveys reveal that most Americans eat too much fat. About 36% of calories in the average adult diet comes from fat, with about 13% from saturated fat. The general recommendation for Americans is to decrease total dietary fat to 30% or less of total calories, with saturated fat decreased to less than 10%. This reduction is consistent with a diet to reduce cardiovascular disease.

Clients with type 2 diabetes often have high triglyceride levels, high low-density lipoprotein (LDL) levels, high very-low-density lipoproteins (VLDL) levels, and low high-density lipoprotein (HDL) levels. This may be the result of increased liver production of triglyceride-rich VLDLs, genetic predisposition, hyperinsulinemia, insulin resistance, or intra-abdominal fat accumulation. Limiting daily cholesterol intake to 300 mg is also recommended. All of these lipid-related dietary modifications are recommended for clients with diabetes as well as for all other Americans.[9]

The guidelines further suggest that people with elevated LDL levels should reduce their intake of saturated fat to 7% of total calories and their intake of total cholesterol to less than 200 mg/day. Whether it is better to increase fiber and carbohydrates or to replace saturated fat with unsaturated fat is still controversial.

Carbohydrates. For most of the 20th century, the most widely held belief about dietary treatment of diabetes was that sugar was to be avoided. Little or no scientific evidence supports this assumption. When fed as a single nutrient, sucrose produces a glycemic response similar to that for bread or pasta. In the United States, the average diet obtains almost half of total carbohydrate intake in the form of simple sugars. Clinical guidelines suggest that 50% to 60% of the diet should consist of carbohydrates, in either simple or complex form. An occasional high-sucrose dessert poses no problem for the client with diabetes when it is accounted for in the day's total caloric and carbohydrate plan. Because some desserts are also high in fat, however, they should be limited.[9]

Working as a team with the client and a nutritionist, make a concrete medical nutrition therapy plan. The following are some helpful questions to ask the client:

- What is your most important goal in managing your diabetes?
- What are some changes you would like to make?
- Of the changes we have talked about, what would you like to work on first?

Team members must remember their roles as providers of information and counselors. Most counseling on nutrition begins with basic overviews of nutrition, diabetes guidelines, and reading of labels. More in-depth counseling on meal planning and calorie counting, for example, can come later. Eating plans vary widely among clients. Consistency within an eating style results in lower levels of glycosylated hemoglobin than does a haphazard eating style.

Diet management for clients with type 1 diabetes. Meals should be adjusted to match insulin action. Breakfast should be eaten within 1 hour after the morning insulin dose and a carbohydrate should be eaten about 3 hours later; lunch should be eaten about 4 to 5 hours after the morning insulin dose. When multiple insulin injections are used, greater flexibility with meal timing is possible.

The following are examples of approaches used successfully to instruct clients with diabetes:

- Handouts available from government sources, such as the USDA's "Food Guide Pyramid"[40] and the USDHHS publication, which uses the four-basic-food-groups approach[39]
- Individualized menus shaped between the client and dietitian
- The exchange system, last revised in 1986, which help with uniform meal planning (available from the ADA

in a simple pamphlet called "Healthy Food Choices," or in an expanded version called "Exchange Lists for Meal Planning")
- Counting components of the diet, such as counting calories and grams of fat
- A point system that utilizes lists of foods with point values and a prescribed number of total points
- The total available glucose system, which looks at foods in terms of their metabolic effects (highly motivated clients who desire flexibility may like this system)

A registered dietitian—preferably a certified diabetes educator—should always be consulted for initial evaluation and teaching of any client with a new diagnosis of diabetes. Each client should receive an individualized meal plan based on ethnic, religious, and cultural background; eating, cooking, and work habits; and food preferences. All clients need to know the dietary basics, which include the following:

- Avoid adding sugar to foods such as coffee and cereal.
- Avoid foods that are sweetened with sugar or honey, such as jellies, jams, cakes, and ice cream.
- Check blood glucose levels regularly.
- Keep periodic appointments with health care providers for evaluation of blood glucose control.
- Be consistent about the amount, distribution, and timing of nutrients.
- Increase the amount of carbohydrate in a meal eaten before sustained exercise.
- Limit intake of saturated fat and cholesterol.

Risk for Ineffective Management of Therapeutic Regimen. A client with diabetes must understand and be able to self-monitor glucose levels and learn self-injection of insulin, leading to the nursing diagnosis of *Risk for Ineffective Management of Therapeutic Regimen (Individuals) related to lack of knowledge and lack of previous experience with testing blood and urine and lack of knowledge and lack of experience with self-injection of insulin.*

Outcomes. The client will state personal goals for urine ketone and blood glucose testing parameters; demonstrate correct techniques for blood glucose testing (including timing), and demonstrate correct technique for urine ketone testing (including timing). The client will test blood glucose at regular times (including during illnesses and when traveling), and will prick the side of the finger, where nerve endings are fewer and more blood is available. The client will test urine for ketones when the glucose level is high (> 250 mg/dl) or during illnesses; keep a record of all tests performed and bring this record to regular, scheduled follow-up visits; and store testing materials away from heat, light, and moisture.

The client will state that insulin lowers blood glucose, and will name the type or types of insulin prescribed and the onset, peak, and duration of each. The client will take injections at regular times, 30 to 60 minutes before meals, every day, even when ill. The client will wash hands before preparing insulin injections, demonstrate proper mixing of insulin, and withdraw prescribed dosage using sterile technique.

When taking two types of insulin, the client will withdraw the prescribed dosage of each insulin into one syringe without contaminating either bottle (regular insulin is drawn up first). The client will demonstrate the correct technique of insulin injection, and inject insulin into the same area to ensure consistency in onset, peak, and duration of action. The client will store at least one extra bottle of insulin in the refrigerator, not use insulin past the expiration date, and will purchase insulin syringes before all of the current supply has been used.

The client will wear medical identification (MedicAlert) bracelet or necklace, or carry a diabetic identification card. The client will state manifestations, describe treatment of hypoglycemia, and will always carry something to treat hypoglycemia.

Interventions

Provide Instruction on Blood Glucose Monitoring. All clients with newly diagnosed diabetes mellitus require teaching about urine and blood glucose monitoring. All clients with diabetes may require review or update of information for self-care. Newer, more accurate blood glucose meters that are easier to use are constantly being made available. Only the basics are covered in this discussion, so you must keep up to date on each meter's advantages and disadvantages.

Many kinds of meters are available. Each client needs to be evaluated so that the proper meter is obtained. The client's ability to calibrate the meter and to visually interpret the digital reading must be considered. Some meters can be connected to a computer, which can convert blood glucose results into bar graphs or other printouts. Glucose meters are available for the visually impaired that give

---

MANAGEMENT AND DELEGATION

Measuring and Recording Blood Glucose Levels

The measurement and recording of blood glucose levels may be delegated to unlicensed assistive personnel. Delegate the data collection only to those who have demonstrated competency in performing this task. Consider the following issues:

- Initial orientation and demonstration of competence in the performance of blood glucose monitoring, including quality control and equipment management requirements.
- Instruction on the time schedule and frequency to obtain blood glucose levels.
- Proper method of recording and reporting of the blood glucose level.
- Rotation of sites from which to obtain samples in order to minimize patient discomfort.

You are responsible for defining those blood glucose levels that are immediately reportable to you (for example, levels outside the range of 70 to 180 mg/dl). Instruct assistive personnel to report any difficulty in obtaining the sample or concerns the client may raise during the process of obtaining a sample.

Verify the competency of assistive personnel in performing blood glucose level testing during orientation and annually thereafter.

Marsha E. Cloud, BSN, RN, Clinician II, Surgical Services, University of Virginia Health System, Charlottesville, Virginia audio commands for use of the device and announce the blood glucose reading.

In addition to demonstrating the techniques of blood glucose self-monitoring, discuss the normal blood glucose range, goals for good control (individualized for each client), when to test, how to record test results, and what to do for abnormal results. Consult a diabetes educator for assistance in helping the client choose an optimal meter.

Clients can use blood glucose strips if they are unable or unwilling to purchase a meter. Make sure the client is not color blind and can read the results accurately. Compare the client's results with blood glucose meter readings to check for accuracy. With some meters and strips, a 15% difference is seen between capillary blood and venous blood glucose levels. The capillary blood reading is lower. When insulin is being adjusted, make sure to account for this difference. As long as the source of blood is consistent, no adjustment is required.

Both health care agencies and clients need to verify the accuracy of their blood glucose determinations. The Joint Commission on Accreditation of Healthcare Organizations (JCAHO) and other regulating bodies dictate the procedure and frequency for quality control of meters used in health care agencies. The usefulness of many glucose meters is technique-dependent. Because treatment is based on results, correct methods of use must be ensured. Clients can perform a self-test and simultaneously send a blood specimen to the laboratory to compare results. Manufacturers of meters also provide quality-control testing solutions, which clients should be instructed to use routinely (weekly, for example). Quality control of glucose monitors is a constantly changing area; nurses and clients must keep up to date (see Management and Delegation).

Provide Instruction on Urine Testing. Urine testing for glucose is rarely done; however, urine can be tested for ketones (beta-hydroxybutyric acid, acetoacetic acid, and acetone). These substances appear in the urine of clients who are fasting, clients with poorly controlled type 1 diabetes, and clients with type 1 or type 2 diabetes who have a secondary illness. Ketones result from fat metabolism and are therefore present during fasting.[37] In a client with diabetes, however, the presence of ketones may indicate the serious complication of diabetic ketoacidosis (see later).

Provide Instruction on Insulin Administration. When administered correctly, insulin acts as a life-saving medication for the insulin-dependent client. When administered incorrectly, it may cause complications ranging from tissue damage to lethal hypoglycemia (*insulin shock*). To administer insulin properly, the client must be familiar with insulin concentrations, syringes, storage, preparation for injection, and techniques for self-injection, as outlined in the Client Education Guide.[5] Insulin inhalers may someday replace insulin injection syringes.

Insulin concentrations. Insulin is prescribed in units. Thus, pharmaceutical companies prepare types of insulin—such as NPH, regular, or Lente—in 10-ml glass vials that contain 100 units/mL. U-100 insulin contains 100 units of insulin per milliliter. It is the insulin of choice for nearly all clients. Those who require large amounts of insulin may benefit from using U-500 insulin, which contains 500 units of insulin per milliliter and is available in the United States only by prescription.[5, 42]

CLIENT EDUCATION GUIDE

Self-Injection of Insulin
Procedure

1. Wash hands.
2. Clean site with soap and water or 70% isopropyl alcohol (optional).
3. Store insulin vial in original carton to keep clean (or wipe top of insulin vial with 70% isopropyl alcohol).
4. Shake or roll insulin vial in palm of hands to resuspend all but short-acting insulins.
5. Inject an amount of air that is equal to each dose into the bottle—short-acting last. Insulin solution should be clear.
6. Aspirate prescribed amount of short-acting insulin into syringe first, intermediate- or long-acting insulin second.
7. Inspect syringe for air bubbles.
8. Pinch up and hold skinfold and inject at 90-degree angle.
9. If you are thin or have loose skin, inject insulin at 45-degree angle to avoid an intramuscular injection, which is absorbed faster.
10. Routine aspiration is not necessary.
11. Inject insulin.
12. If injection is painful or blood or serum oozes from site, apply pressure for 5 to 10 seconds.

Disposal

State laws require that needles and syringes be disposed of as a single unit in a puncture-resistant container. It is unsafe to recap, bend, or break the needle.

Syringe Reuse

The manufacturer intends that the insulin syringe and needle be disposed after one use. Research demonstrates that most people with diabetes reuse the needle and syringe until the needle becomes dull or bent or comes in contact with any surface other than skin. Most insulins have a bacteriostatic agent in them. If you reuse syringes and needles, recap the needle after each use; reusing may carry increased risk for infection, especially if you have poor personal hygiene, acute concurrent illness, or open wounds on hands. Discuss the practice of reuse with your practitioner before initiating:

- Can you safely recap the needle?
- Can you see clearly enough?
- How is your manual dexterity?
- Do you have a visible tremor?

Store syringes at room temperature. The potential benefit of using alcohol on the needle is unknown. It may remove the silicone coat on the needle and contribute to pain at the puncture site.

Insulin syringes. The most commonly used syringe can deliver a maximum of 100 units of insulin in 1 ml. However, insulin syringes are manufactured with capacities of 0.25, 0.30, 0.50, and 1.0 ml. For smaller prescriptions (50 units, 30 units, or less), smaller syringes are used (Fig. 45–5).[5] A smaller syringe enables a more precise insulin dosage. Two lengths of needles are available: short (8 mm) and long (12.7 mm). Short needles are not recommended for obese clients because of variability of insulin absorption when injected into adipose tissue.

FIGURE 45–5 Examples of the sizes of insulin syringes that are available for precise measurement of insulin doses. (Courtesy of Becton Dickinson Consumer Products, Franklin Lakes, NJ.)

Insulin storage. Vials of insulin not in use should be refrigerated. Avoid temperature extremes of less than 36° F or greater than 86° F. Vials in use may be kept at room temperature. A slight loss of potency may occur after 30 days at room temperature. Humalog, regular insulin cartridges, or prefilled regular insulin pens may be kept unrefrigerated for 28 days. Because of potential variations in temperature, insulin should not be left in a car or checked in airline baggage. Mark the date on the vial when it was initially opened. The client should always have a spare vial on hand.[5, 42]

Insulin preparation and injection. Experts once thought that insulin vials should be rolled between the hands to resuspend the insulin without creating air bubbles. Now they believe that vials containing NPH and Lente suspensions should be agitated vigorously to mix the insulin to deliver consistent insulin concentrations.

To minimize the discomfort of subcutaneous insulin injection, administer the insulin at room temperature. The number of bacteria carried through a small-gauge needle is insufficient for infection to occur, and alcohol preparation is no longer considered necessary. If alcohol is used to clean the site, wait until it has evaporated completely. Have the client try to relax. Penetrate the skin quickly. Do not change the direction of the needle once it has entered the subcutaneous tissue or while it is being withdrawn.[5]

Prefilled syringes. Prefilled syringes are chemically stable for up to 3 weeks when stored vertically, needle upward (so that suspended particles do not clog the needle), in the refrigerator. Self-monitoring of blood glucose levels may need to be performed more frequently to check whether storage of the insulin in prefilled syringes alters its effectiveness in achieving glycemic control. Mixing regular and NPH insulins in one syringe is acceptable and convenient. Premixed, fixed-proportion insu-

lins are available commercially. These insulins are not suitable when daily variations are needed in the dose or when short-acting insulin is required.[42]

Site selection and rotation. Certain sites are best used for insulin injection (Fig. 45–6). Insulin absorption varies from site to site. To avoid possibly dramatic changes in daily insulin absorption, instruct the client to give injections in one area, about an inch apart, until the whole area has been used, before changing to another site. Tell the client to avoid sites above muscles that will be exercised heavily that day, because exercise increases the rate of absorption. The client who is taking two injections daily may use one site for the morning insulin and another site for the evening insulin. Some clinicians instruct their clients to use only the abdomen because of its more even and rapid absorption rate. Emphasize the importance of adhering to a definite injection plan for avoiding tissue damage. Rotate injection sites in one area to decrease the variability of absorption.

Techniques for self-injection. Most clients who take insulin learn to give their own injections (see the Client Education Guide on Self-Injection of Insulin). It is primarily your responsibility to instruct clients with diabetes in the techniques for preparing and injecting insulin. The amount of teaching needed depends on the client's familiarity with insulin and the injection equipment.

Equipment that the client will purchase for home use includes insulin of the type prescribed, absorbent cotton,

FIGURE 45–6 Sites used for insulin injection. The injection site can affect the onset, peak, and duration of action of the insulin. Insulin injected into the abdomen (area I) is absorbed fastest, followed by insulin injected into the arm (area II) and the leg (area III).

approved syringes with needles, and 70% ethyl or 91% isopropyl alcohol (optional). As noted, alcohol preparation of the injection site is no longer considered necessary, and cleansing of the top of the insulin vial may increase the risk of infection by transferring resident bacteria from fingers to the vial unless gloves are worn. Storing insulin in its original carton or in a container that will keep it clean may be a more practical option.

Although the prospect of daily injections for life is far from pleasant, the client's attitude toward this intervention may be largely influenced by your own attitude. A matter-of-fact approach helps the client understand and accept responsibility for self-care. Schedule a teaching session for self-injection techniques. Some clients find it difficult to inject the needle into their own skin. For these clients, you might select the site and insert the needle. Then, as the first step in self-injection, have the client push in the plunger and remove the needle. As the client gains confidence, self-injecting will be less traumatic. Jet injectors, which are pen-like devices, can be used.

See the Case Management feature for the diabetic client.

EVALUATION

It is expected that clients with type 1 or type 2 diabetes will learn about the disease process and methods of control. If management is successful, complications of diabetes will be avoided as much as possible. For a client with newly diagnosed type 1 diabetes, return demonstration should be expected for all activities with increasing proficiency over time. The client should not be expected to accomplish complete self-care after a single teaching session. The amount of time required varies from client to client. Follow-up visits must be initiated to make sure that the client is following recommendations and has not experienced problems with the therapeutic regimen. Over time, periodic follow-up visits will help you monitor the client's ability to perform self-care and anticipate any potential difficulties.

Self-Care

Before hospital discharge, the client and family must have a basic understanding of diabetes and its management with blood glucose monitoring, insulin injections, foot care, nutrition, and exercise. Because diabetes is a chronic

CASE MANAGEMENT

DIABETES

Although nurses may care for clients with newly diagnosed diabetes, or clients with diabetic ketoacidosis or hypoglycemia, it is much more common for a client to be admitted with another primary problem and with diabetes as a co-morbid condition. Loss of glycemic control may result in longer lengths of stay and increased cost; because diabetes is a chronic condition with many devastating complications, it is an important focus for case management. Preventing or minimizing complications can help clients maintain a high quality of life even though disease is present.

Assess
Physical
- When was the diagnosis made?
- What are this client's usual medical regimen and blood glucose level?
- What other physical conditions might affect the client's ability to manage diabetes (e.g., retinopathy, peripheral neuropathy, gastroparesis, hypertension, peripheral vascular disease)?
- Are any physical conditions present that show decreased diabetic control (e.g., hyperglycemia, infection, nonhealing wounds or gangrene, poor nutrition)?

Educational
What do the client and family know about diabetes? Assess their knowledge of oral hypoglycemics or other medications, their ability to administer insulin and monitor blood glucose levels, and their knowledge about manifestations of hypoglycemia, hyperglycemia, and the importance of diet and exercise.

Advocate
- Allow the client to continue diabetes management as independently as possible (e.g., with self-administration

of insulin). Remember, consistent timing of meals and medications is important.
- Be aware of sensory deficits: for instance, during teaching, the client may need large-print materials; special equipment or pain management techniques may be needed to maintain mobility.
- Recognize and discuss the client's feelings related to chronic illness, loss, and changes in lifestyle or family role.

Prevent Readmission
- Make sure that diabetic clients have essential "survival skills," such as how to administer insulin and how to obtain help when necessary.
- Explore financial and practical issues around obtaining medications, equipment and food. Determine whether devices to assist vision-impaired clients to draw up insulin or whether prefilled syringes are needed.
- Stress follow-up with the primary care physician.
- Remind the client to keep records on glucose monitoring, diet, and exercise and to bring them to follow-up visits.
- Know when to refer the client to outpatient diabetic programs, including insurance-sponsored disease management programs.
- Consider home nursing follow-up for clients with newly diagnosed diabetes, clients with changes in management (e.g., from oral medications to insulin injections), and older clients for home nursing follow-up.

Summary
Some new diabetic clients will be started on insulin as outpatients, and newer techniques for delivering insulin via pump are changing management. However, weight reduction and control, smoking cessation, blood pressure and lipid control, infection prevention, and foot care remain important strategies to decrease diabetic complications and to avoid readmissions.

Cheryl Noetscher, RN, MS, *Director of Case Management, Cruse Hospital and Community–General Hospital, Syracuse, New York* disorder, the client needs time to adapt to as well as to learn about the many changes that are occurring. The client should be encouraged to anticipate a usual day at work, school, or home and should be taught how and when to give insulin, how to monitor blood glucose, and what types of foods to eat.

Clients with diabetes need ongoing monitoring of their self-care ability. Glycosylated hemoglobin (HbA$_{1C}$) levels are usually checked, as is the client's log of daily glucose levels and insulin. Chronic changes that result from diabetes should also be assessed on an ongoing basis, by checking the client's vision, kidney function, degree of neuropathy, blood pressure, and skin condition. If the client is elderly or debilitated, home nurse visits may be an excellent asset. A referral to a visiting nurse organization or home health care agency should be initiated before discharge.

Modification for Elderly Clients

Diabetes is common among older adults and represents an important health problem for this population. Currently, 6.3 million (19%) of all people over the age of 65 years have diabetes. Many changes that occur with normal aging affect glucose levels. Blood glucose levels increase with age; fasting levels increase by about 1 mg/dl per decade and postprandial values by 6 to 13 mg/dl per decade. It is believed that peripheral receptor sites become less sensitive to insulin with time. A decline also takes place in levels of glucose-regulating hormones (glucagon and epinephrine) and in lean body mass. These changes may be accompanied by decreased physical activity and a poor diet. Elderly people are more susceptible to severe hypoglycemia, which can lead to stroke, myocardial infarction (MI), angina, or seizures. Diminished sensations may mask the manifestations of hyperglycemia. Accompanying changes in liver and kidney function and multi-drug regimens may exacerbate hypoglycemia.

In general, nutritional guidelines for older clients with diabetes are no different than those for older clients without diabetes. However, older people with diabetes are at increased risk for problems that can cause functional limitations, such as:

- Pain
- Urinary incontinence
- Decreased vision (retinopathy, glaucoma, cataracts)
- Decreased proprioception
- Postural hypotension

Impairments in mental status, functional abilities, and sensory function may interfere with the client's ability to understand and follow the treatment plan. In the older client, the risk of acute complications from hypoglycemia may outweigh the benefits of tight glucose control. The older client may enjoy good health and do very well on an individualized treatment plan. A team approach aimed at maximizing health through optimal diet and exercise, may improve the client's quality of life, as well as achieving adequate glucose control.

Surgical Management

PANCREAS AND PANCREAS-KIDNEY TRANSPLANTATION

INDICATIONS. Some clients with type 1 diabetes are now receiving pancreas transplants. The first pancreas transplant was completed in 1966. Eighty per cent of pancreas transplantation procedures are now done concurrently with kidney transplantation. This is usually because the anti-rejection medication cyclosporine has such severe side effects, including hyperglycemia and nephrotoxicity, that adequate renal function unaffected by nephropathy must be present. The client's own pancreas is left intact (98% of its function is exocrine in nature), and the new pancreas is usually anastomosed (attached) to the iliac artery and vein, through which insulin can enter the systemic pathway. The new pancreas is placed in the lower pelvic cavity, and the duct is connected to the urinary bladder. The exocrine secretions of the new pancreas drain into the bladder and are not absorbed. The surgical procedure generally lasts from 4 to 6 hours. Pancreas-after-kidney transplants and pancreas-only transplants account for the remaining 20% of pancreas transplantation procedures.

There has been renewed interest in the surgical technique of anastomosing the transplanted pancreas to the duodenum to allow for exocrine secretions to be absorbed normally through the gastrointestinal tract. This prevents the dehydration that is common with bladder-drained pancreas transplantation. Research is being conducted on the use of transplanted pancreatic islets rather than the entire pancreas.

CONTRAINDICATIONS. Clients with type 1 diabetes must have well-functioning kidneys to receive only a pancreas transplant. If not, the pancreas and kidney must be transplanted simultaneously, or the pancreas must be transplanted following a successful kidney transplant. Other contraindications include problems that make the client unable to withstand the stress of surgery. Clients with type 2 diabetes do not benefit from pancreas transplantation. Type 2 diabetes results from a failure of insulin action, which cannot be improved by adding a pancreas.

COMPLICATIONS. Major complications of pancreas transplantation include vessel thrombosis, rejection, and infection. To help prevent thrombosis, the volume of blood flowing through the pancreas is kept at a high rate for 72 hours. Careful monitoring of laboratory values, fluid and electrolyte status, physical manifestations, and vital sign changes can alert you to possible complications. A sharp and sudden drop in urine amylase levels, rapid increases in serum glucose, gross hematuria (blood in urine), severe pain in the iliac fossa, and tenderness in the graft area are manifestations of vessel thrombosis.

Manifestations of acute and chronic graft rejection include fever, increased serum creatinine and blood urea nitrogen (BUN) levels, weight gain, and graft tenderness. Proteinuria is a primary manifestation of chronic rejection. In addition, fever, decreased urinary amylase levels, increased serum amylase levels, hyperglycemia, and graft tenderness are manifestations of graft rejection. To prevent graft rejection, immunosuppressive therapy with monoclonal antibodies (OKT3) or polyclonal antibody preparations (cyclosporine [Sandimmune], and azathioprine [Imuran] and prednisone) is administered. See Chapter 80 for further discussion of immunosuppressive agents.

Immunosuppressive drugs may be harmful to the transplant recipient. A rise in serum creatinine levels and decreased urine output may be related to the nephrotoxic effects of cyclosporine. Decreased white blood cell counts may be associated with the myelosuppressive effects of azathioprine. Other adverse effects of immunosuppressive agents for which you should monitor are discussed in Chapter 80.

Measures to prevent infection include early removal of invasive lines, adherence to sterile technique with dressing changes and catheter irrigations, pulmonary hygiene measures, and strict hand-washing practices. Antibiotics are used to treat infections.

OUTCOMES. It is expected that the client will recover from the pancreas or pancreas-kidney transplant surgery and will be discharged from the hospital within 7 to 10 days without the need for insulin. Within 3 to 4 months, the client will resume a normal life as long as medication and health care regimens are followed closely. Complications such as rejection and infection will slow postoperative progress. The client's quality of life is improved as a result of freedom from the need for insulin, return to a normal diet, and a less restricted lifestyle. Successful transplantation is indicated by improvement in blood glucose control (levels between 60 and 110 mg/dl) and C-peptide levels.

The survival rate is 91% after transplantation. More than 65% of clients who receive transplants no longer need insulin at 1 year afterward. HLA-DR matching or mismatching affects the results. See Chapter 80 for further discussion of organ transplantation.

■ Nursing Management of the Surgical Client

Once the client has chosen transplantation as an alternative to medical care and is placed on the recipient waiting list, he or she will need to undergo an extensive physical and psychological evaluation (see Chapter 80). Nursing care focuses on assessing the client's needs for knowledge and information.

The nursing care of the client undergoing a pancreas transplantation procedure is similar to that for any client undergoing major abdominal surgery. Postoperative care is directed not only at caring for the client's postsurgical needs but also at addressing the particular needs of a client who has undergone an organ transplant. Care of the client after organ transplantation is discussed in Chapter 80; renal transplantation is discussed briefly in Chapter 36.

The major focus of care is to monitor for rejection, adverse effects of immunsuppressive agents, infection, and occlusion of vessels. Careful monitoring for changes in vital signs, laboratory values, fluid and electrolyte status, and physical manifestations is important to determine the onset of complications—thrombosis, infection, and rejection. Serum glucose levels will range between 60 and 110 mg/dl, without administration of exogenous insulin. Urine amylase levels will remain constant, with urine pH between 7.0 and 8.5.

Immunosuppressive therapy started before surgery must be continued on a regular schedule postoperatively to prevent rejection of the new pancreas. Nursing implications for immunosuppressive agents to prevent rejection and treat rejection are described in Chapter 80.

You are responsible not only for implementing physical care immediately after transplantation but also for

addressing the psychosocial needs of the client and significant others. Keep them informed about the status of the transplanted organ. Allow them to express concerns and ask questions. See Chapter 80 for further discussion of organ transplantation.

■ Self-Care

The self-care regimen following pancreas or pancreas-kidney transplantation is very complex for the client and significant others. Teach the client and significant others about long-term, ongoing care, which includes frequent follow-up to monitor the status of the new organ(s). Discuss self-care involved in managing medications, diet, physical activity, and manifestations of rejection and infection. Explain why continuing the present medication regimen is important and why the client should never miss a dose. Explain the manifestations of rejection and infection if the client cannot remember, needs a review, or did not receive complete information. See Chapter 80 for additional information related to transplantation.

ACUTE COMPLICATIONS OF DIABETES MELLITUS

HYPERGLYCEMIA AND DIABETIC KETOACIDOSIS

Hyperglycemia results when glucose cannot be transported to the cells because of a lack of insulin. Without available carbohydrates for cellular fuel, the liver converts its glycogen stores back to glucose (glycogenolysis) and increases the biosynthesis of glucose (gluconeogenesis). Unfortunately, however, these responses worsen the situation by raising the blood glucose level even higher.[26, 37]

In type 1 diabetes mellitus, as the need for cellular fuel grows more critical, the body begins to draw on its fat and protein stores for energy. Excessive amounts of fatty acids are mobilized from adipose tissue cells and transported to the liver. The liver, in turn, accelerates the rate at which it produces ketone bodies (ketogenesis) for catabolism by other body tissues, particularly muscle. As fat metabolism increases, the liver may produce too many ketone bodies. Ketone bodies accumulate in the blood (ketosis) and are excreted in the urine (ketonuria). Metabolic acidosis develops from the acidic (pH-lowering) effect of the ketones acetoacetate and beta-hydroxybutyrate. This condition is called *diabetic ketoacidosis*. Severe acidosis may cause the diabetic client to lose consciousness, a condition called *diabetic coma*. Diabetic ketoacidosis always constitutes a medical emergency and requires immediate medical attention.[26, 37]

Diabetic ketoacidosis is the most serious metabolic disturbance in type 1 diabetes and is a common cause of hospital admission. Diabetic ketoacidosis is identified in about 40% of clients with previously undiagnosed diabetes and is responsible for more than 160,000 hospital admissions each year. It occurs most frequently in teenagers and older adults.

Etiology and Risk Factors

Diabetic ketoacidosis is primarily a complication of type 1 diabetes mellitus, although it can also affect clients with type 2 diabetes during periods of extreme stress. A precipitating cause can be identified in 80% of clients. Common causes of diabetic ketoacidosis include:

- Taking too little insulin
- Skipping doses of insulin
- Inability to meet an increased need for insulin created by surgery, trauma, pregnancy, stress, puberty, or infection
- Developing insulin resistance through the presence of insulin antibodies

Pathophysiology

Diabetic ketoacidosis is marked by a relative or absolute lack of insulin. Insulin may be present, but not in sufficient amounts for the increased need for glucose due to the stressors present (such as infection). When the body lacks insulin and cannot use carbohydrates for energy, it resorts to using fats and proteins. Excess production of counterregulatory hormones (glucagon, catecholamines, cortisol, and growth hormones) secondary to stress appears to play an important role in the development of diabetic ketoacidosis. These hormones antagonize the effects of insulin and foster diabetic ketoacidosis by promoting hyperglycemia, osmotic diuresis, lipolysis with secondary hyperlipidemia, and acidosis. Figure 45–7 summarizes the pathophysiologic mechanisms involved. The process of catabolizing fats for fuel gives rise to three pathologic events:

- Ketosis and acidosis
- Dehydration
- Electrolyte and acid-base imbalances[37]

KETOSIS

We have already examined the metabolic effect of insufficient insulin on fat metabolism. In diabetic ketoacidosis, buffering of acid by bicarbonate, which is excreted as carbon dioxide and water, fails to compensate for ketosis. Respirations increase in rate and depth (Kussmaul's respirations), and the breath has a "fruity" or acetone-like odor.

The renal system attempts to excrete enough ketone bodies to normalize pH, which leads to osmotic diuresis and hemoconcentration (excessive loss of fluid and electrolytes). Hemoconcentration impedes blood circulation and leads to tissue anoxia and lactic acid production. This rise in lactic acid further acidifies blood pH. The rising tide of ketone bodies eventually overwhelms the body's defenses against hydrogen excess. With its buffer, respiratory, and renal defense systems depleted, the body finally succumbs to its acid overload, and diabetic coma can ensue.

DEHYDRATION

Clients with ketoacidosis lose fluids from several sources. They excrete large amounts of urine in the body's attempt to eliminate excessive glucose and ketones. Second, acidosis can cause severe nausea and vomiting, with further losses of fluid and electrolytes (notably sodium and chloride). Finally, water is lost in the breath as the body attempts to rid itself of excess acetone and carbon dioxide. Typically, clients in diabetic coma lose an amount of water equivalent to 10% of body weight, plus about 40 g of sodium. Severe dehydration resulting from these fluid losses may be followed by hypovolemic shock and lactic acidosis.

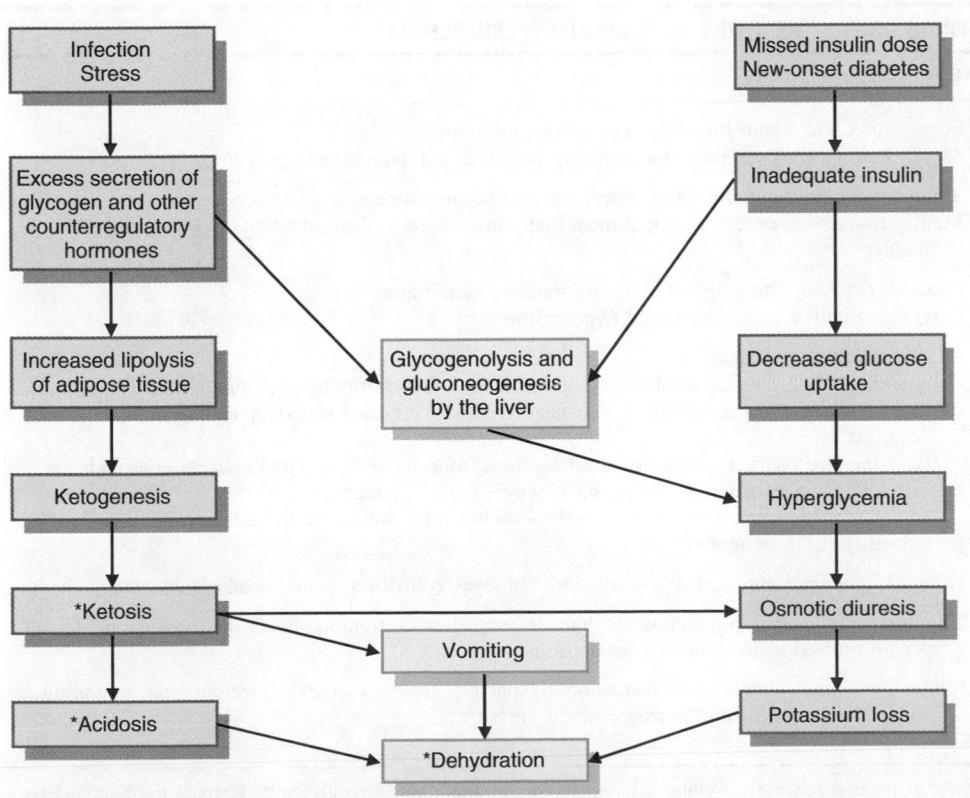

FIGURE 45–7 The pathophysiology of diabetic ketoacidosis. (Adapted from White, N. H., & Henry, D. N. [1996]. Special issues in diabetes management. In D. Haire-Joshu [Ed.], *Management of diabetes mellitus: Perspectives of care across the lifespan* [2nd ed., p. 344]. St. Louis: Mosby–Year Book.)

*Hallmarks of DKA

ELECTROLYTE IMBALANCE

As the pH of the blood decreases (acidosis), the accumulating hydrogen moves from the extracellular fluid to the intracellular fluid. The movement of hydrogen into the cells promotes the movement of potassium out of the cells into the extracellular fluid, which results in severe intracellular potassium depletion. Initially, the intracellular potassium loss may go unrecognized because serum potassium levels are often normal or elevated. As the resulting osmotic diuresis continues, however, much potassium is excreted in the urine. If the client becomes severely dehydrated, hemoconcentration and oliguria may cause the serum potassium levels to rise still higher. In addition to potassium losses, the client in metabolic acidosis loses excessive amounts of sodium, phosphate, chloride, and bicarbonate in the urine and vomitus.

Clinical Manifestations

Common presenting manifestations of the client in diabetic ketoacidosis are listed in Box 45–4.

Outcome Management

▪ Medical Management

Assessment priorities for the client with acute hyperglycemia are presented in Table 45–7. Management of diabetic ketoacidosis usually takes place in a hospital setting, with care managed by the physician, nurse, and pharma-

---

BOX 45–4 **Common Manifestations of Diabetic Ketoacidosis**

Abdominal pain	Polyuria
Anorexia	Somnolence
Dehydration	Tachycardia
Fruity odor of ketones on breath	Thirst
Hyperpnea or Kussmaul's respirations	Visual disturbances
Hypotension	Warm, dry skin
Impaired level of consciousness or coma	Weakness
	Weight loss
Nausea and vomiting	

---

cist. Dehydration resulting in hypovolemic shock, acute tubular necrosis, and uremia are major causes of death in cases of untreated diabetic ketoacidosis. Diabetic ketoacidosis constitutes an emergency. Rapid medical care and nursing intervention are essential to correct the life-threatening abnormalities. Effective therapy is based on an understanding of metabolic changes that occur during diabetic ketoacidosis. The cornerstone of treatment is the administration of fluids, insulin, and electrolytes.

Management outcomes in diabetic ketoacidosis are rehydration, correction of electrolyte and acid-base imbalances, restoration to a state of carbohydrate catabolism from a state of fat catabolism by providing insulin, and identification and correction of those factors that precipitated the ketoacidosis. The measures to achieve these outcomes must be done with great care. Fully correcting all

---

TABLE 45–7	ASSESSMENT FINDINGS FOR THE CLIENT WITH ACUTE HYPERGLYCEMIA
Problem	**Key Assessments**
Hyperglycemia	Finger stick and serum blood glucose levels and ketones Manifestations of hyperglycemia including polyuria, polyphagia, and polydipsia
Hyperosmolality	Serum osmolality, blood urea nitrogen; and serum creatinine Manifestations of neurologic impairment including lethargy, disorientation, and behavioral changes
Dehydration	Flushed, dry skin; "tenting" of skin; dry mucous membranes Polyuria, oliguria, tachycardia, and hypotension
Electrolyte imbalances	Manifestations of imbalances *Hyperkalemia:* Tachycardia, bradycardia, peaked T waves on electrocardiogram, ectopic beats, hypotension, nausea, vomiting, diarrhea, hyperactive bowel sounds, paresthesias, muscle cramps *Hypokalemia:* Nausea, vomiting, diarrhea, ileus, muscle weakness and cramps, ectopic beats, hypotension, flattened T waves and U wave, fatigue, lethargy *Hyponatremia:* Nausea, vomiting, diarrhea, tachycardia, hypotension, lethargy, confusion, seizures, muscle weakness
Metabolic acidosis	Hypotension, arrhythmias, hyperventilation, lethargy, confusion, coma, headache, acetone breath
Hypoglycemia	Diaphoresis, tachycardia, palpitations, hunger, paresthesias, tremors, headache, confusion, slurred speech, blurred vision, shallow respirations
Fluid overload (may develop with insulin treatment for hyperglycemia)	Intake and output, jugular vein distention, dyspnea, pulmonary crackles, weight gain, bounding pulse, edema, confusion, increased blood pressure

Adapted from Reising, D. L. (1995). Acute hyperglycemia: Putting a lid on the crisis; and Acute hypoglycemia: Keeping the bottom from falling out. *Nursing 95, 25*(2), 37, 39, 46.

CRITICAL MONITORING

The Rehydration Process

- The best indication of the degree of dehydration is weight loss, which may be determined if the client's baseline weight is known; loss may be 10% of total body weight.
- Other clinical indices to monitor are tissue turgor, pulse, condition of mucous membranes, level of consciousness, thirst, hematocrit, and positional blood pressure changes (to check for orthostatic hypotension).
- For older adults and clients with heart disease, fluid replacement should be determined according to central venous pressure measurement.
- Too-aggressive fluid replacement (particularly with normal saline) may induce heart failure; frequent auscultation of the lungs is vital.

biochemical abnormalities may take as long as 1 week after the client is able to eat solid food. A comprehensive flow sheet should be kept to record intake and output, body weight, fluids, electrolytes, insulin, and ketones.

REHYDRATE

Intravenous rehydration is required for all clients who are vomiting, are unable to drink, and have acidosis. IV infusions of isotonic or normal saline (0.9% sodium chloride) are started immediately. Usually, the client receives 1000 ml of isotonic solution by the IV route during the first hour (10 to 20 ml/kg), followed by an additional 2000 to 8000 ml of solution over the next 24 hours. Clients with compromised cardiovascular function may require slower IV fluid replacement (see the Critical Monitoring feature and Box 45–5).

A nasogastric tube may be necessary if the client is comatose or is vomiting and likely to aspirate the vomitus. The client's mouth may be dry because of the nasogastric tube and the dehydration. Frequent oral care is important.

Assess bowel sounds frequently for changes. Once the client can tolerate fluids, encourage them. Drinking salted broth is beneficial to replenish needed sodium. Record intake and output accurately. Most clients require a urinary catheter. Because clients with diabetes are susceptible to infection, aseptic catheter care is essential.

REVERSE SHOCK

If the client is in circulatory collapse, the physician may order blood, albumin, or other plasma volume expanders, such as dextran, to be administered alternately with normal saline solution. Also, the client may receive combinations of colloids and saline solution that raise serum levels of both sodium chloride and plasma protein.

RESTORE POTASSIUM BALANCE

Because of the lowered pH in untreated ketoacidosis, potassium leaves the intracellular space, and transient hyperkalemia develops. The total body potassium level is depleted, despite a normal or elevated serum potassium level. Correct potassium replacement requires caution and timely action. Once intervention begins with fluids and insulin, dangerous hypokalemia may develop, manifested by weakness, extreme dyspnea, and even cardiac arrest.

Hypokalemia occurs because potassium reenters the cells (along with glucose) after insulin administration and then is excreted in the urine with rehydration and restoration of renal function. General agreement exists on the following points of assessment and intervention:

- Frequently assess and measure urine output. Do not administer potassium to a client with low urine output; dangerous hyperkalemia may develop. Notify the physician promptly if urine output falls dramatically or is less than 0.5 ml/kg per hour.
- Assess the client continuously for evidence of hyperkalemia (bradycardia, cardiac arrest, weakness, flaccid paralysis, oliguria) or hypokalemia (weakness, flaccid paralysis, paralytic ileus, cardiac arrest). Hyperkalemia may be present during the first 4 hours of intervention. Hypokalemia usually develops 4 to 24 hours after the initial intervention.
- Replace potassium carefully following protocols (Box 45–6).
- Plan to begin potassium administration within 1 to 2 hours after starting insulin therapy and after adequate urine output is ensured.
- When the client has recovered sufficiently to resume eating and drinking, give foods and liquids that are high in potassium, such as bananas or orange juice.
- Monitor sodium chloride and phosphate levels. Sodium is replaced by normal saline. Phosphate levels can also vary to the same degree noted for potassium levels. Sometimes the physician will alternate potassium chloride with potassium phosphate in the IV fluid.

CORRECT pH AND ADMINISTER INSULIN

Clients presenting in diabetic ketoacidosis usually have phosphate depletion from a combination of decreased food intake, excessive catabolism, and increased urinary excretion. As with administration of potassium, adminis-

---

BOX 45–5   Intravenous Fluid Replacement in Diabetic Ketoacidosis*

Hour 1

Provide 15–20 ml/kg of isotonic sodium chloride (0.9%) (normal saline) or full-strength Ringer's lactate (lactated Ringer's solution).

Hour 2

Continue fluid as above at 15 ml/kg. If the client is hypernatremic, in heart failure, or is a child, consider half-strength sodium chloride (0.45% normal saline).

Hour 3

Reduce fluid intake to 7.5 ml/kg in adults. Fluid should be 0.45% normal saline.

Hour 4

Adjust fluid intake to meet clinical need. Consider urine output rate in calculation.

*When blood glucose approaches 250 mg/dl, change fluid to 5% dextrose in half-strength sodium chloride (D_5 0.45% normal saline). Continue intravenous fluids until client can ingest food and drink without vomiting.

Modified from American Diabetes Association. (1998). *Medical management of (type 1) insulin dependent diabetes* (3rd ed.). Alexandria, VA: Author.

BOX 45–6 **Potassium Replacement in Diabetic Ketoacidosis**

In clients with adequate urine output, lead II of the 12-lead electrocardiogram may be used as a guide for plasma potassium (K^+) concentration. Flattening or inversion of the T wave with U wave and prolongation of the QT interval indicate hypokalemia. Peaking of T waves, loss of P wave, and a disrupted QRS complex indicate hyperkalemia. Intravenous replacement of potassium is based on plasma K^+ concentration. If K^+ concentration is:

- <3 mEq/L, infuse ≥0.6 mEq/kg/hr
- 3–4 mEq/L, infuse 0.6 mEq/kg/hr
- 4–5 mEq/L, infuse 0.2–0.4 mEq/kg/hr
- 6 mEq/L, withhold until K^+ concentration is <6.0 mEq/L

Add K^+ to replacement fluid therapy. If concentration is 20–40 mEq/L and infusion into peripheral vein causes irritation, infuse into central vein.

Recheck plasma K^+ concentration every 2 hours if previous value was <4 or >6 mEq/L.

Adapted from American Diabetes Association. (1998). *Medical management of (type 1) insulin dependent diabetes* (3rd ed.). Alexandria, VA: Author.

tration of insulin enhances movement of phosphate into the cells, which further reduces plasma phosphate concentration. However, administering too much phosphate can induce hypocalcemia. Calcium levels should be checked before phosphate (as potassium phosphate) is given.

Clinicians usually administer sodium bicarbonate only to clients with a blood pH of 7.1 or less. Such replacement therapy partially corrects the metabolic acidosis. As the client's condition improves, normal body mechanisms restore the blood pH to normal.

Low-dosage insulin therapy (5 to 10 units/hour) is ordered for the client in diabetic ketoacidosis. Although the blood glucose concentration is usually sharply elevated in diabetic ketoacidosis, a blood glucose level below 300 mg/dl does not exclude the diagnosis. The client in ketoacidosis may receive an initial IV bolus of regular insulin (0.15 unit/kg) in the emergency department. Before starting an infusion of insulin, ask whether the client has already received insulin that day. Insulin should never be given subcutaneously to someone in diabetic ketoacidosis, because the subcutaneous tissues are dehydrated and poorly perfused as a result of dehydration and hypovolemic shock.

Traditionally, the hyperglycemia associated with diabetic ketoacidosis is treated with an IV bolus of regular insulin. Then an insulin drip should be started. Either 0.9% (normal) saline solution or 0.45% saline may be used, depending on the degree of dehydration and concurrent medical problems. Prepare the last amount of insulin in the smallest IV bag available (e.g., 100 units of regular insulin in 100 ml of IV fluid). This gives a 1:1 ratio of regular insulin to IV fluid. Prime the IV tubing with the IV solution first, and then add the regular insulin, because insulin will adhere to the IV tubing. Label the IV bag clearly with the dose and type of insulin added. The IV regular insulin must be administered very meticulously by a control pump and checked frequently.

After the bolus, infuse insulin at a rate of 0.1 unit/kg/hour. If no improvement in the acidosis occurs within 2 to 4 hours, the infusion rate should be doubled. Severe insulin resistance may be precipitated by severe stress. The glucose level is normalized more quickly than pH.

Blood glucose levels need to be monitored every 30 minutes initially, preferably with a blood glucose meter. Rapid blood glucose test results allow you to adjust the insulin infusion rapidly and correctly. When the blood glucose levels approach 250 mg/dl, the insulin infusion should be reduced and 5% dextrose added to the infusion so that the blood glucose level can be maintained at about 250 mg/dl for the first 12 to 24 hours. Faster correction of hyperglycemia can lead to cerebral edema. Monitor the client's level of consciousness closely to assess for this uncommon complication. Monitor blood glucose levels every 1 to 2 hours after reaching 250 mg/dl until they are stable.

As the client improves, decisions must be made about when to discontinue IV insulin and fluids and begin subcutaneous insulin administration. Normalization of the client's vital signs, correction of acidosis, and ability to take oral fluids are important considerations. Short-acting insulin is usually administered subcutaneously every 4 to 6 hours, with the first dose given 15 to 30 minutes before stopping IV insulin. The initial dose is about 0.2 unit/kg. Subsequent doses are determined by blood glucose levels.

While any metabolic abnormalities are being corrected, the cause of the client's diabetic ketoacidosis must be pursued aggressively. Cultures of urine, throat, sputum, and blood; chest x-ray films; and an electrocardiogram (ECG) may reveal the source of stress. Before discharge of the client from the hospital, the health care team reviews the situation that led to diabetic ketoacidosis and institutes teaching for risk factor reduction.

PREVENT RECURRENCE
Primary prevention of diabetic ketoacidosis is through client education. Preventing diabetic ketoacidosis is the long-term goal of good diabetes management. Clients and their families should understand enough about ketoacidosis to avoid potential causes, to recognize its approach, to slow down or minimize its development, and to seek help fast if it begins to occur. To prevent diabetic ketoacidosis, clients with diabetes should learn to:

- Take insulin in appropriate doses at appropriate times
- Monitor blood glucose frequently, at least before each meal and at bedtime
- Monitor urine ketone levels when blood glucose levels rise above 250 mg/dl
- Schedule regular appointments with a health care provider to review blood glucose levels, weight gains or losses, and general state of health and well-being
- Recognize manifestations of infection—a major cause of diabetic ketoacidosis. The first clinical manifestations of infection (upper respiratory tract, urinary tract, or vaginal infection) should be reported immediately to the health care provider; other stressors, such as family or emotional problems, can also precipitate diabetic ketoacidosis[16]

The client should telephone for assistance if any of the following develop:

- Anorexia, nausea, vomiting, or diarrhea
- Ketonuria persisting for more than 8 hours
- Fever or infection
- Any manifestation of acidosis

Emphasize that the greatest weapons against diabetic ketoacidosis are regular, daily self-monitoring of blood glucose; adherence to the diabetes management program; and early recognition of and intervention in mild ketosis.

HYPERGLYCEMIC, HYPEROSMOLAR, NONKETOTIC SYNDROME

Hyperglycemic, hyperosmolar, nonketotic syndrome (HHNS) is a variant of diabetic ketoacidosis characterized by extreme hyperglycemia (600 to 2000 mg/dl), profound dehydration, mild or undetectable ketonuria, and the absence of acidosis. HHNS most commonly occurs in older clients with type 2 diabetes mellitus (Box 45–7).

Mortality with HHNS is higher than with diabetic ketoacidosis (10% to 40%), primarily because clients typically are older and commonly have significant medical problems. HHNS sometimes occurs in people with undiagnosed diabetes and in known diabetic clients after a long period of uncontrolled hyperglycemia. The precipitating factors for HHNS may be the same as those for diabetic ketoacidosis. There is almost always an identifiable precipitating factor.

The major difference between HHNS and diabetic ketoacidosis is the lack of ketonuria with HHNS. Because some residual ability to secrete insulin remains in type 2 diabetes mellitus, the mobilization of fats for energy usually does not occur. In the absence of adequate insulin, the blood becomes loaded with glucose. Glucose molecules are too large to pass into cells; therefore, osmosis of water occurs from the interstitial spaces and cells to dilute the glucose in the blood. Osmotic diuresis occurs. Eventually, the cells become dehydrated.

The client's fluid intake can initially balance the loss of fluid and glucose through the urine. The imbalance gradually becomes more severe as the client cannot match intake to output. In time, the client becomes obtunded and is unable to respond to thirst. At this point, the process is self-perpetuating.

The four major clinical features of HHNS are:

- Severe hyperglycemia (600 to 2000 mg/dl)
- No or only slight ketosis
- Profound dehydration (10% to 15% loss of body water)
- Hyperosmolality (increased concentration) of plasma and elevated blood urea nitrogen

Typically, the client experiences excessive thirst, altered level of consciousness (coma or confusion), and manifestations of dehydration.

The precipitating event should be determined and corrected as soon as possible, even during resuscitation. HHNS is treated with vigorous fluid replacement and administration of insulin and electrolytes. A common initial intervention is infusion of normal saline solution over a 2-hour period, followed by administration of hypotonic (0.45%) saline solution. As in diabetic IV ketoacidosis, potassium, sodium, chloride, and phosphates are administered.

Insulin is given via an infusion pump, but usually at lower dosages, because the client is producing some insulin. Because of severe dehydration, plasma glucose levels fall rapidly with fluid administration. Dextrose is added to the IV fluid when the blood glucose level reaches about 250 mg/dl, to prevent hypoglycemia. Because many clients who have HHNS are older and have other cardiovascular or renal disorders, fluid volume and electrolyte changes must be carefully assessed, especially if acute or chronic renal failure complicates the course.

As the population ages, an increasing number of clients will experience HHNS and you need to be alert for its manifestations. Before discharge, review the causes of HHNS with the client and family, including insulin injection (if necessary) and blood glucose testing techniques. Help the client understand how serious these acute complications are and how to prevent them in the future.

BOX 45–7	**Factors Associated with Hyperglycemic, Hyperosmolar, Nonketotic Syndrome (HHNS)**

Therapeutic Agents

- Glucocorticoids
- Diuretics
- Diphenylhydantoin
- Beta-adrenergic blocking agents
- L-Asparaginase
- Immunosuppressive agents
- Chlorpromazine
- Diazoxide

Therapeutic Procedures

- Peritoneal dialysis
- Hemodialysis
- Hyperalimentation
- Surgical stress

Chronic Illness

- Renal disease
- Heart disease
- Hypertension
- Previous stroke
- Alcoholism
- Psychiatric diagnosis
- Loss of thirst

Acute Illness

- Infection
- Gangrene
- Urinary tract infection
- Septicemia
- Burns
- Gastrointestinal bleeding
- Myocardial infarction
- Pancreatitis
- Cerebrovascular accident (stroke)

From American Diabetes Association. (1998). *Medical management of non-insulin dependent (type 2) diabetes* (4th ed.). Alexandria, VA: Author.

HYPOGLYCEMIA

Hypoglycemia (also known as an *insulin reaction* or hypoglycemic reaction) is a common feature of type 1 diabetes mellitus and can also be seen in clients with type 2 diabetes treated with insulin or oral agents. The precise blood glucose level at which clients have manifestations of hypoglycemia varies, but they usually do not occur until the blood glucose level is less than 50 to 60 mg/dl.

Etiology and Risk Factors

Hypoglycemic reactions may result from the following:

- An overdose of insulin or, less commonly, a sulfonylurea
- Omitting a meal or eating less food than usual
- Overexertion without additional carbohydrate compensation
- Nutritional and fluid imbalances caused by nausea and vomiting
- Alcohol intake

Inadvertent or deliberate errors in insulin dose are a frequent cause of hypoglycemia. Other changes in the schedule of meals or insulin administration, vigorous unexpected exercise, or sleeping later than usual in the morning can also cause hypoglycemia. The effects of alcohol, marijuana, or other drugs can mask a client's awareness of hypoglycemia in its earliest stages.

Hypoglycemia can also occur secondary to administration of an oral hypoglycemic agent. Most recorded cases have been in clients receiving chlorpropamide (Diabinese), which has a duration of action of 24 to 72 hours. Clients at risk for hypoglycemia while taking an oral hypoglycemic are over age 60 years, have poor nutritional intake, use alcohol, have hepatic or renal dysfunction, and are receiving multi-drug regimens. The hypoglycemic reactions can be severe and prolonged.

Pathophysiology

Normally, hypoglycemia triggers counterregulatory hormones, primarily glucagon and epinephrine, to promptly increase blood glucose levels by stimulating glucose release from the liver and inhibiting insulin secretion. Under usual conditions, this leads to normoglycemia.

In contrast, clients with type 1 diabetes have abnormalities in this feedback system. Typically, within the first 2 to 5 years of diabetes, the secretion of glucagon becomes deficient. Later, the secretion of epinephrine may become impaired secondary to subclinical neuropathy. The regulation of insulin absorption from subcutaneous fat also becomes impaired.

The combination of these abnormalities makes the client with type 1 diabetes susceptible to frequent development of hypoglycemia. In this respect, hypoglycemic shock is more dangerous than diabetic ketoacidosis. About one in 10 clients with type 1 diabetes suffer one severe reaction per year that requires emergency treatment. Untreated or prolonged hypoglycemia can cause permanent brain damage, memory loss, decreased learning ability, paralysis, and death.

Clinical Manifestations

Hypoglycemic manifestations are generally divided into two major categories (Box 45–8):

BOX 45–8   **Manifestations of Hypoglycemia**

Adrenergic (increased epinephrine)

- Shakiness
- Irritability
- Nervousness
- Tachycardia, palpitations
- Tremor
- Hunger
- Diaphoresis
- Pallor
- Paresthesias

Neuroglycopenic (decreased glucose to brain)

- Headache
- Mental illness
- Inability to concentrate
- Slurred speech
- Blurred vision
- Confusion
- Irrational behavior
- Lethargy, severe
- Loss of consciousness
- Coma
- Seizure
- Death

---

1. *Adrenergic* (autonomic) manifestations are associated with rising epinephrine levels and are considered "mild" reactions. Cognitive deficits usually do not occur, and affected people are capable of self-treatment. Diaphoresis, although not mediated via adrenergic nerve endings, is usually grouped with the adrenergic manifestations of hypoglycemia. Adrenergic reactions usually occur during rapid decreases in blood glucose. They have been reported by clients with poorly controlled diabetes when the fall in blood glucose level is rapid, even in the absence of hypoglycemia. These manifestations can also occur during other stressful or anxiety-provoking events. These mild reactions may produce only minimal disruptions of daily activities.

2. *Neuroglycopenic* manifestations are associated with lack of glucose availability to the brain and resultant decrease in cognitive functioning. These reactions typically produce longer-lasting and more severe manifestations than those characteristic of mild reactions. Common manifestations are headache, irritability, drowsiness, weakness, and tremor. The client may need assistance in treatment. Severe hypoglycemic reactions render the client unable to self-treat. The client may be awake and alert, semi-comatose, or comatose.

Hypoglycemia can occur at any time of day or night. It seems to occur most commonly during exercise, 8 to 24 hours after strenuous exercise, and in the middle of the night. Severe hypoglycemia seems to occur more often in people who have hypoglycemic unawareness, defective glucose counterregulation, and autonomic neuropathy as well as in clients receiving intensive diabetes therapy.

The period during which the client is most likely to experience an insulin reaction depends on the type of insulin given, the client's response to that type of insulin, and the timing of the insulin injection in relation to food intake. When insulin is given in the morning, short-acting preparations tend to produce reactions before lunch; intermediate-acting insulins, 2 or 3 hours before dinner; and long-acting insulins, between 2:00 AM and breakfast. NPH or Lente insulin injected before dinner (5:00 PM) can cause hypoglycemia around 2:00 AM, when the normal blood glucose level is lowest because of the decrease in metabolism, and again at around 8:00 AM, when the insulin peaks if breakfast is not eaten on time.

Outcome Management

▮ Medical Management

RETURN SERUM GLUCOSE TO NORMAL LEVELS
Management of hypoglycemia depends on the severity of the reaction (Table 45–8). To reverse mild hypoglycemia, 10 to 15 g of simple carbohydrate is given and works quickly to increase blood glucose levels. Reactions that occur during the night should be treated with a carbohydrate followed by a longer-acting mixture of carbohydrate and protein (8 ounces of milk, for example). A blood glucose test (with a glucose meter) should be performed as soon as manifestations begin. If a meter is not available, it is safer to assume and treat hypoglycemia. Blood glucose is retested in 15 to 30 minutes, and treatment is repeated if the level is not over 100 mg/dl. Moderate reactions may need two or more treatments with 10 to 15 g of carbohydrates.

Never force an unconscious or semiconscious client to drink liquids, because fluid may be aspirated into the lungs. The unconscious client with severe hypoglycemia needs glucagon or IV glucose immediately. Family members of clients with diabetes can administer glucagon at home in the event of a serious hypoglycemic reaction. Glucagon, administered intramuscularly or subcutaneously in the amount of 1 mg for adults, may eliminate the need for emergency department intervention. The pharmacy dispenses glucagon in the form of a powder, with the diluent in a separate vial. Instruct family members how and when to mix and inject glucagon, and let them know that the client may experience nausea or vomiting on awakening. Even though glucagon is effective in most clients, its effect is transient and slower than that of dextrose. Hypoglycemia often recurs. Medical assistance is advisable if hypoglycemia recurs, vomiting prevents oral intake, or the client's status does not improve.

A client who experiences severe hypoglycemia in the hospital usually receives 10 to 25 g of IV glucose (as 50% or 25% dextrose) over 1 to 3 minutes. This is followed by an infusion of 5% dextrose at 5 to 10 g/hour until the client is fully recovered and able to eat.

PREVENT HYPOGLYCEMIA
Because insulin reactions are so common, clients with newly diagnosed diabetes must understand the following:

- Why hypoglycemia occurs
- When it is most likely to occur
- The early clinical manifestations of hypoglycemia
- The danger of severe or repeated reactions
- The importance of early intervention
- How to prevent insulin reactions

Whenever administration of insulin or an oral hypoglycemic agent begins, the client must be taught to identify clinical manifestations and to manage hypoglycemia. Once a client experiences and then fully recovers from an episode of hypoglycemia, thoroughly reassess the intervention program. In some cases, insulin reactions develop because the client carelessly prepares insulin dosages, fails to eat, or exercises excessively. Explain the dangers of repeated insulin reactions to a client who is careless in maintaining a normoglycemic balance. These dangers include loss of consciousness, trauma caused by falling after losing consciousness, injury from poor decision-making, seizures, loss of brain cells, and eventual death. Emphasize conscientious adherence to the therapeutic program.

In other cases, hypoglycemia develops because the prescribed insulin dosage is too large or the client's dietary intake is too small. Instruct the client to record the time and probable cause of any hypoglycemic episodes on the blood test record. The health care team and the client can then evaluate the record together, making appropriate changes. Teach the client with type 1 diabetes to adjust diet and insulin by monitoring results. Finally, be certain that the client with diabetes obtains a diabetic identification tag or medical identification bracelet or necklace and a diabetic identification card. Sometimes, a

TABLE 45–8	INTERVENTIONS FOR HYPOGLYCEMIA
Clinical Manifestations	**Interventions**

Mild hypoglycemia
Tremors
Tachycardia
Diaphoresis
Paresthesias
Excessive hunger
Pallor
Shakiness
	10–15 g of carbohydrate,
	    contained in:
	4 oz orange juice
	6 oz regular soda
	6–8 oz 2% milk
	6–8 Life Savers candies
	1 small (2-oz) tube of cake
	    icing
	4 tsp granulated sugar

Moderate hypoglycemia
Manifestations listed
    above plus
Headache
Mood swings
Irritability
Inability to concentrate
Drowsiness
Impaired judgment
Slurred speech
Double or blurred
    vision
	20–30 g of carbohydrate
	Glucagon, 1 mg SC or IM

Severe hypoglycemia Disorientation Seizures Unconsciousness	50% dextrose, 25 g IV Glucagon, 1 mg IM or IV

IM, intramuscularly; IV, intravenously; SC, subcutaneously.

client who is experiencing an insulin reaction behaves as if intoxicated or mentally disturbed. By carrying proper identification, the client can avoid being arrested at a time when emergency care is desperately needed. Table 45–9 compares the data and interventions for diabetic ketoacidosis, HHNS, and hypoglycemia.

As in many chronic disorders, the client needs to develop a positive self-concept and a feeling of control. Help the client and significant others understand the complications associated with diabetes. Equally important, help the client develop and maintain self-care skills that meet emotional and social needs as well as physical ones.

OTHER HYPOGLYCEMIC DISORDERS

Other manifestations of altered counterregulatory mechanisms in type 1 diabetes mellitus are (1) hypoglycemic unawareness, (2) hypoglycemia with rebound hyperglycemia (Somogyi effect), and (3) the dawn phenomenon.

■ HYPOGLYCEMIC UNAWARENESS

Hypoglycemic unawareness refers to a syndrome in which people with diabetes are unaware they are hypoglycemic and therefore do not initiate treatment. In the Diabetes Control and Complications Trial, about a third of all episodes of severe hypoglycemia seen in awake, intensively treated clients were not accompanied by manifestations of sufficient severity that clients could effectively prevent neuroglycopenia. In the past, this condition was incorrectly viewed as being rare and associated only with advanced neuropathy.

Repeated episodes of hypoglycemia seem to blunt the hormonal defense mechanisms that prevent it (blunted epinephrine response) and the client's ability to perceive early manifestations. Beta-adrenergic–blocking agents (such as propranolol) can cause hypoglycemic unawareness and blunt adrenergic (epinephrine) effects in clients with diabetes, because these effects are primarily mediated by beta-adrenergic receptors. Therefore, beta-blockers are contraindicated in clients with diabetes.

Clients with hypoglycemic unawareness (absence of manifestations of hypoglycemia when glucose level is below 55 mg/dl) require consultation with an experienced physician. Increasing the frequency of self-monitored blood glucose levels, particularly before driving and after exercise, should be encouraged. Clients may wish to choose a slightly higher blood glucose target before meals and during the night. Self-management education and follow-up must be intensified for these clients. For clients with type 1 diabetes, maintaining good control is as much of a problem during the night as at any other time of day.

■ HYPOGLYCEMIA WITH REBOUND HYPERGLYCEMIA

Hypoglycemia followed by rebound hyperglycemia, known as the *Somogyi effect* or *Somogyi phenomenon,* may complicate diabetes management. This phenomenon was implicated in the past as a common cause of fasting morning hyperglycemia. Studies have found it to be a rare occurrence. It usually results from excessive evening insulin dosing. The pathophysiology involves hypoglycemia, leading to counterregulatory hormone secretion and

resultant liver production of glucose. This increase in glucose, along with insulin resistance secondary to increased hormone levels, is thought to contribute to rebound hyperglycemia.

Nocturnal rebound hyperglycemia should be investigated by self-monitoring of blood glucose levels between 2:00 and 4:00 AM and again at 7:00 AM. If early-morning levels are less than 50 to 60 mg/dl and those at 7:00 AM are greater than 180 to 200 mg/dl, rebound hyperglycemia may have occurred. Decreasing the intermediate-acting insulin dose at suppertime, moving the intermediate-acting insulin dose to bedtime, or increasing the size of the bedtime snack should prevent this phenomenon.

■ DAWN PHENOMENON

The dawn phenomenon refers to an early-morning (4 to 8 AM) rise in blood glucose level without preceding nocturnal hypoglycemia. Wearing off of insulin does not appear to be the sole cause of this phenomenon. It has been found in people with both type 1 and type 2 diabetes and probably occurs in people without diabetes. Growth hormone, increased insulin clearance, and diurnal variation in counterregulatory hormone levels seem to play a role.

The key clinical implication of the dawn phenomenon is that attempts to normalize pre-breakfast glucose levels often result in early-morning hypoglycemia. Self-monitoring of blood glucose and education about bedtime snacks, manifestations of nocturnal hypoglycemia, and the importance of avoiding hypoglycemia are vital. Investigation has shown positive effects with the use of Ultralente instead of NPH insulin in the elimination of this phenomenon.

CHRONIC COMPLICATIONS OF DIABETES MELLITUS

Clients with diabetes are living longer, with an increased risk for development of chronic complications (Box 45–9). Chronic complications are the major causes of morbidity and mortality in clients with diabetes. These changes affect many body systems and can be devastating to clients and their families; they affect clients with both type 1 and type 2 diabetes. Complications are classified as one of three types[41]:

- *Macrovascular,* including coronary artery disease, cerebrovascular disease, hypertension, peripheral vascular disease, and infection
- *Microvascular,* including retinopathy and nephropathy
- *Neuropathic,* including sensorimotor and autonomic dysfunction

Sustained increases in glucose levels create an imbalance of substances used for making the matrix between cells. Enzyme systems normally convert glucose to other sugars, such as sorbitol and fructose to lower blood glucose. Sorbitol, fructose, and glucose accumulate in the basement membrane of the cell and between the cells. Intracellular accumulations of sorbitol cause intracellular edema and affect function.

The microcirculation is affected by extracellular accumulation of glucose, sorbitol, and fructose. The thickened basement membrane increases the distance over which

TABLE 45–9	ACUTE COMPLICATIONS OF DIABETES		
	Diabetic Ketoacidosis (DKA)	**Hyperglycemic, Hyperosmolar, Nonketotic Syndrome (HHNS)**	**Hypoglycemia**
Type of diabetes	Usually type 1; may occur in type 2	Type 2	Type 1 or type 2
Clinical manifestations	Warm/dry skin, nausea, vomiting, flushed appearance, dry mucous membranes, soft eyeballs, Kussmaul's respirations or tachypnea, abdominal pain, impaired consciousness, hypotension, tachycardia, acetone breath, acute weight loss Polyuria (early) Oliguria/anuria (late)	Same as for DKA except Kussmaul's respirations and acetone breath usually not present Alterations in level of consciousness, severe dehydration Nausea and vomiting not present Tachypnea, shallow respirations	Mild reaction: tremors, palpitations, pallor, sweating, hunger Moderate reaction: headache, irritability, drowsiness, weakness, visual disturbances, decreased mental acuity Severe reaction: loss of consciousness, seizures
Precipitating factors	Undiagnosed diabetes Omission of insulin dose Puberty Infection Cardiovascular disorder Other physical or emotional stress, such as pregnancy or surgery Trauma	Undiagnosed diabetes Infection or other stress Medications: phenytoin sodium (Dilantin), thiazide diuretics, steroids, chlorpromazine Dialysis GI bleed Hyperalimentation, myocardial infarction Acute pancreatitis Central nervous system disorders Major burns rehydrated with high volumes of glucose	Delay or omission of meal Insulin overdosage Excessive exercise Improper timing of insulin and food
Onset of manifestations	Slow (hours to days) or quickly	Slow (hours to days)	Rapid (minutes to hours)
Laboratory findings			
Plasma glucose	300–1500 mg/dl	600–2000 mg/dl	60 mg/dl or less
Serum sodium	Normal or decreased	Normal or increased	Normal
Serum potassium	Normal or elevated at first, then decreased	Same as for DKA	Normal
Blood urea nitrogen	Elevated	Elevated	Normal
Serum ketones	Elevated	Absent	Absent
White blood cells	Elevated	Elevated	Normal or elevated
Hematocrit	Elevated	Elevated	Normal
Urine glucose	Elevated	Elevated	Absent
Urine ketones	Elevated	Absent	Absent
Arterial blood gas	Metabolic acidosis with compensatory respiratory alkalosis	Normal (metabolic acidosis of shock is profound and prolonged)	Normal or slight respiratory acidosis
pH	Less than 7.3	Usually normal or slightly decreased	Normal
Osmolality	300–350 mOsm/L	Usually over 350 mOsm/L	Normal
Acute intervention	IV regular insulin IV fluids such as normal saline or half normal saline Potassium when urine output is adequate Sodium bicarbonate, rarely Phosphate, usually Electrocardiogram Correct underlying problem	Correct underlying problem IV regular insulin IV fluids such as normal saline or half normal saline Potassium when urine output is adequate	Mild reaction: 10–15 g of simple carbohydrate Moderate reaction: one or more simple carbohydrate, glucagon may be needed, 0.5–1 mg Severe reaction: glucagon IM or SC, repeat × 1 in 10 minutes prn, may need IV glucose

Table continued on following page

TABLE 45–9	ACUTE COMPLICATIONS OF DIABETES *Continued*		
	Diabetic Ketoacidosis (DKA)	**Hyperglycemic, Hyperosmolar, Nonketotic Syndrome (HHNS)**	**Hypoglycemia**
Preventive measures	Prompt medical attention when necessary Plan ahead for illness care Frequent SMBG checks during illness or stressful events	Frequent SMBG checks during illness or stressful events Prompt medical attention when necessary	Sleeping late should be planned in advance; if over-sleeping >45 min is planned, changes in insulin or food intake may be necessary Have short-acting carbohydrate available when exercising or reduction of insulin dose before exercise Restricting alcohol intake Double-check insulin type and dosage prior to administration
	→ → → Wearing diabetes identification tag or bracelet. Education for self-care. → → →		

GI, Gastrointestinal; IM, intramuscularly; IV, intravenous; SC, subcutaneously; SMBG, self-monitored blood glucose.

nutrients and waste products must travel to and from the cell. As a result, the cells receive inadequate oxygen and nutrition and cannot rid themselves of waste. Unfortunately, the process starts as early as 2 years after the onset of diabetes.

Clinicians often see clients with diabetes in the hospital with an MI, with loss of cognitive or physical function as a result of a cerebrovascular accident, or with a lower limb amputation necessitated by peripheral vascular disease. Prevention of these all-too-common macrovascular health problems should be a major focus of nurses working with clients with diabetes (Table 45–10).

BOX 45–9 Chronic Complications of Diabetes Mellitus

Macrovascular Complications
- Coronary artery disease
- Cerebrovascular disease
- Hypertension
- Peripheral vascular disease
- Infection

Microvascular Complications
- Retinopathy
- Nephropathy

Neuropathic Complications
- Sensorimotor neuropathy
- Autonomic neuropathy

  - Pupillary
  - Cardiovascular
  - Gastrointestinal
  - Genitourinary

Mixed Vascular and Neuropathic Diseases
- Leg and foot ulcers

MACROVASCULAR COMPLICATIONS

Coronary artery disease, cerebrovascular disease, and peripheral vascular disease are more common, tend to occur at an earlier age, and are more extensive and severe in people with diabetes. Macrovascular disease (disease of large arteries) reflects atherosclerosis with deposits of lipids within the inner layer of vessel walls. The risk for development of macrovascular complications is higher in those with type 1 diabetes than with type 2 diabetes.

Macrovascular disease, especially coronary artery disease, is the most common cause of death in diabetic clients, accounting for 40% to 60% of all cases of diabetes-related macrovascular disease. The most common reason for hospitalization in diabetics is for treatment of macrovascular complications. Diabetes not only is an independent risk factor for these complications but also is a major risk factor for hypertension and hyperlipidemia. Typically, very-low-density and low-density lipoproteins are increased and high-density lipoproteins are decreased. The most characteristic lipid abnormality in diabetes is an elevated triglyceride level. Therefore, the influence of diabetes in these diseases is multiplicative, not additive.

Macrovascular disease tends to occur years before the onset of clinical diabetes and to occur in people with impaired glucose tolerance at a rate similar to that in people with type 2 diabetes. This phenomenon, called *syndrome X,* further establishes the need for disease prevention and health promotion.

Health promotion activities include (1) managing obesity and maintaining ideal body weight, (2) exercising, (3) not smoking, and (4) achieving normal blood lipid levels. Health maintenance actions include (1) prompt recognition and treatment of hyperglycemia with exercise, food, and medication; (2) aggressive management of hypertension, including regular blood pressure checks; and (3)

Clinical Manifestations	Diagnosis	Interventions
CEREBROVASCULAR DISEASE		
Atherothromboembolic infarctions (*transient ischemic attacks and cerebral vascular accidents*) are more severe, have higher mortality rate, have higher recurrence rate	History Manifestations Physical examinations Computed tomography scan Magnetic resonance imaging	Same as for non-diabetics plus: improved glucose control, aspirin, dipyridamole, ticlopidine; ongoing education and support
HEART DISEASE (CORONARY HEART DISEASE)		
Diabetics have a higher incidence of coronary artery changes that influence decreased oxygen and nutrients to myocardium	History Manifestations Physical examination Electrocardiogram Cardiac enzymes Cardiac catheterization Stress test Autopsy	Same as for non-diabetics with cerebrovascular disease plus: improved glucose control, exercise, diet
Clients have more *angina* and higher mortality with *myocardial infarction;* manifestations are often "silent"		Hypertension control: Use of diuretics may worsen hyperglycemia if hypokalemia exists and may adversely affect lipid levels
Clients with a history of diabetes mellitus and myocardial infarction have higher incidence of *congestive heart failure, shock,* and *arrhythmias*		Beta-adrenergic blockers (may cause hypoglycemia), calcium-channel blockers, thrombolytic agents, aspirin, angioplasty, bypass surgery
Cardiomyopathy may occur secondary to small vessel infarctions causing myocardial fibrosis and hypertrophy		
Additional coronary artery disease manifestations:		
Exertional weakness, peripheral edema, orthopnea, fatigue		
Features such as female gender, which normally protects from premature heart disease, do not pertain to individuals with diabetes		
INFECTION		
Diabetics have a higher incidence of *Pseudomonas external otitis* and *monilial skin infections;* common sites of infection in the diabetic include *urinary tract and skin*	History Manifestations Physical examination Laboratory data: serum—increased WBCs and blood sugar; urine—increased WBCs	Improved glucose control; antibiotics, antifungals as required; follow-up with laboratory data; ongoing client education
PERIPHERAL VASCULAR DISEASE (PVD)		
The incidence of *carotid bruits, intermittent claudication, absent pedal pulses* and *ischemic gangrene* is increased in diabetes mellitus	History Manifestations Physical examinations Doppler studies Angiogram Neuropathy identification	Daily foot inspection aimed at prevention and early intervention; meticulous foot care, padded sport socks, well-fitting shoes; weight reduction; smoking cessation; safe exercise programs; ongoing education
PVD and neuropathy augment the morbidity associated with trauma and infection in the lower extremity		
HYPERTENSION		
Usually asymptomatic	History Physical examinations Orthostatic blood pressures with pulse recordings Elevated blood pressure readings at 2–3 recordings Urinalysis: 24-h urine collection for protein, creatinine clearance, and GFR Renal angiogram to evaluate for renal artery stenosis from atherosclerotic disease	Eliminate risk factors; educate client on this silent but deadly disease; diet education: low protein, low salt Pharmacologic intervention dependent on blood pressure readings: diuretics, angiotension-converting enzyme inhibitors, calcium-channel blockers, alphablockers

WBC, white blood cell; GFR, glomerular filtration rate.

screening for high-risk clients (such as those with a family history of diabetes). Health restoration activities involve (1) controlling angina, (2) treating peripheral vascular disease, (3) using blood glucose self-monitoring to keep track of manifestations, (4) controlling risk factors for macrovascular disease, (5) stressing medication compliance and follow-up, and (6) working closely with the client.

Some speculate that type 2 diabetes may be one piece of a syndrome caused by insulin resistance. A well-established association has been demonstrated among hyperglycemia, hyperinsulinemia, dyslipidemia, and hypertension, which leads to coronary artery disease and stroke. The acronym CHAOS (coronary artery disease, hypertension, adult-onset diabetes, obesity, and stress) has been used to remind health care providers to look at the client's entire risk profile for cardiovascular disease when determining treatment for diabetes.

Successful weight reduction with a balanced diet improves lipid profiles, lessens glucose intolerance, lowers blood pressure, and eliminates obesity; otherwise, successful treatment of macrovascular disease in clients with diabetes parallels that in the non-diabetic population.[2, 9, 12]

■ CORONARY ARTERY DISEASE

Clients with diabetes are two to four times more likely than non-diabetic clients to die of coronary artery disease, and the relative risk factor for cardiovascular disease in women with type 2 diabetes is three to four times greater. Female gender does not protect the diabetic woman from premature macrovascular disease. In many clients with diabetes, macrovascular events or processes such as coronary artery disease are atypical or silent, and they often present as indigestion or unexplained heart failure, dyspnea on exertion, or epigastric pain. Coronary artery disease is common in clients under age 40 years if diabetes is of long duration. Clients with diabetes who have had an MI have an increased chance of complications or of having a second infarction, compared with that in non-diabetic clients who have had an MI. After an MI, diabetic clients also experience a higher incidence of heart failure, shock, and dysrhythmias. It has been suggested that insulin therapy in type 2 diabetes may actually increase the incidence of atherosclerotic disease, because such therapy often leads to weight gain and increased blood pressure.

■ CEREBROVASCULAR DISEASE

Prevention of cerebrovascular disease includes the same strategies as for prevention of coronary artery disease, including (1) control of hypertension, lipid levels, and obesity; (2) smoking cessation; (3) exercise; and (4) good nutritional practices.

Cerebrovascular disease, particularly atherothromboembolic infarctions manifested by transient ischemic attacks and cerebrovascular accidents (CVAs), are more common and severe in diabetes. The incidence is two to three times greater in diabetic clients. The relative risk is higher in females, highest in the fifth and sixth decades of life, and much higher in clients with hypertension. In the United States, the southeastern states are often referred to as the "Stroke Belt" because of the sizable black population in that region with its increased prevalence of hypertension. Many clients presenting with CVA have undiagnosed diabetes. In clients with diabetes, CVAs are more serious and carry higher recurrence and mortality rates, especially with type 2 diabetes.

It is speculated that the increased prevalence of CVA in clients with diabetes may be related to the development of diabetic nephropathy and resultant proteinuria, hypertension, and platelet adhesiveness. Clients who present with CVA and high blood glucose levels have a much poorer prognosis than that in clients with normoglycemia. Ticlopidine, a platelet aggregation inhibitor, may be more effective than aspirin in lowering the risk of cerebral infarction, especially in clients with diabetes. This drug may also cause increased cholesterol levels and neutropenia (decreased neutrophils).

■ HYPERTENSION

A 40% increased rate of hypertension has been noted in the diabetic population. Hypertension is a major risk factor for stroke and nephropathy. Inadequately treated hypertension augments the rate at which nephropathy develops. Individualized pharmacologic treatment for hypertension above 140/90 mm Hg is suggested. Angiotensin-converting enzyme (ACE) inhibitors and calcium-channel blockers are the agents of choice for treatment. Beta-blockers and diuretics may increase glucose tolerance and lipid levels.

■ PERIPHERAL VASCULAR DISEASE

In diabetes, the incidence and prevalence of carotid bruits (abnormal sound or murmur), intermittent claudication, absent pedal (foot) pulses, and ischemic gangrene are increased. More than half of nontraumatic lower limb amputations are associated with diabetic changes such as sensory and autonomic neuropathy, peripheral vascular disease, an increased risk and rate of infection, and poor healing. This chain of events, which may lead to amputation, is illustrated in Figure 45–8.

■ INFECTIONS

Clients with diabetes are susceptible to infections of many types. Once infections occur, they are difficult to treat. Three factors that may contribute to the development of an infection are impaired polymorphonuclear leukocyte function, diabetic neuropathies, and vascular insufficiency. Poor glycemic control augments the importance of these factors. Infected areas heal slowly because the damaged vascular system cannot carry sufficient oxygen, white blood cells, nutrients, and antibodies to the injured site. Infections increase the need for insulin and enhance the possibility of ketoacidosis.[43]

Urinary tract infections are the most common type of infections affecting diabetic clients, particularly women. One factor may be the inhibition of polymorphonuclear leukocyte activity while glucosuria is present. Glucosuria is associated with hyperglycemia. The development of a neurogenic bladder, which results in incomplete emptying and urinary retention, may also contribute to the risk of a urinary tract infection.

Diabetic foot infections are very common. Their occurrence is directly related to the three factors just listed, plus hyperglycemia. Up to 40% of diabetic clients with foot infections may require amputation, and 5% to 10% will die despite amputation of the affected area. With proper education and early intervention, foot infections are usually eliminated in a timely manner. The accompanying Care Plan describes prevention of foot infections.[4] Effective foot care can be the initial break in the chain of events that leads to amputation (see Fig. 45–8 and the Bridge to Home Health Care feature).

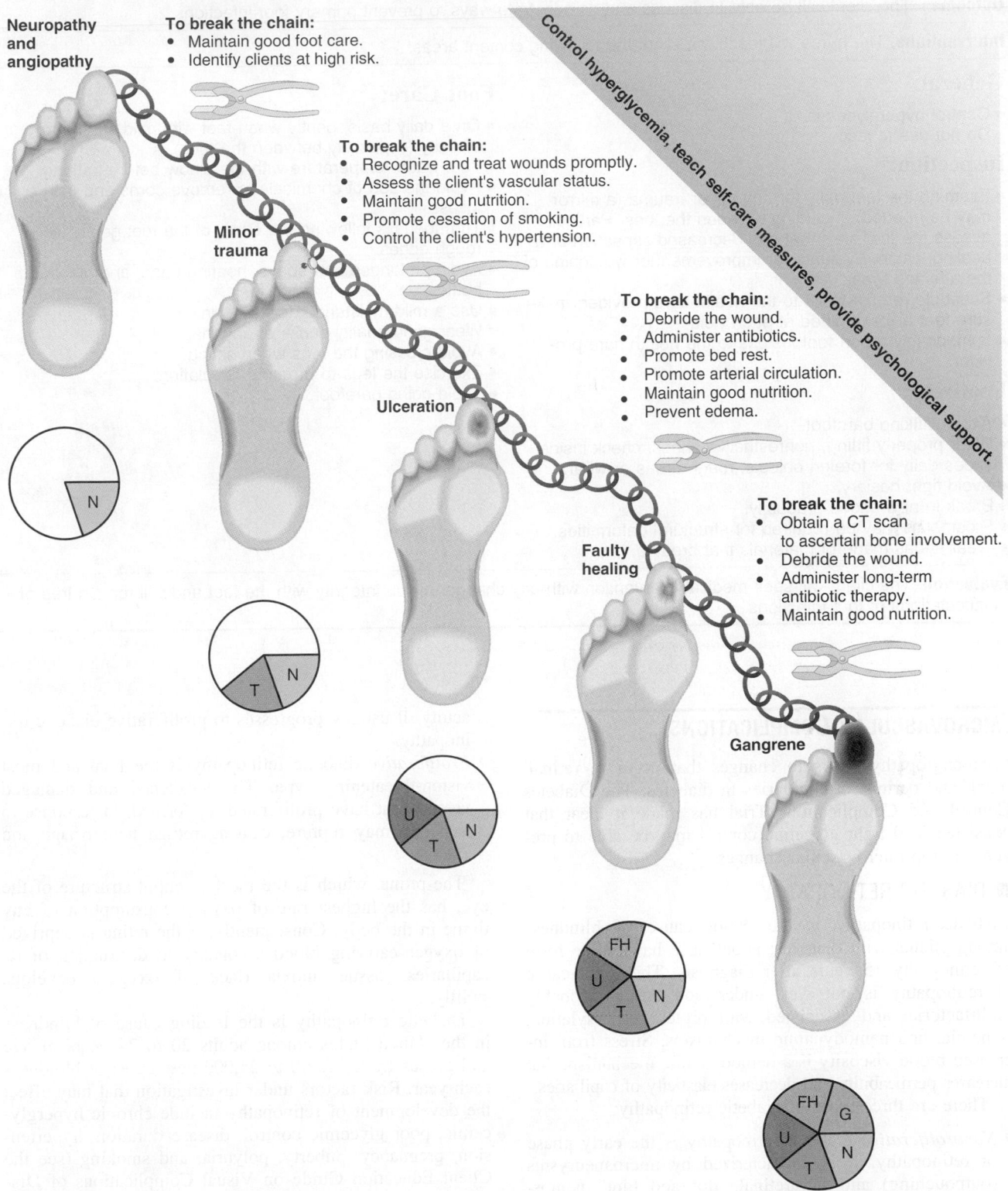

Neuropathy and angiopathy

To break the chain:
- Maintain good foot care.
- Identify clients at high risk.

Control hyperglycemia, teach self-care measures, provide psychological support.

Minor trauma

To break the chain:
- Recognize and treat wounds promptly.
- Assess the client's vascular status.
- Maintain good nutrition.
- Promote cessation of smoking.
- Control the client's hypertension.

Ulceration

To break the chain:
- Debride the wound.
- Administer antibiotics.
- Promote bed rest.
- Promote arterial circulation.
- Maintain good nutrition.
- Prevent edema.

Faulty healing

To break the chain:
- Obtain a CT scan to ascertain bone involvement.
- Debride the wound.
- Administer long-term antibiotic therapy.
- Maintain good nutrition.

Gangrene

FIGURE 45–8 Breaking the chain of events that leads to amputation in high-risk clients with diabetes mellitus. High-risk clients (those with neuropathy, vascular disease, structural deformities, abnormal gait, skin or nail deformities, or a history of previous diabetic ulcers or amputations) need frequent monitoring by the health care team. CT, computed tomography. (Adapted from Pecoraro, R. E., & Burgess, E. M. [1992]. Pathways to diabetic limb amputation: Basis for prevention. *Diabetes Spectrum, 5,* 329–334.)

■ FOOT INFECTIONS IN THE CLIENT WITH DIABETES MELLITUS

Nursing Diagnosis. Altered Peripheral Tissue Perfusion related to neuropathy and atherosclerosis secondary to diabetes mellitus and lack of knowledge related to diabetic foot care and the prevention of diabetic foot infections

Outcomes. The client will be able to discuss and demonstrate ways to prevent primary foot infections.

Interventions. The nurse will teach the client the following content areas:

General:

- Control hyperglycemia.
- Do not use tobacco.

Inspection:

- Examine the feet daily for any minor trauma (a mirror may be needed), including between the toes. Particularly assess the foot area that has decreased sensation or a healing lesion. Evaluate for improvement or worsening of the affected area.
- Schedule regular visits to the health care provider; make sure feet are examined at each visit.
- Immediately report foot lesions to the health care provider.

Footwear:

- Avoid walking barefoot.
- Wear properly fitting, nonrestrictive shoes; check inside shoes daily for foreign objects, rough areas or wear.
- Avoid tight hosiery.
- Break in new shoes gradually.
- Prosthetics may be required for structural deformities.
- Wear shoes made of materials that breathe.

Foot Care:

- On a daily basis, gently wash feet with mild soap and blot dry (especially between the toes).
- Test water temperature with the elbow before bathing.
- Avoid the use of chemicals to remove corns and calluses.
- Trim toenails following the curve of the toe; gently file rough edges.
- Avoid prolonged foot soaks, heating pads, and hot water bottles.
- Use a mild moisturizer for dry skin.
- Wear good-quality socks of any material.
- Avoid crossing the legs when sitting.
- Exercise the legs to promote circulation.
- Avoid going barefoot.

Evaluation. The client will seek medical intervention with any change of skin integrity with the foot and will remain free of manifestations of foot infections.

MICROVASCULAR COMPLICATIONS

Microangiopathy refers to changes that occur in retinal, renal, and peripheral capillaries in diabetes. The Diabetes Control and Complications Trial has made it clear that consistent and tight glycemic control may be able to prevent or stop microvascular changes.

■ DIABETIC RETINOPATHY

Diabetic retinopathy is the major cause of blindness among clients with diabetes; about 80% have some form of retinopathy 15 years after diagnosis. The exact cause of retinopathy is not well understood but is probably multifactorial and associated with protein glycosylation, ischemia, and hemodynamic mechanisms. Stress from increased blood viscosity is a hemodynamic mechanism that increases permeability and decreases elasticity of capillaries.

There are three types of diabetic retinopathy:

- *Nonproliferative* diabetic retinopathy is the early phase of retinopathy. It is characterized by microaneurysms (outpouching) and intraretinal "dot and blot" hemorrhages. It occurs in most clients with long-term diabetes and in many cases it does not progress or affect visual acuity.
- *Preproliferative* diabetic retinopathy involves further progression of the hemorrhages and decreasing visual

acuity. It usually progresses to proliferative diabetic retinopathy.

- *Proliferative* diabetic retinopathy is the final and most vision-threatening type. The weakened and damaged vessels that have proliferated, or formed, in response to ischemia may rupture, causing retinal hemorrhage and exudates.

The retina, which is the most essential structure of the eye, has the highest rate of oxygen consumption of any tissue in the body. Consequently, if the retina is deprived of oxygen-carrying blood secondary to destruction of its capillaries, tissue anoxia (lack of oxygen) develops swiftly.

Diabetic retinopathy is the leading cause of blindness in the United States among adults 20 to 74 years of age and causes from 12,000 to 24,000 new cases of blindness each year. Risk factors under investigation that may affect the development of retinopathy include chronic hyperglycemia, poor glycemic control, disease duration, hypertension, pregnancy, puberty, polyuria, and smoking (see the Client Education Guide on Visual Complications of Diabetes).

Clinical Manifestations

Clinical manifestations of retinopathy typically do not develop until the later stages, when clients have acute vision

BRIDGE TO HOME HEALTH CARE

Diabetic Foot Care

People who have diabetes often develop minor foot problems that progress to major problems, and even amputation. Many foot problems can be prevented or resolved at an early stage. The most important responsibilities of the nurse in diabetic foot care are assessment, education, and direct care measures.

The nurse who initially works with the client in the community needs to do a thorough diabetic assessment that includes evaluation of the client's knowledge, self-care ability, physical status, and needs. Physical assessment of the feet includes:

- Observation of the dermatologic condition, to detect absence of hair, diminished turgor, dry or rough skin, hyperpigmentation, fissures, calluses, ulcers, and lesions or nail problems, such as thickness or discoloration
- Evaluation of the vascular status by checking peripheral pulses, blood return after blanching, and skin temperature, consistency (to rule out edema), and color
- Examination for evidence of orthopedic problems such as hammer toes or bunions
- Evaluation of the neurologic status by testing the deep tendon reflexes and response to pain, vibration, and touch.

Refer the client to a physician if anything abnormal is noted.

Clients who have diabetes must receive very specific education about circulation, self-inspection, protection, and daily foot care. If clients cannot safely perform the necessary tasks independently, it is imperative that other caregivers accept responsibility. Some clients will need a combination of helpers including the home health care nurse, the community health nurse at a foot care clinic, family members, and informal caregivers. Medicare reimbursement for foot care and other home health services is limited. Nurses must advocate for clients and help them obtain the most appropriate and cost-effective services.

Clients who have diabetes need to maximize the circulation of their feet. Teach them to maintain good nutrition and adequate fluid intake. Instruct them not to smoke, cross their legs, or wear restrictive clothing. Demonstrate how to do foot and ankle range-of-motion exercises by writing the alphabet with their feet. Teach them to inspect all areas of their feet daily, looking for open areas, warmth, redness, discharge, formation of calluses or corns, or anything unusual.

Encourage clients to use protective measures, such as (1) always wearing good-fitting, high-quality shoes, (2) avoiding temperature extremes, and (3) seeking immediate medical attention for any injury or problem. Teach daily care of the feet that includes washing with a mild soap; drying thoroughly, especially between the toes; moisturizing feet, except between the toes; and keeping toenails trimmed. If it is necessary to soak feet before trimming toenails, do not soak for longer than 5 to 10 minutes.

Routine foot care performed by nurses in the community may include care of the skin (washing, drying, lubricating, massaging), removal of corns and calluses (shaving to healthy skin with a file or blade), and cutting the toenails. Toenails should be cut straight across or with a slight curve following the shape of the toe and filed smooth to prevent pressure or cutting of adjacent toes.

As with any nursing procedure, appropriate infection control measures should be followed. Cleanse supplies properly, wear gloves and protective eye wear, and dispose of used blades following adequate disposal protocols for sharps.

Debra A. Solomon, RN, MSN, FNP-C, *Clinical Coordinator, Fairview Lakes HomeCaring and Hospice, Chisago City, Minnesota*

---

problems. Blurred vision is a common manifestation that results from an abnormally high blood glucose level. In addition, seeing floaters or flashing lights may indicate hemorrhage or retinal detachment. Because of a lack of early manifestations, it is important to assess the potential for visual problems in all clients with diabetes, including the date of their last dilated pupil examination.

Outcome Management

Major interventions, particularly in the early phases, include achievement of euglycemia and normalization of blood pressure. When retinopathy threatens vision, outpatient laser therapy (photocoagulation) is usually recommended. It halts or slows the decline in vision in most diabetic clients if it is used before too much damage has occurred. Although extensive photocoagulation usually diminishes peripheral vision and may decrease night vision, its success in preserving good visual acuity makes it worthwhile despite these side effects.

If the extent or location of the damage makes photocoagulation ineffective, or if the vitreous is too scarred or clouded with blood, vision may be improved with a vitrectomy, a surgical procedure that removes the vitreous and replaces it with saline solution. About 70% of clients who have vitrectomies notice an improvement in or stabilization of their sight, and some recover enough to resume reading and driving.

■ NEPHROPATHY

Diabetic nephropathy is the single most common cause of end-stage renal disease (ESRD). About 35% to 45% of clients with type 1 diabetes are found to have nephropathy 15 to 20 years after diagnosis. About 20% of clients with type 2 diabetes are found to have nephropathy 5 to 10 years after diagnosis. A consequence of microangiopathy, nephropathy involves damage to and eventual obliteration of the capillaries that supply the glomeruli of the kidney. This damage leads in turn to a complex of pathologic changes and manifestations (intercapillary glomerulosclerosis, nephrosis, gross albuminuria, and hypertension). Risk factors include poor glycemic control, duration of disease, and hypertension. Some clients now self-check microalbumin levels at home. This test can

CLIENT EDUCATION GUIDE

Visual Complications of Diabetes

- Diabetes can cause diabetic retinopathy, which can lead to vision loss.
- There is a relationship between hyperglycemia and diabetic retinopathy. It is extremely important to normalize blood glucose levels.
- Hypertension can worsen diabetic retinopathy. Its diagnosis and aggressive treatment are important.
- If you have diabetic retinopathy, you should know that isometric exercises raise intraocular pressure and can aggravate proliferative retinopathy.
- An ophthalmologist will be brought in to be part of your diabetes management team. If you have any visual impairments, you can be referred to appropriate organizations for assistance.
- If your vision is blurred while reading, you may have hyperglycemia or macular edema. Floaters may indicate hemorrhage, and flashing lights may indicate retinal detachment. If you experience any of these occurrences, you should report them.
- Early laser photocoagulation therapy can reduce risk of vision loss.

Adapted from American Diabetes Association. (1998). *Medical management of non−insulin dependent (type 2) diabetes mellitus* (4th ed.). Alexandria, VA: Author; and Herman, W. H., & Green, D. A. (1996). Microvascular complications of diabetes. In D. Haire-Joshu (Ed.), *Management of diabetes mellitus: Perspectives of care across the life span* (2nd ed.). St. Louis: Mosby−Year Book.

detect very small quantities of urinary albumin, which can indicate very early renal disease. With worsening of the nephrosis, chronic renal failure ensues. Unless the client can be maintained with hemodialysis or receives a renal transplant, uremia eventually causes death.

Clients with nephropathy monitor their blood glucose levels and blood pressure at home. ACE inhibitors can be used to decrease the microalbuminuria. Hypertension should be treated aggressively, as it can be the catalyst for the progression of nephropathy. Clients with nephropathy are taught to eat a low-protein diet and to avoid nephrotoxic drugs (such as gentamicin). If contrast dye is required for radiographic study, mannitol may be ordered, but the client must drink fluids after the test to clear the dye from the kidneys. Serum creatinine levels should be assessed before the administration of the contrast dye or other nephrotoxic agents.

Like diabetic retinopathy, diabetic nephropathy cannot be cured. However, prompt and adequate interventions for renal and bladder infections can prevent these causes of renal failure. Control of hypertension and tight glycemic control can contribute to a delay in the development of nephropathy or a decrease in its progression. Unsuccessfully treated nephropathy progresses to ESRD. Treatment at this point includes hemodialysis, peritoneal dialysis, or a kidney transplant.

■ NEUROPATHY

Neuropathy is the most common chronic complication of diabetes. Nearly 60% of diabetic clients experience it. Because nerve fibers do not have their own blood supply,

they depend on the diffusion of nutrients and oxygen across the membrane. When axons and dendrites are not nourished, their transmission of impulses slows. In addition, sorbitol accumulates in nerve tissue, further diminishing both sensory and motor function. Both temporary and permanent neurologic problems may develop in clients with diabetes during the course of the illness. The neuropathy may be mild (causing minor inconveniences) or so severe that the quality of life is affected. Identified causes of diabetic neuropathy include (1) vascular insufficiency, (2) chronic elevations in blood glucose level, (3) hypertension, and (4) cigarette smoking. Clients may present with mononeuropathy or polyneuropathy and may have sensory or motor impairment, depending on which nerves are involved.

A platelet-derived growth factor, becaplermin (Regranex), that stimulates the body to grow new tissue is being used to promote healing in open wounds associated with lower extremity diabetic neuropathic ulcers that extend into subcutaneous tissue or beyond. The topical agent is applied once daily, spread evenly, and covered with a saline-moistened gauze dressing. After 12 hours, the ulcer is rinsed and re-covered with saline gauze (see Chapter 16).

MONONEUROPATHY

Mononeuropathy, or focal neuropathy, usually involves a single nerve or group of nerves. Mononeuropathies produce sharp, stabbing pains and are usually caused by an infarction of the blood supply. The muscles innervated by nerves affected by focal neuropathies are painful and are at risk for atrophy from disuse. Treatment may include surgical decompression for compression lesions.

POLYNEUROPATHY

Polyneuropathy, or diffuse neuropathy, involves the sensory and autonomic nerves. Sensory neuropathy is the most common type. It is commonly assessed as bilateral, symmetrical, and affecting the lower extremities. The client describes tingling, numbness, burning, and mild to total sensory loss. This complication is a major factor in injuries to the legs.

Treatment includes foot care education to prevent trauma and ulcers. Painful neuropathy may be treated with tricyclic antidepressants, phenytoin, or carbamazepine. Polyneuropathy also may simply resolve spontaneously.

AUTONOMIC NEUROPATHY

Autonomic neuropathy manifests itself in its effect on pupillary, cardiovascular, gastrointestinal, and genitourinary functions.

PUPILLARY. Autonomic neuropathy of the pupil interferes with the pupil's ability to adapt to the dark. Pupil dilation is inadequate. Clients are at risk for accidents when driving at night. The environment should be well lighted at night.

CARDIOVASCULAR. Autonomic neuropathy of the cardiovascular system is evidenced by an abnormal response to exercise. A fixed heart rate may be noted. Orthostatic hypotension may occur, which is dangerous. Resting tachycardia is another possible cardiovascular effect.

GASTROINTESTINAL. Autonomic neuropathy commonly affects the gastrointestinal tract. The client may have dysphagia, abdominal pain, nausea, vomiting, malabsorption, postprandial hypoglycemia, diarrhea, constipation, or fetal incontinence. Gastroparesis (delayed stomach emptying) may give the client the feeling of stomach fullness. This may contribute to anorexia, decreased intake, weight loss, and labile blood glucose levels related to food malabsorption. About 20% to 30% of diabetic clients have gastroparesis, manifestations of which may be alleviated with metoclopramide (Reglan) or cisapride (Propulsid).

GENITOURINARY. Bladder hypotonicity, or neurogenic bladder, is a common manifestation of autonomic neuropathy. Manifestations may include straining with urination, infrequent urge to urinate with long periods of time between voiding, and a decreased urine stream. Urinary stasis may occur, leading to urinary tract infection. In the male client, autonomic neuropathy can contribute to erectile dysfunction and retrograde ejaculation. Penile injections, implantable devices, or sildenafil (Viagra) may improve function (see Chapter 38 on male reproductive problems). Women with autonomic neuropathy may experience painful intercourse, which estrogen-containing lubricants can resolve (see Chapter 39 on female reproductive problems).

Management of a Diabetic Client Having Surgery

Surgery is a stressful experience for anyone; for a client with diabetes, however, surgery imposes several additional stressors. Surgery interrupts the client's usual therapeutic regimen. The diet must be temporarily changed and the dosage of insulin or oral hypoglycemic agent readjusted. The stress of surgery raises serum glucose levels. The client is susceptible to infection. The surgical incision itself becomes a new potential portal of entry for pathogens. Furthermore, postoperative healing in these clients may be slower than normal.

To offset these problems, clients with diabetes require special interventions, both preoperatively and postoperatively. They may vary, depending on whether the client has type 1 or type 2 diabetes and whether the surgery is elective or performed on an emergency basis.

PREOPERATIVE CARE

The goal of preoperative care for clients with diabetes is thorough regulation of blood glucose levels before surgery. Clients with type 1 diabetes need to be closely monitored for several days or even weeks before elective surgery to stabilize their condition and, thereby, to decrease surgical risk. If a client with type 1 diabetes and poor glucose control requires emergency surgery, the surgeon must choose between operating on a hypoglycemic or hyperglycemic client and postponing an emergency operation until the diabetes is controlled. In either case, the client needs constant monitoring of vital signs, frequent laboratory and bedside glucose studies, and vigilant nursing intervention.

In contrast, clients with well-controlled type 2 diabetes usually undergo surgery with only slightly more risk than that for the general population. Typically, preoperative preparation for clients with type 1 and type 2 diabetes includes the following:

- Preoperative laboratory tests, including fasting and preprandial blood glucose levels; glycosylated hemoglobin; serum electrolytes, BUN, and serum creatinine; complete blood count; ECG and cardiac enzymes; and chest radiograph

- Early-morning scheduling of surgery so that the client's diet and insulin regimen undergo as little disruption as possible

- Omission of food, water, and oral hypoglycemic agents on the morning of surgery (one long-acting hypoglycemic agent, chlorpropamide, is discontinued 1 to 2 days before surgery because of its long half-life)

- IV infusion of insulin for insulin-dependent or insulin-requiring clients, usually with glucose (5%) to prevent hypoglycemia (if the surgery is relatively minor, such as for cataract removal, the surgeon may order a 5% dextrose solution infusion and half the usual dose of intermediate-acting insulin; the anesthesiologist can monitor blood glucose levels in the operating room)

- A blood glucose determination performed and reported to the physician within 1 hour before the operation to ensure that the client (who has taken nothing by mouth since midnight) will not develop hypoglycemia during surgery

INTRAOPERATIVE CARE

Once the client arrives in surgery, management again depends on the severity of the diabetes and the extent of the surgery. Regular insulin, in a dose based on the client's blood glucose levels and a sliding scale or an insulin protocol, can be given by the IV route. Subcutaneous insulin should not be given intraoperatively because its absorption is affected by body temperature, circulatory blood volumes, and certain anesthetics.

POSTOPERATIVE CARE

After surgery, the goals of postoperative management are to stabilize the client's vital signs, correct fluid and electrolyte imbalances, reestablish control of the diabetes, prevent wound infection, and promote wound healing. The following are important postoperative interventions:

- Administer prescribed IV infusions and regular insulin until the client can take oral nourishment.

- Once the client can tolerate fluids, offer those that contain calories to prevent hypoglycemia. Once the client can eat, make food available. Discuss the client's calorie level with a dietitian to ensure that enough calories are provided for postoperative wound healing.

- Obtain a blood glucose level four to six times daily.

- Resume the client's prescribed preoperative insulin type and dosage once blood glucose control is reestablished, foods are being consumed at adequate levels, and it has been reordered by the physician.

- Observe for evidence of hypoglycemia after surgery, such as a decrease in blood pressure or an increase in heart rate in a client who is still unresponsive from anesthesia.

- Avoid catheterization, if at all possible, to prevent bladder infection.

- Change wound dressings with meticulous sterile technique to prevent wound infection.

- Assess the client's wound and incision frequently for signs of infection. Be alert for abnormal amounts of drainage or foul-smelling drainage.

- Observe for and treat manifestations of skin breakdown,

especially if the client has peripheral vascular disease or neuropathy.

■ Management of a Sick Diabetic Client

The Client Education Guide presents guidelines for the client to follow during illnesses.

CLIENT EDUCATION GUIDE

Sick Day Management for Diabetes Mellitus*

You should have an individualized plan of care prescribed by the health care team to utilize during illness.

Monitoring is an essential part of diabetes management, but this is even more vital during the stress of illness.

Insulin requirements may be increased secondary to reduced activity and increased secretion of counterregulatory hormones. To prevent diabetic ketoacidosis, you should know the following:

Self-Monitoring of Blood Glucose. It is important to self-monitor blood glucose more frequently during illness, often every 2–4 hours. If premeal blood glucose values stay greater than 250 mg/dl, you should test for urine ketones and contact your health care provider.

Ketones. Urine ketones should be monitored when you feel sick and/or blood glucose is greater than 250 mg/dl. Test for ketones every 2–4 hours.

Insulin. Do not stop taking your insulin, even if you are vomiting and unable to eat. Additional regular insulin may be required, based on self-monitored blood glucose levels.

Nutrition/Fluids. Adequate fluid intake and carbohydrates are essential during illness. Eating 10–15 g of carbohydrate every 1–2 hours and small quantities of fluid every 15–30 minutes is usually sufficient to prevent dehydration and ketoacidosis. Clear broth, tea, and ice chips are usually well tolerated. Examples of foods and beverages containing about 15 g of carbohydrate are as follows:

1 regular whole Popsicle
½ cup applesauce
½ cup regular soft drink
¾ cup ginger ale
½ cup orange or apple juice
1 cup Gatorade
½ cup regular gelatin

Notify your health care provider when you have any of the following problems:

● Illness that persists more than 24 hours
● Severe abdominal pain
● Fever over 100° F, oral
● Persistent diarrhea
● Vomiting with inability to take fluids for more than 4 hours
● Blood glucose levels difficult to control and/or moderate to high levels of ketones in urine
● Shortness of breath or chest pain
● Acute visual loss
● Other unexplained health problems

---

*Most applicable to clients with type 1 diabetes and those with type 2 diabetes receiving insulin therapy.

CONCLUSIONS

Diabetes mellitus is a chronic disease characterized by abnormalities in carbohydrate, fat, and protein metabolism. The two major categories of diabetes mellitus are type 1 and type 2. Meal planning, exercise, and medication are the main forms of treatment. Acute complications include hyperglycemia with diabetic ketoacidosis and hypoglycemia. Chronic complications are relentlessly progressive and result from multiple changes in small and large vessels. Because diabetes is chronic, nursing management focuses on teaching the client and family how to manage the disorder on a day-to-day basis and how to assess for complications.

THINKING CRITICALLY

1. **A client with type 1 diabetes takes 14 units of regular insulin and 32 units of NPH insulin subcutaneously at 7 AM and 5 PM every day. He is now hospitalized for pneumonia and nausea. It is 9:30 AM. On entering his room, you observe the client talking to his plants. What is your priority intervention? How will his confusion be resolved?**

Factors to Consider. When does regular insulin peak? What might be the underlying cause of the client's confusion? How might you confirm the presence of hypoglycemia?

2. **An older woman with type 1 diabetes calls the clinic and tells the nurse that she has the flu. She tells the nurse that she usually takes Humulin N, 12 units, and Humulin R, 8 units, every morning. She has not taken her insulin this morning because of vomiting, nausea, and an inability to eat. She tells the nurse she lives alone. What telephone advice is appropriate? How often should she monitor her blood glucose levels while she is ill?**

Factors to Consider. What learning needs does the client exhibit? When should the insulin be given? Is a clinic visit warranted?

3. **The client is a 72-year-old woman who has a 25-year history of type 2 diabetes. She has managed her care adequately over the years; with the advent of home glucose monitoring, her blood glucose levels have been very well controlled. Her main problem is a history of significant hypertension, controlled with a daily antihypertensive. Lately, she finds that small cuts and bruises take longer than usual to heal. What are the chronic complications of diabetes mellitus? What teaching should you consider for this client?**

Factors to Consider. What risks does this client face as a result of her long-term diabetic history? How would you approach teaching about complications?

BIBLIOGRAPHY

1. American Diabetes Association. (1998). Continuous subcutaneous insulin infusion (position statement). *Diabetes Care, 21* (suppl. 1), S76.

2. American Diabetes Association (1998). Management of dyslipidemia in adults with diabetes (position statement). *Diabetes Care, 21* (suppl. 1), S36–S39.

3. American Diabetes Association (1998). Diabetes mellitus and exercise (position statement). *Diabetes Care, 21* (suppl. 1), S40–S44.

4. American Diabetes Association (1998). Foot care in clients with diabetes mellitus (position statement). *Diabetes Care, 21* (suppl. 1), S54–S55.

5. American Diabetes Association. (1998). Insulin administration (position statement). *Diabetes Care, 21* (suppl. 1), S72–S75.

6. American Diabetes Association. (1998). Magnesium supplementation in the treatment of diabetes (position statement). *Diabetes Care, 21* (suppl. 1), S80–S81.

7. American Diabetes Association. (1998). *Medical management of insulin-dependent (type 1) diabetes* (3rd ed.). Alexandria, VA: Author.

8. American Diabetes Association. (1998). *Medical management of non–insulin-dependent (type 2) diabetes* (4th ed.). Alexandria, VA: Author.

9. American Diabetes Association. (1998). Nutrition recommendations and principles for people with diabetes mellitus (position statement). *Diabetes Care, 21* (suppl. 1), S32–S35.

10. American Diabetes Association. (1998). Prevention of type 1 diabetes mellitus (position statement). *Diabetes Care, 21* (suppl. 1), S83.

11. American Diabetes Association. (1998). Screening for type 2 diabetes (position statement). *Diabetes Care, 21* (suppl. 1), S20–S22.

12. American Diabetes Association (1998). Standards of medical care for patients with diabetes mellitus (position statement). *Diabetes Care, 21* (suppl. 1), S23–S31.

13. American Diabetes Association. (1998). *Diabetes 1998 vital statistics.* Alexandria, VA: Author.

14. Anderson, R. M. (1995). Client empowerment and the traditional medical model: A case of irreconcilable differences? *Diabetes Care, 18*(3), 412–415.

15. Anderson, R. M., et al. (1995). Patients' empowerment: Results of a randomized clinical trial. *Diabetes Care, 18*(7), 943–949.

16. Auslander, W., & Corn, D. (1996). Environmental influences on diabetes management. Family, health care system, and community contexts. In D. Haire-Joshu (Ed.), *Management of diabetes mellitus: Perspectives of care across the life span* (2nd ed., pp. 513–526). St. Louis: Mosby–Year Book.

17. Beaser, R. S. (1995). Putting DCCT into practice. *Client Care, 29*(6), 15–30.

18. Bergenstal, R., & Rubenstein, A. (1995). Diabetes mellitus therapy. In L. J. De Groot (Ed.), *Endocrinology* (3rd ed., pp. 1482–1505). Philadelphia: W. B. Saunders.

19. Carr, S. R. (1998). Screening for gestational diabetes mellitus: A perspective in 1998. *Diabetes Care, 21* (suppl. 2), B14–B18.

20. Coleman, W. C. (1996). Foot care and lower extremity problems of diabetes mellitus. In D. Haire-Joshu (Ed.), *Management of diabetes mellitus: Perspectives of care across the life span* (2nd ed., pp. 309–332). St. Louis: Mosby–Year Book.

21. Couston, D. R., & Carpenter, M. W. (1998). The diagnosis of gestational diabetes. *Diabetes Care, 21* (suppl. 2), B5–B8.

22. Diabetes Control and Complications Trial Research Group. (1993). The effect of intensive treatment of diabetes on the development and progression of long-term complications in insulin-dependent diabetes mellitus. *New England Journal of Medicine, 329*(14), 977–985.

23. Expert Committee on the Diagnosis and Classification of Diabetes Mellitus. (1997). Report of the Expert Committee on the Diagnosis and Classification of Diabetes Mellitus. *Diabetes Care, 20*(7), 1183–1197.

24. Fajans, S. (1995). Diabetes mellitus: Definition, classification, tests. In L. J. DeGroot (Ed.), *Endocrinology* (3rd ed., pp 1411–1422). Philadelphia: W. B. Saunders.

25. Feste, C., & Anderson, R. M. (1995). Empowerment: From philosophy to practice. *Patient Education and Counseling, 26,* 139–144.

26. Foster, D. W., & McGarry, J. D. (1995). Diabetes mellitus: Acute complications, ketoacidosis, hyperosmolar coma, lactic acidosis. In J. L. DeGroot (Ed.), *Endocrinology* (3rd ed., pp 1506–1521). Philadelphia: W. B. Saunders.

27. Franz, M. (1996). Exercise and diabetes. In D. Haire-Joshu (Ed.), *Management of diabetes mellitus: Perspectives of care across the life span* (3rd ed., pp. 162–201). St. Louis: Mosby–Year Book.

28. Funnell, M. M., & Merritt, J. H. (1996). Diabetes and the older adult. In D. Haire-Joshu (Ed.), *Management of diabetes mellitus: Perspectives of care across the life span* (2nd ed., pp. 755–821). St. Louis: Mosby–Year Book.

29. Guyton, A., & Hall, J. C. D. (1997). *Human physiology and mechanisms of disease* (6th ed.). Philadelphia: W. B. Saunders.

30. Jasper, J. B., & Green, A. J. (1995). The neuropathies of diabetes. In L. J. DeGroot (Ed.), *Endocrinology* (3rd ed., pp. 1536–1568). Philadelphia: W. B. Saunders.

31. Klein, R. (1995). Diabetes mellitus: Late complications: Oculopathy. In L. J. DeGroot (Ed.), *Endocrinology* (3rd ed., pp. 1522–1535). Philadelphia: W. B. Saunders.

32. Lernmark, A. (1995). Insulin dependent (type I) diabetes: Etiology, pathogenesis, and natural history. In J. L. DeGroot (Ed.), *Endocrinology* (3rd ed., pp. 1423–1435). Philadelphia: W. B. Saunders.

33. National Diabetes Data Group. (1979). Classification and diagnosis of diabetes mellitus and other categories of glucose intolerance. *Diabetes, 28,* 1039–1057.

34. Olefsky, J. M. (1995). Diabetes mellitus (type II): Etiology and pathogenesis. In J. L. DeGroot (Ed.), *Endocrinology* (3rd ed., pp. 1436–1463). Philadelphia: W. B. Saunders.

35. Peragallo-Dittko, V. (1996). Tight control: A guide to getting started. *Diabetes Self-Management, 13*(5), 20–24.

36. Powers, M. A. (1996). *Handbook of diabetes nutritional management.* Rockville, MD: Aspen Publishers.

37. Ratner, R. E. (1998). Diabetes disease state: Pathophysiology. In M. M. Funnell, et al. (Eds.), *A core curriculum for diabetes educators* (3rd ed., pp. 167–184). Chicago: American Association of Diabetes Educators.

38. Skyler, J. S. (1997). Insulin theory in type II diabetes. *Postgraduate Medicine, 101,* 85–96.

39. U.S. Department of Agriculture, U.S. Department of Health and Human Services. (1995). *Nutrition and your health: Dietary guidelines for Americans* (4th ed) Hyattsville, MD: USDA Human Nutrition Information Service.

40. U.S. Department of Agriculture (1992). *The Food Guide Pyramid.* Hyattsville, MD: USDA Human Nutrition Information Service.

41. Vinicor, F. (1998). Macrovascular disease. In M. M. Funnell, et al. (Eds.), *A core curriculum for diabetes educators* (3rd ed., pp. 787–809). Chicago: American Association of Diabetes Educators.

42. White, J. R., Campbell, R. K., & Yarborough, P. C. (1998). Pharmacologic therapies. In M. M. Funnell, et al. (Eds.), *A core curriculum for diabetes educators* (3rd ed., pp. 295–360). Chicago: American Association of Diabetes Educators.

43. White, N. H., & Henry, D. N. (1996). Special issues in diabetes management. In D. Haire-Joshu (Ed.), *Management of diabetes mellitus: Perspectives of care across the life span* (2nd ed., pp. 342–404). St. Louis: Mosby–Year Book.

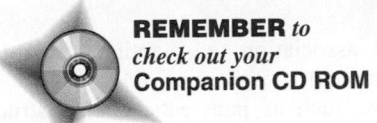
Management of Clients with Exocrine Pancreatic and Biliary Disorders

Dianne Smolen

NURSING OUTCOMES CLASSIFICATION (NOC)
for Nursing Diagnoses—Clients with Exocrine Pancreatic and Biliary Disorders

Altered Nutrition: Less Than Body Requirements
Nutritional Status
Nutritional Status: Food and Fluid Intake
Nutritional Status: Nutrient Intake
Altered Oral Mucous Membrane
Oral Health
Tissue Integrity: Skin and Mucous
  Membrane
Anxiety
Anxiety Control
Coping
Grief Resolution
Psychosocial Adjustment: Life Change
Symptom Control
Effective Management of Therapeutic Regimen: Individual
Adherence Behavior
Compliance Behavior
Family Participation in Professional Care
Knowledge: Treatment Regimen
Participation: Health Care Decisions
Risk Control
Symptom Control
Ineffective Breathing Pattern
Respiratory Status: Airway Patency
Respiratory Status: Ventilation

Vital Signs Status
Knowledge Deficit
Knowledge: Diet
Knowledge: Disease Process
Knowledge: Energy Conservation
Knowledge: Health Behaviors
Knowledge: Health Resources
Knowledge: Illness Care
Knowledge: Medication
Knowledge: Personal Safety
Knowledge: Prescribed Activity
Knowledge: Treatment Procedure(s)
Knowledge: Treatment Regimen
Pain
Comfort Level
Pain Control
Pain: Disruptive Effects
Pain Level
Risk for Fluid Volume Deficit and Electrolyte Imbalance
Bowel Elimination
Cardiac Pump Effectiveness
Electrolyte and Acid/Base Balance
Fluid Balance
Hydration
Knowledge: Disease Process
Knowledge: Health Behaviors

Knowledge: Medication
Knowledge: Treatment Regimen
Nutritional Status: Food and Fluid Intake
Risk Control
Risk Detection
Thermoregulation
Urinary Elimination
Vital Signs Status
Risk for Ineffective Management of Therapeutic Regimen (Individuals)
Compliance Behavior
Knowledge: Disease Process
Knowledge: Treatment Regimen
Participation: Health Care Decisions
Treatment Behavior: Illness or Injury
Risk for Injury
Immune Status
Knowledge: Infection Control
Nutritional Status
Risk Control
Risk Detection
Symptom Control
Treatment Behavior: Illness or Injury
Tissue Integrity: Skin and Mucous
  Membranes
Vital Signs Status
Wound Healing: Primary Intention

Some disorders of the exocrine pancreas and the biliary tract are acute, and others are chronic. Manifestations may be similar to those of other conditions. The nurse plays an important role in assessing the client's manifestations and in managing the outcomes of medical and surgical treatment.

DISORDERS OF THE EXOCRINE PANCREAS

A client with a pancreatic disorder may have problems with both digestion and utilization of glucose. The relative inaccessibility of the pancreas to direct examination and the nonspecificity of manifestations associated with pancreatic disorders make diagnosis of some conditions difficult. In addition, more than 90% of the pancreas must be damaged before fat and protein digestion problems become apparent.

ACUTE PANCREATITIS

Pancreatitis (inflammation of the pancreas) may be acute or chronic. Acute pancreatitis is an inflammation of the pancreas that may result in autodigestion of the pancreas by its own enzymes. Acute pancreatitis is a fairly common but a potentially lethal inflammatory process associated with edema, various amounts of autodigestion, fat necrosis, and sometimes hemorrhage.

Although the frequency is about 5000 new cases per year in the United States, with a mortality rate of about 10%, the number of clients who have recurrent acute pancreatitis or chronic pancreatitis is not known.[18]

The incidence of pancreatitis varies in different countries and depends on the cause (e.g., alcohol, gallstones, metabolic factors, or drugs). In the United States, acute pancreatitis is related to alcohol consumption more commonly than to gallstones; in England, the opposite is true.

Etiology and Risk Factors

There are many causes of acute pancreatitis, such as alcohol (ethanol) abuse, *cholelithiasis* (gallstones), abdominal trauma, and metabolic factors. The mechanisms by which these conditions trigger pancreatic inflammation have not been identified.

In the United States, alcohol abuse is the major cause of acute pancreatitis, with common bile duct stone disease the second most frequent occurrence. Although the exact cause is not known, acute pancreatitis is thought to result from inappropriate intrapancreatic activation of proteases, which causes autodigestion of the pancreas. Exactly how this occurs is not known. It is thought that alcohol-induced pancreatitis may include a physiochemical alteration of protein that results in plugs that block the small pancreatic ductules. Biliary pancreatitis occurs when a stone migrates through the ampulla of Vater, causing diversion of bile into the pancreatic duct and subsequent bile-induced pancreatic parenchymal injury. Other causes include:

- Hyperlipidemia, which may occur secondary to nephritis, castration, or exogenous estrogen administration, or as hereditary hyperlipidemia
- Hypercalcemia arising as a result of hyperparathyroidism
- Familial cases with no definite mechanism defined
- Pancreatic trauma, such as penetrating or blunt external trauma, intraoperative manipulation, or ampullar manipulation and pancreatic ductal overdistention during endoscopic retrograde cholangiopancreatography (ERCP)
- Pancreatic ischemia during episodes of hypotensive shock, cardiopulmonary bypass, visceral atheroembolism, or vasculitis
- Drugs; although azathioprine and estrogens have been directly linked with the disease, many other drugs are believed to have an association (e.g., antibiotics, anticonvulsants, and diuretics)
- Other general causes, such as pancreatic duct obstruction, obesity, duodenal obstruction, viral infection, carcinoma, scorpion venom, and factors still to be determined

Avoidance of alcohol is the best way to promote health and to reduce the risk of pancreatitis. Limiting or completely stopping ingestion of alcohol may be a health promotion, health maintenance, or health restoration activity, depending on a diagnosis or potential diagnosis of pancreatitis. Other risk factors include cholecystitis, cholelithiasis, hyperlipidemia, hypercalcemia, pancreatic tumor, pancreatic ischemia, obesity, certain medications (estrogens, azathioprine), and any condition that causes pancreatic duct obstruction. Correction of these risk factors, such as cholecystectomy for gallstones, are health maintenance or restoration actions.

Pathophysiology

The etiologic mechanism of pancreatic damage remains unclear. The pathologic changes occurring in the pancreas may be due to premature activation of proteolytic and lipolytic pancreatic enzymes. These enzymes are normally activated in the duodenum. The pancreas normally releases protease in an inactive form. Once protease is in the intestine, the action of intestinal enterokinase converts pancreatic trypsinogen (one of the proteases) into trypsin. In pancreatitis, however, activation of the proteases and lipases occurs before secretion into the intestine. When these enzymes are activated before they are secreted into the intestine, pancreatic tissue damage occurs.

Exactly how the enzymes become active in the pancreas is unknown, but they may be triggered by reflux of bile from the duodenum into the pancreatic duct or by pancreatic duct obstruction. The net effect of this enzymatic activation is autodigestion of the pancreas. Once pancreatic inflammation begins, a vicious circle continues the process of further tissue damage and enzyme activation. As the process becomes chronic, the pancreatic parenchyma is destroyed.

In most clients, acute pancreatitis is a mild disease; in 10% to 15% of clients, however, a severe form of illness develops that leads to a lengthy hospitalization, complications, and significant rates of morbidity and mortality. Such clients present a major medical challenge because they require an intensive care setting, hemodynamic monitoring, and frequent laboratory and radiographic evaluation.

One way to predict the severity of attack and overall prognosis is to use the predictive criteria identified by Ranson in 1974 (Box 46–1):

1. Clients with two or fewer prognostic manifestations generally require only supportive care.
2. Clients with three or four manifestations have a mortality rate of approximately 15%.
3. Clients with five or six prognostic manifestations need intensive care, and the mortality rate reaches 40%.[4]
4. Clients with seven or more manifestations have an even higher mortality rate and truly test the limits of modern medicine.

BOX 46-1   Early Prognostic Manifestations of Acute Pancreatitis

At Admission

Age > 55 years
WBC count > 16,000 cells/mm^3
Blood glucose > 200 mg/dl
Serum LDH > 350 units/L
Serum AST > 250 units/L
Base deficit > 4 mEq/L

Indicators of a Worsening Prognosis in the First 48 Hours

Hematocrit fall > 10 percentage points
BUN elevation > 5 mg/dl
Serum calcium falls to < 8 mg/dl
PaO$_2$ < 60 mm Hg
Estimated fluid sequestration > 6 L

AST, aspartate aminotransferase; BUN, blood urea nitrogen; LDH, lactic dehydrogenase; PaO$_2$, partial pressure of arterial oxygen; WBC, white blood cells.

Data from Ranson, J. H. C., et al. (1974) as cited in Friedman, L. S. (1998). Liver, biliary tract, and pancreas. In L. M. Tierney, S. J. McPhee, & M. A. Papadakis (Eds.), *Medical diagnosis and treatment* (37th ed.). Stamford, CT: Appleton & Lange.

Clinical Manifestations

Manifestations in clients presenting with acute pancreatitis are largely the result of activation of proteases and lipases and the resulting autodigestion of the pancreas. Manifestations vary from mild, nonspecific abdominal pain to profound shock with coma and death. The predominant clinical feature is abdominal pain caused by edematous distention of the pancreatic capsule, local peritonitis due to enzyme release into the peritoneum, ductal spasm, or pancreatic autodigestion stimulated by increased enzyme secretion when eating.

Pain normally begins in the midepigastrium and achieves maximal intensity several hours later. In most clients, an extreme epigastric or umbilical pain radiates to the back. In clients with alcohol-associated pancreatitis, pain often begins 12 to 48 hours after an episode of inebriation. Clients with gallstone-associated pancreatitis typically experience pain after a large meal. Nausea and vomiting are frequently present because pain stimulates the vomiting center and gastric and intestinal hypomotility.

Physical examination reveals a distressed, anxious client with abdominal distention and tenderness and with fever caused by paralytic ileus of the small bowel due to localized peritonitis. Severe hemorrhagic pancreatitis may produce two distinctive manifestations: (1) *Turner's sign* (bluish discoloration of the left flank) and (2) *Cullen's sign* (bluish discoloration of the periumbilical area). These manifestations, which occur in fewer than 3% of cases, are the result of tissue catabolism and blood-stained retroperitoneal fluid, respectively. Jaundice, caused by common bile duct obstruction by pancreatic edema, may be present in clients with gallstone-associated pancreatitis but otherwise is uncommon in the initial phase of the disease.

Clients with severe pancreatitis may exhibit severe circulatory complications, such as hypotension; pallor; cool, clammy skin; hypovolemia; hypoperfusion; obtundation; and shock. Shock is not unusual; it may result from:

- Hypovolemia secondary to loss of blood and plasma proteins into the retroperitoneal space
- Increased formation and release of kinins, which cause vasodilation and increased vascular permeability
- Systemic effects of proteolytic and lipolytic enzymes released into the circulation

As many as one third of clients have evidence of left pleural effusion or left hemidiaphragmatic elevation.

Other clinical findings include subcutaneous fat necrosis and cerebral abnormalities, such as belligerence, confusion, psychosis, and coma, that are caused by hyperosmolality, hypoperfusion and hypoxia, cerebral fat embolism, or disseminated intravascular coagulopathy. Transient hyperglycemia is found in 50% of clients, probably as a result of damage to the islets. All of the hormonal (endocrine) functions of the pancreas may be disrupted from tissue damage, and diabetes may develop secondary to the disease. Hypocalcemia occurs in up to 30% of clients, since calcium may be deposited in areas of necrosis and undigested intestinal fat traps calcium in feces.

Serum amylase analysis is the most widely used test for the diagnosis of pancreatitis. In most cases, hyperamylasemia is seen within 24 hours of the onset of manifestations and resolves within 7 to 14 days. Persistent hyperamylasemia may indicate the development of complications.

The measurement of urinary amylase appears to be a sensitive index of pancreatitis. Some support the use of the amylase-creatinine clearance ratio in the diagnosis. Unfortunately, acute pancreatitis may occur with a normal amylase-creatinine clearance ratio.

The serum lipase value is one of the most specific indicators of acute pancreatitis because lipase is solely of pancreatic origin. The duration of hyperlipasemia often exceeds that of hyperamylasemia. However, hyperlipasemia may also be seen in perforated peptic ulcer, acute cholecystitis (inflammation of the gallbladder wall), intestinal ischemia, hereditary hyperlipidemia–associated pancreatitis, or alcohol-induced pancreatitis. Additionally, a white blood cell (WBC) count above 10,000 cells/mm^3 is common; hyperglycemia, mild azotemia, abnormal liver function tests, and hypocalcemia may also be present.

Chest film findings may show left basilar atelectasis, elevated left hemidiaphragm, and left pleural effusion. Abdominal films may reveal nonspecific abnormalities, such as (1) the presence of air in the duodenal loop, indicating duodenal ileus; (2) the "sentinel loop" sign, representing a dilated proximal jejunal loop; (3) the colon "cutoff" sign, indicating distention of the transverse colon; (4) gallstones; or (5) pancreatic calcifications.

Nearly all acute pancreatitis clients have some abnormality on a computed tomography (CT) scan. Pancreatic changes include parenchymal enlargement, edema, or necrosis. A CT scan is also helpful in identifying other structural changes, such as pancreatic pseudocyst, abscess, or phlegmon. A magnetic resonance imaging (MRI) study reveals the same information as CT. Scans with radio pharmaceuticals such as ^{99}mTc-labeled (technetium) N-substituted iminodiacetic acids (HIDA, DIDA, DISIDA) may be useful in acute pancreatitis to evaluate the gallbladder and biliary tree.

Although ERCP has no role in the standard diagnostic evaluation of most clients with acute pancreatitis, it has proved helpful in some clients with recurrent pancreatitis by identifying correctable abnormalities (e.g., duct abnormalities).

Prognosis

The mortality rate for severe acute pancreatitis—more than three Ranson criteria (see Box 46–1)—is high, especially when cardiovascular, renal, or hepatic impairment is present or when pancreatic necrosis develops. Recurrences of acute pancreatitis are common in clients with alcoholic pancreatitis.

Outcome Management

■ Medical Management

REDUCE PAIN

Pain is usually treated with narcotic analgesics, meperidine being the drug of choice. Morphine is contraindicated because it may cause spasm of the sphincter of Oddi, which may then potentiate ongoing pancreatic parenchymal injury.

MAINTAIN VOLUME STATUS, ELECTROLYTE BALANCE, AND NUTRITIONAL STATUS

Acute pancreatitis is commonly associated with fluid loss due to emesis. Fluids can accumulate in the bowel secondary to ileus or in the peripancreatic region because of edema. Management of the client involves replacing lost body fluids, correcting hypovolemia, and restoring electrolyte balance. Normally, the success of fluid and electrolyte restoration is monitored by assessment of heart rate, blood pressure, and urinary output. In clients with pre-existing cardiac, pulmonary, or renal disease or in those with severe pancreatitis, invasive monitoring, including urinary catheterization, central venous pressure monitoring, or monitoring cardiac output and filling via a Swan-Ganz catheter, is indicated. Clients with severe hemorrhagic pancreatitis may require transfusions of blood or clotting factors to correct coagulation problems.

Clients with acute pancreatitis commonly have a variety of electrolyte abnormalities. Clients with severe and persistent vomiting may require saline solutions containing potassium chloride. Serum calcium levels may be depressed secondary to hypoalbuminemia. Mild hyperglycemia is usually corrected with fluid volume replacement, but marked hyperglycemia or glycosuria calls for careful insulin administration.

Treatment may involve attempts to suppress pancreatic exocrine function. Therapy to decrease these enzymes may include nasogastric suction or administration of histamine (H_2)-receptor antagonists, antacids, anticholinergics, glucagon, calcitonin, somatostatin, and proglumide.

Pancreatitis may also be associated with nutritional problems when the client has been allowed nothing by mouth (NPO; *nil per os*), has nausea and vomiting, or has undergone nasogastric suction. Nutritional problems are detailed later in this chapter.

MAINTAIN PANCREATIC REST

Pancreatic rest involves withholding food and liquids by mouth initially, because food ingestion increases pancreatic secretion, which may increase inflammation and pain. No food or fluids should be given orally until the client is largely free of pain and has bowel sounds. Clear liquids are then given, and gradual advancement to a regular low-fat diet is prescribed, guided by the client's tolerance and by the absence of pain. Caution must be taken, because premature return to oral intake has been associated with development of pancreatic abscess and reactivation of inflammation.

Clients with moderate to severe pancreatitis need to be supported nutritionally by total parenteral nutrition (TPN). Administration of a carbohydrate and amino-acid solution along with lipids as a source of calories may be necessary.

TREAT COMPLICATIONS

Complications of pancreatitis include *pancreatic* disorders (e.g., pancreatic abscess, infected necrosis), which may warrant surgery, or *nonpancreatic* disorders (e.g., colonic or bile obstruction or metabolic, renal, or pulmonary disorders). Clients with pulmonary or respiratory complications may require supportive measures, such as endotracheal intubation and positive pressure ventilation.

OTHER MEASURES

Antibiotics are not routinely administered because they are without proven benefit; they are generally reserved for documented infections. Calcium gluconate must be given intravenously if there is evidence of hypocalcemia with tetany. The role of somatostatin in severe acute pancreatitis is unknown, but octreotide and histamine H_2 blocker therapy are thought to be of no benefit.

It may be necessary to perform peritoneal dialysis to rid the peritoneum of potentially toxic compounds commonly found in exudate from acute pancreatitis. Histamine, vasoactive kinins, elastase, prostaglandins, phospholipase A, trypsin, and chymotrypsin may mediate adverse systemic effects, such as hypotension, pulmonary failure, hepatic failure, and altered vascular permeability. This form of therapy is usually reserved for clients who show early clinical deterioration in spite of maximal intensive care support.

■ Nursing Management of the Medical Client
ASSESSMENT

Until a confirmed diagnosis is made, concentrate on preparing clients for diagnostic procedures and on assessing and treating manifestations of disease (see earlier). Assess the location, severity, and character of the pain as well as the onset, duration, and precipitating or relieving factors. Evaluate the client's response to pain and the therapies used to relieve discomfort. Much of your role focuses on educating the client and significant others about procedures and their rationales.

DIAGNOSIS, OUTCOMES, INTERVENTIONS

Pain. A common nursing diagnosis for the client with pancreatitis is *Pain related to inflammation of the pancreas and surrounding tissue, biliary tract disease, obstruction of pancreatic ducts, and interruption of the blood supply.*

Outcomes. The client will demonstrate an absence of or a decrease in pain, as evidenced by verbalizing this fact and resting quietly.

Interventions

Administer Pain Medications. Administer pain medications in a timely manner. Meperidine is the drug of choice because opiate narcotics may stimulate spasm of the ducts and increase pain. Other drugs may be ordered (e.g., anticholinergics, histamine-receptor antagonists) to quiet the pancreas and to decrease enzyme secretion.

Promote Pancreatic Rest. Keeping the client on NPO status (taking nothing by mouth) not only rests the gastrointestinal tract but also decreases pancreatic stimulation and pain. Allowing no oral alimentation and using a nasogastric (NG) tube suction decrease gastrin release from the stomach and prevent gastric contents from entering the duodenum. Nasogastric suctioning removes hydrochloric acid (a powerful stimulant to the release of pancreatic enzymes) and helps to decrease distention, thereby promoting comfort. Check the system frequently to ensure that nasogastric suction is functioning properly. According to some studies, however, nasogastric suction offers only a mild to moderate advantage in the treatment of severe acute pancreatitis and should be considered elective rather than mandatory.

Provide Comfort Measures. Nonpharmacologic measures are often helpful in relieving pain, relaxing the client, and enhancing the effects of narcotics. Correct positioning (particularly a side-lying, knee-chest position with a pillow pressed against the abdomen or a sitting position with the trunk flexed), back rubs, relaxation techniques, and a quiet environment all help to promote comfort and rest.

Risk for Fluid Volume Deficit and Electrolyte Imbalance.
A possible complication of acute pancreatitis is *Risk for Fluid Volume Deficit and Electrolyte Imbalance related to vomiting, nasogastric suctioning, NPO status, shifting of body fluids, fever, and diaphoresis.*

Outcomes. The client will remain normovolemic and maintain electrolyte levels within normal limits.

Interventions. Monitor vital signs for changes in pulse and blood pressure (fluid volume changes) and respiration (acid-base imbalance). If necessary, use hemodynamic monitoring to check for changes in fluid and electrolyte status. Electrocardiographic (ECG) findings of cardiac rhythm changes may be the first indication of electrolyte imbalance.

Check laboratory values for significant changes, and observe for physical manifestations of hyperglycemia, hypocalcemia, and hypokalemia. Monitor the client's response to fluid administration and blood products by monitoring intake and output and assessing for edema, adventitious lung sounds, skin turgor, and mucous membrane alterations. Report significant changes promptly because these clients are at increased risk.

Altered Nutrition: Less Than Body Requirements.
Pancreatitis leads to many gastrointestinal manifestations making *Altered Nutrition: Less Than Body Requirements related to nausea and vomiting, NPO status, and nasogastric suctioning* a common nursing diagnosis for this client.

Outcomes. The client will maintain adequate nutritional status, as evidenced by maintaining normal body weight, keeping blood glucose within normal limits, and showing no evidence of muscle wasting.

Interventions. Depending on the severity of illness, these clients may be kept on NPO status for an extended length of time. When extended fasting is necessary, nutrition is provided through hyperalimentation and lipids (see Chapter 29). Assess the overall nutritional status of the client by checking daily weights, tissue integrity, and the presence of adequate body fat and muscle mass.

Clients with acute pancreatitis are allowed an oral diet when all abdominal pain and tenderness have resolved; however, if oral intake is resumed too soon, reexacerbation of manifestations may occur. Therefore, monitor the client's response to oral intake carefully, and begin intake slowly with liquids before the client progresses to a normal diet. It may be necessary to administer antispasmodics, anticholinergics, histamine-receptor antagonists, and antacids to reduce gastric and pancreatic secretions.

If the pancreas has been severely damaged, it may be necessary to give replacement pancreatic enzymes to replace the enzyme deficit and aid digestion. Monitor the effects of these drugs.

Ineffective Breathing Pattern.
The client with acute pancreatitis has the potential for development of many problems. One appropriate nursing diagnosis is *Ineffective Breathing Pattern related to abdominal distention or ascites, pain, or respiratory complications.*

Outcomes. The client will maintain an effective breathing pattern, as evidenced by a respiratory rate within normal limits, relaxed respiratory effort, absence of cyanosis, and clear lungs.

Interventions. Assess the client's respirations for rate and effort. Your assessment should include lung auscultation for decreased lung sounds (potential for atelectasis), rales or rhonchi (potential for pneumonia and pleural effusion), and cyanosis. Many times, these clients have been given a prescription of bed rest, which precludes the need for prophylactic nursing interventions of pulmonary hygiene (e.g., turning, coughing, deep breathing, and incentive spirometry). Keeping the client comfortable with analgesics enhances full inspiration and normal breathing patterns. Positioning, such as placing the client in the semi-Fowler or a side-lying position, may facilitate normal respiration.

Anxiety.
Because of the uncertainty of the disease and the possibility of recurrence, an appropriate nursing diagnosis is *Anxiety related to change in health status, change in environment, fear of pain returning, and alcohol abuse withdrawal.*

Outcomes. The client will express and demonstrate decreasing manifestations of anxiety, as evidenced by calmly discussing his or her apprehension, stating that anxiety and fear are decreasing, admitting that alcohol is a problem and seeking help with abstinence, and displaying behavior associated with relaxation (e.g., resting quietly).

Interventions. Assess the client's level of anxiety by listening and observing. Reassure the client, and acknowledge that the unknown is frightening. Explain procedures that may cause anxiety for the client. Because clients who are in pain or who have acute anxiety may have a shortened attention span, keep instructions simple and direct. Allow significant others to remain with the client when appropriate for added reassurance and comfort.

The client must be encouraged to face the problem that alcohol is causing if it is the source of the pancreatitis. Spend time with the client to encourage him or her to talk about the problem. Recommend groups such as Alcoholics Anonymous, and encourage the client to join such a program. Discuss supportive services available as necessary with the client and significant others.

EVALUATION

Within a few days of treatment, the client is expected to experience less pain and to gradually resume eating and drinking. For more severe cases, the client must remain on NPO status and rest the pancreas for a much longer time. If this occurs, the client will require TPN to maintain adequate nutrition.

■ Surgical Management

INDICATIONS. Operative intervention is indicated in four specific circumstances:

- Uncertainty of diagnosis
- Treatment of pancreatic necrosis and pancreatic abscess
- Correction of associated biliary tract disease
- Progressive clinical deterioration despite optimal supportive care

If clients with severe pancreatitis do not respond to medical management, operative intervention may be indicated to debride necrosis or, again, to exclude other possible diagnoses as causative factors.

If it is necessary to facilitate drainage of a pancreatic abscess, a laparotomy with sump drainage is usually required. It is usually necessary to resect necrotic tissue because undrained pancreatic abscesses are associated with a high mortality rate.

If the client has extensive disease of the entire gland, a subtotal pancreatectomy may be performed. The operation involves attaching a small remnant of the remaining head of the pancreas to the duodenum. A more extensive procedure, Whipple's operation (pancreaticoduodenectomy), may be necessary if the pancreatitis is confined to the head of the pancreas. In this instance, the distal third of the stomach, the duodenum, common bile duct, gallbladder, and head of the pancreas are removed.

Because it may be difficult to identify acute pancreatitis, exploratory laparotomy may be indicated to eliminate processes such as perforated viscus or acute mesenteric ischemia. If uncomplicated acute pancreatitis is present, no manipulation is needed and the surgery is terminated. In presumed gallstone-associated pancreatitis, cholecystectomy and intraoperative cholangiography are favored. In clients with severe hemorrhagic pancreatitis with necrosis,

debridement of necrotic tissue is performed and retroperitoneal drainage is established.

Treatment of pancreatic abscess combines antibiotic therapy and surgical drainage. Operative debridement is necessary to remove the thick, debris-filled, paste-like collections of infected necrotic material.

CONTRAINDICATIONS. In the past, biliary tract surgery for gallstone-associated pancreatitis was deferred for up to 8 weeks; however, up to 50% of clients awaiting elective surgery experienced a recurrence of pancreatitis. Today most surgeons proceed with surgery as soon as the initial manifestations of pancreatitis resolve.

COMPLICATIONS. Ileus, abdominal distention, and vomiting are possible postoperative complications and require nasogastric suction if they occur. A serious complication of acute pancreatitis is adult respiratory distress syndrome (ARDS), which can occur within 3 to 7 days of the onset of pancreatitis and after the administration of large volumes of fluid and colloids given to sustain blood pressure and adequate urine output. The Critical Monitoring feature presents the findings mandating early intervention in ARDS secondary to acute pancreatitis.

OUTCOMES. Clients are expected to recover from the surgical procedure and not experience postoperative complications. Once bowel sounds have returned approximately 3 days after surgery, the nasogastric tube is discontinued. If tube removal is tolerated and pain is relieved, the client will begin liquids within the next 24 to 72 hours. The client is discharged once a low-fat diet is tolerated.

■ Nursing Management of the Surgical Client
PREOPERATIVE CARE

Preparing a client for pancreatic surgery requires the usual preoperative care. In addition, close monitoring of WBC count, hematocrit, serum electrolytes, serum calcium, serum creatinine, blood urea nitrogen (BUN), aspartate aminotransferase (AST), lactic dehydrogenase (LDH), and arterial blood gases (ABGs) is essential. Other measures may be necessary, depending on the severity of the client's illness, such as insertion of a nasogastric tube, continued replacement of fluids, monitoring of central venous pressure, and blood culture results.

Preoperative nursing management of the client with acute pancreatitis is similar to that described under Nurs-

---

CRITICAL MONITORING

Manifestations of Adult Respiratory Distress Syndrome Secondary to Acute Pancreatitis

Acute respiratory distress: tachypnea, dyspnea, accessory muscle breathing, and cyanosis

Fever and dry cough that develop over a short time period

Fine crackles heard throughout lung fields on auscultation

Possible confusion and agitation

Hypoxemia with partial pressure of oxygen (Po_2) < 50 mm Hg

Early—hypocapnia and respiratory alkalosis

Late—hypercapnia and respiratory acidosis

ing Management of the Medical Client. Pay special attention to the nutritional status of the client as well as to the breathing pattern, fluid volume and electrolyte levels, control of pain, and possible complications as the client is prepared for surgery. The client will require preoperative teaching about the procedure and what to expect postoperatively (see Chapter 15). Encourage clients to ask questions about their condition, treatment, and progress.

POSTOPERATIVE CARE
ASSESSMENT

After pancreatic surgery, you should:

1. Have a clear idea of the surgical procedure performed, its purpose, steps, and dangers.
2. Be aware of the location and purpose of each drain inserted during surgery. If there are multiple drains, especially external drains, assess each for proper function.
3. Continually assess tubes or drains that are in place for decompression. If a T tube or internal stent becomes nonfunctional, alert the surgeon immediately to prevent leakage at the internal insertion site. Leakage may lead to peritonitis or fistula formation. Assess for placement, location (internal or external), and proper function and patency of the drains. If the drains do not appear to be functioning, notify the physician immediately.

After pancreatic excision, it is important to know how much pancreatic tissue was removed. When there is a decrease in endocrine tissue, control of blood glucose with insulin and diet becomes necessary. Exocrine loss does not pose immediate postoperative problems but does necessitate lifelong enzyme replacement when oral ingestion is resumed. Assess the functional ability of remaining pancreatic tissue after excision of the pancreas, determining both endocrine and exocrine functioning and its long-term implications. If the client has lost all endocrine function, insulin administration will be necessary (see Chapter 45). Continue to monitor the client for manifestations of hypoglycemia and hyperglycemia.

With the loss of exocrine function, replacement of pancreatic enzyme function with medications such as pancrelipase (Pancrease) becomes necessary. When the client begins to eat, watch for the development of diarrhea and steatorrhea (fatty stools), which indicate that insufficient pancreatic enzymes are present.

DIAGNOSIS, OUTCOMES, INTERVENTIONS

See the nursing diagnoses discussed under Nursing Management of the Medical Client with acute pancreatitis relating to pain, fluid and electrolyte balance, anxiety, ineffective breathing pattern, and nutrition. All are applicable in the postoperative situation. In addition, the following nursing diagnoses are specifically related to the postoperative period.

Risk for Ineffective Management of Therapeutic Regimen (Individuals). After pancreatectomy, the client will have many and complex learning needs, leading to the nursing diagnosis *Risk for Ineffective Management of Therapeutic Regimen (Individuals) related to care, postoperative nutritional needs, diabetic care, and pancreatic enzyme replacement.*

Outcomes. The client will understand discharge instructions, as evidenced by the ability to describe and demonstrate appropriate wound care, diet, proper diabetes care, and correct administration and side effects of the medication regimen.

Interventions. Assess the knowledge of the client and significant others before providing appropriate learning guidelines before discharge. Provide instructions for wound care. The client will require changes in diet necessitated by diabetes. Provide guidelines for nutritional needs and an appropriate low-fat diet.

Provide the client with important information concerning diabetes, including information about hyperglycemia (polyuria, polydipsia, and polyphagia) and hypoglycemia (see Chapter 45). Explain medication (pancreatic enzymes), including action, side effects, and when to notify the physician.

Effective Management of Therapeutic Regimen: Individual. If the client has an alcohol problem, there will be a need to control it and other potential problems associated with the disease, leading to the nursing diagnosis *Effective Management of Therapeutic Regimen: Individual related to alcohol abuse, surgical procedure, severity of the pancreatitis, and need for follow-up care.*

Outcomes. The client will discuss strategies to address the progression or complications of alcoholism and pancreatitis that challenge his or her continued successful management.

Interventions. The client with loss of pancreatic endocrine function requires extensive education regarding diabetes and its care (see Chapter 45). All clients require instruction on good nutrition to maintain adequate output. The client will need to understand and to follow a nutritious low-fat diet.

Avoidance of alcohol is another area of postoperative education. Explain the problems that alcohol is creating and the importance of stopping drinking before irreversible damage is done.

EVALUATION

If there are no complications, the client can be discharged about a week after surgery. Hence, a visiting nurse may visit the client after discharge to assess the client's ability to follow the postoperative regimen. The client will need to be seen at regular intervals to ensure compliance.

The client's ability to abstain from alcohol should be carefully assessed and further counseling provided, if needed. In the short term, the client should recover from acute pancreatitis without complications. Long-term recovery, however, often depends on the client's willingness and ability to alter one's lifestyle.

■ Self-Care

Because of the complex nature of pancreatitis and the importance of the client's understanding in lowering the risk of recurrence, clients must become knowledgeable about the causes of the disease, treatment, possible complications, and home health care.

Before discharge to the home, ask the client and significant others to verbalize home health care needs related to the diet; medications, including indications, dosage, frequency, and side effects; and the manifestations of recurrence.

MEDICATIONS

Prepare clients for discharge by assessing their level of understanding and their learning needs. Discuss the medication regimen with the client, including its purpose, dosage, frequency, and possible side effects. Explain that an insulin supplement may be required because of pancreatic damage. Begin your teaching as soon as possible to ensure that the client and significant others are fully prepared to cope with glucose monitoring, diet, and insulin administration (see Chapter 45).

DIET MODIFICATIONS

Instruct the client about dietary restrictions, such as avoiding alcohol, tea, coffee, spicy foods, and heavy meals, which stimulate pancreatic secretions and produce attacks of pancreatitis. Clients should understand the benefit of eating small, frequent meals high in protein, low in fat, and moderate to high in carbohydrate.

TEACH MANIFESTATIONS OF RECURRENCE

Ensure that the client is aware of the manifestations of recurrence of pancreatitis and the importance of reporting these manifestations immediately. These manifestations include steatorrhea; severe back or epigastric pain; persistent gastritis, nausea, and vomiting; weight loss; elevated temperature; and evidence of hyperglycemia. If the client has had surgery, routine postoperative teaching (see Chapter 15) and education about care of drains, if still in place, will be needed.

CHRONIC PANCREATITIS

Chronic pancreatitis is a progressive, inflammatory, destructive disease of the pancreas. The incidence in the United States is approximately 4 in 100,000.

Pathophysiology

Chronic pancreatitis involves progressive fibrosis and degeneration of the pancreas. Characteristically, the pancreas is progressively destroyed by repeated flares of usually mild attacks of pancreatitis. After repeated attacks of acute pancreatitis, this inflammatory process results in scarring and calcification of pancreatic tissue. The damage is irreversible, affecting both endocrine and exocrine pancreatic functions.

In the United States and in other industrial countries, chronic alcoholism is the most frequent cause of chronic calcifying pancreatitis. In up to 25% of American adults, chronic pancreatitis is of unknown or idiopathic cause; it may also be hereditary. A gene for hereditary pancreatitis, transmitted as an autosomal dominant trait with variable penetrance, has been identified on chromosome 7. Protein malnutrition is a cause in other parts of the world. Other causes include untreated hyperparathyroidism, congenital anomalies, and pancreatic trauma.

Clinical Manifestations

In chronic pancreatitis, as in acute pancreatitis, dull pain alternates with severe pain, vomiting, constipation, fever, and jaundice. The client may experience some pain relief by sitting in bed with the knees flexed and pressing a pillow to the abdomen. The client generally experiences more pain when supine. Attacks may last only a few days or as long as 2 weeks.

Because food may worsen the pain, the client usually reduces food intake, resulting in weight loss. Reduction in digestive enzyme secretion eventually causes malnutrition and contributes to the weight loss. Ultimately, because of involvement of islet tissue, hyperglycemia develops with manifestations of diabetes. Insulin-dependent diabetes mellitus occurs in up to one third of clients.

The client also suffers from (1) abdominal distention with flatus and cramps and (2) frequent passage of foul fatty stools (steatorrhea). Thus, the clinical group of manifestations that serves as a classic presentation of chronic pancreatitis is abdominal pain, weight loss, diabetes, and steatorrhea. Additionally, many clients present with a history of narcotic analgesic abuse in an effort to control pain. Pain or digestive disturbance may motivate a person with chronic pancreatitis to seek help.

Because clients with chronic pancreatitis have a reduced amount of functioning tissue, pancreatic enzyme analysis may be normal. Blood studies may reveal a mild leukocytosis. Glycosuria may be present. X-ray studies may show reduced bowel motility, calcifications, and adhesions. Both ultrasonography and the more expensive CT study provide useful diagnostic data. Angiography indicates vascular changes. Cholangiography and cholecystography show biliary alterations, which may be either a cause or a consequence of the pancreatic disorder.

Outcome Management

■ Medical Management

RELIEVE PAIN

The control of pain can be a major problem and is generally the sole indication for surgical intervention. Attempts to control pain pharmacologically should begin with nonnarcotic analgesics and should progress to narcotic analgesics, if needed. For alcohol-related pancreatitis, total abstinence from alcohol is imperative and sometimes successful in itself for pain relief. A low-fat diet should be prescribed and may reduce painful stimulation of pancreatitis enzyme secretion.

Steatorrhea may be treated with pancreatic supplements selected for their high lipase activity. Concurrent administration of sodium bicarbonate H_2-receptor antagonists (e.g., ranitidine) or a proton pump inhibitor (e.g., omeprazole) may decrease the inactivation of lipase by acid and thereby may further decrease steatorrhea.

TREATMENT OF ENDOCRINE INSUFFICIENCY

Exogenous insulin therapy may be necessary because of destruction of islet tissue.

TREATMENT OF EXOCRINE INSUFFICIENCY

Exocrine insufficiency is treated with exogenous pancreatic enzyme therapy. This therapy may include lipase, trypsin, or H_2-receptor antagonists.

■ Surgical Management

The three major goals of surgical intervention for chronic pancreatitis are to:

1. Correct the primary tract disease (ampullar procedure)
2. Relieve ductal obstruction (ductal drainage)
3. Alleviate pain (ablative procedure)

Several surgical approaches are available. The major operations are depicted in Figure 46–1.

Endoscopic or surgical drainage is indicated for pseudocysts that cause manifestations. Pancreatic ascites or pancreaticopleural fistulae resulting from a disrupted pancreatic duct can be managed by endoscopic placement of a stent across the disrupted duct. Breaking up stones (calculi) in the pancreatic duct by lithotripsy and endoscopic removal of stones from the duct at ERCP or placement of a stent across pancreatic duct strictures may relieve pain. For clients with chronic pain and nondilated ducts, a percutaneous celiac plexus nerve block may be ordered, although results are often disappointing.

The prognosis for the client with chronic pancreatitis is good if acute attacks decrease in frequency. Replacement therapy for chronic fat indigestion permits a fairly normal life. If the client continues to drink alcohol, the prognosis is poor. Repeated attacks eventually cause death from shock or renal failure.

PANCREATIC PSEUDOCYSTS

Pancreatic pseudocysts are localized collections of pancreatic secretions (high concentrations of amylase, lipase, and trypsin) in a cystic structure usually adjacent to the pancreas rather than within the parenchyma. Pseudocysts account for up to 75% of all cystic lesions of the pancreas. They develop in up to 10% of clients after an attack of acute alcoholic pancreatitis, but they may be associated with acute pancreatitis of other causes, chronic pancreatitis, trauma, and pancreatic neoplasm.

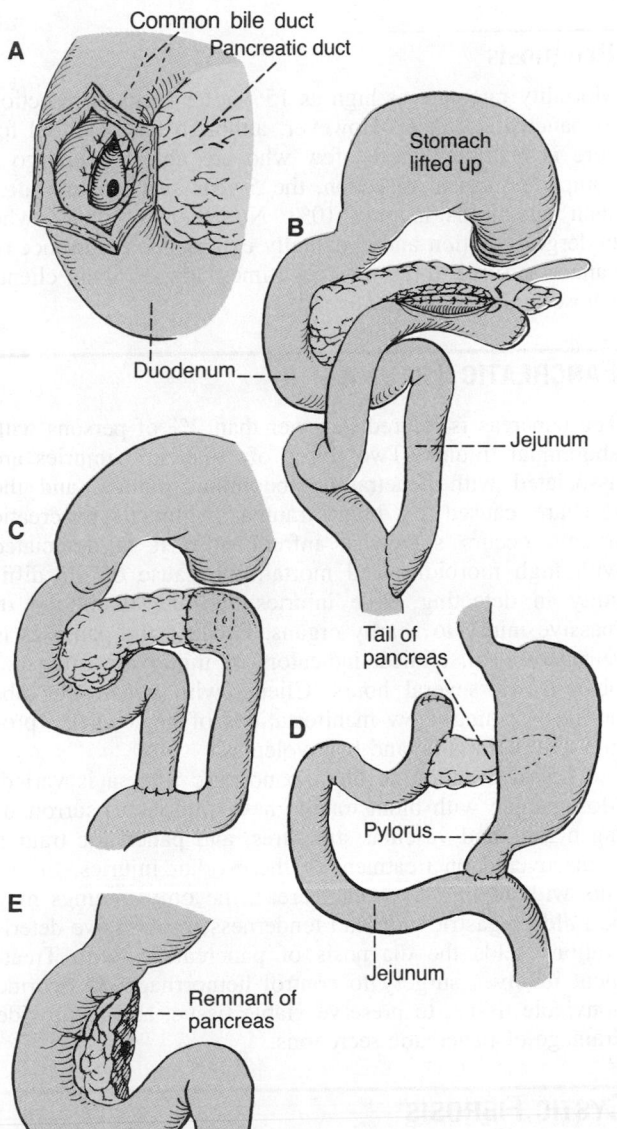

A.   **Sphincteroplasty (ampullary)**
Indicated for stenosis of sphincter of Oddi with dilation of pancreatic duct. This procedure has limited application in pancreatitis, and its use is decreasing.

B.   **Side-to-side pancreaticojejunostomy (ductal drainage)**
Indicated when gross dilation of pancreatic ducts is associated with septa and calculi. The most successful procedure, with rates of 60% to 90%.

C.   **Caudal pancreaticojejunostomy (ductal drainage)**
Indicated for the uncommon cases of isolated proximal pancreatic ductal stenosis not involving the ampulla.

D.   **Pancreaticoduodenal resection (ablative)**
(with preservation of pylorus) (Whipple procedure)
Indicated when major changes are confined to head of pancreas. Preservation of pylorus avoids usual sequelae of gastric resection.

E.   **Subtotal pancreatectomy (ablative)**
Indicated when other operations fail and when ducts are unsuitable for decompression. Because metabolic sequelae are significant, this procedure is declining in popularity.

FIGURE 46–1 Surgical procedures for chronic pancreatitis and pancreatic cancer.

The most common clinical picture of a client with pancreatic pseudocyst involves abdominal pain, early satiety, nausea, and vomiting. Less common manifestations include pruritus, jaundice, sepsis, and hemorrhage. Essentially, diagnosis of pseudocyst is made through the same assessment as that used for pancreatitis.

Treatment is based on the presence or absence of manifestations, the client's age, and the size of the cyst. Cysts smaller than 6 cm in diameter often resolve spontaneously. Clients with such cysts are followed up with frequent ultrasound studies to determine whether the cyst is decreasing in size. Clients with persistent manifestations or pseudocyst-related complications, such as infection, require operative intervention. Erosion of an inflammatory process into a blood vessel can result in a major hemorrhage into the cyst.

Surgical procedures include internal drainage of the pseudocyst (cystojejunostomy, cystogastrostomy, and cystoduodenostomy), pancreatic resection, distal pancreatectomy, and, least often, percutaneous or endoscopic drainage.

PANCREATIC CANCER

Cancer is the most common neoplasm affecting the pancreas. About 75% of cancers occur in the head, and 25% are in the body and tail of the pancreas. Pancreatic cancer is the fifth most common cause of death from cancer, exceeded only by lung, colorectal, breast, and prostate cancer. Of clients with pancreatic cancer, 90% die within the first year of diagnosis. Cancer of the pancreas is more common in blacks than in whites, in smokers, and in men. It appears to be linked to diabetes mellitus, use of alcohol, history of previous pancreatitis, smoking, and ingestion of a high-fat diet and organic chemicals, such as coke, coal gas, and benzidine. Health promotion actions include avoidance of risk factors and pancreatitis. Health maintenance and health restoration activities are limited because of the poor prognosis associated with pancreatic cancer.

Duct cell adenocarcinoma accounts for more than 90% of cell types of malignant pancreatic exocrine tumors. Less common types of pancreatic exocrine cancer include cystadenocarcinoma and acinar cell carcinoma. Periampullary adenocarcinomas originate in the region of the ampulla of Vater. Clients typically present with jaundice, significant unexplained weight loss, and abdominal pain. Many clients are managed operatively by either resection (~30%) or palliative therapy to relieve manifestations such as jaundice.[11]

Carcinomas of the tail and body of the pancreas usually present with significant weight loss and abdominal pain. Because of their location, these tumors generally grow to a large size before manifestations occur and the diagnosis is made. Therefore, the resectability rate is low (<7%), and the prognosis is poor (a 5- to 6-month mean survival). The response to chemotherapy (fluorouracil) has been disappointing.

Cystadenocarcinoma of the pancreas is most frequently seen in women between ages 40 and 60 years, and it accounts for fewer than 2% of all pancreatic exocrine neoplasms. Acinar cell carcinoma of the pancreas is very rare, showing no sex predominance. Surgical treatment is the same as that used for ductal adenocarcinoma.

Outcome Management

■ Medical Management

Medical treatment for pancreatic cancer includes radiation therapy (e.g., high-dose external beam, interstitial seed of iodine 125 or iridium 192, brachytherapy, and intraoperative radiation therapy) and drugs (e.g., 5-fluorouracil alone or with radiation therapy and nitrosourea, mitomycin-C, and doxorubicin). A newer chemotherapeutic agent with success is gemcitabine (Gemzar), which inhibits the movement of cells from the G1 to the S phase of the cell cycle.

■ Surgical Management

Surgical treatment is Whipple's operation, which involves a pancreaticoduodenectomy with removal of the distal third of the stomach, pancreaticojejunostomy, gastrojejunostomy, and choledochojejunostomy (see Fig. 46–1). The nursing care for these clients is similar to that for Nursing Management of the Surgical Client with acute pancreatitis.

Prognosis

Mortality rates are as high as 15% after surgical resection of pancreatic cancer. However, although the potential for cure is restricted to the few who are able to undergo a complete surgical resection, the 5-year survival rate after such operations is only 10%. Nonetheless, clients who undergo resection and eventually experience recurrence of cancer survive three to four times longer than clients whose tumor is not removed.[11]

PANCREATIC TRAUMA

The pancreas is injured in fewer than 2% of persons with abdominal trauma. Two thirds of pancreatic injuries are associated with penetrating abdominal trauma, and the rest are caused by blunt trauma. Although pancreatic trauma occurs somewhat infrequently, it is associated with high morbidity and mortality because of the difficulty in detecting these injuries and the likelihood of massive injury to nearby organs. Because the pancreas is retroperitoneal, clinical indicators of injury are often not obvious for several hours. Clients with penetrating abdominal trauma show manifestations of hemorrhage, progressive peritonitis, and hypovolemia.

The presentation of blunt pancreatic trauma is varied. Most people with blunt trauma have injuries to surrounding organs and vascular structures, and pancreatic trauma is discovered on treatment of these other injuries. In clients without injury to other areas, the only findings may be mild epigastric pain and tenderness; progressive deterioration yields the diagnosis of pancreatic injury. Treatment involves surgery to control hemorrhage, to debride nonviable tissue, to preserve viable tissue, and to provide drainage of pancreatic secretions.

CYSTIC FIBROSIS

Cystic fibrosis (CF) is a hereditary, chronic disease characterized by abnormal secretions of the exocrine glands.

It is genetically transmitted as an autosomal recessive trait. Approximately 4% to 5% of the population are carriers, and the incidence in the United States is about 1 in every 1600 to 2000 births in whites. CF is diagnosed and managed in childhood, but improvements in care have allowed many clients to survive into adulthood.

Pulmonary complications are the most physically visible. Clients have obvious respiratory compromise, with frequent bronchopneumonia and chronic bronchitis. Some improvements in the management of infants and children with CF have led to a greater number of adults with CF. Typically, these adults have a small stature and appear somewhat emaciated. They are barrel-chested and have clubbed fingers. Because the digestive problems encountered with CF are generally managed with diet and oral administration of pancreatic enzymes and fat-soluble vitamins, clients are hospitalized for treatment of respiratory complications rather than for intestinal problems.

In addition to pulmonary problems, clients experience impaired pancreatic exocrine function because of decreased lipase released into the bowel. The result is malabsorption of lipids with blockage of the pancreatic ducts by thick mucus. Pancreatic degeneration, fibrosis, and atrophy of tissues follow, with eventual development of fatty infiltration and loss of function. The intestines have thick, viscous mucus, which may cause a thick mass within the bowel. The lack of pancreatic enzymes causes steatorrhea.

The current trend is to hospitalize the client routinely for thorough pulmonary hygiene with a full course of intravenous (IV) antibiotics, with emphasis on antifungal agents, and respiratory therapy.

Nursing management of the client with CF focuses on two major nursing diagnoses: (1) *Ineffective Airway Clearance* and (2) *Altered Nutrition: Less than Body Requirements*. Interventions for clients with CF include:

- Prophylactic pulmonary support (expectorants, postural drainage, antibiotics)
- Administration of pancreatic enzymes
- A high-protein, high-calorie, high-salt, low-fat diet
- Replacement of fat-soluble vitamins

BILIARY TRACT DISORDERS

Disorders of the gallbladder and ducts are extremely common. In the United States alone, biliary tract disorders account for more than 500,000 hospitalizations annually. Disorders include gallstones, inflammatory conditions, infections, tumors, and congenital malformations.

The two most common conditions are gallstones and associated cholecystitis (inflammation of the gallbladder). Approximately 98% of clients who present with symptomatic gallbladder disease have gallstones. Malignancies and congenital anomalies of the biliary tract are relatively uncommon.

Before beginning this discussion, note the list of terms (Table 46–1) used in association with these conditions.

CHOLELITHIASIS (GALLSTONES)

Approximately 20 million people in the United States have gallstones, and almost 475,000 cholecystectomies

TABLE 46–1	BILIARY TRACT TERMINOLOGY
Term	**Definition**
Chole-	Pertaining to bile
Cholang-	Pertaining to bile ducts
Cholangiography	X-ray study of bile ducts
Cholangitis	Inflammation of bile duct
Cholecyst-	Pertaining to gallbladder
Cholecystectomy	Removal of gallbladder
Cholecystitis	Inflammation of gallbladder
Cholecystography	X-ray study of gallbladder
Cholecystostomy	Incision and drainage of gallbladder
Choledocho-	Pertaining to common bile duct
Choledocholithiasis	Stones in common bile duct
Choledochostomy	Exploration of common bile duct
Cholelith-	Pertaining to gallstones
Cholelithiasis	Presence of gallstones
Cholescintigraphy	Radionuclide imaging of biliary system

are performed every year. The incidence of gallstones increases with age, as do the risks associated with cholelithiasis. In the United States, more than 10% of men and 20% of women have gallstones by age 65 years. Women account for nearly 70% of those treated for gallstones, although the mortality rate may be higher in men. Twice as many white Americans as black Americans are affected, and although gallstones are less common in black people, cholelithiasis attributable to hemolysis occurs in more than one third of people with sickle cell anemia.

The prevalence of gallstones is much the same in Europe and Australia. Clients with diabetes mellitus, obesity, Crohn's disease, and those with cirrhosis show an increased incidence.

Most of our present knowledge of cholesterol gallstones comes from the study of Pima Native American women in south-central Arizona, in whom the occurrence is 75% over age 25 years. Pigment stones are dominant in Asians and in African Americans.

Etiology and Risk Factors

Gallstones are crystalline structures formed by concretion (hardening) or accretion (adherence of particles, accumulation) of normal or abnormal bile constituents. According to various theories, there are four possible explanations for stone formation.

First, bile may undergo a change in composition. Studies of subjects with cholesterol gallstones indicate that their bile is supersaturated with cholesterol but deficient in bile salts. The cholesterol saturation of bile seems to increase with age. Changes in bile composition, however, do not completely explain why gallstones form.

Second, gallbladder stasis may lead to bile stasis. Bile stasis may (1) change the composition of bile, (2) supersaturate bile with cholesterol, and (3) precipitate some bile constituents. Gallbladder stasis may result from decreased contractility and emptying of the gallbladder and spasm of the sphincter of Oddi. Circumstances in which gallbladder stasis occurs (e.g., TPN; low-fat, weight-reduction diets; spinal cord injury, pregnancy) are associated with a high rate of gallstone formation. More specifically, TPN without oral intake for longer than 1 month is associated with gallbladder sludge formation and cholelithiasis. Delayed emptying of the gallbladder may correlate with hormonal factors. In pregnant women, there is an increase in the female sex hormone estrogen. Estrogen increases dietary uptake of cholesterol and increases biliary cholesterol secretion. This may explain why gallstones seem to be associated with pregnancy.

Third, infection may predispose a person to stone formation. Inflammatory debris can form a *nidus* (point of origin) for stone growth. The related tissue injury may alter the composition of bile by increasing the reabsorption of bile salts and lecithin. Certain organisms may also play a part in stone formation by altering the composition of bile. For example, *Escherichia coli* increases the amount of bilirubin available for pigment stones and *Streptococcus faecalis* reduces bile salts.

Fourth, genetics and demography may affect stone formation, as shown by the higher prevalence in Pima and Chippewa Native Americans, Northern Europeans, and South Americans than in Asians.

Health promotion activities to minimize gallstone formation include maintaining a low-fat diet, maintaining ideal body weight, and limiting the number of pregnancies. Clients receiving TPN for longer than 1 month should be monitored closely as health maintenance and restoration actions.

Pathophysiology

Gallstone formation involves several factors:

1. Bile must become supersaturated with cholesterol or calcium.
2. The solute must precipitate from solution as solid crystals.
3. Crystals must come together and fuse to form stones.

Gallstones are generally of three types: (1) cholesterol, (2) pigment, and (3) mixed. Because the incidence of a pure stone formation is rare, stones are generally classified by the predominant substance.

Cholesterol stones are the most common type; the incidence increases with age, and the prevalence is higher in women. Stones are usually smooth and whitish yellow to tan.
Pigment stones are present in about 30% of people with cholelithiasis in the United States. In these people, bile contains an excess of unconjugated bilirubin. Pigment stones may be black (associated with hemolysis and cirrhosis) or earthy calcium bilirubinate (associated with infection in the biliary system).
Mixed stones may be a combination of cholesterol and pigment stones or either of these with some other substance. Calcium carbonate, phosphates, bile salts, and palmitate make up the more common minor constituents.

Most gallstones are formed in the gallbladder, but they may also form in the common duct or hepatic ducts of the liver. The actual incidence is not known, however,

because some stones do not cause manifestations and they pass through the ducts into the bowel unnoticed.

The pathologic findings are best interpreted from the clinical manifestations of the disease, which may be acute or chronic. Once a client becomes symptomatic, treatment and follow-up are essential to prevent progression to a more severe, and sometimes fatal, complication of gallbladder disease. About one third of these complications are due to free perforation, which occurs when a gangrenous area becomes necrotic and bile breaks into the peritoneal cavity. The mortality rate is about 20% for peritonitis with systemic distribution of pepsin.

Pericholecystic abscess accounts for 50% of the complications and is the least severe, with a mortality rate of approximately 15%. Abscess formation occurs while the perforation is walled off by omentum or an adjacent organ (e.g., colon, stomach, or duodenum). Much less frequently, in about 15% of clients, a fistula occurs when the gallbladder becomes attached to a portion of the gastrointestinal tract and perforates it. The duodenum, followed by the colon, is the most common site for this event.

Occasionally, a stone is discharged into the small intestine. If the stone is large enough, it can obstruct the narrow terminal ileum, causing gallstone ileus.

Clinical Manifestations

Manifestations of biliary tract disorders are similar to those of several other conditions. Box 46–2 lists some of the more common diseases that must be differentiated from acute and chronic cholecystitis.

Fewer than half of people with gallstones report any

BOX 46–2   Disorders with Manifestations Similar to Those of Chronic and Acute Cholecystitis

Chronic Cholecystitis

Angina pectoris
Chronic pancreatitis
Esophagitis
Hiatal hernia
Peptic ulcer
Pyelonephritis
Spastic colitis

Acute Cholecystitis

Acute appendicitis
Acute hepatitis
Acute myocardial infarction
Acute pancreatitis
Acute pyelonephritis
Intercostal neuritis
Intestinal obstruction
Perforated ulcer
Pleurisy
Renal calculus
Right lower lobe pneumonia

distress, because gallstones cause no manifestations unless complications develop. The most specific and characteristic manifestation of gallstone disease is pain or biliary colic, which is caused by spasm of the biliary ducts as they try to dislodge the stones. This pain usually follows the temporary obstruction of the gallbladder outlet. Characteristically, the pain starts in the upper midline area. It may radiate around to the back and right shoulder blade, although some clients complain that it passes straight through to the back and substernal areas. The client is often restless, changing positions frequently to relieve the intensity of the pain. Pain may persist for only a few hours or several days, and the interval between attacks is variable.

If the stone is blocking the cystic duct, manifestations of acute cholecystitis (see Acute Cholecystitis) may occur. If the stone lodges in the common duct, gallstones may be complicated by *cholangitis* (inflammation of the bile duct) and pancreatitis. *Jaundice* appears only when common duct obstruction is present.

Nausea and vomiting may occur; occasionally, self-induced vomiting alleviates the manifestations. Assessment may further reveal a history of flatulence, bloating, epigastric pain, belching, intolerance for fatty foods, and vague upper abdominal sensations. Occasionally, clients who have these problems still have them after cholecystectomy.

Assessment of these clients becomes important, in that manifestations of biliary colic and coronary artery disease are remarkably similar. Considering the prevalence of both of these problems, accurate diagnosis is essential. Many times, the diagnosis is based on the manifestations alone. Physical findings are present only during an attack with pain, pain being the cardinal manifestation. The right upper quadrant or epigastric area is tender to palpation with voluntary muscle guarding, but manifestations of peritonitis are absent. The gallbladder is not palpable, and the temperature is normal.

Blood test results are unremarkable. For confirmation of the presence of gallstones, an abdominal ultrasound study is very accurate and has advantages over oral cholecystography. Radionuclide scanning (HIDA, DIDA, or DISIDA) after administration of ^{99m}Tc (technetium) is an accurate test for confirming acute cholecystitis. Other tests may include CT, cholescintigraphy, cholangiography, and, rarely, biliary drainage analysis.

The current trend is to use ERCP and endoscopic retrograde catheterization of the gallbladder (ERCG) in diagnosis, especially for common duct stones (see Chapter 42). Biliary ultrasonography (cholecystosonography) may be the initial study because it is accurate and safe, does not expose the client to ionizing radiation, and can be performed without preparation.

Outcome Management

■ Medical Management
REDUCE PAIN
Pain may arise from contraction of the gallbladder during transient obstruction of the cystic duct by gallstones. Administration of parenteral analgesics, usually meperidine

(Demerol), may be administered intramuscularly (IM) on a schedule or as needed for pain. Antacids are given to neutralize gastric hyperacidity and to reduce associated pain, and antiemetics are given to minimize nausea and vomiting. Antibiotics are administered to reduce the likelihood of infection. Nitroglycerin may reduce biliary colic as well.

MONITOR FLUID AND ELECTROLYTE BALANCE
During an acute attack of biliary colic, the client remains on NPO status, with IV fluids administered to maintain hydration. The client may lose fluids if a nasogastric tube has been inserted for symptomatic relief of vomiting or if pancreatitis is a probable diagnosis.

The diet progresses according to the client's tolerance. The client is advised to avoid foods that precipitate biliary colic. Instructions may include avoiding a fatty meal or a large meal after fasting.

NONSURGICAL APPROACHES TO ERADICATE STONES
ENDOSCOPY. Retrograde endoscopy for stone removal is an important nonsurgical alternative. To remove a gallstone from the common bile duct, the physician passes an endoscope orally into the duodenum, then passes a wire snare into the common bile duct through the ampulla of Vater, securing and removing the obstructing stone (Fig. 46–2). The physician may choose to enlarge the ampulla of Vater by endoscopic papillotomy to allow passage of stones. If stones remain in the common bile duct after cholecystectomy and a T tube is still in place, the physician may pass a stone-retrieving basket or other device through the T tube tract to remove the stone.

GALLSTONE DISSOLUTION (CHOLESTEROL-DISSOLVING AGENTS). The use of oral administration of agents for dissolving cholesterol gallstones is an important nonsurgical intervention. Chenodeoxycholic acid (CDCA), or chenodiol, is not widely used because of its tendency to produce dose-related diarrhea. However, ursodeoxycholic acid, or ursodiol (UDCA) has become popular because it is effective and produces no side effects. Both drugs act to reduce the amount of cholesterol in bile; however, each drug uses a different mechanism. Oral chenodiol is contraindicated in clients with liver disease and in women of childbearing years because of its hepatotoxic effects on the developing fetus. The two drugs, administered together, appear to produce a slightly better effect than when used individually. Diarrhea does not occur when the two drugs are combined.

EXTRACORPOREAL SHOCK WAVE LITHOTRIPSY. Extracorporeal shock wave lithotripsy (ESWL) may be used as an ambulatory treatment in some instances. The client should have symptomatic cholelithiasis with fewer than four stones, each smaller than 3 cm in diameter, and no history of liver or pancreatic disease. Contraindications to the procedure are the presence of common duct stones, recent acute cholecystitis, cholangitis, and pancreatitis.

Up to 1500 shock waves are directed at the stones until they are crushed during the hour-long procedure. The minute particles are then able to travel through the biliary ductal system to be excreted via the intestine (Fig. 46–3). IV conscious sedation with fentanyl citrate (Alfenta) or midazolam hydrochloride (Versed) may be used

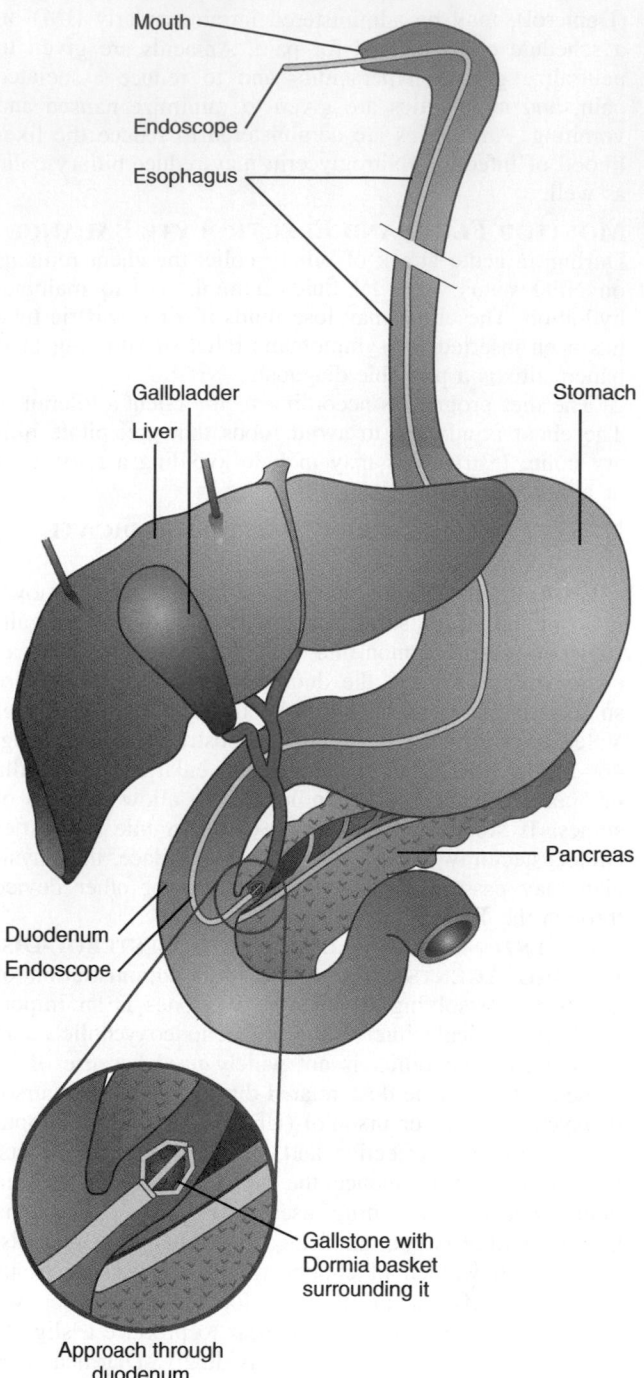

Mouth

Endoscope

Esophagus

Gallbladder

Liver

Stomach

Pancreas

Duodenum

Endoscope

Gallstone with
Dormia basket
surrounding it

Approach through
duodenum

FIGURE 46–2 Cholendoscopic removal of gallstones.

to minimize the mild discomfort that some clients experience while expelling the tiny stone fragments.

After lithotripsy, minor complications may include ecchymosis over the area of entry of the shock waves, gross or microscopic hematuria because of the proximity of the right kidney, and biliary pain when large fragments pass through the cystic duct. About 50% of clients experience a recurrence of gallstones within 5 years of lithotripsy.[6]

MONITOR FOR COMPLICATIONS

Monitoring for complications of gallstone disease includes observing, most commonly, for development of manifes-

tations of biliary colic. Conditions such as bile duct obstruction, cholangitis, pancreatitis, acute calculus, and cholecystitis may occur and cause manifestations consistent with gallbladder disease and subsequent sepsis and death. People with diabetes mellitus and gallstones appear to be somewhat more susceptible to complications of sepsis.

Because the gallbladder is left in place in all interventions except cholecystectomy, recurrence of stones is likely. Investigation continues on long-term prevention of the recurrence of gallstones.

▮ Nursing Management of the Medical Client

ASSESSMENT

If the client is being admitted for evaluation and treatment of manifestations, your assessment should focus on collecting subjective and objective data and noting the client's response to medications. Assess the client's manifestations carefully to help determine the diagnosis. Check vital signs at regular intervals to document inflammation associated with stones. Also assess the client's knowledge of the diagnostic process. Closely monitor the client for manifestations of obstruction from the gallstones.

DIAGNOSIS, OUTCOMES, INTERVENTIONS

Pain. Because one of the major manifestations of the disease is pain, *Pain related to biliary spasms* is the major nursing diagnosis.

Outcomes. The client will demonstrate absence of or a decrease in pain, as evidenced by the client's verbalizing that pain is absent or decreased and that he or she is resting quietly.

Interventions

Administer Pain Medications. Administer pain medication as ordered; document and note the client's response to the medication. Encourage the client to verbalize the effectiveness of the medication by describing whether the pain is absent or decreased. Meperidine is the drug most frequently ordered. Morphine is contraindicated because it may increase spasm of the sphincter of Oddi. Nitroglycerin may be ordered sublingually (under the tongue) to relax smooth muscle and, thereby, to decrease colic.

Provide Comfort Measures. Other comforting measures may be helpful. Providing a quiet environment and using relaxation techniques, such as a back rub, or comfortable positioning may promote rest and enhance the effects of the analgesics.

Risk for Fluid Volume Deficit and Electrolyte Imbalance. Because of the associated gastrointestinal manifestations, write the nursing diagnosis as *Risk for Fluid Volume Deficit and Electrolyte Imbalance related to vomiting and nasogastric suctioning.*

Outcomes. The client will maintain adequate hydration and electrolyte balance, as evidenced by normal skin turgor, moist oral mucous membranes, adequate urinary output, and no manifestations of electrolyte imbalance.

Interventions

Insert a Nasogastric Tube. If the client continues vomiting, obtain an order for a nasogastric (NG) tube with a suction attachment to relieve distention and vomit-

FIGURE 46–3 Ultrasonogram of the gallbladder with a single stone before *(A)*, 1 day after *(B)*, and 6 weeks after *(C)* extracorporeal shock-wave lithotripsy (ESWL). At day 1 after treatment, multiple small fragments are visible that had disappeared 6 weeks after ESWL and adjuvant bile acid dissolution therapy. (From Paumgartner G. [1998]. Nonsurgical management of gallstone disease. In M. Feldman, B. F. Scharschmidt, & M. H. Sleisenger [Eds.], *Sleisinger and Fordtran's gastrointestinal and liver disease* [Vol. 1, 6th ed., p. 989]. Philadelphia: W. B. Saunders.)

ing. Suction also removes the gastric juices that stimulate cholecystokinin, which in turn causes painful contractions of the gallbladder. NG suction is usually maintained on a low intermittent setting when a single-lumen tube (e.g., Levine) is used or on a low continuous setting when a double-lumen (e.g., Salem Sump) tube is used.

Administer IV Fluids and Electrolytes. Assess and document intake, output, and electrolyte laboratory values, communicating discrepancies to the physician. Assess the client for manifestations of dehydration, such as dry mucous membranes, poor skin turgor, and urinary output less than ½ ml/kg/hr.

Risk for Injury. The client undergoing endoscopic retrograde stone removal is assigned the nursing diagnosis *Risk for Injury related to medication during the procedure and possible introduction of bacteria into common bile duct.*

Outcomes. The client will remain free from injury and infection following endoscopic retrograde stone removal, as evidenced by the airway remaining patent without aspiration and absence of manifestations of infection, such as elevated temperature.

Interventions. For the client undergoing endoscopic retrograde papillotomy or stone removal, a local anesthetic solution is sprayed on the back of the throat. This intervention facilitates the passing of the endoscope. After the endoscopic papillotomy, carefully check for the return of the gag reflex before allowing oral intake. If the client receives sedation, raise the side rails on the bed for protection and keep the call light within reach. Antibiotics are often administered during the procedure to minimize the risk of infection from introduction of bacteria from the intestine into the common bile duct.

EVALUATION

Most clients recover from acute cholecystitis in a few days without complications. Once the biliary system is allowed to rest, inflammation decreases and recovery progresses. Clients should be monitored for the development of chronic cholecystitis.

Self-Care

The client and significant others will need to learn about the suggested therapeutic regimen, diet changes, indica-

tions for drugs and their side effects, dosage, and administration instructions, and ways to prevent recurrence. Clients who undergo gallstone dissolution most frequently receive UDCA. Chenodeoxycholic acid (CDCA) administration may result in mild to moderate elevation in liver function test values and serum cholesterol levels. In addition, clients receiving CDCA may experience disabling diarrhea.

MEDICATIONS

After assessing the level of understanding and learning needs, educate the client about the purpose of oral dissolution therapy, expected responses, and possible untoward reactions. Because oral dissolution medication must be taken over a long period of time, help the client devise ways to remember to take the medication daily. For example, a pillbox that is divided into the days of the week clearly indicates whether the client has missed a dose.

The client who is being treated medically may be sent home with oral analgesics or other medications for comfort as well as with an oral dissolution agent. Be sure that the client and significant others can relate all necessary information to the nurse before discharge.

DIET MODIFICATIONS

Diet instructions may be necessary if ingestion of food precipitated the attack; that is, if a fatty food caused the biliary colic, inform the client about the need for a low-fat diet.

PREVENT RECURRENCE

Advise the client about what to do should another attack occur. The client has probably been encouraged by the physician to consider elective cholecystectomy or other surgical intervention before gallbladder disease progresses further. Provide written material on gallbladder disease at this time to aid the client in understanding and decision-making.

Surgical Management

Whether to operate on a client with asymptomatic cholelithiasis ("silent gallstones") is an area for debate. The potential for serious complications (e.g., acute cholecystitis, choledocholithiasis, sepsis) can pose a significant risk. Older people and clients with insulin-dependent diabetes have a high incidence of gallstones. Because such people are at high risk during acute biliary attacks and emergency procedures, surgeons may recommend that they undergo elective cholecystectomy to avoid later emergency surgery. Other procedures that may be performed include percutaneous cholecystolithotomy and laparoscopic cholecystectomy.

PERCUTANEOUS CHOLECYSTOLITHOTOMY

With a percutaneous cholecystolithotomy, surgeons extract stones using cystoscopes, stone baskets, and instruments designed for nephrolithotomy. Stones too large to be extracted manually can be fragmented by means of a lithotriptor or laser fiber. General anesthesia is not necessary for this procedure.

The use of percutaneous insertion of a contact dissolution agent is now being investigated. In this procedure, a catheter is inserted into the gallbladder through the skin and methyl *tert*-butyl ether (MTBE) is instilled directly into the gallbladder to dissolve cholesterol gallstones. When small amounts are infused and withdrawn four to six times per minute, stones dissolve in 1 to 3 days. Early results have been excellent.

LAPAROSCOPIC CHOLECYSTECTOMY

INDICATIONS. Laparoscopic cholecystectomy has become the treatment of choice for symptomatic gallbladder disease. The procedure is suitable for most clients, even those with acute cholecystitis, because there is minimal trauma to the abdominal wall. This makes it possible for clients to go home within 24 hours after the procedure and return to work within a few days instead of a few weeks, as is the case with a cholecystectomy.

With the client under general anesthesia, carbon dioxide is used to create pneumoperitoneum through a needle inserted near the umbilicus. Near the umbilicus, an endoscope is inserted through a small incision to view the gallbladder and to determine the feasibility of success associated with this procedure. Three other small incisions are created: one for grasping the gallbladder, one for suction and irrigation, and one for dissection instruments and applying clips (Fig. 46–4).

CONTRAINDICATIONS. Laparoscopic cholecystectomy is contraindicated if stones are known to exist in the common bile duct. Laparoscopic cholecystectomy does not allow exploration or removal of stones from the common duct.

COMPLICATIONS. Possible complications of surgery or anesthesia include damage to the biliary tract and hemorrhage. However, the advantages of small scars and a short hospital stay have influenced surgeons to opt for this procedure more often. Clients who undergo this procedure are at less risk because they are ambulatory sooner and usually require only oral analgesia. Because of the carbon dioxide pressing on the diaphragm, nausea, vomiting, and shoulder pain are more frequent if the client's head and torso are elevated too soon after surgery.

OUTCOMES. Most clients are discharged the day of surgery or the day after. In most cases, they can resume normal activities and return to work after 3 to 4 days.

CHOLECYSTECTOMY

INDICATIONS. A cholecystectomy consists of excising the gallbladder from the posterior liver wall and ligating the cystic duct, vein, and artery. The surgeon usually approaches the gallbladder through a right upper paramedian or upper midline incision. If necessary, the common duct may be explored through this incision. When stones

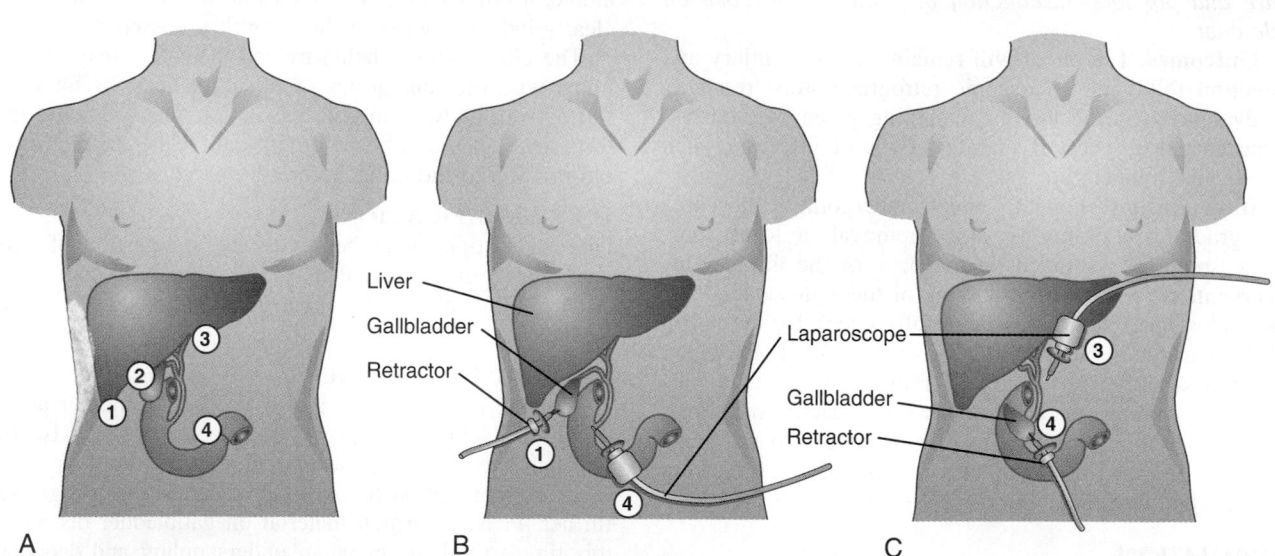

A   B   C

FIGURE 46–4 Laparoscopic cholecystectomy.

A, Standard sites of four ports used in laparoscopic cholecystectomy. 1, The lateral port is used to retract the gallbladder. 2, The subcostal port is used to retract the gallbladder. 3, The superior midline port is used to insert the laparoscope later in the procedure while the gallbladder is being withdrawn from the umbilical port. 4, The umbilical port is most often used to insert the laparoscope for most of the procedure and then is used to withdraw the gallbladder after the laparoscope is moved to the superior midline port.

B, Preparing the gallbladder for removal by ligating it from attachments (e.g., cystic duct, artery, vein). 1, The gallbladder is retracted through the lateral port. 4, A laparoscope is inserted through the umbilical port to visualize the gallbladder.

C, Removal of the gallbladder. 3, Laparoscope through the superior midline port. 4, Removal of the gallbladder through the umbilical port.

are suspected in the common duct, operative cholangiography may be performed (if it has not been ordered pre-operatively). The surgeon may dilate the common duct if it is not already dilated as a result of a pathologic process. Dilation facilitates stone removal. The surgeon passes a thin instrument into the duct to collect the stones, either whole or after crushing them.

After exploring the common duct, the surgeon usually inserts a T tube to ensure adequate bile drainage during duct healing (*choledochostomy*). The T tube also provides a route for postoperative cholangiography or stone dissolution, when appropriate (Fig. 46–5).

A conventional open cholecystectomy is indicated when a laparoscopic cholecystectomy does not allow for retrieval of a stone in the common bile duct and when the client's physique does not allow access to the gallbladder. Occasionally, when a person is very obese, the gallbladder is not retrievable via laparoscopic instruments. Further, a surgeon may have difficulty accessing the gallbladder in an adult with a small frame and may need to perform the conventional open cholecystectomy.

CONTRAINDICATIONS. A client's physical condition may not be able to withstand the stress of surgery, including loss of fluid, electrolytes, and anesthesia. Cholecystotomy, incision and drainage of the gallbladder, may be performed as an alternative procedure.

COMPLICATIONS. After cholecystectomy, monitor the client for the usual postoperative complications, such as hemorrhage, pneumonia, thrombophlebitis, urinary retention, and ileus. The risk of bile leakage into the abdominal cavity is more applicable to surgeries involving the gallbladder. With hemorrhage and bile leakage, the client feels severe pain and tenderness in the right upper quadrant, abdominal girth increases, bile or blood may leak from the wound, blood pressure drops, and tachycardia develops.

OUTCOMES. Cholecystectomy results in immediate cessation of pain in most clients and prevents development of complications such as acute cholecystitis, choledocholithiasis, and cholangitis. Persistence of manifestations after removal of the gallbladder indicates (1) a possible misdiagnosis or functional bowel disorder, such as esophagitis, peptic ulceration, pancreatitis, or irritable bowel syndrome; (2) a technical error; (3) a retained or recurrent common bile duct stone; or (4) spasm of the sphincter of Oddi. Clients must be hospitalized for about 3 days before dismissal. They may be sent home with a T tube in place for 1 to 2 weeks.

▮ Nursing Management of the Surgical Client

PREOPERATIVE CARE

Preoperative care of the client facing gallbladder or biliary surgery is the same as that described in Chapter 15. In addition, preparation involves careful monitoring for early clinical findings that may indicate the onset of complications from infection or obstruction. For laparoscopic cholecystectomy, preoperative preparation involves the same measures taken for other clients going to surgery. They include (1) NPO status after midnight, (2) skin preparation (i.e., showering with bacterial soap, such as Safeguard, Dial, Hibiclens), (3) occasionally an enema to reduce colon mass and to reduce the chance of incontinence contaminating the operative field, and (4) sometimes an antibiotic.

ASSESSMENT

Generally, surgical management of cholelithiasis is elective and is not performed in an emergency situation unless obstruction has occurred. Consequently, although the client is typically knowledgeable about the procedure and the rationale for it, assess client concerning knowledge of preoperative and postoperative care.

DIAGNOSIS, OUTCOMES, INTERVENTIONS

Knowledge Deficit. The preoperative client may not be completely knowledgeable about surgical procedures, particularly gallbladder surgery. The diagnosis, therefore, can be *Knowledge Deficit related to gallbladder surgery and recovery.*

Outcomes. The client will indicate an understanding of the procedure, as evidenced by ability to verbalize information regarding it; will demonstrate an ability to carry out coughing, deep breathing, and leg exercises; and will have knowledge regarding the immediate postoperative course.

Interventions. Reinforce information given to the client about the surgical procedure. Determine the level of understanding and the learning needs of the client and significant others. Provide material, if available, that can be read or viewed at the client's own pace. Give verbal instructions and a demonstration to ensure that the client can perform postoperative exercises (turning, coughing,

T tube in common bile duct
Cystic duct tied off
Hepatic duct
Duodenum
To drainage collection

FIGURE 46–5 Placement of a T tube. The surgeon ties off the cystic duct and sutures the T tube to the common bile duct with the short arms of the T tube toward the hepatic duct and duodenum. The long arm of the T tube exits the body near the incision site. Skin suture and tape secure placement.

deep-breathing, and wound splinting) properly and can understand their importance.

Clients also need some knowledge of what to expect postoperatively, such as IV fluids, T tube placement and drainage, and pain control and activity). Studies have shown that preoperative client education significantly reduces the risk for development of postoperative complications.

Anxiety. Because of the surgery and associated stress, a nursing diagnosis appropriate to these clients is *Anxiety related to the procedure and outcome.*

Outcomes. The client will express and demonstrate feelings of comfort and show decreasing manifestations of anxiety, as evidenced by calmly discussing his or her apprehension, affirming that anxiety is decreasing, and ventilating feelings regarding the surgical procedure and diagnosis.

Interventions. Assess the client's level of anxiety by listening and observing. Reassure the client and acknowledge that the unknown is frightening. Thoroughly explain those topics that may frighten the client, such as diagnostic or preparatory procedures. Allow significant others to stay with the client as appropriate.

POSTOPERATIVE CARE

Respiratory status is carefully monitored after surgery of the gallbladder or biliary tract because of the potential for development of atelectasis and pneumonia. Closely monitor drainage from all biliary tubes and drainage from the incision site, for amount, character, and color. Carefully assess cardiovascular status and manifestations of hemorrhage or shock. Hemorrhage, although rare, may occur if an inflamed gallbladder has adhered to the liver.

Analgesia for pain management is important and should be given on a regular basis to promote comfort and rest as well as to enhance the individual's ability to cough and deep breathe.

Maintain hydration and fluid balance IV until the client is no longer on NPO status and can receive fluids orally. When the client is allowed oral intake, the amount of fluid and food should be sufficient and well balanced enough to maintain renal function and body weight (minimal loss of weight). Clients are generally allowed to progress to a regular diet, with fat content included as tolerated.

ASSESSMENT

Postoperative assessment of the client is important; it includes careful monitoring of vital signs, breath and bowel sounds, and general level of responsiveness to check for complications such as hemorrhage, respiratory problems, or infection. In addition, intake is monitored to reflect renal function and output carefully measured including wound drainage, vomiting, or nasogastric suctioning.

Assess the client's incision for redness or swelling. Monitor the level of pain as well as the location, severity, and the effectiveness of any interventions.

After a laparoscopic cholecystectomy, referred pain to the shoulder is a common postoperative pain pattern. Shoulder pain occurs because of the carbon dioxide that has not been released or absorbed by the body. Carbon dioxide causes irritation of the phrenic nerve and diaphragm and may decrease respiratory excursion.

DIAGNOSIS, OUTCOMES, INTERVENTIONS

Risk for Injury. The postoperative client is at risk for the development of many complications leading to the nursing diagnosis *Risk for Injury related to postoperative complications of hemorrhage, infection, fluid and electrolyte imbalance, pulmonary changes (atelectasis, pneumonia), urinary retention, ileus, and decreased gastrointestinal motility.*

Outcomes. The client will receive appropriate assessments and interventions for early detection and prevention of injury from postoperative complications, as evidenced by stable vital signs; normal pulmonary function; normal gastrointestinal function; laboratory values within normal limits; normal urinary function, which returns within 6 to 8 hours postoperatively; an intact incision that does not exhibit redness, odor, or purulent drainage; and no manifestations of thrombus or embolus.

Interventions

Assess Postoperatively. Take routine postoperative vital signs, and assess for manifestations of shock, such as cyanosis; diaphoresis; cold, clammy skin; decreased blood pressure; and increased pulse. As vital signs are checked, check dressings and drainage tubes at the same time for unusual amounts of bleeding or drainage. If any of the aforementioned manifestations or changes occur, check vital signs frequently and notify the physician.

Prevent Pneumonia. The client should change position at least every 2 hours. While the client is awake for turning, help him or her to cough and deep breathe. Some hospitals use devices such as incentive spirometry to encourage lung expansion and spontaneous coughing. When these devices are used, it is helpful to demonstrate their use before surgery.

Auscultate the lungs for rales, rhonchi, and diminished breath sounds every 4 hours for the first 24 hours and every 8 hours thereafter. If the client had a cholecystectomy, it will be even more difficult to take deep breaths and cough because of the location of the incision. Take extra care to ensure that the client is comfortable enough to breathe normally. Many physicians and nurses believe that smaller doses of narcotics given more frequently are beneficial. Splinting the incision helps as well.

Monitor Fluids and Electrolytes. Measure intake and output every 4 hours or more frequently if ordered. Assess amounts for discrepancies. Since it is not unusual for new postoperative clients to be behind on fluids for the first few hours, do not expect output to equal intake initially. Assess the client for edema along with the lung sounds every 4 hours as another assurance that the client is tolerating the fluids that are being infused.

Unless the client is otherwise compromised, such as being acutely ill at the time of surgery or having a history of other health problems (e.g., heart disease or diabetes), laboratory work will probably not be ordered until the following day. Monitor these values for indications of fluid and electrolyte imbalance (see Chapters 12 and 13).

Monitor Urinary Output. Generally, the client can void within 6 to 8 hours after surgery; if not, assess the bladder for distention. The client may not to be able to void because of pain, discomfort, and position, or absence of feeling the need to void because of the effects of anesthesia and narcotics. The client may need to be catheterized to empty the bladder initially.

Maintain Nasogastric Tube. Occasionally, after gallbladder surgery, the client may return with a nasogastric tube attached to suction. Check the tube frequently to ensure that it is patent and that placement is correct for adequate drainage. A plugged or displaced tube not only causes distention, nausea, and vomiting but also may place undue stress on the surgical site. Auscultate bowel sounds every 8 hours to note return of normal bowel activity. Depending on the surgery, the client may or may not be allowed oral intake before bowel sounds return.

Offer oral care at least every 2 hours while the client is on NPO status. This may consist of rinsing the mouth with water, using mouthwash, swabbing with a moist swab, or assisting the client with brushing the teeth. Assess the oral mucous membranes at least every 8 hours for integrity, color, and moistness. While the client is taking nothing orally, it may be helpful to place a wet washcloth over the lips to humidify the air. Offering ice chips or sips of liquid as soon as allowed also provides much relief.

Advance Diet as Tolerated. For the more involved surgical procedure, such as a cholecystectomy, clients are usually not allowed a normal diet until they have begun to pass flatus and until bowel sounds are heard. After the client is allowed to have fluids or food, continue to assess the client for abdominal distention and normal bowel sounds to ensure that the intake is being tolerated. Early activity also helps the return of intestinal motility, so the client should be encouraged to begin progression of regular activities as soon as possible.

Prevent Infection. If the nurse is to change the dressings, the incision should be checked simultaneously for redness, swelling, drainage characteristics and amounts, and odor. If drains are present, such as a T tube, observe the drainage for its characteristics and amount. Check the client's temperature at least every 4 hours or more frequently if necessary. Keep the dressing and incision clean and dry because moisture enhances bacterial growth. Subjective complaints of increased pain may be the first manifestation that an infectious process is taking place. This is why it is important to document the location, type, and amount of pain routinely so that comparison can be made and a significant change in condition noted immediately. Many times it is your assessment that alerts the physician and facilitates the diagnosis of infection.

Pain. The client may have problems with postoperative pain. Therefore, the following nursing diagnosis, *Pain related to surgical procedure and incision,* is applicable.

Outcomes. The client will feel relief of pain, as evidenced by resting comfortably and quietly; blood pressure and heart rate will be within normal limits, and the client will be able to tolerate postoperative exercises and activities.

Interventions. Assess and document the level, location, and type of pain as well as the client's response to pain medication. You may need to intervene and obtain new medication orders if the medication ordered is ineffective. It may be necessary to administer medication to coincide with activity to keep the client active. Nonpharmacologic measures are helpful as well. Providing a quiet environment (even limiting visitors, if necessary), changing the client's position, and rubbing the client's back all are important in relaxing the client and in enhancing the effects of the pain medication. Assist the client in splinting the incision, and instruct the client on the best way to get out of bed and to lie down.

EVALUATION

The client should heal without difficulty and may be discharged within about 3 to 4 days after cholecystectomy. The client will be able to resume normal activities in 4 to 6 weeks. After laparoscopic cholecystectomy, the client is usually discharged the day of or day after surgery and can return to normal activities within 3 to 4 days.

■ Self-Care

Because the client will be faced with early discharge from the health care setting, the client should be able to verbalize and accurately demonstrate home health care needs and skills, for example, (1) identifying manifestations of infection; (2) demonstrating wound care; (3) naming medications, their purpose, side effects, and administration instructions; and (4) stating activity and dietary restrictions.

Teach the client about home health care as soon after surgery as possible to assess the client's learning potential and learning needs. Instruction should include wound care, dressing changes with a return demonstration, and assessing for manifestations of infection.

TEACH MANIFESTATIONS TO REPORT

Be sure the client is knowledgeable about which manifestations should be reported to the physician and how to contact the physician. Advise the client to report fever, chills, nausea and vomiting, jaundice, dark-colored urine, pale-colored stools, and pruritus. If the client is discharged with a drain or T tube in place, he or she should know the purpose of the tube, how to secure it, how to empty it, what amounts of drainage can be expected, and abnormal characteristics of drainage.

DIET AND ACTIVITY MODIFICATIONS

Explain and reinforce activity and dietary restrictions thoroughly. Advise that heavy lifting (>10 pounds) or strenuous work or sports for as long as prescribed by the physician should be avoided. Instruct and question the client as to the medications he or she is being discharged with, the possible adverse effects, and the dosage and frequencies of the medications. Explain that a low-fat (to be increased gradually), a high-carbohydrate, high-protein diet is needed and that alcohol should be avoided to minimize the risk of pancreatic involvement.

■ Modifications for Elderly Clients

In older clients, gallstones do not necessarily cause pain, fever, or jaundice. Mental confusion, shakiness, and an elevated alkaline phosphatase may be the only manifestations of gallstones in the elderly population. Nonsurgical decompression techniques may be preferred in high-risk older clients.

When the older client undergoes a cholecystectomy, he or she is at greater risk for injury related to anesthesia, pain medications, and sometimes the response to the trauma of surgery. Postoperative care should be modified to prevent injury. Especially in the immediate postoperative period, the side rails should be up, the bed in low position, and the call light within easy reach.

Depending on the client's response to anesthesia and pain medication, frequent reorientation to the environment and circumstances may be necessary. Remind the older client how to summon help and why it is important to not get up alone. Be sure that all IV lines and drainage tubes are secure to prevent the client from inadvertently disconnecting them.

In particular, be alert to the fact that older people tend to become confused after surgery, especially at night. You may need to take precautions by having a physician order soft wrist or vest restraints or a device such as a bed check machine, which is placed under the client and sounds an alarm if it senses weight is no longer on it.

ACUTE CHOLECYSTITIS

Acute cholecystitis refers to acute inflammation of the gallbladder wall. There is an increased incidence of cholecystitis in clients who are overweight, especially those with a sedentary lifestyle. Certain ethnic groups, including Chinese, Jewish, and Italians, have a higher rate of the disease.

Etiology and Risk Factors

Cholecystitis is associated with gallstones and obstruction of the cystic duct by a stone in 90% of cases.[4] Obstruction of a cystic duct by a stone is the usual cause of acute cholecystitis. In 5% to 10% of clients, however, calculi obstructing the cystic duct are not found during surgery (acalculous cholecystitis, or cholecystitis without stones). In more than 50% of such cases, an underlying cause of the inflammation is not found.[6] Hepatic *Helicobacter* bacteria have been implicated in cholecystitis.

The major preventable risk factors are sedentary lifestyle and obesity. If the client increases his or her level of activity and maintains a low-fat diet, the risk of cholecystitis can be reduced. Encourage clients to engage in exercise and to follow healthy dietary habits.

Pathophysiology

Acute calculus cholecystitis, which appears to be caused by obstruction of the cystic duct, in turn causes distention of the gallbladder. Subsequently, (1) venous and lymphatic drainage is impaired, (2) proliferation of bacteria occurs, (3) localized cellular irritation or infiltration, or both, take place, and (4) areas of ischemia may develop. The inflamed gallbladder wall is edematous and thickened, may have areas of gangrene, or necrosis may be present. The term *empyema* describes a gallbladder that contains pus, which is the equivalent of an intra-abdominal abscess and may be associated with severe sepsis. Recurrent episodes of acute cholecystitis cause fibrosis of the wall of the gallbladder.

Complications of untreated acute cholecystitis are usually associated with septic complications. Others are consequences of ischemia, inflammation, adhesions, and gangrene: perforation, pericholecystic abscess, and fistula.

Acalculous cholecystitis (cholecystitis without stones) is far less common than cholecystitis due to gallstones. It apparently can be triggered by (1) multiple blood transfusions, (2) gram-negative bacterial sepsis, or (3) tissue damage after burns, trauma, or extensive surgery. Other possible contributing factors include hyperalimentation, prolonged fasting, hypotension, anesthesia, narcotic analgesics, and mechanical ventilation with positive end-expiratory pressure. Clients with diabetes mellitus and systemic arteritis are also susceptible.

Clinical Manifestations

Inflammation of the gallbladder may be acute or chronic. The most common and reliable finding on physical examination is tenderness in the right upper quadrant, epigastrium, or both. Although clients with chronic and acute cholecystitis may complain of the same type of pain, the distinguishing factor is the severity and persistence of the pain. Chronic cholecystitis rarely lasts more than a few hours, whereas acute cholecystitis may last several days.

Pain in acute cholecystitis may be located in the epigastric, subscapular, or right upper quadrant regions. Sometimes the pain is referred to the right scapula. The pain usually starts suddenly, increases steadily, and reaches a peak in about 30 minutes. Abdominal examination may reveal a tender abdomen with right upper quadrant guarding. Murphy's sign may be elicited when the client is asked to take a deep breath. About 60% to 70% of clients with acute cholecystitis have experienced biliary colic episodes in the past from ductal spasm when a stone moves from the gallbladder into ducts causing waves of pain (biliary colic).

In addition to pain, the following problems may be revealed in clients with acute cholecystitis:

1. Nausea and vomiting occur in 60% to 70% of clients as a result of impulses transmitted to the vomiting center from distention of bile ducts.
2. Approximately 80% of clients have an elevated temperature from the response to inflammation, but this may be absent in older clients, immunocompromised clients, and clients receiving steroidal therapy.
3. Mild jaundice occurs in only 10% of cases.
4. Right upper quadrant tenderness, fever, and leukocytosis suggest acute cholecystitis, particularly if other assessment data support this diagnosis.

The diagnostic examination for acute cholecystitis includes the following:

1. Biliary ultrasonography is often the initial diagnostic procedure. Sonographic findings consistent with acute cholecystitis include (a) cholelithiasis, (b) focal tenderness over the gallbladder (sonographic Murphy's sign), (c) thickening of the gallbladder wall (>3 mm), and (d) distention of the gallbladder lumen (>5 cm).
2. Aminotransferase, alkaline phosphatase, and bromsulfophthalein values may be slightly abnormal.
3. An abdominal x-ray study occasionally reveals the enlarged gallbladder. In 15% of cases, the gallstones contain enough calcium to be visible on film.

4. Radionuclide imaging (cholescintigraphy) can provide additional information (when the diagnosis is clinically obscure) by pinpointing cystic duct obstruction. Confirmation is based on nonvisualization of the gallbladder.

5. The WBC count is elevated in 85% of clients, with the exception of the elderly and those receiving steroid therapy.

Outcome Management

■ Medical Management

Clients thought to have acute cholecystitis may need to be hospitalized, and initial management should include administration of antibiotics effective against organisms found in the bile in approximately 80% of the cases. These organisms include both gram-positive and gram-negative aerobes and anaerobes: *E. coli, Klebsiella aerogenes, S. faecalis, Clostridium welchii, Proteus* species, *Enterobacter* species, *Helicobacter* species, and anaerobic streptococci.

Antibiotics that are effective given singly include ampicillin, cephalosporins, or aminoglycosides. A combination of these drugs may be more effective in clients with diabetes mellitus or with debilitated conditions. Further medical management is the same as for symptomatic cholelithiasis (see Cholelithiasis).

■ Nursing Management of the Medical Client

Assessment becomes extremely important because several other disease entities may produce the same manifestations (see Box 46–2). Collect subjective and objective data, and note the client's response to medications.

Nursing care is the same as for medical management of cholelithiasis except for the certainty that these clients will receive a course of antibiotics. Observe the client for the development of complications, which may include increased pain in the right upper quadrant or jaundice (from an obstruction) and decreased or absent bowel sounds (from peritonitis). For additional information on nursing management, see Nursing Management of the Medical Client under Cholelithiasis.

■ Surgical Management

Once the diagnosis of acute cholecystitis is made, the decision for early or delayed cholecystectomy depends on the risk factors. Delayed surgery is usually the correct decision in those clients who have unstable angina, significant carotid artery disease, congestive heart failure, cirrhosis, and other conditions that would increase their risk.

Cholecystectomy for the client with acute cholecystitis is more difficult than elective surgery because of the distended, inflamed gallbladder. Usually, the gallbladder must be decompressed first to allow complete visualization of all surrounding structures and to avoid injury to the extrahepatic bile ducts.

Cholecystotomy (surgical drainage of the gallbladder) is usually performed only when cholecystectomy is too dangerous, given all the risk factors. Although the procedure relieves the obstruction, the cure depends on the ability of the client's immune system to resolve the inflammatory process. Treatment of complications of chole-

cystotomy is usually cholecystectomy. See Nursing Management of the Surgical Client under Cholelithiasis.

ACUTE ACALCULOUS CHOLECYSTITIS

Acute acalculous cholecystitis (without stones) accounts for approximately 4% to 8% of all cases of acute cholecystitis. Although data are inconclusive, this condition is said to be increasing. It tends to occur after or in association with other conditions, especially major trauma, burns, or surgery. Other pre-existing conditions include the postpartum period after a prolonged childbirth, bacterial sepsis, and debilitating systemic diseases, such as cardiovascular disease, tuberculosis, and sarcoidosis. However, no apparent precipitating factor is present in as many as 50% of the clients.

The pathologic process does not differ from that of the calculous type, although the incidence of gangrene and perforation is higher. It is debatable whether this is an inherent feature of the disease or the result of delayed diagnosis.

Recognition of the disease may be delayed when the client cannot communicate well because of concomitant disease or post-traumatic or postoperative states. The manifestations are the same as those of acute calculous cholecystitis—pain in the right upper quadrant, epigastrium, or both, and vomiting. However, although pain is the cardinal manifestation in the calculous type, it may be obscured or absent in acalculous cholecystitis because of narcotic administration, decreased level of consciousness, or abdominal pain from an incision or from another disease process. Significant physical findings are the same as those in acute calculous cholecystitis, and the same diagnostic procedures are used.

The standard treatment is emergency cholecystectomy because of the increased risk of gangrene and perforation.

CHRONIC CHOLECYSTITIS

Chronic cholecystitis sometimes arises as a sequela to acute cholecystitis. Typically, however, it develops independently of acute cholecystitis. In addition, it is almost always associated with gallstones. Chronic cholecystitis principally affects middle-aged and older obese women. The female-to-male ratio is 3:1.

Assessment data for chronic cholecystitis are similar to those of acute cholecystitis with certain exceptions. In chronic states, (1) the pain is less severe, (2) the temperature is not as high, and (3) the leukocyte count is lower. Vague manifestations of indigestion, epigastric pain, fat intolerance, heartburn, and flatulence accompany chronic cholecystitis. The client has usually experienced these manifestations for a long time as well as repeated attacks (mild or severe) of acute cholecystitis. Eventually, fibrous tissues begin to replace the normal muscle and mucosal tissues of the gallbladder. As a consequence, the gallbladder loses its ability to concentrate bile.

Diagnosis depends largely on ultrasonography, and other diagnostic procedures provide supplementary information. Diagnostic findings include (1) cholelithiasis, (2) gallbladder wall thickening (>3 mm), and (3) delayed visualization or nonvisualization of the gallbladder on radionuclide scanning. Scarring from chronic inflammation may partially or completely obstruct the cystic duct and thus account for this delay in visualization or nonvisualization. It may be difficult to differentiate chronic cholecystitis from other disorders. Conditions that produce manifestations similar to the manifestations of cholecystitis (acute and chronic) are listed in Box 46–2. The diagnostic process serves to rule out these conditions.

Conservative interventions include (1) a low-fat diet, (2) weight reduction, and (3) administration of anticholinergics, sedatives, and antacids. When medical intervention is ineffective, cholecystectomy may be the treatment of choice. About 90% of clients obtain relief of manifestations after cholecystectomy. Of the gallbladders removed, 95% contain stones.

CHOLEDOCHOLITHIASIS AND CHOLANGITIS

Choledocholithiasis is defined as stones in the common duct. Common bile duct calculi can arise from the gallbladder or hepatic ducts. Thus, common duct stones can occur in the absence of a gallbladder and are classified as *primary*. *Cholangitis* is inflammation of the bile duct.

Common duct stones are found in 10% to 15% of clients with cholelithiasis. The incidence increases with age and the frequency of gallstones in the elderly population may be as high as 50%.[3] Frequently, inflammation or bacteria are present, and cholangitis may develop.

Etiology and Risk Factors

The cause is essentially the same as for cholelithiasis. This condition is sometimes combined with a narrowing of the papilla, which traps stones. The risk factor for choledocholithiasis is that a small stone may pass from the gallbladder and lodge in the common bile duct.

Pathophysiology

The pathophysiology is essentially the same as for cholelithiasis. Most bile duct stones are cholesterol or mixed stones. They form in the gallbladder and move into the biliary tree through the cystic duct.

Clinical Manifestations

Common duct calculi may be asymptomatic or cause biliary colic, bile duct obstruction, cholangitis, or pancreatitis. Early manifestations of choledocholithiasis are not easily distinguished from gallbladder colic or acute cholecystitis. Pain may be mild or severe and cannot be differentiated from gallbladder pain. Jaundice is intermittent if obstruction is intermittent but may be progressive if the stone becomes impacted in the cystic duct or bile duct.

Chills and fever, frequently recurring attacks of right upper quadrant severe pain, a history of jaundice, and mild elevation of serum bilirubin are manifestations of *cholangitis.* The WBC count is normal except when cholangitis is present. It is characteristic, however, to see an elevation of serum bilirubin and alkaline phosphatase levels, which result from obstruction. The serum amylase level should always be determined to determine the presence of secondary pancreatitis.

Infrequently, manifestations of cholangitis are accompanied by shock and confusion, coma, or other central nervous system manifestations. These manifestations signal the presence of *acute toxic cholangitis*, a condition in which infected bile or pus is under pressure within the duct system. Emergency decompression of the duct system is necessary to prevent death.

To determine the diagnosis, ultrasonography, CT scan, and radionuclide imaging may be performed. Although they are not reliable for the detection of common duct stones, they can detect common duct dilation. Endoscopic retrograde cholangiography is indicated for clients with bile duct obstruction (as indicated by persistent jaundice) or bile duct dilation on ultrasonography. It allows visualization and endoscopic sphincterotomy when indicated.

Outcome Management

▓ Medical Management

Medical management of pain is based on its severity and frequency and is similar to medical management described for cholelithiasis. Management of inflammation involves antibiotic therapy when cholangitis is present.

▓ Surgical Management

INDICATIONS. Indications for surgical management of common duct calculi may include emergency intervention, which is rare unless severe ascending cholangitis is present. Usually, however, surgical management in some form is necessary for symptomatic choledocholithiasis.

Treatment includes hospitalization, treatment of infection, and removal of stones. The removal of stones may be accomplished surgically in clients with an intact gallbladder by cholecystectomy and choledochotomy. As many as 20% of clients undergoing cholecystectomy will prove to have common bile duct stones in addition to stones in the gallbladder. With the development and refinement of laparoscopic cholecystectomy, the management of common bile duct stones in the presence of gallstones is becoming more easily defined. To remove common bile duct stones, preoperative ERCP with endoscopic papillotomy and stone extraction is the preferred approach. Postoperative ERCP may also be done if necessary. As laparoscopic cholecystectomy becomes more perfected as a technique, the need for preoperative ERCP is expected to decrease.

Common duct stones in a client who has previously had a cholecystectomy is best treated by endoscopic sphincterotomy. The surgeon opens the sphincter of Oddi and allows passage of gallstones up to 1 cm. The success rate is approximately 90%. Extracorporeal shock wave lithotripsy is used when stones are too large to extract via the endoscopic approach. Success can be achieved in 70% to 85% of these complicated cases. Most common duct stones are found and removed at the time of cholecystectomy.

Liver function should be thoroughly evaluated preoperatively by measuring the prothrombin time. If results are abnormal, function should be restored to normal with administration of vitamin K. Antimicrobial agents (e.g., mezlocillin IV along with either metronidazole or gentamicin IV) should be given.

Another procedure, *choledochostomy*, consists of opening the common duct surgically, removing stones, and inserting a T tube for drainage. Choledochostomy may be performed in conjunction with cholecystectomy. Otherwise, cholecystectomy may be necessary at a later date.

Postoperative antibiotics are not usually given after biliary tract surgery unless specimens of the bile obtained for culture during the surgery are positive for organisms.

CONTRAINDICATIONS. Contraindications to surgical management of choledocholithiasis include elderly clients and those who are poor surgical risks.

COMPLICATIONS. Surgical traumas or the presence of stones may result in ductal edema after choledochostomy. Inserting a T tube prevents bile from spilling into the peritoneal cavity and maintains patency of the duct (see Fig. 46–5). T tubes may be attached to continuous gravity drainage or to collapsible bags in the dressing site.

Avoid tension on long tubing and obstruction by kinking. Carefully measure drainage from the T tube. The tube usually drains 300 to 500 ml in the first 24 hours. This amount decreases to less than 200 ml after 3 to 4 days. Record the volume and color of the drainage. To prevent excessive loss of bile, place the drainage bag for the T tube at the level of the abdomen rather than hanging the bag below the bed. At this height, bile flows into the bag only when pressure is high in the biliary tree.

Excessive T tube drainage may indicate obstruction. Occasionally, it signals development of a biliary fistula. Excessive bile losses may necessitate recycling the client's bile drainage. The bile may be returned to the client through a nasogastric tube or orally in fruit juice.

Thick bile or bile containing blood clots may prevent drainage or cause inadequate amounts of drainage from the T tube. Without intervention, bile may begin to leak from the choledochotomy site instead of through the T tube. To prevent this problem, the physician may decide to irrigate the tube with sterile saline.

On rare occasions, tube dislodgment causes failure of the T tube to drain. The tube may dislodge from the common duct when the client moves from a supine to a sitting position. This complication may result from excessive tension during T tube insertion in surgery.

After a few days, the T tube will probably be clamped during meals to aid fat digestion.

The tube remains in place for about 10 days. A T tube cholangiogram should be done on or about the seventh or eighth postoperative day to assess for bile duct obstruction. When the T tube cholangiogram indicates absence of obstruction, the surgeon may decide to remove the T tube. If a retained stone is discovered during cholangiography, the client may go home with the T tube in place. The surgeon may remove the stone through the T tube tract with a catheter at a later time.

OUTCOMES. When stones are extracted, the client is likely to experience a reduction in pain and a general increase in well-being and quality of life. Encourage the client to increase his or her level of activity and maintain a low-fat diet to reduce the risk of forming additional future stones.

▄ Nursing Management of the Surgical Client

Nursing management is the same as for the client with a cholecystectomy.

SCLEROSING CHOLANGITIS

Sclerosing cholangitis is an uncommon, inflammatory disease of the bile ducts that causes fibrosis and thickening of their walls and multiple short, concentric strictures. The disease is progressive and gradually causes cirrhosis, portal hypertension, and death from hepatic failure. It may also predispose the client to the development of cholangiocarcinoma. Some cases are associated with inflammatory bowel disease, especially ulcerative colitis. Sclerosing cholangitis and papillary stenosis are important complications of acquired immunodeficiency syndrome (AIDS). In addition, cytomegalovirus and cryptosporidium are observed frequently in such clients, indicating that these organisms may be involved in causing primary sclerosing cholangitis.

The cause has been linked to altered immunity, toxins, and infectious agents. Clients often have the hepatocompatible antigen HLA-B, suggesting that genetic factors may play a role. The disease is most common in men 20 to 40 years of age. The male-to-female ratio is 3:2.

Usually, clients present with fatigue, anorexia, weight loss, jaundice, and pruritus. They sometimes complain of vague upper abdominal pain. The diagnosis is usually made by endoscopic retrograde cholangiography, clinical findings, and liver biopsy.

Medical management consists of corticosteroids and broad-spectrum antimicrobial therapy when cholangitis is a recurrent problem. Immunosuppressants, bile acid-binding agents, colchicine, and penicillamine have been used with inconsistent and unpredictable results. These agents do not alter the slow, progressive course of the disease. Ursodiol, which improves primary biliary cirrhosis, is now being evaluated in the treatment of sclerosing cholangitis. Cholestyramine may help control the pruritus.

The success of surgical intervention is limited by the progressive nature of the disease and the recurrent cholangitis. Surgery is generally limited to procedures to open the ducts. Cholecystectomy should not be performed unless there is definite evidence of cholecystitis or cholelithiasis. Although surgical therapy may be life-saving in some circumstances, it has to be considered palliative in the overall context of the disease. The definitive management of these clients is liver transplantation, which is the procedure of choice. Survival rates with transplantation are 85% at 3 years.[10]

CARCINOMA OF THE GALLBLADDER

Although cancer of the gallbladder is the most common malignant lesion of the biliary tract, it accounts for only 5% of all cancers at the time of autopsy. Most cancers of the gallbladder develop in conjunction with stones rather than polyps. Of all clients with this malignancy, 91% are over age 50 and the incidence in women is four times that of men. However, the incidence of bile duct cancer is predominant in men. Native Americans, Hispanics, northeastern Europeans, Israelis, and Japanese immigrants to the United States are at greatest risk for cancer of the gallbladder. At least 70% of these clients have gallstones. Adenocarcinoma accounts for 82% of all cases.

The clinical presentation differs according to stage of the disease. There is no distinct pattern because the manifestations depend on the site of the lesion, its extent, and the presence or absence of pre-existing biliary manifestations. Usually, however, the clinical manifestations are unrelenting right upper quadrant pain, weight loss, jaundice, and a palpable right upper quadrant mass.

At this point, treatment modalities and their effectiveness are widely debated. Treatment varies from radical resection, to palliative relief of duct obstruction, to chemotherapy or radiation. None of the treatments have been found to increase survival.

The prognosis for cancer of the gallbladder is poor. About 88% of clients die within the first year, and only about 5% are alive at 5 years. Trials of radiation and chemotherapy in clients with primary gallbladder cancer have been disappointing. The long-term survivors are generally those in whom the diagnosis of cancer had not been made prior to cholecystectomy and was determined by pathologic study.

CONCLUSIONS

Biliary and exocrine pancreatic disorders are common but are extremely complex and diverse. Some of these conditions are treated without further difficulty, such as cholecystitis, whereas others can become chronic and lead to a wide variety of other problems, such as pancreatitis. Teaching is vital to the care of these clients, and the nurse must understand these conditions to initiate appropriate teaching plans.

THINKING CRITICALLY

1. **You are assigned to care for a 35-year-old writer who has been admitted with severe upper abdominal pain radiating to his back and recurrent vomiting. This is his second admission for pancreatitis. He admits to drinking 1 pint of whiskey daily on the weekends and having several drinks nightly on weekdays. His alcohol intake has been greater in the past. Laboratory data include an amylase level of 750 units/L (normal 25 to 125 units); lipase, is 5.6 units/ml (normal, 10 to 140 units); aspartate aminotransferase (AST), 150 units/L (normal, 5 to 40 units) and alanine aminotransferase (ALT), 60 units (normal, 1 to 45 units). How do you feel about caring for this client?**

Factors to Consider. Are you comfortable with the client's lifestyle? Do the biochemical studies support a diagnosis of pancreatitis? What do you need to consider if he complains of pain? What should you do if you discover he is allergic to meperidine? Should a nasogastric tube be inserted?

2. **A 45-year-old woman is admitted to the hospital complaining of colicky pain in the right upper abdominal quadrant. She states that the pain is worse when she eats fried foods. She also states that she has vomited on several occasions and it seems to relieve her manifestations. What are**

your priorities in assessing and caring for the client?

Factors to Consider. What types of diagnostic procedures should be scheduled? Why is an accurate assessment of the clinical manifestations important? What indications warrant insertion of a nasogastric tube?

3. **A 70-year-old woman comes to the emergency department with complaints of recurrent episodes of epigastric pain during the past 9 months. Chills, fever, and jaundice have occurred for the first time and have persisted for 4 days. Her white blood cell count is normal. Serum bilirubin and alkaline phosphatase values are elevated. There is no history of alcoholism, blood transfusions, or hepatitis. The client takes no medications except an occasional "Bufferin for my arthritis." Her past medical history is unremarkable except for a cholecystectomy 10 years ago after an episode of cholecystitis. What are the priorities for care?**

Factors to Consider. What are the client's clinical manifestations? Would surgical treatment alleviate the problem? What might cause stricture of the bile ducts?

BIBLIOGRAPHY

1. Andreoli, R. E., et al. (1996). *Cecil essentials of medicine* (4th ed.). Philadelphia: W. B. Saunders.
2. Copstead, L. C., & Banasik, J. L. (2000). *Pathophysiology: Biological and behavioral perspectives* (2nd ed.). Philadelphia: W. B. Saunders.
3. Frey, C. F. (1993). Management of necrotizing pancreatitis. *Western Journal of Medicine, 159,* 675–680.
4. Friedman, L. S. (1998). Liver, biliary tract, and pancreas. In L. M. Tierney, S. J. McPhee, & M. A. Papadakis (Eds.), *Medical diagnosis and treatment* (37th ed.). Stamford, CT: Appleton & Lange.
5. Greenberger, N. J., Toskes, P.P., & Isselbacher, K. J. (1998). Acute and chronic pancreatitis. In A. S. Fauci, E. Braunwald, K. J. Isselbacher, et al. (Eds.), *Harrison's principles of internal medicine* (14th ed.). New York: McGraw-Hill.
6. Greenberger, N. J., & Isselbacher, K. J. (1998). Diseases of the gallbladder and bile ducts. In A. S. Fauci, E. Braunwald, K. J. Isselbacher, et al. (Eds.), *Harrison's principles of internal medicine* (14th ed.). New York: McGraw-Hill.
7. Guyton, A. C., & Hall, J. E. (1996). *Textbook of medical physiology* (9th ed.). Philadelphia: W. B. Saunders.
8. Hansen, M. (1998). *Pathophysiology: Foundations of disease and clinical intervention.* Philadelphia: W. B. Saunders.
9. Malka, D., et al. (1998). Chronic obstructive pancreatitis due to a pancreatic cyst in a patient with autosomal dominant polycystic kidney disease. *Gut, 42*(1), 131–134.
10. McCance, K. L., & Heuther, S. E. (1998). *Pathophysiology: The biologic basis for disease in adults and children* (3nd ed.). St. Louis: Mosby–Year Book.
11. Mayer, R. J. (1998). Pancreatic cancer. In A. S. Fauci, E. Braunwald, K. J. Isselbacher, et al. (Eds.), *Harrison's principles of internal medicine* (14th ed.). New York: McGraw-Hill.
12. Mergener, K., & Baille, J. (1997). Chronic pancreatitis. *Lancet, 350*(9088), 1379–1385.
13. Noone, J. (1995). Acute pancreatitis: An Orem approach to nursing assessment and care. *Critical Care Nurse, 15*(4), 27–37.
14. Price, T. F., Payne, R. L., & Oberleitner, M. G. (1996). Familial pancreatic cancer in South Louisiana. *Cancer Nursing, 19*(4), 275–282.
15. Soergel, K. H. (1996). Pancreatitis. In J. C. Bennett, & F. Plum. (Eds.), *Cecil textbook of medicine* (20th ed.). Philadelphia: W. B. Saunders.

16. Stabile, B. E. (1998). Laparoscopic cholecystectomy-associated bile duct injuries. *Western Journal of Medicine, 168*(1), 40–41.

17. Stephens, C. D. (1998). Gemcitabine: A new approach to treating pancreatic cancer. *Oncology Nursing Forum, 25*(1), 87–93.

18. Toskes, P. P., & Greenberger, N. J. (1998). Approach to the patient with pancreatic disease. In A. S. Fauci, E. Braunwald, K. J. Isselbacher, et al. (Eds.), *Harrison's principles of internal medicine* (14th ed.). New York: McGraw-Hill.

19. Vaona, B., et al. (1997). Food intake of patients with chronic pancreatitis after onset of the disease. *American Journal of Clinical Nutrition, 65*(30), 851–854.

20. Warsaw, A. L., et al. (1998). Middle segment pancreatectomy: A novel technique for conserving pancreatic tissue. *Archives of Surgery, 133*(3), 327–331.

21. Woodward, J., & Colagiovanni, L. (1998). Feed the patient, fool the pancreas. *Nursing Times, 94*(8), 65–67.

CHAPTER

47

Management of Clients with Hepatic Disorders

Dianne Smolen

NURSING OUTCOMES CLASSIFICATION (NOC)
for Nursing Diagnoses—Clients with Hepatic Disorders

Activity Intolerance
Activity Tolerance
Endurance
Energy Conservation
Self-Care: Activities of Daily Living (ADL)
Self-Care: Instrumental Activities of Daily Living (IADL)
Acute Confusion
Cognitive Ability
Distorted Thought Control
Information Processing
Memory
Neurologic Status: Consciousness
Altered Health Maintenance
Health Belief: Perceived Resources
Health-Promoting Behavior
Health-Seeking Behavior
Knowledge: Health Behaviors
Knowledge: Health Promotion
Knowledge: Health Resources
Knowledge: Treatment Regimen
Psychosocial Adjustment: Life Change
Risk Detection
Self-Direction of Care
Social Support
Treatment Behavior: Illness or Injury
Altered Nutrition: Less Than Body Requirements
Nutritional Status
Nutritional Status: Food and Fluid Intake
Nutritional Status: Nutrient Intake
Weight Control
Altered Protection
Abuse Protection

Immunization Behavior
Infection Status
Altered Tissue Perfusion
Tissue Perfusion: Cardiac
Tissue Perfusion: Pulmonary
Vital Signs Status
Anxiety
Anxiety Control
Coping
Social Interaction Skills
Body Image Disturbance
Body Image
Grief Resolution
Psychosocial Adjustment: Life Change
Self-Esteem
Fatigue
Activity Tolerance
Endurance
Energy Conservation
Nutritional Status: Energy
Psychomotor Energy
Fluid Volume Deficit
Electrolyte and Acid-Base Balance
Fluid Balance
Hydration
Nutritional Status: Food and Fluid Intake
Fluid Volume Excess
Electrolyte and Acid-Base Balance
Fluid Balance
Hydration
Impaired Skin Integrity
Immobility Consequences, Physiologic
Nutritional Status
Risk Control

Tissue Perfusion: Peripheral
Tissue Integrity: Skin and Mucous Membranes
Wound Healing: Primary Intention
Wound Healing: Secondary Intention
Ineffective Breathing Pattern
Respiratory Status: Airway Patency
Respiratory Status: Ventilation
Vital Signs Status
Risk for Impaired Gas Exchange
Electrolyte and Acid-Base Balance
Respiratory Status: Gas Exchange
Respiratory Status: Ventilation
Tissue Perfusion: Pulmonary
Vital Signs Status
Risk for Ineffective Management of Therapeutic Regimen: Families
Family Functioning
Family Participation in Professional Care
Risk for Ineffective Management of Therapeutic Regimen: Individuals
Compliance Behavior
Knowledge: Treatment Regimen
Participation: Health Care Decisions
Treatment Behavior: Illness or Injury
Risk for Injury
Knowledge: Personal Safety
Neurologic Status
Risk Control
Risk Detection
Safety Behavior: Fall Prevention
Safety Status: Physical Injury
Symptom Control

The liver plays a central role in many essential physiologic processes. It is the primary organ of lipid synthesis, and it detoxifies endogenous and exogenous substances such as hormones, drugs, and poisons. When the normal physiologic processes are altered, numerous hepatic and extrahepatic manifestations of liver disease appear. These

manifestations offer the initial clue to liver disease, regardless of the cause.

This chapter describes the clinical features of liver diseases, medical and surgical management, and measures the nurse can take to assist clients with such nursing diagnoses as *Impaired Skin Integrity, Fluid Volume Ex-*

cess, Fatigue, and *Altered Nutrition: Less than Body Requirements.*

JAUNDICE

Jaundice, or icterus, is the yellow pigmentation of the sclerae, skin, and deeper tissues caused by excessive accumulation of bile pigments in the blood. It is a common manifestation of a variety of liver and biliary diseases and serves as a starting point for evaluating many of these disorders. Bilirubin (bile pigment), a product of red blood cell (RBC) breakdown, is deposited in the skin and excreted in the urine when present in the blood in excessive amounts (hyperbilirubinemia). This characteristic makes jaundice a valuable indicator of a variety of disorders involving either hemolysis or biliary obstruction. When there is an obstruction blocking the flow of bile into the intestine, jaundiced clients also may have clay-colored stools owing to lack of bilirubin and its metabolites in the intestine.

Bilirubin is formed from the breakdown of hemoglobin from RBCs by macrophages. This unconjugated bilirubin measured as ("indirect bilirubin") is not water-soluble, cannot be filtered in the kidney, and thus is not excreted in the urine. Normally, the unconjugated bilirubin returns to the liver via the bloodstream and is conjugated with glucuronic acid to form conjugated bilirubin (measured as "direct bilirubin"), which is water-soluble. The conjugated bilirubin travels to the gallbladder and eventually to the intestines. In the bowel, bacterial action converts bilirubin to urobilinogen. A small amount of urobilinogen is absorbed into the bloodstream to be returned to the liver or excreted in the urine.

Etiology and Risk Factors

The cause of jaundice may be described according to the location of the pathologic change. Jaundice may occur because of a problem (1) outside the liver (resulting in unconjugated hyperbilirubinemia, in which the accumulated bilirubin is predominantly of the unconjugated type) or (2) in the liver or biliary tract (resulting in conjugated hyperbilirubinemia, with predominantly conjugated bilirubin). When the problem is in the liver or biliary tract, the cause may be hereditary cholestatic syndromes, hepatocellular dysfunction, or biliary obstruction.

Pathophysiology

The underlying pathophysiologic mechanism in jaundice relates to whether the jaundice results from accumulation of predominantly unconjugated or conjugated bilirubin in the serum.

UNCONJUGATED HYPERBILIRUBINEMIA

Unconjugated hyperbilirubinemia may result from overproduction of bilirubin due to hemolysis, to impaired hepatic uptake of bilirubin caused by certain drugs, or to impaired conjugation of bilirubin by glucuronide, as in Gilbert's syndrome, Crigler-Najjar syndrome, or drug reactions.

CONJUGATED HYPERBILIRUBINEMIA

Conjugated hyperbilirubinemia may result from impaired excretion of bilirubin from the liver due to hepatocellular disease, drugs, sepsis, hereditary disorders such as Dubin-Johnson syndrome, or extrahepatic biliary obstruction.

The pathologic mechanism in conjugated hyperbilirubinemia varies according to the type of jaundice (mechanisms are summarized in Table 47–1).

Hereditary Cholestatic Syndromes

Jaundice related to hereditary cholestatic syndromes or intrahepatic cholestasis (stagnation of bile in liver or bile ducts) results from faulty excretion of bilirubin conjugates, as in conditions such as Dubin-Johnson syndrome or Rotor's syndrome.

Hepatocellular Disease

Hepatocellular jaundice is due to defective uptake, conjugation, or transport of bilirubin by the liver. Liver cell dysfunction or necrosis caused by hepatitis, for example, or defective bile transport in the bile canal and small bile duct can cause hyperbilirubinemia. Unknown channels absorb the pooled bile components into the bloodstream. Although "obstructive jaundice" usually refers to jaundice caused by an obstruction such as a stone, hepatic cellular damage can also result in obstruction sufficient to cause jaundice.

Biliary Obstruction

Biliary obstruction, the cause of obstructive jaundice, results from impaired bilirubin transport and excretion in the biliary system. In this case, the problem arises from obstruction of an extrahepatic bile duct by gallstones.

Clinical Manifestations

Manifestations of jaundice include yellow sclerae, yellowish-orange skin, clay-colored feces, tea-colored urine, pruritus (itching), fatigue, and anorexia. Table 47–1 presents reference values for the laboratory diagnostic tests used to identify the underlying cause and type of jaundice. The following diagnostic test results are consistent with jaundice:

Abnormality	Reason/Result
Increased levels of conjugated serum bilirubin (direct bilirubin >0.4 mg/dl)	Bile excretion is blocked
Increased levels of unconjugated serum bilirubin (indirect bilirubin >0.8 mg/dl)	Liver damage with impaired conjugation of bilirubin; increased hemolysis of red blood cells
Bilirubin in urine	Liver damage or biliary obstruction of conjugated bilirubin
Increased urinary excretion of urobilinogen (>4 mg/24 hr)	Liver's ability to absorb urobilinogen from portal vein is impaired
Reduced fecal excretion of urobilinogen (<40 mg/24 hr)	Urobilinogen does not reach intestine
Increased alkaline phosphatase and cholesterol serum levels	Normal excretion of alkaline phosphatase and cholesterol into bile cannot occur owing to liver cell damage
In extreme cases of liver failure, an unusually low cholesterol level	Liver cannot synthesize cholesterol
Increased levels of serum bile salts	Bile salts are deposited in the skin, causing pruritus
Prolonged prothrombin time (>40 seconds)	Absorption of vitamin K is reduced

TABLE 47-1 TYPES OF JAUNDICE (ICTERUS)

Type of Jaundice	Causes	Assessment	Laboratory Test Results: Reference Values*									
			Conjugated (Direct) Bilirubin (0.1–0.3 mg/dl)	Unconjugated (Indirect) Bilirubin (0.2–0.8 mg/dl)	Total Bilirubin (0.1–1.0 mg/dl)	Urinary Bilirubin (0)	Urinary Urobilinogen (0–4 mg/day)	Fecal Urobilinogen (40–280 mg/day)	AST (5–40 U/L)	ALT (5–35 U/L)	PTT (30–40 sec)	PT (12–15 sec)
Unconjugated hyperbilirubinemia	Increased bilirubin production (hemolytic anemias, hemolytic reactions, hematoma infarction) Impaired bilirubin uptake and storage (post-hepatitis or with Gilbert's syndrome, Crigler-Najjar syndrome, drug reactions) Defective albumin binding	Liver function usually normal; compensates for ↑ bilirubin by ↑ metabolism of bilirubin Weakness or abdominal or back pain may occur with acute, mild jaundice	Normal	↑	↑	None	↑	↑	Normal	Normal	Normal	Normal
■ Hereditary cholestatic syndrome	Faulty excretion of bilirubin conjugates; Dubin-Johnson syndrome	May be asymptomatic May have pruritus, light-colored stools, occasional malaise	↑	↑	↑	↑	↓	↓	↑	↑	Prolonged	Prolonged
■ Hepatocellular disease	Liver's inability to conjugate or transport bilirubin to canaliculi for excretion due to hepatitis, liver congestion, cirrhosis, metastatic cancer, prolonged use of medications metabolized by liver, etc.	Liver may be enlarged Abdomen may be tender May have bruising or bleeding due to vitamin K malabsorption†	↑	↑	↑	↑	⇵	↓	↑	↑	Prolonged	Prolonged

Table continued on following page

TABLE 47-1

TYPES OF JAUNDICE (ICTERUS) Continued

Type of Jaundice	Causes	Assessment	Laboratory Test Results: Reference Values*									
			Conjugated (Direct) Bilirubin (0.1–0.3 mg/dl)	Unconjugated (Indirect) Bilirubin (0.2–0.8 mg/dl)	Total Bilirubin (0.1–1.0 mg/dl)	Urinary Bilirubin (0)	Urinary Urobilinogen (0–4 mg/day)	Fecal Urobilinogen (40–280 mg/day)	AST (5–40 U/L)	ALT (5–35 U/L)	PTT (30–40 sec)	PT (12–15 sec)
▪ Biliary obstruction	Blocked flow of bile into duodenum due to inflammation, scar tissue, stones, or tumors in liver, biliary, or pancreatic system	↑ Level of unconjugated bilirubin if liver cell function is diminished May have bruising or bleeding due to vitamin K malabsorption (bile is necessary for vitamin K absorption)† Abdomen may be tender Stools are clay-colored (bile gives stool its dark color) Urine is brown to foamy (conjugated bilirubin is excreted in urine)	↑	Normal or ↑	↑	↑	↓	Absent or ↓	Normal or slightly ↑	Normal or slightly ↑	Prolonged	Prolonged

ALT, alanine aminotransferase; AST, aspartate aminotransferase; PTT, partial thromboplastin time; PT, prothrombin time; U, units.
*Reference values vary among laboratories.
†Parenteral vitamin K will improve prothrombin time only if jaundice is due to posthepatic cause.
Modified from Friedman, L. S. (1998). Liver, biliary tract, and pancreas. In L. M. Tierney, (Eds.), *Medical diagnosis and treatment manual* (37 ed., pp. 628–630). Stamford, CT: Appleton & Lange.

Outcome Management

■ Medical Management

DETERMINE CAUSE OF JAUNDICE

An early goal in managing jaundice is to determine which category of disease explains the client's jaundice. The clinical evaluation is an important element in this determination. It includes a carefully documented health history, physical examination, basic tests of liver function, and a complete blood count (CBC). Additional tests, such as imaging studies, serologic tests, and laboratory pathologic evaluation, may be required.

The health history should focus on specific manifestations, including presence and character of pain, fever or other manifestations of active inflammation, and changes in appetite, weight, and bowel habits. The clinical evaluation should focus on features of the client's illness that point to hereditary cholestatic syndromes, hepatocellular disease, or biliary obstruction.

REDUCE PRURITUS AND MAINTAIN SKIN INTEGRITY

Pruritus, caused by an accumulation of bile salts in the skin, results from obstructed biliary excretion. Some clients experience only mild itching; others suffer such extreme itching that they tear at their skin or scratch during sleep. If skin lesions develop and become infected, antibiotics may be ordered.

Oral cholestyramine resin provides some relief by binding bile salts in the intestine so that they can be excreted. Antihistamines and phenobarbital (which enhances bile flow) may also relieve itching.

■ Nursing Management of the Medical Client

ASSESSMENT

The client should be observed closely for development of jaundice. Often, the first manifestation the client notices is a change in taste, manifested as a distaste for a food or drink the client previously liked, such as coffee. Pruritus is another early manifestation of incipient jaundice. Check the sclerae daily for the development of yellow coloration.

DIAGNOSIS, OUTCOMES, INTERVENTIONS

Impaired Skin Integrity. The most common nursing diagnosis for the client with jaundice is *Impaired Skin Integrity related to pruritus.*

Outcomes. The client's itching will be controlled, as evidenced by the client's statements of relief, decreased dryness of skin, and a decrease in scratching by the client.

Interventions. Administer antihistamines and phenobarbital as prescribed to relieve the itching. For clients with extreme itching, administer oral cholestyramine resin to bind with bile salts in the intestine so that they can be excreted. Suggest other interventions, including tepid water or emollient baths, avoidance of alkaline soap, and frequent application of lotions. Encourage the client to wear loose, soft clothing. Provide soft bed linens (cotton is best), and change soiled linens as soon as possible. Keep the room cool.

Body Image Disturbance. Clients with jaundice often experience problems associated with the nursing diagnosis *Body Image Disturbance related to yellowing of skin and sclerae.*

Outcomes. Clients will cope with body image disturbance, as evidenced by clients not isolating themselves, verbalizing and demonstrating acceptance of appearance (grooming, dress, posture, eating patterns, and self-presentation), and initiating or reestablishing support systems.

Interventions. Reassure the client that the discoloration is usually temporary. Assist the client in personal hygiene as needed, and promote activity as tolerated. Encourage clients to express their feelings about their self-image.

Altered Health Maintenance. Clients with jaundice may lack understanding of the condition, leading to the nursing diagnosis *Altered Health Maintenance related to lack of knowledge of jaundice.*

Outcomes. The client will understand the cause of jaundice, as evidenced by the client's statements and ability to define the illness.

Interventions. Clients often wonder why they have jaundice, how long the condition will last, and how to cope with the problem. Encourage clients with jaundice to ask questions about their health, treatment, and progress.

EVALUATION

Jaundice should resolve with treatment of the underlying condition. It usually begins to disappear within 4 to 6 weeks. The return of normal stool and urine color is an indication of resolution. As the jaundice lessens, the client's appetite and body image improve and the pruritus subsides.

■ Surgical Management

Surgical exploration of the common bile duct (choledochostomy) enables the diagnostician to differentiate choledocholithiasis (stone in the common bile duct) from tumor. If carcinoma (usually of the head of the pancreas) is discovered during exploration, the surgeon may perform a palliative anastomosis of the gallbladder to the jejunum to bypass the common bile duct. Chapter 46 describes surgical management of the client undergoing a choledochostomy.

HEPATITIS

Simply stated, hepatitis is inflammation of the liver. This inflammation may be caused by viruses, toxins, or chemicals (including drugs). Jaundice usually develops, and the liver is tender. Other manifestations depend on the causative agent and the degree of organ disruption. There are several types of hepatitis, such as viral, toxic, chronic, and alcoholic.

VIRAL HEPATITIS

The development of serologic tests has made it possible to identify a growing number of specific viruses that cause hepatitis. The most common of these are hepatitis A virus, hepatitis B virus, hepatitis C virus, hepatitis D virus (delta agent), and hepatitis E virus—which cause hepatitis A through E, respectively. A sixth agent, hepatitis G virus, has been discovered, but its role in acute viral hepatitis has not been established. Although the manifestations of infection are similar in hepatitis A through E plus G, these conditions differ in incubation period, mode of transmission, and severity (Table 47–2). As noted in

TABLE 47–2   **COMPARISON OF SIX TYPES OF VIRAL HEPATITIS**

Factor	Hepatitis A	Hepatitis B	Hepatitis C	Hepatitis D (Delta Hepatitis)	Hepatitis E	Hepatitis G
Occurrence	Endemic in areas of poor sanitation Common in fall and early winter	Worldwide, especially in drug addicts, homosexuals, people exposed to blood and blood products Occurs all year	Posttransfusion, those working around blood and blood products IV drug users Occurs all year	Hepatitis D virus causes hepatitis only in association with hepatitis B virus and only in presence of HBsAg Endemic in Mediterranean	Parts of Asia, Africa, and Mexico where there is poor sanitation	Associated with chronic viremia lasting 10 years
Incubation period	5–45 days Mean 25 days	30–180 days Mean 60–90 days	15–160 days Mean 50 days	Same as for hepatitis B	14–60 days Mean 40 days	—
Risk factors/high-risk groups	Close personal contact or by handling feces-contaminated wastes Poor sanitation	Health care workers in contact with body secretions, blood, and blood products Hemodialysis and post-transfusion clients Homosexually active males and drug abusers	Similar to that for hepatitis B	Same as for hepatitis B	Traveling or living in areas where incidence is high	Heath care workers in hemodialysis, IV drug users, hemodialysis clients, chronic hepatitis B or C clients
Transmission	Infected feces, fecal-oral route May be airborne if copious secretions Shellfish from contaminated water No carrier state	Parenteral, sexual contact, and fecal-oral route Carrier state	Contact with blood and body fluids Source of infection uncertain in many clients Carrier state	Coinfects with hepatitis B, close personal contact Carrier state	Fecal-oral route, food-borne or water-borne No carrier state	Percutaneous
Severity	Mortality low Rarely causes fulminating hepatic failure	More serious, may be fatal Mortality rate 10%–20%	Can lead to chronic hepatitis	Similar to hepatitis B More severe if occurs with chronic active hepatitis B	Illness self-limiting Mortality rate in pregnant women 10%–20%	Does not appear to cause liver disease
Diagnostic tests	Anti-HAV – IgM-positive in acute hepatitis; IgG-positive after infection	HBsAg or anti-HBc– IgM, HBeAg	Anti-HCV or anti-HDV Recombinant immunoblot assay	HDAg-positive HDV RNA in serum	Anti-HEV	Anti-HGV
Prophylaxis and active or passive immunity	Hygiene Immune globulin (passive) Inactivated hepatitis A vaccine (active)	Hygiene, avoidance of risk factors HBIG (passive) Recombinant hepatitis B vaccine (active)	Hygiene Immune globulin (passive)	Hygiene Hepatitis B vaccine (active)	Hygiene, sanitation No immunity	Hygiene

anti-HAV, antibody to hepatitis A virus; anti-HBc–IgM, antibody to hepatitis B–IgM; HBeAg, hepatitis Be antigen; anti-HCV, antibody to hepatitis C virus; anti-HEV, antibody to hepatitis E virus; HBsAg, hepatitis B surface antigen; anti-HGV, antibody to hepatitis G virus; HBIG, hepatitis B immune globulin; IV, intravenous.

Modified from Friedman, L. S. (1998). Liver, biliary tract, and pancreas. In L. M. Tierney, S. J. McPhee & M. A. Papadakis (Eds.). *Medical diagnosis and treatment* (37th ed.). Stamford, CT: Appleton & Lange.

the Etiology and Risk Factors section, various other viruses can also cause viral hepatitis.

Viral hepatitis occurs worldwide. It is a reportable disease in the United States, with approximately 50,000 cases reported annually to the Centers for Disease Control and Prevention (CDC). Because viral hepatitis is often asymptomatic, it is likely that many cases remain undiagnosed.[12]

HEPATITIS A
Hepatitis A is endemic (prevalent) in some areas of the world, especially areas with poor sanitation. However, epidemics also occur in countries with good sanitation.

HEPATITIS B
Hepatitis B occurs worldwide, even in remote areas. The incidence of hepatitis B increases in areas of high population density and poor hygiene.

HEPATITIS C
Hepatitis C accounts for over 90% of cases of post-transfusion hepatitis and many sporadic cases of hepatitis. Only 4% of cases of hepatitis are caused by the hepatitis C virus; intravenous (IV) drug use accounts for half of these.[10]

HEPATITIS D
Hepatitis D virus (delta agent) is always found with hepatitis B virus. The hepatitis D virus is endemic in some areas, such as in the Mediterranean countries, where up to 80% of hepatitis B carriers may be superinfected with hepatitis D.[10]

HEPATITIS E
Hepatitis E virus is a ribonucleic acid (RNA) virus distinct from hepatitis A virus and the enteroviruses. This agent is a water-borne virus and has been associated with hepatitis outbreaks in India, Burma, Afghanistan, Algeria, and Mexico.

HEPATITIS G
The agent of hepatitis G is a flavivirus that spreads through contact with blood transfusions, contaminated needles, and body fluids.

Etiology and Risk Factors

Agents that may cause viral hepatitis include hepatitis A–E and G viruses, rubella virus, varicella virus, retroviruses, yellow fever virus, adenoviruses, and Marburg virus. Epstein-Barr virus (which causes infectious mononucleosis), cytomegalovirus, and herpes simplex virus are other possible causes of viral hepatitis, especially in immunocompromised people.

HEPATITIS A. Hepatitis A, also known as infectious hepatitis, is caused by an RNA virus of the enterovirus family. Causes of epidemics include infected water, milk, and food, especially raw shellfish from contaminated waters.

People who work with animals imported from areas where hepatitis A is endemic are at increased risk, as are people who eat raw or steamed shellfish. In the general population, children under 15 years of age are at most risk.

Hepatitis A is transmitted primarily by the fecal-oral route. It spreads from person to person by close contact or by the handling of feces-contaminated articles. Because the infected client's feces contain the virus before the onset of manifestations, other household members are at

risk for infection. In addition, hepatitis A may spread in institutions such as day care centers, prisons, or facilities for developmentally disabled people. Spread of the disease is enhanced by crowding and poor sanitation.

HEPATITIS B. Health care workers are at high risk for acquiring hepatitis B because of their close contact with the blood of carriers. Clients who have had multiple blood transfusions or dialysis are also vulnerable. Other high-risk populations are homosexual men, morticians, people who undergo tattooing, and IV drug users.

The major sources of hepatitis B are carriers and clients in the acute phase of the infection. Contact with the serum of an infected person is the major mode of transmission. The virus also may be transmitted by other body fluids such as saliva and semen. Hepatitis B virus can survive on environmental surfaces for at least a week.

HEPATITIS C. Hepatitis C is transmitted parenterally through the blood, by personal contact, and possibly by the fecal-oral route. In contrast to hepatitis A, but like hepatitis B, hepatitis C may be spread by carriers. Because hepatitis C is also parenterally transmitted, the risk factors are similar to those for hepatitis B.

HEPATITIS D. Hepatitis D is transmitted only through blood contact and is thus seen most commonly in clients exposed to blood and blood products, such as IV drug users and people with hemophilia. The risk factors for hepatitis D are the same as for hepatitis B.

HEPATITIS E. The hepatitis E virus is a water-borne virus. This form of hepatitis primarily affects young adults. It has a short incubation, and there is no evidence that it becomes chronic. The risk factors for hepatitis E include travel to countries that have a high incidence of hepatitis E and consuming food or water contaminated with the virus.

HEPATITIS G. Hepatitis G is spread through contact with blood, blood products, and body fluids. Risk factors are the same as those for hepatitis B and hepatitis C.

Prevention

To a great extent, viral hepatitis can be prevented by proper controls within the home, community, and health care facility setting. Table 47–2 describes each disease and contains information on prophylaxis for the hepatitides.

HEPATITIS A
PERSONAL HYGIENE. Because transmission of hepatitis A (and possibly hepatitis C) is by the fecal-oral route, good personal hygiene is important. Strict isolation of clients is not necessary, but hand-washing after a bowel movement is required. Food handlers must wash their hands thoroughly. In some facilities, transmission of the disease occurs because residents are unable to properly perform self-care, including hygiene measures. Care providers must supervise hand-washing by ambulatory residents. Personnel in day care centers need to wash their hands carefully after changing diapers.

WATER SUPPLY. Treatment of municipal water supplies prevents transmission of hepatitis A. Private water supplies can be sources of contamination, and polluted fishing waters pose a threat. Shellfish that come from such waters are a major source of hepatitis A.

RESTAURANTS. It is important for local health authorities to inspect eating establishments consistently and thoroughly. Serologic screening of food handlers for hepatitis A reduces its transmission. Because the disease can be transmitted via food, a person with active hepatitis A should not work in food services.

ANIMAL CARE. Isolating newly imported animals for a 2-month period would reduce the incidence of hepatitis A among people who handle them. If isolation is impossible, these people need to wear protective clothing and use good hand-washing technique. If the risk of contamination is high, some physicians prescribe prophylactic standard immune globulin (see later under prevention of hepatitis A).

ACTIVE IMMUNIZATION. An inactivated hepatitis A vaccine (Havrix) is available commercially. It is recommended for children and adults who travel, work, or live in countries or communities with a high rate of hepatitis A and for people with chronic liver disease, homosexual men, and IV drug users. Children older than 2 years and adolescents receive two doses given 1 month apart, followed by a booster dose 6 to 12 months after the first two doses. Adults receive an initial dose followed by a booster 6 to 12 months later. All injections are intramuscular. Adverse effects include headache, abdominal pain, diarrhea, syncope, fever, fatigue, jaundice, and local soreness.[19]

PASSIVE IMMUNIZATION. Physicians may prescribe standard immune globulin. Adverse effects of intramuscular injection include pain, tenderness, and at times hematoma formation. Administration of immune globulin (gamma globulin [Gammar]) is helpful prophylaxis both before and after exposure. Immune globulin is administered intramuscularly after exposure but not after the development of clinical manifestations. Clients who live in or visit high-risk areas can be protected for up to 3 months by immune globulin. The earlier in the incubation period that the prophylactic immune globulin is given, the greater the protection.

HEPATITIS B

CONTROL OF BLOOD, BLOOD PRODUCTS, AND SKIN-PIERCING INSTRUMENTS. Because hepatitis B is transmitted by the serum of infected people, all blood, blood products, and instruments that pierce the skin and contact the vascular system are potential sources of contamination. Some donor-related precautions that reduce the incidence of hepatitis B are the following:

- Screening of donors' blood for hepatitis B virus surface antigen (HBsAg), antibody to hepatitis B core antigen (anti-HBc), antibody to HbsAg (anti-HBs), hepatitis B, antigen (HbcAg), and hepatitis B virus deoxyribonucleic acid (DNA) (HBVDNA)[10]
- Use of volunteer rather than paid donors
- Registration of carriers
- Sharing of accurate records between institutions
- Testing of all pregnant women for HBsAg

It is possible to reduce the transfusion recipient's exposure to hepatitis B by using blood products only when necessary, using only the necessary amount of blood or blood products, cross-checking laboratory data to reduce errors of reported results, avoiding commercially obtained blood, and encouraging clients who are having elective surgery to donate their own blood (autologous transfusions).

Many health care facilities use disposable equipment, especially needles and syringes, to reduce hepatitis transmission. Nondisposable equipment must be sterilized. All health care workers, of course, must follow CDC standard precautions.

PERSONAL HYGIENE. Good personal hygiene reduces transmission. Clients with hepatitis B and hepatitis B carriers should not share razors, toothbrushes, washcloths, cigarettes, or other personal items.

ACTIVE IMMUNIZATION. Hepatitis B vaccine may provide active immunization before exposure to hepatitis B virus. The injection is best given into the deltoid muscle. Hepatitis B vaccine is given in three doses. The first and second doses must be separated by at least 1 month. The third dose is administered at least 4 months after the initial dose. Adverse reactions include headache, fever, nausea, vomiting, abdominal cramps, local soreness, redness, and swelling. Authorities strongly recommend this killed virus vaccine for all people. Hepatitis B vaccine is now included in the routine vaccination schedule for children (see Chapter 17). It is also recommended for adolescents and adults not previously immunized with the hepatitis B vaccine.

The hepatitis B vaccine is highly recommended for all people in high-risk categories for hepatitis B, including not only health care workers but also dialysis clients and attending personnel, clients requiring repeated transfusions, spouses of HBsAg-positive clients, people who have multiple sex partners (especially homosexual men), prison workers, and handlers of primates. It may be used in conjunction with the preparation *hepatitis B immune globulin* (HBIG) after documented exposure to hepatitis B.

PASSIVE IMMUNIZATION. Standard immune globulin may contain antibodies against hepatitis B. However, HBIG contains much higher levels of antibody. HBIG is given within 24 hours of exposure to hepatitis B or as soon as possible after exposure. Physicians may prescribe HBIG for prophylaxis after percutaneous exposure to blood that contains HBsAg.

HEPATITIS C

Transmission of hepatitis C is similar to that of hepatitis B. Many of the same measures are useful in its prevention, although available evidence suggests that hepatitis C is less readily transmitted through sexual and household contacts than is hepatitis B. Physicians may prescribe standard immune globulin for passive immunization after exposure to hepatitis C. However, the role of this intervention as a preventive measure remains unclear; at present, immune globulin is not officially recommended for prophylaxis. There is no vaccine for active immunization against hepatitis C.

HEPATITIS D

Because hepatitis D must coexist with hepatitis B, the hepatitis B vaccine can help prevent hepatitis D also. The precautions that help prevent hepatitis B also are useful in preventing delta hepatitis.

HEPATITIS E

Because the hepatitis E virus is water-borne and infection occurs by the fecal-oral route in various parts of the world, attention to matters of personal hygiene and sanitation helps prevent the spread of this form of hepatitis, as it does with hepatitis A and hepatitis B.

HEPATITIS G

Hepatitis G virus (HGV) is spread through contact with blood, blood products, and body fluids. HGV has been detected in 50% of IV drug users, 20% of people with hemophilia, and 15% of clients with chronic hepatitis B or C.

Pathophysiology

The pathophysiologic features in viral hepatitis are similar regardless of the cause. Hepatocytes undergo pathologic changes induced by the body's immune response to the virus. Inflammation of the liver with areas of necrosis occurs, and the resultant damage leads to impairment of function. The degree of functional impairment depends on the amount of hepatocellular damage. The endoplasmic reticulum—responsible for protein and steroid synthesis, glucuronide conjugation, and detoxification—is the first cellular organelle (a specialized part of a cell that performs a definite function) to undergo change, and liver functions that depend on these processes are altered. Kupffer cells (fixed phagocytic cells found in sinusoids of liver) increase in size and number. Vascular and ductular tissues undergo inflammatory changes. Healing of the damaged hepatic tissue generally occurs in 3 to 4 months.

Some complications of hepatitis occur, though rarely. (See Complications of Hepatitis below.)

HEPATITIS A

Antibodies to hepatitis A virus (anti-HAV) appear early in the course of the illness. Both immunoglobulin M (IgM) and immunoglobulin G (IgG) anti-HAV are detectable in the serum soon after the onset of illness. IgM anti-HAV titers peak during the first week of the disease and usually disappear within 3 to 6 months. Detection of IgM anti-HAV is a valid test for demonstrating acute hepatitis. IgG anti-HAV peak titers occur 1 month after onset of the disease but may stay elevated for years; this finding is therefore an indicator of past infection.

HEPATITIS B

The hepatitis B virus is a DNA virus that has an inner core and a surface envelope. The body forms antibodies to the viral antigens HBcAg and HBsAg. The presence of HBsAg in the blood denotes (1) a previous or resolving infection with hepatitis B, (2) a continuing, chronic infection, or (3) immunization with immunoglobulin or hepatitis B vaccine.

HEPATITIS C

The hepatitis C virus is a single-stranded RNA virus with properties similar to those of the hepatitis B and hepatitis D viruses. Hepatitis C virus is thought to be a pathogenic factor in conditions such as glomerulonephritis and autoimmune thyroiditis.

HEPATITIS D

Hepatitis D virus is a small defective RNA virus that causes hepatitis only in hepatitis B virus infection, and specifically only in the presence of HBsAg. Hepatitis D virus requires the helper function of hepatitis B virus for its replication and expression. Hepatitis D virus can either infect a person simultaneously with hepatitis B virus (*co-infection*) or infect a person already infected with hepatitis B virus (*superinfection*).

HEPATITIS E

The hepatitis E virus alters hepatocellular function in almost the same way as for the other types of hepatitis viruses. It causes necrosis and liver cell damage.

HEPATITIS G

Hepatitis G virus, like hepatitis C virus, is a blood-borne RNA virus. Current data indicate that a large portion of clients infected with hepatitis G are also infected with hepatitis C. Hepatitis G virus does not alter the severity of hepatitis C, nor is it associated with acute or chronic liver injury, although the latter finding requires continued study.

Clinical Manifestations

Clients with viral hepatitis all experience liver inflammation and other pathologic changes that are similar. Hepatitis B, hepatitis C, and hepatitis D are usually the most severe, although they may be asymptomatic in some clients. The onset of manifestations ranges from abrupt to insidious, according to the incubation period and the degree of infectivity.

Manifestations of viral hepatitis are systemic and vary from client to client. Manifestations occurring during the earlier (prodromal) phase may include jaundice, lethargy, irritability, myalgia, arthralgia, anorexia, nausea, vomiting, abdominal pain (caused by stretching of Glisson's capsule surrounding the liver due to inflammation), diarrhea or constipation, fever, and other flu-like manifestations. Fever is caused by the release of pyrogens in the inflammatory process. Fatigue and malaise are the result of reduced energy metabolism by the liver. Pruritus (itching), the result of bile salt accumulation in the skin, is typically mild and transient and may be more intense at its onset and termination. Jaundice, caused by impaired excretion of conjugated bilirubin, may or may not be present; when it is, it is first seen in the sclerae of the eyes and mucous membranes.

Anicteric (without jaundice) hepatitis may or may not precede jaundice. Children with hepatitis are usually anicteric. Adults often note the appearance of darker urine (the color of tea or mahogany) and clay-colored stools a few days before clinical jaundice develops. The darker urine is from the presence of urobilinogen, which is excreted through the kidneys instead of the bowel as normally occurs. The other manifestations often abate when jaundice appears, but they also may worsen.

If irritability and drowsiness become severe, assess for the possibility of hepatic encephalopathy. Deterioration of handwriting is an early manifestation of hepatic encephalopathy; thus, at each shift ask clients to write their name and observe their writing closely for changes. *Asterixis,* an abnormal muscle tremor sometimes called "liver flap," may accompany encephalopathy. This manifestation is easily elicited by applying a blood pressure cuff on the upper arm and noting whether the tremor is present when the cuff is released. Mild depression is not uncommon because of (1) the nature of the illness (weakness, jaundice, itching, and nausea), (2) its long duration and the expense of treatment, (3) the need for confinement, and (4) forgetfulness and the inability to concentrate on completion of activities of daily living (ADL).

Bleeding tendencies may develop either from reduced prothrombin synthesis by injured hepatic cells or from reduced absorption of the fat-soluble vitamin K due to reduced levels of bile in the intestines. Anemia may occur because of the decreased life span of erythrocytes

(RBCs). Erythrocyte destruction results from liver enzyme alterations. A transient hyperglycemia sometimes develops, and a client with diabetes may need to increase insulin dosage at this time.

The liver is larger than normal in hepatitis and is tender to palpation. Some people with viral hepatitis have spider angiomas, palmar erythema, and gynecomastia, which disappear during the recovery period. A small percentage (5% to 15%) of clients experience splenomegaly or enlargement of the posterior cervical lymph nodes. Occasionally, hepatitis B is accompanied by arthralgias, rash, vasculitis, or glomerulonephritis.

Occasionally, cholestatic viral hepatitis syndrome may develop. This uncommon disease process resembles mechanical obstruction; it is difficult to differentiate cholestatic viral hepatitis from biliary tract obstruction due to gallstones, strictures, and tumors.

The cause and pathophysiology of this hepatitis variant are unclear. Cholestatic viral hepatitis syndrome causes jaundice, itching, and the typical flu-like and gastrointestinal problems of hepatitis, but the manifestations often last longer and are more severe. Serum bilirubin reaches levels of 10 to 15 mg/dl. Diagnostic studies reveal elevations of serum lipoproteins, globulins, cholesterol, and alkaline phosphatase. Rarely, the liver progressively enlarges.

Fulminant viral hepatitis may develop. This life-threatening form resembles acute liver failure with manifestations of encephalopathy (increased excitability, insomnia, somnolence, and impaired mentation). The liver rapidly decreases in size. Other problems include gastrointestinal bleeding, disseminated intravascular coagulation (DIC), fever with leukocytosis and neutrophilia, hepatorenal problems of oliguria and azotemia, edema and ascites, hypotension, respiratory failure, hypoglycemia, bacterial infection of the respiratory or urinary tract or both, and thrombocytopenia and coagulopathy. The prognosis is poor, and death may occur before jaundice appears. Liver transplantation may be performed to save the client's life.

Presence of hepatitis B surface antigen (HBsAg) in the blood usually indicates that the person is infectious. Another antigen, HBeAg, is often associated with progression of acute hepatitis to chronic hepatitis and indicates a highly infectious state.

Levels of serum aminotransferases first rise and then begin to fall as bilirubin starts to increase. Levels that rise, peak, drop, and then rise again indicate severe liver damage and a poor prognosis. Jaundice may not be clinically recognizable until levels are about 3 mg/dl. Bilirubin that rises above 20 mg/dl and remains elevated for a long period may indicate severe liver necrosis, which has a poor prognosis. Mild prolongation of the prothrombin time sometimes occurs. The gamma globulin fraction and alkaline phosphatase are elevated in some clients. If hepatitis B is responsible, detection of HBsAg is possible before the level of aspartate aminotransferase (AST) (formerly serum glutamic-oxaloacetic transaminase [SGOT]) rises.

Prognosis

By 8 to 10 weeks, nearly all clients with acute viral hepatitis demonstrate normal results on liver function tests. However, the clinical course, morbidity, and mortality of viral hepatitis may vary considerably. In most cases, clients recover in 3 to 16 weeks, with abnormal results on liver function testing for a longer time. Most clients recover completely. The mortality rate is less than 1%, with the rate reportedly being higher in older people.[7]

Outcome Management

▪ Medical Management

The acute manifestations of hepatitis generally subside over 2 to 3 weeks. Complete clinical and laboratory recovery occurs in hepatitis A by 9 weeks and in hepatitis B and hepatitis C by 16 weeks. Severe complications develop in fewer than 1% of clients with hepatitis. Clients who have severe nausea and vomiting and have difficulty maintaining normal fluid balance need to be hospitalized if there is progressive deterioration.

REDUCE FATIGUE
Rest is advisable in proportion to the severity of manifestations. Bed rest is usually not necessary but is recommended on an as-needed basis during the initial prodromal, anicteric phase of the disease, when the infection is most active and there is decreased metabolism by the liver. Return to normal activity during the convalescent period should be gradual. If pruritus (itching) disturbs rest, cholestyramine, antihistamines, emollients, and lipid creams may be prescribed.

MAINTAIN NUTRITIONAL AND FLUID BALANCE
No specific dietary measures are indicated, but most clients find a low-fat, high-carbohydrate diet more easily digested and more palatable. During the most severe phase of the illness, when there are changes in the stomach or bowel, anorexia and nausea may be so extreme that oral intake of any kind is greatly reduced. In such cases, IV administration of 10% glucose is indicated. As the client's manifestations abate and appetite improves, food and fluid intake may be resumed as tolerated. All alcoholic beverages should be avoided.

REDUCE EFFECTS OF HEPATITIS
Few medications are available for treating vital hepatitis. Antibiotics are not prescribed. Antiemetics control nausea and vomiting, but phenothiazines should not be used because they are biotransformed in the liver and are therefore potentially toxic. Parenteral vitamin K may be given to clients with prolonged prothrombin time. Antihistamines may provide relief of pruritus but may cause sedation.

STEROIDS. Corticosteroids are not necessary in uncomplicated cases of acute viral hepatitis, and authorities have questioned their use. Although they may reduce serum aminotransferase and bilirubin levels, they have no effect on liver necrosis or regeneration.

ESTROGENS. Estrogens can raise serum bilirubin levels. Therefore, clinicians need to consider the advisability of oral contraceptive use during acute viral hepatitis.

BILE ACID SEQUESTRANTS. The administration of bile acid sequestrants cholestyramine (Questran) or colestipol (Colestid) can relieve pruritus associated with elevated levels of bile acids that may result from severe cholestatic liver disease. Both drugs bind bile acids in the gastrointestinal tract forming an insoluble complex that is excreted in the feces. The result of this action is increased clearance of cholesterol.

IMMUNE GLOBULIN. Immune globulin, although not used to treat viral hepatitis, does provide prophylaxis for family and friends. If given early, standard immune globulin (a preparation of proteins capable of acting as antibodies, formerly termed "immune serum globulin") can prevent hepatitis A or mitigate the severity of manifestations. The hepatitis A virus does not remain in the blood long; therefore, there is no healthy carrier state for hepatitis A as there is for hepatitis B.

VACCINES. Vaccines are available to promote immunity to hepatitis A and hepatitis B. In addition to immune globulin, they may be administered prophylactically in persons exposed to infected clients.

MEDICATIONS TO AVOID. Clinicians administer very few medications to clients with hepatitis. Medications such as chlorpromazine, aspirin, acetaminophen, and a variety of sedatives are given as infrequently as possible because of their hepatotoxic properties.

COMPLICATIONS OF HEPATITIS

Persons with viral hepatitis typically recover completely from the illness in 3 to 16 weeks. Clients who are otherwise healthy usually recover from hepatitis A without major sequelae. Although hepatitis A is associated with a low mortality rate, very rarely fulminant hepatitis may result. The fulminant form, resembling acute liver failure, also occurs with infection due to other hepatitis viruses. Clients with hepatitis B tend to experience more complications. One in 10 persons develops chronic active hepatitis as a result of hepatitis B, often leading to destruction of the liver. Cirrhosis may follow a severe case of hepatitis B or chronic active hepatitis. Primary hepatocellular carcinoma is a potential complication of chronic hepatitis. Other possible complications of hepatitis include chronic persistent hepatitis, chronic carrier state, and aplastic anemia.

FULMINANT HEPATITIS

Fulminant hepatitis (massive hepatic necrosis) is rare and is primarily seen in hepatitis B and hepatitis D as well as in hepatitis E and hepatitis A. Fulminant hepatitis causes severe illness and is fatal in 1% to 2% of all cases and in up to 20% of cases occurring in pregnant women. Fulminant hepatitis involves a progression of manifestations that include jaundice, hepatic encephalopathy, and ascites. The mortality rate varies with age but approaches 90% to 100%, especially in people over 60 years of age.

CHRONIC HEPATITIS

Chronic hepatitis exists when liver inflammation continues beyond a period of 3 to 6 months. This disease may take the form of *chronic persistent hepatitis* (CPH) or *chronic active hepatitis* (CAH). Both CPH and CAH may follow hepatitis B or hepatitis C. Biopsy findings in CPH and CAH are compared in Figure 47–1.

■ CHRONIC PERSISTENT HEPATITIS

CPH is the most common form of chronic hepatitis. Most clients have no manifestations, although some may report fatigue, anorexia, and abdominal pain. Recurrent episodes are not acute in nature, and extrahepatic involvement seldom occurs. The clinical course is benign; fibrotic liver and cirrhosis develop only rarely. Clients with CPH generally have an excellent prognosis.

■ CHRONIC ACTIVE HEPATITIS

CAH is demonstrated by elevation of serum transaminase levels for more than 6 months. It is a complication of hepatitis B and hepatitis C. A more severe illness is caused by CAH than by CPH. CAH leads to hepatic inflammation, hepatic necrosis, and progressive fibrosis, with accompanying manifestations of chronic liver disease such as splenomegaly and spider angiomas. Affected clients are also at risk for hepatocellular carcinoma.

In most instances, CAH results from an autoimmune response or from hepatitis B virus infection with or without superimposed hepatitis D virus infection. Autoimmune CAH is more common in women, whereas hepatitis B CAH is more common in men. The pathogenesis in hepatitis B CAH also indicates an autoimmune response,

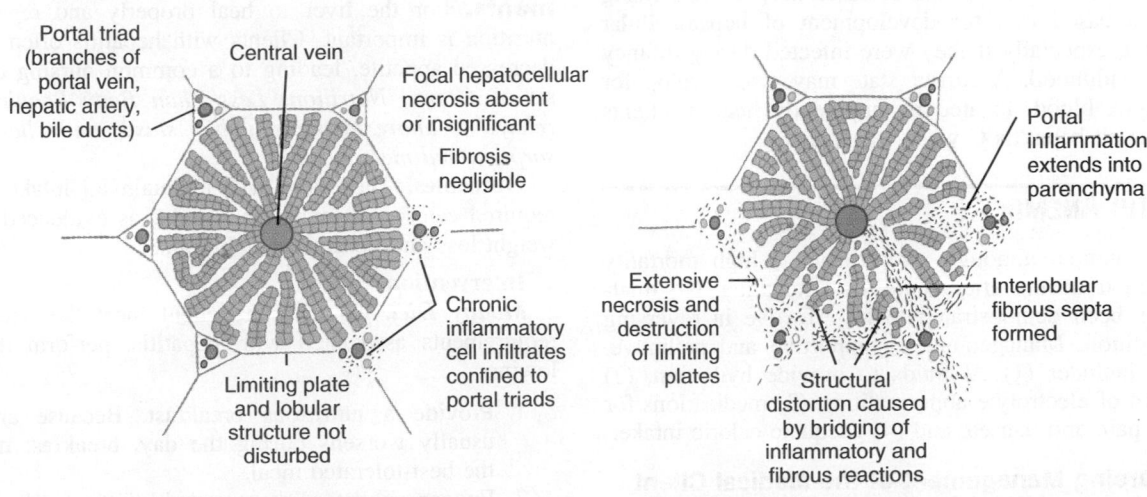

CHRONIC PERSISTENT HEPATITIS   CHRONIC ACTIVE HEPATITIS

FIGURE 47–1 Comparison of biopsy findings in hepatitis. Inflammation is confined to portal triads in chronic *persistent* hepatitis but extends into the parenchyma in chronic *active* hepatitis.

with low-level anti-HBc IgM present in 70% of the clients.

Cytomegalovirus infection during an immunosuppressed state is another viral cause. CAH may also follow acute hepatitis C or post-transfusion hepatitis. When CAH presents in adolescents, it may arise from Wilson's disease, a hereditary disorder. In addition, methyldopa, dantrolene, nitrofurantoin, and isoniazid may cause inflammatory changes consistent with CAH. Discontinuing the medication usually resolves the inflammatory process.

The onset of CAH is gradual. Some clients report the manifestations of acute viral hepatitis, cirrhosis, or extrahepatic problems. Clients come to the acute care setting primarily for liver biopsy and the identification of extrahepatic sequelae, such as thyroiditis, hemolytic anemia, amenorrhea, arthritis, urticaria, or glomerulonephritis.

Treatment of CAH varies. In the past, steroids, with or without azathioprine (Imuran), were often prescribed for treatment of idiopathic CAH. These drugs often reduced manifestations, improved laboratory test results, suppressed the inflammatory response viewed on biopsy, and lowered the short-term and long-term morbidity and mortality. More recently, a combination of two antiviral drugs for treatment of chronic hepatitis C was introduced. A series of ribavirin (Rebetron) capsules and interferon alfacon-1 (Infergen) injections for 6 months has proved very effective in reducing the virus to undetectable levels in about one half of clients who received this treatment.

Clients receiving treatment for CAH require close follow-up. They need periodic liver testing, monitoring for possible side effects of drug treatments, and liver biopsy every 6 months to 1 year. Clients with untreated CAH have a high mortality rate. Death results from hepatic failure, bleeding varices, hepatic encephalopathy, or primary hepatocellular carcinoma. Liver transplantation is a consideration for clients with end-stage liver disease that can no longer be managed medically.

CHRONIC CARRIER STATE

A carrier state is possible in clients who demonstrate persistent HBsAg without clinically evident disease but who are able to transmit the disease. Carriers of HBsAg are at increased risk for development of hepatocellular carcinoma, especially if they were infected during infancy or early childhood. A carrier state may also develop for hepatitis C; blood donated by apparently healthy clients may transmit hepatitis C when transfused.

APLASTIC ANEMIA

Aplastic anemia, although rare, carries a high mortality rate when it occurs after acute viral hepatitis. No treatment has been demonstrated to be effective in reversing this condition. Management is supportive and palliative. Therapy includes (1) IV fluids to provide hydration, (2) correction of electrolyte abnormalities, (3) medications for relief of pain and nausea, and (4) adequate caloric intake.

■ Nursing Management of the Medical Client
ASSESSMENT

To determine the type of hepatitis present, always begin by questioning the client about possible exposure to risk factors. Ask about common manifestations, especially jaundice, and about manifestations of disease progression, such as hepatic encephalopathy (see Hepatic Encephalopathy under Cirrhosis, later on). Assess results of liver function studies, and monitor them to ascertain progression of the disease. Also assess the client's and family's ability to provide home and self-care. Their understanding of the disease and its implications is vital to its successful management in the home setting.

DIAGNOSIS, OUTCOMES, INTERVENTIONS

Fatigue. The client with hepatitis has tremendous metabolic demands, leading to the nursing diagnosis *Fatigue related to decreased metabolic energy production secondary to liver dysfunction.*

Outcomes. The client will convey reduced fatigue and heightened energy, as evidenced by compliance with activity restrictions and a gradual increase in activity to the pre-illness level.

Interventions. Fatigue associated with hepatitis may interfere with ADL. Most clients experience the greatest fatigue during the *anicteric phase* (before jaundice occurs) and begin to feel stronger during the icteric phase. Fatigue may persist, however, even after the jaundice clears. Clients with severe jaundice may suffer pruritus (see Jaundice for nursing interventions for *Impaired Skin Integrity related to pruritus*). During the period of severe fatigue, advise the client to rest in bed. Most clients who feel capable of being up and around can do so without harm if they rest after meals and do not engage in any activity to the point of becoming overly tired. Because prolonged bed rest itself can lead to weakness, a reasonable activity level is more conducive to recovery than enforced bed rest.

Encourage ADL such as exercise of bathroom privileges, performance of personal hygiene measures, and self-feeding unless they cause excessive fatigue. Advise the client to plan rest periods while jaundice is present, especially after meals. Clients who engage in excessive activity too early in the recovery phase sometimes experience a relapse, potentially leading to liver failure.

Altered Nutrition: Less Than Body Requirements. For the liver to heal properly and regenerate, nutrition is important. Clients with hepatitis often have a decreased appetite, leading to a common nursing diagnosis of *Altered Nutrition: Less Than Body Requirements related to anorexia, nausea, bile stasis, and altered absorption and metabolism.*

Outcomes. The client will maintain an intake of the required calories to maintain weight, as evidenced by no weight loss and possible weight gain.

Interventions
Modify Diet. To help the client meet the nutritional requirements associated with hepatitis, perform the following:

1. Provide a nutritious breakfast. Because anorexia usually worsens during the day, breakfast may be the best-tolerated meal.
2. Encourage the client to avoid fatty foods, which can induce nausea.
3. Include the optimal amount of protein and carbohydrates to allow recovery of injured liver cells with-

out overfeeding. If the client has no problem with protein metabolism, a normal intake is helpful for tissue repair. However, clients with very severe hepatitis who are at risk for development of hepatic encephalopathy require a diet low in protein (to prevent the buildup of ammonia in the blood from incomplete clearing of protein metabolic wastes). Alterations in fat metabolism differ according to the degree of interruption of bile production and excretion.

4. Suggest multiple small meals. This approach allows the client with anorexia to ingest a diet of 2500 to 3000 calories more comfortably. Also, candy, juice, sweetened tea, and carbonated drinks can supply calories when nausea is a problem.

Avoid Alcohol. Remind the client to avoid alcohol, which is an extremely hepatotoxic agent.

Provide Vitamin Supplements. Explain that vitamin supplements are not generally necessary in uncomplicated hepatitis if the diet is adequate in nutrients. Vitamin K supplements, as ordered, may be administered if the prothrombin time is longer than normal.

Relieve Nausea and Vomiting. Clients who experience severe nausea and vomiting may obtain relief with antiemetics. However, before administering these medications, review their effect on liver function. Phenothiazines such as prochlorperazine (Compazine) are usually contraindicated. If the client cannot tolerate any oral intake, provide IV nutrition.

Anxiety. It is often difficult to predict the outcome of hepatitis; therefore, the nursing diagnosis *Anxiety related to uncertainty of the effects of hepatitis* is a common one.

Outcomes. The client will experience a decrease in anxiety, as evidenced by the ability to discuss his or her feelings about the disease.

Interventions. Encourage clients with hepatitis to express their feelings concerning the following:

- The illness
- The duration and cost of the illness
- Alterations in home life and in financial status (especially for the parent of young children or for the sole family earner)
- The effect of the illness on future health problems
- The possibility of death in clients who are very ill

Suggest psychosocial and financial counseling for the client who is disturbed. Increase the client's knowledge and understanding of the illness by teaching the facts about the illness and its management. Increased knowledge can reduce anxiety.

Altered Health Maintenance. In order for the client and family members to manage hepatitis at home, the nursing diagnosis of *Altered Health Maintenance related to cause of disease, modes of transmission, and its course* must be addressed.

Outcomes. The client will understand the disease and its treatment, as evidenced by the client's ability to state the causes of the disease and the rationales for treatment.

Interventions
Provide Client Teaching. Teaching for the client with hepatitis varies with the causative agent. Teach the client

how to prevent recurrence and spread. Instruct the client to return to former activity levels slowly in order to avoid a relapse. Provide clear instructions concerning diet.

Administer Medications. Administer medications and provide supportive management. Discontinue any medications that may be causing inflammatory changes. Clients who cannot tolerate large doses of steroids may benefit from azathioprine and smaller steroid doses. Clinicians generally do not recommend steroid therapy for subclinical CAH, especially in older adults.

Promote Rest. Encourage bed rest during the active phase of the disease. The client usually remains at home to convalesce. There may be periods of remission during which liver necrosis continues. Discuss with the client the need for help at home after discharge (such as with housework or shopping), because limits on activity will still have to be maintained. The client will need to see a physician at regular intervals after discharge to ensure that the liver is healing and no further damage has occurred.

EVALUATION
Because the clinical course of acute viral hepatitis varies considerably from client to client, the nurse must assess outcomes carefully to determine whether they have been met. Recovery without permanent liver damage is expected to occur within 1 to 4 months. Permanent damage may result if the therapeutic regimen is not followed.

Self-Care
Most clients recover from acute viral hepatitis, do not require hospitalization, and are appropriately managed at home. However, clinical and biochemical relapses may occur before full recovery. In addition, complications of acute viral hepatitis may develop, necessitating careful monitoring, especially in older clients.

AVOID HEPATOTOXINS
There is no specific ongoing pharmacologic management of clients recovering from acute viral hepatitis. Advise the client to avoid alcohol and medications such as aspirin, acetaminophen, and sedatives because of their hepatotoxicity.

PROMOTE NUTRITION
Encourage clients to continue eating a well-balanced, nutritional diet. A low-fat, high-carbohydrate diet is generally tolerated best. A well-balanced diet promotes liver healing, leading to improved tolerance for activity.

PROVIDE CLIENT TEACHING
One of the primary areas to cover in teaching the client and family members is how to avoid reinfection or possible spread of the infection to others. Caution the client and significant other to avoid sexual activity until there is no longer a chance of disease transmission (generally after liver function tests have returned to normal), and to check with the physician before resuming sexual relations.

PROMOTE REST
Help the client understand the need for adequate rest so that the liver can heal on its own. The client needs to be active enough to prevent complications of immobility but not so active as to risk relapse. The client is also ex-

pected to resume pre-hepatitis activities and to remain free from complications.

PREVENT INFECTION AND REINFECTION
Teach the client to avoid reinfection or possible spread of the infection to other family members. You may recommend vaccination for hepatitis A and B to promote health maintenance.

TOXIC HEPATITIS

Toxins and drugs may produce a wide variety of pathologic lesions in the liver. Some agents may cause toxic hepatitis, whereas others produce necrosis, cholestasis, or neoplasms. The extent and type of hepatitis produced by the toxin depends on the degree of exposure, the chemical properties of the hepatotoxin, and the genetic make-up of the individual. Most commonly, the causative agent is a toxic metabolite formed by the drug-metabolizing enzymes within the liver. Table 47–3 lists some hepatotoxic agents. Liver necrosis occurs within 2 or 3 days after acute exposure to a dose-related hepatotoxin. However, several weeks may pass before manifestations of idiosyncratic reactions appear. People experiencing either type of hepatotoxicity demonstrate abnormal results on liver function testing.

People who are repeatedly exposed to hepatotoxins in minimal amounts but over long periods of time may develop chronic hepatitis or cirrhosis. Clients experiencing a hypersensitivity reaction may demonstrate eosinophilia, fever, arthralgia, and sometimes xanthomatosis (an excessive accumulation of lipids brought about by faulty lipid metabolism).

Nursing intervention begins with obtaining a detailed drug history and information about past exposure and the response to a suspected agent. Ensure removal of the causative agent and adequate rest, promote alleviation of side effects (e.g., with cholestyramine for pruritus), and provide a high-calorie diet with fats and protein as tolerated. Restrict protein intake if there is evidence of impending hepatic encephalopathy. Steroids have not proved of value in treatment of drug-induced liver disease, although they may suppress the manifestations caused by the reaction of the toxic agent.

Renal failure sometimes appears as a complication of toxic hepatitis. Assessment and interventions for renal failure are discussed in Chapter 36.

ALCOHOLIC HEPATITIS

Alcoholic hepatitis may be acute or chronic. It is caused by parenchymal necrosis resulting from heavy alcohol ingestion. Although sometimes reversible, this condition is the most frequent cause of cirrhosis. This fact is important because cirrhosis of the liver is a common cause of death among adults in the United States.

Clinical manifestations of alcoholic hepatitis usually develop after a bout of heavy drinking. Assessment reveals anorexia, nausea, abdominal pain, splenomegaly, hepatomegaly, jaundice, ascites, fever, and encephalopathy. Laboratory studies typically show anemia, leukocytosis, and an elevated serum bilirubin. Liver biopsy reveals fatty hepatic tissue. Hepatitis due to excessive alcohol

TABLE 47–3	SUBSTANCES KNOWN TO BE HEPATOTOXIC	
Type of Hepatotoxicity	Type of Liver Alteration	
	Hepatitis	*Cholestasis*
Dose-related	Acetaminophen	Oxymetholone
	Amanita phalloides (mushroom)	
	Aspirin	
	Benzene	
	Carbon tetrachloride	
	Chloroform	
	Methotrexate	
	Phosphorus	
	Tetracyclines	
	Vitamin A	
Idiosyncratic	Halothane	Allopurinol
	Isoniazid	Anabolic steroids
	Methyldopa	Carbamazepine
	Nitrofurantoin	Chlordiazepoxide
	Oxacillin	Chlorpromazine
	Phenytoin	Chlorpropamide
	Quinidine	Diazepam
	Streptomycin	Erythromycin estolate
	Sulfasalazine	Flurazepam
	Sulfanilamides	Oral contraceptives
	Sulfonamides	Propylthiouracil
	Other sulfa drugs	Thiazides
	Valproic acid	

Data from Di Marin, A. J. (1994). Gastrointestinal diseases. In A. R. Myers (Ed.), *Medicine* (2nd ed.; pp. 225–226). Philadelphia: JB Lippincott.

intake carries a poor prognosis, particularly if the client continues to ingest alcohol.

Nursing interventions include providing a high-vitamin, high-carbohydrate diet and administration of folic acid and thiamine supplements and administration of parenteral fluids as ordered. Administration of liquid formulas may be useful in increasing caloric intake. Steroids sometimes have a beneficial effect, although their use remains controversial.

CIRRHOSIS

Cirrhosis of the liver is a chronic, progressive disease characterized by widespread fibrosis (scarring) and nodule formation. Cirrhosis occurs when the normal flow of blood, bile, and hepatic metabolites is altered by fibrosis and changes in the hepatocytes, bile ductules, vascular channels, and reticular cells.

There are four major types of cirrhosis:

- Alcoholic (historically called "Laënnec's cirrhosis" or micronodular or portal)
- Postnecrotic (macronodular or toxin-induced)
- Biliary
- Cardiac

The types are compared in Table 47–4. The two major clinical problems in cirrhosis are (1) decreased liver func-

Definition	Etiology	Pathology	Assessment Data	Diagnosis and Prognosis	Intervention(s)
POSTNECROTIC (MACRONODULAR) CIRRHOSIS					
Most common world-wide form Massive loss of liver cells, with irregular patterns of regenerating cells	Postacute viral (types B and C) hepatitis Postintoxication with industrial chemicals Some infections and metabolic disorders	Liver small and nodular	As in alcoholic cirrhosis except less muscle wasting and more jaundice	Needle biopsy of liver establishes pathologic processes Within 5 years 75% die of complications ↑ serum aminotransferases ↑ gamma globulins	Treat complications as needed
BILIARY CIRRHOSIS					
Bile flow is decreased with concurrent cell damage to hepatocytes around bile ductules	*Primary* Chronic stasis of bile in intrahepatic ducts Cause unknown Autoimmune process implicated *Secondary* Obstruction of bile ducts outside of liver	Early-stage biopsy reveals inflammatory process with necrosis of cells and ducts Hepatocytes are lost and scar tissue remains End stage similar to postnecrotic type	Generalized pruritus Dark urine Pale stools Jaundice Impaired bile flow Steatorrhea ↓ absorption of fat-soluble vitamins Elevated serum lipids ↑ cholesterol deposits in subcutaneous tissues Signs of portal hypertension	Elevated serum bilirubin levels *Early:* 3–10 mg/100 ml *Late:* >50 mg/100 ml High elevations of alkaline phosphatase ↑ gamma globulins ↑ blood lipids Presence of lipoprotein X ↑ serum bile salts Hypoprothrombinemia ↑ antimitochondrial antibody in primary cases ↑ serum copper in primary cases	*Primary* Treatment is symptomatic, e.g., high-calorie diet, lower intake of fats by 30–40 g/day if problems develop Cholestyramine for pruritus Supplement of fat-soluble vitamins *Secondary* Treatment to relieve mechanical obstruction
CARDIAC CIRRHOSIS					
Chronic liver disease associated with severe right-sided long-term heart failure (fairly rare)	Atrioventricular valve disease Prolonged constrictive pericarditis Decompensated cor pulmonale	*Early* Dark-colored liver enlarged by blood and edema fluid *Late* Liver capsule thickens and nodular scarring occurs	Slight jaundice, enlarged liver, and ascites in person with severe cardiac impairment over 10-year span RUQ pain during acute congestion Cachexia Fluid retention Circulatory problems	↑ conjugated bilirubin in serum ↑ sulfobromophthalein → albumin in serum ↑ serum aminotransferases ↑ alkaline phosphatase Liver biopsy *Prognosis* Depends on course of cardiac disease	Cause of chronic heart failure is treated if possible
ALCOHOLIC CIRRHOSIS					
Alcoholic cirrhosis (Laënnec's, micronodular) Small nodules form as a result of persistence of some offending agent	Associated with alcohol abuse	Scarring and collagen tissue deposits Regenerating nodules are very small Normal lobular structure is destroyed	May produce no symptoms for long periods Onset of symptoms may be insidious or abrupt *Early:* Weakness, fatigue, weight loss *Later:* Anorexia, nausea, and vomiting Abdominal pain Ascites Menstrual irregularities Impotence Enlarged breasts in men Hematemesis Spider angiomas	Liver biopsy; history of alcohol abuse; high AST; high bilirubin (slight); anemia Prognosis depends on presence of complications and continued abuse of alcohol	Correction of vitamin and mineral deficiencies if any (e.g., folate, thiamine, pyridoxine, vitamin K, and minerals [magnesium and phosphate]); treat complications as needed (e.g., ferrous sulfate for anemia, IV vasopressin for esophageal varices, reduce or withhold dietary protein for hepatic encephalopathy or vitamin K for hemorrhagic tendency)

AST, aspartate aminotransferase; IV, intravenous; RUQ, right upper quadrant.
Data from Friedman, L. S. (1995). Liver, biliary tract and pancreas. In L. M. Tierney et al. (Eds.), *Medical diagnosis and treatment manual* (pp. 568–571). Norwalk, CT: Appleton & Lange; and Friedman, L. S. (1996). Cirrhosis of the liver and its major sequelae. In J. C. Bennett & F. Plum (Eds.), *Cecil textbook of medicine* (20th ed.). Philadelphia: W. B. Saunders.

tion and (2) portal hypertension. The latter problem develops in severe cirrhosis.

Cirrhosis is the 11th leading cause of death in the United States, with an age-adjusted mortality rate of 10.4 deaths per 100,000 population. Of those deaths, 45% were alcohol-related.[10] Men are more likely than women to have alcoholic (Laënnec's) cirrhosis. Worldwide, postnecrotic cirrhosis is the most common form; it is also more common in women. Mortality is higher from all types of cirrhosis in men and nonwhites.

Etiology and Risk Factors

The causes of cirrhosis have not been clearly identified, although the relationship between cirrhosis and excessive alcohol ingestion is well established. Countries with the highest incidence of cirrhosis have the greatest per capita consumption of alcohol. Genetic predisposition with a familial tendency, as well as a hypersensitivity to alcohol, is seen in alcoholic cirrhosis.

The primary risk factor for cirrhosis is alcohol ingestion, especially in the absence of proper nutrition. Any client with a family history of alcoholism should avoid alcohol because of the increased risk. Hence, cessation of alcohol consumption may be a health promotion, health maintenance, or health restoration activity. The amount of alcohol consumed daily appears to be a more important factor than the pattern of drinking (binge versus daily) or the type of alcoholic beverage consumed. If the client is in a poor nutritional state, the likelihood of damage is greater and the damage is more severe. Viral hepatitis is the primary risk factor for postnecrotic cirrhosis, which makes prevention of hepatitis through vaccination and good hygiene the most important health promotion activity.

Other risk factors for cirrhosis of the liver are biliary cirrhosis with intrahepatic cholestasis or obstruction of bile ducts; use of drugs (such as acetaminophen, methotrexate, or isoniazid); hepatic congestion from severe right-sided heart failure; constrictive pericarditis; valvular disease; alpha$_1$-antitrypsin deficiency; infiltrative disease (such as amyloidosis, glycogen storage diseases, or hemochromatosis); Wilson's disease; and nutritional deficits related to jejunal bypass.

Pathophysiology

Cirrhosis is the final stage in many types of liver insults. The cirrhotic liver usually has a nodular consistency, with bands of fibrosis (scar tissue) and small areas of regenerating tissue. There is extensive destruction of hepatocytes. This alteration in the architecture of the liver alters flow in the vascular and lymphatic systems and bile duct channels. Periodic exacerbations are marked by bile stasis, precipitating jaundice.

Portal vein hypertension develops in severe cirrhosis. The portal vein receives blood from the intestines and spleen. Thus, an increase of pressure in the portal vein causes (1) a retrograde increase in pressure resistance and enlargement of the esophageal, umbilical, and superior rectus veins, which may result in bleeding varices; (2) ascites (the result of osmotic or hydrostatic shifts leading to fluid accumulation in the peritoneum); and (3) incomplete clearing of protein metabolic wastes, with a resultant increase in ammonia, thus leading to hepatic encephalopathy.

Continuation of the process as a result of unknown causes or of alcohol abuse usually results in death from hepatic encephalopathy, bacterial (gram-negative) infection, peritonitis (bacterial), hepatoma (liver tumor), or complications of portal hypertension. See the algorithm on page 1236 for a summary of pathophysiologic changes, clinical manifestations, and treatment of cirrhosis.

Clinical Manifestations

Manifestations of cirrhosis diminish if the process is arrested at an early stage. Cirrhosis is a disease that initially progresses slowly. Thus, people with cirrhosis often discover the condition incidentally when seeking health care for other problems. In the early stages of cirrhosis, findings include hepatomegaly (enlarged liver), vascular changes, and abnormal results of laboratory tests. Palpation reveals a firm (scarred), lumpy (nodular), usually enlarged liver (although the liver becomes hard and shrunken in late cirrhosis).

In advanced cirrhosis, assessment reveals the following severe complications with their physiologic bases: ascites caused by malnutrition, portal hypertension, hypoalbuminemia, and hyperaldosteronism. Gastrointestinal bleeding arises from esophageal varices (swollen veins), hypoprothrombinemia, thrombocytopenia, and portal hypertension and often results in encephalopathy. Splenomegaly (enlargement of the spleen) indicates severe portal hypertension. Anemia, leukopenia, or thrombocytopenia may result from splenomegaly. Portal hypertension may cause prominent abdominal wall veins and internal hemorrhoids. Infections may be present as a result of an enlarged, overactive spleen, causing leukopenia. In addition, the bacteria that remain in the portal venous blood bypass the liver and are not removed by Kupffer cells and hence may cause infection. Ammonia no longer removed by the liver accumulates to levels toxic to the brain, resulting in encephalopathy. Renal failure occurs with rapidly failing hepatic function. Laboratory determinations reveal impaired hepatocellular function: elevated serum levels of liver enzymes (AST, alanine aminotransferase [ALT], and lactate dehydrogenase [LDH]), hypoalbuminemia, anemia, and prolonged prothrombin time. Liver biopsy allows for definitive diagnosis and demonstrates the associated pathologic changes.

Outcome Management

◼ Medical Management

MONITOR FOR COMPLICATIONS

Ascites, bleeding esophageal varices, and hepatic encephalopathy are discussed in depth later in this chapter. They are the most feared complications of cirrhosis. Renal failure (hepatorenal syndrome) and infection also are deadly. Family members and the client are taught manifestations of progressive liver failure. The family members should know what manifestations they need to report to the physician and when to seek immediate assistance, such as when variceal bleeding or a decrease in the level of consciousness occurs. Clients with encephalopathy may need extensive home care.

MAXIMIZE LIVER FUNCTION

Although cirrhosis is a progressive, degenerative disorder, steps are taken to minimize the risk of trauma and maximize regeneration, thereby slowing the course of the disease and prolonging life. A nutritious diet is recommended for clients with cirrhosis. The diet should be palatable, with adequate calories and protein (75 to 100 g/day) unless hepatic encephalopathy is present, in which case protein is limited. A list of foods to be included in the diet is given to the client and family. Fat intake need not be restricted. If there is edema or fluid retention, restrict sodium and fluids. If the client is receiving a thiazide diuretic, the diet should be high in potassium. The B vitamins and fat-soluble vitamins (vitamins A, D, E, and K) are commonly given to clients with alcoholic cirrhosis. Adequate rest also is important to maximize regeneration of the liver. In postnecrotic or posthepatic cirrhosis, the clinician may prescribe corticosteroids to reduce manifestations of cirrhosis and improve liver function. Other medications may be used to treat the complications.

TREAT THE UNDERLYING CAUSES

It is important that exposure to hepatotoxins be eliminated, that use of alcohol be avoided, and that biliary obstruction be removed. Medications that should be avoided (listed in Table 47–5) are specified to the client. The client should be encouraged to seek help (e.g., from Alcoholics Anonymous) with alcohol abstinence.

PREVENT INFECTION

Prevention of infection is accomplished by adequate rest, appropriate diet, and avoidance of hepatotoxic substances (alcoholic beverages, and medications and chemicals toxic to the liver). Before the discovery of antibiotics, infection was the major cause of mortality in cirrhosis.

TABLE 47–5	CIRRHOSIS AND DRUG-INDUCED LIVER FAILURE
Drugs to Restrict or Avoid	**Rationale**
Acetaminophen	Can cause fatal liver damage
Phenobarbital, phenytoin, chlorpromazine (Thorazine)	Stimulates liver's major drug-metabolizing system; when liver diseased or damaged, drugs may not be metabolized properly and toxicity may occur; may also cause alteration in sensory perception and thought processes related to hepatic encephalopathy
Morphine, paraldehyde, codeine	Can cause spasms and pressure in the biliary tract, thus increasing discomfort
Alcohol	Stimulates liver's major drug metabolizing system; can damage liver further

Nursing Management of the Medical Client

ASSESSMENT

Because the manifestations of cirrhosis are sometimes vague and nonspecific, the client may not be aware of the disease early in its course. Assess the client closely for the presence of early manifestations, such as hepatomegaly, and carefully check the laboratory data for any indication of cirrhosis. As the disease progresses, assess for manifestations of complications of cirrhosis, such as ascites, portal hypertension, or hepatic encephalopathy. These are discussed later in the chapter.

When a client with cirrhosis is hospitalized, use laboratory data and the client's physical and psychosocial assessment data to guide care planning. See the Case Study on cirrhosis for further information about these tests. Also, assess the client and family members for their knowledge of the important aspects of self-care.

DIAGNOSIS, OUTCOMES, INTERVENTIONS

Altered Tissue Perfusion. Because of the increased risk of bleeding in the client with cirrhosis, the nursing diagnosis *Altered Tissue Perfusion related to bleeding tendencies and varices that may hemorrhage* is common.

Outcomes. Hemorrhage will be prevented, as evidenced by absence of bleeding, normal vital signs, and urine output of at least 0.5 ml/kg/hr.

Interventions

Monitor for Hemorrhage. Monitor the client for bleeding gums, purpura, melena, hematuria, and hematemesis. Check vital signs as ordered to assess for signs of shock. In addition, monitor urine output. Report volume that is less than 0.5 ml/kg/hr.

Prevent Hemorrhage. Protect the client from physical injury from falls or abrasions, and give injections only when absolutely necessary, using only small-gauge needles. Be sure to apply gentle pressure after an injection, but do not rub the site because this might cause bruising.

Provide Client Teaching. Instruct the client to avoid vigorous nose-blowing and straining with bowel movements. Sometimes stool softeners may be ordered to prevent straining with rupture of varices. Antidiarrheal agents may be administered to control diarrhea. If bleeding gums are noted, advise the client to use a soft toothbrush and to refrain from flossing until the bleeding has ceased.

Altered Nutrition: Less Than Body Requirements. In order for the liver to regenerate, the client must have adequate levels of vital nutrients; otherwise, the unmet requirements lead to the nursing diagnosis *Altered Nutrition: Less Than Body Requirements related to anorexia, impaired liver function, decreased absorption of fat-soluble vitamins, and diarrhea.*

Outcomes. The client will take in adequate nutrition, as evidenced by no weight loss and no manifestations of malnutrition.

Interventions

Modify Diet. The diet should provide ample protein to rebuild tissue but not enough protein to precipitate hepatic encephalopathy. The diet should supply sufficient carbohydrates to maintain weight and to spare protein

Text continued on page 1239

Understanding Cirrhosis and Its Treatment

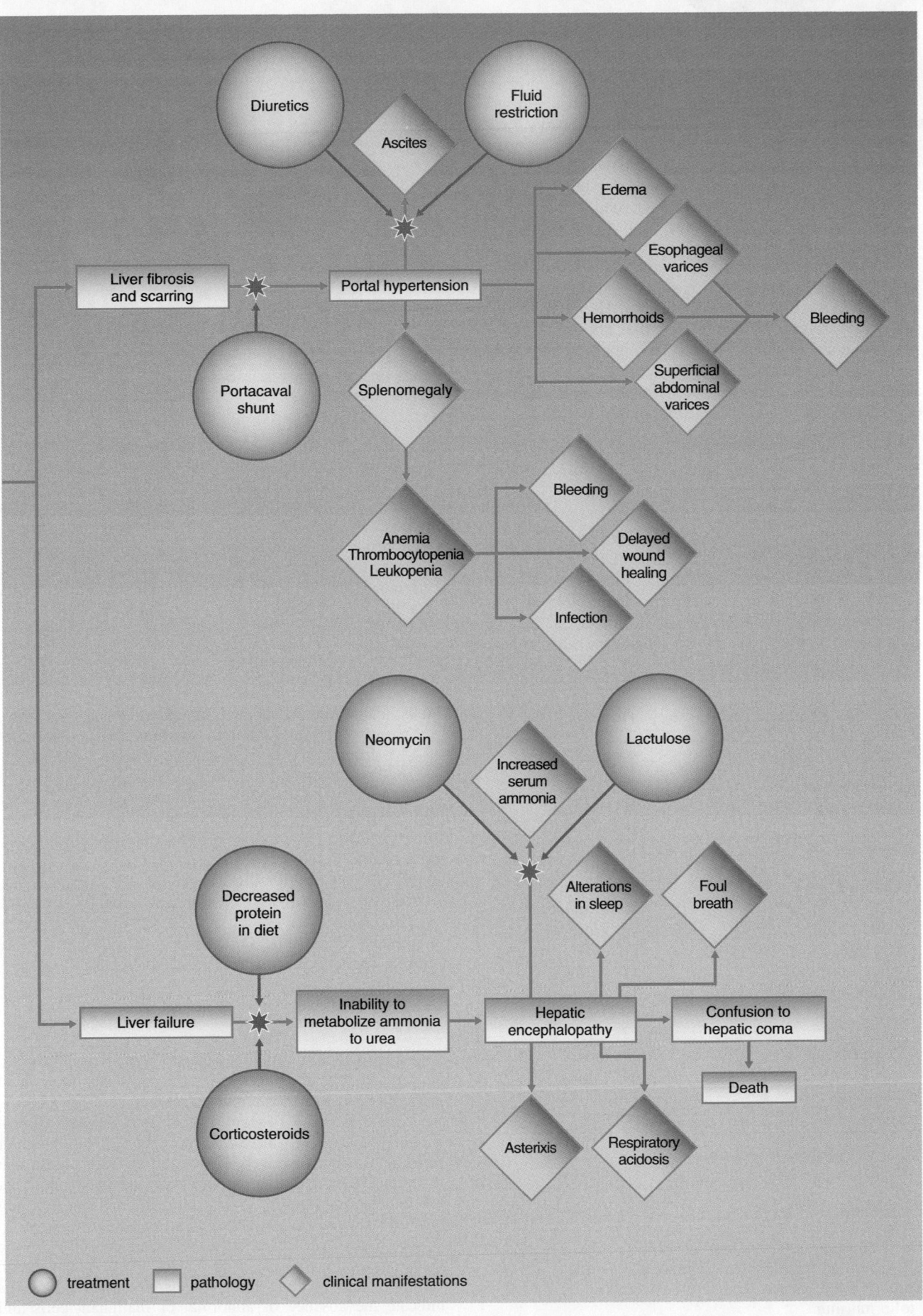

treatment   pathology   clinical manifestations

Cirrhosis

Mr. James is a 53-year-old man on disability from his job as a warehouse forklift driver. He became unable to work after developing idiopathic peripheral neuropathy which resulted in frequent falls and inability to run the controls of the forklift. He uses a cane to ambulate. Mr. James is being admitted with severe abdominal pain and coffee-grounds emesis. He reports that he had been vomiting bright red blood in the 2 days prior to admission. His abdomen is distended, with a measured abdominal girth of 52 inches. Mr. James also states that he has recently gained several pounds and has had shortness of breath and fatigue for the past several weeks. He reports that he smokes cigarettes but says that he does not use alcohol.

Mr. James is scheduled for an upper gastrointestinal endoscopy and paracentesis followed by a CT scan of the abdomen. Review the preprocedure preparations and client teaching required for these diagnostic tests. Also consider the influence of the preprocedure preparations on the order of scheduling these procedures.

Nursing Admission Assessment

Mr. James lives in his own home with his wife of 32 years. His wife works Monday through Friday as a cook in a public school. Mr. James' father died at age 50 years of multiple injuries sustained in an alcohol-related motor vehicle accident. His 75-year-old mother is in good health. The Jameses have three daughters, who are married and live within driving distance.

Selected Admission Laboratory Values	
RBC	2.78 million/mm³
Hb	11.0 g/dl
Hct	30.6%
WBC	12,300/mm³
Sodium	133 mEq/L
Potassium	3.1 mEq/L
Chloride	89 mEq/L
CO_2	32 mEq/L
Total protein	5.0 g/dl
Albumin	2.1 g/dl
Total bilirubin	1.5 mg/dl
Ammonia	79 µg/dl
AST	47 U/L
ALP	178 U/L
Hepatitis panel	Negative
aPTT	62 seconds
Platelets	184,000/mm³
ANA	Negative

Nursing Physical Examination

Height: 5'10"   Weight: 235 lb (106.8 kg)
Vital signs: BP = 110/75
            TPR = 100.3, 95, 25
LOC: Alert and cooperative
EENT: Moon-faced; sclerae are slightly icteric
Cardiac: Regular rate and rhythm with a grade I/VI systolic murmur

● A CT scan of Mr. James' abdomen revealed a shrunken, cirrhotic liver, an enlarged spleen, and ascites *(white arrows)*. There is also a large regenerating nodule *(curved dark arrows)*.

Pulmonary: Slight crackles in the bases bilaterally
Abdominal: Distended and taut; abdominal girth = 52 inches; fluid wave noted; bowel sounds high-pitched and hypoactive
Genitourinary: Voiding infrequently in small amounts; urine is dark amber
Peripheral pulses: 3/3 with pitting pretibial and pedal edema
Skin: Bruising noted on extremities and abdomen

Initial Treatment Plan

Meds: Famotidine (Pepcid) 20 mg IV bid
      Buprenorphine (Buprenex) 0.3 mg IV q 4–6 h prn for pain
      Phytonadione (AquaMEPHYTON) 2 mg IM qod
      Multivitamin preparation with folate and biotin (M.V.I.-12) 1 ampule IV qd
IV: D_5 and 0.5 NS with 40 mEq KCl at 100 ml/hr
Diet: NPO
Activity: Bed rest with BRP, elevate HOB
Additional assessments: Measure abdominal girth and I&O daily weights
Respiratory treatments: O_2 2 L per nasal cannula, albuterol (Ventolin) 2.5 mg in 3 ml NS aerosol qid, spot O_2 oximetry qd
Diagnostic tests: Hb and Hct q 4 h; call if Hb <10 g/dl, aPTT daily

Oozing esophageal varices (see figure) were discovered during Mr. James' endoscopy. The physician notes, as a probable cause, cirrhosis and portal hypertension. During the visit for the CT scan, the nurse tells Mr. James' daughter that liver disease is suspected. The daughter replies, "I'm not surprised. He's been drinking like a fish for years." Upon further inquiry, the daughter states that her father drinks both beer and hard liquor from morning until night while frequently skipping meals.

Mr. James' CT scan reveals a shrunken and cirrhotic liver, splenomegaly, and ascites. During the paracentesis, 60 ml of clear yellow fluid was aspirated. Initial results indicate the absence of abnormal or malignant cells and bacteria. Following diagnostic examinations, the physician discontinues the buprenorphine and orders acetaminophen (Tylenol) 650 mg q 4 h prn. Consider the rationale for this change.

In addition, the physician orders bumetanide (Bumex) 1 mg IV bid. A one-time dose of salt-poor albumin 25 g

● Oozing varix. (Courtesy of Martin Sears, Internal Medicine and Diagnostic Problems, Fremont, NE.)

IV is also ordered. Consider the rationale of using these medications for treatment of ascites. Which of these orders should be implemented first? Why?

Mr. James' hemoglobin level remains stable, and no further bleeding is noted. He is started on an all-cooked, high-carbohydrate, moderate-protein (60–70 g/day) and low-sodium (1–2 g/day) diet. He is to limit his intake of fluids to 1500 ml/day. The intravenous and intramuscular vitamin K preparations are discontinued. Vitamin K (phytonadione) 5 mg PO twice a week and a daily supplement of B vitamins are added to his medication orders. The famotidine is changed from the intravenous route to the oral route of administration. Lansoprazole (Prevacid) 15 mg PO every AM, 30 minutes before breakfast, is added. The bumetanide IV order is discontinued and replaced with an order for spironolactone (Aldactone) 25 mg bid

and potassium (K-Dur) 20 mEq/day. Docusate (Colace) 100 mg/day is also ordered. Discharge is planned for tomorrow morning.

Discharge Criteria

Average length of stay (LOS): 6.6 days
Initiate teaching of client and significant others about diet, medications, drug and alcohol incompatibilities, fluid restriction, and need to report of bleeding and changes in mental status.
Complete community referrals for client and significant others.
What referrals would you make? Why?

Questions to Be Considered

1. Discuss the pathophysiologic changes that have led to Mr. James' ascites, peripheral edema, weight gain, bruising, and esophageal varices.
2. Discuss what further changes in Mr. James' diet and medications might be needed if certain laboratory values suggest progression of the disease process (e.g., serum ammonia levels, bleeding studies, liver enzymes, serum protein, bilirubin, etc.).
3. Mr. James' family decides to confront him about his alcohol consumption. Discuss the nurse's role in supporting the family's decision. Consider the ethical ramifications of your decision.
4. If Mr. James continues to abstain from alcohol, he is at risk of developing delirium tremens (DTs). What are the manifestations of this syndrome, and what treatments are indicated?
5. What is Mr. James' prognosis? Would he be eligible for a liver transplant? What factors would influence the transplant team's decision?
6. Had Mr. James' bleeding not been controlled, what medical and nursing interventions would have been indicated? Consider both medical and surgical management.

Abbreviations: ALP, alkaline phosphatase; ANA, antinuclear antibodies; aPTT, activated partial thromboplastin time; AST, aspartate aminotransferase; BP, blood pressure; BRP, bathroom privileges; CO_2, carbon dioxide; CT, computed tomography; D_5, 5% dextrose; EENT, eye-ear-nose-throat; Hb, hemoglobin; Hct, hematocrit; HOB, head of bed; IM, intramuscularly; I&O, intake and output; IV, intravenously; KCl, potassium chloride; L, liter; LOC, level of consciousness; LOS, length of stay; Meds, medications; NPO, *nil per os* (nothing by mouth); NS, normal saline; O_2, oxygen; PO, *per os* (orally); prn, as needed; qd, once daily; RBC, red blood cell(s); TPR, temperature/pulse/respirations; WBC, white blood cell(s).

stores. Fat restriction is not necessary. Total daily calories should range between 2000 and 3000. Place the client on daily weight, intake and output, and calorie counts to assess fluid and nutritional balance.

Closely monitor the laboratory and nutritional panels for manifestations of improvement or further deterioration. If ammonia levels rise (normal levels are 70 to 200 mg/dl in whole blood and 56 to 150 mg/dl in plasma), foods high in protein may be restricted.

If the client has ascites or edema, sodium and fluids should be restricted in the diet. Small, frequent meals make it easier for clients with anorexia to eat enough food. Adequate rest and a stable environmental temperature should be ensured to allow optimal use of calories. Administer prescribed medications such as antacids, anti-

emetics, antidiarrheals, or cathartics to decrease gastric distress, but avoid antiemetics such as phenothiazines.

Provide Vitamin Supplements. The physician usually prescribes a maintenance multivitamin preparation or, in severe malnutrition, therapeutic levels of vitamins. Also, vitamins A, D, E, and K are supplied if fat absorption is adequate. The client with severe malabsorption may require IV vitamins with calcium gluconate supplementation. Encourage family or friends to provide desirable foods as permitted.

Activity Intolerance. The client with cirrhosis often experiences severe fatigue, leading to the nursing diagnosis *Activity Intolerance related to bed rest, fatigue, lack of energy, and altered respiratory function secondary to ascites.*

Outcomes. The client will maintain a balance between rest and activity, as evidenced by the absence of fatigue and problems associated with immobility.

Interventions. Clinicians often prescribe rest for clients with cirrhosis, but how much rest is necessary is debated. During periods of acute malfunction, rest reduces metabolic demands on the liver and increases circulation. Long-term planning should include counseling the client to rest frequently and to avoid unnecessary fatigue.

Risk for Injury. Because the liver is in a very precarious state, intake of alcohol or other hepatotoxins should cease immediately. Otherwise, the nursing diagnosis *Risk for Injury related to continued intake of hepatotoxins* becomes appropriate.

Outcomes. The client will not suffer injury from continued intake of hepatotoxins as evidenced by cessation of drinking and avoidance of medications that may cause further damage.

Interventions. Ensure that all known hepatotoxic medications (including alcohol) are removed from therapeutic regimens, and that dosages of all drugs thought to be metabolized by the liver have been lowered. Avoid administration of sedatives and opiates.

Altered Protection. Because of portal hypertension and decreased filtering capability of the liver, the nursing diagnosis *Altered Protection related to alcohol abuse and inadequate nutrition* may be appropriate.

Outcomes. The client will not experience systemic infection or spontaneous bacterial peritonitis with ascites.

Interventions. Clients with cirrhosis may experience spontaneous bacterial peritonitis with ascites. Mortality is high when this occurs. Your role as nurse is to monitor for manifestations of infection and to administer antibiotics as prescribed. Antibiotics may be required to control intestinal flora that aggravate encephalopathy.

Altered Health Maintenance. The client with cirrhosis must become involved in self-care if the treatment is to be successful. Therefore, *Altered Health Maintenance related to lack of knowledge of the disease and long-term treatment is an important nursing diagnosis.*

Outcomes. The client with cirrhosis will understand the disease and the implications of long-term management, as evidenced by the client's statements.

Interventions. Provide the client and significant others with information to manage care at home. Clients with cirrhosis will live longer if they get adequate rest, abstain from alcohol, and eat nutritious meals.

Encourage clients with a history of alcohol abuse to seek assistance from support groups such as AA to stop drinking. Even if cirrhotic changes have begun in the liver, it is vital for the client to stop drinking before irreparable damage occurs. See Chapter 24 for further information on alcoholism.

EVALUATION

The outcome in cirrhosis depends on the client's ability to stop intake of alcohol, or any other substances toxic to the liver, early enough to prevent irreparable liver damage. If biliary obstruction is the cause of the cirrhosis, the client must seek further medical or surgical treatment. Once extensive damage has occurred, the client will not recover and the disease will progress with manifestations of liver failure.

◼ Self-Care

Clients with cirrhosis are managed at home unless they encounter complications or are in the end stage of the disease process. Hence, it is important to teach them how to maintain adequate nutrition, to alternate rest and activity, and to avoid hepatotoxic substances. Refer the client to the appropriate agency or support group for assistance with alcohol cessation such as AA, Al-Anon, or Al-Ateen. Provide referrals to community nursing support agencies as needed. If the client is exposed to hepatotoxic agents in the workplace, suggest that the client try to change jobs. Emphasize that regular check-ups and blood tests to follow the progress of the disease are needed.

COMPLICATIONS OF CIRRHOSIS

PORTAL HYPERTENSION

Portal hypertension exists when there is a persistent increase in blood pressure in the portal venous system occurring as a result of increased resistance to or obstruction of blood flow through the portal venous system into the liver.

Etiology and Risk Factors

Most cases of portal hypertension in the United States are associated with cirrhosis. The portal vein is likely to be obstructed by a thrombus; a tumor is the next most common cause. Box 47–1 lists factors that may cause portal hypertension.

Pathophysiology

The normal blood flow to and from the liver depends on proper functioning of the portal vein (70% of inflow), the hepatic artery (30% of inflow), and the hepatic veins (outflow). Disease processes that damage the liver or its

---

BOX 47–1 **Factors in the Pathogenesis of Cirrhotic Portal Hypertension**

1. *Presinusoidal obstruction*
   a. Outside liver
      (1) Portal vein thrombosis
   b. Within liver
      (1) Schistosomiasis
2. *Postsinusoidal obstruction*
   a. Distal to liver
      (1) Budd-Chiari syndrome
      (2) Right-sided heart failure
   b. Within liver
      (1) Veno-occlusive disease
3. *Increased inflow beyond vessel capacity*
   a. Arterial–portal venous fistulas
   b. Splenomegaly

Adapted from Friedman, S. L. (1996). Cirrhosis of the liver and its major sequelae. In J. C. Bennett & F. Plum (Eds), *Cecil textbook of medicine* (20th ed.). Philadelphia: W. B. Saunders.

major vessels or alter the flow of blood through these structures are responsible for the development of portal hypertension. Portal hypertension may result either from increased blood flow in the portal vein or from an increased resistance to flow within the portal venous system.

The most common cause of portal hypertension is cirrhosis. The pathophysiologic mechanism in cirrhosis is increased resistance, which is intrahepatic and primarily sinusoidal. Portal hypertension may also arise from presinusoidal obstruction, either outside the liver (as in portal vein thrombosis) or within it (as in schistosomiasis). In addition, lesions leading to portal hypertension may be postsinusoidal, either within the liver (as in veno-occlusive disease) or distal to it (as in Budd-Chiari syndrome or right-sided heart failure). Rarely, portal hypertension can occur in the normal liver from markedly increased inflow beyond the capacity of the compliant portal vessels to absorb. Arterial–portal venous fistulas and massive splenomegaly due to infection or neoplasm are examples of causes of this type of portal hypertension. The degree of liver dysfunction varies with the causative process, the duration of the process, and individual client characteristics.

Normal portal venous blood pressure is 5 to 10 mm Hg. Portal hypertension exists when the pressure rises 5 mm Hg higher than the inferior vena cava pressure. Collateral vessels develop in an effort to equalize pressures between the two venous systems. The spleen and other organs that empty into the portal venous system also begin to undergo the effects of congestion.

Clinical Manifestations

In clients with portal hypertension, assessment reveals a network of slightly tortuous epigastric vessels that branch off the area of the umbilicus and lead toward the sternum and ribs (caput medusae); an enlarged, palpable spleen; internal hemorrhoids; bruits, which may be heard over the upper abdomen; and ascites, which typically appears when there is concurrent liver disease.

Direct measurement of portal venous blood pressure is possible only during laparotomy. The diagnosis of portal hypertension often relies on indirect measurements of portal pressure—obtained at liver scanning, splenoportography, abdominal angiography, or liver biopsy—and on other laboratory data (see Chapter 42). Radiography and endoscopy procedures may be used to differentiate variceal hemorrhage from other types of gastrointestinal bleeding.

Outcome Management

■ Medical Management

One of the most serious disabling complications of portal hypertension is dilatation of the superior rectal veins, abdominal wall veins, and esophagogastric veins. With conditions such as cirrhosis, portal venous blood pressure increases, causing esophageal veins to swell and distend. These swollen, dilated veins are called *varices*. Several factors can contribute to the rupturing of varices (Fig. 47–2): increased portal venous blood pressure, increased

FIGURE 47–2 A bleeding esophageal varix. (Courtesy of Martin Sears, M.D., Internal Medicine and Diagnostic Problems, Fremont, NE.)

intrathoracic pressure (coughing and straining at stools), irritation by food or alcohol, and erosion by gastric juices. The veins of the stomach and esophagus are most subject to rupture; when rupture occurs, it constitutes a medical emergency.

Another mechanism that leads to hemorrhage involves the spleen. The splenic vein merges with the superior mesenteric vein to form the portal vein. When pressure increases in the portal venous system, damage to the spleen occurs. Damage to the spleen is not proportional to the increase in portal venous blood pressure. As the spleen enlarges, it destroys blood cells, especially platelets, which increases the risk of hemorrhage and anemia.

Hepatic encephalopathy is an extremely dangerous complication of portal hypertension. This problem usually arises following a period of bleeding into the gastrointestinal tract. Digestion of this blood takes place in the intestines. Because blood is a protein, this process increases ammonia in the gut and bloodstream. In turn, the excessive ammonia disturbs brain function. The Critical Monitoring feature lists assessment findings that mandate early intervention in esophageal bleeding secondary to portal hypertension. Hepatic encephalopathy is discussed later in this chapter.

Death often follows rupture of esophageal varices if the hemorrhage is not immediately controlled. To stop hemorrhage, health practitioners perform emergency measures: administration of vasopressin, balloon tamponade, injection sclerotherapy, endoscopic electrocautery, direct ligation of the bleeding varices, transhepatic embolization

---

CRITICAL MONITORING

Esophageal Bleeding Secondary to Portal Hypertension

Blood pressure ≤ 90/60 mm Hg
Heart rate ≥ 100 BPM
Cool, clammy skin
Distal pulses <2+ on a 0–4+ scale
Slowed capillary refill (>2 seconds)
Diminished orientation to person, place, and time
Restlessness

of the left gastric vein, or even urgent portacaval shunt surgery. Cold saline lavage is probably ineffective but is occasionally done while the client is awaiting transport to surgery or the gastrointestinal laboratory. Fluids, especially volume expanders and blood products, are administered to maintain volume.

CONTROL HEMORRHAGE

SCLEROTHERAPY. To perform sclerotherapy, the operator passes an endoscope into the esophagus and injects a sclerosing agent (e.g., morrhuate sodium) that flows into the varices. The sclerosing agent initially causes inflammation of the vein wall and then fibrosis. The operator may give repeated injections over a period of weeks until the varices are no longer prominent.

TRANSJUGULAR INTRAHEPATIC PORTOSYSTEMIC SHUNT. For years, surgical decompression procedures were used to lower portal pressure in clients with bleeding esophageal varices. However, survival rates in clients with hepatitis were not improved with portal vein–systemic (portosystemic) shunt surgery. Decompression can now be accomplished without surgery through the percutaneous placement of a portosystemic shunt, called a transjugular intrahepatic portosystemic shunt (TIPS). With the use of fluoroscopy, an expandable metal stent is used to keep open a parenchymal tract created between the hepatic vein and the intrahepatic portion of the portal vein. Physiologically, the TIPS is similar to a side-to-side surgical shunt. Placement is successful in more than 90% of the clients and bleeding is controlled in 90 to 95% of clients.

VASOPRESSIN. When varices rupture, IV vasopressin is routinely administered to stop variceal bleeding. Administration of vasopressin achieves temporary lowering of portal pressure. These agents reduce portal venous blood flow by constricting afferent arterioles. Direct infusion of vasopressin into the superior mesenteric artery is most effective. Serious side effects include hypothermia, myocardial and gastrointestinal tract ischemia, and acute renal failure. It is therefore contraindicated in clients with a recent myocardial infarction. Vasopressin may be given in conjunction with nitroglycerin, which is administered intravenously, sublingually, or by patch to minimize vasoconstrictive side effects. Alternatively, somatostatin is at least as effective as vasopressin. Drug therapy may stop bleeding, but it has no effect on survival.

BETA-ADRENERGIC–BLOCKING AGENTS. The effectiveness of beta-adrenergic–blocking agents (e.g., propranolol [Inderal], metoprolol [Lopressor] or nadolol [Corgard]) in the management of acute variceal bleeding is limited, because they reduce the heart rate (and hence the blood pressure) and mask the early manifestations of hypoglycemia. However, studies suggest that such therapy has been effective in preventing a first episode of variceal bleeding or subsequent episodes after an initial bleed.

BALLOON TAMPONADE. Applying pressure to ruptured varices via balloon tamponade may stop the hemorrhage. For this intervention, the clinician inserts a Sengstaken-Blakemore or Minnesota tube into the stomach and inflates the esophageal and gastric balloons (Fig. 47–3). The pressure of the esophageal balloon against the varices may stop the bleeding. It is important to release this pressure periodically to prevent tissue necrosis. The esophageal balloon is not left inflated for more than 24

hours. Also, it is important to remove secretions and saliva that accumulate above the balloon to prevent aspiration. The Minnesota tube has an additional port for aspiration of secretions above the esophageal balloon. Ensure that the gastric balloon is inflated to prevent migration of the tube. You should also have scissors at the bedside in order to be able to remove the tube in an emergency. Complications of balloon tamponade may occur in 15% or more of clients and include aspiration pneumonitis as well as esophageal rupture. This intervention is performed less frequently today now that other treatment is available.

◼ Nursing Management of the Medical Client
ASSESSMENT

The major assessment for you to make is for the presence of hemorrhage. The other important aspect of assessment is to check for indicators of the client's clinical status after any intervention to treat the hemorrhage, such as in assessing tube function after placement of a Sengstaken-Blakemore or Minnesota tube. Monitor the client's vital signs continuously for any significant changes.

DIAGNOSIS, OUTCOMES, INTERVENTIONS

Altered Tissue Perfusion. With rupture of varices, the nursing diagnosis that must be addressed immediately is *Altered Tissue Perfusion related to portal hypertension and rupture and hemorrhage of esophageal varices.*

Outcomes. Hemorrhage will be controlled, as evidenced by the return of vital signs to normal and no further bleeding.

Interventions. The client can learn activities to help reduce the risk of rupture of esophageal varices.

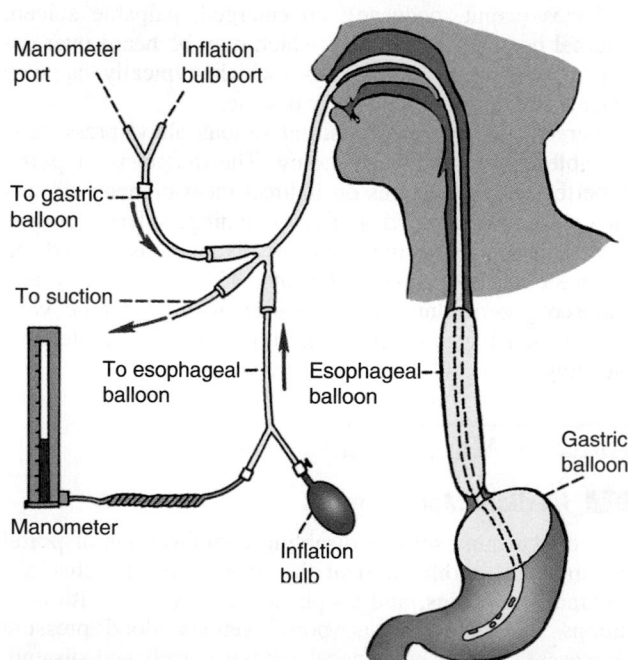

FIGURE 47–3 A Sengstaken-Blakemore tube may be used to control ruptured esophageal varices, a potential complication of portal hypertension.

Prevent Hemorrhage. The nurse should instruct the client as follows:

- Avoid straining maneuvers that increase intra-abdominal or intrathoracic pressure.
- Avoid rough foods, which may traumatize the esophagus, and spicy foods, which may irritate the esophageal mucosa.
- Develop an emergency plan in case severe esophageal varices should rupture. Include in this plan a list of all emergency telephone numbers. Discuss the plan with both the client and family members.

Monitor for Hemorrhage. If hemorrhage from ruptured varices occurs, monitor blood pressure, pulse, respiration, and urine output continuously, and assist with interventions to restore circulating blood volume. Monitor vital signs closely throughout this period. This is a critical time for nursing intervention and can be a very stressful time for the client, family members, and nurse. Further information on the assessment and treatment of shock and hemorrhage can be found in Chapter 81.

Risk for Impaired Gas Exchange. The client
with ruptured varices is prone to many problems. A major potential problem is addressed in the nursing diagnosis *Risk for Impaired Gas Exchange related to decreased oxygen supply secondary to aspiration pneumonitis or obstruction occurring after balloon tamponade with the Sengstaken-Blakemore tube.*

Outcomes. The client will not suffer injury related to the Sengstaken-Blakemore tube, as evidenced by no respiratory distress, absence of aspiration, and absence of esophageal ischemia.

Interventions
Prevent Esophageal Necrosis. The pressure of the esophageal balloon on the esophagus not only stops hemorrhage but also may cause esophageal necrosis. As noted earlier, you must release the pressure on the esophagus periodically to prevent tissue damage. Consult the physician on how often to release balloon pressure, because practices vary widely.

Prevent Aspiration Pneumonia. Aspiration pneumonia is another complication of balloon tamponade. The inflated balloon in the esophagus prevents saliva and secretions from reaching the stomach. Ascertain whether the tube used for tamponade has a suction port above the esophageal balloon. If not, insert a nasogastric tube to the upper balloon level or perform suctioning frequently to remove accumulating fluid.

Prevent Nares Erosion. Tubes inserted through the nose may cause erosion of the nares, especially if traction is applied to the tamponading tube (practices differ). To prevent this complication, clean and lubricate the external nares. Provide padding if necessary.

Prevent Airway Obstruction. Airway obstruction, another complication of balloon tamponade, occurs when the gastric balloon deflates or breaks and traction on the tube pulls the esophageal balloon up into the oropharynx. Keep scissors at the bedside. If this emergency arises, cut the tube and pull it out to restore airway patency. To prevent airway obstruction, label each port of the tube to prevent accidental deflation of the gastric balloon.

Acute Confusion. Because of the potential buildup
of ammonia, the client with bleeding varices is likely to have the nursing diagnosis *Acute Confusion related to portosystemic encephalopathy and hepatic coma occurring in conjunction with gastrointestinal bleeding and accumulation of ammonia.*

Outcomes. The client will be oriented to person, place, and time. Serum ammonia levels will not increase, and level of consciousness will not decrease.

Interventions
Monitor Level of Consciousness. Assess the client's level of consciousness and orientation on a regular basis (after performing a baseline assessment). Ask clients to write their name each day, and assess for writing deterioration and possible rising ammonia levels. Also assess the client regularly for the development of asterixis (liver flap or flapping tremor). Monitor for evidence of gastrointestinal bleeding, including melena or hematemesis, because bleeding can precipitate hepatic coma. Report the bleeding promptly to the physician.

Protect from Injury. Protect the client from injury by keeping the side rails up and the bed in the lowest position. Assist the client with ambulation as needed. Use caution when administering sedatives, antihistamines, and other agents that affect the central nervous system (CNS).

EVALUATION
Although the acute episode of bleeding from esophageal varices can usually be controlled, the development of varices is a sign of deterioration of the liver and increasing portal hypertension. The client will need careful and continued follow-up to prevent recurrence or further complications.

■ Surgical Management

PORTOSYSTEMIC SHUNT
Several surgical procedures can be used to reduce the danger of hemorrhage from varices caused by portal hypertension. These procedures involve anastomosing the high-pressure portal venous system to the low-pressure systemic venous system. This creates a portosystemic shunt.

Surgical creation of a portosystemic shunt reduces portal hypertension by sending portal venous blood directly into the inferior vena cava, bypassing the liver. Other vessels may be altered, depending on the type of shunt selected. Such a procedure lowers portal venous blood pressure, thus decreasing the risk of rupture of esophageal varices. Figure 47-4 illustrates some of the many possible portosystemic (portal vein–vena cava) shunt procedures.

Overall, clients who require portosystemic shunts are poor surgical candidates because of their suboptimal nutritional status, increased risk of infection, and deteriorating liver function. The role of portosystemic shunt surgery in the management of bleeding esophageal varices after initial medical control of bleeding is uncertain.

INDICATIONS. Although surgical shunting reduces the risk of recurrent hemorrhage, the overall mortality of clients undergoing such surgery is comparable with that of

FIGURE 47-4 Some types of portacaval or portosystemic shunt procedures used to reduce portal hypertension.

clients managed medically. The similarity of outcomes is related to the increased incidence of encephalopathy in surgically managed clients when the shunted blood is not cleared of toxic substances, and to the higher incidence of death from progressive liver failure with their increased longevity. For these reasons, surgical creation of a portosystemic shunt is reserved for clients who have not responded to other treatment, and who, despite periodic endoscopic sclerotherapy, continue to bleed.

CONTRAINDICATION. The main contraindication to portosystemic shunt procedures is poor general health, so that the client is not able to withstand the trauma, blood and fluid loss, and anesthesia of surgery.

COMPLICATIONS. Major complications after a shunt procedure are bacteremia and DIC, heart failure, shunt clotting, and hepatic encephalopathy. Clients must he monitored closely to detect the onset of these complications, and corrective measures implemented quickly if they arise.

OUTCOMES. Clients who undergo portosystemic shunt procedures require surgery because other methods of controlling bleeding have been unsuccessful. The goal of these procedures is (1) to reduce portal venous blood flow enough to prevent variceal hemorrhage, (2) to preserve enough blood inflow to the liver to prevent hepatic encephalopathy and hepatic failure, and (3) to increase client comfort (the shunting is a palliative procedure).

▪ Nursing Management of the Surgical Client
PREOPERATIVE CARE

Preoperative management of the client undergoing a portosystemic shunt procedure includes an appraisal of the client's general physical condition and readiness for surgery along with assessment of the client's neurologic, respiratory, and renal systems to establish a baseline. Blood and urine may be examined for the presence of infectious organisms and an arterial blood gas analysis may be performed to assess general respiratory function.

Blood clotting mechanisms are analyzed, as well as the client's fluid and electrolyte status and levels of ammonia, protein, bilirubin, and liver enzymes. If the client has an inappropriate level of any one of these substances, measures are taken to correct the problem. If the hemoglobin and hematocrit are low, the client may receive a blood transfusion. The client's general nutritional status is important, and protein hydrolysates are administered by total parenteral nutrition (TPN) if indicated.

POSTOPERATIVE CARE
ASSESSMENT

After portosystemic shunt surgery, assess the client's respiratory, renal, and hemodynamic status. In addition, observe the client and inspect the operative site carefully for any manifestations of shunt clotting, such as pain, distention, or nausea. Assess the client after portosystemic shunt surgery by monitoring for the following:

- Presence of hemorrhage, hypovolemia, and oliguria
- Fluid and electrolyte imbalance (dilutional hyponatremia, ascites)
- Respiratory rate and rhythm (rales, atelectasis, labored breathing, pneumonia)
- Hypoalbuminemia
- Hypoglycemia
- Manifestations of infection (fever, increased white blood cells [WBCs])
- Pain levels
- Mental status (alertness)

DIAGNOSIS, OUTCOMES, INTERVENTIONS

Nursing diagnoses associated with care of the client after portosystemic shunt surgery include *Altered Tissue Perfusion, Impaired Gas Exchange,* and *Acute Confusion* (see Nursing Management of the Medical Client). In addition, *Fluid Volume Excess* is a pertinent nursing diagnosis for the client undergoing portosystemic shunt surgery.

Fluid Volume Excess. The client who has undergone portosystemic shunt surgery often retains excess fluid, leading to the nursing diagnosis *Fluid Volume Excess related to retention of fluids secondary to portal hypertension, liver failure, and hemodilution of blood related to the new portosystemic shunt.*

Outcomes. A normovolemic state will be maintained, as evidenced by a stable or decreasing abdominal girth and a regular respiratory rate and rhythm.

Interventions

Assess for Fluid Volume Excess. Assess the client for retention of fluid, which is likely to occur because of hemodynamic fluid shifts. Measure abdominal girth to obtain a baseline, and then recheck daily or every shift, as appropriate, to detect development of ascites. Also, monitor weight and intake and output. Output should not be less than intake. Assess for the presence of edema and document its degree, from 1+ (barely noticeable) to 4+ (deep and pitting). Be sure to check for clinical indicators of pulmonary edema, including dyspnea and orthopnea. See that appropriate pulmonary and respiratory therapy is initiated if the client has any respiratory involvement.

Monitor and Treat Postprocedure Complications. Assess the client for hepatic encephalopathy. If portal hypertension is due to liver disease, carefully monitor for postoperative hemorrhage, because bleeding tendencies often arise from liver cell malfunction. Assess cardiovascular function carefully, because the shunt increases venous return to the heart, thus increasing the workload of the heart and placing the client at risk for heart failure.

After surgery, carefully monitor laboratory data, including hemoglobin, hematocrit, prothrombin time, ammonia level, blood urea nitrogen (BUN) level, bilirubin level, blood gas concentrations, and fluid and electrolyte levels. If the hemoglobin and hematocrit are below normal, you may need to administer a blood transfusion. However, many times the low hematocrit and hemoglobin levels occur because of hemodilution that results after the shunt is completed. If clotting time (prothrombin time) is not within normal limits, administer vitamin K. If the client is having difficulty breathing because of ascites, it is doubly important after surgery to implement measures that improve respirations (turning, coughing, and deep-

breathing; respiratory treatments; and maintaining any chest drainage system). Other areas in which you may need to intervene for clients who have undergone portosystemic shunt surgery include the following:

- Administering IV fluids plus blood or volume expanders such as dextran and maintaining line patency and prescribed flow rates
- Monitoring blood and urine values and noting any manifestations of infection (such as increased WBCs and elevated erythrocyte sedimentation rate)
- Eliminating medications that sedate, depress the CNS, or are known hepatotoxins (e.g., acetaminophen)
- Maintaining nutrition: while client is receiving nothing by mouth, i.e., is on *nil per os* (NPO) status, usually for several days postoperatively, administer TPN; when food intake begins, protein intake may be limited and increased slowly if BUN and ammonia levels and mental status remain within normal limits
- Maintaining sterile technique when changing dressing(s)
- Maintaining patency if a gastrointestinal tube is in place
- Assisting the client and family to cope with postoperative discomfort and with issues pertinent to chronic liver disease and its sequelae

When emergency shunt surgery is performed, there may be little time to complete preoperative teaching of appropriate information to the client and significant others. Present careful explanations postoperatively to compensate for the lack of preoperative teaching.

EVALUATION

Although shunt procedures may decrease the bleeding, the long-term prognosis for the client is poor. Severe encephalopathy often develops, followed by coma and death.

ASCITES

Etiology and Risk Factors

Ascites is the accumulation of fluid in the peritoneal cavity that results from the interaction of several pathophysiologic changes. Portal hypertension, lowered plasma colloidal osmotic pressure, and sodium retention all contribute to this condition. Disease processes that lead to these events include cirrhosis of the liver, right-sided heart failure, tuberculous peritonitis, cancer, and complications of pancreatitis.

Pathophysiology

Any process that blocks the flow of blood through the liver sinusoids to the hepatic veins and vena cava causes an increase in hydrostatic pressure in the portal venous system. Most commonly, this problem develops in cirrhosis of the liver or right-sided heart failure. As portal pressure increases, plasma leaks directly from the liver capsule and the congested portal vein into the peritoneal cavity. Congestion of lymph channels occurs, leading to the leakage of more plasma into the peritoneal cavity. Loss of plasma proteins into ascitic fluid from the portal venous system reduces oncotic pressure in the vascular compartment. Reduction in oncotic pressure limits the vascular system's ability to hold onto or collect water.

In addition, hepatocellular damage reduces the liver's ability to synthesize normal amounts of albumin. Decreased albumin synthesis leads to hypoalbuminemia, which is exacerbated by leakage of protein into the peritoneal cavity. The circulating blood volume decreases from loss of colloid osmotic pressure. The secretion of aldosterone increases to stimulate the kidneys to retain sodium and water. As a result of hepatocellular damage, the liver is unable to inactivate aldosterone. Thus, sodium and water retention continue. More fluid is held, and the volume of ascitic fluid grows.

Clinical Manifestations

Ascitic fluid typically produces abdominal distention, bulging flanks, and a downward-protruding umbilicus. Figure 47–5 depicts a client with ascites. Although large accumulations of ascitic fluid are obvious, small or moderate amounts may be more difficult to detect.

Diagnostic tests to confirm the presence of ascites include paracentesis, abdominal x-ray studies, ultrasonography, and computed tomography (CT) scan. These tests may locate fluid in the peritoneal cavity. Paracentesis provides samples of fluid for analysis. Findings help determine the underlying cause of the ascites; for example, the finding of malignant cells may indicate a tumor.

Outcome Management

■ Medical Management

CORRECT FLUID AND ELECTROLYTE IMBALANCE
Fluid and electrolyte balance is corrected by improving renal sodium excretion and restricting sodium and water intake. This involves discontinuing medications that inhibit prostaglandin synthesis and thus impair renal sodium excretion (e.g., aspirin, ibuprofen, indomethacin).

PARACENTESIS. Repeated large-volume paracentesis, in combination with IV administration of albumin to maintain plasma volume, is used to manage clients with ascites resulting from cirrhosis. However, repeated removal of fluid, protein, and electrolytes from the body causes severe disturbances in homeostasis. It is becoming more common to remove the least amount of fluid, such as 100 ml, sufficient to relieve manifestations such as shortness of breath. Clients must be monitored for rupture of the umbilicus.

ALBUMIN. The physician may prescribe IV administration of albumin to replace each liter of ascitic fluid removed.

DIET MODIFICATIONS. The diet is low in sodium with restriction of fluids. Protein intake is moderate unless the client has manifestations of hepatic encephalopathy.

PROMOTE EFFECTIVE BREATHING PATTERN
Edema in the form of ascites, besides compressing the liver and thus affecting its function, may also cause shallow breathing and impaired gas exchange, resulting in respiratory compromise. When ascites is present, potassium-sparing diuretics (e.g., spironolactone) are prescribed. Oxygen may be prescribed, and arterial blood gas analysis and pulse oximetry may be ordered. Semi-Fowler or high Fowler position, as well as daily or every-shift measurement of abdominal girth, is often prescribed.

MAINTAIN SKIN INTEGRITY
When edema is present in liver disease, the client is at increased risk for development of skin impairment and possibly infected skin lesions. If jaundice is present, tepid water or emollient baths may be ordered, along with use of non-alkaline soaps and application of emollient lotions. If antihistamines are prescribed, observe for excessive sedation.

■ Nursing Management of the Medical Client

ASSESSMENT
Some simple assessments to perform at the bedside are the following:

- Percussion of the abdomen; if the client has ascites, the sound will be dull
- Measurement of circumference (abdominal girth)

Standing

Supine

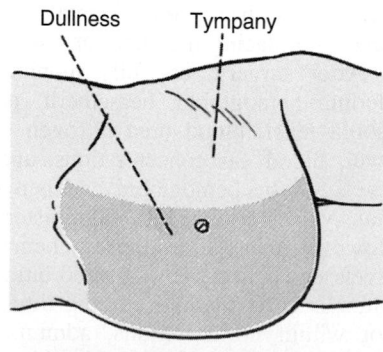
Right lateral

FIGURE 47–5 Assessment of fluid levels in ascites.

- Turning the client laterally and percussing the abdomen (see Fig. 47–5). Because ascitic fluid flows to the lowest point in the abdomen, it will move downward when the client turns; this causes a shift in the area where dullness is heard
- Tapping the abdomen to elicit a fluid wave

Assess the amount of distress caused by the ascites. Ask whether the fluid is interfering with sleeping, eating, and breathing. Assess for the presence of a hydrothorax or misplaced point of maximal impact (PMI). See the Care Plan on Management of the Client with Hepatic Failure.

DIAGNOSIS, OUTCOMES, INTERVENTIONS

Fluid Volume Excess and Fluid Volume Deficit. The client with ascites has a combination of volume problems leading to the nursing diagnoses *Fluid Volume Excess* and *Fluid Volume Deficit related to fluid shifts secondary to portal hypertension, hypoalbuminemia, and hyperaldosteronism.*

Outcomes. A normal balance of fluid between the intracellular and extracellular spaces will be maintained, as evidenced by absence of hypovolemia, normal serum albumin, decreased abdominal girth, and normal blood pressure.

Interventions

Restrict Fluids. The client's fluid restriction must be strictly followed. Give medications with meals, if possible, so that mealtime fluids can be used for taking medications.

Monitor Intake and Output. Measure abdominal girth daily (sometimes twice a day), and weigh the client daily. Monitor intake and output daily. Output should be equal to or exceed intake.

Administer Albumin and Diuretics. Administer albumin and diuretics as ordered. Give the albumin first to pull fluid back into the blood vessels. Give the diuretics second to promote excretion of the extra fluid. Assess the client for electrolyte imbalance and heart failure.

Avoid Hepatotoxins. Avoid administering aspirin and nonsteroidal anti-inflammatory drugs (NSAIDs), because they inhibit prostaglandin synthesis and, as noted previously, impair sodium excretion by the kidney.

Monitor after Paracentesis. Monitor the client closely after a paracentesis procedure. Check vital signs frequently to ensure that the client has tolerated the procedure well, and check the dressing carefully to ensure that excessive amounts of fluid are not lost. Sometimes a pouch is placed to collect leaking fluid. If too much fluid is lost, the physician may suture the site closed to prevent excess loss.

Ineffective Breathing Pattern. Ascites leads to many other problems. *Ineffective Breathing Pattern related to increased intra-abdominal pressure on the diaphragm* is a common nursing diagnosis in clients with ascites.

Outcomes. The client will not experience an ineffective breathing pattern, as evidenced by the absence of shortness of breath and the presence of normal respiratory excursion.

Interventions. Position the client in the high Fowler position to facilitate breathing, and monitor respiratory status for the development of atelectasis or pneumonia. Ask the client to cough and take a deep breath hourly to maintain adequate respiratory function. The client may need to use an incentive spirometer or receive ultrasound treatments if the cough does not loosen and bring up respiratory secretions.

Risk for Impaired Skin Integrity. In clients with ascites, severe edema as well as other problems may develop, leading to the nursing diagnosis *Risk for Impaired Skin Integrity related to immobility, edema, and pressure from the abdomen.*

Outcomes. The client will maintain skin integrity.

Interventions. Turn the client frequently, providing adequate support for the distended abdomen. If the client is on bed rest, recommend a specialty mattress used to prevent skin breakdown. Inspect the client's skin carefully daily, and apply lotions and creams as necessary. Keep the skin cool, and change soiled bed linens as soon as possible.

Altered Health Maintenance. Once the acute problems associated with ascites are controlled, the client and family members are faced with long-term control of the problem, often leading to the nursing diagnosis *Altered Health Maintenance related to lack of knowledge about ascites, treatment, and self-care.*

Outcomes. The client will understand ascites, its treatment, and self-care after discharge, as evidenced by the client's statements, compliance with the treatment regimen, and abstinence from alcohol.

Interventions. Help the client to understand ascites, its treatment, and self-care needs after discharge. Discuss the causes of ascites with the client, making sure that the client understands ways to slow the recurrence. Ensure that the client understands the need for dietary modifications, fluid restrictions, and home health care measures. Help the client to understand that all alcohol intake must be stopped. Refer the client to AA and other support groups for assistance with abstinence if necessary.

EVALUATION

The client's ascites may be controlled to an extent, but once cirrhosis is advanced, it is difficult to control. The optimal outcome is that the client will stop drinking, thereby preventing further liver damage.

Surgical Management

PERITONEOVENOUS SHUNT

The client with refractory and disabling chronic ascites may obtain relief from the insertion of a peritoneovenous (LeVeen or Denver) shunt.

INDICATIONS. Insertion of a peritoneovenous shunt may be indicated for clients whose ascites is not responding to medical management. As Figure 47–6 shows, a properly functioning shunt moves fluid from the peritoneal (abdominal) cavity into the superior vena cava. Resolution of ascites may be dramatic after implantation of a peritoneovenous shunt. The shunt contains a one-way valve that prevents back-flow of ascitic fluid.

CONTRAINDICATION. The main contraindication to placement of a peritoneovenous shunt is a state of health too poor for the client to withstand the trauma of surgery.

COMPLICATIONS. Complications of shunt implantation include infection, hemodilution, DIC, heart failure, and shunt clotting. For additional information, see the earlier discussion of surgical management of portal hypertension.

■ MANAGEMENT OF THE CLIENT WITH HEPATIC FAILURE

Nursing Diagnosis. Activity Intolerance related to fatigue, anemia from poor nutrition and bleeding, ascites, dyspnea from pressure of ascites on diaphragm, muscle wasting.

Outcomes. Client will feel rested, with fewer complaints of fatigue and increased tolerance for activity.

Interventions	Rationales
1. Alternate rest and activity.	1. Conserves energy and reduces demands on liver.
2. Monitor hemoglobin and hematocrit.	2. Allows detection of gastrointestinal bleeding.
3. Assist with activities of daily living (ADL).	3. Conserves energy and reduces demands on liver.
4. Administer iron supplements or blood transfusions as ordered to treat anemia.	4. Increases activity tolerance.
5. Assist with measures to decrease edema and ascites (see Fluid Volume Excess below).	5. Increases lung capacity.

Evaluation. Within a day after paracentesis or shunting surgery, the client will have decreased volume of ascitic fluid, tolerate activity better, perform more ADL, and experience less dyspnea and tachycardia. If ascitic fluid reaccumulates after paracentesis, the activity intolerance will return. Continued improvement will be seen after various shunting procedures. Blood transfusions will immediately improve hemoglobin and hematocrit levels, while iron replacement therapy will take longer to be effective.

Nursing Diagnosis. Altered Nutrition: Less than Body Requirements related to impaired utilization and storage of nutrients, increased pressure on stomach and intestines, feeling full, anorexia, nausea, loss of nutrients from vomiting.

Outcomes. Client will maintain or increase body weight to ideal weight and will consume adequate nutrients.

Interventions	Rationales
1. Weigh daily.	1. Monitors weight loss or gain
2. Provide oral hygiene before meals.	2. Improves taste of food.
3. Administer antiemetics as ordered.	3. Relieves nausea and vomiting.
4. Provide small, frequent meals.	4. Prevents feeling of fullness and ensures adequate nutritional intake.
5. Determine food preferences and assist in selection of those that contain low or no protein and/or low salt, as ordered.	5. Allows preferred foods, when possible, to encourage nutrition.
6. Prevent constipation.	6. Reduces abdominal pressure.

Evaluation. With interventions, the client will maintain weight (not fluid) or begin to gain weight by consuming adequate nutrients and following diet restrictions.

Nursing Diagnosis. Altered Protection related to decreased filtering of bacteria by liver and impaired synthesis of clotting factors.

Outcomes. Client will remain free of infection and will have no bruising or hemorrhage.

Interventions	Rationales
1. Monitor for manifestations of hemorrhage.	1. Decreased synthesis of clotting factors can lead to hemorrhage.
2. Provide assistance with ambulation and ADL.	2. Minimizes risk of trauma and injury.
3. Use small-gauge needles for injections and apply prolonged pressure after injection.	3. Minimizes risk of bleeding into tissues.
4. Recommend soft-bristle toothbrush.	4. Reduces injury to oral tissues.
5. Teach to avoid vigorous blowing of nose or straining at stool.	5. Reduces risk of hemorrhage.
6. Administer vitamin K as ordered.	6. Necessary for synthesis of clotting factors.
7. Follow infection control procedures.	7. Minimizes risk of infection.
8. Monitor for manifestations of infection (temperature, leukopenia).	8. Promotes identification and treatment of infection.

Evaluation. If interventions are successful, the client will not experience hemorrhage or infection.

Nursing Diagnosis. Confusion related to portal systemic encephalopathy occurring in conjunction with gastrointestinal bleeding and accumulation of ammonia in the bloodstream.

Outcomes. Client will be oriented to person, place, and time. Serum ammonia levels will not increase, and level of consciousness will not decrease.

Interventions	Rationales
1. Monitor for manifestations of encephalopathy such as disorientation, changes in handwriting or speech, or coma.	1. Liver is unable to convert ammonia to urea for excretion.
2. Encourage fluids (unless restricted).	2. Promotes excretion of ammonia and urea.
3. Give laxatives and enemas.	3. Decreases serum ammonia.
4. Provide low-protein diet.	4. Reduces generation of ammonia, which is a by-product of protein metabolism.

5. Limit activity.
6. Treat gastrointestinal bleeding as ordered.

5. Reduces generation of ammonia, a by-product of metabolism.
6. Reduces generation of ammonia, a by-product of bacterial action on blood.

Evaluation. Within 1 or 2 days of treatment, the client's serum ammonia levels will decrease and the client will become oriented to person, place, and time.

Nursing Diagnosis. Body Image Disturbance related to yellowing of skin and sclerae (jaundice), ascites, and edema.

Outcomes. Client will cope with body image disturbance; avoid isolation, and initiate or reestablish support systems.

Interventions	Rationales
1. Assess client's response to changes in body.	1. Determines extent of body image disturbance.
2. Promote accepting and nonjudgmental attitude.	2. Respects client's sensitivity to body image changes.
3. Listen and encourage ventilation of feelings.	3. Helps client feel valued.
4. Suggest clothing colors and options and make-up suggestions.	4. Enhances self-esteem.

Evaluation. Within 1 to 2 days of beginning treatment, some of the body changes will be corrected. Jaundice usually resolves in about 3 weeks. The volume of ascitic and edematous fluid can be reduced in a few days. Some degree of ascites and muscle wasting is irreversible, and the client will learn to accept the altered body image. In addition, it is expected that the client will maintain or establish new interpersonal relationships and activities.

Nursing Diagnosis. Fluid Volume Excess related to retention of fluids secondary to decreased serum albumin, increased sodium and water, portal hypertension, and possible shunting procedures causing hemodilution of blood.

Outcomes. Client will maintain a normovolemic state and adequate respirations and will have a decreased abdominal girth.

Interventions	Rationales
1. Follow sodium and fluid restrictions.	1. Helps decrease ascites and edema.
2. Administer diuretics as ordered.	2. Promotes excretion of fluid.
3. Weigh daily.	3. Evaluates treatment measures.
4. Measure abdominal girth every day or shift.	4. Evaluates treatment measures.
5. Monitor intake and output.	5. Evaluates treatment measures.
6. Monitor electrolytes, hemoglobin, and hematocrit.	6. Diuretics may cause electrolyte imbalances; shunting may cause hemodilution.
7. Implement measures to prevent skin breakdown (see Impaired Skin Integrity below).	7. Edema causes skin to break down faster.
8. Administer albumin as ordered.	8. Albumin pulls fluid into blood vessels, where the action of diuretics can remove the excess fluid.
9. Assist with paracentesis procedure.	9. Paracentesis removes a liter or more of fluid.

Evaluation. If some liver function is restored, the client will produce more albumin to promote return of fluid into blood vessels. Administration of albumin and diuretics will promote diuresis within hours, but repeated administration may be necessary because their effect is temporary. Paracentesis is a temporary solution; ascitic fluid will accumulate again if albumin levels remain low and portal hypertension is untreated.

Nursing Diagnosis. Ineffective Breathing Pattern related to pressure on diaphragm and reduced lung capacity secondary to ascites.

Outcomes. Client will breathe with minimal difficulty; there will be no manifestations of hypoxia.

Interventions	Rationales
1. Place the client in the semi-Fowler or Fowler position with arms supported with pillows.	1. Relieves pressure on diaphragm.
2. Assess for manifestations such as crackles or increased respirations.	2. Identifies fluid in lungs.
3. Administer oxygen as needed.	3. Improves gas exchange.

Evaluation. Treatment of ascites will enable the client to breathe with minimal difficulty.

Nursing Diagnosis. Impaired Skin Integrity related to pruritus (itching), edema, ascites, decreased mobility.

Outcomes. Client will maintain skin integrity and obtain relief from pruritus.

Interventions	Rationales
1. Limit bathing to every 2–3 days, with sponge baths in between.	1. Keeps skin moist and minimizes itching.
2. Use warm (95–100° F) rather than hot water.	2. Cool water minimizes vasodilation and itching.

Care Plan continued on following page

continued

■

3. Avoid alkaline soaps.
4. Apply emollients (mineral oil, lanolin, baby oil).
5. Use cool, light cotton clothing, which promotes evaporation.
6. Keep clothing and bedding dry.
7. Keep the environment cool (65–70° F).
8. Avoid activities that promote sweating.
9. Keep nails short and smooth.
10. Administer cholestyramine as ordered.

11. Administer diphenhydramine hydrochloride (Benadryl) at night.
12. Encourage diversional activities.
13. Encourage the client to avoid trauma.

14. Monitor manifestations.

15. Restrict sodium intake.
16. Restrict fluids as ordered.
17. Administer prescribed diuretics.
18. Monitor intake and output.
19. Weigh daily.
20. Reposition every 2 hours.
21. Use special mattress such as alternating air mattress or eggcrate mattress.

3. Soaps dry skin.
4. Emollients reduce evaporation and keep skin moist.
5. Minimizes irritation and itching.
6. Minimizes itching.
7. Minimizes vasodilation and itching.
8. Minimizes vasodilation and itching.
9. Prevents breaking skin integrity when scratching.
10. Combines with bile salts and promotes intestinal elimination to decrease itching.
11. Antihistamine that has antipruritic and sedative effect; itching is worse at night.
12. Decreases perception of itching and improves coping.
13. May have impaired clotting activity, which will result in bruises with trauma.
14. Observes for changes that suggest improvement or worsening of condition.
15. Prevents additional fluid retention.
16. Reduces fluid retention.
17. Reduces fluid retention and promotes diuresis.
18. Assesses renal function and fluid retention.
19. Assesses fluid retention.
20. Relieves pressure over bony prominences.
21. Reduces likelihood of skin breakdown.

Evaluation. After jaundice resolves in about 3 weeks, the client will have relief from pruritus, be able to sleep without interruption, and maintain skin integrity.

■ ## Nursing Management of the Surgical Client

Pre-and postoperative management of a client with ascites is similar to that of a client who has undergone surgery for portal hypertension and esophageal varices. See the discussion of nursing care of the client with surgical treatment of a hepatic problem.

HEPATIC ENCEPHALOPATHY

Etiology and Risk Factors

Hepatic encephalopathy constitutes a spectrum of CNS disturbances. These disturbances may appear in conjunction with severe liver injury or liver failure or after porto-

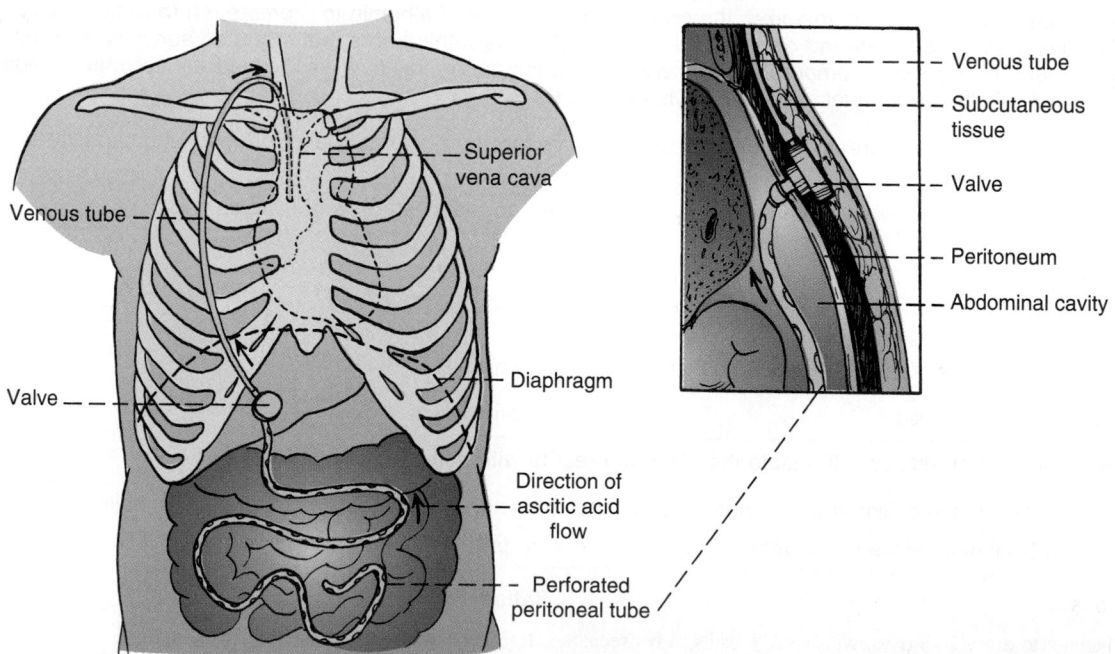

FIGURE 47–6 LeVeen peritoneovenous shunt for chronic ascites moves fluid from the peritoneal (abdominal) cavity into the superior vena cava.

BOX 47–2   Hepatic Encephalopathy: Causes or Precipitating Factors

- Decrease in hepatocellular function
- Hypoxia
- Infection
- Diuretics (produce hypokalemia, alkalosis, and hypovolemia)
- Depressants: (produce phenobarbital, narcotics, tranquilizers, and sedatives)
- Gastrointestinal bleeding
- Medications containing ammonium or amino compounds
- Paracentesis
- Increased protein intake
- Constipation
- Dehydration
- Hypokalemia
- Portosystemic and portacaval shunts

systemic shunt surgery. The cause of this disorder is the liver's inability to metabolize ammonia to form urea, so that it can be excreted. Ammonia is a CNS depressant. Changes during the initial stages of hepatic encephalopathy include reduced mental alertness, confusion, and restlessness. Loss of consciousness, seizures, and irreversible coma occur in the terminal stage.

Pathophysiology

The specific cause of hepatic encephalopathy is unknown, but it is characterized by elevations of ammonia levels in the blood and cerebrospinal fluid (CSF). Ammonia is produced in the gastrointestinal tract when protein is broken down by bacteria, by the liver, and, in lesser amounts, by gastric juices and peripheral tissue metabolism. The kidneys are another source of ammonia in the presence of hypokalemia. More recently implicated as a cause of encephalopathy are false neurotransmitters, elevated levels of mercaptans (organic chemicals that contain the sulfhydryl radical, formed when the oxygen of an alcohol molecule is replaced by sulfur), and fatty acids.

Normally, the liver converts ammonia into glutamine, which is stored in the liver and is later converted to urea and excreted through the kidneys. Blood ammonia rises when the liver cells are unable to perform this conversion. Failure of the liver to perform this function may be due to liver cell damage and necrosis. It also may result from the shunting of blood from the portal venous system directly into the systemic venous circulation (bypassing the liver). In either case, as blood ammonia levels rise, many unusual compounds begin to form. Some of these (e.g., octopamine) apparently act as false neurotransmitters in the CNS. Ammonia also is a CNS toxin, affecting glial and nerve cells; it leads to altered CNS metabolism and function.

Any process that increases protein in the intestine, such as increased dietary protein or gastrointestinal bleeding, causes elevated blood ammonia levels and possible manifestations of hepatic encephalopathy in clients with hepatocellular failure or who have undergone portosystemic shunt surgery (Box 47–2).

Clinical Manifestations

The manifestations of hepatic encephalopathy are primarily neurologic and range from mild mental confusion to deep coma. The neurologic changes occur with cerebral accumulation of ammonia or gastrointestinal bleeding. Hepatic encephalopathy impairs memory, attention, concentration, and rate of response. Sleep pattern reversal often occurs, with the client awake at night and sleepy during the day. Handwriting and speech show significant changes as intellectual deterioration occurs. Asterixis may be present. In some clients with hepatic encephalopathy, hyperventilation with respiratory alkalosis develops because high ammonia levels stimulate the respiratory center. The presence of methylmercaptan causes a characteristic odor on the breath called *fetor hepaticus*.

As the client's condition deteriorates, characteristic delta waves appear on the electroencephalogram (EEG). As the syndrome progresses, the client's level of consciousness slowly diminishes, and confusion becomes more severe. However, the level of CNS depression commonly fluctuates. Coma may eventually ensue, which deepens until there is no pain response and the reflexes, including the corneal reflex, are completely absent. Box 47–3 lists the stages of hepatic encephalopathy.

Laboratory results show elevated blood ammonia and CSF glutamine. Although these findings help to confirm the diagnosis of encephalopathy, they are not specific to it. Monitor serum ammonia levels, electrolytes, blood gases, and hepatic function test results (bilirubin, albumin, prothrombin, and enzymes) throughout the course. These

BOX 47–3   Stages of Hepatic Encephalopathy

Stage 1
Fatigue
Restlessness
Irritability
Decreased intellectual performance
Decreased attention span
Diminished short-term memory
Personality changes
Sleep pattern reversal

Stage 2
Deterioration in handwriting
Asterixis
Drowsiness
Confusion
Lethargy
Fetor hepaticus

Stage 3
Severe confusion
Inability to follow commands
Deep somnolence, but arousable

Stage 4
Coma
Unresponsive to painful stimuli
Possible decorticate or decerebrate posturing

findings help determine the degree of imbalance and the extent of hepatic injury (see Chapter 42).

Prognosis

Although intervention usually alleviates hepatic encephalopathy, the client may succumb to circulatory or respiratory complications, infection, or delirium and convulsions. Mortality is high among clients who progress into coma with hepatic failure. Health practitioners often use dramatic measures to reduce toxic levels of ammonia in the blood. Such measures include hemodialysis and exchange transfusions, which involve removal and replacement of approximately 80% of the client's blood. A liver transplant may be performed in cases of fulminant liver failure.

Outcome Management

■ Medical Management

IDENTIFY AND TREAT PRECIPITATING CAUSES

Factors that may precipitate or severely aggravate hepatic encephalopathy in clients with severe liver disease include gastrointestinal bleeding, increased dietary protein, constipation, infection, CNS-depressant drugs (e.g., opiates, benzodiazepines), and dehydration. Gastrointestinal bleeding and increased protein intake may lead to increased bacterial formation of nitrogenous compounds that induce encephalopathy. The use of CNS-depressant drugs should be avoided in these clients.

Protein may be totally eliminated from the diet, with an intake of only fruit juices and IV fluids, although this radical restriction leads to catabolism of the client's own protein stores. The usual protein restriction is 20 to 40 g/day. The client with chronic hepatic encephalopathy may need to adjust to a long-term, low-protein diet (50 to 60 g/day), which can be difficult. Vegetable and dairy protein may be better tolerated than meats. These proteins contain fewer ammonia-forming amino acids than those in meat. A diet high in vegetables and dairy products also helps prevent constipation, thus further reducing ammonia production.

REDUCE NITROGENOUS WASTE (AMMONIA) IN BLOOD AND BACTERIA IN COLON

Neomycin and lactulose are given to reduce bacteria in the intestinal tract. Because it is not absorbed into the circulation, neomycin exerts a powerful effect on the intestinal bacteria that are responsible for ammonia production. Undesirable side effects result from the depletion of intestinal flora (e.g., diarrhea, vitamin K deficiency). Also, because neomycin is nephrotoxic, its use must be avoided in clients with renal insufficiency. Lactulose, which helps decrease blood ammonia levels by reducing absorption of ammonia, is given to clients to produce two to four stools a day. Antibiotics are administered to inhibit growth of gastrointestinal bacteria, and oral magnesium sulfate or enemas are given after hemorrhage to clean out the intestines.

MAINTAIN FLUID VOLUME BALANCE

With the accumulation of fluid in the abdominal area (ascites), bleeding, and decreased fluid intake, the client may experience a fluid volume deficit. This deficit, along with electrolyte imbalances that may occur, should be corrected. IV fluids are administered, with the quantity and rate of administration carefully monitored.

■ Nursing Management of the Medical Client

ASSESSMENT

When working with a client susceptible to hepatic encephalopathy, use interviewing and assessment techniques to evaluate psychophysiologic status. For example, has the client's normally neat handwriting become sloppy and difficult to read? Is speech slow and slurred? Observe the client for personality changes with labile feeling states, and elicit liver flap or flapping tremor (asterixis) by asking the client to dorsiflex the hand with the rest of the arm resting on the bed. (In asterixis, the hand cannot be held steady.)

The nurse who is with the client over time is often the best person to assess a change in level of mental functioning. Early detection of a depressed or confused level of consciousness greatly improves the client's chances of recovery. To make nursing progress notes relevant, describe behavior vividly and objectively, as in "States pigeons are pecking at his bedclothes," rather than offering interpretations that may have a different meaning for each reader, such as "Seems more confused." As the client progresses into coma, make ongoing neurologic checks to determine the level of consciousness. See Unit 15 for neurologic assessment of comatose clients.

DIAGNOSIS, OUTCOMES, INTERVENTIONS

Risk for Ineffective Management of Therapeutic Regimen: Individuals and Risk for Ineffective Management of Therapeutic Regimen: Families. The client and family members are vital players in the control of encephalopathy. Thus, the nursing diagnoses *Risk for Ineffective Management of Therapeutic Regimen: Individuals,* and *Risk for Ineffective Management of Therapeutic Regimen: Families, related to reduction in protein in the diet and long-term pharmacologic intervention with neomycin* are common with hepatic encephalopathy.

Outcomes. The client will understand and comply with the reduction of protein in the diet and long-term pharmacologic intervention with neomycin, as evidenced by the client's following a low-protein diet and stating reasons why neomycin should be taken.

Interventions
Promote Low-Protein Diet. It is important that the client understand the importance of the reduced protein diet in order to have the motivation to remain on this diet.

Monitor for Gastrointestinal Hemorrhage. In addition to ensuring a low-protein diet, assess for manifestations of gastrointestinal bleeding, checking for bright red blood in the stool or for black, tarry stools. As previously noted, bleeding results in protein accumulation in the gastrointestinal tract, which exacerbates hepatic encephalopathy. To reverse the progression of manifestations, constipation must be prevented. Administer cathartics and enemas to hasten the exit of protein material from the intestine.

Encourage Bowel Cleansing. The client may need to learn to manage diarrhea, a possible side effect related to the laxative action of lactulose or neomycin sulfate. Intervention in severe hepatic encephalopathy commonly combines neomycin therapy with protein restriction and bowel cleansing. Administer the prescribed maintenance doses of neomycin and provide a low-protein diet for clients with chronic hepatic encephalopathy. In addition, administer oral lactulose, a combination of galactose and fructose that passes through the intestine unchanged, to decrease ammonia by trapping ammonium ions and allowing their evacuation from the bowel. As noted earlier, the appropriate lactulose dosage causes two to four soft stool evacuations daily. If severe diarrhea occurs, the dosage is reduced to prevent further electrolyte imbalance.

Fluid Volume Deficit. The client often has difficulties with fluid volume, leading to the nursing diagnosis *Fluid Volume Deficit related to bleeding, decreased intake, and ascites.*

Outcomes. The client will maintain a balanced fluid volume, as evidenced by normal blood pressure, absence of edema, absence of ascites, and balanced intake and output.

Interventions. Hypovolemia often precipitates hepatic encephalopathy by reducing hepatocellular perfusion. Fluid balance must be achieved, maintained, and monitored to prevent further hepatic injury and reduced renal perfusion. Deliver IV fluids evenly over time. Monitor vital signs frequently. If necessary, measure urine output hourly.

Electrolyte and acid-base disturbances such as hypokalemia and alkalosis may precipitate hepatic encephalopathy or may develop during its course. Laboratory tests indicate which replacement therapy is necessary.

Risk for Injury. Because of the multitude of problems faced by the client with encephalopathy, the nursing diagnosis *Risk for Injury related to loss of protective mechanisms secondary to hepatic coma* is common.

Outcomes. Injury or complications of immobility will be prevented or will be identified early, as evidenced by the absence of problems related to immobility.

Interventions. Hepatic coma may create a multitude of problems for the client with encephalopathy.

Prevent Hypoxemia. Hypoxemia may precipitate hepatic encephalopathy by damaging the hepatic cell. To prevent and treat hypoxemia, attend to respiratory interventions (e.g., maintain a patent airway).

Prevent Infection. Concurrent infection, with accumulation of protein from tissue catabolism, necessitates rapid intervention. The client is particularly vulnerable to nosocomial (hospital-acquired) infections. Wash your hands thoroughly, and take other measures to prevent cross-contamination.

Prevent Ammonia Toxicity and Hypokalemia. Be alert to possible harmful accumulations of ammonia due to diuretic therapy. Hypokalemia from the use of diuretics contributes to hepatic encephalopathy by increasing ammonia production in the kidney.

Avoid Sedation. Agents with CNS-depressant effects may precipitate coma, and their use should thus be avoided. If agitation occurs in early encephalopathy, administer agents that are excreted partially through the kidney, instead of the liver (e.g., phenobarbital). *Administer phenobarbital with caution!* Know which narcotics, tranquilizers, and sedatives are biotransformed by the liver; they are often contraindicated in clients with decreased hepatic function.

Prevent Complications of Immobility. The immobile client who lacks protective reflexes (blink or gag reflex) is vulnerable to numerous complications. Preventing complications requires intensive nursing intervention. Measures for intervention are discussed further in Chapter 68 on the care of the client in a coma. Prevent pneumonia and skin breakdown by turning the client frequently and promoting lung aeration.

As the body accumulates metabolic substances, physiologic disturbances develop that may produce a state of agitation. Therefore, protect the client from self-injury, for example, by lowering the bed and padding the side rails. See Chapter 68 for further discussion of the comatose client and the client with neurologic disturbances.

EVALUATION

The prognosis for the client with hepatic encephalopathy is poor. Generally, the best outcome that can be hoped for is maintenance with slowed deterioration.

■ Self-Care

As the acute stages of cirrhosis subside, the ongoing care of the client continues. If the care plan includes discharge from the hospital, provide extensive discharge teaching for the client with cirrhosis who has experienced complications. Family members and significant others need to know how to reduce the incidence of complications from cirrhosis. Review the potential complications with the caregivers as well as how to prevent and treat them.

MEDICATIONS

Review all medications, along with scheduled times of administration and their intended and adverse side effects. Potential medications include lactulose, diuretics, and vitamin supplements.

DIET MODIFICATIONS

Explain the importance of a well-balanced, nutritional diet to the client, with specific information about limitations on dietary protein, sodium, and water. Teach family members and significant others about the need to encourage eating and still maintain food intake within prescribed limits.

HOME MODIFICATIONS

Teach that the client's home may need to be altered to adjust for limitations in mobility. Safety precautions should be taken to help prevent injury to the client. The client's bedroom should be near the bathroom if the client is receiving diuretics.

FOLLOW-UP ASSESSMENTS

The client's status should be followed closely. Be sure that the client's caregivers are aware of any changes that require immediate medical attention. They should also know that diagnostic testing at regular intervals is continued to monitor the status of the liver.

FATTY LIVER (HEPATIC STENOSIS)

Lipid infiltration may lead to hepatic stenosis, or "fatty liver," one of the more common metabolic diseases of the liver. This pathologic process causes liver enlargement and increased firmness and may result in decreased function. Liver biopsy establishes the diagnosis. Laboratory studies reveal that triglyceride is the major lipid involved, but small amounts of cholesterol and phospholipid also may have infiltrated the liver.

Major causes of lipid infiltration include chronic alcoholism, protein malnutrition in early life, diabetes mellitus, obesity, Cushing's syndrome (natural or induced), jejunoileal bypass, prolonged IV hyperalimentation, chronic illnesses that involve impaired nutrition or malabsorption, some hepatotoxins (carbon tetrachloride and DDT [dichlorodiphenyltrichloroethane]), and Reye's syndrome in children.

The manifestations of fatty liver are related to the degree of fat infiltration, the amount of time fat has been accumulating, and the underlying cause. Clients with moderate to severe lipid infiltration are frequently asymptomatic. However, clients with massive infiltration experience anorexia, abdominal pain, and sometimes jaundice. Laboratory studies demonstrate elevated serum alkaline phosphatase and bilirubin levels.

Recovery begins after the source of the problem is removed and metabolic balance and adequate nutrition are restored. Residual damage, if it occurs, usually follows persistent fatty infiltration and chronic alcoholism. Fat embolization may occur and can cause death.

Nursing intervention for clients with fatty infiltration of the liver includes the following:

- Directing attention to correction of the cause (abstinence from alcohol, control of diabetes, weight loss, or correction of the intestinal absorptive defect)
- Preparing the client for diagnostic procedures
- Giving emotional support by allowing verbalization of concerns and fears
- Giving supportive physical care including adequate nutritional intake
- Designing teaching guidelines that promote proper diet and prevent a recurrence

LIVER NEOPLASMS

Tumors of the liver are either primary or metastatic. Primary liver tumors may arise from hepatocytes, connective tissue, blood vessels, or bile ducts. These tumors are either benign or malignant (Fig. 47–7). Figure 47–8 presents a classification of the primary liver neoplasms. Metastatic malignant tumors arise from the gastrointestinal tract (particularly the colon), the breasts, and the lungs.

BENIGN HEPATIC TUMORS

Hepatic adenomas are benign tumors of the liver occurring most commonly in women in their 20s and 30s. Nearly 90% of cases are associated with oral contraceptive use. The fact that the tumors occur more commonly in women, especially women who take oral contraceptives, suggests a hormonal influence in their pathogenesis.

Although these tumors are classified as benign, they are nevertheless dangerous because of their vascularity. A benign adenoma may rupture, with consequent hemorrhage. Diagnosis is made by a combination of tests including sonography, CT scanning, selective hepatic arteriography, and radionuclide scanning. Liver biopsy is not warranted because the tumors are hypervascular.

Intervention for benign adenoma depends on its cause. Discontinuation of oral contraceptives or androgens, when a tumor appears to be hormone-dependent, may correct the condition. Otherwise, treatment may include surgical excision of the involved liver segment. If acute hemorrhage calls for surgery, the surgeon may perform a hepatic lobectomy. Benign hepatic tumors are associated with an excellent prognosis if they can be removed surgically before they rupture and cause death from hemorrhage.

MALIGNANT HEPATIC TUMORS

PRIMARY HEPATOCELLULAR CANCER

Primary hepatocellular cancer (malignant hepatoma) is one of the most common tumors worldwide. It is four times more common in men than in women. About 15,300 new cases of liver cancer were expected in the United States in 2000, which represents a 71% increase from the mid-1970s.[1, 2] Etiologic factors that may contribute to hepatoma are hepatitis B, hepatitis C, cirrhosis,

FIGURE 47–7 Benign liver tumor *(A)* and metastatic malignant liver tumor *(B)*.

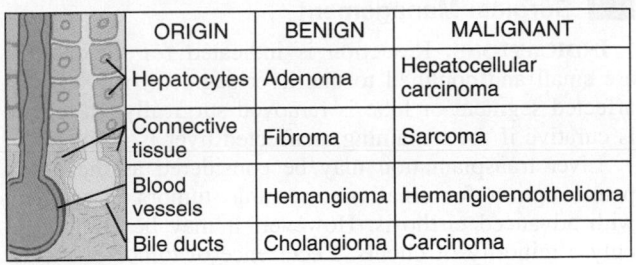

ORIGIN	BENIGN	MALIGNANT
Hepatocytes	Adenoma	Hepatocellular carcinoma
Connective tissue	Fibroma	Sarcoma
Blood vessels	Hemangioma	Hemangioendothelioma
Bile ducts	Cholangioma	Carcinoma

FIGURE 47–8 Classification of primary liver neoplasms.

chronic liver disease, hemochromatosis, ingestion of certain mycotoxins (aflatoxins), anabolic steroid use, and long-term androgen therapy. Primary hepatocellular carcinoma is the main cause of death from cancer in many areas of the world, including sub-Saharan Africa and parts of Asia.

After the diagnosis of liver cancer and if intervention fails to terminate the neoplastic process, the client usually dies of hepatic failure within 3 to 6 months. Surgical resection of the tumor is the only method of cure and may be attempted if the tumor is confined to one lobe. Many clients, however, do not have a resectable tumor because of underlying cirrhosis and involvement of both lobes.

METASTATIC HEPATIC CANCERS

The liver is one of the common sites of metastasis for all cancers. In the United States, metastatic cancers of the liver are 20 times more common than primary liver tumors.

Etiology and Risk Factors

The liver is a common site of metastasis because of the liver's high rate of blood flow, its size, and portal venous drainage from the major abdominal organs. Tumors of the gastrointestinal tract, lung, and breast metastasize to the liver more frequently than do tumors of the prostate or thyroid.

Pathophysiology

Metastatic cancers spread to the liver in three ways: by direct extension from adjacent organs (stomach and gallbladder), via the hepatic arterial system, or via the portal venous system. Also, as a result of cell migration, the surface of the liver may become seeded with metastatic cells.

Clinical Manifestations

Clients with primary (benign and malignant) and secondary (metastatic) tumors often present with similar manifestations. Early indicators of liver neoplasm are usually vague. Many clients with metastatic malignancy of the liver present with the following three types of manifestations:

- Manifestations that are specific only to the primary tumor, hepatic involvement being discovered incidentally in the course of a diagnostic evaluation

- Nonspecific manifestations of anorexia, diaphoresis, fever, weight loss, and weakness
- Manifestations of active liver disease, such as abdominal pain, ascites, and hepatomegaly

Diagnostic studies and physical examination may reveal the following: elevated alkaline phosphatase, hepatomegaly, a liver mass, a friction rub or bruit over the liver, angiographic evidence of neoplasm hypoproteinemia, blood-tinged ascitic fluid, decreased liver function, and reversal of the albumin-globulin (A/G) ratio. The A/G ratio is a calculation of the distribution of two major protein fractions, albumin and globulin. The value of the A/G ratio is > 1.0, albumin divided by globulin (A ÷ G). A high ratio is considered insignificant. However, a low ratio occurs in liver and renal diseases.

Some clients also may have metabolic derangements such as in polycythemia, blood glucose disorders, and high levels of calcium. Other clients may present with marked leukocytosis and anemia. Jaundice occurs more often when a bile duct is the site of a primary tumor or when the tumor mass obstructs a major outflow duct. Other manifestations may be present, depending on the concurrent pathologic condition. At times, the tumor process causes elevation of the diaphragm and some respiratory problems.

Although neoplasms of the liver create numerous clinical manifestations, many pathologic features may not appear until the tumors have grown quite large. Malignant tumor cells may have replaced as much as 90% of normal liver tissue before liver insufficiency becomes clinically evident.

In primary hepatocellular cancers, diagnostic tests often reveal high levels of alpha-fetoprotein (AFP). This substance is sometimes present in clients who have metastatic tumors, but levels rarely reach those found in clients with primary tumors.

A diagnosis of liver cancer is suggested by an elevated serum alkaline phosphatase level and by abnormal findings on ultrasonography, CT, liver scanning, or magnetic resonance imaging (MRI). Cytologic examination of aspirated fluid can also be used to establish the diagnosis.

Liver biopsy is very helpful in establishing the diagnosis. The route of access may be percutaneous, direct via laparotomy, or through a peritoneoscope. Each method has its limitations. Percutaneous procedures may cause seeding of tumor cells along the biopsy needle pathway as it is withdrawn. Laparotomy requires anesthesia, which may be too dangerous. Peritoneoscopy may be impossible if there are extensive adhesions. Because all of these biopsy procedures require internal membrane puncture, be sure the client has an acceptable prothrombin time (PT) because of the risk of hemorrhage if the time is too prolonged.

Prognosis

Because hepatic tumors may be far advanced before clinical manifestations or laboratory data indicate their presence, and because severe liver disease (e.g., cirrhosis) frequently coexists, liver cancer carries a poor prognosis. In the United States, median survival from the time of diagnosis is about 6 months.

Outcome Management

■ Medical Management

RELIEF OF MANIFESTATIONS AND PROMOTION OF PALLIATION

As noted previously, treatment of liver cancer is aimed at relieving manifestations and supporting the client physically and emotionally. The treatment options for medical management include chemotherapy, radiation therapy, and other approaches such as cryoablation.

CHEMOTHERAPY. Regional perfusion of the liver with infusions given directly into the hepatic artery to relieve pain or slow tumor growth may be useful and may produce fewer side effects than those incurred with systemic chemotherapy. Various chemotherapeutic agents have been used singly or in combination with other agents infused into the hepatic artery, or have been given by regional infusion with other agents given systemically.

During surgery, the surgeon may implant a chemotherapy infusion pump. Such pumps, filled percutaneously, deliver medication continuously into the hepatic artery. With metastatic growths, the oncologist may prescribe systemic chemotherapy to reduce tumor size and pain.

Chemotherapeutic agents used to induce regression of primary and metastatic tumors of the liver include 5-fluorouracil (5-FU) and doxorubicin. (Adriamycin) for single-dose therapy and 5-FU with carmustine (BCNU), semustine (methyl CCNU), or streptozocin for combination therapy.

RADIATION THERAPY. Radiation therapy has produced disappointing results. Irradiation of liver tumors may provide temporary pain relief but does not promote survival.

OTHER APPROACHES. Some of the other approaches that have been used for treatment of primary hepatic tumor include alcohol ablation via ultrasound-guided percutaneous injection, ultrasound-guided cryoablation, and gene therapy with retroviral vectors containing genes that express cytotoxic agents. Biliary drainage achieved percutaneously or through an internal stent placed surgically helps increase the passage of bile into the duodenum, decreasing jaundice and discomfort.

■ Nursing Management of the Medical Client

Nursing diagnoses and interventions for clients with liver neoplasms vary according to the amount of liver dysfunction and the treatment modalities. Plan to assess the client for metabolic malfunctions, pain, bleeding problems, ascites, edema, inability to biotransform endogenous and exogenous (drug) wastes, hypoproteinemia, jaundice, and endocrine complications.

Take time to prepare the client in the diagnostic stage for the various procedures, and assess carefully for postprocedure complications. If pain is a problem, administer medication at the prescribed time and dosage. In addition, assist the client and family members to gain knowledge about the condition and offer support necessary for them to cope with the uncertainty and fear associated with cancer. See Chapters 18 and 19 for detailed discussions of nursing care of clients with malignant tumors. See also the Care Plan on Management of the Client with Hepatic Failure.

■ Surgical Management

INDICATIONS. Resection is indicated for tumors that are small and confined to one liver segment or lobe. The affected segment or lobe is removed surgically. Resection is curative if the remaining unaffected liver is normal.

Liver transplantation may be considered as the therapeutic option for small unresectable tumors in a client with advanced cirrhosis. However, it may be curative in only a minority of clients. Recurrence of tumor or metastasis after transplantation has limited its usefulness.

CONTRAINDICATIONS. The client may not be able to withstand the stress of surgery. An additional contraindication to surgery is the presence of liver disease too extensive for surgery to be beneficial.

COMPLICATIONS. Tumor rupture, gastrointestinal hemorrhage from varices, progressive cachexia, and hepatic failure are the primary complications of hepatic tumors. Management of the client with these complications is supportive and palliative and will vary according to the client's overall condition, degree of liver impairment, and extent of surgery.

OUTCOMES. Prognosis is poor. Most clients with hepatic carcinoma have a median survival time of 3 to 6 months.

■ Nursing Management of the Surgical Client

Nursing management of the client preoperatively and postoperatively includes many responsibilities. See the discussion of nursing management of the client who has undergone surgery for complications of portal hypertension, earlier in the chapter.

LIVER TRANSPLANTATION

■ Surgical Management

Liver transplantation is now considered a feasible form of intervention for a variety of end-stage liver diseases. The number of liver transplants has continued to grow each year. In 1995, more than 3700 people in the United States received liver transplants. The demand for livers for transplantation continues to outpace availability. As many as 6000 clients in the United States remain on a donor liver waiting list.

The duration of the surgical procedure is generally 8 hours but can be from 6 to 18 hours. The surgery may be *orthotopic,* involving removal of the diseased liver and insertion of the donor liver. Anastomoses of the vena cava, portal vein, hepatic artery, and bile duct are performed. In the *heterotopic* approach, the diseased liver is left in and the transplanted liver is inserted alongside. Orthotopic surgery is by far the more common of the two. Because excessive bleeding may occur, large amounts of blood, blood products, and volume expanders are needed.

INDICATIONS. The most appropriate candidates for liver transplant are people who, in the absence of contraindications, have severe, irreversible liver disease for which alternative medical or surgical treatments have not been successful or are not available. Ideally, transplantation should be considered in clients with end-stage liver disease who are experiencing life-threatening complications of liver dysfunction, whose quality of life has increasingly deteriorated, or who are predicted to experience neurologic effects of liver damage. If the surgery is performed sufficiently early, contraindications and extrahepatic deterioration are less likely.[12]

Some of the most common conditions warranting transplantation are as follows:

- Primary and secondary biliary cirrhosis (adult)
- Hepatitis—chronic with cirrhosis, chronic viral or fulminant (usually adult)
- Primary sclerosing cholangitis (adult)
- Biliary atresia (pediatric)
- Alpha$_1$-antitrypsin deficiency (usually pediatric)
- Confined hepatic malignancy (adult or pediatric)
- Wilson's disease
- Budd-Chiari syndrome (hepatic vein obstruction)
- Alcoholic cirrhosis

Choosing clients with alcoholic cirrhosis, chronic viral hepatitis, and primary hepatocellular malignancies as liver transplant recipients may be questionable. Clients with any one of these conditions are considered to be high-risk surgical candidates, but liver transplantation may be offered to carefully selected individuals. The alcoholic client, for example, must be willing to adhere to certain guidelines such as abstinence and a substance abuse treatment program in order to be eligible for the procedure. The client must be psychologically stable and have good support systems for the complex postoperative course.

CONTRAINDICATIONS. Contraindications include (1) life-threatening systemic diseases; (2) uncontrolled extrahepatic bacterial or fungal infections; (3) pre-existing advanced cardiovascular or pulmonary disease; (4) multiple, uncorrectable, life-threatening congenital anomalies; (5) metastatic malignancy; (6) active alcoholism or drug abuse; (7) cholangiocarcinoma; and (8) human immunodeficiency virus (HIV) infection. See Chapter 80 for other contraindications to transplantation.

COMPLICATIONS. Postoperative complications can be *hepatic* and *nonhepatic*. They may include cardiovascular and pulmonary problems as well as infection, rejection, hemorrhage, atelectasis, failure of anastomosis, and acute renal failure. Rejection occurs most commonly between postoperative days 4 and 10. Manifestations of acute rejection include fever, tachycardia, right upper quadrant or flank pain, and increasing jaundice. Drugs including azathioprine, cyclosporine, FK506, OKT3, and steroids such as prednisone and methylprednisolone are used to stop or prevent rejection; otherwise, liver function rapidly deteriorates. Chapter 80 describes management of clients undergoing transplantation.

OUTCOMES. It is expected that the client will recover from the liver transplant surgery, be discharged from the hospital in 1 week, and within 3 to 4 months be able to resume a normal life as long as medication and health care regimens are followed closely. Complications such as rejection and infection will slow the progress of affected clients.

The survival rate after liver transplantation has improved steadily since 1983, approximately 70% in the early 1980s to 80% to 90% in the mid-1990s. The 5-year survival rate is about 60%. Survival rate is higher and quality of life better after transplantation in people who

had less hepatic damage before surgery and in those who had fewer extrahepatic manifestations.

■ Nursing Management of the Surgical Client
PREOPERATIVE CARE
Once the client has chosen transplantation as an alternative to care and is placed on the recipient waiting list, an extensive physical and psychological evaluation is required (see Chapter 80). The client must undergo a variety of tests, including blood analysis, hepatic angiogram, abdominal CT scan, chest and hip x-ray studies, electrocardiogram (ECG), bone density studies, and nutritional assessment. The client may also have the opportunity to meet the transplant team. Matching donor and recipient organ size and blood and tissue type are important considerations in donor selection.

Focus on assessing the client's needs in relation to the amount of knowledge and information he or she has. Ascertain how the client and family members are coping with the situation. In addition, the needs dictated by the extent of organ failure will guide care. The specific nursing care needs of clients during the waiting period for a liver transplant depend on the degree of end-stage liver disease.

POSTOPERATIVE CARE
The major focus of care is to monitor for rejection, infection, and occlusion of vessels. Immunosuppressive therapy, which is started before surgery, must be continued on a regular schedule postoperatively to prevent rejection of the new liver. The client requires constant monitoring of respiratory, cardiovascular, neurologic, and hemodynamic status. Liver function is monitored through assessment of serum transaminases (ALT, AST), bilirubin, albumin, and clotting factors. Monitor fluid and electrolyte status, serum glucose, and pH. Clients are always somewhat fluid-overloaded from receiving extensive volumes of blood products during the long surgical procedure. This overload can lead to pulmonary edema and heart failure. Serum potassium will be decreased as a result of transplantation, and serum glucose will be increased. The serum pH will be normal to acidic.

Monitor wound drains and bile drains for patency, and note bile characteristics (amount, color, consistency). Obstruction of wound drains causes increased intra-abdominal pressure from accumulation of ascitic fluid and blood. Obstruction of bile flow can cause damage to the liver and biliary system.

Assess the needs of family members and significant others, who may have traveled long distances from home and may be feeling powerless, stressed, and anxious. Much of the care and many of the nursing diagnoses for a client who undergoes liver transplantation are the same as for a client after any other type of surgery. See Chapter 80 for care of the client after transplantation.

LIVER ABSCESS

A liver abscess is a localized collection of pus and organisms within the parenchyma of the liver. Liver abscess usually develops in association with one of the following three conditions:

- *Bacterial cholangitis,* which results from obstruction of the bile ducts by stone or stricture
- *Portal vein bacteremia,* which may develop following bowel inflammation or organ perforation
- *Amebiasis* (infestation with amebae from tropical or subtropical areas)

Other predisposing factors are diabetes mellitus, infected hepatic cysts, metastatic liver tumors with secondary infection, and diverticulitis.

The client commonly reports right upper quadrant pain and abdominal and right shoulder pain. Assessment may also reveal liver enlargement, tenderness, nausea, vomiting, weight loss, anorexia, fever, and diaphoresis. Sometimes a right pleural effusion may develop. The liver's proximity to the base of the right lung contributes to this process.

Liver scanning is extremely valuable in diagnosis. Other useful diagnostic modalities include ultrasonography, CT, and arteriography. Laboratory data reflect slight to marked elevations of aminotransferases, alkaline phosphatase, and bilirubin. High levels indicate the presence of concurrent obstruction. Blood culture yields positive results in some cases.

Intervention in hepatic abscess consists of (1) percutaneous drainage of the abscess with antimicrobial therapy, (2) surgical drainage of large abscesses with postoperative antimicrobial therapy, or (3) antimicrobial therapy without drainage for a few months. Abscesses due to amebic infestation (such as by *Entamoeba histolytica*) call for treatment with metronidazole (Flagyl) or chloroquine phosphate (Aralen phosphate) instead of broad-spectrum antibiotics. Early diagnosis and therapy for uncomplicated amebic liver abscess result in less than 1% mortality.

When caring for the client with liver abscess, assess vital signs regularly. High temperature and rapid pulse may indicate the presence of general sepsis, a likely complication. Encourage movement, coughing, and deep breathing to prevent or limit pulmonary complications related to hepatic abscess. Increase the client's fluid intake and provide skin care in the event of hyperpyrexia. Dispose of feces carefully, and wash your hands to prevent transmission of amebic infestations.

HEMOCHROMATOSIS

Hemochromatosis is an uncommon disorder of iron metabolism that is often associated with portal hypertension and hepatomegaly. It affects men more often than women. *Primary* hemochromatosis, a recessive inherited metabolic defect, causes increased iron absorption from the gastrointestinal tract. *Secondary* hemochromatosis is caused by alcoholism, excessive dietary intake of iron, or conditions in which repeated blood transfusions have been required, such as chronic anemias.

Total body iron in most clients ranges from 2 to 5 g. Clients with hemochromatosis often have levels of 20 g or higher. The excess iron travels to parenchymal cells, where it is deposited as ferritin (form in which iron is stored in the liver) or hemosiderin (an iron-containing pigment derived from hemoglobin breakdown and one way iron is stored until needed for hemoglobin synthesis). The liver and pancreas are most at risk for iron deposi-

tion and its untoward effects. The heart, spleen, kidney, and skin undergo less damage. As these organs become fibrotic in response to iron deposition, loss of function occurs. As a result, the more common problems associated with hemochromatosis include diabetes, enlarged liver, cirrhosis, cardiac disease, increased skin pigmentation, and arthritis. Pseudogout, a form of arthritis in which calcium phosphate crystals accumulate in large joints, is also associated with hemochromatosis. It is often the arthritis that prompts clients to seek medical attention.

Diagnosis depends on the presence of (1) elevated plasma iron levels (>150 mg/ml), (2) more than 60% saturation of iron-binding protein (transferrin), and (3) manifestations of specific organ dysfunction. Liver biopsy provides the definitive diagnosis.

Intervention involves phlebotomy (a surgical opening of a vein to withdraw blood) performed on a biweekly or weekly basis over a 1- or 2-year period (2 ml of blood = 1 mg of iron). Once the excess iron has been removed from the body, two or three maintenance phlebotomies per year keep the level of body iron normal. If hemochromatosis is diagnosed before cirrhosis develops, phlebotomy can reverse or prevent all of the manifestations except arthropathy and hepatocellular carcinoma. Desferrioxamine mesylate, a chelating agent, also facilitates the removal of iron from the body.

AMYLOIDOSIS

Amyloid is a proteinaceous, starch-like substance that can infiltrate the liver and other organs. Accumulation of amyloid deposits causes tissues to cease functioning. Clinicians classify amyloidosis according to the type of protein that forms the amyloid deposits. In the most common form of amyloidosis (*primary*), light-chain amyloid formed from immunoglobins is deposited. This abnormal protein material causes the most damage to tissues of cardiac, smooth muscle, skin, kidney, and liver origin. However, light-chain amyloid can accumulate in every organ or system except the CNS.

Amyloidosis due to deposition of protein A is associated with chronic inflammation in conditions such as tuberculosis, rheumatoid arthritis, osteomyelitis, and bronchiectasis. Tissues most disturbed by this type of amyloidosis include those of the spleen, kidney, and liver. Although many organs may be affected, the liver incurs the greatest damage. Assessment reveals that hepatomegaly is the most noticeable effect of this pathologic process. Liver function remains relatively unaffected. Clinical jaundice rarely appears. Liver biopsy provides excellent diagnostic data, but there is a high incidence of post-biopsy hemorrhage or liver rupture.

Chemotherapy may be prescribed to provide symptomatic relief of inflammation and pain for the client with light-chain amyloidosis.

CONGENITAL CONDITIONS

Three congenital conditions affecting the liver are Wilson's disease, Caroli's syndrome, and congenital hepatic fibrosis.

WILSON'S DISEASE

Wilson's disease leads to an accumulation of copper in the tissue of the liver, brain, and kidney. The primary manifestations of this disorder are abnormal liver function and neurologic changes. Hepatic manifestations may occur from early childhood to adulthood. This disease is usually chronic but also may be acute. The acute form is often fatal unless transplantation can be performed. One of the hallmarks of this disease is the presence of Kayser-Fleischer rings encircling the corneas. These greenish-yellow–pigmented rings are due to copper deposits. Copper deposits also can be seen on liver biopsy. Penicillamine is the drug of choice to treat this problem.

CAROLI'S SYNDROME

Caroli's syndrome is characterized by dilated bile ducts and cyst formations. The condition may be localized or widespread. Clinical manifestations usually present soon after birth, but the syndrome may not be diagnosed until early adulthood. Fever and bacterial cholangitis are usually the two manifestations that lead to diagnosis. Other manifestations may include right upper quadrant pain and jaundice, both of which may be caused by obstruction of the biliary tract by one or more cysts or stones. Treatment consists of antibiotics, external biliary drainage, or even liver transplantation.

CONGENITAL HEPATIC FIBROSIS

Congenital hepatic fibrosis is characterized by portal hypertension caused by portal vein fibrosis. It usually presents as upper gastrointestinal bleeding from gastric or esophageal varices. Treatment ranges from blood transfussions and sclerotherapy to portacaval shunting.

LIVER TRAUMA

Liver injury usually results from a penetrating injury or blunt trauma. Either may lead to laceration and hemorrhage. Penetrating injuries are usually knife or missile (gunshot) wounds. A knife wound generally is superficial and leaves a sharp clear edge, whereas missile wounds cause perforations through the liver tissue, that is, the entrance and exit points. The greater the velocity of the missile, the greater the damage. Often, a close-range missile injury is fatal because of the large amount of damage. Blunt trauma (e.g., from a steering wheel or a fall) can have various effects, ranging from small hematomas that remain under the liver capsule to large, star-like lacerations from severe impact forces.

Management of liver injuries consists of control of the hemorrhage, debridement, and drainage. Surgical resection of liver lobes may be necessary, but more often the major goal of surgical intervention is to control hemorrhage. Monitor victims of trauma carefully for falling blood pressure and tachycardia, which may indicate hemorrhage. The problem is more difficult when the liver's blood vessels or bile ducts are damaged as well. Later complications include bile peritonitis and abscess formation.

CONCLUSIONS

Hepatic disorders are complex and difficult for all involved. You should have a thorough understanding of the liver and its functions to care for these clients. Many hepatic disorders are the result of the client's lifestyle, further complicating an already difficult problem. The nurse must therefore consider both the physiologic and psychosocial problems associated with many hepatic disorders. Helping the client make appropriate lifestyle changes is an important nursing function.

THINKING CRITICALLY

1. **A 37-year-old man is admitted to the hospital with a 10-day history of anorexia, fatigue, malaise, low-grade fever, dark urine, and upper abdominal discomfort. There is no history of jaundice, IV drug use, or blood transfusions. He is homosexual. Alcohol intake consists of several mixed drinks nightly and wine with dinner. Findings on physical examination include temperature of 99.6° F, jaundice, blood pressure of 150/80 mm Hg, and no spider nevi. The liver measures 12 cm in the midclavicular line and is moderately tender. The spleen is not palpable. Initial laboratory data: total bilirubin, 6.8 mg/dl (normal, 0.2 to 1.2 mg/dl); alkaline phosphatase, 240 units (U)/L (normal, 20 to 90 U/L); AST, 980 U/L (normal, 5 to 40); ALT, 1200 U/L (normal, 5 to 35 U/L). The WBC count is 5600/mm³, with a normal differential count. What are the priorities for care in this situation? What interventions might be used?**

Factors to Consider. Without further data, what would appear to be the major organ systems involved? What additional information do you, as his nurse, think it is necessary to obtain? If you are caring for this client and you inadvertently sustain a needle-stick from a syringe used to give an injection to this client, what action would you take?

2. **A 48-year-old man arrives in the emergency department. He felt well until 2 hours previously, when he became nauseated and subsequently vomited a large amount of red blood and clots. He reports a long history of heavy alcohol use and cigarette smoking. He takes no medications. Laboratory data: hemoglobin, 9.6 g/dl; hematocrit, 28.4%; platelet count, 92,000/mm³; prothrombin time, 16.5 seconds (normal, 11 to 15); alkaline phosphatase, 120 U/L (normal, 20 to 90); AST, 265 U/L; ALT, 112 U/L. What is likely to be a major underlying cause of this client's problem? Is it reversible? Can further damage be stopped? With the client vomiting blood, what should your priority interventions be?**

Factors to Consider. What gastrointestinal disorders can be manifested in people who consume large quantities of alcohol? What risks does the client face in the present situation?

3. Your client is a 68-year-old man with cirrhosis. He is admitted for treatment of ascites and acute upper right abdominal pain. His abdomen is very large, and the ascitic fluid shifts from side to side whenever he moves. Diagnostic studies reveal that the cause of his pain is cholelithiasis, and surgery is scheduled. What are the client's priority needs on admission? What complications might he face following surgery?

Factors to Consider. What are the clinical manifestations of cirrhosis? Is the client with cirrhosis a good candidate for abdominal surgery?

BIBLIOGRAPHY

1. Alexander, I. M. (1998). Viral hepatitis: Primary care diagnosis and management. *American Journal of Primary Care Health, 23*(10), 13–20.
2. American Cancer Society. (2000). *Cancer facts and figures.* Atlanta: Author.
3. Bass, N. M. (1996). Toxic and drug-induced liver disease. In J. C. Bennett & F. Plum (Eds.), *Cecil textbook of medicine* (20th ed., pp. 772–776). Philadelphia: W. B. Saunders.
4. Burke, W., et al. (1998). Hereditary hemochromatosis. *Journal of the American Medical Association, 280*(2), 172–178.
5. Caregaro, L., et al. (1996). Malnutrition in alcoholic and virus-related cirrhosis. *American Journal of Clinical Nutrition, 63*(4), 602–609.
6. Chappell, S. M. (1997). Anxiety in liver transplant patients. *MED-SURG Nursing, 6*(2), 98–103.
7. Dienstag, J. (1998). Liver transplantation. In A. S. Fauci, et al. (Eds.), *Harrison's principles of internal medicine* (14th ed.). New York: McGraw-Hill.
8. Feldman, M., Scharschmidt, B.F., & Sleisenger, M. H. (Eds.) (1998). *Sleisenger and Fordtran's gastrointestinal and liver disease: Pathophysiology, diagnosis, management* (6th ed., pp. 1721–1725). Philadelphia: W. B. Saunders.
9. Friedman, L. S. (1996). Cirrhosis of the liver and its major sequelae. In J. C. Bennett & F. Plum (Eds.), *Cecil textbook of medicine* (20th ed., pp. 788–796). Philadelphia: W. B. Saunders.
10. Friedman, L. S. (1998). Liver, biliary tract, and pancreas. In L. M. Tierney, S. J. McPhee, & M. A. Papadakis (Eds.), *Current medical diagnosis and treatment 1998* (37th ed., pp. 628–665). Stamford, CT: Appleton & Lange.
11. Gubby, L. (1998). Assessment of quality of life and related stressors following liver transplantation. *Journal of Transplant Coordination, 8*(2), 113–118.
12. Hansen, M. (1998). *Pathophysiology: Foundations of disease and clinical intervention.* Philadelphia: W. B. Saunders.
13. Isselbacher, K. J., & Dienstag, J. L. (1998). Tumors of the liver and biliary tract. In A. S. Fauci, et al. (Eds.), *Harrison's principles of internal medicine* (14th ed., pp. 578–581). New York: McGraw-Hill.
14. Jonsen, E., Athlin, E., & Suhr, O. (1998). Familial amyloidotic patients' experience of the disease and liver transplantation. *Journal of Advanced Nursing, 27*, 52–58.
15. Kaplan, L. M., & Isselbacher, K. J. (1998). Jaundice. In A. S. Fauci, et al. (Eds.), *Harrison's principles of internal medicine* (14th ed., pp. 249–254). New York: McGraw-Hill.
16. Kelvin, J. F., & Scagliola, J. (1998). Metastases involving the gastrointestinal system. *Seminars in Oncology Nursing, 14*(3), 87–98.
17. King, R. (1997). Hepatitis C: Past, present and future issues. *Advances for Nurse Practitioners, 5*(3), 51–56.
18. Lee, W. M. (1997). Hepatitis B virus infection. *New England Journal of Medicine, 337*(24), 1733–1745.
19. Lerner-Durjava, L. (1998). Nurse's guide to immunizations. *Nursing 98, 28*(7), 10–12.
20. LoBiondio-Wood, G., et al. (1997). Impact of liver transplantation on quality of life: A longitudinal perspective. *Applied Nursing Research, 10*(1), 27–32.
21. Maddrey, W. C. (1996). Parasitic, bacterial, fungal, and granulomatous liver disease. In J. C. Bennett & F. Plum (Eds.), *Cecil textbook of medicine* (20th ed.). Philadelphia: W. B. Saunders.
22. Marx, J. F. (1998). A, B, C, D, E, and G: Understanding the varieties of viral hepatitis. *Nursing 98, 28*(7), 43–49.
23. McEwen, D. R. (1996). Management of alcoholic cirrhosis of the liver. *AORN Journal, 64*(2), 209–220.
24. Moyer, L. A., & Mast, E. E. (1998). Hepatitis A through E. *Journal of Intravenous Nursing, 21*(5), 286–290.
25. Ockner, R. K. (1996). Chronic hepatitis. In J. C. Bennett & F. Plum (Eds.), *Cecil textbook of medicine* (20th ed., pp. 776–781). Philadelphia: W. B. Saunders.
26. Podolsky, D. K., & Isselbacher, K. J. (1998). Major complications of cirrhosis. In A. S. Fauci, (Eds.), *Harrison's principles of internal medicine* (14th ed.). New York: McGraw-Hill.
27. Reed, S. L. (1998). Amebiasis and infection with free-living amebas. In A. S. Fauci, et al. (Eds.), *Harrison's principles of internal medicine* (14th ed., pp. 1176–1180). NY: McGraw-Hill.
28. Sabiston, D. C., Jr. (1997). *Textbook of surgery: The biologic basis of modern surgical practice* (15th ed.). Philadelphia: W. B. Saunders.
29. Schaffner, W. (1998). The bright spot: Immunizations in 1998. *Patient Care, 32*(13), 123–126, 135–138, 141–144.
30. Scharschmidt, B. F. (1996). Acute and chronic hepatic failure and hepatic encephalopathy. In J. C. Bennett & F. Plum (Eds.), *Cecil textbook of medicine* (20th ed., pp. 797–800). Philadelphia: W. B. Saunders.
31. Scharschmidt, B. F. (1996). Hepatic tumors. In J. C. Bennett & F. Plum (Eds.), *Cecil textbook of medicine* (20th ed., pp. 802–805). Philadelphia: W. B. Saunders.
32. Scharschmidt, B. F. (1996). Bilirubin metabolism and hyperbilirubinemia. In J. C. Bennett & F. Plum (Eds.), *Cecil textbook of medicine* (20th ed., pp. 755–759). Philadelphia: W. B. Saunders.
33. Thanassi, W. T. (1998). Topics in primary care medicine: Immunization for international travelers. *Western Journal of Medicine, 168*(3), 197–202.
34. Wong, J. C., et al. (1998). Pretreatment evaluation of chronic hepatitis C: Risks, benefits, costs. *JAMA, 280*(24), 2088–2093.
35. Zakim, D., & Boyer, T. D. (1996). *Hepatology: A textbook of liver disease* (3rd ed.). Philadelphia: W. B. Saunders.
36. Zollo, A. J. (1997). *Medical secrets.* Philadelphia: Hanley & Belfus, Inc.
37. Zollo, A. J. (1998). Infectious diseases in the United States: A snapshot. *Patient Care, 32*(13), 188–194.
38. Zollo, A. (1998). Understanding hepatitis C. *Patient Care Nurse Practitioner, 1*(8), 32.

Index

Note: Page numbers in *italics* indicate illustrations; those followed by t indicate tables; and those followed by b indicate boxed material.

A

Abacavir (Ziagen), 2196t
ABCDE mnemonic, 274
Abciximab, for myocardial infarction, 1592t
Abdomen, auscultation of, 652–655, 655b,
    742, 754, 1075–1077
  in cardiac assessment, 1462
  computed tomography of, 657, *657*, 746
  examination of, 169t–170t, 652–655, *654*,
    742–743
    in cardiac assessment, 1462
    in lower gastrointestinal disorders, 742–
      743
    in metabolic disorders, *1073*, 1075–1078,
      1076t
    in upper gastrointestinal disorders, 650–
      652
    in urinary tract disorders, 754–755
  inspection of, 652, 754
  palpation of, 655, 655b, 744, 1077–1078
  percussion of, 655, 655b, 742–743, 1077
    in ascites, 1247
  quadrants of, *654*
  radiography of, 656–657, 746
  regions of, *654*
  ultrasonography of, 657, 746
Abdominal angina, 791
Abdominal aortic aneurysm, 1416–1419, *1417*
  case study of, 884–885
  dissecting, 1419–1420, 1449t
Abdominal aortic pulse, assessment of, 1373,
    1374
Abdominal bruit, 654–655, 742, 1462
Abdominal films, 195, 746
Abdominal pain, 472, 705. See also *Pain.*
  assessment of, 743, 1073, *1073*
  characteristics of, 646t
  rebound tenderness and, 743
  rigidity and, 743
  sources of, 646t
Abdominal reflexes, 1889, 1891t
Abdominal rigidity, 743
Abdominal thrusts, 2268, *2268*
Abdominal trauma, 798–799
Abdominal-perineal resection, for colon can-
    cer, 783
  colostomy in, 783. See *Colostomy.*
  postoperative care in, 784–787
  preoperative care in, 784
Abdominoplasty, 1320, *1320*
Abducens nerve, 1870t
  assessment of, 1884
Abduction pillow, in total hip replacement,
    560, *560*
A-beta fibers, in pain transmission, 469
Ablative endocrine procedures, for breast can-
    cer, 1036
ABO blood group, 2087
Abortion, government funding for, 73
Abrasion, corneal, prevention of, 1976
Abscess, anorectal, 797
  brain, 1946
  crypt, 772

Abscess (Continued)
  liver, 1257–1258
  lung, 1716
  pancreatic, treatment of, 1198
  pelvic, *987*, 988
  perinephric, 858
  peritonsillar, 1679
  renal, 857–858
  subdiaphragmatic, 1743–1744
  thyroid, 1106
Absence seizures, 1925
Absolute neutrophil count (ANC), 392, 2171,
    2171b
Absolute refractory period, 1867
Absorption. See *Intestinal absorption; Malab-
    sorption.*
Abuse, domestic, 39
    assessment for, 918
  elder, 57, 57b
Acalculous cholecystitis, 1212, 1213
Acarbose (Precose), for diabetes mellitus,
    1161t
Acceleration injury, 2039, *2041*
Acceleration-deceleration injury, 2039, *2041*
Accidents, emergency care for. See *Emergency
    care.*
  prevention of, 37, 153t–154t, 157t. See also
    Safety measures.
Accolate (zafirlukast), for asthma, 1689, 1690,
    1691t, *1692, 1694*
Accommodation, 1791
Accreditation, for ambulatory care, 92
Accreditation surveys, 102
Accutane (isotretinoin), for acne, 1294
ACE inhibitors, for heart failure, 1538t, 1540
Acetaminophen (Tylenol), 486
  dosage of, 487t
  for osteoarthritis, 554, 555t
  reference values for, 2307t
Acetic acid, 327t, 332
Acetoacetate plus acetone, reference values
    for, 2303t
Acetone, urine, reference values for, 2306t
Acetylcholine, 1871
Acetylsalicylic acid. See *Aspirin.*
Achalasia, 691–695
  clinical manifestations of, 691–692
  etiology of, 691
  in elderly, 694
  medical management of, 692
  pathophysiology of, 691
  self-care in, 694
  surgery for, 692–694
Achilles tendon reflex test, thyroid function
    and, 1079
Acid(s), fatty, 14
  fixed, 260–261
  volatile, 260
Acid hemolysis test, 2302t
Acid perfusion test, 659
Acid phosphatase, reference values for, 2303t
Acid-base balance, 259–271
    assessment of, arterial blood gas analysis in,
      264, 264b, 269–271, 270t

Acid-base balance (Continued)
  compensation in, 263
  correction in, 263–264
  disorders of, 264–271. See also *Acidosis;
    Alkalosis.*
    clinical manifestations of, 270t
    in diabetic ketoacidosis, 1175–1186
    in shock, 2236–2237
    mixed, 268
    nursing management in, 271
    risk factors for, 268–269
    triple, 268
  regulation of, 259–264
    buffer systems in, 259–260, 261, *261,
      262, 263,* 263–264
    kidneys in, 260–261, 263, *263,* 735–
      736
    lungs in, 260, *260,* 263, *263,* 1621–
      1622
Acid-base map, *269*
Acid-fast bacillus smear and culture, for tuber-
    culosis, 1720
Acidosis. See also *Acid-base balance, disor-
    ders of.*
  lactic, in shock, 2236, *2238*
  metabolic. See *Metabolic acidosis.*
  respiratory, 265–266
    in mechanical ventilation, 1756
    in shock, 2236–2237
Acne rosacea, 1294
Acne vulgaris, *1293,* 1293–1294
  benzoyl peroxide for, 1280t, 1294
Acoustic nerve, assessment of, 1885–1886
Acoustic neuroma, 1840, 1933. See also *Brain
    tumors.*
Acquired immunodeficiency syndrome. See
    Human immunodeficiency virus infection.
Acral lentiginous melanoma, 1307–1309,
    1308t
Acromegaly, *1139,* 1141t
ACTH. See *Adrenocorticotropic hormone
    (ACTH).*
Actinic keratosis, 1303–1305
Action potential, 1437
Activated charcoal, for poisoning, 2281
Activated clotting time, 2099t
Activities of daily living, hepatitis and,
    1230
  in elderly, 52, 52–53, *53*
Activity and exercise, after myocardial infarc-
    tion, 1596–1605
  barriers to, 35t
  benefits of, 33
    for young/middle-aged adults, 33–35
  Borg perceived exertion scale for, 33, *34*
  cardiovascular adjustment to, 1367
  fluid intake in, 224
  health promotion/risk management for,
    151t
  in cardiac rehabilitation, 1527–1529
  in chronic conditions, 25
  in chronic obstructive pulmonary disease,
    1698
  in coronary artery disease, 1517

Activity and exercise (Continued)
  in diabetes mellitus, 1158–1159, 1164–1165
  in elderly, 49–51
  in heart disease, 1454–1455, 1517
  in hypertension, 1387, 1394
  in lower back pain, 1986
  in multiple sclerosis, 2015
  in osteoarthritis, 552, 554
  in osteoporosis prevention, 570
  in peripheral arterial occlusive disease, 1402
  intensity of, 33, 34t
  myocardial infarction during, 1585
  postoperative, cholelithiasis and, 1211
  promotion of, 33–35, 35t
Activity Pyramid, 33, 34
Acupressure, 498
Acupuncture, 28, 74b, 498
  for anesthesia, 298
  for urge incontinence, 833b
Acute arterial occlusion, 1415–1416
Acute care nursing, 95–106. See also Hospitals.
  access to, 102
  case management in, 99–100
  client education in, 98
  client management in, 98–99
  cross-training in, 101
  cultural aspects of, 104
  delegation in, 100, 100b
  direct care in, 98
  efficiency measures in, 96
  ethical issues in, 104
  functional, 99
  future of, 106
  history of, 95
  legal issues in, 102–104
  levels of care in, 98b
  nurse roles in, 98–99
  nursing intensity classification in, 101–102, 103t
  primary, 99
  quality assurance in, 100–102
  risk management in, 105
  skill-mix in, 100
  staffing issues in, 100, 101–102
  subacute care in, 96–98, 98b
  team, 99
  total care in, 99
  unlicensed assistive personnel in, 100, 100b. See also Unlicensed assistive personnel.
  work redesign in, 100
Acute leukemia. See Leukemia.
Acute phase reactants, 323
Acute phase response, 2081
Acute renal failure (ARF). See Renal failure, acute.
Acute respiratory distress syndrome. See Adult respiratory distress syndrome (ARDS).
Acute respiratory irritation, occupational, 1739–1740, 1740t
Acute stress disorder, 413–416, 414b
Acute tubular necrosis, causes of, 876
Acyclovir, for genital herpes, 1045t, 1052
Adaptation, 1868
  to chronic conditions, 17–20
    family, 20
    physiologic, 17, 23
    psychological, 17–18, 23–24
    social, 18–20, 24
  to failing vision, 1819b
  to stress, 6t
Addiction, 508–509
  definition of, 463
  to opioid analgesics, 463, 485

Addison's disease, 1120–1126
  assessment in, 1124
  clinical manifestations of, 1120, 1121t
    in addisonian crisis, 1125
  diagnosis of, 1120, 1122t–1123t
  etiology of, 1120
  follow-up monitoring in, 1126
  in elderly, 1126
  medical management of, 1122–1124, 1124t
    in addisonian crisis, 1120–1122
  nursing management of, 1124–1125
    in addisonian crisis, 1124
  pathophysiology of, 1120, 1120
  risk factors for, 1120
  self-care in, 1125–1126
A-delta fibers, in pain perception, 466
Adenocarcinoma, 350t. See also Cancer.
  pancreatic, 1202
  thyroid, 1108, 1108t
Adenohypophysis. See Pituitary gland, anterior.
Adenoidectomy, 1678–1679
Adenoids, 1612
Adenoma, ACTH-secreting, radiation therapy for, 1132
  hepatic, 1254, 1254, 1255
Adenosine (Adenocar), for decreased cardiac output, 2275
Adenosine triphosphate (ATP), synthesis of, 2236
ADH. See Antidiuretic hormone (ADH).
Adhesions, intestinal, 790
Adipose layer, 1263, 1263–1264
Admission, 96, 96b
Adolescents. See also Children.
  immunizations for, 342t
  skin problems in, 1265t, 1265–1266
Adrenal blocking agents, for hypercortisolism, 1132
Adrenal cortex, 1063
  disorders of, 1119–1135
  function of, 1066–1067
    diagnostic tests of, 1122t–1123t
  hyperfunction of, 1126–1135. See also Hyperaldosteronism; Hypercortisolism.
  hypofunction of. See Adrenal insufficiency.
Adrenal function, 1066–1067
  assessment of, 1079–1080
Adrenal glands, anatomy of, 1063, 1064
  disorders of, 1119–1137
  in shock, 2239
Adrenal hyperplasia. See Hypercortisolism.
Adrenal insufficiency, 1119–1126
  hypopituitarism and, 1143
  postoperative, hyperpituitarism and, 1140
  primary, 1120–1126. See also Addison's disease.
Adrenal medulla, 1063
  disorders of, 1135t, 1135–1137
  function of, 1067
Adrenalectomy, for Cushing's syndrome, 1130
  for pheochromocytoma, 1136–1137
  self-care after, 1133, 1137
Adrenergic fibers, 1872
Adrenergic receptors, 1443–1444
Adrenocorticotropic hormone (ACTH), 1138t
  adrenal function and, 1079, 1122t, 1123t
  cortisol and, 1067, 1126. See also Hypercortisolism.
  in stress response, 408
  reference values for, 2303t
Adrenocorticotropic hormone (ACTH) reducing agents, for hypercortisolism, 1132
Adriamycin (doxorubicin), for breast cancer, 1032, 1033, 1034, 1036
Adson's maneuver, 544t
Adult day care, 65, 125, 2008

Adult respiratory distress syndrome (ARDS), 1761–1764, 1763, 1764, 1764b
  in acute pancreatitis, 1198, 1198b
  shock and, 2236
Adult-onset diabetes. See Diabetes mellitus, type 2.
Advance directives, 67–68, 2009
  emergency care and, 2264–2265
Adventitious breath sounds, 1633, 1634t
  in pneumonia, 1713
Advil. See Ibuprofen (Advil, Motrin).
Adynamic ileus. See Paralytic ileus.
Aerobic metabolism, 2236
Aerosols, 1281t
  for hypersensitivity disorders, 2133, 2135
Aerotitis media, 1842
Affect, assessment of, 143, 1881
Afferent neurons, 1869
African Americans. See also Cultural issues.
  cancer in, 353, 353, 368
  hypertension in, 1380, 1381, 1391b
  keloids in, 333, 334
Afterload, 1441, 1442, 1530, 1530t
  reduction of, 1538t, 1540, 1748
    in pulmonary edema, 1748
Age Discrimination and Employment Act, 104
Ageism, 55
Agency for Health Care Policy and Research (AHCPR), 73
Agenerase (amprenavir), 2197t
Aging. See also Elderly.
  cellular changes in, 211, 212t
  chronic conditions and, 14
  cultural aspects of, 47–48
  definition of, 52
  disease and, 14
  functional status and, 52–57
  health promotion and, 45–70
  normal changes in, 50t, 52
  presentation of illness and, 52
  psychosocial issues in, 55–58
  theories of, 211
Agnosia, in stroke, 1957t, 1959–1960, 1976
Agranulocytes, 2080–2081
Agranulocytosis, 2119
  antithyroid drugs and, 1101
AIDS. See Human immunodeficiency virus infection.
AIDS dementia, 2206
Air plethysmography, 1376
Airborne precautions, 344
Airborne transmission, 335
Airway, artificial, 304, 306
  lower, 1613–1617, 1614–1616
  upper, 1612–1613, 1613
Airway burns, 1332, 1335, 1338
Airway management, in asthma, 1690–1691
  in balloon tamponade, 1243
  in burns, 1341, 1349–1351
  in coma, 1910, 1912–1913
  in emergency care, 2267–2270
  in head trauma, 2045
  in laryngectomy, 1666–1667, 1667
  in obstructive sleep apnea, 435–436
  in pulmonary edema, 1748
  in shock, 2244, 2252
  in spinal cord injury, 2053, 2055, 2059, 2062
  postoperative, 303, 303, 304, 306, 308, 308
    in esophageal surgery, 701
    in oral surgery, 688–689
Airway obstruction, emergency care for, 2267–2268
  in tracheostomy, 1654–1655
  upper airway, 1681–1683
Airway resistance, 1617
Akinesia, in Parkinson's disease, 2017

Alanine aminotransferase (ALT), 1082t
  in jaundice, 1221t–1222t
  reference values for, 2303t
Albright's hereditary osteodystrophy, 1114
Albumin, ascites and, 1246, 1247
  fluid balance and, 216
  glycosylated, in diabetes mellitus, 1157
  preoperative measurement of, 277t
  serum, reference values for, 2303t, 2305t
    liver function and, 1082t
      reference ranges for, 656t
  urine, reference values for, 2306t
Albumin/globulin ratio, 1082t
  in liver metastasis, 1255
Albuterol (Proventil), for asthma, 1690, 1691t,
    1692, 1694
  for hyperkalemia, 247
Alcohol Use Disorders Identification Test
    (AUDIT), for alcohol abuse, 39, 40t
Alcohol use/abuse, 513–516
  acute intoxication in, 515
  addiction in, 508–509
  breast cancer and, 1013, 1014
  by elderly, 58–60
  by health care professionals, 524b, 524–525
  causes of, 508–509
  cirrhosis due to, 1233t, 1234. See also Cir-
    rhosis.
  client teaching in, 519, 522b
  delirium tremens (DTs) in, 515, 524
  disease and, 15
  disulfiram for, 519, 522b
  drug treatment for, 515–516
  health promotion/risk management for,
    151t
  heart disease and, 1455
  hepatitis due to, 1232
  hypertension and, 1381, 1387
  hypomagnesemia in, 255, 256
  intoxication in, 515
  medical complications of, 516t
  pancreatitis due to. See also Pancreatitis.
    acute, 1194, 1199
    chronic, 1200
  physical effects of, 515, 516t, 520t–521t
  physiologic effects of, 510t
  poisoning in, antidote for, 2281t
  preoperative assessment for, 274–275
  prevention of, 37
  reference values in, 2309t
  relapse in, prevention of, 522–523, 524b
  resources for, 523b
  terminology for, 509t, 509–511
  therapeutic intervention in, 519
  treatment of, 519–522, 523t
  urinary elimination and, 754
  withdrawal in, 514t, 515–516
Aldactone. See Spironolactone (Aldactone).
Aldolase A, 549t
Aldomet (methyldopa), for hypertension,
    1389t
  perioperative use of, 275t
Aldosterone, 1066–1067
  adrenal function and, 1079, 1123t
  deficiency of, 1121t. See also Addison's dis-
    ease.
  excess of, 1133–1135, 1134, 1135b
  in blood pressure regulation, 1383, 1383
  in fluid balance, 217, 218
  plasma, reference values for, 2303t
  urine, reference values for, 2306t
Alendronate (Fosamax), for osteoporosis, 571t,
    572
  for Paget's disease, 575
Alkaline phosphatase (ALP), 1082t
  in parathyroid disorders, 1111t
  in prostate cancer, 941

Alkaline phosphatase (ALP) (Continued)
  normal values for, 549t
  reference values for, 2302t, 2303t
Alkaline reflux gastritis, postoperative, 721
Alkalosis. See also Acid-base balance, disor-
    ders of.
  metabolic, 266–267
  respiratory, 264–265
    in mechanical ventilation, 1756
    in shock, 2236–2237
Allen's test, 269, 1374, 1641, 1642
Allergen, avoidance of, 2133
  identification of, 2133
Allergic contact dermatitis, 1286, 1291,
    1291
Allergic reactions, 2135–2138, 2136b, 2137t.
    See also Hypersensitivity disorders.
  anaphylactic, 2130, 2137t, 2137–2138,
    2233–2234. See also Anaphylactic
    shock.
    diphenhydramine for, 2251
    epinephrine for, 2251
  chemical mediators of, 2131t
  definition of, 1267
  ear manifestations of, 1799–1800
  eye manifestations of, 1789
  health promotion/risk management for,
    150t
  in asthma, 1685–1686
  in surgical clients, 302
  skin tests for, 1291, 2101
  to chemotherapy drugs, 387–388
  to contrast agents, 196b
  to fluorescein, 1798
  to food, 648, 2135, 2136b
    in atopic dermatitis, 1288
    tests for, 2101–2102
  to insect stings, 2127t, 2137–2138
  to latex, 302, 2137, 2138
  to lipids, in total parenteral nutrition, 670
  vs. irritation, 1267
Allergic rhinitis, 1679–1680, 2138
Alopecia, 1271–1722
  in chemotherapy, 394
ALP. See Alkaline phosphatase (ALP).
Alpha₁-antitrypsin, deficiency of, in emphy-
    sema, 1695–1696
Alpha-adrenergic blocking agents, for benign
    prostatic hyperplasia, 947
Alpha-adrenergic receptors, 1443–1444
Alpha-fetoprotein (AFP), liver function and,
    1083
Alpha-glucosidase inhibitors, for diabetes mel-
    litus, 1159, 1161t
Alpha-hydroxy acids, 1283
Alpha-hydroxy acid peel, 1318
Alprostadil, for erectile dysfunction, 974
Alternative therapies, 27t, 27–28
  for Alzheimer's disease, 2005
  for benign prostatic hyperplasia, 946b, 948–
    949
  for cancer, 390
  for cardiovascular disease, 1525b
  for chronic conditions, 27t, 27–28
  for dysmenorrhea, 980
  for dyspnea, 452
  for ear disorders, 1799
  for endocrine disorders, 1072
  for heart disease, 1453, 1525b
  for HIV infection, 2200
  for irritable bowel syndrome, 794b
  for male reproductive disorders, 935
  for menstrual disorders, 916
  for metabolic disorders, 1072
  for neurologic disorders, 1879
  for osteoarthritis, 554
  for pain, 496–500

Alternative therapies (Continued)
  for respiratory disorders, 1626
  for rheumatoid arthritis, 2153, 2154b
  for skin disorders, 1267, 1283, 1287b
  for vascular disorders, 1370, 1405
  herbal. See Herbal remedies.
  in health history, 136
  interest in, 27–28
  nutritional supplements in, 647–648, 648t
  perioperative use of, 282
  safety and effectiveness of, 28
  spirituality and, 413
  traditional healers and, 74b–75b
  types of, 27t
Aluminum intoxication, in hemodialysis,
    894
Alveolar surface tension, 1617
Alveoli, 1614, 1615–1616, 1616
Alzheimer's disease, 57–58, 2002–2009. See
    also Dementia.
  clinical manifestations of, 2003b, 2003–
    2004
  diagnosis of, 2004
  epidemiology of, 2003
  etiology of, 2003
  family needs in, 2007–2009, 2008b, 2010t–
    2011t
  medical management of, 2004–2005,
    2005t
  nursing management of, 2005–2009
  pathophysiology of, 2003, 2003
  progression of, 2003b, 2003–2004
  risk factors for, 2003
  self-care in, 2006–2007
  sleep problems in, 438
Amantadine (Symmetrel), for Parkinson's dis-
    ease, 2019t
Amaurosis, 1797
Ambulation, in hemiplegia, 1972–1973
  postoperative, 286, 308
    preoperative teaching for, 286
Ambulatory care, 83–93
Ambulatory care nursing, accreditation in, 92
  certification in, 91–92
  challenges of, 84
  characteristics of, 83
  clinical model for, 84
  competence in, 91
  conceptual framework for, 85–86, 86
  definition of, 83
  expert practice in, 91
  holistic care in, 84
  in emergency departments, 88
  in HMOs, 88
  in outpatient departments, 87
  in physician offices, 87
  interdisciplinary team in, 91
  licensure in, 92
  nursing roles in, 89, 90
  patient population in, 88, 88–89, 89
  practice settings for, 86–88
  research in, 89
  standards of care for, 91
  telephone practice in, 89–91
  trends in, 84, 92
Ambulatory esophageal pH monitoring, 659
Ambulatory surgery. See also under Intraoper-
    ative; Perioperative; Postoperative; Pre-
    operative; Surgery.
  case management for, 283
Amebiasis, 767
  liver abscess and, 1258
Amenorrhea, 982–983, 983
Americaine (benzocaine), 297t
American Association of Retired Persons
    (AARP), 76
American Hospital Association (AHA), 76

American Nurses Association (ANA), health definition of, 10
  policy statements of, on health promotion, 10
Americans with Disabilities Act, 104
Amidate (etomidate), for rapid-sequence induction, 2268
Amikacin, reference values for, 2307t
Amiloride (midamor), for hypertension, 1389t
Amino acids, hormones derived from, 1061
  in parenteral nutrition, 668
  plasma levels of, 1067
Aminolevulinic acid, urine, reference values for, 2306t
Aminophylline, for asthma, 1690, 1691t, *1692, 1694*
Aminosalicylates, for inflammatory bowel disease, 773
Amiodarone, reference values for, 2308t
Amitriptyline, perioperative use of, 275t
  reference values for, 2308t
Ammonia, as buffer, 261, *262*
  in cirrhosis, 1239
    and confusion, 1243
  in hepatic encephalopathy, 1251, 1252, 1253
  plasma levels of, 1082t
Ammonia nitrogen, reference values for, 2303t
Ammonia trapping, 736
Ammonium, formation of, 736
Amoxapine, perioperative use of, 275t
Amphetamines, abuse of, 510t, 514t, 516, 520t–521t
Amphotericin B, for fungal pulmonary infections, 1724
Amprenavir (Agenerase), 2197t
Amputation, 1410–1415
  gait training in, 1413–1414
  level of, 1410, *1411*
  lower extremity, 1410–1415
  phantom limb sensation and, 473
  postoperative care in, 1412–1414
  preoperative assessment for, 1410–1415
  preoperative care in, 1410–1412
  prosthesis for, 1412–1413, *1413,* 1414b
  psychosocial aspects of, 1410, 1414
  stump care in, 1414b
  stump wrapping in, *1412,* 1413
  traumatic, 1328, 1415
    emergency care for, 2279
  types of, 1410–1415
Amsler grid, 1794
Amylase, serum, 1081t
  in acute pancreatitis, 1195
  reference values for, 2303t
  urine, 1081t
    after pancreas transplantation, 1172
    in acute pancreatitis, 1195
    reference values for, 2306t
Amylase/creatinine clearance ratio, urine, reference values for, 2306t
Amyloidosis, 1258
Amyotrophic lateral sclerosis (ALS), 2023–2024
Anaerobic metabolism, 2236
Anal examination, 172t, 743, *744*
Anal fissure, *795,* 797
Anal fistula, 797
Anal reflex, 1889, 1891t
Anal sphincter, examination of, 743
Anal tumors, 797
Analgesia. See also *Pain management.*
  effectiveness of, factors affecting, 492–494
  nerve block, 496
  nurse-administered (demand), 494
  patient-controlled, 311, *311,* 494–495
  postoperative, preoperative teaching for, 286–287
  principles of, 493b

Analgesic block, 496
Analgesics, addiction to, 463, 485
  adjuvant, 450–451, 451t
  adjuvant medications for, 491–492
  administration of, 480–481
    by patient, 311, *311,* 494–495
    epidural, 495
    intramuscular, 495
    intravenous, 495
    on prn basis, 494
    oral, 495
    rectal, 495
    spinal, 495
    transdermal, 495
    transmucosal, 495
  ceiling effect of, 485
  definition of, 483
  dependence on, 485
  dosage of, 450, 451, 487t, 489t–490t, 493–494
    equianalgesic, 289t–290t, 487t, 489t–490t, 492–493
  drug interactions of, 493
  duration of action of, 489t–490t, 492
  effectiveness of, factors affecting, 492–494
  for osteoarthritis, 554, 555t
  mechanism of action of, 469–470
  mu agonist, 450
  nephrotoxicity of, 854
  non-opioid, 485–486
    dosage of, 487t
    types of, 485–486
  opioid. See *Opioid analgesics.*
  oral potency of, 492–493
  peak effect of, 489t–490t, 492
  preoperative, 290t
  reference ranges for, 2307t
  relative potency of, 489t–490t, 492
  selection of, 484–485, *485,* 488t
  tolerance to, 485
  types of, 485–491
  urinary, 805t, 806
Anaphylactic shock. See also *Shock.*
  etiology of, 2233–2234
Anaphylaxis, 2130, 2137t, 2137–2138
  diphenhydramine for, 2251
  epinephrine for, 2251
Anaplastic, definition of, 350t
Anaplastic carcinoma, thyroid, 1108, 1108t
Anasarca, 225, 1535
Anastrozole (Arimidex), in breast cancer, 1036
Anatomic dead space, 1614
Androgens, 1067
  deficiency of, 1121t. See also *Addison's disease.*
Anectine (succinylcholine), 295t
  for rapid-sequence induction, 2268
Anemia, 2103–2116
  aplastic, 2115
    after viral hepatitis, 1230
  assessment of, 2109
  classification of, 2104
  clinical manifestations of, 2104
  etiology of, 2103
  folic acid deficiency and, 2113, 2114–2115
  hemolytic, 2115–2116
  in cancer, 393
  in chronic renal failure, 883, 886
    treatment of, 894
  in elderly, 2111
  iron deficiency, 2112–2113
  medical management of, 2104–2109, 2106t–2108t
  megaloblastic, 2113
  nursing management of, 2109–2111, 2112t
  pathophysiology of, 2104

Anemia *(Continued)*
  pernicious, 2113–2114
  screening for, 157t
  sickle cell, *2104, 2116,* 2116–2118
  urinary tract involvement in, 752
Anesthesia, 483–484
  acupuncture for, 298
  balanced, 293
  Bier block, 298
  caudal, *295,* 296
  client teaching for, 282, 292
  cryothermia for, 298
  epidural, *295,* 295–296
  field block, 298
  general, 292t, 292–293, 483
  inhalation, 293, 294t–295t, *295*
  intravenous, 293, *295*
  local, 296–298, 297t, 483, 484, 492
  malignant hyperthermia and, 301–302
  monitored, 298
  neuroleptic, 293
  preoperative teaching for, 282, 292
  recovery from, 303–307. See also *Post-anesthesia care unit (PACU); Postoperative period.*
  regional, 298, 483, 496
  renal injury in, 854
  reversal of, 304
  risk assessment for, 282, 284b
  spinal, 293–295, *295, 296,* 296t
  topical, 296–298, 297t, 484
    for wound care, 2280
Aneuploidy, 350t, 1017
Aneurysm, 1416–1419, *1417*
  abdominal aortic, 1416–1419, *1417*
    case study of, 884–885
    dissecting, 1419–1420, 1449t
  intracranial, 1940–1944, *1941*
    stroke and, 1953, *1954,* 1954–1955, 1956
    subarachnoid hemorrhage and, 1940–1944, *1941*
  peripheral, 1422
  thoracic aortic, 1416, 1420
    dissecting, 1419–1420, 1449t
Angelchick prosthesis, 697, *697*
Angina, abdominal, 791
  nocturnal, 439
  Vincent's, 684–685
Angina decubitus, 1581
Angina pectoris, 1448–1451, 1579–1585
  assessment of, 1448–1451, 1582
  characteristics of, 1581
  clinical manifestations of, 1581
  diagnosis of, 1581
  differential diagnosis of, 1624
  epidemiology of, 1580
  etiology of, 1580
  medical management of, 1581–1582, 1583t–1584t
  nursing management of, 1582–1585
  pathophysiology of, 1580–1581
  patterns of, 1581
  risk factors for, 1580
  self-care in, 1582–1583
Angiocardiography, 1475–1476, 1476t
Angiogenesis, in cancer, 360
  in wound healing, 318, 320
Angiogenesis factor, 318
Angiography, 198, *198,* 1376–1377
  cerebral, 1899–1901, *1900*
  coronary, 1476, 1476t
  fluorescein, of eye, *1797,* 1797–1798
  in peripheral arterial occlusive disease, 1401
  liver disorders and, 1080, 1083
  magnetic resonance, 1376
  of ear, 1804
  procedure for, 198

Angiography (Continued)
  pulmonary, 1647, 1706, *1706*
  renal, 759
Angiomas, 1372
Angioplasty, percutaneous transluminal, 1405–1406
  renal artery, 870
Angioscopy, 1377
Angiotensin, in blood pressure regulation, 1383, *1383*
  in shock, 2239
Angiotensin-converting enzyme (ACE) inhibitors, for heart failure, 1538t, 1540
Animals, handling of, hepatitis A and, 1226
Anion gap, reference values for, 2303t
Anisocoria, 1884
Ankle, sprains of, 621–622, *622*
Ankle reflex, 1889, 1891t, *1892*, 1893b
Ankle-brachial index, 1401
Ankylosing spondylitis, 2160–2161, *2161*
Anorectal abscess, 797
Anorectal disorders, 795–798
Anorectal tumors, 797
Anorexia, 705
  in cancer, 394
Anorexia nervosa, 679–681, *680*
Anosmia, 1636
Antabuse (disulfiram), 519, 522b
Antacids, for gastroesophageal reflux disease, 696
  for peptic ulcers, 711t, 715
Anterior cervical fusion, *1992*, 1992–1993
Anterior chamber, 1791
Anterior cord syndrome, 2051, *2052*
Anterior cruciate ligament, *535*
  injuries of, 623, *623*
  tests for, 545, *546*
Anterior drawer test, 545t, *546*
Anthropometric measurements, 649–650, *650*, 651b, 651t, *652*
Antiandrogens, for prostate cancer, 962
Antianxiety agents, 415b
Antiarrhythmics, 1562t–1563t
  emergency administration of, 2275t
  for myocardial infarction, 1591
  perioperative use of, 275t
Antibiotics. See also specific drugs.
  for acne, 1294
  for acute cholecystitis, 1213
  for bacterial meningitis, 1945
  for chlamydia, 1044t, 1048
  for ear infection, 1844–1845, *1845*
  for gonorrhea, 1044t, 1049
  for inflammatory bowel disease, 773
  for prostatitis, 963
  for pyelonephritis, 855–856
  for septic shock, 2248–2250
  for urinary tract infection, 803, 804t–805t
  in home care, 1487
  nephrotoxicity of, 853–854
  perioperative use of, 275t
  prophylactic, in HIV infection, 2199
  reference ranges for, 2307t
  resistance to, 339, 341b
  sensitivity studies for, 189
  topical, 327t, 332–333, 1280t
  for burns, 1347–1348, 1348t
Antibodies, 2083–2085, *2084*, 2084t
  complement fixation and, 2085, *2085*
  monoclonal, 2085
    for cancer, 389
    for transplant immunosuppression, 2224t
  polyclonal, for transplant immunosuppression, 2224t
  production of, 2083, *2083*

Anticholinergics, for asthma, 1690, 1691t, *1692, 1694*
  for hypersensitivity disorders, 2133–2134
  for inflammatory bowel disease, 773
  for pain, 451, 451t
  for Parkinson's disease, 2019t
  for urinary incontinence, 836, 837t
  preoperative, 290t
Anticoagulants, for coronary heart disease, 1521
  for peripheral arterial occlusive disease, 1406
  for pulmonary embolism, 1706
  for venous thrombosis, in prevention, 1424
    in treatment, 1426
  in arterial bypass surgery, 1407
  natural, 2080
  perioperative use of, 275t
  postoperative, in total hip replacement, 561–562
  prophylactic, for stroke, 1965
Anticonvulsants. See Antiepileptics.
Antidepressants, 422
  for pain, 450, 451t, 491, 492
  perioperative use of, 275t
Antidiabetic agents, 1159, 1160t–1161t. See also Insulin therapy.
  combined with insulin therapy, 1162
  perioperative use of, 275t
Antidiarrheals, 773
Antidiuretic hormone (ADH), 1065, 1138t, 1143. See also Vasopressin.
  diabetes insipidus and, 1143, 1144t–1145t. See also Diabetes insipidus.
  in cardiac regulation, 1444
  in fluid balance, 217, *218*
  in shock, 2239
  inappropriate secretion of. See Syndrome of inappropriate antidiuretic hormone (SIADH).
  release of, *1146*
Antidotes, 2281t
Antidysrhythmics, 1562t–1563t
  emergency administration of, 2275t
  for myocardial infarction, 1591
  perioperative use of, 275t
Antiembolism stockings, 286
Antiemetics, for chemotherapy, 394
  for hepatitis, 1231
Antiepileptics, 1927t, 1927–1928.
  emergency administration of, 2277
  for elderly, 1928
  for pain, 450, 451t, 492
  for status epilepticus, 1931
  for trigeminal neuralgia, 1996
  reference ranges for, 2307t
Antiestrogens, for breast cancer, 1035–1036
Antifungals, topical, 1280t
Antigen(s), blood group, 2087–2088
  definition of, 350t
  epitopes of, 2081, *2081*
  histocompatibility, 2088
  human leukocyte. See under HLA.
  in primary immune response, 2082
  in secondary immune response, 2082–2083
  processing of, skin in, 1264
  prostate-specific. See Prostate-specific antigen (PSA).
  tumor-specific, 358, 361
  types of, 2082
Antigen-presenting cells (APCs), 2072
  in primary immune response, 2082
  in secondary immune response, 2083
Antiglobulin tests, 2096
Antihemophilic factor, 2127

Antihistamines, for hypersensitivity disorders, 2133
  for pruritus, 1286
Antihypertensives, 1387–1391, 1389t–1390t
  compliance with, 1394–1395
  for hypertensive crisis, 1395, 1396t
  perioperative use of, 275t
  stepped-care therapy with, 1391–1392, 1392b
Antileukotrienes, for hypersensitivity disorders, 2134
Antilymphocyte globulin, for transplant immunosuppression, 2224t
Antimanic agents, 422
Antimicrobial antibody, 1083t
Antimicrobials. See Antibiotics; Antifungals.
Antinuclear antibodies, test for, 549t
Antioxidants, 15
Antipruritics, 1280t
Antipsychotics, adverse effects of, 418–419
  for schizophrenia, 417–418, 419t
Antireflux prosthesis, 697, *697*
Antiresorption agents, for hyperparathyroidism, 1110, 1112t
Antiretrovirals, for HIV infection, 2191, 2195–2199, 2196t–2198t
  client teaching for, 2200–2202, 2201t
Antirheumatic drugs, slow-acting, for rheumatoid arthritis, 2150
Antiseizure agents. See Antiepileptics.
Antiseptics, 327t
  topical, 327t, 332–333
Antispasmodics, for urinary incontinence, 836, 837t
  for urolithiasis, 825
Antithrombotic therapy. See Thrombolytics.
Antithymocyte globulin, for transplant immunosuppression, 2224t
Antithyroid antibody tests, 1079
Antithyroid drugs, 1096t, 1100–1101
Antitubercular drugs, 1720, 1721t
Antivenin, snake, 2282
Antral irrigation, 1676–1677
Antrectomy, 720. See also Gastric surgery.
Anuria, 747, 831
  definition of, 876
Anus. See under Anal.
Anxiety, assessment of, 409
  definition of, 407
  in acute pancreatitis, 1197–1198
  in cholelithiasis, 1210
  in hepatitis, 1231
  management of, 409, 409b
  manifestations of, 407b, 408t
  pain and, 451, 451t, 476
  preoperative, 285
  stress and, 407–408
Anxiety disorders, 412–416, 414b, 416b
Anxiolytics, 415b
  abuse of, 511t, 515t, 519, 520t–521t
  for dyspnea, 452
  for pain, 451, 451t, 492
Aorta, abdominal, examination of, 169t
Aortic aneurysms, abdominal, 1416–1419, *1417*
  case study of, 884–885
  dissecting, 1419–1420, 1449t
  thoracic, 1416, 1420
Aortic dissection, 1419–1420
  chest pain in, 1449t
Aortic regurgitation, *1494*, 1499–1500
Aortic stenosis, *1494*, 1499–1500
Aortic valve, 1434t, 1435, *1436, 1437*
Aortic valve disease, *1494*, 1499–1500, 1501
  surgery for, 1501–1502. See also Cardiac surgery.
Aortoiliac disorders, 1401, *1401*

APCs. See *Antigen-presenting cells (APCs)*.
Aphakia, correction of, 1816
Aphasia, in stroke, 1956–1958, 1957t, 1975–1976
Apheresis, for leukemia, 2169
Aphthous stomatitis, 684
Aplastic anemia, 2115
    after viral hepatitis, 1230
Apley's scratch test, 544t
Apnea, *184*
    central, 436
    obstructive, 435–436, 436b
        hypertension and, 439
    sleep, 435–436
Apneustic breathing, *184*
Apocrine glands, 1262
Apoptosis, *361*, 361–362
Appearance, assessment of, 138–139
Appendicitis, 768–769
    peritonitis and, 769–770
Appendicular skeleton, 530, *533*
Appetite, loss of, 705
    in terminal illness, 455, 456t
    stimulation of, 664
Apraxia, 1887
    in stroke, 1957t, 1958
Apresoline (hydralazine), for hypertension, 1389t
    for hypertensive emergencies, 1396t
Aqueous humor, 1778–1779
Arachnoid, 1862, *1862*
Arachnoid space, 1862, *1862*
Arbovirus encephalitis, 1947
Arcus senilis, 1456, 1782
ARDS. See *Adult respiratory distress syndrome (ARDS)*.
Aredia (pamidronate), for bone metastases, in breast cancer, 1036
Areola, 907
    examination of. See *Breast, examination of*.
ARF. See *Renal failure, acute*.
Arginine vasopressin. See *Antidiuretic hormone (ADH); Vasopressin*.
Argyll Robertson pupil, 1995
Aricept (donepezil), for Alzheimer's disease, 2004–2005
Arimidex (anastrozole), in breast cancer, 1036
Arm edema, postmastectomy, 1025, 1429–1430, *1430*
Arm exercises, after mastectomy, 1027b, 1028
Arnold-Chiari malformation, syringomyelia and, 1993–1994
Aromatase inhibitors, for breast cancer, 1036
Arrector pili muscle, 1263, *1263*
Arrhythmias. See *Dysrhythmias*.
Arsenic, reference values for, 2309t
Artane (trihexyphenidyl), for Parkinson's disease, 2019t
Arterial aneurysms, 1416–1419
Arterial baroreceptors, 2234
Arterial blood gas analysis, 264, 264b, 269–271, 270t, 1641–1642, *1642*. See also *Gas exchange*.
    errors in, 269–271, 270t
    in shock, 2243
    in tracheostomy, 1657
    interpretation of, 269
Arterial blood gases, in respiratory control, 1618
Arterial blood sampling, 191, 1641–1642, *1642*
    Allen's test for, 269, 1374, 1641, *1642*
Arterial bypass surgery, for peripheral arterial occlusive disease, 1404–1410
Arterial disorders, assessment in. See *Vascular assessment*.
    clinical manifestations of, 1368, 1369t
    home care in, 1428b

Arterial embolism, 1415–1416
Arterial embolization, for gastrointestinal bleeding, 717
Arterial occlusion, acute, 1415–1416
Arterial occlusive disease. See *Peripheral arterial occlusive disease*.
Arterial oxygen saturation. See *SaO₂*.
Arterial pressure, 1364, *1365*, 1365–1366, 1442. See also *Blood pressure*.
    diastolic, 1442
    systolic, 1442
Arterial steal, 1400
Arterial thoracic outlet syndromes, 1422
Arterial thrombosis, 1415–1416
    thrombolytics for, 1406
Arterial ulcers, 1416, *1417*
Arteries, structure and function of, 1362, *1363, 1364*
Arteriography. See *Angiography*.
Arterioles, 1362, *1363, 1364*
Arteriovenous fistula, in hemodialysis, 892, *893*
Arteriovenous graft, in hemodialysis, 892
Arteriovenous malformations, 1944
Arthritis, degenerative. See *Osteoarthritis (OA)*.
    gouty, 575–576
    herbal remedies for, 539
    in rheumatic fever, 1482
    post-traumatic, 601
    rheumatoid. See *Rheumatoid arthritis (RA)*.
    secondary, 2163
    septic, 579–580
Arthrocentesis, 548
Arthrodesis, for osteoarthritis, 555
    for rheumatoid arthritis, 2154
    spinal, 1987–1991, *1988*
        anterior cervical, *1992*, 1992–1993
Arthrography, 546
Arthroplasty, in rheumatoid arthritis, 2154–2156, *2155*
    total hip, 555–564. See also *Total hip replacement (THR)*.
    total knee, *564*, 564–565, *565*
Arthroscopy, 200, 548
Articulations. See *Joints*.
Artificial airway, 304, *306*
Artificial larynx, 1669, *1670*
Artificial pacemakers. See *Pacemaker(s), artificial*.
Artificial rectal sphincter, 798
Artificial urinary sphincter, 840, *840*
Ascariasis, 767
Ascending pathways, 1860–1861, *1862t*
Ascites, 1462
    assessment for, 742–743, 1075, 1077, *1246*, 1246–1247
    care plan for, 1248b–1250b
    clinical manifestations of, 1246, *1246*
    etiology of, 1245
    in cirrhosis, 1245–1250
    medical management of, 1246
    nursing management of, 1246–1247
    pathophysiology of, 1245–1246
    percussion in, 742–743
    risk factors for, 1245
    self-care in, 1247
    surgery for, 1247, 1250, *1250*
        nursing management in, 1250
Ascitic fluid, drainage of, 1086–1087
Ascorbic acid. See *Vitamin C*.
Asepsis, surgical, maintenance of, 300
Aspartate aminotransferase (AST), 549t, 1082t
    in jaundice, 1221t–1222t
    in myocardial infarction, 1589
    reference values for, 2303t

Aspiration, 200, 374. See also *Biopsy*.
    airway, in stroke, 1965, 1971
        prevention of, in burns, 1342
        in coma, 1913
        in enteral nutrition, 676
        in tracheostomy, 1658–1659, 1666–1667
    diagnostic joint, 548
    of pericardial fluid, 1490, *1490*
Aspiration biopsy, 200, 374
    of bone marrow, 2098–2100
    of liver, 1084–1085
    of thyroid gland, 1095t
Aspiration pneumonia, balloon tamponade and, 1243
Aspirin, 486
    dosage of, 487t
    for angina, 1582, 1584t
    for coronary heart disease, 1521, 1522t
    for myocardial infarction, 1592t
    for rheumatoid arthritis, 2148
    perioperative restriction of, 275t, 282
Assessment, cultural, 145, 146–147, 412b
    diagnostic, 187–203. See also *Diagnostic assessment*.
    functional, for elderly, 52–53
    mental health, 153t, 409–411, 410t, 511–513
    preoperative, 274–276
    psychological, rating scales for, 417b
    psychosocial, 137–144, 139b, 140t–143t, 409–411, 410t. See also *Psychosocial assessment*.
    sexual, 418b
Assisted living facilities, 125
Assistive listening devices, 1836
Assistive personnel. See *Unlicensed assistive personnel*.
AST. See *Aspartate aminotransferase (AST)*.
Asterixis, 1227
Asthma, 1685–1691. See also *Chronic obstructive pulmonary disease (COPD)*.
    assessment in, 1689–1690
    cardiac, 1534
    client teaching in, 1693b
    clinical manifestations of, 1686–1688, *1687*
    critical monitoring in, 1689
    diagnosis of, 1687
    emergency management of, 1689
    etiology of, 1685
    medical management of, *1687*, 1689–1690
        action plan for, *1693*
        problems in, 1693t
        stepwise approach in, 1690–1691, *1692*
    nocturnal, 438
    nursing management of, 1689–1690
    occupational, 1739–1740, 1740t
    pathophysiology of, 1685, *1687*
    peak flowmetry in, 1637, *1639*
    risk factors for, 1685
    self-care in, 1690–1691, 1693b, *1694*
    severity of, 1688t
    status asthmaticus in, 1687–1688
Astigmatism, *1827*, 1828
Astrocytes, *1865*, 1866
Astrocytoma, 1932b. See also *Brain tumors*.
Atelectasis, 1710–1711, 1711
    crackles in, 1634t
Atenolol, for angina, 1582, 1583t
    for heart failure, 1539t, 1540
    perioperative use of, 275t
Atherectomy, directional coronary, 1523, *1523*
Atheroma, 1518
Atherosclerosis, angina pectoris in, 1448–1451, 1579–1586. See also *Angina pectoris*.
    arterial aneurysms in, 1416

Atherosclerosis (Continued)
  arterial occlusion in, 1399–1415. See also
    Peripheral arterial occlusive disease.
  clinical manifestations of, 1520
  collateral circulation in, 1518–1520
  coronary heart disease and, 1518–1520,
    1519t–1520t. See also *Coronary heart
    disease (CHD).*
  directional coronary atherectomy for, 1522,
    1522
  in chronic renal failure, 883
  laser ablation for, 1523
  pathogenesis of, 1518–1520, 1519t–1520t
  percutaneous transluminal coronary angio-
    plasty for, *1521,* 1521–1522
  progression of, 1520
  renal artery disease in, 869–870
  stent placement for, 1522, *1522*
Atherosclerotic plaque, 1518–1520, 1519t–
  1520t
  rupture of, 1585
  stroke and, 1954
Atonic seizures, 1926
Atopic dermatitis, 1286, 1287–1290, *1288,*
  2135–2136
Atopic hypersensitivity, 2081
Atria, anatomy and physiology of, 1434,
  1434t, 1435
Atrial baroreceptors, 2234
Atrial dysrhythmias, 1552–1553, *1554*
Atrial fibrillation, *1555,* 1556
Atrial flutter, *1555,* 1556
Atrial kick, 1552
Atrial systole, 1440, *1441*
Atrioventricular block, first-degree, 1557, *1558*
  second-degree, 1558, *1558,* 1558–1559
  third-degree, *1558,* 1559
Atrioventricular dissociation, *1558,* 1559
Atrioventricular dysrhythmias, 1556–1559
Atrioventricular node (junction), 1439, *1440*
  as escape pacemaker, 1550
Atrioventricular valves, 1434t, 1435, *1436,*
  1437
Atrophic gastritis, 709
Atrophic vaginitis, 985, 1003
Atrophy, 211
  skin, *1272*
Atropine, for decreased cardiac output, 2275
  preoperative, 290t
Atrovent (ipratropium), for asthma, 1690,
  1691t, *1692, 1694*
Attending physician, 96
Attention span, assessment of, 143
Attentional disorders, 1919
Audiography, 1804–1805, *1805*
Audiometric tests, 1804–1806, *1805*
AUDIT test, for alcohol abuse assessment, 39,
  40t
Auditory acuity, testing of, 1802–1804, *1803*
Auditory agnosia, in stroke, 1957t, 1960, 1976
Auditory system. See also *Ear; Hearing.*
  function of, 1785–1786
    assessment of, 1804–1806, *1805, 1806*
  structure of, 1782–1785, *1783, 1784*
Aura, seizure, 1925
Aural rehabilitation, 1836
Auricle, 1782, *1783,* 1800
  traumatic injuries of, 1842
Auscultation, 178–179, *179*
  of abdomen, 652–655, 655b, 742, 754,
    1075–1077
    in cardiac assessment, 1462
  of chest, in cardiac assessment. See also
    Heart sounds.
    in respiratory assessment, *1631,* 1632–
      1633. See also *Breath sounds.*
  of head and neck vessels, 1883

Auscultation (Continued)
  of heart sounds, 1459–1461
  of lungs, 1632–1633, *1633,* 1634t
    in cardiac assessment, 1461
  sounds on, 178–179, *179*
Auscultatory gap, 185
Autoimmune disorders, 2140–2164. See also
  specific disorders.
  ankylosing spondylitis, 2160–2161
  chronic active hepatitis, 1229–1230
  cranial arteritis, 2163
  dermatomyositis, 2162
  fibromyalgia syndrome, 2161
  hypothyroidism due to, 1091
  Lyme disease, 2163
  mixed connective tissue disease, 2163
  outcomes classification for, 2140b
  polymyalgia rheumatica, 2163
  polymyositis, 2162
  Reiter's syndrome, 2163
  rheumatoid arthritis, 2142–2156
  scleroderma, 2159–2160
  secondary arthritis, 2163
  Sjögren's syndrome, 2161
  spectrum of, 2141
  systemic lupus erythematosus, 2156–2159
  theories of autoimmunity and, 2141–2142,
    2142
  vasculitis, 2162
Autoinoculation, 1052
Autolytic debridement, 329, 1296
Automated external defibrillator, 1568
Automated implantable cardioverter-defibrillator, 1568
  quality of life and, 1607–1609
Automatic bladder, 2049
Automaticity, cardiac, 1438–1439
  disturbances in, 1560–1565. See also *Dys-
    rhythmias.*
Automatisms, in seizures, 1925
Autonomic dysreflexia, 2050–2051, 2064b,
  2064–2065
  in spinal cord injury, 2045–2046
  neurogenic bladder and, 843–844
Autonomic nervous system, age-related
  changes in, 50t
  assessment of, 1892. See also *Neurologic
    assessment.*
  functional effects of, 1870, 1871t
  in cardiac regulation, 1442–1443
  structure of, 1870–1872, *1872*
Autonomic neuropathy, in diabetes mellitus,
  1188–1189
Autonomous neurogenic bladder, *842,* 843–
  846
Autonomy, for elderly, 65–66
Autotransfusion, in emergency care, 2274
  in shock, 2248
  of mediastinal drainage, 1508
Autotransplantation, parathyroid, 1113
Avandia. See *Rosiglitazone (Avandia).*
Avascular necrosis, of femoral head, 601
  of talus, 2960
Avonex (interferon β₁ₐ), for multiple sclerosis,
  2014
Avulsion fracture, 595t
Axial skeleton, 530, *533*
Axilla, examination of, 168t
  in breast examination. See *Breast examina-
    tion.*
Axillary dissection, for breast cancer, 1020–
  1021
Axillary lymph nodes, palpation of, 921, *921,*
  2094, 2095t
Axillofemoral artery bypass surgery, 1406–
  1410, *1407*
Axon, in nerve regeneration, 1873, *1873*

Azathioprine (Imuran), for transplant immuno-
  suppression, 2224t
Azoospermia, 969
AZT (zidovudine), 2195, 2197t
Aztreonam (Azactam), for urinary tract infec-
  tion, 804t, 805t

B

B cells, 2081
  activation of, 2083, *2083*
Babinski's reflex, 1890, 1891t, *1893*
Bacille Calmette-Guérin (BCG), for bladder
  cancer, 810–811
  for interstitial cystitis, 808
Bacitracin, 327t
  for burns, 1348t
Bacitracin and polymyxin B (Polysporin),
  1280t
Back brace, for lower back pain, 1986
  in spinal cord injury, 2058
  postoperative, 1990
Back pain, 1983–1991. See also *Lower back
  pain.*
  in spinal cord compression, 397
Back rubs, 498, *498*
Back strain, 1984
Baclofen, 492
  intravesical, for neurogenic bladder, 844
Bacteremia, 189
  nosocomial, 338t, 339
  portal vein, liver abscess and, 1258
Bacterial arthritis, 579–580
Bacterial endocarditis, 1484–1487, *1485*
Bacterial flora, normal, 336–337
Bacterial infections, cell damage in, 213
  characteristics of, 337t
  pathogenesis of, 337t
Bacterial meningitis, 1944–1945, *1945*
Bacterial pneumonia, 1711–1716, 1712t
Bacterial vaginosis, 1055
Bacteriuria, asymptomatic, 803
  screening for, 157t
Balance, age-related changes in, 53–54, 1849
  assessment of, 182–183
  disorders of, 1847–1853. See also specific
    disorders.
  inner ear in, 1786, 1799
    assessment of, 1804, 1806, *1806*
Balanced anesthesia, 293
Balanitis, 970, *971*
Balloon angioplasty, 1405–1406
  renal artery, 870
Balloon dilation, of prostate, 955, *955*
Balloon tamponade, for bleeding esophageal
  varices, 1242, *1242*
  and gas exchange, 1243
Bandaging, compression, for venous thrombosis, 1425
  compressive, for amputation stump, *1412,*
    1413
Bands in white blood cell count, 318
Barbiturates, for increased intracranial pres-
  sure, 2031
  for rapid-sequence induction, 2268
Barium enema, 746
Barium swallow, 656–657
  modified, 657
Baroreceptors, arterial, 2234
  atrial, 2234
  in blood pressure regulation, 1366, 1381,
    1382, 2234
  in heart rate regulation, 1442, *1444,* 2234
Barotrauma, otalgia due to, 1841–1842
Barrel chest, 1629, *1630*
Barrett's esophagus, 701

Barrier precautions, 343–344
Bartholinitis, 1008
Bartholin's glands, *905, 906t*
  palpation of, *923, 924*
Baruch-doktor, 75b
Basal cell carcinoma, 1306, *1306.* See also
  Skin cancer.
  of eyelid, 1826
  of oral cavity, 687–690
Basal cell secretion test, 658–659
Basal energy expenditure (BEE), 663, 663t
Basal ganglia, 1857–1858
Base excess, in arterial blood, reference values
  for, 2303t
Basic activities of daily living, in elderly, *52,
  52–53*
Basiliximab (Simulect), for transplant immuno-
  suppression, 2224t
Basophils, 2080
  in wound healing, 319
BCG. See *Bacille Calmette-Guérin (BCG).*
Beau's line, 1273t
Becker's muscular dystrophy, 583t, 584
Beclomethasone (Vanceril), for asthma, 1690,
  1691t, *1692, 1694*
Beds, pressure reducing, *1300, 1914, 1914*
  Roto-Rest, 2064
Bed-to-wheelchair transfer, *1972, 2061*
Bed-wetting, 437
Bee stings, allergy to, 2137t, 2137–2138
Behavior, assessment of, 139
Behavior modification, for urinary inconti-
  nence, 838
Behavioral changes, in stroke, 1957t, 1960,
  1976
Belching, 706
Bell's palsy, *1996, 1996–1997*
Belsey repair, 697
Benadryl (diphenhydramine), for Parkinson's
  disease, 2019t
  for phenothiazine overdose, 2281t
Bench surgery, 869
Benign breast disease, 1036–1037
  cancer and, 1012
Benign paroxysmal positional vertigo, 1848
Benign prostatic hyperplasia (BPH), 945–958
  alternative therapies for, 946b
  clinical manifestations of, 946–947
  complications of, 946, *947*
  etiology of, 946
  incidence of, 946
  medical management of, 947–948
  nursing management of, 948–949
  pathophysiology of, 946
  risk factors for, 946
  screening for, 159t
  surgery for, 949–964
    complications of, 956
    postoperative care in, 956–958
    preoperative care in, 956
    procedures in, 949–956
Benign tumors, 349, 362–363, 363t. See also
  Tumor(s).
Bentiromide test, 2310t
Bentyl (dicyclomine), for peptic ulcer disease,
  710t, 715
Benzocaine (Americaine), 297t
Benzodiazepines, for alcohol withdrawal, 515
  for insomnia, 455
Benzoyl peroxide, 1280t, 1294
Benztropine (Cogentin), for Parkinson's dis-
  ease, 2019t
Bereavement, 18, 457–459, 459t. See *Grief.*
Berger's disease, 864t
Bernard and Cannon's homeostasis theory, 5t
Bernstein test, 659
Beta-adrenergic receptors, 1443–1444

Beta-blockers, for asthma, 1689, 1690, 1691t,
  1692, 1694
  for bleeding esophageal varices, 1242
  for heart failure, 1539t, 1540
  in hyperthyroidism, 1101
  overdose of, antidote for, 2281t
  perioperative use of, 275t
Betadine (povidone-iodine), 327t
Betapace (sotalol), for dysrhythmias, 1563t
Betaseron (interferon β_{1b}), for multiple sclerosis, 2014
Bethanechol (Urecholine), for gastroesophageal
  reflux disease, 696
  for urinary incontinence, 837t
Biaxin (clarithromycin), for peptic ulcer disease, 710t, 715
Bicarbonate, as buffer, 259–260, 261, *261.*
  See also *Acid-base balance.*
  fluid concentration of, 234t
  in respiratory control, 1618. See also under
    Arterial blood gas.
  reference values for, 2303t
Biceps reflex, 1889, 1891t, *1892,* 1893b
Bicipital tendinitis, 1999t
Bicycle ergometry, 1470–1472
Bier block, 298
Biguanides, for diabetes mellitus, 1159, 1160t
Bile, collection of, 1086
  drainage of, choledocholithiasis and, 1215
  liver transplantation and, 1257
Bile acid sequestrants, for hepatitis, 1228
Bile acids, 635t, 635–636
  reference values for, 2303t
Bile duct, common, stones in, 1214–1215
Biliary cirrhosis, 1233t. See also *Cirrhosis.*
Biliary colic, 1205. See also *Cholelithiasis.*
Biliary drainage analysis, 1086
Biliary pancreatitis, 1194. See also *Pancreatitis.*
  treatment of, 1198
Biliary tract. See also *Gallbladder.*
  disorders of, 1203t, 1203–1216. See also
    specific disorders.
  function of, assessment of, 1086
  obstruction of, jaundice due to, 1220, 1222t
  ultrasonography of, in acute cholecystitis,
    1212
Bilirubin, 1220
  conjugated, 1220
  in biliary cirrhosis, 1233t
  in cholestatic viral hepatitis syndrome, 1228
  in jaundice, 1220, 1221t–1222t
  serum, 1081t
    reference values for, 2303t
  unconjugated, 1220, 1221t
  urine, 1081t
    reference values for, 2306t
Billroth procedures, 720, *720.* See also *Gastric
  surgery.*
Bimanual palpation, 174, *177*
  in pelvic examination, 924–925, *925*
Binocular vision, 1781
Biofeedback, for irritable bowel syndrome,
  794b
  for pain, 499–500
  for urinary incontinence, 836, 838
Biologic dressings, for burns, 1350t
Biologic response modifiers, for cancer, 388–
  389
Biomedical model, 3, 5t
Biopsy, 200–201
  aspiration, 200, 374
  bone, 548
  bone marrow, 2098–2100
  breast, 933–934, 1016
  cervical, *930,* 930–931, 996
  closed, 200

Biopsy *(Continued)*
  ear tissue, 1807
  endometrial, 931, *931*
    in menorrhagia, 984
  excisional, 374, *1277,* 1278
    of actinic keratosis, 1305
  frozen sections for, 201
  incisional, 374
  liver, 1084–1085, *1085,* 1255
  lung, 1649
  muscle, 548, 1904
  needle, 200, 374
  open, 200–201
  permanent sections for, 201
  pleural, 1649
  prostate, 761, 942
  punch, *1277,* 1277–1278
  renal, *761,* 761–762
  sentinel node, in breast cancer, 1021
  shave, 1277, *1277*
    of actinic keratosis, 1305
  skin, *1277,* 1277–1278
  thyroid, 1095t
  transurethral, 761
  tumor, 371–373, 374
  types of, 200–201
Biorhythms, 432
  disturbances of, sleep disorders and, 437
  drug effects and, 432
  sleep and, 432
Biosynthetic dressings, for burns, 1350t
Biotherapy, for cancer, 388
Biot's breathing, *184*
Bipolar disorder, assessment in, 426–428
  care plan for, 427b
  causes of, 421–422
  client/family teaching in, 428
  clinical manifestations of, 421b
  drug therapy for, 422b
  manic episodes in, 420
  nursing management in, 426–428
  referral for, 428
Bisphosphonates, for osteoporosis, 571t
  for Paget's disease of bone, 575
Bivalved cast, 604
Blacks. See *African Americans.*
Bladder, age-related changes in, 737–738
  anatomy of, *732,* 734
  automatic, 2049
  closed irrigation of, 956, 957, *957*
  congenital anomalies of, 751, 847
  cord, 2049
  decompression drainage of, 832
  diverticula of, 829
  dysplasia of, 809
  imaging of, 758–760
  injuries of, 751
  neurogenic, 841–846, *842*
    in diabetes mellitus, 852, 1189
    in spinal cord injury, 841–846, 2049,
      2059, 2063, 2066–2067
  pain in, 750
  palpation of, 755
  percussion of, 754, *755*
  prolapse of, 998, *998*
  spasms of, after prostate surgery, 958
  transurethral resection of, 812
  traumatic injuries of, 846
Bladder atony, in spinal cord injury, 2063
Bladder cancer, 809–821
  assessment in, 811
  chemotherapy for, 810–811
  clinical manifestations of, 810
  epidemiology of, 809
  etiology of, 809
  metastasis in, 810
  nursing management in, 811–812

Bladder cancer (Continued)
pathophysiology of, 809–810
radiation therapy for, 811
risk factors for, 809
staging of, 810, 810
surgery for, 812–821
palliative, 814–815
partial cystectomy, 812
percutaneous nephrostomy in, 814–815
percutaneous pyelostomy in, 814–815
postoperative care in, 816–821
preoperative care in, 815–816
radical cystectomy, 812–813
transurethral resection, 812
ureterostomy in, 815
urinary diversion in, 813, 813–814, 814.
See also Urinary diversion.
urine cytology in, 758
Bladder diary, 835
Bladder distention, in spinal cord injury, 2063
Bladder hyperreflexia, in multiple sclerosis, 2013
Bladder irrigation, closed, 956, 957, 957
Bladder neck incision, for neurogenic bladder, 844
Bladder neck repair, 832
Bladder neck support prosthesis, 837, 837
Bladder neck suspension, 839
Bladder outlet obstruction, in benign prostatic hyperplasia, 946, 947, 947
reflux and, 829
Bladder training, 836, 836, 838
in spinal cord injury, 2066–2067
Blanch test, 1272
Blast cells, in leukemia, 2166, 2167
Blast crisis, in chronic leukemia, 2166–2167, 2169, 2170
Bleeding. See also Hemorrhage.
abnormal uterine, 982–984
leiomyomas and, 991–994
postmenopausal, 986, 987
gastrointestinal, 706, 715–717. See also Gastrointestinal bleeding.
in cancer, 392, 396
in chronic gastritis, 709
in cirrhosis, 1235, 1241–1243
in hepatitis, 1227–1228
in leukemia, 2170, 2171–2172
in renal trauma, 867, 868, 869
intestinal, 765
intracranial, in head trauma, 2041, 2041–2043, 2042
nasal, 1672–1676, 1676
postoperative, in oral surgery, 689
rectal, from hemorrhoids, 795
in colon cancer, 781–782
in ulcerative colitis, 772–773
thrombolytics and, 1964–1965, 1971
variceal, in cirrhosis, 1241, 1241b, 1241–1243
Bleeding disorders, 2122–2127. See also specific disorders.
classification of, 2122b
screening for, 2096t
surgery in, 282
Bleeding time, 2099t
reference values for, 2302t
Blepharitis, 1827t
Blepharoplasty, 1317, 1318
Blindness. See Vision impairment.
Blink response, 1790
Blinking, absence of, 1827t
Blisters, 1271
in pemphigus, 1310
Blood, 2074–2081
components of, 2106t–2108t
composition of, 2074–2080

Blood (Continued)
coughing of, 1452, 1462, 1624
in pulmonary embolism, 1426
fecal occult, 744t, 745
functions of, 2074
HIV transmission via, 2186–2189
in sputum, 1452, 1462, 1624
in urine. See Hematuria.
pH of, measurement of, 1641–1642. See also Arterial blood gas analysis.
reference values for, 2304t
reference values for, 2303t–2305t
Blood alcohol level, 515
Blood assays, in hypersensitivity disorders, 2133
Blood bank, release from, 2110
Blood cultures, 189
Blood flow, 1364
in exercise, 1367
regulation of, local, 1367
systemic, 1364–1365
Blood glucose. See also Glucose.
diabetic ketoacidosis and, 1176
fasting, 1155, 1157b
in cardiac disease, 1465
postprandial, 1155
random, 1155, 1157t
Blood groups, ABO, 2087
Rh, 2088
Blood pressure, 1442. See also Hypertension; Hypotension.
in coronary heart disease, 1521
in shock, 2242–2243, 2252
maintenance of, in coma, 1910
in spinal cord injury, 2053
in stroke, 1964
in thrombolytic therapy, 1964, 1971
measurement of, 183b, 184–185, 1385b, 1456–1457
alternative methods of, 2252–2253
intra-arterial pressure monitoring for, 1479–1480
paradoxical, 1457
postoperative maintenance of, 304–305
in cardiac surgery, 1506–1507
postural, 1457, 1457
regulation of, 1365, 1365–1366, 2234–2235
self-measurement of, 1397
treatment of, 1385–1392
Blood products. See also Transfusion(s).
pretransfusion testing of, 2105–2109
Blood specimen, arterial, 191, 1641–1642, 1642
Allen's test for, 269, 1374, 1641, 1642
collection of, 189, 190b, 190–191, 192
arterial, 191, 1641, 1642, 1642
microcapillary, 190
sequence for, 191
serial port, 190
venipuncture for, 190b, 190–191, 192
Blood tests, fecal occult, for colorectal cancer, 43
specimen collection for, 189, 190b, 192
Blood typing, 2087–2088
Blood urea nitrogen (BUN), 758
in cardiac disease, 1465
preoperative measurement of, 277t
Blood vessels, structure and function of, 1362–1377, 1363, 1364
Blood volume, regulation of, 2234
Blood-borne pathogens standard, 345
Blood-brain barrier, 1863–1864
Blue Cross/Blue Shield, 77, 78b
Blunt trauma, abdominal, 798–799
chest, 1764–1765
head, 2039–2040, 2041
liver, 1259
pancreatic, 1202

BMD. See Bone mineral density (BMD).
Body frame size, calculation of, 649, 650
Body image, colostomy and, 785
ileostomy and, 777
in burns, 1353, 1356
in cancer, 398
in eating disorders, 680
in mastectomy, 1024
jaundice and, 1223
plastic surgery and, 1314–1316, 1315b
rheumatoid arthritis and, 2152–2153
urinary diversion and, 815–816
Body language, 147
Body lice, 1311t
Body mass index, 31, 649–650
Body plethysmography (body box), 1637, 1640
Body substance isolation, 343
Body temperature. See Temperature.
Body weight. See Weight.
Bone, abnormalities of, in chronic renal failure, 881, 883
age-related changes in, 536
biopsy of, 548
cancellous, 588
cells in, 532
compact, 531, 533
composition of, 531–532
cortical, 588
function of, 535–536
healing of, 536, 588, 589t–590t
infection of, 578–580
metastasis to, 581–582
in breast cancer, 1035–1036
Paget's disease of, 572–575, 575
remodeling of, 535–536, 567, 567
spongy, 531, 533
structure of, 530–531, 534
tumors of, 580t, 580–582
types of, 530
Bone hearing devices, 1841
Bone marrow, 535
biopsy of, 2098–2100
erythropoiesis in, 2075–2077
harvesting of, 2179
hematopoiesis in, 2074
structure and function of, 2074
Bone marrow aspiration, 2098–2100
Bone marrow suppression, for multiple myeloma, 2120
Bone marrow transplantation, 2179–2180
allogenic, 389
autologous, 389, 2179
for aplastic anemia, 2115
for cancer, 389
for leukemia, 2173
graft-versus-host disease and, 2180t, 2180–2182
syngeneic, 2179
Bone mineral density (BMD), in osteoporosis, 566, 566
measurement of, 568–569, 569
normal, 566, 566
Bone scans, 546–548
Bony labyrinth, 1784, 1784–1785
Bony orbit, 1778, 1779
Borborygmi, 742
Borg perceived exertion scale, 33, 34
Bottoming out, of support surfaces, 1301, 1301
Bouchard's nodes, 552, 553
Bougienage, 692, 693, 693–694
Boutonnière deformity, in rheumatoid arthritis, 2145, 2145, 2156
Bowel elimination, assessment of, 739–747
diagnostic tests in, 743–747, 744t
history in, 739–742
in neurologic assessment, 1878t

Bowel elimination (Continued)
  laboratory tests in, 744t, 745–746
  physical examination in, 742–743
  in coma, 1917
  in spinal cord injury, 2063–2064
Bowel incontinence, 797–798
  in coma, 1917
  in spinal cord injury, 2063–2064, 2067
  in stroke, 1960
Bowel preparation, 282
  for barium enema, 746
  for colorectal surgery, 784
Bowel retraining, in spinal cord injury, 2066–2067, 2067
Bowel sounds, auscultation of, 652–654, 742
  in cardiovascular disease, 1462
Bowlegs, 540, 541
Bowman's capsule, 733, 733
Brace, back, for lower back pain, 1986
  in spinal cord injury, 2058
  postoperative, 1990
Brachial plexus, 1869
Brachial plexus injury, rheumatoid arthritis and, 2155, 2155b
Brachial pulse, assessment of, 1373, 1374
  in blood pressure measurement, 2252–2253
Brachioradialis reflex, 1891t
Brachytherapy, 377–378
  for endometrial cancer, 995
  for prostate cancer, 961
Braden scale, for pressure ulcer risk, 1298, 1299
Bradycardia, 183, 1442
  definition of, 1551
  in increased intracranial pressure, 2028, 2028
  sinus, 1553, 1554
Bradykinesia, in Parkinson's disease, 2017
Bradykinin, 319
  in pain, 468
  in shock, 2239
Bradypnea, 184
Brain. See also under Cerebral; Intracranial.
  blood supply of, 1864, 1864–1865
    compensatory reduction of, 2027
  contusion of, 2041
  infratentorial lesions of, clinical manifestations of, 1907t, 1908
  structure of, 1856–1859, 1857, 1858, 1859t
  supratentorial lesions of, clinical manifestations of, 1907t, 1907–1908
  swelling of, 2028. See also Cerebral edema; Increased intracranial pressure (ICP).
Brain abscess, 1946
Brain attack, 1954
Brain death, organ donation and, 2215, 2221
Brain injury, traumatic. See Head trauma.
Brain stem, 1858, 1858–1859, 1859t, 1860
Brain stem auditory evoked responses, 1806
Brain stem contusions, 2041, 2043–2044
Brain surgery. See Cranial surgery.
Brain tumors, 1931–1939
  chemotherapy for, 1937–1939
  classification of, 1931–1932
  clinical manifestations of, 1933–1935, 1934b
  diagnosis of, 1935
  etiology of, 1932
  imaging of, 1935, 1935
  medical management of, 1935
    postoperative, 1937–1939
  metastatic, 1933
  nursing management of, 1936
  pathophysiology of, 1932–1933
  radiation therapy for, 1937, 1940t
  surgery for, 1935–1937, 1936t
  types and locations of, 1932–1933, 1933

Braucher, 75b
BRCA mutation, in breast cancer, 1012–1013
Breast, biopsy of, 933–934, 1016
  blood supply of, 907
  disorders of, 1011–1039
    benign, 1036–1039
    history in, 917
    malignant. See Breast cancer.
  duct ectasia of, 1037
  examination of, 168t, 919–922
    by client, 41, 42, 369t, 1014
    normal findings on, 921b
    positioning for, 921
  fibroadenoma of, 1037
  fibrocystic, 1037
  hyperplasia of, 1037
  inspection of, 919–920, 920
  intraductal papilloma of, 1037
  lymphatic drainage of, 907, 907
  male, 907
    cancer of, 1036
    enlarged, 1037
    examination of, 936
  painful, 1037
  palpation of, 920–922, 921
  structure and function of, 906t, 906–907, 907
  ultrasonography of, 933
Breast augmentation, 1037–1038, 1038
Breast cancer, 1011–1036
  ablative endocrine procedures for, 1036
  carcinoma in situ, 1015–1016, 1019
  chemotherapy for, 1019, 1031–1033, 1034
    in metastatic disease, 1036
  clinical manifestations of, 1016
  diagnosis of, 1016
  epidemiology of, 1011–1012
  estrogen replacement therapy and, 571t, 571–572
  etiology of, 1012–1015
  genetic factors in, 1012–1013
  grading of, 1018
  health promotion/risk management for, 149t
  hormonal therapy for, 1035–1036
  hormone receptor status in, 1020, 1035
  incidence of, 1011
  invasive, 1016
  lobular carcinoma in situ, 1015–1016, 1019
  male, 1036
  medical management of, 1019–1020
    nursing management in, 1033–1034
  metastatic, 1035–1036
  outcome classification for, 1011
  overview of, 1011–1012
  pathophysiology of, 1015–1016
  pretreatment assessment in, 1019
  prevention of, 369, 1013–1014
  prognosis in, 1016–1019, 1018t, 1020
  radiation therapy for, 1019, 1025, 1031, 1032
  recurrence of, 1034–1035
    disseminated, 1035–1036
    local, 1034–1035
    surveillance for, 1034
  risk factors for, 369, 1012–1013, 1013t
  screening for, 41, 158t, 369, 369t, 932, 932–933, 933, 1012, 1014, 1015
    mammography in, 932, 932–933, 933
  sites of, 1016
  surgery for, 1020–1031. See also Mastectomy.
    axillary dissection, 1020–1021
    breast-conserving, 1019, 1020
    nursing management in, 1021–1029
    postoperative care in, 1024–1029
    preoperative care in, 1021–1024
  treatment planning in, 1019–1020, 1021–1022

Breast cancer (Continued)
  tumor markers in, 931–932, 1018
  types of, 1015–1016
Breast implants, cosmetic, 1037–1038, 1038
  in postmastectomy reconstruction, 1029–1031
Breast prosthesis, 1028–1029
Breast reconstruction, 1029, 1029–1031, 1030
  postmastectomy, 1029, 1029–1031, 1030
Breast reduction, 1038, 1038
Breast self-examination, 41, 42, 369t, 1014
Breast-conserving surgery, 1019, 1020
Breath sounds, adventitious, 1633, 1634t
  in pneumonia, 1713
  in cardiac assessment, 1462
  normal, 1632, 1633, 1633t
Breathing. See also Respiration.
  apneustic, 184
  Biot's, 184
  Cheyne-Stokes, 184, 1462
    in heart failure, 1462, 1534
  diaphragmatic, preoperative teaching of, 285–286, 286
  glossopharyngeal, 2059
  Kussmaul's, 184
  mechanics of, 1616, 1616–1617
  pursed-lip, in asthma, 1689, 1690
  relaxation, 27, 36
    for pain, 499
  rescue. See also Cardiopulmonary resuscitation (CPR).
    chin lift in, 2267, 2267–2268
    jaw thrust in, 2267, 2267–2268
    through stoma, 1656
  rhythmic, for pain, 499
  work of, 1618
Breathing pattern, acute pancreatitis and, 1197
  ascites and, 1246, 1247
Brief Pain Inventory, 478, 482
Brittle diabetes. See Diabetes mellitus, type 1.
Broca's aphasia, 1856, 1956
Broca's area, 1856, 1858
Bromides, reference values for, 2309t
Bromocriptine (Parlodel), for Parkinson's disease, 2019t
  for premenstrual syndrome, 982
  growth hormone levels and, 1080
Bromsulphalein excretion, liver function and, 1082t
Bronchi, structure of, 1613, 1614, 1614
Bronchial breath sounds, 1632, 1633t
Bronchiectasis, 1705–1706
Bronchioles, terminal, 1614, 1614
Bronchitis, acute, 1705–1706
  chronic, 1695–1705. See also Chronic bronchitis.
Bronchodilators, 2134
  for asthma, 1689, 1690–1691, 1691t
  for chronic obstructive pulmonary disease, 1691t, 1697
  for dyspnea, 452
  for ventilatory failure, 1750
  metered-dose inhaler for, 1691, 1693, 1693b
  reference ranges for, 2308t
Bronchophony, 1635
Bronchopleural fistula, 1743
Bronchopneumonia, 1713, 1714. See also Pneumonia.
Bronchopulmonary segments, 1615
Bronchoscopy, 200
Bronchovesicular breath sounds, 1632, 1633t
Brown-Séquard syndrome, 2051, 2052
Brudzinski's sign, 1945, 1945
Bruit, abdominal, 654–655, 742, 1462
  carotid artery, 1458
  renal, 742
Bruxism, sleep, 437
Buerger's disease, 1421–1422

Buffalo hump, 1127
Buffer systems, blood, 259–260
  urinary, 261, *261, 262*
Bulbocavernosal reflex, 756
Bulbourethral glands, 911, 911t
Bulimia nervosa, 679–681, *680*
Bulla, *1271*
Bumetanide (Bumex), for hypertension, 1389t
BUN. See *Blood urea nitrogen (BUN)*.
Bundle branch block, 1559
Bundle of His, 1439, *1440*
Bunions, 582, *582*
Bupivacaine (Marcaine), 297t, 484
Buprenorphine (Buprenex), 490t
Bupropion, reference values for, 2308t
Burch culposuspension, 839, 999
Burn diagram, 1339, *1340*
Burns, 1331–1359
  airway, 1332, 1335, 1338
  airway management in, 1341, 1344
  carbon monoxide poisoning in, 1335, 1337,
    1337t
  cardiac function in, 1335, 1338
  chemical, 1332
  circumferential, 1343
  classification of, 1341t
  clinical manifestations of, 1335–1338
  compartment syndrome in, 1343
  contractures in, 1349
  debridement of, 1347
  depth of, 1335–1337, *1336*
    assessment of, 1339, *1340*
  dressings for, 1348, 1350t
  edema in, 1337, *1337*
  electrical, 1332
  emergency care for, 1338–1346, 2274
  escharotomy for, 1343, *1344,* 1345
  esophageal, 701
  etiology of, 1331–1332
  extent of, assessment of, 1339, *1339, 1340*
  first-degree, 1335, *1336*
  fluid management in, 1341–1342, 1342t,
    1344
  fluid shifts in, 1334, *1334*
  fourth-degree, *1335,* 1336, *1336*
  full-thickness, 1336, *1336*
  home care in, 1355b
  hydrotherapy for, 1347, *1347*
  immunosuppression in, 1335
  infection of, 1345, 1346, 1346b, 1352
  inhalation injury in, 1332, 1335, 1337–1338
  medical management of, in acute phase,
    1344–1349
    in emergent phase, 1338–1344
    in rehabilitation phase, 1354
  minor, classification of, 1341t
    treatment of, 1341
  nursing management of, in acute phase,
    1349–1353
    in emergent phase, 1344–1346
    in rehabilitation phase, 1355–1357
  nutritional support in, 1346, 1346t, 1352
  outcome classifications for, 1331
  pain in, 1338, 1343, 1352, 1355–1356
  partial-thickness, *1335,* 1335–1336, *1336*
  pathophysiology of, 1333–1335
  physical therapy for, 1348–1349, 1355
  prevention of, 1332–1333, 1333b
  psychological response to, 1335, 1338, 1349
  radiation, 1332
  renal dysfunction in, 1334, 1344
  respiratory function in, 1332, 1334–1335,
    1335, 1337–1338
  risk factors for, 1332–1333
  rule of nines for, 1337, *1337*
  scald, 1332
  scarring in, minimization of, 1354, *1356*

Burns *(Continued)*
  second-degree, 1335, *1335, 1336*
  self-care in, 1355
  severity of, 1335–1337, *1336*
    assessment of, *1339,* 1339–1341, *1340,*
      1341t
  shock in, 2232–2233. See also *Hypovolemic
    shock.*
  solar, 1302–1303
  surgery for, 1353–1354
  systemic effects of, 1334–1335
  thermal, 1331
  third-degree, *1335,* 1335–1336, *1336*
  tissue injury in, *1333,* 1333–1334
  topical antimicrobials for, 1347–1348, 1348t
  transport to burn facility for, 1343–1344
  wound care in, in acute phase, 1347–1349
    in emergent phase, 1343
Burr holes, 2045–2046, *2046*
Bursae, 533, *535*
Burst fracture, 592t
Business and industry, in health care system,
  76, 80
Butorphanol (Stadol), 490t
Butterfly needle, for specimen collection, 191,
  193
Bypass grafting, arterial, 1406–1410, *1407*

C

C fibers, in pain perception, 466
CA 15-3, in breast cancer, 1018
CA-125, in breast cancer, 1018
  in ovarian cancer, 1001–1002
CABG. See *Coronary artery bypass grafting
  (CABG).*
Cachexia-anorexia syndrome, 455, 456t
Caffeine, 510t, 514t, 517, 520t–521t
  cardiac effects of, 1455
  hypertension and, 1381, 1387
CAGE mnemonic, for alcohol abuse assessment, 39
Calamine lotion, 1280t
Calan (verapamil), for dysrhythmias, 1563t
  for hypertension, 1389t, 1396t
Calcitonin (Miacalcin), 535, 1068
  for osteoporosis, 571t, 572
  for Paget's disease, 575
Calcium, deficiency of, 150t–151t, 641t
  dietary sources of, 250, 251b, 252
  food sources of, 641t
  functions of, 248–249
  imbalances of, 249–254. See also *Hypercal-
    cemia; Hypocalcemia.*
  in acid-base balance, 262–263
  in cardiac assessment, 1465
  metabolism of, 535
  normal values for, 235b, 248, 250, 549t,
    1111t
  osteoporosis and, 569–570, 570b
  parathyroid hormone and, 1068
  pharmaceutical, for hypermagnesemia, 257
    for hypocalcemia, 250–251, 252
    for hypoparathyroidism, 1115, 1116
    for premenstrual syndrome, 982
    for shock, 2251
    hypercalcemia and, 252, 253
  plasma levels of, 235b, 248, 250, 1068
  recommended intake of, 569–570, 570b
  regulation of, 249, *249*
  serum, reference values for, 2303t
  urinary, 1111t
    reference values for, 2306t
  vitamin D and, 1068
Calcium balance, preoperative assessment of,
  277t

Calcium channel blockers, overdose of, antidote for, 2281t
Calcium chloride, for calcium channel blocker
  overdose, 2281t
Calcium ions, in pain, 468, 469
Calculi, common bile duct, 1214–1215
  gallbladder. See *Cholelithiasis.*
  renal, 854
    hypercalcemia and, 253
  salivary, 690
  urinary, 821–829. See also *Urinary calculi.*
Calculous cholecystitis, acute, 1212–1213
Caldwell-Luc procedure, 1677–1678
Calix, renal, 733, *733*
Callus, foot, 1273
  fracture, 589t
Caloric requirements, determination of, 663,
  663t
  in diabetes mellitus, 1165, 1166t
Caloric testing, 1903, 1909, *1909*
Campylobacter gastroenteritis, 766, 768
Canaliculi, in bone, 531, *534*
Cancellous bone, 588
Cancer. See also specific sites and types.
  absolute neutrophil count in, 2171, 2171b
  age and, 355
  angiogenesis in, 360
  apoptosis in, *361,* 361–362
  body image in, 398
  cachexia-anorexia syndrome in, 455, 456t
  carcinogenesis and, 355–362. See also *Car-
    cinogenesis.*
  carcinogens in, 15, 354t, 354–355, 355t
  cardiac tamponade in, 397
  case management in, 376b
  cellular changes in, 211, 356–360, 357t
  chemicals and, 354t, 354–355
  client needs and problems in, 397–398,
    398b, 400b, 400–401, 401b
  clinical manifestations of, 371
  coping with, 398b, 399b, 399–400, 400b
  definition of, 349
  diagnosis of, 371–373, 372t
    biopsy in, 371–373, 374. See also
      Biopsy.
    client response to, 398b, 399b, 399–400
    cytologic specimens in, 374
    laboratory tests in, 371, 372t
  diet and, 15, 355
  disseminated intravascular coagulation in,
    396
  early detection of, 368, 369t
  emergent complications in, 395–397
  environmental factors in, 15–16, 28, 354t,
    354–355
  epidemiology of, 349–353
  familial, 362
  family needs in, 397–398, 398b, 399
  financial concerns in, 390
  free radicals and, 15
  gender and, *352, 353,* 355
  genetic factors in, 350t, 362
  grading of, 358, 373
  health promotion in, 370
  hereditary, 362
  hospice care for, 401–402
  host factors in, 355
  hypercalcemia in, 252, 395–396
  immune system in, 360–361
  in HIV infection, 1309–1310, *1310,* 2205–
    2206
  in pregnancy, 395
  incidence of, 350, 351t, *353*
  lifestyle factors in, 353
  metastasis in, 359–360, *360*
    surgery for, 375
  mortality in, 350, *352,* 401–402

Cancer (Continued)
occupational factors in, 354t, 355
oncogenes and, 350t, 356
opportunistic infections in, 2171
outcomes classification for, 367
pain in, 371, 395, 466, 466t, 471, 471b
palliative care in, 375, 401
pathogenesis of, 355–362. See also Carcinogenesis.
pathophysiology of, 353–362
post-transplantation, 2225
prevalence of, 350, 351t
prevention of, 367–370, 369t
progression of, 359–360, 401
psychosocial aspects of, 397–398, 397–402
race and ethnicity and, 353, 353, 368t
radiation and, 354
recurrence of, 401
rehabilitation in, 370–371
resources for, 400, 401b
risk factors for, 354t, 354–355, 355t, 369–370
screening for, 40–43, 41t, 368, 369t, 369–370. See also Screening.
self-care in, 390
smoking and, 354t, 354–355
spinal cord compression in, 396–397
spread of, 359–360
staging of, 373, 373t
surgery for, 374–375
TNM system for, 373, 373t, 1279b, 1728, 1728b
superior vena cava syndrome in, 397
survivorship in, 400–401
syndrome of inappropriate antidiuretic hormone in, 396
telephone medicine in, 392
terminal phase of, 401–402. See also Death and dying.
terminology for, 349, 350t
treatment of, adjuvant, 377
alternative therapies in, 390
biotherapy in, 388–389
bone marrow transplantation in, 389
chemotherapy in, 380–388. See also Chemotherapy.
clinical trials for, 389–390
complementary, 390
complications of, 391–397
evaluation of, 390–391
financial aspects of, 390
goals for, 373
home care in, 390
late effects of, 400
multimodal, 373
nursing management in, 391–397
palliative, 375, 401, 448–449
performance status and, 373, 374t
psychosocial aspects of, 385
radiation therapy in, 377–380. See also Radiation therapy.
response to, 390–391
selection of, 373
side effects of, 379–380, 391b
care plan for, 383–387
home care for, 390
management of, 383–387, 390, 391–396
surgery in, 373–377
diagnostic, 374
for recurrence and metastasis, 375
nursing management in, 375–376
palliative, 375
preventive, 375
reconstructive, 375
staging, 374–375

Cancer (Continued)
therapeutic, 375
trends in, 350–353
tumor characteristics in, 362–363, 363t
tumor growth in, 359
tumor lysis syndrome in, 247
tumor markers in, 350t
tests for, 372t
viruses and, 355, 355t
tumor lysis syndrome in, 396, 2169
tumor markers in, 350t, 372t
Candidiasis, 1311t
in HIV infection, 2203–2204
oral, 685, 685–686
renal, 856
Canker sores, 684
Cannabis, 510t, 514t, 517, 520t–521t
Cannon's homeostasis theory, 5t
Cantor tube, 706t, 707
Capillary beds, 1362–1364, 1363, 1365
Capillary blood pressure, in shock, 2241
Capillary exchange, 1365–1366
Capillary fragility test, 2099t
Capillary refill time, 1371, 1372, 1456, 1629
Capitation, 78b, 80–81
Capnography, 1639–1641
Capreomycin, for tuberculosis, 1720, 1721t
Capsaicin, 492, 539
for osteoarthritis, 554
Captopril (Capoten), for angina, 1582, 1583t
for heart failure, 1538t, 1540
for hypertension, 1389t, 1396t
perioperative use of, 275t
Captopril test, 1123t
Carafate (sucralfate), for peptic ulcers, 711t, 715
Carbamazepine (Tegretol), for epilepsy, 1927–1928
for trigeminal neuralgia, 1996
reference values for, 2307t
Carbidopa-levodopa (Sinemet), for Parkinson's disease, 2018, 2019t
Carbohydrates, digestion and absorption of, 636
in diabetes mellitus, 1166, 1166t
and hypoglycemia, 1179, 1179t
before exercise, 1165
in parenteral nutrition, 668
Carbon dioxide, accumulation of, in shock, 2238
in acid-base balance, 260, 260, 263
in respiratory control, 1618
partial pressure of, 1619, 1620
preoperative measurement of, 277t
reference values for, 2303t
transport of, 1619, 1620
Carbon monoxide poisoning, 1770, 2281t
carboxyhemoglobin levels in, 2309t
in burns, 1335, 1337, 1337t
Carboxyhemoglobin, reference values for, 2309t
Carbuncle, 1311t
Carcinoembryonic antigen (CEA), 744t, 745
in breast cancer, 1018
Carcinogenesis, 355–362
cellular changes in, 356–360, 357t
stages of, 355–356, 356
Carcinogens, 15, 354t, 354–355, 355t
Carcinoma, 350t, 363. See also Cancer.
Carcinoma in situ, 350t, 363
of breast, 1015–1016, 1019
Cardiac arrest, intraoperative, 302
Cardiac arrhythmias. See Dysrhythmias.
Cardiac assessment, 1447–1480
diagnostic tests in, 1463–1480
history in, 1447–1455

Cardiac assessment (Continued)
normal findings in, 1456b
physical examination in, 1455–1463
risk factor analysis in, 1447–1448, 1448t
Cardiac asthma, 1534
Cardiac automaticity, 1438–1439
Cardiac cachexia, 1535
Cardiac catheterization, 1475
cineangiography in, 1476, 1476t
in electrophysiologic studies, 1472
Cardiac cells, depolarization of, 1436–1438, 1438
Cardiac cirrhosis, 1233t, 1535. See also Cirrhosis.
Cardiac compensation, 1531–1532
Cardiac conduction, disturbances in, 1551
Cardiac contractility, 1439
Cardiac cycle, 1439–1440, 1440–1441, 1441
ejection phase of, 1440, 1441
isovolumic contraction phase of, 1440, 1441
isovolumic relaxation phase of, 1440, 1441
refractory period in, 1439
Cardiac dysrhythmias. See Dysrhythmias.
Cardiac enzymes, 1464–1465
in myocardial infarction, 1588–1589
Cardiac function, in burns, 1335, 1338
Cardiac glycosides, for heart failure, 1536, 1537b, 1539t
Cardiac index, 1441, 2253–2254
Cardiac monitoring, in shock, 2253
Cardiac muscle, 530
Cardiac output, 1434, 1441
decreased, causes of, 1479t
compensatory mechanisms for, 1531–1532
emergency care for, 2275
in burns, 1335, 1338
in dysrhythmias, 1552
in myxedema, 1096–1097
intra-aortic balloon pump counterpulsation for, 1509, 1510b
in dehydration, 219
in exercise, 1367
increased, causes of, 1479t
monitoring of, 1478b, 1479
in shock, 2253–2254
Cardiac pacemaker, artificial. See Pacemaker(s), artificial.
sinoatrial node as, 1438–1439, 1440
Cardiac pressures, 1442, 1443
Cardiac refractoriness, 1439
Cardiac rehabilitation, 1527–1529
after myocardial infarction, 1596–1605
Cardiac standstill, 1565
Cardiac stress testing, 1376, 1470–1472
first-past cardiac study in, 1475
myocardial scintigraphy in, 1474
Cardiac surgery, 1500–1513
assisted circulation in, 1504
client teaching in, preoperative, 1505–1506, 1506b
extracorporeal circulation in, 1504–1505
home care in, 1512b, 1512–1513
in elderly, 1513
respiratory care in, 1774–1776
mechanical hearts in, 1504
open heart, 1504–1505
postoperative care in, 1506–1512
preoperative care in, 1505–1506, 1506b
self-care after, 1512–1513
temporary pacing in, 1570, 1570, 1572, 1572–1573
transplantation, 1502–1504
valvular, 1501–1502
Cardiac tamponade, 1435, 1489–1490, 1509
emergency care for, 2275, 2276
heart failure and, 1531

Cardiac tamponade (Continued)
  in cancer, 397
  shock and, 2233
Cardiac transplantation, 1502–1504, 1503b,
    1503t, 1504, 1506b, 1505t, 1546, 2226.
    See also Cardiac surgery.
  complications of, 1511
Cardiac valves, 1434t, 1435
  aortic, 1434t, 1435, 1436, 1437
  atrioventricular, 1434t, 1435, 1436, 1437
  disease of, 1495–1501. See also Valvular
      heart disease.
  mitral, 1434t, 1435, 1436, 1437
  prosthetic, 1502, 1503
  pulmonic, 1434t, 1435, 1436, 1437
  regurgitant, 1435
  semilunar, 1434t, 1435, 1436, 1437
  stenotic, 1435
  tricuspid, 1434t, 1435, 1436, 1437
Cardiogenic shock, 2231. See also Shock.
  clinical manifestations of, 2243
  etiology of, 2233
  in myocardial infarction, 1591, 1594–1595
  medical management of, 2249t
Cardiomyopathy, 1490–1495
  dilated, 1490–1492, 1491, 1492t
  hypertrophic, 1491, 1492t, 1492–1493
  restrictive, 1491, 1492t, 1493–1495
Cardiomyoplasty, 1546
Cardiopulmonary bypass, 1504–1505
Cardiopulmonary resuscitation (CPR), advance
    directives and, 66–67
  chin lift in, 2267, 2267–2268
  defibrillation in, 1566–1568, 1567
  jaw thrust in, 2267, 2267–2268
  rescue breathing in, through stoma, 1656
  termination of, 1567–1568
Cardiopulmonary stretch receptors, 1442, 1444
Cardiotonic drugs, for shock, 2251
Cardiovascular disability, 1532b
Cardiovascular disorders, dysphagia in, 690
  renal function in, 852–853
  sleep problems in, 439
Cardiovascular drugs, reference ranges for,
    2308t
Cardiovascular system. See also Heart; Vascu-
    lar system.
  age-related changes in, 50t, 212t
  autonomic neuropathy of, in diabetes melli-
      tus, 1188
  epinephrine effects on, 1135t
  exercise adaptation in, 1367
  in shock, 2237–2239, 2242
  norepinephrine effects on, 1135t
  preoperative assessment of, 276
Cardioversion, 1568–1569
Carditis, rheumatic, 1482, 1482t
Cardizem (diltiazem), for angina, 1582,
    1584t
  for hypertension, 1389t, 1396t
Cardura (Doxazosin), for hypertension, 1389t
Care map. See Clinical pathway.
Care plan, 99
  for arterial bypass surgery, 1408b–1409b
  for atopic dermatitis, 1289b–1290b
  for bipolar disorder, 427b
  for cardiomyopathy, 1494b–1495b
  for chemotherapy, 383–385
  for chronic obstructive pulmonary disease
      (COPD), 1702b–1704b
  for depression, 423, 425
  for graft-versus-host disease, 2181b
  for heart failure, 1542b–1545b
  for hepatic failure, 1248b–1250b
  for long-term care facilities residents, 121,
      121b
  for myocardial infarction, 1599b–1605b

Care plan (Continued)
  for osteoporosis, 574
  for panic disorder, 416b
  for relocation stress syndrome, 56
  for schizophrenia, 420b
  for thoracic surgery, 1733b–1736b
  for traction, 610–611
Caregiver needs, in Alzheimer's disease,
    2007–2009, 2008b, 2010t–2011t
Caries, dental, 683–684
Carina, 1613, 1614
Caroli's syndrome, 1259
β-Carotene, reference values for, 2303t,
    2310t
Carotid artery, examination of, 168t, 1458,
    1458
  postoperative rupture of, 1666
Carotid endarterectomy, for transient ischemic
    attacks, 1979
  procedure for, 1979, 1980
Carotid pulse, assessment of, 1373, 1374
Carotid vein, examination of, 168t
Carpal tunnel syndrome, 1998, 1999t,
    2000b
Cartilage, 534
  ear canal, 1783
  elastin, 534
  epiphyseal, 531, 534
  fibrocartilage, 534
  hyaline, 532, 534, 535
  in osteoarthritis, 552
Cartilaginous joints, 533
Case management. See also Clinical pathway.
  for cancer, 376
  for chronic obstructive pulmonary disease,
      1686b
  for elderly, 65
  for heart failure, 1547b
  for hip fracture, 615–616
  for myocardial infarction, 1593b
  for Parkinson's disease, 2020b
  for pneumonia, 1715b
  for pressure ulcers, 1302b
  for stroke, 1970b
  in acute care, 99–100
Case manager, perioperative, 291b
Cast(s), application of, 602
  assessment of, 605
  bivalving of, 604
  care of, 602–606
  compartment syndrome and, assessment for,
      604, 604t
  drying of, 602–603
  neurovascular assessment for, 604, 604t,
      605, 605b
  nursing management for, 606
  types of, 602, 603
  urine, 750, 750
  windowing of, 604
Cast syndrome, 601, 601
  assessment for, 604, 604t, 605, 605b
  management of, 606
Cataplexy, narcolepsy and, 435
Catapres (clonidine), for hypertension,
    1389t
Cataract, 1782, 1814–1817, 1815, 1817b
Catarrhal exudate, 323, 323t
Catecholamines, adrenal medulla and, 1063,
    1067
  pheochromocytoma and, 1135, 1135t
  in pain, 469
  in shock, 2239
  in sleep, 432, 437–438
  plasma, reference values for, 2303t
  urinary, adrenal function and, 1079
    pheochromocytoma and, 1136
    reference values for, 2306t

Catheter, central venous, dressings for, 671
  for total parenteral nutrition, 669, 669,
      670, 670t
  maintenance of, 670, 670t
  condom, 831–832, 832, 839
  peripherally inserted central, for chemother-
      apy, 386, 386
  peritoneal dialysis, 888, 888
  pulmonary artery, 1476
  Tenckhoff, 888, 888
  urinary, insertion of, 845
    specimen collection from, 190
    types of, 950t–953t
  ventricular, in intracranial pressure monitor-
      ing, 2030, 2032b–2033b
Catheter infection, 338, 339
  urinary, 832
Catheterization, cardiac, 1475
  cineangiography in, 1476, 1476t
  in electrophysiologic studies, 1472
  in peritoneal dialysis, 889–890, 890
  of Kock pouch, 779
  of urinary reservoir, 819–820
  pulmonary artery, 1476, 1477b–1478b
  umbilical vein, 1084
  urinary. See Urinary catheterization.
Cations, 233
Cauda equina syndrome, 1989, 2051, 2052
Caudal anesthesia, 295, 296. See also Anesthe-
    sia.
Cavomesenteric shunt, 1244
CD4+ cells, in HIV infection, 2190–2191,
    2193
Cecum, 630
Ceftriaxone, for gonorrhea, 1044t
Celecoxib (Celebrex), 486t
Cell(s). See also specific type.
  age-related changes in, 211, 212t
  alterations in, 211
    in shock, 2238
  atrophy of, 211
  cancer, characteristics of, 356–360, 357t
  communication between, 209
  connective tissue, 211
  damage to, 212–214
  death of, 214, 361, 361–362
  development of, 208
  differentiation of, 357–358
  epithelial, 211
  eukaryotic, 206
  hypertrophy of, 211
  in tissues and organs, 210–211
  muscle, 211
  neoplastic changes in, 211
  nerve. See Neuron(s).
  nucleus of, 206, 207t, 209
  precancerous changes in, 211
  prokaryotic, 206
  replication of, 209–210, 210
  structure of, 206, 206–208, 207t
Cell cycle, 210, 210, 356–357, 358
Cell membrane, 206, 207t, 208–209, 209
CellCept (mycophenolate), for transplant im-
    munosuppression, 2224t
Cell-mediated immunity, 2081, 2085–2087,
    2086
Cellulitis, 1310, 1312
Centers for Disease Control and Prevention
    (CDC), 73
Central auditory dysfunction, 1833
Central cord syndrome, 2051, 2052
Central lobe, 1857, 1858
Central nervous system, age-related changes
    in, 50t, 1873
  cells of, 1865, 1865–1867
  structure of, 1856–1861, 1857, 1858, 1859t,
      1860, 1861

Central sleep apnea, 436
Central tentorial herniation, 2029, *2029*
Central venous catheterization, catheter maintenance in, 670, 670t
  dressings for, 671
  for total parenteral nutrition, 669, *669,* 670, 670t
Central venous pressure (CVP), neck vein distention and, 1457–1458, *1458*
Central venous pressure (CVP) monitoring, 1476–1479, 1478t
  after cardiac surgery, 1507
  in shock, 2253
Centrioles, *206,* 207t
c-erbB2, in breast cancer, 1018, 1020, 1033
Cerebral aneurysms, 1940–1944, *1941*
Cerebral angiography, 1899–1901, *1900*
Cerebral artery spasm, stroke and, 1955
Cerebral circulation, *1864,* 1864–1865
Cerebral compliance, 2027
Cerebral contusion, 2041, 2043
Cerebral cortex, 1856, *1857, 1858*
Cerebral edema, 228–229, 2028, 2034t. See also *Increased intracranial pressure (ICP)*.
  definition of, 2028
  in hyponatremia, 237
  in water intoxication, 228–229
  stroke and, 1965
Cerebral hemispheres, 1856, *1857, 1858*
Cerebral herniation, 2027
  central tentorial, 2029, *2029*
  cingulate, *2029,* 2029–2030
  infratentorial, *2029,* 2030
  lateral tentorial, 2029, *2029*
  supratentorial, 2029, *2029*
Cerebral perfusion pressure (CPP), decreased, ischemic stroke and, 1955
  definition of, 2027
  in shock, 2242–2243
  in subarachnoid hemorrhage, 1942, 1943t
  maintenance of, 2038
Cerebral perfusion studies, 1901
Cerebrospinal fluid (CSF), 1863
  abnormal findings in, 1898t
  circulation of, 1863, *1864*
  collection of, via cisternal puncture, 1896–1899, *1897*
    via lumbar puncture, 1896–1899, *1897*
  displacement of, 2027
  drainage of, ventriculostomy for, 1965
  ear examination and, 1807
  reference values for, 1898t, 2309t
  ventriculoperitoneal shunt for, in increased intracranial pressure, 2038–2039, *2039*
Cerebrovascular accident. See *Stroke*.
Cerebrovascular disease, in diabetes mellitus, 1183t, 1184
Cerebrum, structure of, 1856–1857, *1857, 1858*
Certificate of need (CON) review, 79
Certification, for ambulatory care nursing, 91–92
Certified registered nurse anesthetist, 291b
Ceruloplasmin, reference values for, 2303t
Cerumen, 1783, 1785, 1802
Cervical biopsy, *930,* 930–931
Cervical cancer, 995–998
  in HIV infection, 2206
  prevention of, 370
  risk factors for, 370
  screening for, 158t, 200, 369t, 370, 926–928, *927,* 995, 996
Cervical collar, 1992, *1992*
Cervical culture, *927,* 928
Cervical disc disorders, 1991–1993
Cervical dysplasia, 995

Cervical fusion, *1992,* 1992–1993
Cervical intraepithelial neoplasia, 995
Cervical lymph nodes, dissection of. See *Radical neck dissection*.
  palpation of, 2094, 2095t
Cervical plexus, 1869
Cervical polyps, 1000, *1000*
Cervical spine, fusion of, *1992,* 1992–1993, 2057, *2057*
  immobilization of, emergency, 2269, *2269*
Cervical spine injuries, 2047, *2048*
  compression, 2047, *2048*
  dislocation, 2047, *2048*
  emergency care for, 2269, *2269*
  flexion-rotation, 2047, *2048*
  fracture, 2047, *2049*
  fracture-dislocation, 2047, *2048*
  hyperextension, 2047, *2048*
  spinal cord injury in. See *Spinal cord injury (SCI)*.
  surgical management of, 2057, *2057*
Cervical syndrome, 1999t
Cervicitis, chlamydial, 1044t, 1047
Cervix, cold conization of, 996
  examination of, 924, *925*
Cestodes, 767
Chalazion, 1827t
Challenge diet, 2101–2102
Chancre, in syphilis, 1050, *1050*
Chancroid, 1053, *1053*
CHAOS association, in diabetes mellitus, 1184
Charcot's disease, 2023–2024
Charcot's joint, 1995
Charting, in neurologic assessment, 2036–2037
CHD. See *Coronary heart disease (CHD)*.
Chemical burns, 1332. See also *Burns*.
  esophageal, 701
Chemical injury, cell damage in, 213
Chemicals, cancer and, 354t, 354–355
Chemonucleolysis, 1987
Chemoreceptor trigger zone, 706
Chemoreceptors, 2234
  in blood pressure regulation, 1381, *1382,* 2234–2235
  in heart rate regulation, 1442, *1444,* 2234–2235
  in respiratory regulation, 1618
Chemotaxis, in inflammation, 318, 319
Chemotherapy, 380–388
  adjuvant, 380
  administration of, 383–388
  agents for, 381, 382b
    handling and disposal of, 388
  alopecia in, 394
  anemia in, 393
  anorexia in, 394
  assessment in, 381–382
  care plan for, 383–385
  client teaching for, 382
  clinical trials of, 389–390
  combination, 381, 381b
  constipation in, 394
  diarrhea in, 394
  dosage in, 381
    verification of, 382
  extravasation in, 387–388
  for bladder cancer, 810–811, 812
  for brain tumors, 1937–1939
  for breast cancer, 1019, 1020, 1031–1033, 1034
    in metastatic disease, 1036
  for colorectal cancer, 782
  for esophageal cancer, 700
  for Hodgkin's disease, 381b, 2175–2176
  for laryngeal cancer, 1663–1664
  for leukemia, 2169

Chemotherapy *(Continued)*
  for liver cancer, 1256
  for lung cancer, 1730
  for multiple myeloma, 2120
  for non-Hodgkin's lymphoma, 2178
  for oral cancer, 687
  for pancreatic cancer, 1202
  for prostate cancer, 962
  for renal cancer, 859–860
  for testicular cancer, 965
  hypersensitivity to, 387
  in pregnancy, 395
  infection in, 383–384, 392–393, 395, 396
  intravenous, 382–388
  mechanism of action of, 381
  myelosuppression in, 392–393
  nausea and vomiting in, 393–394, 1034
  neoadjuvant, 380
  nursing management in, 381–388
  regional, 387
  reproductive effects of, 395
  side effects of, 381–382, 387, 391b
    management of, 383–387, 390, 391–396
  skin problems in, 395
  stomatitis in, 394, 1034
  syndrome of inappropriate antidiuretic hormone in, 396
  thrombocytopenia in, 393
  tumor lysis syndrome in, 2169
  vascular access devices for, 386, *386*
Chenodeoxycholic acid, for cholelithiasis, 1205, 1207
Chest. See also under *Thoracic*.
  auscultation of, in cardiac assessment, 1459–1461. See also *Heart sounds*.
    in respiratory assessment, *1631,* 1632–1633. See also *Breath sounds*.
  barrel, 1629, *1630*
  deformities of, 1629, *1630*
  examination of, 167t–169t
    in cardiac assessment, 1458
    in respiratory assessment, 1627–1629
  flail, 1768–1769, *1769*
    emergency care for, 2272, *2272*
  funnel, 1629, *1630*
  landmarks for, *1628*
  movements of, assessment of, 1629, *1630,* 1631, *1631*
  palpation of, 1630–1631, *1631*
    in cardiac assessment, 1458
  percussion of, *1631,* 1631–1632
  pigeon, 1629, *1630*
  structure of, 1616
Chest drainage. See also *Chest tubes*.
  in hemothorax, 1768
  postoperative, in cardiac surgery, 1508
Chest pain. See also *Pain*.
  assessment of, 1448–1451, 1449t–1450t, 1625
  characteristics of, 1448–1451
  gender and, 1451t
Chest physiotherapy, for chronic obstructive pulmonary disease, 1698
Chest radiography, 195
  in acute pancreatitis, 1195
  in cardiac assessment, 1472
  in respiratory assessment, 1643–1645, *1644*
Chest thrusts, 2268, *2268*
Chest trauma, 1764–1770
  assessment in, 1765, 1765b
  management of, 1765, 1765b
  mechanisms of, 1764–1765
  nonpenetrating (blunt), 1764–1765
  penetrating, 1764–1765
  pneumothorax in, 1765–1768. See also *Pneumothorax*.

Chest tubes, 1731, 1732
  clamping of, 1738
  emergency placement of, 2272
  for closed pneumothorax, 1767
  for open pneumothorax, 1767
  for simple pneumothorax, 1767
  for tension pneumothorax, 1768
  in closed chest drainage, 1731–1738
  in surgery, 1731, 1732
  insertion of, 1731
  mediastinal, 1508
  milking of, 1738, 1738
  removal of, 1738–1739
  stripping of, 1738, 1738
Chest wall, diameters of, 1627, 1628
Chewing reflex, 1891
Cheyne-Stokes breathing, 184, 1462
  in heart failure, 1534
Chickenpox, immunization for, 342, 342t
Children. See also Adolescents.
  consent for, 286
  health promotion/risk appraisal for, 155,
    156t–159t
  pain in, 476
    rating scale for, 477, 481
Chin lift, 2267, 2267–2268
Chlamydial infection, 1044t, 1047–1048
Chloramphenicol, reference values for, 2307t
Chloride, fluid concentration of, 234t
  in acid-base balance, 262
  plasma levels of, 235b
  serum, reference values for, 2303t
  urine, reference values for, 2306t
Chloride balance, preoperative assessment of,
    277t
Chloride ions, in pain, 467, 469
Chloride shift, 260
Chlorprocaine (Nesacaine), 297t
Chlorpropamide (Diabinese), for diabetes mel-
    litus, 1161t
  and hypoglycemia, 1178
  perioperative use of, 275t
Chocolate cyst, 989
Cholangiography, 1086
  T tube, 1215
Cholangiopancreatography, 1086
Cholangitis, 1214–1215
  bacterial, liver abscess and, 1258
  sclerosing, 1215
Cholecystectomy, for acute cholecystitis, 1213
  for choledocholithiasis, 1214
  for cholelithiasis, 1208–1209, 1209
  laparoscopic, 1208, 1208
Cholecystitis, acute, 1212–1213
  acalculous, 1213
  chronic, 1213–1214
  clinical manifestations of, 1204b
Cholecystography, oral, 1085–1086
Cholecystolithotomy, percutaneous, 1208
Cholecystotomy, for acute cholecystitis, 1213
Choledocholithiasis, 1214–1215
Choledochostomy, for choledocholithiasis, 1215
  for cholelithiasis, 1209, 1209
Choledochotomy, for choledocholithiasis, 1214
Cholelithiasis, 636, 1203–1212
  assessment of, 1206
  clinical manifestations of, 1204b, 1204–
    1205
  complications of, 1206
  epidemiology of, 1203
  etiology of, 1203–1204
  in elderly, 1211–1212
  medical management of, 1205–1206, 1206,
    1207
  nursing management of, 1206–1207
  pancreatitis and, 1195. See also Pancreatitis.
    treatment of, 1198

Cholelithiasis (Continued)
  pathophysiology of, 1204
  recurrent, prevention of, 1207
  risk factors for, 1203–1204
  self-care in, 1207
    postoperative, 1211
  surgery for, 1207–1209, 1208, 1209
    nursing management in, 1209–1211
    postoperative care in, 1210–1211
Cholendoscopy, 1205, 1206
Cholera, 337t
Cholestasis, hepatotoxicity and, 1232t
  hereditary syndromes of, 1220, 1221t
Cholestatic viral hepatitis syndrome, 1228
Cholesteatoma, 1843
Cholesterol, 15
  dietary, in diabetes mellitus, 1166
    restriction of, 32–33
    in hypertension, 1393–1394
  elevated, coronary heart disease and, 1516–
    1517
  reference values for, 2303t
  serum, liver function and, 1081t
    reference ranges for, 1517
    thyroid function and, 1079
Cholesterol-dissolving agents, for cholelithia-
    sis, 1205
Cholestyramine (Questran), for hepatitis,
    1228
Choline magnesium trisalicylate, 486, 487t
Choline salicylate, 486, 487t
Cholinergic crisis, 2022, 2022b
Cholinergic fibers, 1871
Chondrocytes, 552
Chondrosarcoma, 580t, 581–582
Chordae tendineae, 1435
Chordee, 756, 971
Choroid, 1779
Choroid plexus, 1863
Christmas disease, 2126t
Chromosome analysis, 1904
Chromosomes, 207t
Chronic bronchitis, 1692–1705
  care map for, 1700b
  care plan for, 1702b–1704b
  case management in, 1686b
  clinical manifestations of, 1696, 1696, 1697,
    1698b
  complications of, 1696, 1697
  epidemiology of, 1693
  etiology of, 1693
  in elderly, 1700
  medical management of, 1691t, 1696–1699
  nursing management of, 1699–1700
  oxygen conservation strategies in, 1705b
  pathophysiology of, 1693–1695
  radiographic findings in, 1696, 1697
  risk factors for, 1693
  self-care in, 1700–1705
  sleep problems in, 438–439
Chronic conditions, 13–24
  adaptation to, 17–20, 23–24
    family, 20
    physiologic, 17, 23
    psychological, 17–18, 18t, 23–24
    social, 18–20, 24
  aging and, 14, 14
  client education in, 22–24
  client strengths in, identification of, 21
  clinical manifestations of, control of, 23
  complementary therapies for, 27t, 27–28
  coping behaviors in, 18, 26–27
  costs of, 13
  cultural aspects of, 19b
  economic aspects of, 13, 20–21, 21t
  empowerment in, 25
  environmental factors in, 14, 15–16, 28

Chronic conditions (Continued)
  evaluation in, 22
  exercise in, 25
  expected outcomes in, 22
  genetic factors in, 13–14, 14
  health promotion and prevention in, 24–28
  interventions in, 22–24
  management of, 20–24
  mind-body interactions in, 16
  mortality in, 14t
  multifactorial aspects of, 13
  nursing diagnoses for, 21, 22b
  nutrition and, 14, 14–15, 24–26
  nutrition in, 24–25
  overview of, 13
  risk factors for, 13, 14
  self-actualization in, 25, 25–26
  self-help groups for, 26
  sick role and, 19–20
  social support in, 26
  stages of, 16–17
  stress and, 3, 5t–7t, 16, 26–27
Chronic constrictive pericarditis, 1489
Chronic fatigue syndrome, 442
Chronic gastritis, 709–712, 710t–711t
Chronic leukemia. See Leukemia.
Chronic obstructive pulmonary disease
    (COPD), 1692–1705
  asthma in, 1685–1691
  care map for, 1700b
  care plan for, 1702b–1704b
  case management in, 1686b
  chronic bronchitis in, 1695
  clinical manifestations of, 1696, 1696, 1697
  complications of, 1696, 1697, 1698–1699
  emphysema in, 1695–1696
  epidemiology of, 1693
  etiology of, 1693
  in elderly, 1700
  medical management of, 1696–1699
  nursing management of, 1699–1700
  oxygen conservation strategies in, 1705b
  pathophysiology of, 1693–1696
  radiographic findings in, 1696, 1697
  risk factors for, 1693
  self-care in, 1700–1705
  sleep problems in, 438–439
  surgery for, 1700
Chronic pain, 465–466. See also Pain.
  intermittent, 466
  malignant, 466
  nonmalignant, 465–466
Chronic renal failure (CRF). See Renal failure,
    chronic.
Chronic venous insufficiency, 1427, 1427–
    1429
Chronobiology, 432
Chronopharmacology, 432
Chvostek's sign, 250, 251, 251
  hypoparathyroidism and, 1115
  thyroidectomy and, 1105
Chyme, 630, 634
  movement of, 632–634
Cigarette smoking. See Smoking.
Cilia, 207t, 1614, 1614
Ciliary body, 1778–1779
  age-related changes in, 1782
Cimetidine (Tagamet), preoperative, 290t
Cineangiography, in cardiac catheterization,
    1476, 1476t
Cingulate herniation, 2029, 2029–2030
Cinobac (cinoxacin), for urinary tract infection,
    804t
Cinoxacin (Cinobac), for urinary tract infec-
    tion, 804t
Ciprofloxacin (Cipro), for urinary tract infec-
    tion, 805t

Circadian rhythms, 432
disturbances of, sleep disorders and, 437
Circulating nurse, 291b
Circulation. See also under *Vascular.*
cerebral, *1864,* 1864–1865
collateral, in atherosclerosis, 1518–1520
D enterohepatic, 635–636
pulmonary, 1362, *1363*
systemic, 1362, *1363*
Circulatory support, in shock, 2245–2246
Circumcision, *938,* 970, *970*
female, 1008
Cirrhosis, 1232–1253, *1236–1237*
ascites in, 1245–1250. See also *Ascites.*
assessment in, 1235
cardiac, 1535
case study of, 1238–1239
clinical manifestations of, 1234
complications of, 1240–1253. See also specific complications.
monitoring for, 1234–1235
epidemiology of, 1234
etiology of, 1234
hepatic encephalopathy in, 1250–1253. See also *Hepatic encephalopathy.*
hepatotoxins and, 1235, 1235t
medical management of, 1234–1235, 1235t
nursing management of, 1235–1240, *1236–1239*
pathophysiology of, 1234
portal hypertension in, 1240–1245. See also *Portal hypertension.*
risk factors for, 1234
self-care in, 1240, 1253
types of, 1232, 1233t
Cisapride (Propulsid), for gastroesophageal reflux disease, 696
Cisterna magna, 1863
Cisternal puncture, 1899
Civil Rights Act of 1964, 102–104
CK. See *Creatine kinase (CK).*
Clarithromycin (Biaxin), for peptic ulcer disease, 710t, 715
Clean-catch urine specimen, 189–190
Clicks, 1460
Client teaching, 12–13. See also specific disorders.
for discharge, 312, 312b
for elderly, 51, 51b
for hospitalized clients, 98
for role changes, 24
in chronic conditions, 22–24
postoperative, 312, 312b
preoperative, 282, 284–287, 291b
Climacteric, 910
Clinical model, for health care, 84
Clinical nurse specialist, 291b
Clinical pathway, 99. See also *Case management.*
for chronic obstructive pulmonary disease, 1700b, 1701b
for coronary artery bypass grafting, 1528b
for gastrointestinal hemorrhage, 715b, 716b
for hip fracture, 615–616
for mastectomy, 1021b, *1022–1023*
for pneumonia, 1716b, 1717b
for stroke, 1968b, 1969b
for total hip replacement, 562, 563
Clinical trials, 389–390
Clitorectomy, 1008
Clitoris, *905,* 906t
examination of, 924
Clodronate (Ostac), for bone metastases, in breast cancer, 1036
Clonic seizures, 1925
Clonidine (Catapres), for hypertension, 1389t
Clonotypes, 2073

Clonus, 1891
Closed pneumothorax, 1765–1767, *1766*
Closed-chest drainage, 1732–1738, *1737*
Closed-circuit helium method, for lung volumes, 1637
Clostridial gastroenteritis, 766–767, 768
Clot. See also *Coagulation.*
formation of, 316
Clot retraction test, 2099t
Clotting. See under *Coagulation.*
Clubbing, of fingers, 1273, 1273t, 1453, 1456, 1629, *1630*
of nails, 1273, 1273t, 1453, 1456
Cluster headaches, 1948, *1949*
Coagulation. See also *Hemostasis.*
disseminated intravascular. See *Disseminated intravascular coagulation (DIC).*
in wound healing, 316
process of, 2078–2080, *2079*
Coagulation disorders, 2122b, 2123–2127, 2124b, *2125,* 2126t
screening for, 1096–1098
Coagulation factors, in hemophilia, 2126b, 2126–2127
in thyroid storm, 1100
reference values for, 2302t
Coagulation pathways, extrinsic, 2079, *2079*
intrinsic, *2079,* 2080
Coagulation tests, in cardiac assessment, 1465
reference values for, 2302t
Coagulation time, reference values for, 2302t
Cobalamin. See *Vitamin B₁₂.*
Cocaine, 510t, 514t, 517, 520t–521t
for topical anesthesia, 297t, 297–298
Coccidioidomycosis, 1723–1724
in HIV infection, 2204
Cochlea, *1784,* 1784–1785
Cochlear implants, 1840, *1841*
Cochlear nerve, 1870t
assessment of, 1885–1886
Codeine, 489t
Cogentin (benztropine), for Parkinson's disease, 2019t
Cognex (tacrine), for Alzheimer's disease, 2004–2005
Cognitive function, age-related changes in, 57–58, 59t
assessment of, 143. See also *Neurologic assessment.*
in hepatic encephalopathy, 1252
neuropsychological tests for, 1902–1903
postoperative, 280, 308–309
preoperative, 280
impaired, in Alzheimer's disease, 2003–2004
in confusional states, 1918–1922
in Creutzfeldt-Jakob disease, 2009
in Huntington's disease, 2011
in hypercortisolism, 1132
in stroke, 1976
sensory overload and, 443
Cognitive reappraisal, 36
Cognitive theory, of mood disorders, 421
Colchicine, for gout, 576
Cold, cellular injury from, 213
Cold application, for pain, 498, 614b
Cold conization, 996
Cold injury. See also *Hypothermia.*
emergency care for, 2282–2283
Cold shock, 2243
Colds, 1679–1680
Cold-spot imaging, 199
Colestid. See *Colestipol (Colestid).*
Colestipol (Colestid), for hepatitis, 1228
Colic, biliary, 1205. See also *Cholelithiasis.*
renal, 750
ureteral, 750

Colitis, pseudomembranous, 766–767, 768
ulcerative, 770–780
Collagen, 531–532
in wound healing, 320
Collateral circulation, in atherosclerosis, 1518–1520
Colles' fracture, 596t, 618
Colloid osmotic pressure, 216, *1365*
Colloid solutions, for shock, 2247
in emergency care, 2274
Colon. See also under *Colorectal; Gastrointestinal; Intestinal.*
function of, 634
in digestion, 634
obstruction of, 790–793
polyps of, cancer and, 781
structure of, 630
Colonization, 338
Colonoscopy, 747
Colony-stimulating factors, 2087t
for cancer, 388
in hematopoiesis, 2075
in wound healing, 320
Color vision, 1794
Colorectal cancer, 780–787
chemotherapy for, 782
clinical manifestations of, 781–782
diagnosis of, 781–782
etiology of, 780–781
obstruction in, 790
pathophysiology of, 781, *781*
prevention of, 369–370
prognosis in, 782
radiation therapy for, 782
risk factors for, 42–43, 369, 780–781
screening for, 42–43, 158t, 369t, 370, 781, 782
carcinoembryonic antigen in, 744t, 745
fecal occult blood test in, 744t, 745
staging of, 781, *781*
surgery for, *782,* 782–787, *783.* See also *Colostomy.*
postoperative care in, 784–787
preoperative care in, 784
procedures in, *782,* 782–783, *783*
Colostomy, complications of, 783
contraindications to, 783
double-barrel, *782,* 783
flatus and, 786
indications for, 783
irrigation of, 785–786, 786b
loop, *782,* 783
nursing management in, 784–787
outcome of, 783
resources for, 786b
self-care for, 785–787, 787b
single-barrel, *782,* 783
stoma care in, 784–786, *785,* 786b
supplies for, 786b
Colposcopy, 928, *929*
Coma, 1905–1918
characteristics of, 1906
clinical manifestations of, 1907t, 1907–1908
complications in, prevention of, 1911
critical monitoring in, 1912b
definition of, 1906
diabetic, 1172
diagnostic testing in, *1909,* 1909–1910
emergency care in, 2276
etiology of, *1906,* 1906–1907
family needs in, 1917, 1917b
hepatic, 1251
complications of, 1253
in elderly, 1918
increased intracranial pressure in. See *Increased intracranial pressure (ICP).*
infratentorial lesions and, 1907, 1907t

Coma *(Continued)*
  level of involvement in, 1910
  long-term care in, 1918
  medical management of, 1910–1911
  metabolic, 1906–1907, 1907t
  motor assessment in, 1887–1888, *1909,*
    1909–1910
  myxedema, 1091, 1093
    medical management of, 1093, 1095
    risk of, 1097
  neurologic assessment in, 1909–1910, 1911,
    1912b
  nursing management of, 1911–1918
  nutritional support in, 1915b, 1915–1916
  outcomes in, 1911
  pathophysiology of, 1907, *1907*
  prognosis in, 1911
  reflex assessment in, 1887–1888, *1909,*
    1909–1910
  respiratory patterns in, 1908, *1908*
  reversal of, 1910–1911
  safety measures in, 1916–1917
  stroke and, 1965
  supratentorial lesions and, 1907, 1907t
Combivir (lamivudine-zidovudine), 2196t
Comedone, 1293, *1293*
Comminuted fracture, 592t
Common bile duct, calculi in, 1214–1215
Common cold, 1679–1680
Common vehicle transmission, 335
Communicable infection, 338
Communication, after total laryngectomy, 1669
  assessment of, 143, 1882–1883
  cultural aspects of, 147
  hearing impairment and, 1837, 1837b
  in mental health problems, 410–411, 419,
    426, 428
  in tracheostomy, 1659
  intercellular, 209
  language barriers in, 147
  nonverbal, 147, 410–411
  patient-centered, 202–203
  with dying patient, 456
  with long-term care facilities residents, 123
  with stroke clients, 1975–1976
  with tracheostomy patient, 689
Community health nursing, 109. See also
    Home health care.
  substance abuse and, 512
Community resources, for elderly, 54t, 61–63,
    63b
Community-acquired infection, 338
Compact bone, 531, *533*
Compartment syndrome, after arterial bypass
    surgery, 1409
  assessment for, 604, 604t, 605, 605b
  fractures and, 599–600, *600*
  in burns, 1343
  Volkmann's contracture and, 600
Complement, 2085, *2085*
Complement assays, 2100, 2101t
Complement system, in inflammation, 319
Complementary therapies. See *Alternative ther-
    apies.*
Complete blood count (CBC), 2094–2096
  components of, 2094–2096
  disorders and conditions affecting, 2097t
  in cardiac assessment, 1464
  in lower gastrointestinal assessment, 744t
  reference values for, 2096t, 2097t
Complete fracture, 592t
Complex regional pain syndrome, 602
Compliance, pulmonary, 1617
Compression fracture, 595t
Computed tomography (CT), *195,* 195–196
  abdominal, 657, *657,* 746
  electron-beam, in angina evaluation, 1581

Computed tomography (CT) *(Continued)*
  in coma, 1909
  in musculoskeletal assessment, 546
  in neurologic assessment, 1894–1895, *1895*
  in pancreatitis, 1080, *1083,* 1195–1196
  in reproductive assessment, in females, 928
  in respiratory assessment, 1645
  in vascular assessment, 1376
  of adrenal glands, 1122t
  of ear, 1804
  of thyroid gland, 1095t
  of urinary tract, 759
  procedure for, 195–196
Concussion, 2041
  headache after, 1950
Condom catheter, 831–832, *832,* 839
Condoms, client teaching for, 1046, 1046b
Condylar fractures, 616
Condylomata acuminata, 1053–1054, *1054*
Condylomata lata, in syphilis, 1050
Cones, retinal, 1780, 1781
Confusional states, 1918–1922
  emergency care for, 2276–2277
  hepatic encephalopathy and, 1251
  in stroke, 1957t, 1960, 1976
  postoperative, 612
  variceal bleeding and, 1243
Congenital heart disease, 1500
Congestive heart failure. See *Heart failure.*
Conization, cold, 996
  for cervical cancer, 996, 997
Conjugate gaze, 1885
Conjunctiva, 1778, *1779,* 1790
  disorders of, 1827t
Conjunctivitis, 1827t
Connecting peptide (C-peptide), in diabetes
    mellitus, 1157
Connective tissue, 2140, 2141b
  cells of, 211
Connective tissue disorders. See *Autoimmune
    disorders;* specific disorder.
Conn's syndrome, 1133
Conscious sedation, in emergency care, 2276
Consciousness, altered. See also *Coma.*
    causes of, *1906*
    level of, 1908
      assessment of, 1875t, 1880–1881
        in coma, 1910
        in increased intracranial pressure, 2031
        in mental status assessment, 139
        postoperative, 1393
    properties of, 1905–1906
    regulation of, 1907
Consent, 287, *288*
  competence and, 66–67
  for emergency care, 2262–2263
Constipation, 766
  in cancer, 394
  in chronic renal failure, 886, 896
  in hyperparathyroidism, 1113
  in hypothyroidism, 1098
  in multiple sclerosis, 2013, 2014
  in spinal cord injury, 2063–2064
  opioid analgesics and, 450, 490–491
  postoperative, in hip surgery, 613, 615
Constrictive pericarditis, heart failure and,
    1531
Consultation, telephone, 90
Contact bone, 531
Contact dermatitis, 1286, 1291, *1291*
Contact lenses, for aphakia, 1816
Contact precautions, 344
Contact transmission, 335
Continent ileostomy, 775, *775*
  postoperative care in, 779
Continent urinary diversion. See *Urinary di-
    version.*

Continuous ambulatory peritoneal dialysis,
    887. See also *Dialysis, peritoneal.*
Continuous cyclic peritoneal dialysis, 887. See
    also *Dialysis, peritoneal.*
Continuous passive motion (CPM) machine,
    565, *565,* 624
Continuous positive airway pressure (CPAP),
    in mechanical ventilation, 1754–1755
  in obstructive sleep apnea, 435–436
Continuous renal replacement therapy, for
    acute renal failure, 879
Continuous subcutaneous analgesia, 495
Continuous suture, *301*
Contraception, vasectomy for, 967, *967*
Contraceptive history, 917
Contractile state, 1439, 1441–1442, *1442*
Contraction, muscle, *532,* 534
Contractures, 320
  Dupuytren's, 2000
  in burns, 1349
  prevention of. See also *Exercises.*
    in comatose patients, 1914–1915
    in spinal cord injury, 2062–2063
    in stroke, 1973–1974
  Volkmann's, 600
Contrast agents, 196b
  nephrotoxicity of, 854
Contrecoup injury, 2040, *2041*
Contusion, brain stem, 2041, 2043–2044
  cerebral, 2041, 2043
  renal, *867,* 867–869
Conus medullaris, 1859, *1860*
Conus medullaris syndrome, 2051, *2052*
Coombs' test, 2096
  reference values for, 2302t
Coordination, assessment of, 1886–1887
Coping behaviors, 18, 26–27, 36, 399b, 408b,
    408–409. See also *Psychosocial concerns.*
  defense mechanisms and, 408b
  emotion-focused, 408
  in cancer, 399–400, 400b, 499b
  in hearing impairment, 1838
  problem-focused, 408
Copper, deficiency of, 641t
  excess of, Wilson's disease and, 1259
  food sources of, 641t
  serum, reference values for, 2303t
  urine, reference values for, 2306t
Coproporphyrin, urine, reference values for,
    2307t
Cord bladder, 2049
Core-needle biopsy, 200, 374. See also *Biopsy.*
  of breast, 933
Corn, 1273
Cornea, 1778
  age-related changes in, 1782
  in Wilson's disease, 1259
  infection of, *1823,* 1823–1824
  physical examination of, 1791
  transplantation of, *1822,* 1822–1823
  ulcer of, 1823, *1823*
Corneal abrasion, prevention of, in stroke,
    1976
Corneal dystrophies, 1821–1823, *1822*
Corneal reflex, 1790–1791, 1889, 1891t
  assessment of, 1885
Corneal reflex test, 1791
Coronal sulcus, 911
Coronary angiography, 1476, 1476t
Coronary arteries, 1435–1436, *1436, 1437*
Coronary arteritis, 1580
Coronary artery bypass grafting (CABG),
    1524–1526, *1526*
  care map for, 1528b
  in elderly, 1526–1527
Coronary artery disease. See *Coronary heart
    disease (CHD).*

Coronary atherectomy, 1523, *1523*
Coronary heart disease, in diabetes mellitus, 1182, 1183t, 1184
Coronary heart disease (CHD), angina in, 1448–1451, 1579–1585. See also *Angina pectoris.*
    antiplatelet therapy in, 1521, 1522t
    coronary artery bypass grafting for, 1524–1526, *1526*
    directional coronary atherectomy for, 1522, *1522*
    laser ablation for, 1523
    percutaneous transluminal coronary angioplasty for, 1521–1522, *1522*
    prevention of, 1520–1521
    stent placement for, 1522, *1522*
    transmyocardial revascularization for, 1526
Corpus callosotomy, for epilepsy, 1929, *1929,* 1930
Corpus callosum, 1856, *1857*
Corpus luteum, 904, 909–910
    involution of, 910
Corpus luteum cysts, 1001
Cortical bone, 588
Cortical discrimination, assessment of, 1888–1889
Cortical resection, for epilepsy, 1929, *1929,* 1930
Corticospinal tract, 1861, 1862t
Corticosteroids. See *Steroids.*
Corticotropin-releasing hormone (CRH), 1067
    stimulation of, adrenocortical function and, 1123t
Cortisol, 1067
    deficiency of, 1121t. See also *Addison's disease.*
        diagnosis of, 1122t, 1123t
    diurnal variation in, 1130
    excess of, 1126–1133. See also *Hypercortisolism.*
        diagnosis of, 1122t, 1123t
    plasma, reference values for, 2303t
    urine, reference values for, 2306t
Cortisol suppression test, 1079
Cosmetic surgery. See *Plastic surgery.*
Cost containment, 79–81
Costovertebral angle, percussion over, 754, *755*
Costovertebral pain, 750
Cosyntropin test, 1122t
Cotswold staging, of Hodgkin's disease, 2175t
Cough, herbal remedies for, 1626
    quad-assisted, 2062
Coughing, assessment of, 1624
    in heart failure, 1534
    incision splinting for, 1731, *1732*
    of blood, 1452, 1462, 1624
        in pulmonary embolism, 1426
    physiology of, 1618, 1618t
    preoperative teaching of, 286
Coumadin (warfarin), for venous thrombosis, 1425
Counterpulsation device, for shock, 2246
Coup-contrecoup injury, 2040, *2041*
Cover-uncover test, in eye examination, 1791–1792
Cowper's glands, 911, 911t
COX-1 inhibitors, 486
COX-2 inhibitors, 486
    for osteoarthritis, 554, 555t
CPAP. See *Continuous positive airway pressure (CPAP).*
C-peptide. See *Connecting peptide (C-peptide).*
CPP. See *Cerebral perfusion pressure (CPP).*
Crabs, 1056
Crack cocaine, 510t, 514t, 517, 520t–521t
Crackles, 1461, 1633, 1634t

Cramps, nocturnal leg, 437
Cranberry juice, for urinary tract infection, 833b
Cranial arteritis, 2163
Cranial nerves, *1869,* 1869t, 1869–1870
    disorders of, 1995–1997
    distribution of, *1884*
    examination of, 1883–1886
Craniotomy, care plan for, 1938b–1940b
    for aneurysm, 1943
    for brain tumors, 1935, 1936t
    for epilepsy, 1929, *1929,* 1929–1930
    in head trauma, 2045–2046
    postoperative care in, 1937
    preoperative care in, 1936–1937
Cranium, structure of, 1861
C-reactive protein, test for, 549t
Creams, 1281t
Creatine, reference values for, 2303t
Creatine clearance test, 758
Creatine kinase, reference values for, 2304t
Creatine kinase (CK), 549t, 1464
    in myocardial infarction, 1588, *1589*
Creatinine, preoperative measurement of, 277t
    serum, 758
        reference values for, 2304t
    urine, reference values for, 2306t
Credé maneuver, 843, 2066
Cremasteric reflex, 1889, 1891t
CREST constellation, in scleroderma, 215
Creutzfeldt-Jakob disease, 2009
CRH. See *Corticotropin-releasing hormone (CRH).*
Cricothyroidotomy, 2268, *2269*
Crimes, evidence collection and preservation for, 2263, 2263t, 2264t
Crixivan (indinavir), 2197t
Crohn's disease, 770–780
    clinical manifestations of, 771t, 772
    etiology of, 771
    medical management of, 773–774
    nursing management of, 774
    pathophysiology of, 771t, 772
    prognosis in, 771t, 772–773
    surgery for, 774–780. See also *Ileostomy.*
        postoperative care in, 776–780
        preoperative care in, 776–780
    vs. ulcerative colitis, 771t
Cross-matching, for transplantation, 2223
    of bone marrow, 2179
Cross-training, 101
Crust, *1272*
Crutchfield tongs, 2053, *2053*
Crutch-walking, client teaching for, 2279, 2279t
Cryosurgery, for cervical cancer, 996, 997–998
    of cervical cancer, 996, 997–998
    of hemorrhoids, 796
Cryotherapy, for actinic keratosis, 1304, *1305*
Cryothermia, for anesthesia, 298
Crypt abscess, 772
Cryptococcosis, 1947
    in HIV infection, 2204
Cryptorchidism, 967–968
    infertility and, 968, 969
    testicular cancer and, 964, 967
Cryptosporidiosis, 767
    in HIV infection, 2204–2205
Crystalloid solutions, for shock, 2247
    in emergency care, 2274
CSF. See *Cerebrospinal fluid (CSF).*
Culdocentesis, *988*
Cullen's sign, in pancreatitis, 1195
Culposuspension, 839, 999

Cultural assessment, 145, 146, 412b
Cultural diversity, 424b
Cultural factors, in acute care nursing, 104
    in aging, 47–48
    in cancer, 368t
    in chronic disease, 19b
    in communication, 147
    in death and dying, 457b
    in elder care, 47–48
    in female genital mutilation, 1008
    in health beliefs and practices, 19b, 424b
    in menstrual disorders, 979–980
    in mental health problems, 424b
    in nutrition, 643b–645b
    in pain, 474–476, 475b
    in transplantation, 2216t–2217t
    overview of, 146
Cultural sensitivity, 424b
Culture, definition of, 146
Cultures, 189–190
    blood, 189
    cervical, *927,* 928
    definition of, 424b
    ear drainage, 1807
    for tuberculosis, 1720
    nasal, 1648
    skin, 1276
    specimen collection for, 188b, 188–189
    stool, 744t, 745
    throat, 1648
    urine, 189–190, 758
        in urinary tract infection, 803
        specimen collection for, 189–190, 191–192
    wound, 189
Culturette, 189
Cumulative trauma disorders, 1998, 1999t
Curandero, 74b
Curettage, for actinic keratosis, 1304, *1305*
Cushing's disease, 1126, *1128–1129*
    surgery for, 1130–1131
    treatment of, 1130–1131, 1133t
Cushing's syndrome, 1126–1133. See also *Hypercortisolism.*
    iatrogenic, 1126–1127
    laboratory studies in, 1130
    pathophysiology of, 1127, *1127*
    treatment of, 1133t
Cushing's triad, 2028, *2028*
    in increased intracranial pressure, 2028, 2038
Cutaneous pain, 471, 471t
Cutaneous stimulation, in pain management, 496–498
Cutaneous T-cell lymphoma, 1309
CVP. See *Central venous pressure (CVP).*
Cyanosis, 1456
    in heart disease, 1452
Cyclodestructive procedures, for glaucoma, 1813
Cyclooxygenase inhibitors, 486
    for osteoarthritis, 554, 555t
    for rheumatoid arthritis, 2148
Cyclophosphamide, for breast cancer, 1032, 1033, 1034, 1036
Cyclosporine (Neoral, Sandimmune), for transplant immunosuppression, 2224t
Cyst, breast, 1037
    chocolate, 989
    corpus luteum, 1001
    cutaneous, *1271*
    follicular, 1001
    ganglion, 2000
    ovarian, 989, *1000,* 1001
    pancreatic pseudocyst, 1201–1202
    pilonidal, 797
Cystadenocarcinoma, pancreatic, 1202

Cystectomy, partial, 812
    postoperative care in, 816
    preoperative care in, 815–816
    radical, 812–813
        urinary diversion in. See *Urinary diversion.*
Cystic fibrosis, 1202–1203, 1724–1725
Cysticercosis, 1948
Cystine stones, 824
Cystitis, 802–807. See also *Urinary tract in-fection (UTI).*
    clinical manifestations of, 803
    etiology of, 802
    honeymoon, 802
    interstitial, 750, 807–808
    medical management of, 803–805, 805t
    nosocomial, 338, 339t
    nursing management in, 805–806
    pathophysiology of, 802
    risk factors for, 802
    surgery for, 806–807
Cystocele, 756
    examination for, 924–925
    management of, 999–1000
Cystogram, 759
Cystolitholapaxy, for urinary calculi, 826
Cystolithotomy, 828
Cystometrography, 762
Cystoscopy, for urinary calculi, 826
    in male reproductive assessment, 942
Cystourethrography, 760, *760*
Cytokines, 2087, 2087t
    in B-cell activation, 2083, *2083*
    in inflammation, 2081
    in wound healing, 318, 319–320
Cytologic specimens, in cancer, 374. See also *Biopsy.*
Cytologic studies, 200–201
Cytomegalovirus infection, in HIV infection, 2205
Cytomegalovirus retinitis, 1829
Cytoskeleton, 207t
Cytotec (misoprostol), for peptic ulcer disease, 710t, 715
Cytotoxic hypersensitivity, 2130, 2131t

D

d4T (stavudine), 2196t
Dacliximab (Zenapax), for transplant immuno-suppression, 2224t
Dacryocystitis, 1827t
Dakin's solution, 327t
Dalgan (dezocine), 490t
Danazol (Danocrine), for endometriosis, 990
Dark, adaptation to, aging and, 1782
Darvon (propoxyphene), 489t
ddC (zalcitabine), 2196t
ddI (didanosine), 2196t
D-dimer test, 1424, 2099t
    reference values for, 2302t
De Quervain's thyroiditis, 1106
Deafness. See *Hearing impairment.*
Death and dying, advance directives and, 67–68
    cachexia-anorexia syndrome in, 454, 456t
    caregiver support in, 456–457
    causes of, 14t
        in young/middle-aged adults, 30, 31t
    communication in, 456
    cultural aspects of, 457b
    definition of, organ donation and, 2215
    delirium in, 452, 452t
    depression in, 452–453
    disease trajectory in, 448
    durable power of attorney for health care and, 67

Death and dying *(Continued)*
    dyspnea in, 451–452
    family support in, 457–459, 458b
    fatigue in, 453
    grief in, 457–459, 459t
    hospice care in, 65, 447–448, 449b
    imminent, signs of, 456, 456t
    in cancer, 401–402
    living wills and, 67
    pain management in, 449–451, 451t
    palliative care in, 375, 447, 448–449, 449b
    quality of life in, 448–449
    religious beliefs and practices for, 2216t–2217t
    sleep problems in, 453–454
    symptom management in, 447, 449–455
    treatment withholding/withdrawal in, 527–528
    unexpected, in emergency department, 2264
    unmet needs in, 448
    weakness in, 453
DEATH mnemonic, 52
Debridement, 325, *328*, 328–330
    autolytic, 329, 1296
    enzymatic, 329, 1296, 1347
    mechanical, *328*, 328–329, 1296, 1347
    of burns, 1347
    of pressure ulcers, 1296
    sharp (surgical), 325, 1296, 1347
Decadron. See *Dexamethasone (Decadron).*
Deceleration injury, 2039, *2041*
Decerebrate posturing, 1888
Decibels, 1800
Decompression, gastric, 706–708. See also *Gastrointestinal intubation.*
    intestinal, 792
Decompression drainage, of bladder, 832
Decompressive laminectomy, for disc hernia-tion, 1987, *1987,* 1989–1991
    for spinal cord injury, 2057
Decongestants, for hypersensitivity disorders, 2133
    nasal, rhinitis and, 1679, 1680
Decorticate posturing, 1888
Decortication, 1743
Decubitus ulcers. See *Pressure ulcers.*
Deep pain, 471t, 471–472
Deep tendon reflexes, 1863, *1863,* 1889, 1891t, *1892.* See also *Reflex(es),*
        assessment of, 1889, 1891t, *1892,* 1893b.
        See also *Reflex(es).*
Deep vein thrombosis, 1422. See also *Venous thrombosis.*
Deep-breathing exercises, preoperative teach-ing of, 285–286, *286*
Defecation. See *Bowel elimination.*
Defense mechanisms, 408b
Deferoxamine, for iron overload, 2281t
Defibrillation, 1566–1568, *1567*
    automated external defibrillator in, 1568
    automated implantable cardioverter-defi-brillator in, 1568
    cardioversion in, 1568–1569
Degenerative neurologic disease, 2002–2024
Dehiscence, 309, *309,* 333
Dehydration, 215
    assessment in, 222–223
    clinical manifestations of, 219–220
    diagnosis of, 220
    diarrhea and, 218
    emergency care for, 2273–2274
    etiology of, 217–218
    fluid replacement in, 220–222, 221t
    hypernatremia in, 239–242
    in diabetic ketoacidosis, 1173, 1174t

Dehydration *(Continued)*
    in hyperglycemic, hyperosmolar, nonketotic syndrome, 1177
    nursing management in, 223–225
    pathophysiology of, 218–219
    self-care in, 225
    shock in, 2233. See also *Hypovolemic shock.*
    treatment of, 220–222, 221t
    vomiting and, 218
Dehydration test, 1080
Dehydroepiandrosterone, urine, reference val-ues for, 2306t
Delavirdine (Rescriptor), 2198t
Delayed hypersensitivity, 2130, 2131t, 2132
    skin testing for, 2101
Delegation. See *Unlicensed assistive person-nel.*
Delirium, 453, 1918–1922
    assessment in, 453
    definition of, 453
    diagnostic criteria for, 453
    etiology of, 453, 453t
    in dying patients, 453
    in elderly, 58, 59t
    management of, 453, 453t
    postoperative, 306
    sleep problems in, 440
Delirium tremens (DTs), 515, 524
Delta hepatitis. See *Hepatitis D.*
Deltasone. See *Prednisone (Deltasone).*
Delusions, in confusional states, 1919
Dementia, 57–58, 1918–1922
    AIDS-related, 2206
    Alzheimer's. See *Alzheimer's disease.*
    classification of, 1918
    features of, 1918
    sensory disturbances in, 442–443
    sleep problems in, 438
    vs. delirium, 58, 59t
    vs. depression, 58, 59t
Demerol. See *Meperidine (Demerol).*
Demyelination, in multiple sclerosis, 2012, *2013*
Denial, 408, 408b
    in cancer, 399
Dental care, 156t
Dental disorders, 683–684
Denver shunt, for ascites, 1247
Deoxyribonucleic acid (DNA), 209, 210
Depakote (valproate), for epilepsy, 1927–1928
    reference values for, 2307t
Dependence, on opioid analgesics, 485
Dependent edema. See *Edema.*
Dependent rubor, 1369, 1371, *1371,* 1400
Depolarization, 1867
    membrane, 467
    of cardiac cells, 1437, *1438*
Deprenyl (selegiline), for Parkinson's disease, 2018, 2019t
Depression, assessment in, 422–423, 424–426, 454
    care plan for, 423, 425
    causes of, 421–422
    chest pain in, 1450t
    client/family teaching in, 423, 426
    clinical manifestations of, 421b
    cultural aspects of, 424b
    drug-related, 411t
    in dying patients, 453–454
    in elderly, 58, 59t
    in seasonal affective disorder, 437
    medical conditions and, 421, 424–426, 425b
    menopausal, 985
    nursing management in, 423–426
    referral for, 423–424, 426
    sleep problems in, 438

Depression *(Continued)*
   suicide and, 421, 421b
   treatment of, 422, 422b, 454
DeQuervain's tenosynovitis, 1999t
Dermatitis, 1286–1291
   acute, 1286
   allergic contact, 1286
   atopic, 1286, 1287–1290, *1288,* 2135–2136
   chronic, 1286
   contact, 1286, 1291, *1291*
   irritant, 1286, 1291
   seborrheic, 1286
   stasis, 1286, 1290–1291, *1291, 1427,* 1427–1428
   subacute, 1286
   types of, 1286–1291
Dermatologic assessment, 1267–1277. See also *Skin assessment.*
Dermatomyositis, 2162
Dermatoses. See *Dermatitis; Skin disorders.*
Dermis, 1263, *1263*
Dermoepidermal junction, 1263
DES. See *Diethylstilbestrol (DES).*
Descending pathways, 1860–1861, 1862t
Desensitization therapy, 2134
Desipramine, reference values for, 2308t
Desmopressin, in dehydration test, 1080
Desmosomes, 1262
Detrusor instability, incontinence and, 834. See also *Urinary incontinence.*
Detrusor muscle, 734
Development, psychosocial, assessment of, 144
Deviated nasal septum, 1682–1683
Device-related infections, 338, 339
DEXA scan, 545–546
Dexamethasone (Decadron), for Addison's disease, 1124t
   perioperative use of, 275t
Dexamethasone suppression test, 1122t, 1130
Dextrose, for hypoglycemia, in diabetes mellitus, 1179t
Dextrose in water (5%), 221t
   for hypernatremia, 240
Dezocine (Dalgan), 490t
Diabetes insipidus, 1143, 1144t–1145t
   after pituitary surgery, 1937
   diagnosis of, 1080
   postoperative, hyperpituitarism and, 1142
   post-traumatic, 2034t
Diabetes mellitus, 1149–1190, *1152*
   activity and exercise in, 1158–1159
      program planning for, 1164–1165
   assessment in, 1164
   atherosclerosis in, 1517
   case management in, 1170b
   cerebrovascular disease in, 1183t, 1184
   classification of, 1149–1150, 1150b, 1156t
   client teaching in, 1163, 1164b
      and illness, 1190b
      and insulin injection, 1168b, 1168–1170, *1169*
      and ketoacidosis prevention, 1176–1177
   clinical manifestations of, 1155, 1156t
   complications of, 1150
      acute, 1172–1180, *1173,* 1174b–1178b, 1174t, 1179t, 1181t–1182t
      chronic, 1180, 1182–1189
         classification of, 1180, 1182, 1182b
         macrovascular, 1182–1185, 1183t, *1185,* 1186b, 1187b
         microvascular, 1186–1189, 1188b
      coronary artery disease in, 1182, 1183t, 1184
   dawn phenomenon in, 1180
   diagnosis of, 1155, 1157b, 1157t, 1157–1158
   diet in, 1158, *1165,* 1165–1167, 1166t

Diabetes mellitus *(Continued)*
   epidemiology of, 1150
   fasting blood glucose in, 1155, 1157b
   foot care in, 1184–1185, *1185,* 1186b, 1187b, 1188
   gestational, 1149–1150
   health promotion/risk management for, 148t, 1073
   heart disease in, 1517
   honeymoon period in, 1151
   hypercortisolism and, 1131
   hyperglycemic, hyperosmolar, nonketotic syndrome in, 1177, 1177b, 1181t–1182t
   hypertension in, 1183t, 1184
   hypoglycemia in, 1177–1180, 1178b, 1179t, 1181t–1182t
      unawareness of, 1180
   illness in, 1190b
   in elderly, 1171
   infections in, 1183t, 1184–1185, 1186b, 1187b
   ketoacidosis in. See *Diabetic ketoacidosis.*
   medical management of, 1158–1162, 1160t–1162t, *1163.* See also *Insulin.*
      self-management and, 1167b, 1167–1170, 1168b, *1169,* 1170b
   nursing management of, 1162–1170
      altered health maintenance and, 1164–1167, *1165,* 1166t
      client teaching in, 1163, 1164, 1164b
   outcomes classification for, 1149
   pathophysiology of, 1151–1155, *1152, 1155*
      client teaching about, 1164
   peripheral vascular disease in, 1183t, 1184, *1185*
   pneumonia and, case study of, *1153,* 1153–1154
   renal disease in, 851–852
   secondary, 1149, 1150b
   self-care in, 1170–1171
      insulin therapy and, 1168b, 1168–1170, *1169*
      pancreas transplantation and, 1172
   self-monitoring in, 1158, 1167b, 1167–1168
      before exercise, 1165
   sleep problems in, 438
   Somogyi effect in, 1180
   surgery for, 1171–1172
      nursing management in, 1172
   surgery in, special considerations for, 1189–1190
   type 1, 1149
      diet management for, 1166–1167
      distinguishing features of, 1156t
      epidemiology of, 1150
      etiology of, 1150
      pancreas transplantation for, 1171–1172
      pathophysiology of, 1151
      risk factors for, 1150–1151
   type 2, 1149
      distinguishing features of, 1156t
      epidemiology of, 1150
      etiology of, 1151
      pathophysiology of, 1151, 1154–1155, *1155*
      risk factors for, 1151
   wound healing in, 332
Diabetic coma, 1172
Diabetic ketoacidosis, 1172–1177, 1181t–1182t
   assessment in, 1174t
   clinical manifestations of, 1174b
   critical monitoring in, rehydration and, 1175b
   epidemiology of, 1172
   etiology of, 1172–1173

Diabetes ketoacidosis *(Continued)*
   hyperglycemic, hyperosmolar, nonketotic syndrome vs., 1177
   insulin administration in, 1176
   medical management of, 1174–1177, 1175b, 1176b
   pathophysiology of, *1172,* 1172–1173
   pH correction in, 1175–1176
   potassium imbalance in, 1174, 1174t
      correction of, 1175, 1176b
   recurrence of, prevention of, 1176–1177
   rehydration in, 1175, 1175b
   risk factors for, 1172–1173
   shock in, reversal of, 1175
Diabetic nephropathy, 851–852, 1187–1188
   insulin dosage in, 882
Diabetic neuropathy, 1188–1189
Diabetic retinopathy, 1186–1187, 1188b, 1820, *1820*
Diabetic ulcers, eschar in, *328*
   healing of, 332
Diabinese. See *Chlorpropamide (Diabinese).*
Diagnosis-related groups (DRGs), 80
Diagnostic assessment, cytologic studies in, 200–201
   imaging studies in, 192–200
   tests in, 187–192
Diagnostic imaging, 192–200. See also specific studies.
Diagnostic tests, 187–192. See also specific tests.
   blood, 190–191
   by unlicensed assistive personnel, 188b
   false-negative results of, 187, 188
   false-positive results of, 187
   guidelines for, 188–189
   International System of Units for, 188
   microbiology, 189–190
   nursing management in, 187
   reference values for, 188, 2301–2310
   specificity and sensitivity of, 187–188
   specimen collection for, 188b, 188–191
   urine, 191–192
Dialysis, assessment in, 895–896
   diffusion in, 888
   for acute renal failure, 878–879
   hemodialysis, 888–895
      arteriovenous fistula in, 892, *893*
      arteriovenous graft in, 892
      complications of, 894
      dialyzers for, *892, 893*
      diet in, 894–895
      history of, 891
      medications for, 894
      procedure for, 891–893, *892*
      schedule for, 893
      therapeutic effects of, 893–894
   in acute pancreatitis, 1196
   in home care, 890b, 898
   in systemic lupus erythematosus, 2158
   nursing management in, 893–899
   peritoneal, 888–895
      automated, 889
      catheters for, 889, *890*
      complications of, 891
      continuous ambulatory, 889
      continuous cyclic, 889
      contraindications to, 889
      dialysate in, 889–890
      dwell time in, 889–890
      in acute pancreatitis, 1196
      indications for, 889
      intermittent, 889
      procedures for, 889–890
   quality of life in, 895
   self-care in, 899
   ultrafiltration in, 888

Dialysis equilibrium syndrome, 894
Diapedesis, 318, *318*
Diaphragm, disorders of, 1743–1744
    structure of, *1614, 1616,* 1616–1617
Diaphragmatic breathing, preoperative teaching
    of, 285–286, *286*
Diaphragmatic hernia, 697–698, *698*
    gastroesophageal reflux disease and, 695
Diaphragmatic paralysis, 1744
Diarrhea, 706, 766
    dehydration and, 218
    drug therapy for, 773
    in cancer, 394
    in hepatic encephalopathy, 1252–1253
    in inflammatory bowel disease, 771t, 772,
        773, 774
    infectious, 766, 767, 768
    management of, 768
    pathogenesis of, 337t
    rectal pouch for, 799
Diastasis recti, 652, 742
Diastole, atrial, 1440
    ventricular, 1440
Diastolic pressure, 1442
Diazepam (Valium), emergency administration
    of, 1931
    for status epilepticus, 1931
    preoperative, 290t
DIC. See *Disseminated intravascular coagula-
    tion (DIC).*
Diclofenac, 486, 487t
Dicyclomine (Bentyl), for peptic ulcer disease,
    710t, 715
Didanosine (Videx, ddI), 2196t
Didronel (etidronate disodium), for hypercal-
    cemia, 253
Diencephalon, 1858
Diet. See also *Feeding; Food; Nutrition.*
    acne and, 1293
    assessment of. See *Nutritional assessment.*
    atherosclerosis and, 1517, 1521
    bowel elimination and, 741
    breast cancer and, 1013, 1014
    calorie requirements in, determination of,
        663, 663t
    cancer and, 15, 355, 394
    challenge, 2101–2102
    colon cancer and, 780–781
    coronary heart disease and, 1517, 1521
    cultural variations in, 634b–645b
    disease and, *14,* 14–15, 24–26
    diverticular disease and, 789
    elimination, 2101–2102
    goitrogens in, 1090
    health promotion/risk management for,
        150t–151t
    heart disease and, 1455
    in acute pancreatitis, 1197, 1200
    in acute renal failure, 879, 880
    in alcoholic hepatitis, 1232
    in ascites, 1246
    in atopic dermatitis, 1288
    in cancer, 394
    in cholelithiasis, 1207, 1211
    in chronic renal failure, 894–895, *897*
    in cirrhosis, 1235, 1239, 1253
    in diabetes mellitus, 1158, *1165,* 1165–
        1167, 1166t
        and exercise, 1165
    in dumping syndrome, 721b
    in edema, 227, 228
    in gastroesophageal reflux disease, 696
    in gout, 576
    in hemodialysis, 892
    in hepatic encephalopathy, 1252
    in hiatal hernia, 699
    in hyperkalemia, 245b, 248

Diet *(Continued)*
    in hypermagnesemia, 256b, 257
    in hypernatremia, 238b, 241
    in hyperphosphatemia, 254
    in hypertension, 1383, 1387, 1388t
    in hyperthyroidism, 1101
    in hypocalcemia, 250, 251b, 252
    in hypokalemia, 244, 245b, 246
    in hypomagnesemia, 256, 256b
    in hyponatremia, 238b, 239
    in hypoparathyroidism, 1115, 1116
    in ileostomy, 779
    in inflammatory bowel disease, 772, 774
    in irritable bowel syndrome, 793, 794
    in leukemia, 2172
    in peptic ulcer disease, 715, 718
    in peripheral arterial occlusive disease,
        1402
    in premenstrual syndrome, 981–982
    in prostate cancer, 959
    in renal disease, 241
    in urinary tract infection, 803–804, 806
    in viral hepatitis, 1230–1231
    low-fat, 32–33, 1393b, 1517, 1521
        in atherosclerosis, 1521
        in coronary heart disease, 1521
        in hypertension, 1387, 1393b
    low-sodium, 238b
        in edema, 227, 228
        in heart failure, 1536, 1538t, 1541
        in hypernatremia, 241
        in hypertension, 1387, 1393
        in renal disease, 241
    potassium in, 244, 245b, 246, 248
    recommended dietary allowances for, 638
    reference daily intakes for, 638
    sodium in, 238b, 239
    urinary elimination and, 753, 753t
    urolithiasis and, 825
    weight-loss, 32
Diet history, 649
Diethylstilbestrol (DES), testicular cancer and,
    964
    vaginal cancer and, 1004–1005
Diffuse axonal injury, 2041
Diffuse toxic goiter, *1090.* See also *Graves'
    disease.*
Diffusion, 216, 888
    in capillary exchange, 1365, *1366*
Diffusion capacity, assessment of, 1637
Diflunisal, 486, 487t
Digestion, age-related changes in, 637
    carbohydrate, 636
    enzymes in, 634, 635t
    esophageal, 633, *633*
    gastric, 633–634
    gastroduodenal, 634
    lipid, 636
    lubricants in, 634–635, 635t
    peristalsis in, 632–633
    physiology of, 630, 632–636
    protein, 636
    regulation of, 631
    swallowing in, 633, *633*
Digital rectal examination, 743, *744,* 756
    in pelvic examination, 743
Digital venous angiography, 1900
Digitalis, in hypokalemia, 245
    parathyroidectomy and, 1113
Digitoxin, reference values for, 2308t
Digoxin, administration of, 1537b
    dosage of, 1537b
    drug interactions with, 1537b
    for dysrhythmias, 1563t
    for heart failure, 1536, 1539t
        in emergency care, 2274–2275
    pharmacokinetics of, 1537b

Digoxin, administration of *(Continued)*
    reference values for, 2308t
    toxicity of, 1537b
Dilantin. See *Phenytoin (Dilantin).*
Dilantin (phenytoin), gingival hyperplasia and,
    1930
Dilated cardiomyopathy, 1490–1492, *1491,
    1492t*
Dilaudid (hydromorphone), 489t
Diltiazem (Cardizem), for angina, 1582, 1584t
    for hypertension, 1389t, 1396t
Diluting segment, 735
Diphenhydramine (Benadryl), for anaphylaxis,
    2251
    for Parkinson's disease, 2019t
    for phenothiazine overdose, 2281t
Diphtheria, 1680–1681
    immunization for, 342, 342t
Diploidy, 1017
Diplopia, 1885
    in myasthenia gravis, 2020
Diprivan (propofol), for rapid-sequence induc-
    tion, 2268
Dipyridamole thallium 201 scintigraphy, in
    cardiac assessment, 1474
Direct antiglobulin test, 2096
Direct bilirubin, 757, 757t
Directional coronary atherectomy, 1523, *1523*
Disability, cardiovascular, 1532b
Disc herniation, cervical, 1991–1993, *1992*
    lumbar, 1984–1985, *1985*
    surgery for, *1987,* 1987–1991
Discectomy, percutaneous, 1987, 1989–1991
Discharge, from post-anesthesia care unit,
    307b, 307–308
Discography, 1985
Discoid lupus erythematosus, 2156
Disconjugate gaze, 1885
Disconnection syndrome, 1929
Disease, causation of, theories of, 3, 4t–7t, 8
    chronic. See *Chronic conditions.*
    cultural aspects of, 19b
    health and wellness and, 8–9
    personality types and, 7t
    presentation of, in elderly, 52
    risk factors for, 10, 13–16, *14*
    stress and, 3, 5t–7t, 16, 26–27
    terminal. See *Death and dying.*
Dislocations, 619
    emergency care for, 2279
Disopyramide, reference values for, 2308t
Displaced fracture, 593t
Displacement, 408b
Dissecting aortic aneurysm, 1419–1420
    chest pain in, 1449t
Disseminated intravascular coagulation (DIC),
    2123–2126, 2124b, *2125,* 2126t
    in cancer, 396
    in shock, 2237–2238
Distraction, for pain, 500
Distributive (vasogenic) shock, 2231. See also
    Shock.
    clinical manifestations of, 2243
    etiology of, 2233–2234
    medical management of, 2250t
Disulfiram (Antabuse), 519, 522b
Disuse syndrome, 17
Ditropan (oxybutynin), for urinary inconti-
    nence, 837t
Diuresis, 217
Diuretics, for ascites, 1247
    for chronic renal failure, 894
    for edema, 227
    for heart failure, 1536, 1538t, 1541
        in emergency care, 2274
    for hemodialysis, 892
    for hypertension, 1389t

Diuretics (Continued)
  for nephrotic syndrome, 863
  nephrotoxicity of, 854
  perioperative use of, 275t
  potassium-sparing, hypermagnesemia and, 256
  thiazide, hypercalcemia and, 252
Diverticulitis, 789–790
Diverticulosis, 789–790
Diverticulum, bladder, 829
  esophageal, 698–699
  intestinal, 789–790
  Meckel's, 790
Dizziness, 1799, 1847, 1849–1850. See also Balance; Vestibular system.
  etiology of, 1847b
  risk factors for, 1847
DNA, 209, 210
DNA ploidy, 1017
Dobutamine, for heart failure, 1537b
Documentation, in acute care nursing, 104
  in health history, 160
  in neurologic assessment, 2036–2037
  of consent, 287, 288
  of emergency care, 2267
  of pain management, 502, 503
  of physical examination, 185
  photographic, in plastic surgery, 1316
  postoperative, 304, 305
Doll's eye reflex, assessment of, 1909, 1909
Dolophine (methadone), 488–490, 489t
Domestic violence, 39
  assessment for, 918
Donepezil (Aricept), for Alzheimer's disease, 2004–2005
Donovanosis, 1053
Dopamine (Intropin), for acute renal failure, 878
  for heart failure, 1537b
Dopamine hypothesis, for schizophrenia, 417
Doppler scanning, in neurologic assessment, 1896
Doppler ultrasonography, in neurologic assessment, 1896
  in skin graft assessment, 1323
  in vascular assessment, 1375–1376
  in venous thrombosis, 1424
Dorsal horn, in pain perception, 469–471, 470
Dorsal recumbent position, 181, 299, 300
Dorsalis pedis pulse, assessment of, 1373, 1374
Double vision, 1885
Douching, 1002
Dowager's hump, 578
Down syndrome, Alzheimer's disease in, 2003
Doxazosin (Cardura), for hypertension, 1389t
Doxepin, perioperative use of, 275t
Doxorubicin (Adriamycin), for breast cancer, 1032, 1033, 1034, 1035
Drainage, chest, closed, 1732–1738, 1737
  postoperative, in cardiac surgery, 1508
  decompression, of bladder, 832
  from incision, 324
  in hemothorax, 1768
  of cerebrospinal fluid, 1965
  postural, for chronic obstructive pulmonary disease, 1698
  wound, 300, 324
    postoperative management of, 307
    preoperative teaching for, 287
Drains, surgical, 300
  postoperative care of, 307, 309, 310b, 310–311
  preoperative teaching for, 287
Draping, for physical examination, 180, 181
Drawer tests, 545t, 546

Dressings, biologic, 1350t
  biosynthetic, 1350t
  disposal of, 330, 331
  for burns, 1348, 1350t
  for central venous catheter, 671
  for incisions, 324
  for skin tears, 1295
  in debridement, 328, 328–329
  occlusive, 1281t
  postoperative care of, 307, 309, 310b
  removal of, 330, 331
  selection of, 330
  tracheostomy, 1658, 1659
  types of, 329t
  wet, 1280t, 1283, 1283
  wet-to-dry, 328–329, 329
    in debridement, 328–329, 329, 1347
  wet-to-moist, 326, 329t
  wound, 1282, 2280
Dressler's syndrome, 1596
DRGs (diagnosis-related groups), 80
Drop arm test, 544t
Droperidol (Inapsine), preoperative, 290t
Droplet precautions, 344
Droplet transmission, 335
Drowning, 1770
Drug(s). See also specific drugs and drug families.
  administration of, via feeding tube, 676, 676b
  anaphylaxis due to, 2137t, 2137–2138
  biorhythms and, 432
  delirium and, 453t
  for elderly, 60–61, 62t
  for surgical client, 274–275, 275t, 284
  goiter due to, 1090
  hepatotoxic, 1232, 1232t, 1235t
    ascites and, 1247
    hepatitis and, 1229, 1230
  lupus-like syndrome due to, 2157, 2157b
  nebulized, metered-dose inhaler for, 1691, 1693, 1693b
  nephrotoxic, 853t, 853–854
  ototoxic, 1799, 1800b
  overdose of, antidotes for, 2281t
  pharmacokinetics and pharmacodynamics of, in chronic renal failure, 886
    in elderly, 60–61
  psychiatric side effects of, 409–410, 411t
  sensitivity studies for, 189
  side effects of, gastrointestinal, 740–741
  therapeutic monitoring of, reference values for, 2307t–2308t
  urinary elimination and, 752, 752t
Drug abuse. See Substance abuse.
Drug history, in preoperative assessment, 275, 275t, 282
Drug-resistant microorganisms, 339, 341b
Drusen, 1821
Dry eye syndrome, 1826
Dry skin, management of, 1286
DTs. See delirium tremens.
Dual-energy absorptiometry (DXA), 566, 568–569, 569
Dual-energy X-ray absorptiometry (DEXA), 545–546
Duchenne's muscular dystrophy, 583t, 583–584
Duct ectasia, of breast, 1037
Ductal carcinoma in situ, 1015
Ductal hyperplasia, of breast, 1037
Dullness, on percussion, 177, 742–743
Dumping syndrome, 721, 721b
Duodenal drainage analysis, 1086
Duodenal ulcers, 712, 713t. See also Peptic ulcer disease.
  drug-induced, 712
  stress, 712

Duodenum, function of, 633
  assessment of, 1086
  structure of, 630
Duplicate ureter, 846
Dupuytren's contracture, 2000
Dura mater, 1862, 1862
Durable power of attorney for health care, 67, 2009
Dust diseases, occupational, 1739–1740, 1740t
DXA. See Dual-energy absorptiometry (DXA).
D-xylose absorption test, 656
Dysarthria, in stroke, 1957t, 1958, 1975–1976
Dysentery, 766–767, 768
Dysfunctional uterine bleeding, 982–984
  leiomyomas and, 991–994
  postmenopausal, 986, 987
Dysmenorrhea, 980–981
  in endometriosis, 989
Dyspareunia, after hysterectomy, 998
Dyspepsia, 706
Dysphagia, 690–691
  achalasia and, 691
  assessment of, 652
  causes of, 690–691
  feeding in, 223, 1974–1975, 1975t
  fluid management in, 223
  in cardiovascular disease, 690
  in esophageal cancer, 700, 701
  in gastroesophageal reflux disease, 695
  in Huntington's disease, 2012
  in neurologic disease, 690–691
  in stroke, 1957t, 1958
  malnutrition and, 667
  management of, 667
  obstructive, 690
Dysplasia, 211
  definition of, 350t
Dyspnea, 451–452
  acute, 1451–1452
  assessment of, 452, 1623–1624, 1624, 1624t
  chronic, 1452
  etiology of, 452
  exertional, 1452
  in asthma, 1689
  in chronic obstructive pulmonary disease, 1696, 1698t
  in diaphragmatic paralysis, 1744
  in dying patients, 451–452
  in heart disease, 1451–1452, 1534
  in mechanical ventilation, 1507
  management of, 452
  paroxysmal nocturnal, 1452, 1534
Dysrhythmias, 1550–1577
  ablative procedures for, 1569
  atrial, 1552–1553, 1554
  atrioventricular, 1556–1559
  automaticity disturbances in, 1550–1551
  clinical manifestations of, 1552
  conduction disturbances in, 1551
  defibrillation for, 1566–1568, 1567
  diagnosis of, 1552, 1553b. See also Electrocardiography (ECG).
  drug therapy for, 1562t–1563t
  electrocardiography in, 1466–1472. See also Electrocardiography (ECG).
  electrophysiologic testing in, 1472
  emergency care for, 2275
  etiology of, 1550–1551
  in hyperkalemia, 244, 247, 248
  in hypokalemia, 243–244, 244
  in hypomagnesemia, 256
  management of, 1552
  pathophysiology of, 1552
  postinfarction, 1591, 1594–1595
  post-traumatic, 2034t
  reentry, 1551

Dysrhythmias (Continued)
    risk factors for, 1551–1552
    ventricular, 1559–1566
Dyssomnias, 434–437
Dysuria, 748

E

Ear. See also Hearing.
    anatomy of, 1782–1785, 1783, 1784
    assessment of, 1798–1807
        chief complaint in, 1799
        diagnostic tests in, 1804–1807, 1805,
            1806
        history in, 1798b, 1798–1800, 1799t,
            1800b
        laboratory studies in, 1806–1807
        physical examination in, 1800–1804,
            1801b, 1801–1803
        symptom analysis in, 1799
    biopsy of, 1807
    drainage from, 1799
        culture of, 1807
    examination of, 165t
    external, 1782–1783, 1783, 1785
        examination of, 1800
        infection of, 1842
        traumatic injuries of, 1842
    foreign bodies in, 1842, 1845
    infection of, 1832, 1842–1843
        antibiotics for, 1844–1845, 1845
        surgery for, 1846, 1846–1847, 1847b
    inner, 1784, 1784–1786
    irrigation of, 1844, 1844
    middle, 1783, 1783–1784, 1785
        implants for, 1841
        infection of, 1842–1843
        prosthetic, 1846, 1846–1847
    obstruction of, 1832
    pain in, 1799, 1840–1847, 1844–1846
    physiology of, 1785–1786
    swimmer's, 1842
    tumors of, 1833, 1843
        surgery for, 1840
Ear canal, 1783, 1783
    physical examination of, 1801, 1801–1802,
        1802
Ear wax, 1783, 1785
Eardrum. See Tympanic membrane.
Eating disorders, 677–681
Eaton-Lambert syndrome, 2023
Eccrine glands, 1262, 1263
ECG. See Electrocardiography (ECG).
Echocardiography, 198, 198–199, 1473, 1473–
    1474
    in myocardial infarction, 1590
    transesophageal, 1473–1474
        in myocardial infarction, 1590
Economic aspects, of chronic conditions, 13,
    20–21, 21t
    of chronic disease, 13
    of hospital care, 96
Ectopic ACTH syndrome, 1126
    treatment of, 1133t
Ectopic pregnancy, 1000
Ectopic testis, 967–968
Ectopic ureter, 846
Eczema, 1286, 1287–1290, 1288
    xerotic, 1290
Eczematous disorders, 1286–1291. See also
    Dermatitis.
Edema, 225–228, 1274, 1365. See also
    Lymphedema.
    arm, postmastectomy, 1025
    assessment in, 227
    assessment of, 1371–1372, 1372

Edema (Continued)
    cerebral, 228–229, 2028, 2034t. See also In-
        creased intracranial pressure (ICP).
        definition of, 2028
        in hyponatremia, 237
        in water intoxication, 228–229
        stroke and, 1965
    clinical manifestations of, 225–226
    etiology of, 225, 225t
    hyponatremia and, 237
    hypothyroidism and. See Myxedema.
    in burns, 1337, 1337, 1351
    in heart disease, 1452, 1456, 1534–1535
        treatment of, 1536, 1538t, 1541
    in inflammation, 322, 323
    in nephrotic syndrome, 863
    in vascular disorders, 1369, 1371–1372,
        1372
    laryngeal, 1681
    medical management of, 227
    nursing management of, 227–228, 323
    of spinal cord, 2047–2048, 2049
    pathophysiology of, 225, 226
    pulmonary. See Pulmonary edema.
    self-care in, 228
Education, client. See Client teaching.
Educational assessment, preoperative, 282
Efavirenz (Sustiva), 2198t
Efferent neurons, 1869
Efudex (5-fluorouracil), for actinic keratosis,
    1304
Ego defense mechanisms, 408b
Egophony, 1635
Ejaculation, 911
Ejaculatory cord, 912
Ejaculatory problems, in infertility, 969
Ejection click, 1461
Elastic stockings, in chronic venous insuffi-
    ciency, 1428
Elastic wraps, for venous thrombosis, 1425
Elastin cartilage, 534
Elbow, examination of, 543, 544t
    fractures of, 618
    golfer's, 621, 1999t
    replacement of, in rheumatoid arthritis, 2156
    tennis, 621, 1999t
        test for, 544t
Elbow breadth method, for body frame size
    calculation, 650b
Elderly. See also Aging and specific disorders.
    abuse of, 57, 57b
    achalasia in, 694
    acid-base disorders in, 268
    activities of daily living in, 52, 52–53, 53
    acute care for, 64
    adult day care for, 65, 125
    ageism and, 55
    autonomy of, 65–66
    balance disorders in, 1849
    cardiac function in, 1444
    cardiovascular function in, 212t
    care alternatives for, 125
    case management for, 65
    cholelithiasis in, 1211–1212
    chronic conditions in, 14, 14
    cognitive function in, 57–58, 59t
    competence of, 66–67
    definitions of, 47
    dehydration in, 218
    delirium in, 58, 59t
    dementia in, 57–58, 59t
    depression in, 58, 59t
    diabetes mellitus in, 1171
    economic status of, 46–47
    edema in, 228
    educational status of, 47
    ethical issues affecting, 65–68

Elderly (Continued)
    ethnicity of, 46
    exercise and activity in, 49–51
    falls in, 55, 626–627
    family support for, 47–48
    functional status in, 52–57
    gastrointestinal function in, 212t, 637
    health care delivery for, 61–65
    health promotion for, 48t, 48–70, 149t–
        150t, 155, 156t–159t
    health trends in, 46–47
    hearing impairment in, 50t, 53, 1786, 1799t,
        1832
    hip fractures in, 607–616. See also Hip,
        fractures of.
    home care for, 65
    home modifications for, 54t
    hospice care for, 65
    hyperparathyroidism, 1114
    hyperthyroidism in, 1106
        case study of, 1102
    hypothyroidism in, 1098–1099
    immune function in, 212t
    increasing population of, 45, 46
    influenza vaccine for, 342
    intermittent self-catheterization by, 845
    legal issues affecting, 65, 66t
    living/housing options for, 54t, 62–63, 64–
        65, 125
    long-term care for, 62–63, 64–65, 118–
        126. See also Long-term care facilities.
        alternatives to, 54t, 62–63, 64–65, 125
    malnutrition in, 661
    managed care for, 63–64
    marital status of, 46
    medication use by, 60–61, 62t
    mental health disorders in, 57–60
    metabolic assessment in, 1076t, 1078
    metabolic function in, 1068–1069
    multiple losses of, 55–57
    musculoskeletal system in, 212t, 536
    neglect of, 57, 57b
    neurologic function in, 212t
    nosocomial infections in, 340, 340b, 344–
        346
    opioid analgesics for, 493
    pain in, 476, 493
    postoperative confusion in, 612
    preoperative teaching for, 287
    presentation of illness in, 52
    rehabilitation for, inpatient, 64
        outpatient, 654
    relocation stress syndrome in, care plan for,
        56
        outcomes for, 45
    renal function in, 212t, 737–738
    respiratory function in, 212t, 1622
    respite care for, 65
    screening and prevention for, 149t–150t
    self-care and self-responsibility by, 49
    self-determination for, 67
    sensory function in, 212t
    sexuality of, 46
    skin in, 212t, 1265t, 1265–1266
    sleep in, 53, 433
    subacute care for, 64–65
    substance abuse by, 58–60
    support services for, 54t, 61–63, 63b
    surgery in, 280, 281t
    urinary diversion in, 821
    urinary function in, 212t
    urinary incontinence in, 840
    urinary system in, 737–738
    urinary tract infection in, 807
    vision impairment in, 50t, 53, 1781–1782,
        1814–1817, 1821, 1821
    wound healing in, 331

Elective surgery. See also under *Intraoperative; Perioperative; Postoperative; Preoperative; Surgery.*
  case management for, 283
Electrical burns, 1332. See also *Burns.*
Electrical injury, cell damage in, 213
Electrical safety, during surgery, 299–300
Electrical stimulation, for urinary incontinence, 836, *836*
  for wound healing, 333
Electrocardiography (ECG), 1466–1472. See also specific dysrhythmias.
  continuous ambulatory, 1470
  exercise, 1470–1472
  in angina, 1581
  in Holter monitoring, 1470
  in hyperkalemia, *244,* 247
  in hypokalemia, 243–244, *244*
  in myocardial infarction, 1469, 1469t, 1587, *1589*
  in shock, 2253
  indications for, 1468
  interpretation of, 1553b
  lead placement in, *1466,* 1466–1467, *1468,* 1468–1470
  lesion location on, 1469, 1469t
  normal tracings on, *1467,* 1467–1468
  of paced beats, 1574, *1575*
  postprocedure care in, 1466
  preprocedure care in, 1466
  signal-averaged, 1470
  sounds, after cardiac surgery, 1508
  12-lead, *1468,* 1468–1470, *1469*
Electrocochleography, 1806
Electroconvulsive therapy, 422
Electrodesiccation, for actinic keratosis, 1304, *1305*
Electroencephalography (EEG), *1901,* 1901–1902, *1902*
  in coma, 1909
Electrolyte(s). See also *Fluid and electrolyte balance* and specific electrolytes.
  definition of, 233
  fluid concentrations of, 234t
  food sources of, 233
  imbalances of, 234–257
    as collaborative problems, 235
    critical monitoring in, 236b
    diagnosis of, 234–235
    etiology of, 234
    in acute pancreatitis, 1196, 1197
    in acute renal failure, 878
    in addisonian crisis, 1121
    in burns, 1334, *1334,* 1337
    in chronic renal failure, 883
    in diabetic ketoacidosis, 1174, 1174t
    in tumor lysis syndrome, 396
    of calcium, 248–254
    of magnesium, 255–257
    of phosphorus, 254
    of potassium, 242–248
    of sodium, 235–242
    pathophysiology of, 234, *235*
    risk factors for, 234
  in acid-base balance, 259–262, *260–262*
  in intracellular vs. extracellular fluid, *234*
  in parenteral nutrition, 668, 668t
  intake of, 233
  intestinal absorption of, 636–637
  intracellular, 206
  plasma concentrations of, 235b
  regulation of, 233. See also *Fluid and electrolyte balance.*
    kidney in, 735, 736t
  serum, in cardiac assessment, 1465
Electromyography, 548, 1903, *1903*
  sphincter, 762, *762*

Electron-beam computed tomography, in angina evaluation, 1581
Electronic pacemakers. See *Pacemaker(s), artificial.*
Electronystagmography, 1806
Electrophysiologic studies, in cardiac assessment, 1472
Electroretinography (ERG), 1797
Electrosurgical unit, 300
Elevation pallor, 1372, *1373*
Elimination. See *Bowel elimination; Urinary elimination.*
Elimination diet, 2101–2102
Elliptical incisions, 1314
Emancipated minor, 286
Embolectomy, for pulmonary embolism, 1708
Embolism, arterial, 1415–1416
  fat, 600–601, 605
  in infective endocarditis, 1486
  postoperative, 308
    prevention of, 286, 308
  pulmonary. See *Pulmonary embolism.*
  stroke and, 1594, 1953, *1954.* See also *Stroke.*
Embolization, arterial, for gastrointestinal bleeding, 717
  for intracranial aneurysms, 1943
  renal artery, 861
Emergency care, 2261–2283
  airway management in, 2266–2268, *2267,* 2267–2270, *2268*
  client disposition in, 2267
  components of, 2265–2267
  conscious sedation in, 2276
  consent for, 2262–2263
  cricothyroidotomy in, 2268, *2269*
  diagnosis in, 2266–2267
  documentation of, 2267
  Emergency Medical Services and, 2261
  endotracheal intubation in, 2268–2269
  ethical issues in, 2264–2265
  evaluation in, 2267
  evidence collection and preservation in, 2263, 2263t, 2264t
  federal regulation of, 2262
  fluid management in, 2273–2275
  for asthma, 1689
  for burns, 2274
  for cardiac tamponade, 2275, *2276*
  for confusional states, 2276–2277
  for decreased cardiac output, 2275
  for dysrhythmias, 2275
  for flail chest, 2272, *2272*
  for fractures, 590–596
  for frostbite, 2283
  for gas exchange abnormalities, 2270–2271
  for head injuries, 2044
  for head trauma, 2276–2277
  for heart failure, 2274–2275
  for heat stroke, 2282
  for hyperthermia, 2282
  for hyperventilation, 2269–2270
  for hypervolemia, 2274–2275
  for hypothermia, 2282–2283
  for hypoventilation, 2270
  for hypovolemia, 2273–2274
  for infection, 2278
  for myocardial infarction, 2275
  for narcotic overdose, 2276–2277
  for poisoning, 2281t, 2281–2282
  for seizures, 2277
  for snake bite, 2282
  for spinal cord injury, 2053–2054, 2279
  for status epilepticus, 1931
  for stroke, 1960–1964, 2277
  for sucking chest wound, 1767
  for traumatic amputation, 2279

Emergency care *(Continued)*
  for unconscious patient, 2276–2277
  for vision impairment, 2277–2278
  Heimlich maneuver in, 2266, 2268, *2268*
  legal issues in, 2261–2264
  nursing assessment in, *2265,* 2265–2266
  outcome management in, 2267
  outcomes classification for, 2261
  oxygen administration in, 2270
  pain management in, 2275–2276
  pericardiocentesis in, 2275, *2276*
  psychosocial aspects of, 2283
  restraints in, 2263
  spinal immobilization in, 2269
  triage in, 2265, 2265t
  wound care in, 2280–2281
Emergency departments, nursing care in, 88
Emergency Medical Services, 2261
Emergency nursing, 2261
Emollients, 1283, 1286
Empacho, 19b
Emphysema, pulmonary, 1692–1705
  care map for, 1700b
  care plan for, 1702b–1704b
  case management in, 1686b
  centrilobular, 1695, *1695*
  clinical manifestations of, 1696, *1696, 1697,* 1698t
  complications of, 1696, *1697*
  epidemiology of, 1693
  etiology of, 1693
  in elderly, 1700
  medical management of, 1691t, 1696–1699
  nursing management of, 1699–1700
  oxygen conservation strategies in, 1705b
  panlobular, 1695, 1695–1696
  paraseptal (panacinar), *1695,* 1696
  pathophysiology of, 1695–1696
  radiographic findings in, 1696, *1697*
  risk factors for, 1693
  self-care in, 1700–1705
  sleep problems in, 438–439
  surgery for, 1700
  types of, *1695*
  subcutaneous, in tracheostomy, 1655
Empowerment, in chronic conditions, 25
Empyema, in cholecystitis, 1212
Enalapril (Vasotec), for hypertension, 1389t, 1396t
Enalaprilat, for hypertension, 1396t
Encapone, for Parkinson's disease, 2018, 2019t
Encephalitis, viral, 1947
Encephalopathy, hepatic, 1065, 1250–1253, 1251b
  after paracentesis, 1087
  cirrhosis and, 1241
  viral hepatitis and, 1227
Enchondroma, 580t, 580–581
Endemic goiter, 1089–1090
Endocardial (transvenous) pacing, 1572, *1572*
Endocarditis, infective, 1484–1487, *1485*
Endocardium, 1435, *1436*
Endocrine ablation, for breast cancer, 1036
Endocrine disorders. See also specific disorders.
  assessment of, 1070–1073, 1070–1087
    diagnostic tests in, 1078–1080
    history in, 1070–1073
    laboratory studies in, 1080, 1081t–1083t
    physical examination in, *1073,* 1073–1078
      of abdomen, *1073,* 1075–1078, 1076t
      of neck, 1074, *1075,* 1075b
    symptom analysis in, 1070–1071
  hypertension and, 1383
  in chronic renal failure, 887
  sleep problems in, 438

Endocrine system. See also *Hormones; specific glands; specific hormones.*
  age-related changes in, 50t
  anatomy of, 1060–1064, *1062–1064*
  function of, 1065–1067
  in shock, 2239–2240, *2240,* 2242–2243
  preoperative assessment of, 280
Endocrine therapy. See *Hormonal therapy.*
End-of-life care, 447–459
Endolymph, 1785
Endolymphatic sac, surgery of, 1851
Endometrial ablation, for menorrhagia, 984
Endometrial biopsy, 931, *931*
  in menorrhagia, 984
Endometrial cancer, *994,* 994–995
  screening for, 369t, 370
Endometrial uterine lavage, *931*
Endometrioma, 989
Endometriosis, 989–991, *990, 1000*
Endometrium, 905
Endoplasmic reticulum, *206,* 207t
Endoscopic retrograde cholangiopancreatography (ERCP), 1086
  in choledocholithiasis, 1214
Endoscopic sphincterotomy, for choledocholithiasis, 1214
Endoscopic thoracotomy, 1647
Endoscopy, 200, *200*
  gastrointestinal, 657–658, *658,* 746–747
  in reproductive assessment, in females, 928–930
  retrograde, for gallstone removal, 1205, *1206*
  urinary tract, 760
Endoskeleton, 530
Endosteum, 531
Endotoxins, 213
Endotracheal intubation, cuff deflation in, 1752
  cuff inflation in, 1750–1751
  cuff leaks in, 1752
  emergency, 2268–2269
  extubation in, in mechanical ventilation, 1761
    postoperative, 304
  in general anesthesia, 293, *295*
  in mechanical ventilation, 1750, *1751.* See also *Mechanical ventilation.*
  in shock, 2244
  tube insertion in, 1750, *1751*
  tube securing in, 1750, *1751*
Endovascular procedures, for aneurysms, 1418
  for peripheral vascular disease, 1405
End-stage renal disease, 880, 881
  transplantation in, 899–901
Enema, barium, 746
  preoperative, 284
Enflurane (Ethrane), 294t
Enkephalin, in pain, 469
Enteral nutrition, 671–677
  administration of, by unlicensed assistive personnel, 1915b
    methods of, 673, 675–676, 693, *693*
    routes of, 673, *673*
  aspiration in, prevention of, 676
  assessment in, 673–675
  bolus, 673
  client teaching for, 676, 678b
  continuous, 673
  delegation in, 677b
  fluid intake in, 224
  formulas for, 671–672, 672t
    dilution of, 224
  in coma, 1915b, 1915–1916
  in esophageal surgery, 693, *693,* 694
  indications for, 671, 671b
  infection control in, 675
  intermittent, 673

Enteral nutrition *(Continued)*
  medication administration via, 676, 676b
  monitoring in, 676, 678t
  nursing management in, 673–677
  preoperative, 284
  self-care in, 676, 678b
  tube insertion in, 707. See also *Gastrointestinal intubation.*
    errors in, 728–729
  tube maintenance in, 708
  tube patency in, maintenance of, 676
  tube position in, assessment of, 675, 728–729
Enteric infections, sexually transmitted, 1056
Enteric nervous system, 630, 631
Enterobiasis, 767
Enterocele, 999
Enterococcus, vancomycin-resistant, 339, 341b
Entropion, 1827t
Enucleation, for ocular melanoma, 1825
Enuresis, sleep, 437
Environmental factors, in disease, *14,* 15–16, 28
  in hypersensitivity, 2133, *2134*
Environmental risks, 153t–154t
Environmental structuring, 443
Enzymatic debridement, 329, 1296
  of burns, 1347
Enzymes, cardiac, 1464–1465
    in myocardial infarction, 1588–1589, *1589*
  digestive, 633, 635t, 635–636
  liver, 1082t
  lysosomal, in shock, 2238–2239
  muscle, 549t
  pancreatic, 635t, 636, 1081t
    in acute pancreatitis, 1194
Eosinophils, 2080
  Cushing's syndrome and, 1130
  in white cell count and differential, 322t
  in wound healing, 319
Ependymal cells, *1865,* 1866
Ependymomas, 1932. See also *Brain tumors.*
Epicardial (transthoracic) pacing, 1572
Epicondylitis, medial, 621, 1999t
  test for, 544t
Epidemiology, 10–11
Epidermal appendages, 1262–1263
Epidermal growth factor, in wound healing, 320
Epidermis, 1262, *1263*
Epididymis, 911t, 912, *912*
  pain in, 750–751
  palpation of, 938
Epididymitis, 966
Epidural analgesia, 495
Epidural anesthesia, *295,* 295–296. See also *Anesthesia.*
Epidural blood patch, 1898–1899
Epidural hematoma, *2041,* 2041–2042
Epidural space, 1862, *1862*
Epiglottis, 1613, *1613*
Epilepsy, 1923–1930. See also *Seizures.*
  classification of, 1924
  diagnosis of, 1926
  epidemiology of, 1923
  etiology of, 1923–1924
  medical management of, 1926–1928
  nursing management of, in medical management, 1928
    in surgical management, 1930
    self-care in, 1930
  pathophysiology of, *1924,* 1924–1925
  risk factors for, 1923–1924
  sleep deprivation and, 439
  status epilepticus in, 1931
  surgery for, 1928
  vs. seizures, 1923

Epinephrine, 1067
  excess of, 1135t, 1135–1137
  for anaphylaxis, 2251
  in regional anesthesia, 293
  plasma, reference values for, 1136, 2303t
  urine, reference values for, 2306t
Epiphyseal cartilage, 531, *534*
Episcleritis, in rheumatoid arthritis, 2145
Epispadias, 756, 971, *971*
Epistaxis, 1672–1676, *1676*
Epithelial autografting, for burns, 1353–1354
Epithelial cells, 211
Epithelialization, in wound healing, 320
Epithelium, 1262
Epitopes, 2081, *2081*
Epivir (lamivudine), 2196t
Epley maneuvers, in vestibular rehabilitation, 1850
Epoprostenol, for pulmonary hypertension, 1708–1709
Equianalgesic dosage, 289t–290t, 492–493
Equilibrium, age-related changes in, 53–54
  assessment of, 1885
Equipment, surgical, safety measures for, 299–300
ERCP. See *Endoscopic retrograde cholangiopancreatography (ERCP).*
Erectile dysfunction, 972–974
  after prostate surgery, 956, 958
Erection, nocturnal, 439
  penile, 911
  prolonged, 972
ERG. See *Electroretinography (ERG).*
Erosion, *1272*
ERT. See *Estrogen replacement therapy (ERT).*
Erysipelas, 1310
Erythema multiforme, in coccidioidomycosis, 1723
Erythrocyte(s), 2075–2078
  abnormalities of, 2096, 2098t
  destruction of, 2075–2077, *2078*
  life span of, 2075
  production of, 2075–2077, *2076*
  reference ranges for, 2096t
Erythrocyte count, 2094, 2096t
  disorders and conditions affecting, 2097t
  in cardiac assessment, 1464
  reference values for, 2302t
Erythrocyte indices, 2095–2096, 2097t
  disorders and conditions affecting, 2097t
Erythrocyte sedimentation rate (ESR), 322–323
  in thyroiditis, 1107t
  measurement of, 549t
  reference values for, 2302t
Erythroplakia, 686
Erythropoiesis, *1077,* 2075–2077, *2076*
  nutrition and, 2077–2078
Erythropoietin, 737
  for anemia, 2104
  for cancer, 388
  for chronic renal failure, 894
Escape pacemaker, 1550
Escape phenomenon, in hyperaldosteronism, 1134
Eschar, removal of, 325, *328,* 328–330
Escharotomy, for burns, 1343, *1344,* 1345
Escherichia coli gastroenteritis, 766–767, 768
Esmolol, for hypertensive emergencies, 1396t
Esophageal diverticula, 698–699
Esophageal manometry, 659
Esophageal pH monitoring, 659
Esophageal speech, 1669

Esophageal varices, in cirrhosis, *1241,* 1241b,
    1241–1242
  confusion and, 1243
  gas exchange and, 1243
  hemorrhage prevention and, 1242–1243
Esophagectomy, 701
Esophagitis, in achalasia, 691, *691*
  reflux, 695–697, *695–697*
  sleep problems in, 439
Esophagoenterostomy, 701
Esophagogastroduodenoscopy, 658, *658*
Esophagogastrostomy, 701
Esophagomyotomy, 692–694, *693*
Esophagoscopy, 658
Esophagus, anatomy of, *690*
  Barrett's, 701
  cancer of, 699–702
  dilation of, 692, *693,* 693–694
  disorders of, 690–702
  function of, 633, *634*
  in digestion, 633, *634*
  injuries of, 701
  structure of, 630
  surgery of, 701–702
Espiritulista, 74b
ESR. See *Erythrocyte sedimentation rate
    (ESR).*
Estrogen(s), 907–908, 1067
  hepatitis and, 1228
  in menstrual cycle, 908–910
  natural, 908
  pharmaceutical, for menopausal symptoms,
      985–986
    for prostate cancer, 961
    for urinary incontinence, 837t
  urine, reference values for, 2306t
Estrogen receptors, in breast cancer, 1020, 1035
Estrogen replacement therapy (ERT), after hys-
    terectomy, 993
  breakthrough bleeding in, 984
  breast cancer and, 571–572
  for endometriosis, 990
  for menopause, 985–986
  for osteoporosis, 570–572, 571t
  heart disease and, 1518, 1521
Ethanol, for ethylene glycol poisoning, 2281t
  for methanol poisoning, 2281t
Ethical issues, advance directives, 67–68
  autonomy, for elderly, 65–66
  competence, for elderly, 66–67
  elderly and, 65–68
  end-of-life, 67–68
  in acute care nursing, 104
  in emergency care, 2264–2265
  in transplantation, 2215
  living wills, 67
  placebos, 477
  self-determination, for elderly, 67
Ethionamide (Trecator-SC), for tuberculosis,
    1720, 1721t
Ethnicity. See also *Race and ethnicity.*
  definition of, 146
Ethnocentrism, definition of, 146
Ethnopharmacology, 1391b
Ethopropazine (Parsidol), for Parkinson's dis-
    ease, 2019t
Ethosuximide (Zarotin), for epilepsy, 1927t,
    1927–1928
  reference values for, 2307t
Ethrane (enflurane), 294t
Ethyl chloride spray, 297t
Ethylene glycol poisoning, antidote for, 2281t
Etidronate disodium (Didronel), for hypercal-
    cemia, 253
Etodolac, 486, 487t
Etomidate (Amidate), for rapid-sequence in-
    duction, 2268

Etretinate (Tegison), for psoriasis, 1292
Eukaryotic cell, 206
Euploidy, 1017
Eupnea, *184*
Eustachian tube, *1783,* 1783–1784, 1785
  disorders of, 1842
Evidence, collection and preservation of, 2263,
    2263t, 2264t
Evil eye, 19b
Evisceration, 309, *309,* 333
Evista (raloxifene), for breast cancer preven-
    tion, 1014
Evoked potential studies, 1902
Ewing's sarcoma, 580t, *581,* 581–582
Excisional biopsy, 374. See also *Biopsy.*
  of actinic keratosis, 1305
  of skin, *1277,* 1278
Excoriation, *1272*
Excretory urography, 758–759
Exercise. See *Activity and exercise.*
Exercise prescription, 33
Exercise stress testing, 1376, 1470–1472
  first-past cardiac study in, 1475
  myocardial scintigraphy in, 1474
Exercise testing, 1376, 1470–1472
  first-past cardiac study in, 1475
  myocardial scintigraphy in, 1474
Exercises, after mastectomy, 1027b, 1028
  coughing, preoperative teaching of, 286
  deep-breathing, preoperative teaching of,
      285–286, *286*
  extremity, preoperative teaching for, 286
  for burn patients, 1349
  for comatose patients, 1914–1915
  for lower back pain, 1986
  in immobility, 618b
  in musculoskeletal trauma, 624
  in rheumatoid arthritis, 2147–2148, 2152,
      2152
  in spinal cord injury, 2062–2063
  in stroke, 1968, 1971, 1973–1974
  neck, hyperthyroidism and, 1105–1106
  pelvic muscle (Kegel), 836, 838, 958,
      1000
  postoperative, for total knee replacement,
      565
    in radical neck dissection, *1673–1675*
    in total hip replacement, 559
  range of motion, 624
    by assistive personnel, 573
    in rheumatoid arthritis, 2147–2148
  turning, preoperative teaching for, 286
Exfoliative cytologic analysis, 658
Exophthalmometry, 1796
Exophthalmos, in hyperthyroidism, 1099–
    1100, *1100,* 1828, *1828*
Exotoxins, 213
Expiration, mechanics of, *1616,* 1616–1618
Expiratory reserve volume, 1615, *1615*
  measurement of, 1637, 1638t
External counterpulsation device, for shock,
    2246
External fixation, of fractures, 598, *598*
  nursing management in, 606–607
External (transcutaneous) pacing, 1571–1572
External sphenoethmoidectomy, 1677–1678
External sphincterotomy, for neurogenic blad-
    der, 844
Extinction phenomenon, assessment of, 1889
Extracellular fluid, 215
Extracellular fluid volume deficit, 217–224.
    See also *Dehydration.*
Extracellular fluid volume excess, 225–228.
    See also *Edema.*
Extracellular fluid volume shift, 229–230
Extracorporeal circulation, in cardiac surgery,
    1504–1505

Extracorporeal membrane oxygenation
    (ECMO), 1540
  for shock, 2244
Extracorporeal renal surgery, 869
Extracorporeal shock wave lithotripsy, 826–
    827, *827*
  for choledocholithiasis, 1214
  for cholelithiasis, 1205–1206, *1207*
Extraocular movements, assessment of, 1885
Extrapyramidal disease, movement abnormali-
    ties in, 1887b
Extrapyramidal side effects, 418
Extravasation, of chemotherapy drugs, 387–
    388
Extremity exercises, preoperative teaching for,
    286
Extrinsic coagulation pathway, 2079, *2079*
Extrinsic factor, 2077
Exudates, 1743
Eye. See also *Vision.*
  accessory structures of, 1778, *1779*
  anatomy of, 1778–1780, *1779*
  assessment of, 1787–1798
    chief complaint in, 1787
    diagnostic tests in, *1796,* 1796–1798,
        1797
    history in, 1787–1789, 1788b
    physical examination in, 1789–1796,
        1790b
      of central area blindness, 1794
      of color vision, 1794
      of external eye, 1789–1791
      of internal eye, 1794–1796, *1795*
      of ocular motility, 1791–1792, *1792*
      of visual acuity, 1792–1793, *1793*
      of visual fields, 1793, *1793*
    symptom analysis in, 1787–1788, 1788b
  disorders of, 1809–1830. See also specific
      disorders.
  emergency care for, 2277–2278
  drugs affecting, 1788
  dry, 1826
  examination of, 164t–165t
  in diabetes mellitus, 1186–1187, 1188b,
      1820, *1820*
  in glaucoma, 1809–1814. See also *Glau-
      coma.*
  in Graves' disease, 1099–1100, *1100,* 1828,
      1828
  in HIV infection, 1829
  in hyperthyroidism, 1099–1100, *1100,* 1103,
      1828, *1828*
  in Lyme disease, 1829–1830
  in myasthenia gravis, 1829
  in rheumatoid arthritis, 2145
  in Sjögren's syndrome, 1829
  in systemic lupus erythematosus, 1829
  in Wilson's disease, 1259
  inner, 1778–1780
  irrigation of, 2278
  magnetic resonance imaging of, 1796,
      1796
  muscles of, 1778, *1780,* 1791, *1792*
  pain in, 1788
  physiology of, 1780–1781, *1781*
  position of, 1790
  prosthetic, 1825, *1826*
  red, 1787, 1788b
  tumors of, 1825–1826
  ultrasonography of, 1797, *1797*
Eye drops, for corneal infection, 1824
  for exophthalmos, 1100
  for glaucoma, 1813, 1813t
Eyeball, 1778, *1779,* 1790
Eyebrows, 1790
Eyeglasses, for aphakia, 1816
Eyelashes, 1790

Eyelid, 1778, 1790
  disorders of, 1826, 1827t
  plastic surgery of, *1317,* 1318
  tumors of, 1826

F

Face lift, 1316–1318, *1317*
Faces Pain Rating Scale, 477, *481*
Facial fractures, *1325,* 1326–1328, *1327*
Facial lacerations, 1326
Facial nerve, 1870t
  assessment of, 1885
  paralysis of, *1996,* 1996–1997
Facial resurfacing, 1318–1319
Factor evaluation method, 101, 103t
Fainting, 1397
  in heart disease, 1452
Fallopian tubes, infection of. See *Salpingitis.*
  structure and function of, 904, *905,* 906t
Falls, hip fractures and, 608, 626–627
  in elderly, 55, 626–627
  prevention of. See *Safety measures.*
False-negative results, 187
False-positive results, 187
Famciclovir, for genital herpes, 1045t
Family, in chronic illness, 20
  in terminal illness, 456–459, 458b
  respite care for, 65, 2008, 2008b
Family history, 137, *138*
Family support, for elderly, 47–48, 65
  in chronic illness, 20
Far vision, 1781
Farsightedness, *1827,* 1827–1828
Fascia, 530
Fasciculi, 530
Fasciotomy, for burns, 1343, *1344,* 1345
  in compartment syndrome, 600
Fat, body, surgical removal of, 1319–1321
  dietary, cancer and, 15
    digestion and absorption of, 636–637
    disease and, *14,* 14–15
    in diabetes mellitus, 1166, 1166t
    in hypertension, 1387
    restriction of, 32–33, 1393b, 1517, 1521
      in atherosclerosis, 1521
      in hypertension, 1387, 1393b
  fecal, 744t, 745–746
    reference values for, 2310t
Fat embolism, 600–601, 605
Fat emulsions, in parenteral nutrition, 668
  allergy to, 670
Fat metabolism, in diabetes mellitus, 1155
  liver in, 1064–1065
Fatigue, 442
  in cancer, 384, 393
  in chronic renal failure, 896–897
  in cirrhosis, 1239–1240
  in dying clients, 454
  in heart disease, 1452
  in hepatitis, 1228, 1230
  in HIV infection, 2209–2210
  in hyperthyroidism, 1103
  in hypothyroidism, 1097–1098
  in leukemia, 2172
  in multiple sclerosis, 2013
  in myasthenia gravis, 2020, 2022
  in post-polio syndrome, 1993
  in rheumatoid arthritis, 2152
  steroid-related, 1132
Fatty acids, 14
  free, 1067–1068
Fatty liver, 1253–1254
Fecal analysis, 744t, 745
  reference values for, 2310t
Fecal fat, 744t, 745–746

Fecal incontinence. See *Bowel incontinence.*
Fecal lipids, tests for, 745–746
Fecal occult blood test, 43, 158t, 369t, 370,
  744t, 745
Fecal urobilinogen, 1081t
Federal government, in health care system, 73,
  77–80
Feedback, in homeostasis, 5t
Feeding. See also *Diet; Food; Nutrition.*
  in coma, 1913, 1915–1916
  in dysphagia, 223, 1974–1975, 1975t
  in Huntington's disease, 2012
  in laryngectomy, 1668, 1669
  in spinal cord injury, 2055–2056
  in stroke, 1974–1975, 1975t
  in tracheostomy, 1658–1659
  tube. See *Enteral nutrition.*
Feeding tube. See also *Enteral nutrition.*
  care of, 675, 694
  drug administration via, 676, 676b
  irrigation of, 675
  patency of, access sites for, 673, *673*
  position of, assessment of, 675
Felty's syndrome, rheumatoid arthritis and,
  2146
Female genital mutilation, 1008
Femoral artery bypass surgery, 1406–1410,
  1407
Femoral head, avascular necrosis of, 601
Femoral hernia, 787–789, *788*
  palpation for, *937,* 939
Femoral pulse, assessment of, 1373, *1374*
Femoropopliteal disorders, 1401
Femura (letrozole), in breast cancer, 1036
Fenamates, 486, 487t
Fenoldopam mesylate, for hypertensive emer-
  gencies, 1396t
Fenoprofen, 486, 487t
Fentanyl (Sublimaze), 489t, 492
  for rapid-sequence induction, 2268
  preoperative, 290t
  transcutaneous administration of, 495
Fentanyl citrate–droperidol (Innovar), 294t
Ferritin, reference values for, 2304t
Ferrous gluconate (Fergon), for anemia, 2104
Ferrous sulfate (Feosol), for anemia, 2104
Fetor hepaticus, 1251
Fever, in HIV infection, 2209
  in infectious mononucleosis, 2121
  in inflammation, 321
  management of, 322, 2285–2287
  systemic effects of, 322
Fiber, dietary, colon cancer and, 780–781
  diabetes mellitus and, 1166t
  diverticular disease and, 789
Fibrin clot, formation of, *2079,* 2079–2080
Fibrin degradation test, 2099t
Fibrin split products, 2099t
  reference values for, 2302t
Fibrinogen, reference values for, 2302t, 2304t
Fibrinogen level, 2099t
Fibrinolysis, 2080
Fibrinolytics. See *Thrombolytics.*
Fibroadenoma, breast, 1037
Fibroblasts, in wound healing, 320
Fibrocartilage, 534
Fibrocystic breast, 1037
Fibroids, uterine, 362, *991,* 991–994, *1000*
Fibromas, 362
Fibromuscular dysplasia, renal artery disease
  in, 869–870
Fibromyalgia, 2161, *2162*
  sleep problems in, 439
Fibrosarcoma, 363, 580t, 581–582
Fibrothorax, 1743
Fibrous joints, 533
Fibula, fractures of, 596t, 617

Field block anesthesia, 298. See also *Anesthesia.*
Filariasis, 1430
Filter, vena cava (umbrella), 1426, 1708, *1708*
Filtration, 215–216
  in capillary exchange, *1336,* 1365
Filum terminale, 1862
Finasteride (Proscar), for benign prostatic hyperplasia, 947
Fine-needle aspiration biopsy, 200, 374. See
  also *Biopsy.*
  of breast, 933, 1016
  of liver, 1084–1085
  of thyroid gland, 1095t
Fingers, clubbing of, 1273, 1273t, 1453, 1456,
  1629, *1630*
  fractures of, 619
Finkelstein's test, 544t
First-pass cardiac study, 1475
Fissure, *1272*
Fistula, anal, 797
  arteriovenous, in hemodialysis, 892, *893*
  bronchopleural, 1743
  gastrojejunocolic, postoperative, 721
  tracheoesophageal, in tracheostomy, 1654
    assessment for, 1658
  vaginal, *1003,* 1003–1004
Flagella, 207t
Flagyl (metronidazole), for bacterial vaginosis,
  1055
  for peptic ulcer disease, 710t, 715
  for trichomoniasis, 1054–1055
Flail chest, 1768–1769, *1769*
  emergency care for, 2272, *2272*
Flaps, 1322–1325, *1323,* 1324b
  free, *1323,* 1323–1325
  muscle, *1323,* 1324b
    in breast reconstruction, *1029,* 1029–
      1030, *1030*
  musculocutaneous, 1322–1323, *1323,* 1324b
Flat bones, 530
Flat plate of abdomen, 195, 656, 746
Flatness, on percussion, 177
Flatulence, 706
  rectal tube for, 799
  with colostomy, 786
Flecainide, reference values for, 2308t
Floaters, 1782
Floating ribs, 1616
Flora, normal, 336–337, 637
Fludrocortisone (Florinef), for Addison's disease, 1124t
Fluid, extracellular, 215
  hyperosmolar, 216
  hypoosmolar, 216–217
  interstitial, 215
  intracellular, 215
  intravascular, 215
  lymphatic, 216
  movement of, 215–217, *216*
  renal reabsorption of, 735
  renal secretion of, 735
  third-space, 229
  transcapillary exchange of, 735
Fluid and electrolyte balance, absorption in,
  216t, 636–637
  diffusion in, 216
  disturbances of, 217–230. See also under
    *Electrolyte(s), imbalances of; Fluid vol-
    ume.*
  critical monitoring in, 236b
  in addisonian crisis, 1121
  in ascites, 1246
  in cholelithiasis, 1205, 1206–1207
  fluid movement and, 215–217, *216*
  hormonal regulation of, 217
  intracapillary pressure and, 215–216, *216*
  kidney in, 735–736, 736t

Fluid and electrolyte balance *(Continued)*
  osmolality in, 216–217
  postoperative monitoring of, in cardiac surgery, 1508
  preoperative assessment of, 281
  reabsorption in, 216, 216t
  resorption in, 216t
Fluid compartments, 215
Fluid intake, 215–230. See also *Fluid management; Intravenous therapy; Transfusion(s).*
  in diabetic ketoacidosis, 1175b
  in hyperparathyroidism, 1112
  in third-spacing, 230
  measurement of, 219, 222
  recommendations for, 217
Fluid management. See also *Intravenous therapy; Transfusion(s).*
  colloid solutions in, 2247, 2274
  crystalloid solutions in, 2247, 2274
  in acute pancreatitis, 1196, 1197
  in acute renal failure, 878, 879–880
  in addisonian crisis, 1121
  in ascites, 1247
  in burns, 1342, 1342t
  in cardiac surgery, 1510
  in cholelithiasis, 1207, 1210
  in chronic renal failure, 896
  in coma, 1910, 1915, 1916
  in dehydration, 220t, 220–222, 221t, 223–224
  in diarrhea, 768
  in dysphagia, 223
  in edema, 227–228
  in emergency care, 2273–2275
  in enteral feeding, 224
  in gastrointestinal bleeding, 715–717
  in glomerulonephritis, 866
  in heart failure, 1536, 1538t, 1541
  in hepatic encephalopathy, 1252, 1253
  in hepatitis, 1228
  in hyperkalemia, 248
  in hypernatremia, 240–241
  in hyponatremia, 238–239
  in ileostomy, 779
  in intermittent self-catheterization, 843
  in multiple myeloma, 2120
  in pulmonary edema, 1748
  in shock, 2246–2248
  in syndrome of inappropriate antidiuretic hormone, 396
  in tracheostomy, 1657
  in urinary incontinence, 836–837, 838
  in urinary tract infection, 804, 806
  in urolithiasis, 824, 825–826
  postoperative, 307, 309–310
  preoperative, 281
Fluid overload. See *Hypervolemia.*
Fluid resuscitation, 2273–2274
  for burns, 2274
Fluid shifts, 229–230
  in burns, 1334, *1334,* 1336
  third-space, 218
Fluid volume deficit, emergency care for, 2273–2274
  extracellular, 217–224. See also *Dehydration; Hypovolemia.*
  hyperosmolar, 219
  hypotonic, 219
  intracellular, 225
  iso-osmolar, 219
Fluid volume excess, extracellular, 225–228. See also *Edema; Hypervolemia.*
  intracellular, 228–229
Fluid volume shift, extracellular, 229–230
Fluid wave test, 1077
Fluorescein, in slit-lamp examination, 1796

Fluorescein angiography, *1797,* 1797–1798
Fluorescent treponemal antibody absorption (FTA-ABS) test, for syphilis, 1051
Fluoroscopy, 195
  in musculoskeletal assessment, 546
  in respiratory assessment, 1645
5-Fluorouracil, for breast cancer, 1032, 1033, 1034, 1036
  topical, for actinic keratosis, 1304
Fluothane (halothane), 294t
Flurbiprofen, 486, 487t
Focal glomerular sclerosis, 864, 864t
Folate, deficiency of, 641t–642t, 2113, 2114–2115
  food sources of, 641t
  in erythropoiesis, 2077
  reference values for, 2304t
Foley catheters, *951.* See also *Urinary catheterization.*
  for urinary retention, 831–832
Folic acid. See *Folate.*
Folk medicine, 19b, 27t. See also *Alternative therapies.*
Follicle-stimulating hormone (FSH), 1138t
  deficiency of, 1143
  excess of, 1142
  in female, 908, *909*
  in male, 913
  reference values for, 2304t
Follicular adenocarcinoma, thyroid, 1108, 1108t
Follicular cyst, 1001
Folliculitis, 1311t
Fomites, 1052
Food. See also *Diet; Nutrition.*
  allergy to, 648, 2135, 2136b
    atopic dermatitis and, 1288
    tests for, 2101–2102
  calcium content of, 251b
  digestion of, 631–636. See also *Digestion.*
  handling of, hepatitis A and, 1225–1226
  magnesium content of, 256b
  nutrient content of, 641t–642t
  potassium content of, 245b
  sodium content of, 238b, 1541b
Food diary, 649
Food Guide Pyramid, 30, *31,* 638, *639*
Food labeling, 30, *32*
Food poisoning, 766–767, 768
Foot, disorders of, *582,* 582–583, *583*
    in diabetes mellitus, 1184–1185, *1185, 1186b, 1187b,* 1188
  fractures of, 617
    stress, 620
  plantar fasciitis of, 620
Foot care, in peripheral arterial occlusive disease, 1403, 1403b
Foot drop, prevention of, 1973–1974
Foot ulcers, arterial, 1416
  diabetic, 1184–1185, *1185,* 1186b, 1187b, 1188
    eschar in, *328*
    healing of, 332
  venous. See *Venous ulcers.*
Forane (isoflurane), 294t
Forced expiratory flow, measurement of, 1637, 1638t
Forced expiratory volume, measurement of, 1637, 1638t
Forced spirometry, 1637, *1639*
Forced vital capacity, measurement of, 1637, 1638t
Forearm, fractures of, 618
Foreign bodies, in ear, 1842, 1845
Foreskin, 911
  in paraphimosis, 970, *970*
  inflammation of, 970, *971*

Formulas, enteral, 671–672, 672t
  dilution of, 224
  parenteral, 668t, 668–669, 669t
Fortovase (saquinavir), 2198t
Fosamax (alendronate), for osteoporosis, 571t, 572
  for Paget's disease, 575
Fosfomycin (Monurol), for urinary tract infection, 803
Fosinopril (Monopril), for hypertension, 1389t
Fossae, cranial, 1861
Fracture(s), 587–619
  arthritis after, 601
  assessment of, initial, 590–596
  avascular necrosis and, 601
  avulsion, 595t
  blowout, 1327
  burst, 592t
  casts for, 602–606. See also *Cast(s).*
  classification of, 592t–596t
  clinical manifestations of, 588–590, *591*
  closed, 590
  Colles,' 596t
  comminuted, 592t
  compartment syndrome in, 599–600, *600*
  complete, 592t
  complications of, 599–602
  compression, 595t
  condylar, 616
  definition of, 587
  delayed union of, 602
  displaced, 593t
  elbow, 618
  emergency care for, 2279
  etiology of, 587–588
  external fixation of, 598, *598*
    nursing management in, 606–607
  facial, *1325,* 1326–1328, *1327*
  fat embolism and, 600–601
  fibrous union of, 602
  fibular, 596t, 617
  finger, 619
  foot, 617
  greenstick, 596t
  hand, 619
  healing of, 536, 588, 589t–590t
  hip, 607–616. See also *Hip, fractures of.*
  humeral, 617–618
  impacted, 596t
  in hypercortisolism, 1131
  in hyperparathyroidism, 1111–1112
  in osteoporosis, 566, *566,* 567, 568, 572
  incomplete, 593t
  internal fixation of, *597,* 597–598
  Le Fort, 1326–1328, *1327*
  linear, 593t
  longitudinal, 594t
  malunion of, 602
  management of, emergency, 590–596
  medical management of, 590–602
  nasal, 1327, 1682
  nerve injury in, 599
  neurovascular assessment in, 604, 604t
  nondisplaced, 594t
  nonunion of, 602
  nursing management in, 602–607
  oblique, 594t
  open, 590
    infection of, 601, 605, 605b
  outcomes classification for, 587
  patellar, 617
  pathophysiology of, 588
  pelvic, 616–617
  Pott's, 596t
  radial, 618
  reduction of, 596–598

Fracture(s) (Continued)
  closed, 597, 597
  open, 597, 597–598
  renal, 867, 867–869
  risk factors for, 587–588
  skull, 2040–2041, 2043
  spiral, 594t
  stellate, 595t
  stiffness after, 601
  stress, 620
  tibial, 617
  toe, 619
  traction for, 598–599, 599b, 599t
    nursing management in, 607
  transverse, 595t
  ulnar, 618
  upper extremity, 617–618
  weight-bearing status in, 614b
  wrist, 596t, 618–619
Fracture board, 2269, 2269
Frank-Starling law, 1441–1442, 1442
Free fatty acids, 1067–1068
Free flaps, 1322, 1323, 1323–1325, 1324b
Free prostate-specific antigen (PSA), 959
Free radicals, disease and, 15
  in wound healing, 319
Free thyroxine (FT$_4$) concentration, 1094t
  in thyroiditis, 1107t
Free water clearance, 736
Friction rub, abdominal, 654–655, 1077
Frostbite, emergency care for, 2283
Frozen sections, 201
FSH. See Follicle-stimulating hormone (FSH).
FT$_4$ (free thyroxine) concentration, 1094t
Fuchs' dystrophy, 1821–1823, 1822
Functional assessment, for elderly, 52–53
Functional endoscopic sinus surgery, 1677, 1677
Functional health patterns, 160b
  in health history, 160b, 2298–2300
Functional incontinence, 749. See also Urinary incontinence.
Functional nursing, 99
Functional residual capacity, 1615, 1615
  measurement of, 1637, 1638t
Functional status measurement, 102
Fundus photography, 1796, 1796
Fungal infections, central nervous system, 1947
  in HIV infection, 2203–2204
  mode of infection in, 337t
  pathogenesis of, 337t
  pulmonary, 1723–1724
Fungal pneumonia, 1723–1724
Funnel chest, 1629, 1630
Furosemide (Lasix), for heart failure, 1538t
  in emergency care, 2274
  for hypertension, 1389t
  perioperative use of, 275t
Furuncles, 1311t

G

G$_0$ phase, of cell cycle, 356, 358
G$_1$ phase, of cell cycle, 356, 358
G$_2$ phase, of cell cycle, 356–357, 358
GABA (gamma-aminobutyric acid), in pain, 469
Gag reflex, 1886, 1889, 1891t
Gait, assessment of, 540–541, 541, 1887
Gait disturbances, in Parkinson's disease, 2017, 2107
  terminology for, 1887b
Gait training, for amputee, 1413–1414
Gallbladder, carcinoma of, 1215–1216
  function of, 636
    assessment of, 1085–1086
  inflammation of. See Cholecystitis.

Gallium nitrate, for hypercalcemia, 253
Gallium scans, in respiratory assessment, 1645
Gallops, 1460–1461
Gallstones. See Cholelithiasis.
Gamma globulin (Gammar), in hepatitis A prevention, 1226
Gamma-aminobutyric acid (GABA), in pain, 469
Gamma-glutamyltransferase, 1082t
Gammar. See Gamma globulin (Gammar).
Ganglion, 2000
Gardner-Wells tongs, 2053, 2053
Gas exchange. See also Arterial blood gas analysis.
  esophageal varices and, bleeding, 1243
  in respiration, 1618, 1619
Gas exchange abnormalities, emergency care for, 2270–2271
Gas transport, in respiration, 1620
Gas-bloat syndrome, 697
Gastrectomy. See also Gastric surgery.
  subtotal, 720, 720
  total, 720, 720
Gastric acid stimulation test, 659
Gastric acids, 635t, 635–636
  measurement of, 658–659
Gastric analysis, 658–659
Gastric cancer, 724–726
  surgery for, 725. See also Gastric surgery.
Gastric decompression. See also Gastrointestinal intubation.
  intubation for, 706–707
Gastric ischemia, in mechanical ventilation, 1756
Gastric lavage, 706–708. See also Gastrointestinal intubation.
  for poisoning, 2281
Gastric motility, 633–634
Gastric outlet obstruction, in peptic ulcer disease, 717
  postoperative, 721–722
Gastric residuals, in enteral nutrition, 676
Gastric secretions, 635t, 635–636
  measurement of, 658–659
Gastric surgery, 719–724
  case study of, 723–724
  complications of, 720–722
  contraindications to, 719
  for cancer, 725
  for perforated ulcer, 723–724
  indications for, 719
  nursing management in, 722–724
  types of, 719, 719–720, 720
Gastric ulcers, drug-induced, 712, 713
  in peptic ulcer disease, 712, 713t. See also Peptic ulcer disease.
  in Zollinger-Ellison syndrome, 714
  marginal, 720–721
  stress-induced, 712, 714
Gastrics, measurement of, reference values for, 2310t
Gastrin, reference values for, 2304t
Gastritis, acute, 708–709
  alkaline reflux, postoperative, 721
  chronic, 709–712, 713t–714t
Gastroduodenal junction, 634
Gastroenteritis, 766–767, 768
  sexually transmitted, 1056
Gastroenterostomy, 719, 720. See also Gastric surgery.
Gastroesophageal reflux disease (GERD), 695–697, 695–697
  laryngitis in, 1680
  sleep problems in, 439
Gastrointestinal assessment, lower tract, 739–747. See also Bowel elimination, assessment of.
  upper tract. See Nutritional assessment.

Gastrointestinal bleeding, 706. See also Bleeding; Hemorrhage.
  clinical pathway for, 715b
  emergency care for, 2273–2274
  in chronic gastritis, 709
  in hepatic encephalopathy, 1252
  in peptic ulcer disease, 714, 715
  in shock, 2248
  management of, 715b, 715–717, 716b
  postoperative, in gastric surgery, 721
  shock in, 715–716
  transfusion for, 716–717
Gastrointestinal disorders. See also Intestinal disorders.
  chest pain in, 1450t
  clinical manifestations of, 705–706
  digestive, 705–726
  ingestive, 683–703
  pain in, 472, 705
  sleep problems in, 439
Gastrointestinal endoscopy, 200, 200
Gastrointestinal intubation, for decompression, 706–707, 792
  in enteral nutrition. See Enteral nutrition.
  nursing management in, 708
  suctioning in, 707–708
  tube insertion in, 707
    errors in, 728–729
  tube irrigation in, 708
  tube types for, 706t, 706–707
Gastrointestinal lubricants, 635t, 635–636
Gastrointestinal preparation, preoperative, 282
Gastrointestinal secretions, 634–636, 635t
Gastrointestinal system, age-related changes in, 50t, 212t, 637
  assessment of. See Gastrointestinal assessment.
  autonomic neuropathy of, in diabetes mellitus, 1188–1189
  blood supply of, 630–631
  function of, 632–637
  in shock, 2240–2241
  lymphatic drainage of, 631
  neural regulation of, 630, 631
  preoperative assessment of, 279
  smooth muscle of, 632–634
  structure of, 630–631, 631, 632
Gastrojejunocolic fistula, postoperative, 721
Gastroparesis, in diabetes mellitus, 1189
Gastroscopy, 658
Gastrostomy feeding, 673, 673, 693, 693. See also Enteral nutrition.
Gate control theory, 470–471
  of pain, 470, 470–471
Gauze dressings, 329t, 329–330. See also Dressings.
Gavage feeding. See Enteral nutrition.
Gaze, 1778, 1780, 1791, 1792
  assessment of, 1885
G-CSF (granulocyte colony-stimulating factor), for cancer, 388
  in hematopoiesis, 2075
Gels, dressings, 1281t
Gender identity, 418b
Gender role, 418b
Gene therapy, 14, 210
General adaptation syndrome, 5t
  in shock, 2239
General anesthesia, 292t, 292–293, 294t–295t, 483. See also Anesthesia.
Generalized anxiety disorder, 413–416, 414b
Genetic disorders, 14, 14
  screening and prevention for, 148t–149t
Genetic factors, in chronic conditions, 13–14, 14
Genetic mutations, 210
Genetics, cancer, 350t, 362

Genital herpes, 1045t, 1051–1053, *1052*
Genital mutilation, 1008
Genital warts, 1045t, 1053–1054, *1054*
Genitals. See also *Reproductive system.*
  examination of, in urinary tract disorders, 755–756
    female, examination of, 173t, 922–926, *923*
      normal findings on, 921b
      structure and function of, 904–906, *905,* 906t
    imaging of, 758–760
    male, examination of, 172t, 936–939, *937, 940*
      normal findings on, 921b
      structure and function of, *910,* 910–913, 911t
Genogram, *138*
Gentamicin, perioperative use of, 275t
  reference values for, 2307t
  topical, 327t
Genu valgum, 540, *541*
Genu varum, 540, *541*
GERD. See *Gastroesophageal reflux disease (GERD).*
Geriatric nursing, 46
Geriatrics, 45–46. See also *Elderly.*
Germ cells, 904
Germ theory, 3, 5t
Gerontological nursing, 46
Gerontology, 46
Gerota's fascia, 733
Gestational diabetes, 1149–1150
GFR. See *Glomerular filtration rate (GFR).*
GH. See *Growth hormone (GH).*
Giant cell arteritis, 2163
Giant cell tumor of bone, 580t, 580–581, *581*
Giardiasis, 767
Gigantism, 1139, *1140*
Gingivitis, 683, 684
  necrotizing ulcerative, 684–685
Glabella reflex, 1891
Glans penis, 911, *912*
  inflammation of, 970, *971*
Glare, aging and, 1782
Glasgow Coma Scale, 2031, 2035b, 2266t
Glaucoma, 1809–1814
  after cataract extraction, 1816
  assessment of, 1812
  classification of, 1809–1810, *1810*
  clinical manifestations of, 1811
  epidemiology of, 1809
  etiology of, 1810
  in elderly, 1813
  medical management of, *1811,* 1811–1812
  nursing management of, 1812–1813, 1813t
  pathophysiology of, 1810–1811
  risk factors for, 1810
  self-care in, 1814
  surgery for, 1813
    nursing management in, 1813–1814
Glial cells, *1865,* 1865–1866
Glial tumors, 1932, 1932b. See also *Brain tumors.*
Glipizide (Glucotrol), for diabetes mellitus, 1161t
  perioperative use of, 275t
Globulin(s), serum. See also *Albumin/globulin ratio.*
  liver function and, 1082t
  reference values for, 2305t
Glomerular filtrate, transport of, 735
Glomerular filtration, 732, 734, 735
  fluid balance and, 236
  in shock, 2241
Glomerular filtration rate (GFR), 734, 735
  hyperparathyroidism and, 1109

Glomerulonephritis, 862–867
  acute, 865
  assessment in, 866
  chronic, 865
  classification of, 863t
  clinical manifestations of, 865
  idiopathic membranous, 864t
  latent, 865
  medical management of, 865–866
  membranoproliferative, 864t
  membranous, 864t
  minimal change, 864t
  nephritic syndrome in, 863
  nephrotic syndrome in, 862–863
  nursing management of, 866–867
  pathophysiology of, 864, *865*
  poststreptococcal, 864t
  primary, 863t
  rapidly progressive, 864t
  secondary, 863t
  self-care in, 867
  subacute, 865
Glomerulosclerosis, in diabetic nephropathy, 851, 852
Glomerulus, 733, *733*
Glossopharyngeal breathing, 2059
Glossopharyngeal nerve, 1870t
  assessment of, 1886
Glottis, 1613, *1613*
Glucagon, 1066
  for beta-blocker overdose, 2281t
  for hypoglycemia, in diabetes mellitus, 1179t
Glucocorticoids. See *Steroids.*
Gluconeogenesis, 737
Glucophage. See *Metformin (Glucophage).*
Glucosamine, for osteoarthritis, 554, 555t
Glucose. See also *Hyperglycemia; Hypoglycemia.*
  blood, in cardiac disease, 1465
  decreased utilization of, in diabetes mellitus, 1154
  fasting, impaired, 1149
    in diabetes mellitus diagnosis, 1155, 1157b
    preoperative measurement of, 277t
    reference values for, 2304t
  in parenteral nutrition, 668
  plasma, 1067, *1068*
    reference values for, 2304t
  postprandial, in diabetes mellitus diagnosis, 1157
  random, in diabetes mellitus diagnosis, 1157, 1157t
  serum, reference values for, 2304t
  urine, reference values for, 2306t
Glucose control, 1158–1162, 1160t–1162t, *1163*
  in elderly, 1171
  ineffective, risk for, 1167b, 1167–1168
  nutrition therapy for, *1165,* 1165–1167, 1166t
Glucose metabolism, 1067, *1068*
  kidney in, 737
Glucose monitoring, in diabetes mellitus, after pancreas transplantation, 1172
  by client, 1158
    before exercise, 1165
    in ketoacidosis, 1176
  in total parenteral nutrition, 670
Glucose tolerance, impaired, 1149
Glucose tolerance test, oral, in diabetes mellitus, 1157b, 1157–1158
Glucosuria, 757, 757t, 1154
Glucotrol (glipizide), for diabetes mellitus, 1161t
  perioperative use of, 275t

Glutamyltransferase, reference values for, 2304t
Gluteal muscle flap, in breast reconstruction, 1030
Glyburide, perioperative use of, 275t
Glycopyrrolate (Robinul), preoperative, 290t
Glycosylated albumin, in diabetes mellitus, 1157
Glycosylated hemoglobin, in diabetes mellitus, 1155, 1157
GM-CSF (granulocyte-macrophage colony-stimulating factor), for cancer, 388
GnRH. See *Gonadotropin-releasing hormone (GnRH).*
Goeckerman regimen, 1284
Goiter, 1089–1090, *1090.* See also *Hyperthyroidism; Hypothyroidism.*
Goitrogens, 1090
Golfer's elbow, 621
Golgi complex, *206,* 207t
Gonadal development, 904
Gonadal function, 1067
  disorders of, 1143, 1145
Gonadotropin-releasing hormone (GnRH), 913, 1067
  pharmaceutical, for prostate cancer, 961–962
Gonads, 904. See also *Ovary; Testis.*
Goniometer, 542, *542*
Gonioscope, 1796
Gonorrhea, 1044t, 1048–1049
  pathogenesis of, 337t
Gordon's functional health patterns, 160b
Gout, 575–576, *576,* 576t
Graafian follicle, 904, 906t, 908–909, *909*
Grading, tumor, 358, 373
Grafts, arteriovenous, in hemodialysis, 892
  coronary artery bypass, 1524–1526, *1526*
  skin, 325, 1321–1322
Graft-versus-host disease (GVHD), 2132, 2180t, 2180–2182, 2181b
Granulation tissue, in wound healing, 320
Granulocyte colony-stimulating factor (G-CSF), for cancer, 388
  in hematopoiesis, 2075
Granulocyte-macrophage colony-stimulating factor (GM-CSF), for cancer, 388
Granulocytes, 2080
Granuloma, 324
Granuloma inguinale, 1053
Granulomatous thyroiditis, subacute, 1106–1107, 1107t
Graphism, 1888–1889
Grasp reflex, 1891
Graves' disease. See also *Hyperthyroidism.*
  clinical manifestations of, 1099–1100, *1100, 1828, 1828*
  complications of, 1100
  diagnosis of, 1100
  medical management of, 1100–1101
Gravity test, 545t
Gray matter, 1867
Greenstick fracture, 596t
Grey Turner's sign, 867
Grief, 457–459, 459t
  stages of, 18
Growth factors, for wound healing, 333
  hematopoietic, for cancer, 388
  in hematopoiesis, 2075
  in wound healing, 320
Growth hormone (GH), 1065, 1138t
  deficiency of, 1143
  excess of, 1139, *1140*
  pituitary function and, 1080
  reference values for, 2304t
Guanadrel (Hylorel), for hypertension, 1389t

Guided imagery, 36
  for pain, 499
Guillain-Barré syndrome, 2016–2017
Gurgles, 1633, 1634t
GVHD. See *Graft-versus-host disease (GVHD)*.
Gynecologic history, 916–917
Gynecomastia, 935, 1037

H

H₂ receptor antagonists, for gastroesophageal reflux disease, 696
  for gastrointestinal bleeding, 717
  for shock, 2251
  preoperative, 290t
Hair, age-related changes in, 50t
  distribution of, in vascular disorders, 1371
  examination of, normal findings on, 1269b
  excess body, 1271
  growth of, 1263
  in chronic renal failure, 887
  pubic, examination of, in female, 922–923
    in male, 936
  structure and function of, 1263
Hair loss, 1271–1272
  in chemotherapy, 394
Hallucinations, hypnogogic, in narcolepsy, 435
  in confusional states, 1919
Hallucinogens, 510t, 514t, 517–518, 520t–521t
Halo jacket, 2054, *2054*
Halothane (Fluothane), 294t
Ham test, 2302t
Hammer toe, 583, *583*
Hand, deformities of, in rheumatoid arthritis, 2145, *2145*, 2156
  examination of, *543*, 544t
  fractures of, 619
  replacement of, in rheumatoid arthritis, 2156
Hand-washing, 341, 343
  hepatitis A and, 1225
Hanging cast, *603*
Hangman's fracture, 2047, *2049*
Haptoglobin, reference values for, 2302t, 2304t
Harmonic acceleration, in vestibular testing, 1806
Harris tube, 706t, 707
Harris-Benedict equation, 663
Hashimoto's disease, 1091, 1106, 1107, 1107t
Haversian canal, 531, *534*
Haversian system, 531, *534*
Havrix. See *Hepatitis A, immunization for*.
Hazards of immobility, 17
HBsAg (hepatitis B surface antigen), 1228, 1230
Head and neck, examination of, 164t–166t
  in neurologic assessment, 1883
Head and neck cancer. See also *Larynx, cancer of*.
  prevention of, 370
Head lice, 1272
Head trauma, 2039–2046
  acceleration injury in, 2039, *2041*
  blunt, 2039–2040, *2041*
  brain injury in, mechanisms of, 2039–2040, *2041*
    pathophysiology of, 2043
    types of, *2041*, 2041–2043, *2042*
  brain stem contusions in, 2041, 2043–2044
  cerebral contusions in, 2041, 2043
  client education in, 2046, 2046b
  clinical manifestations of, 2043–2044
  coma in. See *Coma*.
  complications of, 2031, 2034t
  concussions in, 2041, 2043
  coup-contrecoup injuries in, 2040, *2041*

Head trauma (*Continued*)
  deceleration injury in, 2039, *2041*
  deformation injury in, 2039, *2041*
  diffuse axonal injury in, 2041
  emergency care in, 2276
  epidural hematoma in, *2041*, 2041–2042
  headache after, 1950
  in elderly, 2046
  intracerebral hematoma in, *2041*, 2042–2043
  mechanisms of injury in, 2039–2040, *2041*
  medical management of, 2044–2045
  nursing management of, 2045
  penetrating, 2040
  primary injuries in, 2040–2041
  prognosis in, 2045
  rehabilitation in, 2046
  scalp injuries in, 2040
  self-care in, 2046
  skull fractures in, 2040–2041, 2043
  sleep problems in, 438
  subdural hematoma in, *2041*, 2042, *2042*
  surgery for, 2045–2046, *2046*
Headache, 1948–1950
  brain tumors and, 1934
  cancer, 471, 471b
  cluster, 1948, *1949*
  in autonomic dysreflexia, 2051, 2064, 2064b, 2065
  in spinal anesthesia, 296t
  in subarachnoid hemorrhage, 1941
  lumbar puncture, 1898, 1950
  migraine, 1948–1949, *1949*
  pain in, 471
  postconcussion, 1950
  tension, 1948, *1949*
Head-to-toe examination, periodic, 163, 173b
  preoperative, 279b
Health, concepts and definitions of, 3–7, 8t
  wellness and, 8–9
Health Belief Model, 12, 12b
Health beliefs and practices, cultural aspects of, 19b, 424b, 2291–2297
  religious aspects of, 2291–2297
Health care, ambulatory, 83–93
  chronic vs. acute, 20
  clinical model for, 84
  funding for, 73
  history of, 3–9, 4t–7t
  medical model for, 84
  models of, 85, 85b
  primary, 85
  trends in, 92
Health care delivery, 73–81
  for elderly, 61–65
Health care funding, 77–81
  health care expansion and, 77–79
  health care reform and, 81
  modes of, 78b
  regulation and cost containment and, 79–81
Health care providers, HIV infection in, 345, 2188–2189
  immunizations for, 342t, 343
  infection control measures for, 343–346
  radiation safety for, 378–379
  substance abuse by, 524b, 524–525
  traditional, 74b–75b
  violence against, 2263–2264
Health care reform, 77, 81
Health care system, business and industry in, 76, 80
  chronic conditions and, 13, 20–21, 21t
  government in, 73
  hospital administrators/boards in, 76
  nurses in, 76–77
  physicians in, 75
  public's role in, 76
  stakeholders in, 73–77

Health history, 129–145
  accuracy of, 129–130
  biographical and demographic information in, 135–136
  chief complaint in, 136
  client preparation for, 130–135
  complementary therapies in, 136
  components of, 135–145
  current, 136–137
  data organization in, 160, 160b
  depth of, 130
  documentation of, 160
  environment for, 130
  family, 137, *138*
  functional health patterns in, 160b, 2298–2300
  guidelines for, 130–135
  interviewer preparation for, 135
  long format (exhaustive), 130, 131b–135b
  nursing process in, 160, 161b
  past, 137
  psychosocial, 137–145. See also *Psychosocial assessment*.
  review of systems in, 131b–135b, 145
  risk appraisal in, 145–155, 148t–154t, 155b
  short format (episodic), 130, 135b
  stereotyping in, 129–130, 130b
  symptom analysis in, 136–137
Health insurance, 77–81
  access to, 76
  for cancer survivors, 401
  for home care, 108, 109b
  private, 77, 78b
  sources of, 77–81, 78b
Health maintenance organizations (HMOs), 78b, 80–81
  nursing care in, 88
Health promotion, 9–13, 145–155
  across life span, 155, 156t–159t
  alternative therapies in, 19b, 27t, 27–28
  client education and motivation in, 12–13. See also *Client education*.
  conceptual development of, 9–10
  definition of, 9
  empowerment and, 9, 25
  environmental factors in, 28
  epidemiologic concepts in, 10–11
  exercise in, 25
    in elderly, 49
  for children, 155, 156t–159t
  for elderly, 48t, 48–70
  for young and middle-aged adults, 30–43
  goals of, 9–10
  guidelines for, 148t–154t
  in chronic conditions, 24–28
  models of, 11–12, 12b
  nutrition in, 24–25, 30–33
    in elderly, 49–51, 51b
  prevention and, 10–11, 24–28, 36–40
  risk appraisal and, 145–155, 148t–154t, 155b
  screening in. See *Screening*.
  self-actualization in, *25*, 25–26
  self-help groups and, 26
  stress management in, 26–27, 35–36
    in elderly, 51
  wellness and, 7–8
Health Promotion Model, 12
Health risks. See *Risk factors*.
Healthy People 2000, 9–10, 30, 31t
  diabetes mellitus and, 1073
Hearing, 1785–1786. See also *Ear*.
  age-related changes in, 50t, 53, 1786, 1799t, 1832
  assessment of, 1802–1804, *1803*
    audiometric tests in, 1804–1806, *1805*
  noise exposure and, 1800, 1801t
Hearing aids, 1835–1836, *1836*, 1839, 1839b

Hearing impairment, 1831–1847
  assessment of, 1799, 1837
  behavioral clues to, 1798b
  clinical manifestations of, 1834–1835, 1835t
  conductive, 1804, 1831
    clinical manifestations of, 1835t
    etiology of, 1832, *1832*
    surgery for, 1840
  congenital, 1832–1833
  epidemiology of, 1831
  etiology of, 1831–1833, *1832*
  health promotion/risk management for, 149t, 156t
  medical management of, 1835–1836, *1836*
  mixed, 1833
  noise-induced, 1833
  nursing management of, 1837b–1839b, 1837–1839
  pathophysiology of, 1834
  risk factors for, 1831–1833
  screening for, prevention and, 1833–1834
  sensorineural, 1804, 1831–1832
    clinical manifestations of, 1835t
    etiology of, 1832–1833
  sudden, 1832–1833
  surgery for, 1840, *1841*
  types of, 1833b
Hearing tests, in neurologic assessment, 1885
Heart. See also under *Cardiac; Cardiovascular.*
  age-related changes in, 1444
  anatomy and physiology of, 1434–1444
  autoregulation of, 1442–1444
  blood supply of, 1435–1436, *1436, 1437*
  chambers of, 1434, 1435, 1435t
  electrophysiologic properties of, 1436–1440
  examination of, 168t
  imaging of, 1472–1475
  in shock, 2237–2239
  layers of, 1435
  mechanical, 1504
Heart attack. See *Myocardial infarction (MI).*
Heart disease, clinical manifestations of, 1448b, 1448–1453
  congenital, 1500
  cyanotic, 1452–1453
  diet and, 1455
  disability in, 1532b
  emergency care in, 2275
  exercise and, 1454–1455
  exercise testing in, 1470–1472
  health promotion/risk management for, 148t–149t
  heart failure in, 1530t, 1531
  hyperthyroidism and, 1100
  in diabetes mellitus, 1182, 1183t, 1184
  infectious, 1481–1490
  preoperative assessment in, 276
  renal function in, 852–853
  rheumatic, 1482, 1482t
    prevention of, 1484
  screening for, 158t
  sleep problems in, 439
  structural, 1481–1514
  surgery for, 1500–1513. See also *Cardiac surgery.*
  valvular, 1495–1501. See also *Valvular heart disease.*
Heart failure, 1529–1547
  acute, 1535
  after myocardial infarction, 1591–1592
  backward, 1535
  care plan for, 1542b–1545b
    nursing management in, 1542b–1545b
  case management for, 1547b
  chronic, 1535
  clinical manifestations of, 1520, 1532–1535, *1533*

Heart failure *(Continued)*
  compensated, 1531–1532
  decompensated, 1532
  diagnosis of, 1535
  disability in, 1532b
  emergency care for, 2274–2275
  epidemiology of, 1515, 1529
  etiology of, 1515–1516, 1529, 1530t, 1531
  forward, 1535
  heart transplant for, 1546–1549
  high-output, 1535
  home care in, 1546b
  hypervolemia and, 225
  in elderly, 1546–1547
  in extracardiac disease, 1531
  left ventricular, 1531–1534, *1533*
  low-output, 1535
  medical management of, 1520–1524, 1535–1541
  nursing management of, 1524, 1541
  overview of, 1529
  pathogenesis of, 1518–1520
  pathophysiology of, 1531–1532
  remodeling in, 1532
  right ventricular, 1531–1533, *1533,* 1534–1535
  risk factors for, 1515–1518
    minimization of, 1520–1521
  self-care in, 1527–1529
  surgery for, 1524–1527. See also *Cardiac surgery.*
    in elderly, 1526–1527
    nursing management in, 1527
  terminology for, 1529, 1530t
Heart rate, 1434, 1442
Heart rhythm, abnormalities of, 1451. See also *Dysrhythmias.*
Heart sounds, 1459–1461, *1460*
  abnormal, 1459–1461, *1460*
  after cardiac surgery, 1508
  auscultation of, 1459
  extra, 1440
  in mitral valve disease, 1497–1498
  normal, 1459, *1460*
  types of, 1463t
Heart transplantation, 1502–1504, *1504,* 1504b, 1505t, 1546, 2226. See also *Cardiac surgery.*
  complications of, 1511
Heartburn, 691
  in gastroesophageal reflux disease. See *Gastroesophageal reflux disease (GERD).*
Heat, cellular injury from, 213
Heat application, for pain, 498, 614b
Heat stroke, 2282
Heaves, 1458
Height, measurement of, 182, 649
Heimlich maneuver, 2268, *2268*
Helicobacter pylori infection, antibiotics for, 710t, 715
  chronic gastritis and, 709
  peptic ulcers and, 712–713, 715
Helium method, for lung volumes, 1637
Heller's procedure, 692–694, *693*
Helminthic infections, 767–768
  pathogenesis of, 337t
Hemarthrosis, in hemophilia, 2127
Hematocrit, 2074–2075, 2094–2096, 2096t
  in cardiac assessment, 1464
  preoperative measurement of, 278t
  reference values for, 2096t, 2302t
Hematologic disorders, 2103–2128. See also specific disorders.
  of red blood cells, 2103–2118
  of white blood cells, 2119–2122
  outcomes classification for, 2103b

Hematologic system, age-related changes in, 50t
  assessment of, 2089–2102. See also *Hematopoietic assessment.*
  preoperative assessment of, 282
Hematologic tests, reference values for, 2302t
Hematoma, epidural, *2041,* 2041–2042
  intracerebral, *2041,* 2042–2043
  perichondrial, 1842
  subdural, *2041,* 2042, *2042*
Hematomyelia, 1994
Hematopoiesis, 2075
  in bone marrow, 2074
  liver in, 2078–2079
  regulation of, 2075
  spleen in, 2078–2079
  steps in, *2076*
Hematopoietic assessment, 2089–2102
  diagnostic tests in, 2094–2102
  history in, 2089–2093
  normal findings in, 2094b
  physical examination in, 2093–2094
Hematopoietic growth factors, for cancer, 388
Hematopoietic stem cells, 2075
Hematopoietic system. See also *Immune system.*
  anatomy and physiology of, 2072–2088
Hematuria, 759
  in glomerulonephritis, 865
  in renal cancer, 859
  in renal trauma, 868
  postoperative, 816
Hemilaryngectomy, 1665, *1665*
Hemiparesis, in stroke, 1956, 1957t
Hemiplegia, in stroke, 1956, 1957t, *1958*
  nursing management for, 1971–1973, *1972*
Hemisensory loss, in stroke, 1960
Hemispherectomy, for epilepsy, 1929, *1929,* 1930
Hemoccult test, 744t, 745
Hemochromatosis, 1258
Hemodialysis. See *Dialysis.*
Hemodynamic monitoring, 1476–1479
  in shock, 2244, 2253
  postoperative, 304–305, 306–307
    in cardiac surgery, 1507
Hemodynamic studies, 1475–1480
Hemoglobin, glycosylated, in diabetes mellitus, 1155, 1157
  in anemia, 2104
  in oxyhemoglobin dissociation curve, 1620, *1620*
  preoperative measurement of, 278t
  production of, 2078
  reference values for, 2302t
  urine, reference values for, 2306t
Hemoglobin electrophoresis, in sickle cell anemia, 2117
Hemoglobin level, 2094, 2096t
Hemoglobinuria, in burns, 1334, 1344–1345
Hemolytic anemia, 2115–2116
Hemolytic-uremic syndrome, 864t
Hemophilia, 2126t, 2126–2127
Hemopneumothorax, 1768
Hemoptysis, 1452, 1462
  assessment of, 1624
  causes of, 1624
  in pulmonary embolism, 1426
Hemorrhage. See also *Bleeding.*
  cirrhosis and, 1241–1242
  emergency care for, 2273–2274
  gastrointestinal. See *Gastrointestinal bleeding.*
  intracranial, in head trauma, *2041,* 2041–2043, *2042*
    thrombolytics and, 1964, 1971

Hemorrhage (Continued)
  renal, traumatic, 867, 868, 869
  shock in, 2232, 2232t. See also Hypovolemic shock.
  splinter, 1273t
  subarachnoid, 1940–1944
    head trauma and, 2034t
    stroke and, 1954, 1954–1959
  thyroidectomy and, 1105
Hemorrhagic exudate, 323, 323t
Hemorrhagic stroke, 1953, 1954, 1954–1955, 1956. See also Stroke.
Hemorrhoidectomy, 796–797
Hemorrhoids, 795, 795–797
Hemostasis, 2078–2080, 2079. See also Coagulation.
  disorders of, 2122b, 2122–2127, 2124b, 2125, 2126t
  liver function and, 1082t
  vasoconstriction in, 2079
Hemothorax, 1617, 1768
  emergency care for, 2271, 2271–2272
Henderson-Hasselbalch equation, 263
Heparin, for interstitial cystitis, 808
  for myocardial infarction, 1592t
  for shock, 2251
  for total hip replacement, 561–562
  for venous thrombosis, 1425
  low-molecular-weight, 1425
  perioperative use of, 275t
  postoperative, in abdominal-perineal resection, 785
  prophylactic, for stroke, 1965
Heparin lock, 310
Hepatic artery, 1060, 1061
Hepatic coma, 1251
  complications of, 1253
Hepatic disorders. See also Liver and specific disorders.
  congenital, 1258–1259
  outcomes classification for, 1219
Hepatic encephalopathy, 1065
  after paracentesis, 1087
  assessment of, 1252
  cirrhosis and, 1241
  clinical manifestations of, 1251–1252
  etiology of, 1250–1251, 1251b
  medical management of, 1252
  nursing management of, 1252–1253
  pathophysiology of, 1251
  prognosis of, 1252
  risk factors for, 1250–1251, 1251b
  self-care in, 1253
  stages of, 1251b
  viral hepatitis and, 1227
Hepatic failure, care plan for, 1248b–1250b
Hepatic fibrosis, congenital, 1259
Hepatic sinusoids, 1060, 1061
Hepatic stenosis, 1253–1254
Hepatitis, 1223–1232
  alcoholic, 1232
  chronic, 1229, 1229–1230
  chronic carrier state and, 1230
  toxic, 1232, 1232t
  viral, 1223–1229. See also specific type.
    aplastic anemia after, 1230
    assessment in, 1230
    clinical manifestations of, 1227–1228
    complications of, 1229
    epidemiology of, 1225
    etiology of, 1225
    fulminant, 1228, 1229
    medical management of, 1228–1229
    nursing management of, 1230–1231
    pathophysiology of, 1227
    prevention of, 1225–1227
    prognosis of, 1228

Hepatitis (Continued)
    risk factors for, 1225
    self-care in, 1231–1232
    types of, 1223–1225, 1224t
  Hepatitis A, 1224t
    chronic carrier state and, 1230
    epidemiology of, 1225
    immunization for, 342t, 1226, 1229
    pathophysiology of, 1227
    prevention of, 1225–1226
    risk factors for, 1225
    sexually transmitted, 1056
  Hepatitis antibodies, 1083t
  Hepatitis antigens, 1083t
  Hepatitis B, 1224t
    chronic carrier state and, 1230
    epidemiology of, 1225
    immunization for, 342t, 343, 1226, 1229
    in health care providers, prevention of, 345
    nosocomial, 340
    pathophysiology of, 1227
    prevention of, 1226
    risk factors for, 40t, 1225
    sexually transmitted, 1056
  Hepatitis B surface antigen (HBsAg), 1228, 1230
  Hepatitis C, 1224t
    chronic carrier state and, 1230
    epidemiology of, 1225
    pathophysiology of, 1227
    prevention of, 1226
    risk factors for, 1225
  Hepatitis D, 1224t
    epidemiology of, 1225
    pathophysiology of, 1227
    prevention of, 1226
    risk factors for, 1225
  Hepatitis E, 1224t
    epidemiology of, 1225
    pathophysiology of, 1227
    prevention of, 1226
    risk factors for, 1225
  Hepatitis G, 1224t
    epidemiology of, 1225
    pathophysiology of, 1227
    prevention of, 1226–1227
    risk factors for, 1225
  Hepatocellular carcinoma, 1254, 1254–1255, 1255
  Hepatocellular jaundice, 1220, 1221t
  Hepatocytes, 1060, 1061
  Hepatotoxicity, ascites and, 1247
    cirrhosis and, 1235, 1235t, 1240
    hepatitis and, 1229, 1230, 1232, 1232t
  HER-2/NEU protein, in breast cancer, 1018, 1020, 1033
  Herbal remedies, 27t. See also Alternative therapies.
    for ear disorders, 1799
    for heart disease, 1453
    for hematologic disorders, 2091
    for immunologic disorders, 2091
    for irritable bowel syndrome, 794b
    for musculoskeletal disorders, 539
    for neurologic disorders, 1879
    for reproductive disorders, in female, 916
      in male, 935
    for respiratory disorders, 1626
    for vascular disorders, 1370, 1425
    gastrointestinal upset due to, 741
    metabolic effects of, 1072
    nutritional, 647–648, 648t
  Herbalists, 74b
  Herceptin (trastuzumab), for breast cancer, 1033
  Herd immunity, 341

Hernia(s), abdominal, assessment for, 742
  femoral, 787–789, 788
    palpation for, 937, 939
  hiatal, 697–698, 698
    gastroesophageal reflux disease and, 695
  incisional (ventral), 787–788
  inguinal, 787–789, 788
    palpation for, 937, 939
  intestinal obstruction and, 790
  umbilical, 787–789, 788
Herniation, cerebral. See Cerebral herniation.
Herpes genitalis, 1045t, 1051–1053, 1052
Herpes labialis, 684, 685
Herpes simplex virus encephalitis, 1947
Herpes simplex virus infection, central nervous system and, 1947
  cutaneous, 1312t
  genital, 1045t, 1051–1053, 1052
  in HIV infection, 2205
  oral, 684, 685
Herpes zoster, 1310–1313, 1313
  chest pain in, 1450t
Heterosexuality, 418b
Heterotopic ossification, in spinal cord injury, 2060
Hiatal hernia, 696, 697–698, 698
  gastroesophageal reflux disease and, 695
High-density lipoproteins (HDLs), 15, 1517
  target levels for, 15
High-potassium diet, 244, 245b
High-sodium diet, 238b, 239
Hill operation, 697
Hill-Burton Act, 77–79
Hilus, 733, 733, 1617
Hip, avascular necrosis of, 601
  fractures of, 607–616
    clinical manifestations of, 608
    diagnosis of, 608
    epidemiology of, 607–608
    etiology of, 608
    in osteoporosis, 566, 566, 567
    medical management of, 608
    mobility in, 613–614, 614b
    mortality in, 608
    pathophysiology of, 608
    risk factors for, 608
    self-care in, 614
    surgery for, 611–612
      postoperative care in, 612–616
      preoperative care in, 611–612
    traction for, 608
    types of, 608, 609
  total replacement of, 555–564. See also Total hip replacement (THR).
Hip spica cast, 603
Hippocampus, 1857, 1858
Hippus, 1885
Hirschberg's test, 1791
Hirsutism, 1271
Hispanics. See also Cultural factors.
  elder care by, 47–48
Histamine, in inflammation, 318, 319
  in pain, 468
  in shock, 2239
Histamine H$_2$ receptor antagonists. See H$_2$ receptor antagonists.
Histocompatibility antigens, 2088
Histocompatibility testing, for bone marrow transplant, 2088
Histoplasmosis, 1723–1724
  in HIV infection, 2204
History, contraceptive, 917
  family, 137, 138
  health. See Health history.
  menstrual, 917
  obstetric, 917

History (Continued)
  psychosocial, 137–144, 139b, 140t–143t.
      See also Psychosocial assessment.
  sexual, 145
      female, 917, 918t
      male, 918t, 935
      social, 139b
History taking, in emergency care, 2266
HIV infection. See Human immunodeficiency
      virus infection.
HIV wasting syndrome, 2206
Hives, 2136–2137
Hivid (zalcitabine), 2196t
HLA matching, for transplantation, 2223
  of bone marrow, 2179
HLA system, 2074, 2088
HMOs, 78b, 80–81
  ambulatory nursing care in, 88
Hoarseness, in laryngeal cancer, 1661
  in laryngitis, 1680
  thyroidectomy and, 1105
Hodgkin's disease, 2173–2176
  chemotherapy for, 381b, 2175–2176
  complications of, 2176, 2176t
  Cotswold staging of, 2175t
  radiation therapy for, 2175, 2176
  breast cancer after, 1013
Holistic care, 84
  in long-term care facilities, 123, 124b
Holmes and Rahe's theory of life change and
      illness onset, 6t
Holter monitoring, 1470
Homans' sign, 605, 1374–1375, 1424
Home health care, 107–116. See also specific
      conditions.
  care delivery systems in, 111–116
  community focus in, 110–111
  dialysis in, 895, 898b
  discharge instructions and care in, 312, 312b
  dysphagia in, 667
  economic aspects of, 107–108, 108b, 109b
  education and training for, 111
  for elderly, 125
      elder abuse and, 57b
      medication management in, 60b
  guidelines for, 110–111
  historical perspective on, 109–110
  infection control measures in, 345b, 346
  information resources for, 125b
  intravenous therapy in, 242b
  OASIS data set for, 108, 113
  Omaha System for, 111–116. See also
      Omaha System.
  overview of, 109–110
  pain management in, 484b
  postoperative, 312, 312b
  reimbursement for, 107, 108, 109, 109b
  resources for, 111
  safety issues in, 111
  software systems for, 116
  standards of care for, 109–110
  trends in, 107–108
Homeostasis, integumentary system in, 1264
  theory of, 5t
Homocysteine, elevated, coronary heart disease
      and, 1517
Homonymous hemianopia, 1959, 1959
Homosexuality, 418b
Honeymoon cystitis, 802
Hordeolum, 1827t
Hormonal therapy, for benign prostatic hyper-
      plasia, 948
  for breast cancer, 1035–1036
  for prostate cancer, 961–962
Hormone ablation, for breast cancer, 1036
Hormone receptor status, in breast cancer,
      1020, 1035

Hormone replacement therapy (HRT), after
      hysterectomy, 993
  breakthrough bleeding in, 984
  breast cancer and, 571–572
  for endometriosis, 990
  for menopause, 985–986
  for osteoporosis, 570–572, 571t
  heart disease and, 1518, 1521
Hormones. See also Endocrine disorders; En-
      docrine system and specific hormones.
  classification of, 1060–1061
  hypothalamic, 1065
  in fluid and electrolyte balance, 217, 218
  pituitary, 1065
  sex, 1067
Horner's syndrome, in stroke, 1959
Horseshoe kidney, 871, 871
Hospice care, 65, 125, 401–402, 447–448,
      449b
Hospital(s), acute care in, 95–106. See also
      Acute care nursing.
  admission to, 96, 96b
  ambulatory care in, 87
  efficiency measures in, 96
  for-profit, 96
  funding for, 77–79
  government-owned, 95
  history of, 95
  levels of care in, 98b
  magnet, 96
  nonprofit, 96
  performance improvement for, 104–105,
      105b
  personnel and departments in, 97b
  regulation of, 102–104
  risk management for, 105
  service lines of, 96
  subacute care in, 96–98, 98b
  support services in, 97b
  transitional care in, 98, 98b
Hospital administrators/boards, 76
Hospital-acquired infection, 338t, 338–340
  prevention of, 343–346
Hospital-acquired sleep disorders, 439
Hospitalization, sensory deprivation in, 443
  sensory overload in, 443
Hot flashes, 984–985
Hot-cold theory of illness, 19b
Hot-spot imaging, 199, 199
Hougan, 74b
Housing, for elderly, 54t, 62–63
HPV infection. See Human papillomavirus in-
      fection.
Hruby lens, 1796
Huffing, 510t, 514t, 518, 520t–521t
Humalog insulin analog, 1159, 1162t
Human immunodeficiency virus, 2185–2186,
      2189–2190
  as retrovirus, 2189
  discovery of, 2185–2186
  genetic promiscuity of, 2185–2186, 2199
  structure of, 2189, 2190
  subtypes of, 2186
Human immunodeficiency virus infection,
      2185–2212
  AIDS indicator conditions in, 2202
  alternative therapy for, 2200
  assessment in, 2199–2200
  cancer in, 1309–1310, 1310, 2205–2206
  case study of, 2207b–2208b
  clinical manifestations of, 2191–2193,
      2192b
  course of, 2191
  diagnosis of, 2193
  drug therapy for, 2195–2199, 2196t–2198t
      client teaching for, 2200–2202, 2201t
  epidemiology of, 2185

Human immunodeficiency virus infection
      (Continued)
  etiology of, 2185–2186
  eye infections in, 1829
  fatigue in, 2209–2210
  fever in, 2209
  health maintenance in, 2195
  historical perspective on, 2185–2186
  home care in, 2208b
  in health care providers, prevention of, 343–
      345
  in health care workers, 345, 2188–2189
  in minorities, 2186, 2187b–2188b
  in older adults, 2186
  in pregnancy, 2189
  Kaposi's sarcoma in, 1309–1310, 1310
  long-term nonprogressors in, 2191
  long-term survivors in, 2191
  medical management of, in early stages,
      2193–2199
      in late stages, 2202–2206
  nursing diagnoses in, 2209b
  nursing management of, in early stages,
      2199
      in late stages, 2206–2212
  nutrition in, 2210
  opportunistic infections in, 2202–2205
      prevention of, 2199, 2201–2202
      treatment of, 2202–2205
  outcomes classification for, 2185
  pain in, 474
      management of, 2210–2211
  pathogenesis of, 337t
  pathophysiology of, 2189–2191
  primary infection in, 2191–2193
  psychosocial concerns in, 2200
  risk factors for, 2186–2189
      assessment for, 2194b
  sclerosing cholangitis in, 1215
  seroconversion in, 2193
  sexually transmitted diseases in, 1055–1056
  transfusions and, 2105
  transmission of, 2186–2189
  tuberculosis in, 1718, 2202–2203
  vaccine for, 2189
  viral load testing in, 2193, 2195
  weight loss in, 2206
Human leukocyte antigens, 2074, 2088
Human papillomavirus infection, 1045t
  cervical cancer and, 995
  warts and, 1312t
Human potential, development of, 25, 25–26
Humectants, 1283
Humerus, fractures of, 617–618
Humor, in pain management, 499
Humoral immunity, 2081
Humpback, 578
Hungry bones syndrome, 1114
Huntington's disease, 2009–2012
Hyaline cartilage, 532, 535
Hydralazine (Apresoline), for hypertension,
      1389t
  for hypertensive emergencies, 1396t
Hydrocele, 966, 966
Hydrocephalus, post-traumatic, 2034t
Hydrochloric acid, gastric secretion of, 635–
      636
  measurement of, 658–659
Hydrochlorothiazide (Hydrodiuril), for hyper-
      tension, 1389t
  perioperative use of, 275t
Hydrocodone, 489t
Hydrocortisone, for addisonian crisis, 1122
  for Addison's disease, 1124t
  perioperative use of, 275t
Hydrodiuril. See Hydrochlorothiazide (Hydro-
      diuril).

Hydrogen, fluid concentration of, 234t
  in acid-base balance, 259–262, *260–262*
Hydrogen ions, in pain, 467, 468, 469
Hydrogen peroxide, 327t, 332
Hydromorphone (Dilaudid), 489t
Hydronephrosis, 858
Hydrostatic pressure, 215–216, *1365*
Hydrotherapy, for burns, 1347, *1347*
17-Hydroxycorticosteroids, urine, reference
      values for, 2306t
5-Hydroxyindoleacetic acid, urine, reference
      values for, 2306t
17-Hydroxysteroids, adrenocortical function
      and, 1122t
Hylorel (guanadrel), for hypertension, 1389t
Hymen, 904
Hyperaldosteronism, 1133–1135, *1134,* 1135b
Hyperamylasemia. See also *Amylase.*
  in acute pancreatitis, 1195
Hyperbaric oxygen, complications of, 1842
  for shock, 2244
  for wound healing, 333
Hypercalcemia, 252–254
  clinical manifestations of, 1110
  diet in, 1113
  hyperparathyroidism and, 1110
  in cancer, 395–396
  in cardiac disease, 1465
  treatment of, 1110, 1112t
      in multiple myeloma, 2120–2121
Hypercalciuria, stone formation and, 823
  variants of, 823
Hypercapnia, 1621
  in shock, 2238
Hypercholesterolemia. See also *Hyperlipid-
      emia.*
  coronary heart disease and, 1516–1517
  definition of, 1517
  health promotion/risk management for, 150t,
      1521
Hypercortisolism, 1126–1133, *1128–1129*
  client teaching in, 1131
  clinical manifestations of, 1130
  epidemiology of, 1126
  etiology of, 1126–1127
  in elderly, 1133
  medical management of, 1132, 1133t
  pathophysiology of, 1127, *1127*
  risk factors for, 1126–1127
  self-care in, 1133
  surgery for, 1130–1131
      nursing management in, 1131–1132
Hyperglycemia, health promotion/risk manage-
      ment for, 150t
  in cardiac disease, 1465
  in diabetes mellitus, 1155. See also *Diabetes
      mellitus.*
      ketoacidosis and, 1172–1177, 1174t. See
      also *Diabetic ketoacidosis.*
  rebound, hypoglycemia with, 1180
Hyperglycemic, hyperosmolar, nonketotic syn-
      drome, 1177, 1177b, 1181t–1182t
Hyperkalemia, 246–248
  in acute renal failure, 878
  in addisonian crisis, 1121
  in cardiac disease, 1465
  in chronic renal failure, 878, 892
  in diabetic ketoacidosis, 1174t
Hyperlipasemia. See also *Lipase.*
  in acute pancreatitis, 1195
Hyperlipidemia, coronary heart disease and,
      1516–1517
  definition of, 1517
  health promotion/risk management for, 150t,
      1521
  in chronic renal failure, 883
      hemodialysis and, 893

Hyperlipidemia *(Continued)*
  management of, drug therapy in, 1402
      in peripheral arterial occlusive disease,
      1402
      lifestyle modifications in, 1402
  screening for, 158t
Hyperlipoproteinemia, definition of, 1517
  health promotion/risk management for, 150t,
      1521
Hypermagnesemia, in acute renal failure, 878
  in cardiac disease, 1465
Hypernatremia, 239t, 239–242
  in cardiac disease, 1465
Hyperopia, *1827,* 1827–1828
Hyperosmolality, in diabetic ketoacidosis,
      1174t
Hyperosmolar nonketotic syndrome, hypergly-
      cemic, 1177, 1177b, 1181t–1182t
Hyperparathyroidism, 1109–1114
  altered nutrition in, 1113
  assessment in, 1110–1111
  clinical manifestations of, 1109–1110,
      1110
  constipation in, 1113
  critical monitoring in, 1109b
  diagnosis of, 1110, 1111t
  epidemiology of, 1109
  etiology of, 1109
  fractures in, 1111–1112
  hypercalcemia and, 252
  in chronic renal failure, 881
      treatment of, 892
  in elderly, 1114
  medical management of, 1110, 1112t
  nursing management of, 1110–1113
  pathophysiology of, 1109
  primary, 1109
  risk factors for, 1109
  secondary, 1109
  surgery for, 1113
      nursing management in, 1113–1114
  tertiary, 1109
Hyperphosphatemia, 254
  in cardiac disease, 1465
  in chronic renal failure, 881
Hyperpigmentation, in chemotherapy, 395
Hyperpituitarism, hyperprolactinemia and,
      1139, 1139–1142, *1140,* 1141t
Hyperplasia, 211
  definition of, 350t
Hyperprolactinemia, hyperpituitarism and,
      1139, 1139–1142, *1140,* 1141t
  sexual disturbances and, 1142
Hyperresonance, on percussion, 177
Hypersensitivity. See also *Allergic reactions.*
  delayed, 2130, 2131t, 2132
      skin testing for, 2101
  type I, 2081
Hypersensitivity disorders, 2129–2135. See
      also *Allergic reactions.*
  assessment of, 2134–2135
  classification of, 2130, 2131t
  clinical manifestations of, 2132–2133
  etiology of, 2129–2130
  medical management of, 2133–2134, *2134*
  nursing management of, 2134–2135
  pathophysiology of, 2130–2132, 2133t
  risk factors for, 2129–2130
Hypersensitivity pneumonitis, 1739–1740,
      1740t
Hypersplenism, 2121–2122
Hypertension, 184, 1379–1398
  assessment in, 1384, 1386t
  classification of, 1384, 1386t
  clinical manifestations of, 1383–1384
  community care for, 1395–1396
  coronary heart disease and, 1516

Hypertension *(Continued)*
  cultural factors in, 1391
  diagnosis of, 1384
  diet in, 1383, 1387, 1388t
  drug therapy for, 1387–1392, 1388t–1390t
  epidemiology of, 1379–1380
  health promotion/risk management for, 148t
  heart disease and, 1380
  in autonomic dysreflexia and, 2051, 2064,
      2064b, 2065
  in diabetes mellitus, 1183t, 1184
  in elderly, 1394–1395
  in hypercortisolism, 1131
  in increased intracranial pressure, 2028, *2028*
  in pheochromocytoma, 1136
  intracranial. See *Increased intracranial pres-
      sure (ICP).*
  isolated systolic, 1380, 1380t
  labile, 1383
  lifestyle modifications for, 1386
  malignant, 1380, 1380t, 1395–1397
  nursing management of, 1392–1395
  obstructive sleep apnea in, 439
  pathophysiology of, 1381–1383, *1382, 1383*
  persistent severe, 1395
  portal. See *Portal hypertension.*
  postoperative, 305
  primary (essential), 1380, 1380t
  pulmonary, 1708–1709
  racial factors in, 1380, 1381, 1391b
  renal, 852, 882–883, 1383
      treatment of, 892
  risk factors for, 1380–1381
  risk stratification for, 1384, 1386t
  screening for, 158t, 1397
  secondary, 1380, 1380t, 1384b
  staging of, 1384, 1386t
  treatment of, compliance with, 1394
      emergency, 1395–1397
  trends in, 1379–1380
  types of, 1380, 1380t
  vessel changes in, 1383
  weight reduction for, 1386–1387
  white coat, 1380, 1380t
Hypertensive crisis, 1395–1397, 1396t
Hypertensive retinopathy, 1829
Hyperthermia, emergency care for, 2282
  for benign prostatic hyperplasia, 956
  in HIV infection, 2209
  in hyperthyroidism, 1103
  in increased intracranial pressure, 2028,
      2038
  in stroke, 1965, 1973
  malignant, 301–302
Hyperthyroidism, 1099–1106
  activity intolerance in, 1103
  altered nutrition in, 1103
  assessment in, 1101
  case study of, 1102
  clinical manifestations of, 1092t, 1099–
      1100, *1100*
  complications of, 1100
  critical monitoring in, 1099b
  epidemiology of, 1099
  etiology of, 1099
  eye in, 1099–1100, *1100,* 1103, 1828
  hyperthermia in, 1103
  in elderly, 1106
  medical management of, 1096t, 1100–1101
  nursing management of, 1101–1103
  pathophysiology of, 1099
  psychosocial issues in, 1103
  risk factors for, 1099
  self-care in, 1105–1106
  sleep problems in, 438
  surgery for, 1103–1105, 1104t
      nursing management in, 1105

Hypertriglyceridemia, 1517, 1521. See also
  Hyperlipidemia.
Hypertrophic cardiomyopathy, *1491,* 1492t,
  1492–1493
Hypertrophic gastritis, 709
Hypertrophy, 211
Hyperuricemia, in gout, 575–576
Hyperventilation, *184*
  emergency care for, 2269–2270
  in burns, 1334–1335, 1337
Hypervolemia, 225t, 225–228, *226.* See also
  Edema.
  after portosystemic shunt surgery, 1245
  emergency care for, 2274–2275
  fluid shift and, 229–230
  hypernatremia and, 239t
  hyponatremia and, 236–239
  in ascites, 1247
  in diabetic ketoacidosis, 1174t
Hypnogogic hallucinations, in narcolepsy, 435
Hypnosis, for pain, 499
Hypnotics, abuse of, 511t, 515t, 519, 520t–
  521t
Hypocalcemia, 249–252
  health promotion/risk management for,
    150t–151t
  hypermagnesemia and, 257
  hypomagnesemia and, 255
  in cardiac disease, 1465
  in chronic renal failure, 883
    treatment of, 894
  parathyroidectomy and, 1113–1114. See
    also *Hypoparathyroidism.*
  thyroidectomy and, 1105
Hypocapnia, 1621
Hypodermis, 1262, *1263,* 1263–1264
Hypoglossal nerve, 1870t
  assessment of, 1886
Hypoglycemia, in addisonian crisis, 1122
  in diabetes mellitus, 1177–1180, 1178b,
    1179t, 1181t–1182t
    and diabetic ketoacidosis, 1174t
    exercise and, 1158–1159
Hypoglycemic unawareness, in diabetes mellitus, 1180
Hypogonadism, 1143, 1145
Hypogonadotropic hypogonadism, 1143
Hypokalemia, 243–246
  hypomagnesemia and, 255
  in acute renal failure, 878
  in cardiac disease, 1465
  in diabetic ketoacidosis, 1174t, 1175, 1176b
  in hepatic encephalopathy, 1253
  in hyperaldosteronism, 1134
Hypomagnesemia, in cardiac disease, 1465
Hyponatremia, 236t, 236–239
  in acute renal failure, 878
  in cardiac disease, 1465
  in chronic renal failure, 881
  in diabetic ketoacidosis, 1174t
  in syndrome of inappropriate antidiuretic
    hormone, 396
Hypoosmolar, 216–217
Hypoparathyroidism, 1114–1116
  acute, 1114
  after thyroidectomy, 1104–1105
  assessment in, 1115
  chronic, 1114–1115
  clinical manifestations of, 1114–1115
  complications of, 1115
  critical monitoring in, 1109b
  diagnosis of, 1111t, 1115
  epidemiology of, 1114
  etiology of, 1114
  hypocalcemia and, 249, 250
  iatrogenic, 1114
  idiopathic, 1114

Hypoparathyroidism *(Continued)*
  medical management of, 1115
  nursing management of, 1115–1116
  pathophysiology of, 1114
  risk factors for, 1114
  self-care in, 1116
Hypopharynx, 1612, *1613*
Hypophosphatemia, 254
  in cardiac disease, 1465
Hypophysis. See *Pituitary gland.*
Hypopituitarism, 1142–1143
Hypoprothrombinemia, 2123
Hyposmia, 1636
Hypospadias, 756, 971, *971*
Hypotension, 184
  in dehydration, 219
  in shock, 2242
  in spinal anesthesia, 296t
  in spinal cord injury, 2054, 2055
  opioid analgesics and, 491
  orthostatic (postural), 1397, 1849
    in dehydration, 219
    opioid analgesics and, 491
  postoperative, 304–305
  renal function in, 852
Hypothalamic-pituitary-adrenal axis dysfunction, adrenal insufficiency in, 1126
Hypothalamo-hypophyseal portal system, 1062
Hypothalamus, 1858, *1858*
  anatomy of, 1061, 1062, *1063*
  hormones regulated by, *1063,* 1065
Hypothermia, emergency care for, 2282–2283
  in burns, 1351–1352
  in myxedema, 1097
  in shock, 2252, 2253
  in spinal cord injury, 2057
  intraoperative, 300–301
  postoperative, 306
Hypothyroidism, 1090–1099
  activity intolerance in, 1097–1098
  altered nutrition in, 1097
  assessment in, 1097
  central, 1091
  clinical manifestations of, 1091–1093,
    1092t, *1093*
  constipation in, 1098
  critical monitoring in, 1097b
  diagnostic tests in, 1093, 1094t
  epidemiology of, 1091
  etiology of, 1091
  hypopituitarism and, 1143
  in elderly, 1098–1099
  medical management of, 1093, 1095, 1096t,
    1098b
  mild, 1091–1092
  nursing management of, 1097b, 1097–1098
  pathophysiology of, 1091
  primary, 1091
  risk factors for, 1091
  secondary, 1091
  self-care in, 1098, 1098b
  sleep problems in, 438
  subclinical, 1091, 1098–1099
  tertiary, 1091
Hypoventilation, 1621
  emergency care for, 2270
  postoperative, 304, 306
Hypovolemia, 217–224. See also *Dehydration.*
  emergency care for, 2273–2274
  fluid shift and, 229–230
  in acute pancreatitis, 1196, 1197
  in ascites, 1247
  in hepatic encephalopathy, 1253
Hypovolemic shock, 230, 2231. See also
  Shock.
  clinical manifestations of, 2243
  etiology of, 2232–2233

Hypovolemic shock *(Continued)*
  in gastrointestinal hemorrhage, 715–716
  medical management of, 2249t
  postoperative, 304–305, 306–307
Hypoxemia, in hepatic encephalopathy, 1253
  in pulmonary edema, 1746–1749
Hypoxemic respiratory failure, 1746–1748
Hypoxia, 212–213
  tissue, in shock, 2236, *2238*
Hysterectomy, *992,* 992–994
  dyspareunia after, 998
  for endometriosis, 990
  for leiomyomas, 992–994
  for uterine prolapse, 999–1000
  postoperative care in, 993–994
  preoperative care in, 992–993
  radical, 992–994
  surgical menopause in, 984
  total, *992,* 992–994
Hysteroscopy, 928–929, *929*

I

IBD. See *Inflammatory bowel disease (IBD).*
Ibuprofen (Advil, Motrin), 486
  dosage of, 487t
Ice application, for pain, 498, 614b
ICP. See *Increased intracranial pressure
  (ICP).*
Icterus (jaundice), 1220–1223, 1221t–1222t
IDDM (insulin-dependent diabetes mellitus).
  See *Diabetes mellitus, type 1.*
Idiopathic membranous glomerulonephritis,
  864t
Idiopathic thrombocytopenic purpura, 2122–
  2123
IgA, 2083–2084, *2084,* 2084t
  reference values for, 2304t
  serum levels of, 2100, 2100t
IgA nephropathy, 864t
IgD, *2084,* 2084t, 2084–2085
  reference values for, 2304t
  serum levels of, 2100, 2100t
IgE, 2083–2084, *2084,* 2084t
  reference values for, 2304t
  serum levels of, 2100, 2100t
IgG, 2083, *2084,* 2084t
  reference values for, 2304t
  serum levels of, 2100, 2100t
IgM, 2083–2084, *2084,* 2084t
  reference values for, 2304t
  serum levels of, 2100, 2100t
Ileal conduit, 813, *813.* See also *Urinary diversion.*
  catheterization of, 819–820
  pouch application for, 818, *819*
  self-care for, 817–821, 818b
Ileal pouch–anal anastomosis, 775–776, *776*
  postoperative care in, 779
Ileal W-bladder, *813,* 814. See also *Urinary
  diversion.*
Ileocecal valve, 630
Ileorectal anastomosis, 775
  postoperative care in, 779
Ileostomy, 776–780
  body image and, 777
  continent, 775, *775*
    postoperative care in, 779
  delegation for, 788
  diet in, 779
  drug therapy and, 778
  nursing management in, 776
  odor control in, 778
  pouches for, 777–778, 778b
  resources for, 786b
  self-care in, 777–779, 780

Illeostomy (Continued)
  sexual function and, 779–780
  skin care in, 777–778
  stoma care in, 776–778, 778b
  supplies for, 786b
  urolithiasis and, 779
Ileum, structure of, 630
Ileus, adynamic. See Paralytic ileus.
Illness. See also Disease.
  chronic. See Chronic conditions.
  cultural aspects of, 19b, 424b
  health and wellness and, 8–9
  natural vs. unnatural, 19b
  presentation of, in elderly, 52
  terminal. See Death and dying.
Illusions, in confusional states, 1919
Imagery, for pain, 499
  guided, 36
Imaging studies, 192–200. See also specific studies.
  contrast agents for, 196b
  cytologic, 200–201
Imipramine, reference values for, 2308t
Immersion syndrome, 1770
Immobility, complications of, 17, 612. See also Contractures; Pressure ulcers.
  hepatic encephalopathy and, 1253
  in coma, 1914–1915
  in stroke, 1973–1974
  disuse syndrome and, 17
  exercises in, 618b
  home care in, 618b
  in elderly, 53–55, 612–614
  in rheumatoid arthritis, 2151–2152, 2152
  pressure ulcers and, 605, 612, 1295. See also Pressure ulcers.
  skin care in, 612, 613, 618b
  venous thrombosis and, 605–606, 612
Immune cascade, 2082
Immune complex hypersensitivity, 2130–2132, 2131t
Immune globulin, in hepatitis prevention, 1226, 1229
Immune response, 336–338
  host defenses in, 336–338
  in transplantation, 2223
  primary, 2081–2082, 2082
  secondary, 2082, 2082–2085
Immune system, age-related changes in, 50t, 212t
  anatomy and physiology of, 2072–2088
  assessment of, 2089–2102. See also Hematopoietic assessment.
  disorders of, 2129–2138
    outcomes classification for, 2129b
  in cancer, 360–361
  in chronic renal failure, 886
  in HIV infection, 2190–2191
  in shock, 2240
  lungs in, 1622
  organs of, 2072–2074, 2073
  preoperative assessment of, 281–282
  skin in, 1264
  surface defenses in, 2072
Immunity, 2081–2088
  acquired, 2081–2082
  active, 2081
  artificial, 2081
  cell-mediated, 2081, 2085–2087, 2086
  herd, 341
  humoral, 2081
  innate, 2072–2081
  mucosal, 2081
  natural, 2081
  passive, 2081
Immunization(s), 40, 341–343. See also under specific disease.
  active, 341, 1226

Immunization(s) (Continued)
  for adolescents, 342t
  for adults, 342t
  for HIV infection, 2189
  influenza, 1711
  passive, 341, 1226
  schedule for, 157t
  tetanus, 40, 342, 342t
    for burns, 1343, 1345
Immunoglobulins, 2083–2085, 2084, 2084t. See also Antibodies.
  reference values for, 2304t
  serum levels of, 2100, 2100t
  surface, 2073
Immunosuppression, for bone marrow transplant, 2180
  for heart transplant, 1503–1504, 1505t
  for inflammatory bowel disease, 773
  for transplantation, 2223, 2224t
    compliance with, 2228
  in burns, 1335
  in chronic renal failure, 882
  in pancreas transplant, 1171–1172
  nutrition and, 2136b
Immunotherapy, for hypersensitivity disorders, 2134
  for renal cancer, 859–860
Impacted fracture, 596t
Impedance plethysmography, 1376
Impetigo, 1311t
Impingement syndromes, 620–621
Implantable cardioverter-defibrillator, 1568
  quality of life and, 1607–1609
Impotence, 972–974
  after prostate surgery, 956, 958
Imuran (azathioprine), for transplant immunosuppression, 2224t
Inactivity. See also Activity and exercise; Immobility.
  management of, 33–35
Inapsine (droperidol), preoperative, 290t
Incentive spirometry, postoperative, 308, 308
  preoperative teaching for, 286
Incision(s). See also Wound(s).
  assessment of, 324
  care of, 324
  closure of, 300, 301
  drainage of, 324
  dressings for, 324
  elliptical, 1314
  opening of, 309, 309
  skin lines and, 1314
  splinting of, 286, 1731, 1732
Incisional biopsy, 374
Incisional hernia, 787–788
Incomplete fracture, 593t
Incontinence. See Bowel incontinence; Urinary incontinence.
Incontinence pads, 839
Increased intracranial pressure (ICP), 2026–2039. See also Cerebral edema.
  brain tumors and, 1932, 1934
  clinical manifestations of, 1934, 1970b, 2028
  compensatory mechanisms in, 2027
  complications of, 2031, 2034t
  Cushing's triad in, 2028, 2028
  definition of, 2027
  diagnostic studies in, 2029
  etiology of, 2027
  in head trauma, 2045
  in hyponatremia, 237
  in stroke, 1965, 1969–1971, 1970b
  in subarachnoid hemorrhage, 1942, 1943t
  in water intoxication, 228–229
  neurologic assessment in, 2031–2038. See also Neurologic assessment.

Incision(s) (Continued)
  nursing management in, 1969–1971
  pathophysiology of, 2027–2028
  postoperative, hyperpituitarism and, 1140
  pressure monitoring in, 2030b, 2030–2031, 2032b–2033b
  risk factors for, 2027
  ventriculostomy for, 1965
Incubation period, 338
Incus, 1783, 1783. See also Ossicles.
Inderal (propranolol), for hypertension, 1389t
  perioperative use of, 275t
  reference values for, 2308t
Indiana pouch, 813, 813–814, 814. See also Urinary diversion.
Indigestion, 706
Indinavir (Crixivan), 2197t
Indirect antiglobulin test, 2096
Indomethacin, 486, 487t
Indwelling catheter, for urinary retention, 831–832
Infarction, mesenteric, 791
Infection, 335–346. See also specific sites and types.
  bacterial, cell damage in, 213
    characteristics of, 337t
    pathogenesis of, 337t
  by drug-resistant organisms, 339, 341b
  carrier of, 336
  catheter, 338, 339
  cell damage in, 213
  cholelithiasis and, 1204, 1211
  cirrhosis and, 1235
  colonization in, 338
  communicability period in, 338
  community-acquired, 338
  device-related, 339
  emergency care for, 2278
  environmental factors in, 336
  hepatic encephalopathy and, 1253
  historical perspective on, 335
  host factors in, 336–338, 340, 340b
  in cancer, 383–384, 392–393, 395, 396
  in chemotherapy, 383–384, 392–393, 395
  in diabetes mellitus, 1183t, 1184–1185, 1186b, 1187b
  in health care providers, prevention of, 343–346
  in HIV infection, 2202–2205
    prevention of, 2199, 2201–2202
    treatment of, 2202–2205
  in leukemia, 2171
  in transplant recipients, 1512, 2225, 2225t
  incubation period in, 338
  latent period in, 338
  nosocomial. See Nosocomial infection.
  of open fractures, 601
  pathogenic factors in, 335, 337t
  phases of, 338
  portal of entry in, 335
  portal of exit in, 335
  preoperative management of, 281–282
  prevention of, 340–346. See also Infection control measures.
  process of, 335–338
  shock in, 2234. See also Septic shock.
  steroid replacement and, in hypercortisolism, 1132
  subclinical, 338
  susceptibility to, 336–338, 340, 340b
  transfusion-related, 340
  transmission of, 336
  wound, 331–333
    nosocomial, 338t, 339
    pathogenesis of, 337t
    postoperative, 309

Infection control measures, 340–346. See also *Immunization(s).*
  delegation in, 344b
  in community-based settings, 345b, 346
  in home health care, 345b, 345–346
  in hospitals, 343–346
  in long-term care facilities, 346
Infectious arthritis, 579–580
Infectious mononucleosis, 2121
Infective endocarditis, 1484–1487, *1485*
Inferior petrosal sinus sampling test, in hypercortisolism, 1130
Infertility, female, chlamydial infection and, 1047
    endometriosis and, 989–991, *990*
    pelvic inflammatory disease and, 987
  male, 968–970
    cryptorchidism and, 967
Infibulation, 1008
Inflammation, 316–319, 2081
  acute, 321–324
  assessment in, 323
  chemotaxis in, 318, 319
  chronic, 324
  clinical manifestations of, 323
  complement in, 319
  edema in, 322
  fever in, 321
  in wound healing, 316–318, *317, 318*
  kinins in, 319
  lymphocytes in, 318
  macrophages in, 318
  management of, medical, 321–323
    nursing, 323–324
  mast cells in, 319
  mediators of, *317, 318,* 319–320
  monocytes in, 318
  neutrophils in, 317–318, *318*
  oxygen free radicals in, 319
  pain in, 472–473
  phagocytosis in, *317,* 317–318, *318*
  process of, *317,* 317–319
  self-care in, 324
  walling off in, 319
  white blood cells in, 317–319, *318*
Inflammatory bowel disease (IBD), 770–780
  clinical manifestations of, 771t, 772–773
  etiology of, 771–772
  medical management of, 773–774
  nursing management of, 774
  pathophysiology of, 771t, 772
  prognosis in, 771t, 772–773
  surgery for, 774–780. See also *Ileostomy.*
    postoperative care in, 776
    preoperative care in, 776
    procedures in, 774–776, *775, 776*
  vs. ulcerative colitis, 771t
Inflammatory exudates, 323, 323t
Influenza, 1711
  immunization for, 342, 342t
Influenzal pneumonia, 1711–1716, 1712t
Informed consent, 287, *288*
  competence and, 66–67
  for emergency care, 287, *288*
Infratentorial herniation, *2029,* 2030
Infusion pumps, for home care, 242b
Ingram method, 1284
Ingrown nail, 1328
Inguinal area, examination of, 169t
Inguinal hernia, 787–789, *788*
  palpation for, *937,* 939
Inhalants, 510t, 518, 520t–521t
Inhalation anesthesia, 293, 294t. See also *Anesthesia.*
Inhalation injury, 1332
  in burns, 1332, 1335, 1337–1338, 1341, 1349

Inhalers, for allergic disorders, 2133, 2135
Inhibin, 913
Inhibitory neurons, 469
Initial Pain Assessment Tool, 477, *480*
Injection, intramuscular, 495
  trigger point, 496
Innovar (fentanyl citrate–droperidol), 294t
Insect stings, allergy to, 2137t, 2137–2138
Insight, assessment of, 143–144, 1882
Insomnia, 434
  benzodiazepines for, 455
Inspection, 174, *175, 176*
Inspiration, mechanics of, *1616,* 1616–1618
Inspiratory capacity, 1615, *1615*
  measurement of, 1637, 1638t
Inspiratory reserve volume, 1615, *1615*
  measurement of, 1637, 1638t
Instrumental activities of daily living, in elderly, 52–53, *53*
Insula lobe, 1857, *1858*
Insulin, 1066, 1159, 1161–1162, 1162t, *1163*
  client management and, 1167b, 1167–1170, 1168b, *1169,* 1170b
  concentrations of, 1168
  diet management and, 1166–1167
  dosage of, 1159, *1163*
    in renal failure, 882
  endogenous, reference values for, 2304t
  growth hormone levels and, 1065, 1080
  in hyperglycemic, hyperosmolar, nonketotic syndrome, 1177
  in ketoacidosis, 1176
  injection sites for, preparation of, 1169
    selection and rotation of, 1169, *1169*
  intensive therapy with, 1161–1162
  perioperative use of, 275t
  preparations of, 1159, 1162t, 1169
  self-injection of, instruction in, 1168b, 1168–1170, *1169*
    techniques for, 1169–1170
  storage of, 1169
  syringes for, 1168, *1169*
    prefilled, 1169
  with oral antidiabetic agents, 1162
Insulin pumps, 1159, 1161, *1163*
Insulin reaction, 1177–1180, 1178b, 1179t, 1181t–1182t
Insulin resistance, 1154, *1155,* 1184
Insulin-dependent diabetes mellitus (IDDM). See *Diabetes mellitus, type 1.*
Insurance. See *Health insurance.*
Intake and output. See also *Fluid intake; Urine output.*
  measurement of, 219, 222
Integrated sensory functions, assessment of, 1883
Integumentary assessment, 1267–1277. See also *Skin assessment.*
Integumentary system. See also *Hair; Nails; Skin.*
  age-related changes in, 50t, 212t
Intellectual performance, assessment of, 1881–1882
Intellectualization, 408b
Intelligence. See *Cognitive function.*
Intensive care unit (ICU), postoperative transport to, 302
Intercellular communication, 209
Intercostal muscles, 1617–1618
Interferon(s), extrinsic, for cancer, 388
  for multiple sclerosis, 2014
  intrinsic, 2087t
Interleukins, extrinsic, for cancer, 389
  in wound healing, 319–320
  intrinsic, 2087, 2087t
Intermediate care facilities, 63, 65

Intermittent claudication, 1368, 1400, 1404
Intermittent pneumatic compression, 1423, *1424*
Intermittent self-catheterization. See also *Urinary catheterization.*
  for neurogenic bladder, 844, 845b, 846
  in benign prostatic hyperplasia, 948b
Internal capsule, 1857–1858
Internal carotid arteries, *1864,* 1865
Internal jugular vein, assessment of, 1457, *1458*
International Normalized Ratio, 2098
International System of Units (SI system), 188
Interneurons, in pain, 469
Interrupted suture, *301*
Interstate Compact, 92
Interstitial cystitis, 750, 807–808
Interstitial fluid compartment, 215
Interstitial lung disease, 1725–1726
Interstitial nephritis, 862
Interstitial radiation therapy, 378
Intertrigo, 1291–1292
Intervention Scheme, in Omaha System, 114–115, 115b
Interventional angiography, cerebral, 1900
Intervertebral disc disease, cervical, 1991–1993, *1992*
  lumbar, 1984–1985, *1985*
  surgery for, *1987,* 1987–1991
Intestinal absorption, carbohydrate, 636
  fluid and electrolyte, 216t, 636–637
  impaired. See *Malabsorption.*
  lipid, 636
  protein, 636
Intestinal decompression, 792. See also *Gastrointestinal intubation.*
Intestinal disorders, assessment of, 739–747
    diagnostic tests in, 743–747, 744t
    history in, 739–742
    laboratory tests in, 744t, 745–746
    physical examination in, 742–743
  bleeding in, 765
  clinical manifestations of, 765–766
  constipation in, 766
  diarrhea in, 766
  distention in, 766
  fecal abnormalities in, 766
  infectious, 766–770
  inflammatory, 766–780
  nausea and vomiting in, 766
  outcomes classification for, 765
  pain in, 765–766
Intestinal distention, 766
Intestinal flora, normal, 336–337, 637
Intestinal ischemia, in shock, 2240
Intestinal motility, 632–633
Intestinal obstruction, *790,* 790–793
Intestinal parasites, 767–768
Intestinal volvulus, *790,* 790–793
Intra-aortic balloon pump, for shock, 2245–2246
Intra-aortic balloon pump counterpulsation, 1510b, 15098
Intra-arterial chemotherapy, 387
Intra-arterial pressure monitoring, 1479–1480
Intracapillary pressure, fluid movement and, 215–216, *216*
Intracavitary chemotherapy, 387
Intracavitary radiation therapy, 378
Intracellular fluid, 215
Intracellular fluid volume deficit, 225
Intracellular fluid volume excess, 228–229
Intracerebral hematoma, *2041,* 2042–2043
Intracoronary stents, 1523, *1523*
Intracranial aneurysms, 1940–1944, *1941*
Intracranial bleeding, in head trauma, *2041,* 2041–2043, *2042*

Intracranial compartments, *2027*
Intracranial hemorrhage, 1940–1944
  subarachnoid, head trauma and, 2034t
  thrombolytics and, 1964, 1971
Intracranial pressure, autoregulation of, 2028
  definition of, 2026
  increased. See *Increased intracranial pressure (ICP).*
  maintenance of, 2038
  measurement of, 2026–2027
  monitoring of, 2030b, 2030–2031, 2032b–2033b, 2038
  reference values for, 2027
Intracranial surgery. See *Craniotomy.*
Intracranial vault, components of, *2027*
Intradermal allergy tests, 2101
Intramuscular injection, 495
Intraocular lens, for aphakia, 1816
  implantation of, 1815–1816
Intraocular pressure, assessment of, *1795,* 1795–1796
  in glaucoma. See *Glaucoma.*
  reduction of, *1811,* 1811–1812
Intraoperative period, allergic reactions in, 302
  anesthesia in, 292–298. See also *Anesthesia.*
  cardiac arrest in, 302
  diabetes mellitus and, 1189
  documentation for, 302
  emergencies in, 301–302
  malignant hyperthermia in, 301–302
  monitoring in, 300–302
  nursing roles in, 291b, 292
  positioning in, 299, 299b, *300*
  respiratory arrest in, 302
  safety measures in, 298–300
  surgical asepsis in, 300
  wound closure in, 300
Intraperitoneal chemotherapy, 387
Intraspinal analgesia, 495
Intraspinal anesthesia, 293–295, *295, 296,* 296t
Intrathecal chemotherapy, 387
Intravascular fluid compartment, 215
Intravascular ultrasonography, 1377
Intravenous analgesia, 495
Intravenous anesthesia, 293, 294t–295t. See also *Anesthesia.*
Intravenous drug use, HIV transmission via, 2188
Intravenous pyelography, 758–759
Intravenous regional extremity block, 298
Intravenous therapy. See also *Fluid management.*
  fluid volume excess in, 228–229
  for dehydration, 220, 221t, 223–224
    in diabetic ketoacidosis, 1175, 1175b
    in hyperglycemic, hyperosmolar, nonketotic syndrome, 1177
  for hyponatremia, 238, 239
  heparin lock in, 310
  in home care, 242b
  in hypokalemia, 244, 245–246
    in diabetic ketoacidosis, 1175, 1176b
  monitoring in, 309–310
  postoperative, 309–310
  preoperative teaching for, 287
  solutions for, 220, 221t, 2247, 2274
Intraventricular catheter, in intracranial pressure monitoring, 2030, 2032b–2033b
Intrinsic coagulation pathway, *2079,* 2080
Intrinsic factor, 2077
Intrinsic sphincter deficiency, 835
  sling procedure for, 839
Introitus, examination of, 924
Intropin (dopamine), for acute renal failure, 878
  for heart failure, 1537b

Intubation. See also *Tube(s).*
  chest. See *Chest tubes.*
  endotracheal. See *Endotracheal intubation.*
  gastrointestinal, 706–708. See also *Gastrointestinal intubation.*
  nasogastric, in shock, 2248
    postoperative, 722
    in esophageal surgery, 699
  rectal, 799
Intussusception, *790,* 790–793
Inverse ratio ventilation, 1762
Invirase (saquinavir), 2198t
Iodine, deficiency of, 641t–642t
  food sources of, 641t
  for goiter, 1090
  for hyperthyroidism, 1101
  radioactive, for hyperthyroidism, 1096t, 1101
  uptake of, 1079, 1094t
    in thyroid cancer, 1108
    in thyroiditis, 1107t
Ion(s), 233
  absorption of, 637
Ion channels, 208–209, *209*
  in pain transmission, 467, 468, 469
Ipecac syrup, for poisoning, 2281
Ipratropium (Atrovent), for asthma, 1690, 1691t, *1692, 1694*
Iridectomy, 1813
Iridium implants, for breast cancer, 1031, *1032*
Iris, 1778, 1791
  age-related changes in, 1782
Iron, deficiency of, 641t–642t, 2112–2113
  essential, 2078
  food sources of, 641t
  in hemoglobin production, 2078
  reference values for, 2304t
  replacement of, for anemia, 2104–2105, 2114
  total body, 2078
Iron overload, 1258
Iron poisoning, antidote for, 2281t
Iron-binding capacity, reference values for, 2304t
Irregular bones, 530
Irrigation, antral, 1676–1677
  bladder, closed, 956, 957, *957*
  for urinary calculi, 826
  of colostomy, 785–786, 786b
  of eye, 2278
  of feeding tube, 675, 676
  of nasogastric tube, 708
  of urinary reservoir, 820
  wound, 326, 328
Irritable bowel syndrome, 793–794
Irritant dermatitis, 1286, 1291
Irritation, vs. allergy, 1267
Ischemia, clinical manifestations of, 1368, 1369t
  definition of, 1368
  gastric, in mechanical ventilation, 1756
  in burns, 1343, 1344–1345
  intermittent claudication and, 1368, 1369t
  myocardial, 1580–1581
    damage from, 1585–1587, *1586, 1587.* See also *Myocardial infarction (MI).*
    pain in. See *Angina pectoris.*
  renal, 869–870
    in shock, 2240
  rest pain in, 1368
Ischemic stroke, 1953–1954, 1954, *1954,* 1955. See also *Stroke.*
Islets of Langerhans, 1062–1063, 1066
Isoflurane (Forane), 294t
Isolated systolic hypertension, 1380, 1380t
Isolation procedures, 343

Isoniazid, for tuberculosis, 1720, 1721t
  overdose of, antidote for, 2281t
Isosorbide (Ismotic), in intraocular pressure reduction, 1811–1812
Isosporiasis, in HIV infection, 2205
Isotretinoin (Accutane), for acne, 1294
Itching. See *Pruritus.*
Itch-scratch-itch cycle, 1284–1285, 1286

J

Jaundice, 1220–1223, 1221t–1222t
  in hepatitis, 1227
Jaw, wiring of, 1327–1328
Jaw reflex, 1891
Jaw thrust, *2267,* 2267–2268
Jefferson fracture, 2047, *2049*
Jejunostomy feeding, 673, *673,* 683. See also *Enteral nutrition.*
Jejunum, structure of, 630
Jet lag, 437
Joint(s), 532–533
  aspiration of, 548
  cartilaginous, 533
  examination of, 542, *542, 543,* 544t–545t, *546*
  fibrous, 532–533
  protection of, in rheumatoid arthritis, 2147, 2149t
  range of motion of, assessment of, 542, *542, 543,* 544t–545t
  stiffness of, assessment of, 538
  suture, 532
  syndesmosis, 533
  synovial, 532, *533*
Joint contractures. See *Contractures.*
Joint fusion, for osteoarthritis, 555
Jones criteria, for rheumatic fever, 1483b
Judgment, assessment of, 143, 1882
Jugular vein, examination of, 168t–169t, 1457, *1458, 1462*
Jumper's knee, 620
Junctional rhythms, 1557, *1557*
Juvenile-onset diabetes. See *Diabetes mellitus, type 1.*

K

Kallmann's syndrome, 1143, 1145
Kanamycin, for tuberculosis, 1720, 1721t
Kaposi's sarcoma, in HIV infection, 1309–1310, *1310,* 2205–2206
Karnofsky scale, 374t
Kayexalate (sodium polystyrene sulfonate), for hyperkalemia, 247–248
  in addisonian crisis, 1121
Kayser-Fleischer rings, 1259
Kegel exercises, 836, 838, 958, 1000
Keloids, 333, *334*
Kemadrin (procyclidine), for Parkinson's disease, 2019t
Kenalog (triamcinolone), 1280t
Keratectomy, photorefractive, 1828
Keratin, 1262
Keratinocytes, 1262
Keratitis, *1823,* 1823–1824
Keratoconjunctivitis sicca, 1826, 1829
Keratoplasty, *1822,* 1822–1823
Kernig's sign, 1945, *1945*
Ketamine (Ketalar), 294t
  for rapid-sequence induction, 2268
Ketoacidosis, diabetic, 1172–1177, *1173,* 1174b–1176b, 1174t
Ketones, formation of, in diabetes mellitus, 1155

Ketonuria, 757, 757t
  in diabetes mellitus, 1156t, 1158, 1168
Ketoprofen, 486, 487t
Ketorolac, 486, 487t
Ketosis, 214
  in diabetic ketoacidosis, 1173
Ketosteroids, 1079
  adrenocortical function and, 1122t
17-Ketosteroids, urine, reference values for, 2306t
Kidney. See also under *Renal*.
  aplastic, 871
  benign tumors of, 858
  biopsy of, *761*, 761–762
  blood flow in, *733*, 734
  congenital anomalies of, 751
  contusion of, *867*, 867–869
  ectopic, 870–871
  endocrine functions of, 737
  examination of, 167t–168t, 169t
  fractured, *867*, 867–869
  function of, 735–738
    age-related changes in, 737–738
  horseshoe, 871, *871*
  imaging of, 758–760
  in acid-base regulation, 260–261, 263, *263*, 736
  in blood pressure regulation, 1383, *1383*, 2235
  in cardiac regulation, 1444
  in electrolyte balance, 235–236
  in fluid balance, 217, *218*, 735–736, 736t
  in heart failure, 1531
  in shock, 852, 2241, 2243, 2254
  in sodium balance, 235–236
  laceration of, *867*, 867–869
  medullary sponge, 872
  metabolic functions of, 737
  pain in, 750
  palpation of, 755, *755*
  percussion of, 754, *755*
  polycystic, *871*, 871–872
  structure of, *732*, 732–733, *733*
  supernumerary, 870
  vascular injury of, *867*, 867–869
Kidney stones, 821–828. See also *Renal calculi; Urinary calculi*.
Kidney-ureter-bladder (KUB) film, 195, 758
Kinins, in inflammation, 319
Klinefelter's syndrome, 1143
Knee, examination of, *543*, 545t, *546*
  jumper's, 620
  ligaments of, 534, *535*
    examination of, 545t, *546*
    injuries of, 623, *623*
  meniscal injuries in, 623, *623*
  motion of, *564*
  total replacement of, *564*, 564–565, *565*
Knee-jerk reflex, 1863, *1863*, 1889, 1891t, *1892*, 1893b
Knock-knee, 540, *541*
Kobasa's hardiness model, 7t
Kock pouch, 775, *775*
  postoperative care in, 779
KUB film, 195
Kupffer cells, 1060, 2078
Kussmaul's respiration, *184*
Kwashiorkor, 640t, 661. See also *Malnutrition*.
Kwell (lindane), 1280t
Kyphoscoliosis, 540, *541*, 577, 577–578, 1629, *1630*
  restrictive lung disease in, 1740, *1741*
Kyphosis, 540, *541*, 578
  in osteoporosis, 568, *568*

L

Labels, food, 30, *32*
Labetalol (Normodyne), for hypertension, 1389t, 1396t
Labia majora and minora, *905*, 906t
  examination of, 923
Labile diabetes. See *Diabetes mellitus, type 1*.
Labile hypertension, 1383
Laboratory studies, preoperative, 277t–278t
  reference ranges for, 2301–2310
Labyrinth, *1784*, 1784–1785
Labyrinthectomy, 1851
Labyrinthitis, 1832, 1848
Lacerations, emergency care for, 2280–2281
  facial, 1326
  renal, *867*, 867–869
Lachman's test, 545t, *546*
Lacrimal apparatus, 1778, 1790
Lacrimal gland, 1778, *1779*
  disorders of, 1826, 1827t
Lactate, reference values for, 2304t
Lactate dehydrogenase (LDH), 549t, 1082t, 1464
  in myocardial infarction, 1588–1589, *1589*
  reference values for, 2304t
Lactated Ringer's solution, 221t
Lactic acidosis, in shock, 2236, *2238*
Lactose intolerance, 648
Lactulose, for hepatic encephalopathy, 1252
  and diarrhea, 1253
Lacuna, in bone, 531, *534*
Lacunar stroke, 1954
Laënnec's cirrhosis, 1233t. See also *Cirrhosis*.
Lagophthalmos, 1827t
Lamellae, in bone, 531, *534*
Lamellar keratoplasty, 1822
Laminectomy, decompressive, 1987, *1987*, 1989–1991
Laminectomy position, *300*
Laminotomy, 1987
Lamivudine (Epivir, 3TC), 2196t
Lamivudine-zidovudine (Combivir), 2196t
Lamotrigine, for epilepsy, 1927–1928
Langerhans cells, 1264
Language, assessment of, 1875t–1876t, 1882–1883
  impaired, in Alzheimer's disease, 2004, 2006
  in stroke, 1956–1958, 1957t, 1975–1976
Language barriers, 147
Lansoprazole (Prevacid), for gastroesophageal reflux disease, 696
Laparoscopic cholecystectomy, 1208, *1208*
Laparoscopic nephrectomy, 860–861
Laparoscopy, in female reproductive assessment, 929–930, *930*
Large intestine. See *Colon*.
Laryngectomy, 1664–1672
  partial, 1664–1665, *1665*
    nursing management in, 1666–1669
  rescue breathing in, 1656
  supraglottic, 1665
  total, 1664–1666
    communication after, 1669, *1670*
    nursing management in, 1669–1672
Laryngitis, 1680
Laryngopharynx, 1612, *1613*
Laryngoscopy, 1661, *1664*
Laryngospasm, 1681
  after extubation, 304
  hypoparathyroidism and, 1115
Larynx, anatomy of, 1613, *1613*
  artificial, 1669, *1670*
  benign tumors of, 1660
  cancer of, 1661–1672
    chemotherapy for, 1663–1664

Larynx (*Continued*)
  clinical manifestations of, 1661, 1662b, 1663b, 1671
  diagnosis of, 1661–1663
  epidemiology of, 1661
  etiology of, 1661
  metastasis in, *1663*
  pathophysiology of, 1661
  radiation therapy for, 1663
  recurrence of, 1671
  risk factors for, 1661
  staging of, 1663
  surgery for, 1664–1672. See also *Laryngectomy*.
  edema of, 1681
  examination of, endoscopic, 1661, *1664*
  injuries of, 1682
  paralysis of, 1681–1682
Lasègue's sign, 544t
Laser lithotripsy, for urinary calculi, 826
Laser resurfacing, facial, 1318–1319
Laser therapy, for actinic keratosis, 1305, *1305*
  for benign prostatic hyperplasia, 955–956
  for cervical cancer, 997–998
  for coronary heart disease, 1523
  for diabetic retinopathy, 1187
  for glaucoma, 1813
  for laryngeal cancer, 1664
  for lung cancer, 1730
  for refractive errors, 1828
  for skin lesions, 1326
  of hemorrhoids, 796
LASIK procedure, 1828
Lasix. See *Furosemide (Lasix)*.
Latent infection, 338
Lateral corticospinal tract, 1861, 1862t
Lateral epicondylitis, 1999t
Lateral position, 299, *300*
Lateral tentorial herniation, 2029, *2029*
Latex allergy, 302, 2137, 2138
Lavage, endometrial, *931*
  gastric, 706–708. See also *Gastrointestinal intubation*.
    for poisoning, 2281
  peritoneal, diagnostic, 2273, *2273*
Lazarus' stress response theory, 5t
LDH. See *Lactate dehydrogenase (LDH)*.
Le Fort fractures, 1326–1327, *1327*
Lead, reference values for, 2309t
Left bundle branch, 1439, *1440*
Left bundle branch block, 1564
Left heart filling pressure, after cardiac surgery, 1507
Left ventricular failure, 1531–1534, *1533*
Leg bag, 831–832, *832*
Leg cramps, nocturnal, 437
Leg ulcers, arterial, 1416
  venous. See *Venous ulcers*.
Legal issues, advance directives, 6, 2009
  competence, 66–67
  durable power of attorney for health care, 67, 2009
  elderly and, 65, 66t, 67
  hospital regulation, 102–104
  in ambulatory care nursing, 91–92
  in emergency care, 2261–2264
  informed consent, 66–67, 287, *288*
  living wills, 67, 2009
Legionnaire's disease, 1711–1716, 1712t
Leiomyomas, 362, *991*, 991–994, *1000*
Lens, 1780
  age-related changes in, 1782, 1814–1817, *1815*, 1817b
Lente insulin, 1162t. See also *Insulin therapy*.
Lentigo maligna melanoma, 1307–1309, 1308t
LES. See *Lower esophageal sphincter (LES)*.
Letrozole (Femura), in breast cancer, 1036

Leucine aminopeptidase, 1082t
Leukapheresis, 2169, *2170*
Leukemia, 2166–2173
  acute lymphoblastic, 2166, *2167*
  acute nonlymphocytic, 2166, *2167*
  bone marrow transplant for, 2173
  chemotherapy for, 2169
  chronic lymphocytic, 2166–2167, *2167*
  chronic myelogenous, 2166–2167, *2167*
  classification of, 2166, 2167t
  clinical manifestations of, 2167–2168, *2168*
  diagnostic findings in, 2168
  epidemiology of, 2166
  etiology of, 2166
  medical management of, 2168–2169
  nursing management of, 2169–2173
  outcomes classification for, 2165
  pathophysiology of, 2166–2167, *2167*
  radiation therapy for, 2169
  risk factors for, 2166
Leukocyte esterase, 757, 757t
Leukocytes. See *White blood cells.*
Leukocytosis, in inflammation, 322
Leukopenia, in agranulocytosis, 2119
  in cancer, 383–384
Leukoplakia, 686, *686, 687*
Leukorrhea, 1002
Leukotriene inhibitors, for asthma, 1689, 1690,
  1691t, *1692, 1694*
Leukotrienes, 319
  in pain, 468
Leuprolide (Lupron), for endometriosis, 990
LeVeen shunt, for ascites, 1247, *1250*
Level of consciousness, assessment of, 1875t,
  1880–1881
    in coma, 1910
    in increased intracranial pressure, 2031
    in mental status assessment, 139
    postoperative, 1393
Levin tube, 706t, 707
Levodopa, for Parkinson's disease, 2018
  growth hormone levels and, 1080
Levorphanol (Levo-Dromoran), 489t
Levothyroxine sodium, for hypothyroidism,
  1093, 1096t
    self-care and, 1098, 1098b
    for myxedema, 1093
    side effects of, 1098b
Leydig's cells, 912
LH. See *Luteinizing hormone (LH).*
Libido, reduced. See also *Sexual function.*
  after hysterectomy, 993
Lice, body, 1311t
  head, 1272
  lindane for, 1280t
  pubic, 1056
Licensure, for ambulatory care nursing, 92
  multi-state, 92
Lichen sclerosus, vulvar cancer and, 1005,
  1006
Lichenification, *1272*
Lidocaine (Xylocaine), 297t, 484
  for dysrhythmias, 1562t, 2277
  reference values for, 2308t
Lifestyle, assessment of, 144–145
  screening and prevention and, 152t–153t
Lifts, 1458
Ligaments, 534
  of knee, *535*
    examination of, 545t, *546*
    injuries of, 623, *623*
    sprains of, 621–622
Ligation, of hemorrhoids, 796
Light, adaptation to, aging and, 1782
  transmission of, vision and, 1780–1781
Light therapy, for seasonal affective disorder,
  437

Limb girdle muscular dystrophy, 583t, 584
Limbic system, 1858
Lindane (Kwell), 1280t
Linear fracture, 593t
Lingual tonsils, 1612, *1613*
Lip, herpes simplex of, 684, *685*
Lipase, reference values for, 2304t
  serum, 1081t
    in acute pancreatitis, 1195
Lipectomy, 1319–1320, *1320*
Lipids, 14
  digestion and absorption of, 636
  fecal, tests for, 745–746
  in parenteral nutrition, 668
    allergy to, 670
  reference values for, 2304t
  serum, in cardiac assessment, 1465
Lipoid nephrosis, 864, 864t
Lipomas, 362
Lipoproteins, 14–15
  high-density, 15, 1517
    target levels for, 15
  low-density, 15, 1517
    target levels for, 15
  very low-density, 15, 1517
    target levels for, 15
Liposuction, 1319–1320, *1320*
Liquid nitrogen. See *Cryotherapy.*
Lithium, reference values for, 2308t
Lithotomy position, 299, *300*
Lithotripsy, 826–828, *827*
  extracorporeal shock wave, 826–827, *827*
    for choledocholithiasis, 1214
    for cholelithiasis, 1205–1206, *1207*
Lithotrite, for urinary calculi, 826
Liver. See also under *Hepatic.*
  abscess of, 1257–1258
  anatomy of, 1060, *1061*
  examination of, 169t
    in metabolic disorders, 1076t, 1077–1078
  fatty, 1253–1254
  in amyloidosis, 1258
  in hematopoiesis, 2078–2079
  in shock, 2240–2241
  iron deposition in, hemochromatosis and,
    1258
  metastasis to, 1255
  size of, 1077
  transplantation of, 1256–1257
    sclerosing cholangitis and, 1215
  traumatic injuries of, 1259
  tumors of, *1254*, 1254–1256, *1255*
Liver biopsy, 1084–1085, *1085*, 1255
Liver enzymes, 1082t
Liver flap, hepatitis and, 1227
Liver function, 1064–1065
  age-related changes in, 1068–1069
  assessment of, 1080–1085, 1081t–1083t
    after liver transplantation, 1257
    biopsy in, 1084–1085, *1085*
    peritoneoscopy in, 1083–1084
    portal pressure measurements in, 1084
  in heart failure, 1534–1535
  maximization of, in cirrhosis, 1235
  preoperative assessment of, 280
Liver tap, 1078
Liver transplant, 2226
Living wills, 67, 2009
Lobectomy, 1730, *1731.* See also *Thoracic
  surgery.*
Lobular carcinoma in situ, 1015–1016, 1019
Local adaptation syndrome, 5t
Local anesthesia, 296–298, 297t, 483, 484,
  492. See also *Anesthesia.*
Logrolling, 2053
Long bones, 530, *534*
Long leg cast, *603*

Longitudinal fracture, 594t
Long-term care, for elderly, 62–63, 64–65
  in Alzheimer's disease, 2009
Long-term care facilities, 118–126
  alternatives to, 125
  environment in, 121–123
  historical perspective on, 118–119, 119t
  information resources for, 125b
  levels of care in, 125
  Minimum Data Set for, 121, *122*
  nurse managers in, 123–125
  nurse-physician collaboration in, 123
  nursing care in, 121–125
  reimbursement issues and, 119
  residents of, adjustment of, 121–123, 124b
    assessment for, 121
    care planning for, 121, 121b
    caregiving for, 121
    communication with, 123
    holistic care for, 123, 124b
    independence of, 123
    nursing needs of, 119–121
    rights of, 119, 120b
  staff of, 121
  standards of care for, 119, 120b
  telephone medicine in, 123
Loop electrocautery excision procedure
  (LEEP), 996, 997–998
Loop of Henle, *733, 735*
Lopressor (metoprolol), for dysrhythmias,
  1563t
  for hypertension, 1389t
Lorazepam, for status epilepticus, 1931
Lordosis, 540, *541*, 578, 1984
Losses, of elderly, 55–56
Lotions, 1281t
Lou Gehrig's disease, 2023–2024
Low-density lipoproteins (LDLs), 15, 1517
  target levels for, 15
Lower airway, structures of, 1613–1617,
  1614–1616
Lower back pain, client teaching for, 1991,
  1991b
  clinical manifestations of, 1984–1985
  diagnostic findings in, 1985
  etiology of, 1983–1984
  medical management of, 1985–1986
    nursing management in, 1986–1987
  pathophysiology of, 1984
  self-care in, 1991, 1991b
  surgery for, 1987–1988
    nursing management in, 1988–1991
Lower esophageal sphincter (LES), dilation of,
  692, *693*
  in achalasia, 691
  in gastroesophageal reflux disease, 691
  in hiatal hernia, 697–698
  regurgitation and, 691
Lower extremity, examination of, 170t
Lower gastrointestinal series, 195
Lower motor neuron, 1860
Lower motor neuron lesions, 1997
  in amyotrophic lateral sclerosis, 2023
  neurogenic bladder and, 840, 842
Low-fat diet, 32–33, 1393b, 1517, 1521
  in atherosclerosis, 1521
  in hypertension, 1387, 1393b
Low-molecular-weight heparin, 1425
Low-potassium diet, 245b, 248
Low-protein diet, in chronic renal failure, 886,
  894, *894*
Low-sodium diet, 238b
  in edema, 227, 228
  in heart failure, 1536, 1538t, 1541
  in hypernatremia, 241
  in hypertension, 1387, 1393
  in renal disease, 241

LSD, 510t, 517–518, 520t–521t
Lubricants, gastrointestinal, 634–635, 635t
skin, 1283
Lugol's solution, for hyperthyroidism, 1101
Lumbar disc herniation, 1984–1985, *1985*
surgery for, *1987*, 1987–1991
Lumbar nerve root compression, assessment of, *1986*
Lumbar puncture, 1896–1899, *1897*
headache after, 1898, 1950
in coma, 1909
Lumbar spine, examination of, *543*, 544t
Lumbosacral plexus, 1869
Lumpectomy, 1020
Lung, abscess of, 1716
age-related changes in, 1627
anatomy of, 1614–1616, *1614–1616*
auscultation of, 1632–1633, *1633*, 1634t
benign tumors of, 1739
blood supply of, 1615
burns of, 1335, 1338
compliance of, 1617
defense mechanisms in, 1622
examination of, 167t, 168t
floppy, 1617
in acid-base balance, 260, *260*, 263, *263*, 1621
in cystic fibrosis, 1203
repair process in, 1621
stiff, 1617
structure of, *1628*
surface tension of, 1617
uremic, 886
Lung biopsy, 1649
Lung cancer, 1726–1739
chemotherapy for, 1730
clinical manifestations of, 1727
diagnosis of, 1727–1728
etiology of, 1726
metastasis of, 1729
nursing management of, 1730
pathophysiology of, 1726, 1727t
prevention of, 369
radiation therapy for, 1729–1730
risk factors for, 369, 1726
staging of, 1728, 1728b, 1729b
surgery for, 1730–1739. See also *Thoracic surgery.*
types of, 1726, 1727t
warning signs of, 1727b
Lung diffusion capacity, assessment of, 1637
Lung disorders. See also *Respiratory disorders.*
occupational, 1739–1740, 1740t
restrictive, 1740–1741, 1741b
surgery for, 1730–1739. See also *Thoracic surgery.*
Lung scan, ventilation-perfusion, 1642–1643
for pulmonary embolism, 1707
Lung sounds. See *Breath sounds.*
in cardiac assessment, 1462
Lung surgery. See also *Thoracic surgery.*
types of, 1730–1732, *1732*
Lung transplantation, 1741–1742, 2226–2227
Lung volume reduction surgery, for emphysema, 1700
Lung volumes and capacities, 1615, *1615*
measurement of, 1637, 1638t, *1640*, 1640t
Lupron (leuprolide), for endometriosis, 990
Lupus erythematosus, systemic. See *Systemic lupus erythematosus (SLE)*
Lupus-like syndrome, drug-induced, 2157, 2157b
Luteinizing hormone (LH), 1067, 1138t
deficiency of, 1143
excess of, 1142
in female, 908, *909*
in male, 913
reference values for, 2304t

Luteinizing hormone–releasing hormone (LNRH), pharmaceutical, for prostate cancer, 961–962
Lyme disease, 337t, 1829–1830, 2163
Lymph, 1364
Lymph nodes, axillary, palpation of, 921, *921*
removal of, in breast cancer, 1020–1021
biopsy of, in breast cancer, 1021
cervical, removal of. See *Radical neck dissection.*
palpation of, 921, *921*, 2094, 2095t
structure and function of, 2072, *2073*
superficial, 2072
Lymph nodules, 2072–2073, *2073*
Lymphangiography, 2100–2101
Lymphatic disorders, 1429–1431
home care in, 1428b
Lymphatic drainage, of gastrointestinal system, 631
Lymphatic fluid, movement of, 216
Lymphatics, 1364, *1365*
Lymphedema, 1429–1431, *1430*, *1431*
postmastectomy, 1025, 1429–1430, *1430*
Lymphocyte(s), 2081
B, 2081
activation of, 2083, *2083*
Cushing's syndrome and, 1130
in white cell count and differential, 322t
in wound healing, 319
T. See *T cells.*
Lymphocyte immunophenotyping, 2100, 2100t
Lymphocytic thyroiditis, 1106–1107, 1107t
Lymphogranuloma venereum, 1053
Lymphography, 198
Lymphokines, in wound healing, 319
Lymphoma, cutaneous, 1309
Hodgkin's, 2173–2176
non-Hodgkin's, 2176–2179
in HIV infection, 2206
Rappaport staging of, 2177t
outcomes classification for, 2165
radiation therapy for, breast cancer after, 1013
Lysergic acid diethylamide (LSD), 510t, 517–518, 520t–521t
Lysophosphatidic acid, in ovarian cancer, 1002
Lysosomal enzymes, in shock, 2238–2239
Lysosomes, *206*, 207t

M

M phase, of cell cycle, 357, *358*
Maceration, 332
Macrophages, in inflammation, 318, *318*
Macrovascular disease. See also specific type.
in diabetes mellitus, 1182–1185, 1183t, *1185*, 1186b, 1187b
Macular degeneration, age-related, 1821, *1821*
Macule, *1271*
Mafenide, for burns, 1348t
Magissa, 75b
Magnesium, dietary sources of, 256b
functions of, 255
imbalances of, 255–257. See also *Hypermagnesemia; Hypomagnesemia.*
in cardiac assessment, 1465
plasma levels of, 235b, 255
replacement, for hypomagnesemia, 256
indications for, 256
serum, reference values for, 2304t
urine, reference values for, 2306t
Magnesium salicylate, 486, 487t
Magnet hospitals, 96
Magnetic resonance angiography, 1376

Magnetic resonance imaging (MRI), 196–197, *197*
cardiac, 1472
in musculoskeletal assessment, 546, *548*
in myocardial infarction, 1590
in neurologic assessment, *1895*, 1895–1896
in reproductive assessment, in females, 928
in respiratory assessment, 1645
in vascular assessment, 1376
of adrenal glands, 1122t
of ear, 1804
of eye, 1796, *1796*
of spine, 1985, *1985*
of thyroid gland, 1095t
of urinary tract, 759
procedure for, 196–197
Magnets, for pain, 500
Major histocompatibility complex (MHC), 2073–2074, 2082–2083
Mal ojo, 19b
Malabsorption, 636
lipid, 636
Malar fractures, 1327
Malaria, 337t
Malignant fibrosarcoma, 363
Malignant hypertension, 1380, 1380t, 1395–1397
Malignant hyperthermia, 301–302
Malignant melanoma, 1307, *1307*, *1308*, 1308t. See also *Skin cancer.*
ocular, 1825–1826
Malignant tumors, 349, 363, 363t. See also *Cancer; Tumor(s).*
Malleus, 1783, *1783*. See also *Ossicles.*
Malnutrition, 661–677
clinical manifestations of, 641t–642t, 662, 663t
cognitive impairment and, 666
dysphagia and, 667
energy needs in, determination of, 663, 663t
etiology of, 662
fatigue and, 666–667
in chronic pancreatitis, 1200
in elderly, 49–51, 51b, 661
in heart failure, 1534–1535
in inflammatory bowel disease, 772, 774
inadequate intake and, 639–640
ketosis in, 214
medical management of, 662–663. See also *Nutritional support.*
neuromuscular impairment and, 666
nursing management in, 663–677
nutrient goals in, 662–663, 663t
obesity and, 640. See also *Obesity.*
outcomes classification for, 661
pathophysiology of, 662, 663t
postgastrectomy, 721
pressure ulcers and, 1295–1297, 1298
primary, 639, 661
protein-energy, 639, 640t, 661–662
risk factors for, 662
secondary, 639, 661
self-care deficit and, 664–667
sensory-perceptual deficits and, 666
surgery and, 281, 284
Mammography, 369, 369t, *932*, 932–933, *933*, 1012, 1014, *1015*
Mammoplasty, augmentation, 1037–1038, *1038*
reduction, 1038, *1038*
Managed care, 78b, 80–81, 85b
for elderly, 63–64
HMOs in, 78b
PPOs in, 78b
Mandibular fractures, 1326–1328, *1327*
Mandibular nerve, 1870t
Manganese, deficiency of, 642t
food sources of, 642t

Mania, 420, 422b, 426–428. See also *Bipolar disorder.*
Mannitol, in intraocular pressure reduction, 1812
Manometry, esophageal, 659
 splenic pulp, 1084
Mantoux test, *1719,* 1719–1720
MAP. See *Mean arterial pressure (MAP).*
Marasmus, 640t, 661. See also *Malnutrition.*
Marcaine (bupivacaine), 297t, 484
Marginating, 318, *318*
Marie-Strumpell disease, 2160–2161, *2161*
Marijuana, 510t, 514t, 517, 520t–521t
Mason's stress response theory, 5t
Massage, for pain, 497–498
Mast cells, in inflammation, 319
MAST garment, for shock, 2245, *2246*
Mastalgia, 1037
Mastectomy, axillary dissection with, 1020–1021
 breast prosthesis after, 1028–1029
 breast reconstruction after, *1029,* 1029–1031, *1030*
 care map for, *1022–1023*
 case study of, 1026–1027
 chemotherapy after, 1031–1032
 clinical pathway for, 1021b
 complications of, 1020
 contraindications to, 1020
 exercises for, 1027b, 1028
 lymphedema after, 1025, 1429–1430, *1430*
 modified radical, 1020
 nursing management in, 1021–1029
 partial, 1020
 postoperative care in, 1024–1029
 preoperative care in, 1021–1024
 prophylactic, 1014
 radiation therapy after, 1031, *1032*
 Reach for Recovery program for, 1028
 recurrence after, 1035–1036
 self-care in, 1024
 simple, 1020
 total, 1020
Mastication, 634
Mastodynia, 1037
Mastoid bone, 1784, 1785
Mastoidectomy, 1847
Mastoiditis, 1843
Mastopexy, 1039
Mattresses, for pressure ulcer prevention, *1300,* 1301
Maturity-onset diabetes of the young (MODY), 1151
Maxillary fractures, 1326–1328, *1327*
Maxillary nerve, 1870t
Maximal expiratory pressure, measurement of, 1637, 1638t
Maximal inspiratory pressure, measurement of, 1637, 1638t
Maximal voluntary ventilation, measurement of, 1637, 1638t
McBurney's point, 655, 768
McGill-Melzack Pain Questionnaire, 477, *479*
MCH. See *Mean corpuscular hemoglobin (MHC).*
MCHC. See *Mean corpuscular hemoglobin concentration (MCHC).*
McMurray's test, 545t
M-CSF, in hematopoiesis, 2075
MCV. See *Mean corpuscular volume (MCV).*
Mean arterial pressure (MAP), 2027
 maintenance of, 2235
Mean corpuscular hemoglobin (MCH), 2095, 2097t
 reference values for, 2302t
Mean corpuscular hemoglobin concentration (MCHC), 2095, 2097t
 reference values for, 2302t

Mean corpuscular volume (MCV), 2095, 2097t
 reference values for, 2302t
Measles, immunization for, 342, 342t
Meatus, urethral, 735
Mechanical debridement, 328–329, *329,* 1296, 1347
Mechanical ventilation, 1750–1761
 capnography in, 1639–1641
 care plan for, 1757b–1760b
 complications of, 1755–1756
 continuous positive airway pressure in, 1754–1755
 endotracheal intubation in, cuff deflation in, 1752
  cuff inflation in, 1750–1751
  cuff leaks in, 1752
  extubation in, 1761
  tube insertion in, 1750, *1751*
  tube securing in, 1750, *1751*
 in cardiac surgery, 1507
 in home care, 1762b
 in shock, 2244
 modes of, 1754, 1755t
 nursing management in, 1756–1761
 physiologic changes in, 1755–1756
 positive end-expiratory pressure in, 1754–1755
 tracheostomy for, 1651–1660. See also *Tracheostomy.*
 triggering mechanisms in, 1754
 ventilators for, *1752,* 1752–1754
  control panels of, *1752,* 1753b–1754b
 weaning in, 1655–1656, 1759–1761, 1761b
Meckel's diverticulum, 790
Meclofenamate, 486, 487t
Medial collateral ligament, injuries of, *623*
Medial epicondylitis, 621, 1999t
 test for, 544t
Median nerve, examination of, *547*
Mediastinal flutter, in open pneumothorax, 1767
Mediastinal shift, in open pneumothorax, 1767
 in tension pneumothorax, 1767–1768
Mediastinal tubes, 1508
Mediastinum, 1615
Medical model, for health care, 84
Medicare/Medicaid, 73, 78b, 79, 80, 81
 for home care, 107, 108, 109, 109b
Medication history, in preoperative assessment, 275, 275t, 282
Medications. See *Drug(s).*
Medicine, history of, 3–9, 4t–7t
Meditation, 27, 36
 for pain, 499
Medrol. See *Methylprednisolone (Solu-Medrol).*
Medulla oblongata, 1858–1859, 1859t, *1860*
Medullary carcinoma, thyroid, 1108, 1108t
Medullary polycystic disease, 872
Medullary sponge kidney, 872
Mefenamic acid, 486, 487t
Megakaryocytes, 2078
Megaloblastic anemia, 2113
Megaureter, 846
Meglitinides, for diabetes mellitus, 1159, 1161t
Meibomian glands, 1778, *1779*
Meiosis, 210
Melanin, 1262
Melanoma, *1307,* 1307–1309, *1308,* 1308t. See also *Skin cancer.*
 ocular, 1825–1826
Melanosomes, 1262
Meloxicam (Vioxx), 486t
Membrane, cell, *206,* 207t, 208–209, *209*
Membrane channels, 208–209, *209*
Membrane depolarization, 467
Membrane potential, 1867, *1867*

Membrane proteins, 208
Membrane transport, 208, 208t
Membranoproliferative glomerulonephritis, 864t
Membranous glomerulonephritis, 864t
Membranous labyrinth, 1785
Memory, assessment of, 143, 1881
Memory loss, in Alzheimer's disease, 2003–2004, 2006
 in confusional states, 1919
Menarche, 908
Menghini's technique, in liver biopsy, 1084
Ménière's disease, balance disorders in, 1848
 hearing loss in, 1833
Meninges, 1861–1862
Meningiomas, 1932–1933. See also *Brain tumors.*
Meningitis, bacterial, 1944–1945, *1945*
 fungal, 1947
 pathogenesis of, 337t
 viral, 1946–1947
Meniscus, injuries of, 623, *623*
Menopause, 910, 984–986
 atrophic vaginitis and, 985, 1003
 coronary heart disease after, 1518
 osteoporosis and, 566–567
  hyperthyroidism and, case study of, 1102
 sleep problems in, 438
 surgical, 984
Menorrhagia, 983–984
Menstrual cycle, 908–910, *909*
 menstruation in, 908, *909,* 910. See also *Menstruation.*
 ovulation in, 908–909, *909*
 premenstrual (ischemic) phase of, *909,* 910
 proliferative phase of, 908, *909*
 secretory (luteal) phase of, 909, *909*
Menstrual disorders, 979–986
 complementary therapies for, 916
 cultural aspects of, 979–980
 psychosocial aspects of, 980
Menstrual history, 917
Menstruation, 910
 absence of, 982–983, *983*
 cessation of. See *Menopause.*
 cultural attitudes toward, 979–986
 excessive bleeding in, 983–984
 onset of, 908
 painful, 980–981
  in endometriosis, 989
 tampon use in, toxic shock syndrome and, 1003
Mental health assessment, components of, 513t
 in substance abuse, 138–144, 140t–143t, 409–411, 410t, 512, 513t
 tools for, 417b
Mental health problems, 405–428. See also *Psychosocial concerns.*
 anxiety disorders, 412–416, 414b
 assessment of, 138–144, 140t–143t, 409–411, 410t
 client/family teaching in, 411, 414b
 communication in, 410–411, 419, 426, 428
 cultural aspects of, 424b
 drug-related, 409–410, 411t
 in elderly, 57–60
 in hypercortisolism, 1127
 mood disorders, 420–426, 421b. See also *Bipolar disorder; Depression.*
 outcomes classification for, 405
 referral for, 411
 resources for, 414b
 risk factors for, 409
 sexuality and, 418b
 sleep problems in, 438
 spirituality and, 425b
 terminology for, 410b

Mental status assessment, 139–144, 1875t, 1880–1883
Mental status changes, in brain tumors, 1933–1934
in confusional states, 1918–1922
Meperidine (Demerol), 490
dosage of, 489t
preoperative, 290t
Mercury, reference values for, 2309t
Mesalamine, for inflammatory bowel disease, 773
Mescaline, 510t, 517–518
Mesenteric infarction, 791
Metabolic acidosis, 267–268. See also *Acid-base balance.*
assessment in, arterial blood gas analysis in, 264, 264b, 269–271, 270t
clinical manifestations of, 270t
in chronic renal failure, 883
treatment of, 894
in diabetic ketoacidosis, 1174t. See also *Diabetic ketoacidosis.*
nursing management of, 271
risk factors for, 268–269
Metabolic alkalosis, 266–267, 270t. See also *Acid-base balance.*
Metabolic bone disorders, 565–576
Metabolic disorders. See also specific disorders.
assessment of, 1070–1087
diagnostic tests in, 1078–1080
history in, 1070–1073
laboratory studies in, 1080, 1081t–1083t
physical examination in, *1073,* 1073–1078
of abdomen, *1073,* 1075–1078, 1076t
of neck, 1074, *1075,* 1075b
symptom analysis in, 1070–1071
coma in, *1906,* 1906–1907
Metabolic equivalent test (MET), 1597
Metabolic substrates, 1067–1068, *1068*
Metabolic system(s). See also *Endocrine system.*
age-related changes in, 50t
anatomy and physiology of, 1060–1069, *1061–1064, 1068*
epinephrine effects on, 1135t
norepinephrine effects on, 1135t
Metabolism, aerobic, 2236
anaerobic, 2236
Metamorphopsia, 1821
Metaplasia, 211
definition of, 350t
Metarterioles, 1363
Metastasis, 359–360, *360.* See also specific cancers.
in breast cancer, 1035–1036
in laryngeal cancer, *1663*
in lung cancer, 1729
surgery for, 375
to bone, 581–582
in breast cancer, 1035–1036
to brain, 1933
to liver, 1255
Metered-dose inhaler, 1691, *1693,* 1693b
Metformin (Glucophage), for diabetes mellitus, 1160t
Methadone (Dolophine), 488–490, 489t
Methanol poisoning, antidote for, 2281t
Methemoglobin, reference values for, 2302t
Methicillin-resistant *S. aureus,* 339, 341b
Methimazole (Tapazole), for hyperthyroidism, 1101
Methotrexate, for breast cancer, 1032, 1033, 1034
for psoriasis, 1292, 1293

Methylcellulose eye drops, for exophthalmos, 1100
Methyldopa (Aldomet), for hypertension, 1389t
perioperative use of, 275t
Methylprednisolone (Solu-Medrol), for Addison's disease, 1124t
for asthma, 1690, 1691t, *1692, 1694*
for spinal cord injury, 2053, 2279
for transplant immunosuppression, 2224t
Methylxanthines, for asthma, 1690, 1691t, *1692, 1694*
Metoclopramide (Reglan), for gastroesophageal reflux disease, 696
Metoprolol (Lopressor), for dysrhythmias, 1563t
for hypertension, 1389t
Metronidazole (Flagyl), for bacterial vaginosis, 1055
for peptic ulcer disease, 710t, 715
for trichomoniasis, 1054–1055
Metrorrhagia, 984
Mexiletine, reference values for, 2308t
MI. See *Myocardial infarction (MI).*
Miacalcin. See *Calcitonin (Miacalcin).*
Micelles, 636
Microbiology studies, 189–190
Microbodies, 207t
Microcapillary blood collection, 191
Microcirculation, regulation of, 2234
Microdiscectomy, cervical, 1992
lumbar, 1987, 1989–1991
Microfilaments, *206,* 207t
Microglia, *1865,* 1866
Microorganisms, drug-resistant, 339, 341b
Microtubules, *206,* 207t
Microvascular disease. See also specific type.
in diabetes mellitus, 1186–1189, 1188b
Micturition, 737. See also *Urination.*
age-related changes in, 737–738
Midamor (amiloride), for hypertension, 1389t
Midarm muscle circumference, 650, *653*
Midazolam, preoperative, 290t
Midbrain, 1858–1859, 1859t, *1860*
Midwives, lay, 75b
Migraine headaches, 1948–1949, *1949,* 1949b
Migrating myoelectric complex, 634
Milking, of chest tubes, 1738, *1738*
Miller-Abbott tube, 706t, 707
Mind-body interactions. See also *Complementary therapies.*
disease and, 16, 27–28
Mineralocorticoids. See *Steroids.*
Minerals, deficiency of, 641t–642t
food sources of, 641t–642t
in parenteral nutrition, 668, 669t
Minimal leak technique, for tracheostomy cuff inflation, 1653
Minimal occlusion technique, for tracheostomy cuff inflation, 1751
Mini-Mental State Examination (MMSE), in confusional states, 1919–1920
in delirium, 453
Minimum Data Set, 121, *122*
Minipress (prazosin), for hypertension, 1389t
Minnesota tube, in balloon tamponade, for bleeding esophageal varices, 1242
Minors, consent for, 286
Misoprostol (Cytotec), for peptic ulcer disease, 710t, 715
Mitochondria, *206,* 207t
Mitosis, 210, *210,* 356–357, *358*
Mitral regurgitation, 1494–1498, *1496, 1498*
Mitral stenosis, 1494–1498, *1496*
Mitral valve, 1434t, 1435, *1436, 1437*
Mitral valve disease, 1494–1498, *1496*
surgery for, 1501–1502. See also *Cardiac surgery.*

Mitral valve prolapse, 1494–1498, *1496, 1498*
chest pain in, 1449t
Mittelschmerz, 909
Mixed connective tissue disease, 2163
Mixed incontinence, 749. See also *Urinary incontinence.*
Mnemonic, ABCDE, 274
CAGE, for alcohol abuse assessment, 39
DEATH, 52
PQRST, for pain assessment, 2266
RICE, 322
SHAFT, 52
6 Ps, 604, 1415b
Vowels-TIP, 2276
Mobility, age-related changes in, 53–54
impaired. See *Immobility.*
promotion of, by assistive personnel, 573
Mobitz type I block, 1558, *1558*
Mobitz type II block, *1558,* 1558–1559
Modified barium swallow, 657
Modified Trendelenburg position, in shock, 2246, *2246*
MODY. See *Maturity-onset diabetes of the young (MODY).*
Mohs' surgery, 1307
Mole, in SI system, 188
Moles, malignant transformation in, 370, 1306b, 1307
Moniliasis. See *Candidiasis.*
Monitored anesthesia, 298
Monoclonal antibodies, 2085
for cancer, 389
for transplant immunosuppression, 2224t
Monoclonal antiendotoxin, for shock, 2250–2251
Monocytes, in inflammation, 318, *318*
in white cell count and differential, 322t
Mononeuropathy, in diabetes mellitus, 1188
Monopril (fosinopril), for hypertension, 1389t
Mons pubis, *905,* 906t
Monurol (fosfomycin), for urinary tract infection, 803
Mood, assessment of, 143
Mood and affect, assessment of, 1881
Mood disorders, 420–426, 421b. See also *Bipolar disorder; Depression.*
Morphine. See also *Opioid analgesics.*
dosage of, 489t, 492–494
duration of action of, 492
for angina, 1582, 1584t
for dyspnea, 452
oral potency of, 492
preoperative, 290t
side effects of, 450. See also *Opioid analgesics.*
Mortality. See also *Death and dying.*
causes of, 14t
in young/middle-aged adults, 30, 31t
Morton's neuroma, 582–583
Motivation, assessment of, 144
Motor assessment, 1876t–1877t. See also *Neurologic assessment.*
in spinal cord injury, 2055, 2055t
in unconscious patients, 1887–1888
Motor examination, 171t
Motor neurons, 1869
Motor paralytic bladder, *841,* 842–845
Motor pathways, in spinal cord, 1860, 1862t
Motrin. See *Ibuprofen (Advil, Motrin).*
Mourning, 18, 457–459, 459t
Mouth. See under *Oral.*
Movements. See also under *Motor.*
abnormal, in extrapyramidal disease, 1887b
in Huntington's disease, 2011, 2012
in multiple sclerosis, 2015
in Parkinson's disease, 2017, *2017*
Mu agonists, 450

Mucin deficiency, in dry eye syndrome, 1826
Mucociliary blanket, respiratory tract, 1614, *1614*, 1621
Mucormycosis, 1947
Mucosa, gastrointestinal, 630, *631*
Mucosal immunity, 2081
Mucositis, oral, in cancer, 394
Multiple gated acquisition scanning (MUGA), 1474–1475
Multiple myeloma, 2120–2121
Multiple organ dysfunction syndrome, 2255–2258
Multiple sclerosis, 2012–2016
  optic neuritis in, 1829
Multiple sleep latency test, 440
Multi-state licensure, 92
Mumps, immunization for, 342, 342t
  surgical, 690
Murmurs, 1460
  characteristics of, 1462t
  grading of, 1462b
  in aortic valve disease, 1499
  in mitral valve disease, 1498
  in pulmonic valve disease, 1500
  in tricuspid valve disease, 1500
  types of, 1463t
Muromonab CD3 (Orthoclone OKT3), for transplant immunosuppression, 2224t
Muscle(s), biopsy of, 548, 1904
  cardiac, 530
  cells of, 211
  contraction of, *532,* 534
  examination of, 541t, 541–542
  eye movements and, 1778, *1780,* 1791, *1792*
  function of, 534
  gastrointestinal, 632–633
  of respiration, 1617–1618
  skeletal, 530, *531*
  smooth, 530, 534–535
  strains of, 621
Muscle contraction headache, 1948, *1949*
Muscle coordination, assessment of, 1886–1887
Muscle enzymes, measurement of, 549t
Muscle fibers, 530
Muscle flaps, 1322–1325, *1323,* 1324b
  in breast reconstruction, 1029, *1029,* 1029–1030, *1030*
Muscle relaxants, for general anesthesia, 293, 294t
  for pain, 491, 492
Muscle relaxation, progressive, 27, 36
  for pain, 498–499
Muscle spasms, in multiple sclerosis, 2015
  in spinal cord injury, 2049, 2050
Muscle strength, assessment of, 541t, 542, 1886
Muscle tone, assessment of, 542, 1886
Muscle weakness, in diabetes mellitus, 1156t
  in dying clients, 454
  in myasthenia gravis, 2020, 2022
  in post-polio syndrome, 1993
Muscular dystrophy, 583t, 583–584
Musculocutaneous flaps, 1322–1323, *1323,* 1324b
Musculoskeletal assessment, 537–549
  chief complaint in, 537
  diagnostic tests in, 545–548
  history in, 537–540
  imaging studies in, 545–548, *548*
  laboratory studies in, 548, 549t
  neurovascular assessment in, 542
  peripheral nerve assessment in, 542, *547*
  physical examination in, 540–543
    of bones, 542
    of gait and posture, 540–541, *541*

Musculoskeletal assessment *(Continued)*
  of general condition, 540–541, *541*
  of joints, 542, *542, 543,* 544t–545t, *546*
  of muscles, 541–542
  symptom analysis in, 537–538
Musculoskeletal disorders, chest pain in, 1450t
  emergency care for, 2278–2279
Musculoskeletal system, age-related changes in, 50t, 212t, 536
  anatomy and physiology of, 530–536, *531–535*
  functions of, 534–536
  preoperative assessment of, 279
Musculoskeletal trauma, 587–624
  dislocations in, 619
  fractures in, 587–619. See also *Fracture(s).*
  remobilization after, 623 624
  sports injuries in, 619–623
  subluxations in, 619
  weight-bearing status in, 614b
Music therapy, for pain, 498
Mutations, 210
Mutual Recognition Model, 92
Myasthenia gravis, 2020–2023
  ocular manifestation in, 1829
Myasthenic crisis, 2022, 2022b
Myasthenic syndrome, 2023
Mycobacterial infection, nontuberculous, 1723
  in HIV infection, 2199, 2203
Mycobacterium avium complex infection, 1723
  in HIV infection, 2199, 2203
Mycophenolate (CellCept), for transplant immunosuppression, 2224t
Mycoplasma tuberculosis, culture of, 1720
  drug resistance of, 1718
Mycoplasmal pneumonia, 1711–1716, 1712t
Mycosis fungoides, 1309
Mycostatin (nystatin), 1280t
Myelin, 1867–1868
Myelography, 546, 1899, *1899*
Myeloma, multiple, 2120–2121
Myelomalacia, 1994
Myelosuppression, in cancer, 392
Myocardial cells, depolarization of, 1436–1438, *1438*
Myocardial contractility, 1439, 1441–1442
Myocardial depressant factor, in shock, 2232, 2237, 2239
Myocardial depression, in burns, 1335, 1338
Myocardial infarction (MI), 1585–1605
  angina after, 1581
  angina preceding, 1581
  cardiac enzymes in, 1588–1589, *1589*
  care plan for, 1599b–1605b
  case management for, 1593b
  case study of, 1594–1596
  chest pain in, 1449t, 1587, *1588*
    management of, 1590–1591
  clinical manifestations of, 1587
  complications of, 1591–1592
  depth of, 1587, *1587, 1598*
  diagnosis of, 1587–1590
  electrocardiography in, 1469, 1469t, 1587, *1589*
  emergency care for, 2275
  epidemiology of, 1585
  etiology of, 1585
  heart failure after, 1530, 1530t
  home care in, 1598b
  imaging studies in, 1589–1590
  medical management of, *1586,* 1590–1598
  necrosis in, 1593–1596
  nursing management of, 1598–1606, 1599b–1605b
  outcomes classification for, 1585–1605
  pathophysiology of, 1585–1587, *1586*
  recurrent, 1593

Myocardial infarction (MI) *(Continued)*
  rehabilitation after, 1596–1605
  risk factors for, 1585
  shock in. See *Cardiogenic shock.*
  sites of, 1587, *1588*
  surgery for, 1596
  transmural, 1587, *1587, 1589*
Myocardial ischemia, 1580–1581
  damage from, 1585–1587, *1586, 1587.* See also *Myocardial infarction (MI).*
  pain in. See *Angina pectoris.*
Myocardial necrosis, 1593–1596
Myocardial rupture, 1593
Myocardial scintigraphy, 1474–1475
Myocarditis, 1487–1488
Myocardium, 530, 1435, *1436*
Myoclonic seizures, 1925
Myocutaneous flaps, 1322–1323, *1323,* 1323–1325, 1324b
Myofibrils, 530
Myofibroblasts, in wound healing, 320
Myoglobin, 1464
  in myocardial infarction, 1588, *1589*
  urine, reference values for, 2306t
Myomectomy, 992
Myopathy, in hyperparathyroidism, 1109
Myopia, 1827, *1827*
Myringoplasty, 1846
Myringotomy, 1847
Myxedema, 1091
  assessment in, 1095
  clinical manifestations of, 1093, *1093*
  decreased cardiac output in, 1096–1097
  hypothermia in, 1097
  medical management of, 1093, 1095, 1096t
  nursing management of, 1095–1097

N

Nabumetone, 486, 487t
Nafarelin (Synarel), for endometriosis, 990
Nails, age-related changes in, 50t
  capillary refill in, 1371, *1372,* 1456, 1629
  clubbing of, 1273, 1273t, 1453, 1456, 1629, *1630*
  disorders of, 1328–1329
  examination of, 1272–1273, 1273t
    in respiratory assessment, 1629
    normal findings on, 1269b
  fungal infection of, 1329
  in chronic renal failure, 883
  ingrown, 1328
  spoon-shaped, 1273t
  structure and function of, 1263
Nalbuphine (Nubain), 490t
Naloxone (Narcan), for comatose patients, 1910, 2277
  for narcotic overdose, 1910, 2277, 2281
  for poisoning, 1910, 2277, 2281
  for shock, 2251
Naltrexone (ReVia), for alcoholism, 515–516
Naproxen, 486, 487t
Narcan. See *Naloxone (Narcan).*
Narcolepsy, 434–435
Narcotic analgesics. See *Opioid analgesics.*
Nares, 1612, *1613*
  erosion of, balloon tamponade and, 1243
Nasal airway, 304, *306*
Nasal cavity, assessment of, 1635–1636, *1636*
  structure of, 1612, *1613, 1636*
Nasal culture, 1648
Nasal decongestants, rhinitis and, 1679, 1680
Nasal drip pad, 1678, *1678*
Nasal fracture, 1327, 1682
Nasal packing, 1675, 1676, *1676*
Nasal polyps, 1682

Nasal septum, deviated, 1682–1683
Nasal speculum, 1635–1636, *1636*
Nasal surgery, 1319
Nasal vestibule, 1612, *1613*
Nasogastric intubation, for feeding, 673, *673.*
    See also *Enteral nutrition.*
  in shock, 2248
  postoperative, 722
    in esophageal surgery, 699
Nasogastric suctioning, in acute pancreatitis, 1197
  in cholelithiasis, 1206–1207, 1211
Nasointestinal feeding, 673, *673.* See also *Enteral nutrition.*
Nasolacrimal duct, 1778, *1779*
Nasopharynx, 1612, *1613*
  examination of, 1636
National Institute for Nursing Research, 73
National Institutes of Health (NIH), 73
National Organ Transplant Act of 1984, 2215, 2219
Natural illnesses, 19b
Natural killer cells, 2081
Nausea, 705–706
  in brain tumors, 1934
  in chemotherapy, 393–394, 1034
  in hepatitis, 1231
  in intestinal disorders, 766
  in peptic ulcer disease, 714
  in spinal anesthesia, 296t
  opioid analgesics and, 450, 491
  postoperative, 311b, 311–312
Near vision, 1781
Near-drowning, 1770
Nearsightedness, 1827, *1827*
Nebulized drugs, metered-dose inhaler, 1691, *1693*, 1693b
Neck. See also under *Cervical.*
  examination of, 166t
    in thyroid disorders, 1074, *1075,* 1075b
  exercises of, hyperthyroidism and, 1105–1106
Neck veins, assessment of, 1457–1458, *1458*
Necrotizing ulcerative gingivitis, 684–685
Needle biopsy, 200, 374. See also *Biopsy.*
Needle-stick injuries, HIV transmission via, 2189
  prevention of, 345
Negative pressure wound therapy, 333
Neglect, elder, 57, 57b
Nelfinavir (Viracept), 2197t
Nembutal (pentobarbital), for increased intracranial pressure, 2031
  preoperative, 290t
Neobladder, *813,* 814. See also *Urinary diversion.*
Neocortex, 1856
Neomycin, for burns, 1348t
  for hepatic encephalopathy, 1252
    diarrhea and, 1253
Neonate, HIV infection in, 2189
Neoplasia, 211. See also *Cancer; Tumor(s).*
  definition of, 349
Neoral (cyclosporine), for transplant immunosuppression, 2224t
Neosporin, 327t
Neostigmine (Prostigmin), for myasthenia gravis, 2021–2022
Nephrectomy, 860–861
  for cancer, 860–861
  for trauma, 869
Nephritic syndrome, in glomerulonephritis, 863
Nephritis, interstitial, 862
Nephroblastoma, 858–862. See also *Renal cancer.*
Nephrolithiasis, 821–828, 854. See also *Urinary calculi.*
  hypercalcemia and, 253

Nephrolithotomy, for urinary calculi, *827,* 828
Nephron, 733, *733*
Nephropathy. See also *Renal disease.*
  diabetic, 1187–1188
Nephrosclerosis, in diabetic nephropathy, 851
Nephroscopy, 760
  for urinary calculi, 826, *827*
Nephrostomy, percutaneous, *813,* 814–815
Nephrotic syndrome, in glomerulonephritis, 862–863
Nephrotoxins, 853t, 853–854
Nephrourectomy, 860
Nerve(s), cranial, *1869,* 1869t, 1869–1870
  regeneration of, 1872–1873, *1873*
  spinal, *1868,* 1869
Nerve block. See also *Anesthesia.*
  analgesic, 483, 496
  peripheral, 298
  regional, 293–296
Nerve cells. See *Neuron(s).*
Nerve conduction velocity study, 1903–1904
Nerve fibers, adrenergic, 1872
  cholinergic, 1871
  myelinated, 1867
  unmyelinated, 1867
Nerve growth factor, in pain, 468
Nerve impulses, 1867, *1867*
Nerve injury, 2026
  emergency care for, 2276–2277
  in compartment syndrome, 599–600, *601*
  in fractures, 599
  nerve regeneration in, 1872–1873, *1873*
Nerve root compression, assessment of, *1986*
Nervous system, age-related changes in, 50t, 1873
  assessment of. See also *Neurologic assessment.*
  autonomic, age-related changes in, 50t
    assessment of, 1892
    structure of, 1870–1872, *1872*
  central. See *Central nervous system.*
  enteric, 630, 631
  epinephrine effects on, 1135t
  functional effects of, 1870, 1871t
  in cardiac regulation, 1442–1443
  in pain perception, 466–468
  in pain transmission, 468
  in shock, 2239
  norepinephrine effects on, 1135t
  parasympathetic, effects of on organs, 1870, 1871t
    functional effects of, 1871t
    gastrointestinal function and, 631, 1871t
    in cardiac regulation, 1443
    structure of, 1870–1872, *1872*
  peripheral, *1868, 1869,* 1869–1870, 1870t
  structure of, 1870–1872, *1872*
  sympathetic, effects of on organs, 1870, 1871t
    functional effects of, 1871t
    gastrointestinal function and, 631
    in cardiac regulation, 1443
    structure of, 1870–1872, *1872*
Nesacaine (chloroprocaine), 297t
Neumega (oprelvekin), for cancer, 388, 393
Neural stalk, 1062
Neurilemma, *1865,* 1866
Neuritis, optic, in multiple sclerosis, 1829
Neuroendocrine system, in shock, 2239–2240, *2240,* 2242–2243
Neurofibrillary tangles, in Alzheimer's disease, 2003, *2003*
Neurofibrils, 1866, *1866*
Neurofibromas, 2001
Neurofibromatosis, 2001

Neurogenic bladder, 841–846, *842*
  in diabetes mellitus, 852, 1189
  in spinal cord injury, 841–846, 2049, 2059, 2063, 2066–2067
Neurogenic shock, 2051, 2055–2056, 2232. See also *Shock.*
  clinical manifestations of, 2243
  etiology of, 2234
Neuroglia, *1865,* 1865–1866
Neurohypophysis. See *Pituitary gland, posterior.*
Neuroleptic anesthesia, 293
Neuroleptic malignant syndrome, 419
Neurologic assessment, 170t–171t, 1874–1904
  autonomic nervous system assessment in, 1892
  bowel and bladder function in, 1878t
  charting in, *2036–2037*
  clinical applications of, 1893–1894
  cranial nerve examination in, 1883–1886
  diagnostic tests in, 1894–1904
  functional, 1875t–1878t, 1893
  Glasgow Coma Scale in, 2031, 2035b
  guidelines for, 1875t–1878t
  head, neck and back examination in, 1883
  history in, 1874–1879
  in comatose patients, 1909–1910, 1911, 1912b
  in emergency care, 2266, 2276
  in increased intracranial pressure, 2031–2038
  in spinal cord injury, 2055, 2055t
  initial, 1881b
  level of consciousness in, 1875t, 1880–1881
  mental status, 1880–1883
  mentation in, 1875t
  motor, 1876t–1877t, 1886–1888
  normal findings in, 1882b
  physical examination in, 1879–1894
  postoperative, 306, 308–309
    in cardiac surgery, 1508–1509
  preoperative, 280
  reflexes in, 1889–1892
  sensory, 1877t–1878t, 1888–1892
  speech and language in, 1875t–1876t
  vital signs in, 1880, 2035
Neurologic complications, of spinal anesthesia, 296t
Neurologic disorders, alternative therapies for, 1879
  chest pain in, 1450t
  clinical manifestations of, 1880t
  degenerative, 2002–2024
  dysphagia in, 690–691
Neurologic function, age-related changes in, 212t
  in hepatic encephalopathy, 1251
Neurolytics, for pain, 483–484
Neuroma, acoustic, 1840, 1933
  Morton's, 582–583
Neuromuscular blocking agents, for general anesthesia, 293, 294t
  for increased intracranial pressure, 2031
  for mechanical ventilation, 1756, *1760*
Neuromuscular junction, *532*
Neuron(s), 211
  in pain perception/transmission, 466, 467, 469–470, *470*
  motor (efferent), 1869
  nociceptive-specific, 469
  of autonomic nervous system, 1870
  sensory (afferent), 1869
  somatic, 1870
  structure of, *1866,* 1866–1867
Neuronitis, vestibular, 1848
Neuropathy, diabetic, 1188–1189
  pain in, 473

Neuropsychological testing, 1902–1903
Neurosyphilis, 1995
Neurotransmitters, 1866b, 1867
  in pain, 466, *466*, 468, 469
  in sleep, 432, 437–438
Neurovascular assessment, components of, 604t
  for casts, 604, 604t, 605, 605b
  in musculoskeletal assessment, 542
  postoperative, in hip fracture, 615
Neutropenia, in cancer, 392–393
Neutrophils, 392, 2080
  banded, 318, 322t, 392
  deficiency of, in cancer, 392–393
  in inflammation and infection, 317–318, *318*, 392
  measurement of, 392
  segmented, 318, 322t, 392
Nevi, malignant transformation in, 370, 1306b, 1307
Nevirapine (Viramune), 2198t
Niacin, deficiency of, 642t
  food sources of, 642t
Nicardipine, for hypertension, 1396t
Nicotine, 510t, 514t, 518
NIDDM (non-insulin-dependent diabetes mellitus). See *Diabetes mellitus, type 2.*
Nifedipine (Procardia), for hypertension, 1389t
Night sweats, 985
Night vision, 1781
Nightingale, Florence, 4t
Nightingale Tracker, 116
Nightmares, 437
Nipple, 907
  examination of. See *Breast, examination of.*
Nipple-areola reconstruction, 1030, *1030*
Nipride (sodium nitroprusside), for hypertensive emergencies, 1396t
Nissen fundoplication, *696*, 696–697
Nitric oxide, for adult respiratory distress syndrome, 1762–1763
Nitrites, in urine, 757, 757t
Nitrogen balance, nutritional status and, 656
Nitrogen method, for lung volumes, 1637
Nitroglycerin, for angina, 1582, 1583t
  for heart failure, 1538t, 1540
    in emergency care, 2274
  for hypertensive emergencies, 1396t
Nitroprusside, for heart failure, 1538t, 1540
Nitrous oxide, 294t
Nociceptive-specific neurons, 469
Nociceptors, 466–468
Nocturia, 748
Nocturnal angina, 1581
Nocturnal erections, 439
Nocturnal penile tumescence studies, 973
Nocturnal rebound hyperglycemia, 1180
Nodes, Bouchard's, 552, *553*
Nodular melanoma, 1307–1309, 1308t
Nodules, *1271*
  rheumatoid, 2145, *2146*
  thyroid, 1108
  vocal cord, 1660
Noise exposure, 1800, 1801t
  hearing loss due to, 1833
Nolvadex (tamoxifen), for breast cancer, 1014, 1032, 1035–1036
Nondisplaced fracture, 594t
Non-Hodgkin's lymphoma, 2176–2179
  in HIV infection, 2206
  Rappaport staging of, 2177t
Non-insulin-dependent diabetes mellitus (NIDDM). See *Diabetes mellitus, type 2.*
Non-native English speakers, communication with, 147
Non-nucleoside reverse transcriptase inhibitors, for HIV infection, 2195–2199, 2198t

Non-REM sleep, 432, *433*, 433–434
Nonsteroidal anti-inflammatory drugs (NSAIDs), 486
  for dysmenorrhea, 981
  for osteoarthritis, 554, 555t
  for pain, 450, 451t
  for rheumatoid arthritis, 2147, 2148t, 2148–2149
  in HIV infection, 474
  perioperative use of, 275t
  side effects of, 486
Nonverbal communication, 147, 410–411
Norcuron (vecuronium), 295t
Norepinephrine, 1067
  excess of, 1135t, 1135–1137
  in pain, 469
  plasma, reference values for, 1136, 2303t
  urine, reference values for, 2306t
Normal flora, 336–337
Normal saline, 221t
  for wound irrigation, 326, 327t
  infusion of. See *Saline infusion.*
  recipe for, 330
Normodyne (labetalol), for hypertension, 1389t, 1396t
Nortriptyline, reference values for, 2308t
Norvir (ritonavir), 2198t
Nose. See also under *Nasal.*
  assessment of, 1635–1636, *1636*
  examination of, 165t–166t
  structure of, 1612, *1613*, *1636*
Nosebleed, 1672–1676, *1676*
Nosocomial infections, prevention of, 338–340, 339t, 343–346
  in community-based settings, 345b, 346
  in health care providers, 345–346
  in home health care, 345b, 346
  in hospitals, 343–346
  in long-term care facilities, 344–346
  prevention of, 343–346
NPH insulin, 1162t, *1163*. See also *Insulin therapy.*
NPO status, preoperative, 284
NSAIDs. See *Nonsteroidal anti-inflammatory drugs (NSAIDs).*
Nubain (nalbuphine), 490t
Nucleolus, 207t
Nucleoside reverse transcriptase inhibitors, for HIV infection, 2195–2199, 2196t–2197t
5'-Nucleotidase, 1082t
Nucleus, cell, *206*, 207t, 209
Null lymphocytes, 2081
Nummular eczema, 1286
Numorphan (oxymorphone), 489t
Nurse(s), certification of, for ambulatory care nursing, 91–92
  circulating, 291b
  delegation by. See *Unlicensed assistive personnel.*
  distribution of, 76–77
  first assistant, 291b
  immunizations for, 342t, 343
  in health care system, 76–77
  infection control measures for, 345–346
  on surgical team, 291b, 292
  Oncology Certified, 381
  perioperative, 273
  political influence of, 77
  scrub, 291b
Nurse anesthetist, 291b
Nurse extender, 100
Nurse manager, in long-term care facilities, 123–125
  operating room, 291b
Nurse-Managed Center, 88

Nursing, acute care, 95–106
  ambulatory care, 83–93
  community health, 109
  definition of, 10
  demographics of, 76–77
  emergency, 2261
  functional, 99
  gerontic, 46
  gerontological, 46
  holistic, 84
  home health. See *Home health care.*
  perioperative, 273–274. See also under *Intraoperative; Postoperative; Preoperative.*
  primary, 99
  subacute care, 96–98, 98b
  team, 99
  total care, 99
Nursing care classification, 101–102, 103t
Nursing care intensity, levels of, 101–102, 103t
Nursing care plans. See *Care plans.*
Nursing Center, 88
Nursing diagnoses, for chronic conditions, 21, 22b
Nursing education, for home care, 111
Nursing Home Reform Act, 65
Nursing homes. See *Long-term care facilities.*
Nursing intensity classification, 101–102, 103t
Nursing's Agenda for Health Care Reform, 77
Nutrients, recommended intake of, 638–639
Nutrition. See also *Diet; Feeding; Food.*
  cancer and, 15
  cultural aspects of, 643b–645b
  disease and, *14*, 14–15, 24–26
  enteral. See *Enteral nutrition.*
  erythropoiesis and, 2077–2078
  Food Guide Pyramid for, 30, *31*, 638, *639*
  food labels and, 30, *32*
  guidelines for, 24–25
    for young/middle-aged adults, 30–33, *31*, 31t
  health promotion/risk management for, 150t–151t
  immunosuppression and, 2136b
  in acute pancreatitis, 1196, 1197
  in alcoholic hepatitis, 1232
  in anemia, 2111
  in anorexia nervosa, 680
  in burns, 1346, 1346t
  in cancer, 384, 394
  in chemotherapy, 384
  in chronic conditions, 24–25
  in chronic obstructive pulmonary disease, 1699
  in diabetes mellitus, 1158, *1165*, 1165–1167, 1166t
    and exercise, 1165
  in eating disorders, 680
  in elderly, 49–51, 51b
  in HIV infection, 2210
  in hyperparathyroidism, 1113
  in hyperthyroidism, 1103
  in hypothyroidism, 1097
  in inflammatory bowel disease, 772, 774
  in oral cancer, 688, 689
  in stress management, 35–36
  in terminal illness, 455, 456t
  in viral hepatitis, 1228, 1230–1231
  in wound healing, 321, 321t, 330, 331
  inadequate. See *Malnutrition.*
  outcomes classification for, 661
  preoperative, 284
  pressure ulcers and, 1295–1297, 1298
  promotion of, 664–667
  recommended dietary allowances in, 638
  reference daily intakes in, 638
  renal function and, 738

Nutritional assessment, 638–639
  abdominal examination in, 652–655, 654
  acid perfusion test in, 659
  anthropometric measurements in, 649–650, 650, 651b, 651t, 652
  diabetes mellitus and, 1165, 1165
  diagnostic tests in, 655–659
  esophageal manometry in, 659
  esophageal pH monitoring in, 659
  exfoliative cytologic analysis in, 658
  gastric analysis in, 658–659
  history in, 645–649
  imaging studies in, 656–658
  in obesity, 32
  laboratory tests in, 655–656, 656t
  oral examination in, 650–652, 653
  physical examination in, 649–655
    abdominal, 650–652, 653
    oral, 650–652, 653
  preoperative, 280–281
  screening in, 640, 642b, 663, 666b
  symptom analysis in, 645–646
Nutritional health, components of, 638–639
Nutritional requirements, determination of, 663, 663t
Nutritional screening, 640, 642b, 663, 666b
Nutritional supplements, 647–648, 648t. See also Minerals; Vitamin(s).
  for premenstrual syndrome, 981–982
  pharmaceutical, 981–982
Nutritional support, costs of, 662
  enteral nutrition in, 671–677. See also Enteral nutrition.
  in burns, 1346, 1346t, 1352
  in chronic obstructive pulmonary disease, 1699
  in coma, 1915b, 1915–1916
  in eating disorders, 680
  in inflammatory bowel disease, 774
  oral supplements in, 663, 664t, 665
  parenteral nutrition in, 668–671. See also Total parenteral nutrition (TPN).
  routes of administration for, 663, 665
Nystagmus, 1791, 1885
  in caloric testing, 1903, 1909
  testing for, 1804, 1806
Nystatin (Mycostatin), 1280t

O

OA. See Osteoarthritis (OA).
OASIS data set, 108, 113
Obesity, 30–32, 677–679
  abdominoplasty in, 1320
  body mass index and, 31
  coronary heart disease and, 1517, 1521
  health risks of, 15
  hypertension and, 1381, 1386–1387
  lipectomy in, 1319–1320
  malnutrition and, 640
  management of, 32
  panniculectomy in, 1320–1321
  surgery and, 281, 284, 309
Object loss theory, 421
Oblique fracture, 594t
Obsessive-compulsive disorder, 413–416, 414b
Obstetric history, 917
Obstructive shock, 2231. See also Shock.
Obstructive sleep apnea, 435–436, 436b
  hypertension and, 439
Occipital lobe, 1856, 1858
Occlusive dressings, 1281t
Occlusives, topical, 1283
Occult blood test, for colorectal cancer, 43
Occupational Health and Safety Administration (OSHA), 104
  infection control standards of, 343, 345–346

Occupational lung disease, 1739–1740, 1740t
Occupational risk factors, 153t–154t
Occupational therapy, in rheumatoid arthritis, 2148
  in stroke rehabilitation, 1968
Ocular adnexa, 1778, 1779
Ocular motility, assessment of, 1791–1792, 1792
Ocular muscles, 1778, 1780
Oculocephalic reflex, assessment of, 1909, 1909
Oculomotor nerve, 1870t
  assessment of, 1884
Oculovestibular reflex, assessment of, 1903, 1909, 1909
Odontoid fracture, 2047, 2049
Odynophagia, 691
  in esophageal cancer, 700, 701
Ointments, 1281t
  antibiotic, 327t
  for skin disorders, 1283
Older adults. See Elderly.
Olfaction, assessment of, 1636, 1636b, 1883
  in physical examination, 179
Olfactory nerve, 1870t
  assessment of, 1883
Oligodendrocytes, 1865, 1866
Oligodendrogliomas, 1932. See also Brain tumors.
Oligospermia, 969
Oliguria, 747, 831
  definition of, 876
  in acute renal failure, 877–878
  in dehydration, 219
  in shock, 2248
Omaha System, 111–112, 112, 114t
  Intervention Scheme in, 114–115, 115b
  Nightingale Tracker and, 116
  Problem Classification Scheme in, 112–114, 113b, 114b, 114t
  Problem Rating Scale for Outcomes in, 115–116, 116t
Omental flap, 1323, 1323–1325
Omeprazole (Prilosec), for peptic ulcer disease, 710t, 711t, 715
Ommaya reservoir, 388, 388
Oncogenes, 350t, 356
Oncologic emergencies, 395–396
Oncology, definition of, 349
Oncology Certified Nurses, 381
Oncotic pressure, 215–216
Onychomycosis, 1329
Open fractures, 590
  infection of, 601
Open pneumothorax, 1766, 1766, 1767
  conversion of tension pneumothorax to, 1768
  emergency care for, 2271, 2271–2272
Open-circuit nitrogen method, for lung volumes, 1637
Opening snap, 1461
  in mitral stenosis, 1497
Operating room, transport from, 302
  transport to, 289, 298
Ophthalmic nerve, 1870t
Ophthalmic radiography, 1796
Ophthalmodynamometry, 1797, 1896
Ophthalmoscope, 176
Ophthalmoscopy, direct, 1794, 1794b, 1795
  indirect, 1795
Opiate receptors, 488
Opiates, endogenous, 469
  pharmaceutical. See Opioid analgesics.
Opioid analgesics, 450, 486–491. See also Analgesics; Pain management.
  abuse of, 510t, 514t, 518, 520t–521t
  addiction to, 463, 485
  adjuvant medications for, 491–492

Opioid analgesics (Continued)
  adverse effects of, 450, 490–491
  dependence on, 485
  dosage of, 450, 451, 493–494
    equianalgesic, 289t–290t, 489t–491t, 492–493
    inadequate, 461–462, 462b, 494
  duration of action of, 489t–490t, 492–493
  effectiveness of, factors affecting, 492–494
  for dyspnea, 452
  during shock, 2251, 2252
  mechanism of action of, 488
  misconceptions about, 463, 464b
  opiate receptors and, 488
  opioid agonist, 488
  opioid agonist-antagonist, 488
  opioid antagonist, 488
  oral potency of, 489t–490t, 492
  peak effect of, 489t–490t, 492
  relative potency of, 489t–490t, 492
  selection of, 488t
  side effects of, 450
  tolerance to, 485
Opportunistic infections, in cancer, 383–384, 392–393, 395, 396
  in chemotherapy, 383–384, 392–393, 395
  in diabetes mellitus, 1183t, 1184–1185, 1186b, 1187b
  in HIV infection, 2202–2205
    prevention of, 2199, 2201–2202
    treatment of, 2202–2205
  in leukemia, 2171
  in transplant recipients, 2225, 2225t
Oprelvekin (Neumega), for cancer, 388, 393
Optic disc, swelling of, 2028
  in brain tumors, 1934
Optic nerve, 1780, 1870t
  assessment of, 1883–1884
Optic neuritis, in multiple sclerosis, 1829
Oral airway, 304, 306
Oral cancer, 686–690
  assessment in, 687
  basal cell, 687
  biopsy of, 687
  causes of, 686
  chemotherapy for, 687
  clinical manifestations of, 687, 687
  medical management of, 687
  nursing management in, 687–689
  prevention of, 686–687
  prognosis in, 687
  radiation therapy for, 687
  screening for, 158t
  self-care in, 689–690
  squamous cell, 687, 687
  surgery for, 688–690
Oral candidiasis, 685, 685–686
Oral care, in cancer, 394
  in coma, 1913–1914
  in dehydration, 224
  in hypernatremia, 241
  in oral cancer, 688
  in phenytoin therapy, 1930
  postoperative, cholelithiasis and, 1211
Oral cavity, age-related changes in, 50t
  anatomy of, 653
  disorders of, 684–690
  examination of, 166t, 650–652, 653
  tumors of, benign, 686
    malignant, 686–690, 687. See also Oral cancer.
    premalignant, 686, 686
Oral cholecystography, 1085–1086
Oral contraceptives, breast cancer and, 1012
  for dysmenorrhea, 981
  for endometriosis, 990
  hepatic adenoma and, 1254

Oral glucose tolerance test, in diabetes mellitus, 1157b, 1157–1158
Oral mucositis, in cancer, 394
Oral rehydration, in diarrhea, 768
  solutions for, 220, 221t
Oral surgery, 688–690
Oral ulcers, 684
  chemotherapy and, 394, 1034
  herpetic, 684, 685
Orbit, 1778, 1779
  fractures of, 1326–1327, 1327
Orchiectomy, for prostate cancer, 961
  for testicular cancer, 965
Orchitis, 966
Organ Donation Request Act, 2219
Organ of Corti, 1785
Organ Procurement and Transplant Network, 2219
Organ transplantation. See Transplantation.
Organelles, 206, 206, 207t
Orientation, assessment of, 143, 1881
    postoperative, 306, 308–309
    preoperative, 280
Orientation measures, for confusional states, 1920
Oropharynx, 1612, 1613
Orthoclone OKT3 (muromonab-CD3), for transplant immunosuppression, 2224t
Orthopnea, 1452
  in heart failure, 1534
Orthostatic hypotension, 1397, 1849
  in dehydration, 219
  opioid analgesics and, 491
Osmolality, 216–217
  reference values for, 2304t
  urine, reference values for, 2306t
Osmolarity, 216
  urine, 736–737, 756, 757t
Osmotic pressure, 215–216
Ossicles, ear, 1783, 1783
  in sound wave conduction, 1785
Ossiculoplasty, 1846, 1846–1847
Ostac (clodronate), for bone metastases, in breast cancer, 1036
Osteitis deformans, 572–575, 575
Osteoarthritis (OA), 551–565
  clinical manifestations of, 552–554, 553, 553t
  diagnosis of, 552–554, 553t
  drug therapy for, 554, 555t
  etiology of, 551–552
  herbal remedies for, 539
  management of, medical, 554, 555t
    nursing, 554–555
    surgical, 555–565. See also Total hip replacement (THR); Total knee replacement (TKR).
  pain management in, 554, 555t
  pathophysiology of, 552, 552, 553t
  primary, 551
  risk factors for, 551–552
  secondary, 551
Osteoblast, 532
Osteoblastoma, 580t, 580–581
Osteochondroma, 580t, 580–581
Osteoclast, 532, 567, 567
Osteoclastoma, 580t, 580–581
Osteocyte, 532, 534
Osteodystrophy, hereditary, 1114
  renal, 886–887
    treatment of, 894
Osteogenic sarcoma, 580t, 581, 581–582
Osteoid osteoma, 580t, 580–581
Osteomalacia, 757
Osteomyelitis, 578–579
Osteon, 531, 534
Osteopenia, 566
Osteoporosis, 536, 566–572
  care plan for, 574

Osteoporosis (Continued)
  definition of, 566
  diet and, 569–570, 570b
  etiology of, 566–567
  fractures in, 566, 566, 567, 568, 572
  glucocorticoid-induced, 1123–1124, 1127
  hyperthyroidism and, case study of, 1102
  medical management of, 569–572
  menopause and, 985
  parathyroidectomy and, 1114
  pathophysiology of, 567, 567
  prevention of, 569–572
  risk factors for, 567
  self-care in, 572
Osteosarcoma, 580t, 581, 581–582
Osteotomy, for osteoarthritis, 555
  for rheumatoid arthritis, 2153–2154
Ostomy care, in colostomy, 785–787
  in ileostomy, 777–779
Otalgia, 1799, 1840–1847
  clinical manifestations of, 1843–1844
  etiology of, 1841–1843
  medical management of, 1844, 1844–1845, 1845
  nursing management of, 1845–1846, 1846b
  pathophysiology of, 1843
  risk factors for, 1841–1843
  surgery for, 1846, 1846–1847
    nursing management in, 1847, 1847b
Otitis externa, 1842
  treatment of, 1844, 1845
Otitis media, 1842–1843
  treatment of, 1844–1845
Otoacoustic emissions, 1806
Otosclerosis, 1832, 1832, 1840
Otoscope, 176
Otoscopy, 1801, 1801–1802, 1802
Ototoxicity, 1799, 1800b
Outcome monitoring, 102
Outpatient departments, in community hospitals, 87
  in teaching hospitals, 87
Outpatient surgery. See also under Intraoperative; Perioperative; Postoperative; Preoperative; Surgery.
  case management for, 283
Oval window, of ear, 1783, 1783
Ovarian cancer, 1001–1002
  genetic factors in, 1012–1013
Ovarian cycle, 908–909, 909
Ovarian cyst, 989, 1000, 1001
Ovarian follicles, 904, 906t, 908, 909
Ovarian suppression, for endometriosis, 990
Ovary, benign tumors of, 1000–1001
  examination of, 924
  structure and function of, 904, 905, 906t
Overflow incontinence, 749, 834. See also Urinary incontinence.
  urinary retention and, 829
Overhydration, 225–228
  emergency care for, 2274–2275
Overuse syndromes, 619b, 619–621, 621t
  lower extremity, 620
  upper extremity, 620–621
Ovulation, 908–909, 909
Oxalate stones, 823
Oxaprozin, 486, 487t
Oxybutynin (Ditropan), for urinary incontinence, 837t
Oxycodone, 489t
Oxygen, arterial, reference values for, 2304t
  partial pressure of. See PaO₂.
  transport of, 1620, 1620
Oxygen administration, flow rate in, 1699, 1699t
  for anemia, 2104

Oxygen administration (Continued)
  for chronic obstructive pulmonary disease, 1698, 1699, 1699t
  for dyspnea, 452
  for heart failure, 1536
  for ventilatory failure, 1750
  hyperbaric, complications of, 1842
    for shock, 2244
    for wound healing, 333
  in emergency care, 2270
  postoperative, 304
Oxygen conservation strategies, for chronic obstructive pulmonary disease, 1705b
Oxygen free radicals, disease and, 15
  in wound healing, 319
Oxygen saturation, arterial. See SaO₂.
Oxygen toxicity, in mechanical ventilation, 1756
Oxyhemoglobin dissociation curve, 1620, 1620
Oxymorphone (Numorphan), 489t
Oxytocin, 1065, 1138t

P

Pacemaker(s), artificial, 1569–1576. See also Pacing.
  classification of, 1574b
  demand, 1573, 1573–1574
  design of, 1570, 1570–1571
  failure of, 1571t, 1575, 1575
  fixed-rate, 1573
  permanent, 1570, 1570
  pulse generator in, 1570, 1570–1571
  temporary, 1570
  transtelephone monitoring of, 1576
  intrinsic, ectopic, 1551
    escape, 1550
Pachymeter, 1796
Pacing, client teaching for, 1576b, 1576–1577
  demand, 1573, 1573–1574
  electrocardiography in, 1574, 1575
  endocardial (transvenous), 1572, 1572
  epicardial (transthoracic), 1572
  external (transcutaneous), 1571–1572
  fixed-rate, 1573
  in home care, 1576b, 1576–1577
  nursing management in, 1575–1576
  permanent, 1573b, 1573–1576
  problems in, 1571t, 1575, 1575
  self-care in, 1576b, 1576–1577
  temporary, 1570, 1572, 1572–1573, 1573
  transvenous temporary endocardial, 1570, 1570
Packed red cell volume, 2074–2075, 2075
Packing, nasal, 1675, 1676, 1676
  wound, 326–328
Paclitaxel, for breast cancer, 1033
PaCO₂, in respiratory failure, 1746
  measurement of, 1641–1642. See also Arterial blood gas analysis.
PACU. See Post-anesthesia care unit (PACU).
Paget's disease of bone, 572–575, 575
Pain, 461–503
  abdominal, 472, 705
    assessment of, 1073, 1073
    characteristics of, 646t
    rebound tenderness and, 743
    rigidity and, 743
    sources of, 646t
  acute, 464–465
  adaptation to, 463
  age and, 476
  anxiety and, 451, 451t, 476
  assessment of, 137, 477b, 477–478, 478–482, 483b, 537–538
    in emergency care, 2266
  back, in spinal cord compression, 397

Pain *(Continued)*
  behavioral indicators of, 450, 450t
  behavioral response to, 450, 450t
  bladder, 750
  breast, 1037
  cancer, 466, 466t
  chest, anginal. See *Angina pectoris.*
    assessment of, 1448–1451, 1449t–1450t
    characteristics of, 1448–1451
    gender and, 1451t
  chronic, 465–466
    intermittent, 466
    malignant, 466, 466t
    nonmalignant, 465–466
  costovertebral, 750
  cutaneous, 471, 471t
  deep, 471t, 471–472
  definition of, 462–463
  descriptive terms for, 483b
  distress from, 478
  ear, 1799, 1840–1847, *1844–1846*
  epididymal, 750–751
  eye, 1788
  factors affecting, 474–477
  gate control theory of, *470,* 470–471
  gender and, 476
  headache, 471
  in acute cholecystitis, 1212
  in acute pancreatitis, 1195, 1196, 1197
  in appendicitis, 768, 769
  in bone cancer, 582
  in burns, 1338, 1343, 1346–1347, 1352, 1356
  in cancer, 371, 395
  in children, 476
    rating scale for, 477, *481*
  in cholelithiasis, 1205, 1206, 1211
  in chronic pancreatitis, 1200
  in complex regional pain syndrome, 602
  in elderly, 476
  in endometriosis, 989
  in fibromyalgia, 2161
  in fractures, 590, 605
  in gastroesophageal reflux disease, 695
  in gastrointestinal disorders, 472, 646t, 705
  in herpes zoster, 1312
  in HIV infection, 474, 2210–2211
  in inflammation, 472–473
  in intermittent claudication, 1368, 1400, 1408
  in interstitial cystitis, 808
  in intestinal disorders, 765–766
  in myocardial infarction, 1449t, 1587, *1588*
    management of, 1590–1591
  in oral candidiasis, 686
  in osteoarthritis, 552, 553t, 554
  in peptic ulcer disease, 714, 717, 718
  in pericarditis, 1488–1489
  in peritoneal dialysis, 889
  in pulmonary embolism, 1706
  in reflex sympathetic dystrophy, 602
  in respiratory disorders, 472
  in sickle cell anemia, 2118
  in spinal cord injury, 2060, 2064
  in trigeminal neuralgia, 1995
  in urinary tract disorders, 750–751
  in urolithiasis, 824, 825
  in vertebral compression fractures, 572
  intensity of, assessment of, 478, *482*
  location of, 478
  lower back, 1983–1991. See also *Lower back pain.*
  lower extremity, differential diagnosis of, 1401
  meaning of, 476
  menstrual, 980–981

Pain *(Continued)*
  myths and misconceptions about, 463–464, 464b
  negative effects of, 496
  neuropathic, 473
    analgesics for, 491
  nursing diagnoses for, 483b
  nursing management in, 478–483. See also *Pain management.*
  on intercourse, after hysterectomy, 998
  on swallowing, 691
    in esophageal cancer, 700, 701
  ovulatory, 909
  past experience with, 476–477
  pattern of, 478
  perception of, 463
    assessment of, 1888
    physiologic factors in, 463, 466–470
    psychological factors in, 463
  phantom limb, 473, 1412–1413
  physiology of, 466–471
  pleural, 1450t, 1742
  postamputation, 1411, 1412
  postoperative, in hip surgery, 558, 613
    pheochromocytoma and, 1137
  preoperative assessment for, 280
  prostate, 750
  quality of, 478, 483b
  rating scales for, 477–478, *479–482*
  receptors for, 466–468
  referred, 472, *472,* 766
  renal, 750
  rest, 1368, 1400
  situational factors in, 474
  sociocultural factors in, 474–476, 475b
  somatic, 471t, 471–472, 766
  sources of, 471–474
  superficial, 471, 471t
  testicular, 750
  transmission of, 468–470
    inhibition of, 469
  types of, 464–466
  undertreatment of, 461–462, 462b, 494
  urethral, 751
  urinary tract, 750–751
  visceral, 472, 766
Pain attack, 464
Pain ladder, 485, *485*
Pain management. See also *Analgesia; Anesthesia.*
  acupressure in, 498
  acupuncture in, 498
  algorithm for, *501*
  biofeedback in, 499–500
  clinical practice guidelines for, 465
  cold application in, 498, 614b
  complementary therapies in, 496–500
  cutaneous stimulation in, 496–498
  deep breathing in, 499
  distraction in, 500
  documentation of, *502,* 503
  evaluation of, 500–503, *502*
  flow sheet for, *502,* 503
  for chronic intractable pain, 483
  for progressive pain, 483
  guided imagery in, 499
  heat application in, 498, 614b
  humor in, 499
  hypnosis in, 499
  in cancer, 471b
  in emergency care, 2275–2276
  in HIV infection, 474
  in home care, 484b
  in rheumatoid arthritis, 2147, 2148t, 2150–2151, 2151b, 2152b
  in terminal illness, 449–451
  inadequate, 461–462, 462b, 494

Pain management *(Continued)*
  magnets in, 500
  massage in, 497–498, *498*
  meditation in, 499
  misconceptions about, 463, 464b
  music in, 498
  neurolytics in, 483–484
  nonpharmaceutical, 496–500
  outcomes classification for, 459
  patient-controlled analgesia in, 311, *311*
  pharmaceutical, 483–496. See also *Analgesics; Anesthesia.*
  physiology of, 469–470
  placebo effect in, 477
  postoperative, 307, 311, *311*
    preoperative medication for, 290t
    preoperative teaching for, 286
  principles of, 493b
  progressive muscle relaxation in, 498–499
  rescue dosing in, 451
  rhythmic breathing in, 499
  therapeutic relationship in, 481–483
  Therapeutic Touch in, 500
  transcutaneous electrical nerve stimulation in, 497, *497*
Pain threshold, 463
Pain tolerance, 463
Palatal reflex, 1891t
Palatine tonsils, 1612, *1613*
Palliative care, 375, 401, 447, 448–449, 449b
  symptom management in, 447
Palliative surgery, 375, 401
Pallor, elevation, 1372, *1373*
Palm-chin reflex, 1891
Palmomental reflex, 1891
Palpation, 174–177, *175, 177*
  abdominal, 652–655, 655b, 743, 755, *755,* 1077–1078
  bimanual, 174, *177*
    in pelvic examination, 924–925, *925*
  deep, 174, *177*
  light, 174, *177*
  of Bartholin's glands, *923,* 924
  of bladder, 755
  of breast, 920–922, *921*
  of chest, 1630–1631, *1631*
    in cardiac assessment, 1458
  of ear, 1800
  of epididymis, 938
  of head and neck, 1883
  of kidney, 743, 755, *755*
  of liver, 1077–1078
  of lymph nodes, 2094, 2095t
    axillary, 921, *921*
  of nose, 1635
  of paranasal sinuses, 1636
  of penis, 938
  of pulses, 1373, *1374*
  of rectum, 743, *744,* 756
  of scrotum, 938
  of Skene's glands, *923,* 924
  of spleen, 1077
  of testis, 938
  of trachea, 1629
  of urethra, 756
Palpitations, 1451, 1452b
Pamidronate (Aredia), for bone metastases, in breast cancer, 1036
Pancoast's tumor, 1728
Pancreas, abscess of, treatment of, 1198
  anatomy of, 1062–1063
  cancer of, *1201,* 1202
  disorders of, 1193–1203
  function of, 1066
    age-related changes in, 1069
  in cystic fibrosis, 1202–1203
  traumatic injuries of, 1202

Pancreas transplant, 2226
  for diabetes mellitus, 1171–1172
Pancreas-kidney transplant, 2226
Pancreatectomy, subtotal, for acute pancreatitis, 1198
  for chronic pancreatitis, *1201*
  for pancreatic cancer, 1202
Pancreatic enzymes, 635t, 636, 1081t
  in acute pancreatitis, 1194
Pancreatic function, assessment of, 1078, 1081t, 1086
Pancreatic pseudocysts, 1201–1202
Pancreatic rest, 1196, 1197
Pancreaticoduodenectomy, for acute pancreatitis, 1198
  for chronic pancreatitis, *1201*
Pancreaticojejunostomy, for chronic pancreatitis, *1201*
Pancreatitis, acute, 1194–1200
  adult respiratory distress syndrome and, critical monitoring for, 1198b
  assessment in, 1196
  clinical manifestations of, 1195–1196
  complications of, 1196
  computed tomography in, 1195–1196
  epidemiology of, 1194
  etiology of, 1194
  medical management of, 1196
  nursing management of, 1196–1198
  pancreatic pseudocysts and, 1201
  pathophysiology of, 1194
  prognosis of, 1194, 1195b, 1196
  recurrent, 1200
  risk factors for, 1194
  self-care in, 1199–1200
  surgery for, 1198
    nursing management in, 1198–1199
  chronic, 1200–1201, *1201*
    computed tomography in, 1080, *1083*
Pancuronium (Pavulon), 295t
Panic disorder, 412–416, 414b, 426b
Panniculectomy, 1320–1321
PaO₂, in oxyhemoglobin dissociation curve, 1620, *1620*
  measurement of, 1641–1642. See also *Arterial blood gas analysis.*
  reference values for, 2304t
  vs. SaO₂, 1637, 1641t
Papanicolaou smear, 200, 369t, 370, 926–928, *927*, 995, 996
Papaverine, for erectile dysfunction, 974
Papillae, 1263
Papillary adenocarcinoma, thyroid, 1108, 1108t
Papilledema, 2028
  in brain tumors, 1934
Papilloma, intraductal, 1037
  laryngeal, 1660
Papule, *1271*
Paracentesis, 1086–1087
  for ascites, 1246, 1247
Paradoxical blood pressure, 1457
Paralysis, diaphragmatic, 1744
  in spinal cord injury. See *Spinal cord injury.*
  in stroke, 1956, 1957t, *1958*
  of facial nerve, *1996*, 1996–1997
  respiratory, in spinal anesthesia, 296t
  sleep, 435, 437
Paralytic ileus, 791, 792
  postoperative, in cardiac surgery, 1511
  in spinal surgery, 1990–1991
Paranasal sinuses, 1612, *1613*
  examination of, 165t–166t, 1636
Paraphimosis, 970, *970*
Parasinusitis, 1676–1678

Parasitic infections, central nervous system, 1948
  intestinal, 767–768
  pathogenesis of, 337t
  stool examination in, 744t, 745
Parasomnias, 437
Parasympathetic nervous system, effects of on organs, 1870, 1871t
  gastrointestinal function and, 631
  in cardiac regulation, 1443
  structure of, 1870–1872, *1872*
Parathyroid glands, 1062
  disorders of, 1109–1116. See also *Hyperparathyroidism; Hypoparathyroidism.*
    outcomes classification for, 1089
  function of, 1066
    diagnostic tests of, 1111t
Parathyroid hormone (PTH), 535, 1066. See also *Hyperparathyroidism; Hypoparathyroidism.*
  calcium and, 1068
  deficiency of, hypocalcemia and, 249, 250
  in calcium regulation, 249, *249*
  replacement of, 1115
Parathyroid hormone (PTH) radioimmunoassay, 1111t
Parathyroidectomy, 1113–1114
Paraurethral glands, palpation of, *923, 924*
Parenteral nutrition, 668–671. See also *Total parenteral nutrition (TPN).*
Paresthesias, opioid analgesics and, 491
Parietal lobe, 1856, *1858*
Parietal pleura, *1614*, 1617
Parkinson's disease, *2017*, 2017–2020, 2020b, 2021b
Parlodel (bromocriptine), for Parkinson's disease, 2019t
  for premenstrual syndrome, 982
  growth hormone levels and, 1080
Paronychia, 1273t, 1328
Parotitis, 690
Paroxysm, risk factors for, in pheochromocytoma, 1136
Paroxysmal atrial tachycardia, *1555*, 1555–1556
Paroxysmal junctional tachycardia, 1557
Paroxysmal nocturnal dyspnea, 1452, 1534
Pars intermedia, 1061
Parsidol (ethopropazine), for Parkinson's disease, 2019t
Partial thromboplastin time (PTT), 2096–2098, 2099t
  in cardiac assessment, 1465
  in jaundice, 1221t–1222t
  preoperative measurement of, 278t
  reference values for, 2302t
Passive smoking, 39
Pasteur's germ theory, 3, 5t
Past-pointing test, 1804
Patch, for analgesics, 495
Patch tests, 1276–1277, 2101
  for contact dermatitis, 1291
Patella, fractures of, 617
Patellar reflex, 1889, 1891t, *1892*, 1893b
Patellar tendinitis, 620
Pathogens, 335, 337t
  drug-resistant, 339, 341b
  transmission of, 335
Pathologic fractures, in osteoporosis, 566, *566*, 567, 568, 572
Patient care classification, 101–102, 103t
Patient positioning. See *Position; Positioning.*
Patient satisfaction surveys, 102
Patient Self-Determination Act, 67
Patient teaching. See *Client teaching.*
Patient transfer, to intensive care unit, 302

Patient transport, from operating room, 302
  to operating room, 289
Patient-centered communication, 202–203
Patient-controlled analgesia (PCA), 311, *311*, 494–495
Pavementing, cellular, 318, *318*
Pavulon (pancuronium), 295t
PCA. See *Patient-controlled analgesia (PCA).*
PCO₂, 1618, *1619*
  in respiratory control, 1618
  measurement of. See also *Arterial blood gas analysis.*
PCP (phencyclidine), 510t, 514t, 515t, 518–519, 520t–521t
PCWP. See *Pulmonary capillary wedge pressure (PCWP).*
PE. See *Pulmonary embolism (PE).*
Peak bone mass, 566
Peak expiratory flow rate, measurement of, 1637, 1638t
Peak flowmeter, 1637, *1639*
Pediculosis, 1311t
  lindane for, 1280t
Pediculosis capitis, 1272
Pediculosis pubis, 1056
PEEP. See *Positive end-expiratory pressure (PEEP).*
PEG. See *Percutaneous endoscopic gastrostomy (PEG).*
PEJ. See *Percutaneous endoscopic jejunostomy (PEJ).*
Pelvic abscess, *987*, 988
Pelvic examination, 172t, 922–926, *923*
  rectal examination in, 743
Pelvic exenteration, 997, *997*
Pelvic fractures, 616–617
Pelvic inflammatory disease (PID), 986–989. See also *Sexually transmitted diseases.*
  chlamydial, 1047
  chronic, 989
  gonococcal, 1044t, 1049
Pelvic muscle exercises, 836, 838, 958, 1000
Pemphigus, 1310
Penetrating keratoplasty, 1822
Penetrating trauma, to head, 2040
  to liver, 1259
  to pancreas, 1202
Penicillin, for syphilis, 1044t, 1051
  perioperative use of, 275t
Penile clamp, for urinary incontinence, 839, *839*
Penile erection, 911
Penile prostheses, 974, *975*
Penis, cancer of, 972
  circumcised vs. uncircumcised, *938, 970*
  curvature of, 971
  disorders of, 970–972
  examination of, 755–756, 936–938, *937, 938*
  fibrous plaques of, 971–972
  structure and function of, 910–911, 912t, *913*
  traumatic injuries of, 972
Pentazocine (Talwin), 490t
Pentobarbital (Nembutal), for increased intracranial pressure, 2031
  preoperative, 290t
Pentothal (thiopental), 294t
  for rapid-sequence induction, 2268
Peppermint oil, for irritable bowel syndrome, 794b
Pepsin, gastric secretion of, measurement of, 658–659
Peptic ulcer disease (PUD), 712–724
  assessment in, 718
  bleeding in, 715b, 715–717, 716b
  case study of, 723–724

Peptic ulcer disease (Continued)
  chronic gastritis in, 709
  client teaching in, 718–719
  clinical manifestations of, 714
  drug therapy for, 711t–712t, 715
  duodenal ulcers in, 712, 713t
  etiology of, 712–713
  gastric acids and, 636
  gastric ulcers in, 712, 713t
  medical management in, 714–717
  nursing management in, 718–719
  obstruction in, 717
  pathophysiology of, 713–714
  perforation in, 717, 717
  risk factors for, 713
  surgery for, 717, 719–724. See also Gastric
    surgery.
    case study of, 723–724
Peptides, 1061
Perceptual deficits, in stroke, 1957t, 1958–
  1960, 1959, 1976–1977
Percocet (Oxycodone), 489t
Percussion, 177–178, 178
  direct, 177, 178
  indirect, 177–178, 178
  of abdomen, 652–655, 655b, 742–743, 754,
    755, 1077
    in ascites, 1247
  of bladder, 754, 755
  of chest, 1631, 1631–1632
  of kidney, 754, 755
  of liver, 1077
  of spleen, 1077
  sounds on, 177–178
Percutaneous cholecystolithotomy, 1208
Percutaneous discectomy, 1987, 1989–1991
Percutaneous endoscopic gastrostomy (PEG),
  673, 673, 693, 693. See also Enteral nu-
  trition.
Percutaneous endoscopic jejunostomy (PEJ),
  673, 693
Percutaneous lithotripsy, 828
Percutaneous liver biopsy, 1084, 1085
Percutaneous nephrostomy, 813, 814–815
Percutaneous pyelostomy, 814–815
Percutaneous transhepatic cholangiography,
  1086
Percutaneous transluminal angioplasty (PTA),
  1405–1406
Percutaneous transluminal coronary angioplasty
  (PTCA), 1521, 1521–1522
Percutaneous transluminal renal angioplasty,
  870
Perforins, 2081
Performance improvement, 104–105, 105b
Performance status, cancer treatment and, 373,
  374t
Perfusion, ventilation and, 1620–1621, 1621
Pergolide (Permax), for Parkinson's disease,
  2019t
Pericardial effusion, 1489
  aspiration of, 1490, 1490
  cardiac tamponade and, 1489–1490
  in cancer, 397
Pericardial friction rub, 1460, 1489
Pericardial tamponade, shock and, 2233
Pericardiocentesis, 1490, 1490
  emergency, 2275, 2276
Pericarditis, 1488b, 1488–1490
  chest pain in, 1449t
  constrictive, heart failure and, 1531
  in chronic renal failure, 883
  postinfarction, 1596
Pericardium, 1435, 1436
Perilymph, 1785
Perimenopausal period, 910
Perineal prostatectomy, 954, 955

Perinephric abscess, 858
Perineum, 904
Periodic limb movement disorder, 436
Periodontal disease, 683, 684
Perioperative nursing, 273–274. See also under Intraoperative; Postoperative; Preoperative.
  definition of, 273
  nursing outcomes classification for, 273
  principles of, 273–274
Periosteum, 531, 534
Peripheral aneurysms, 1422
Peripheral arterial disorders, 1421–1422
Peripheral arterial occlusive disease, 1399–
  1415
  clinical manifestations of, 1400–1401
  etiology of, 1399
  in elderly, 1404
  medical management of, 1401–1402
  nursing management in, 1402–1404
  pathophysiology of, 1399–1400, 1400
  risk factors for, 1399
  surgery for, 1404–1407
    arterial bypass in, 1406–1407, 1407
    complications, 1409
    endovascular procedures in, 1404–1405
    nursing management in, 1407–1415
    percutaneous transluminal angioplasty in,
      1405–1406
    postoperative care in, 1407–1409, 1408b–
      1409b
    preoperative care in, 1407
    self-care in, 1409
Peripheral blood smear, 2096, 2098t
Peripheral nerve assessment, in musculoskeletal assessment, 542, 547
Peripheral nerve block. See also Anesthesia.
Peripheral nerve injuries, 2000–2001
Peripheral nerve stimulator, in mechanical ventilation, 1756, 1760
Peripheral nerve tumors, 2001
Peripheral nervous system, age-related changes
  in, 1873
  structure of, 1868, 1869, 1869–1870, 1870t
Peripheral neuropathy, 1997–2001
  in chronic renal failure, 883
Peripheral stem cells, harvesting of, 2180
Peripheral vascular disease, 1399–1431
  arterial, 1399–1422
  definition of, 1399
  home care in, 1428b
  in diabetes mellitus, 1183t, 1184, 1185
  lymphatic, 1429–1431
  outcome classifications for, 1399
  renal function in, 853
  venous, 1422–1429
Peripherally inserted central catheter, for
  chemotherapy, 386, 386
Peristalsis, 632–633
Peritoneal dialysis. See Dialysis, peritoneal.
Peritoneal friction rub, 1474
Peritoneal lavage, diagnostic, 2273, 2273
Peritoneal tap (paracentesis), 1086–1087
Peritoneoscopy, 1083–1084
Peritoneovenous shunt, for ascites, 1247, 1250,
  1250
Peritonitis, 769–770
  in peritoneal dialysis, 891
Peritonsillar abscess, 1679
Permanent sections, 201
Permax (pergolide), for Parkinson's disease,
  2019t
Pernicious anemia, 2113–2114
Peroneal nerve, examination of, 547
PERRLA/PERL, 1884–1885, 2034
Personal habits, screening and prevention and,
  150t–152t

Personal resources, assessment of, 144
Personality, assessment of, 144
  disease and, 7t
Pertussis, immunization for, 342t
Pessary, for urinary incontinence, 838
  vaginal, 1000
PET. See Positron emission tomography
  (PET).
Petechiae, 1372
Petrosal sinuses, ACTH levels in, hypercorti-
  solism and, 1130
Peyote, 510t, 517–518, 520t–521t
Peyronie's disease, 971–972
pH, 259
  arterial blood, measurement of, 1641–1642.
    See also Arterial blood gas analysis.
  reference values for, 2304t
  esophageal, ambulatory monitoring of, 659
  regulation of, 259–264. See also Acid-base
    balance.
  urine, 756, 757t
    reference values for, 2306t
Phacoemulsification, for cataract, 1815
Phagocytosis, 317, 317–318, 318
Phalen's test, 544t, 1998, 2000
Phantom limb sensation, 473, 1411, 1412
Pharmacodynamics, in elderly, 61
Pharmacokinetics, in elderly, 60–61
Pharyngeal reflex, 1886, 1889, 1891t
Pharyngitis, 1678
  herbal remedies for, 1626
  in chronic tonsillitis, 1679
  streptococcal, rheumatic heart disease and,
    1484
Pharynx, anatomy of, 1612–1613, 1613
  examination of, 166t
Phenazopyridine (Pyridium), for urinary tract
  infection, 805t, 806
Phencyclidine (PCP), 510t, 514t, 515t, 518–
  519, 520t–521t
Phenobarbital, for epilepsy, 1927t, 1927–1928
  reference values for, 2307t
Phenothiazines, for pain, 491
  overdose of, antidote for, 2281t
Phentolamine, for erectile dysfunction, 974
  for hypertensive emergencies, 1396t
Phenylalanine, reference values for, 2304t
Phenylpyruvic acid, urine, reference values for,
  2306t
Phenytoin (Dilantin), 1927t, 1927–1928
  for status epilepticus, 1931
  gingival hyperplasia and, 1930
  reference values for, 2307t
Pheochromocytoma, 1135t, 1135–1137
Philadelphia chromosome, in chronic leukemia,
  2166–2167
Philadelphia collar, 2269, 2269
Phimosis, 970–972
Phlebotomy, for hemochromatosis, 1258
Phobias, 413–416, 414b
Phonocardiography, 1474
Phosphate, as buffer, 261, 262
  imbalances of, 254. See also Hyperphospha-
    temia; Hypophosphatemia.
  plasma levels of, 235b, 254
  serum, reference values for, 2304t
  urine, reference values for, 2306t
Phosphorus, in cardiac assessment, 1465
  in parathyroid disorders, 1111t, 1115,
    1116
  reference values for, 549t, 2304t
Photochemotherapy, 1284
Photocoagulation, for diabetic retinopathy,
  1187
Photodamage, 1302
Photodynamic therapy, for esophageal cancer,
  700

Photographic documentation, in plastic surgery, 1316
Photoplethysmography, 1325
Photorefractive keratectomy, 1828
Photosensitivity, in chemotherapy, 395
Physical examination, 163–185
  accuracy of, 163
  auscultation in, 178–179, *179*
  balance assessment in, 182–183
  branching, 163
  client preparation for, 180, *181*
  comparison of findings in, 185
  complete, 163
  data processing for, 185
  documentation of, 185
  draping for, 180, *181*
  equipment for, *176*
    preparation of, 179–180
  general survey in, 164t, 180
  guidelines for, 179–180
  health teaching in, 185
  height and weight in, 182
  inspection in, 174
  levels of, 163
  motor examination in, 171t
  neurologic examination in, 170t–171t
  nursing process in, 163–174
  of abdomen, 169t–170t
  of aorta, 169t
  of axillae, 168t
  of breast, 168t
  of carotid vessels, 168t
  of ear, 164t–165t
  of eye, 164t–165t
  of genitals, in female, 173t
    in male, 171t
  of head and neck, 164t–166t
  of jugular veins, 168t–169t
  of kidneys, 167t–168t, 169t
  of liver, 169t
  of lower extremities, 170t
  of lungs, 167t, 168t
  of mouth, 166t
  of neck, 166t
  of pharynx, 166t
  of prostate, 172t–173t
  of rectum and anus, 172t–173t
  of sinuses, 165t
  of spine, 167t, 170t–171t
  of spleen, 169t
  of upper extremities, 167t
  olfaction in, 179
  palpation in, 174–177, *175*
  percussion in, 177–178, *178*
  periodic head-to-toe, 163, 173b
  positioning for, 180, *181*
  preoperative, 276–282, 279b
  preparation for, client, 180, *181*
    environmental, 179
    equipment, 179
    examiner, 180
  purpose of, 163
  regional, 163, 164t–173t
  screening, 163, 180–185. See also *Screening.*
  sensory examination in, 170t–171t
  skin color in, 185
  suspected problem areas in, 185
  techniques of, 174–179, *175*
  termination of, 185
  vital signs in, 183b, 183–185
Physical therapy, for burns, 1348–1349
  in stroke rehabilitation, 1968, 1971, 1973–1974
Physician, attending, 96
  in health care system, 75
Physician group practices, nursing care in, 87
Pia mater, 1862, *1862*

PID. See *Pelvic inflammatory disease (PID).*
Pigeon chest, 1629, *1630*
Pigmentation, of skin, 1262
Pilocarpine, perioperative use of, 275t
Pilonidal cyst, 797
Pinna, 1782, *1783*, 1800
  traumatic injuries of, 1842
Pinocytosis, 1366
Pinworms, 767–768
Piroxicam, 486, 487t
Pitting edema, 1371–1372, *1372*
Pituitary, tumors of, 1932. See also *Brain tumors.*
Pituitary function, assessment of, 1080
Pituitary gland, ACTH oversecretion by, hypercortisolism due to, 1130
  radiation therapy in, 1132
  anatomy of, 1061, 1062, *1063*
  anterior, 1062, *1063*
    disorders of, 1137–1143. See also *Hyperpituitarism; Hypopituitarism.*
  hormones regulated by, *1063*, 1065, 1138t.
    See also specific hormones.
  in shock, 2239–2240
  posterior, 1062, *1063*
    disorders of, 1138t, 1143, 1144t–1145t
  tumors of, hypercortisolism due to, 1130–1131
    hyperpituitarism due to, hyperprolactinemia and, *1139*, 1139–1142, *1140*, 1141t
Pituitary surgery, 1935–1937, *1936*
Placebo effect, in pain management, 477
Plantar fasciitis, 620
Plantar neuroma, 582–583
Plantar reflex, 1889, 1891t
Plaque(s), amyloid, in Alzheimer's disease, 2003, *2003*
  atherosclerotic, 1518–1520, 1519t–1520t
    rupture of, 1585
    stroke and, 1954
  fibrous penile, 971–972
  myelin sheath, in multiple sclerosis, 2012, *2013*
  skin, *1271*
Plasma, 2074–2075, *2075*
  reference values for, 2303t–2305t
Plasma membrane, *206*, 207t, 208–209, *209*
Plasmapheresis, for myasthenia gravis, 2022
Plastic surgery, 1313–1326
  aesthetic, 1313–1321
  blepharoplasty in, *1317*, 1318
  body-contouring, 1319–1321
  client motivations for, 1314–1316
  client selection for, 1314
  for breast augmentation, 1037–1038, *1038*
  for breast reduction, 1038, *1038*
  photographic documentation in, 1316
  postoperative care in, by unlicensed assistive personnel, 1320b
  reconstructive, 375, 1313, 1321–1326
    flaps in, *1323*, 1323–1325, 1324b
    for burns, 1353–1354
    grafts in, 1322–1323, *1324*
    implants in, 1325, *1325*
    in breast cancer, *1029*, 1029–1031, *1030*
    skin expansion in, 1029, 1325–1326
  rhinoplasty in, 1319
  rhytidectomy in, 1316–1318, *1317*
  technical aspects of, 1314, *1314*
Platelet(s), 2078
  deficiency of, in cancer, 393
    in disseminated intravascular coagulation, 2124
  disorders of, 2122–2123
  in hemostasis, 2079, *2079*
  liver function and, 1082t
  production of, 2078
  reference ranges for, 2096t, 2302t

Platelet count, 2099t
Platelet-derived growth factor, in wound healing, 320
Platform posturography, 1806, *1806*
Plethysmography, in venous thrombosis, 1424–1425
  volume, 1637, *1640*
Pleurae, *1614*, 1617
Pleural biopsy, 1649
Pleural effusion, 226, 1742–1743
Pleural friction rub, 1633, 1634t
Pleural pain, 1450t, 1742
Pleural space, 1617
Pleural stripping, 1743
Pleural tumors, metastatic, 1743
Pleurectomy, 1743
Pleurisy, 1450t, 1742
Pleurodesis, 1743
Plexuses, 1869
PLISSIT model, 395
PMS. See *Premenstrual syndrome (PMS).*
Pneumatic antishock garment, 2245, *2246*
Pneumatic compression devices, 1423, *1424*
Pneumaturia, 750
Pneumococcal pneumonia, 1711–1716, 1712t
  immunization for, 342, 342t
Pneumoconioses, 1739–1740, 1740t
Pneumocystis carinii pneumonia, in HIV infection, 2199, 2202, 2204
Pneumocytes, 1616
Pneumonectomy, 1730, *1731*. See also *Thoracic surgery.*
Pneumonia, 1711–1716
  aspiration, balloon tamponade and, 1243
  bacterial, in HIV infection, 2203
  case management in, 1715b
  chest pain in, 1450t
  classification of, 1713, *1714*
  clinical manifestations of, 1712t–1713t, 1713
  clinical pathway for, 1716b, 1717b
  diabetes mellitus and, case study of, *1153*, 1153–1154
  diagnosis of, 1713
  etiology of, 1711, 1712t–1713t
  in chronic obstructive pulmonary disease, 1696
  in tracheostomy, 1655
  lung abscess and, 1716
  medical management of, 1712t–1713t, 1713–1714
  nosocomial, 338–339, 338t
  nursing management of, 1714–1715
  P. carinii, in HIV infection, 2199, 2202, 2204
  pathogenesis of, 337t
  pathophysiology of, 1713
  pneumococcal, 1711–1716, 1712t
    immunization for, 342, 342t
  postoperative, cholelithiasis and, 1210
  prevention of, 1715b
  risk factors for, 1711–1713
  self-care in, 1715b–1716b
  types of, 1712t–1713t, 1713–1714, *1714*
Pneumonitis, hypersensitivity, 1739, 1740t
Pneumothorax, 1617
  chest pain in, 1450t
  clinical manifestations of, 1766–1767
  closed, 1765–1766, *1766*
  emergency care for, *2271*, 2271–2272
  in chronic obstructive pulmonary disease, 1696
  in thoracic surgery, 1731
  open, 1766, *1766*, 1767
    conversion of tension pneumothorax to, 1768
  severity of, 1766–1767

Pneumothorax *(Continued)*
  tension, *1766, 1767*–1768. See also *Pneumothorax.*
    emergency care for, *2271, 2271*–2272
    open pneumothorax conversion to, 1767
    shock and, 2233
  traumatic, 1766–1768
PO₂, 1618, *1619*
  in oxyhemoglobin dissociation curve, 1620, *1620*
  in respiratory control, 1618
  measurement of, 1641–1642. See also *Arterial blood gas analysis.*
Podofilox, for genital warts, 1054
Podophyllin, for genital warts, 1054
Poietins, 2075
Point of maximum intensity, 1458
Point-to-point testing, 1887
Poisoning, 2281t, 2281–2282
  reference values in, 2309t
Polio, immunization for, 342t
  post-polio syndrome and, 1993
Polyclonal antibodies, for transplant immunosuppression, 2224t
Polycystic kidney disease, *871,* 871–872
Polycythemia vera, 2118
Polydipsia, in diabetes mellitus, 1156t
Polymenorrhea, 996
Polymorphonuclear neutrophils (polys). See *Neutrophils.*
Polymyalgia rheumatica, 2163
Polymyositis, 2162
Polymyxin B, for burns, 1348t
Polymyxin B–bacitracin (Polysporin), 327t
Polyneuropathy, in diabetes mellitus, 1188
Polypeptides, 1061
Polyphagia, in diabetes mellitus, 1156t
Polypharmacy, in elderly, 60b, 61
Polyps, colonic, cancer and, 781
  genital, 1000
  laryngeal, 1660
  nasal, 1682
  uterine, 1000
Polysomnography, 440, *441*
Polysporin, 327t
Polyuria, 747
  in acute renal failure, 877
  in diabetes mellitus, 1156t
Pons, 1858–1859, 1859t, *1860*
Pontocaine (tetracaine), 297t
Popliteal pulse, assessment of, 1373, *1374*
Porphobilinogen, urine, reference values for, 2306t
Porphyrins, urine, reference values for, 2306t
Port, implanted, for chemotherapy, 386, *386*
Portacaval shunt, 1243, *1244*
Portal hypertension, assessment in, 1242
  bleeding in, *1241,* 1241b, 1241–1242, *1242*
    prevention of, 1243
  clinical manifestations of, 1241
  confusion and, 1243
  critical monitoring in, 1241b
  diagnosis of, 1084
  etiology of, 1240
  gas exchange and, 1243
  in cirrhosis, 1234, 1240b, 1240–1245, *1241, 1241b, 1242, 1244*
  medical management of, *1241,* 1241b, 1241–1242, *1242*
  nursing management of, 1242–1243
  pathophysiology of, 1240–1241
  risk factors for, 1240, 1240b
  surgery for, 1243–1244, *1244*
    nursing management in, 1244–1245
Portal of entry, 336
Portal of exit, 336
Portal pressure, measurements of, 1084

Portal vein, 1060, *1061*
Portal vein bacteremia, liver abscess and, 1258
Porter-Silber reaction, 1122t
Portosystemic shunt, for bleeding esophageal varices, 1242
  for portal hypertension, 1243–1245, *1244*
Position, dorsal recumbent, *181,* 299, *300*
  knee chest, *181*
  laminectomy, *300*
  lateral, 299, *300*
  lithotomy, *181,* 299, *300*
  prone, *181*
  Sims', *181*
  sitting, *181*
  standing, *181*
  supine, *181,* 299, *300*
  Trendelenburg, 299, *300*
Positioning, for breast examination, *921*
  for burn patients, 1349, 1351t
  for lumbar puncture, 1897, *1897*
  for pelvic examination, 922
  for physical examination, 180, *181*
  for pressure ulcer prevention, 612, 613
  for spinal anesthesia, *296*
  for surgery, 299, 299b, *300*
  in adult respiratory distress syndrome, 1763, *1764*
  in heart failure, 1536
  in lower back pain, 1986
  in peripheral vascular disease, 1402, 1403
  in pulmonary edema, 1748
  in shock, 2246, *2246*
  in total hip replacement, 558, 560, *560*
  postoperative, 303, *303*
Positive end-expiratory pressure (PEEP), in mechanical ventilation, 1754–1755
  in shock, 2244
Positron emission tomography (PET), *197,* 197–198
  in cardiac assessment, 1472–1473
  in myocardial infarction, 1590
  in neurologic assessment, 1896
  procedure for, 197–198
Post-anesthesia care unit (PACU). See also *Postoperative period.*
  admission to, 303, 303b
  airway management in, 303, *303,* 304, *306*
  assessment in, 303–304
  blood pressure maintenance in, 304–305
  discharge from, 307b, 307–308
  documentation in, 304, *305*
  equipment in, 303b
  nursing care in, 303–307
  patient monitoring in, 304–307
  records needed in, 303, 303b
Postconcussion headache, 1950
Postconcussion syndrome, 1950
Posterior cruciate ligament, *535*
Posterior drawer test, 545t, *546*
Posterior plug, for epistaxis, 1675, 1676, *1676*
Posterior sag sign, 545t
Posterior tibial pulse, assessment of, 1373, *1374*
Posthitis, 970, *971*
Postictal state, 1924
Postoperative period, 302–313
  airway management in, 303, *303,* 304, *306,* 308, *308*
  ambulation in, 286, 308
  assessment in, 308–312
    immediate, 303–304
  breathing exercises for, 285–286, *286,* 308, *308*
  circulatory assessment in, 304–305, 308
  confusion in, 612
  coughing in, 286
  diabetes mellitus and, 1189–1190

Postoperative period *(Continued)*
  discharge from post-anesthesia care unit in, 307b, 307–308
  discharge instructions and care in, 312, 312b
  documentation in, 304, *305*
  extremity exercises in, 286
  fluid management in, 307, 309–310
  home care in, 312, 312b
  hypertension in, 305
  hypotension in, 304–305
  hypothermia in, 306
  immediate assessment in, 303–304
  monitoring in, 302–304, 308–311
  nausea and vomiting in, 311b, 311–312
  neurologic assessment in, 306, 308–309
  nursing care in, 308–312
    immediate, 303–304
  orientation in, 306
  pain management in, 286–287, 307, 311, *311*
    preoperative medication for, 290t
  patient positioning in, 303, *303*
  post-anesthesia care in. See also *Post-anesthesia care unit (PACU).*
  safety concerns in, 307
  turning exercises in, 286
  wound care in, 307, 309, *309*
Postphlebitic syndrome, *1427,* 1427–1429
Post-polio syndrome, 1993
Postprandial renal hyperemia, 738
Poststreptococcal glomerulonephritis, 864t
Post-trauma response, 2034t
Post-traumatic arthritis, 601
Post-traumatic stress disorder, 413–416, 414b
Post-traumatic vessel disease, 1324
Postural blood pressure, 1457, *1457*
Postural drainage, for chronic obstructive pulmonary disease, 1698
Postural hypotension, 1397, 1849
  in dehydration, 219
  opioid analgesics and, 491
Posture, assessment of, 540–541, *541*
Postvoid residual, 748, 831
Potassium, dietary restriction of, in hemodialysis, 895
  dietary sources of, 245b
  fluid concentration of, 234t
  in acid-base balance, 261
  in cardiac assessment, 1465
  plasma levels of, 235b
  recommended intake of, 242–243
  replacement of, in diabetic ketoacidosis, 1175, 1176b
    in hypokalemia, 244, 245–246
  serum, reference values for, 2304t
  supplemental, for hypertension, 1387
  urine, reference values for, 2307t
Potassium balance, disturbances of, 243–248. See also *Hyperkalemia; Hypokalemia.*
  in diabetic ketoacidosis, 1174, 1174t, 1175, 1176b
  preoperative assessment of, 277t
  regulation of, 242–243
Potassium hydroxide test, 1276
Potassium iodide, for hyperthyroidism, 1101
Potassium ions, in pain, 467
Potassium-sparing diuretics, hypermagnesemia and, 256
Pott's fracture, 596t
Pouch, colostomy, 774–776, 786b
  ileal, with anal anastomosis, 775–776, *776*
  ileostomy, 777–778, 778b, 786b
  Indiana, *813,* 813–814, *814.* See also *Urinary diversion.*
  Kock, 775, *775*
  rectal, 799
Povidone-iodine (Betadine), 327t, 332

Powders, 1281t
Power of attorney for health care, 67, 2009
PPOs (preferred provider organizations), 78b, 80–81
PQRST mnemonic, for pain assessment, 2266
Prandin. See *Repaglinide (Prandin).*
Prazosin (Minipress), for hypertension, 1389t
Prealbumin, preoperative measurement of, 278t
  serum, normal values for, 656t
    reference ranges for, 656t
Precancerous changes, 211
Precapillary sphincters, 1362
Precautions, barrier, 343–344
Precordium, auscultation of, 1459–1461
  inspection of, 1458
Precose. See *Acarbose (Precose).*
Prednisone (Deltasone), for asthma, 1690, 1691t, *1692, 1694*
  for myasthenia gravis, 2022
  perioperative use of, 275t
Pre-excitation syndromes, 1565–1566
Preferred provider organizations (PPOs), 78b, 80–81
Prefrontal cortex, 1856
Pregnancy, cervical cancer in, 996
  chemotherapy in, 395
  diabetes mellitus in, 1149–1150
  diagnosis of, 983
  ectopic, *1000*
  HIV transmission in, 2189
  renal function in, 8533
Pregnanediol, reference values for, 2307t
Pregnanetriol, reference values for, 2307t
Preload, 1441, *1442,* 1530, 1530t
  reduction of, 1538t, 1546, 1748
    in pulmonary edema, 1748
Premature atrial contractions, 1554, *1554*
Premature junctional contractions, 1557, *1557*
Premature ventricular contractions, 1560–1562, *1561*
Premenstrual syndrome (PMS), 981–982
  sleep problems in, 438
Preoperative period, 274–290
  anesthesia concerns in, 282, 284b
  anxiety in, 285
  assessment in, 274–276
  client teaching in, 282, 284–287
  diabetes mellitus and, 1189
  drug administration in, 289, 290t
  family needs in, 289–290
  final patient preparation in, 289, 289b
  laboratory studies in, 277t–278t
  NPO status in, 284
  nursing diagnoses for, 282
  patient transport in, 289
  physical examination in, 276–282
  risk assessment in, 282, 284b
  room preparation in, 289
  skin preparation in, 282
  surgery-day care in, 288–290
Presbycusis, 1786, 1832
Presbyopia, 1782
Presbystasis, 1849
Pressure flow study, 762, *762*
Pressure garments, for burns, 1354, *1356*
Pressure reducing devices/surfaces, *1300,* 1914, *1914*
Pressure ulcers, 612, 1295–1302
  Braden scale for, 1298, *1299*
  case management for, 1302b
  clinical manifestations of, 1296
  debridement of, 1296
  etiology of, 1295–1296
  home care for, 1303b
  infection of, 1296
  medical management of, 1296–1298
  nursing management of, 1298–1302

Pressure ulcers *(Continued)*
  nutritional support for, 1296–1297, 1298
  pathophysiology of, 1296
  prevention of, 612, 613, 618b, 1300b, 2059
    in comatose patients, 1914
    in spinal cord injury, 2064
  risk factors for, 1295–1296, 1298, *1299*
  self-care for, 1301–1302
  staging of, *1297*
  surgery for, 1302
Prevacid (lansoprazole), for gastroesophageal reflux disease, 696
Prevention, 10–11, 24–28, 36–40. See also *Health promotion.*
  in chronic conditions, 24–28
  levels of, 10–11, 11t, 84–85, 85b
  primary, 84, 85b
  secondary, 85, 85b
  tertiary, 85, 85b
Priapism, 972
Priftin (rifapentine), for tuberculosis, 1720, 1721t
Prilosec (omeprazole), for peptic ulcer disease, 710t, 711t, 715
Primary care, 85
Primary nursing, 99
Primary prevention, 10, 11t, 84–85, 85b
Primidone, reference values for, 2307t
Prisoners, as organ donors/recipients, 2215
Problem Classification Scheme, in Omaha System, 112–114, 113b, 114b, 114t
Problem Rating Scale for Outcomes, in Omaha System, 115–116, 116t
Procainamide, perioperative use of, 275t
  reference values for, 2308t
Procaine, 484
Procardia (nifedipine), for hypertension, 1389t
Proctocolectomy, total, 775
Proctosigmoidectomy, *783*
Proctosigmoidoscopy, 746–747
Procyclidine (Kemadrin), for Parkinson's disease, 2019t
Progesterone, 908
  in menstrual cycle, 908–910
  pharmaceutical, 908
    for premenstrual syndrome, 982
    in hormone replacement therapy, 985–986
Progesterone receptors, in breast cancer, 1020, 1035
Programmed cell death, *361,* 361–362
Progressive multifocal leukoencephalopathy, in HIV infection, 2205
Progressive muscle relaxation, 27, 36, 498–499
Progressive systemic sclerosis, 2159–2160, *2160*
Project PACE, 33
Projection, 408b
Prokaryotic cell, 206
Prolactin, 1065, 1138t. See also *Hyperprolactinemia.*
  hypopituitarism and, 1143
  reference values for, 2305t
Prolapse, bladder, 998, *998*
  urethral, 998, *998*
  uterine, *999,* 999–1000
  vaginal, *999,* 999–1000
Promethazine, preoperative, 290t
Pronator drift, 1886
Prone position, *181*
Propafenone (Rhythmol), for dysrhythmias, 1562t
Propantheline bromide (Pro-Banthine), for urinary incontinence, 837t
Propofol (Diprivan), for rapid-sequence induction, 2268

Propoxyphene (Darvon), 489t
Propranolol (Inderal), for hypertension, 1389t
  perioperative use of, 275t
  reference values for, 2308t
Proprietary hospitals, 96
Proprioception, assessment of, 1887, 1888
  in stroke, 1960
Propulsid (cisapride), for gastroesophageal reflux disease, 696
Propylthiouracil (PTU), for hyperthyroidism, 1096t, 1100–1101
Proscar (finasteride), for benign prostatic hyperplasia, 947
Prospective payment systems (PPSs), 80
Prostaglandin(s), 319
  in pain, 468
  intrarenal, 737
Prostaglandin E, for erectile dysfunction, 974
Prostaglandin synthesis inhibitors, for dysmenorrhea, 981
Prostate, balloon dilation of, 955, *955*
  benign hyperplasia of. See *Benign prostatic hyperplasia (BPH).*
  biopsy of, 761, 942
  disorders of, 945–964
  examination of, 172t–173t, 939, *940*
  imaging of, 758–760
  pain in, 750
  structure and function of, 735, 911t, *912,* 912–913
  transurethral incision of, 955
  ultrasonography of, 758–760, 941
Prostate cancer, 958–962
  alkaline phosphatase in, 941
  prevention of, 370
  risk factors for, 370, 959
  screening for, 41, 159t, 358, 369t, 370, 940–941
Prostate intraepithelial neoplasia, 960
Prostate surgery, self-care in, 958
Prostatectomy, for benign prostatic hyperplasia, 949
  perineal, *954,* 955
  radical, 960–961
  retropubic, *954, 955*
  suprapubic, 949–954, *954*
Prostate-specific antigen (PSA), 358
  in prostate cancer, 41, 159t, 358, 369t, 370, 940–941, 959–960
  test for, 940–941
Prostate-specific antigen density, 941, 959
Prostate-specific antigen velocity, 941
Prostatic fluid, 913
Prostatic massage, 939, *940*
Prostatic stent, for benign prostatic hyperplasia, 956
Prostatic urethra, 912–913
Prostatitis, 962–964, *963*
Prosthesis, antireflux, 697, *697*
  bladder neck support, 837, *837*
  breast, 1028–1029
  limb, 1412–1413, *1413,* 1414b
  middle ear, *1846,* 1846–1847
  ocular, 1825, *1826*
  penile, 974, *975*
Prosthetic heart valves, 1502, *1503*
Protease, in acute pancreatitis, 1194
Protease inhibitors, for HIV infection, 2195–2199, 2197t–2198t
Protective reflexes, 1883
Protein(s), 1061
  deficiency of, ketosis in, 214
  dietary restriction of, in chronic renal failure, 886, 894, *894*
  digestion and absorption of, 636
  in fluid balance, 216

Protein(s) (Continued)
  membrane, 208
  renal function and, 738
  serum, 655, 655t
    reference values for, 655, 655t, 2305t
    urine, reference values for, 2307t
Protein intake, in diabetes mellitus, 1165–
  1166, 1166t
Protein metabolism, in diabetes mellitus, 1155
  liver in, 1065
  tests of, 1082t
Protein osmotic pressure, 216
Protein restriction, in hepatic encephalopathy,
  1252
Protein-energy malnutrition, 639, 640t, 661–
  662. See also Malnutrition.
Proteinuria, 757, 757t
  in chronic renal failure, 881–882
  in diabetes mellitus, 1158
  in nephrotic syndrome, 863
Prothrombin, deficiency of, 2123
Prothrombin time (PT), 2096–2098, 2099t
  in cardiac assessment, 1465
  in jaundice, 1220, 1221t–1222t
  liver function and, 1082t
  preoperative measurement of, 278t
  reference values for, 2302t
Prototype evaluation method, 102, 103t
Protozoal infections, intestinal, 767
Proventil (albuterol), for asthma, 1690, 1691t,
  1692, 1694
  for hyperkalemia, 247
Pruritus, drugs for, 1280t
  in atopic dermatitis, 1287–1288
  in chronic renal failure, 887, 888
  in jaundice, 1223
  in skin disorders, 1284–1285, 1286
  vaginal, 1002
PSA. See Prostate-specific antigen (PSA).
Pseudoaneurysm, in angiography, 1376
Pseudocysts, pancreatic, 1201–1202
Pseudoephedrine (Sudafed), for urinary incon-
  tinence, 837t
Pseudogout, hemochromatosis and, 1258
Pseudohypertrophic muscular dystrophy, 583t,
  583–584
Pseudohypoparathyroidism, 1114
Pseudomembranous colitis, 766–767, 768
Pseudopregnancy, for endometriosis, 990
Pseudoseizures, 1931
Psilocybin, 510t, 517–518, 520t–521t
Psoralen plus ultraviolet light (PUVA) therapy,
  1284
Psoriasis vulgaris, 1292, 1292–1293
Psychedelic drugs, 510t, 514t, 517–518
Psychiatric disorders. See Mental health prob-
  lems.
Psychiatric referral, 411
  for anxiety disorders, 416
  for bipolar disorder, 428
  for depression, 423–424
  for schizophrenia, 419–420
Psychiatric treatment, levels of, 417t
  referral for. See Psychiatric referral.
Psychoanalytic view, of mood disorders, 421
Psychological assessment, 138–144, 140t–
  143t, 409–411, 410t
  rating scales for, 417b
Psychopharmacologic drugs, reference ranges
  for, 2308t
Psychosocial assessment, 137–145, 139b,
  140t–143t, 409–410, 410t
  cultural component of, 145, 146–147
  mental status assessment in, 139–144
  psychological component of, 138–144,
    140t–143t, 409–411, 410t
  social component of, 140t–143t, 144–145

Psychosocial concerns, 405–428. See also
  Mental health problems.
  anxiety as, 407, 407b, 408t
  examples of, 406–407
  in aging, 55–58
  in amputation, 1410, 1414
  in breast cancer, 1024–1025
  in burns, 1335, 1338, 1349, 1354
  in cancer, 385, 397–398, 397–402
  in chronic conditions, 17–18, 18t
  in chronic renal failure, 887, 897
  in emergency care, 2283
  in epilepsy, 1930
  in erectile dysfunction, 972–974
  in hearing impairment, 1838
  in HIV infection, 2200
  in hyperthyroidism, 1103
  in irritable bowel syndrome, 793
  in lower back pain, 1983–1984
  in mastectomy, 1024–1025
  in menopause, 910
  in menstrual disorders, 980
  in radical vulvectomy, 1007
  in reproductive history, in female, 919
  in spinal cord injury, 2060, 2065–2066
  in stroke, 1977
  in transplantation, 2219
  nursing diagnoses for, 406b
  self-esteem as, 409, 410t
  stress as, 407b, 407–408
  universal, 407–409
Psychosocial development, assessment of, 144
Psychosocial history, 137–144, 139b, 140t–
  143t
Psychosocial risk factors, 138, 139b
Psychosocial theories, of disease causation, 3,
  5t–6t
Psychotherapy. See Psychiatric treatment.
PT. See Prothrombin time (PT).
PTA. See Percutaneous transluminal angio-
  plasty (PTA).
PTCA. See Percutaneous transluminal coro-
  nary angioplasty (PTCA).
PTH. See Parathyroid hormone (PTH).
Ptosis, 1827t, 1885
  in myasthenia gravis, 2020
PTT. See Partial thromboplastin time (PTT).
PTU. See Propylthiouracil (PTU).
Puberty, in male, 908
  menarche and, 908
Pubic hair, examination of, in female, 922–
  923
  in male, 936
Pubic lice, 1056
PUD. See Peptic ulcer disease (PUD).
Pudendum, 904
Pulmonary angiography, 1647, 1706, 1706
Pulmonary artery catheterization, 1476,
  1477b–1478b
Pulmonary capillary wedge pressure (PCWP),
  1442, 1476
  after cardiac surgery, 1442, 1476
  in shock, 2253
Pulmonary circulation, 1362, 1363
Pulmonary compliance, 1617
Pulmonary defense mechanisms, 1621–1622
Pulmonary edema, 225–226, 1746–1749
  cardiogenic, 1531, 1534, 1747
  in adult respiratory distress syndrome,
    1761–1762
  in heart failure, 1531, 1534
  neurogenic, 1747, 2034
  noncardiac, emergency care for, 2270
  noncardiogenic, 1747, 1747b
Pulmonary embolism (PE), 1706–1708
  after myocardial infarction, 1591–1592
  chest pain in, 1449t

Pulmonary embolism (PE) (Continued)
  clinical manifestations of, 606
  diagnosis of, 606
  monitoring for, 1425–1426
  shock in, 2233. See also Cardiogenic shock.
  venous thrombosis and, 1423
Pulmonary fibrosis, rheumatoid arthritis and,
  2145–2146
Pulmonary function tests, 1637, 1638t, 1640,
  1640t
  in asthma, 1687
  in hypersensitivity disorders, 2133
  in restrictive lung disease, 1741
Pulmonary gases, partial pressures of, 1618,
  1619
  transport of, 1620
Pulmonary hygiene, for chronic obstructive
  pulmonary disease, 1698
Pulmonary hypertension, 1708–1709
Pulmonary injury, in burns, 1332
Pulmonary rehabilitation, 1700–1705
Pulmonary resection, types of, 1730–1731.
  See also Thoracic surgery.
Pulmonary vasculature, disorders of, 1706–
  1709
Pulmonic valve, 1434t, 1435, 1436, 1437
Pulmonic valve disease, 1494, 1500
  surgery for, 1501–1502. See also Cardiac
  surgery.
Pulse(s), amplitude of, 183, 183b
  assessment of, 183, 183b, 1373, 1374, 1457
  after cardiac surgery, 1507
  rate of, 183
Pulse oximetry, 183b, 1637–1639, 1641,
  1641t
  in SaO$_2$ measurement, 1772–1773
  in skin graft assessment, 1324
Pulsed galvanic stimulation (Diapulse), for
  wound healing, 333
Pulseless electrical activity, 1565
Pulsus paradoxus, 1457
Punch biopsy, 200, 1277, 1277–1278. See also
  Biopsy.
Pupil, 1791
  Argyll Robertson, 1995
  autonomic neuropathy of, in diabetes melli-
    tus, 1188
  examination of, in increased intracranial
    pressure, 2031–2034
    in neurologic assessment, 1884–1885,
    2031–2034
Pupillary light reflex, assessment of, 1885,
  2033–2034
Purkinje's fibers, 1439–1440, 1440
Purpura, 2122b, 2122–2123
Pursed-lip breathing, in asthma, 1689, 1690
Purulent exudate, 323, 323t, 324
Pustule, 1271
PUVA therapy, 1284
Pyelolithotomy, for urinary calculi, 827, 828
Pyelonephritis, bacterial, 854–856
  fungal, 856
  in diabetic nephropathy, 851–852
  reflux and, 829
Pyelostomy, percutaneous, 814–815
Pyloric obstruction, in peptic ulcer disease,
  717
  postoperative, 721–722
Pyloroplasty, 719, 720. See also Gastric sur-
  gery.
Pyogenic arthritis, 579–580
Pyramidal tract, 1861, 1862t
Pyridostigmine (Mestinon), for myasthenia
  gravis, 2021–2022
Pyridoxine, deficiency of, 641t
  food sources of, 641t
  for isoniazid overdose, 2281t

Pyrosis, 691
   in gastroesophageal reflux disease. See *Gastroesophageal reflux disease (GERD)*.
Pyruvate, reference values for, 2305t
Pyuria, 749t, 750, 757, 757t, 809

Q

Q-tip test, 834, *834*
Quad-assisted cough, 2062
Quadriceps reflex, 1889, 1891t, *1892*, 1893b
Quadruple heart rhythms, 1461
Quality assurance, functional status measurement in, 102
   in acute care nursing, 100–102
   nursing intensity classification in, 101–102, 103t
   outcome monitoring in, 102
   patient satisfaction surveys in, 102
Quality of life, in chronic renal failure, 895
   post-transplant, 2228, 2288–2289
Quantitative spectral phonoangiography, 1896
Questran. See *Cholestyramine (Questran)*.
Quinidine, for dysrhythmias, 1562t
   perioperative use of, 275t
   reference values for, 2308t
Quinsy, 1679

R

RA. See *Rheumatoid arthritis (RA)*.
Rabies prophylaxis, 2280–2281
Race and ethnicity, cancer and, 353, *353*, 368t
   cholecystitis and, 1212
   cholelithiasis and, 1203
   gallbladder carcinoma and, 1215
   HIV infection and, 2186, 2187b–2188b
   hypertension and, 1380, 1381, 1391b
   screening and prevention and, 148t
   sickle cell anemia and, 2117, 2118
Radial nerve, examination of, *547*
Radial pulse, assessment of, 1373, *1374*
   in blood pressure measurement, 2252–2253
Radiation, cancer and, 354
   cellular injury from, 213
   risks of, 194
   solar, skin cancer and, 15
Radiation burns, 1332. See also *Burns*.
Radiation recall, 395
Radiation therapy, 377–380
   brachytherapy in, 961, 995
   breast cancer due to, 1013
   client teaching in, 380
   dosage in, 379
   effectiveness of, 379
   external beam, 377
   for adrenal hyperplasia, 1132
   for bladder cancer, 811
   for brain tumors, 1937, 1940t
   for breast cancer, 1019, 1020, 1025, 1031, *1032*, 1033
   for cervical cancer, 996
   for colorectal cancer, 782
   for endometrial cancer, 995
   for esophageal cancer, 700
   for Hodgkin's disease, 2175, *2176*
      breast cancer after, 1013
   for laryngeal cancer, 1663–1664
   for leukemia, 2169
   for lung cancer, 1729–1730
   for non-Hodgkin's lymphoma, 2178
   for oral cancer, 687
   for pancreatic cancer, 1202
   for prostate cancer, 961

Radiation therapy *(Continued)*
   for renal cancer, 859
   for testicular cancer, 965
   for vaginal cancer, 1005
   fractionation of, 379
   internal beam, 377–378
   interstitial, 378
   intracavitary, 378
   mechanism of action of, 377
   nursing management in, 379–380
   radiosensitivity and, 377
   safety standards for, 378–379
   sealed-source, 377–378
   side effects of, 379–380
   skin care in, 380, 380b
   skin changes in, 395
   types of, 377
   unsealed-source, 378
Radical cystectomy, 812. See also *Urinary diversion*.
   postoperative care in, 816
   preoperative care in, 815–816
Radical hysterectomy, 992–994. See also *Hysterectomy*.
Radical neck dissection, 688
   exercises after, *1673–1675*
   in laryngeal cancer, 1666
   nursing management in, 1672
   self-care in, 1666
Radical prostatectomy, *954*, 960–961
Radical vulvectomy, *1006*, 1006–1008
Radioactive iodine, for hyperthyroidism, 1096t, 1101
Radioactive iodine uptake, 1079, 1094t
   in thyroid cancer, 1108
   in thyroiditis, 1107t
Radioallergosorbent test, 2133
Radiofrequency ablation, 1569
Radiography. See also specific techniques.
   abdominal, 195, 656–657, 746
   chest, 195
      in acute pancreatitis, 1195
      in cardiac assessment, 1472
   contrast, 195
   contrast agents for, 196b
      nephrotoxicity of, 854
   in hematopoietic assessment, 2100–2101
   in musculoskeletal assessment, 545–546
   in neurologic assessment, 1894
   lower gastrointestinal series in, 195
   of fractures, 588, *591*
   ophthalmic, 1796
   procedure for, 192–194
   safety measures for, 194
   skeletal, 195
   upper gastrointestinal series in, 195
Radiolucent tissue, 193, 194
Radionuclide scanning, *199*, 199–200
   Doppler, in neurologic assessment, 1896
   in metabolic assessment, 1083t
   in musculoskeletal assessment, 546–548
   in myocardial infarction, 1589–1590
   in respiratory assessment, 1645
   of lung, 1642–1643
      in pulmonary embolism, 1706
   of thyroid gland, 1095t
   of urinary tract, 759–760
   procedure for, 199–200
Radiopaque tissue, 193, 194, *194*
Radiosensitivity, 377
Radius, fractures of, 618
Rales, 1633, 1634t
Raloxifene (Evista), for breast cancer prevention, 1014
   for osteoporosis, 571t, 572
Range of motion (ROM), assessment of, 542, *542*, *543*, 544t–545t

Range of motion (ROM) exercises, 624. See also *Exercises*.
   active, 624
   by assistive personnel, 573
   in rheumatoid arthritis, 2147–2148
   passive, 624
Ranitidine (Zantac), for peptic ulcer disease, 710t, 715
Rape, 1056
   evidence collection and preservation for, 2263, 2263t, 2264t
Rapid alternating movements, 1886
Rapid eye movement (REM) sleep, 432, *433*, 433–434
Rapidly progressive glomerulonephritis, 864t
Rapid-sequence induction, 2268–2269
RAS. See *Reticular activating system (RAS)*.
Rash. See also *Skin lesions*.
   in atopic dermatitis, 1287
   in syphilis, 1050
Rational emotive therapy, 36
Rationalization, 408b
Raynaud's disease, 1421
Raynaud's syndrome, 1421
Reabsorption, 216, 216b
Reach for Recovery, 1028
Reactive airway disease. See *Asthma*.
Rebound tenderness, 743
Receptors, 1868
   pain, 466–468
Recommended dietary allowances (RDAs), 638
Reconstructive surgery, 375, 1321–1327
   flaps in, 1322–1325, *1323*, 1324b
   for burns, 1353–1354
   implants in, 1325, *1325*
   in breast cancer, *1029*, 1029–1031, *1030*
   skin expansion in, 1029, 1325–1326
   skin grafts in, 1321–1322, *1323*
Rectal bleeding, from hemorrhoids, 795
   in colon cancer, 781–782
   in ulcerative colitis, 772–773
Rectal disorders. See under *Anorectal; Colorectal*.
Rectal pouch, 799
Rectal sphincter, artificial, 798
Rectal stretch, 2066
Rectal tube, 799–800
Rectocele, 756, *998*, *999*
   examination for, 925
Rectoprostatic examination, 939, *940*
Rectovaginal examination, 925–926, *926*
Rectovaginal fistula, *1003*, 1003–1004
Rectum, 630
   examination of, 172t–173t, 743, *744*, 756
   palpation of, 743, *744*
Red blood cell count, in cardiac assessment, 1464
Red blood cells. See *Erythrocyte(s)*.
   disorders affecting, 2103–2118. See also specific disorders.
   normal, *2104*
Red eye, 1787, 1788b
Red marrow, 2074
Reduced renal reserve, 881
Reentry, in dysrhythmias, 1551, 1554–1556
Reference daily intakes, 638
Reference values, 188
Referral, psychiatric, 411
   for anxiety disorders, 411
   for bipolar disorder, 428
   for depression, 423–424
   for schizophrenia, 419–420
Referred pain, 472, *472*, 766

Reflex(es), 1863, *1863*
  abdominal, 1889, 1891t
  abnormal, 1890–1891
  Achilles tendon, 1079
  anal, 1889, 1891t
  ankle, 1889, 1891t, *1892,* 1893b
  assessment of, 1889–1892
    in coma, *1909,* 1909–1910
  Babinski's, 1890, 1891t, *1893*
  baroreceptor, 1366, 1381, *1382*
  biceps, 1889, 1891t, *1892,* 1893b
  blink, 1790
  brachioradialis, 1891t
  bulbocavernosal, 756
  chemoreceptor, 1381, *1382*
  chewing, 1891
  corneal, 1790–1791, 1889, 1891t
    assessment of, 1885
  cough, 1618, 1618t
  cremasteric, 1889, 1891t
  deep tendon, 1863, *1863,* 1889, 1891t, *1892*
    assessment of, 1889, 1891t, *1892,* 1893b
  gag, 1886, 1889, 1891t
  glabella, 1891
  grading of, 1891–1892
  grasp, 1891
  jaw, 1891
  micturition, 737
  normal, 1889
  oculocephalic, assessment of, 1909, *1909*
  oculovestibular, assessment of, 1903
  palatal, 1891t
  palm-chin (palmomental), 1891
  patellar (knee-jerk), 1863, *1863,* 1889, 1891t, *1892,* 1893b
  plantar, 1889, 1891t
  protective, 1883
  pupillary light, assessment of, 1885, 2033–2034
  rooting, 1891
  snout, 1891
  sucking, 1891
  superficial (cutaneous), 1889
  triceps, 1889, 1891t, *1892,* 1893b
  ureterorenal, 737
  vomiting, 633
  withdrawal, 1863, *1863*
Reflex incontinence, 749. See also *Urinary incontinence.*
Reflex neurogenic bladder, *841,* 842–845
Reflex sympathetic dystrophy, 602
Reflux, gastroesophageal, 695–697, *695–697.* See *Gastroesophageal reflux disease (GERD).*
  laryngitis in, 1680
  sleep problems in, 439
  urinary, 829
  vesicoureteral, 734
Reflux esophagitis, 695–697, *695–697*
  sleep problems in, 439
Reflux gastritis, postoperative, 721
Refractive errors, 1826–1828, *1827*
Refractoriness, cardiac, 1439
Regional anesthesia, 293–296, 298, 483. See also *Anesthesia.*
  Bier block, 293–296
Regional enteritis. See *Crohn's disease.*
Registered nurse anesthetist, 291b
Registered nurse first assistant, 291b
Reglan (metoclopramide), for gastroesophageal reflux disease, 696
Regression, 408b
Regurgitation, 691
Rehabilitation, aural, 1836
  cardiac, 1527–1529
    after myocardial infarction, 1596–1605
  for elderly, inpatient, 64

Rehabilitation *(Continued)*
  outpatient, 65
  in burns, 1354–1357
  in cancer, 370–371
  in head injury, 2046
  in musculoskeletal trauma, 623–624
  in spinal cord injury, 2057–2060
  in stroke, 1965–1968, 1968, 1971, 1973–1974, 1978
  pulmonary, 1700–1705
  vestibular, 1850
Rehabilitation Act of 1973, 104
Rehabilitation centers, for elderly, 64
Rehabilitation home visit, 1978
Reimplantation surgery, after traumatic amputation, 1328
Reiter's syndrome, 2163
Relative refractory period, 1867
Relaxation techniques, 27, 36
  for pain, 27, 36, 498–499
Religious beliefs and practices. See also *Spirituality.*
  cultural aspects of, 146
  dietary, 634b–645b
  health care implications of, 2291t–2297t
  in death and dying, 2216t–2217t
  transplantation and, 2216t–2217t
Relocation stress syndrome, care plan for, 56
  outcomes for, 45
REM sleep, 432, *433,* 433–434
Renal abscess, 857–858
Renal agenesis, 751, 870
Renal angiography, 759
Renal aplasia, 871
Renal artery, balloon angioplasty of, 870
Renal artery bypass graft surgery, 870
Renal artery disease, 869–870
Renal artery embolization, 861
Renal bruit, 742
Renal calcium leak, 823
Renal calculi, 854. See also *Urinary calculi.*
  hypercalcemia and, 253
Renal calyx, 733, *733*
Renal cancer, 858–862
  chemotherapy for, 859–860
  clinical manifestations of, 859
  etiology of, 859
  immunotherapy for, 860
  nephrectomy for, 860–861
  nursing management in, 861
  pathophysiology of, 859
  radiation therapy for, 859
  risk factors for, 859
  self-care in, 862
  staging of, 859, *860*
Renal candidiasis, 856
Renal cell carcinoma, 858–862. See also *Renal cancer.*
Renal clearance, 736
Renal colic, 750
  in urolithiasis, 824, 825
Renal cortex, 733, *733*
Renal disorders, clinical manifestations of, 750–751
  congenital, 870
  cystic, *871,* 871–872
  edema in, 225
  gastrointestinal manifestations of, 750–751
  in burns, 1334, 1344–1345
  in diabetes mellitus, 851–852, 1187–1188
  in extrarenal conditions, 851–853
  in HIV infection, 853
  in hyperparathyroidism, 1109–1110
  in systemic lupus erythematosus, 2158
  infectious, 854–858
  inflammatory, 862–867

Renal disorders *(Continued)*
  neoplastic, 858
  obstructive, 858
  outcome classification for, 851
  traumatic, *867,* 867–869
  tubulointerstitial, 862
  vascular, 869–870
Renal failure, acute, 876–882
  abdominal aortic aneurysm repair in, case study of, 880–881
  assessment in, 879
  clinical manifestations of, 877–878
  definition of, 876
  etiology of, 876–877
  hyperkalemia in, 246–248
  intrarenal, 876, *876*
  medical management of, 878–879, 892–893
  nonoliguric, 877
  nursing management of, 879–882
  oliguric, 877–878
  pathophysiology of, 877
  postrenal, *876,* 876–877
  prerenal, 876, *876*
  prognosis in, 878
  self-care in, 882
  chronic, 882–901
    clinical manifestations of, 882–887
      cardiovascular, 886
      electrolyte, 883
      endocrine, 887
      gastrointestinal, 886
      hematologic, 883
      immunologic, 886
      integumentary, 887
      metabolic, 883, 886
      musculoskeletal, 886–887
      neurologic, 887
      psychosocial, 887
      pulmonary, 886
      reproductive, 887
    definition of, 882
    dialysis for, 888–894. See also *Dialysis.*
    drug metabolism in, 883
    end-stage renal disease in, 882, 883
    etiology of, 882
    incidence of, 882
    medical management of, 887–895, *890, 892–893*
    nursing management of, 895–899, *897*
    pathophysiology of, 882
    patient/family teaching in, 898–899
    prognosis in, 887
    quality of life in, 895
    renal transplantation for, 899–901, *899*
    risk factors for, 881–882
  in rhabdomyolysis, 852
  outcome classification for, 875
Renal function, age-related changes in, 212t
  in cardiovascular disease, 852–853
  in extrarenal conditions, 851–853
  in heart failure, 1534
  in hypotension, 852
  in peripheral vascular disease, 853
  in pregnancy, 853
  in sepsis, 853
  in shock, 852
  postoperative assessment of, 307
  postoperative monitoring of, in cardiac surgery, 1508
  preoperative assessment of, 279–280
Renal hemorrhage, traumatic, 867, 868, 869
Renal hypertension, 852, 1383, 1384b
  treatment of, 892
Renal hypoplasia, 871
Renal insufficiency, 883

Renal ischemia, 869–870
  in shock, 2240
Renal medulla, 733, *733*
Renal osteodystrophy, 886–887
  treatment of, 894
Renal pelvis, 733, *733*
Renal perfusion pressure, 737
Renal pyramids, 733, *733*
Renal reserve, reduced, 881
Renal surgery, extracorporeal (bench), 869
  nephrectomy, for cancer, 860–861, 869
    for trauma, 869
  percutaneous transluminal renal angioplasty,
    870
  slush technique, 869
Renal transplant, 899–901, 2225–2226
  for diabetes mellitus, 1171–1172
Renal transport, 735–736
Renal trauma, *867*, 867–869
Renal tuberculosis, 857
Renal tubules, in fluid balance, 735–736, 736t
Renal tumors, benign, 858
  malignant. See *Renal cancer.*
Renal vascular disease, 869–870
Renal vein thrombosis, 870
Renin, 737
  adrenocortical function and, 1123t
Renin-angiotensin system, in fluid balance,
    217, *218*
  in heart failure, 1531
Renin-angiotensin-aldosterone system, in blood
    pressure regulation, 1383, *1383*, 2235
  in cardiac regulation, 1444
  in electrolyte balance, 235–236
Renovascular disease, 869–870
Reorientation, for confusional states, 1920
Repaglinide (Prandin), for diabetes mellitus,
    1161t
Repatterning, 19b
Repetitive strain injuries, 1998, 1999t
Repolarization, 1867
  of cardiac cells, 1437
Reporting, mandatory, 2263
Reproductive assessment, female, 915–934
    diagnostic tests in, 926–931
    history in, 915–919
    normal findings on, 921b
    physical examination in, 919–926
  male, 934
    diagnostic tests in, 939–942
    history in, 934–936
    normal findings on, 941b
    physical examination in, 936–939, *937,
      940*
Reproductive disorders, female, 979–1009
  in chronic renal failure, 887
  male, 945–976
    prevention of, 942
Reproductive system, age-related changes in, 50t
  assessment of. See *Reproductive assessment.*
  chemotherapy effects on, 395
  female, anatomy and physiology of, 904–
    910, *905, 906t*
    blood supply of, 905
    hormones of, 907–908
    innervation of, 906
    lymphatic drainage of, 906
  in hypopituitarism, 1143
  male, anatomy and physiology of, *910*,
    910–913, 911t
RES. See *Reticuloendothelial system (RES).*
Rescriptor (delavirdine), 2198t
Rescue breathing. See also *Cardiopulmonary
    resuscitation (CPR).*
    chin lift in, *2267*, 2267–2268
    jaw thrust in, *2267*, 2267–2268
    through stoma, 1656

Reservoir, infectious, 336
Residual volume, 1615, *1615*
  measurement of, 1637, 1638t
Resilience, 69–70
Resonance, on percussion, 177
Resorption, 216b
Respiration. See also *Breathing; Ventilation.*
  assessment of, 183b, 183–184
  Cheyne-Stokes, *184*, 1462
    in heart failure, 1462, 1534
  external, 1618
  gas exchange and transport in, 1618–1620
  infratentorial lesions and, 1908, *1908*
  internal, 1618
  mechanics of, *1616*, 1616–1617
  muscles of, 1616–1617, 1617–1618
  physiology of, 1617–1620, *1619*
  postoperative monitoring of, in cardiac sur-
    gery, 1507–1508
  rapid, *184*, 1461
    in pneumonia, 1714
  regulation of, 1618
  ventilation in, 1617–1618
Respiratory acidosis, 265–266, 270t. See also
    Acid-base balance.
  in mechanical ventilation, 1756
  in shock, 2236–2237
Respiratory alkalosis, 264–265, 270t. See also
    Acid-base balance.
  in mechanical ventilation, 1756
  in shock, 2236–2237
Respiratory arrest, intraoperative, 302
  tetany and, hypoparathyroidism and, 1115
Respiratory assessment, 1623–1649
  acute pancreatitis and, 1197
  diagnostic tests in, 1637–1645
  history in, 1623–1627
  normal findings on, 1629b
  physical examination in, 1627–1635
  postoperative, 303, *303*, 304, *306*, 308
  preoperative, 276–279
Respiratory care, postoperative, for elderly,
    1774–1776
Respiratory depression, opioid analgesics and,
    450, 491
Respiratory disorders, assessment in. See *Res-
    piratory assessment.*
  infectious, 1711–1726
  lower airway, 1685
  obstructive, 1692–1705
    emergency care for, 2270–2271
    pulmonary function tests in, 1640t
  pain in, 472
  parenchymal, 1710–1745
  pleural, 1710–1745
  restrictive, pulmonary function tests in,
    1640t
  sleep problems in, 438–439
  upper airway, 1651–1683
  vascular, 1706–1709
Respiratory distress, 1761–1764, *1763, 1764,*
    1764b
  in acute pancreatitis, 1198, 1198b
  in Guillain-Barré syndrome, 2106, 2106b
  in obstructive sleep apnea, 435–436
  in spinal cord injury, 2053
  shock and, 2236
Respiratory failure, 1746–1761
  acute, 1746
  definition of, 1746
  hypoxemic, 1746–1749
    in pulmonary edema, 1746–1749
  overview of, 1746
  ventilatory, 1746, 1749
Respiratory infections, in tracheostomy, 1655
Respiratory membrane, 1615–1616, *1616*
Respiratory paralysis, in spinal anesthesia, 296t

Respiratory patterns, assessment of, 183–184,
    184
Respiratory rate, decreased, *184*
  increased, *184*, 1461
    in pneumonia, 1714
  measurement of, 183b, 183–184
Respiratory system, age-related changes in,
    50t, 212t, 1622
  epinephrine effects on, 1135t
  filtration in, 1621
  function of, 1617–1622
  in acid-base balance, 260, *260*, 263, *263*,
    1621
  in burns, 1332, 1334–1335, 1337–1338
  in cystic fibrosis, 1203
  in shock, 2236–2237, 2241–2242
  mucociliary blanket in, 1614, *1614*, 1621
  structure of, 1612–1617
    lower airway, 1613–1617, *1614–1616*
    upper airway, 1612–1613, *1613*
Respiratory zone, 1615, *1616*
Respite care, 2008, 2008b
  for elderly, 65
Rest, in stress management, 36
Rest pain, 1368, 1400
Resting membrane potential, 1867, *1867*
Restless legs syndrome, 436
Restraints, in confusional states, 1920, 1921b
  in emergency care, 2263
Restrictive cardiomyopathy, *1491*, 1492t,
    1493–1495
Restrictive lung disease, 1740–1741, 1741b
Resuscitation, advance directives and, 66–67
  cardiopulmonary, defibrillation in, 1566–
    1568, *1567*
    termination of, 1567–1568
  fluid. See also *Fluid management.*
    in burns, 1342, 1342t
Retention suture, *301*
Reteplase, for myocardial infarction, 1592t
Reticular activating system (RAS), 1907, *1907*
  in sleep, 432
Reticulocyte count, 2096
Reticulocytes, reference values for, 2302t
Reticuloendothelial system (RES), 2072, 2080
  in shock, 2238–2239
Retina, 1780
  detachment of, *1817*, 1817–1820, *1818*, 1819b
  visual receptors of, 1780, 1781
Retinal artery, occlusion of, 1821
Retinitis, cytomegalovirus, 1829
Retinitis pigmentosa, 1821
Retinoblastoma, 1826
Retinoids, for acne, 1294
Retinol-binding protein, 656t
Retinopathy, diabetic, 1186–1187, 1188b,
    1820, *1820*
  hypertensive, 1829
Retractile testis, 967–968
Retrograde endoscopy, for gallstone removal,
    1205, *1206*
Retrograde pyelography, 759
Retrograde urethrography, 759
Retrograde urography, 759
Retroperitoneal lymph node dissection, for tes-
    ticular cancer, 965
Retropubic prostatectomy, *954*, 955
Retropulsion, of gastric contents, 634
Retrovir (zidovudine), 2195, 2197t
Retroviruses, human immunodeficiency virus
    as, 2189–2190
ReVia (naltrexone), for alcoholism, 515–516
Review of systems, 131b–135b, 145
Rewarming, in hypothermia, 2282–2283
Rh blood group, 2088
Rhabdomyolysis, in burns, 1334, 1344
  renal injury from, 852, 876

Rheumatic fever, 1481–1484
Rheumatic heart disease, prevention of, 1484
Rheumatoid arthritis (RA), 2142–2156, *2143*
  assessment of, 2150
  clinical manifestations of, 2144–2146, *2145, 2146*
  diagnosis of, *2146*, 2146–2147
  epidemiology of, 2142
  etiology of, 2142
  herbal remedies for, 539
  in elderly, 2153, 2156
  medical management of, 2147–2150, 2148t, 2149t
  nursing management of, 2150–2153, 2151b, *2152*, 2152b, 2154b
  pathophysiology of, 2142–2144, *2144*
  risk factors for, 2142
  surgery for, 2153–2156, *2155*
    critical monitoring in, 2155b
  vs. osteoarthritis, 553t
Rhinitis, 1679–1680
  allergic, 2138
Rhinitis medicamentosa, 1679, 1680
Rhinoplasty, 1319, 1682–1683
Rhinosinusitis, 1676–1678
Rhonchi, 1633, 1634t
Rhythmic breathing, for pain, 499
Rhythmol (propafenone), for dysrhythmias, 1562t
Rhytidectomy, 1316–1318, *1317*
Rib fractures, 1769
  in flail chest, 1768–1769, *1769*, 2272, *2272*
Riboflavin, deficiency of, 642t
  food sources of, 642t
Ribonucleic acid (RNA), 209
Ribosomes, 207t
Ribs, 1616
RICE mnemonic, 322
Rifampin, for tuberculosis, 1720, 1721t
Rifapentine (Priftin), for tuberculosis, 1720, 1721t
Right bundle branch, 1439, *1440*
Right bundle branch block, 1561–1564
Right ventricular failure, 1531–1533, *1533*, 1534–1535
Riluzole (Rilutek), for amyotrophic lateral sclerosis, 2023
Rimantadine, for influenza, 1711
Rinne test, *1803*, 1803–1804
Risk appraisal, 145–155, 148t–155t
  for surgery, 282, 284b
Risk factors, 10, 13–16, *14*
  age-related, 14, *14*, 149t–150t
  biologic, 150t
  environmental/occupational, *14*, 15–16, 153t–154t
  for chronic conditions, 13, *14*
  for young/middle-aged adults, 30, 31t
  genetic, 13–14, *14*
  genetic/family-related, 148t–149t
  interrelationship of, 16
  lifestyle-related, 152t–153t
  nutritional, *14*, 14–15
  personal habits and, 150t–152t
  race-related, 148t
  socioeconomic, 154t
Risk management, 105
Ritonavir (Norvir), 2198t
RNA, 209
Rods, retinal, 1780, 1781
Rofecoxib (Vioxx), for osteoarthritis, 554, 555t
Role changes, client education for, 24
ROM. See *Range of motion (ROM)*.
Romberg test, 182, 1804
R-on-T phenomenon, *1560*, 1560–1561
Room preparation, preoperative, 289
Root canal therapy, 683, 684

Rooting reflex, 1891
Rosenbaum pocket vision screener, *1793*
Rosiglitazone (Avandia), for diabetes mellitus, 1161t
Rotary chair assessment, 1806
Rotator cuff tears, 622–623
Roto-Rest bed, 2064
Rough endoplasmic reticulum, *206*, 207t
Round window, of ear, 1783, *1783*
Roundworms, 767–768
Roy's adaptation model, 6t
Rubber band ligation, of hemorrhoids, 796
Rubella, immunization for, 40, 342, 342t
Rubor, dependent, 1369, 1371, *1371*, 1400
Rule of nines, 1337, *1337*
Rumpel-Leede test, 2099t
Running suture, *301*

S

S_1 heart sound, 1459, *1460*
S_2 heart sound, 1459, *1460*
  splitting of, 1459–1460, *1460*
S_3 heart sound, *1460*, 1460–1461
S_4 heart sound, 1460, *1460*, 1461
Sabador, 74b
Safe sex practices, 40, 152t, 2186
Safety, health promotion/risk management for, 151t
Safety measures, for falls by elderly, 626–627
  for seizures, 1926, 1930
  in Alzheimer's disease, 2006, 2007b
  in burns, 1332–1333, 1333b
  in chemotherapy, 388
  in coma, 1916–1917
  in confusional states, 1920
  in drug therapy, for elderly, 62t
  in epilepsy, 1926, 1930
  in home care, 111
  in radiation therapy, 378–379
  in radiography, 194
  in spinal cord injury, 2065
  in stroke, 1974
  intraoperative, 298–300
  postoperative, 307
Salem sump tube, 706t, 707
Salicylate, reference values for, 2307t
Salicylate salts, 486
Saline, normal, recipe for, 330
Saline infusion. See also *Intravenous therapy*.
  for diabetic ketoacidosis, 1175, 1175b
  for hyperglycemic, hyperosmolar, nonketotic syndrome, 1177
  for hyponatremia, 238, 239
  hypernatremia and, 239, 239t
  solutions for, 221t
Saline irrigation. See *Irrigation*.
Saliva, 635, 635t
Salivary glands, calculi of, 690
  inflammation of, 690
  tumors of, 690
Salmonellosis, 766–767, 768
  in HIV infection, 2203
Salpingitis, chlamydial, 1047
  gonococcal, 1044t, 1049
  in pelvic inflammatory disease, 987, *988*
Salsalate, 486, 487t
Salt. See also *Sodium*.
  iodized, 1090
Same-day surgery. See also under *Intraoperative; Perioperative; Postoperative; Preoperative; Surgery*.
  case management for, 283
Sandimmune (cyclosporine), for transplant immunosuppression, 2224t

Sanguineous exudate, 323, 323t
SaO_2, measurement of, 1641–1642. See also *Arterial blood gas analysis*.
  by pulse oximetry, 1772–1773
  reference values for, 2304t
  vs. PO_2, 1637, 1641t
Saquinavir (Invirase), 2198t
Sarcoidosis, pulmonary, 1726
Sarcoma, 350t, 363. See also *Cancer*.
  Kaposi's, in HIV infection, 1309–1310, *1310*, 2205–2206
  osteogenic, 580t, *581*, 581–582
Sarcomeres, 530
Saw palmetto, for benign prostatic hyperplasia, 946b
Scabies, 1056, 1311t
  lindane for, 1280t
  scraping for, 1276
Scald burns, 1332. See also *Burns*.
Scale, *1272*
Scalene muscles, 1617–1618
Scalp, injuries of, 2040
  inspection of, 1272
  psoriasis of, 1292
Scars, *1272*
  burn, minimization of, 1354, *1356*
  contracture of, 320
  formation of, 320
  hypertrophic, 333, *334*
  minimization of, 1314
Schistosomiasis, 767–768
Schizophrenia, 416–420
Schwartz's brain adaptation model, 6t
SCI. See *Spinal cord injury (SCI)*.
Sciatica, 1984
Scintigraphy, myocardial, 1474–1475
Sclera, 1778, 1790
Scleral buckling, for retinal detachment, 1818, *1818*
Scleroderma, 2159–2160, *2160*
Sclerosing cholangitis, 1215
Sclerotherapy, for bleeding esophageal varices, 1242
  for hemorrhoids, 796
  for varicose veins, 1427
Scoliosis, 540, *541, 577*, 577–578, 1629, *1630*
  restrictive lung disease in, 1740, *1741*
Scotoma, 1794
Scratch tests, 2101
Screening, 40–43
  age-appropriate, 155, 156t–159t
  for alcohol abuse, 39, 40t
  for breast cancer, 41, *42*, 369, 369t, *932*, 932–933, *933*, 1012, 1014, *1015*
    mammography in, *932*, 932–933, *933*
  for cancer, 368, 369t, 369–370
  for cervical cancer, 200, 369t, 370, 926–928, *927*, 995, 996
  for coagulation disorders, 1096–1098
  for colorectal cancer, 42–43, 369t, 370, 781, 782
    carcinoembryonic antigen in, 745
    fecal occult blood test in, 744t, 745
  for domestic abuse, 39
  for endometrial cancer, 369t, 370
  for malignant hyperthermia, 302
  for prostate cancer, 41, 159t, 358, 369t, 370
  for skin cancer, 370
  for substance abuse, 512, 512b
  for suicide risk, 426t
  for testicular cancer, 41, *43*
  nutritional, 640, 642b, 663, 666b
  physical examination in, 163, 180–185. See also *Physical examination*.
  recommendations for, 40, 41t, 148t–154t

Scrotum, structure and function of, 911, 912t, *913*
  transmillumination of, *938,* 938–939
  traumatic injuries of, 972
Scrub nurse, 291b
Seasonal affective disorder, 437
Sebaceous glands, 1262–1263, *1263*
Seborrheic dermatitis, 1286
Sebum, 1262
Secobarbital (Seconal), preoperative, 290t
Secondary prevention, 10–11, 11t, 84–85, 85b
Sedative-hypnotics, abuse of, 510t
Sedatives, abuse of, 511t, 515t, 519, 520t–521t
  for insomnia, 455
  for mechanical ventilation, 1756
  hepatic encephalopathy and, 1253
  preoperative, 290t
Segmental resection, pulmonary, 1730, *1731.* See also *Thoracic surgery.*
Segmented urine specimens, 963
Segs in white blood cell count, 318
Seizures, absence, 1925
  atonic, 1925
  clonic, 1925
  definition of, 1923
  diagnosis of, 1926
  emergency care for, 2277
  generalized, 1925–1926
  hypoparathyroidism and, 1115
  in brain tumors, 1934
  in epilepsy, 1923–1930. See also *Epilepsy.*
  injury prevention in, 1926
  medical management of, 1927t, 1927–1928
  myoclonic, 1925
  nonepileptic, 1931
  partial, 1907, 1925
  pathophysiology of, *1924,* 1924–1925
  post-traumatic, 2034t
  sleep deprivation and, 439
  tonic, 1925
  tonic-clonic, 1925
  types of, 1925–1926
  vs. epilepsy, 1923
Selective estrogen receptor modulators, for osteoporosis, 571t, 572
Selegiline (Deprenyl), for Parkinson's disease, 2018, 2019t
Selenium, as antioxidant, 15
Self-actualization, in chronic conditions, *25,* 25–26
Self-care, guidelines for, 148t–154t
  health promotion/risk management for, 151t–152t
Self-care and self-responsibility, by elderly, 49
Self-determination, for elderly, 67
Self-esteem, 409, 410t
Self-help groups, for chronic conditions, 26
Selye's general adaptation syndrome, 5t
Semen, 913
Semen analysis, 941, 968–969
  reference values for, 2310t
Semicircular canals, 1785, 1786
Semilunar valves, 1434t, 1435, *1436, 1437*
Seminal vesicles, structure and function of, 911t, *912,* 913
Sengstaken-Blakemore tube, in balloon tamponade, for bleeding esophageal varices, 1242, *1242*
  gas exchange and, 1243
Sensitivity, test for, 187–188
Sensitivity studies, 189
Sensory assessment, 170t–171t, 1877t–1878t, 1888–1889. See also *Neurologic assessment.*
  postoperative, 306

Sensory deficits, 442–443
  in stroke, 1957t, *1959,* 1960
  patterns of, *1890*
  types of, 1889
Sensory deprivation, 443
Sensory function, age-related changes in, 50t, 53, 212t
Sensory neurons, 1869
Sensory neuropathy, in diabetes mellitus, 1188
Sensory overload, 443
Sensory paralytic bladder, *841,* 842–845
Sensory pathways, in spinal cord, 1860, 1862t
Sensory receptors, 1868
Sepsis, emergency care for, 2278
Septic arthritis, 579–580
Septic shock. See also *Shock.*
  antibiotics for, 2248–2250
  clinical manifestations of, 2243
  emergency care for, 2278
  etiology of, 2234
Septicemia, 189
Serial port sampling, 191
Serosanguineous exudate, 323, 323t
Serotonin, in inflammation, *318,* 319
  in pain, 468, 469
Serous exudate, 323, 323t
Sertoli's cells, 913
Serum, reference values for, 2303t–2305t
Serum creatinine, 758
Serum proteins, 655, 655t
  nutritional status and, 655, 656t
  reference ranges for, 655t
Service lines, 96
Sex hormones, 1067
Sexual assault, 1056
  evidence collection and preservation for, 2263, 2263t, 2264t
Sexual assessment, 418b
Sexual development, female, 908
  male, 913
Sexual function, after bladder surgery, 816, 820–821
  after hysterectomy, 993, 998
  after myocardial infarction, 1597
  after radical vulvectomy, 1007
  assessment of, PLISSIT model for, 395
  in cancer, 395
  in osteoarthritis, 554–555
  in spinal cord injury, 2059–2060, 2060t, 2067–2068
  in vaginal cancer, 1005
  with colostomy, 785
  with ileostomy, 779–780
  with urinary diversion, 820–821
Sexual history, 145
  female, 917, 918t
  male, 918t, 935
Sexual intercourse, painful, after hysterectomy, 998
Sexual orientation, 418b
Sexual practices, safe, 40, 152t, 2186
Sexual precocity, pituitary disorders and, 1142
Sexuality, assessment of, 145
  mental health problems and, 418b
  of elderly, 46
Sexually transmitted diseases, assessment in, 1043–1044
  client teaching for, 1045b, 1045–1046
  clinical manifestations of, 1043
  definition of, 1041
  etiology of, 1042, 1042b
  health promotion for, 1043
  health promotion/risk management for, 152t
  HIV as, 2186. See also *Human immunodeficiency virus infection.*
  in HIV infection, 1055–1056

Sexually transmitted diseases *(Continued)*
  medical management of, 1043, 1044t–1045t
  nursing management of, 1043–1047
  outcomes classification for, 1041
  overview of, 1041–1042
  pathophysiology of, 1043
  pelvic inflammatory disease and, 986–989
  prevalence of, 1042
  prevention of, 40, 1043
  risk factors for, 1042–1043
  screening for, 159t
SHAFT mnemonic, 52
Shaman, 75b
Sharp debridement, 325, 1296, 1347
  of burns, 1347
Sharpey's fibers, 531, *534*
Shave biopsy, 200, 1277, *1277.* See also *Biopsy.*
  of actinic keratosis, 1305
Shellfish, hepatitis A and, 1225
Shift to the left, 1620, *1620*
Shift to the right, 1620, *1620*
Shift work sleep disorder, 437
Shin splints, 620
Shingles, 1310–1313, *1313*
  chest pain in, 1450t
Shock, 2231–2255
  anaphylactic, 2232
    clinical manifestations of, 2243
    etiology of, 2233–2234
  cardiogenic, 2231
    clinical manifestations of, 2243
    etiology of, 2233
    in myocardial infarction, 1591, 1594–1595
    medical management of, 2249t
  cardiovascular system in, 2237–2239, 2242
  client teaching for, 2255b
  clinical manifestations of, 2241–2243
  cold, 2243
  compensatory mechanisms in, 2235, *2235*
  complications in, prevention of, 2254
  critical monitoring in, 2242b
  definition of, 2231
  diagnostic assessment in, 2243–2244
  distributive (vasogenic), 2231–2232
    clinical manifestations of, 2243
    etiology of, 2233
    medical management of, 2250t
  etiology of, 2232–2234
  family needs in, 2255
  gastrointestinal system in, 2240–2241
  hepatic function in, 2240–2241
  hypovolemic, 230, 2231
    clinical manifestations of, 2243
    etiology of, 2232t, 2232–2233
    in gastrointestinal hemorrhage, 715–716
    medical management of, 2249t
    postoperative, 304–305, 306–307
  immune system in, 2240
  in acute pancreatitis, 1195
  in burns, 1341–1342
  in diabetic ketoacidosis, 1175
  neuroendocrine system in, 2239–2240, 2242–2243
  neurologic system in, 2239
  nursing diagnoses for, 2254b
  obstructive, 2231
  outcomes classification for, 2231
  overview of, 2231–2232
  pathophysiology of, 2234–2235
  postoperative, 304–305, 306–307
    pheochromocytoma and, 1137
  renal system in, 852, 2241, 2243
  respiratory system in, 2236–2237, 2241–2242

Shock *(Continued)*
  septic, 2232
    antibiotics for, 2248–2250
    clinical manifestations of, 2243
    emergency care for, 2278
    etiology of, 2234
    spinal (neurogenic), 2051, 2056–2057, 2232
    etiology of, 2234
    stages of, *2235,* 2235–2236
    systemic effects of, 2236–2244
    warm, 2243
Shock wave lithotripsy, 826–827, *827*
  for choledocholithiasis, 1205–1206, *1207*
  for cholelithiasis, 1205–1206, *1207*
Short arm cast, *603*
Short bones, 530
Short leg cast, *603*
Short stature, in hypopituitarism, 1143
Shoulder, examination of, *543,* 544t
  impingement in, 620–621
  replacement of, in rheumatoid arthritis, 2155, *2155*
  rotator cuff tears in, 622–623
Shunt, peritoneovenous, for ascites, 1247, 1250, *1250*
  portosystemic, for bleeding esophageal varices, 1242
    for portal hypertension, 1243–1245, *1244*
  splenorenal, *1244*
  ventriculoperitoneal, 2038–2039, *2039*
SI system (International System of Units), 188
SIADH. See *Syndrome of inappropriate antidiuretic hormone (SIADH).*
Sick care, principles of, 246
Sick role, 19–20
Sickle cell anemia, *2104, 2116,* 2116–2118
  urinary tract involvement in, 752
Sickle cell crisis, 2117
Sickle cell trait, 2116
Sildenafil (Viagra), for erectile dysfunction, 974
Silver nitrate solution, for burns, 1348t
Silver sulfadiazine, 327t
  for burns, 1348t, *1349*
Sims' position, *181*
Simulect (basiliximab), for transplant immunosuppression, 2224t
Simvastatin, 1521, 1522t
Sinemet (carbidopa-levodopa), for Parkinson's disease, 2018, 2019t
Single-photon emission computed tomography (SPECT), 1896
Sinoatrial arrest, 1554–1555
Sinoatrial node, 1438–1439, *1440*
  abnormalities of, 1550–1551. See also *Dysrhythmias.*
  conduction defects of, 1554–1555
Sinography, 546
Sinus(es), paranasal, 1612, *1613*
  examination of, 165t–166t, 1636
Sinus bradycardia, 1442, 1553, *1554*
Sinus dysrhythmia, 1554
Sinus exit block, 1554–1555
Sinus lavage, 1676
Sinus rhythm, normal, 1550, *1551,* 1551t
Sinus tachycardia, 1442, 1552, *1554*
Sinusitis, 1676–1678
Sitting position, *181*
6 Ps mnemonic, 604, 1415b
Sjögren's syndrome, 2161
  rheumatoid arthritis and, 2145
Skeletal muscle, 530, *531.* See also *Muscle.*
Skeletal radiography, 195
Skeletal system. See also under *Musculoskeletal.*
Skeleton, appendicular, 530, *533*
  axial, 530, *533*

Skene's glands, palpation of, *923,* 924
Skilled care facilities, 63–64, 65
Skin, age-related changes in, 50t, 212t, 1265t, 1265–1266
  atrophy of, *1272*
  biopsy of, *1277,* 1277–1278
  color of, 1262, 1274
    assessment of, 185
    in vascular disorders, 1370–1371, *1371,* 1400
  disorders of, in chemotherapy, 395
    in diabetes mellitus, 1156t
    in jaundice, 1223
  dry, management of, 1286
  examination of, 1269–1272
    by client, 1276
    by unlicensed assistive personnel, 1295b
  homeostatic function of, 1264
  immunologic function of, 1264
    in chronic renal failure, 887
    in myxedema, 1097
    in thermoregulation, 1264
  maceration of, 332
  moisture content of, 1274
  odor of, 1274
  photodamage to, 1302
  precancerous changes in, 1302–1305
  preoperative assessment of, 279
  protective function of, 1264
  psychosocial aspects of, 1265
  sensory function of, 1264
  sensory reception in, 1264
  structure and function of, 1262–1266, *1263*
  temperature of, 1274
  texture of, 1274
  vitamin D production in, 1264
Skin assessment, history in, 1267–1269, 1268t
  normal findings on, 1269b
  physical examination in, 1269–1272
Skin cancer, 1305–1310
  basal cell, 1306, *1306*
  etiology of, 1305–1306
  Kaposi's sarcoma, 1309–1310, *1310*
  medical management of, 1307
  melanoma, 1307, *1307, 1308,* 1308t
  mycosis fungoides, 1309
  precancerous changes and, 1302–1305
  prevention of, 370
  risk factors for, 370, 1305–1306
  screening for, 370
  self-examination for, 1285, *1285*
  squamous cell, 1306, *1306*
  sun exposure and, 15
  surgery for, 1307–1309
Skin care, client teaching for, 1265
  in ascites, 1246, 1247
  in chronic renal failure, 897
  in colostomy, 785
  in coma, 1914
  in healed burns, 1356
  in hypercortisolism, 1132
  in ileostomy, 777–778
  in immobility, 612, 613, 618b
  in radiation therapy, 380, 380b
  in spinal cord injury, 2064
  in total hip replacement, 561
  in tracheostomy, 1656, 1658, *1659*
  in urinary diversion, 818, 820
  in urinary incontinence, 839
  in venous insufficiency, 1429
Skin, culture and sensitivity, 1276
Skin disorders, bullous, 1310
  complementary therapies for, 1267, 1287b
  dressings for, 1282
  eczematous, 1286–1291. See also *Dermatitis.*
  infectious, 1310–1313, 1311t–1312t

Skin disorders *(Continued)*
  laser therapy for, 1326
  lubricants for, 1283
  neoplastic, 1305–1310. See also *Skin cancer.*
  outcomes classification for, 1279
  photochemotherapy for, 1284
  pruritus in, 1284–1285, 1286
  psychosocial aspects of, 1265
  PUVA therapy for, 1284
  soaks and wet wraps for, 1282–1283, *1283*
  terminology for, 1269, 1270t
  topical therapy for, 1279–1282, 1280t. See also *Topical therapy.*
  ultraviolet light therapy for, 1283–1284
Skin expansion, in reconstructive surgery, 1325–1326
  of breast, 1029
Skin flaps, *1323,* 1323–1325, 1324b
Skin grafts, 325, 1321–1322
  for burns, *1353,* 1353–1354
Skin lesions, arrangement of, 1275, *1275*
  assessment of, 1274–1275
  configuration of, 1275t, 1276
  terminology for, 1275t
  types of, 1269, *1271*
Skin lines, surgical incisions and, 1314
Skin patch, for analgesics, 495
Skin peels, 1318
Skin preparation, preoperative, 282
Skin self-examination, 1276, 1285, *1285*
Skin strips, *301*
Skin substitutes, for burns, 1348, 1350t
Skin tears, 1294–1295
Skin temperature, in vascular disorders, 1373
Skin tests, 1291, 2101
  for allergens, 1291, 2101
  for delayed type hypersensitivity, 2101
  for hypersensitivity disorders, 2132–2133
  tuberculin, *1719,* 1719–1720
Skin turgor, 1274, 1456
  assessment of, 222–223, *223*
Skull, fractures of, 2040–2041, 2043
  radiography of, 1894
  structure of, 1861
SLE. See *Systemic lupus erythematosus (SLE).*
Sleep, 431–444
  age-related changes in, 53
  assessment of, 440–441
  chronobiology of, 432
  definition of, 431
  erections during, 439
  in elderly, 433
  in stress management, 36
  need for, 433
  non-REM, 432, *433,* 433–434
  physiology of, 432–434
  purposes of, 433
  REM, 432, *433,* 433–434
  stages of, *433,* 433–434
Sleep apnea, 435–436
  central, 436
  obstructive, 435–436, 436b
    hypertension and, 439
Sleep bruxism, 437
Sleep deprivation, in hospitalized clients, 440
  seizures and, 439
Sleep disorders, 433–442
  arousal, 437
  circadian rhythm, 437
  classification of, 432t
  diagnosis of, 440–441, *441*
  dyssomnias, 434–437
  extrinsic, 436–437
  fatigue in, 442
  health promotion/risk management for, 150t
  hospital-acquired, 439–440

Sleep disorders (Continued)
in cardiovascular disorders, 439
in confusional states, 1920–1921
in delirium, 440
in dementia, 438
in depression, 438
in dying clients, 454–455
in elderly, 433
in endocrine disorders, 438
in gastrointestinal disorders, 439
in head trauma, 438
in respiratory disorders, 438–439
intrinsic, 433–436
neurotransmitter imbalances and, 437–438
nursing management in, 441–442, 455
parasomnias, 437
sleep hygiene and, 455
sleep-wake transition, 437
Sleep enuresis, 437
Sleep hygiene, 455
Sleep maintenance disturbance, in hospitalized clients, 439–440
Sleep onset difficulty, in hospitalized clients, 439
Sleep paralysis, 435, 437
Sleep pattern disturbances, 431–432, 441
Sleep starts, 437
Sleep terrors, 437
Sleeptalking, 437
Sleep-wake cycle, 432, 433, 433–434
Sleep-wake patterns, irregular, 437
Sleep-wake transition disorders, 437
Sleepwalking, 437
Sling procedure, for intrinsic sphincter deficiency, 839
Slit-lamp examination, 1796
Slough, removal of, 325, 328, 328–330
Slush technique, 869
Small intestine. See also under Gastrointestinal; Intestinal.
cancer of, 780
function of, 634
obstruction of, 790–793
resection of, for inflammatory bowel disease, 776–780. See also Ileostomy.
structure of, 630
transplantation of, 776
Smear, 189
acid-fast bacillus, for tuberculosis, 1720
Papanicolaou, 200, 369t, 370, 926–928, 927, 995, 996
Tzanck's, 1276
wet vaginal, 927, 928
Smegma, 911
Smell, assessment of, 1636, 1636b, 1883
impairment of, 1636
in physical examination, 179
Smoke inhalation, 1332, 1335, 1338
in burns, 1341, 1349
Smoking, cancer and, 354t, 354–355
cessation of, 37–39, 39t
chronic obstructive pulmonary disease and, 1693
coronary heart disease and, 1516
head and neck cancer and, 370
health promotion/risk management for, 151t
heart disease and, 1455
hypertension and, 1381, 1387
in peripheral arterial occlusive disease, 1402, 1403
laryngeal cancer and, 1661
nicotine effects in, 510t, 514t, 518
osteoporosis and, 570
passive, 39
preoperative assessment for, 274–275
urinary elimination and, 754
wound healing and, 332

Smooth endoplasmic reticulum, 206, 207t
Smooth muscle, 530, 534–535
Snake bite, 2282
Snellen chart, 1792, 1793
Snoring, in obstructive sleep apnea, 435, 436
primary, 437
Snout reflex, 1891
Soaks, 1282–1283, 1283
Social adaptation, to chronic conditions, 18–20
Social assessment, 140t–143t, 144–145
Social Cognitive Theory, 11–12
Social history, 139b
Social learning theory, 422
Social network, assessment of, 144
Social support, health benefits of, 26
Socioeconomic status, assessment of, 144
screening and prevention and, 154t
Sodium. See also Salt.
dietary restriction of, 238b
in edema, 227, 228
in heart failure, 1536, 1538t, 1541
in hypernatremia, 241
in hypertension, 1387, 1393
in renal disease, 241
dietary sources of, 238b
fluid concentration of, 234t
hypertension and, 1381, 1387
in acid-base balance, 262
in cardiac assessment, 1465
plasma levels of, 235b
replacement of, in hyponatremia, 238, 239
serum, reference values for, 2305t
urine, reference values for, 2307t
Sodium balance, disturbances of, 236–242. See also Hypernatremia; Hyponatremia.
preoperative assessment of, 277t
regulation of, 235–236
Sodium bicarbonate, for hemodialysis, 894
Sodium ions, in pain, 467, 469
Sodium nitroprusside (Nipride), for hypertensive emergencies, 1396t
Sodium polystyrene sulfonate (Kayexalate), for hyperkalemia, 247–248, 892
in addisonian crisis, 1121
Soft tissue injuries, emergency care for, 2279–2280
Solar radiation, skin cancer and, 15
Solu-Medrol. See Methylprednisolone (Solu-Medrol).
Solutions, colloid, for shock, 2247
in emergency care, 2274
crystalloid, for shock, 2247
in emergency care, 2274
intravenous, 220, 221t
administration of. See Intravenous therapy.
oral rehydration, 220, 221t
Solvent abuse, 510t, 514t, 518, 520t–521t
Somatic neurons, 1870
Somatic pain, 471t, 471–472, 766
Somatostatin, 1066
Somatotropin. See Growth hormone.
Somnambulism, 437
Somogyi effect, 1180
Sorbitol, for acute renal failure, 878
Sore throat, 1678
herbal remedies for, 1626
in chronic tonsillitis, 1679
Sotalol (Betapace), for dysrhythmias, 1563t
Sound waves, conduction of, 1785. See also Hearing.
Spasm, laryngeal, 1681
Spasticity, in multiple sclerosis, 2015
in spinal cord injury, 2049, 2050, 2058–2059
Specificity, test for, 187–188

Specimens, collection of, 188b, 188–189
for blood tests, 189, 190b, 190–191, 192
for stool analysis, 745
for urine tests, 189–190
for wound culture, 189
cytologic, in cancer, 374. See also Biopsy.
recovery and analysis of, 1647–1649
Speculum, nasal, 1635–1636, 1636
vaginal, 924, 925
Speech, assessment of, 143, 1875t–1876t, 1882–1883
esophageal, 1669
impaired, in stroke, 1957t, 1958, 1975–1976
Speech evaluation, 1805
Speech reading, 1836
Speech reception threshold, 1835
Speech therapy, in stroke rehabilitation, 1968
Sperm, 911t, 912
abnormalities of, in infertility, 968–969
examination of, 941, 968–969
Spermatocyte, 913
Spermatogenesis, 913
Spermatogonia, 913
Sphenoethmoidectomy, external, 1677–1678
Sphincter, anal, examination of, 743
artificial rectal, 798
artificial urinary, 841, 841
lower esophageal. See Lower esophageal sphincter (LES).
precapillary, 1362
Sphincter electromyography, 762, 762
Sphincteroplasty, for chronic pancreatitis, 1201
Sphincterotomy, endoscopic, for choledocholithiasis, 1214
Spinal accessory nerve, 1870t
assessment of, 1886
Spinal analgesia, 495
Spinal anesthesia, 293–295, 295, 296, 296t. See also Anesthesia.
Spinal cord, blood supply of, 1865
dorsal horn of, in pain perception, 469–471, 470
structure of, 1859–1861, 1860–1862
tumors of, 1994
vascular lesions of, 1994–1995
Spinal cord compression, in cancer, 396–397
signs of, 1994
Spinal cord injury (SCI), 2046–2068
airway management in, 2053, 2055, 2059, 2062
anterior cord syndrome in, 2051, 2052
autonomic dysreflexia in, 2050–2051, 2064b, 2064–2065
bladder dysfunction in, 840–845, 2049, 2059, 2063
bladder retraining in, 2066–2067
bowel retraining in, 2066–2067
Brown-Séquard syndrome in, 2051, 2052
case study of, 2056
cauda equina syndrome in, 2051, 2052
central cord syndrome in, 2051, 2052
conus medullaris syndrome in, 2051, 2052
diagnostic findings in, 2051
emergency care for, 2269, 2269, 2279
etiology of, 2047
family needs in, 2066
functional impairment in, 2049, 2050
heterotopic ossification in, 2060
immobilization for, 2269, 2269
impairment in, 2049, 2050
in elderly, 2068
initial management of, 2053–2054
level of, 2049, 2050
mechanisms of, 2047, 2048
medical management of, 2054
mobility in, 2058, 2061–2062
neurologic assessment in, 2055, 2055t

Spinal cord injury (SCI) (Continued)
  nursing management of, initial, 2054–2057
    ongoing, 2060–2068
  pain in, 2060, 2064
  pathophysiology of, 2047–2049
  psychosocial aspects of, 2060, 2065–2066
  reflex changes in, 2049–2050
  rehabilitation in, 2057–2060
  risk factors for, 2047
  self-care in, 2068
  sexual function in, 2059–2060, 2060t, 2067–2068
  shock in, 2234. See also Neurogenic shock.
  skin care in, 2064
  spasticity in, 2049, 2050, 2058–2059
  spinal shock in, 2051, 2055–2056. See also Neurogenic shock.
  surgery for, 2057, 2057
Spinal fusion, 1987–1991, 1988
  cervical, 1992, 1992–1993, 2057, 2057
Spinal manipulation, 1986
Spinal nerves, 1868, 1869
Spinal reflexes, 1863, 1863
Spinal shock, 2051, 2055–2056, 2232. See also Shock.
  clinical manifestations of, 2243
  etiology of, 2234
Spinal stenosis, 1984, 1985, 1985
Spinal tap, 1896–1899, 1897
  headache after, 1898, 1950
  in coma, 1909
Spine. See also Vertebrae.
  cervical, disc disorders in, 1991–1993
    fusion of, 1992, 1992–1993, 2057, 2057
    immobilization of, emergency, 2269, 2269
    injuries of. See Cervical spine, injuries of; Spinal cord injury.
  curvature of, 540, 541, 576–578, 577, 577–578, 1629, 1630
    in osteoporosis, 568, 568
    restrictive lung disease in, 1740, 1741
  examination of, 167t, 170t–171t, 543, 544t
  fractures of, in osteoporosis, 567, 568, 568, 572
  immobilization of, 2269, 2269
    emergency, 2269
  in ankylosing spondylitis, 2160, 2161
  radiography of, 1894
  structure of, 1861
  tumors of, 1994
Spine board, 2269, 2269
Spinocerebellar tract, 1861, 1862t
Spinothalamic tract, 1861, 1862t
Spiral fracture, 594t
Spiritualists, 74b
Spirituality. See also Religious beliefs and practices.
  assessment of, 144
  health and, 413
  mental health problems and, 425b
Spironolactone (Aldactone), for hyperaldosteronism, 1134–1135
  for hypertension, 1389t
  for premenstrual syndrome, 982
  side effects of, 1135b
Spleen, examination of, 169t
  in metabolic disorders, 1076t, 1077
  in cirrhosis, 1241
  in hematopoiesis, 2078–2079
  rupture of, 2121–2122
  size of, 1077
  structure and function of, 2073, 2073
Splenectomy, 2121–2122
Splenic pulp manometry, 1084
Splenorenal shunt, 1244
Splinter hemorrhage, 1273t
Splinting, of incision, 286, 1731, 1732

Splints, care of, by assistive personnel, 573
  for burn patients, 1349
  nursing management for, 573
Split-ejaculate technique, for infertility, 969
Spondylolisthesis, 1984, 1984
Spondylolysis, 1984, 1984
Spongy bone, 531, 533
Sporadic goiter, 1090
Sports injuries, overuse, 619b, 619–621, 621t
  prevention of, 620b
  risk factors for, 619–620
Spousal abuse, 39. See Domestic violence.
Sprains, 621–622
  emergency care for, 2279
Sputum, assessment of, 1624
  blood in, 1452, 1462, 1624
  collection of, 1647
Squamous cell carcinoma, of eyelid, 1826
  of oral cavity, 687, 687–690
  of skin, 1306, 1306. See also Skin cancer.
Stable angina, 1581
Stadol (butorphanol), 490t
Staffing issues, in acute care, 100, 101–102
  unlicensed assistive personnel and, 100, 100b. See also Unlicensed assistive personnel.
Staghorn calculi, 823, 823
Staging, cancer, 373, 373t
  surgery for, 374–375
  TNM system for, 373, 373t, 1728, 1728b, 1729b
Stain, 189
Standard precautions, 344
Standards of care, for ambulatory care nursing, 91
  for home health care, 109–110
Standing position, 181
Stapedectomy, 1832, 1840
Stapedial otosclerosis, 1832, 1832, 1840
Stapes, 1783, 1783. See also Ossicles.
Staphylococcal food poisoning, 766–767, 768
Staphylococcal pneumonia, 1711–1716, 1712t
Staphylococcus aureus, drug-resistant, 339, 341b
Staples, 301
Stasis dermatitis, 1286, 1290–1291, 1291, 1427, 1427–1428
Stasis ulcers. See Venous ulcers.
Stature, short, in hypopituitarism, 1143
Status asthmaticus, 1687–1688
Status epilepticus, 1931
Stavudine (Zerit, d4T), 2196t
Steatorrhea, in chronic pancreatitis, 1200
  test for, 744t, 745–746
Stellate fracture, 595t
Stem cells, 2075
Stents, intracoronary, 1523, 1523
  prostatic, for benign prostatic hyperplasia, 956
Stereognosis, 1888
Stereotactic needle-guided biopsy, of breast, 1016
Stereotyping, in health history, 129–130, 130b
  of elderly, 55
Sternal fracture, 1770
Sternocleidoid muscles, 1617–1618
Steroid hormones, 1060–1061, 1067. See also specific hormones.
  adrenal cortical, 1063, 1066–1067
    deficiency of, 1120, 1120–1126, 1121t–1124t, 1126
Steroids, Cushing's syndrome due to, 1126–1127
  for Addison's disease, 1122–1123, 1124t
    in addisonian crisis, 1122
    self-care and, 1125
  for asthma, 1690, 1691t, 1692, 1694

Steroids (Continued)
  for chronic obstructive pulmonary disease, 1691t, 1697–1698
  for dyspnea, 452
  for hypersensitivity disorders, 2133
  for inflammatory bowel disease, 773
  for myasthenia gravis, 2022
  for pain, 492
  for rheumatoid arthritis, 2149
  for shock, 2251
  for transplant immunosuppression, 2224t
  hepatitis and, 1228
  infection risk and, 1132
  perioperative use of, 275t
  side effects of, 1123–1124, 1124t
  topical, 1280t, 1282
    for atopic dermatitis, 1288
  wound healing and, 332
Stethoscope, 178–179, 179
Stiffness, joint, assessment of, 538
Stings, insect, allergy to, 2137t, 2137–2138
Stockings, antiembolism, 286
  support, in chronic venous insufficiency, 1428
Stoma care, in colostomy, 784–786, 785, 786b
  in ileostomy, 776–778, 778b
    delegation of, 778b
  in tracheostomy, 1656, 1658, 1659, 1669
  in urinary diversion, 816, 817–818
Stomach. See also under Gastric; Gastrointestinal.
  function of, 633–634
  in digestion, 633–634
  structure of, 630
Stomatitis, 684–685
  aphthous, 684
  chemotherapy and, 394, 1034
  herpetic, 684, 685
Stones. See Calculi.
Stool, analysis of, 744t, 745
  blood in, 744t, 745
  culture of, 744t, 745
  lipids in, 744t, 745
  ova and parasites in, 744t, 745
Stool specimen, collection of, 745
Strabismus, 1791
Straight leg raising test, 544t
Strain, 621
  back, 1984
  emergency care for, 2279
Strain void, 820
Strength, assessment of, 541t, 542, 1886
Streptococcal sore throat, rheumatic heart disease and, 1484
Streptokinase, 1406. See also Thrombolytics.
  for peripheral arterial occlusive disease, 1404
  for venous thrombosis, 1425
  in arterial bypass surgery, 1407
Stress, 35
  coronary heart disease and, 1517
  disease and, 3, 5t–7t, 16, 26–27
  health promotion/risk management for, 151t
  hypertension and, 1381, 1387
  in inflammatory bowel disease, 774
  in myxedema, 1093
  physiologic response to, 408
  theories of, 3, 5t–7t
Stress fractures, 620
Stress incontinence, 749. See also Urinary incontinence.
Stress management, 18, 26–27, 35–36, 408b, 408–409
  nutrition in, 35–36
Stress resistance, 35–36

Stress response, Lazarus' theory of, 5t
   Mason's theory of, 5t
   mediators of, 7t
Stress testing, 1376, 1470–1472
   first-past cardiac study in, 1475
   myocardial scintigraphy in, 1474
Stress ulcers, 712, 714, 2034t
   prevention of, 2251
Stretching, pre-exercise, 620, 620b
Stridor, assessment of, 1624
Stripping, of chest tubes, 1738, *1738*
Stroke, 1953–1978
   case management for, 1970b
   case study of, 1966b–1967b
   clinical manifestations of, 1956b, 1956–
      1960, 1957t
   clinical pathway for, 1968b, 1969b
   death in, 1965
   diagnosis of, 1960
   early identification of, 1956, 1960–1964
   emergency care for, 2277
   epidemiology of, 1953
   etiology of, 1953–1955
   hemorrhagic, 1953, 1954–1955, *1955,*
      1956
   in diabetes mellitus, 1183t, 1184
   in elderly, 1977
   initial assessment in, 1960–1964, 1961t–
      1963t
   ischemic, 1953, 1954, *1954,* 1955
   lacunar, 1954
   medical management of, 1953–1954, 1960–
      1968
   nursing management of, 1968–1977
   outcomes classification for, 1953
   overview of, 1953–1954
   pathophysiology of, 1955–1956
   prevention of, 1955
      carotid endarterectomy for, 1979, *1980*
   recurrence of, prevention of, 1965
   rehabilitation for, 1965–1968, 1968, 1971,
      1973–1974, 1978
   risk factors for, 1955
   self-care in, 1974, 1978
   surgery for, 1977
   thrombolytic therapy for, bleeding in, 1964–
      1965, 1971
      complications of, 1964–1965
      contraindications for, 1964
      indications for, 1960–1964, 1961t–1963t
      timing of, 1964
   transient ischemic attacks and, 1978–1980
Stroke volume, 1434, 1441, *1442,* 2234
Struvite stones, 823
Stump care, 1414b
Stump wrapping, *1412,* 1413
Stye, 1827t
Subacute care, 96–98, 125
Subacute care facilities, 64–65
Subarachnoid bolt, in intracranial pressure
   monitoring, 2030, 2032b–2033b
Subarachnoid hemorrhage, 1940–1944
   head trauma and, 2034t
   stroke and, *1954,* 1954–1959
Subarachnoid space, 1862, *1862*
Subclavian steal syndrome, 1422
Subclinical infection, 338
Subcutaneous emphysema, in tracheostomy,
   1655
Subcutaneous layer, *1263,* 1263–1264
Subdiaphragmatic abscess, 1743–1744
Subdural hematoma, *2041,* 2042, *2042*
Subdural space, 1862, *1862*
Subepidermal basement membrane zone,
   1263
Sublimaze. See *Fentanyl (Sublimaze).*
Subluxations, 619

Substance abuse, 507–528. See also *Alcohol*
   use/abuse; Smoking.
   addiction in, 508–509
   assessment in, 511–513, 513b, 513t
   biological model of, 508
   by elderly, 58–60
   by health care professionals, 524b, 524–525
   by surgical client, 274–275, 275t
   causes of, 508–509
   client teaching in, 519, 522b
   community health nursing and, 512
   disease concept of, 508
   health promotion/risk management for, 151t,
      157t
   history in, 513, 513b
   HIV transmission via, 2188
   intoxication in, 513–519
   nursing diagnoses for, 522b
   nursing management in, 519
   outcomes classification for, 507
   overdose in, coma in. See *Coma.*
      emergency care for, 2276–2277
      naloxone for, 1910, 2277
   physical effects of, 510t–511t, 515–519,
      520t–521t
   preoperative assessment for, 274–275
   prevention of, 37
   psychological model of, 508–509
   relapse in, prevention of, 522–523, 524b
   resources for, 523–524
   sociocultural model of, 509
   surgery and, 523–524
   terminology for, 509t, 509–511
   therapeutic intervention in, 519
   treatment of, 519–522, 523t
   withdrawal in, 513, 514t–515t. See also
      Withdrawal.
Substance P, in pain, 468
Substrates, metabolic, 1067–1068, *1068*
Subtotal gastrectomy, 720, *720.* See also *Gas-*
   tric surgery.
Succinylcholine (Anectine), 295t
   for rapid-sequence induction, 2268
Sucking chest wound, 1766, *1766,* 1767
Sucking reflex, 1891
Sucralfate (Carafate), for peptic ulcers, 711t,
   715
Suction-assisted lipectomy, 1319–1320, *1320*
Suctioning, in acute pancreatitis, 1197
   in chest drainage, 1736–1737
   in cholelithiasis, 1206–1207, 1211
   in gastric decompression, 707–708
   of tracheostomy tube, 1656–1657, 1667–
      1668
   tracheobronchial, in coma, 1913
Sudafed (pseudoephedrine), for urinary inconti-
      nence, 837t
Suicide, 421
   risk factors for, 421b
   screening for, 426b
Sulfonylureas, for diabetes mellitus, 1159,
   1160t
   combined with insulin therapy, 1162
Sulindac, 486, 487t
Sulkowitch test, 1111t
Summation gallop, 1460
Sun exposure, actinic keratosis and, 1303–
   1305
   skin cancer and, 15, 1305–1306
   sunburn and, 1302–1303
Sunburn, 1302–1303
Sundowning, 1918
Sunna, 1008
Superficial gastritis, 709
Superficial pain, 471, 471t
Superficial spreading melanoma, 1307–1309,
   1308t

Superficial thrombophlebitis, 1422–1426. See
   also *Venous thrombosis.*
Superior vena cava syndrome, 397
Superoxide radicals, disease and, 15
   in wound healing, 319
Supine position, *181,* 299, *300*
Support groups, for chronic conditions, 26
Support services, for elderly, 54t, 61–63,
   63b
Support stockings, in chronic venous insuffi-
   ciency, 1428
Suppuration, 324
Suppurative arthritis, 579–580
Suppurative thyroiditis, 1106, 1107, 1107t
Suprapubic catheterization, 832–833
Suprapubic prostatectomy, 949–954, *954*
Supraspinatus tendinitis, 1999t
Supratentorial herniation, 2029, *2029*
Supraventricular tachycardia, 1557
Surface immunoglobulins, 2073
Surfactant, 1617
Surgery. See also under *Intraoperative; Laser*
   therapy; Perioperative; Postoperative;
   Preoperative and specific types and disorders.
   anesthesia in, 292–298. See also *Anesthesia.*
   cardiac, 1500–1513
   elective, case management for, 283
   gastric, 719–724
   in diabetic client, 1189–1190
   in elderly, 280, 281t
   in substance abusers, 523–524
   informed consent for, 287, *288*
   intracranial. See *Craniotomy.*
   palliative, 375, 401
   plastic, 1313–1326. See also *Plastic sur-*
      gery.
   positioning for, 299, 299b, *300*
   reconstructive, 375, 1321–1327
   reimplantation, 1328
   risk assessment for, 282, 284b
   thoracic, 1730–1739
   transport for, 298, 302
   types of, 283t
Surgical debridement, 325, 1296, 1347
   of burns, 1347
Surgical drains, 300
   postoperative care of, 307
   preoperative teaching for, 287
Surgical equipment, safety measures for, 299–
   300
Surgical excision biopsy, 374
   of skin, *1277,* 1278
Surgical mumps, 690
Surgical team, 290–292, 291b
Surveys, accreditation, 102
   patient satisfaction, 102
Sustiva (efavirenz), 2198t
Susto, 19b
Suture(s), continuous (running), *301*
   cranial, 1861
   interrupted, *301*
   materrupted, *301*
   retention, *301*
Suture joints, 532
Suture materials, selection of, 2280t
Suturing, in emergency care, 2280, 2280t
   techniques of, 1314
SVO₂, measurement of, in shock, 2253
SVR. See *Systemic vascular resistance (SVR).*
Swallowing, 633, *633*
   after partial laryngectomy, 1668b
   evaluation of, 652
      after coma reversal, 1913
   impaired. See *Dysphagia.*
   painful, 691
      in esophageal cancer, 700, 701

Swan-Ganz monitoring, 1477b
  in shock, 2253
Swan-neck deformity, in rheumatoid arthritis, 2145, *2145*, 2156
Swayback, 578
Swelling, assessment of, 538
  of brain, 2028. See also *Cerebral edema; Increased intracranial pressure (ICP).*
Swimmer's ear, 1842
Symmetrel (amantadine), for Parkinson's disease, 2019t
Sympathetic nervous system, effects of on organs, 1870, 1871t
  gastrointestinal function and, 631
  in cardiac regulation, 1443
  structure of, 1870–1872, *1872*
Symphyses, 533
Symptom management, in palliative care, 447
Synapses, *1866*, 1866–1867
Synchondroses, 533
Syncope, 1397
  in heart disease, 1452
Syndesmosis joints, 533
Syndrome of inappropriate antidiuretic hormone (SIADH), 228, 229, 1143, 1144t–1145t
  in cancer, 396
  post-traumatic, 2034t
Syndrome X, 1182
Synovectomy, for rheumatoid arthritis, 2154
Synovial fluid, 532
  sampling of, 548
Synovial joints, 532, *533*
Synthroid. See *Levothyroxine sodium.*
Syphilis, 1044t, *1050*, 1050–1051
  neurosyphilis and, 1995
Syringomyelia, 1993–1994
Syrup of ipecac, for poisoning, 2281
Systemic circulation, 1362, *1363*
Systemic lupus erythematosus (SLE), 2156–2159, *2157*, 2157b, *2158*
  eye in, 1829
Systemic vascular resistance (SVR), in shock, 2242, 2253
  measurement of, 2253–2254
Systole, atrial, 1440
  ventricular, 1440
Systolic pressure, 1442

T

T cells, *2073*, 2073–2074, 2081, 2085–2087, *2086*
  helper, 2086
    in HIV infection, 2190–2191
  suppressor, 2086
T tube, in cholangiography, 1086, 1215
  in cholecystectomy, 1209, *1209*
  in choledochostomy, 1215
T_3. See *Triiodothyronine (T_3).*
T_4. See *Thyroxine (T_4).*
Tabes dorsalis, 1995
Tachycardia, 183, 1442, 1451
  definition of, 1551
  in shock, 2242
  paroxysmal atrial, *1555*, 1555–1556
  paroxysmal junctional, 1557
  sinus, 1552, *1554*
  supraventricular, 1557
  ventricular, *1560*, 1565
Tachypnea, *184*, 1461
  in pneumonia, 1714
Tacrine (Cognex), for Alzheimer's disease, 2004–2005
Tacrolimus (FK506), for transplant immunosuppression, 2224t
Tactile fremitus, 1631

Tactile sensation, 1264
Tagamet (cimetidine), preoperative, 290t
TAH-BSO. See *Total hysterectomy with bilateral salpingo-oophorectomy (TAH-BSO).*
Talk test, 33
Talking tracheostomy, 1653
Talwin (pentazocine), 490t
Tamoxifen (Nolvadex), for breast cancer, 1014, 1032, 1035–1036
Tamponade, balloon, for bleeding esophageal varices, 1242, *1242*
    and gas exchange, 1243
  cardiac, 1435, 1489–1490
    emergency care for, 2275, *2276*
    heart failure and, 1531
    in cancer, 397
  pericardial tamponade, shock and, 2233
Tampons, toxic shock syndrome and, 1003
Tapazole. See *Methimazole (Tapazole).*
Tape, for endotracheal tube, 1750, *1751*
  for wound closure, *301*
Tapeworms, 767–768
Tardive dyskinesia, 418
Tarsal tunnel syndrome, 1998
Tarsorrhaphy, for corneal infection, 1824
Taste, assessment of, 1885
T-cell lymphoma, cutaneous, 1309
TDD (Telecommunication Device for the Deaf), 1836
Teaching, patient. See *Client teaching.*
Teaching hospitals, ambulatory care nursing in, 87
Team nursing, 99
Tear film, 1778
  inadequate production of, 1826
Technetium 99m ventriculography, 1474–1475
Teeth, disorders of, 683–684
Tegison (etretinate), for psoriasis, 1292
Tegretol (carbamazepine). See *Carbamazepine (Tegretol).*
Telecommunication Device for the Deaf (TDD), 1836
Telephone medicine, in cancer, 392
  in long-term care facilities, 123
Telephone nursing practice, 89–91
Temperature, measurement of, 183, 183b
  monitoring of, in shock, 2253
    intraoperative, 300–301
    postoperative, 306
  postoperative monitoring of, in cardiac surgery, 1507
  skin, in vascular disorders, 1373
Temperature sensation, assessment of, 1888
Temporal arteritis, 2163
Temporal bone, 1782
Temporal bone stimulators, 1841
Temporal lobe, 1856–1857, *1858*
Temporal lobectomy, for epilepsy, 1929, *1929*, 1930
Temporal pulse, assessment of, 1373, *1374*
Temporomandibular joint (TMJ), pain in, ear pain and, 1842, 1845, 1846
TEN (total enteral nutrition). See *Enteral nutrition.*
Tenckhoff catheter, 888, *888*
Tendinitis, 621
  bicipital, 1999t
  supraspinatus, 1999t
Tendon, 530
Tendon sheath, 533
Tendon transfer, for rheumatoid arthritis, 2153–2154
Tennis elbow, 621, 1999t
  test for, 544t
TENS. See *Transcutaneous electrical nerve stimulation.*
Tensilon test, 2021

Tension headache, 1948, *1949*
Tension neck syndrome, 1999t
Tension pneumothorax, *1766*, 1767–1768. See also *Pneumothorax.*
  emergency care for, *2271*, 2271–2272
  open pneumothorax conversion to, 1767
  shock and, 2233
Tentorium, 1862
Terminal bronchioles, 1614, *1614*
Terminal illness. See *Death and dying.*
Tertiary prevention, 11, 11t, 84–85, 85b
Testicular dysfunction, 1143
Testicular self-examination, 41, *43*
Testis, cancer of, *964*, 964–965
  screening for, 41, *43*, 159t
  ectopic, 967–968
  examination of, 938
  inflammation of, 966
  malposition of, 967–968
  pain in, 750
  retractile, 967–968
  structure and function of, 911–912, 912t, *913*
  torsion of, 966, *966*
  traumatic injuries of, 972
  undescended, 967–968
    infertility and, 968, 969
    testicular cancer and, 964, 967
Testosterone, 912, 913, 1067
  pharmaceutical, for erectile dysfunction, 973
  for infertility, 969
  reference values for, 2305t
Tetanus, 1945–1946
  immunization for, 40, 342, 342t, 2280, 2280t
  for burns, 1343, 1345
Tetany, in hypocalcemia, 251, *251*
  parathyroidectomy and, 1113–1114. See also *Hypoparathyroidism.*
  thyroidectomy and, 1105, 1115–1116
  in hypomagnesemia, 256
Tetracaine (Pontocaine), 297t
Thalamus, 1858, *1858*
Thallium 201 scintigraphy, in cardiac assessment, 1474
Theophylline (Theo-Dur), for asthma, 1690, 1691t, *1692*, *1694*
  reference values for, 2308t
Therapeutic passes, 1978
Therapeutic relationship, in pain management, 481–483
Therapeutic Touch, 500
Thermal therapy, for benign prostatic hyperplasia, 956
Thermodilution method, for cardiac output measurement, 1478b, 1479
Thermoregulation, in shock, 2252, 2253
  integumentary system in, 1264
Thiamine, deficiency of, 641t
  food sources of, 641t
Thiazide diuretics, hypercalcemia and, 252
  perioperative use of, 275t
Thiazolidinediones, for diabetes mellitus, 1159, 1161t
Thinking. See *Cognitive function.*
Thiopental (Pentothal), 294t
  for rapid-sequence induction, 2268
Third-space fluid shifts, 218
Third-spacing, 229–230
Thirst, 217–218, *218*
  in fluid restriction, 239
Throat culture, 1648
Thoracentesis, 1648–1649, *1648*
  for pneumothorax, 2272
Thoracic aortic aneurysm, 1420
  dissecting, 1419–1420, 1449t
Thoracic excursion, assessment of, 1629, *1630*, 1631, *1631*

Thoracic landmarks, *1628*
Thoracic outlet syndrome, 1422, 1999t
Thoracic surgery, 1730–1739
  care plan for, 1733b–1736b
  closed-chest drainage in, 1732–1738, *1737*
  in elderly, respiratory care in, 1774–1776
  laser, 1730
  postoperative care in, 1731–1739
  preoperative care in, 1731
  pulmonary resection in, 1730–1731
Thoracolumbar orthosis, in spinal cord injury, 2058
Thoracotomy, endoscopic, 1647
Thorax. See *Chest.*
Thought processes. See *Cognitive function.*
Thought stopping, 36
THR. See *Total hip replacement (THR).*
3-log, dietary, 32
  exercise, 33
3TC (lamivudine), 2196t
Thrills, 1458–1459
Thrombin time, 2099t
Thromboangiitis obliterans, 1421–1422
Thrombocytapheresis, for leukemia, 2169
Thrombocytes. See *Platelet(s).*
Thrombocytopenia, in cancer, 393
Thrombocytopenic purpura, idiopathic, 2122–2123
Thromboembolism, postoperative, 308
  in total hip replacement, 286, 308
  prevention of, 286, 308
Thrombolytics, 1406
  bleeding and, 1964–1965, 1971
  for myocardial infarction, 1591, 1592t
  for peripheral arterial occlusive disease, 1404
  for pulmonary embolism, 1706
  for stroke, 1953–1954
    contraindications for, 1964
    indications for, 1960–1964, 1961t–1963t
    timing of, 1964
  for venous thrombosis, 1425
  in arterial bypass surgery, 1406, 1407
Thrombophlebitis, in spinal cord injury, 2065
  superficial, 1422–1426. See also *Venous thrombosis.*
Thromboplastin generation test, 2099t
Thrombosis, arterial, 1415–1416
  thrombolytics for, 1406
  renal vein, 870
  stroke and, 1594, 1953, *1954.* See also *Stroke.*
  venous. See *Venous thrombosis.*
Thrombo-Welco test, reference values for, 2302t
Thrush, *685,* 685–686
Thymectomy, for myasthenia gravis, 2023
Thymus, structure and function of, *2073,* 2073–2074
Thyroglobulin, reference values for, 2305t
Thyroid antibodies, 1094t
  in thyroiditis, 1107t
Thyroid cartilage, 1613, *1613*
  fracture of, 1682
Thyroid disorders, 1089–1109. See also *Hyperthyroidism; Hypothyroidism.*
  outcomes classification for, 1089
  physical examination in, of neck, 107b, 1074, *1075*
Thyroid function, assessment of, 1078–1079, 1094t
Thyroid gland, abscess of, 1106
  anatomy of, 1062, *1064*
  cancer of, 1107–1109, 1108t
  enlargement of, 1089–1090, *1090*
  hormones secreted by, 1065–1066
  imaging of, 1095t
  palpation of, 1074, *1075,* 1075b

Thyroid hormone, 1065–1066. See also *Hyperthyroidism; Hypothyroidism; Thyroxine (T₄); Triiodothyronine (T₃)*
Thyroid scan, 1095t
Thyroid storm, 1100
  thyroidectomy and, 1105
  treatment of, 1101
Thyroid supplements, 1093, 1096t
  self-care and, 1098, 1098b
Thyroidectomy, for hyperthyroidism, 1103–1105
  for thyroid cancer, 1108t, 1109
  hypoparathyroidism after. See *Hypoparathyroidism.*
  postoperative care in, 1104t, 1104–1105
Thyroiditis, 1106–1107, 1107t
Thyroid-stimulating hormone (TSH), 1066, 1138t
  in thyroiditis, 1107t
  reference values for, 2305t
  serum, 1079
Thyroid-stimulating hormone (TSH) assay, 1094t
Thyroplasty, for vocal cord paralysis, 1681
Thyrotoxicosis, 1100, 1101
  clinical manifestations of, 1097
  thyroidectomy and, 1105
Thyrotropin-releasing hormone (TRH), 1066
Thyrotropin-releasing hormone (TRH) stimulation test, 1079, 1094t
Thyroxine (T₄), 1065–1066
  in thyroid disorder diagnosis, 1094t
  in thyroiditis, 1107t
  reference values for, 2305t
  serum, 1078
Thyroxine-binding globulins (TBGs), 1094t
TIA. See *Transient ischemic attack (TIA).*
Tibial fractures, 617
Tibial nerve, examination of, *547*
Tidal volume, 183, 1615, *1615*
  measurement of, 1637, 1638t
Time zone change syndrome, 437
Tinea, 1311t
Tinel's sign, 1998, *2000*
Tinnitus, 1799, 1834–1835
  medical management of, 1836
Tissue expanders, in reconstructive surgery, 1325–1326
  of breast, 1029
Tissue hypoxia, in shock, 2236, *2238*
Tissue load, management of, 1296, 1300b
Tissue-type plasminogen activator. See also *Thrombolytics.*
  for peripheral arterial occlusive disease, 1404
  in arterial bypass surgery, 1407
TKR. See *Total knee replacement.*
TMJ. See *Temporomandibular joint (TMJ).*
TNM staging system, 373, 373t, 1279b, 1728b
Tobacco use. See *Smoking.*
Tobramycin, reference values for, 2307t
Tocainide, reference values for, 2308t
Toe, fracture of, 619
  hammer, 583, *583*
Tolcapone, for Parkinson's disease, 2018, 2019t
Tolerance, to opioid analgesics, 485
Tolmetin, 486, 487t
Tomography, 195
  computed. See *Computed tomography (CT).*
  in musculoskeletal assessment, 546
  positron emission. See *Positron emission tomography (PET).*
Tongue, examination of, 651–652
Tonic seizures, 1925
Tonic-clonic seizures, 1925–1926, *1926*
Tonometry, *1795,* 1795–1796
Tonsillectomy, 1678–1679

Tonsillitis, 1678–1679
  chronic, 1679
  peritonsillar abscess and, 1679
Tonsils, 1612, *1613*
Topical anesthesia, 296–298, 297t. See also *Anesthesia.*
Topical therapy, 1279–1282, 1280t
  antibiotic, 327t, 332–333, 1280t
  for burns, 1347–1348, 1348t
  for skin disorders, 1280–1283
  for wounds, 327t, 332–333
  lubricants in, 1283
  occlusive dressings in, 1281t
  soaks in, 1282–1283
  steroids in, 1280t, 1281–1282
  Unna boot in, 1282
  vehicles for, 1280–1281, 1281t
  wet wraps in, 1282–1283, *1283*
  wound dressings in, 1282
Torsades de pointes, *1564,* 1565
Total care nursing, 99
Total free catecholamines, urinary, reference values for, 2306t
Total gastrectomy, 720, *720.* See also *Gastric surgery.*
Total hip replacement (THR), 555–563
  assessment in, 557
  cemented vs. noncemented, 555–556
  client teaching in, 557–558
  clinical pathway for, 562, *563*
  complications in, 557
    management and prevention of, 557–562
  components for, *556,* 556–557
  contraindications to, 556
  exercises for, 559
  indications for, 555–556
  infection in, 560–561
  mobility after, 559
  nursing management in, 557–562
  outcomes in, 557
  positioning in, 558, 560, *560*
  postoperative care in, 558–563
  self-care in, 562–563
  skin care in, 561
  surgical technique in, 556–557
  venous thrombosis in, 561–562
Total hysterectomy, 992, *992.* See also *Hysterectomy.*
Total hysterectomy with bilateral salpingo-oophorectomy (TAH-BSO), 992
  for ovarian cancer, 1002
Total knee replacement (TKR), *564,* 564–565, *565*
Total lung capacity, 1615, *1615*
  measurement of, 1637, 1638t
Total lymphocyte count, nutritional status and, 655–656
Total metanephrines, urinary, reference values for, 2306t
Total parenteral nutrition (TPN), 668–671
  administration of, 669, *669,* 670, 670t
  client teaching for, 676, 678b
  delegation in, 677b
  formulas for, 668t, 668–669, 669t
  in inflammatory bowel disease, 774
  indications for, 668, 668b
  monitoring in, 676, 678t
  preoperative, 284
  self-care in, 676, 678b
Total peripheral resistance, 1364–1365
Total proctocolectomy, 775
Total protein, 1082t
Total shoulder replacement, in rheumatoid arthritis, 2155, *2155*
Touch, 1264
  assessment of, 1888
Tourniquet test, 2099t

Toxic goiter, diffuse, *1090*. See also *Graves' disease.*
Toxic megacolon, 772
Toxic shock syndrome, 1003
Toxicology, 2281t, 2281–2282
    reference values in, 2309t
Toxoplasmosis, 1948
    in HIV infection, 2204
    pathogenesis of, 337t
TPN. See *Total parenteral nutrition (TPN).*
Trabeculectomy, 1813
Trabeculoplasty, laser, 1813
Trace elements, in parenteral nutrition, 668, 669t
Trachea, disorders of, in tracheostomy, 1654
    palpation of, 1629
    structure of, 1613–1614, *1614*
Tracheal stenosis, in tracheostomy, 1654
Tracheobronchial suctioning, in coma, 1913
Tracheobronchial tree, structure of, 1613–1617, *1614–1616*
Tracheobronchitis, 1705
Tracheoesophageal fistula, in tracheostomy, 1654
    assessment for, 1658
Tracheoesophageal puncture, 1669, *1671*, 1671b
Tracheostomy, 1651–1660
    arterial blood gas analysis in, 1657
    communication in, 689
    complications of, 1654–1655
    decannulation in, 1656, 1666–1667, 1669
        accidental, 1655
    definition of, 1651
    dressings for, 1658, *1659*
    in laryngectomy, *1665*, 1665–1668, *1667*
    incision in, *1652*
    indications for, 1651–1652
    infection control in, 1655, 1657
    nursing care in, 1656–1660
        postoperative, 1656–1660, 1666–1667, 1668
        preoperative, 1656
    permanent, in total laryngectomy, 1669
    tube for, 1654
    rescue breathing in, 1656
    self-care for, 1659–1660, 1660b, 1669–1670, *1671, 1672*
    talking, 1653
    weaning in, 1655–1656
Tracheostomy button, 1653–1654
Tracheostomy tube, changing of, 1655, *1658*
    cuff inflation and deflation for, 1653b
    cuff pressure for, 1654
    dislodgement of, 1655
    obstruction of, 1654–1655
    parts of, 1652, *1654*
    problems with, 1654–1655
    removal of, 1656
    securing of, 1657
    selection of, 1652
    suctioning of, 1656–1657, 1667
    types of, 1652–1654
Tracheotomy, definition of, 1651
Traction, 598–599, 599b, 599t
    care plan for, 610–611
    Crutchfield tongs for, 2053, *2053*
    for hip fractures, 608
    for spinal cord injury, *2053*, 2053–2054
    Gardner-Wells tongs for, 2053, *2053*
    halo, 2054, *2054*
    nursing management in, 607, 610
Traditional healers, 74b–75b. See also *Alternative therapies.*
Tranquilizers, preoperative, 290t
Transcapillary fluid exchange, 735
Transcription, 209

Transcultural nursing. See also *Cultural factors.*
    concepts in, 146
    health beliefs and practices and, 19b
Transcutaneous electrical nerve stimulation (TENS), 497, *497*
Transcutaneous oxygen determination, 1325
Transdermal analgesia, 495
Transesophageal echocardiography, 1473–1474
    in myocardial infarction, 1590
Transfer, bed-to-wheelchair, *1972, 2061*
    for hemiplegic, *1972*
    to intensive care unit, 302
Transferrin, 656t
Transforming growth factors, in wound healing, 318, 320
Transfusion(s), acute reactions to, 2111, 2112t
    blood acceptability for, 2110
    blood infusion in, 2110
    blood release request for, 2110
    complications of, delayed, 2109
    consent for, 287, *288*
    for anemia, 2105–2109, 2106t–2108t
    for hemophilia, 2127
    for leukemia, 2169
    for shock, 2247–2248
    HIV transmission via, 2186–2188
    in hyperkalemia, 248
    infection transmission via, 340, 1226
    monitoring during, 2110–2111
    venous access for, 2109–2110
Transient ischemic attack (TIA), 1978–1980
    balance disorders in, 1849
    diabetes mellitus and, 1184
    stroke and, 1955, 1978–1980
Transillumination, of scrotum, *938*, 938–939
    of sinuses, 1636
Transitional care unit, 98, 98b
Transjugular intrahepatic portosystemic shunt, for bleeding esophageal varices, 1242
Translation, 209
Transmission, of infections, 336
Transmission-based precautions, 344
Transmucosal analgesia, 495
Transmyocardial revascularization, 1526
Transplantation, bone marrow, 2179–2180
    allogenic, 389
    autologous, 389, 2179
    for aplastic anemia, 2115
    for cancer, 389
    for leukemia, 2173
    graft-versus-host disease and, 2180t, 2180–2182
    syngeneic, 2179
    cardiac, 1502–1504, 1503t, *1504*, 1504b, 1505t, 1546, 2226. See also *Cardiac surgery.*
        complications of, 1511–1512
    client teaching for, 2227b, 2227–2228
    commercialization of, 2215
    complications of, 2223–2225
    contraindications to, 2221b
    corneal, *1822*, 1822–1823
    costs of, 2214–2215
    cultural aspects of, 2216t–2217t
    donors for, brain death determination for, 2215, 2221
        ethical considerations in, 2215
        medical management of, 2221–2222
        payment of, 2215
        prisoners as, 2215
        selection of, 2221–2222, 2222b
        shortage of, 2215
    government regulation of, 2215, 2218–2221
    historical perspective on, 2213–2214, *2214*
    HLA matching for, 2179, 2223
    immunologic aspects of, 2223

Transplantation (*Continued*)
    immunosuppression for, 2223, 2224t
        compliance with, 2228
    infection in, 2225, 2225t
    inter-species, 2215
    liver, 1256–1257, 2226
        for sclerosing cholangitis, 1215
    lung, 1741–1742, 2226–2227
    malignancy after, 2225
    nurse's role in, 2221–2222
    nursing diagnoses for, 2228b
    organ harvesting for, *2221*, 2222
    organ procurement organizations in, 2219–2221
    pancreas, 2226
        for diabetes mellitus, 1171–1172
    pancreas-kidney, 2226
    parathyroid, 1113
    postoperative care in, 2222–2223
    psychosocial aspects of, 2219
    quality of life after, 2228, 2288–2289
    recipients of, postoperative care for, 2222–2223
        preparation of, 2222
        prisoners as, 2215
        selection of, 2215–2217, *2218*, 2219t, *2220*
    rejection in, 2223–2225
        acute, 2223–2224
        chronic, 2224–2225
        hyperacute, 2224
    religious beliefs and, 2216t–2217t
    renal, 899–901, 2225–2226
        for diabetes mellitus, 1171–1172
    self-care in, 2227b, 2227–2228
    small intestinal, 776
    waiting for, 2217–2218
Transport, from operating room, 302
    to operating room, 289
Transrectal prostate biopsy, 761
Transsexuality, 418b
Transsphenoidal hypophysectomy, 1935–1937, *1936*
Transtheoretical Model, 12–13
Transudates, 1743
Transurethral biopsy, 761
Transurethral incision of prostate (TUIP), 955
Transurethral resection of prostate (TURP), 949–954, *954*
Transurethral ultrasound-guided laser incision of prostate (TULIP), 955
Transverse fracture, 595t
Transverse rectus abdominis flap, in breast reconstruction, 1029, *1029*
Trastuzumab (Herceptin), for breast cancer, 1033
Trauma, abdominal, 798–799
    auricular, 1842
    bladder, 846
    chest, 1764–1770
    head, 2039–2046
    laryngeal, 1682
    liver, 1259
    pancreatic, 1202
    penile, 972
    renal, *867*, 867–869
    scrotal, 972
    spinal, 2046–2068
    tympanic membrane, 1832
    ureteral, 847
    urethral, 846–847
    urinary tract, 751
Traumatic amputation, 1328, 1415
    emergency care for, 2279
Traumatic brain injury. See *Head trauma.*
Treadmill testing, 1376, 1470–1472
    first-past cardiac study in, 1475
    myocardial scintigraphy in, 1474

Treatment, withholding/withdrawal of, in emergencies, 2264–2265
in terminal illness, 527–528
termination of resuscitation and, 1567–1568
Trecator-SC (ethionamide), for tuberculosis, 1720, 1721t
Tremor, in Parkinson's disease, 2017
Trench mouth, 684–685
Trendelenburg position, 299, *300*
modified, in shock, 2246, *2246*
Trendelenburg test, 1373
TRH. See *Thyrotropin-releasing hormone (TRH)*.
Triage, 2265, 2265t. See also *Emergency care*.
telephone, 90
Triamcinolone (Kenalog), 1280t
Triceps reflex, 1889, 1891t
Trichinosis, 767
Trichloroacetic acid peels, 1318
Trichomoniasis, 1054–1055
Tricuspid valve, 1434t, 1435, *1436, 1437*
Tricuspid valve disease, *1494*, 1500
surgery for, 1501–1502. See also *Cardiac surgery*.
Tricyclic antidepressants, 422
for pain, 450, 451t, 491, 492
perioperative use of, 275t
Trigeminal nerve, 1870t
assessment of, 1885
distribution of, 1995, *1995*
Trigeminal neuralgia, 1995–1996
Trigger point injection, 496
Triglycerides, 14
elevated, 1517. See also *Hyperlipoproteinemia*.
reference values for, 2305t
target levels for, 15
Trigone, 734
Trihexyphenidyl (Artane), for Parkinson's disease, 2019t
Triiodothyronine (T$_3$), 1065–1066
reference values for, 2305t
serum, 1078
in thyroiditis, 1107t
Triiodothyronine (T$_3$) radioimmunoassay, 1094t
Triiodothyronine (T$_3$) resin uptake, 1078–1079, 1094t
Trimethoprim-sulfamethoxazole (Bactrim), for urinary tract infection, 804t
Trochanter roll, 1974
Trochlear nerve, 1870t
assessment of, 1884
Troponin, 1464–1465
in myocardial infarction, 1588–1589, *1589*
Trousseau's sign, 250, 251, *251*
hypoparathyroidism and, 1115
thyroidectomy and, 1105
TSH. See *Thyroid-stimulating hormone (TSH)*.
Tube(s), chest. See *Chest tubes*.
endotracheal. See *Endotracheal intubation*.
gastrointestinal, 706t, 706–708. See also *Feeding tube; Gastrointestinal intubation*.
in balloon tamponade, for bleeding esophageal varices, 1242
and gas exchange, 1243
rectal, 799
Sengstaken-Blakemore, in balloon tamponade, for bleeding esophageal varices, 1242, *1242*, 1243
tracheostomy. See *Tracheostomy tube*.
types of, 1652–1654
venipuncture, 192t–193t
Tube feeding. See *Enteral nutrition*.

Tuberculin converter, 1720
Tuberculin skin test, *1719*, 1719–1720
Tuberculosis, 1716–1723
client teaching for, 1722, 1722b
clinical manifestations of, 1718–1719
diagnosis of, *1719*, 1719–1720
drug-resistant, 340, 1718
epidemiology of, 1717
etiology of, 1718
extrapulmonary, 1722–1723
in health care providers, prevention of, 345–346
in HIV infection, 1718, 2202–2203
prevention of, 2199
medical management of, *1719*
miliary, 1722
nosocomial, 340
nursing management of, 1720–1722
pathogenesis of, 337t
pathophysiology of, 1718
prevention of, 1720–1722
primary infection in, 1718
renal, 857
risk factors for, 1718
secondary infection in, 1718
self-care in, 1722
urinary tract involvement in, 752
Tubuloglomerular feedback, 737
Tubulointerstitial disease, 862
Tumor(s). See also specific sites and types.
benign, 349, 362–363, 363t
biopsy of, 371–373, 374. See also *Biopsy*.
bone, 580t, 580–582
characteristics of, 363t
definition of, 349
grading of, 358, 373
growth of, 359, *359*, 363t
malignant, 349, 362, 363t. See also *Cancer*.
metastatic, 359–360, *360*
skin, *1271*
Tumor burden, 359
Tumor doubling time, 359, *359*
Tumor lysis syndrome, 247, 396, 2169
Tumor markers, 350t, 372t
in breast cancer, 931–932, 1018
Tumor necrosis factor, 2087, 2087t
Tumor-specific antigens, 358, 361
Tunica adventitia, 1362, *1364*
Tunica intima, 1362, *1364*
Tunica media, 1362, *1364*
Turgor, skin, assessment of, 222–223, *223*
Turner's sign, in pancreatitis, 1195
Turning, after spinal fusion, 1989, *1990*
logrolling for, 2053
Turning exercises, preoperative teaching for, 286
Twenty-four-hour recall, for activity, 33
for diet, 32
Twenty-four-hour urine collection, 191–192
in nitrogen balance assessment, 656
Two-point stimulation, assessment of, 1889
Tylenol. See *Acetaminophen (Tylenol)*.
Tylox (Oxycodone), 489t
Tympanic membrane, 1783
in sound wave conduction, 1785
infection of, 1842
physical examination of, 1802, *1802*
traumatic injuries to, 1832
Tympanometry, 1805–1806
Tympanoplasty, 1846
Tympanosclerosis, 1802, 1832, 1842
Tympany, on percussion, 177–178, 742
Type A personality, 7t
Type B personality, 7t
Tzanck's smear, 1276

U

Ulcer(s), *1272*. See also *Wound(s)*.
arterial, 1416, *1417*
corneal, 1823, *1823*
diabetic, 1184–1185, *1185*, 1186b, 1187b, 1188
eschar in, *328*
healing of, 332
duodenal, drug-induced, 712
in peptic ulcer disease. See *Peptic ulcer disease (PUD)*.
stress, 712
gastric, drug-induced, 712, *713*
in peptic ulcer disease, 712, 713t. See also *Peptic ulcer disease (PUD)*.
in Zollinger-Ellison syndrome, 714
marginal, 720–721
stress-induced, 712, 714
in syphilis, 1050, *1050*
oral, 684
chemotherapy and, 394, 1034
herpetic, 684, *685*
in aphthous stomatitis, 684
pressure, 1295–1302. See also *Pressure ulcers*.
stasis. See *Venous ulcers*.
stress, 712, 714, 2034t
prevention of, 2251
venous. See *Venous ulcers*.
assessment for, 1372, *1373*
Ulcerative colitis, 770–780
clinical manifestations of, 771t, 772–773
etiology of, 771–772
medical management of, 773–774
nursing management of, 774
pathophysiology of, 771t, 772
prognosis in, 771t, 772–773
surgery for, 774–780
postoperative care in, 776–780
preoperative care in, 776–780
vs. Crohn's disease, 771t
vs. ulcerative colitis, 771t
Ulnar drift, in rheumatoid arthritis, 2145, *2145*, 2156
Ulnar fractures, 618
Ulnar nerve, examination of, *547*
Ulnar nerve syndrome, 1998, 1999t
Ulnar pulse, assessment of, 1373, *1374*
Ultradian cycles, 432
Ultrafiltration, 888
Ultralente insulin, 1162t, *1163*. See also *Insulin therapy*.
Ultrasonography, *198*, 198–199
abdominal, 657, 746
Doppler, in neurologic assessment, 1896
in skin graft assessment, 1324
in vascular assessment, 1375–1376
in venous thrombosis, 1424
in reproductive assessment, in females, 928
in respiratory assessment, 1645
intravascular, 1377
of breast, 933
of eye, 1797, *1797*
of gallbladder, in acute cholecystitis, 1212
of prostate, 941
imaging of, 758–760
of thyroid gland, 1095t
of urinary tract, 759
Ultraviolet light therapy, 1283–1284
Ultraviolet radiation, skin cancer and, 15
Umbilical hernia, 787–789, *788*
Umbilical vein catheterization, 1084
Umbrella filter, 1426, 1708, *1708*
Unconsciousness, 1906. See also *Coma*.
emergency care in, 2276
motor assessment in, 1887–1888

Undescended testis, 967–968
  infertility and, 968, 969
  testicular cancer and, 964, 967
Unguis incarnatus, 1328
Uniform Anatomical Gift Act, 2215, 2218–2219
Unilateral neglect, 1977
  in stroke, 1957t, 1960
Uninhibited neurogenic bladder, 841, 841–845
Universal precautions, 343
Unlicensed assistive personnel, 100, 100b. See
    also Health care providers.
  diagnostic testing by, 188b
  enteral nutrition administration by, 1915b
  fluid management by, 222b
  heat and cold application by, 614b
  ileostomy care by, 778b
  infection control by, 344b
  mobility promotion by, 573
  nutritional support by, 677b
  postoperative care by, in plastic surgery,
      1320b
  postoperative wound care by, 310b
  pressure ulcer care by, 1301b
  rectal pouch application by, 799
  rectal tube insertion by, 799
  respiratory care by, 1657b
  restraint use by, 1921b
  skin inspection by, 1295b
  vital signs measurement by, 183b
Unna boot, 1282, 1429
Unnatural illnesses, 19b
Unstable angina, 1581, 1582
Upper airway, disorders of, 1651–1683
  structures of, 1612–1613, 1613
Upper extremity, examination of, 167t
Upper gastrointestinal series, 195, 656–657
Upper motor neuron, 1860
Upper motor neuron lesions, 1997
  in amyotrophic lateral sclerosis, 2023
  neurogenic bladder and, 840, 842
Urates, serum, reference values for, 2305t
  urine, reference values for, 2307t
Urea, reference values for, 2305t
Urecholine (bethanechol), for gastroesophageal
    reflux disease, 696
  for urinary incontinence, 837t
Uremia, 875–876. See also Renal failure.
Uremic lung, 886
Uremic syndrome, 875–876. See also Renal
    failure.
Ureter, abnormal dilation of, 846
  anatomy of, 732, 734
  congenital anomalies of, 751, 846
  duplicate, 846
  ectopic, 846
  imaging of, 758–760
  injuries of, 751
  pain in, 750
  traumatic injuries of, 847
  tumors of, 821
Ureteral catheterization. See Urinary catheteri-
    zation.
  in urolithiasis, 828
Ureteral colic, 750
  in urolithiasis, 824, 825
Ureteritis, 809
Ureteropelvic obstruction, congenital, 846
Ureterorenal reflex, 737
Ureterorenoscopy, 760
Ureteroscopy, 760
  for urinary calculi, 826
Ureterostomy, 813, 815. See also Urinary di-
    version.
Ureterolithotomy, 828
Urethra, anatomy of, 732, 734–735
  cavernous (penile), 735

Urethra (Continued)
  congenital anomalies of, 847
  examination of, 755–756
  injuries of, 751
  membranous, 735
  pain in, 751
  palpation of, 756
  prolapse of, 998, 998
  prostatic, 912–913
  traumatic injuries of, 846–847
Urethral catheterization. See Urinary catheteri-
    zation.
Urethral meatus, examination of, in female, 924
  in male, 936–938
Urethral pressure profile, 763
Urethral stricture, 971
Urethritis, 809
  chlamydial, 1044t, 1047
  gonococcal, 1044t, 1049
Urethrocele, 998, 998
Urethroscopy, 760
Urethrovaginal fistula, 1003, 1003–1004
Urge incontinence, 749, 834. See also Urinary
    incontinence.
  alternative therapy for, 833b
  in Alzheimer's disease, 2007
Urgency, urinary, 748
Uric acid stones, 823
Urinalysis, 191, 756–758, 757t
  normal findings on, 193t
  reference values for, 2306t–2307t
  specimen collection for, 189–190, 191–192,
      757–758
Urinary bladder. See Bladder.
Urinary buffer systems, 261, 261, 262
Urinary calculi, 821–829
  calcium, 822–823
  clinical manifestations of, 824
  cystine, 824
  epidemiology of, 822
  etiology of, 822
  hypercalcemia and, 253
  ileostomy and, 779
  in spinal cord injury, 2063
  medical management of, 824–825
  oxalate, 823
  pathophysiology of, 822
  prevention of, 825–826, 826b
    in hyperparathyroidism, 1112–1113
  recurrent, 825
  risk factors for, 822
  staghorn, 823, 823
  struvite, 823
  surgery for, 825–826, 826b
  types of, 822–824
  uric acid, 823
  xanthine, 824
Urinary catheterization, catheter insertion in,
    845b
  catheter types in, 950–953
  for urinary retention, 831–832
  in benign prostatic hyperplasia, 948b, 949
  in spinal cord injury, 2059, 2063
  in urolithiasis, 828
  infection in, 802, 803
  intermittent self, in benign prostatic hyper-
      plasia, 948b
    in neurogenic bladder, 844, 845b, 846
  postoperative, in bladder surgery, 816–817
    in prostate surgery, 956–958
  suprapubic, 832–833
Urinary catheters, specimen collection from,
    190
  types of, 190
Urinary diversion, in elderly, 821
  monitoring after, 817b
  odor control in, 818

Urinary diversion (Continued)
  postoperative care in, 816–821, 817b
  pouch application in, 818, 819
  preoperative care in, 815–816
  reservoir catheterization in, 819–820
  reservoir irrigation in, 820
  self-care in, 817–821, 818b
  skin care in, 818
  stoma in, care of, 817–818
    postoperative assessment of, 816
    stenosis of, 816
Urinary elimination, assessment of, 747–763
  diagnostic tests in, 756–763
  history in, 747–754
  in neurologic assessment, 1878t
  physical examination in, 754–756
  Symptom Index for, 748, 748
  disorders of, 747–751, 829–846
    in hyperparathyroidism, 1112–1113
    in urinary tract infection, 803
    irritative, 748
    obstructive, 748. See also Urinary tract
        obstruction.
  drug effects on, 752t
  in shock, 2248
  in spinal cord injury, 841–846, 2049, 2059,
      2063, 2066–2067
  in systemic disease, 751
  strain void in, 820
  with urinary diversion, 816–821. See also
      Urinary diversion.
Urinary frequency, 748
Urinary hesitancy, 748
Urinary incontinence, 749, 833–846
  after prostate surgery, 58, 956
  clinical manifestations of, 835
  etiology of, 834–835
  in Alzheimer's disease, 2007
  in elderly, 737–738, 841
  in multiple sclerosis, 2013, 2014
  in spinal cord injury, 841–846, 2049, 2059,
      2063, 2066–2067
  in stroke, 1960
  medical management of, 835–837, 837t
  neurogenic bladder and, 841–846. See also
      Neurogenic bladder.
  nursing management in, 837–839
  overflow, 749, 834
  pathophysiology of, 835
  postmenopausal, 985, 986
  risk factors for, 834–835
  self-care in, 841
  stress, 749, 834
  surgery for, 839, 841
  types of, 749
  urge, 749, 834
    alternative therapy for, 833b
  urinary retention and, 829
Urinary output, in shock, 2248, 2254
Urinary reflux, 829
Urinary retention, 748, 829–833
  autonomic dysreflexia and, 2050–2051,
      2064b, 2064–2065
  in benign prostatic hyperplasia, 946, 948
  in neurogenic bladder, 843
  intermittent self-catheterization for, 844,
      845b, 846, 948b
  opioid analgesics and, 491
Urinary sphincter, artificial, 841, 841
  intrinsic deficiency of, 835, 839
Urinary system, in shock, 2241, 2243
Urinary tract, age-related changes in, 212t,
    737–738
  structures of, 732, 732
Urinary tract disorders, 801–847
  assessment of, 747–763
    diagnostic tests in, 756–763

Urinary tract disorders (Continued)
history in, 747–754
physical examination in, 754–756
Symptom Index for, 748, 748
clinical manifestations of, 750–751
congenital, 751, 846
drug-related, 752, 752t
gastrointestinal manifestations of, 750–751
imaging studies in, 758–760
in diabetes mellitus, 1189
infectious/inflammatory, 802–809. See also
Urinary tract infection (UTI).
irritative, 748
diet and, 753, 753t
obstructive. See Urinary tract obstruction.
outcome classification for, 801
pain in, 750–751
traumatic, 751, 845–846
voiding, 829–845
Urinary tract infection (UTI), 802–807
alternative therapy for, 833b
antibiotics for, 803, 804t–805t
assessment in, 805
catheter-related, 802, 803
clinical manifestations of, 803
complications of, 804–805, 806
diagnosis of, 803
epidemiology of, 802
etiology of, 802
in diabetes mellitus, 1184
in elderly, 807
medical management of, 803–805, 805t
microbiology of, 802
nosocomial, 338, 338t
pathophysiology of, 802
prevention of, 806
pyuria in, 750
recurrent, 803
risk factors for, 802
self-care in, 807
urinary retention and, 829, 832
urosepsis and, 809–810
Urinary tract obstruction, 748, 809–829
effects of, 830
hydronephrosis and, 858
in benign prostatic hyperplasia, 946, 947,
947
in urolithiasis. See Urolithiasis.
postrenal failure in, 876
reflux and, 829
sites of, 734
urinary retention and, 829–833
Urinary urgency, 748
Urinary volume, changes in, 747–748
Urination, 737
age-related changes in, 737–738
mechanism of, 737
stimulation of, for neurogenic bladder, 843,
2066–2067
Urine, amylase in, 1081t
after pancreas transplantation, 1172
in acute pancreatitis, 1195
bilirubin in, 1081t
jaundice and, 1220
blood in. See Hematuria.
calcium in, 1111t
catecholamines in, adrenal function and,
1079
pheochromocytoma and, 1136
characteristics of, 749–750
clarity of, 749t, 750
color of, 749t, 749–750
hepatitis and, 1227
concentration of, 736–737
tests for, 758
cortisol in, Cushing's syndrome and, 1130
dilution of, 736–737

Urine (Continued)
tests for, 758
formation of, 735–737
regulation of, 737
gas in, 750
glucose in, 757, 757t
ketones in, 757, 757t
diabetes mellitus and, 1156t, 1158, 1168.
See also Diabetic ketoacidosis.
nitrites in, 757, 757t
odor of, 750
osmolality of, 756, 757t
reference values for, 2306t
osmolarity of, 736–737
pH of, 756, 757t
reference values for, 2306t
post-void residual of, 831
production of, 737
protein in. See Proteinuria.
reference values for, 2306t–2307t
specific gravity of, 756, 757t, 2307t
urobilinogen in, 1081t
jaundice and, 1220
white blood cells in, 749t, 750, 757, 757t
Urine casts, 750, 750, 757, 757t
Urine clearance studies, 758
Urine culture, 189–190, 758
in urinary tract infection, 803
specimen collection for, 189–190, 191–192
Urine cytology, 758
Urine output, decreased, in dehydration, 219
in acute renal failure, 877–878
in burns, 1337
in urolithiasis, 828
increased, in dehydration, 219
measurement of, 219, 222
normal values for, 876
postoperative, cholelithiasis and, 1210–
1211
reduced, in dehydration, 219
Urine specimen, clean-catch, 189–190
collection of, 189–190, 191–192, 757–758
segmented, 963
12/24-hour, 191–192
24-hour, in nitrogen balance assessment,
656
Urine urea nitrogen, 656
Urobilinogen, fecal, 1081t
in jaundice, 1220, 1221t–1222t
urine, 1081t, 2307t
Urodynamic assessment, in male reproductive
assessment, 942
Urodynamic studies, 762–763, 835
Uroflowmetry, 762, 762
in benign prostatic hyperplasia, 947
Urogenital displacement, 998, 998–1000,
999
Urokinase, 1406. See also Thrombolytics.
for peripheral arterial occlusive disease,
1404
for venous thrombosis, 1425
in arterial bypass surgery, 1407
Urolithiasis. See Urinary calculi.
Uroporphyrin, reference values for, 2307t
Urosepsis, 808–809
Ursodeoxycholic acid, for cholelithiasis, 1205,
1207
Urticaria, 2136–2137
Uterine bleeding, abnormal, 982–984
leiomyomas and, 991–994
postmenopausal, 986, 987
Uterine cancer, 994, 994–995
screening for, 369t, 370
Uterine fibroids, 362, 991, 991–994, 1000
Uterine lavage, 931
Uterine polyps, 1000
Uterine prolapse, 999, 999–1000

Uterus, benign tumors of, 362, 991, 991–994,
1000
disorders of, 989–1000
examination of, 924
in menstrual cycle, 908, 909
structure and function of, 904–905, 905,
906t
UTI. See Urinary tract infection (UTI).
Uveal tract, 1778–1779
disorders of, 1824
Uveitis, 1824
Uvulopalatopharyngoplasty, for obstructive
sleep apnea, 436

V

Vaccination, 40. See Immunization(s).
Vaccine, human immunodeficiency virus, 2189
Vacuoles, 206, 207t
Vacuum devices, for erectile dysfunction, 974
Vagal nerve stimulator implantation, for epi-
lepsy, 1929–1930
Vagina, examination of, 924
structure and function of, 905, 905, 906t
Vaginal cancer, 1004–1005
Vaginal cone, 836
Vaginal discharge, 1002
in bacterial vaginosis, 1055
in trichomoniasis, 1054–1055
in vaginitis, 1002
Vaginal disorders, 1002–1005
Vaginal fistula, 1003, 1003–1004
Vaginal pessary, 1000
for urinary incontinence, 838
Vaginal pool, aspiration of, 988
Vaginal prolapse, 999, 999–1000
Vaginal pruritus, 1002
Vaginal smear, wet, 927, 928
Vaginal speculum examination, 924, 925
Vaginitis, 1002–1003, 1003b
atrophic, 1003
menopausal, 985
Vaginosis, bacterial, 1055
Vagotomy, 719, 719–720. See also Gastric
surgery.
Vagus nerve, 1870t
Valium (diazepam), emergency administration
of, 1931
for status epilepticus, 1931
preoperative, 290t
Valproate (Depakote), for epilepsy, 1927–1928
reference values for, 2307t
Valsalva maneuver, eustachian tube and, 1785
for urination, 2066
Values and beliefs. See also Religious beliefs
and practices.
assessment of, 144
Valvular heart disease, 1495–1501
aortic valve, 1496, 1498–1500
mitral valve, 1495–1498, 1496, 1498
pulmonic valve, 1496, 1500–1501
surgery for, 1501–1502. See also Cardiac
surgery.
tricuspid valve, 1496, 1500
Valvuloplasty, cardiac, 1502, 1502
Vanceril (beclomethasone), for asthma, 1690,
1691t, 1692, 1694
Vancomycin, reference values for, 2307t
Vancomycin-resistant Enterococcus, 339, 341b
Vanillylmandelic acid (VMA), pheochromocytoma and, 1136
urine, reference values for, 2307t
Variant angina, 1581
Varicella, immunization for, 342, 342t
Varices, esophageal, in cirrhosis, 1241, 1241b,
1241–1243

Varicocele, *966*, 966–967
Varicose veins, 1369, *1426*, 1426–1427
Vas deferens, 911t, 911–912, *912*
Vascular access, for total parenteral nutrition, 669, *669*, 670, 670t
Vascular access devices, for chemotherapy, 386, *386*
Vascular assessment, 1368–1378
    diagnostic tests in, 1375–1377
    history in, 1368–1370
    normal findings in, 1370b
    physical examination in, 1370–1375
Vascular disorders, 1399–1431
    alternative therapy for, 1405
    arterial, 1399–1422
    complementary therapies for, 1405
    lymphatic, 1429–1431
    outcomes classification for, 1399
    venous, 1422–1429
Vascular endoscopy, 1377
Vascular resistance, 1364–1365
Vascular system, post-traumatic changes in, 1323
    structure and function of, 1362–1377, *1363–1366*
Vasculitis, 2162
    rheumatoid arthritis and, 2145
Vasectomy, 967, *967*
Vasoactive polypeptides, in shock, 2239
Vasoactive substances, in shock, 2239
Vasoconstriction, in hemostasis, 2079
    in shock, 2238
Vasoconstrictors, for shock, 2244t, 2244–2245
Vasodilators, for heart failure, 1538t, 1540
    for peripheral arterial occlusive disease, 1402
    for pulmonary hypertension, 1708–1709
    for shock, 2244t, 2245
Vasogenic shock. See *Distributive shock.*
Vasomotor instability, in menopause, 984–985
Vasomotor rhinitis, 1680
Vasopressin. See also *Antidiuretic hormone (ADH).*
    for bleeding esophageal varices, 1242
    for gastrointestinal bleeding, 717
    in dehydration test, 1080
Vasospasm, cerebral artery, stroke and, 1955
    in subarachnoid hemorrhage, 1941–1942
Vasotec (enalapril), for hypertension, 1389t, 1396t
VDRL test, for syphilis, 1051
Vector transmission, 335
Vecuronium (Norcuron), 295t
Vein(s), incompetent, 1369
    structure and function of, *1363*, 1364, *1364*
    varicose, 1369, *1426*, 1426–1427
Vein ligation and stripping, 1427
Vena cava filter, 1426, 1708, *1708*
Venereal Disease Research Laboratory (VDRL) test, for syphilis, 1051
Venipuncture, 190–191
    for blood sampling, 190–191
    procedure for, 190b
    tubes for, 192t–193t
Venography, 198, 1377
Venous access, for transfusion, 2109–2110
Venous disorders, 1422–1429
    acute, 1422–1426
    assessment in. See *Vascular assessment.*
    chronic, 1426–1429
    clinical manifestations of, 1368–1369, 1369t
    home care in, 1428b
Venous hum, abdominal, 654–655
Venous stasis, management of, 1423
    ulcers and. See *Venous ulcers.*
Venous thoracic outlet syndrome, 1422

Venous thrombosis, 1422–1426
    assessment for, 605–606
    chronic venous insufficiency after, *1427*, 1427–1429
    clinical manifestations of, 605, 1424–1425
    etiology of, 1422–1423, 1423b
    immobilization and, 605, 612
    in hip fracture, 612
    medical management of, 1425–1426
    nursing management of, 1425–1426
    pathophysiology of, 1423, *1423*
    postoperative, 308
        in total hip replacement, 561–562
        prevention of, 286, 308
    prevention of, 1423–1424
    pulmonary embolism and, 1423, 1706. See also *Pulmonary embolism.*
    renal vein, 870
    risk factors for, 1422–1423
    surgical management of, 1426
    thrombolytics for, 1406
Venous ulcers, 1291, 1400, *1401*, 1429, *1429*
    assessment for, 1372, *1373*
    healing of, 328
    in postphlebitic syndrome, *1427*, 1427–1428
    prevention of, 1403b
    stasis, 1291
    Unna boot for, 1282, 1429
Ventilation, 1617–1618
    inverse ratio, 1762
    mechanical. See *Mechanical ventilation.*
    perfusion and, 1620–1621, *1621*
Ventilation-perfusion balance, 1620, *1621*
Ventilation-perfusion (V/Q) scan, 1642–1643
    for pulmonary embolism, 1707
Ventilators. See also *Mechanical ventilation.*
    control panels of, *1752, 1753*, 1753b–1754b
    types of, 1752–1754
    weaning from, 1655–1656, 1759–1761, 1761b
Ventilatory failure, acute, 1749–1761
    clinical manifestations of, 1750
    etiology of, 1749
    mechanical ventilation in, 1750–1761. See also *Mechanical ventilation.*
    medical management of, 1750
    pathophysiology of, 1749–1750
    risk factors for, 1749, 1749t
Ventral hernia, 787–788
Ventricles, anatomy and physiology of, 1434, 1434t, 1435
Ventricular assist devices, 1540
Ventricular asystole, *1564*, 1565
Ventricular catheter, in intracranial pressure monitoring, 2030, 2032b–2033b
Ventricular diastole, 1440, *1441*
Ventricular dilation, in heart failure, 1531
Ventricular dysrhythmias, 1559–1566, *1560, 1564*
Ventricular failure, eight-, 1531–1534, *1533*
    left-sided, 1531–1534, *1533*
    right-sided, 1531–1533, *1533*, 1534–1535
Ventricular fibrillation, *1564*, 1564–1565
    defibrillation for, 1566–1568, *1567*
Ventricular independence, 1533
Ventricular premature beats, 1559–1561, *1560*
Ventricular system, 1863, *1864*
Ventricular systole, 1440, *1441*
Ventricular tachycardia, *1560*, 1565
Ventriculoperitoneal shunt, 2038–2039, *2039*
Ventriculostomy, for increased intracranial pressure, 1965
Venules, *1363*, 1364
Verapamil (Calan), for dysrhythmias, 1563t
    for hypertension, 1389t, 1396t

Vertebrae. See also *Spine.*
    fractures of, in osteoporosis, 567, 568, *568*, 572
    radiography of, 1894
Vertebral arteries, 1864, *1864*
Vertebral column. See also *Spine.*
    structure of, 1861
Vertical partial laryngectomy, 1665, *1665*
Vertigo, 1799, 1847. See also *Balance; Vestibular system.*
    benign paroxysmal positional, 1848
    care plan for, 1852b–1853b
    etiology of, 1847, 1847b
    physiologic, 1849
    presbystasis and, 1849
    risk factors for, 1847
    types of, 1849, 1849t
Very low-density lipoproteins (VLDLs), 15, 1517
    target levels for, 15
Vestibulocochlear nerve, 1870t
    assessment of, 1885–1886
Vesicle, *1271*
Vesicoureteral reflux, 734, 829
Vesicovaginal fistula, *1003*, 1003–1004
Vesicular breath sounds, 1632, 1633t
Vestibular bulbs, *905*, 906t
Vestibular nerve, 1870t
    assessment of, 1885
    resection of, 1851
Vestibular rehabilitation, 1850
Vestibular system, disorders of, 1847–1853
    assessment of, 1850–1851
    central, 1849
    clinical manifestations of, 1849t, 1849–1850
    medical management of, 1850
    nursing management of, 1850–1851, 1851b
    pathophysiology of, 1849
    peripheral, 1848–1849
    surgery for, 1851
    systemic disorders and, 1849
    testing of, 1804, 1806, *1806*
Vestibule, nasal, 1612, *1613*
    vaginal, *905*, 906t
Viagra (sildenafil), for erectile dysfunction, 974
Vibration sense, assessment of, 1888
Video-fluoroscopic urodynamics, 763
Videx (didanosine), 2196t
Vincent's angina, 684–685
Violence, domestic, 39
    assessment for, 918
Violent patients, management of, 2263–2264
Vioxx (meloxicam), 486t
Viracept (nelfinavir), 2197t
Viral encephalitis, 1947
Viral hepatitis, 1223–1229, 1224t. See also *Hepatitis.*
Viral infections, cancer and, 355, 355t
    cell damage in, 213
    central nervous system, 1946–1947
    pathogenesis of, 337t
Viral load testing, in HIV infection, 2193, 2195
Viral meningitis, 1946–1947
Viral pneumonia, 1711–1716, 1712t
Viramune (nevirapine), 2198t
Virchow's triad, 1422
Visceral pain, 472, 766
Visceral pleura, *1614*, 1617
Viscosity, serum, reference values for, 2305t
Vision. See also *Eye.*
    age-related changes in, 50t, 53, 1781–1782, 1821, *1822*
    assessment of, 1792–1794, *1793*

Vision (Continued)
  double, 1885
  light transmission in, 1780–1781
  peripheral, aging and, 1782
  refractive disorders of, 1826–1828, 1827
  retinal receptors in, 1780, 1781
Vision assessment, in neurologic assessment, 1883–1885
Vision impairment. See also specific eye disorders.
  adaptations for, 1819b
  emergency care for, 2277–2278
  health promotion/risk management for, 149t, 156t
  in diabetes mellitus, 1156t, 1186–1187, 1188b
  in stroke, 1957t, 1958–1960, 1959, 1976–1977
  preparation for, glaucoma and, 1812
Visual acuity, testing of, 1792–1793, 1793
Visual agnosia, in stroke, 1957t, 1959–1960, 1976
Visual Analog Scale, for pain, 477, 481
Visual cortex, 1781, 1781
Visual evoked response, 1797
Visual field defects, in stroke, 1957t, 1959, 1959
Visual field testing, 1793, 1793
Visual fields, assessment of, 1884
Visual laser ablation of prostate (VLAP), 956
Visual system. See also Eye.
  disorders of, 1809–1830. See also specific disorders.
  function of, 1780–1781, 1781
  structure of, 1778–1780, 1779
Vital capacity, 1615, 1615
  measurement of, 1637, 1638t
Vital signs, assessment of, 183b, 183–185
  in neurologic assessment, 1880, 2035
  in shock, 2252
Vitamin(s), absorption of, 637
  antioxidant, 15
  cancer and, 15
  deficiency of, 641t–642t
  food sources of, 641t–642t
  in cirrhosis, 1239
  in parenteral nutrition, 668, 669t
  supplemental, for hemodialysis, 894
Vitamin A, as antioxidant, 15
  deficiency of, 641t
  food sources of, 641t
  reference values for, 2305t
Vitamin B₆, deficiency of, 641t
  food sources of, 641t
  for isoniazid overdose, 2281t
Vitamin B₁₂, deficiency of, 641t, 2113–2114
  food sources of, 641t
  in erythropoiesis, 2077
  reference values for, 2305t
Vitamin C, as antioxidant, 15
  deficiency of, 641t
  food sources of, 641t
  reference values for, 2303t
Vitamin D, calcium and, 1068
  calcium metabolism and, 570
  deficiency of, 15, 641t
    hypocalcemia and, 250
  food sources of, 641t
  replacement, for hypocalcemia, 252
    in hypoparathyroidism, 1115, 1116
  supplemental, 570
  synthesis of, skin in, 1264
Vitamin E, as antioxidant, 15
  deficiency of, 641t
  food sources of, 641t

Vitamin K, deficiency of, 641t–642t
    hypoprothrombinemia and, 2123
  food sources of, 641t
  liver function and, 1065
Vitreous body, 1780
  age-related changes in, 1782
Vocal cords, nodules on, 1660
  paralysis of, 1681–1682
Voice, thyroidectomy and, 1105
Voice box. See Larynx.
Voice sounds, 1635
Voiding. See also Urinary elimination; Urination.
Voiding cystourethrogram, 759
Voiding disorders, 829–845
Voiding schedule, 836, 838
Volkmann's canals, 531, 534
Volkmann's contracture, 600
Volume plethysmography (body box), 1637, 1640
Voluntary effort, 80
Voluntary emotional dissociation, 1996
Voluntary health agencies, 96
Volvulus, intestinal, 790, 790–793
Vomiting, 634, 705–706
  dehydration and, 218
  in brain tumors, 1934
  in bulimia nervosa, 679
  in chemotherapy, 393–394, 1034
  in hepatitis, 1231
  in inflammatory bowel disease, 772, 773
  in intestinal disorders, 766
  in peptic ulcer disease, 714
  in spinal anesthesia, 296t
  opioid analgesics and, 450, 491
  postoperative, 311b, 311–312
Von Recklinghausen's disease, 2001
Von Willebrand's disease, 2126t
Voodoo, 74b
Vowels-TIP mnemonic, 2276
V/Q lung scan, 1642–1643
  for pulmonary embolism, 1707
Vulva, cancer of, 1005–1008
  disorders of, 1005–1009
  structure and function of, 904, 905, 906t
Vulvectomy, radical, 1006, 1006–1008
  simple, 1006

W

Wada's test, 1929
Waist-to-hip proportions, 650
Walking. See Ambulation; Gait.
Warfarin, for total hip replacement, 561–562
  perioperative use of, 275t
  prophylactic, for stroke, 1965
Warfarin (Coumadin), for venous thrombosis, 1425
Warm shock, 2243
Warts, 1312t
  genital, 1053–1054
Water. See also under Fluid.
Water intoxication, 228–229
Water supply, hepatitis A and, 1225
Water-in-oil, 1281t
Weakness, in diabetes mellitus, 1156t
  in dying clients, 454
  in myasthenia gravis, 2020, 2022
  in post-polio syndrome, 1993
Weaning, ventilator, 1655–1656, 1759–1761, 1761b
Weber test, 1803, 1803
Wedge resection, pulmonary, 1730, 1731. See also Thoracic surgery.
Wedged hepatic venous pressure, 1084

Weight, body mass index and, 31
  ideal, 649, 651t
  measurement of, 182, 649
Weight gain, in heart disease, 1452
Weight loss, 1535
  for hypertension, 1386–1387, 1393
  for peripheral arterial occlusive disease, 1401–1402
  in cancer, 394
  in dehydration, 219
  in diabetes mellitus, 1156t
  in HIV infection, 2206
  strategies for, 32, 1393b
Weight-bearing status, 614b
Wellness, 8–9. See also Health promotion.
  Dunn's model of, 7–8
  health and disease and, 8–9
  Travis' model of, 8, 9
Wenckebach phenomenon, 1558, 1558
Wernicke's aphasia, 1956
Westergren test, reference values for, 2302t
Wet dressings, 1280t
Wet smear, vaginal, 927, 928
Wet wraps, 1280t, 1283, 1283
Wet-to-dry dressings, in debridement, 328–329, 329, 1347
Wet-to-moist dressings, 326, 329t
Wheal, 1271
Wheelchair transfer, 1972, 2061, 2061
Wheelchair use, in spinal cord injury, 2058, 2059
Wheezing, 1633, 1634t
  assessment of, 1624
  in asthma, 1687
Whipple's disease, 2163
Whipple's operation, for acute pancreatitis, 1198
  for chronic pancreatitis, 1201
  for pancreatic cancer, 1202
Whispered pectoriloquy, 1635
White blood cell(s), 2080–2081
  disorders affecting, 2119–2122. See also specific disorders.
  in inflammation, 317–319, 318, 2081
  in urine, 749t, 750, 757, 757t
  types of, 2080–2081
White blood cell count and differential, 2096, 2096t
  disorders and conditions affecting, 2097t
  in acute pancreatitis, 1195
  in cancer, 392
  in cardiac assessment, 1464
  in Cushing's syndrome, 1130
  in ear disorders, 1806
  in infectious mononucleosis, 2121
  interpretation of, 322t
  nadir of, 392
  preoperative measurement of, 278t
  propylthiouracil and, 1101
  reference values for, 2302t
White coat hypertension, 1380, 1380t
White matter, 1867
Wide dynamic range neurons, 469
Wilms' tumor, 858–862. See also Renal cancer.
Wilson's disease, 1259
Window, cast, 604
Wintrobe test, reference values for, 2302t
Wire fixation, of jaw, 1327–1328
Withdrawal, 513, 514t–515t
  alcohol, 514t, 515–516, 516t
  amphetamine, 514t, 516
  caffeine, 514t, 517
  cocaine, 514t, 517
  hallucinogen, 514t, 518
  inhalant, 514t, 518
  marijuana, 514t, 517
  nicotine, 514t, 518
  opioid, 514t, 518

Withdrawal reflex, 1863, *1863*
Wolff-Parkinson-White syndrome, 1565–1566
Wolff's stress theory, 6t
Wolf's disease concept, 6t
Wood's light examination, 1276
Workers' compensation, 78b
Worms, intestinal, 767–768
Wound(s), assessment of, 325–326, 326b
  postoperative, 307, 309
  color of, 328
  dressings for. See *Dressings.*
  irrigation of, 326, 328
  skin grafts for, 325
  topical agents for, 327t
Wound care, 324–330
  assessment in, 325–326, 326b
  delegation of, 310b
  emergency, 2280–2281
  for incisions, 324
  for pressure ulcers, 1299–1301
  medical management in, 324–325
  nursing management in, 326–330
  postoperative, 307, 309, 310b, 310–311
  self-care in, 330, *331*
  topical anesthesia for, 2280
Wound closure, intraoperative, 300
  methods of, 300, *301*
Wound contraction, 320
Wound cultures, 189
Wound debridement, 325, *328,* 328–330. See also *Debridement.*
Wound dehiscence, 309, *309,* 333
Wound drainage, 300, 324
  postoperative management of, 307
  preoperative teaching for, 287
Wound evisceration, 309, *309,* 333
Wound exudate, 323, 323t
Wound healing, 315–324
  acceptable, 315
  angiogenesis in, 318, 320
  assessment of, 325–326, 326b
  by primary intention, 320, *321*
  by secondary intention, 321, *321*
  by tertiary intention, 321, *321*
  collagen in, 320

Wound healing (*Continued*)
  cytokines in, 319–320
  delayed, 330–332
  electric stimulation for, 333
  epithelialization in, 320
  extrinsic factors in, 330, 331
  factors affecting, 315
  granulation in, 320
  growth factors for, 333
  growth factors in, 320
  hyperbaric oxygen for, 333
  ideal, 315
  in diabetes mellitus, 332
  in incisions, 324
  intrinsic factors in, 330, 331
  minimal, 315
  moist environment for, 326, *327*
  negative pressure therapy for, 333
  normal, 315–324
  nutrition and, 321, 321t
  nutrition in, 321, 321t, 330, 331
  outcomes classification for, 315
  oxygen free radicals in, 319
  phagocytosis in, 317–318, *318*
  phases of, 316–320
    inflammation, *316,* 316–319. See also *Inflammation.*
    maturation, *316,* 320
    proliferative, *316,* 319–320
    vascular response, 316, *316*
  promotion of, 333
  scar formation in, 320
  tissue oxygenation in, 318
  tissue type and, 315, 316
  under occlusive dressing, *327*
  wound contraction in, 320
Wound infection, 331–333
  nosocomial, 338t, 339
  pathogenesis of, 337t
  postoperative, 309
Wound packing, 326–328
Wrist, circumference of, in body frame size calculation, 649, *650*
  examination of, *543,* 544t
  fractures of, 596t, 618–619
Wrist compression test, 1998, *2000*

X

Xanthelasma, 1456
Xanthine stones, 824
Xenotransplantation, 2215
Xerosis, management of, 1286
Xerotic eczema, 1290
X-ray studies. See *Radiography.*
Xylocaine. See *Lidocaine (Xylocaine).*
D-Xylose absorption test, 656

Y

Yellow marrow, 2074
Yerbero, 74b
Yin and yang, 19b
Yohimbe, for erectile dysfunction, 973

Z

Zafirlukast (Accolate), for asthma, 1689, 1690, 1691t, *1692, 1694*
Zalcitabine (Hivid, ddC), 2196t
Zantac (ranitidine), for peptic ulcer disease, 710t, 715
Zarotin (ethosuximide), for epilepsy, 1927t, 1927–1928
  reference values for, 2307t
Zenapax (dacliximab), for transplant immuno-suppression, 2224t
Zenker's diverticulum, 698–699
Zerit (stavudine), 2196t
Ziagen (abacavir), 2196t
Zidovudine (Retrovir, AZT), 2195, 2197t
Zinc, deficiency of, 642t
  food sources of, 642t
Zoladex (goserelin), for breast cancer, 1036
Zollinger-Ellison syndrome, 714
Zona fasciculata, 1063, *1064*
Zona glomerulosa, 1063, *1064*
Zona reticularis, 1063, *1064*